SPECIAL FEATURE
ON ENCLOSED
DVD

THE GENERAL AND SCREENING MUSCULOSKELETAL EXAMINATION BY GEORGE LAWRY

Kelley's
TEXTBOOK OF
Rheumatology

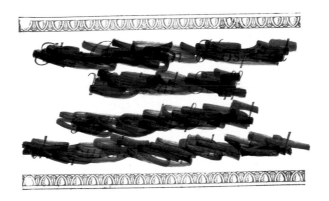

Kelley's

TEXTBOOK OF
Rheumatology

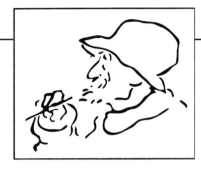

EDITORS

Edward D. Harris, Jr., MD
George DeForest Barnett Professor
 of Medicine, Emeritus
Stanford University School of
 Medicine
Academic Secretary to Stanford
 University
Stanford, California

Ralph C. Budd, MD
Professor of Medicine
Chief of Clinical Services
Division of Immunology and
 Rheumatology
University of Vermont College of
 Medicine
Burlington, Vermont

Mark C. Genovese, MD
Associate Professor of Medicine
Chief of Clinical Services
Division of Immunology and
 Rheumatology
Stanford University
Stanford, California

Gary S. Firestein, MD
Professor of Medicine
Chief, Division of Rheumatology,
 Allergy and Immunology
University of California, San Diego
School of Medicine
La Jolla, California

John S. Sargent, MD
Professor of Medicine and
 Senior Associate Dean for
 Clinical Affairs
Vanderbilt University School of
 Medicine
Chief Medical Officer
Vanderbilt University Medical
 Center
Nashville, Tennessee

Clement B. Sledge, MD
John B. and Buckminster Brown
 Professor Emeritus of
 Orthopedic Surgery
Harvard Medical School
Chairman Emeritus, Department
 of Orthopedic Surgery
Brigham and Women's Hospital
Boston, Massachusetts

ELECRONIC
EDITOR

Shaun Ruddy, MD
Elam C. Toone Professor Emeritus
 of Internal Medicine,
 Microbiology and Immunology
Chairman Emeritus, Division of
 Rheumatology, Allergy, and
 Immunology
Department of Internal Medicine
Virgina Commonwealth University
School of Medicine
Richmond, Virginia

ELSEVIER
SAUNDERS

ELSEVIER
SAUNDERS

The Curtis Center
170 S Independence Mall W 300 E
Philadelphia, Pennsylvania 19106

Kelley's Textbook of Rheumatology, Seventh
Edition

ISBN: 0-7216-0141-3

Notice

Surgery is an ever-changing field. Standard safety precautions must be followed, but as new research and clinical experience broaden our knowledge, changes in treatment and drug therapy may become necessary or appropriate. Readers are advised to check the most current product information provided by the manufacturer of each drug to be administered to verify the recommended dose, the method and duration of administration, and contraindications. It is the responsibility of the licensed prescriber, relying on experience and knowledge of the patient, to determine dosages and the best treatment for each individual patient. Neither the publisher nor the author assumes any liability for any injury and/or damage to persons or property arising from this publication.

Previous editions copyrighted 1981, 1985, 1989, 1993, 1997, 2001

International Standard Book Number: 0-7216-0141-3

Library of Congress Cataloging-in-Publication Data

Kelley's textbook of rheumatology / edited by Edward D. Harris, Jr. ...[et al.].–7th ed.
  p.; cm.
 Includes bibliographical references and index.
 ISBN 0-7216-0141-3
  1. Rheumatism. 2. Arthritis. I. Title: Textbook of rheumatology. II. Harris, Edward D.,
1937-III. Kelley, William N., 1939-
  [DNLM: 1. Rheumatic Diseases. 2. Arthritis. WE 544 K29 2005]
RC927.T49 2005
616.7'23—dc22   2004052586

Printed in the United States

Last digit is the print number: 9 8 7 6 5 4 3 2 1

Kelley's

TEXTBOOK OF

Rheumatology

The Aultman Hospital
Medical Staff
generously funded
the purchase of this book

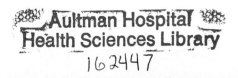

The editors are proud to dedicate this seventh edition of Textbook of Rheumatology to our mentors, colleagues in research and the clinics, and family and loved ones. Our mentors showed us the way, giving us focus and a sense of what questions were truly important to answer. Our colleagues amplified our work, gave us course correction, and through their own hard efforts and successes, invigorated our own efforts. To our wives and loved ones (including those dear children and grandkids) we owe deep and abundant thanks for nurture and sustenance in good times and, especially, on those days when all seems bleak. We all agree that we would choose the paths we have taken once again, so long as those mentioned above would be there to join us.

Ted Harris: Many thanks to my mentor, Steve Krane, and for the support of the Harris boys and Eileen...and for the happy smiles of the grandkids—Andrew, Eliza, Maeve, and Liam.

Ralph C. Budd: Sincere thanks to the kind mentoring from Edward D. Harris, Jr., H. Robson MacDonald, and C. Garrison Fathman, as well as to the support of my wife, Lenore, and my children, Graham and Laura.

Gary S. Firestein: Thanks to Linda and our children, David and Cathy, for their patience and support, as well as to Nathan Zvaifler for his guidance for over two decades.

Mark C. Genovese: To my wife Nancy and our daughters, Alexandra, Danielle, and Lauren, for their patience and support, and to Ted Harris for his guidance and mentorship.

Shaun Ruddy: To my wife, Millie; our children, Christi and Candace; and our grandchildren, Kevin, Matthew and Katharine.

John S. Sergent: To Carole and our children, Ellen and Katie, and to our grandchildren, Kathryn, Henry, and Emmaline.

Clement Sledge: To my wife, Georgia; our children, Mego, John, Matthew, and Claire; and our grandchildren, Matthew, Kaitlyn, Kevin, and Brian Tracy; Alexa and Jake Sledge; and Mollie, Reid, and Elsa Smith.

Contributors

Anthony J. Abene, M.D., M.B.A.
Fellow
Sports, Orthopaedics and Rehabilitation
Redwood City, California
Hip and Knee Pain

Steven B. Abramson, M.D.
Professor of Medicine and Pathology
New York University School of Medicine
Division of Rheumatology
New York, New York
Neutrophils and Eosinophils; Pathogenesis of Osteoarthritis

Leena Ala-Kokko
Professor, Department of Medicine
Center for Gene Therapy
Tulane University Health Sciences Center
New Orleans, Louisiana
Collagen and Elastin

Roy D. Altman, M.D.
Professor of Medicine
Division of Rheumatology
David Geffen School of Medicine at the
University of California at Los Angeles
Los Angeles, California
Hypertrophic Osteoarthropathy

William P. Arend, M.D.
Scoville Professor of Rheumatology Medicine
University of Colorado School of Medicine
Denver, Colorado
Antigen-Presenting Cells

Erin L. Arnold, M.D.
Rheumatologist
Center for Arthritis and Osteoporosis
Illinois Bone and Joint Institute, LTD
Morton Grove, Illinois
Arthroscopy

William J. Arnold, M.D., F.A.C.P., F.A.C.R.
Rheumatologist
Center for Arthritis and Osteoporosis
Illinois Bone and Joint Institute, LTD
Morton Grove, Illinois
Arthroscopy

Leyla Alparslan, M.D.
Associate Professor
Department of Radiology
Florence Nightingale Hospital
Kadir Has University School of Medicine
Istanbul, Turkey
Imaging

John P. Atkinson, M.D.
Samuel B. Grant Professor of Medicine
Professor of Molecular Microbiology
Department of Medicine/Rheumatology Division
Washington University School of Medicine
Physician
Internal Medicine
Barnes-Jewish Hospital
St. Louis, Missouri
Complement System

Stanley P. Ballou, M.D.
Associate Professor of Medicine
Case Western Reserve University
Director of Rheumatology
Metro Health Medical Center
Cleveland, Ohio
Laboratory Evaluation of Inflammation

N. Nichole Barry, M.D.
Sports Medicine
Stanford University
Palo Alto, California
Hip and Knee Pain

Robert M. Bennett, M.D., FRCP, FACP
Professor of Medicine
Oregon Health and Science University
and Portland, Oregon
Mixed Connective Tissue Disease and Other Overlap Syndromes

Johannes W.J. Bijlsma, M.D., Ph.D.
Professor and Head
Department of Rheumatology and Clinical
    Immunology
University Medical Center Utrecht
Utrecht, The Netherlands
Glucocorticoid Therapy

Joseph J. Biundo, Jr., M.D.
Emeritus Professor of Medicine
Louisiana State University Health Science Center
New Orleans, Louisiana
Medical Director of Rehabilitation
Kenner Regional Medical Center
Kenner, Louisiana
  Rehabilitation of Patients with Rheumatic Diseases

Juergen Braun, M.D., Ph.D.
Medical Director
Professor of Rheumatology
Rheumazentrum Ruhrgebiet
Herne, Germany
  Ankylosing Spondylitis

Michael B. Brenner, M.D.
Theodore B. Bayles Professor of Medicine
Harvard Medical School
Chief, Division of Rheumatology, Immunology and
  Allergy
Brigham and Women's Hospital
Boston, Massachusetts
  Synoviocytes

Doreen B. Brettler, M.D.
Professor of Medicine
University of Massachusetts Medical School
Director
New England Hemophilia Center/Staff Hematologist
Hematology/Oncology
University of Massachusetts Memorial Healthcare
Worcester, Massachusetts
  Hemophilic Arthropathy

Lenore M. Buckley, M.D., M.P.H.
Professor of Internal Medicine and Pediatrics
Virginia Commonwealth University School of
  Medicine
Attending Physician
Internal Medicine and Pediatrics
Medical College of Virginia Hospitals
Richmond, Virginia
  Development, Execution, and Analysis of Clinical Trials

Ralph C. Budd, M.D.
Professor of Medicine
Director, Immunobiology Program
The University of Vermont College of Medicine
Burlington, Vermont
  T Lymphocytes

Nathalie D. Burg, M.D.
Postdoctoral Fellow
Coller Lab
Rockefeller University
Clinical Instructor
Department of Medicine
New York University School of Medicine
New York, New York
  Neutrophils and Eosinophils

Jennifer Burkham, M.D., Ph.D.
Department of Rheumatology
University of California, San Francisco
San Francisco, California
  Fibromyalgia: A Chronic Pain Syndrome

Leonard H. Calabrese, B.S., D.O.
Department of Rheumatic and Immunologic Disease
Head, Section of Clinical Immunology
R.J. Fasenmyer Chair of Clinical Immunology
Cleveland Clinic Foundation
Cleveland, Ohio
  Antineutrophil Cytoplasmic Antibody–Associated Vasculitis

Dennis A. Carson, M.D.
Professor of Medicine
University of California San Diego
La Jolla, California
  Rheumatoid Factor

Steve Carsons, M.D.
Professor of Medicine
SUNY Health Science Center at Stony Brook
Stony Brook, New York
Chief, Division of Rheumatology, Allergy and
  Immunology
Winthrop University Hospital
Meneola, New York
  Sjögren's Syndrome

James T. Cassidy, M.D.
Professor and Chief of Pediatric Rheumatology
Department of Child Health
University of Missouri Health Sciences
Columbia, Missouri
  *Juvenile Rheumatoid Arthritis; Systemic Lupus
  Erythematosus, Juvenile Dermatomyositis, Scleroderma,
  and Vasculitis*

Eliza F. Chakravarty, M.D.
Assistant Professor
Division of Immunology and Rheumatology
Stanford University School of Medicine
Palo Alto, California
  Musculoskeletal Syndromes in Malignancy

Doyt L. Conn, M.D.
Professor of Medicine
Director Division of Rheumatology
Department of Medicine
Emory University School of Medicine
Grady Health System
The Emory Clinic
Atlanta, Georgia
  *Alternative Care for Arthritis and Related Musculoskeletal
  Diseases; Cutaneous Small-Vessel Vasculitis*

Paul P. Cook, M.D.
Associate Professor of Medicine
Division of Infectious Diseases
Department of Infectious Diseases
Department of Internal Medicine
Brody School of Medicine at East Carolina University
Greenville, North Carolina
Arthritis Caused by Bacteria or Their Components

Joseph E. Craft, M.D.M.D.
Professor of Medicine and Immunobiology
Chief, Section of Rheumatology
Department of Medicine
Yale School of Medicine
Attending and Chief of Rheumatology
Yale-New Haven Hospital
New Haven, Connecticut
Antinuclear Antibodies

Leslie J. Crofford, M.D.
Associate Professor
Internal Medicine, Division of Rheumatology
University of Michigan
Ann Arbor, Michigan
Nonsteroidal Anti-Inflammatory Drugs

Jody A. Dantzig, Ph.D.
Senior Research Investigator
Physiology/Pennsylvania Muscle Institute
School of Medicine
University of Pennsylvania
Philadelphia, Pennsylvania
Muscle: Anatomy, Physiology, and Biochemistry

Devin K. Datta, M.D.
Brevard Orthopaedic Clinic
Melbourne, Florida
Low Back Pain

Jeroen DeGroot, Ph.D.
Head
Matrix Biology Research Group
Division of Biomedical Research
TNO Prevention and Health
Netherlands Organization for Applied Scientific
  Research
Leiden, the Netherlands
Biological Markers

Betty Diamond, M.D.
Professor of Microbiology and Immunology, Medicine
Albert Einstein College of Medicine
Bronx, New York
B Cells

Federico Díaz-González, M.D.
Staff of Rheumatology
Rheumatology Service
Hospital Universitario de Canarias
La Laguna, Spain
Platelets and Rheumatic Diseases

Paul E. DiCesare, M.D.
Associate Professor of Orthopaedic Surgery and Cell
  Biology
New York University School of Medicine
Director, Musculoskeletal Research Center
Chief, Adult Reconstructive Surgery
Hospital for Joint Disease
New York, New York
Pathogenesis of Osteoarthritis

Michael F. Dillingham, M.D.
Adjunct Clinical Professor
Division of Orthopedic Surgery
Stanford University School of Medicine
Director and Team Physician
Orthopedics
Stanford University Medical Center
San Francisco, California
Hip and Knee Pain

Maxime Dougados, M.D.
Professor of Rheumatology
Rene(') Descartes University
Chief and Professor
Department of Rheumatology
Hospital Cochin
Paris, France
Clinical Features of Osteoarthritis

Joost P.H. Drenth, M.D., Ph.D.
Research Fellow
Department of Medicine
Division of Gastroenterology and Hepatology
University Medical Center St. Radboud
Nijmegen, The Netherlands
Familial Autoinflammatory Syndromes

George F. Duna, M.D., F.A.C.P.
Associate Professor of Medicine
Baylor College of Medicine
Chief of Rheumatology
St. Luke's Episcopal Hospital
Houston, Texas
Antineutrophil Cytoplasmic Antibody–Associated Vasculitis

Steven M. Edworthy, B.Sc., M.D., F.R.C.P.C.
Associate Professor of Medicine and Community
  Health Sciences
Department of Medicine
University of Calgary
Associate Professor of Medicine
Foothills Hospital
Calgary, Alberta, Canada
Clinical Manifestations of Systemic Lupus Erythematosus

Keith B. Elkon, M.D.
Professor of Medicine
Division of Rheumatology
University of Washington
Seattle, Washington
Apoptosis

Peng Thim Fan, M.D.
Clinical Professor of Medicine
David Geffen School of Medicine
University of California at Los Angeles
Los Angles, California
*Reiter's Syndrome, Undifferentiated Spondyloarthropathy,
and Reactive Arthritis*

Barbara K. Finck, M.D.
Vice President
Clinical Development
Eos Biotechnology, Inc.
San Francisco, California
Development, Execution, and Analysis of Clinical Trials

Gary S. Firestein, M.D.
Professor of Medicine and Chief
Division of Rheumatology, Allergy and Immunology
University of California San Diego School of Medicine
Director
University of California San Diego Clinical
     Investigation Institute
La Jolla, California
Etiology and Pathogenesis of Rheumatoid Arthritis

Karen A. Fortner, Ph.D.
Research Associate
Immunobiology Program, Department of Medicine
The University of Vermont College of Medicine
Burlington, Vermont
T Lymphocytes

Andrew G. Franks, Jr., M.D.
Clinical Professor of Dermatology
New York University School of Medicine
Attending Physician in Rheumatology
Hospital for Joint Diseases
New York University Medical Center
New York, New York
The Skin and Rheumatic Diseases

Sherine E. Gabriel, M.D., M.Sc.
Professor of Medicine Rheumatology and
     Epidemiology
Mayo Clinic
Chair, Department of Health Sciences Research
Mayo Clinic College of Medicine
Rochester, Minnesota
Epidemiology of the Rheumatic Diseases

Rachel A. Garton, M.D.
Chief Resident in Dermatology
Department of Dermatology
Wake Forest School of Medicine
Winston-Salem, North Carolina
Behcet's Disease

Mark C. Genovese, M.D.
Associate Professor of Medicine
Chief of Clinical Services
Division of immunology and Rheumatology
Stanford University
Palo Alto, California
*Treatment of Rheumatoid Arthritis; Musculoskeletal
Syndromes in Malignancy*

Danielle M. Gerlag, M.D.
Assistant Professor of Medicine
Division of Clinical Immunology and Rheumatology
Academic Medical Center
University of Amsterdam
Amsterdam, The Netherlands
*Synovial Fluid Analyses, Synovial Biopsy, and Synovial
Pathology*

Jayashri V. Ghate, M.D.
Department of Dermatology
Wake Forest University School of Medicine
Winston-Salem, North Carolina
Behcet's Disease

Allan Gibofsky, M.D., J.D., F.A.C.P., F.C.L.M.
Professor
Medicine and Public Health
Weill Medical College of Cornell University
Attending Rheumatologist
Hospital for Special Surgery
New York, New York
Acute Rheumatic Fever and Poststreptoccocal Arthritis

Mark H. Ginsberg, M.D.
Professor of Cell Biology
The Scripps Research Institute
La Jolla, California
Adjunct Professor
University of California School of Medicine
San Diego, California
Platelets and Rheumatic Diseases

Dafna O. Gladman, M.D., F.R.C.P.C.
Professor of Medicine/Rheumatology
University of Toronto
Senior Rheumatologist
University Health Network, Toronto Western Hospital
Toronto, Ontario, Canada
Psoriatic Arthritis

Joseph Golbus, M.D.
Associate Professor
Department of Medicine
Northwestern University Medical School
Chicago, Illinois
Head, Division of Rheumatology
Evanston Northwestern Healthcare
Evanston, Illinois
Monarticular Arthritis

Yale E. Goldman, M.D., Ph.D.
Professor, Institute Director
Physiology/Pennsylvania Muscle Institute
School of Medicine, University of Pennsylvania
Philadelphia, Pennsylvania
Muscle: Anatomy, Physiology, and Biochemistry

Mary B. Goldring, Ph.D.
Associate Professor of Medicine (Cell Biology)
Division of Medical Sciences
Harvard Medical School
Associate Professor of Medicine
Department of Medicine/Division of Rheumatology
Beth Israel Deaconess Medical Center
Boston, Massachusetts
Biology of the Normal Joint; Chondrocytes

Steven R. Goldring, M.D.
Professor of Medicine
Harvard Medical School
Chief of Rheumatology
Department of Medicine/Division of Rheumatology
Beth Israel Deaconess Medical Center
Boston, Massachusetts
Biology of the Normal Joint

Emilio B. Gonzalez, M.D.
Clinical Associate Professor
Internal Medicine
Emory University School of Medicine
Chief, Rheumatology Section
Atlanta Medical Center
Atlanta, Georgia
Cutaneous Small-Vessel Vasculitis

Duncan A. Gordon, M.D., M.A.C.R.
Professor
Department of Medicine
University of Toronto
Senior Rheumatologist
Division of Rheumatology
University Health Network, Toronto Western Hospital
Toronto, Ontario, Canada
Second Line Agents

Peter K. Gregersen
Professor of Medicine and Pathology
Department of Medicine and Pathology
New York University School of Medicine
New York, New York
Director
Robert S. Boas Center for Genomics and Human
   Genetics
North Shore Long Island Jewish Research Institute
Manhasset, New York
Genetics of Rheumatic Diseases

Christine Grimaldi, Ph.D.
Instructor, Microbiology and Immunology
Albert Einstein College of Medicine
Bronx, New York
B Cells

Bevra Hannahs Hahn, M.D.
Chief of Rheumatology and Professor of Medicine
Department of Medicine
David Geffen School of Medicine
University of California, Los Angeles
Los Angeles, California
Pathogenesis of Systemic Lupus Erythematosus;
Management of Systemic Lupus Erythematosus

J. Timothy Harrington, M.D.
Associate Professor
Rheumatology Section, Department of Medicine
University of Wisconsin Medical School
Madison, Wisconsin
Mycobacterial and Fungal Infections

Edward D. Harris, M.D.
George DeForest Barnett Professor of Medicine,
   Emeritus
Stanford University School of Medicine
Academic Secretary to Stanford University
Stanford, California
Biological Markers; Fibromyalgia:
A Chronic Pain Syndrome;
Clinical Features of Rheumatoid Arthritis;
Treatment of Rheumatoid Arthritis

Dick Heinegärd, M.D., Ph.D.
Professor
Department of Cell and Molecular Biology
Lund University
Lund, Sweden
Matrix Glycoproteins and Proteoglycans in Cartilage

David B. Hellman, M.D.
Mary Betty Stevens Professor of Medicine
Johns Hopkins University School of Medicine
Chairman and Physician-in-Chief, Department of
   Medicine
Johns Hopkins Bayview Medical Center
Baltimore, Maryland
Giant Cell Arteritis and Polymyalgia Rheumatica

George Ho, Jr., M.D.
Professor of Medicine
Division of Allergy, Immunology, and Rheumatology
Department of Internal Medicine
Brody School of Medicine at East Carolina University
Greenville, North Carolina
Arthritis Caused by Bacteria or Their Components

Jeffrey D. Horn, M.D.
Assistant Professor of Ophthalmology
Department of Ophthalmology and Visual Services
Vanderbilt University Medical Center
Nashville, Tennessee
The Eye and Rheumatic Disease

Gene G. Hunder, M.D.
Professor Emeritus
Department of Medicine
Mayo Medical School
Rochester, Minnesota
History and Physical Examination of the Musculoskeletal
System; Giant Cell Arteritis and Polymyalgia Rheumatica

Johannes W.G. Jacobs, M.D., Ph.D.
Associate Professor
Department of Rheumatology and Clinical
   Immunology
University Medical Center Utrecht
Utrectht, The Netherlands
   Glucocorticoid Therapy

Charles A. Janeway, Jr., M.D. (Deceased)
Professor
Section of Immunobiology and Howard Hughes
   Medical Institute
Yale University School of Medicine
New Haven, Connecticut
   Innate Immunity

Joseph L. Jorizzo, M.D.
Professor and Former (Founding) Chair
Department of Dermatology
Wake Forest University School of Medicine
Winston-Salem, North Carolina
   Behcet's Disease

Sue Joan Jue, M.D.
Associate Professor of Pediatrics
Section of Infectious Diseases
Greenville Hospital Systems
Greenville, South Carolina
   Arthritis Caused by Bacteria or Their Components

George A. Karpouzas, M.D.
Clinical Instructor, Assistant Researcher
Department of Medicine
David Geffen School of Medicine
University of California, Los Angeles
Los Angeles, California
   Pathogenesis of Systemic Lupus Erythematosus

Arthur Kavanaugh, M.D.
Professor of Medicine
Director of the Center for Innovative Therapy
Division of Rheumatology, Allergy and Immunology
University of California, San Diego
San Diego, California
   Anticytokine Therapies

William N. Kelley, M.D.
Professor
Department of Medicine
University of Pennsylvania
Philadelphia, Pennsylvania
   Gout and Hyperuricemia

Edward Keystone, M.D., F.R.C.P.(C).
Professor of Medicine
Department of Medicine
University of Toronto
Rheumatologist
Mount Sanai Hospital
Toronto, Ontario, Canada
   Emerging Therapies in Rheumatoid Arthritis

Hans P. Kiener, M.D.
Research Fellow
Harvard Medical School
Research Fellow
Brigham and Women's Hospital
Boston, Massachusetts
   Synoviocytes

Alice V. Klinkhoff, M.D., F.R.C.P.
Clinical Associate Professor
Department of Medicine
University of British Columbia
Medical Director
Mary Pack Arthritis Program
Vancouver General Hospital
Vancouver, British Columbia, Canada
   Second Line Agents

Alisa E. Koch, M.D.
William D. Robinson and Frederick Huetwell
   Endowed Professor
University of Michigan
Ann Arbor, Michigan
   *Endothelial Cell Biology, Angiogenesis, and Recruitment
   of Cells*

Joseph H. Korn, M.D.
Alan S. Cohen Professor of Medicine in Rheumatology
Director, Arthritis Center
Boston University School of Medicine
Boston, Massachusetts
   Fibroblast Function and Fibrosis

Brian L. Kotzin, M.D.
Professor of Medicine and Immunology
Co-Head, Division of Clinical Immunology
University of Colorado Health Sciences Center
Denver, Colorado
   Autoimmunity

Joel M. Kremer, M.D.
Clinical Professor of Medicine
Department of Medicine, Division of Rheumatology
Albany Medical College
Albany, New York
   Nutrition and Rheumatic Diseases

Hilal Maradit Kremers, M.D., M.Sc.
Assistant Professor of Epidemiology
Mayo Medical School
Rochester, Minnesota
Research Associate, Department of Health Sciences
   Research
Mayo Clinic College of Medicine
Rochester, Minnesota
   Epidemiology of the Rheumatic Diseases

Irving Kushner, M.D.
Professor of Medicine and Pathology
Case-Western Reserve University
Attending Physician
MetroHealth Medical Center
Cleveland, Ohio
   Laboratory Evaluation of Inflammation

Robert Lafyatis, M.D.
Associate Professor of Medicine
Rheumatology Section
Boston University School of Medicine
Associate Professor of Medicine
Department of Rheumatology
Boston University Medical Center
Boston, Massachusetts
  Fibroblast Function and Fibrosis

R. Elaine Lambert, M.D.
Adjunct Clinical Associate Professor
Department of Internal Medicine
Stanford School of Medicine
Palo Alto, California
  Iron Storage Disease

Nancy E. Lane, M.D.
Associate Professor of Medicine in Residence
Department of Medicine
University of California at San Francisco
Department of Medicine and Division of
  Rheumatology
San Francisco General Hospital
San Francisco, California
  Metabolic Bone Disease

Daniel M. Laskin, DDS, MS
Professor and Chairman Emeritus
Department of Oral and Maxillofacial Surgery
Virginia Commonwealth University School of
  Dentistry
Attending Oral and Maxillofacial Surgeon
Medical College of Virginia/Virginia Commonwealth
  University Hospital
Richmond, Virgina
  Temporomandibular Joint Pain

Meryl S. LeBoff
Associate Professor
Department of Internal Medicine
Harvard Medical School
Director
Skeletal Health and Osteoporosis
Division of Endocrine, Diabetes and Hypertension
Brigham and Women's Hospital
Boston, Massachusetts
  Metabolic Bone Disease

David M. Lee, M.D., Ph.D.
Instructor of Medicine
Harvard Medical School
Division of Rheumatology, Immunology and Allergy
Department of Medicine
Brigham and Women's Hospital
Boston, Massachusetts
  Synoviocytes

Michael D. Lockshin, M.D.
Professor of Medicine and Obstetrics and Gynecology
Joan and Sanford Weill Medical College of Cornell
  University
Attending Physician
Hospital for Special Surgery
New York, New York
  Antiphospholipid Antibody Syndrome

Pilar Lorenzo, Ph.D.
Cell and Molecular Biology
Lund University
Rheumatology
Lund University Hospital
Lund, Sweden
  Matrix Glycoproteins and Proteoglycans in Cartilage

Kate R. Lorig, RN, DrPH
Professor
Department of Medicine
Stanford University
Palo Alto, California
  Education of Patients

Carlos J. Lozada, M.D.
Associate Professor of Medicine
Director, Rheumatology Fellowship Program
Division of Rheumatology and Immunology
University of Miami School of Medicine
Director
Rheumatology Fellowship Training Program and
Rheumatology Clinical Services
Jackson Memorial Hospital
Miami, Florida
  Management of Osteoarthritis

Maren Lawson Mahowald, M.D.
Professor of Medicine
University of Minnesota
Rheumatology Section Chief
Minneapolis VA Medical Center
Minneapolis, Minnesota
  Chronic Musculoskeletal Pain

Scott David Martin, M.D.
Assistant Professor of Orthopedics
Harvard Medical School
Brigham and Women's Hospital
Boston, Massachusetts
  Shoulder Pain

W. Joseph McCune, M.D.
Professor of Medicine
Department of Internal Medicine/Rheumatology
University of Michigan Medical Center
Ann Arbor, Michigan
  Monarticular Arthritis

Iain B. McInnes, MRCP, Ph.D.
Professor
Division of Immunology, Infection and Inflammation
University of Glasgow
Consultant Rheumatologist
Centre for Rheumatic Diseases
Glasgow Royal Infirmary
Glasgow, Scotland, United Kingdom
Cytokines

Richard T. Meehan, M.D., FACP, FACR
Chief of Rheumatology
Associate Professor of Medicine
National Jewish Medical and Research Center
Associate Clinical Professor of Medicine
Rheumatology, Department of Medicine
University of Colorado Health Sciences Center
Denver, Colorado
Sarcoidosis

Sohail K. Mirza, M.D.
Associate Professor
Department of Orthopaedics and Sports Medicine
Harborview Medical Center
University of Washington
Seattle, Washington
Low Back Pain

Kevin G. Moder, M.D.
Assistant Professor
Division of Rheumatology
Department of Internal Medicine
Mayo Clinic
Rochester, Minnesota
History and Physical Examination of the Musculoskeletal System

Stanley J. Naides, M.D.
Thomas B. Hallowell Professor of Medicine
Chief, Division of Rheumatology
Medicine, Microbiology and Immunology and Pharmacology
Pennsylvania State University College of Medicine
Professor and Chief
Division of Rheumatology
The Milton S. Hershey Medical Center
Hershey Pennsylvania
Viral Arthritis

Kenneth K. Nakano, M.D.
Clinical Professor of Medicine
Albany Medical College
Director of Research
The Center for Rheumatology
Attending Physician
Albany Medical Center Hospital
Albany, New York
Neck Pain

Lee S. Newman, M.D., MA, FCCP
Professor of Medicine
Professor of Preventive Medicine and Biometrics
University of Colorado Health Sciences Center
Professor of Medicine
Head, Division of Environmental and Occupational
    Health Sciences
National Jewish Medical and Research Center
Denver, Colorado
Sarcoidosis

Urs E. Nydegger, M.D.
Titularprofessor
Faculty of Medicine
University of Bern
Leitender Arzt
University Clinic for Cardiovascular Surgery
Universitätsklinik für Herzund Gefässchirurgie
    Inselspital
Bern, Switzerland
Immune Complexes

Denis M. O'Day, M.D., F.A.C.S.
Professor of Ophthalmology
Department of Ophthalmology and Visual Sciences
Vanderbilt University School of Medicine
Nashville, Tennessee
The Eye and Rheumatic Disease

James R. O'Dell, BS, M.D.
Professor of Medicine
Chief, Section of Rheumatology and Immunology
Vice-Chairman, Department of Internal Medicine
University of Nebraska Medical Center
Omaha, Nebraska
Methotrexate, Leflunomide, and Combination Therapies

Yasunori Okada, M.D., Ph.D.
Professor and Chairman
Department of Pathology
School of Medicine
Keio University
Tokyo, Japan
Proteinases and Matrix Degradation

Richard S. Panush, M.D.
Clinical Professor
Department of Medicine
Mount Sinai School of Medicine
Chair
Department of Medicine
Saint Barnabas Medical Center
Livingston, New Jersey
Occupational and Recreational Musculoskeletal Disorders

Stanford L. Peng, M.D., Ph.D.
Assistant Professor
Department of Internal Medicine, Division of
    Rheumatology
Washington University School of Medicine
Assistant Professor
Department of Internal Medicine, Division of
    Rheumatology
Barnes-Jewish Hospital
St. Louis, Missouri
Antinuclear Antibodies

Jean-Charles Piette, M.D.
Medecine Interne 2
Hospital Pitie-Salpetriere
Paris, France
Relapsing Polychondritis

Lorenzo Pilar, Ph.D.
Department of Cell and Molecular Biology
Lund University
Lund, Sweden
Matrix Glycoproteins and Proteoglycans in Cartilage

Michael H. Pillinger, M.D.
Assistant Professor
Department of Medicine and Pharmacology
New York University School of Medicine
    Section Chief, Rheumatology
New York Harbor Veterans Health Care System,
    Manhattan Campus
New York, New York
Neutrophils and Eosinophils

Robert S. Pinals, M.D.
Professor and Vice-Chairman
Department of Medicine
University of Medicine and Dentistry of New Jersey
Robert Wood Johnson Medical School
Chief, Rheumatology Service
Robert Wood Johnson University Hospital
New Brunswick, New Jersey
Felty's Syndrome

Steven A. Porcelli, M.D.
Associate Professor
Department of Microbiology and Immunology
Department of Medicine
Albert Einstein College of Medicine
Bronx, New York
Innate Immunity

Darwin J. Prockop, M.D., Ph.D.
Director and Chairman
Center for Gene Therapy
Tulane University Health Sciences Center
New Orleans, Louisiana
Collagen and Elastin

Eric L. Radin, M.D.
Adjunct Professor
Orthopaedic Surgery
Tufts University School of Medicine
Boston, Massachusetts
Biomechanics of Joints

Jaya K. Rao, M.D., MHS
Medical Epidemiologist
Health Care and Aging Studies Branch
Centers for Disease Control and Prevention
Adjunct Clinical Associate Professor
Division of Rheumatology
Department of Medicine
Emory University School of Medicine
Atlanta, Georgia
*Alternative Care for Arthritis and Related Musculoskeletal
Diseases*

John D. Reveille, M.D.
George S. Bruce Professor in Arthritis and Other
    Rheumatic Diseases
Rheumatology, Internal Medicine
The University of Texas Health Science Center at
    Houston
Director, Division of Rheumatology
Hermann Hospital
Houston, Texas
*Rheumatic Manifestations of Human Immunodeficiency
Virus Infection*

Marco Rizzo, M.D.
Assistant Professor
Division of Orthopaedic Surgery
Duke University Medical Center
Durham, North Carolina
Osteonecrosis

W. Neal Roberts, Jr., M.D.
Director
Rheumatology Training Program
C.W. Thomas Associate Professor of Medicine
Virginia Commonwealth University
Medical College of Virginia
Richmond, Virginia
Psychosocial Management of the Rheumatic Diseases

Andrew E. Rosenberg, M.D.
Associate Professor
Department of Pathology
Harvard Medical School;
Associate Pathologist
Department of Pathology
Massachusetts General Hospital
Boston, Massachusetts
Tumors and Tumor-like Lesions of Joints

Keith T. Rott, M.D., Ph.D.
Assistant Professor
Division of Rheumatology and Immunology
Department of Medicine
Emory University School of Medicine
Atlanta, Georgia
Cutaneous Small-Vessel Vasculitis

David Rowe, M.D.
University of Connecticut Health Science Center
Heritable Disorders of Structural Proteins

Clinton T. Rubin, Ph.D.
Professor and Chair
Department of Biomedical Engineering
Director, Center for Biotechnology
State University of New York
Stony Brook, New York
Biology, Physiology, and Morphology of Bone

Janet E. Rubin, M.D.
Professor of Medicine
Division of Endocrinology and Metabolism
Emory University School of Medicine
Physician
Endocrinology and Metabolism
Atlanta Veterans Affairs Medical Center
Atlanta, Georgia
Biology, Physiology, and Morphology of Bone

Perry J. Rush, M.D.
Assistant Professor
Department of Medicine
University of Toronto
Chief Physiatrist
Department of Medicine
St. John's Rehabilitation Hospital
Toronto Ontario Canada
Rehabilitation of Patients with Rheumatic Diseases

Tore Saxne, M.D., Ph.D.
Professor
Department of Rheumatology
Lund University
Lund, Sweden
Matrix Glycoproteins and Proteoglycans in Cartilage

H. Ralph Schumacher, Jr., M.D.
Professor of Medicine
University of Pennsylvania School of Medicine
Chief of Rheumatology
VA Medical Center
Philadelphia, PA
Hemoglobinopathies and Arthritis

Edward M. Schwarz, Ph.D.
Associate Professor
Department of Orthopaedics
University of Rochester School of Medicine and
   Dentistry
Rochester, New York
Signal Transduction in Rheumatic Diseases

James R. Seibold, M.D.
Professor of Medicine
Director, Scleroderma Program
University of Medicine and Dentistry of New Jersey
Robert Wood Johnson Medical School Attending
   Physician
Internal Medicine andand Rheumatology
Robert Wood Johnson University Hospital
New Brunswick, New Jersey
Scleroderma

David C. Seldin, M.D., Ph.D.
Associate Professor of Medicine and Microbiology
Boston University School of Medicine
Attending Physician, Section of Hematology-Oncology
Department of Medicine
Boston Medical Center
Boston, Massachusetts
Amyloidosis

John S. Sergent, M.D.
Professor of Medicine
Vanderbilt University School of Medicine
Vice Chairman for Education
Department of Medicine
Vanderbilt Medical Center
Nashville, Tennessee
*Polyarticular Arthritis; Polyarteritis and Related
   Disorders; Arthritis Accompanying Endocrine and
   Metabolic Disorders*

Jay R. Shapiro, M.D.
Professor
Department of Medicine
Uniformed Services University
Bethesda, Maryland
Director
Osteogenesis Imperfecta Program
Kennedy Krieger Institute
Baltimore, Maryland
Heritable Disorders of Structural Proteins

Leonard H. Sigal, M.D., FACP, FACR
Clinical Professor
Departments of Medicine
Department of Pediatrics
Department of Molecular Genetics and Microbiology
University of Medicine and Dentistry of New Jersey
Robert Wood Johnson Medical School
Attending, Rheumatology Service
Robert Wood Johnson University Hospital
New Brunswick, New Jersey
Lyme Disease

Anna Simon, M.D.
Resident
Department of Medicine
Division of General Internal Medicine
University Medical Center St. Radboud
Nijmegen, The Netherlands
Familial Autoinflammatory Syndromes

Sheldon R. Simon, M.D.
Professor of Clinical Orthopaedics
Albert Einstein School of Medicine
Bronx, New York
Chief Division of Pediatric Orthopaedics
Department of Orthopaedics
Beth Israel Medical Center
New York, New York
Biomechanics of Joints

Martha Skinner, M.D.
Professor
Department of Medicine
Boston University School of Medicine
Director, Amyloid Program
Boston Medical Center
Boston, Massachusetts
Amyloidosis

Clement B. Sledge, M.D.
John B. and Buckminster Brown
Professor of Orthopedic Surgery, Emeritus
Harvard Medical School
Chairman, Department of Orthopedic Surgery,
    Emeritus
Brigham and Women's Hospital
Boston, Massachusetts
*Introduction to Surgical Management of Patients with
    Arthritis*
Principles of Reconstructive Surgery for Arthritis

Nicholas A. Soter, M.D.
Professor of Dermatology
The Ronald O. Perelman Department of Dermatology
New York University School of Medicine
Attending Physician
Tisch Hospital
The University Hospital of NYU
New York, New York
The Skin and Rheumatic Diseases

Timothy M. Spiegel, M.D., MPH
Department of Medicine/Rheumatology
Cottage Hospital
Santa Barbara, California
Ankle and Foot Pain

Paul A. Sponseller, M.D.
Professor and Vice-Chair
Department of Orthopaedics
Head, Pediatric Orthopaedics
Johns Hopkins University
Boston, Massachusetts
Heritable Disorders of Structural Proteins

C. Michael Stein, M.D.
Associate Professor of Medicine
Associate Professor of Pharmacology
Vanderbilt University School of Medicine
Nashville, Tennessee
Immunoregulatory Drugs

John H. Stone, M.D., MPH
Associate Professor of Medicine
Division of Rheumatology
Johns Hopkins University
Director
The Johns Hopkins Vasculitis Center
Baltimore, Maryland
The Classification and Epidemiology of Systemic Vasculitis

Vibeke Strand, M.D.
Adjunct Clinical Professor
Division of Immunology and Rheumatology
Stanford University School of Medicine
Palo Alto, California
Emerging Therapies in Rheumatoid Arthritis

Stephanie Studenski, M.D., MPH
Professor
Department of Medicine
University of Pittsburgh
Staff Physician
Geriatric Research Education and Clinical Center
Virgina Pittsburgh Healthcare System
Pittsburgh, Pennsylvania
Pharmacology and the Elderly

Carrie R. Swigart, M.D.
Assistant Clinical Professor
Department of Orthopaedics and Rehabilitation
Yale University School of Medicine
Associate
Yale–New Haven Hospital
New Haven, Connecticut
Hand and Wrist Pain

Zoltan Szekanecz, M.D., Ph.D., DSC
Associate Professor of Medicine, Rheumatology and
    Immunology
Head of Rheumatology Division
Third Department of Medicine
Rheumatology Division
Debrecen, Hungary
*Endothelial Cell Biology, Angiogenesis, and Recruitment
Cells*

Paul P. Tak, M.D., Ph.D.
Professor of Medicine
Director, Division of Clinical Immunology and
    Rheumatology
Academic Medical Center
University of Amsterdam
The Netherlands
*Synovial Fluid Analyses, Synovial Biopsy, and Synovial
Pathology; Biological Markers*

Johan M. TeKoppele, Ph.D.
Head, Division of Biomedical Research
TNO Prevention and Health
Netherlands Organization for Applied Scientific
    Research
Leiden, The Netherlands
Biological Markers

Jerry Tenenbaum, M.D., FRCPC
Professor of Medicine
University of Toronto;
Director
Ontario International Medical Graduate Program
Mount Sinai Hospital
Toronto, Ontario, Canada
Hypertrophic Osteoarthropathy

Robert Terkeltaub, M.D.
Professor of Medicine in Residence
Director, Rheumatology Training Program
University of California at San Diego
Chief, Rheumatology Section
VA Medical Center
San Diego, California
  *Diseases Associated with Articular Deposition of Calcium
  Pyrophosphate Dihydrate and Basic Calcium Phosphate
  Crystals*

Ranjeny Thomas, M.D.
Associate Professor
Centre for Immunology and Cancer Research
University of Queensland
Consultant Rheumatologist
Princess Alexandra Hospital
Brisbane, Australia
  Antigen-Presenting Cells

Thomas S. Thornhill, M.D.
John B. and Buckminster Brown
Professor of Orthopaedics
Harvard Medical School
Orthopaedist-in-Chief
Brigham and Women's Hospital
Boston, Massachusetts
  Shoulder Pain

Helen Tighe, Ph.D.
Associate Professor of Medicine
University of California San Diego
La Jolla, California
  Rheumatoid Factor

Betty P. Tsao, Ph.D.
Professor of Medicine
David Geffen School of Medicine University of
  California at Los Angeles
Los Angeles, California
  Pathogenesis of SLE

Zuhre Tutuncu, M.D.
Assistant Clinical Professor of Medicine
Center for Innovative Therapy
Division of Rheumatology
University of California at San Diego
San Diego, California
  Anticytokine Therapies

Katherine S. Upchurch, M.D.
Associate Professor of Medicine
University of Massachusetts Medical School
Associate Chief, Division of Rheumatology
University of Massachusetts Memorial Medical Center
Worcester, Massachusetts
  Hemophilic Arthropathy

James R. Urbaniak, M.D.
Virginia Flowers Baker Professor of Orthopedic
  Surgery
Duke University Medical Center
Durham, North Carolina
  Osteonecrosis

Désirée van der Heijde, M.D., Ph.D.
Professor of Rheumatology
Department of Internal Medicine
Division of Rheumatology
University Hospital Maastvicht
Maastvicht, The Netherlands
  Ankylosing Spondylitis

Sjef van der Linden, M.D., Ph.D.
Professor of Rheumatology
Department of Internal Medicine
Division of Rheumatology
University Hospital Maastvicht
Maastvicht, The Netherlands
  Ankylosing Spondylitis

Jos W.M. van der Meer, M.D., Ph.D., FRCP
Professor of Internal Medicine
Department of Medicine
Division of General Internal Medicine
University Medical Center St. Radboud
Nijmegen, The Netherlands
  Familial Autoinflammatory Syndromes

Philippe Vinceneux, M.D.
Medecine Interne 2
Hospital Pitie-Salpetriere
Paris, France
  Relapsing Polychondritis

Michael M. Ward, M.D., MPH
Senior Investigator, Intramural Research Program
National Institute of Arthritis and Musculoskeletal and
  Skin Diseases
National Institutes of Health
U. S. Department of Health and Human Services
Bethesda, Maryland
  *Assessment of Health Outcomes; Pharmacology and the
  Elderly*

Yasmine Wasfi, M.D.
Instructor, Parker B. Francis Fellow
Department of Medicine
National Jewish Medical and Research Center
Instructor, Division of Pulmonary Sciences and Critical
  Care Medicine
University of Colorado Health Sciences Center
Denver, Colorado
  Sarcoidosis

Barbara N. Weissman, M.D.
Professor
Harvard Medical School
Radiology
Brigham and Women's Hospital
Boston, Massachusetts
Imaging

Augustus A. White, III, M.D., Ph.D.
Ellen and Melvin Gordon Professor of Medical
    Education
Professor of Orthopaedic Surgery
Harvard Medical School
Orthopedic Surgeon-In-Chief, Emeritus
Beth Israel Deaconess Medical Center
Boston, Massachusetts
Low Back Pain

Christopher M. Wise, M.D.
W. Robert Irby Professor, Internal Medicine
Division of Rheumatology, Allergy, and Immunology
Virginia Commonwealth University Health System
Medical College of Virginia
Richmond, Virginia
Arthrocentesis and Injection of Joints and Soft Tissues

Scott W. Wolfe, M.D.
Professor of Orthopedic Surgery
Weill Medical College of Cornell University
Chief of Hand Surgery
Hospital for Special Surgery
New York, New York
Hand and Wrist Pain

Frank A. Wollheim, M.D., Ph.D., FRCP
Professor of Rheumatology
Department of Rheumatology
University of Lund
Lund University Hospital
Lund, Sweden
Enteropathic Arthritis

Anthony D. Woolf, BSc, MB, BS, FRCP
Honorary Professor of Rheumatology
Institute of Health and Social Care Research
Peninsula Medical School
Universities of Exeter and Plymouth
Consultant Rheumatologist
Department of Rheumatology
Royal Cornwall Hospital
Truro, United Kingdom
Economic Burden of Rheumatic Diseases

Robert L. Wortmann, M.D.
Professor and Chair
Department of Internal Medicine
The University of Oklahoma College of Medicine
Tulsa, Oklahoma
*Inflammatory Diseases of Muscle and Other Myopathies;
Gout and Hyperuricemia*

David Tak Tan Yu, M.D., B.S.
Professor of Medicine
David Geffen School of Medicine
University of California at Los Angeles
Los Angeles, California
*Reiter's Syndrome, Undifferentiated Spondyloarthropathy,
and Reactive Arthritis*

Joseph S. Yu, M.D.
Chief of Musculoskeletal Division
Department of Radiology
Ohio State University Medical Center
Columbus, Ohio
Imaging

John B. Zabriskie, M.D.
Professor Emeritus
Laboratory of Clinical Microbiology/Immunology
Rockefeller University
Senior Scientist, Research Division
Hospital for Special Surgery
New York, New York
Acute Rheumatic Fever and Poststreptoccocal Arthritis

Robert B. Zurier, M.D.
Professor of Medicine
Chief of the Division of Rheumatology
University of Massachusetts Memorial Health Care
Worcester, Massachusetts
Prostaglandins, Leukotrienes, and Related Compounds

International Reviewers

The Publisher wishes to acknowledge the following individuals, who previewed advance materials from Kelley's Textbook of Rheumatology, 7th Edition

Sang-Cheol Bae, MD, PhD, MPH
Professor and Head,
Division of Rheumatology,
Department of Internal Medicine,
The Hospital for Rheumatic Diseases, Hanyang
University,
Seoul, Korea

Pradeep Bambery, MD
Professor,
Department of Internal Medicine/Rheumatology,
Postgraduate Institute of Medical Education and
Research,
Chandigarh, India

Prof. Em. Dr. Jan Dequeker
Department of Rheumatology,
University Hospital of Leuven,
Leuven, Belgium

Katsuyuki Fujii, MD, PhD
Professor,
Department of Orthopaedic Surgery,
The Jikei University School of Medicine,
Tokyo, Japan

Rajiva Gupta, MD, DNB, MRCP
Assistant Professor of Medicine,
All India Institute of Medical Sciences,
New Delhi, India

Soo-Kon Lee, MD, PhD
Division of Rheumatology,
Department of Internal Medicine,
Yonsei University College of Medicine,
Seoul, Korea

Caio Moreira
Rheumatologist,
Hospital das Clínicas,
Federal University of Minas Gerais,
Brazil. President,
Brasilian Society of Rheumatology 2002/2004

Prakash K. Pispati, MD, FRSM (Lon.)
Consultant Rheumatologist,
Jaslok Hospital & Research Centre,
Bombay, India.
President,
Asia Pacific League of Associations for Rheumatology.
Past President, Indian Rheumatology Association

C. Panchapakesa Rajendran, MBBS, DCH, MD, DM
Professor and Head,
Department of Rheumatology,
Madras Medical College and
Government General Hospital,
Chennai, India

Morton Scheinberg, MD, PhD, FACP
Physician and Research Associate,
Hospital Israelita Albert Einstein,
Sao Paulo, Brazil

Yeong-Wook Song, MD, PhD
Professor and Chief,
Division of Rheumatology,
Department of Internal Medicine,
Seoul National University Hospital,
Seoul, Korea

Preface

Twenty-three years have passed since Bill Kelley, Clem Sledge, Shaun Ruddy, and I met with Jack Hanley at W.B. Saunders to plan production of *The Textbook of Rheumatology*. Our goal was to equal or better any current text that described clinical entities and their treatment, but to exceed by far the depth and breadth of existing text in the detail and explication of basic sciences that provide the infrastructure of rheumatology and orthopedic surgery. That first edition, thanks to the diligent writing of many contributors, exceeded our expectations. It became the best-seller of rheumatology texts.

The template for that first edition proved successful, and there has been no reason to change it for subsequent editions. When Bill Kelley stepped down as an active editor, we recognized the importance of "name recognition" and kept the title as *Kelley's Textbook of Rheumatology* while adding John Sergent and Ralph Budd as associate editors in the sixth edition published in 2001. Recognizing as well the reality that new and younger minds should be involved for the present as well as future editions, this seventh edition has seven editors. We added Gary Firestein and Mark Genovese to the group, and the result is highly amplified brain power. Supplementing Shaun, and Ted, and Clem is the basic science knowledge of Gary and Ralph and the clinical science backgrounds of John and Mark. The future of *Kelley's Textbook of Rheumatology* is secure.

This seventh edition was planned with full awareness that we are in the midst of remarkable change in the sciences that form the base of rheumatology. Over the past 70 years we have seen the birth and growth of immunology, biochemistry, cell biology, and genetics. Each of these specialties grew with remarkable independence from the others until recent years. The future of our specialty is now intimately associated with integrative science. Recombinant technology now links genetics with biochemistry, and more important, the translational science that has evolved often enables us to leapfrog directly over traditional basic science to understanding of clinical disease states. Just as in neu-robiology, where studies of the basis of consciousness involve psychology, philosophy, mathematics, and computer science, the unraveling of complex diseases such as systemic lupus erythematosus will require collaborative ventures by immunologists, immunogeneticists, biochemists, and cell biologists. Ironically, each of these specialists is using the same molecular tools, and so added to the team must be those who are developing the next methods that will supplant the micro-arrays, Western and Southern blots, and knock-out mice.

It is with the likelihood that this integrative collaboration that can bring true synergism to the understanding of rheumatic disease that this edition of *Kelley's Textbook of Rheumatology* has been planned. Each of the chapters in the section on the basic sciences describes well both the present and future opportunities for application of these specialized data to specific diseases, and each chapter on pathogenesis of specific diseases refers frequently to the advances that science brings to clinical science.

In this seventh edition an accompanying DVD, organized and edited by Shaun Ruddy, provides expansion of clinical photographs, histopathology, and detailed videos of the musculoskeletal system and arthroscopic views of diseased joints.

The corollary of this burst of basic science that can be clearly integrated with clinical science is the need for frequent updates for our readers, updates that fill the gaps between subsequent editions. In response, we are providing "e-ditions" in the format of a web site that will provide every reader with the latest data and their interpretations that will enable basic scientists to plan new experiments, and clinicians to better diagnose and treat their patients.

While we recognize that the future of paper texts is indeterminate amidst the electronic revolution, we are satisfied that this seventh edition of *Kelley's Textbook of Rheumatology* will serve readers better than any other source of information about rheumatology, orthopedic approaches to rheumatic diseases, and the science that drives understanding of the pathogenesis and treatment of the afflictions that our patients suffer from.

Contents

VOLUME 2

Kelley's
TEXTBOOK OF
Rheumatology

Rheumatoid Arthritis

65 Etiology and Pathogenesis of Rheumatoid Arthritis

GARY S. FIRESTEIN

Rheumatoid arthritis (RA) is the most common inflammatory arthritis, affecting from 0.5 to 1 percent of the general population worldwide. Although the prevalence is surprisingly constant across the globe, regardless of geographic location and race, there are some exceptions. For instance, in China the occurrence of RA is somewhat lower (about 0.3 percent), whereas it is substantially higher in other groups, such as the Pima Indians in North America (about 5 percent). Because of its prevalence and the ready accessibility of joint samples for laboratory investigation, RA has served as a useful model for the study of all inflammatory and immune-mediated diseases. As such, the information gleaned from these studies has provided new and unique insights into the mechanisms of normal immunity.

Although RA is properly considered a disease of the joints, it can cause a variety of extra-articular manifestations. These manifestations clearly show that RA has features of a systemic disease capable of involving a variety of major organ systems. In some cases, rheumatoid factor (RF) production with the formation of immune complexes that fix complement contribute to these extra-articular findings. Moreover, one of the great mysteries of RA is why the synovium is the primary target. Keys to understanding these phenomena lie in comprehension of the arthrotropism of antigens and inflammatory cells and in learning what specific receptors and chemotactic gradients focus the inflammation to the joints.

Despite intensive work, only modest progress has been achieved in determining the cause of RA. Clues have been provided by detailed studies of immunogenetics of the class II major histocompatibility complex (MHC) loci and the usage of specific RF genes, but the truth is we still simply do not know what causes the disease. It is in the area of pathogenesis that most progress has been made since the early 1990s: The role of small-molecule mediators of inflammation (e.g., arachadonic acid metabolites), cytokines, growth factors, chemokines, adhesion molecules, and matrix metalloproteinases (MMPs) has been carefully defined. These products attract and activate cells from the peripheral blood and evoke proliferation and activation of synoviocytes. Proteases can subsequently lead to behavior resembling a localized tumor, which invades and destroys articular cartilage, subchondral bone, tendons, and ligaments (Fig. 65–1). New appreciation of these pathogenic mechanisms has increased awareness that irreversible loss of articular cartilage begins relatively early in the course of RA; therapies to suppress the synovitis must be effective early if joint destruction is to be avoided.

Susceptibility to Development of Rheumatoid Arthritis

Although the etiology of RA remains a mystery, a variety of studies suggest that a blend of environmental and genetic factors is responsible; a contribution of either one is necessary but not sufficient for full expression of the disease. The most compelling example for a genetic component is in monozygotic twins, in whom the concordance rate is perhaps 30 to 50 percent when one twin is affected, compared to 1 percent for the general population. The risk for a fraternal twin of a patient with RA also high (about 2 to 5 percent), but this is not more than the rate for other first-degree relatives. Although the immunogenetics is, at best, incompletely understood, the dominant risk factor (albeit not the only one) is the class II MHC haplotype of an individual.[1]

ROLE OF HLA-DR IN THE SUSCEPTIBILITY TO AND SEVERITY OF RHEUMATOID ARTHRITIS

The structure of class II surface molecules on antigen-presenting cells is of great importance in the susceptibility and severity of RA and accounts for about 40 percent of the genetic influence. Chapter 17 presents a detailed discussion of class I and II MHC antigens and of the insights provided by intensive study of the molecular genetics of RA. Initiation of certain T cell immune responses is dependent, in part, on the presence or absence of particular MHC (in this case DR) allelic products. The MHC also helps determine the T cell repertoire

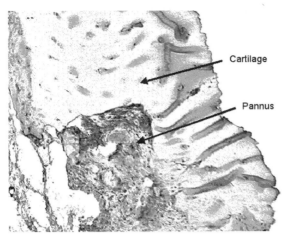

FIGURE 65–1 · Pannus-Cartilage Junction. The invasive front of pannus burrows into cartilage matrix in rheumatoid arthritis (RA) joints. The pannus is primarily composed of macrophages and mesenchymal cells. Immunostaining with anti-CD68 antibody shows the distribution of macrophages in the invasive tissue. (Courtesy of Dr. Paul-Peter Tak.)

in a given individual; those T cells that cannot recognize the endogenous MHC antigens are eliminated in fetal development through thymic deletion. At the same time, autoreactive T cells are eliminated. The end result in the thymus is a fine balance in discrimination between self and non-self; it is not surprising in light of the complexity of this process that autoantibodies can occur to various antigens, to a variable extent, in all of us. The role of the MHC in shaping T cell receptor (TCR) gene usage is not a trivial point because, as will be discussed later, characterization of specific T cell repertoires in the joint or blood of RA patients has been a subject of intense scrutiny, and a bias in the usage of TCR genes has been assumed to be de facto evidence of ongoing T cell activation. Because HLA-DR haplotypes are not randomly distributed among RA patients compared to healthy controls, it is only natural to expect that the T cell repertoire in these patients is skewed as well.

A genetic link between HLA-DR and RA was initially described in the 1970s, with the observation that HLA-DR4 occurred in 70 percent of RA patients, compared to about 30 percent of controls, giving a relative risk of having RA to those with HLA-DR4 of approximately 4 to 5. Careful study of the MHC using complementary DNA (cDNA) probes directed against specific α- and β-chains of the DR loci have revealed "susceptibility cassettes," or shared epitopes on the β-chains of DR that predispose to the development of RA.

The susceptibility to RA is associated with the third hypervariable region of DRβ-chains, from amino acids 70 through 74.[2] The susceptibility epitope is glutamine-leucine-arginine-alanine-alanine (QKRAA), a sequence found in DR4 and DR14 (in which RA is more prevalent), in addition to some DR1β-chains. Current nomenclature attempts to clarify these ambiguities by including information on the specific DRβ sequences. For instance, the DR4β-chains with the greatest association with RA are

referred to as DRB*0401, DRB*0404, DRB*0101, and DRB*1402 (Table 65–1). Individuals with DRβ-chains exhibiting other substitutions in this region have no increased susceptibility to RA. Once the structure of this sequence is considered, up to 96 percent of patients with RA exhibit the appropriate HLA-DR locus, in some populations.[3] In certain ethnic and racial groups, the association with DR4 or QKRAA is not as prominent or is not associated, including Greeks, Pakistanis, Chileans, and African Americans.[4,5]

The QKRAA epitope might also predict the severity of established RA.[6] In one study, all patients who inherited two DRB*04 alleles had rheumatoid nodules, compared to fewer than two thirds of patients with only one allele. Major organ system involvement was observed in 61 and 11 percent of these patients, respectively. These data suggest a "dose response" effect of the HLA genes and imply that severity, rather than susceptibility, is the major contribution of HLA-DR to the disease. This notion is not universally true, and the interpretation depends greatly on the inclusion of patients with transient, self-limited arthritis and varies with race and ethnic background. If transient, self-limited patients (who frequently lack HLA-DR4) are included in the analysis, the correlations between DR4 and RA severity are less striking.[7] The influence of HLA on disease severity also can be influenced by treatment. Early, aggressive administration of corticosteroids, methotrexate, and sulfasalazine prevents enhanced radiographic progression in HLA-DR4–positive patients.

What is so special about the shared epitope? The dose effect of the QKRAA epitope argues against a role for binding of a specific rheumatoid antigen, because DR surface density usually does not alter T cell responses. Based on the crystal structure of HLA-DR molecules, one can infer that the region associated with RA (QKRAA)

TABLE 65–1 · NOMENCLATURE FOR HLA-DR ALLELES AND ASSOCIATIONS WITH RHEUMATOID ARTHRITIS

Old Nomenclature (HLA-DRB1* Alleles)	New Nomenclature	Association with Rheumatoid Arthritis
HLA-DR1	0101	+
HLA-DR4 Dw4	0401	+
HLA-DR4 Dw14	0404/0408	+
HLA-DRw14 Dw16	1402	+
HLA-DR4 Dw10	0402	–
HLA-DR2	1501, 1502, 1601, 1602	–
HLA-DR3	0301, 0302	–
HLA-DR5	1101–1104, 1201, 1202	–
HLA-DR7	0701, 0702	–
HLA-DRw8	0801, 0803	–
HLA-DR9	0901	–
HLA-DRw10	1001	–
HLA-DRw13	1301–1304	–
HLA-DRw14 Dw9	1401	–

From Weyand CM, Hicok KC, Conn DL, Goronzy JJ: The influence of HLA-DRB1 genes on disease severity in rheumatoid arthritis. Ann Intern med 117:801, 1992.

primarily faces away from the antigen-binding cleft of the DR molecule that determines the specificity of peptides presented to CD4+ helper T cells. Attempts to elute peptides from the binding pocket of RA-associated alleles have not revealed a specific antigen that is either unique to or associated with RA.[8] The negative findings in RA contrast with type I diabetes mellitus, in which fragments of a key putative autoimmune target, glutamic acid decarboxylate 65 (GAD65), are bound to the diabetes-associated MHC molecules.

There are several additional caveats: (1) Other genes must be involved, because many healthy individuals carry the QKRAA motif and do not develop RA; (2) the converse hypothesis is also plausible, that is, QKRAA might create a "hole" in the immune response due to a DR topography that prevents an arthrotropic agent from binding, thereby preventing an appropriate T cell–mediated response; (3) the association between the shared epitope and RA might have little to do with antigen recognition and might function by shaping the T cell repertoire in the thymus; and (4) specific DR sequences might alter intracellular MHC trafficking and antigen loading, thereby indirectly affecting antigen presentation in a nonspecific fashion. A reinterpretation of the shared-epitope hypothesis suggests that disease-associated alleles are not involved with presentation of organ-specific autoantigens but rather fail to provide protection against escape from tolerance.[9]

HLA-DQ ASSOCIATIONS

Additional associations with HLA molecules implicate the DQ locus as a key MHC protein that can display arthritogenic peptides, although certain HLA-DR genes are actually protective.[10] This hypothesis is based on the observation that the presentation of collagen II peptide by the H-2Aq molecule (equivalent to DQB1) in mice determines the susceptibility to collagen arthritis, but H-2Eb gene (equivalent to DRB1) confers protection. Perhaps the DQ/DR haplotype is responsible for RA predisposition in humans and the polymorphism of the HLA-DR4 allele determines the degree of protection. This observation is supported by the fact that HLA-DQB1*0302 and HLA-DQB1*0301 are in linkage disequilibrium with most DR4 haplotypes, and the majority of HLA-DR4+ RA patients express one of these alleles.[11] However, a recent study failed to confirm a specific association between HLA-DQ and disease susceptibility in a cohort of Dutch patients.[12]

One possible mechanism for protection is through the presentation of DRB1-derived peptides by RA-associated DQ molecules. To investigate this, DQ8-transgenic mice were produced that express a functional DQB1*0302/DQA1*0301 dimeric molecule in the absence of endogenous mouse class II molecules.[13] These mice were immunized with a series of DRB1 peptides corresponding to most HLA-DRB1 alleles, and in vitro T cell responses against the immunizing peptides were assessed. Although the peptides derived from nonassociated DRB1 molecules were highly immunogenic in DQ8-transgenic mice, those derived from RA-associated DRB1 alleles failed to induce a T cell response.

IMMUNOGLOBULINS

The class II MHC associations described previously primarily implicate cellular immune responses in RA. Associations have also been noted in the humoral system, albeit not as striking. For example, a particular immunoglobulin kappa genotype appears to confer a risk of RA. Although it cannot be considered an immunogenetic determinant, strictly speaking, deficient galactosylation of immunoglobulin might also be a risk factor for the development of autoimmune diseases, including RA. The immunoglobulin G (IgG) glycosylation defect is present before the onset of RA and is especially prominent on the IgG_1, IgG_2, and IgG_4 isotypes of RF.[14] The cause might be reduced galactosyl transferase activity in RA B cells. Deficient galactosylation is also thought to be predictive, in some settings, for patients with early synovitis who will progress ultimately to full-blown RA. Autoantibodies lacking galactose are more pathogenic than those with a normal glycosylation in murine collagen arthritis; passive transfer of arthritis in T cell–primed mice is exacerbated by infusions of IgG fractions that lack galactose, whereas the galactosylated fraction is nonpathogenic.[15]

CYTOKINE POLYMORPHISMS AND OTHER GENETIC ASSOCIATIONS

The clear genetic influences on RA naturally directed considerable attention toward additional non-MHC genes. Single nucleotide polymorphisms (SNPs) in promoter regions or coding regions have been extensively investigated in RA. The former could lead to altered gene regulation due to variable binding of transcription factors to promoters, whereas the latter directly changes the amino acid sequence of the encoded protein. A second method for assessing genetic associations involves the evaluation of microsatellite sequences near key genes that are implicated in the disease. Microsatellites are tandem repeated sequences in the DNA that are primarily (but not exclusively) located in noncoding regions. Considerable heterogeneity exists in the length of each microsatellite, which can indirectly alter gene expression or be in linkage disequilibrium with other undefined genetic polymorphisms. Table 65–2 shows some of the SNPs and microsatellites that have been studied in with RA. The relative contribution of each is still poorly defined, and variations in technique, stage of disease, and patient populations result in some disagreement among various reports.

Given the importance of cytokines in RA (see following), it is not surprising that many studies have focused on these genes. The most intriguing evidence relates to tumor necrosis factor-alpha (TNF-α) (see also Chapter 25). This proinflammatory factor is thought to be a major cytokine in the pathogenesis of RA, and the TNF genes are located in the MHC locus on chromosome 6 in humans. Several polymorphisms of the TNF-α promoter, including two at positions −238 and −308, can alter gene transcription. Associations among the TNF polymorphisms and RA susceptibility and radiographic progression have been reported, although there is not uniform agreement.

TABLE 65–2 • NON–CLASS II MAJOR HISTOCOMPATIBILITY COMPLEX (MHC) ASSOCIATIONS IN RHEUMATOID ARTHRITIS

Gene	Region Studied	Association with Susceptibility	Association with Severity
TNF-α	Promoter	+	+/–
IL-1	Coding region; association with IL-1β strongest	+/–	+
IL-1Ra	Coding region	–	+
IL-3	Promoter	+	
IL-4	Intron	+	
	Promoter	–	
IL-6	Promoter	–	
IL-10	Promoter	–	
IL-12	3′ untranslated region	–	
IFNγ	Intron microsatellite	+/–	+/–
CCR5	CCRδ32 allele	–	+
RANTES	Promoter	+	
MIF	Promoter		+
RAGE	Ligand binding domain	+	
CTLA4	3′ untranslated region	+	
TGF-β	Coding region	+	
FcRγIII	Coding region	+	

Abbreviations: +, association observed; –, no association observed; +/–, association observed in some studies but not in others; CCR5, chemokine receptor 5; FcRγIII, Fc receptor γIII; IFN-γ, interferon-gamma; IL, interleukin; IL-1Ra, interleukin-1 receptor antagonist; MIF, macrophage inhibitory factor; RAGE, receptor for advanced glycosylation end products; RANTES, regulated on activation normal T expressed secreted; TGF-ß, transforming growth factor-beta; TNF-α, tumor necrosis factor-alpha.

Associations with other polymorphisms or microsatellites have been identified for several other cytokines, inflammatory mediators, and chemokines, including interleukin-1 (IL-1), CCR5, and RANTES. One SNP for the T cell costimulatory molecule CTLA4 is also associated with susceptibility.[16] The contribution of each gene is relatively small compared to class II MHC, but combinations might provide an appropriate genetic background to influence the course of arthritis. No linkage has been noted with other cytokines that might play a role in RA, such as IL-6 and IL-12.

GENDER

RA is one of many chronic inflammatory diseases that predominates in women. The ratio of female to male patients (2:1 to 4:1) is significant yet not nearly as high as in Hashimoto's thyroiditis (25:1 to 50:1), systemic lupus erythematosus (9:1), or even autoimmune diabetes mellitus (5:1). The basis of the gender differences is not known but presumably is related to effects of the hormonal milieu on immune function.

Pregnancy is often associated with remission of the disease in the last trimester. More than three quarters of pregnant patients with RA improve, starting in the first or second trimester; but 90 percent of these experience a flare of disease associated with a rise in RF titers in the weeks or months after delivery. The mechanism of protection is not defined but might be due to the expression of suppressive cytokines such as IL-10 during pregnancy or alterations in cell-mediated immunity. A possible relationship between the alleviation of RA symptoms during the last trimester of pregnancy and immunogenetics may be supported by the observation that during pregnancy, alloantibodies in the maternal circulation develop against paternal HLA antigens. Maternal-fetal disparity in HLA class II phenotypes can correlate with pregnancy-induced remission. Over three fourths of pregnant women with maternal-fetal disparity of HLA-DRB1, DQA, and DQB haplotypes have significant improvement, whereas disparity is only observed in one fourth of women whose pregnancy is characterized by continuous active arthritis.[17] Therefore, suppression of maternal immune responses to paternal HLA haplotypes might be protective. This question remains unsettled because a recent study failed to find a correlation between the HLA disparity and clinical improvement during pregnancy.[18]

OTHER ENVIRONMENTAL INFLUENCES

A number of environmental factors clearly must be related to RA susceptibility, although no specific exposure has been definitively identified as a pivotal agent. Considerable effort has been expended on case-controlled and retrospective studies to determine the influence of oral contraceptives. Although some suggestive data exist for a protective effect, the effect (if it exists) is probably very small and is temporary (i.e., delaying rather than preventing disease). Other endocrine influences, including corticotrophin-releasing hormone or estrogen synthase, have been linked with RA. Nulliparity has also been described as a risk factor, but not all studies confirm this. Smoking is associated with RA and the generation of RF. Of the many studies that have been performed, most suggest a relatively small independent risk posed by smoking in patients that are seropositive for RF.

Possible Direct Causes of Rheumatoid Arthritis

One or multiple genetic factors probably predispose an individual to developing RA. However, attempts to identify specific infectious agents as the etiology have generally met with disappointment. A guess, based on available data, is that several environmental stimuli, possibly viruses or retroviruses, infect an individual with the appropriate genetic background, and through some mechanism, the inflammatory response is focused in joints (Table 65–3). After gaining a toehold there, the synovitis persists—even in the absence of the offending agent—because of local autoimmunity and other influences that enable the disease to become self-perpetuating. This hypothesis will be discussed in greater detail at the end of this chapter.

INFECTIOUS AGENTS

Bacteria, Mycobacteria, Mycoplasma, and Their Components

Although animal models of arthritis in which immunization with bacterial cell walls (e.g., streptococcal cell wall arthritis in Lewis rats) or killed mycobacteria (e.g., adjuvant arthritis in Lewis rats) exhibit many clinical and histologic features of RA, active infection of synovial tissue by pyogenic bacteria is an unlikely cause of RA. Extensive searches for a unique or specific organism in synovial tissue or joint effusions have been negative. Antibodies to certain organisms, such as *Proteus*, are reportedly elevated in the blood of patents with RA, but this could represent an epiphenomenona or a result of nonspecific B cell activation.[19] Sensitive polymerasechain reaction techniques to identify the bacterial genome in synovial tissue demonstrate that a high percentage of RA and reactive arthritis patients contain bacterial DNA sequences.[20] The bacteria identified are not unique and generally represent a cross section of skin and mucosal bacteria, including *Acinetobacter* and *Bacillus* spp. It is possible that the synovium functions as an adjunct to the reticuloendothelial system in arthritis, allowing local macrophages to accumulate circulating bacterial products.

Bacterial proteoglycans have also been detected in RA synovial tissue using immunohistochemistry, and antigen-presenting cells containing these products express proinflammatory cytokines such as TNF-α. Although the bacteria or their proteoglycans might persist in the joint, this is likely a secondary phenomenon that can contribute to established synovitis.[21] An alternative hypothesis is that nonspecific activation of innate immunity by bacterial products through Toll-like receptors can serve as an initiating event that permits local establishment of cytokine networks or autoimmunity. The same might be true for DNA from many bacterial species, including *Mycobacteria.* Specific nucleotide sequences found in prokaryotic cells can activate Toll-like receptors and stimulate innate immune responses. Chronic synovitis can then potentially persist through independent mechanisms (see following).

Considerable attention has been directed at a potential role for *Mycoplasma* and *Chlamydia* in arthritis. *Mycoplasma*-derived superantigens, such as from *Mycoplasma arthritidis*, can directly induce T cell–independent cytokine production by macrophages and can exacerbate or trigger arthritis in mice immunized with type II collagen.[22] Despite this and other circumstantial evidence, most efforts to identify *Mycoplasma* organisms or DNA in joint samples have been negative, and there is no direct evidence to support these organisms as etiologic agents.[23] The situation is similar with *Chlamydia*; a synovitis can be explained by this organism in a small minority of patients at best.[24]

The striking similarity of histopathologic changes in RA and in joints of occasional patients with Lyme disease, caused by the spirochete *Borrelia burgdorferi*, leaves open the possibility that an as-yet-unappreciated or unknown organism is causative. Lyme arthritis provides a clear example of an infectious arthritis caused by an organism that can be very difficult to detect or grow from joint tissue. It is not known if chronic Lyme arthritis requires continued antigen exposure or whether, as might occur in RA, the inciting organism can be eradicated without necessarily curing the synovitis.

Epstein-Barr Virus, dnaJ Proteins, and Molecular Mimicry

Epstein-Barr virus (EBV) has been indirectly implicated in the pathogenesis as well as the etiology of RA.[25] EBV is a polyclonal activator of B lymphocytes that increases the production of RF, and rheumatoid macrophages and T cells have defective suppression of EBV proliferation in human B cells. Rheumatoid patients appear to have higher levels of EBV shedding in throat washings, an increased number of virus-infected B cells in the circulating blood, higher levels of antibodies to the EBV antigens, and abnormal EBV-specific cytotoxic T cell responsiveness compared to controls. Patients with RA have problems with the control and elimination of EBV-transformed lymphocytes; this has fueled speculation that a lymphocyte defect is a principal triggering event in this disease and that abnormal control of EBV is pathogenic. More recent studies suggest that EBV DNA is present more frequently in RA synovial tissue compared to controls, especially if the patient expresses the RA-associated susceptibility epitope on class II MHC molecules. Patients with a low frequency of T cell precursors that respond to EBV glycoprotein gp110 have more severe disease, perhaps because they have less effective immunity to the virus.[26]

Additional intriguing data implicating EBV in RA are derived from sequence homology between the susceptibility cassette in HLA-DR proteins and the EBV glycoprotein gp110. Like DRB*0401, gp110 contains the QKRAA motif, and patients with serologic evidence of a previous EBV infection have antibodies against this epi-

---

TABLE 65–3 • ETIOLOGY OF RHEUMATOID ARTHRITIS: POSSIBLE INFECTIOUS CAUSES

Infectious Agent	Potential Pathogenic Mechanisms
Mycoplasma	Direct synovial infection; superantigens
Parvovirus B19	Direct synovial infection
Retroviruses	Direct synovial infection
Enteric bacteria	Molecular mimicry (QKRAA)
Mycobacteria	Molecular mimicry (proteoglycans, QKRAA), immunostimulatory DNA
Epstein-Barr virus	Molecular mimicry (QKRAA)
Bacterial cell walls	Macrophage activation

tope.[27] An inference from these data can be that T cell recognition of EBV epitopes in some patients with HLA-DR4, -DR14, or -DR1 may cause an immune response directed at innocent bystander cells through "molecular mimicry," whereas in those with other class II MHC alleles, no cross-reactivity with EBV proteins would exist. This hypothesis could potentially account for disease perpetuation in the absence of active infection in patients with a specific MHC genotype, a scenario that is consistent with many observations in the chronic rheumatoid joint. Nevertheless, the data are primarily circumstantial, and gp110 is only one of many xenoproteins that contain QKRAA. The *E. coli* dnaJ protein, which is a bacterial heat-shock protein (HSP), also contains the cassette and also represents a potential link between gut bacteria and chronic arthritis. RA T cells, especially synovial fluid T cells, but not normal peripheral blood cells, have increased proliferative responses to this protein, perhaps supporting the molecular-mimicry link between any of a variety of QKRAA-containing proteins and arthritis.[28]

Parvovirus

Antecedent infection with parvovirus B19 has been suggested in some patients with RA based on serologic evidence.[29] Anti–human parvovirus (IgG) levels later decline but are still present 8 months or more after the onset of symptoms. Despite these cases, it is important to point out that very few rheumatoid patients have evidence of such a coincident infection, and only about 5 percent have evidence of recently acquired parvovirus B19 infection at the time of disease onset. Using polymerase chain reaction methods to detect B19 genes in synovial tissue, however, 75 percent of RA synovium samples were positive compared to about 20 percent of non-RA controls.[30] Many of the B19-positive RA patients did not have serum anti-B19 antibodies. More recently, immunohistochemical evidence of the B19 protein VP-1 was detected in patients with RA but not other forms of arthritis.[31] Sublining mononuclear cells, rather than the intimal lining, exhibited the most intense staining. The majority of the patients also had detectable B19 DNA in their synovium. Furthermore, evidence of infective B19 virus was provided by coculture experiments with uninfected cell lines and RA synovial cells. In other studies, however, no evidence of the B19 genome in joint samples was detected, or the presence of B19 DNA was not specific for RA.[32]

The mechanisms of B19-induced synovitis, when it does occur, could be related to alterations in the function of fibroblast-like synoviocytes.[33] In a cell-culture model of synoviocyte invasion into cartilage, infection with the parvovirus significantly increased the migration of cells into the matrix. Because this phenotype has also been described in RA, local infection could increase to the aggressive nature of synoviocytes. Based on current data, however, it is likely that parvovirus B19 accounts for only a small subset of patients with RA-like disease.

Other Viruses

Because rubella virus and the rubella vaccine can cause synovitis in humans, the virus has attracted some atten-

tion as a possible triggering agent. Live rubella virus can be isolated from synovial fluid in some patients with chronic inflammatory oligoarthritis or polyarthritis in the absence of firm clinical evidence of rubella. However, the rubella patients do not have the classic polyarticular involvement seen so often in RA; most have an oligoarthritis involving large joints. As with B19 infection, it is possible that a subset of patients with chronic polyarthritis have disease due to direct infection with wild-type or attenuated rubella virus.

Studies of synovial tissue in a variety of inflammatory and noninflammatory arthropathies have also demonstrated DNA of other viruses, such as cytomegalovirus and herpes simplex, but not adenovirus or varicella zoster.[34] As with bacterial DNA, parvovirus, and EBV, the localization of viral DNA to the inflamed joint might be related to the migration of inflammatory cells containing the viral genome or other nonspecific mechanisms rather than due to active infection. Although the hypothesis that one or more of these viral infections might serve as a triggering agent in the genetically susceptible host is both appealing and intellectually satisfying, the pathogenic role of these agents remains uncertain.

Lentiviruses are a subfamily of retroviruses that derive their name from the slow time course of the infections they cause in humans and animals. Pathologic changes in lentivirus infections are, for the most part, indirectly mediated by the immune and inflammatory responses of the host. For example, an epidemic deforming arthritis in goats and sheep is caused by the Visna lentivirus. The pathogenesis of the disease appears to be infection of monocytes that subsequently migrate to the synovium; resultant cytokine production leads to the accumulation of lymphocytes and other cells. Of interest, the cytokine profile of this disease is very similar to RA in that T cell products are relatively low and macrophage cytokines are abundant.[35] Hence, a "Trojan horse" mechanism can be invoked; the viral genome can be concealed within monocytes and transported without detection to other sites.

Although similar retroviral infections have been suggested many times as the cause of RA, extensive searches for potential agents have not been fruitful. This does not rule out the possibility that difficult-to-detect agents might be present, or even that endogenous retroviruses might play a role. In fact, endogenous retroviruses are abundant in inflamed and normal synovium, although certain transcripts are differentially expressed in RA cells.[36] Some indirect studies are suggestive of retroviral infection, such as the demonstration of zinc-finger transcription factors in cultured synoviocytes. In addition, the pX domain of one human retrovirus, human T lymphotropic virus-1 (HTLV-1), causes synovitis in transgenic mice, and synoviocytes from patients infected with HTLV-1 express some features of a transformed phenotype, with increased proliferation and cytokine production.[37]

AUTOIMMUNITY

The idea that aberrant immune responses are directed toward self antigens in RA was recognized with the discovery of RF in the blood of patients with the disease. Initially described by Waaler and later by Rose, it was not until the mid 1950s that Kunkel and colleagues firmly established that RF is an autoantibody. This ultimately led to the notion that RA is an autoimmune disease. Synovial inflammation was thought to be mediated by local immune-complex formation and complement consumption. Although the understood nature of the autoantigens has changed over the years, and the relative contributions of cellular and humoral immunity have been debated, emphasis on the role of autoantibodies in RA has had a resurgence over the last few years. Patterns of autoantibodies and autoimmune cellular responses initiated by activation of the innate immune system might be more important than a particular antigen.

Rheumatoid Factor: The First Evidence of Autoimmunity in Rheumatoid Arthritis

The identification and characterization of RF as a self antibody was the first direct evidence that auto-immunity might play a role in RA. For many years, immune complexes comprising RF and other immunoglobulins were thought to be solely responsible for RA (see Chapter 19). Although it is now generally accepted that RF can contribute to acute inflammatory synovitis, RF and even B cells might not be required for expression of a rheumatoid-like arthritis described in patients with agammaglobulinemia caused by inactive B lymphocytes.[38] Nevertheless, the presence of RF and its resultant pathogenic consequences are still considered a cardinal feature of RA.

Longitudinal studies of patients with a high risk of RA, such as Native Americans, show that RF production often precedes the onset of RA by many years. One confounding feature is that pinpointing the actual date of disease onset is not always readily discernable. In animal models of arthritis, the preclinical phase can be marked by synovial inflammation, cytokine production, and transcription-factor activation long before clinical signs of arthritis are apparent. The same is probably true in RA because the synovial biopsies of asymptomatic joints in patients with established disease can have the typical appearance of rheumatoid synovitis. Although some patients are initially "seronegative" for RA and subsequently convert to "seropositive," this is rather unusual, and any seroconversion typically occurs during the first year of disease activity. Some patients who are seronegative but otherwise have a clinical diagnosis consistent with RA have "hidden" RFs in their 19-S or 7-S serum fractions, and these can be identified by antibody specific for the major RF cross-reactive idiotype.[39] Cross-reactive idiotypes among monoclonal IgM proteins with anti-IgG activity, and the possible expression of this germline by many individuals, suggests that antibodies against IgG might contribute to the triggering event.

The role of RF in the initiation, amplification, and perpetuation of the process is well supported. For instance, although some patients with virtually no circulating IgG develop RA, patients with a positive test result for RF in blood have more severe clinical disease and complications than seronegative patients. RF is also able to fix and activate complement by the classic pathway, and there is clear evidence of local complement production and consumption in the rheumatoid joint. Large quantities of IgG RF are produced by rheumatoid synovial tissue and form complexes through self-association. RF-containing immune complexes are readily detected in RA synovial tissue as well as the surface layers of cartilage. The latter is especially relevant because immobilized complexes can facilitate complement fixation with resultant release of chemotactic peptides. In experiments performed in patients with RA, a marked inflammatory response was elicited when RF from the patient was injected into a joint, but not when normal IgG was given.[40] Although this type of experiment is clearly difficult to reproduce today, it provides clear evidence that RF has phlogistic properties that can either initiate or exacerbate synovial inflammation.

Despite the evidence for antigen-mediated responses as regulators of RF, the driving force behind RF production has not been fully elucidated and must be considered in light of the observation that RF production can precede the onset of RA (see Chapter 19). Enhanced helper T cell function has been correlated with the spontaneous production of RF, although mainly for the IgM isotype.[41] The natural killer (NK) cells and the cytokine profile of the joint (especially IL-6), which have well-described B cell stimulating properties, can also support nonspecific B cell activation. In addition, terminally differentiated plasma cells that spontaneously secrete RF are present in RA synovial fluid, and RF production has markedly increased when the cells were cultured in the presence of fibroblast-like synoviocytes and IL-10.[42] These CD20$^-$ CD38$^+$ cells also can be demonstrated in other forms of arthritis, but they do not release significant amounts of RF.

Several hypotheses have been advanced to explain how IgG could become immunogenic. First, new determinants on IgG might be exposed after polymerization of molecules or formation of IgG complexes with specific antigens. Second, structural anomalies in the IgG of rheumatoid patients may render it immunogenic, such as a possible defect in the hinge region of rheumatoid IgG that could increase the binding affinity to membrane fragment crystallizable (Fc) receptors on B lymphocytes. Finally, autoantigenic reactivity of IgG could be related to demonstrated changes in the relative extent of galactosylation, as mentioned previously. Breaking tolerance for immunoglobulin determinants recognized by RF has a genetic influence as well, because first-degree relatives of seropositive patients with RA frequently are seropositive themselves.

Three quarters of patients with RA are seropositive using standard tests for RF, although the percentage can be as high as 90 percent when assayed for IgM RF with enzyme-linked immunosorbent assays. Although IgG and IgM RFs are thought to be the most abundant and most pathogenic in RA, IgE RF has also been demonstrated in some patients, especially those with extra-articular manifestations. IgE RF can potentially complex with aggregated IgG in synovial tissue, and the subsequent complexes then could degranulate synovial mast cells through activation of Fc receptors in the synovium. IgA RFs are also produced in RA, including patients who are seronegative as determined by standard clinical tests that primarily detect IgM RF.

The RFs produced in RA differ from those produced by in healthy individuals or from patients with paraproteins.[43] The avidity of RF for the Fc portion of IgG is several orders greater in RA than in Waldenström's macroglobulinemia or in cryoglobulins. The germline-derived RFs are produced by immature CD5-positive B cells, and many paraproteins expressed by malignant B cells (such as Waldenström's macroglobulinemia) are derived from the germline. In addition, some normal B cells in adult human tonsil tissue express and synthesize germline-encoded RFs, although they do not secrete the protein. RFs produced by RA B cells are distinct in that these proteins are often not encoded by germline sequences. Instead, their sequence appears to be derived through rearrangements and somatic mutations. RF analysis in synovial membrane cultures from patients with a variety of diseases have indicated that only cells from patients with seropositive RA synthesize RF spontaneously.[44] IgM RF represents about 7 percent of the total IgM produced by cells, and IgG RF represents 3 percent of IgG synthesized in the synovial cultures.

The expression of any particular idiotype on RFs (or other immunoglobulins, for that matter) is under genetic control. This limited response is related to restriction of the number of relevant or expressible variable (V) genes available in the germline.[45] RF in RA primarily use the variable heavy 3 (VH3) gene and a variety of variable light (VL) genes, whereas natural antibodies use VH1 or VH4 and the Vκ3 genes. The kappa light chain repertoire expressed in RF-producing cells isolated from a patient with chronic RA are enriched for two specific Vκ genes, known as Humkv325 and Humkv328, which are also frequently associated with RF paraproteins.[46] However, the κ-variable domains contained many somatic mutations and non–germline-encoded nucleotides. Based on the extent of substitutions, the selection and production of these specific RFs was likely due to antigenic drive rather than derived directly from the germline, as is the case with many paraproteins. Additional RFs have been identified with characteristics similar to an antigen-driven response, although some examples of germline RFs have also been isolated from RA synovium. A crystal structure of one IgM RF bound to IgG showed a key contact residue of the RF with the Fc portion of IgG containing a somatic mutation, thereby supporting the notion that the mutations are related to affinity maturation.[47] Of interest, only a few amino acid contact points were identified, suggesting that this antibody might have arisen in response to another, as-yet-unidentified antigen, and the reactivity with IgG Fc was due to cross-reactivity. The binding site did not include any contacts with carbohydrates, as might have been predicted if abnormal galactosylation was responsible for breaking tolerance.

The ability to generate high-affinity RFs similar to those found in RA is tightly controlled. Transgenic mice engineered to produce RFs indicate that high-affinity RFs are deleted in the thymus, whereas the low-affinity RFs are not.[48] Therefore, mechanisms for inactivation of higher-affinity RF B cell clones must exist. Exposure of transgenic mice expressing a human IgM RF to soluble human IgG in the absence of T cell help causes antigen-specific B cell deletion in 2 to 3 days.[49] However, B cell activation and sustained RF secretion does occur if T cell help is provided simultaneously. This suggests that the high-affinity RF production, as occurs in RA, is associated with T cell activation, whereas these RF-producing cells are deleted in normal individuals. It is still a matter of conjecture whether the antigen-driven affinity maturation and the escape from B cell deletion that occurs in RA is a primary event due to loss of tolerance or whether it is secondary to acquired conformation changes of immunoglobulin caused by RA. In either case, there is little question that the ability to produce high-affinity RF and create a milieu that favors intra-articular complement fixation can participate in the synovial inflammatory process.

Autoimmunity to Cartilage-Specific Antigens

Because synovial tissue inflammation is a hallmark of RA, it is only natural to assume that certain joint-specific antigens might play an etiologic or pathogenic role. The number of potential antigens is extensive, and there is no convincing evidence to date that one specific "rheumatoid" antigen exists. In contrast, the emerging picture of autoimmunity in RA tends to implicate patterns of self-directed responses, rather than a single epitope that encompasses all patients at all times during the disease. It is quite possible that articular autoimmunity could vary with the stage of disease, the clinical manifestations, and treatment.

Type II Collagen

The discoveries that immunization with type II collagen can cause arthritis in rats and mice and that the disease can be passively transferred by IgG fractions containing anticollagen antibodies or by transfer of lymphocytes from affected animals have spawned extensive experiments that illustrate the antigenicity of collagen, the arthrotropic nature of the disease produced, and the dependence of experimental animals on class II MHC genes for reactivity. It is clear that functional T cells are necessary to initiate a collagen-induced arthritis and that a major immunogenic and arthritogenic epitope on type II collagen resides in a restricted area of the type II collagen chains.

Most data in humans are consistent with the hypothesis that RA is not caused by the development of antibodies to type II collagen but that the inflammatory response is amplified by their production (Table 65–4). Sera from patients with RA contain antibody titers to denatured bovine type II collagen that are significantly higher than those found in control sera[50]; however, there is no difference in antibody titers to native collagen, suggesting that the denatured form generated after the breakdown of connective tissue might serve as the immunogen. Antibodies that bind collagen have pathogenic potential in RA, especially among the IgG$_3$

TABLE 65–4 • POTENTIAL AUTOANTIGENS IN RHEUMATOID ARTHRITIS

Cartilage antigens
- Type II collagen
- gp39
- Cartilage link protein
- Proteoglycans
- Aggrecan
Citrullinated peptides
Glucose-6-phosphoisomerase
HLA-DR (QKRAA)
Heat-shock proteins
Heavy-chain binding protein (BiP)
hnRNP-A2
Immunoglobulins (IgG)

subclass.[51] Anticollagen antibodies purified from the sera of patients with RA can activate complement, generating C5a when they bind to cartilage. This adds relevance to the observations that anticollagen antibodies can be eluted from rheumatoid articular cartilage.[52] In addition, isolated synovial-tissue B lymphocytes actively secrete anti–type II collagen antibodies in almost all patients with seropositive RA, whereas articular cells from non-RA patients do not.[53] Synovial fluid T cells also recognize and respond to type II collagen, and 3 to 5 percent of RA synovial fluid–derived T cell clones are autoreactive to the protein. Of interest, T cell responses to type II collagen, especially a dominant epitope at amino acid 263-270, is much greater if the epitope is glycosylated.[54] This could explain why traditional approaches using nonglycosylated antigen have not consistently shown increased reactivity to type II collagen in RA.

gp39 and Other Cartilage-Specific Antigens

Several other cartilage components besides type II collagen have been implicated as potential autoantigens in RA. Among the most provocative is cartilage glycoprotein gp39. Several gp39 peptides can bind to the HLA-DR*0401 molecule and stimulate proliferation of T cells from patients with RA.[55] BALB/c mice, which are often resistant to experimental arthritis, develop a polyarticular inflammatory arthritis after immunization with gp39 and complete Freund's adjuvant. Although anti-gp39 antibodies are only detected in a small percentage of patients, it appears to be highly specific for RA.[56] Other examples of potential cartilage autoantigens include proteoglycans, aggrecan, cartilage-link protein, and other types of collagen. T cell clones derived from RA peripheral blood can proliferate in response to aggrecan, and most of these cells had a T helper type 1 (Th1) cytokine profile, suggesting that they contribute to the Th1 bias in synovial tissue.[57]

Autoimmunity to Nonarticular Antigens

Increasing attention has been focused on autoimmune responses that are not specific for components unique to articular structures.[58] Although their role in etiology is not always clear, at least some autoantibodies (such as

RF) can appear before the onset of clinical disease. In other cases, the antigen-antibody system might participate in a pattern of autoimmune responses that can lead to synovial inflammation.

Citrullinated Peptides

Antibodies directed against keratin were first described in the 1970s and the primary target antigen was later discovered to be the filament-aggregating protein, filaggrin. These antibodies actually bind to epitopes on filaggrin that contain citrulline, which is derived from post-translational modification of arginine by peptidylarinine deiminase. Anticitrulline antibodies recognize many proteins that contain this modified amino acid and have been reported in the serum of more than 90 percent of RA patients.[59] IgG and IgM anticitrulline antibodies are produced by B cells in rheumatoid synovial tissue and synovial fluid. Although their pathogenic role is not certain, they are produced in early RA as well as during the preclinical phase in some patients. The antibodies, therefore, might have some diagnostic utility and have also been described as useful as predictors of severity. Certain isoforms of the enzyme that citrullinate peptides are increased in RA synovium, and its polymorphisms may be associated with the disease.[59a]

Glucose-6-Phosphoisomerase

An interesting spontaneous arthritis model demonstrated that antigen-specific immunity against a seemingly irrelevant nonarticular antigen can lead to destructive arthritis.[60] A transgenic mouse strain was developed by breeding nonobese diabetic mice (which develop autoimmune diabetes) with a strain that expressed a transgenic T cell receptor recognizing bovine pancreas ribonuclease. The cross-bred animals developed spontaneous polyarticular inflammatory arthritis after 1 month that required both CD4+ T cells and B cells for its initiation but was independent of these elements after the disease was established. Hence, joint-specific disease can occur in a host with a predisposition to autoimmunity and systemic self-reactivity. The mechanism of disease relates to the fortuitous formation of antibodies to the ubiquitous enzyme glucose-6-phosphate isomerase (GPI), and the disease can be transferred to normal mice with the serum of affected animals. The passive arthritis model is dependent on the alternate complement pathway, Fc receptors (especially FcRγIII), and mast cells, but not T or B cells. IL-1 appears to be more important than TNF-α in this model, and the IL-1 knockout mice are almost completely protected from disease. Histochemical studies indicate that GPI adheres to the surface of cartilage, hence permitting local antibody binding and complement fixation.

Although the model appears on first blush to be due to a ubiquitous antigen, articular homing of the antigen suggests that it behaves like other arthritis models with "joint-specific" antigens. Although initial data suggested some specificity for RA, anti-GPI antibodies are detected in a relatively small percentage of RA patients and are not specific for the disease.[61] Nevertheless, it might, along with several other antibody systems, contribute to local complement fixation and inflammation.

Heterogeneous Nuclear Ribonuceloprotein-A2 and Heavy chain Binding Protein

Several other autoantigens have been characterized in RA that are expressed in synovium, although they are also produced in many other locations. For instance, antibodies directed against the heterogeneous nuclear ribonuceloprotein-A2 (hnRNP-A2), sometimes called RA33, occur in about one third of RA patients, as well as patients with other systemic autoimmune diseases. However, there may be some specificity for RA when compared to osteoarthritis (OA) and seronegative spondyloarthropathies. Autoantibodies that bind to stress-protein immunoglobulin heavy-chain binding protein (BiP) have also been observed.[62] About 60 percent of RA patients have anti-BiP antibodies, and the specificity is reportedly more than 90 percent. In addition to humoral responses, RA T cells can proliferate in response to this protein. Immunization of mice with BiP does not cause arthritis, but it can cross-tolerize mice and prevent collagen-induced arthritis if administered before immunization with type II collagen.[63] BiP is normally expressed in many tissues but is markedly increased in RA synovium.

Heat-Shock Proteins

The HSPs are a family of mainly medium-sized (60 to 90 kD) proteins produced by cells of all species in response to stress. These proteins have conserved amino-acid sequences; for example, certain HSPs of *Myobacterium tuberculosis* have considerable homology with HSPs of humans. The HSPs may facilitate intracellular folding and translocation of proteins as they protect cells from insults induced by heat, bacteria, and oxygen radicals. Immunity against HSPs contributes directly to synovitis and joint destruction in the adjuvant arthritis model in rats in which T lymphocytes recognize an epitope of mycobacterial HSP65 (amino acids 180 through 188). Some of these cells also recognize cartilage proteoglycan epitopes,[64] perhaps explaining the targeting of joints.

Some patients with RA have elevated levels of antibodies to mycobacterial HSPs, especially in synovial fluid.[65] The majority of T cell clones isolated from RA synovial fluid with specificity to mycobacterial components express the γδ–T cell receptor (instead of the more common αβ form) and do not display CD4 or CD8 surface antigens. Freshly isolated synovial fluid T cells from patients with RA briskly proliferate in response to both the acetone-precipitable fraction of *M. tuberculosis* and recombinant 65-kD HSP.[66] However, proliferation to other recall antigens, such as tetanus toxoid, is not increased. Synovial-fluid mononuclear cells activated by 60-kD mycobacterial HSP inhibit proteoglycan production by human cartilage explants.[67] This effect is dependent on the generation of cytokines such as IL-1 and TNF-α by the activated cells. Human 60-kD HSP is expressed in the synovium, although the amount expressed per cell appears to be similar in OA, RA, and normal tissue.

THE RISE AND FALL OF RHEUMATOID ARTHRITIS

Any proposed causative mechanism for RA should incorporate one additional key element: RA might be a relatively new disease in Europe and Northern Africa. Examination of ancient skeletal remains in Europe and Northern Africa fails to reveal convincing evidence of RA, even though other rheumatic diseases, such as OA, ankylosing spondylitis, and gout, are readily discernable. In contrast, typical marginal erosions and rheumatoid lesions are present the skeletons of Native Americans found in Tennessee, Alabama, and Central America from thousands of years ago. The first clear descriptions of RA in Europe appeared in the seventeenth century, and the disease was distinguished from gout and rheumatic fever by Garrod in the mid-nineteenth century. Although still controversial, at least one school of thought suggests that the disease migrated from the New World to the Old World coincident with opening the trade and exploration routes. Because genetic admixture was relatively limited, an undefined environmental exposure potentially caused RA in susceptible Europeans. The most obvious explanation would, of course, be that an infectious agent is responsible.

Equally intriguing, the severity and incidence of RA seems to be decreasing[68] (Fig. 65–2). Whereas the former could be related to the advent of new treatments, the latter could be due to a "birth cohort" effect. In certain well-defined populations, including Native Americans, the incidence of RA has gradually declined by as much as half over the last half of the twentieth century. The birth-cohort theory suggests that the earlier high incidence of disease was cause by an etiologic agent, and the exposure decreased with each succeeding generation. Changes in hygiene and other lifestyle modifications related to industrialization might contribute, and an infectious agent might be less prevalent secondary to these societal changes, as with many other infectious diseases. Perhaps the incidence of RA will continue to

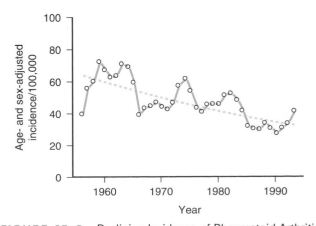

FIGURE 65–2 · Declining Incidence of Rheumatoid Arthritis (RA). Population studies in Minnesota have demonstrated a gradually decreasing incidence of RA over the last 50 years. Similar results have been observed in Native American populations. (From Doran, et al: Arthritis Rheum 46:635, 2002.)

decline over the next half century and will cease to be a serious cause of disability.

Synovial Pathology and Biology

The primary site of immune activation in RA is the synovium. Infiltration of the synovium with mononuclear cells, especially T cells and macrophages, and synovial intimal lining hyperplasia are hallmarks of the disease (Fig. 65–3). In this section, histopathologic and functional aspects of the inflamed joint are reviewed.

SYNOVIAL INTIMAL LINING

The synovial intimal lining is a loosely organized collection of cells that form an interface between the synovium and the synovial fluid space. The synovial intimal lining cells lack tight junctions and a definite basement membrane. The increase in cell number in RA can be quite substantial. In the normal joint, the lining is only one to two cell layers deep, whereas in RA it is often four to 10 cells deep (and sometimes more than

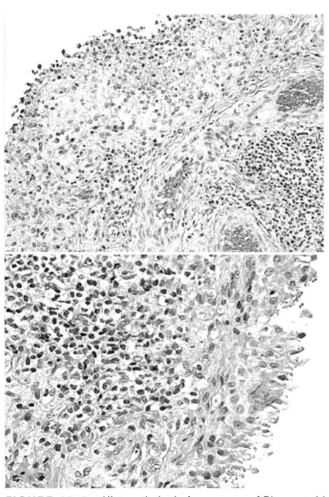

FIGURE 65–3 · Histopathologic Appearance of Rheumatoid Arthritis (RA) Synovium. Intimal lining hyperplasia, angiogenesis, and a prominent mononuclear cell infiltrate are present. Top panel is magnified ×200 and the bottom panel is ×400. (Courtesy of Dr. Paul-Peter Tak.) (See color plate 30.)

20). Two major cell types are found in the lining: a macrophage-like cell known as a type A synoviocyte and a fibroblast-like cell called a type B synoviocyte. The former are derived from the bone marrow and express macrophage surface markers such as CD68, Fc receptors, and CD14, as well as abundant HLA-DR, whereas the latter express little if any class II MHC antigens, are devoid of macrophage markers, and have a scant endoplasmic reticulum. The type B cells also express certain proteins that are unusual for mesenchymal cells, including vascular cell adhesion molecule-1 (VCAM-1), CD55 (decay activating factor [DAF]), cadherin 11, and the proteoglycan-synthesis enzyme uridine diphosphoglucose dehydrogenase (UDPGD). The numbers of type A and B cells are relatively equal in normal synovium. There is an absolute increase in both cell types in RA, although the percentage increase in macrophage-like cells is often greater. In addition, the type A synoviocytes tend to accumulate in the more superficial regions of the intimal lining.

Synovial macrophages are terminally differentiated cells that presumably do not divide in the joint, and the accumulation of cells in RA is likely from the ingress of new bone marrow–derived precursors. Mesenchymally derived type B synoviocytes can divide locally in response to the proliferative factors generated by the activated immune response. Platelet-derived growth factor (PDGF), transforming growth factor-beta (TGF-ß), TNF-α, and IL-1 produced by many different cells combine with products of arachadonic acid metabolism to induce proliferation of these cells. In addition, pluripotential mesenchymal stem cells that arise in the bone marrow and circulate through the blood can migrate into the synovium and differentiate into type B synoviocytes.

Although local proliferation of cells in the intimal lining likely occurs, rheumatoid synovium rarely shows mitotic figures, and thymidine uptake occurs in only a very small percentage of synovial cells. Using a monoclonal antibody that recognizes dividing cells, an even lower rate of cell division (approximately 0.05 percent) is apparent.[69] A somewhat higher percentage of cells that express the cell cycle–specific antigen proliferating cell nuclear antigen (PCNA) are present in RA lining compared to OA.[70] This correlates with the lining-cell expression of the protooncogene c-*myc*, a gene that is intimately linked with fibroblast proliferation.

After rheumatoid synovium is enzymatically dispersed in vitro, two major populations of adherent cells can be readily identified.[71] As might be expected from studies of intact tissue, one type of cell is macrophage-like; these cells have DR antigens, Fc receptors, and monocyte lineage–differentiation antigens and are capable of phagocytosis. They have a limited life span in vitro, rarely surviving more than a few weeks even in the presence of exogenous growth factors or colony-stimulating factors. A second type is defined by the presence of antigens expressed primarily on fibroblasts and by the absence of phagocytic capability, demonstrable DR antigens, or antigens of the monocytic lineage. When the enzymatically dispersed cells are cultured for several passages, it is this last cell type that ultimately survives and proliferates, resulting in a relatively homogeneous population of fibroblast-like cells that are presumed (but not proved) to be derived from the type B synoviocytes in the intimal lining. Additional less-abundant adherent-cell populations are also present in early cultures, including dendritic cells and endothelial cells.

Ultrastructural studies and cell-cloning experiments of dissociated rheumatoid synovial cells have supported this classification.[72] Macrophage-like and fibroblast-like cells grow slowly, with a doubling time of 5 to 7 days. A dendritic or stellate cell population has also been identified; this phenotype may be derived from fibroblast-like cells that can generate a dendritic appearance when incubated with prostaglandin E_2 (PGE_2).[73] After removal of the prostaglandin, the cells revert to normal fibroblast appearance. The fibroblast-like cells grown from the dispersed cells can be passaged for several months in vitro. Their doubling rate is rapid at first, perhaps due to the presence of cytokines produced by contaminating macrophages in the culture or a carry-over effect from the synovial milieu. Over time, proliferation slows, and after 12 to 15 passages, the cells gradually become senescent and ultimately cease to grow. Although it has not been proven that these cells originate solely from the synovial intimal lining, the fact that a significant percentage of cells express VCAM-1 and CD55 suggests that at least some are derived from this region. Synovial fibroblasts from RA have some characteristics reminiscent of tumors or transformed cells, a notion that is consistent with the concept that RA can resemble a locally invasive mesenchymal tumor (see following).

SYNOVIAL T LYMPHOCYTES

Immunohistologic Patterns

In chronic RA, the synovium contains a collection of T lymphocytes that can lead to an organizational structure that resembles a lymph node. The distribution of lymphocytes in the tissue varies from discrete lymphoid aggregates to diffuse sheets of mononuclear cells, with the most prominent location for T cells being the perivascular region. These collections consist of small, $CD4^+$ memory T cells ($CD45RO^+$) with scant cytoplasm. Even though few $CD8^+$ T cells accumulate in the aggregates, formation of ectopic germinal centers in RA synovial tissue may be dependent on them. In a severe combined immunodeficiency (SCID) mouse model of RA using synovial tissue explants, depletion of the CD8+ population causes disintegration of the follicles.[74] Peripheral to these foci is a transitional zone with a heterogeneous mixture of cells, including lymphocytes, occasional undifferentiated blast cells, plasma cells, and macrophages (see Fig. 65–3). Intercellular communication by soluble mediators and direct cell-cell contact occurs here via adhesion molecules, including the lymphocyte function–associated antigens.

Considerable heterogeneity exists in the histologic patterns within a single joint, as well as from patient to patient. In some patients, a more intense inflammatory histopathologic appearance correlates with systemic anergic T cell responses to recall antigens. In other cases, the presence of granulomatous lesions might be associated with extra-articular disease and production of both Th1 and Th2 cytokines in the synovium. In contrast, abundant lymphoid follicles are associated primarily with Th1 cytokines.

T cells constitute about 50 percent or more of cells in most RA synovia, and most are CD4+; only 5 percent or fewer of cells are B lymphocytes or plasma cells. The B cells are located primarily within reactive lymphoid centers, whereas plasma cells and macrophages are often found outside these centers. This arrangement is consistent with T cell–dependent B lymphocyte activation; plasma cells, the main immunoglobulin producers, migrate away from the germinal centers after differentiation. CD4 cells in RA synovium are in intimate contact with B lymphocytes and HLA-DR–positive dendritic cells.

RA synovial T lymphocytes display an activated surface phenotype, with high expression of HLA-DR antigens and CD27. CD27+ CD4+ T cells provide B cell help that can potentially increase synovial antibody production. For maximal T cell responses, a second signal, in addition to antigen stimulation, is usually required. CD28 is one of these costimulatory molecules on T lymphocytes and is highly expressed by synovial T cells in RA.[75] Its ligands, CD80 and CD86 (also called B7-1 and B7-2), are also displayed on antigen-presenting cells in the joint, thereby providing an excellent environment for T cell activation. One unusual phenotype of synovial T cells in RA is a population that expresses CD4 but lacks CD28. Oligoclonal expansion of CD4+CD28-T cells has been described in the peripheral blood and joint samples of patients with RA.[76] The cells can be cytotoxic and can respond to autoantigens but are inefficient B cell stimulators. This population of T cells also occurs more frequently in patients with extra-articular manifestations of RA.

CD40, another costimulatory molecule, and its ligand on T cells, CD40L, are also expressed in RA synovium.[77] CD40L can synergize with IL-1 for the production of cytokines such as granulocyte macrophage-colony stimulating factor (GM-CSF) by CD40-bearing synoviocytes.[78] Synovial lymphocytes also bear adhesion molecules of the very late activation antigen (VLA) and lymphocyte function–associated antigen (LFA) superfamily of integrins, which may enable the inflammatory response to localize and persist within the synovium. A high level of telomerase activity is also present in synovial lymphocytes in RA, but not in OA or trauma patients. Telomerase activity level in the synovial T cells correlates with the intimal lining hyperplasia, angiogenesis, and local lymphocyte accumulation.

T cell activation and the induction of adhesion molecules and other "activation markers" may not actually occur within the joint; rather, this T cell phenotype could enter the synovium and then remains within the joint under the influence of locally expressed chemotactic factors and their armamentarium of adhesion molecules. The cytokine milieu of the joint induces adhesion molecules like intercellular adhesion molecule-1 (ICAM-1), VCAM-1, and connecting segment-1 (CS-1) fibronectin on vascular endothelium. These, in conjunction with chemokines and other chemoattractants, call the cells to the joint based precisely on this phenotype. Furthermore, synovial T cells in RA express characteristic receptors to specific chemokines. The chemokine receptor CCR5 is the ligand for macrophage inhibitory protein-1α and -β and is highly expressed in the infiltrating RA T cells.[79] This particular receptor is preferentially found on Th1 T cells, which might explain accumulation of this phenotype in the rheumatoid synovium. Expression of nonfunctional CCR5 alleles might protect from RA, perhaps by diminishing T lymphocyte ingress into the joint. The chemotactic factor stromal cell–derived factor-1 (SDF-1) is also produced by synovial tissue, and its specific receptor, CXCR4, is displayed by rheumatoid synovial T cells.[80]

These data suggest that the local accumulation of T cells in the joint is not necessarily related to a particular antigen. Instead, antigen-independent processes related to the expression of chemokines and adhesion molecules on vascular endothelium and circulating lymphocytes help determine the mononuclear cell infiltrate. Although local antigen-specific expansion might occur, it is probably is responsible for a small component of the T cell infiltrate. Those cells that encounter their appropriate antigen in the correct cytokine and antigen-presenting cell environment can potentially activate other local cells through direct cell-cell contact or the elaboration of lymphokines.

Synovial T Cell Immune Response

The histopathologic appearance of RA, with exuberant infiltration of the synovium with T lymphocytes, is often pointed to as evidence of a T cell–mediated disease because this is also characteristic of antigen-specific responses. However, the synovium can only respond to inflammation in a limited number of ways. In fact, the histologic appearance of chronic arthritides that are clearly not mediated by T cells (e.g., chronic tophaceous gout) exhibits many of the same features. Progressive destruc-

tion in RA patients despite acquired immunodeficiency syndrome (AIDS) suggests that non–T cell mechanisms are also important.[81]

More direct evidence for synovial T cell activation is often cited from experimental therapeutics. Fistula of the thoracic duct that removes T lymphocytes from the body was shown in 1970 have some efficacy in RA, and leukapheresis has been associated with brief improvement associated with the return toward normal in vitro anergy of peripheral blood mononuclear cells. Total nodal irradiation and high-dose chemotherapy are also very effective means of suppressing systemic helper T cell function. In clinical studies, these procedures did offer some benefit, although symptoms often returned despite persistent suppression of delayed-type hypersensitivity. Treatment with antibodies that deplete T cells, including anti-CD4, anti-CD5, and anti-CD52, has been reported at various times. The responses, if any, were usually very modest and transient despite profound and sometimes prolonged lymphopenia and immunosuppression. In some cases, as with anti-CD4 antibodies, synovial T cells were depleted even though clinical improvement was not observed. However, it is still possible that small numbers of antigen-specific memory T lymphocytes might persist despite an overall decrease in synovial tissue infiltration. Blockade of T cell co-stimulation with the CTLA4-Ig fusion protein has demonstrated some efficacy in RA, supporting the role of T cell activation.

Nevertheless, T cell responses and autoimmunity have been implicated in the pathogenesis of RA, and many sites in the synovium resemble those of a classic delayed-type hypersensitivity reaction. In the subsynovial areas around the small capillaries and high endothelial venules in synovium, tissue macrophages and dendritic cells that express HLA-DR antigens are available to process and present antigen to T lymphocytes (Fig. 65–4). Normal synovial-lining cells can mediate T lymphocyte prolif-

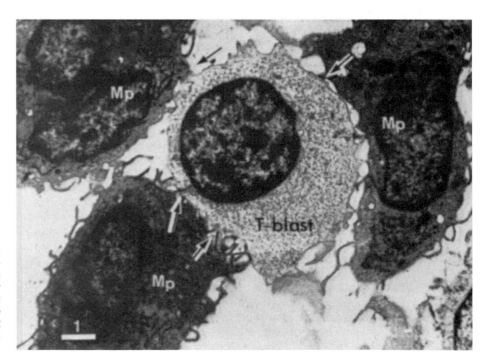

FIGURE 65–4 · T Lymphoblast in Rheumatoid Synovial Tissue Surrounded by Three Macrophages (Mp). The *arrows* point to probable intercellular bridging. This may be the morphologic manifestation of presentation of antigen to the helper T cell by the antigen-presenting cells. (Courtesy of Dr. H. Ishikawa and Dr. M. Ziff.)

eration, but their activating ability appears to be lower than that of epidermal Langerhans' cells, which stand as barriers to the entrance of antigen through the skin. Rheumatoid synovial dendritic cells, however, are extremely efficient in allogeneic T cell activation.[82] In addition to professional antigen-presenting cells, interferon-gamma (IFN-γ)–stimulated fibroblast-like synoviocytes can present antigen to T cells.[83] The microheterogeneity of the rheumatoid synovial tissue, with different numbers and proportions of cell lineages in each area, suggests that antigens presented at each location might also differ, with type II collagen presented to T cells one place, proteoglycans presented elsewhere, and responses to HSPs or viral antigens in yet another region.

Although synovial T cells are generally considered activated, proliferative and cytokine responses are often less than normal peripheral blood cells or even autologous peripheral blood T cells. Spontaneous and stimulated cytokine production, including Th1 factors such as IFN-γ and IL-2, are relatively low. Responses directed toward recall antigens are also deficient, although RA synovial T cells can proliferate briskly to certain HSPs. The mechanisms of decreased responsiveness in the synovial tissue compartment have not been as extensively studied as in synovial fluid or peripheral blood, but they likely include exposure to suppressive factors (e.g., TGF-β), abnormal redox potential that suppresses T cell receptor signal transduction, or induction of anergy. Another contributor to local anergy is the relative lack of the costimulatory molecule CD80 on HLA-DR+ fibroblast-like synoviocytes because coculture of T cells with the synoviocytes suppresses subsequent allogenic responses.[84]

Synovial T cells in RA functionally resemble resting peripheral blood T lymphocytes that have been activated by cytokines rather than antigen.[85] Both synovial and blood T lymphocytes are able to stimulate macrophages to produce TNF-α in a cell contact–dependent manner. This process is dependent on nuclear factor kappa B (NFκB) and is mechanistically distinct from T cell activation via the T cell receptor, which is independent of NFκB. Therefore, the contribution of T cell to the proinflammatory cytokine milieu may be unrelated to antigen-mediated events and could result from passive activation after exposure to the cytokine environment.

T Cell Oligoclonality

Another approach to evaluate T cell activation is to perform detailed analysis of TCR expression. The vast majority of T cells express αβ TCR heterodimers. The receptor antigen specificity is determined by genetic rearrangement of variable (V), diversity, and joining segments of germline sequences that are then combined with constant regions. Antigen recognition and the specificity of T cell responses results from the many permutations of these segments and the occurrence of deletion or point mutations during rearrangement. In theory, the TCR repertoire in immune-mediated diseases could lead to the expansion of cells with similar α-and β-chains.

Dozens of studies were published in the late 1990s reporting a variety of specific TCR genes that were over-represented in the joint (either synovial fluid or tissue) compared to blood of patients with RA. Conflicting data led to the general conclusion that a specific TCR gene profile could not be identified for in RA.[86] In some patients, however, a pattern emerged, suggesting an increased number of T cells expressing Vβ3, -14, and -17, especially in synovial tissue. These particular Vβ genes are structurally related and are unusually susceptible to activation by superantigens. This supports the hypothesis that specific T cells are activated by bacterial or mycoplasmal superantigens, leading to oligoclonal expansion and release of cytokines. Other studies have either not found evidence for the restricted clonality of T cells in RA synovial fluid, synovial tissue, and blood, nor have they identified expansion of different Vβ or Vα genes.

Even if a specific TCR predominated, it might not necessarily reflect the initiating autoimmune event or even the T cells that are pathogenic in the synovium. The best opportunity for detecting the appropriate pathogenic T cell clones in RA is in very early RA, because disease chronicity causes T cells to accumulate in an antigen-independent manner. This is best exemplified in the experimental allergic encephalitis model in rats, which is caused by autoimmunity against myelin basic protein. In the earliest phases, there is a strong bias in the central nervous system for a few antigen-specific pathogenic TCR genes.[87] As the disease progresses, this bias is rapidly overwhelmed by the continued influx of nonspecific cells recruited into the brain by chemokines and adhesion molecules, not by antigen. The same situation likely occurs in RA and other chronic inflammatory arthritides, and the study of TCRs in chronic disease might not give accurate information on the inciting populations.

SYNOVIAL B CELLS

Synovial B cells and plasma cell hyperreactivity are increasingly viewed as key participants in the perpetuation and initiation phases of RA. This notion has been fueled by the descriptions of novel spontaneous models of arthritis in mice, like the K/B×N model, in which loss of tolerance leads to autoantibody production, activation of innate immunity, and chronic synovitis. Furthermore, B cell–directed therapies, such as anti-CD20 antibody, have demonstrated efficacy in RA.

Although many rheumatoid synovial tissues exhibit a diffuse infiltration with mononuclear cells, a significant percentage also have discrete lymphoid follicles populated by B cells in the sublining region. Follicular dendritic cells, B cells, plasma cells, and T lymphocytes collect in these aggregates. The germinal centers are highly organized structures where affinity maturation occurs. B cells are present in the aggregates and express the maturation marker CD20 as well as proliferation antigens such as Ki67. The formation of these structures is dependent on several soluble and membrane-bound cytokines, including lymphotoxin. Recently, a member of the TNF superfamily of cytokines known as B lymphocyte stimulator (BlyS) was identified as a key molecule that regulates B cell differentiation. BlyS binds to transmembrane activator and CAML interactor (TACI), which is present on both B and T cells. If this system is blocked using recombinant TACI-Ig, then the number of B cells is dramatically reduced and antibody production is decreased. The same construct is effective as a therapeutic agent in collagen-induced arthritis, a model that is dependent on autoantibody production.[88] B cells accumulate in lymphoid aggregates in RA synovium under the influence of a variety of chemotactic factors, including B cell–attracting chemokine-1 (CXCL13). This cytokine is expressed in RA synovial lymphoid follicles, especially by follicular dendritic cells.[89]

B cells isolated directly from germinal centers of RA synovium demonstrate a heterogeneous pattern of V-gene usage and rearrangement. The majority of VH genes are not mutated, suggesting that they are recent immigrants from the peripheral blood and are activated locally.[90] For rheumatoid factor-producing cells, shared mutations containing an identical sequence throughout the variable domain of immunoglobulins have been identified in synovial tissue.[91] Preferential utilization of a limited number of VH and DH gene segments and marked preference for a DH reading frame encoding particular hydrophilic residues has also been observed, suggesting antigen-related selection and maturation. Analysis of expressed heavy-chain variable domains supports the notion that the B cell response in RA synovium is oligoclonal.

B cells associated with follicular dendritic cells in the rheumatoid synovium then further differentiate and develop additional mutations, suggesting antigen-driven selection. Plasma cells in other areas of the synovium have distinct rearrangements compared to the B lymphocytes associated with dendritic cells. This raises the question of whether the plasma cells arise locally or migrate from the blood. Although plasma cell rearrangements are not similar to the B cells, groups of plasma cells used similar genes, albeit with distinct mutations. Therefore, the plasma cells likely were derived from a synovial B cell clone that mutated and whose progeny proliferated and differentiated into plasma cells.

What is not yet certain is whether this process represents an ectopic lymphoid organ performing normal functions or whether it is related to autoimmunity. The presence of abundant autoantibody-producing cells in the synovium supports the latter hypothesis, although normal immune responses might also occur in the joint. Cells that produce rheumatoid factors, anti–type II collagen antibody, and anti–citrulline-containing peptide antibody populate the RA synovium. However, not all B cells in the joint are activated. As with T cells, some populations have blunted responses. A population of CD20+ CD38 - B cells with impaired receptor-induced signaling as previously observed in anergic cells also infiltrates the synovium.[92] Some B cells also serve a more active role in synovial immune responses. For instance, in a SCID mouse model using synovial explants, T cell activation and cytokine production was dependent on B cells.[93] These data indicate that, as in T lymphocytes, considerably heterogeneity exists among B cell subsets in RA.

B cell maturation and survival is dependent on stromal cells and cells with "nurse-like" properties that support lymphocyte maturation in the thymus. The bone marrow and synovium of patients with RA also contain nurse-like cells, which can increase expression of CD40 and class II MHC proteins on B cells.[94] B cell survival is supported by this population of cells, whereas autoreactive clones evade deletion and produce autoantibodies. A variety of cytokines, including GM-CSF, IL-6 and IL-8, are produced by RA nurse-like cells, and direct contact with B cells is critical for maximal proliferation and antibody production.[95] Of interest, cultured B cells spontaneously migrate beneath ordinary fibroblast-like synoviocytes, which permits them to survive in vitro for prolonged periods of time. The process is dependent on the interaction of the integrin $\alpha 4/\beta 1$ on B cells with synoviocytes expressing CD106 (VCAM-1).[96] The chemokine SDF-1 also is constitutively expressed by synoviocytes and contributes to the process. Interference with the B cell–synoviocyte interaction decreases B cell survival and is one potential mechanism by which therapeutic interventions targeted at integrins might suppress autoreactivity and inflammation in RA.

OTHER CELL TYPES

Dendritic cells are potent antigen-presenting cells that are readily detected in synovial tissue and synovial effusions of patients with RA. Cytokines that are abundant in RA, such as GM-CSF, influence the proliferation and maturation of these antigen-presenting cells. Dendritic cells can comprise up to 5 percent of synovial fluid mononuclear cells, which is almost tenfold higher than in peripheral blood.[97] RA synovial tissue contains dendritic cells that display the costimulatory molecule CD86, are located near dense lymphoid aggregates and high endothelial venules, and can respond abnormally to cytokines. For instance, IL-10 normally suppresses dendritic cell function, in part by decreasing expression of CD86 and class II MHC molecules. However, RA dendritic cells isolated from the joint are resistant to this effect, possibly because they express lower amounts of the IL-10 receptor.[98] Fibroblast-like synoviocytes also possess the ability to differentiate into cells similar to dendritic cells. However, only synoviocytes derived from RA samples can bind to germinal-center B cells and suppress B cell apoptosis.[99]

Despite the abundance of neutrophils in RA synovial effusions, only rare polymorphonuclear leukocytes (PMNs) infiltrate the synovium. NK cells have, however, been identified in RA synovium.[100] Cytotoxic NK cells contain large amounts of granzymes, which are serine proteases. One potentially important immunoregulatory role of NK cells is that they can stimulate B cells to produce RFs.

Mast cells are present in the synovial membranes of patients with RA and, in some patients, are located at sites of cartilage erosion. Rheumatoid synovial membranes contain more than 10 times as many mast cells in histologic sections than do control synovial samples from patients undergoing surgery for meniscectomy. Patients with high numbers of mast cells have more intense clinical synovitis in the affected joints. Mast cells and histamine are also found in a majority of synovial fluid specimens from inflammatory synovitis. A detailed analysis of several indicators of proliferation and the enumeration of synovial mast cells has demonstrated strong positive correlations between the number of mast cells in synovial tissue and the degree of lymphocyte infiltration.[101] Mast cells from RA synovium express significantly higher amounts of the C5a receptor, compared to OA synovium.[102]

What is the contribution of mast cells to rheumatoid synovitis? They could be responding to cytokines that stimulate mast cell growth and chemotaxis. Extracts of mast cells can induce adherent rheumatoid synovial cells to increase production of PGE_2 and collagenase. Heparin, however, does have significant effects on connective tissue. In particular, it may modulate the effects of hormones on osseous cells and thereby alter the balance of bone synthesis toward degradation. The role of mast cells in the initiation phase of synovitis was confirmed in the passive K/B×N model in which the absence of mast cells prevented disease.[103] It is not certain if the cells are required once synovial inflammation has been established and other cell types, such as neutrophils, supplant the mast cells.

SYNOVIAL HISTOPATHOLOGY IN EARLY VERSUS LATE RHEUMATOID ARTHRITIS

Some observations suggested that the earliest phases of RA, that is, during the first few weeks of symptoms, exhibit distinct histopathology with a paucity of lymphocyte infiltration in the presence of endothelial cell injury, tissue edema, and neutrophil accumulation. More recent reports, however, suggest that the histologic appearance of RA is similar regardless of the duration of clinical symptoms.[104] The extent of lymphoid aggregation, T cell infiltration, and synovial-lining hyperplasia can resemble chronic disease even when symptoms have been present for a very short period of time. The cytokine patterns of these biopsies as determined by immunohistochemical analysis indicated similar levels of T cell (such as IFN-γ) and non–T cell factors (such as IL-1 and TNF-α). The tumor suppressor gene p53 is also expressed in early RA, most likely due to the intensely genotoxic environment generated by hypoxia and oxygen radicals (see following).

Biopsies of asymptomatic joints from patients with early or late RA also have lymphocyte infiltration, cytokine production, and p53 expression.[105] Although IFN-γ, IL-1, and TNF-α levels are increased compared to those of normal synovium, they are modestly lower than those of clinically active joints. One difference might be the relative abundance of some cytokines, such as IL-8, and the number of macrophages, which are higher in the painful joints. Some aspects of synovial histology in early RA, such as macrophage and plasma cell infiltration, might predict more erosive or severe disease. Of interest, studies in animal models of arthritis also demonstrate increased expression of proinflammatory transcription factors such as activator protein-1 (AP-1) and NFκB before clinically evident arthritis.[106] These studies suggest that patients with "early" RA, as defined by the duration of symptoms, might, in fact, already have chronic disease and that evaluation of truly early disease might require assessment of patients long before the onset of symptoms (if this is even possible).

RHEUMATOID ARTHRITIS SYNOVIUM AND SEVERE COMBINED IMMUNODEFICIENCY MICE

SCID mice, which lack a functional immune system, have been utilized to evaluate the biology of rheumatoid synovium. Several variations of this model have been developed, and in each case explanted synovium can successfully engraft. A blood supply develops over a period of weeks, and many of the resident human cells remain in the synovium. When coimplanted with cartilage, synoviocytes from the explant attach to and invade cartilage matrix. CD4+ and CD8+ lymphocytes in the synovium produce a variety of cytokines, including IFN-γ. CD8+ T cells in the explant produce IL-16, which appears to be an endogenous suppressor of CD4+ T cell function. Despite the appeal of these models, it is important to recognize their limitations, especially when evaluating T cell function. Although the SCID mice lack an immune system, the explanted synovium contains functional human lymphocytes and antigen-presenting cells that, when implanted into mice, can respond to host of murine proteins. Hence, the cytokine profile of the explant could also reflect that of human T cells exposed to xenoantigens.

A second SCID model utilizes enzymatically dispersed synovial tissue cells that have been coimplanted into the mice with cartilage explants. The rheumatoid cells invade into the cartilage matrix, looking very much like destructive pannus.[107] Perhaps more important, this phenomenon still occurs even if pure populations of long-term cultured RA fibroblast-like synoviocytes are used[108] (Fig. 65–5). Because these synoviocytes are devoid of T cells and macrophages, there is no contribution from an immune response to murine antigens. The invading cells express VCAM-1, which could potentially facilitate adhesion to cartilage or chondrocytes, as well as proteases that digest the cartilage matrix. Control synoviocytes from OA patients and normal dermal fibroblasts do not invade the cartilage, indicating that the activity is unique to rheumatoid fibroblast-like synoviocytes.

Using viral vectors to introduce cytokine genes into this explanted synoviocyte, one can evaluate their respective role in cartilage invasion. Interleukin-1 receptor antagonist (IL-1Ra), a natural antagonist to IL-1, has no effect on synoviocyte invasion but decreases perichondrocyte matrix loss.[109] In contrast, IL-10 decreases invasion but does not alter matrix loss. Finally, overexpression of soluble TNF receptors has no consistent effect in this model. These studies suggest that excessive production of IL-1 and underexpression of IL-10 contribute to the invasive properties of RA synoviocytes. In another study, transfecting normal synoviocytes with the human papilloma virus gene encoding E6 induced the rheumatoid phenotype.[110] The E6 protein leads to the inactivation and degradation of the p53 tumor suppressor protein. Although this is not the sole explanation for the altered adhesion and invasion properties of RA synoviocytes, loss of p53 function through somatic mutation can potentially contribute.

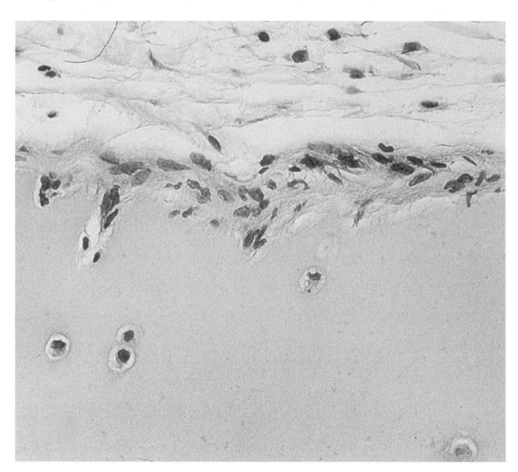

FIGURE 65-5 · Invasion of Rheumatoid Arthritis (RA) Synoviocytes into Cartilage Explants in Severe Combined Immunodeficiency Syndrome (SCID) Mice. RA fibroblast-like synoviocytes were been coimplanted with normal human cartilage into the renal capsule of SCID mice. Note that the synoviocytes attached to the cartilage and invaded into the matrix. Several chondrocytes in lacunae are also present. (Courtesy of Dr. S. Gay.)

■ Peripheral Blood and Synovial Fluid Immune Responses

PERIPHERAL BLOOD LYMPHOCYTES

Although peripheral lymphocytes are the most accessible, most investigators believe there is greater value studying cells isolated from the site of disease. Nevertheless, a number of early studies demonstrated functional and phenotypic differences between RA and normal peripheral blood cells. The number of CD4+ helper T cells is mildly increased in the circulation of patients with RA, with a concomitant decrease in CD8+ lymphocytes (and an increased CD4 to CD8 ratio). The surface phenotype of circulating T cells in RA suggests activation in some studies, but not in others. For instance, an increased percentage of $\alpha\beta$ and $\gamma\delta$ TCR–bearing cells might express HLA-DR and the adhesion protein VLA-4 ($\alpha_4\beta_1$-integrin). The latter is especially critical in that VLA-4 plays an important role in the recruitment of cells to the synovium through interactions with counterreceptors VCAM-1 and CS-1 fibronectin on endothelial cells. Other markers of activation are not necessarily elevated on RA T cells, including IL-2 receptors, the costimulatory molecule B7, and VLA-1. Elevated levels of soluble IL-2 receptors, which are shed by activated T cells, are found in sera of rheumatoid patients, and the levels appear to correlate with disease activity. Therefore, peripheral-blood T cells express some phenotypic characteristics of

partial activation. It is not clear whether this process occurs in the periphery or whether cells are activated in the synovium and reenter the circulation via the synovial lymphatics.

Immunoregulatory dysfunction in RA has been described in the blood cells of some patients. One of the primary observations was the inadequate control of EBV-infected B lymphocyte growth due to a defect in T cell function in RA. The abnormal T cell response could be correlated somewhat with disease activity, but it was also noted that the abnormality was present in T cells of some patients with inflammatory arthropathies other than RA.[111] A more-specific defect was apparent in the autologous mixed lymphocyte reaction, in which T cells proliferate and produce cytokines in response to class II MHC antigens expressed on autologous antigen-presenting cells.[112] IFN-γ production is significantly suppressed in these RA cultures, and the abnormality is corrected by the addition of indomethacin. Peripheral blood T lymphocytes from rheumatoid patients also express unusually low amounts of IL-2. Unlike lymphocytes from normal individuals, recombinant IL-2 has minimal effect on IFN-γ production by peripheral blood lymphocytes from patients with active RA.

In contrast to synovial tissue, where there is a Th1 bias of T cell cytokines (see following), a mixed population of cells is present in the peripheral circulation in RA. Cells that do not fit neatly into the Th1 or Th2 paradigm and instead express IL-10 but not IL-2 or IL-4 are decreased in RA compared to OA or normal individuals. It is possible that the relative lack of IL-10 could contribute to the proinflammatory milieu.

T cell diversity and maturation is abnormal in RA. Whereas thymic output normally decreases with age, this process appears to be accelerated in RA.[113] The presence of T cell receptor rearrangement excision circles (TREC) is a measure of thymic release of mature T cells. Using this parameter, the thymic output in RA may decline prematurely. Similarly, telomere attrition suggests inappropriate "aging" of the T cells. This could be due to a primary defect in peripheral T cell homeostasis or due to impaired thymic function with increased T cell turnover due to chronic immune stimulation.

Activated B lymphocytes are also present in the peripheral blood of patients with RA. The number of circulating B cells that spontaneously produce RF is significantly higher in RA compared to normal individuals. A B cell subset that is enriched in autoantibody production is characterized by a surface determinant CD5.[114] This antigen is normally expressed by T cells, but it is also displayed by fetal B cells as well as a small number of immature B cells in adults. RA patients with normal circulating numbers of lymphocytes show an abnormal kappa-to-lambda–chain analysis compared to controls, implying oligoclonal B cell proliferation.[115] It is not known whether this reflects expansion of the restricted number of clones capable of producing RF or whether an inciting antigen is something other than IgG and related specifically to RA. On the other hand, normal and RA peripheral blood B cells have equal numbers of B cells that produce IgM anti–type II collagen antibodies. The B cells that accumulate in the synovial fluid, however, produce IgG antibodies that are more likely to be pathogenic.[116]

SYNOVIAL FLUID LYMPHOCYTES

The cell mix in synovial fluid differs from that of peripheral blood as well as synovial tissue. Therefore, analysis of synovial fluid cells is not necessarily an accurate reflection of the synovium. Even though synovial effusions contain an abundance of T cells, the CD4-to-CD8 ratio is actually reversed compared to that of blood or synovial tissue, with an excess of CD8+ suppressor cells relative to CD4+ lymphocytes. In addition, synovial tissue is nearly devoid of neutrophils, which often constitute 50 to 75 percent of synovial fluid cells. Hence, the synovial fluid does not contain a random distribution of cells shed from synovial tissue.

Synovial fluid contains T cells express high levels of surface HLA-DR antigens. Other activation antigens not increased on peripheral blood cells are increased on synovial fluid lymphocytes, including VLA-1. Surprisingly, IL-2 receptor expression is not increased. Of CD4+ cells in rheumatoid synovial fluid, most are memory cells and express CD45RO on their surface.[117] Despite the phenotypic appearance of activation, synovial-fluid T cell function is rather deficient when compared with that of peripheral blood cells. For instance, synovial-fluid lymphocyte proliferation in response to mitogens or most recall antigens, such as tetanus toxoid, is significantly less than paired blood T lymphocytes. Mycobacterial

antigens and the 60-kD HSP appear to be exceptions because proliferation is greater in cells isolated from rheumatoid effusions. Cytokine production by synovial-fluid T cells in vitro is also low, including mitogen-induced expression of IFN-γ and IL-1.[118]

A possible mechanism that explains defective T cell responses by synovial fluid mononuclear cells from rheumatoid patients is the presence of local inhibitors of cell activation. IL-1Ra and TGF-β are possible T cell suppressants and have been identified as components of synovial effusions that can suppress thymocyte proliferation.[119] Nonspecific components of joint effusions such as hyaluronic acid can be toxic to cells and can indirectly suppress T cell activation. The mechanism of diminished T cell activation could be related to abnormalities in TCR signaling. Articular T cells have diminished tyrosine phosphorylation of proteins after stimulation, especially the key signal transduction pathway p38 mitogen-activated protein (MAP) kinase.[120] Furthermore, tyrosine phosphorylation of the TCR zeta chain, an early event in TCR signaling, is low compared to peripheral blood T cells. Decreased levels of the zeta protein are also observed, suggesting that the TCR apparatus is abnormal in RA. The hyporesponsiveness of synovial-fluid T cells correlates with a significant decrease in the levels of the intracellular redox-regulating agent glutathione.[121] Restoration of the intracellular glutathione enhances mitogenic-induced proliferative responses and IL-2 production in RA synovial fluid T cells. These data suggest that oxidative stress in the articular environment can suppress antigen-specific T cell responses.

▌ T cell Cytokines

Cytokines are hormone-like proteins that enable immune cells to communicate. They can either interact with cells after being released in a soluble form or can be involved with direct cell-cell communication through membrane-bound factors such as TNF-α. In addition to participating in normal immune responses, they play an integral role in the initiation and perpetuation of synovitis. The cytokine milieu in RA is not random, although early studies suggested an unrestricted abundance of cytokines. Factors produced by T lymphocytes are surprisingly low in RA, whereas those generated by macrophages and by synovial fibroblasts are markedly increased[122] (Table 65–5).

Helper T cells have been divided into cytokine-specific subsets. Th1 cells produce IFN-γ, IL-2, and IL-17, but not IL-4, IL-5, or IL-10. In contrast, Th2 cells produce the opposite profile (IL-4+ IL-5+, IL-10+, IL-2−, IFN-γ−). Some cytokines are produced by both subsets, including TNF-α, IL-3, and GM-CSF. A third subset with an unrestricted cytokine profile is called Th0,[123] whereas Th3 cells produce TGF-β. Other phenotypes have since been reported, and, although Th0, Th1, and Th2 cells predominate, some T cells do not fit into well-defined categories (especially in humans). Th1 cells primarily mediate delayed-type hypersensitivity in vivo, whereas Th2 cells are more prominent regulators of isotype switching and antibody production. Some cytokines produced by Th2 cells are

TABLE 65–5 • LEVEL OF PRODUCTION OF SYNOVIAL CYTOKINES IN RHEUMATOID ARTHRITIS ACCORDING TO CELLULAR SOURCE*

Cellular Source	Level of Production in Rheumatoid Arthritis Synovium
T cells	
Interleukin-2	−
Interleukin-3	−
Interleukin-4	−
Interleukin-6	±
Interleukin-13	±
Interleukin-17	+
Interferon-γ	±
TNF-α	−
TNF-β	−
GM-CSF	−
Macrophages†/Fibroblasts ‡	
Interleukin-1	+++
Interleukin-1Ra	+
Interleukin-6	+++
Interleukin-10	+
Interleukin-15	++
Interleukin-18	++
TNF-α	++
M-CSF (CSF-1)	+
GM-CSF	++
TGF-β	++
Chemokines (IL-8, MCP-1, etc.)	+++
Fibroblast growth factor	++

† Tissue macrophages or type A synoviocytes
‡ Tissue fibroblasts or type B synoviocytes

Abbreviations: −, absent or very low concentrations; +, present; GM-CSF, granulocyte macrophage colony stimulating factor; MCP-1, monocyte chemoattractant; M-CSF, macrophage colony-stimulating factor TGF-β, transforming growth factor-β; TMF, tumor necrosis factor.

immunosuppressive, because IL-4 and IL-10 downregulate Th1 cell differentiation and activation, as well as delayed-type hypersensitivity.

T HELPER TYPE 1 CELL CYTOKINES

Extensive investigations into the cytokine profile of RA suggest a Th1 bias to the synovium. Considerable data has accrued on the relative abundance and function of the prototypic Th1 cytokine, IFN-γ, which is the most potent inducer of MHC class II antigen on many cell types. IFN-γ also induces adhesion molecules such as VCAM-1 and ICAM-1 on the surface of endothelial cells and can help recruit inflammatory cell accumulation at sites of injury. One of the most important functions of IFN-γ is its capacity to alter the balance of extracellular matrix synthesis and degradation by decreasing collagen synthesis and inhibiting (MMP) production by cytokine-stimulated cultured fibroblast-like synoviocytes.[124]

Despite the evidence for T cell activation in the rheumatoid synovium, only relatively low concentrations of IFN-γ have been detected,[125] far below the amounts needed to induce HLA-DR expression on monocytes. The relative lack of IFN-γ in rheumatoid joints has been observed at the level of mRNA using a variety of techniques, including reverse transcriptase-polymerase chain reaction (PCR).[126] The difficulty detecting IFN-γ in RA does not appear to be due to methodologic problems, because it is easily measured in other diseases known to be mediated by T cells, such as tuberculous pleuritis, in which IFN-γ levels can be several orders of magnitude higher than in RA synovium. Although immunohistochemical analysis clearly demonstrates IFN-γ in a small percentage of RA synovial T cells, the percentage is far less than in chronically inflamed tonsils.[127]

Another major Th1 cytokine, IL-2, is a T cell–derived cytokine that serves as an autocrine or paracrine T cell growth factor. Although it was originally reported to be present in synovial fluid using biologic assays, specific monoclonal antibodies that block the IL-2 receptor do not interfere with this activity.[128] More specific immunoassays showed that IL-2 is detected in only a small percentage of RA synovial effusions and synovial tissues and, when present, is only found in low concentrations.[129] Results of studies of IL-2 gene expression in synovial tissue are mixed, and some studies detect specific IL-2 mRNA, whereas others do not. The possible presence of IL-2 mRNA without protein production could suggest that the T cells are anergic.

The recently described Th1 cytokine IL-17 is present in low, but functionally relevant, concentrations in RA synovial effusions.[130] IL-17 mimics many of the activities of IL-1 and TNF-α with respect to fibroblast-like synoviocyte function, including induction collagenase and cytokine production.[131] More important, T cell–derived IL-17 in synovial tissue can synergize with IL-1 and TNF-α by activating synoviocytes to produce matrix MMPs as well as other proinflammatory cytokines. Specific IL-17 receptors are expressed by synoviocytes and, when engaged, can activate the transcription factor NFκB and initiate an inflammatory cascade. In addition to its effect on mesenchymal cells, IL-17 can participate in bone erosion by enhancing osteoclast activation.[132] Bone resorption in an in vitro model using synovial explants and bone showed that blockade of IL-17, IL-1, and TNF-α was more effective than blocking the individual factors. Because immunoreactive IL-17 can be detected near the erosive front of pannus, it could also participate in this process in RA.[133]

TNF-α, GM-CSF, and IL-6 can be expressed by Th1 and Th2 cells. All three are present in synovial fluid and produced by RA synovial tissue. However, the primary sources of these cytokines in the rheumatoid joint are macrophages and fibroblasts rather than T cells (see following).

T HELPER TYPE 2 CELL CYTOKINES

Whereas Th1 cytokines have been detected (albeit in relatively low concentrations), Th2 cytokine levels are exceedingly low in RA. Using immunoassays, IL-4 and TNF-β are generally not detected in RA synovial fluid. In situ hybridization also shows little or no IL-4 in RA synovial tissue, even though a small amount of IFN-γ is detected using the same method. When extremely sensitive nested RT-PCR techniques are used on synovial biopsies, Th2 cytokines IL-4 and IL-13 are absent in RA, whereas both IFN-γ and IL-12 (a cytokine that induces T cell maturation toward the Th1 phenotype) are present. In another study, IL-13 protein was detected in RA synovial effusions. IL-10, which has potent anti-inflammatory activities, is expressed in RA synovium. However, macrophages, not T cells, are the major producers of IL-10 in RA.

T CELL SUBSETS IN RHEUMATOID ARTHRITIS: T HELPER CELL TYPES 1 AND 2 IMBALANCE

As noted previously, Th1 cytokine mRNA, such as IFN-γ, can be detected in RA synovial tissue using very sensitive techniques. T cell clones from RA joints tend to confirm the Th1 bias, and in vitro stimulation of synovial fluid mononuclear cells also demonstrates a Th1 phenotype compared to peripheral blood.[134] Most T cells in RA synovial fluid and synovial tissue express chemokine receptors that are preferentially displayed by Th1 cells.[135] Cytokines that bias T cell differentiation toward the Th1 phenotype, such as IL-12 and IL-18, are produced by macrophages and NK cells in the joint and can contribute to the preferential differentiation of Th1 cells.

The relative abundance of Th1 cells and cytokines suggests that the synovium participates in an unregulated Th1-like delayed type hypersensitivity reaction. Th2 cytokines and cellular responses that normally suppress Th1 activation are nearly absent, thereby raising the possibility that the lack of T cell activation along the Th2 pathway in RA contributes to disease perpetuation. For example, addition of exogenous IL-10 or IL-4 to cultures of synovial tissue cells or synovial tissue explants suppresses synthesis of proinflammatory cytokines such as IL-6, IL-1, TNF-α, and GM-CSF, as well as MMPs by cultured RA synovial tissue explants.[136] The inhibitory action of IL-4 might be mediated by decreased c-*jun* and c-*fos* expression, which is required for efficient production of MMPs and cytokines. In addition, IL-10 and IL-4 increase the release of other anti-inflammatory cytokines, like IL-1Ra, by synovial cells. Although IL-10 protein is present in RA synovial fluid and the gene is expressed by synovial tissue cells,[137] in vitro studies of cultured synovial cells suggest that not enough IL-10 is produced to suppress IFN-γ production.

The notion that Th1 cytokines initiate and perpetuate arthritis, whereas Th2 cytokines are suppressive is supported by studies in animal models. For instance, administration of IL-10 to mice with collagen-induced arthritis is modestly effective.[138] In a second study, IL-4 and IL-10 were administered individually or in combination in the same model.[139] The cytokines had modest or no benefit when used separately, but together the effect was impressive. Clinical improvement correlated with decreased synovial IL-1, TNF-α, and cartilage destruction. Anti–IL-10 antibody therapy in collagen-induced arthritis accelerated disease. The complexity of cytokine networks in inflammatory arthritis is underscored by studies on the role of IL-12 in collagen-induced arthritis. In early arthritis, IL-12 administration increases the incidence of collagen-induced arthritis, whereas anti–IL-12 is beneficial.[140] However, in late disease, IL-12 administration suppresses arthritis, and anti–IL-12 causes an exacerbation.

Therefore, synovial inflammation in RA may be a complex process involving macrophage- and fibroblast-cytokine networks in combination with defective T cell responses. Animal models support the concept that ineffective or insufficient Th2 cell activation might be permissive in RA. Although this hypothesis is attractive, the use of a single Th2 cytokine, IL-10, as a therapeutic agent in RA was unimpressive.[141] It is possible that combinations will be required to coordinate a maximum effect.

ACTIVATION OF SYNOVIAL CELLS BY CELL-CELL CONTACT WITH T LYMPHOCYTES

Even though T cell activation is unexpectedly modest in rheumatoid synovium, alternative mechanisms permit these cells to participate in synovial cytokine networks and matrix destruction. A second process by which T cells can activate macrophages and fibroblasts in RA is through direct cell-cell contact. Membranes prepared from activated T cells can directly stimulate macrophages and fibroblast-like synoviocytes to produce cytokines and MMPs.[142] The membrane constituents that regulate this process vary, depending on the particular culture conditions, but include adhesion molecules such as LFA-1 and membrane-bound TNF-α. Hence, a T cell displaying these proteins, even if the cell is no longer functional, can potentially contribute to macrophage and fibroblast activation in an antigen-independent fashion. One of the best-characterized consequences of this pathway is the ability of T cells to enhance synovial macrophage TNF-α production in a contact-dependent manner after exposure to macrophage-derived IL-15.[143]

The notion that lymphocytes can activate cells in the environment through direct contact suggests an unanticipated role for T cells in RA. The traditional paradigm assumes that T cells in the joint respond to a pathogenic stimulus and subsequently drive an antigen-specific response. However, cell-cell contact influences can be entirely antigen-independent and only require colocalization of memory T cells with synoviocytes or macrophages. Because T cells with a memory phenotype accumulate into the joint due to the release of synovial chemoattractants, there is no requirement for a specific arthritogenic antigen to initiate the process. Instead, activation of innate immunity by nonspecific stimuli permits subsequent ingress of the correct T cell phenotype to engage resident synovial lining cells.

▌ The Role of Macrophage and Fibroblast Cytokines

Although the production of T cell cytokines is relatively low in RA, the same is not true for products of macrophages and fibroblasts. Virtually every macrophage and fibroblast proinflammatory mediator investigated in the RA synovium is abundant. In this section, some of the major cytokines and effectors produced in the joint are enumerated, with an emphasis on the prevalence of macrophage and fibroblast products as driving forces during the perpetuation phase of RA. Macrophages, in particular, are the most vigorous producers of cytokines. These cells, which are present in small numbers in normal synovium, increase in number by migration from extrasynovial sites (e.g., the bone marrow) after inflammation begins. Their responses include secretion of more than

100 substances and regulation of a biologic array of activity from the induction of cell growth to cell death.

PROINFLAMMATORY MACROPHAGE AND FIBROBLAST CYTOKINES

Interleukin 1 Family

IL-1 family is a ubiquitous group of polypeptides with a wide range of biologic activity; they include IL-1α, IL-1β, IL-18, and IL-1Ra, which is a natural inhibitor of IL-1 (see following section, Suppressive Cytokines and Cytokine Antagonists, for a description of IL-1Ra). The proinflammatory actions of IL-1α and -β allow them to serve as major amplifiers and translators of the inflammatory response of RA into a destructive one. Abundant animal data indicate that IL-1 can serve as a key regulatory factor in inflammatory arthritis. For instance, recombinant IL-1β induces the accumulation of PMNs and mononuclear leukocytes in the joint space and the loss of proteoglycan from articular cartilage when injected directly into rabbit knee joints.[144] Transgenic mice that overexpress IL-1 also develop inflammatory arthritis, whereas mice that lack the natural IL-1 antagonist IL-1Ra have increased susceptibility to collagen-induced arthritis.

The effect of IL-1 inhibition, using either monoclonal antibodies or administration of exogenous IL-1Ra, has been evaluated in many animal models of arthritis. By and large, IL-1 blockade modestly decreases synovial inflammation while markedly diminishing bone and cartilage destruction. In contrast, TNF-α inhibition is mainly anti-inflammatory with less effect on extracellular matrix destruction (see following). One exception to this paradigm is the passive model using anti-GPI antibodies, in which the inflammatory response is profoundly dependent on IL-1.

IL-1 has been implicated in RA, and inhibition of this mediator using IL-1Ra has modest anti-inflammatory activities in humans. IL-1 activity has been detected in culture supernatants of rheumatoid synovial biopsies, and in one study the amount produced correlated with joint destruction found on roentgenograms.[145] IL-1 production by peripheral blood monocytes in RA is much greater when cells are isolated from rheumatoid patients who had recent onset of disease or an exacerbation compared to cells from patients with stable arthritis or from controls.[146] Concentrations of the cytokine sufficient to stimulate collagenase and PGE$_2$ production from synovial lining fibroblasts are generated by synovial fluid macrophages from patients with RA, and the synoviocytes that respond express high-affinity receptors for IL-1α and IL-1β. Even PMNs stimulated by phagocytosis or by other activating substances produce IL-1. Thus, the macrophages, synovial fibroblasts, PMNs, and endothelial cells can be induced to generate this powerful mediator within the rheumatoid joint.

Synovial macrophages are the most prolific source of IL-1 gene expression in the joint, and nearly half of all macrophages in the RA synovium contain significant amounts of IL-1β mRNA.[147] Immunohistologic studies confirm this, with especially abundant IL-1 protein in synovial lining macrophages adjacent to type B synovio-cytes and in sublining macrophages near blood vessels. The IL-1 in the lining can subsequently activate type B synoviocytes to proliferate and secrete a variety of mediators. A broad range of stimuli are capable of inducing IL-1 production by macrophages; for example, immunoglobulin Fc fragments and, to a lesser extent, immune complexes, can generate IL-1 production by rheumatoid synovial macrophages. Collagen fragments can induce IL-1 production, and type IX collagen, which has been found only in articular cartilage and localized into intersections of collagen fibrils, is a potent inducer of IL-1 by human monocyte.

Within the rheumatoid joint, IL-1 induces fibroblast proliferation, stimulates the biosynthesis of IL-6, IL-8, and GM-CSF by synovial cells, and enhances collagenase and prostaglandin production.[148] It increases glycosaminoglycan release in human synovial fibroblast cultures, although the effect of IL-1 on the production of intact proteoglycan molecules by intact articular cartilage explants can be the opposite. IL-1 induces a number of adhesion molecules on fibroblast-like synoviocytes and endothelial cells, including VCAM-1 and ICAM-1, and enhances bone resorption.

In addition to IL-1α and -β, a homologous protein in the IL-1 family known as IL-18 has been implicated in RA. This cytokine was originally defined by its ability to bias the immune response toward the Th1 phenotype, especially in the presence of IL-12. In collagen-induced arthritis, IL-18 inhibition significantly attenuates disease.[149] Of particular interest, the same effect was observed in IFN-γ knockout mice, indicating that other non–Th1-related activities of IL-18 might be important. Subsequent studies showed that IL-18 induces GM-CSF, nitric oxide production, and TNF-α expression by synovial macrophages.[150] Although IL-18 can, along with IL-12 or IL-15, increase IFN-γ production by synovial tissues in vitro, the relative importance of this activity is uncertain compared with the IL-1–like activities of the cytokine. IL-18 is expressed by RA synovial tissue, especially by synovial fibroblasts and macrophages, and its production is markedly increased by TNF-α and IL-1β. A natural inhibitor, the IL-18 binding protein, can potentially be used as a therapeutic agent to block both the proinflammatory effects and pro-Th1 effects of IL-18.

Tumor Necrosis Factor-α

TNF-α is a pleiotropic cytokine that has been implicated as a key proinflammatory cytokine in RA and detected in rheumatoid synovial fluid and serum. It is produced as a membrane-bound protein that is released from the cell surface after proteolytic cleavage by a TNF convertase, a membrane MMP. IL-1 and TNF-α have many similar activities, including the ability to enhance cytokine production, adhesion-molecule expression, proliferation, and MMP production by cultured synoviocytes. In some systems, the effects of these two agents are synergistic. Although they share many functions and signal transduction pathways, IL-1 and TNF utilize distinct surface receptors. One TNF receptor, p75, has been engineered with an Fc fragment of immunoglobulin to create etanercept, one of the TNF inhibitors that is an effective therapeutic agent in RA. The clearly defined efficacy of TNF inhibitors in RA demonstrates its critical role in the disease; heterogeneity of the rheumatoid process is also apparent because only about one third of patients have a dramatic response to TNF inhibitors.[151] Efficacy requires continuous therapy because cessation leads to a flare of disease.

TNF-α, like IL-1, stimulates collagenase and PGE$_2$ production by human synovial cells, induces bone resorption, inhibits bone formation in vitro, and stimulates resorption of proteoglycan and inhibits its biosynthesis in explants of cartilage.[152] In situ hybridization and immunohistochemical studies show that TNF-α is primarily produced by synovial macrophages in RA. Animal models have also supported the general role played by TNF-α in inflammatory arthritis. For instance, overexpression of TNF-α in transgenic mice leads to an aggressive and destructive synovitis. In fact, the arthritis also spontaneously occurs in transgenic mice that express only a membrane-bound form of TNF-α on T cells.[153] TNF blockade is an effective anti-inflammatory agent in animal models of arthritis, such as collagen-induced arthritis in mice,[154] although the effects on bone and cartilage destruction are less prominent than with IL-1 inhibitors. Of interest, TNF inhibition in RA significantly decreases extracellular-matrix destruction as measured by radiographic progression.[155] It is not clear why the bone-protective effects are more prominent in humans than in the animal models. TNF blockade is also more effective in animal models when combined with an IL-1 inhibitor, supporting the additive or synergistic relationship between the two cytokines.

Interleukin-6 Family

IL-6 is an IL-1–inducible protein produced by T cells and monocytes and is spontaneously expressed by cultured fibroblast-like synoviocytes.[156] Originally defined by its B cell–stimulating properties, it induces immunoglobulin synthesis in B cell lines, is involved in the differentiation of cytotoxic T lymphocytes, and is a major factor in the regulation of acute-phase response proteins by the liver. A striking correlation between serum IL-6 activity and serum levels of acute-phase reactants like C-reactive protein, α_1-antitrypsin, fibrinogen, and haptoglobin occurs in patients with RA.[157] Very high levels of IL-6 are present in RA synovial fluid, and synovial cells in culture from diverse inflammatory arthropathies produce IL-6.[158] In situ hybridization of frozen sections of synovial tissue also shows IL-6 mRNA in the intimal lining, and immunoperoxidase studies show IL-6 protein in the lining and sublining regions.[159] Although many synovial macrophages express the IL-6 gene, the majority of IL-6 appears to be produced by type B synoviocytes.

Cytokines with structural similarity to IL-6 and that share surface-receptor subunits have also been implicated in RA. Several of these, IL-11, leukemia inhibitory factor (LIF), and oncostatin M, are expressed by rheumatoid synovium and can be detected in synovial effusions. The biologic effects of these factors are complex and can be either protective (e.g., by increasing expression of protease inhibitors such as tissue inhibitors of metalloproteinase [TIMP]) or proinflammatory (e.g., by increasing expression of chemokines or MMPs) depending on the culture conditions or the specific model evaluated. This dichotomy among the family members is demonstrated by the fact that IL-11 administration ameliorates collagen-induced arthritis,[160] whereas antibodies to oncostatin M are protective.[161]

Interleukin-15

IL-15 is an IL-2–like cytokine that can induce T cell proliferation. Although it can serve as an IL-2–independent mechanism for activating T cells, its role in RA is more likely related to its key role in TNF-α regulation. Macrophages are the primary source of IL-15 in RA, and the cytokine is able to induce a cell-contact mechanism of macrophage TNF-α production that requires T cells. Although T lymphocytes, or at least their membranes, are required for this process, the macrophages actually produce the TNF-α. This network provides a potential mechanism whereby local IL-15 production in the synovium can lead to autocrine production of TNF-α in a T cell–dependent, but antigen-independent, fashion. IL-15 is has been demonstrated in RA synovial macrophages cells using immunohistochemical techniques.[162] Soluble IL-15 receptors can function as an IL-15 inhibitor, and when used in vivo can decrease joint inflammation in collagen–induced arthritis.[163] The mechanism of action probably includes TNF-α inhibition, although decreased IFN-γ production and immune responses to type II collagen indicate that IL-15 also regulates antigen-dependent responses.

Colony-Stimulating Factors

GM-CSF supports the differentiation of bone marrow precursor cells to mature granulocytes and macrophages. As with other major colony-stimulating factors, GM-CSF also participates in normal immune responses. It is a potent macrophage activator, including the induction of HLA-DR expression, tumoricidal activity, IL-1 secretion, intracellular parasite killing, and priming for enhanced release of TNF-α and PGE$_2$. Neutrophil function is also regulated by GM-CSF, which enhances antibody-dependent cytotoxicity, phagocytosis, chemotaxis, and the production of oxygen radicals.

RA synovial fluid contains GM-CSF, which is produced by RA synovial tissue cells.[164] The major source in the synovium is macrophages, although IL-1– or TNF-α–stimulated fibroblast-like synoviocytes also express the GM-CSF gene.[165] In situ hybridization studies show little or no GM-CSF mRNA in synovial T cells. Its ability to induce HLA-DR gene expression on macrophages might be of particular importance in RA: GM-CSF, not IFN-γ, is the major DR-inducing cytokine in RA synovial fluid and in supernatants of cultured synovial tissue cells. Collagen-induced arthritis in mice is less severe in animals that lack a functional GM-CSF gene or are treated with anti–GM-CSF antibody, which supports the hypothesis that GM-CSF is an important proinflammatory mediator.[166]

Macrophage colony-stimulating factor (M-CSF) is also expressed by RA synovium and is present in synovial effusions. Its primary pathogenic role in RA probably relates to its osteoclast-differentiating capacity. As will be described later, this factor cooperates with RANKL to facilitate bone erosions.

Chemokines

Chemokines are a family of related chemoattractant peptides that, with the assistance of adhesion molecules, summon cells into inflammatory sites. They are generally divided into two major families, known as C-C and C-X-C, based on the position of characteristic cysteine residues. In the former, two conserved cysteines are adjacent to one another, whereas in the C-X-C family, the cysteines are separated by a nonconserved amino acid. The families are also encoded on different chromosomes, with C-C chemokines found on chromosome 17 and C-X-C factors on chromosome 4. Each individual factor has the ability to attract specific lineages of cells after interacting with specific surface receptors. Many chemokines have been identified in the rheumatoid joint. IL-8, a C-X-C chemokine that was originally characterized as a potent chemoattractant for neutrophils, along with immune complexes and other chemotactic peptides such as C5a, contributes to the large influx of PMNs into the joint. Immunohistochemical analysis of synovial tissue demonstrates IL-8 protein in sublining perivascular macrophages, as well as in scattered lining cells.[167] Cultured synovial tissue macrophages constitutively produce IL-8, and fibroblast-like synoviocytes express the gene if they are stimulated with IL-1 or TNF-α. Although proinflammatory cytokines IL-1 and TNF-α induce the expression of a large number of chemokines by cultured synoviocytes, IL-8 accounts for the majority of neutrophil-attracting activity. The addition of anti–IL-8 neutralizing antibodies eliminate about 40 percent of the neutrophil chemoattractant activity in synovial fluid. IL-8 has a number of other activities: It activates neutrophils through G-protein–coupled receptors and is a potent angiogenesis factor.

Many other chemoattractant proteins are implicated in RA. Macrophage-inhibitory protein-1α, macrophage-inhibitory protein-1β, macrophage chemoattractant protein-1 (MCP-1), and regulated on activation, normally T cell expressed and secreted (RANTES)—members of the C-C subfamily—are produced by RA synovium.[168] Epithelial neutrophil-activating peptide-78 (ENA-78), which is a C-X-C chemokine, is also abundant.[169] ENA-78 accounts for about 40 percent of the chemotactic activity for neutrophils in RA synovial fluid. In each case, the source of the chemokine appears to be synovial macrophages or cytokine-stimulated type B synoviocytes. The regulation of each chemokine appears to be distinct in fibroblast-like synoviocytes. The concentrations of chemokines are higher in RA synovial effusions compared to samples from noninflammatory arthritides such as OA. Although the chemokines can also be detected in the blood, the levels are considerably lower than in the joint, thereby providing a gradient that signals cells to migrate into the synovium.

More recently characterized lymphocyte-specific factors might contribute to the germinal center architecture of RA. The C-X-C factor B cell–activating chemokine-1 (BCA-1) binds to specific CXCR5 receptors on B cells. BCA-1 is expressed in the RA synovial tissues, especially by follicular dendritic cells in germinal centers and likely accounts for B cell migration to these regions. Another chemokine, SDF-1, is expressed by synoviocytes and endothelial cells and can play a major role as a chemoattractant for T cells in synovium via its receptor CXCR4. Unlike other chemokine receptors that can bind multiple members of the family, CXCR4 is highly specific for SDF-1 and is expressed by memory CD4+ lymphocytes.

Platelet-Derived Growth Factor and Fibroblast Growth Factor

PDGF is a potent growth factor that is both chemoattractant and mitogenic for fibroblasts and induces collagenase expression. It is the most potent stimulator of long-term growth of synovial cells in culture.[170] PDGF is expressed in vascular endothelial cells and other synovial sublining cells in rheumatoid synovium, compared to healthy tissue.[171] Its receptor also is expressed in the same regions of RA synovium, suggesting the presence of an autocrine or paracrine system.

Fibroblast growth factors (FGFs) are a family of peptide growth factors with pleiotropic activities. In rheumatoid patients, it is likely that heparin-binding growth factor, the precursor of acidic fibroblast growth factor, is a major mitogen for many cell types and stimulates angiogenesis. An interaction between FGF and proteoglycans is required for biologic activity.[172] It induces capillary endothelial cells to invade a three-dimensional collagen matrix, organizing themselves to form characteristic tubules that resemble blood capillaries. FGF is present in RA synovial fluid, and the genes are expressed by synovial cells. Synovial fibroblasts express FGF receptors and proliferate after exposure to the growth factor.

SUPPRESSIVE CYTOKINES AND CYTOKINE ANTAGONISTS

The proinflammatory cytokine network in RA is offset by a variety of suppressive and anti-inflammatory factors that attempt to reestablish homeostasis. Underproduction of these suppressive cytokines could potentially contribute to the perpetuation of the synovitis. As described previously, relative deficiency of some T cell–derived mediators such as IL-4 might lead to unopposed activation of synoviocytes by TNF-α or other cytokines. However, in addition to these, there are many other cytokine antagonists or natural immunosuppressives that represent potential therapeutic targets for the treatment of inflammatory diseases.

Interleukin-1 Receptor Antagonist

IL-1Ra is a naturally occurring IL-1 inhibitor that binds directly to types I and II IL-1 receptors and competes with IL-1 for the ligand-binding site. Interaction of

IL-1Ra with the IL-1 receptors does not result in signal transduction, and, in contrast to IL-1α or -β, the receptor-ligand complex is not internalized after it binds to the IL-1 receptor. Even though IL-1Ra has high affinity for the IL-1 receptor, it is a relatively weak inhibitor because IL-1 can activate cells even if only a small percentage of IL-1 receptors are occupied. Because of this, a substantial excess of the inhibitor is required to saturate the receptor and thereby block IL-1–mediated stimulation (usually 10- to 100-fold excess of IL-1Ra). Recombinant IL-1Ra inhibits a variety of IL-1–mediated events in cultured cells derived from the joint, including the induction of MMP and prostaglandin production by chondrocytes and synoviocytes. It can block synovitis in rabbits induced by direct intra-articular injection of recombinant IL-1.[173] Two major structural variants of IL-1Ra have been described: (1) secretory IL-1Ra, which is synthesized with a signal peptide that allows it to be transported out of cells; and (2) intracellular IL-1Ra, which lacks a leader peptide due to alternative splicing of mRNA and, therefore, remains intracellular. Secretory IL-1Ra is a major product of mononuclear phagocytes, particularly mature tissue macrophages, and intracellular IL-1Ra is the dominant form in cultured fibroblast-like synoviocytes, as well as keratinocytes and epithelial cells.

Abundant IL-1Ra is present in rheumatoid synovial effusions; much of it is produced by neutrophils and macrophages.[174] Immunohistochemical studies of rheumatoid synovium reveal IL-1Ra protein especially in perivascular mononuclear cells and the synovial intimal lining. The IL-1Ra protein and mRNA can be detected in synovial macrophages and, to a lesser extent, in type B synoviocytes (Fig. 65–6). The presence of IL-1Ra in synovium is not specific to RA, because OA synovial tissue also contains IL-1Ra, albeit in lesser amounts; normal synovium contains little, if any, IL-1Ra protein. Despite the presence of significant amounts of IL-1Ra in synovial tissue, its importance as an IL-1 antagonist can only be evaluated in the context of the IL-1 to IL-1Ra ratio. Studies of synovial cell culture supernatants show that the amount of IL-1Ra is insufficient to antagonize synovial IL-1.[175] Therapeutic doses of IL-1Ra have been used successfully to treat RA. Its efficacy is less than observed with TNF inhibitors, perhaps because of its short half-life and its relative inefficiency as a direct competitive inhibitor of IL-1.

Interleukin-10

IL-10 is a major immunosuppressive cytokine that was originally characterized as an inhibitor of T cell cytokine production. Its immunosuppressive actions might be important in pregnancy to suppress an immune response directed against paternal MHC antigens, and it might regulate susceptibility to some parasitic infections. As noted previously, IL-10 protein is present in RA synovial fluid, and the gene is expressed by synovial tissue macrophages. Serial synovial biopsies in RA patients who were treated with recombinant IL-10 did not show any significant histologic improvement, and clinical responses were not impressive in a limited study.

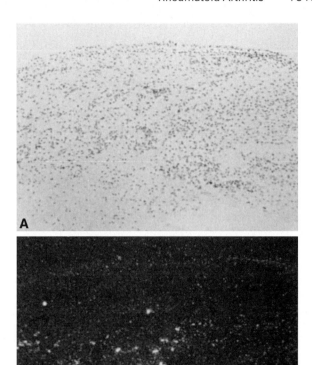

FIGURE 65–6 · Localization of Interleukin-1 Receptor Antagonist (IL-1Ra) Messenger RNA in RA Synovial Tissue by in Situ Hybridization. The specific RNA transcript was detected in perivascular cells, especially macrophages. A, Bright field view. B, Same area using a dark field filter. Silver grains in the dark field view show the location of IL-1Ra–positive cells.

Transforming Growth Factor-ß

TGF-β is widely distributed in different tissues and produced by many cells, including T cells, monocytes, and platelets. It suppresses the production of collagenase and induces the expression of TIMP. TGF-ß accelerates the healing of incisional wounds and induces both fibrosis and angiogenesis in experimental animal models. Substantial amounts of TGF-β are present in synovial fluid (although it is mainly present in an inactive, latent form), and the mRNA can be detected in RA synovial tissue.[176] Although typically considered an immunosuppressive cytokine with wound-healing properties, the role of TGF-β in RA is quite complex as demonstrated by the conflicting results of its administration in various animal models. In RA, TGF-β is one of the factors responsible for blunted responses of T cells that have been exposed to synovial fluid. TGF-β also downregulates IL-1 receptor expression on some cell types, including chondrocytes. When it is injected directly into the knees of animals, fibrosis and synovial lining hyperplasia develop.[177] In streptococcal cell wall arthritis, parenteral administration or systemic gene therapy with the TGF-β gene ameliorates the disease.[178] However, intra-articular administration of anti–TGF-β antibody decreases arthritis in the injected joint but not in the contralateral joint in the same model.

Soluble Cytokine Receptors and Binding Proteins

Soluble cytokine receptors and binding proteins can absorb free cytokines and prevent them from engaging functional receptors on cells. Although these obviously could inhibit cytokine action, it should be kept in mind that they also could act as carrier proteins that protect cytokines from proteolytic degradation or deliver them directly to cells. For instance, the IL-1 type II receptor is present in RA synovial fluid, along with lesser amounts of the type I receptor.[179] These soluble receptors can bind to IL-1 or IL-1Ra in synovial effusions.

TNF receptors are normally expressed as membrane-bound proteins and can be released from the cell surface after proteolytic cleavage. Soluble p55 and p75 TNF receptors have been detected in RA synovial fluid, sometimes in very high concentrations.[180] Soluble TNF receptor levels can be considerably higher than the concentration of TNF-α in blood or synovial fluid and probably explains why biologically active TNF is difficult to detect in RA synovial fluid despite the presence of immunoreactive protein. Synovial membrane mononuclear cells have increased surface expression and mRNA levels of both TNF receptors compared to OA synovial tissue cells or peripheral blood cells.[181] Cultured fibroblast-like synoviocytes express TNF receptors and shed them into culture supernatants.

Many other soluble receptors and binding proteins are produced in RA, albeit in concentrations too low effectively suppress the exuberant proinflammatory cytokine milieu of the joint. Soluble receptors to IL-15 and IL-17 have been characterized, and an IL-18 binding protein also can inhibit cytokine activity. In some cases, a soluble receptor can protect a cytokine from degradation or transport it to the cells, as with the IL-6 receptor.

PERPETUATION OF SYNOVITIS BY MACROPHAGE-FIBROBLAST CYTOKINE NETWORKS

To incorporate information on the cytokine profile into current concepts of RA, a variety of models have been proposed. One recurrent theme is that the chronic inflammatory process might achieve a certain degree of autonomy that permits inflammation to persist after a T cell response has been downregulated. This could occur if the inflammation is sustained by factors produced by neighboring macrophages and synovial fibroblasts in the joint lining in paracrine or autocrine networks (Fig. 65–7). Several cytokines that have been identified in the synovium or synovial fluid can participate in this system and might explain lining cell hyperplasia, HLA-DR and adhesion-molecule induction, and synovial angiogenesis. The list of potential candidates in this highly redundant system is very long. For example, one can assume that at least two, IL-1 and TNF-α, play particularly central roles. Both are produced by synovial

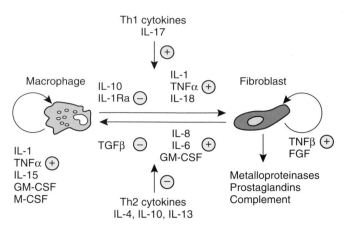

FIGURE 65–7 · Cytokine Networks in Rheumatoid Arthritis (RA). Paracrine and autocrine pathways can lead to activation of fibroblast-like and macrophage-like synoviocytes in the synovial intimal lining. Both positive (+) and negative (−) feedback loops are present, although in RA the former predominate. T helper type 1 (Th1) cytokines can potentially enhance the network, whereas Th2 cytokines are suppressive.

macrophages and stimulate synovial fibroblast proliferation and secretion of IL-6, GM-CSF, and chemokines, as well as effector molecules such as MMPs and prostaglandins. GM-CSF, which is produced by both synovial macrophages and IL-1β– or TNF-α–stimulated synovial fibroblasts, can, in turn, induce IL-1 secretion to form a positive feedback loop. GM-CSF, especially in combination with TNF-α, also increases HLA-DR expression on macrophages. Macrophage and fibroblast cytokines could also indirectly contribute to the evidence for local T cell and B cell activation, including RF production.

This model for the perpetuation of RA does not eliminate the requirement for an initiating event, perhaps involving a specific arthritogenic antigen. In fact, it certainly requires an external stimulus to initiate the process, along with periodic restimulation. T cell–mediated responses, directed against either an inciting antigen or a secondary target-like type II collagen or proteoglycan can occur along with this macrophage-fibroblast cytokine network and might enhance the local inflammatory response. Although the factors released by macrophages and fibroblasts are reasonably well defined, the precise function of synovial T cells remains less well characterized and might involve antigen-independent processes (e.g., cell contact with or without IL-15) or traditional antigen-specific stimulation.

▌ Signal Transduction and Transcription Factors

Intracellular signal transduction systems transmit extracellular stimuli initiated from the cell surface to the cytoplasm or nucleus, where they are subsequently integrated at the level of transcription factor activity. The transcription factors bind to specific DNA sites in promoter regions and regulate the expression of the appropriate genes. The remarkable diversity of signaling pathways and transcription factors provides a selective mechanism for orchestrating activation and repression for appropriate arrays of genes in response to an extracellular stress. Many of the inflammatory responses observed in RA synovium, including the activation of cytokine and adhesion-molecule genes, can be traced to specific transcription factors and signal transduction pathways. Although an extensive description of these mechanisms is beyond the scope of this chapter, they are reviewed in Chapter 18 and reference 182. Considerable enthusiasm abounds for targeting signal transduction pathways. One recurrent theme is that these pathways play a role in normal cells and host defense, thereby increasing the issues of balancing efficacy with toxicity.

NUCLEAR FACTOR KAPPA B

NFκB is a ubiquitous transcription factor that plays a key role in the expression of many genes central to RA, including IL-1β in monocytes, as well as ICAM-1, TNF-α, IL-6, and IL-8 in rheumatoid synoviocytes. NFκB normally resides as an inactive hetero- or homodimer in the cell cytoplasm associated with an inhibitory protein called IκB that regulates the DNA binding and subcellular localization of NFκB proteins by masking a nuclear localization signal. Extracellular stimuli initiate a signaling cascade leading to activation of two IκB kinases (IKKα and IKKß), which phosphorylate IκB at specific NH_2-terminal serine residues. Phosphorylated IκB is then selectively ubiquitinated and degraded by the 26S proteasome. This process permits NFκB to migrate to the cell nucleus, where it binds its target genes to initiate transcription.

NFκB is abundant in rheumatoid synovium, and immunohistochemical analysis demonstrates p50 and p65 NFκB proteins in the nuclei of cells in the synovial intimal lining.[183] Although the proteins can also be detected in OA synovium, NFκB activation is much greater in RA because of phosphorylation and degradation of IκB in RA intimal lining cells (Fig. 65–8). Nuclear translocation of NFκB in cultured fibroblast-like synoviocytes occurs rapidly after stimulation by IL-1 or TNF-α through the activation of the IKK signaling complex. Both IKKα and IKKβ are constitutively expressed by synoviocytes, and IKK functional activity increases 10- to 20-fold within 10 minutes of cytokine exposure. IKKß is the primary path by which NFκB is activated in synoviocytes after cytokine stimulation because selective inhibition of this kinase in vitro with dominant negative adenoviral constructs completely abrogates cytokine-mediated induction of IL-6, IL-8, and ICAM-1.[184] Aberrant NFκB function might occur in RA synovial cells because high constitutive IL-6 production in RA synoviocyte clones is associated with increased NFκB activation involving p50 and p65 subunits.[185]

The relevance of NFκB to inflammatory arthritis has been tested in several animal models. Synovial NFκB is rapidly activated, often long before clinical arthritis is evident. Adjuvant arthritis in rats is ameliorated using intra-articular gene therapy with the dominant negative IKKß construct that blocks the IKK pathway,[186] whereas streptococcal cell-wall arthritis is blocked with decoy oligonuclcotides or a dominant negative IκB adenovirus. NFκB inhibition was associated with decreased synovial cellular infiltration, as well as increased apoptosis. The role of this transcription factor in murine

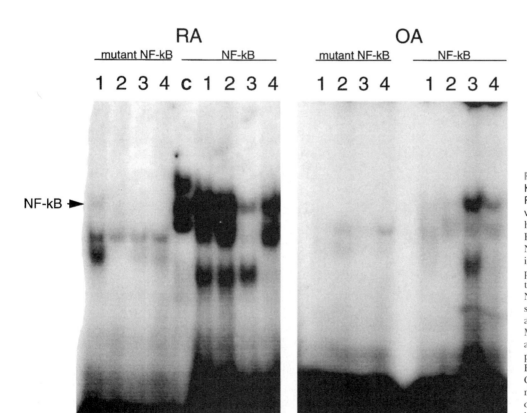

FIGURE 65–8 · Nuclear Factor Kappa B (NFκB) Activation in Rheumatoid Arthritis (RA) Synovium. Electromobility shift assays have been performed on extracts of RA and osteoarthritis (OA) synovium. NFκB activity is significantly higher in RA synovial tissue extracts compared to those of OA. This is consistent with increased expression of NFκB-driven genes in RA synovium, such as proinflammatory cytokines and vascular adhesion molecules. Mutant probe is shown on the left as a negative control, and C is a positive control. (From Han Z, Boyle DL, Manning AM, Firestein GS: AP-1 and NF-κB regulation in rheu-matoid arthritis and murine collagen-induced arthritis. Auto-immunity 28:197, 1998.)

collagen-induced arthritis has been demonstrated using a selective NFκB inhibitor, IKKβ inhibitors on mice that lack certain NFκB proteins in T cells. In each case, synovial inflammation was significantly ameliorated.

One of the primary concerns with NFκB-directed therapy is that it participates in so many cellular functions, especially those involved with host defense. Blockade could potentially impair both innate and adaptive immune responses. In addition, NFκB activation prevents apoptosis in many cell lineages, especially after exposure to proinflammatory cytokines such as TNF-α. By interfering with this pathway, increased apoptosis can potentially damage major organs. Although NFκB inhibition has great potential, balancing the risks and benefits will be crucial.

MITOGEN-ACTIVATED PROTEIN KINASES

MAP kinases, which are signal-transduction enzymes activated in response to cellular stress, are composed of parallel protein-kinase cascades that regulate cytokine and MMP gene expression. There are three different families of MAP kinases known as c-Jun N-terminal kinase (JNK), p38, and extracellular signal-regulated kinase (ERK). MAP kinases phosphorylate selected intracellular proteins, including transcription factors, that subsequently regulate the expression of various genes by transcriptional and post-transcriptional mechanisms. MAP kinases are activated by phosphorylation at conserved threonine and tyrosine residue by a cascade of dual-specificity kinases. These are, in turn, activated by MAP kinase kinase kinases. The relative hierarchy of the individual MAP kinases is dependent on the cell type and inflammatory stimulus.

The MAP kinases are widely expressed in synovial tissue and are activated in rheumatoid synovium. Phosphorylated ERK, p38, and JNK can be detected by immunohistochemistry or western blot analysis.[187] All three kinases are constitively expressed by cultured fibroblast-like synoviocytes and can be activated within minutes after exposure to cytokines such as IL-1 and TNF-α. Once phosphorylated, each initiates an interlocking series of additional kinases or transcription factors. Cytokine-gene expression, especially IL-1 and TNF-α, are induced by p38, whereas JNK can activate AP-1 by phosphorylating c-Jun, which, in turn, increases MMP gene expression. The p38 and ERK pathways can also regulate MMPs in many cells types, such as synoviocytes and chondrocytes.

The p38 inhibitors are effective anti-inflammatory agents in murine collagen-induced arthritis and rat adjuvant arthritis, possibly by decreasing the production of proinflammatory cytokines.[188] Treated animals also had improved bone-mineral density and decreased histologic evidence of joint inflammation. JNK2, which is one of the three JNK isoforms, is constitively expressed by RA synoviocytes and appears to be the primary JNK in this cell type. JNK inhibition blocks collagenase-gene expression in the cultured synoviocytes. Using a selective JNK inhibitor, marked protection of bone destruction was observed in the adjuvant arthritis model, along with decreased synovial AP-1 activation and collagenase-

3–gene expression.[189] As with the NFκB pathway, the ubiquitous expression and critical role of these kinases in normal homeostasis suggests that development of agents for clinical use will be challenging. Because many of these enzymes have multiple isoforms and splice variants, it is possible that some specificity can be achieved by inhibiting certain forms of the enzyme to minimize potential for toxicity. This question was partially addressed in passive collagen-induced arthritis using JNK2 knockout mice.[190] Although some joint protection was observed, the decrease in cartilage and bone damage was less impressive than when all isoforms were blocked with a small-molecule inhibitor.

ACTIVATOR PROTEIN-1

Like NFκB, AP-1 regulates many genes implicated in RA, including TNF-α and the MMPs. AP-1 activity can be induced by extracellular signals including cytokines, growth factors, tumor promoters, and the Ras oncoprotein. AP-1 includes members of the Jun and Fos families of transcription factors, which are characterized by leucine zipper DNA-binding domains. AP-1 proteins bind to DNA and activate transcription as Jun homodimers, Jun-Jun heterodimers, or Jun-Fos heterodimers. Multiple Jun and Fos family members (c-Jun, JunB, JunD, c-Fos, FosB, Fra-1, Fra-2) are expressed in different cell types that mediate the transcription of both unique and overlapping genes.

AP-1 proteins and mRNA, including c-jun and c-fos, are expressed in RA synovium, especially in the nuclei of cells in the intimal lining layer.[191] c-Jun and c-Fos proteins are also expressed in the sublining inflammatory infiltrate, albeit to a lesser degree. Localization of AP-1 to the intimal lining correlates with the site where most protease and cytokine genes are overexpressed in RA. AP-1 proteins are usually not detected in normal synovium, although modest amounts have also been detected in OA. Electromobility shift assays (EMSAs) demonstrate very high levels of AP-1–binding activity in nuclear extracts from RA synovium compared to OA tissue.[192]

Cytokines such as IL-1 and TNF-α probably contribute to the activation of AP-1 in RA synovium. These factors are potent inducers of AP-1 nuclear binding in cultured fibroblast-like synoviocytes. This is accompanied by increased c-jun and c-fos mRNA and enhanced collagenase-gene transcription.[193] The specific Jun family genes that constitute AP-1 in synoviocytes have a clear effect on function. For instance, c-Jun increases the production of proinflammatory mediators, whereas JunD suppresses cytokine and MMP production.[194] AP-1 decoy oligonucleotides suppress collagen-induced arthritis and inhibit IL-1, IL-6, TNF-α, MMP-3, and MMP-9 production by synovial tissue.[195]

SIGNAL TRANSDUCERS AND ACTIVATORS OF TRANSCRIPTION

The signal transducers and activators of transcription (STATs) are a family of latent cytoplasmic transcription factors that are activated in response to cytokine stimulation of cells. STAT proteins contain domains that promote docking to the appropriate tyrosine-phosphorylated cytokine receptor. STATs have been implicated in the expression of many proinflammatory genes. Active STAT3 has been detected in cells from inflamed joints,[196] and synovial fluid from RA patients can activate STAT3, but not STAT1, in monocytes.[197] The induction of STAT translocation in the joint is independent of IFN-γ and appears to be regulated primarily by IL-6. STAT3 is also strongly phosphorylated in RA synovium and supports the hypothesis that IL-6 plays a pathogenic role in the disease. In an animal model of arthritis, treatment with the suppressor of cytokine signaling repressor (SOCS3), which blocks the activation of certain STATs, suppresses arthritis.[198] This inhibitor is also expressed in the synovium of patients with RA, although it appears to be insufficient to block STAT3 phosphorylation.

■ Life and Death in the Rheumatoid Synovium

Studies defining the life cycle of cells have opened a new door to understanding the pathogenesis of neoplastic and inflammatory diseases. Although most investigators previously focused on cell proliferation as a mechanism of synovial hyperplasia, increasing attention has been paid to the other side of the equation (i.e., whether insufficient cell death could also contribute to this process). In this section, the role of oxidative damage, programmed cell death, and permanent changes in the genome are discussed, as they can alter the natural history of RA.

REACTIVE OXYGEN AND NITROGEN

Oxidative stress in the joints of RA patients results from a confluence of several stimuli, including increased pressure in the synovial cavity, reduced capillary density, vascular changes, an increased metabolic rate of synovial tissue, and locally activated leukocytes. The generation of reactive oxygen species can also be facilitated by repetitive ischemia reperfusion injury in the joint. Tissue injury releases iron and copper ions and heme proteins that are catalytic for free-radical reactions. Electron transport chains are also disrupted in the mitochondria and endoplasmic reticulum, leading to leakage of electrons to form superoxide.

Evidence for increased production of reactive oxygen species in RA patients includes elevated levels of lipid peroxidation products, degradation of hyaluronic acid by free radicals, decreased levels of ascorbic acid in serum and synovial fluid, and increased breath pentane excretion. Moreover, the levels of thioredoxin, which is a marker of oxidative stress, are significantly higher in synovial fluid from RA patients compared to other forms of arthritis.[199] Peripheral blood lymphocyte DNA from RA patients contains significantly increased levels of the mutagenic 8-oxohydrodeoxyguanosine,[200] which is a product of oxidative damage to DNA, pointing to the genotoxic effects of oxidative stress.

Nitric oxide (NO) production is also high in rheumatoid synovial tissue.[201] Low levels of NO are constitutively produced by endothelial or neuronal synthases, and this is substantially increased by inducible NO synthase after stimulation by cytokines or bacterial products. The nitrite levels in synovial fluid are elevated in RA patients, indicating local NO production.[202] In addition, the urinary nitrate-to-creatinine ratio is increased and inducible NO synthase is present in the synovium.

APOPTOSIS

Programmed cell death, or apoptosis, is a process by which cells can be safely eliminated in the midst of living tissue. This stereotypic response provides a mechanism for tissue development, remodeling, or cell deletion without instigating an inflammatory response. Apoptosis is a normal process that is tightly regulated and can be initiated by withdrawal of hormones and growth factors. It is evident in the elimination of autoreactive cells such as thymocytes in the thymus gland and the loss of cells after DNA damage. It also plays a critical role in immune response by deleting activated T cells and terminating an inflammatory response by rapidly removing neutrophils.

The accumulation of cells in RA is typically considered as a process involving in situ cell proliferation or recruitment of cells from the blood stream. However, it is equally tenable that increased cell numbers could collect in the synovium due to insufficient cell deletion. T cell apoptosis in RA synovial effusions, for instance, is significantly less than lymphocytes from crystal-induced arthropathy.[203] The RA T cells show high Fas (CD95) expression, high Bax, and low Bcl-2, which is a phenotype typically associated with increased susceptibility to apoptosis. This contrasts with synovial tissue cells in which high Bcl-2 expression is found in lymphoid aggregates and protects synovial T cells from programmed cell death. Resistance to apoptosis in vitro is prolonged if the RA T cells are cocultured with fibroblast-like synoviocytes or IL-15. The specific adhesion molecules involved are not defined, although the integrin-binding RGD motif (arginine-glycine-asparagine) could block the protective effects of synoviocytes.

Fas and its counterreceptor Fas ligand (FasL) are potent regulators of cell death for many cell types, including synovial T cells and synoviocytes. Fas is expressed by rheumatoid synovial fluid T cells, and the number of Fas+ cells in the peripheral blood of RA patients is greater than in healthy controls.[204] Anti-Fas antibody, which cross-links Fas on cell surfaces, rapidly causes apoptosis in synovial fluid B and T lymphocytes in RA, although peripheral-blood T cells are more resistant. The presence of the natural ligand to Fas, FasL, is uncertain, with some groups detecting FasL whereas others do not.

Studies of apoptosis in RA synovial tissue have relied on a number of techniques that label damaged DNA. Using the most stringent methods, a small number of apoptotic nuclei have been detected in both the intimal lining and sublining.[205] Electron microscopic studies only show rare cells that exhibit the typical findings of programmed cell death. Surprisingly, less-specific techniques that detect any DNA damage show abundant cells in the intimal lining with nuclear fragmentation.[206]

Hence, there is an unexpected discrepancy between the cytologic evidence of DNA damage and the rarity of typical morphologic changes of apoptosis, even using ultrastructural criteria.[207] One explanation for synovial macrophages is that they express high levels of the caspace 8 inhibitor FLIP (FLICE-like inhibitory protein), which can inhibit Fas-mediated apoptosis.[208] Despite the dearth of apoptotic cells in the lining, Bcl-2 expression (which inhibits apoptosis) is low in this region. The mechanisms for inducing apoptosis in fibroblast-like synoviocytes can involve several pathways, including induction of JNK and AP-1 activation, inhibition of the kinase Akt, or suppression of NFκB.[209] p53, which typically induces cell-cycle arrest and either DNA repair or apoptosis, is also expressed in the synovial lining and sublining. Notably, abnormal p53 function could also permit the persistence of DNA damage without significant apoptosis.

Because of these unexpected findings, the regulation of apoptosis has been evaluated in cultured fibroblast-like synoviocytes in RA. Fas is constitutively expressed by cultured synoviocytes, and programmed cell death is initiated in a minority of cells (generally 20 percent or less) when it is cross-linked by anti-Fas antibody. Most investigators find that RA and OA synoviocytes are equally susceptible to anti-Fas–mediated death. TGF-β decreases Fas-antigen expression, upregulates Bcl-2, and increases resistance to anti-Fas–mediated apoptosis in synoviocytes.[210] Fas-mediated synoviocyte death appears to utilize the JNK signal transduction pathway and involves activation of the transcription factor AP-1.[211] Synoviocyte apoptosis can also be initiated by oxidative stress, such as hydrogen peroxide, or by exposure to NO, both of which are tightly regulated by p53 and are produced by the rheumatoid synovium.

The potential relevance of Fas-induced death as a therapeutic modality has been demonstrated in murine collagen-induced arthritis, in which high levels of Fas and low levels of FasL are expressed by synovial cells.[212] Mice treated with an intra-articular injection of an adenoviral vector encoding Fas ligand had decreased synovial inflammation. DNA-labeling studies showed that the construct increased synovial apoptosis. Anti-Fas antibody also induces synovial cell death in RA synovial tissue explanted in SCID mice.

Other targets that regulate apoptosis have also demonstrated potential utility in animal models. For instance, NFκB blockade in streptococcal cell-wall arthritis induces synovial apoptosis and suppresses arthritis. p53 gene therapy in rabbit antigen-induced arthritis induces synovial apoptosis and decreases inflammation. The pleiotropic activities of p53 were demonstrated in collagen-induced arthritis because p53 knockout mice with the disease developed increased inflammation and greater joint destruction in association with decreased apoptosis. Joint damage was mediated by increased collagenase-gene expression in the knockout mice, most likely because p53 directly suppresses MMP gene transcription.[213]

SYNOVIOCYTE TRANSFORMATION

Although RA fibroblast-like synoviocytes often appear and behave like normal fibroblasts, they also exhibit certain characteristics that suggest partial transformation. Certainly, the dichotomy between the extent of DNA fragmentation in the synovial lining and the lack of effective apoptosis is consistent with this notion. Several properties of cell transformation have been evaluated in RA and have led to the notion that synoviocytes might be permanently altered by their environment. For instance, adherence to plastic or extracellular matrix is generally required for normal fibroblasts to proliferate and survive in culture. Although fibroblast-like synoviocytes typically grow and thrive under conditions that permit adherence, RA synoviocytes can also proliferate in an anchorage-independent manner.[214] In addition, cultured RA synoviocytes can exhibit defective contact inhibition and express a variety of transcription factors, such as c-Myc, that are typically abundant in tumor cells. Poorly regulated cell growth likely occurs in vivo as well, and studies examining X-linked genes demonstrate oligoclonality in the synoviocyte population from RA, but not OA, synovium.[215] This is especially true of cells derived from the invading pannus, which is the most aggressive region of the synovium. Increased telomerase activity, another feature of transformed tissue, is also present in RA synovium and can be observed in FGF-stimulated RA synoviocytes.

The most compelling data indicating permanent changes in RA synoviocyte function were demonstrated in the SCID mouse model where only RA synoviocytes invade cartilage. In toto, these studies provide strong evidence that fibroblast-like synoviocytes are irreversibly altered in RA and that an autonomous process allows them to remain activated even after removal from the articular inflammatory milieu. However, RA synoviocytes are not truly transformed or immortalized; they do not form tumors and, after multiple passages in vitro, they ultimately senesce.

Tumor Suppressor Genes and Mutations: Mechanisms for Autonomous Activation

The p53 tumor suppressor is a key regulator of DNA repair and cell replication. Although not an oncogene itself, p53 is under the transcriptional control of oncogenes like c-*myc* and provides critical signals that arrest cell growth, induce apoptosis, or both. p53 has several domains that serve distinct functions. A transactivation region stimulates transcription of a number of genes, including p21[waf] and the ribosomal gene cluster. In contrast, a transrepression region decreases expression of proteins such as retinoblastoma gene-1 (RB1) and PCNA. Many of the suppressed genes regulate cell proliferation, and downregulation arrests the cell cycle at the G1 phase. This is especially prominent after cells are transformed by oncogenes such as *ras* or sustain DNA damage, thereby leading to apoptosis or providing sufficient time for DNA repair.

p53 protein expression is significantly greater in the rheumatoid synovium compared to OA and normal tissue. In long-standing disease marked by joint destruction, immunostaining localizes the protein to sublining mononuclear cells as well as the intimal lining.[216] Of interest, p53 protein can also be detected in RA synovium from patients with very early RA as well as asymptomatic rheumatoid joints.[217] However, its expression is much lower in other inflammatory arthropathies such as reactive arthritis, which might reflect the generally greater amount of DNA damage and oxidative stress in RA. Fibroblast-like synoviocytes from RA patients constitutively express significantly greater amounts of p53 compared to skin fibroblasts or OA synoviocytes.

The possibility that somatic mutations in the p53 gene might explain, in part, the unusual phenotype of RA synoviocytes and inadequate apoptosis in rheumatoid synovial tissue has been carefully investigated.[218] p53 mutations have been identified in RA synovial tissue and synoviocytes by several independent groups. The mutations are not found in the skin or blood from the same patients, indicating that they are somatic rather than germline. Transition mutations, which are characteristic of damage induced by reactive oxygen or nitric oxide, account for more than 80 percent of the base changes.

Almost all the mutations identified in the rheumatoid samples are similar to those previously identified in neoplastic diseases, suggesting that they are functionally relevant. At least some of them exhibit dominant negative characteristics and suppress the function of the wild-type allele.[219] The effect of losing p53 function in fibroblast-like synoviocytes was investigated by transducing fibroblast-like synoviocytes expressing wild-type p53 with the human papilloma virus 18 E6 gene, which inactivates p53.[220] The loss of p53 function enhanced synoviocyte proliferation, anchorage-independent growth, and invasiveness into cartilage extracts, as well as impairing apoptosis. Thus, cells with p53 mutations might have a selection advantage, because these mutations produce resistance to p53-dependent apoptosis. Furthermore, loss of p53 function induced a rheumatoid synoviocyte phenotype in normal synoviocytes that were tested in the SCID mouse model of cartilage invasion by markedly increasing fibroblast adherence and invasion into cartilage.

In RA, local mutagenesis could provide a mechanism for the creation of partially transformed synoviocyte clusters in the synovium marked by increased invasive potential.[221] Microdissection studies confirmed the presence of mutant islands, and the loss of p53 function in a region of RA synovium was associated with increased IL-6 gene expression in the same location. Based on the current data, it is likely that the mutations do not cause RA but, instead, are the result of the longstanding oxidative stress (Fig. 65–9). The somatic gene alterations can then potentially increase the aggressive nature of the synovium and alter the natural history of RA.

Other Mutations in Rheumatoid Arthritis

Mutations in other genes have also been reported in RA. For instance, synovial T cells in RA have an increased incidence of mutations in the hprt gene.[222] Although not functionally significant, these act as a marker for oxida-

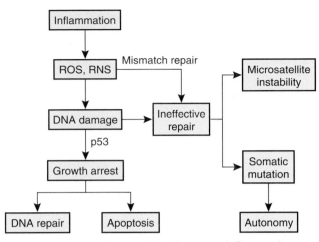

FIGURE 65–9 · Relationship Between Inflammation and Somatic Mutation in RA. Inflammatory processes can increase reactive oxygen and nitrogen species, which, in turn, can damage DNA and induce the p53 gene. Normally, this results in cell cycle arrest and either DNA repair or cell deletion through apoptosis. These same conditions can paradoxically suppress DNA repair enzymes and permit mutations in microsatellites or important regulatory genes like p53. Abbreviations: RNS, reactive nitrogen species; ROS, reactive oxygen species.

tive damage that occurs in the synovial milieu. Some of these abnormal lymphocytes also can be detected in the peripheral blood, suggesting that articular T cells can migrate out of the joint to other parts of the body. Abnormalities of the ras gene, which is involved in many signal transduction pathways, have also been noted in some patients. The ras family of oncogenes includes three genes (H-ras, K-ras, and N-ras) that encode guanine-binding proteins. The H-ras gene is expressed in the synovium of patients with a variety of arthritides,[223] and mutations have been identified in both RA and OA synovium.[224] Microsatellite instability, which is marked by mutations in mono- and dinucleotide repeat sequences in noncoding DNA, is also significantly greater in RA than OA synovial tissue. This process may be facilitated in RA by suppressed DNA-repair mechanisms. Therefore, the mutagenic potential of the synovial environment is amplified by a combination of reactive oxygen and nitrogen species with inadequate mismatch repair.

Dedifferentiation and Expression of Embryonic Genes

Because the rheumatoid synovium exhibits properties of less-differentiated neoplasias, the possibility that the tissue contains immature cells or embryonic genes has been explored. The embryonic growth factors from the wingless (wnt) and frizzled (fz) gene families have been demonstrated in RA synovium.[225] Normally, these proteins participate in bone marrow progenitor differentiation and limb bud mesenchyme. Wnt5a and Fz5, in particular, are markedly elevated in RA tissues and cultured synoviocytes. When normal fibroblasts are transfected with the wnt5a gene, cytokine expression, such as IL-6, increases significantly. Antisense wnt-5A and dominant negative wnt-5A vectors diminish IL-6 and IL-15 expression by synoviocytes.[226] These data raise the possibility that immature mesenchymal cells populate the synovium in RA, either as a primary event or as a repair mechanism. Similar primitive mesenchymal cells circulate in the peripheral blood of RA and normal individuals, and in collagen-induced arthritis they infiltrate the synovium before clinically apparent synovial inflammation.

Blood Vessels in Arthritis

Blood vessels were once thought of as passive conduits through which red blood cells and leukocytes circulated while en route to an inflammatory site. This is now known to be far from the truth: The microvasculature plays an active role in such processes, not only as the means of selecting which cells should enter the tissue but also as a determinant of tissue growth and nutrition through the proliferation of new capillaries.

ANGIOGENESIS IN RHEUMATOID ARTHRITIS: FEEDING THE STARVED SYNOVIUM

From the vantage of new blood-vessel proliferation in the synovium, synovitis in RA resembles both tumor growth and wound healing. The importance of luxurious new capillary growth early in the development of synovitis has been recognized for many years (Fig. 65–10). The absolute number of blood vessels is increased in RA synovium, with a rich network of sublining capillaries and postcapillary venules in histologic sections stained with endothelium-specific antibodies. However, the mass of tissue outstrips angiogenesis in RA as determined by the number of blood vessels per unit area and causes local tissue ischemia.[227] Synovial fluid oxygen tensions are remarkably low, lactate measurements are frequently high, and the pH can be as low as 6.8. The mean rheumatoid synovial fluid PO_2 in samples from rheumatoid

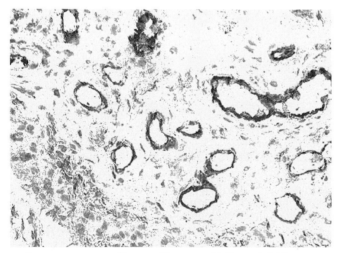

FIGURE 65–10 • Human Rheumatoid Synovial Membrane Stained with Antibody to Von Willebrand Factor to Delineate Blood Vessels. Virtually all of these blood vessels have formed in response to angiogenic stimuli after the rheumatoid process had been initiated. (Courtesy of Dr. Paul-Peter Tak.) (See color plate 31.)

knees is approximately 30 mm Hg, and occasionally less than 15 mm Hg. Another cause of diminished blood flow is increased positive pressure exerted by synovial effusions within the joint, a process that obliterates capillary flow while producing ischemia-reperfusion injury in the joint. Clearance values generated by the kinetics of iodine-123 removal from synovial fluid have shown that small-solute removal from rheumatoid synovial effusions is less than in normal individuals or in patients with other rheumatic diseases.[228] Patients with the lowest synovial iodine clearance have the lowest synovial fluid pH, the lowest synovial fluid glucose–to–serum glucose ratios, the highest synovial fluid lactate levels, and the highest numbers of synovial fluid neutrophils. Thus, the most seriously affected rheumatoid joints may be both hypoperfused and ischemic. Altered vascular flow may not be the only cause of hypoxia in joints; oxygen consumption of the rheumatoid synovium (per gram of tissue) is 20 times normal.[229]

Hypoxia is a potent stimulus for angiogenesis. One of the mechanisms by which this occurs is through the production of angiogenic factors such as vascular endothelial growth factor (VEGF).[230] VEGF is a specific endothelial cell mitogen and is present in high concentrations in rheumatoid synovial fluid and tissue. Elevated serum concentrations in early disease correlate with subsequent radiographic progress, although it is not clear if there is a causal relationship.[231] VEGF is also able to stimulate the expression of collagenase, which can degrade the extracellular matrix to make room for the advancing vasculature and pannus.[232] VEGF expression is especially high in the synovial intimal lining, and the angiogenesis factor is produced by cultured fibroblast-like synoviocytes that have been exposed to hypoxia and IL-1.[233]

In addition to the hypoxia-driven stimulus for blood-vessel growth, the inflammatory cytokine milieu of the joint also encourages angiogenesis. Several proinflammatory factors expressed by the rheumatoid joint, including IL-8, FGF, and TNF-α, are angiogenic. Many of these cytokines, including TNF-α, further enhance angiogenesis by increasing expression of angiopoietins (Ang-1 and Ang-2) by synoviocytes, which can then bind to their tyrosine kinase receptor, Tie-1, on RA capillary endothelial cells.[234] Additional angiogenesis factors, such as soluble E-selectin and soluble VCAM, are released by activated endothelium in RA synovium and contribute to vascular proliferation.[235] Limited quantities of some antiangiogenic mediators that inhibit capillary proliferation, such as platelet factor-4 and thrombospondin, are also produced by the joint.[236]

Vascular remodeling is an active process that involves the continuous creation and resorption of blood vessels. In RA, new capillaries that form under the influence of proangiogenic factors can be identified by the expression of integrins such as $\alpha_v\beta_3$. Endothelial proliferation is especially prominent in synovial tissue regions containing VEGF. Synovial blood vessel involution can also be detected as evidenced by apoptosis of the endothelium in other synovial locations. An index comparing proliferation and death of blood vessels is significantly higher in RA compared to OA or normal synovium.

The importance of new blood-vessel formation in inflammatory arthritis was elegantly demonstrated in the collagen-induced arthritis model. The disease was markedly attenuated in animals pretreated with an angiostatic compound similar to fumagillin, which is derived from *Aspergillus*.[237] This compound is cytotoxic to proliferating, but not resting, endothelial cells. In addition, there was regression of established arthritis if treatment was initiated well into the course of the disease. Hence, angiogenesis is essential for the establishment and progression of inflammatory arthritis, because of the need for blood vessels either to recruit leukocytes or to provide nutrients and oxygen to starved tissue.

Several other antiangiogenesis approaches are effective in animal models of arthritis. For instance, direct intra-articular administration of a cyclic RGD peptide was used in a rabbit model to block $\alpha_v\beta_3$ integrin.[238] As with RA synovium, $\alpha_v\beta_3$ is expressed by proliferating blood vessels in inflamed rabbit synovial tissue. The cyclic peptide decreased joint inflammation, increased endothelial cell apoptosis, and suppressed bone and cartilage destruction. More recently, the ability of RGD to bind selectively to proliferating blood vessels was used to home a proapoptotic agent to synovial neovasculature in murine collagen-induced arthritis.[239] The cyclic RGD peptide was administered systemically and accumulated in inflamed synovium but not normal joints or other organs. Apoptosis was induced in synovial blood vessels and arthritis regressed. The potent angiogenesis inhibitor endostatin has been tested in the SCID mouse model, and it decreased synovial explant inflammatory cell infiltration and capillary density.[240]

ADHESION MOLECULE REGULATION

The formation of new capillaries is only one aspect of blood vessel involvement in the rheumatoid process. Endothelial cells are also activated by cytokines to express adhesion molecules that bind to counterreceptors on mononuclear cells and neutrophils from the circulation and facilitate their transfer from the blood into the subsynovial tissue (see Chapter 24). There are two main categories of vascular adhesion molecules. The selectins (E-, L-, and P-selectin) are a family of adhesion molecules whose primary ligands are carbohydrates, especially sialyl Lewis$_x$, and related oligosaccharides. The second family is integrins, which are heterodimers that include an α- and a β-chain. The counterreceptors depend on the specific combination of these chains and are frequently proteins in the immunoglobulin supergene family (e.g., the combination of ICAM-1 and $\alpha_M\beta_2$) or extracellular matrix proteins (e.g., the combination of fibronectin and $\alpha_5\beta_1$ or vitronectin and $\alpha_v\beta_3$). Adhesion molecules specific for synovial vasculature have not been identified, but phage-display peptide libraries demonstrate localization of constrained RGD-containing sequences to inflamed synovium in mice. Several novel peptides have been described that bind to the blood vessels of human synovial explants in SCID mice.[241]

As one might expect, adhesion-molecule expression is increased in the RA synovium (Table 65–6). This is almost certainly due to exposure of the vasculature to the rich cytokine milieu, especially IL-1 and TNF-α. IFN-γ and IL-4 also increase adhesion-molecule expression, but their role is less certain due to relatively low production in RA. Immunohistochemical techniques localize high levels of ICAM-1 to sublining macrophages, macrophage-like synovial lining cells, and fibroblasts, compared to normal tissue.[242] Significant amounts are also present on the majority of vascular endothelial cells, although the ICAM-1 levels are quantitatively similar to those of vessels in normal endothelium. Cultured fibroblast-like synoviocytes also constitutively express ICAM-1, which can be markedly increased by TNF-α, IL-1, and IFN-γ. Maintenance of ICAM-1 expression on synoviocytes requires continuous cytokine exposure, and levels decline to baseline if the cytokine is removed. ICAM-1 on synoviocytes might serve as a counterreceptor to leukocyte integrins or act as a barrier to cells trying to migrate through the tissue to the synovial fluid space. Alternatively, integrin counterreceptors are costimulatory molecules that participate in the activation of T lymphocytes through $\alpha_1\beta_2$ (LFA-1).

Adhesion of $\alpha_4\beta_1$-expressing mononuclear cells, such as memory T cells or monocytes, to cytokine-activated endothelial cells can be mediated by VCAM-1. Under some culture conditions, VLA-4 mediates CD18-independent monocyte transendothelial migration. VLA-4, which is predominately expressed on lymphocytes, monocytes, and eosinophils, but not on neutrophils, serves as a receptor for both the six- and seven-domain forms of VCAM-1 and a 25–amino acid sequence in an alternatively spliced region of fibronectin (FN) known as CS-1. A role for VLA-4 in arthritis has been suggested by a number of experimental observations. In adjuvant

TABLE 65–6 · MAJOR ADHESION MOLECULE INTERACTIONS WITH RHEUMATOID ARTHRITIS SYNOVIAL ENDOTHELIUM

Endothelial Cell Adhesion Molecule	Leukocyte Counterreceptors	Leukocytes Expressing Counterreceptor
ICAM family	β_2 integrins	Neutrophils, lymphocytes, monocytes
VCAM-1	$\alpha4\beta1$ (VLA-4); $\alpha4\beta7$	Lymphocytes, monocytes
CS-1 fibronectin	$\alpha4\beta1$ (VLA-4)	Lymphocytes, monocytes
E-selectin, P-selectin	L-selectin; sLex	Neutrophils, lymphocytes, monocytes
PECAM-1	$\alpha v\beta3$	Lymphocytes, monocytes
Hyaluronate	CD44	Neutrophils, lymphocytes, monocytes

Abbreviations: ICAM, Intercellular adhesion molecule; SLex, sialyl Lewis$_x$; VCAM-1, vascular cell adhesion molecule-1.

arthritis in rats, anti-α_4 antibody decreases lymphocyte accumulation in the joint but not lymph nodes, suggesting that VLA-4 is more important in recruitment to inflamed sites than to noninflamed sites.[243] In streptococcal cell-wall arthritis, intravenous injection of CS-1 peptide decreases the severity of acute and chronic arthritis.[244] T lymphocytes isolated from the synovial fluid and synovial membrane of RA patients exhibit increased VLA-4–mediated adherence to both CS-1 and VCAM-1, relative to autologous peripheral blood lymphocytes.[245] These studies also suggest that leukocytes expressing functionally activated VLA-4 are selectively recruited to inflammatory sites in RA.

Moderate amounts of VCAM-1 are expressed in RA synovial blood vessels. Surprisingly, the intimal lining is the location of the most intense staining with anti–VCAM-1 antibodies on histologic sections. Even normal synovial tissue expresses VCAM-1 in the lining, albeit less than in RA. Cultured fibroblast-like synoviocytes constitutively express small amounts of VCAM-1, and the level is increased by IL-1, TNF-α, IFN-γ, and IL-4. VCAM-1 on synoviocytes is functionally active and can support T cell binding. VCAM-1 also contributes to T cell adhesion to high endothelial venules in frozen sections of RA synovium.[246] The other VLA-4 counterreceptor, CS-1–containing forms of FN, is restricted to inflamed RA vascular endothelium and the synovial intimal lining.[247] Normal synovial tissue contains little, if any, CS-1 fibronectin. RA synovial endothelium binds activated T lymphocytes; this can be blocked by anti-α_4 antibody and synthetic CS-1 peptide but not anti–VCAM-1 antibody, suggesting that the CS-1–VLA-4 interaction is critical to lymphocyte homing to the joint. Binding studies confirmed this in vitro, because a portion of VLA-4–mediated T cell adhesion to cultured synoviocytes is blocked by CS-1 peptides.

The integrin $\alpha_4\beta_7$, which can also bind to VCAM-1, is a specific adhesion molecule involved in lymphocyte homing to Peyer's patches. Most intraepithelial and lamina propria lymphocytes express $\alpha_4\beta_7$; this molecule is rarely identified in other lymphoid tissues. The expression of $\alpha_4\beta_7$ on peripheral blood lymphocytes from patients with RA is low (similar to normal individuals), but up to a quarter of synovial fluid lymphocytes, mostly CD8+ T lymphocytes, express this adhesion molecule.[248] This observation reinforces a putative linkage between the gastrointestinal epithelium and the joint that has been especially prominent when considering the pathogenesis of reactive arthritis.

E-selectin expression is also elevated in rheumatoid synovium, although the increase is less dramatic than for the integrins and their counterreceptors.[249] This might be due, in part, to the kinetics of E-selectin expression on endothelial cells. The protein is not found on resting endothelial cells and peaks after about 3 hours of cytokine stimulation. However, even in the continued presence of cytokines, E-selectin expression declines to near-basal levels after about 6 hours. In one study, E-selectin expression was decreased in synovial biopsies after patients were treated with injectable gold and corticosteroids.[250]

The therapeutic potential for antiadhesion therapy has been studied in the SCID mouse model. Labeled human peripheral mononuclear cells were injected into engrafted mice, and migration into the tissue was examined.[251] If the mice were treated with TNF-α, ICAM-1 expression and trafficking into synovium was significantly increased. Anti–ICAM-1 antibody blocked leukocyte migration into the explant under these conditions. In another study, tonsil mononuclear cells also migrated into the RA synovial grafts in SCID mice.[252] However, leukocyte accumulation was mainly blocked by anti–LFA-1 antibody (a counterreceptor for ICAM-1). RA clinical trials using anti–ICAM-1 therapy have been reported using anti–ICAM-1 antibody or antisense ICAM-1 oligonucleotides. Although there are some caveats with regard to the reagents used, dramatic clinical benefit was not observed.[253]

▎ Cartilage and Bone Destruction

CARTILAGE DESTRUCTION AND THE PANNUS-CARTILAGE JUNCTION

In RA, the cartilage is often covered by a layer of tissue composed of mesenchymal cells, which might represent the progenitor of the aggressive, mature pannus. In the established lesion, numerous areas are seen in which macrophage-like and fibroblast-like cells penetration into cartilage matrix far from lymphocytes.[254] However, some regions show relatively acellular pannus tissue, suggesting that there is little if any enzyme-mediated tissue destruction in these areas. Invasive pannus is more commonly found in metatarsophalangeal joints, compared to hip and knee joints in which a layer of resting fibroblasts appeared to separate pannus from cartilage, perhaps explaining why erosions occur more often around small joints. In contrast, joint-space narrowing without erosions is more common in knees.

A more-primitive cell type might play a role in RA, especially at the cartilage-pannus junction. This less-differentiated cell type could, then, be responsible for the aggressive degradation of the extracellular matrix and help drive the destructive phase of the disease. Fibroblast-like synoviocytes from the intimal lining exhibit some characteristics of transformed cells but are not necessarily alone in their ability to degrade articular structures. Other cells in the joint, especially from the pannus that erodes directly into cartilage, could also be responsible for cartilage, whereas osteoclasts mediate bone erosions. Despite differences in morphologic appearance and cellular content, direct comparisons of erosion and nonerosion synovial tissue reveal more similarities than differences with regard to cytokine and protease expression.

Primitive mesenchymal cells isolated directly from the cartilage pannus junction express phenotypic and functional features of both synoviocytes and chondrocytes and have been referred to as *pannocytes*.[255] They exhibit a distinctive rhomboid morphology and can grow in culture for a prolonged time without becoming senescent. In addition, VCAM-1 surface expression is constitutive and very high compared with synoviocytes or chondrocytes. Pannocytes exhibit some features of chondrocytes in that both express inducible lymphocyte antigen, which is a surface receptor in the TNF–nerve growth factor family, and inducible NO synthase. These genes are not usually expressed by fibroblast-like synoviocytes. Interestingly, pannocytes, like synoviocytes, do not produce NO synthase even though they contain NO-synthase mRNA. Pannocytes are more fibroblast-like in that they produce type I but not type II collagen and, like synoviocytes, contain intracellular vimentin. Others have suggested that pannus-derived cells can express the type II collagen gene or produce proteoglycans that stain positively with safranin O.[256]

Cartilage is destroyed in RA by both enzymatic and mechanical processes. The enzymes induced by factors such as IL-1, TNF-α, phagocytosis of debris by synovial cells and mechanic trauma cause the joint destruction. Early in synovitis, proteoglycans are depleted from the tissue, most likely due to the catabolic effect of cytokines such as IL-1 on chondrocytes with the production of MMPs and aggrecanases, and this leads to mechanical weakening of cartilage. As proteoglycans are depleted (Fig. 65–11), cartilage loses the ability to rebound from a deforming load and thereby becomes susceptible to mechanical fragmentation and fibrillation. Eventually the tissue loses functional integrity concurrent with its complete dissolution by collagenase and stromelysin. Some of the MMPs responsible for this process are also derived from the chondrocytes themselves. Both stromelysin and collagenase mRNA levels are increased in RA cartilage, and in situ hybridization studies confirm the presence of the specific RNA transcripts within chondrocytes.[257]

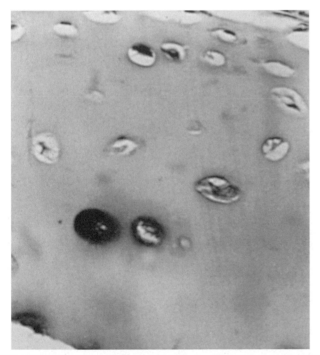

FIGURE 65–11 · Human Articular Cartilage from Active RA Removed at Joint Arthroplasty and Stained for Metachromasia. The only metachromatic stain surrounds a few chondrocytes that, presumably, are actively making proteoglycan only to have it broken down by proteinases derived from synovial fluid, chondrocytes, or synovial tissue. The form of this depleted cartilage is normal; however, its functional capacity to rebound from a deforming load is seriously impaired.

Hence, the cartilage is under attack from a multitude of sources: It being bathed in protease-rich synovial fluid, is under extrinsic attack from the invasive pannus, and the chondrocytes themselves contribute to destruction from within.

Enzymes released from PMNs in synovial fluid also contribute to cartilage loss. Immune complexes containing rheumatoid factors are embedded in the superficial layers of cartilage and can attract and activate neutrophils. Electron microscopic examinations of articular cartilage in RA reveal amorphous-appearing material and evidence of breakdown of collagen and proteoglycan consistent with superficial diffuse activity of joint-fluid enzymes.[258] However, in a rabbit model of arthritis in which IL-1 was injected directly into the joint, the degree of cartilage damage as measured by proteoglycan levels in synovial fluid correlated best with the stromelysin concentrations in synovial effusions (presumably derived from synoviocytes). Neutrophil depletion of animals did not interfere with subsequent destruction of extracellular matrix, suggesting that synovium-derived MMPs are more important.

By and large, most animal studies indicate that IL-1 is a key regulator of matrix degradation in arthritis.[259] This has been true across a broad range of arthritis models, including zymosan-induced arthritis, collagen-induced arthritis, antigen-induced arthritis, and streptococcal cell wall–induced arthritis. Although TNF-α blockade has clear anti-inflammatory effects, chondroprotection is less prominent. This does not mean that TNF-α cannot mediate joint destruction; the TNF transgenic mice that develop polyarticular arthritis have severe erosions and deformities. The prominent bone and cartilage protection observed in patients receiving TNF inhibitors reminds us that animal models are imperfect predictors of RA responses.

The rate-limiting step in cartilage loss is the cleavage of collagen, because proteoglycans are degraded very soon after inflammation begins. MMPs, released into the extracellular space and active at neutral pH, are probably responsible for most of the effective proteolyses of articular-cartilage proteins, but other classes of enzymes may contribute to joint destruction. Enzymes such as cathepsins B, D, G, K, L, and H may play a role within and outside cells in degrading noncollagenous matrix proteins. Serine proteinases (e.g., elastase and plasmin) and aggrecanases are doubtless involved as well.

PROTEASES—KEY MEDIATORS OF JOINT DESTRUCTION

Matrix Metalloproteinases

The MMPs are a family of enzymes that participate in extracellular-matrix degradation and remodeling (see Chapter 4). MMPs are usually secreted as inactive proenzymes, and their proteolytic activity requires limited cleavage or denaturation to reveal a zinc cation at the core. Their activation can be mediated by other proteases, including trypsin, plasmin, or tryptase. The substrates for MMPs are varied but quite specific for individual members of the family. Collagenases degrades native collagen types I, II, III, VII, and X, whereas gelatinases are able to degrade denatured or cleaved collagen. Stromelysins have broader specificity and can digest proteoglycans in addition to proteins. They also process procollagenase to the active form, thereby serving as a positive-feedback signal for matrix destruction. Many different families of proteinases are found in the joint (Table 65–7), but the MMPs are thought to play a pivotal role in joint destruction.

The cytokine milieu has the capacity to induce the biosynthesis of MMPs by synovial cells and alter the balance between extracellular matrix production and degradation. IL-1 and TNF-α, in particular, directly induce MMP gene expression by many cells, including fibroblast-like synoviocytes and chondrocytes. These two cytokines are additive or synergistic when used in combination. Many other cytokines implicated in rheumatoid synovitis can also induce MMP expression, including IL-17 and LIF.

MMP induction is mediated by both a change in gene transcription and mRNA stabilization. Increased cyclic AMP levels, such as by activation of A2b adenosine receptors, in synoviocytes can suppress collagenase expression by decreasing mRNA half-life.[260] Culture medium from rheumatoid synovium stimulates cartilage degradation in vitro, and this can be inhibited by an antibody against IL-1; these data implicate rheumatoid synovium as a source of IL-1 that activates chondrocytes to produce proteases.[261] IL-6 does not induce MMP production by synovial cells but instead increases the production of TIMP-1, a naturally occurring inhibitor of MMPs.[262] TGF-β inhibits collagenase synthesis in vitro and enhances the production of TIMP by fibroblasts and chondrocytes.[263] TGF-β also increases collagen production, shifting the balance to matrix repair.

Substances other than cytokines are capable of inducing synovial cells to produce MMPs in vitro, and it is probable that many have a role in vivo as well. Proteinases, soluble iron, collagens, monosodium urate monohydrate crystals, and various calcium crystals are found in joints at one time or another and stimulate col-lagenase biosynthesis. The crystals, and perhaps other substances in this group, stimulate MMP production by triggering IL-1 (and possibly other cytokine) production. Excessive shear force and physical trauma can also induce MMP gene expression in synovial tissue. Some proteases, such as the 92-kD gelatinase, are constitutively released by early-passage RA synoviocytes.[264]

Although multiple upstream regulatory sequences are involved in the regulation of MMP gene transcription, the dominant element in the promoter is AP-1. Other regulatory sites, such as an NFκB-like region, can also contribute to collagenase expression.[265] AP-1 activity is markedly increased in fibroblast-like synoviocytes by proinflammatory cytokines, and its transcriptional activity is mediated by increased expression of components such as c-Jun and post-translational modification by phosphorylation. The MAP kinases are especially important for this activity, and JNK is the most efficient upstream activator. Glucocorticoid-mediated inhibition of collagenase gene expression is due to interference with the Fos-Jun complex by the glucocorticoid receptor.

Collagenases and stromelysins have the capacity to degrade all the important structural proteins in the extracellular tissues within joints. Collagenase-1 (MMP-1) is an MMP with maximal activity in a range between pH 7 and 8. It cleaves through the triple-helical collagen molecule at a single glycine-isoleucine bond approximately three quarters of the distance from the NH_2 terminus of the 300-nm protein. This enzyme has the capability to degrade only the interstitial helical collagens (e.g., types I, II, III, and X). It has little or no activity against types IV, V, and IX and other nonhelical collagens or denatured collagen; the degradation of the latter is primarily accomplished by the gelatinases. MMP-1, however, is a relatively inefficient enzyme, and the more recently characterized collagenase-3 (MMP-13) has more favorable kinetics. Like collagenase-1, collagenase-3 has an AP-1–binding site in the promoter that is an important regulator of MMP-13 gene transcription. Neutrophil collagenase, or MMP-8, is constitutively stored in neutrophil granules and is released into the milieu after degranulation. The relative importance of this enzyme in inflammatory arthritis is uncertain, and neutrophil depletion does not necessarily prevent cartilage damage in animal models. Of note, rodents lack the collagenase-1 gene, whereas the collagenase-3 gene is preserved. This is especially important to note when evaluating effects of MMP inhibitors in animal models.

The collagenase-1 and collagenase-3 genes are produced by RA synovial tissue, and the latter is highly expressed by chondrocytes in cartilage. In situ hybridization studies show that the primary location of collagenase-1 gene expression in the synovium, like many other MMPs, is the intimal lining, especially in fibroblast-like cells.[266] Subchondral bone is another region in which proteinase expression occurs in RA and could participate in bone resorption. Increased MMP gene expression is an early feature of RA and occurs during the first few weeks or months of disease.[267] This underscores the need for early therapy to prevent joint destruction. High expression of collagenase-1, as well as gelatinases such as MMP-2, early in disease correlates with rapidly progres-

TABLE 65–7 • KEY PROTEASES AND INHIBITORS IN RHEUMATOID ARTHRITIS SYNOVIUM

Protease	Inhibitor
Metalloproteinases	TIMP family; α2 macroglobulin
Collagenase-1	
Collagenase-3	
Stromelysin-1	
92-kD gelatinase	
Serine proteases	SERPINs; α2 macroglobulin
Trypsin	
Chymotrypsin	
Tryptase	
Cathepsins	α2 macroglobulin
Cathepsin B	
Cathepsin L	
Cathepsin K	

Abbreviations: SERPIN, Serine protease inhibitors; TIMP, tissue inhibitor of metalloproteinases.

sive erosions. Similarly, increased blood levels of the proenzymes also are associated with more severe disease.

Stromelysin-1 (MMP-3) and the other members of the stromelysin family have no activity against interstitial collagens but effectively degrade type IV collagen, fibronectin, laminin, proteoglycan core protein, and type IX collagen. Stromelysin removes the NH_2-terminal propeptides from type I procollagen and is integrally involved in the activation of procollagenase. Like collagenase, stromelysin gene expression is almost exclusively in the synovial intimal lining (Fig. 65–12).

Most data indicate a cascade of activation of the MMPs. Once prostromelysin is activated, it is subsequently essential for the activation of procollagenase. Prostromelysin from human synovial cells can be activated by other proteases, including cysteine proteases (the cathepsins), trypsin, chymotrypsin, plasma kallikrein, plasmin, and mast cell tryptase. Despite the putative importance of this enzyme in matrix destruction, stromelysin knockout mice are susceptible to collagen-induced arthritis and develop as much joint destruction as mice with functional stromelysin.[268] MMP inhibitors are effective in animal models of arthritis and can suppress bone destruction as well as the inflammatory synovitis.[269] However, clinical trials in RA using nonselective inhibitors have had less success and significant side effects, possibly related to decreased matrix turnover.

Cysteine Proteases—The Cathepsins

Cathepsins are an extensive family of cysteine proteases that have broad proteolytic activity, including activity on types II, IX, and XI collagen and proteoglycans.[270] Like MMPs, the cathepsins are regulated by cytokines and by protooncogenes such as ras. IL-1 and TNF-α induce cathepsin L expression in cultured fibroblast-like synoviocytes.[271] In situ hybridization studies demonstrate expression of cathepsin B and L in RA synovium, especially at sites of erosion. A novel cysteine protease called cathepsin K has been implicated in bone resorption by osteoclasts. It is unique among the cathepsins in its ability to degrade native type I collagen.[272] Cathepsin K is expressed in RA synovial tissue by both macrophages and fibroblasts and is present in significantly higher concentrations than in OA.[273] A potential role of cathepsins as mediators of bone destruction in arthritis was confirmed in studies in which a cysteine protease inhibitor significantly decreased joint damage in the rat adjuvant arthritis model.[274]

Aggrecanases

In addition to type II collagen, aggrecan is a critical component of cartilage as one of the major proteoglycan components. Because of its large size and negative charge, it contains a considerable amount of water, which serves to increase compressibility. Two proteolytic sites are available on aggrecan in its globular domain. One site is susceptible to MMP cleavage, including MMP-1, -2, -3, -7, -8, -9, and -13, whereas the other, located 32 amino acids toward the carboxyterminus, is the site for cleavage by a new family of enzymes known as aggrecanases. The two sites can be identified in tissues using monoclonal antibodies after cleavage when specific neoepitopes are revealed. Normal cartilage contains a surprising amount of aggrecanase neoepitope, suggesting continuous matrix turnover, and the level of aggrecanase cleavage product increases with age.[275] Two aggrecanase genes, aggrecanase-1 and aggrecanase-2, have been cloned and are members of the "a disintegrin and metalloproteinase with thrombospondin motif" (ADAMTS) family of proteins.[276] They are expressed in OA and RA cartilage, and their proteolytic activity can be detected in synovial fluids using bioassays. High levels of the neoepitope are present in arthritic cartilage.[277] IL-1 increases aggrecanase expression in cartilage explants as well as cultures of chondrocytes. Aggrecanase-1 and aggrecanase-2 are constitutively expressed by RA and OA fibroblast-like synoviocytes and synovial tissues. Aggrecanase-1 is induced in synoviocytes by cytokines, especially TGF-β, whereas aggrecanase-2 expression remains constant despite TGF-β or IL-1 stimulation.

INHIBITORS OF PROTEASE ACTIVITY

α_2-Macroglobulin (α_2M) accounts for more than 95 percent of collagenase inhibitory capacity in serum. The mechanism of inhibition by α_2M involves hydrolysis by the proteinase of a susceptible region in one of the four polypeptide chains of α_2M (sometimes called the "bait"), with subsequent trapping of the proteins within the interstices of the α_2M. Ultimately, the protease is covalently linked to a portion of the α_2M molecule. The serine protease inhibitors (SERPINs) are also abundant in synovial effusions and plasma and can serve a dual purpose of directly blocking serine protease function and indirectly decreasing MMP activity by preventing serine proteases from activating

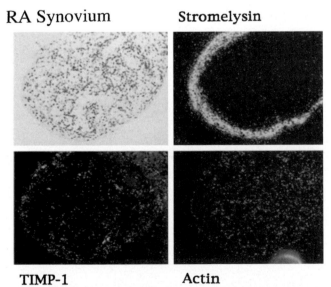

RA Synovium   Stromelysin

TIMP-1   Actin

FIGURE 65–12 · Localization of Stromelysin, Tissue Inhibitor of metalloproteinases-1 (TIMP-1), and Actin mRNA in Rheumatoid Arthritis (RA) Synovial Tissue by in Situ Hybridization. Stromelysin is mainly expressed in the synovial intimal lining, presumably by cytokine-stimulated type B synoviocytes. Bright field and dark field views are shown. (Courtesy of D. Boyle.)

MMP proenzymes. One SERPIN, α_1-antitrypsin, has been well characterized in synovial fluid and is frequently inactivated after oxidation by reactive oxygen species.[278]

A family of proteins that specifically block MMP activity, called TIMPs, has been cloned and characterized. Each member has distinctive pattern of affinity for members of the MMP family. The TIMP proteins block proteinase activity by binding directly to MMPs in a 1:1 molar ratio. TIMP generally binds only to the active enzyme, although there are some exceptions, such as TIMP-2, which can interact with a progelatinase (MMP-2). The inhibitors bind to MMPs with extremely high avidity. Even though the interaction does not result in new covalent bonds, it is essentially irreversible.

TIMP proteins are present in RA synovial fluid in excess. It is, in fact, very difficult to detect free active collagenase or stromelysin, as they are usually complexed with the inhibitors.[279] The majority of MMP, however, is not unbound and is in the proenzyme form. Immunohistochemical and in situ hybridization studies have localized the TIMPs in hyperplastic synovial lining cells in rheumatoid synovium, but not in the cells of normal synovium. TIMP gene expression is not significantly altered by IL-1 or TNF-α but it is increased by IL-6, oncostatin M, and TGF-ß.

Given the important role of MMPs in tissue destruction, the relative balance between MMPs and TIMPs ultimately determines the fate of the extracellular matrix. The ratio in RA, with its more destructive potential, favors degradation, whereas OA has a lower MMP:TIMP ratio. The levels of TIMP gene expression are very similar in the two diseases and may well be maximal. The higher ratio in RA results from increased MMP production. This balance between protease and inhibitor can be modified in vivo with drug therapy. For instance, intra-articular corticosteroid injections markedly decrease synovial collagenase, stromelysin, and TIMP gene expression. In contrast, chronic low-dose methotrexate therapy specifically decreases collagenase but not TIMP-1 mRNA.[280] Suppressed collagenase gene expression suggests that a low collagenase-to-TIMP ratio is one mechanism of decreased bone destruction observed in a patients treated with methotrexate.

REGULATION OF BONE DESTRUCTION BY THE RECEPTOR ACTIVATOR OF NUCLEAR FACTOR κB -RANK LIGAND SYSTEM

Although synoviocytes have been extensively investigated as primary mediators of joint destruction in RA, more recent data suggest that osteoclasts are the major cells responsible for bone degradation. Receptor activator of NFκB ligand (RANKL), which was originally described for its role in T cell–dendritic cell interactions as well as lymphocyte and lymph node development, is perhaps the single most important factor that modulates bone resorption.[281] Osteoclast development is complex and involves the differentiation of monocytes under the influence of cytokines such as M-CSF in combination with RANKL. Subsequent osteoclast activation can involve several pathways, most of which also depend on the presence of RANKL. The receptor for RANKL, known as RANK, is expressed by the osteoclast precursors; RANKL is produced by many cell types, including activated T cells and fibroblast-like synoviocytes. RANKL knockout mice have abnormally dense bones due to a nearly complete lack of osteoclasts. When osteoclasts or their precursors are activated by soluble RANKL or by direct contact with cells displaying RANKL on their surface, bone resorption can then occur through the elaboration of MMPs and cathepsin K. The RANKL-RANK system is antagonized by a soluble decoy receptor, osteoprotegerin (OPG), which binds to RANK and competes with RANKL.

Abundant evidence implicates this powerful mechanism for bone destruction in inflammatory arthritis. For instance, administration of OPG to rats with adjuvant arthritis inhibits bone destruction but has almost no effect on inflammation or clinical signs of arthritis.[282] RANKL knockout mice are also protected from bone erosions in the passive K/BxN model of arthritis, although cartilage destruction still occurs.[283]

RANK, RANKL, and OPG (as well as M-CSF) have been detected in the synovium and synovial fluid of patients with RA. The ratio of RANKL to OPG is significantly higher in RA synovial effusions than in either OA or gout, which is consistent with the more destructive nature of RA.[284] Osteoclasts expressing tartrate-resistant acid phosphatase (TRAP), capable of forming resorption lacunae, can be generated from cultured RA synovial cells[285] (Fig. 65–13). This activity is blocked by the addition of exogenous OPG. RA synoviocytes and synovial membrane T cells that display RANKL can also induce differentiation of osteoclasts from peripheral blood cells.[286]

▮ Synovial Fluid

Although it would be of great interest to examine synovial tissue from each patient with RA to compare histologic changes with those from previous specimens and perhaps assay for T cell subsets, RF production, and cytokine production by synovial cells, this is impractical (although

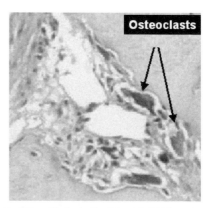

FIGURE 65–13 · Tartrate Resistant Acid Phosphatase (TRAP)-Positive Osteoclasts are shown Invading Bone in Rheumatoid Arthritis (see *arrows* for examples). This process is regulated by RANKL in the presence of other cytokines such as macrophage colony-stimulating factor (M-CSF) and tumor necrosis factor -alpha (TNF-α). (Courtesy of Dr. Steven Goldring, Dr. Ellen Gravallese, and Dr. Allison Pettit.)

miniarthroscopy might someday permit one to "stage" RA in this manner to determine the prognosis and appropriate therapy). As stressed previously, blood is far removed from the site of disease and the focus of inflammatory activity. Despite some limitations, synovial fluid has been a reasonable compromise; by examination of its characteristics, some appreciation for the extent of inflammation can be gained, and by using synovial fluid, investigators can learn about events within the synovium itself. Components of the inflammatory and proliferative response that can be dissected by examination of synovial fluid from patients are discussed in the following sections.

It has been known for many years that there is an inverse relationship between the molecular weight of proteins and their concentrations in minimally inflamed synovial fluid; the high-molecular-weight serum proteins gain access more easily to synovial fluid in inflamed joints, and the relatively high concentration of IgG in RA synovial fluid is good evidence for local (synovial) synthesis of IgG. Protein traffic in human synovial effusions has been measured by determining the clearance of proteins from synovial fluid and gives a useful measure of afferent synovial lymph flow. A markedly increased permeance of proteins in rheumatoid patients confirms the severity of the microvascular lesion in rheumatoid synovitis.

POLYMORPHONUCLEAR LEUKOCYTES

The number of PMNs remains one of the most consistent indices of inflammation within a particular joint. These cells truly amplify inflammatory responses and contribute to the perpetuation of the inflammation within joints. The articular cavity serves as a depository for PMNs; they enter the synovial fluid by direct passage from postcapillary venules in the synovium. Neutrophils adhere to activate synovial microvasculature because of the action of selectins and the β_2 integrins. After adherence, however, agents such as IL-8 and other chemotactic factors produced by endothelium and fibroblasts may facilitate egress through the capillaries along the chemoattractant gradients of the synovium. Thus, considering the survival time of PMNs in synovial fluid, it has been estimated that the breakdown of an average (30 ml) rheumatoid effusion containing 25,000 PMNs per mm^3 may well exceed 1 billion cells each day. The ultimate fate of many of these cells is apoptosis.

The strong attraction of chemotactic agents within the synovial fluid in RA is responsible for the large number of cells found there. Few PMNs are seen in the pannus itself and subsynovial tissue; once in the synovium they move rapidly to the synovial fluid, drawn by the activated component of cleavage of the fifth component of complement (C5a), leukotriene B$_4$ (LTB$_4$), platelet-activating factor, and chemokines. The reason neutrophils can move into the articular cavity without resistance, whereas mononuclear cells collect in the sublining, is not clear. It might be related to the fact that neutrophils express very little VLA-4 compared to mononuclear cells and, therefore, are unimpeded by VCAM-1 and CS-1 fibronectin in the intimal lining. In the synovial fluid, PMNs come in contact with immune complexes and particulate material (i.e., fibrin, cell membranes, cartilage fragments). Phagocytosis occurs, especially to particles coated with IgG, and

the PMNs are activated. The neutrophils degranulate, generate products of oxygen metabolism, metabolize arachadonic acid, and develop the capacity for aggregation. In addition, PMNs from synovial fluid in RA release de novo synthesized proteins, including fibronectin, neutral proteinases, and IL-1. Neutrophils also secrete IL-1Ra as a major product. Although the amount of IL-1Ra each neutrophil produces is low compared to that produced by macrophages, the sheer number of PMNs allows them to produce massive amounts in synovial effusions.

IMMUNE COMPLEXES

The significance of immunoglobulin complexes circulating in blood and in synovial fluid was appreciated several decades ago. However, it was not until more reliable assays for immune complexes were available that broad studies correlating disease activity and immune complexes could be generated. By and large, the most relevant data relate to the production of such complexes in the joint rather than the blood, except in the unusual case of systemic rheumatoid vasculitis. Nevertheless, circulating IgM immune complexes, are elevated in both RA and systemic lupus erythematosus. In studies designed to identify the components of immune complexes in the circulation of rheumatoid patients, most data have indicated no specific antigen other than IgG complexed with RF. Using more sensitive techniques, circulating immune complexes in RA contained as many as 20 polypeptides, including albumin, immunoglobulin, complement, and acute-phase reactants.

Most relevant to the pathogenesis of joint destruction in RA has been the identification of immunoglobulins and complement in articular collagenous tissues from RA patients. Almost all cartilage and meniscus samples from rheumatoid patients have evidence of these components in the avascular connective tissue. Electron microscopic morphology of immunoglobulin aggregates show that there are pathologic changes in the matrix of cartilage in the microenvironment of the aggregates themselves. Immune complexes are absent under areas of cartilage invaded actively by synovial pannus, suggesting that phagocytic cells in the invasive synovium ingest the immune complexes. This possibility lends credence to the notion that immune complexes deposited in the avascular superficial layers of cartilage in the joint may serve as chemoattractants for the pannus. Immune complexes have been extracted from cartilage of RA and OA patients. Rheumatoid cartilage contains more than 40-fold more IgM and more than 10-fold more IgG than healthy cartilage extracts. IgM RF is found in the majority RA cartilage extracts but not in OA or healthy control extracts. In addition, more than 60 percent of the RA cartilage extracts are positive for native and denatured collagen type II antibody.

These observations support the hypothesis that the presence of cartilage itself, and perhaps these complexes, contributes to the chronicity and persistence of rheumatoid inflammation. Orthopedic surgeons have noted for many years that joints from which all cartilage is removed do not participate in general flares of rheumatoid disease after surgery. The localization of immune complexes, either due to in situ formation or absorption from the synovial fluid, could be required for the full expression of RA.

ARACHIDONATE METABOLITES

Accompanying activation of PMNs is the increased mobilization of membrane phospholipids in these cells to arachadonic acid and its subsequent oxidation by cyclooxygenases (COX) to prostaglandins and thromboxanes, or by lipoxygenases to leukotrienes. Although the stable prostaglandins, especially PGE_2, produce vasodilation, cause increased vascular permeability, and are involved centrally in fever production, there is increasing evidence that they have significant antiinflammatory activities as well. For example, stable prostaglandin can retard the development of adjuvant arthritis, and the drug misoprostol, a prostaglandin analogue, may have significant anti-inflammatory or immunomodulatory effects. Physiologic concentrations of PGE_2 inhibit IFN-γ production by T cells, HLA-DR expression by macrophages, and T cell proliferation. Certain arachadonic acid metabolites, such as 15-deoxy-delta(12,14)-PGJ(2) can bind to peroxisome proliferators-activate receptors (PPARs) and inhibit cytokine production, as well as adjuvant arthritis.[287] Cyclopentenone prostaglandins can also inhibit NFκB by blocking IKK, thereby suppressing the NFκB-driven array of proinflammatory genes.[288]

Production of prostaglandins in RA is dependent on two distinct COX enzymes, COX-1 and COX-2 (see Chapter 23). The former is constitutively expressed and is responsible for the normal endogenous production of prostaglandins in the joint as well as in other tissues. COX-2, on the other hand, is an inducible enzyme responsible for increased prostaglandin synthesis in inflamed tissue. Cytokines such as IL-1 and TNF-α induce COX-2 gene expression by cultured synoviocytes and macrophages. COX-2 mRNA and immunoreactive protein are increased in RA synovium.[289] Most nonsteroidal anti-inflammatory drugs, including indomethacin and ibuprofen, inhibit both COX-1 and COX-2. Much of the anti-inflammatory activity (and analgesia) results from inhibition of the latter. Clinical experience using similar compounds in patients with OA or RA indicates that COX-2 blockade is sufficient for the therapeutic benefit.

LTB_4 has also received considerable attention as a proinflammatory product of neutrophil activation. It is chemotactic for neutrophils, eosinophils, and macrophages and promotes neutrophil aggregation and adherence to endothelium. Peripheral blood PMNs from rheumatoid patients have an enhanced capacity for the production of LTB_4 compared with similar cells from control groups.[290] In murine collagen-induced arthritis, a specific LTB_4 antagonist significantly decreased paw swelling and joint destruction, suggesting a pivotal role for this potent chemoattractant.[291] However, LTB4 blockade in RA has been less impressive.

COMPLEMENT

The liver is the major source of complement synthesis in humans, and passive transfer of serum proteins into effusions accounts for much of the complement proteins found there. However, synovial tissue also actively produces complement proteins.[292] Macrophages and fibroblasts produce complement proteins under the influence of cytokines such as IFN-γ, IL-1, and TNF-α. In situ hybridization shows that C2 is expressed in the synovial intimal lining, whereas C3 appears to be produced by synovial sublining macrophages. Northern blot analysis of synovial tissue shows that all complement genes from the classic pathway are expressed in RA synovium, as well as in healthy synovium. Despite the local production of complement components, the activities of C4, C2, and C3 and total hemolytic complement in rheumatoid synovial effusions are lower than in synovial fluids from patients with other joint diseases.[293]

Using a sensitive solid-phase radioimmunoassay to quantify the activation of the classic pathway of complement by RF, IgM RF appears to be a much more important determinant of complement activation than IgG RF in both serum and synovial fluid.[294] Combined with other data showing accelerated catabolism of C4 in RA and that the presence of C4 fragments in the plasma of rheumatoid patients correlates with titers of IgM RF, the weight of evidence indicates a role in vivo for IgM RF in complement activation.

The biologically active products of complement activation are probably the most important consequence of intra-articular complement consumption. Like proteases from PMNs, these inflammatory components accumulate in synovial fluid during acute inflammation. The potential for interaction between PMNs and the complement system is substantial. Neutrophil lysosomal lysates contain enzymatic activity capable of generating chemotactic activity (probably C5a) from fresh serum. C5a, in addition to being a principal chemotactic factor in inflammatory effusions, mediates lysosomal release from human PMNs. This sets up one of many amplification loops in inflammatory synovial fluid.

Complement activation as a potential therapeutic target has received increasing attention. In rat antigen-induced arthritis, for instance, intra-articular treatment with a soluble complement receptor (sCR1) inhibits joint swelling.[295] Knockout mice lacking various complement components also provide evidence for the utility of this approach. C5-deficient mice have decreased joint inflammation in collagen-induced arthritis and the passive K/BxN model.[296] Absence of C3 or factor B also inhibits collagen-induced arthritis. Unlike the C5 knockout mice, which had normal antibody responses, the C3- and factor B–null animals had lower levels of anti–type II collagen antibodies.[297] Therefore, both classic and alternative complement pathways are implicated in inflammatory arthritis. The mechanisms of action can be either by inhibiting the innate immune responses or the adaptive immune responses, depending on the specific model and complement components targeted.

EXTRAVASCULAR COAGULATION

Fibrin accumulation in synovial fluid, especially on the surface of synovium, frequently occurs in RA and suggests dysregulated fibrinogen metabolism. Production of fibrin is mediated by neutral proteases such as thrombin and can result from activation of the coagulation cascade. Indeed, tissue factor, thrombin, and many other elements of coagulation are present in inflammatory synovial fluid. Accumulation of fibrin and its degradation products can impair normal diffusion of nutrients and oxygen to cartilage, increase vascular permeability, enhance cytokine production, and induce leukocyte chemotaxis.[298] Plasmin, which degrades fibrin and is expressed by fibroblast-like synoviocytes, can also contribute directly to extracellular matrix destruction by activating MMPs or latent cytokines (i.e., TGF-β). In antigen-induced arthritis, mice lacking urokinase or plasminogen genes have increased fibrin deposition and more aggressive disease. However, in other models, absence of urokinase can suppress disease. Therefore, the contribution of the coagulation cascade and fibrinolysis depends on whether fibrinolysis or activation of other substrates is dominant.

Interactions Between Innate and Adaptive Immunity

Many mechanisms of disease have been considered in this chapter. Innate immunity, which is a primitive pattern-recognition system that can lead to rapid inflammatory responses, has been implicated through the engagement of Fc receptors by immune complexes and perhaps Toll-like receptors by bacterial products. Antigen-driven T cell and B cell responses may also participate due to either xenoantigen reactivity or, more likely, responses directed at a number of autoantigens described earlier in the chapter. Cytokine networks clearly participate, with paracrine and autocrine loops that maintain cellular activation in the synovial intimal lining. Finally, permanent alterations in some cell types might occur during the evolution of disease that can accelerate destruction.

One potential synthesis of these data suggests that an induction phase, initiated by innate immunity, can then "prepare" the joint for subsequent recruitment of inflammatory and immune cells[299] (Fig. 65–14). This process probably occurs often in normal individuals but is self-limited. Once the cell recruitment begins, a genetically susceptible host in the appropriate environment can develop a primary response to a arthrotropic antigen, secondary immune responses to articular antigens, or overactive cytokine networks due to gene polymorphisms that increase the production of proinflammatory factors. The typical clinical picture of RA ensues, driven by lymphocytes, macrophages, and other antigen-presenting cells. Ultimately, a destructive phase proceeds, which can be antigen dependent and independent and supported by mesenchymal elements such as fibroblasts and synoviocytes. Bone erosions are subsequently caused by osteoclasts, whereas cartilage dissolution results from proteolytic enzymes produced by synoviocytes in the pannus or synovial fluid neutrophils.

Although not proven, this general hypothesis takes into account many of the elements described by investigators in the field. The heterogeneity of mechanisms provides an explanation for the unpredictable response to therapeutic agents and also allows clinicians to envision new therapeutic targets to either prevent RA or interfere with the immunologic, inflammatory, or destructive components as separate but interrelated entities.

Summary

Understanding the etiology and pathogenesis of RA remains a complex problem, although the level of understanding has progressed considerably in recent years. Both T cell–dependent and –independent processes might contribute to disease initiation and perpetuation. Moreover, it might be important to appreciate differences in disease pathogenesis at various stages of the

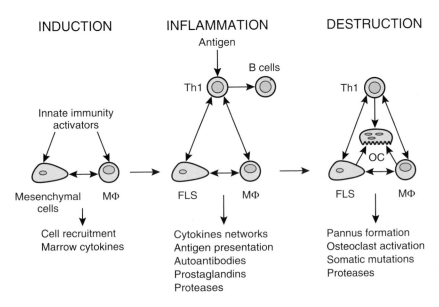

INDUCTION   INFLAMMATION   DESTRUCTION

FIGURE 65–14 · Schematic Diagram of Disease Mechanisms that Likely Occur in Various Phases of Rheumatoid Arthritis. Innate Immunity Activates Mesenchymal Cells and Macrophages (Mφ) in the Earliest Phases, which can Focus a Subsequent Immune Response to the Synovium. Antigen-specific responses, although not proven, are probably most important in the inflammatory phases, eventhough macrophage and fibroblast-like synoviocyte (FLS) cytokines dominate. Direct T cell contact can also activate other cells in an antigen-independent manner. In the latter phases of disease, many cell types activate osteoclasts through the receptor activator of NFκB/receptor activator of NFκB ligand (RANK/RANKL) system, although FLSs likely provide the greatest stimulus. Autonomous activation of FLS might contribute to this process. (From Firestein GS, Zvaifler NJ: How important are T cells in chronic rheumatoid arthritis. Arthritis Rheum, 46:298-308, 2002.)

process. These hypotheses have unveiled many novel therapeutic targets and interventions that might lead to significant clinical benefit. Such was the case with the TNF inhibitors that have joined the pharmacopoeia for the treatment of RA; initial observations that defined the cytokine profile in arthritis and that delineated the biology of macrophage cytokines led to this breakthrough. Similarly, it is possible that understanding of apoptotic pathways, abnormalities in tumor-suppressor genes, the function of the susceptibility cassette, or the mechanisms of Th1-Th2 balance might have unexpected rewards.

REFERENCES

1. Silman AJ, Pearson JE: Supplement review: Epidemiology and genetics of rheumatoid arthritis. Arthritis Res 4:S265, 2002.
2. Nepom GT, Byers P, Seyfried C, et al: HLA genes associated with rheumatoid arthritis: Identification of susceptibility alleles using specific oligonucleotide probes. Arthritis Rheum 32:15, 1989.
3. Weyand CM, Hicok KC, Conn DL, Goronzy JJ: The influence of HLA-DRB1 genes on disease severity in rheumatoid arthritis. Ann Intern Med 117:801, 1992.
4. Boki KA, Drosis AA, Tzioufas GA, et al: Examination of HLA-DR4 as a severity marker for rheumatoid arthritis in Greek patients. Ann Rheum Dis 52:517, 1993.
5. Hameed K, Bowman S, Kondeatis E, et al: The association of HLA-DRB genes and the shared epitope with rheumatoid arthritis in Pakistan. Br J Rheumatol 36:1184, 1997.
6. Calin A, Elswood J, Klouda PT: Destructive arthritis, rheumatoid factor, and HLA-DR4: Susceptibility versus severity, a case control study. Arthritis Rheum 32:1221, 1989.
7. Thomson W, Pepper L, Payton A, et al: Absence of an association between HLA-DRB1*04 and rheumatoid arthritis in newly diagnosed cases from the community. Ann Rheum Dis 52:539, 1993.
8. Kirschmann DA, Duffin KL, Smith CE, et al: Naturally processed peptides from rheumatoid arthritis and non-associated HLA-DR alleles. J Immunol 155:5655, 1995.
9. Zanelli E, Breedveld FC, de Vries RRP: HLA association with autoimmune disease: A failure to protect? Rheumatology 39:1060, 2000.
10. Zanelli E, Gonzalez-Gay MA, David CS: Could HLA-DRB1 be the protective locus in rheumatoid arthritis? Immunol Today 16:274, 1995.
11. Doherty DG, Vaughan RW, Donalson PT, Mowat AP: HLA DQA, DQB, and DRB genotyping by oligonucleotide analysis: Distribution of alleles and haplotypes in British caucasoids. Hum Immunol 34:53, 1992.
12. de Vries N, van Elderen C, Tijssen H, et al: No support for HLA-DQ encoded susceptibility in rheumatoid arthritis. Arthritis Rheum 43:946, 2000.
13. Zanelli E, Krco CJ, Baisch JM, et al: Immune response of HLA-DQ8 transgenic mice to peptides from the third hypervariable region of HLA-DRB1 correlates with predisposition to rheumatoid arthritis. Proc Natl Acad Sci U S A 93:1814, 1996.
14. Tsuchiya N, Endo T, Shiota M, et al: Distribution of glycosylation abnormality among serum IgG subclasses from patients with rheumatoid arthritis. Clin Immunol Immunopathol 70:47, 1994.
15. Rademacher TW, Williams P, Dwek RA: Agalactosyl glycoforms of IgG autoantibodies are pathogenic. Proc Natl Acad Sci U S A 91:6123, 1994.
16. Rodriguez MR, Nunez-Roldan A, Aguilar F, et al: Association of the CTLA4 3' untranslated region polymorphism with the susceptibility to rheumatoid arthritis. Hum Immunol 63:76, 2002.
17. Nelson JL, Hughes KA, Smith AG, et al: Maternal-fetal disparity in HLA class II alloantigens and the pregnancy-induced amelioration of rheumatoid arthritis. N Engl J Med 329:466, 1993.
18. Brennan P, Barrett J, Fiddler M, et al: Maternal-fetal HLA incompatibility and the course of inflammatory arthritis during pregnancy. J Rheumatol 27:2843, 2000.
19. Rashid T, Darlington G, Kjeldsen-Kragh J, et al: Proteus IgG antibodies and C-reactive protein in English, Norwegian and Spanish patients with rheumatoid arthritis. Clin Rheumatol 18:190, 1999.

20. Gerard HC, Wang Z, Wang GF, et al: Chromosomal DNA from a variety of bacterial species is present in synovial tissue from patients with various forms of arthritis. Arthritis Rheum 44:1689, 2001.
21. van der Heijden IM, Wilbrink B, Tchetverikov I, et al: Presence of bacterial DNA and bacterial peptidoglycans in joints of patients with rheumatoid arthritis and other arthritides. Arthritis Rheum 43:593, 2000.
22. Cole BC, Griffiths MM: Triggering and exacerbation of autoimmune arthritis by the Mycoplasma arthritidis superantigen MAM. Arthritis Rheum 36:994, 1993.
23. Hoffman RW, O'Sullivan FX, Schafermeyer KR, et al: Mycoplasma infection and rheumatoid arthritis: Analysis of their relationship using immunoblotting and an ultrasensitive polymerase chain reaction detection method. Arthritis Rheum 40:1219, 1997.
24. Wilkinson NZ, Kingsley GH, Sieper J, et al: Lack of correlation between the detection of Chlamydia trachomatis DNA in synovial fluid from patients with a range of rheumatic diseases and the presence of an antichlamydial immune response. Arthritis Rheum 41:845, 1998.
25. Blaschke S, Schwarz G, Moneke D, et al: Epstein-Barr virus infection in peripheral blood mononuclear cells, synovial fluid cells, and synovial membranes of patients with rheumatoid arthritis. J Rheumatol 27:866, 2000.
26. Toussirot E, Wendling D, Tiberghien P, et al: Decreased T cell precursor frequencies to Epstein-Barr virus glycoprotein Gp110 in peripheral blood correlate with disease activity and severity in patients with rheumatoid arthritis. Ann Rheum Dis 59:497, 2000.
27. Roudier J, Petersen J, Rhodes GH, et al: Susceptibility to rheumatoid arthritis maps to a T-cell epitope shared by the HLA-Dw4 DR beta-1 chain and the Epstein-Barr virus glycoprotein gp 110. Proc Natl Acad Sci U S A 86:5104, 1989.
28. Albani S, Ravelli A, Mass M, et al: Immune responses to the Escherichia coli dnaJ heat shock protein in juvenile rheumatoid arthritis and their correlation with disease activity. J Pediatr 124:561, 1994.
29. Cohen BJ, Buckley MM, Clewley JP, et al: Human parvovirus infection in early rheumatoid and inflammatory arthritis. Ann Rheum Dis 45:832, 1986.
30. Saal JG, Steidle M, Einsele H, et al: Persistence of B19 parvovirus in synovial membranes of patients with rheumatoid arthritis. Rheumatol Int 12:147, 1992.
31. Takahashi Y, Murai C, Shibata S, et al: Human parvovirus B19 as a causative agent for rheumatoid arthritis. Proc Natl Acad Sci U S A 95:8227, 1998.
32. Nikkari S, Luukkainen R, Mottonen T, et al: Does parvovirus B19 have a role in rheumatoid arthritis? Ann Rheum Dis 53:106, 1994.
33. Ray NB, Nieva DR, Seftor EA, et al: Induction of an invasive phenotype by human parvovirus B19 in normal human synovial fibroblasts. Arthritis Rheum 44:1582, 2001.
34. Stahl HD, Hubner B, Seidl B, et al: Detection of multiple viral DNA species in synovial tissue and fluid of patients with early arthritis. Ann Rheum Dis 59:342, 2000.
35. Lechner F, Vogt HR, Seow HF, et al: Expression of cytokine mRNA in lentivirus-induced arthritis. Am J Pathol 151:1053, 1997.
36. Nakagawa K, Brusic V, McColl G, Harrison LC: Direct evidence for the expression of multiple endogenous retroviruses in the synovial compartment in rheumatoid arthritis. Arthritis Rheum 40:627, 1997.
37. Nakajima T, Aono H, Hasunuma T, et al: Overgrowth of human synovial cells driven by the human T cell leukemia virus type I tax gene. J Clin Invest 92:186, 1993.
38. Pipitone N, Jolliffe VA, Cauli A, et al: Do B cells influence disease progression in chronic synovitis? Lessons from primary hypogammaglobulinaemia. Rheumatology (Oxford) 39:1280, 2000.
39. Bonagura VR, Wedgwood JF, Agostino N, et al: Seronegative rheumatoid arthritis, rheumatoid factor cross reactive idiotype expression, and hidden rheumatoid factors. Ann Rheum Dis 48:488, 1989.
40. Rawson AJ, Hollander JL, Quismorio FP, Abelson NM: Experimental arthritis in man and rabbit dependent upon serum antiimmunoglobulin factors. Ann N Y Acad Sci 168:188, 1969.
41. Patel V, Panayi GS: Enhanced T helper cell function for the spontaneous production of IgM rheumatoid factor in vitro in rheumatoid arthritis. Clin Exp Immunol 57:584, 1984.

42. Reparon-Schuijt CC, van Esch WJ, van Kooten C, et al: Functional analysis of rheumatoid factor–producing B cells from the synovial fluid of rheumatoid arthritis patients. Arthritis Rheum 41:2211, 1998.

43. Carson DA, Chen PP, Kipps TJ: New roles for rheumatoid factor. J Clin Invest 87:379, 1991.

44. Wernick RM, Lipsky PE, Marban-Arcos E, et al: IgG and IgM rheumatoid factor synthesis in rheumatoid synovial membrane cell cultures. Arthritis Rheum 28:742, 1985.

45. Bouvet JP, Xin WJ, Pillot J: Restricted heterogeneity of polyclonal rheumatoid factor. Arthritis Rheum 30:998, 1987.

46. Lee SK, Bridges SL Jr., Koopman WJ, Schroeder HW Jr.: The immunoglobulin kappa light chain repertoire expressed in the synovium of a patient with rheumatoid arthritis. Arthritis Rheum 35:905, 1992.

47. Sutton BJ, Corper AL, Sohi MK, et al: The structure of a human rheumatoid factor bound to IgG Fc. Adv Exp Med Biol 435:41, 1998.

48. Wang H, Shlomchik MJ: High affinity rheumatoid factor transgenic B cells are eliminated in normal mice. J Immunol 159:1125, 1997.

49. Tighe H, Warnatz K, Brinson D, Corr M, et al: Peripheral deletion of rheumatoid factor B cells after abortive activation by IgG. Proc Natl Acad Sci U S A 94:646, 1997.

50. Rowley M, Tai B, Mackay IR, et al: Collagen antibodies in rheumatoid arthritis. Significance of antibodies to denatured collagen and their association with HLA-DR4. Arthritis Rheum 29:174, 1986.

51. Watson WC, Cremer MA, Wooley PH, Townes AS: Assessment of the potential pathogenicity of type II collagen autoantibodies in patients with rheumatoid arthritis. Arthritis Rheum 29:1316, 1986.

52. Jasin HE: Autoantibody specificities of immune complexes sequestered in articular cartilage of patients with rheumatoid arthritis and osteoarthritis. Arthritis Rheum 28:241, 1985.

53. Tarkowski A, Klareskog L, Carlsten H, et al: Secretion of antibodies to types I and II collagen by synovial tissue cells in patients with rheumatoid arthritis. Arthritis Rheum 32:1087, 1989.

54. Bäcklund J, Carlsen S, Höger T, et al: Predominant selection of T cells specific for the glycosylated collagen type II epitope (263–270) in humanized transgenic mice and in rheumatoid arthritis. Proc Natl Acad Sci U S A 10:1073, 2002.

55. Verheijden GF, Rijnders AW, Bos E, et al: Human cartilage glycoprotein-39 as a candidate autoantigen in rheumatoid arthritis. Arthritis Rheum 40:1115, 1997.

56. Sekine T, Masuko-Hongo K, Matsui T, et al: Recognition of YKL-39, a human cartilage related protein, as a target antigen in patients with rheumatoid arthritis. Ann Rheum Dis 60:49, 2001.

57. Li NL, Zhang DQ, Zhou KY, et al: Isolation and characteristics of autoreactive T cells specific to aggrecan G1 domain from rheumatoid arthritis patients. Cell Res 10:39, 2000.

58. Steiner G, Smolen J: Autoantibodies in rheumatoid arthritis and their clinical significance. Arthritis Res 4:S1, 2002.

59. Union A, Meheus L, Humbel RL, et al: Identification of Citrullinated rheumatoid arthritis-specific epitopes in natural filaggrin relevant for antifilaggrin autoantibody detection by line immunoassay. Arthritis Rheum 46:1185, 2002.

59a.Suzuki A, Yamada R, Chang X, et al: Functional haplotypes of PADIH encoding citrullinating enzyme peptidylar ginine deiminase 4 are associated with rheumatoid arthritis. Nat Genetics 34:395, 2003.

60. Kouskoff V, Korganow AS, Duchatelle V, et al: Organ-specific disease provoked by systemic autoimmunity. Cell 87:811, 1996.

61. Corr M, Firestein GS: Innate immunity as a .hired gun: But is it rheumatoid arthritis? J Exp Med 195:F33, 2002.

62. Blass S, Union A, Raymackers J, et al: The stress protein BiP is overexpressed and is a major B and T cell target in rheumatoid arthritis. Arthritis Rheum 44:761, 2001.

63. Corrigall VM, Bodman-Smith MD, Fife MS, et al: The human endoplasmic reticulum molecular chaperone BiP is an autoantigen for rheumatoid arthritis and prevents the induction of experimental arthritis. J Immunol 166:1492, 2001.

64. Van Eden W, Holoshitz J, Nevo Z, et al: Arthritis induced by a T-lymphocyte clone that responds to *Mycobacterium tuberculosis* and to cartilage proteoglycans. Proc Natl Acad Sci U S A 82:5117, 1985.

65. Oda A, Miyata M, Kodama E, et al: Antibodies to 65Kd heat-shock protein were elevated in rheumatoid arthritis. Clin Rheumatol 13:261, 1994.

66. Gaston JSH, Life PF, Bailey LC, Bacon PA: In vitro responses to a 65-kilodalton mycobacterial protein by synovial T cells from inflammatory arthritis patients. J Immunol 143:2494, 1989.

67. Wilbrink B, Holewijn M, Bijlsma JW, et al: Suppression of human cartilage proteoglycan synthesis by rheumatoid synovial fluid mononuclear cells activated with mycobacterial 60-kd heat-shock protein. Arthritis Rheum 36:514, 1993.

68. Doran MF, Pond GR, Crowson CS, et al: Trends in incidence and mortality in rheumatoid arthritis in Rochester, Minnesota, over a forty-year period. Arthritis Rheum 46:625, 2002.

69. Revell PA, Mapp PI, Lalor PA, Hall PA: Proliferative activity of cells in the synovium as demonstrated by a monoclonal antibody, Ki67. Rheumatol Int 7:183, 1987.

70. Qu Z, Garcia CH, O'Rourke LM, et al: Local proliferation of fibroblast-like synoviocytes contributes to synovial hyperplasia: Results of proliferating cell nuclear antigen/cyclin, c-myc, and nucleolar organizer region staining. Arthritis Rheum 37:212, 1994.

71. Burmester GR, Dimitriu-Bona A, Waters SJ, Winchester RJ: Identification of three major synovial lining cell populations by monoclonal antibodies directed to Ia antigens associated with monocytes/macrophages and fibroblasts. Scand J Immunol 17:69, 1983.

72. Goto M, Sasano M, Yamanaka H, et al: Spontaneous production of an interleukin 1–like factor by cloned rheumatoid synovial cells in long-term culture. J Clin Invest 80:786, 1987.

73. Baker DG, Dayer JM, Roelke M, et al: Rheumatoid synovial cell morphologic changes induced by a mononuclear cell factor in culture. Arthritis Rheum 26:8, 1983.

74. Kang YM, Zhang X, Wagner UG, et al: CD8 T cells are required for the formation of ectopic germinal centers in rheumatoid synovitis. J Exp Med 195:1325, 2002.

75. Liu MF, Kohsaka H, Sakurai H, et al: The presence of costimulatory molecules CD86 and CD28 in rheumatoid arthritis synovium. Arthritis Rheum 39:110, 1996.

76. Warrington KJ, Takemura S, Goronzy JJ, Wayland CM: CD4+, CD28– T cells in rheumatoid arthritis patients combine features of the innate and adaptive immune systems. Arthritis Rheum 44:13, 2001.

77. MacDonald KP, Nishioka Y, Lipsky PE, Thomas R: Functional CD40 ligand is expressed by T cells in rheumatoid arthritis. J Clin Invest 100:2404, 1997.

78. Rissoan MC, Van Kooten C, Chomarat P, et al: The functional CD40 antigen of fibroblasts may contribute to the proliferation of rheumatoid synovium. Clin Exp Immunol 106:481, 1996.

79. Patel DD, Zachariah JP, Whichard LP: CXCR3 and CCR5 ligands in rheumatoid arthritis synovium. Clin Immunol 98:39, 2001.

80. Nanki T, Hayashida K, El-Gabalawy HS, et al: Stromal cell-derived factor-1-CXC chemokine receptor 4 interactions play a central role in CD4+ T cell accumulation in rheumatoid arthritis synovium. J Immunol 165:6590, 2000.

81. Muller-Ladner U, Kriegsmann J, Gay RE, et al: Progressive joint destruction in a human immunodeficiency virus–infected patient with rheumatoid arthritis. Arthritis Rheum 38:1328, 1995.

82. Poulter LW, Janossy G: The involvement of dendritic cells in chronic inflammatory disease. Scand J Immunol 21:401, 1985.

83. Tsai C, Diaz LA Jr., Singer NG, et al: Responsiveness of human T lymphocytes to bacterial superantigens presented by cultured rheumatoid arthritis synoviocytes. Arthritis Rheum 39:125, 1996.

84. Corrigall VM, Solau-Gervais E, Panayi GS: Lack of CD80 expression by fibroblast-like synoviocytes leading to anergy in T lymphocytes. Arthritis Rheum 43:1606, 2000.

85. Brennan FM, Hayes AL, Ciesielski CJ, et al: Evidence that rheumatoid arthritis synovial T cells are similar to cytokine-activated T cells: Involvement of phosphatidylinositol 3-kinase and nuclear factor kappaB pathways in tumor necrosis factor alpha production in rheumatoid arthritis. Arthritis Rheum 46:31, 2002.

86. Fox DA: The role of T cells in the immunopathogenesis of rheumatoid arthritis: new perspectives. Arthritis Rheum 40:598, 1997.

87. Karin N, Szafer F, Mitchell D, et al: Selective and nonselective stages in homing of T lymphocytes to the central nervous system during experimental allergic encephalomyelitis. J Immunol 150:4116, 1993.

88. Wang H, Marsters SA, Baker T, et al: TACI-ligand interactions are required for T cell activation and collagen-induced arthritis is mice. Nat Immunol 2:632, 2001.

89. Shi K, Hayashida K, Kaneko M, et al: Lymphoid chemokine B cell-attracting chemokine-1 (CXCL13) is expressed in germinal center of ectopic lymphoid follicles within the synovium of chronic arthritis patients. J Immunol 166:650, 2001.

90. Kim H-J, Berek C: B cells in rheumatoid arthritis. Arthritis Res 2:126, 2000.

91. Clausen BE, Bridges SL Jr., Lavelle JC, et al: Clonally-related immunoglobulin VH domains and nonrandom use of DH gene segments in rheumatoid arthritis synovium. Mol Med 4:240, 1998.

92. Reparon-Schuijt CC, van Esch WJ, van Kooten C, et al: Presence of a population of CD20+, CD38− B lymphocytes with defective proliferative responsiveness in the synovial compartment of patients with rheumatoid arthritis. Arthritis Rheum 44:2029, 2001.

93. Takemura S, Klimiuk PA, Braun A, et al: T cell activation in rheumatoid synovium is B cell dependent. J Immunol 167:4710, 2001.

94. Shimaoka Y, Attrep JF, Hirano T, et al: Nurse-like cells from bone marrow and synovium of patients with rheumatoid arthritis promote survival and enhance function of human B cells. J Clin Invest 102:606-618, 1998.

95. Takeuchi E, Tomita T, Toyosaki-Maeda T, et al: Establishment and characterization of nurse cell-like stromal cell lines from synovial tissues of patients with rheumatoid arthritis. Arthritis Rheum 42:221, 1999.

96. Burger JA, Zvaifler NJ, Tsukada N, et al: Fibroblast-like synoviocytes support B-cell pseudoemperipolesis via a stromal cell-derived factor-1- and CD106 (VCAM-1)-dependent mechanism. J Clin Invest 107:305, 2001.

97. Tsai V, Zvaifler NJ: Dendritic cell–lymphocyte clusters that form spontaneously in rheumatoid arthritis synovial effusions differ from clusters formed in human mixed leukocyte reactions. J Clin Invest 82:1731, 1988.

98. MacDonald KP, Pettit AR, Quinn C, et al: Resistance of rheumatoid synovial dendritic cells to the immunosuppressive effects of IL-10. J Immunol 163:5599, 1999.

99. Lindhout E, van Eijk M, van Pel M, et al: Fibroblast-like synoviocytes from rheumatoid arthritis patients have intrinsic properties of follicular dendritic cells. J Immunol 162:5949-5956, 1999.

100. Tak PP, Kummer JA, Hack CE, et al: Granzyme-positive cytotoxic cells are specifically increased in early rheumatoid synovial tissue. Arthritis Rheum 37:1735, 1994.

101. Malone DG, Wilder RL, Saavedra-Delgado AM, Metcalfe DD: Mast cell numbers in rheumatoid synovial tissues. Arthritis Rheum 30:130, 1987.

102. Kiener HP, Baghestanian M, Dominkus M, et al: Expression of the C5a receptor (CD88) on synovial mast cells in patients with rheumatoid arthritis. Arthritis Rheum 41:233, 1998.

103. Lee DM, Friend DS, Gurish MF, et al: Mast cells: A cellular link between autoantibodies and inflammatory arthritis. Science 297:1689, 2002.

104. Smeets TJ, Dolhain RJEM, Miltenburg AM, et al: Poor expression of T cell–derived cytokines and activation and proliferation markers in early rheumatoid synovial tissue. Clin Immunol Immunopathol 88:84, 1998.

105. Kraan MC, Versendaal H, Jonker M, et al: Asymptomatic synovitis precedes clinically manifested arthritis. Arthritis Rheum 41:1481, 1998.

106. Han Z, Boyle DL, Manning AM, Firestein GS: AP-1 and NF-κB regulation in rheumatoid arthritis and murine collagen-induced arthritis. Autoimmunity 28:197, 1998.

107. Geiler T, Kriegsmann J, Keyszer GM, et al: A new model for rheumatoid arthritis generated by engraftment of rheumatoid synovial tissue and normal human cartilage into SCID mice. Arthritis Rheum 37:1664, 1994.

108. Muller-Ladner L, Kriegsmann J, Franklin BN, et al: Synovial fibroblasts of patients with rheumatoid arthritis attach to and invade normal human cartilage when engrafted into SCID mice. Am J Pathol 149:1607, 1996.

109. Muller-Ladner U, Roberts CR, Franklin BN, et al: Human IL-1Ra gene transfer into human synovial fibroblasts is chondroprotective. J Immunol 158:3492, 1997.

110. Pap T, Aupperle KR, Gay S, et al: Invasiveness of synovial fibroblasts is regulated by p53 in the SCID mouse in vivo model of cartilage invasion. Arthritis Rheum 44:676, 2001.

111. Gaston JSH, Rickinson AB, Yao QY, Epstein MA: The abnormal cytotoxic T cell response to Epstein-Barr virus in rheumatoid arthritis is correlated with disease activity and occurs in other arthropathies. Ann Rheum Dis 45:932, 1986.

112. Hasler F, Bluestein HG, Zvaifler NJ, Epstein LB: Analysis of the defects responsible for the impaired regulation of EBV-induced B cell proliferation by rheumatoid arthritis lymphocytes. II. Role of monocytes and the increased sensitivity of rheumatoid arthritis lymphocytes to prostaglandin E. J Immunol 131:768, 1983.

113. Goronzy JJ, Weyand CM: Thymic function and peripheral T-cell homeostasis in rheumatoid arthritis. Trends Immunol 22:251, 2001.

114. Burastero SE, Casali P, Wilder RL, Notkins AL: Monoreactive high affinity and polyreactive low affinity rheumatoid factors are produced by CD5+ B cells from patients with rheumatoid arthritis. J Exp Med 168:1979, 1988.

115. Fox DA, Smith BR: Evidence for oligoclonal B cell expansion in the peripheral blood of patients with rheumatoid arthritis. Ann Rheum Dis 45:991, 1986.

116. He X, Kang AH, Stuart JM: Anti-Human type II collagen CD19+ B cells are present in patients with rheumatoid arthritis and healthy individuals. J Rheumatol 28:2168, 2001.

117. Lasky HP, Bauer K, Pope RM: Increased helper inducer and decreased suppressor inducer phenotypes in the rheumatoid joint. Arthritis Rheum 31:52, 1988.

118. Nouri AME, Panayi GS: Cytokines and the chronic inflammation of rheumatic disease. III. Deficient interleukin-2 production in rheumatoid arthritis is not due to suppressor mechanisms. J Rheumatol 14:902, 1987.

119. Firestein GS, Berger AE, Tracey DE, et al: IL-1 receptor antagonist protein production and gene expression in rheumatoid arthritis and osteoarthritis synovium. J Immunol 149:1054, 1992.

120. Maurice MM, Lankester AC, Bezemer AC, et al: Defective TCR-mediated signaling in synovial T cells in rheumatoid arthritis. J Immunol 159:2973, 1997.

121. Maurice MM, Nakamura H, van der Voort EA, et al: Evidence for the role of an altered redox state in hyporesponsiveness of synovial T cells in rheumatoid arthritis. Immunology 158:1458, 1997.

122. Firestein GS, Zvaifler NJ: How important are T cells in chronic rheumatoid synovitis? Arthritis Rheum 33:768, 1990.

123. Firestein GS, Roeder WD, Laxer JA, et al: A new murine CD4+ T cell subset with an unrestricted cytokine profile. J Immunol 143:518, 1989.

124. Unemori EN, Bair MJ, Bauer EA, Amento EP: Stromelysin expression regulates collagenase activation in human fibroblasts. Dissociable control of two metalloproteinases by interferon-gamma. J Biol Chem 266:23, 477, 1991.

125. Firestein GS, Zvaifler NJ: Peripheral blood and synovial fluid monocyte activation in inflammatory arthritis. II. Low levels of synovial fluid and synovial tissue interferon suggest that γ-interferon is not the primary macrophage activating factor. Arthritis Rheum 30:864, 1987.

126. Chen E, Keystone EC, Fish EN: Restricted cytokine expression in rheumatoid arthritis. Arthritis Rheum 36:901, 1993.

127. Smeets TJ, Dolhain RJ, Breedveld FC, Tak PP: Analysis of the cellular infiltrates and expression of cytokines in synovial tissue from patients with rheumatoid arthritis and reactive arthritis. J Pathol 186:75, 1998.

128. Firestein GS, Xu WD, Townsend K, et al: Cytokines in chronic inflammatory arthritis. I. Failure to detect T cell lymphokines (interleukin 2 and interleukin 3) and presence of macrophage colony-stimulating factor (CSF-1) and a novel mast cell growth factor in rheumatoid synovitis. J Exp Med 168:1573, 1988.

129. Miossec P, Navillat M, Dupuy d'Angeac A, et al: Low levels of interleukin-4 and high levels of transforming growth factor beta in rheumatoid arthritis. Arthritis Rheum 145:2514, 1990.

130. Chabaud M, Durand JM, Buchs N, et al: Human interleukin-17: A T cell-derived proinflammatory cytokine produced by the rheumatoid synovium. Arthritis Rheum 43:963, 1999.

131. Chabaud M, Fossiez F, Taupin JL, Miossec P: Enhancing effect of IL-17 on IL-1–induced IL-6 and leukemia inhibitory factor

production by rheumatoid arthritis synoviocytes and its regulation by Th2 cytokines. J Immunol 161:409, 1998.

132. Lubberts E, Joosten LA, Chabaud M, et al: IL-4 gene therapy for collagen arthritis suppresses synovial IL-17 and osteoprotegerin ligand and prevents bone erosion. J Clin Invest 105:1697, 2000.

133. Chabaud M, Lubberts E, Joosten L, et al: IL-17 derived from juxta-articular bone and synovium contributes to joint degradation in rheumatoid arthritis. Arthritis Res 3:168, 2001.

134. Kusaba M, Honda J, Fukuda T, Oizumi K: Analysis of type 1 and type 2 T cells in synovial fluid and peripheral blood of patients with rheumatoid arthritis. J Rheumatol 25:1466, 1998.

135. Qin S, Rottman JB, Myers P, et al: The chemokine receptors CXCR3 and CCR5 mark subsets of T cells associated with certain inflammatory reactions. J Clin Invest 101:746, 1998.

136. Chomarat P, Banchereau J, Miossec P: Differential effects of interleukins 10 and 4 on the production of interleukin-6 by blood and synovium monocytes in rheumatoid arthritis. Arthritis Rheum 38:1046, 1995.

137. Katsikis KD, CQ Chu, FM Brennan, et al: Immunoregulatory role of interleukin 10 in rheumatoid arthritis. J Exp Med 179:1517, 1994.

138. Walmsley M, Katsikis PD, Abney E, et al: Interleukin-10 inhibition of the progression of established collagen-induced arthritis. Arthritis Rheum 39:495, 1996.

139. Joosten LA, Lubberts E, Durez P, et al: Role of interleukin-4 and interleukin-10 in murine collagen-induced arthritis: Protective effect of interleukin-4 and interleukin-10 treatment on cartilage destruction. Arthritis Rheum 40:249, 1997.

140. Joosten LAB, Lubberts E, Helsen MMA, van den Berg WB: Dual role of IL-12 in early and late stages of murine collagen type II arthritis. J Immunol 159:4094, 1997.

141. Smeets TJ, Kraan MC, Versendaal J, et al: Analysis of serial synovial biopsies in patients with rheumatoid arthritis: Description of a control group without clinical improvement after treatment with interleukin 10 or placebo. J Rheumatol 26:2089, 1999.

142. Burger D, Rezzonico R, Li JM, et al: Imbalance between interstitial collagenase and tissue inhibitor of metalloproteinases 1 in synoviocytes and fibroblasts upon direct contact with stimulated T lymphocytes: Involvement of membrane-associated cytokines. Arthritis Rheum 41:1748, 1998.

143. McInnes IB, Leung BP, Sturrock RD, et al: Interleukin-15 mediates T cell-dependent regulation of tumor necrosis factor-alpha production in rheumatoid arthritis. Nat Med 3:189-195, 1997.

144. Pettipher ER, Higgs GA, Henderson B: Interleukin 1 induces leukocyte infiltration and cartilage proteoglycan degradation in the synovial joint. Proc Natl Acad Sci U S A 83:8749, 1986.

145. Miyasaka N, Sato K, Goto M, et al: Augmented interleukin-1 production and HLA-DR expression in the synovium of rheumatoid arthritis patients: Possible involvement in joint destruction. Arthritis Rheum 31:480, 1988.

146. Shore A, Jaglal S, Keystone EC: Enhanced interleukin 1 generation by monocytes in vitro is temporally linked to an early event in the onset or exacerbation of rheumatoid arthritis. Clin Exp Immunol 65:293, 1986.

147. Firestein GS, Alvaro-Gracia JM, Maki R: Quantitative analysis of cytokine gene expression in rheumatoid arthritis. J Immunol 144:3347, 1990.

148. Postlethwaite AE, Lachman LB, Kang AH: Induction of fibroblast proliferation by interleukin-1 derived from human monocytic leukemia cells. Arthritis Rheum 27:995, 1984.

149. Joosten LA, van De Loo FA, Lubberts E, et al: An IFN-gamma-independent proinflammatory role of IL-18 in murine streptococcal cell wall arthritis. J Immunol 165:6553, 2000.

150. Gracie JA, Forsey RJ, Chan WL, et al: A proinflammatory role for IL-18 in rheumatoid arthritis. J Clin Invest 104:1393, 1999.

151. Elliott MJ, Maini RN, Feldmann M, et al: Randomised double-blind comparison of chimeric monoclonal antibody to tumour necrosis factor (CA^2) versus placebo in rheumatoid arthritis. Lancet 344:1105, 1994.

152. Saklatvala J: Tumour necrosis factor α stimulates resorption and inhibits synthesis of proteoglycan in cartilage. Nature 322:547, 1986.

153. Georgopoulos S, Plows D, Kollias G: Transmembrane TNF is sufficient to induce localized tissue toxicity and chronic inflammatory arthritis in transgenic mice. J Inflamm 46:86,1996.

154. Williams RO, Mason LJ, Feldmann M, Maini RN: Synergy between anti-CD4 and anti-tumor necrosis factor in the amelioration of established collagen-induced arthritis. Proc Natl Acad Sci U S A 91:2762, 1994.

155. Lipsky PE, van der Heijde DM, St Clair EW, et al: Infliximab and methotrexate in the treatment of rheumatoid arthritis. Anti-tumor necrosis factor trial in rheumatoid arthritis with concomitant therapy study group. N Engl J Med 343:1594, 2000.

156. Guerne PA, Zuraw BL, Vaughan JH, et al: Synovium as a source of interleukin 6 in vitro. Contribution to local and systemic manifestations of arthritis. J Clin Invest 83:585, 1989.

157. Houssiau FA, Devogelaer J-P, van Damme J, et al: Interleukin-6 in synovial fluid and serum of patients with rheumatoid arthritis and other inflammatory arthritides. Arthritis Rheum 31:784, 1988.

158. Guerne PA, Zuraw BL, Vaughan JH, et al: Synovium as a source of interleukin 6 in vitro: Contribution to local and systemic manifestations of arthritis. J Clin Invest 83:585, 1989.

159. Field M, Chu C, Feldman M, Maini RN: Interleukin-6 localisation in the synovial membrane in rheumatoid arthritis. Rheumatol Int 11:45, 1991.

160. Walmsley M, Butler DM, Marinova-Mutafchieva L, Feldmann M: An anti-inflammatory role for interleukin-11 in established murine collagen-induced arthritis. Immunology 95:31, 1998.

161. Plater-Zyberk C, Buckton J, Thompson S, et al: Amelioration of arthritis in two murine models using antibodies to oncostatin M. Arthritis Rheum 44:2697, 2001.

162. Thurkow EW, van der Heijden IM, Breedveld FC, et al: Increased expression of IL-15 in the synovium of patients with rheumatoid arthritis compared with patients with *Yersinia*-induced arthritis and osteoarthritis. J Pathol 181:444, 1997.

163. Ruchatz H, Leung BP, Wei XQ, et al: Soluble IL-15 receptor alpha-chain administration prevents murine collagen-induced arthritis: A role for IL-15 in development of antigen-induced immunopathology. J Immunol 160:5654, 1998.

164. Xu WD, Firestein GS, Taetle R, et al: Cytokines in chronic inflammatory arthritis. II. Granulocyte-macrophage colony-stimulating factor in rheumatoid synovial effusions. J Clin Invest 83:876, 1989.

165. Alvaro-Gracia JM, Zvaifler NJ, Brown CB, et al: Cytokines in chronic inflammatory arthritis. VI. Analysis of the synovial cells involved in granulocyte-macrophage colony-stimulating factor production and gene expression in rheumatoid arthritis and its regulation by IL-1 and tumor necrosis factor-alpha. J Immunol 146:3365, 1991.

166. Cook AD, Braine EL, Campbell IK, et al: Blockade of collagen-induced arthritis post-onset by antibody to granulocyte-macrophage colony-stimulating factor (GM-CSF): requirement for GM-CSF in the effector phase of disease. Arthritis Res 3:293, 2001.

167. Koch AE, Kunkel SL, Burrows JC, et al: Synovial tissue macrophage as a source of the chemotactic cytokine IL-8. J Immunol 147:2187, 1991.

168. Koch AE, Kunkel SL, Harlow LA, et al: Enhanced production of monocyte chemoattractant protein-1 in rheumatoid arthritis. J Clin Invest 90:772, 1992.

169. Koch AE, Kunkel SL, Harlow LA, et al: Epithelial neutrophil activating peptide-78: A novel chemotactic cytokine for neutrophils in arthritis. J Clin Invest 94:1012, 1994.

170. Remmers EF, Lafyatis R, Kumkumian GK, et al: Cytokines and growth regulation of synoviocytes from patients with rheumatoid arthritis and rats with streptococcal cell wall arthritis. Growth Factors 2:179, 1990.

171. Remmers EF, Sano H, Lafyatis, et al: Production of platelet derived growth factor B chain (PDGF-B/c-sis) mRNA and immunoreactive PDGF B–like polypeptide by rheumatoid synovium: Coexpression with heparin binding acidic fibroblast growth factor-1. J Rheumatol 18:7, 1991.

172. Yayon A, Klagsbrun M, Esko JD, et al: Cell surface, heparin-like molecules are required for binding of basic fibroblast growth factor to its high affinity receptor. Cell 64:841, 1991.

173. Henderson B, Thompson RC, Hardingham T, Lewthwaite J: Inhibition of interleukin-1-induced synovitis and articular cartilage proteoglycan loss in the rabbit knee by recombinant human interleukin-1 receptor antagonist. Cytokine 3:246, 1991.

174. Malyak M, Swaney RE, Arend WP: Levels of synovial fluid interleukin-1 receptor antagonist in rheumatoid arthritis and other

arthropathies: Potential contribution from synovial fluid neutrophils. Arthritis Rheum 36:781, 1993.

175. Firestein GS, Boyle DL, Yu C, et al: Synovial interleukin-1 receptor antagonist and interleukin-1 balance in rheumatoid arthritis. Arthritis Rheum 37:644, 1994.

176. Fava R, Olsen N, Keski-Oja J, et al: Active and latent forms of transforming growth factor beta activity in synovial effusions. J Exp Med 169:291, 1989.

177. Allen JB, Manthey CL, Hand AR, et al: Rapid onset synovial inflammation and hyperplasia induced by transforming growth factor beta. J Exp Med 171:231, 1990.

178. Song XY, Gu M, Jin WW, et al: Plasmid DNA encoding transforming growth factor-beta1 suppresses chronic disease in a streptococcal cell wall–induced arthritis model. J Clin Invest 101:2615, 1998.

179. Arend WP, Malyak M, Smith MF Jr., et al: Binding of IL-1 alpha, IL-1 beta, and IL-1 receptor antagonist by soluble IL-1 receptors and levels of soluble IL-1 receptors in synovial fluids. J Immunol 153:4766, 1994.

180. Cope AP, Aderka D, Doherty M, et al: Increased levels of soluble tumor necrosis factor receptors in the sera and synovial fluid of patients with rheumatic diseases. Arthritis Rheum 35:1160, 1992.

181. Brennan FM, Gibbons DL, Mitchell T, et al: Enhanced expression of tumor necrosis factor receptor mRNA and protein in mononuclear cells isolated from rheumatoid arthritis synovial joints. Eur J Immunol 22:1907, 1992.

182. Firestein GS, Manning AM: Signal transduction and transcription factors in rheumatic diseases Arthritis Rheum 42:609, 1999.

183. Sioud M, Mellbye O, Forre O: Analysis of the NF-kappa B p65 subunit, Fas antigen, Fas ligand and Bcl-2–related proteins in the synovium of RA and polyarticular JRA. Clin Exp Rheumatol 16:125, 1998.

184. Aupperle K, Bennett B, Han Z, et al: NF-kappaB regulation by I kappa B kinase-2 in rheumatoid arthritis synoviocytes. J Immunol 166:2705, 2001.

185. Miyazawa K, Mori A, Yamamoto K, Okudaira H: Constitutive transcription of the human interleukin-6 gene by rheumatoid synoviocytes: Spontaneous activation of NF-kappaB and CBF1. Am J Pathol 152:793, 1998.

186. Tak PP, Gerlag DM, Aupperle KB, et al: Inhibitor of nuclear factor kappaB kinase beta is a key regulator of synovial inflammation. Arthritis Rheum 44:1897, 2001.

187. Schett G, Tohidast-Akrad M, Smolen JS, et al: Activation, differentiatial localization, and regulation of the stress-activated protein kinases, extracellular signal-regulated kinase, c-JUN N-terminal kinase, and p38 mitogen-activated protein kinase, in synovial tissue and cells in rheumatoid arthritis. Arthritis Rheum 43:2501, 2000.

188. Badger AM, Bradbeer JN, Votta B, et al: Pharmacological profile of SB 203580, a selective inhibitor of cytokine suppressive binding protein/p38 kinase, in animal models of arthritis, bone resorption, endotoxin shock and immune function. J Pharmacol Exp Ther 279:1453, 1996.

189. Han Z, Boyle DL, Chang L, et al: c-Jun N-terminal kinase is required for metalloproteinase expression and joint destruction in inflammatory arthritis. J Clin Invest 108:73, 2001.

190. Han Z, Chang L, Yamanishi Y, et al: Joint damage and inflammation in c-Jun N-terminal kinase 2 knockout mice with passive murine collagen-induced arthritis. Arthritis Rheum 46:818, 2002.

191. Kinne RW, Boehm S, Iftner T, et al: Synovial fibroblast-like cells strongly express Jun-B and C-Fos proto-oncogenes in rheumatoid- and osteoarthritis. Scand J Rheumatol Suppl 101:121, 1995.

192. Han Z, Boyle DL, Manning AM, Firestein GS: AP-1 and NF-kB regulation in rheumatoid arthritis and murine collagen-induced arthritis. Autoimmunity 28:197, 1998.

193. Boyle DL, Han Z, Rutter J, et al: Post-transcriptional regulation of collagenase gene expression in synoviocytes by adenosine receptor stimulation. Arthritis Rheum 40:1772, 1997.

194. Wakisaka S, Suzuki N, Saito N, et al: Possible correction of abnormal rheumatoid arthritis synovial cell function by jun D transfection in vitro. Arthritis Rheum 41:470, 1998.

195. Shiozawa S, Shimizu K, Tanaka K, Hino, K: Studies on the contribution of c-fos/AP-1 to arthritic joint destruction. J Clin Invest 99:1210-1216, 1997.

196. Wang F, Sengupta TK, Zhong Z, Ivashkiv LB: Regulation of the balance of cytokine production and the signal transducer and

activator of transcription (STAT) transcription factor activity by cytokines and inflammatory synovial fluids. J Exp Med 182:1825, 1995.

197. Sengupta TK, Chen A, Zhong Z, et al: Activation of monocyte effector genes and STAT family transcription factors by inflammatory synovial fluid is independent of interferon. J Exp Med 181:1015, 1995.

198. Shouda T, Yoshida T, Hanada T, et al: Induction of the cytokine signal regulator SOCS3/CIS3 as a therapeutic strategy for treating inflammatory arthritis. J Clin Invest 108:1781, 2001.

199. Maurice MM, Nakamura H, van der Voort EAM, et al: Increased expression of thioredoxin in rheumatoid arthritis. Arthritis Rheum 41:S319, 1998.

200. Bashir S, Harris G, Denman MA, et al: Oxidative DNA damage and cellular sensitivity to oxidative stress in human autoimmune diseases. Ann Rheum Dis 52:659, 1993.

201. Sakurai H, Kohsaka H, Liu MF, et al: Nitric oxide production and inducible nitric oxide synthase expression in inflammatory arthritides. J Clin Invest 96:2357, 1995.

202. Farrell AJ, Blake DR, Palmer RM, Moncada S: Increased concentrations of nitrite in synovial fluid and serum samples suggest increased nitric oxide synthesis in rheumatic diseases. Ann Rheum Dis 51:1219, 1992.

203. Salmon M, Scheel-Toellner D, Huissoon AP, et al: Inhibition of T cell apoptosis in the rheumatoid synovium. J Clin Invest 99:439, 1997.

204. Chou CT, Yang JS, Lee MR: Apoptosis in rheumatoid arthritis: Expression of Fas, Fas-L, p53, and Bcl-2 in rheumatoid synovial tissues. J Pathol 193:110, 2001.

205. Catrina AI, Ulfgren AK, Lindblad S, et al: Low levels of apoptosis and high FLIP expression in early rheumatoid arthritis synovium. Ann Rheum Dis 61:934, 2002.

206. Firestein, GS, Yeo M, Zvaifler NJ: Apoptosis in rheumatoid arthritis synovium. J Clin Invest 96:1631, 1995.

207. Matsumoto S, Muller-Ladner U, Gay RE, et al: Ultrastructural demonstration of apoptosis, Fas and Bcl-2 expression of rheumatoid synovial fibroblasts. Rheumatology 23:1345, 1996.

208. Perlman H, Pagliari LJ, Liu H, et al: Rheumatoid arthritis synovial macrophages express the Fas-associated death domain-like interleukin 1beta-converting enzyme-inhibitory protein and are refractory to Fas-mediated apoptosis. Arthritis Rheum 44:21, 2001.

209. Zhang HG, Wang Y, Xie JF, et al: Regulation of tumor necrosis factor alpha-mediated apoptosis of rheumatoid arthritis synovial fibroblasts by the protein kinase Akt. Arthritis Rheum 44:1555, 2001.

210. Kawakami A, Eguchi K, Matsuoka N, et al: Inhibition of Fas antigen-mediated apoptosis of rheumatoid synovial cells in vitro by transforming growth factor beta 1. Arthritis Rheum 39:1267, 1996.

211. Okamoto K, Fujisawa K, Hasunuma T, et al: Selective activation of the JNK/AP-1 pathway in Fas-mediated apoptosis of rheumatoid arthritis synoviocytes. Arthritis Rheum 40:919, 1997.

212. Zhang H, Yang Y, Horton JL, et al: Amelioration of collagen-induced arthritis by CD95 (Apo-1/Fas)-ligand gene transfer. J Clin Invest 100:1951, 1997.

213. Yamanishi Y, Boyle DL, Pinkoski MJ, et al: Regulation of joint destruction and inflammation by p53 in collagen-induced arthritis. Am J Pathol 160:123, 2002.

214. Lafyatis R, Remmers EF, Roberts AB, et al: Anchorage-independent growth of synoviocytes from arthritis and normal joints: Stimulation by exogenous platelet-derived growth factor and inhibition by transforming growth factor-beta and retinoids. J Clin Invest 83:1267, 1989.

215. Imamura F, Aono H, Hasunuma T, et al: Monoclonal expansion of synoviocytes in rheumatoid arthritis. Arthritis Rheum 41:1979, 1998.

216. Firestein GS, Nguyen K, Aupperle K, et al: Apoptosis in rheumatoid arthritis: p53 overexpression in rheumatoid arthritis synovium. Am J Pathol 149:2143, 1996.

217. Tak PP, Smeets TJM, Boyle DL, et al: p53 overexpression in synovial tissue from patients with early and chronic rheumatoid arthritis. Arthritis Rheum 42:948, 1999.

218. Firestein GS, Echeverri F, Yeo M, et al: Somatic mutations in the p53 tumor suppressor gene in rheumatoid arthritis synovium. Proc Natl Acad Sci U S A 94:10895, 1997.

219. Han Z, Boyle DL, Shi Y, et al: Dominant negative p53 mutations in rheumatoid arthritis. Arthritis Rheum 42:1088, 1999.

220. Aupperle KR, Boyle DL, Hendrix M, et al: Regulation of synoviocyte proliferation, apoptosis, and invasiveness by the p53 tumor suppressor gene. Am J Pathol 152:1091, 1998.

221. Tak PP, Zvaifler NJ, Green DR, Firestein GS: Rheumatoid arthritis and p53: how oxidative stress might alter the course of inflammatory diseases. Immunol Today 21:78, 2000.

222. Cannons JL, Karsh J, Birnboim HC, Goldstein R: HPRT⁻ mutant T cells in the peripheral blood and synovial tissue of patients with rheumatoid arthritis. Arthritis Rheum 41:1772, 1998.

223. Cannons JL, Karsh J, Birnboim HC, Goldstein R: HPRT⁻ mutant T cells in the peripheral blood and synovial tissue of patients with rheumatoid arthritis. Arthritis Rheum 41:1772, 1998.

224. Roivainen A, Jalava J, Pirila L, et al: H-ras oncogene point mutations in arthritic synovium. Arthritis Rheum 40:1636, 1997.

225. Sen M, Lauterbach K, ElGabalawy H, et al: Expression and function of wingless and frizzled homologs in rheumatoid arthritis. Proc Natl Acad Sci U S A 97:2791, 2000.

226. Sen M, Chamorro M, Reifert J, et al: Blockade of Wnt-5A/frizzled 5 signaling inhibits rheumatoid synoviocyte activation. Arthritis Rheum 44:772, 2001.

227. Stevens CR, Blake DR, Merry P, et al: A comparative study by morphometry of the microvasculature in normal and rheumatoid synovium. Arthritis Rheum 34:1508, 1991.

228. Wallis WJ, Simkin PA, Nelp WB: Low synovial clearance of iodide provides evidence of hypoperfusion in chronic rheumatoid synovitis. Arthritis Rheum 28:1096, 1985.

229. Dingle JTM, Page-Thomas DP: In vitro studies in human synovial membrane: A metabolic comparison of normal and rheumatoid disease. Br J Exp Pathol 37:318, 1956.

230. Shweiki D, Itin A, Soffer D, Keshet E: Vascular endothelial growth factor induced by hypoxia may mediate hypoxia-initiated angiogenesis. Nature 359:843, 1992.

231. Fava RA, Olsen NJ, Spencer-Green G, et al: Vascular permeability factor/endothelial growth factor (VPF/VEGF): Accumulation and expression in human synovial fluids and rheumatoid synovial tissue. J Exp Med 180:341, 1994.

232. Unemori EN, Ferrara N, Bauer EA, Amento EP: Vascular endothelial growth factor induces interstitial collagenase expression in human endothelial cells. J Cell Physiol 153:557, 1992.

233. Jackson JR, Minton JA, Ho ML, et al: Expression of vascular endothelial growth factor in synovial fibroblasts is induced by hypoxia and interleukin 1beta. Rheumatol 24:1253, 1997.

234. Scott BB, Zaratin PF, Colombo A, et al: Constitutive expression of angiopoietin-1 and -2 and modulation of their expression by inflammatory cytokines in rheumatoid arthritis synovial fibroblasts. J Rheumatol 29:230, 2002.

235. Koch AE, Halloran MM, Haskell CJ, et al: Angiogenesis mediated by soluble forms of E-selectin and vascular cell adhesion molecule-1. Nature 376:517, 1995.

236. Koch AE, Friedman J, Burrows JC, et al: Localization of the angiogenesis inhibitor thrombospondin in human synovial tissues. Pathobiology 61:1, 1993.

237. Peacock DJ, Banquerigo ML, Brahn E: Angiogenesis inhibition suppresses collagen arthritis. J Exp Med 175:1135, 1992.

238. Storgard CM, Stupack DG, Jonczyk A, et al: Decreased angiogenesis and arthritis in rabbits treated with an $\alpha_v\beta_3$ antagonist. J Clin Invest 103:47, 1998.

239. Gerlag DM, Borges E, Tak PP, et al: Suppression of murine collagen-induced arthritis by targeted apoptosis of synovial neovasculature. Arthritis Res 3:357, 2001.

240. Matsuno H, Yudoh K, Uzuki M, et al: Treatment with the angiogenesis inhibitor endostatin: A novel therapy in rheumatoid arthritis. J Rheumatol 29:890, 2002.

241. Lee L, Buckley C, Blades MC, et al: Identification of synovium-specific homing peptides by in vivo phage display selection. Arthritis Rheum 46:2109, 2002.

242. Hale LP, Martin ME, McCollum DE, et al: Immunohistologic analysis of the distribution of cell adhesion molecules within the inflammatory synovial microenvironment. Arthritis Rheum 32:22, 1989.

243. Issekutz TB, Issekutz AC: T lymphocyte migration to arthritic joints and dermal inflammation in the rat: Differing migration patterns and the involvement of VLA-4. Clin Immunol Immunopathol 61:436, 1991.

244. Wahl SM, Allen JB, Hines KL, et al: Synthetic fibronectin peptides suppress arthritis in rats by interrupting leukocyte adhesion and recruitment. J Clin Invest 94:655, 1994.

245. Laffon A, Garcia-Vicuna R, Humbria A, et al: Upregulated expression and function of VLA-4 fibronectin receptors on human activated T cells in rheumatoid arthritis. J Clin Invest 88:546, 1992.

246. Van Dinther-Janssen AC, Pals ST, Scheper RJ, Meijer CJ: Role of the CS1 adhesion motif of fibronectin in T cell adhesion to synovial membrane and peripheral lymph node endothelium. Ann Rheum Dis 52:672, 1993.

247. Elices MJ, Tsai V, Strahl D, et al: Expression and functional significance of alternatively spliced CS1 fibronectin in rheumatoid arthritis microvasculature. J Clin Invest 93:405, 1994.

248. Jorgensen C, Travaglio-Encinoza A, Bologna C: Human mucosal lymphocyte marker expression in synovial fluid lymphocytes of patients with rheumatoid arthritis. J Rheumatol 21:1602, 1994.

249. Koch AE, Burrows JC, Haines GK, et al: Immunolocalization of endothelial and leukocyte adhesion molecules in human rheumatoid and osteoarthritic synovial tissues. Lab Invest 64:313, 1991.

250. Corkill MM, Kirkham BW, Haskard DO, et al: Gold treatment of rheumatoid arthritis decreases synovial expression of the endothelial leukocyte adhesion receptor ELAM-1. J Rheumatol 18:1453, 1991.

251. Jorgensen C, Couret I, Canovas F, et al: Mononuclear cell retention in rheumatoid synovial tissue engrafted in severe combined immunodeficient (SCID) mice is up-regulated by tumour necrosis factor-alpha (TNF-alpha) and mediated through intercellular adhesion molecule-1 (ICAM-1). Clin Exp Immunol 106:20, 1996.

252. Jorgensen C, Couret I, Canovas F, et al: In vivo migration of tonsil lymphocytes in rheumatoid synovial tissue engrafted in SCID mice: Involvement of LFA-1. Autoimmunology 24:179, 1996.

253. Haraoui B, Strand V, Keystone E: Biologic agents in the treatment of rheumatoid arthritis. Curr Pharm Biotechnol 1:217, 2000.

254. Annefeld M: The potential aggressiveness of synovial tissue in rheumatoid arthritis. J Pathol 139:399, 1983.

255. Zvaifler NJ, Tsai V, von Kempis J, et al: Pannocytes: Distinctive cells found in articular cartilage erosions from the joints of patients with rheumatoid arthritis. Am J Pathol 150:1125, 1997.

256. Xue C, Takahashi M, Aono H, et al: Characterization of alternative fibroblast-like cells sharing the properties of fibroblasts and chondrocytes in RA pannus lesions. Arthritis Rheum 38:S344, 1995.

257. Wolfe GC, MacNaul KL, Buechel FF, et al: Differential in vivo expression of collagenase messenger RNA in synovium and cartilage: Quantitative comparison with stromelysin messenger RNA levels in human rheumatoid arthritis and osteoarthritis patients and in two animal models of acute inflammatory arthritis. Arthritis Rheum 36:1540, 1993.

258. Cooke TD, Hurd ER, Jasin HE, et al: Identification of immunoglobulins and complement in rheumatoid articular collagenous tissues. Arthritis Rheum 18:541, 1975.

259. Kuiper S, Joosten LA, Bendele AM, et al: Different roles of tumour necrosis factor alpha and interleukin 1 in murine streptococcal cell wall arthritis. Cytokine 10:690, 1998.

260. Boyle DL, Han Z, Rutter J, et al: Post-transcriptional regulation of collagenase gene expression in synoviocytes by adenosine receptor stimulation. Arthritis Rheum 40:1772, 1997.

261. Yodlowski ML, Hubbard JR, Kispert J, et al: Antibody to interleukin 1 inhibits the cartilage degradative and thymocyte proliferative actions of rheumatoid synovial culture medium. J Rheumatol 17:1600, 1990.

262. Lotz M, Guerne PA: Interleukin-6 induces the synthesis of tissue inhibitor of metalloproteinases-1/erythroid potentiating activity (TIMP-1/EPA). J Biol Chem 266:2017, 1991.

263. Gunther M, Haubeck HD, van de Leur E, et al: Transforming growth factor beta 1 regulates tissue inhibitor of metalloproteinases-1 expression in differentiated human articular chondrocytes. Arthritis Rheum 37:395, 1994.

264. Unemori EN, Hibbs MS, Amento EP: Constitutive expression of a 92-kD gelatinase (type V collagenase) by rheumatoid synovial fibroblasts and its induction in normal human fibroblasts by inflammatory cytokines. J Clin Invest 88:1656, 1991.

265. Mengshol JA, Vincenti MP, Coon CI, et al: Interleukin-1 induction of collagenase 3 (matrix metalloproteinase 13) gene expression in chondrocytes requires p38, c-Jun N-terminal kinase, and nuclear factor kappaB: differential regulation of collagenase 1 and collagenase 3. Arthritis Rheum 43:801, 2000.

266. Firestein GS, Paine MM, Littman BH: Gene expression (collagenase, tissue inhibitor of metalloproteinases, complement, and

HLA-DR) in rheumatoid arthritis and osteoarthritis synovium: Quantitative analysis and effect of intraarticular corticosteroids. Arthritis Rheum 34:1094, 1991.

267. Zvaifler NJ, Boyle D, Firestein GS: Early synovitis: Synoviocytes and mononuclear cells. Semin Arthritis Rheum 23 (Suppl 2):11, 1994.

268. Mudgett JS, Hutchinson NI, Chartrain NA, et al: Susceptibility of stromelysin 1–deficient mice to collagen-induced arthritis and cartilage destruction. Arthritis Rheum 41:110, 1998.

269. Hamada T, Arima N, Shindo M, et al: Suppression of adjuvant arthritis of rats by a novel matrix metalloproteinase-inhibitor. Br J Pharmacol 131:1513, 2000.

270. Muller-Ladner U, Gay RE, Gay S: Cysteine proteinases in arthritis and inflammation. Perspect Drug Discovery Design 6:87, 1996.

271. Lemaire R, Huet G, Zerimech F, et al: Selective induction of the secretion of cathepsins B and L by cytokines in synovial fibro-blast-like cells. Br J Rheumatol 36:735, 1997.

272. Garnero P, Borel O, Byrjalsen I, et al: The collagenolytic activity of cathepsin K is unique among mammalian proteinases. J Biol Chem 273:32,347, 1998.

273. Hou WS, Li W, Keyszer G, et al: Comparison of cathepsins K and S expression within the rheumatoid and osteoarthritis cynovium. Arthritis Rheum 46:663, 2002.

274. Esser RE, Angelo RA, Murphey MD, et al: Cysteine proteinase inhibitors decrease articular cartilage and bone destruction in chronic inflammatory arthritis. Arthritis Rheum 37:236, 1994.

275. Lark MW, Gordy JT, Weidner JR, et al: Cell-mediated catabolism of aggrecan: Evidence that cleavage at the "aggrecanase" site (Glu373-Ala374) is a primary event in proteolysis of the inter-globular domain. J Biol Chem 270:2550, 1995.

276. Tortorella MD, Burn TC, Pratta MA, et al: Purification and cloning of aggrecanase-1: A member of the ADAMTS family of proteins. Science 284:1664, 1999.

277. Lark MW, Bayne EK, Flanagan J, et al: Aggrecan degradation in human cartilage: Evidence for both matrix metalloproteinase and aggrecanase activity in normal, osteoarthritic, and rheuma-toid joints. J Clin Invest 100:93, 1997.

278. Abbink JJ, Kamp AM, Nuijens JH, et al: Proteolytic inactivation of alpha 1-antitrypsin and alpha 1-antichymotrypsin by neu-trophils in arthritic joints. Arthritis Rheum 36:168, 1993.

279. Clark IM, Powell LK, Ramsey S, et al: The measurement of col-lagenase, tissue inhibitor of metalloproteinases (TIMP), and collagenase-TIMP complex in synovial fluids from patients with osteoarthritis and rheumatoid arthritis. Arthritis Rheum 36:372, 1993.

280. Firestein GS, Paine MM, Boyle DL: Mechanisms of methotrexate action in rheumatoid arthritis: Selective decrease in synovial col-lagenase gene expression. Arthritis Rheum 37:193, 1994.

281. Goldring SR, Gravallese EM: Mechanisms of bone loss in inflam-matory arthritis: Diagnosis and therapeutic implications. Arthritis Res 2:33, 2000.

282. Kong YY, Feige U, Sarosi I, et al: Activated T cells regulate bone loss and joint destruction in adjuvant arthritis through osteo-protegerin ligand. Nature 402:304-9, 1999.

283. Pettit AR, Ji H, von Stechow D, et al: TRANCE/RANKL knock-out mice are protected from bone erosion in a serum transfer model of arthritis. Am J Pathol 159:1689, 2001.

284. Feuerherm AJ, Borset M, Seidel C, et al: Elevated levels of osteo-protegerin (OPG) and hepatocytes growth factor (HGF) in rheumatoid arthritis. Scand J Rheumatol 30:229, 2001.

285. Haynes DR, Crotti TN, Loric M, et al: Osteoprotegerin and receptor activator of nuclear factor kappaB ligand (RANKL) regulate osteoclast formation by cells in the human rheumatoid arthritis joint. Rheumatology (Oxford) 40:623, 2001.

286. Kotake S, Udagawa N, Hakoda M, et al: Activated human T cells directly iduce osteoclastogenesis from human monocytes: Possible role of T cells in bone destruction in rheumatoid arthri-tis patients. Arthritis Rheum 44:1003, 2001.

287. Kawahito Y, Kondo M, Tsubouchi Y, et al: 15-deoxy-delta(12,14)-PGJ(2) induces synoviocyte apoptosis and suppresses adjuvant-induced arthritis in rats. J Clin Invest 106:189, 2000.

288. Rossi A, Kapahi P, Natoli G, et al: Anti-inflammatory cyclopen-tenone prostaglandins are direct inhibitors of IkappaB kinase. Nature 403:103, 2000.

289. Siegle I, Klein T, Backman JT, et al: Expression of cyclooxygenase 1 and cyclooxygenase 2 in human synovial tissue: Differential ele-vation of cyclooxygenase 2 in inflammatory joint diseases. Arthritis Rheum 41:122, 1998.

290. Elmgreen J, Haagen N, Ahnfelt-Ronne I: Enhanced capacity for release of leukotriene B_4 by neutrophils in rheumatoid arthritis. Ann Rheum Dis 46:501, 1987.

291. Griffiths RJ, Pettipher ER, Koch K, et al: Leukotriene B4 plays a critical role in the progression of collagen-induced arthritis. Proc Natl Acad Sci U S A 92:517, 1995.

292. Neumann E, Barnum SR, Tarner IH, et al: Local production of complement proteins in rheumatoid arthritis synovium. Arthritis Rheum 46:934, 2002.

293. Pekin TJ Jr, Zvaifler NJ: Hemolytic complement in synovial fluid. J Clin Invest 43:1372, 1964.

294. Sabharwal UK, Vaughan JH, Fong S, et al: Activation of the clas-sical pathway of complement by rheumatoid factors: Assessment by radioimmunoassay for C4. Arthritis Rheum 25:161, 1982.

295. Goodfellow RM, Williams AS, Levin JL, et al: Local therapy with soluble complement receptor 1 (sCR1) suppresses inflammation in rat mono-articular arthritis. Clin Exp Immunol 110:45, 1997.

296. Wang Y, Kristan J, Hao L, et al: A role for complement in anti-body-mediated inflammation: C-5 deficient DBA/1 mice are resistant to collagen-induced arthritis. J Immunol 164:4340, 2000.

297. Hietala MA, Jonsson IM, Tarkowski A, et al: Complement defi-ciency ameliorates collagen-induced arthritis in mice. J Immunol 169:454, 2002.

298. Busso N, Hamilton JS: Extravascular coagulation and plasmino-gen activator/plasmin system in rheumatoid arthritis. Arthritis Rheum 46:2268, 2002.

299. Firestein GS, Zvaifler NJ: How important are T cells in chronic rheumatoid synovitis? II. T cell-independent mechanisms from beginning to end. Arthritis Rheum 46:298, 2002.

66 Clinical Features of Rheumatoid Arthritis

EDWARD D. HARRIS, JR.

First Appearance

Medical historians disagree about the first references to rheumatoid arthritis (RA) in lay and medical writings. Some have concluded that RA developed only recently as a clear-cut entity, whereas others interpret writings of Soranus in the second century as referring to a patient with RA.[1] Sir Alfred Garrod, an astute English clinician and geneticist, first introduced the term *rheumatoid arthritis* in 1876.[2] Storey and colleagues have published an excellent historic review of the subject and have searched records of hospitals in the United Kingdom for descriptions of symmetric inflammatory arthritis.[3] Their evidence suggests that in England, the disease can be traced at least to descriptions by Sydenham in the 1600s. Paleopathologic studies have identified bone erosions consistent with RA in many Native American skeletons dating as far back as 6500 years ago in a circumscribed area of the Mississippi Basin.[4]

The question "When did rheumatoid arthritis first appear?" is not trivial. If its origins are in antiquity, it implies that humans have long had a capacity to react to multiple antigens by developing chronic inflammatory arthritis. In contrast, if RA has afflicted humans for only 300 to 400 years, the implication is that the disease has developed in response to the appearance of a relatively specific environmental agent, probably infectious.

Although the natural course of RA has changed minimally (except for a decreased incidence worldwide) what is changing is the understanding of pathophysiology, the new therapies that have become available, and the costs of these treatments. A 1999 paper demonstrated clearly that in persons with RA, poor and declining function is associated with much higher cumulative costs of care.[5] The correlative argument can be made that the most effective treatments for aggressive disease should be available to patients early in their disease to save on costs years later.

Epidemiology and the Burden of Disease

In past years most investigators accepted a prevalence of RA in most populations of around 1 percent, with an incidence in women twice that in men. This number was based on many studies of population samples[6-10] that varied among the surveys from 0.3 to 1.5 percent. This figure of 1-percent prevalence of RA in most populations may be changing, however, as incidence rates in different decades are studied. The incidence of RA in Rochester, Minnesota, declined 50 percent between 1950 and 1974.[11] The differences between incidence and prevalence are enhanced by realizing that as the population ages, the prevalence of RA may increase or stay the same, even though the incidence stays the same or is decreasing, simply because people with RA are living longer.

The incidence of RA rises dramatically during adulthood; the exception is men in their 40s through 60s. In Olmstead County, Minnesota, this increase in incidence with increasing age continues until age 85, after which the incidence declines.[12] In a 10-year extension of this study, making it a 40-year population-based history of RA, the age- and sex-adjusted incidence per 100,000 population fell from 62 in the 1955 to 1964 decade to 32.7 in the years from 1985 to 1994.[13] The fall was more prominent in women than in men, and the average age at onset of the disease shifted upward. Most intriguing were the cyclic patterns of incidence within decades, suggesting the influence of an environmental (infectious?) factor. One obvious explanation for both the decline in incidence and shift toward an older age at onset is a birth cohort effect, whose greatest impact is early in life.[14]

Throughout the world, there are pockets of ethnic groups that have a much higher incidence of RA. North American Indians are one of these. In one geographic area, for instance, non-Indian populations had an RA prevalence of 1.1 to 0.9 percent between 1986 and 1994, whereas the prevalence in Algonquian Indians in the same region ranged from 2 to 2.1 percent, and the disease onset was 12 years earlier in the Indian population.[15] In Pima Indians, who bear a very high incidence of RA, a decline in incidence has been correlated with a decrease in seropositivity for rheumatoid factor (RF). The highest likelihood of seropositivity was in those born at the turn of the 20th century and has decreased ever since. This is additional supportive evidence for a birth cohort effect.[16] Although newer, more effective therapy for rheumatoid patients has reduced morbidity and disability from the disease, there are still substantial dollar costs for RA. In a panel of 1156 persons with RA in San Francisco followed for up to 15 years, medical care costs for RA averaged $5919/year with an additional $2582 incurred for medical but non-RA reasons.[18] More than half of the costs were for hospitalizations, with some patients bearing costs of more than $85,000/year, as their function declined. In another cohort of 4258 patients with RA followed for 17,085 patient-years, lifetime direct medical-care costs were estimated to be $93,296.[19]

Risk Factors

When one considers that 1) few identical twins have RA, even though it is much more likely that there is concordance for the disease in twins than in the normal population; 2) despite the powerful influence of the "shared epitope" on HLA-DRB chains in predisposing to the severity of disease, this susceptibility cassette is not present in many patients in certain population studies (see Chapter 17); and 3) certain polymorphisms in the genes for T cell receptors or for immunoglobulins[20] are risk factors for RA, we must conclude that a predisposition to RA is multifactorial. A reasonable hypothesis is that all of the population would be susceptible to developing inflammatory synovitis caused by an environmental agent, but whether this is self limiting or goes on to persistent disease depends on genetic factors regulating antigen presentation, T and B cell reactivity, and cytokine profiles.[21] The National Institutes of Health (NIH) is sponsoring a consortium of medical centers that is collecting the genetic material of sibling pairs with RA to search for additional genes that can be linked with phenotypes of the disease (narac@hshs.edu). Initial data from this study reported results of a genome-wide screen of multiplex families with RA gathered in the United States. Using microsatellite markers, it was shown that there was a significant overlap of allele sharing between RA and other immune diseases such as systemic lupus erythematosus (SLE), inflammatory bowel disease, multiple sclerosis (MS), and ankylosing spondylitis.[22]

RHEUMATOID FACTOR AND ANTICYCLIC CITRULLINATED PEPTIDE ANTIBODIES

Since 1948, when the studies of Rose and colleagues[23] confirmed the findings of Waaler linking a factor in sera of patients with RA to agglutination of normal and sensitized sheep red blood cells,[24] the presence or absence of RF in serum has occupied the attention of epidemiologists in this field. RF is found more frequently (in 3 to 5 percent) than is RA in population studies; in the general population, the prevalence of seropositivity is approximately equal between men and women. As shown in Table 66–1, many pathologic states—particularly those associated with chronic infection—are associated with positive tests for RF. It has been estimated that the risk of morbidity or future disease associated with seropositivity in an otherwise healthy individual is less than 5 percent.[25]

Citrulline is formed by deimination of the amino acid arginine. Antibodies directed against citrullinated peptides have been found in serum of many patients with RA. Recombinant fillagrin protein deiminated in vitro appears to be a particularly useful substrate to detect these autoantibodies. Sensitivities of this test in clinically diagnosed rheumatoid patients is in the range of 70 percent, and specificities as high as 98 percent have been reported.[26] The measurement of antibodies against citrullinated peptides must be tested head-to-head against assays for RF to determine which of the two is more likely to provide early diagnosis of active, persistent, and erosive arthritis.

TABLE 66–1 • DISEASES COMMONLY ASSOCIATED WITH RHEUMATOID FACTOR

Category	Diseases
Rheumatic diseases	Rheumatoid arthritis, systemic lupus erythematosus, scleroderma, mixed connective tissue diseases, Sjögren's syndrome
Viral infections	Acquired immunodeficiency syndrome, mononucleosis, hepatitis, influenza, and many others; after vaccination (may yield falsely elevated titers of antiviral antibodies)
Parasitic infections	Trypanosomiasis, kala-azar, malaria, schistosomiasis, filariasis, and others
Chronic bacterial infections	Tuberculosis, leprosy, yaws, syphilis, brucellosis, subacute bacterial endocarditis, salmonellosis
Neoplasms	After irradiation or chemotherapy
Other hyperglobulinemic states	Hypergammaglobulinemic purpura, cryoglobulinemia, chronic liver disease, sarcoid, other chronic pulmonary diseases

From Carson DA: Rheumatoid factor. *In* Kelley WN, Harris ED Jr, Ruddy S, Sledge CB (eds): Textbook of Rheumatology, 4th ed. Vol 1. Philadelphia, WB Saunders, 1993, p 155.

TWIN STUDIES AND OTHER GENETIC FACTORS

After controlling for age and gender, there remains an eightfold increased relative risk for a monozygotic twin to develop RA if the other twin is affected.[27,28] For a dizygotic twin, the relative risk to the unaffected twin is estimated to range from 2 to 3.4. That having been said, concordance for the disease is about 30 percent in monozygotic twins,[28] a fact that attests to the powerful role of environmental factors in development.

It is estimated that one third to one half of the genetic influence for concordance in twins is accounted for by polymorphisms for HLA-DRB chains coded within major histocompatibility complex (MHC) genes[29]; this is reviewed in Chapter 17. However, increasingly detailed studies indicate that in addition to susceptibility-associated genes, protection-associated alleles can be found among HLA class II genes and that loci outside DR/DQ may contribute to development of RA.[30] In a study of identical twins from Manchester, England, it was demonstrated that in the absence of the "shared epitope" on HLA-DRB chains, concordance for RA is rare and that homozygosity for the shared epitope is the most important factor in determining concordance for RA.[31] Only HLA-DRB1*0404 may be associated with susceptibility to RA, whereas other shared epitope–bearing alleles are likely to be involved with disease progression.[32] Tempering the focus on HLA-DRB1 alleles is the information from a study of 777 rheumatoid patients in whom the shared epitope (SE) was associated with a younger age at symptom onset and increased pain, swelling, and deformity of RA in men, but not in women.[33] The relative risk ratio for developing RA for first-degree relatives of a person with RA is much less than that for twins and is estimated to be no more than 1.6.[34] In summary, certain genetic factors (e.g., the sequences of amino acids in HLA-DRB chains) may be necessary but are not sufficient to result in the expression of RA.

SEX AND THE REPRODUCTIVE CYCLE

It is assumed that the link for the higher incidence of RA among women is related to sex hormones. Estrogens have a generally stimulatory effect on the immune system, and this may be a factor in the increased female-to-male ratio. The published data on the relationships of sex hormones (including dehydroepiandrosterone sulfate, testosterone, and estradiol) have been extensively reviewed, but no unifying or convincing mechanism is available to explain the differences between the sexes in susceptibility to this disease.[35] Another relationship is that RA exhibits a lower penetrance in men; in one series 49 percent of affected men carried two disease-associated HLA-DR alleles, in contrast to only 29 percent of the women.[36] In the same population, men were more likely to have erosive disease, although joint surgery (particularly of the hands and feet) was performed more frequently in women than in men. Nodules and rheumatoid lung were typical manifestations in men, whereas women typically developed the sicca syndrome.

The relative risks of developing RA in women appear to fluctuate with different stages of the reproductive cycle through their lives, from menarche to menopause.

Puberty Until Pregnancy

There are several publications demonstrating that oral contraceptives may protect women from developing more severe disease.[37,38] These are supported by another study of women with RA and at least one child,[39] and are reviewed in Chapter 65.

Pregnancy

At least 75 percent of women with RA find substantial relief of symptoms during pregnancy, although in the postpartum state the disease activity often recurs. The remission of RA during pregnancy has been linked to differences in maternal-fetal HLA antigens, although there is still some controversy. Disparities in the mother and fetus for HLA-DRB1, -DQA, and -DQB were found in 26 of 34 pregnancies (76 percent) in women whose RA went into remission or improved during pregnancy, against a 25 percent disparity (3 of 12) in those whose RA remained active.[40]

Along with the benefit conferred on those already with the disease, there appears to be a slight reduction in the risk of developing RA during pregnancy but an increased risk of developing RA during the first 3 months or more after delivery.[41,42] Interestingly, multiparity may be a risk factor for severe disease. Having more than three children has been shown in one study to increase the risk of developing severe RA by a factor of close to five.[39] No difference in adverse outcomes of pregnancy (including spontaneous abortions) has been found in women who later developed arthritis.[43]

OTHER ENVIRONMENTAL RISK FACTORS

Education Level

RA shares with several other chronic diseases the fact that there is an increased mortality and morbidity from RA in patients, particularly women, who have had less formal education.[44] RA is one of several chronic diseases in which the patient can have a major role in improving the outcome through self-help programs. Not intuitive, but interesting, are data showing that young women in the Netherlands with RA who had low and medium levels of education had more initial joint erosions and poorer functional scores compared with those who had higher levels of education, even though the symptoms had been present for the same length of time in both groups.[45] Callahan and Pincus make a good argument for reassessing health policy on the basis of associations between formal educational levels and clinical health status when considering RA.[46]

Tobacco Smoking and Other Habits

In a survey of 377,841 women who were health professionals, the duration of smoking was associated with significantly increased risk of both RA and seropositive RA using multivariate analyses controlling for age, education, reproductive history, and race.[47] In women, smoking was associated with the most severe disease in patients who carried the glutathione S-transferase M1-null polymorphism, which is also associated with RF production in smokers.[48] One study has generated hope for current younger smokers; in a large prospective study of women in Iowa aged 55 to 69, it was found that women who had quit smoking more than 10 years before entry to the study did not share the increased risk of developing RA with their smoking peers.[49] Additional data generated in the same study showed that decaffeinated coffee intake is independently and positively associated with RA onset, whereas there was an inverse association with disease onset in tea drinkers.[50]

Coexisting Gout

Still inadequately understood is the apparent negative association between gout and RA. It has been estimated that there should be almost 150 times more cases of coexistent RA and gout than have been reported. In one study, 12 of 160 seropositive RA patients were found to have hyperuricemia. Eleven of the 12 had quiet disease; indeed, the onset of hyperuricemia and the improvement in RA appeared to coincide. In patients with fluctuations in uric acid levels, there was a statistically significant correlation between an increase in serum uric acid concentration and improvement in disease activity.[51] Thus, the hypothesis stands: The hyperuricemic state may be anti-inflammatory.

Silicone Breast Implants

Large population studies have demonstrated no increase in the risk of developing RA in those who have had silicone breast implants.[52] In a prospective study generated in 1985 and reported in 1998, a group of reconstructive surgeons found no statistic increase in clinical or laboratory test findings among nonimplanted women, women with saline implants, or those with polysiloxane gel implants.[53]

Diet

Although there are indications that certain diets (e.g., those that replace animal fats with fish oils) may alleviate inflammation in patients with already existing RA (see Chapter 54), there are no solid data to implicate any diet or food additive as a potential cause of RA or in its prevention.

Atopy

With the realization that an imbalance between T cells producing interferon-γ (IFN-γ) and those producing interleukin-4 (IL-4) may be important in RA (see Chapter 65), population studies of coexisting manifestation of atopy and RA have been done. In a Japanese study, atopy (T helper type 2 [Th2] cell driven) was negatively correlated with skin test positivity to mycobacterial antigens (T helper type 1 [Th1] cell driven).[54] In a study from Europe, the prevalence of hay fever was lower in RA patients (4 percent) than in non-RA patients (8 percent), yielding a relative risk for RA patients to develop hay fever of 0.48 percent. Those patients with RA who had hay fever had lower indices of disease activity than those without hay fever. There was a lower IFN-γ–to–IL-4 ratio in blood in the RA patients with hay fever.[55] Two inferences from these data are possible: 1) If it is accurate that atopy is increasing in incidence in developed countries, this could be reflected in the decreased incidence of RA described in some subpopulations; and 2) immune deviation from Th1 to Th2 could be a valid therapeutic goal for RA.[17]

Other Predisposing Factors

Much more diffuse, subjective, and difficult to study are possible precipitating factors of arthritis in the susceptible host. Trauma, including surgery, is a prelude to arthritis that is often identified by patients in retrospect. Other stimuli, including infections, vaccine inoculations, and emotional trauma, have been implicated by many patients as causes of their problems. The increased awareness of the effects of the central nervous system on inflammation in joints makes it essential for physicians to be aware of these "nonscientific" associations and to be sensitive to patients' concerns about them.

▌ Clinical Syndromes of Early Rheumatoid Arthritis

In the Northern Hemisphere, the onset of RA is more frequent in winter than in summer. In several series, the onset of RA from October to March in the Northern Hemisphere was found to be twice as frequent as in the other 6 months.[56] Data suggest that the appearance of

RF may be more likely to precede symptoms of arthritis in patients than was previously recognized. In 30 patients whose frozen sera were available from a time before symptoms of RA began, half had a positive latex fixation test,[57] and many more of these were men than women.

PATTERNS OF ONSET

Insidious Onset

RA usually has an insidious, slow onset over weeks to months. Fifty-five to 65 percent of cases begin this way.[58] The initial symptoms may be systemic or articular. In some individuals, fatigue, malaise, puffy hands, or diffuse musculoskeletal pain may be the first nonspecific complaints, with joints becoming involved later. Involvement of tendon sheaths early in the process can focus attention on periarticular structures. In retrospect, the patient often can identify one joint that was involved first, quickly followed by others. Asymmetric presentations (often with more symmetry developing later in the course of disease) are not unusual. The reason for the symmetry of joint involvement may be related to the bilateral release of neuropeptides (e.g., substance P) at terminal nerve endings in joints.

Morning stiffness can appear even before pain and is related to the accumulation of edema fluid within inflamed tissues during sleep. The morning stiffness dissipates as edema and products of inflammation are absorbed by lymphatics and venules and returned to the circulation by motion accompanying the use of muscles and joints. To be specific for joint inflammation, morning stiffness, (e.g., "difficulty moving around") should persist for at least 30 to 45 minutes before disappearing.

It is rare for symptoms to remit completely in one set of joints while developing in another. This quality of arthritis sets RA apart from rheumatic fever, in which a true migratory pattern of arthritis is common. A subtle, early change in RA is the development of muscle atrophy around affected joints. This diminishes efficiency and strength. As a result, weakness develops that can be out of proportion to pain. Opening doors, climbing stairs, and doing repetitive work rapidly become more demanding. A low-grade fever without chills is rarely present. Depression and both focused and nonspecific anxiety accentuate symptoms. A small but significant weight loss is common and reflects the catabolic effects of cytokines and an associated anorexia.

Acute or Intermediate Onset

Eight to 15 percent of patients have an acute onset of symptoms that peak within a few days. Rarely, a patient can pinpoint the onset of symptoms to a specific time or activity, such as opening a door or driving a golf ball. Symptoms mount, with pain developing in other joints, often in a less-symmetric pattern than in patients who have an insidious onset. Diagnosis of acute-onset RA is difficult to make, and sepsis or vasculitis must be ruled out. Fever, suggesting an infectious process, can be a prominent sign. Fifteen to 20 percent of patients have an intermediate type of onset, in which symptoms develop over days or weeks. Systemic complaints are more noticeable than in the insidious type of onset.

Joint Involvement

The joints most commonly involved first in RA are the metacarpophalangeal (MCP) joints, proximal interphalangeal (PIP) joints, metatarsophalangeal joints, and wrists.[59] Larger joints generally become symptomatic after small joints. It is likely that synovitis in large joints remains asymptomatic for a longer time than in smaller ones. One anatomic study correlated the area, in square centimeters, of synovial membrane with that of hyaline cartilage in each joint. The joints with the highest ratio of synovium to articular cartilage correlated positively with the joints most frequently involved in the disease.[60] (Table 66–2)

UNUSUAL PATTERNS OF DISEASE

Adult-Onset Still's Disease

Significant fever present at the onset of definite RA in adults is unusual. Later in the course, if vasculitis or serositis is present, or if there are intense exacerbations of disease, it is more common. Adult Still's disease, in contrast, usually presents with fever. Adult Still's disease was first described in 14 patients by Bywaters.[61] Women and men are affected equally. It usually appears during the third or fourth decade of life. Serologic studies (RF and antinuclear antibody) are negative, and patients do not have subcutaneous nodules. Most are febrile, and fevers can develop before arthritis. Fever patterns in these patients are often quotidian (i.e., reaching normal levels at least once each day). Occasionally, evanescent salmon-colored or pink macules appear on the trunk and extremities that become more prominent when patients are febrile. The cervical spine is involved, and loss of neck motion may be striking. Pericarditis, pleural effusions, abnormal liver function tests consistent with hepatitis, and severe abdominal pain can be present and may confound attempts at diagnosis. Unlike active SLE with nephritis, the serum complement level is normal or high. Serum ferritin levels can be enormously elevated, well beyond those expected when compared with other acute-phase reactants in the same individual.[62] Levels in serum as high as 30,000 ng/ml have been reported in some with highly active disease, and when levels are higher than 10,000 ng/ml, they can incline physicians strongly in the direction of adult Still's disease as the diagnosis. It has been reported that T cell receptor $\gamma\delta^+$ T cells in peripheral blood are significantly increased in active phases of adult-onset Still's disease.[63]

The diagnosis of adult-onset Still's disease still remains one of exclusion, despite the unusually elevated ferritin levels in serum. Systemic infection, malignancy (e.g., lymphoma), and diffuse vasculitis are usually entertained as diagnoses, searched for, and then discarded before a diagnosis of adult-onset Still's disease is made.

Yamaguchi and associates have developed criteria for establishing the diagnosis of adult Still's disease that, in numerous series, have more than 90-percent sensitivity[64] (Table 66–3). After excluding other diseases, adult Still's should be considered if five criteria (more than two being major ones) are met. It is not known yet whether adding hyperferritinemia would increase the specificity of diagnosis.

What happens to patients with a diagnosis of adult-onset Still's disease? In one series, 11 patients (all of whom were Caucasian women), followed for a mean of 20.2 years after disease onset, had the following characteristics[65]:

- Ten had a polycyclic pattern (characterized by remissions and exacerbations).
- Patterns of exacerbations were similar to, but less severe than, the original presentations.
- Loss of wrist extension was the most common clinical abnormality, and carpal ankylosis was present in 10 patients.
- Five of 11 patients had distal interphalangeal (DIP) joint involvement.
- Biopsy of the characteristic skin rash of Still's disease showed perivascular infiltrate of neutrophils in the superficial dermis.

TABLE 66–2 • DISTRIBUTION OF JOINTS INVOLVED IN ATTACKS BASED UPON A CUMULATIVE EXPERIENCE WITH 227 PATIENTS

Joint Involvement	Mean % of Patients	Range of % of Patients
MCP, PIP	91	74-100
Wrists	78	54-82
Knees	64	41-94
Shoulders	65	33-75
Ankles	50	10-67
Feet	43	15-73
Elbows	38	13-60
Hips	17	0-40
Temporomandibular	8	0-28
Spine	4	0-11
Sternoclavicular	2	0-6
Para-articular sites	27	20-29

Abbreviations: MCP, Metacarpophalangeal; PIP, proximal interphalangeal. Modified from Guerne P-A, Weisman MH: Palindromic rheumatism: part of or apart from the spectrum of rheumatoid arthritis. Am J Med 16:451-460, 1992. Copyright 1992, with permission from Excerpta Medica, Inc.

TABLE 66–3 • CRITERIA FOR DIAGNOSIS OF STILL'S DISEASE

Major Criteria	Minor Criteria
Temperature of >39°C for >1 wk	Sore throat
Leukocytosis >10,000/mm³ with >80% PMNs	Lymph node enlargement
Typical rash	Splenomegaly
Arthralgias >2 wk	Liver dysfunction (high AST/ALT)
	Negative ANA, RF

Abbreviations: ALT, alanine transaminase; ANA, antinuclear antibody; AST, aspartate transaminase; PMN, polymorphonuclear leukocyte; RF, rheumatoid factor.

In another group, 20 percent showed significant functional deterioration from erosive joint disease.[66] Functional class III/IV (Steinbrocker's classification) was usually related to hip disease. The overall long-term prognosis of adult-onset Still's disease is good for systemic manifestations, but less so for articular disease. The incidence of amyloidosis may be as high as 30 percent within 10 years of onset of the illness, perhaps reflecting the sustained high titers of acute-phase reactants found in this disease.

Therapy must be aggressive. Full doses of aspirin or nonsteroidal anti-inflammatory drugs (NSAIDs) should be prescribed soon after diagnosis. Oral glucocorticoids are often needed to control systemic symptoms. It is reasonable to prescribe weekly methotrexate (MTX) to help control the inflammation and serve as a steroid-sparing drug. Because of the high likelihood that this is an example of a cytokine-driven disease, use of etanercept or infliximab to neutralize tumor necrosis factor-α (TNF-α) has been used and proved effective.

Palindromic Pattern of Onset

Palindromic rheumatism was described by Hench and Rosenberg in 1942.[67] Pain usually begins in one joint or in periarticular tissues; symptoms worsen for several hours to a few days and are associated with swelling and erythema. Then, in reverse sequence, symptoms resolve, leaving no residua. Joints involved in a series of 227 patients are listed in Table 66–4. An intercritical period, similar to that of gout, is asymptomatic. Up to half of patients with palindromic rheumatism go on to develop RA, particularly those with HLA-DR4. It is significant that in a compilation of 653 patients from nine series, only 15 percent became asymptomatic after at least 5 years with a palindromic syndrome[68] (Table 66–4). In the remainder, multiple joints became involved, swelling did not subside completely between attacks, and tests for RF became positive. Neither the characteristics of joint fluid nor the pathologic findings of synovial biopsies allow the prediction that RA will evolve from palindromic rheumatism,[69] although in the future, it will be interesting to measure anticyclic citrullinated peptide antibodies in these individuals. Those who do not develop RA rarely have constitutional symptoms, and the involved joints have no erosions because the synovitis does not become chronic. Of 51 patients with palindromic rheumatism, 41 experienced marked improvement in frequency and duration of attacks during treatment with antimalarials.[70]

Effect of Age on Onset

RA developing in older persons (65 years of age and older) often presents as stiffness, limb girdle pain, and diffuse boggy swelling of the hands, wrists, and forearms. A clinical onset that mimics polymyalgia rheumatica is also common. Those with the onset at 60 years of age or older are less likely to have subcutaneous nodules or RF at the onset of disease, despite the high prevalence of RF in the general population in this age-group. In general, elderly individuals who develop RA tend to have a more benign course than younger patients; there is a lower frequency of positive tests for RF, but there is a strong association with HLA-DR4. The onset is slow, but the stiffness is often incapacitating.

Rheumatoid Arthritis and Paralysis: Asymmetric Disease

Being relatively common, RA is likely to occur with many other types of chronic disease. A striking asymmetry or even unilateral involvement has been described in patients with poliomyelitis, meningioma, encephalitis, neurovascular syphilis, strokes, and cerebral palsy.[71] Joints are spared on the paralyzed side, and the degree of protection demonstrates a rough correlation with the extent of paralysis. The protective effect on the affected side is less if a neurologic deficit develops in a patient who already has RA.

TABLE 66–4 • EVOLUTION OF PATIENTS WITH PALINDROMIC RHEUMATISM IN NINE SERIES TOTALING 653 PATIENTS*

Series of Patients	Number of Cases	Remission or Cure (%)	Persistent PR (%)	PR-RA (%)	Other Diseases (%)
1	34	15	85	0	0
2	140	8	52	36	4
3	179	10	47	38	5
4	39	0	56	44	0
5	70	24	34	30	12
6	38	8	66	15	11
7	43	23	23	49	5
8	50	0	46	54	0
9	60	43	21	35	2
Total or average	653	15	48	33	4

*In each series, the number of patients undergoing a remission or a cure, remaining palindromic, evolving toward rheumatoid arthritis (PR-RA), or developing another disease is expressed as a percentage.

Abbreviations: PR, Palindromic rheumatism; RA, rheumatoid arthritis.

Modified from Guerne P-A, Weisman MH: Palindromic rheumatism: part of or apart from the spectrum of rheumatoid arthritis. Am J Med 16:451-460, 1992. Copyright 1992, with permission from Excerpta Medica, Inc.

Arthritis Robustus

Arthritis robustus is not so much an unusual presentation of disease as an unusual reaction of patients to the disease.[72] Men dominate this group. Their disease is characterized by proliferative synovitis that appears to cause little pain and even less disability. Patients are athletic and invariably keep working (often at physical labor). Periarticular osteopenia is unusual, whereas new bone proliferation at joint margins near significant erosions of bone and cartilage are common. Bulky subcutaneous nodules develop. Subchondral cysts also develop, presumably from the excessive pressure developed from synovial fluid within a thick joint capsule during muscular effort.

■ Course and Complications of Established Rheumatoid Arthritis

INVOLVEMENT OF SPECIFIC JOINTS: EFFECTS OF DISEASE ON FORM AND FUNCTION

The effects of rheumatoid synovitis on joints are a complex function of the intensity of the underlying disease, its chronicity, and the stress put on individual joints by the patient. A majority of the well-documented observations of specific joint involvement and of complications of the disease were reported in the decades before 1980. Since then, there have been refinements on these observations, but few new data. A full bibliography for this section can be found on the CD-ROM for this edition. Despite the advances in understanding the pathophysiology of RA, including delineations of the cellular and enzymatic pathways that destroy joints, it must be emphasized that guidelines for the practicing physician—so that in an individual patient the probability that he or she will go on to develop erosive disease and therefore needs aggressive treatment can be determined—are only in early stages of development.[73] Therefore, in the following discussion of the patterns of involvement of individual joints, no attempt to estimate the time of appearance of disease from onset of disease is made.

Cervical Spine

Unlike other nonsynovial joints, such as the manubriosternal joint or symphysis pubis, the diskovertebral joints in the cervical spine often manifest osteochondral destruction in RA, and on lateral radiographs may be found to be narrowed (see Chapter 51). There is significant pain, but passive range of motion in the absence of muscle spasm may be normal. There are two possible mechanisms for this process: 1) extension of the inflammatory process from adjacent neurocentral joints (the joints of Luschka), which are lined by synovium, into the diskovertebral area; and 2) chronic cervical instability initiated by apophyseal joint destruction leading to vertebral malalignment or subluxation. This may produce microfractures of the vertebral end plates, disk herniation, and degeneration of disk cartilage.

The atlantoaxial joint is prone to subluxation in several directions:

1. The atlas can move anteriorly on the axis (most common). This results from laxity of the ligaments induced by proliferative synovial tissue developing in adjacent synovial bursa or from fracture or erosion of the odontoid process.
2. The atlas can move posteriorly on the axis. This can occur only if the odontoid peg has been fractured from the axis or destroyed.
3. The atlas can sublux vertically in relation to the axis (least common). This results from destruction of the lateral atlantoaxial joints or of bone around the foramen magnum. It is apparent now that vertical (superior) migration of the odontoid can develop from unattended anterior or posterior subluxation.

The earliest and most common symptom of cervical subluxation is pain radiating up into the occiput. Two other serious, but less common, clinical patterns are as follows:

1. Slowly progressive spastic quadriparesis, frequently with painless sensory loss in the hands
2. Transient episodes of medullary dysfunction associated with vertical penetration of the dens and probable vertebral artery compression; paresthesias in the shoulders or arms may occur during movement of the head

Physical findings suggestive of atlantoaxial subluxation include a loss of occipitocervical lordosis, resistance to passive spine motion, and abnormal protrusion of the axial arch felt by the examining finger on the posterior pharyngeal wall. Radiographic views (lateral, with the neck in flexion) reveal more than 3 mm of separation between the odontoid peg and the axial arch. In symptomatic patients, the films in flexion should be taken only after radiographs (including an open-mouth posteroanterior view) have ruled out an odontoid fracture or severe atlantoaxial subluxation. Studies have indicated that computed tomography (CT) is useful for demonstrating spinal cord compression by a loss of posterior subarachnoid space in patients with C1 to C2 subluxation. Magnetic resonance imaging (MRI) has proved particularly valuable in determining pathologic anatomy in this syndrome.[108]

Neurologic symptoms often have little relationship to the degree of subluxation and may be related to individual variations in the diameter of the spinal canal. Symptoms of spinal cord compression that demand intervention include:

- A sensation of the head falling forward on flexion of the cervical spine
- Changes in the level of consciousness
- "Drop" attacks
- A loss of sphincter control
- Dysphagia, vertigo, convulsions, hemiplegia, dysarthria, or nystagmus
- Peripheral paresthesias without evidence of peripheral nerve disease or compression

Some of these symptoms may be related to compression of the vertebral arteries, which must wind through foramina in the transverse processes of C1 and C2, rather than to compression of the spinal cord.

The progression of peripheral joint erosions parallels cervical spine disease in RA. The two coincide in severity and timing; the development of cervical subluxation is more likely in patients with erosion of the hands and feet. In a series of 113 patients with RA referred for hip or knee arthroplasty, 61 percent had roentgenographic evidence of cervical spine instability.[75]

Is mortality increased in patients with atlantoaxial subluxation? Neurologic signs do not inevitably develop in patients with large subluxations. On the other hand, when signs of cervical cord compression do appear, myelopathy progresses rapidly, and 50 percent of these patients die within a year.[76] These patients are at risk from even small falls, whiplash injuries, and general anesthesia with intubation. Cervical collars should be prescribed for stability. Operative stabilization may be considered if symptoms are progressive.

Some data support the hypothesis that early C1 to C2 fusion for atlantoaxial subluxation before the development of superior migration of the odontoid decreases the risk of further progression of cervical spine instability.[77] However, the incidence of sustained neurologic deterioration related to surgery may be as high as 6 percent, and this emphasizes the importance of a skilled surgical team and the careful assessment of each patient.

Vertical atlantoaxial subluxation is important and may follow anterior or posterior subluxation. Symptoms associated with this collapse of the lateral support system of the atlas occur in patients with severe erosive disease. Neurologic findings have included decreased sensation in the distribution of cranial nerve V, sensory loss in the C2 area, nystagmus, and pyramidal lesions.

Thoracic, Lumbar, and Sacral Spine

The thoracic, lumbar, and sacral portions of the spine usually are spared in RA. The exceptions are the apophyseal joints; rarely, synovial cysts at the apophyseal joint can impinge as an epidural mass on the spinal cord, causing pain, neurologic deficits, or both.

Temporomandibular Joint

The temporomandibular joint (TMJ) is commonly involved in RA. Histories reveal that 55 percent of patients have jaw symptoms at some time during the course of their disease. Radiographic examination reveals structural alterations in 78 percent of the joints examined. An overbite may develop as the mandibular condyle and the corresponding surface of the temporal bone, the eminentia articularis, are eroded. Physical examination of the rheumatoid patient should include palpation of the TMJ for tenderness and auscultation for crepitus. Occasionally, patients have acute pain and an inability to close the mouth, necessitating intra-articular glucocorticoid therapy to suppress the acute process.

It is important to remember that TMJ abnormalities are very common in nonrheumatoid populations. The only specific findings for RA in the TMJ are erosions and cysts of the mandibular condyle detected by CT or MRI. There is no correlation between clinical and CT findings of the TMJ in RA.[78]

Cricoarytenoid Joints

The cricoarytenoid joints are small diarthrodial joints with an important function: They rotate with the vocal cords as they abduct and adduct to vary the pitch and tone of the voice. Careful histories may reveal hoarseness in up to 30 percent of rheumatoid patients. This is not disabling in itself, but there is a danger that the cricoarytenoid joints may become inflamed and immobilized, with the vocal cords adducted to the midline, causing inspiratory stridor. Autopsy examinations have demonstrated cricoarytenoid arthritis in almost half the patients with RA, suggesting that much significant disease of the larynx may be asymptomatic. This is borne out by the finding that although CT scans detected laryngeal abnormalities in 54 percent of patients with moderately severe RA, no symptoms suggested that these abnormalities would be found.[79] In contrast, findings with indirect laryngoscopy, which detected mucosal and gross functional abnormalities (including rheumatoid nodules), were abnormal in 32 percent of the same patients and correlated with symptoms of sore throat and difficult inspiration. It follows that the latter examination should be obtained in symptomatic rheumatoid patients. Asymptomatic cricoarytenoid synovitis may occasionally lead to aspiration of pharyngeal contents, particularly at night.

Ossicles of the Ear

Many rheumatoid patients experience a decrease in hearing. In general, this has been ascribed to salicylate toxicity, and it is believed to be reversible when the drug is discontinued. On the other hand, conductive hearing loss in patients not taking salicylates was reported by Copeman.[80] Studies using otoadmittance measurements have been carried out in patients with RA in an attempt to determine whether the interossicle joints were involved.[81] The data showed that 38 percent of "rheumatoid ears" and only 8 percent of controls demonstrated a pattern characteristic of increased flaccidity of a clinically normal tympanic membrane. This is consistent with erosions and shortening of the ossicles produced by the erosive synovitis, not with ankylosis.

Sternoclavicular and Manubriosternal Joints

Sternoclavicular and manubriosternal joints, both possessing synovium and a large cartilaginous disk, are often involved in RA. Because of their relative immobility, there are few symptoms. However, patients occasionally complain of experiencing pain in sternoclavicular joints while lying on their sides in bed. When symptoms do occur, the physician must be concerned about superimposed sepsis. CT or MRI is useful for careful delineation of the sternoclavicular joint. Manubriosternal involvement is almost never clinically important, although by tomographic criteria it is common in RA.

Shoulder

RA of the shoulder not only affects synovium within the glenohumeral joint but also involves the distal third of the clavicle, various bursae and the rotator cuff, and multiple muscles around the neck and chest wall. Involvement of the rotator cuff in RA has been recognized as a principal cause of morbidity. The function of the rotator cuff is to stabilize the humeral head in the glenoid. Weakness of the cuff results in superior subluxation. Rotator cuff tears or insufficiency from other causes can be demonstrated by shoulder arthrography or MRI. In a series of 200 consecutive patients with RA studied by arthrography, 21 percent had rotator cuff tears and an additional 24 percent had evidence of frayed tendons.[82] One likely mechanism behind tears is that the rotator cuff tendon insertion into the greater tuberosity is vulnerable to erosion by the proliferative synovitis that develops there. Previous injury and aging may predispose to the development of tears. Sudden tears may be accompanied by pain and inflammation so great as to suggest sepsis.

Standard radiographic examinations of the shoulder in RA reveal erosions and superior subluxation. Arthrograms, in addition to showing tears of the rotator cuff, can demonstrate diffuse nodular filling defects, irregular capsular attachment, bursal filling defects, adhesive capsulitis, and dilation of the biceps tendon sheath (perhaps unique to RA).[83] High-resolution CT or MRI may provide much of this information without invasive techniques.

Marked soft tissue swelling of the anterolateral aspect of the shoulders in RA may be caused by chronic subacromial bursitis rather than by glenohumeral joint effusions. In contrast to rotator cuff tears, bursal swelling is not necessarily associated with a decreased range of motion or pain. Synovial proliferation within the subdeltoid bursa may explain the resorption of the undersurface of the distal clavicle seen in this disease. Rarely, the shoulder joint may rupture, with symptoms resembling those of obstruction of venous return from the arm.[84]

Elbow

Severe pain in the elbow, perhaps because it is a stable hinge joint, is rarely manifest in RA. Nevertheless, involvement of the elbow is common, and if lateral stability at the elbow is lost as the disease progresses, disability can be severe.

The frequency of elbow involvement varies from 20 to 65 percent, depending on the severity of disease in the patient populations studied. One of the earliest findings, often unnoticed by the patient, is a loss of full extension. Because the elbow is principally a connecting joint between the hand and the trunk, the shoulder and wrists can compensate partially for the loss of elbow motion.

Hand and Wrist

The hand and wrist should be considered together because they form a functional unit. There are data, for example, linking disease of the wrist to ulnar deviation of the MCP joints.[85] The hypothesis is that weakening of the extensor carpi ulnaris muscle leads to radial deviation of the wrist as the carpal bones rotate (the proximal row in an ulnar direction, the distal ones in a radial direction). In response to this, ulnar deviation of the fingers (a "zigzag" deformity) occurs to keep the tendons to the phalanges in a normal line with the radius. Other factors, including the tendency for a power grasp to pull the fingers into an ulnar attitude and inappropriate intrinsic muscle action, are involved (Fig. 66–1). It is important to note that erosion of bone or articular cartilage is not essential for the development of ulnar deviation (Fig. 66–2). Significant, although reducible, ulnar deviation can result from repeated synovitis or muscle weakness in the hands (e.g., in SLE and Parkinson's disease).

Dorsal swelling on the wrist within the tendon sheaths of the extensor muscles is one of the earliest signs of disease. Typically, the extensor carpi ulnaris and extensor digitorum communis sheaths are involved. Rarely, cystic structures resembling ganglia are early findings of RA.[86]

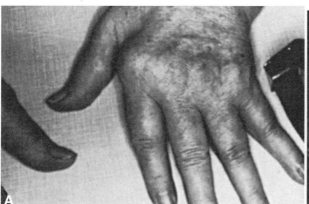 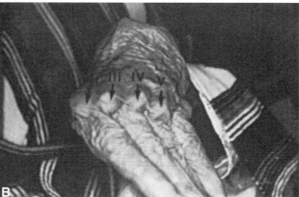

FIGURE 66–1 · *A*, Early ulnar deviation of the metacarpophalangeal joints without subluxation. Extensor tendons have slipped to the ulnar side. The fifth finger, in particular, is compromised with weak flexion, causing a loss of power grip. *B*, Complete subluxation with marked ulnar deviation at the metacarpophalangeal joints of a 90-year-old woman with rheumatoid arthritis (RA). *Arrows* mark the heads of the metacarpals, now in direct contact with the joint capsule instead of the proximal phalanges. (Courtesy of James L. McGuire, MD.)

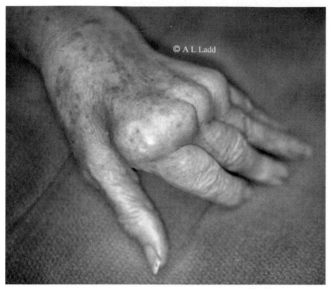

FIGURE 66–2 · Ulnar Deviation and Subluxation. This left hand shows typical manifestations of end-stage erosive changes about the metacarpophalangeal (MP) joints, with volar dislocation and ulnar drift of the fingers. (Copyright A.L. Ladd) (See color plate 32.)

As the synovial proliferation develops within the wrist, pressure increases within the relatively nondistensible joint spaces. Proliferative synovium develops enzymatic machinery sufficient to destroy ligaments, tendons, and the articular disk distal to the ulnar head. Pressure and enzymes combine to produce communications among radiocarpal, radioulnar, and midcarpal joints. Integrity of the distal radioulnar joint is lost. The ulnar collateral ligament, stretched by the proliferative synovium of the radioulnar joint, finally either ruptures or is destroyed, and the ulnar head springs up into dorsal prominence, where it "floats" and is easily depressed by the examiner's fingers.

On the volar side of the wrist, synovial protrusion cysts develop; they can be palpated, and their origins can be confirmed by arthrography. The thick transverse carpal ligament provides significant resistance to decompression, however, and the hyperplastic synovium can compress the median nerve and cause carpal tunnel syndrome, often bilaterally.

Progression of disease in the wrist is characterized either by loss of joint space and bone or by ankylosis. Disintegration of the carpus has been quantified in terms of a carpal-to-metacarpal (C/MC) ratio (length of the carpus divided by that of the third metacarpal). There is a linear decrease in the C/MC ratio with progressive disease.[87] This is caused by compaction of bone at the radiolunate, lunate-capitate, and capitate–third metacarpal joints, which usually accompanies severe disease. One study has confirmed the usefulness of the C/MC ratio for quantifying joint destruction and making correlations with anatomic progression over time.[88] Early detection of carpal bone involvement by RA is possible using MRI, which reveals early synovial proliferation and carpal bone erosions. Bony ankylosis is associated with both the duration and the severity of

disease and is found in joints that have been relatively immobilized by pain, inflammation, treatment, or all of these.

The hand may have many joints involved in RA. A sensitive index of hand involvement is grip strength. The act of squeezing puts stress on all hand joints. Muscular contraction causes ligamentous tightening around joints, compressing inflamed synovium. The immediate result is weakness, with or without pain; the reflex inhibition of muscular contraction due to pain may be a primary factor in this weakness. Quantitative radiographic scores for joint space narrowing, erosion, and malalignment correlate well with loss of motion but do not correlate with joint count tenderness scores[89]; these data support the concept that inflammatory synovitis and the erosive-destructive potential of proliferative synovitis in RA are not one and the same, but rather reflect different aspects of the same disease.

The swan neck deformity is one of flexion of the DIP and MCP joints with hyperextension of the PIP joint. The lesion probably begins with shortening of the interosseous muscles and tendons. Shortening of the intrinsic muscles exerts tension on the dorsal tendon sheath, leading to hyperextension of the PIP joint[90] (Fig. 66–3). Deep tendon contracture or, rarely, DIP joint involvement with RA leads to the DIP joint flexion. Marginal erosive changes in the DIP joints occur more often in patients with RA who have coexisting osteoarthritis (OA).[91]

If, during chronic inflammation of a PIP joint, the extensor hood stretches or is avulsed, the joint may pop up in flexion, producing a boutonnière deformity (Fig. 66–3). The DIP joint remains in hyperextension.

The most serious result of rheumatoid involvement of the hand is resorptive arthropathy, which is defined as severe resorption of bone that begins at the articular cartilage and spreads along the diaphysis of the involved phalanges. Digits appear shortened, excess skin folds are present, and phalanges can be retracted (telescoped) into one another and then pulled out into abnormally long extension, often without pain. With the availability of more effective therapy for RA, resorptive arthropathy is less common and should become rare.

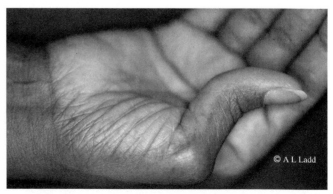

FIGURE 66–3 · Boutonnière Deformity. This is a right thumb demonstrating typical soft tissue imbalance found in rheumatoid arthritis (RA). The metacarpophalangeal (MP) joint is hyperflexed, and the interphalangeal (IP) joint is hyperextended. (Copyright A.L. Ladd) (See color plate 33.)

Three types of deformity have been described for the thumb:

Type I: MCP inflammation leads to stretching of the joint capsule and a boutonnière-like deformity
Type II: Inflammation of the carpometacarpal (CMC) joint leads to volar subluxation during contracture of the adductor hallucis
Type III: After prolonged disease of both MCP joints, exaggerated adduction of the first metacarpus, flexion of the MCP joint, and hyperextension of the DIP joint result from the patient's need to provide a means to pinch

One of the most common manifestations of RA in hands is tenosynovitis in flexor tendon sheaths, and this can be a major cause of hand weakness.[92] This is manifested on the volar surfaces of the phalanges as diffuse swelling between joints or a palpable grating within flexor tendon sheaths in the palm and may occur in up to half of the patients.

It is particularly important to diagnose de Quervain's tenosynovitis because it causes severe discomfort and yet is relatively easily treated; it represents tenosynovitis in the extensors of the thumb. Pain originating from these sheaths can be demonstrated by Finkelstein's test: ulnar flexion at the wrist after the thumb is maximally flexed and adducted.

Not infrequently, rheumatoid nodules or less well-differentiated fibrin deposits develop within tendon sheaths and may "lock" the finger painfully into fixed flexion. When they are chronic and recurrent, it may be necessary to inject the tendon sheath, or if that fails, remove it surgically.

Hip

The hip is less frequently involved early in RA than in juvenile RA. Hip joint involvement must be ascertained by a careful clinical examination; symptoms of hip synovitis are pain in the lower buttock or groin. Pain on the lateral aspect of the hip is often a manifestation of trochanteric bursitis rather than synovitis.

About half the patients with well-established RA have radiographic evidence of hip disease. The femoral head may collapse and be resorbed, and the acetabulum is remodeled and pushed medially, leading to protrusio acetabuli. Significant protrusion occurs in about 5 percent of all patients with RA.[93] Loss of internal rotation on physical examination correlates best with radiographic findings. Like the situation in other weight-bearing joints, the femoral head may develop cystic lesions that communicate with the joint space.

Knees

In contrast to the hips, synovial inflammation and proliferation in the knees are readily demonstrated on physical examination. Early in knee disease, often within a week after the onset of symptoms, quadriceps atrophy is noticeable and leads to the application of more force than usual through the patella to the femoral surface. Another early manifestation of knee disease in RA is a loss of full extension, a functional loss that can become a fixed flexion contracture unless corrective measures are undertaken.

Many patients have a genu varum or valgus that precedes the onset of RA. In these individuals, it is the medial or lateral compartment that bears the most stress from the malalignment that is first symptomatic and is likely to have radiographic evidence of erosion of bone and thinning of cartilage.

Flexion of the knee that has a moderate to large effusion markedly increases the intra-articular pressure. This may cause an outpouching of posterior components of the joint, producing a popliteal or Baker's cyst. Jayson and Dixon have demonstrated that fluid from the anterior compartments of the knee may enter a popliteal cyst but does not readily return.[94] This one-way valve may generate pressures so high in the popliteal space that it may rupture down into the calf or, less often, superiorly into the posterior thigh. Rupture occurs posteriorly between the medial head of the gastrocnemius and the tendinous insertion of the biceps. Clinically, popliteal cysts and their complications have several manifestations. The intact popliteal cyst may compress superficial venous flow to the upper part of the leg, producing dilatation of superficial veins, edema, or both.[95] Rupture of the joint posteriorly with dissection of joint fluid into the calf may resemble acute thrombophlebitis with swelling and tenderness, as well as producing systemic signs of fever with leukocytosis. One helpful sign in identifying joint rupture may be the appearance of a crescentic hematoma beneath one of the malleoli of the ankle.[96] Although arthrography will clearly define the abnormal anatomy of a Baker's cyst, this invasive procedure has been replaced by ultrasonography and, when necessary, MRI.

Ankle and Foot

The ankle is rarely involved in mild or oligoarticular RA but often is damaged in severe progressive forms of the disease. Clinical evidence for ankle involvement is a cystic swelling anterior and posterior to the malleoli. Much of the stability of the ankle depends on the integrity of the ligaments holding the fibula to the tibia, and of these two bones to the talus. In RA, inflammatory and proliferative disease may loosen these connections by stretching and eroding the collagenous ligaments. The result is incongruity, which progresses to pronation deformities and eversion of the foot.

The Achilles tendon is a major structural component and kinetic force in the foot and ankle. Rheumatoid nodules develop in this collagenous structure, and spontaneous rupture of the tendon has been reported when diffuse granulomatous inflammation is present.[97] The subtalar joint controls eversion and inversion of the foot on the talus; patients with RA invariably have more pain while walking on uneven ground, and this is related to the relatively common subtalar joint involvement in RA. Progressive eversion at the subtalar joint, combined with foot pain, leads also to a lateral subluxation beginning in the mid-foot and the development of a "rocker bottom" deformity.

More than one third of patients with RA have significant disease in the feet[98] (Fig. 66–4). Metatarsophalangeal (MTP) joints are often involved, and gait is altered as pain develops during push-off in striding. Downward subluxation of the metatarsal heads occurs soon after the MTP joints become involved, producing "cock-up" toe deformities of the PIP joints. Hallux valgus and bunion or callus formation appear if disease continues. Cystic collections representing outpouchings of flexor tendon sheaths often develop under the MTP joints.[99] Patients with subluxation of metatarsal heads can develop pressure necrosis of the plantar surfaces. Alternatively, patients who have subluxation of MTP joints often develop ulceration over the PIP joints that protrude dorsally (hammer toes).

The sequence of changes as disease progresses in the foot is as follows:[100]

1. Intermetatarsal joint ligaments stretch in response to inflammation.
2. Spread of the forefoot occurs.
3. The fibrofatty cushion on the plantar surface migrates anteriorly.
4. Subluxation of toes occurs dorsally, and extensor tendons shorten.
5. Subluxation of metatarsal heads to a subcutaneous site on the plantar surface develops.
6. Concurrently, a hallux valgus results in "stacking" of the second and third toes on top of the great toe.

It is important to note that DIP joints of the foot are rarely affected in RA, but a functional rigid hallux caused by muscle spasm of the great toe intrinsic muscles in an effort to relieve pressure on the lesser metatarsal heads can be very painful and require surgical intervention.[101]

Another cause of foot pain in rheumatoid patients is the tarsal tunnel syndrome. In a group of 30 patients with RA, radiographically demonstrated erosions in the feet and foot pain, four (13 percent) were shown by electrodiagnostic techniques to have slowing of medial or lateral plantar nerve latency, or both.

▌Extra-articular Complications of Rheumatoid Arthritis

In general, the number and severity of extra-articular features vary with the duration and severity of the disease. A number of these features may be related to extra-articular foci of an immune response,[102] based on evidence of independent and qualitatively different production of RF in the pleural space, pericardium, muscle, and even meninges. These patients with "spillover" immune responses have true rheumatoid disease, not just RA. Other unusual proteins and protein complexes in the circulation of patients with active rheumatoid disease can include antiphospholipid antibodies, circulating immune complexes, and cryoglobulins. Physicians must remember that extra-articular manifestations of RA are associated with an excess mortality.[103]

SKELETON

The skeleton has two anatomically and functionally separate components, cortical and trabecular bone, which respond differently to systemic and local diseases and to drugs. Three questions about bones are of great interest to those studying and caring for patients with RA:

Does RA produce a generalized osteopenia?
What are the influences of sex and age on the skeleton in patients with RA?
Can glucocorticoid-induced osteoporosis be effectively treated, and can new therapies help build new bone?

Because postmenopausal women are more at risk both for RA and osteoporosis, this group must be

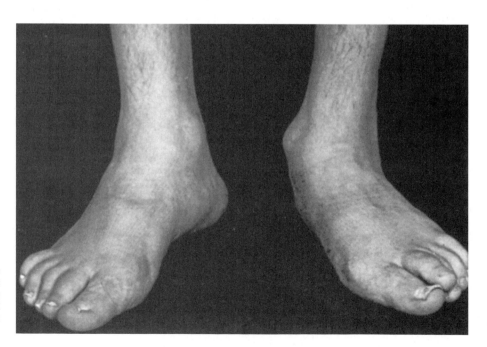

FIGURE 66–4 · Valgus of ankle, pes planus, and forefoot varus deformity of the left foot related to painful synovitis of the ankle, forefoot, and metatarsophalangeal joint in a 24-year-old man with severe rheumatoid arthritis (RA).

treated early and aggressively. At least one study indicates that adequate management of patients with RA that addresses both RA and osteoporosis can protect against bone loss.[104] There appears to be a two-phase loss of bone induced by glucocorticoids: a first rapid phase when up to 12 percent of bone mass disappears in the first 6 to 12 months of therapy, followed by a subsequent chronic phase that has a slower rate of bone loss.[105] It is encouraging, however, that the axial bone loss in patients with RA induced early by glucocorticoids can be reversed.[106] It also is encouraging that after the initial rapid loss of bone in RA patients, not considering various therapies used, the bone loss in the next decade is lower than expected.[107] The available data on these topics are reviewed extensively in Chapters 89 and 90. Although the focus on the relationship between RA and bone is, appropriately, on osteoporosis, physicians should remember that the diffuse loss of bone in RA, whether or not it is related to glucocorticoid therapy, leads to the high incidence of stress fractures of long bones in RA.[108] The fibula is the most common fracture site. Acute leg pain in the thin, elderly rheumatoid patient, even without a history of trauma, should generate suspicion of a stress fracture. Geodes (i.e., subchondral cysts developed by synovial penetration of the cortex or subchondral plate and subsequent proliferation) weaken bone and can predispose bone to fracture.

MUSCLE

Clinical weakness is common in RA, but is it caused by muscle involvement in the rheumatoid inflammation or is it a reflex weakness response to pain? Most rheumatoid patients have muscle weakness, but few have muscle tenderness. An exception to this is the occasional patient with a severe flare of disease activity; such a patient may cry out in severe pain, unable to move either muscles or joints. These symptoms resemble those of vascular insufficiency (ischemic pain) in their intensity.

In an early autopsy series, focal accumulations of lymphocytes and plasma cells with some contiguous degeneration of muscle fibers were found in all rheumatoid patients, a condition termed *nodular myositis*. More recent studies have pointed to at least five different stages of muscle disease in RA[109]:

1. Diminution of muscle bulk with atrophy of type II fibers
2. Peripheral neuromyopathy, usually due to a mononeuritis multiplex
3. Steroid myopathy
4. Active myositis and muscle necrosis with foci of endomysial mononuclear cell infiltration
5. Chronic myopathy resembling a dystrophic process, probably the end stage of inflammatory myositis

In biopsy specimens, atrophy of type II fibers is most common. Active myositis and focal necrosis are found occasionally on biopsy specimens of patients with active disease, particularly in an interesting subset with mild synovitis and a disproportionately high erythrocyte sedimentation rate (ESR).[109] In some patients, the lymphocytes in biopsied muscle have been shown to synthesize immunoglobulin M (IgM) rheumatoid factor, emphasizing the systemic nature of RA. Thus, the patchy "nodules of myositis" contain plasma cells as well as lymphocytes.

SKIN

The most frequently recognized skin lesion in RA is the rheumatoid nodule (discussed in the section "Rheumatoid Nodules"), but there are several other manifestations as well. Perhaps related to the underlying synovitis, skin—particularly over the hands and fingers—becomes thin and atrophic. Palmar erythema is common, but Raynaud's syndrome is rare. Manifestations of vasculitis can range from occasional nail fold infarcts to a deep, erosive, scarring pyoderma gangrenosum. Palpable purpura in rheumatoid patients is often related to a reaction to a drug that the patient is taking but can be primary and a direct function of the severity of articular disease (see Chapter 45). Livido reticularis, the lacy, dusky purple, asymptomatic discoloration seen on the extremities, is believed to signify a deep dermal vasculopathy. It can be present in any or all diffuse connective tissue diseases and is associated often with antiphospholipid antibodies in the circulation.[110]

EYE

Virtually all ocular manifestations of RA can be considered complications of the disease (see Chapter 44). Keratoconjunctivitis sicca is a component of Sjögren's syndrome and is discussed in Chapter 69. More directly related to the rheumatoid process and seen in the synovium and within rheumatoid nodules are scleritis and episcleritis. The highly differentiated connective tissues in the eye make rheumatoid manifestations particularly interesting and, when they occur in aggressive form, very serious.

The episclera of the eye is highly vascular compared to the dense sclera. Scleritis, episcleritis, or both, occur in less than 1 percent of rheumatoid patients.[111] In episcleritis, the eye becomes red within minutes. Unlike conjunctivitis, episcleritis results in no discharge other than tearing in response to the gritty discomfort. Loss of vision does not occur as a direct result of the episcleritis, but a keratitis or cataract developing secondarily can cause visual loss. Scleritis causes severe ocular pain and a dark red discoloration (Fig. 66–5). No discharge is present. Depending on the intensity of the process, scleritis can be localized and superficial or generalized, with or without granulomatous resorption of the sclera down to the uveal layer; when this complication occurs, it is known as scleromalacia perforans. Rarely, perilimbic ischemic ulcers can be caused by cryoproteins (RF-IgG complexes) and if untreated can result in perforation of the anterior chamber.[111] Patients with RA that have an associated keratoconjunctivitis sicca secondary to Sjögren's syndrome have pruritic and painful eyes, sometimes leading to chronic blepharitis.

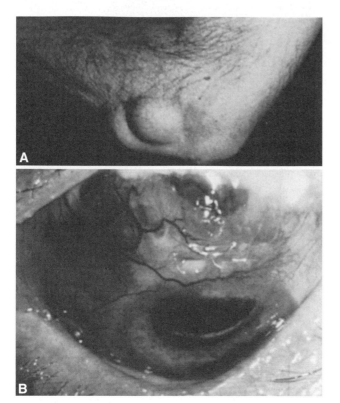

FIGURE 66-5 · Manifestations of increased reactivity of mesenchymal tissue in RA appearing *(A)* as nodules on the elbow and *(B)* within the sclera of the eye. The eye lesion represents scleral perforation associated with a granulomatous scleral reaction. Treatment was placement of a scleral patch graft. Note the increase in vascularity of the sclera. The dark areas represent scleral thinning with exposure of uveal pigment. (Patient of Drs. S. Arthur Bouchoff and G.N. Fouhls. Photograph courtesy of Marty Schener.)

RHEUMATOID NODULES

The mature rheumatoid nodule has a central area of necrosis rimmed by a corona of palisading fibroblasts that is surrounded in turn by a collagenous capsule with perivascular collections of chronic inflammatory cells. The earliest nodules, nests of granulation tissue, have been identified at a size of less than 4 mm.[112] The nodules grow by accumulating cells that expand centrifugally, leaving behind central necrosis initiated by vasculopathy and compounded by protease destruction of the connective tissue matrix. Occurring in 20 to 35 percent of patients with definite or classic RA, nodules are found most often on extensor surfaces such as the olecranon process and the proximal ulna. They are subcutaneous and vary in consistency from a soft, amorphous, entirely mobile mass to a hard, rubbery mass attached firmly to the periosteum.

The appearance of nodules in unusual sites may lead to confusion in diagnosis. Sacral nodules may be mistaken for bedsores if the overlying skin breaks down. Occipital nodules also occur in bedridden patients. In the larynx, rheumatoid nodules on the vocal cords may cause progressive hoarseness. Nodules found in the heart and lungs are discussed later. Nodules on the sclera can produce perforation of this collagenous tissue. There have been multiple reports of rheumatoid

nodule formation within the central nervous system, involving leptomeninges more than parenchyma.[113] Some patients develop rheumatoid nodules within vertebral bodies, resulting in bone destruction and signs of myelopathy.

Careful histologic study of early lesions[114] suggests that development of the nodule is mediated through affected small arterioles and resulting complement activation and terminal vasculitis. This immunologic response is linked to proliferation of resident histiocytes and fibroblasts, as well as to an influx of macrophages from the circulation. The proliferation of both cells and the supporting scaffold of connective tissue is mediated by cytokines expressed in patterns very similar to those found in rheumatoid synovium. Data from studies using monoclonal antibodies against receptors for complement C3b and C3bi, monocytes, activated macro-phages, and HLA-DR molecules suggest that mononuclear phagocytes are constantly being recruited into the peripheral layers and subsequently migrate into the palisade to constitute most of the cell population in this area.[117] Other studies, using cytochemical markers (nonspecific esterase and CD68—a protein associated with lysosomes—for macrophages, and prolyl hydroxylase for fibroblasts), indicate that a mixture of macrophages and nonsynoviocyte fibroblasts make up the cellular content of nodules.[118] This evidence fits with data from nodule tissue in organ culture; like synovial tissue, the cells in the palisading region have the capacity to produce collagenase and proteases in large quantity.[119]

RF is almost always found in the serum of patients with rheumatoid nodules. Rarely, such nodules are present in the absence of obvious arthritis. The presence of multiple nodules on the hands and a positive test for RF associated with episodes of acute intermittent synovitis and subchondral cystic lesions of small bones of the hands and feet represent a condition that has been called rheumatoid nodulosis.[120] Many clinicians have noted that during MTX therapy that is successful in downregulating synovitis, existing nodules may enlarge and new ones may develop; the pathophysiology underlying this phenomenon is not known, although it may relate to the effects of MTX or adenosine (see Chapter 59).

The differential diagnosis of rheumatoid nodules includes the following:

1. *"Benign" nodules:* These usually are found in healthy children without RF or arthritis. They are nontender; appear often on the pretibial regions, feet, and scalp; increase rapidly in size; and are histologically identical to rheumatoid nodules.
2. *Granuloma annulare:* These nodules are intracutaneous but histologically identical to rheumatoid nodules. They slowly resolve and are not associated with other disease.
3. *Xanthomatosis:* These nodules usually have a yellow tinge, and patients have abnormally high plasma lipoprotein and cholesterol levels. There is no underlying bone involvement.
4. *Tophi:* These collections of monosodium urate crystals in patients with gout are associated with small, punched-out bone lesions and are rarely found in

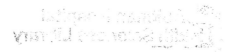

patients with a normal serum urate concentration. A search for crystals with a polarizing microscope will reveal the classic needle-shaped, negatively birefringent crystals.

5. *Miscellaneous nodules:* The nodules of multicentric reticulohistiocytosis contain large lipid-filled macrophages. Numerous proliferative disorders that affect cutaneous tissue, including erythema elevatum diutinum, acrodermatitis chronica atrophicans, bejel, yaws, pinta, and leprosy, can resemble rheumatoid nodules. A rheumatoid nodule, particularly when it occurs on the face, may simulate basal cell carcinoma.

FISTULA DEVELOPMENT

Cutaneous sinuses near joints develop rarely in sero-positive patients with long-standing disease and positive tests for RF. These fistulas can be either sterile or septic and connect the skin surface with a joint, with a para-articular cyst in bone or soft tissues, or with a bursa. The pathogenesis of fistulas without a septic origin is particularly difficult to understand because the rheumatoid process usually is so clearly centripetal (i.e., progressing toward the center of the joint) rather than centrifugal.

INFECTION

The incidence of infections as a complication of RA has paralleled the use of glucocorticoids and immunosuppressive agents, including biologic agents, particularly infliximab and etanercept. Pulmonary infections, skin sepsis, and pyarthrosis are most common sites of infection in RA.[121,122] Difficulty in diagnosis is accentuated by the similarity of aggressive RA to infection, particularly in joints; a "pseudoseptic" arthritis in rheumatoid patients, associated with fever, chills, and grossly purulent synovial fluid, can be part of a severe exacerbation of RA and clearly must be distinguished from infection.[123] A retrospective longitudinal cohort study has been completed that compared the frequency of infections in a population-based incidence cohort of RA patients to that in a group of individuals without RA from the same population; this study looked at more than 7900 to 9100 person-years.[124] There were 609 RA patients and 609 non-RA patients; 73 percent were women, and the mean age was 58 years. Hazard ratios for RA patients versus controls after adjustment for age, sex, smoking status, leukopenia, corticosteroid use, and diabetes mellitus were as follows:

- Objectively confirmed infections = 1.7:1
- Infections requiring hospitalization = 1.83:1

Bone, joints, skin, respiratory tract, and soft tissues were the organs with highest hazard ratios. In a subsequent study it was shown that, in this cohort, the predictors of infection were as follows:

- Increasing age
- Extra-articular manifestations of RA
- Leukopenia
- Comorbidities such as chronic lung disease, alcoholism, diabetes mellitus, and the use of glucocorticoids

DMARD use was not associated with an increased incidence with infection.[125,126] It is apparent that physicians must have a low threshold of concern for infection in rheumatoid patients.

CANCER

There appears to be an increased risk for malignancy in all RA patients, with a markedly increased risk, particularly for lymphoma, in certain patient subsets. Interstitial fibrosis may be a risk factor for lung carcinoma, particularly of the bronchoalveolar variety.[127] One exception is cancer of the gastrointestinal tract, for which there appears to be a reduced risk for RA patients.[128] It is possible that NSAIDs lower the risk of this form of cancer, as supported by evidence that these drugs can diminish the occurrence and numbers of colonic polyps.

RA patients confront a risk of Hodgkin's disease, non-Hodgkin's lymphoma, and leukemia two to three times that of the normal population; this is independent of immunosuppressive therapy. Of the lymphomas arising in RA, about half are low grade and half high grade; most of these are B cell lymphomas, although there is no evidence that these originate from clonally proliferated lymphocytes associated with RA. In contrast, although the relative risk for total cancer in patients with Felty's syndrome is only 2, the relative risk for non-Hodgkin's lymphoma in this complication of RA is near 13,[129] similar to that associated with Sjögren's syndrome. Detailed discussions are given in Chapter 69.

HEMATOLOGIC ABNORMALITIES

The majority of patients with RA have a mild normocytic hypochromic anemia that correlates with ESR elevation and the activity of the disease. Anemia has mixed causes in RA. One deficiency may mask evidence of others. A useful guide is that three quarters of rheumatoid patients with anemia have the anemia of chronic disease, whereas one quarter respond to iron therapy. Patients in both groups may have superimposed B_{12} or folate deficiencies.[130]

The following guidelines may be helpful in diagnosing the cause of anemia in rheumatoid patients:

1. Anemia of chronic disease is associated with significantly higher serum ferritin concentration than is found in isolated iron deficiency.
2. Folate and B12 deficiency may mask iron deficiency by increasing the mean cell volume and mean cell hemoglobin level of erythrocytes.
3. The ESR correlates inversely with hemoglobin levels in RA, as expected in anemia of chronic disease.
4. Erythropoietin levels are more elevated in patients with iron-deficiency anemia than in those with anemia of chronic disease; rheumatoid patients also have a diminished response to erythropoietin.[131]

In patients with the anemia of chronic disease, the total erythroid heme turnover is slightly reduced, and ineffective erythropoiesis accounts for a much higher than normal percentage of total heme turnover. In contrast to anemia associated with blood loss, the ineffective erythropoiesis will return to normal in RA if remission can be induced.[132] Red blood cell aplasia, immunologically mediated, is a rare finding in RA. However, because erythropoiesis in animals has been shown to be dependent on T lymphocytes, it is logical to search for immunologic factors that can induce anemia in RA. Serum from RA patients can profoundly suppress erythroid colony formation,[133] but T lymphocytes from bone marrow of rheumatoid patients have not been shown to inhibit erythroid development in vitro.

Eosinophilia and thrombocytosis are often associated with RA. Eosinophilia (5 percent of total white blood cell [WBC] count) was observed in 40 percent of patients with severe seropositive disease.[134] Similarly, there is a significant relationship between thrombocytosis and extra-articular manifestations of rheumatoid disease and disease activity.[135]

An interesting subset of patients with RA has increased numbers of large granular lymphocytes (LGLs) in the peripheral blood, bone marrow, and liver. The lymphocytes contain many azurophilic granules in the cytoplasm and may account for more than 90 percent of mononuclear cells in blood. They are increased in certain viral infections. The cells are E rosette–positive, are fragment crystallizable (Fc) receptor–positive, do not produce IL-2, respond poorly to mitogens, and have either antibody-dependent cell-mediated cytotoxicity activity (expressing cell determinant 3 [CD3], CD8, and CD57) or natural killer (NK) cells (expressing CD16 and CD56).[136,137] Of previously described patients with LGL proliferation, almost one third have had RA.[173] Because the LGL syndrome in patients with RA has the same HLA-DR4 association seen in Felty's syndrome, the proposal has been made that both Felty's and the LGL syndrome represent different variants of a broader syndrome comprising RA, neutropenia, LGL expansions, HLA-DR4 positivity, and variable splenomegaly.[138]

Paraproteinemia, typified by monoclonal gammopathies, has a poor prognostic significance when it appears in rheumatoid patients. This evidence for monoclonal B cell proliferation carries with it a high frequency of malignant transformation to lymphoma or myeloma.[139]

VASCULITIS

In one sense, it is redundant to think of vasculitis as a complication of RA, because the initial pathologic change in RA may include inflammatory changes in small blood vessels. However, it is useful to use the term *vasculitis* to group those extra-articular complications related not to proliferative granulomas but rather to inflammatory vascular disease. Systemic rheumatoid vasculitis, one of the most feared complications of this disease, has become increasingly uncommon in the last decade. This likely relates to the marked improvement in therapy due to widespread use of MTX and the new biologic agents.

Variables associated with the development of rheumatoid vasculitis have included the following[140]:

- Male gender
- High titers of RF in serum
- Joint erosions
- Subcutaneous nodules and other extra-articular features
- The number of disease-modifying drugs previously prescribed
- Current treatment with glucocorticoids
- Circulating cryoglobulins

Clinical vasculitis usually takes one of the following forms:

- Distal arteritis (ranging from splinter hemorrhage to gangrene) (Fig. 66–6)
- Cutaneous ulceration (including pyoderma gangrenosum)
- Peripheral neuropathy
- Arteritis of viscera, including heart, lungs, bowel, kidney, liver, spleen, pancreas, lymph nodes, and testis
- Palpable purpura

The pathologic finding in rheumatoid vasculitis is a panarteritis. All layers of the vessel wall are infiltrated with mononuclear cells. Fibrinoid necrosis is seen in active lesions. Intimal proliferation may predispose to thrombosis. Obliterative endarteritis of the finger is one of the most common manifestations of vasculitis, and immune complex deposits have been demonstrated in those vessels.[141] When larger vessels are involved, the pathologic changes resemble those of polyarteritis nodosa. In addition, a venulitis associated with RA has been described.[142] In patients with hypocomplementemia, the cellular infiltrate around the vessels contains neutrophils. In normocomplementemic patients, lymphocytes predominate.

It is unusual for vasculitis to be active in any but the sickest patients: those with severe deforming arthritis and high RF titers[143]; this subgroup represents less than 1 percent of patients with RA. Although RA is more common in women than in men, vasculitis is more often seen in men than in women with RA. Supporting the

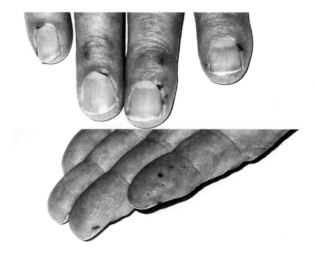

FIGURE 66–6 • Digital vasculitis in a 65-year-old man with seropositive rheumatoid arthritis (RA). (Courtesy of Eileen Moynihan, M.D.) (See color plate 34.)

hypothesis that vascular injury is mediated by deposition of circulating immune complexes are 1) depressed levels of C2 and C4; 2) hypercatabolism of C3[144]; 3) deposition of IgG, IgM, and C3 in involved arteries; and 4) the presence of large amounts of cryoimmunoglobulin in the serum of occasional patients with vasculitis.

Neurovascular disease may be the only manifestation of vasculitis. The two common clinical patterns are a mild distal sensory neuropathy and a severe sensorimotor neuropathy (mononeuritis multiplex).[145] The latter form is characterized by severe arterial damage on nerve biopsy specimens. Symptoms of the milder form may be paresthesias or "burning feet" in association with decreased touch and pin sensation distally. Patients with mononeuritis multiplex have weakness (e.g., footdrop) in addition to sensory abnormalities. Symptoms and signs are identical to those found in polyarteritis. Rheumatoid pachymeningitis is a rare complication of RA; confined to the dura and pia mater, this process may be limited to certain areas (e.g., lumbar cord or cisternae).[146] Elevated levels of IgG (including IgM and IgG RFs and low-molecular-weight IgM) and immune complexes are found in the cerebrospinal fluid. In addition, there appears to be a real entity of autonomic nervous system disease in RA that is isolated from other peripheral or central nervous system damage.[147,148]

Visceral lesions occur generally as claudication or infarction of the organ supplied by the involved arteries. Intestinal involvement with vasculitis presents as abdominal pain, at first intermittent and progressing often to continuous pain and a tender, quiet belly on examination. If infarction develops, resection must be accomplished promptly. The presence of gangrene of digits and extremities, the development of intestinal lesions with bleeding or perforation, cardiac or renal involvement, and mononeuritis multiplex indicate extensive vasculitis and are associated with a poor prognosis.[149]

Current practice is to treat organ-specific vasculitis aggressively when it occurs in rheumatoid patients, similar to the treatment for patients with polyarteritis. This therapeutic approach may be responsible for the rather small excess mortality in rheumatoid vasculitis patients compared to "controls" with RA alone. In 61 patients with rheumatoid vasculitis, after allowance for general risk factors such as age and sex, the risk of death was only 1.26 times that of rheumatoid patients without vasculitis.[150]

RENAL DISEASE

The kidney is an example of an organ that is rarely involved directly in RA but often is compromised indirectly by therapy. Amyloidosis is a complication of chronic RA, and particularly of Still's disease. Phenacetin abuse causes renal papillary necrosis, and salicylates and other NSAIDs may cause abnormalities as well. A membranous nephropathy is the pathologic lesion related to therapy with gold salts and D-penicillamine. Rarely, a focal necrotizing glomerulitis is seen in patients dying with RA and disseminated vasculitis.

PULMONARY DISEASE

There are at least six forms of lung disease in RA:

- Pleural disease
- Interstitial fibrosis
- Nodular lung disease
- Bronchiolitis
- Arteritis, with pulmonary hypertension
- Small airways disease

It is not surprising, perhaps, that lung disease is associated with RA, considering that the drugs used to treat the disease, such as MTX can also cause pulmonary problems. In some cases, it may be difficult to distinguish pulmonary fibrosis related to RA from MTX pulmonary toxicity. Reactivation of tuberculosis by anti–TNF-α biologic agents is of particular concern to rheumatologists.

Pleural Disease

Pleuritis is commonly found on autopsy of patients with RA, but clinical disease during life is seen less frequently. In about 20 percent of patients it develops concurrently with the onset of the arthritis. Pleuritic pain is not usually a major complaint. Effusions can be large enough to cause dyspnea. Characteristics of the exudative rheumatoid effusions are as follows: glucose, 10 to 50 mg/dl; protein, more than 4 g/dl; cells (mononuclear), 100 to 3500/mm^3; lactic dehydrogenase, elevated; and CH_{50}, depressed. The low glucose concentrations are of interest. Sepsis (particularly tuberculosis) is the only other condition that commonly has such a low pleural fluid glucose level. An impaired transport of glucose into the pleural space appears to be the cause of this.[151]

Interstitial Pneumonitis and Fibrosis

The increased reactivity of mesenchymal cells in RA is believed to be the cause of pulmonary fibrosis in this disease. Like the findings in scleroderma, physical findings are of fine, diffuse, dry rales. Radiographs show a diffuse reticular (interstitial) or reticulonodular pattern in both lung fields; these can progress to a honeycomb appearance on plain radiographs and a characteristic lattice network seen on high-resolution CT scans. The pathologic findings are those of diffuse fibrosis in the midst of a mononuclear cell infiltrate (Fig. 66–7). The principal functional defect is impairment of alveolocapillary gas exchange with decreased diffusion capacity, best measured using single-breath carbon monoxide diffusion capacities.[152] It is likely that RA patients who smoke are at a higher risk for fibrotic complications in the lungs than are those in the general population. It has been reported that bronchoalveolar lavage may reveal increased numbers of lymphocytes, even in those with only mildly abnormal chest radiographs and normal pulmonary function test results.[153] In more aggressive disease, a higher proportion of neutrophils can be found in bronchoalveolar lavage. Lymphoid interstitial pneumonitis has been described in patients with rheumatoid arthritis and Sjögren's syndrome. This is a relatively indolent disorder and is associated with elevated serum globulin levels. Bronchoalveolar lavage reveals a primarily lymphocytic response.[154]

Nodular Lung Disease

Pulmonary nodules may appear singly or in clusters that coalesce. Single ones appear as coin lesions and, when significant peripheral arthritis and nodules are present, can be diagnosed by needle biopsy without thoracotomy. Caplan's syndrome,[155] in which pneumoconiosis and RA are synergistic, producing a violent fibroblastic reaction with obliterative granulomatous fibrosis, has become a rare occurrence as the respiratory environment in mining operations has improved. Nodules may cavitate, creating a bronchopleural fistula. In several cases, solitary pulmonary nodules in RA patients have proved to be a rheumatoid nodule and a coexistent bronchogenic carcinoma,[156] a finding that suggests caution in interpreting "benign" results from fine-needle aspiration biopsy in such patients.

Bronchiolitis

A rare finding is an interstitial pneumonitis that progresses to alveolar involvement and bronchiolitis, respiratory insufficiency, and death. Pathologic studies show a cellular loose fibrosis and proteinaceous exudate in bronchioles and alveoli; interstitial infiltrations of lymphocytes attest to the immunogenic aspects of the disease (Fig. 66–7).

Pulmonary Hypertension

Pulmonary hypertension is more common than previously appreciated in RA. Noninvasive echocardiograms have suggested that mild pulmonary hypertension can be detected in more than 30 percent of patients with RA.[157] Most of these patients are asymptomatic.

Small Airways Disease

Defined by a reduced maximal midexpiratory flow rate and maximal expiratory flow rate at 50 percent of functional vital capacity, small airways disease was observed in 50 percent of 30 RA patients, compared to 22 percent of a control population.[158] The study was adjusted for pulmonary infections, α_1-antitrypsin deficiency, penicillamine treatment, environmental pollution, and smoking. Other investigations have not found small airways dysfunction in RA and have suggested that, if present, it probably is related to factors other than RA.[159] If real, this phenomenon may be part of a generalized exocrinopathic process in the disease, expressed most flagrantly, of course, in Sjögren's syndrome.

CARDIAC COMPLICATIONS

Cardiac disease in RA can take many forms related to granulomatous proliferation or vasculitis. Advances in echocardiography have made the diagnosis of pericarditis and endocardial inflammation easier and more specific. Myocardial biopsy through vascular catheters

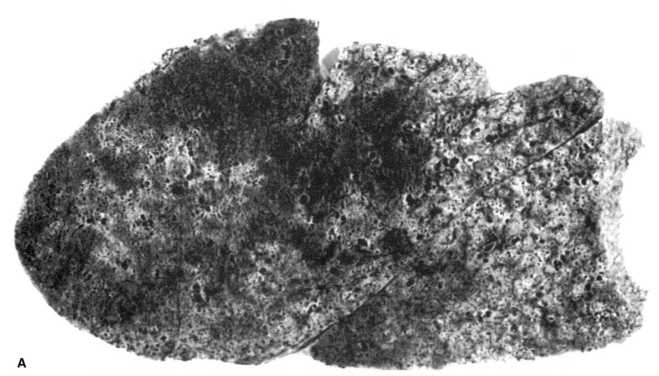

A

FIGURE 66–7 • Severe, Subacute Interstitial Pneumonitis in Rheumatoid Arthritis (RA). This complication proved fatal in 5 weeks in this 66-year-old woman with severe, active seropositive RA. *A*, The gross photograph of the left lung shows dense interalveolar thickening by a fibrofibrinous exudate. Air sacs are becoming obliterated. Lungs were heavy and incompressible, but there was only a trace of excess fluid.

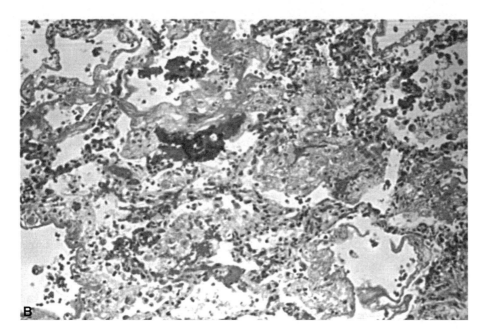

FIGURE 66–7 CONT'D · *B*, Microscopic sections showed thickened alveolar septa with a rich fibrinous exudate present. (Courtesy of Charles Faulkner III, M.D.)

has facilitated diagnosis and classification of myocarditis. In a detailed study of rheumatoid patients using echocardiography, Holter monitors, and electrocardiogram (ECG), it is reported that 70 percent of patients with nodular disease and 40 percent of those with nonnodular RA have some cardiac involvement, including valve thickening or incompetence.[160]

Pericarditis

Infrequently diagnosed on the basis of history and physical examination in RA, pericarditis is present in up to 50 percent of patients at autopsy. In one study, 31 percent of patients with RA had echocardiographic evidence of pericardial effusion. The same study revealed only rare evidence of impaired left ventricular function in prospectively studied outpatients with RA.[161] Although unusual, cardiac tamponade with constrictive pericarditis develops in RA and may require pericardectomy. Almost all patients have a positive test for RF, and half have nodules. The preservation of good ventricular function on echocardiography in the face of deteriorating clinical myocardial function should raise a high index of suspicion of constrictive pericarditis.[162]

Myocarditis

Myocarditis can take the form of either granulomatous disease or interstitial myocarditis. The granulomatous process resembles subcutaneous nodules and could be considered specific for the disease. Diffuse infiltration of the myocardium by mononuclear cells, on the other hand, may involve the entire myocardium and yet have no clinical manifestations, but it could possibly be suggested by echocardiography.

Endocardial Inflammation

Echocardiographic studies have reported evidence of previously unrecognized mitral valve disease diagnosed by a reduced E-F slope of the anterior leaflet of the mitral valve. Although aortic valve disease and arthritis are generally associated through ankylosing spondylitis, a number of patients with granulomatous nodules on the valve have been reported.[163]

Conduction Defects

Atrioventricular block is unusual in RA but is probably related to direct granulomatous involvement. Pathologic examination may reveal proliferative lesions or healed scars. Complete heart block has been described in more than 30 patients with RA. It generally occurs in patients with established erosive nodular disease.[164] It usually is permanent and is caused by rheumatoid granulomas in or near the atrioventricular node or bundle of His. Rarely, amyloidosis is responsible for heart block.

Coronary Arteritis

Patients with severe RA and active vasculitis who develop a myocardial infarction are likely to have coronary arteritis as a basis for the process.

Granulomatous Aortitis or Valvular Disease

In severe rheumatoid heart disease, granulomatous disease can spread to involve even the base of the aorta. Occasionally, granulomatous disease associated with RA necessitates urgent valve replacement for aortic incompetence.[165]

Diagnosis

Diagnosis of RA must be by established criteria that are based on an effective clinical history and examination, laboratory tests, and diagnoses that exclude it. No single feature allows a definite diagnosis. The 1988 ACR criteria for classification should not be used in individual cases for diagnosis; however, the requirement that objective evidence for synovitis must be present for at least 6 weeks is an important one (Table 66–5). A physician should not make a premature diagnosis of RA in a patient who may have a self-limited synovitis. On the other hand, to attempt preventing irreversible damage to joints, the diagnosis of RA should be confirmed or ruled out within 2 months after the onset of synovitis.

The characteristic patient with RA complains of pain and stiffness in multiple joints. The joint swelling is boggy and includes both soft tissue and synovial fluid. These joints are tender to the touch, especially the small joints of the hands and feet. Palmar erythema and prominent veins on the dorsum of the hand and wrist indicate increased blood flow. DIP joints are rarely involved. The temperature over the involved joints (except the hip) can be elevated, but the joints are not usually red. The range of motion is limited, and muscle strength and function around inflamed joints are diminished. Soft, poorly delineated subcutaneous nodules are often found in the extensor surface of the forearm. Findings on general physical examination are normal, except for a possible low-grade fever (38°C) and a pulse more rapid than normal for that individual. Soft, small lymph nodes are found occasionally in epitrochlear, axillary, and cervical areas. Movement is guarded, and apprehension often dominates the facial expression. Initial laboratory tests often show the following (essential tests are indicated with an asterisk (*); the others are largely of academic interest):

- Slight leukocytosis with a normal differential white blood cell (WBC) count*
- Thrombocytosis*
- Slight anemia (hemoglobin 10 g/dl), normochromic and either normocytic or microcytic*
- Normal urinalysis*
- An ESR of 30 mm/hour or more (Westergren method) and a C-reactive protein (CRP) level of more than 0.7 pg/ml*

- Normal renal, hepatic, and metabolic function*
- A normal serum uric acid level (before the initiation of salicylate therapy)
- A positive RF test and negative antinuclear antibody test (A negative test for RF in serum is found in up to 30 percent of patients early in the illness. In the seropositive patents and in some of these "seronegative" patients there will be a positive test for anticyclic citrullinated peptides.)*
- Elevated levels of α_2- and α_1-globulins
- A normal or elevated serum complement level
- A "typical" arthrocentesis, when obvious fluid is present, in early RA reveals the following:
  - The joint fluid is straw colored, slightly cloudy and contains many flecks of fibrin
  - A clot forms in fluid left standing at room temperature
  - There are 5000 to 25,000 WBC/mm^3, and at least 50 percent of these are polymorphonuclear leukocytes
  - Some large polymorphonuclear leukocytes with granules staining positively for immunoglobulins (IgG and IgM) and complement C3 can often be found; no crystals are present
  - Complement C4 and C2 levels are depressed, but the C3 level can be normal
  - IgG in synovial fluid may approach serum concentrations
  - The synovial fluid glucose level is usually normal but can be depressed, occasionally to less than 25 mg/dl
  - Cultures are negative
  - Routinely, the cell count and differential, along with culture and examination for crystals are the only essential tests on synovial fluid in this clinical situation

DIAGNOSIS OF EARLY RHEUMATOID ARTHRITIS

This is the most important time to make a diagnosis of RA, and it is the most difficult task. It is especially important in the twenty-first century because there are

---

TABLE 66–5 • 1988 REVISED AMERICAN RHEUMATISM ASSOCIATION CRITERIA FOR CLASSIFICATION OF RHEUMATOID ARTHRITIS*

Criterion	Definition
1. Morning stiffness	Morning stiffness in and around the joints lasting at least 1 hr before maximal improvement
2. Arthritis of three or more joint areas	At least three joint areas simultaneously having soft tissue swelling or fluid (not bony overgrowth alone) observed by a physician (the 14 possible joint areas are [right or left] PIP, MCP, wrist, elbow, knee, ankle, and MTP joints)
3. Arthritis of hand joints	At least one joint area swollen as above in wrist, MCP, or PIP joint
4. Symmetric arthritis	Simultaneous involvement of the same joint areas (as in criterion 2) on both sides of the body (bilateral involvement of PIP, MCP, or MTP joints is acceptable without absolute symmetry)
5. Rheumatoid nodules	Subcutaneous nodules over bony prominences or extensor surfaces, or in juxta-articular regions, observed by a physician
6. Serum rheumatoid factor	Demonstration of abnormal amounts of serum "rheumatoid factor" by any method that has been positive in less than 5 percent of normal control subjects
7. Radiographic changes	Changes typical of RA on PA hand and wrist radiographs, which must include erosions or unequivocal bony decalcification localized to or most marked adjacent to the involved joints (osteoarthritis changes alone do not qualify)

* For classification purposes, a patient is said to have RA if he or she has satisfied at least four of the seven criteria. Criteria 1 through 4 must be present for at least 6 weeks. Patients with two clinical diagnoses are not excluded. Designation as classic, definite, or probable rheumatoid arthritis is not to be made.
Abbreviations: MCP, Metacarpophalangeal; MTP, metatarsophalangeal; PA, posteroanterior; PIP, proximal interphalangeal; RA, rheumatoid arthritis.

such powerful and effective therapies for RA available. On the one hand, rheumatologists should not be giving patients who do not have RA these drugs, and on the other, no one wants to miss a true rheumatoid in the early phases for lack of a good diagnostic algorithm. Follow-up studies in Europe have indicated that after a 2-year period, the 1987 ACR criteria in combination with an office-based rheumatologist were effective in differentiating among patients with and without RA. However, the criteria were not useful for predicting RA in patients with the onset of symptoms within the previous year.[166] The sensitivity and specificity of each of the ACR criteria applied at the first visit for identifying patients who would have a diagnosis of RA 2 years later in 172 patients were as follows:

ACR Criterion	Sensitivity (%)	Specificity (%)73
Morning stiffness	68	65
Arthritis of >3 areas	80	43
Arthritis of the hand joints	81	46
Symmetric arthritis	77	37
Rheumatoid nodules	3	100
Rheumatoid factor	59	93
Radiographic change	22	98

A prediction model for persistent (erosive) polyarthritis (e.g., RA) has been developed,[167] recognizing that the ACR criteria were designed for classification, not diagnosis. The final prediction model consists of seven variables. In the following table, both odds ratios, as well as a weighted score, are given for each measurable variable to help a physician put the patient into one of three groups: 1) self-limiting arthritis; 2) persistent nonerosive arthritis; or 3) persistent erosive arthritis.

The total score ranged from 0 to 13 for the prediction of persistent arthritis and from 0 to 9 for the prediction of erosive arthritis. For example, in testing erosive versus nonerosive arthritis (given persistence) a total score of 1 in a patient gave a probability of 0.16 that the patient would develop erosions, whereas a total score of 8 gave a probability of 0.92 of developing erosions. Similarly, in testing persistent arthritis versus self-limiting arthritis, a total score of 9 gave a probability of developing persistent but nonerosive arthritis of 0.92.

This system appears to work well. In a study of 524 consecutive patients it was possible to discriminate, at the first visit, between what would be persistent nonerosive disease and persistent erosive disease, and to separate these two from self-limiting disease. The discrimination ability of this criteria set is higher than that of the ACR classification criteria, using the same patients.

DIFFERENTIAL DIAGNOSIS

Other diseases must be excluded before the diagnosis of RA is made.[168] One of the most difficult challenges is the adult presenting with polyarthritis and fever; for this patient, a full workup may be required to define the underlying cause[169] (Table 66–6). The following sections on various diseases are listed in alphabetic order, and the illness' relative frequency is specified as common, uncommon, or rare.

Acute Relapsing Symmetric Seronegative Synovitis and Peripheral Edema (Rare)

Acute relapsing symmetric seronegative synovitis and peripheral edema (RS_3PE), a condition of elderly persons, presents as joint swelling, especially in the hands and feet, associated with pitting edema. It may herald several different and distinct diseases (e.g., polymyalgia rheumatica, dermato- or polymyositis, or late-onset peripheral spondyloarthropathy). The course is benign, but relapses may be noted. Evolution into RA is rare, if it occurs at all.

Amyloidosis (Rare)

Deposits of amyloid can be found in synovial and periarticular tissues and are presumably responsible for the joint complaints of some patients. The synovial fluid in amyloid arthropathy is noninflammatory, and particulate material with apple-green fluorescence after Congo red staining may be found in the fluid. Amyloid formed of β_2-microglobulin is found in joints of patients with chronic renal failure, usually those who are on dialysis (see Chapter 104).

Angioimmunoblastic Lymphadenopathy (Rare)

Nonerosive symmetric seronegative polyarthritis involving large joints can be an initial complaint in angioim-

Clinical or Laboratory variable		Persistent nonerosive vs.	Self-limiting	Persistent erosive vs.	Persistent nonerosive
		Odds Ratio	Score	Odds Ratio	Score
Symptom duration at first visit	>6 weeks, <6 months	2.49	2	0.96	0
	>6 months	5.49	3	1.44	0
Morning stiffness longer than 1 hour		1.96	1	1.96	1
Arthritis in three or more joints		1.73	1	1.73	1
Bilateral MTP compression pain		1.65	1	3.78	2
Rheumatoid factor positivity		2.99	2	2.99	2
Anticitrullinated peptide antibody positivity		4.58	3	4.58	3
Radiographic erosions (hands or feet)		2.75	2	infinite	infinite

TABLE 66–6 • DISCRIMINATING FEATURES IN PATIENTS PRESENTING WITH POLYARTHRITIS AND FEVER

Symptom or Sign	Possible Diagnoses
Temperature >40°C	Still's disease Bacterial arthritis Systemic lupus erythematosus
Fever preceding arthritis	Viral arthritis Lyme disease Reactive arthritis Still's disease Bacterial endocarditis
Migratory arthritis	Rheumatic fever Gonococcemia Meningococcemia Viral arthritis Systemic lupus erythematosus Acute leukemia Whipple's disease
Effusion disproportionately greater than pain	Tuberculous arthritis Bacterial endocarditis Inflammatory bowel disease Giant cell arteritis Lyme disease
Pain disproportionately greater than effusion	Rheumatic fever Familial Mediterranean fever Acute leukemia Acquired Immunodeficiency syndrome
Positive test for rheumatoid factor	Rheumatoid arthritis Viral arthritis Tuberculous arthritis Bacterial endocarditis Systemic lupus erythematosus Sarcoidosis Systemic vasculitis
Morning stiffness	Rheumatoid arthritis Polymyalgia rheumatica Still's disease Some viral and reactive arthritides
Symmetric small joint synovitis	Rheumatoid arthritis Systemic lupus erythematosus Viral arthritis
Leukocytosis (>15,000/mm³)	Bacterial arthritis Bacterial endocarditis Still's disease Systemic vasculitis Acute leukemia
Leukopenia	Systemic lupus erythematosus Viral arthritis
Episodic recurrences	Lyme disease Crystal-induced arthritis Inflammatory bowel disease Whipple's disease Mediterranean fever Still's disease Systemic lupus erythematosus

From Pinals RS: Polyarthritis and fever. N Engl J Med 330:769, 1999.

munoblastic lymphadenopathy.[170] Typical clinical features are lymphadenopathy, hepatosplenomegaly, rash, and hypergammaglobulinemia. It can resemble Still's disease in adults if the arthritis precedes other manifestations. Diagnosis is based on the characteristic appearance of a lymph node or skin biopsy specimen, which includes effacement of lymph node architecture, proliferation of small vessels, and a cellular infiltrate (immunoblasts, plasma cells, T lymphocytes, and histiocytes) within amorphous acidophilic interstitial material. It is believed that symptoms may be related to excessive production of IL-2 by helper T cells in this process.

Ankylosing Spondylitis, Seronegative Spondyloarthropathy, and Reactive Arthritis (Common)

Ankylosing spondylitis, seronegative spondyloarthropathy, and reactive arthritis are often referred to as the B27-associated diseases. The problem in differentiating them from RA arises with the patient (particularly a woman) who has minimal back pain and definite peripheral joint involvement. Indications against RA include noninvolvement of small joints, asymmetric joint disease, and lumbar spine involvement (see Chapter 70).

In some cases, the conclusion is inescapable that RA and ankylosing spondylitis are present in the same patient. In one series, nine patients with RF in serum had spinal ankylosis and symmetric erosive polyarthritis; eight of the nine carried HLA-B27.[171] If these two diseases occur completely independently of each other, simultaneous appearance in the same patient should occur once in every 50,000 to 200,000 adults.

In distinguishing patients with Reiter's syndrome from those with RA, a careful search for heel pain or tenderness and ocular or urethral symptoms is of great importance. Polyarthritis persists chronically in more than 80 percent of patients with Reiter's syndrome. The characteristics of enthesopathy in patients with Reiter's syndrome (i.e., "sausage" digits indicating periarticular soft tissue inflammation, insertional tendinitis, periostitis, and peri-insertional osteoporosis or erosions) may point to the diagnosis.

The differential diagnosis between RA with psoriasis and psoriatic arthritis may be artificial (see Chapter 72). Some patients with DIP joint involvement and severe skin involvement obviously have a disease that is not RA. Others, however, have a seropositive symmetric polyarthritis that appears to be RA, yet they also have psoriasis. These patients can be treated with the same disease-modifying drugs as those with progressive RA, including TNF-α inhibitors

A syndrome described extensively in the French literature, acne pustulosis hyperostosis osteitis,[172] may resemble psoriatic arthritis and, occasionally, when peripheral arthritis is present, RA. As the name implies, these patients variably express severe acne, palmar and plantar pustules, hyperostotic reactions (particularly in the clavicles and sternum), sacroiliitis, and peripheral inflammatory arthritis.

Inflammatory bowel disease (ulcerative colitis and Crohn's disease) is associated with arthritis in 20 percent of cases (see Chapter 73). Peripheral arthritis occurs more commonly than spondylitis in many series.[173] Ankles, knees, and elbows are the most typically involved peripheral joints, with PIP joints and wrists next in frequency. Simultaneous attacks of arthritis and the development of erythema nodosum are not uncommon. Only two or three joints are affected at once. Involvement is usually asymmetric, and erosions are uncommon. The occurrence of peripheral arthritis in inflammatory bowel disease is not related to HLA-B27.

Behçet's syndrome is marked by asymmetric polyarthritis in 50 to 60 percent of cases (see Chapter 86).[174] It is rare, with a prevalence of less than 1 in 25,000 in the United States. In more than half the cases, the attacks of arthritis are monarticular. Knees, ankles, and wrists are affected most often; synovial fluid usually contains more than 5000 but less than 30,000 WBC/mm^3. Joint deformity is unusual. Painful oral and genital ulcers and central nervous system involvement are characteristic. Uveal tract involvement in Behçet's syndrome must be differentiated from the scleritis characteristic of RA in patients with ocular and joint disease.

Enteric infections are complicated occasionally by inflammatory joint disease resembling RA. The joint disease associated with *Yersinia enterocolitica* infections occurs several weeks after the gastrointestinal illness.[175] Knees and ankles are the joints most commonly involved, and the majority of patients (even those with peripheral arthritis and no spondylitis) have HLA-B27. Reactive arthritis also has been reported after salmonella, shigella, and *Campylobacter (Helicobacter) jejuni* infection.

Arthropathy may precede other findings of Whipple's disease (see Chapter 73). The pattern is that of a migratory poly- or oligoarthritis involving ankles, knees, shoulders, elbows, and fingers, as with inflammatory bowel disease. Remission may occur when diarrhea begins. Joint destruction in Whipple's disease is rare, presumably because the synovitis lacks sustained chronicity.

Arthritis Associated with Oral Contraceptives (Uncommon)

A syndrome of persistent arthralgias, myalgias, and morning stiffness with occasional development of polyarticular synovitis has been described in women, usually in their twenties, who have been taking oral contraceptives (estrogens and progestins). Positive tests for antinuclear antibody are common, and patients may have circulating RF. Symptoms resolve after the contraceptive therapy is discontinued.

Arthritis of Thyroid Disease (Uncommon)

In hypothyroidism (see Chapter 109), synovial effusions and synovial thickening that simulate RA have been described.[176] The ESR may be elevated because of hypergammaglobulinemia, but the CRP is normal. The joint fluid is noninflammatory and may have increased viscosity. Knees, wrists, hands, and feet are involved most often, and coexisting calcium pyrophosphate dihydrate (CPPD) deposition disease is not infrequently found.

The syndrome of thyroid acropachy complicates less than 1 percent of cases of hyperthyroidism. This represents periosteal new bone formation, which may be associated with a low-grade synovitis similar to hypertrophic osteoarthropathy. Patients with coexisting RA and hyperthyroidism have pain from their arthritis that, although impossible to quantify, appears to exceed that expected from the degree of inflammation.

Bacterial Endocarditis (Uncommon)

Arthralgias, arthritis, and myalgias occur in approximately 30 percent of patients with subacute bacterial endocarditis.[177] Symptoms typically occur in one or several joints, usually large, proximal ones. This synovitis is probably caused by the deposition of circulating immune complexes. Confusion with RA may arise because more than half the patients with endocarditis are seropositive for RF. Fever out of proportion to joint findings in the setting of leukocytosis should lead to a consideration of infective endocarditis as a diagnostic possibility, even in the absence of a significant heart murmur. Peripheral emboli with digital infarctions may be found, simulating palpable purpura when they occur on the lower legs. It is wise to obtain blood cultures in all patients with polyarthritis and significant fever. Embolic phenomena with constitutional symptoms, including arthralgias, can be presenting symptoms of atrial myxoma, but this process usually mimics systemic vasculitis or subacute bacterial endocarditis more than it does RA.

Calcium Pyrophosphate Dihydrate Deposition Disease (Common)

CPPD deposition disease is a crystal-induced synovitis that takes many forms, ranging from a syndrome of indolent osteoarthrosis to that of an acute, hot joint. About 5 percent of patients have a chronic polyarthritis (sometimes referred to as pseudorheumatoid arthritis) associated with proliferative erosions of subchondral bone. Although radiographs are of great help when chondrocalcinosis is present, CPPD deposition may be present in the absence of calcification on radiographs.[178] Diagnosis then can be made only by arthrocentesis. One of the radiographic signs of CPPD deposition that helps to differentiate it from RA is the presence of unicompartmental disease in the wrists (see Chapter 88).

Diffuse Connective Tissue Disease: Systemic Lupus Erythematosus, Scleroderma, Dermatomyositis-Polymyositis, Vasculitis, Mixed Connective Tissue Disease (Common)

The entities constituting diffuse connective tissue disease, discussed in depth in other chapters, may begin with a syndrome of mild systemic symptoms and minimal polyarthritis involving the PIP and MCP joints, along with a "puffy hand syndrome." The following list contains rules of thumb for characterizing joint disease of the various entities:

1. In SLE, an organized synovitis that causes erosions is rare. Soft tissue and muscle inflammation may lead to reversible subluxation of the PIP and MCP joints with ulnar deviation.
2. Limitation of joint motion in scleroderma is due to taut skin bound to underlying fascia. The same holds for dermatomyositis and polymyositis; proliferative synovitis is rarely sustained in these processes.

3. In reports of mixed connective tissue disease (i.e., patients with arthralgias, arthritis, hand swelling, sclerodactyly, Raynaud's phenomenon, esophageal hypomotility, and myositis with circulating antibody to ribonucleoprotein), 60 to 70 percent of patients have arthritis. Although few have significant titers in serum of RF, many are given an initial diagnosis of RA. Numerous studies of mixed connective tissue disease have revealed deforming, erosive arthritis. In one series, for example, 8 of 17 patients had a presentation similar to that of RA.[179] Articular and periarticular osteopenia alone was found in eight. Six had a loss of joint space, and five had erosions typical of RA (see Chapter 78).

Calcific Periarthritis (Uncommon)

Although usually involving single joints, calcific periarthritis can be confused with polyarthritis. The skin is red over and around the affected joints; the tissues are boggy and tender, but no joint effusion is present. Passive motion is easier than active motion. Periarticular calcification is visible on radiographs. Unless the periarthritis can be differentiated from true arthritis, the findings may mimic those of palindromic rheumatism or early monarticular RA.

Chronic Fatigue Syndrome (Common)

Numerous physicians prefer to separate chronic fatigue syndrome from fibromyalgia because of the possibility that the former is caused by a slow virus infection (e.g., Epstein-Barr virus). However, because of the great overlap between the two, the best approach is to consider both as forms of "a diffuse pain and fatigue syndrome" and manage them in similar ways. The finding of true synovitis essentially rules out the diagnosis of both chronic fatigue syndrome and fibromyalgia (see Chapter 36).

Congenital Camptodactyly and Arthropathy (Rare)

Congenital camptodactyly and arthropathy is a deformity that begins in utero and produces synovial cell hypertrophy and hyperplasia without inflammatory cells.[180] Clinical manifestations include contractures of the fingers; flattening of the metacarpal heads; and short, thick femoral necks. This can present as oligoarticular seronegative RA.

Familial Mediterranean Fever (Uncommon)

The articular syndrome in familial Mediterranean fever is an episodic monarthritis or oligoarthritis of the large joints that appears in childhood or adolescence, mimicking oligoarthritic forms of juvenile RA. The disease is caused by a genetic abnormality due to a mutation in the pyrin gene, and 60 percent of reported cases have been in Sephardic Jews. Episodes of arthritis begin acutely with fever and other signs of inflammation (e.g., peritonitis or pleuritis) and can precede other manifestations of the disease. Although usually limited to days or weeks, attacks occasionally last for months and are associated with radiographic changes of periarticular osteopenia without erosions. The abdominal pain that

these patients experience can be a key to diagnosis. Amyloidosis (type AA) is a late complication of this syndrome in a number of patients. This and related forms of periodic inflammatory syndromes are discussed fully in Chapter 112).

Fibromyalgia (Common)

In fibromyalgia, there is no evidence of synovitis. Although no specific diagnostic tests define this entity, certain nonarticular locations of pain are common to different patients. In an analysis contrasting the pain properties with those of RA,[181] the fibromyalgia patients used diverse adjectives to describe their pain, the most common being pricking, pressing, shooting, gnawing, cramping, splitting, and crushing. A majority in both groups defined the pain as aching and exhausting. Evidence is accumulating that patients with diffuse connective tissue diseases, including RA, may develop a superimposed fibromyalgia, adding to the difficulty of treating the arthritis. Rheumatoid patients have fewer psychologic disturbances than patients with fibromyalgia, and RA patients who develop fibrositis score higher on testing scales for hypochondriasis, depression, and hysteria than those with RA who do not have fibrositis (see Chapter 36).

Glucocorticoid Withdrawal Syndrome (Common)

Often confused with RA are the symptoms of glucocorticoid withdrawal. Patients on glucocorticoid therapy who are being treated for nonrheumatic diseases may have diffuse polyarticular pain, particularly in the hands, if the glucocorticoid dose is tapered too rapidly.

Gout (Common)

Before a diagnosis of chronic erosive RA is made, chronic tophaceous gout must be ruled out. The reverse applies as well. Features of gouty arthritis that can mimic those of RA include polyarthritis, symmetric involvement, fusiform swelling of joints, subcutaneous nodules, and a subacute presentation of attacks. Conversely, certain aspects of RA that suggest gouty arthritis include hyperuricemia after treatment with low doses of aspirin, periarticular nodules, and seronegative disease (particularly in men).[182] Radiographic findings may be similar, with the appearance of the subcortical erosions of RA resembling small osseous tophi in gout. Although large asymmetric erosions with ballooning of the cortex are more likely to be caused by gout than by RA, this is not always the case. Serologic test results may be misleading as well; RF has been found in as many as 30 percent of patients with chronic tophaceous gout who have no clinical or radiographic signs of RA.[183]

Hemochromatosis (Uncommon)

The characteristic articular feature of hemochromatosis that is almost diagnostic is firm bony enlargement of the MCP joints, particularly the second and third, with associated cystic degenerative disease and large hook-like osteophytes on radiographs and, not infrequently, chondrocalcinosis. Marginal erosions, juxta-articular osteoporosis, synovial proliferation, and ulnar deviation are not seen in the arthropathy of hemochromatosis but are common in RA. Wrists, shoulders, elbows, hips, and knees are involved less often than the MCP joints. Arthritis leads the list of diagnoses provided to patients to explain their symptoms before their diagnosis of hemochromatosis.[184] In this series, persons with symptoms received a diagnosis of hemo-chromatosis only after the symptoms had been present, on average, for an extended period (10 years) and after visiting an average of 3.5 physicians (see Chapter 106).

Hemoglobinopathies (Uncommon)

In homozygous (SS) sickle cell disease, the most common arthropathy is associated with crisis and is believed to be a result of microvascular occlusion in articular tissues. However, in some cases, a destructive arthritis with a loss of articular cartilage that resembles severe RA has been reported.[185] In most patients with sickle cell disease and joint complaints, periosteal elevation, bone infarcts, fishmouth vertebrae, and avascular necrosis can be found on radiographs. In a series of 37 patients with SS disease, from which those with gout or avascular necrosis of the femoral head were excluded, 12 complained of a monarthritis or oligoarthritis associated with painful crises; tenderness was most marked over the epiphyses rather than the joint space, and synovial fluid was noninflammatory. Another 12 patients had arthritis of the ankle associated with a malleolar ulcer; this arthritis was chronic and resolved with improvement of the leg ulcer.[186] Episodic polyarthritis and noninflammatory synovial effusions are also found in sickle cell–β-thalassemia (see Chapter 108).

Hemophilic Arthropathy (Uncommon)

A deficiency of factor VIII or, less frequently, factor IX, sufficient to produce clinical bleeding frequently results in hemarthroses. The iron overload in the joint generates a proliferative synovitis that often leads to joint destruction. Because iron stimulates metalloproteinase production by synovial cells, when feasible, large hemarthroses should be aspirated and the joint immobilized and wrapped well. The clotting abnormality is rarely overlooked, however, and it is unlikely that a diagnosis of RA would be made in the setting of hemophilia A or B (see Chapter 107).

Human Immunodeficiency Virus Infection (Common)

Several types of arthropathy have been described in association with human immunodeficiency virus (HIV) infection[187]:

1. Brief, acute arthralgias concurrent with the initial HIV viremia
2. Acquired immunodeficiency syndrome (AIDS)-associated arthritis, lower extremity oligoarthritis, or a persistent polyarthritis[187]

3. Seronegative spondyloarthropathy, resembling Reiter's syndrome, psoriatic arthritis, or reactive arthritis, often more severe than in patients without HIV infection[188]

The importance of ruling out HIV in any patient with an acute polyarthritis and fever is crucial: HIV-positive patients do not do well on immunosuppressive drugs (see Chapter 101). HIV-positive patients can also present with syndromes of vasculitis.

Hyperlipoproteinemia (Uncommon)

Achilles tendinitis and tenosynovitis can be presenting symptoms in familial type II hyperlipoproteinemia and may be accompanied by arthritis. Synovial fluid findings may resemble those of mild RA, and the tendon xanthomas may be mistaken for rheumatoid nodules or gouty tophi. Conversely, bilateral pseudoxanthomatous rheumatoid nodules have been described. The treatment of hyperlipoproteinemia with with "statins" may cause an acute or subacute muscular syndrome that resembles myositis or polymyalgia rheumatica more than RA (see Chapters 80 and 82).

Hypertrophic Osteoarthropathy (Uncommon)

Hypertrophic osteoarthropathy may present as oligoarthritis involving the knees, ankles, or wrists. The synovial inflammation accompanies periosteal new-bone formation that can be seen on radiographs. Correction of the inciting factor (e.g., cure of pneumonia in a child with cystic fibrosis) will likely alleviate the synovitis. The synovium is characterized primarily by an increased blood supply and synovial cell proliferation. Little infiltration by mononuclear cells is seen. Pain in the bones that increases when extremities are dependent is characteristic, although it is not always present. If clubbing is not present or is not noticed, this entity is easily confused with RA (see Chapter 110).

Idiopathic Hypereosinophilic Syndrome with Arthritis (Rare)

The poorly defined idiopathic hypereosinophilic syndrome often includes myalgias and arthralgias and evolves into a clinical picture of hepatomegaly with or without pericarditis, pulmonary hypertension, subcutaneous nodules, and cardiomyopathy. Synovitis, characterized by inflammatory joint fluid, is rarely erosive or deforming. The similarities between this and toxic oil syndrome and eosinophilia-myalgia syndrome, both of which are caused by the ingestion of toxic substances, suggest a basic hypersensitivity reaction.

Infectious Arthritis, Including Viral Causes (Common)

Bacterial sepsis may be superimposed on RA. Viral infections, however, may present as arthritis, with many characteristics of RA. Arthritis complicates rubella more often in adults than in children and may affect the small joints of the hands. Lymphocytes predominate in synovial effusions.

Arthritis often precedes jaundice in viral hepatitis and is associated with the presence of circulating hepatitis B surface antigen and hypocomplementemia. The surface antigen has been found in synovial tissues with the use of direct immunofluorescence, and this supports the concept that this synovitis is mediated by immune complexes.[189] A relatively acute onset of diffuse polyarthritis with small joint effusions and minimal synovial swelling, often accompanied by urticaria, should prompt the physician to obtain liver function tests in the patient with a history of exposure to hepatitis. With the onset of icterus, the arthritis usually resolves without a trace.

The increasing recognition of the RNA virus hepatitis C as a cause of joint complaints is related to the availability of specific serologic tests for this virus. About one third of individuals infected with hepatitis C virus will have arthralgias or arthritis, and in a Korean series, the prevalence of cryoglobulins (mean concentration of 9.8 g/liter) was 59 percent.[190] Such individuals can present with palmar tenosynovitis, small joint synovitis, carpal tunnel syndrome, and positive tests for RF. Other findings, including the mixed cryoglobulinemia syndrome, glomerulonephritis, and cutaneous vasculitis, round out the clinical spectrum of rheumatic complaints associated with this viral infection. Because exacerbation of hepatitis can be associated with both the use and the cessation of MTX therapy, a good case has been made for testing for hepatitis C in every patient with RA scheduled to be started on therapy with this drug.[191]

Fever, sore throat, and cervical adenopathy followed by symmetric polyarthritis are compatible with infection due to hepatitis B, rubella, adenovirus type 7, echovirus type 9, *Mycoplasma pneumoniae*, or Epstein-Barr virus, as well as acute rheumatic fever or adult-onset Still's disease.

In Japan, many more patients with RA have circulating antibodies against human T lymphotropic virus-1 (HTLV-1). Multiple nodules within tendon sheaths associated with inflammation resembling rheumatoid tenosynovitis have been described in a patient with HTLV-1 arthropathy.[192]

A chronic polyarthritis resembling RA has been described after serologic proof of parvovirus infection. Usually the process is self limited and does not progress to a destructive synovitis (see Chapter ***). Adults, often those involved in child care, present with a history of a viral-like illness, sometimes with desquamating finger involvement and a diffuse, red facial rash ("slapped cheeks") that is followed by arthralgias and synovitis.

Intermittent Hydrarthrosis (Common)

Intermittent hydrarthrosis is a syndrome of periodic attacks of benign synovitis in one or few joints, usually the knee, beginning in adolescence. The difference between this and oligoarticular juvenile RA or RA is one of degree, not kind. In contrast to palindromic rheumatism, in which acute synovitis may occur in different joints during successive attacks, the same joint or joints are affected during each attack in intermittent hydrarthrosis. Joint

destruction does not occur because there is no chronic, persistent, proliferative synovitis.

Lyme Disease (Common in Some Areas)

Lyme disease can closely simulate RA in adults or children because of its intermittent course with the development of chronic synovitis. A proliferative, erosive synovitis necessitating synovectomy has evolved in several cases. The histopathologic appearance of the proliferative synovium is not different from that of RA (see Chapter 99) and the Lyme synovial cells produce a similar excess of metalloproteinases.

Malignancy (Rare)

Direct involvement by cancer of synovium usually presents as a monarthritis. However, non-Hodgkin's lymphoma can present as seronegative polyarthritis without hepatomegaly or lymphadenopathy. Intravascular lymphoma can present as a symmetric polyarthritis.[193] In children, acute lymphocytic leukemia can present as a polyarticular arthritis. Paraneoplastic syndromes and others related to direct involvement with cancer are described in detail in Chapter 111.

Multicentric Reticulohistiocytosis (Rare)

Multicentric reticulohistiocytosis is particularly interesting because it causes severe arthritis mutilans with an opera-glass hand (main en lorgnette).[194] Other causes of arthritis mutilans are RA, psoriatic arthritis, erosive OA treated with glucocorticoids, and gout (after tophi are resorbed by treatment with allopurinol). The cell that effects damage to tissues is the multinucleate lipid-laden histiocyte, which appears to release degradative enzymes sufficient to destroy connective tissue. These cells in aggregates produce multiple small nodules around joints of the hands.

Osteoarthritis (Common)

Although OA begins as a degeneration of articular cartilage and RA begins as inflammation in the synovium, each process approaches the other as the diseases progress (Table 66–7). In OA, as cartilage deteriorates and joint congruence is altered and stressed, a reactive synovitis often develops. Conversely, as the rheumatoid pannus erodes cartilage, secondary osteoarthritic changes in bone and cartilage develop. In end stages of both degenerative joint disease and RA, the involved joints appear the same. Therefore, to differentiate clearly between the two, the physician must delve into the early history and functional abnormalities of the disease.

Erosive OA occurs frequently in middle-aged women (more frequently than in men) and is characterized by inflammatory changes in PIP joints with destruction and functional ankylosis of the joints. The PIP joints can be red and hot, yet there is almost no synovial proliferation or effusion; joint swelling involves hard, bony tissue and not synovium. The ESR may be slightly elevated, but RF is not found[134] (see Chapter 92).

TABLE 66–7 · FACTORS USEFUL FOR DIFFERENTIATING EARLY RHEUMATOID ARTHRITIS FROM OSTEOARTHROSIS (OSTEOARTHRITIS)

	Rheumatoid Arthritis	Osteoarthritis
Age at onset	Childhood and adults, peak incidence in 50s	Increases with age
Predisposing factors	HLA-DR4, -DR1	Trauma, congenital abnormalities (e.g., shallow acetabulum)
Symptoms, early	Morning stiffness	Pain increases through the day and with use
Joints involved	Metacarpophalangeal joints, wrists, proximal interphalangeal joints most often; distal interphalangeal joints almost never	Distal interphalangeal joints (Heberden's nodes), weight-bearing joints (hips, knees)
Physical findings	Soft tissue swelling, warmth	Bony osteophytes, minimal soft tissue swelling early
Radiologic findings	Periarticular osteopenia, marginal erosions	Subchondral sclerosis, osteophytes
Laboratory findings	Increased erythrocyte sedimentation rate, rheumatoid factor, anemia, leukocytosis	Normal

Parkinson's Disease (Common)

Although the tremor or rigidity of Parkinson's disease is rarely confused with symptoms of RA, Parkinson's patients have a predilection for developing swan neck deformities of the hands, a phenomenon generally unappreciated by rheumatologists. This abnormality was first described in 1864,[195] and its pathogenesis is still unknown (Fig. 66–8).

Pigmented Villonodular Synovitis (Rare)

Pigmented villonodular synovitis is a nonmalignant but proliferative disease of synovial tissue that has many functional characteristics similar to those of RA and usually involves only one joint. The histopathologic appearance is characterized by proliferation of histiocytes, multinucleate giant cells, and hemosiderin and lipid-laden macrophages. Clinically, this is a relatively painless chronic synovitis (most often of the knee) with joint effusions and greatly thickened synovium. Subchondral bone cysts and cartilage erosion may be associated with the bulky tissue. It is not clear whether this should be classified as an inflammation or a neoplasm of synovium (see Chapter 113).

Polychondritis (Uncommon)

Polychondritis can mimic infectious processes, vasculitis, granulomatous disease, or RA. Patients with RA and ocular inflammation (e.g., scleritis) usually have active joint disease before ocular problems develop; the reverse is true in polychondritis. In addition, polychondritis is not associated with RF. The joint disease is usually episodic. Nevertheless, erosions can develop that are not unlike those of RA. In affected tissues of the external ears, nose, larynx, trachea, and costochondral areas, this disease may represent a true immune response against cartilage (see Chapter 94).

Polymyalgia Rheumatica and Giant Cell Arteritis (Common)

Although joint radionuclide imaging studies have indicated increased vascular flow in the synovium of patients with classic polymyalgia rheumatica (PMR), it remains appropriate to exclude PMR as a diagnosis if significant synovitis (soft tissue proliferation or effusions) is detected. Otherwise, many patients who actually have RA would be diagnosed as having PMR and treated with potentially harmful doses of glucocorticoids. A careful history can usually differentiate shoulder or hip-girdle muscle pain from shoulder or hip joint pain. Examination of synovial biopsy specimens from PMR patients indicates that the synovitis is much

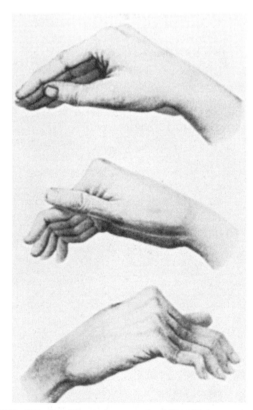

FIGURE 66–8 · These swan neck deformities are a result of Parkinson's disease, not rheumatoid arthritis (RA). (From Ordenstein L: Sur la Paralysie Agitante et la Sclérose en Plaques Generalisée. Paris, Imprimerie de E Martinet, 1864.)

more mild than that found in RA. RA and PMR probably coexist in numerous patients, but careful descriptions of such patients are rare.

Several patients have been described whose initial symptom of giant cell arteritis was a peripheral polyarthritis clinically indistinguishable from RA.[196] In 19 such patients in a group of 522 with biopsy-proven giant cell arteritis, however, only three were positive for RF. The interval between the onsets of each set of symptoms was 3 years or less in 15 of the 19, which also suggests a relationship between the two (see Chapter 82), and it is known that patients with giant cell arteritis often have HLA-DR4 alleles.

Rheumatic Fever (Uncommon)

Rheumatic fever is much less common than it once was but still must be considered in adults with polyarthritis. In adults, the arthritis is the most prominent clinical finding of rheumatic fever; carditis is less common than in children, and erythema marginatum, subcutaneous nodules, and chorea are rare. The presentation is often that of an additive, symmetric, large joint polyarthritis (involving lower extremities in 85% of patients), developing within a week and associated with a severe tenosynovitis. This extremely painful process is often dramatically responsive to salicylates. Unlike Still's disease in the adult, rheumatic fever generally has no remittent or quotidian fevers and shows evidence of antecedent streptococcal infection. It also has a less protracted course than Still's disease. There are many similarities between rheumatic fever in adults and "reactive" postinfectious synovitis developing from *Shigella*, *Salmonella*, *Brucella*, *Neisseria*, or *Yersinia* infections. The latter processes do not respond well to salicylates, however. As rheumatic fever becomes less common, and as penicillin prophylaxis effectively prevents recurrence of the disease, Jaccoud's arthritis (chronic post–rheumatic fever arthritis) is now quite rare. This entity, described nicely by Bywaters in 1950,[197] results from severe and repeated bouts of rheumatic fever and synovitis, which stretches joint capsules and produces ulnar deformity of the hands without erosions. The same deformity can develop in SLE characterized by recurrent synovitis and soft tissue inflammation and in Parkinson's disease. Differentiating rheumatic fever from RA is particularly difficult when subcutaneous nodules are present with rheumatic fever).

Sarcoidosis (Uncommon)

The two most common forms of sarcoid arthritis are usually easily differentiated from RA. In the acute form with erythema nodosum and hilar adenopathy (Löfgren's syndrome), the articular complaints are usually related to periarthritis affecting large joints of the lower extremities. Differential diagnosis may be complicated because many of these patients have RF in serum. Joint erosions and proliferative synovitis do not occur in this form of sarcoidosis.

In chronic granulomatous sarcoidosis, cystlike areas of bone destruction, mottled rarefaction of bone, and a reticular pattern of bone destruction with a lacelike appearance on radiographs may simulate destructive RA. This form of sarcoidosis is often polyarticular, and biopsy of bone or synovium for diagnosis may be essential, because there is often no correlation between joint disease and clinical evidence for sarcoid involvement of other organ systems. Poncet's disease (tuberculous rheumatism) might actually represent granulomatous "idiopathic" arthritis (i.e., sarcoidosis)[198] (see Chapter 105).

Sweet's Syndrome (Rare)

Sweet's syndrome is also called acute febrile neutrophilic dermatosis. It has been described in adults, often following an influenza-like illness. The three major features are an acute illness with fever; leukocytosis; and raised, painful plaques on the skin that show neutrophilic infiltration of the dermis on biopsy. Joint disease occurs in 20 to 25 percent of cases and is characterized by acute, self-limited polyarthritis. Because of the skin lesions, Sweet's syndrome is confused with SLE, erythema nodosum, and erythema elevatum diutinum more often than with RA. It has been treated effectively with indomethacin and glucocorticoids.

Thiemann's Disease (Rare)

Thiemann's disease is a rare form of idiopathic vascular necrosis of the PIP joints of the hands with occasional involvement of other joints. Bony enlargement begins relatively painlessly, and the digits (one or more may be involved) become fixed in flexion. The primary lesion is in the region of the epiphysis and generally begins before puberty, distinguishing it from erosive OA, which it resembles radiographically. It is clearly a heritable disease, but the genetic factors have not been defined.

Whipple's Disease (Common)

Since the identification of the uncultured bacillus of Whipple's disease in 1992,[199] numerous proven cases of this process that resemble adult Still's disease, in particular, have been described. Eight times as many men as women develop Whipple's disease. Many have a low-grade, intermittent fever; 80 percent or more have arthralgias in large joints. Diarrhea, abdominal pain, and weight loss are more common than in Still's disease, but the Whipple patients do not have a characteristic skin rash.[200]

▌ Course of Disease: with and without Therapy

Epidemiologists have pointed out the multiple difficulties in attempting to establish a change in patterns of RA in different time periods or different communities. The best data suggest that patients currently admitted to the hospital for RA are likely to have fewer joint contractures and less ankylosis of peripheral joints at admission than patients admitted 20 years ago, whereas the prevalence of RF and subcutaneous nodules and the mean number of affected joints have, if anything, increased slightly.[201] These and other findings suggest that the disease is not changing, but that earlier, more effective treatment has perhaps diminished the morbidity. As with other chronic diseases, both physicians and patients are eager to know the prospects for remission and are anxious about the threat of severe morbidity or death.

There are now well-tested criteria for a clinical remission.[202] Six have yielded optimal discrimination (Table 66–9). Few patients achieve five of these six criteria, and most fail to achieve a true remission. It is probable that less than 25 percent of patients will achieve a true remission of disease during the first 5 years. There is a better chance of remission in men and in those older than 60 years.

With an increased number of effective therapies available, and more in phase 2 and 3 clinical trials, it becomes increasingly important for physicians to be able to determine which patients will be most at risk for progressive destructive disease, and which ones will have a more benign illness that is not erosive and responsive to moderate intervention. A clinical model to predict, at the first visit, three forms of arthritis outcome—self limiting, persistent nonerosive, and persistent erosive arthritis[167]—has been discussed in the previous section on diagnosis, but this must be subjected to more validation testing in the clinics. Cautionary data about this model have been published; a large study of patients in the Norfolk Arthritis Register (UK) has revealed that many patients with erosive disease develop their first erosions more than 2 years after the onset of disease.[203]

In addition to predicting which patients may or may not develop erosions, it is equally important to identify which patients who already have erosions are more likely to progress rapidly to joint destruction. One study of an inception cohort of patients newly presenting with inflammatory polyarthritis confirmed the fact that although the initial radiographic score is, as expected, a powerful predictor of subsequent radiographic damage, a high titer of RF continues to be a powerful predictor of deteriorating radiographic damage in subjects receiving conventional therapy.[204]

Using a measure of both limited motion and joint deformity, a good correlation was found in one study with the C-reactive protein and also with DQB1*301 and DR4 alleles.[205] In the current days of emphasizing cost cutting in health care, it is interesting to note that in one study an instrument that listed the number of deformed joints (the NJD) was found to correlate well with the Sharp score of radiographic damage, although not with most functional assays.[206]

It is important to emphasize that joint erosions and deformity may not be the most important aspects of disease to the patients, and it has been demonstrated in several studies that the Health Assessment Questionnaire (HAQ) is an excellent predictor of both work disability and mortality[207] and is discrepant from damage measured by radiographs and from HLA-DR4 genes.

In future years, with proteomics and proteopharmacology helping to identify subsets of patients who are at very high risk of developing aggressively destructive disease, it will become important to learn the most about what is happening, biochemically and immunologically, in the synovium. Serial small joint arthroscopic biopsies, as well as using the same procedure on the knee, will become more routine, and it is probable that what is found in the synovium of one joint is representative of that in other inflamed joints.[208] It seems apparent that combinations of the following baseline parameters: swollen joints, RF (or, more recently, anticitrullated peptides), the presence of erosions at baseline, and the HAQ, can be used effectively in predicting disability, in the long term, of rheumatoid patients.[209]

MORTALITY

In well-established RA, the median life expectancy is less than in control populations.[210,211] In one study, a 25-year prospective follow-up of 208 patients, the median life expectancy was shortened by 7 years in males and 3 years in females. Infection, renal disease, and respiratory failure have traditionally been the primary factors contributing to excess mortality in RA patients. One study published in 1990 revealed that of 100 patients with RA followed for 25 years, 63 had died—an excess mortality of approximately 40 percent.[212] Although it is apparent that disability develops most rapidly during the first 2 years of RA,[213,214] the current focus of interest is on this increased mortality.

Careful epidemiologic studies have indicated that, in addition to infection and gastrointestinal hemorrhage secondary to NSAIDs, cardiovascular mortality is increased in RA. In the Norfolk Arthritis Register, a primary care–based inception cohort, patients who were seropositive for RF died within the first 7 years of disease at an excess rate from cardiovascular causes (men 1.34, women 2.02) of controls.[215] This increased incidence of cardiovascular events in RA patients is independent of traditional risk factors, such as age, sex, smoking status, diabetes mellitus, hypercholesterolemia, systolic blood pressure, and body mass index.[216] The generally accepted explanation for this is that inflammatory cytokines that are produced in excess in RA (e.g., TNF-α, platelet-derived growth factor [PDGF]) have the capacity to activate endothelial and subendothelial myofibroblasts, and numerous inflammatory cells are found in atheromatous plaques. Considering that nonrheumatoid patients who have higher levels of CRP than control groups have higher incidences of coronary disease, these data are consistent with hypotheses. Ultrasonography has shown that RA patients have greater thickness of both the common carotid and femoral arteries than do healthy controls, a finding that was independent of glucocorticoid therapy but related to the duration and severity of RA.[217] Platelet-derived microparticles, the small vesicles that are released from the plasma membrane when these cells are activated, are elevated in RA in proportion to disease activity.[218] It has been suggested that all of the following factors and pathobiologic mechanisms could contribute to atherosclerosis in RA[219]:

- Immune complex–mediated endothelial damage
- Acute-phase reactants (C-reactive protein and serum amyloid A, both of which have proinflammatory activity)
- Inflammatory cytokines
- Upregulation of endothelial cell leukocyte adhesion molecules
- Medications (e.g., steroids and MTX)
- Prothrombotic factors (e.g., increased platelets, fibrinogen, and thromboxane)
- Endothelial cell dysfunction induced by inflammation

It is becoming increasingly obvious that considerations of therapy in rheumatoid patients must factor in the effects on atherogenesis. These might include, in those patients with an unfavorable vascular profile, supplementation with Ω-3 fatty acids in the diet, early use of HMG-CoA reductase inhibitors ("statins" that, in addition to lipid-lowering effects, lower CRP), attempts to lower elevated levels of homocysteine induced by MTX, avoidance of cyclosporine, and certainly aggressive weight-loss disciplines and smoking cessation.

In addition to cardiovascular causes of death associated with RA are those due to the complications (both articular and extra-articular) of RA and to side effects of therapy. The probability of death varies directly with the severity of complications. Potentially morbid articular complications include the various forms of atlantoaxial subluxation, cricoarytenoid synovitis, and sepsis of involved joints. Extra-articular complications directly causing a higher mortality include Felty's syndrome, Sjögren's syndrome, pulmonary complications, and diffuse vasculitis.

One of the largest and best-documented studies of survival, prognosis, and causes of death in RA was published by Mitchell and associates.[220] In this prospective study of 805 patients including 12 years of observation, 233 died during the course of the study; survivorship was only 50 percent of that in population controls. The increased mortality associated with RA is impressive and equals that of all patients with Hodgkin's disease, diabetes mellitus, or stroke (age adjusted). In another group of 107 patients followed for 8 years, each of whom had extra-articular disease or needed hospitalization for some aspect of the disease,[221] those with cutaneous ulcers, vasculitic rash, neuropathy, and scleritis had a higher mortality than those whose disease was confined to joints. Of great concern to all health care workers is the correlation of a lack of formal education with increased mortality in RA.[222]

VARIABLES RELATED TO PROGNOSIS

In attempting to sort out the relative roles of disease manifestations, compared to nondisease factors, in generating disability in RA, investigators have generated hypothetic models of the disablement process in RA using the demographic, sociocultural, and clinical characteristics of a consecutive cohort of RA patients.[223] Although their methods were unable to explain the dynamics of disability in 41 percent of cases, disease-related factors explained 33 percent, and nondisease

factors (e.g., depression and psychologic status, education) accounted for 26 percent of the disability.

Other studies have emphasized the following disease factors that correlate with a poorer prognosis and greater likelihood of joint destruction:

- Positive RF in serum[224,225]
- IgA RF[226]
- Rheumatoid nodules[227]
- Being a young woman
- Synovial fluid abnormalities[228]
- WBC count greater than 50,000/mm^3
- Synovial fluid acidosis

ASSESSMENT OF THE INDIVIDUAL PATIENT

Assessment of disease activity and its progression is different from prognosis. Prognosis extrapolates from a known set of indices (as noted earlier) and the degree of measured activity of disease to a prediction of the outcome. Assessment is the accurate evaluation of disease progression over time. Although the indices listed in the previous section are useful as a way to predict the outcome from one-time measurements, having three or more assessment measures provides the physician with a graph of progression in an individual patient that he or she can try to flatten out by therapy.[229] It is important that whatever assessment index is used, it be used for the first time early in the patient's disease so that values before a significant loss of function are recorded.

For most patients, a self-report questionnaire based on degrees of difficulty in performing activities of daily living correlates well with the joint count, radiographic score, acute-phase reactants, grip strength, walking time, functional class estimates, and global self-assessment. One useful self-report includes only eight items from the much longer Stanford Health Assessment Questionnaire[230] (Table 66–8). The limitation of this form, failure to detect clinical improvement in patients with relatively few impairments in activities of daily living, may be offset by its acceptability to patients within busy office practices.

There are situations in which more comprehensive joint counts are needed. These include points when large changes in drug therapy are about to be instituted and when patients are to undergo joint reconstruction by orthopedic or hand surgeons. The Thompson index[231] uses a relatively few number of joints and weights data from each joint to reflect the joint surface area, giving a better measure of the "burden of synovitis." Particularly inclusive, and appropriate for clinical trials, is the ACR core set of disease activity measures for RA clinical trials[232] (Table 66–9).

The choice of imaging techniques and measures remains a very important one in the assessment of the destructive lesions of RA. The inflammatory lesion in RA is reflected reasonably well by heat, pain, swelling, and tenderness. Joint destruction can occur with minimal inflammation, however. MRI provides a way to visualize pannus development and the loss of cartilage (see Chapter 51). It will be extraordinarily important for rheumatologists and radiologists to come to a consensus on cost-benefit analyses for MRI. For which patients is it appropriate to order this procedure?

TABLE 66–8 • ACTIVITIES OF DAILY LIVING AND VISUAL ANALOGUE QUESTIONNAIRE

A. How often is it PAINFUL for you to:	Never	Sometimes	Most of the Time	Always
I Dress yourself?	___	___	___	___
I Get in and out of bed?	___	___	___	___
I Lift a cup or glass to your lips?	___	___	___	___
I Walk outdoors on flat ground?	___	___	___	___
I Wash and dry your entire body?	___	___	___	___
I Bend down to pick up clothing from the floor?	___	___	___	___
I Turn faucets on or off?	___	___	___	___
I Get in and out of a car?	___	___	___	___

B. How much pain have you had in the PAST WEEK (mark the scale)

No pain _____ Pain as bad as it could be
0   100

From Callahan LF, Brooks RH, Summey JA, et al: Quantitative pain assessment for routine care of rheumatoid arthritis patients, using a pain scale based on activities of daily living and a visual analog pain scale. Arthritis Rheum 30:630, 1987.

TABLE 66–9 • WEIGHTED AND SELECTIVE INDEX FOR ACTIVITY OF SYNOVITIS

Joint	Weighted Factor (Related to Joint Surface Area)	Degree of Tenderness and Swelling (Scale: 0 to 3)	= Joint Score
Elbow			
R	48	___	___
L	48	___	___
Wrist			
R	32	___	___
L	32	___	___
MCP (separately)			
R	5	___	___
L	5	___	___
PIP (separately)			
R	5	___	___
L	5	___	___
Knee			
R	95	___	___
L	95	___	___
Ankle (mortise)			
R	32	___	___
L	32	___	___
1st MTP			
R	8	___	___
L	8	___	___
2nd to 5th MTP (separately)			
R	5	___	___
L	5	___	___
	TOTAL	___	___

From Thompson PW, Silman A, Kirwan JR, et al: Articular indices of joint inflammation in rheumatoid arthritis. Arthritis Rheum 30:618, 1987.

In each patient, when the diagnosis of RA is reasonably certain, these measures of assessment and estimates of prognosis should be recorded. They should be major determinants of what therapies are instituted. Therapy is discussed in the following chapter.

REFERENCES

1. Soranus of Ephesus: On Acute Diseases and on Chronic Diseases. Translated into Latin by Caelius Aurelianus (5th century). English translation by IE Drabkin. Chicago, University of Chicago Press, 1950.
2. Garrod A: A Treatise on Gout and Rheumatic Gout. London, Longman Green, 1876.
3. Storey GO, Comer M, Scott DL: Chronic arthritis before 1876: early British cases suggesting rheumatoid arthritis. Ann Rheum Dis 53:557, 1994.
4. Rothschild BM, Turner KR, DeLuca MA: Symmetrical erosive peripheral polyarthritis in the late Archaic period of Alabama. Science 241:1498, 1988.
5. Yelin E, Wanke LA: An assessment of the annual and long-term direct costs of rheumatoid arthritis. Arthritis Rheum 42:1209, 1999.
6. Wolfe AM: The epidemiology of rheumatoid arthritis: a review. I. Surveys. Bull Rheum Dis 19:518-523, 1968.
7. Engel A, Roberts J, Burch TA: Rheumatoid arthritis in adults in the United States, 1960-1962. In Vital and Health Statistics, Series 11, Data from the National Health Survey, Number 17. Washington, DC, National Center for Health Statistics, 1966, pp ***.
8. Mikkelsen WM, Dodge HJ, Duff IF, et al: Estimates of the prevalence of rheumatic disease in the population of Tecumseh, Michigan, 1959-1960. J Chronic Dis 20:351-369, 1967.

9. O'Brien WM, Bennet PH, Burch TA, et al: A genetic study of rheumatoid arthritis and rheumatoid factor in Blackfeet and Pima Indians. Arthritis Rheum 10:163-179, 1967.

10. Wood WJ, Kato H, Johnson KG, et al: Rheumatoid arthritis in Hiroshima and Nagasaki, Japan. Arthritis Rheum 10:21, 1967.

11. Gabriel SE, Crowson CS, O'Fallon WM: The epidemiology of rheumatoid arthritis in Rochester Minn, 1955-1985. Arthritis Rheum 1989; 32: Abst 1950.

12. Linos A, Worthington JW, O'Fallon WM, et al: The epidemiology of rheumatoid arthritis in Rochester, Minnesota: a study of incidence, prevalence and mortality. Am J Epidemiol 111:87, 1980.

13. Doran MF, Pond GR, Crowson CS, et al: Trends in incidence and mortality in rheumatoid arthritis in Rochester, Minnesota, over a forty-year period. Arthritis Rheum. 46:625-631, 2002.

14. Silman AJ: The changing face of rheumatoid arthritis: why the decline in incidence. Arthritis Rheum 46:579-581, 2002.

15. Peschken CA, El-gabalawy HS, Roos LL, et al: Algonkian Indians have twice the frequency of rheumatoid arthritis with a younger age of onset. Arthritis Rheum 1998, 41: supplement 9 Abst #558.

16. Enzer I, Dunn G, Jacobsson L: An epidemiologic study of trends in prevalence of rheumatoid factor seropositivity in Pima Indians. Arthritis Rheum 46:1729-1734, 2002.

17. Gaston JSH: Will the increasing prevalence of atopy have a favorable impact on rheumatoid arthritis? Ann Rheum Dis 57:265, 1998.

18. Yelin E, Wanke LA: An assessment of the annual and long-term direct costs of rheumatoid arthritis: the impact of poor function and functional decline. Arthritis Rheum 42:1209-1218, 1999.

19. Wong JB, Ramey DR, Singh G: Long-term morbidity, mortality and economics of rheumatoid arthritis. Arthritis Rheum 44: 2746-2749, 2001.

20. Moxley G: Variable-constant segment genotype of immunoglobulin kappa is associated with increased risk for rheumatoid arthritis. Arthritis Rheum 35:19, 1992.

21. Huizinga TWJ, Machold KP, Breedveld FC: Criteria for early rheumatoid arthritis: from Bayes' law revisited to new thoughts on pathogenesis. Arthritis Rheum 46:1155-1159, 2002.

22. Jawaheer D, Seldin MF, Amos CI: A genomewide screen in multiplex rheumatoid arathritis families suggests genetic overlap with other autoimmune diseases. Am J Hum Genet 68: 927-936, 2001.

23. Rose HM, Ragan C, Pearce E, et al: Differential agglutination of normal and sensitized sheep erythrocytes by sera of patients with rheumatoid arthritis. Proc Soc Exp Biol Med 68:1, 1948.

24. Waaler E: On the occurrence of a factor in human serum activating the specific agglutination of sheep blood corpuscles. Acta Pathol Microbiol Scand 17:172, 1940.

25. He X, Gorony JJ, Weyand CM: The repertoire of rheumatoid factor-producing cells in normal subjects and patients with rheumatoid arthritis. Arthritis Rheum 36:1061, 1993.

26. Vincent C, Nogueira L, Sebbag M, et al: Detection of antibodies to deiminated recombinant rat filaggrin by enzyme-linked immunosorbent assay: a highly effective test for the diagnosis of rheumatoid arthritis. Arthritis Rheum 46:2051-2058, 2002.

27. Jarvinen P, Aho K: Twin studies in rheumatic diseases. Semin Arthritis Rheum 24:19, 1994.

28. Silman AJ, MacGregor AJ, Thomson W, et al: Twin concordance rates for rheumatoid arthritis: a natonwide study. Br J Rheumatol 32:903, 1993.

29. Rigby AS, Silman AJ, Voelm L, et al: Investigating the HLA component in RA: an additive (dominant) mode of inheritance is rejected, a recessive mode is preferred. Genet Epidemiol 8:153, 1991.

30. Tuokko J, Nejentsev S, Luukkainen R, et al: HLA haplotype analysis in Finnish patients with rheumatoid arthritis. Arthritis Rheum 44:315-322, 2001.

31. Jawaheer D, Thomson W, MacGregor AJ, et al: "Homozygosity" for the HLA-DR shared epitope contributes the highest risk for rheumatoid arthritis concordance in identical twins. Arthritis Rheum 37:681, 1994.

32. Thomson W, Harrison B, Ollier B, et al: Quantifying the exact role of HLA-DRB1 alleles in susceptibility to inflammatory polyarthritis. Arthritis Rheum 42:757-762, 1999.

33. del Rincón ***, Battafarano DF, Arroyo RA, et al: Heterogeneity between men and women in the influence of the HLA-DRB1

34. Jones MA, Silman AJ, Whiting S, et al: Occurrence of rheumatoid arthritis is not increased in the first degree relatives of a population based inception cohort of inflammatory polyarthritis. Ann Rheum Dis 51:943, 1992.

shared epitope on the clinical expression of rheumatoid arthritis. Arthritis Rheum 46:1480-1488, 2002.

35. Masi AT, Feigenbaum SL, Chatterton RT: Hormonal and pregnancy relationships to rheumatoid arthritis: convergent effects with immunologic and microvascular systems. Semin Arthritis Rheum 25:1, 1995.

36. Weyand CM, Schmidt D, Wagner U, et al: The influence of sex on the phenotype of rheumatoid arthritis. Arthritis Rheum 41:817, 1998.

37. Spector TD, Hochberg MC: The protective effect of the oral contraceptive pill on rheumatoid arthritis: an overview of the analytic epidemiological studies using meta-analysis. J Clin Epidemiol 43:1221, 1990.

38. Van Zeben D, Hazes JMW, Vandenbroucke JP, et al: Diminished incidence of severe rheumatoid arthritis associated with oral contraceptive use. Arthritis Rheum 33:1462, 1990.

39. Jorgensen C, Picot MC, Bologna C, et al: Oral contraception, parity, breast feeding, and severity of rheumatoid arthritis. Ann Rheum Dis 55:94, 1996.

40. Nelson JL, Hughes KA, Smith AG, et al: Maternal-fetal disparity in HLA class II alloantigens and pregnancy-induced amelioration of rheumatoid arthritis. N Engl J Med 329:466, 1993.

41. Hazes JMW, Dijkmans BAC, Vandenbroucke JP, et al: Pregnancy and the risk of developing rheumatoid arthritis. Arthritis Rheum 33:1770, 1990.

42. Silman A, Kay A, Brennan P: Timing of pregnancy in relation to the onset of rheumatoid arthritis. Arthritis Rheum 35:152, 1992.

43. Nelson JL, Voigt LF, Koepsell TD, et al: Pregnancy outcome in women with rheumatoid arthritis before disease onset. J Rheumatol 19:18, 1992.

44. Pincus T, Callahan LF: Formal education as a marker for increased mortality and morbidity in rheumatoid arthritis. J Chron Dis 38:973, 1985.

45. Vlieland TPMV, Buitenhuis MA, van Zeben D, et al: Sociodemographic factors and the outcome of rheumatoid arthritis in young women. Ann Rheum Dis 53:803, 1994.

46. Callahan LF, Pincus T: Formal education level as a significant marker of clinical status in rheumatoid arthritis. Arthritis Rheum 31:1346, 1988.

47. Karlson EW, Lee M, Cook MR, et al: A retrospective cohort study of cigarette smoking and risk of rheumatoid arthritis in female health professionals. Arthritis Rheum 42:910, 1999.

48. Mattey DL, Hutchinson D, Dawes PT, et al: Smoking and disease severity in rheumatoid arthritis. Arthritis Rheum 46:640-646, 2002.

49. Criswell LA, Merlino LA, Cerhan JR, et al: Cigarette smoking and the risk of rheumatoid arthritis among postmenopausal women: results from the Iowa Women's Health Study. Am J Med 112:465-471, 2002.

50. Mikuls TR, Cerhan JR, Criswell LA: Coffee, tea, and caffeine consumption and risk of rheumatoid arthritis. Arthritis Rheum 46:83-91, 2002

51. Wallace DJ, Klinenberg JR, Morham D, et al: Coexistent gout and rheumatoid arthritis: case report and literature review. Arthritis Rheum 22:81-86, 1979.

52. Janowsky EC, Kupper LL, Hulka BS: Meta-analyses of the relation between silicone breast implants and the risk of connective-tissue diseases. New Engl J Med 342:781, 2000.

53. Miller AS III, Willard V, Kline K: Absence of longitudinal changes in rheumatologic parameters after silicone breast implantation: a prospective 13-year study. Plast Reconstr Surg 102:2299, 1998.

54. Shirakawa T, Enomoto T, Shimazu S: The inverse association between tuberculin responses and atopic disorder. Science 275:77, 1997.

55. Verhoef CM, van Roon JAG, Vianen ME: Mutual antagonism of rheumatoid arthritis and hay fever: a role for type 1/type 2 T cell balance. Ann Rheum Dis 57:275, 1998.

56. Jacoby RK, Jayson MI, Cosh JA: Onset, early stages, and prognosis of rheumatoid arthritis: a clinical study of 100 patients with 11-year follow-up. BMJ 2:96-100, 1973.

57. Aho K, Palosuo T, Raunio V, et al: When does rheumatoid disease start? Arthritis Rheum 28:485-489, 1985.

58. Fleming A, Crown JM, Corbett M: Early rheumatoid disease. 1. Onset. Ann Rheum Dis 35:357-360, 1976.

59. Fleming A, Benn RT, Corbett M, et al: Early rheumatoid disease. II. Patterns of joint involvement. Ann Rheum Dis 35:361-364, 1976.

60. Mens JM: Correlation of joint involvement in rheumatoid arthritis and in ankylosing spondylitis with the synovial: cartilaginous surface ratio of various joints [letter]. Arthritis Rheum 30:359-360, 1987.

61. Bywaters EGL: Still's disease in the adult. Ann Rheum Dis 30:121-133, 1971.

62. Van Reeth C, Le Moel G, Lasne Y: Serum ferritin and isoferritins are tools for diagnosis of active adult Still's disease. J Rheumatol 21:890, 1994.

63. Hoshino T, Ohta A, Nakao M: TCR gamma delta+ T cells in peripheral blood of patients with adult Still's disease. J Rheumatol 23:124, 1996.

64. Yamaguchi M, Ohta A, Tsunematsu T, et al: Preliminary criteria for classification of adult Still's disease. J Rheumatol 19:424, 1992.

65. Elkon KB, Hughes GR, Bywaters EG, et al: Adult-onset Still's disease: twenty-year followup and further studies of patients with active disease. Arthritis Rheum 25:647-654, 1982.

66. Cush JJ, Medsger TA Jr., Christy WC, et al: Adult-onset Still's disease: clinical course and outcome. Arthritis Rheum 30:186-194, 1987.

67. Hench PS, Rosenberg EF: Palindromic rheumatism: new oft-recurring disease of joints (arthritis, periarthritis, para-arthritis) apparently producing no articular residues—report of 34 cases. Proc Mayo Clin 16:808, 1942.

68. Guerne P-A, Weisman MH: Palindromic rheumatism: part of or apart from the spectrum of rheumatoid arthritis. Am J Med 93:451-460, 1992.

69. Schumacher HR: Palindromic onset of rheumatoid arthritis: clinical, synovial fluid, and biopsy studies. Arthritis Rheum 25:361-369, 1982.

70. Youssef W, Yan A, Russell AS: Palindromic rheumatism: a response to chloroquine. J Rheumatol 18:35-37, 1991.

71. Yoghmai I, Rooholamini SM, Faunce HF: Unilateral rheumatoid arthritis: protective effects of neurologic deficits. Am J Roentgenol 128:299-301, 1977.

72. De Haas WHD, de Boer W, Griffioen F, et al: Rheumatoid arthritis of the robust reaction type. Ann Rheum Dis 33:81-85, 1974.

74. Glew KD, Watt I, Dieppe PA, et al: MRI of the cervical spine: rheumatoid arthritis compared with cervical spondylosis. Clin Radiol 44:71, 1991.

75. Smith PH, Benn RT, Sharp J: Natural history of rheumatoid cervical luxations. Ann Rheum Dis 31:431-439, 1972.

76. Collins DN, Barnes CL, FitzRandolph RL: Cervical spine instability in rheumatoid patients having total hip or knee arthroplasty. Clin Orthop 272:127-135, 1991.

77. Agarwal AK, Peppelman WC, Kraus DR, et al: Recurrence of cervical spine instability in rheumatoid arthritis following previous fusion: can disease progression be prevented by early surgery? J Rheumatol 19:1364-1370, 1992.

78. Goupille P, Fouquet B, Cotty P, et al: The temporomandibular joint in rheumatoid arthritis: correlations between clinical and computed tomography features. J Rheumatol 17:1285-1291, 1990.

79. Lawry GV, Finerman ML, Hanafee WN, et al: Laryngeal involvement in rheumatoid arthritis: a clinical, laryngoscopic, and computerized tomographic study. Arthritis Rheum 27:873-882, 1984.

80. Copeman WSC: Rheumatoid oto-arthritis. BMJ 2:1536, 1963.

81. Moffat DA, Ramsden RT, Rosenberg JN, et al: Otoadmittance measurements in patients with rheumatoid arthritis. J Laryngol Otol 91:917-927, 1977.

82. Ennevaara K: Painful shoulder joint in rheumatoid arthritis: a clinical and radiological study of 200 cases, with special reference to arthrography of the glenohumeral joint. Acta Rheumatol Scand 11:1-116, 1967.

83. Huston KA, Nelson AM, Hunder GG: Shoulder swelling in rheumatoid arthritis secondary to subacromial bursitis. Arthritis Rheum 21:145-147, 1978.

84. DeJager JP, Fleming A: Shoulder joint rupture and pseudothrombosis in rheumatoid arthritis. Ann Rheum Dis 43:503-504, 1984.

85. Hastings DE, Evans JA: Rheumatoid wrist deformities and their relation to ulnar drift. J Bone Joint Surg Am 57:930-934, 1975.

86. Martin LF, Bensen WG: An unusual synovial cyst in rheumatoid arthritis. J Rheumatol 14:139-141, 1987.

87. Trentham DE, Masi AT: Carpometacarpal ratio: a new quantitative measure of radiologic progression of wrist involvement in rheumatoid arthritis. Arthritis Rheum 19:939-944, 1976.

88. Alarcon GS, Koopman WJ: The carpometacarpal ratio: a useful method for assessing disease progression in rheumatoid arthritis. J Rheumatol 12:846-848, 1985.

89. Fuchs HA, Callahan LF, Kaye JJ, et al: Radiographic and joint count findings of the hand in rheumatoid arthritis: related and unrelated findings. Arthritis Rheum 31:44-51, 1988.

90. Brewerton DA: Hand deformities in rheumatoid disease. Ann Rheum Dis 16:183, 1957.

91. Abbott GT, Bucknall RC, Whitehouse GH: Osteoarthritis associated with distal interphalangeal joint involvement in rheumatoid arthritis. Skeletal Radiol 20:495-497, 1991.

92. Gray RG, Gottlieb NL: Hand flexor tenosynovitis in rheumatoid arthritis: prevalence, distribution, and associated rheumatic features. Arthritis Rheum 20:1003-1008, 1977.

93. Hastings DE, Parker SM: Protrusio acetabuli in rheumatoid arthritis. Clin Orthop 108:76-83, 1975.

94. Jayson MIV, Dixon A St J: Valvular mechanisms in juxta-articular cysts. Ann Rheum Dis 29:415-420, 1970.

95. Hench PK, Reid RT, Reames PM: Dissecting popliteal cyst stimulating thrombophlebitis. Ann Intern Med 64:1259-1264, 1966.

96. Kraag G, Thevathasan EM, Gordon DA, et al: The hemorrhagic crescent sign of acute synovial rupture (letter). Ann Intern Med 85:477-478, 1976.

97. Rask MR: Achilles tendon rupture owing to rheumatoid disease: case report with a nine-year follow-up. JAMA 239:435-436, 1978.

98. Vidigal E, Jacoby R, Dixon A St J, et al: The foot in chronic rheumatoid arthritis. Ann Rheum Dis 34:292-297, 1975.

99. Bienenstock H: Rheumatoid plantar synovial cysts. Ann Rheum Dis 34:98-99, 1975.

100. Calabro JJ: A critical evaluation of the diagnostic features of the feet in rheumatoid arthritis. Arthritis Rheum 5:19, 1962.

101. Clayton ML, Ries MD: Functional hallux rigidus in the rheumatoid foot. Clin Orthop 271:233-238, 1991.

102. Halla JT, Schrohenloher RE, Koopman WJ: Local immune responses in certain extra-articular manifestations of rheumatoid arthritis. Ann Rheum Dis 51:698-701, 1992.

103. Turesson C, O'Fallon WM, Crowson CS, et al: Occurrence of extraarticular disease manifestations is associated with excess mortality in a community based cohort of patients with rheumatoid arthritis. J Rheumatol 29:62-67, 2002.

104. Haugeberg G, Ørstavik RE, Uhlig T: Bone loss in patients with rheumatoid arthritis: results from a population-based cohort of 366 patients followed up for two years. Arthritis Rheum 46:1720-1728, 2002.

105. Manolagas SC, Weinstein RS: Perspective: New developments in the pathogenesis and treatment of steroid-induced osteoporosis. J Bone Mineral Res 14:1061-1066, 1999.

106. Laan RF, van Riel PL, van de Putte LB, et al: Low-dose prednisone induces rapid reversible axial bone loss in patients with rheumatoid arthritis: a randomized, controlled study. Ann Intern Med 119:963-968, 1993.

107. Kroot E-JJA, Nieuwenhuizen MG, de Waal Malefijt MC: Change in bone mineral density in patients with rheumatoid arthritis during the first decade of the disease. Arthritis Rheum 44:1254-1260, 2001.

108. Maddison PJ, Bacon PA: Vitamin D deficiency, spontaneous fractures and osteopenia in rheumatoid arthritis. BMJ 4:433-435, 1974.

109. Halla JT, Koopman WJ, Fallahi S, et al: Rheumatoid myositis: clinical and histologic features and possible pathogenesis. Arthritis Rheum 27:737-743, 1984.

110. Wolf P, Gretler J, Aglas F, et al: Anticardiolipin antibodies in rheumatoid arthritis; their relation to rheumatoid nodules and cutaneous vascular manifestations. Br J Dermatol 131:48-51, 1994.

111. Watson PG, Hayreh SS: Scleritis and episcleritis. Br J Ophthalmol 60:163-191, 1976.

112. Ziff M: The rheumatoid nodule. Arthritis Rheum 33:761-767, 1990.

113. Jackson CG, Chess RL, Ward JR: A case of rheumatoid nodule formation within the central nervous system and review of the literature. J Rheumatol 11:237-240, 1984.

114. Sokoloff L: The pathophysiology of peripheral blood vessels in collagen diseases. In Orbison JL, Smith DE (eds): The Peripheral Blood Vessels. Baltimore, Williams & Wilkins, 1963, p 297.

115. Mellbye OJ, Forre O, Mollnes TE, et al: Immunopathology of subcutaneous rheumatoid nodules. Ann Rheum Dis 50:909-912, 1991.

116. Wikaningrum R, Highton J, Parker A, et al: Pathogenic mechanisms in the rheumatoid nodule. Arthritis Rheum 41:1783, 1998.

117. Palmer DG, Hogg N, Highton J, et al: Macrophage migration and maturation within rheumatoid nodules. Arthritis Rheum 30:728-736, 1987.

118. Edwards JCW, Wilkinson LS, Pitsillides AA: Palisading cells of rheumatoid nodules: comparison with synovial intimal cells. Ann Rheum Dis 52:801-805, 1993.

119. Harris ED Jr: A collagenolytic system produced by primary cultures of rheumatoid nodule tissue. J Clin Invest 51:2973-2976, 1972.

120. Ginsberg MH, Genant HK, Yu TF, et al: Rheumatoid nodulosis: an unusual variant of rheumatoid disease. Arthritis Rheum 18:49-58, 1975.

121. Baum J: Infection in rheumatoid arthritis. Arthritis Rheum 14:135-137, 1971.

122. Huskisson EC, Hart FD: Severe, unusual and recurrent infections in rheumatoid arthritis. Ann Rheum Dis 31:118-121, 1972.

123. Singleton JD, West SG, Nordstrom DM: "Pseudoseptic" arthritis complicating rheumatoid arthritis: a report of six cases. J Rheumatol 18:1319-1322, 1991.

124. Doran MF, Crowson CS, Pond GR, et al: Frequency of infection in patients with rheumatoid arthritis compared with controls. Arthritis Rheum 46:2287-2293, 2002.

125. Doran MF, Crowson CS, Pond GR: Predictors of infection in rheumatoid arthritis. Arthritis Rheum 46:2294-2300, 2002

126. Cash JM, Klippel JH: Second-line drug therapy for rheumatoid arthritis. N Engl J Med 330:1368-1375, 1994.

127. Samet JM. Does idiopathic pulmonary fibrosis increase lung cancer risk? Am J Respir Crit Care Med 161:1-2, 2000.

128. Gridley G, McLaughlin JK, Ekbom A, et al: Incidence of cancer among patients with rheumatoid arthritis. J Natl Cancer Inst 85:307-311, 1993.

129. Gridley G, Klippel JH, Hoover RN, et al: Incidence of cancer among men with the Felty syndrome. Ann Intern Med 120:35-39, 1994.

130. Peeters HRM, Jongen-Lavrencic M, Raja AN, et al: Course and characteristics of anaemia in patients with rheumatoid arthritis of recent onset. Ann Rheum Dis 55:162, 1996.

131. Vreugdenhil G, Wognum AW, van Eijk HG, et al: Anaemia in rheumatoid arthritis: the role of iron, vitamin B_{12}, and folic acid deficiency, and erythropoietin responsiveness. Ann Rheum Dis 49:93-98, 1990.

132. Williams RA, Samson D, Tikerpae J, et al: In-vitro studies of ineffective erythropoiesis in rheumatoid arthritis. Am J Rheum Dis 41:502-507, 1982.

133. Reid CD, Prouse PJ, Baptista LC, et al: The mechanism of anaemia in rheumatoid arthritis: effects of bone marrow adherent cells and of serum on in vivo erythropoiesis. Br J Haematol 58:607-615, 1984.

134. Winchester RJ, Koffler D, Litwin SD, et al: Observations on the eosinophilia of certain patients with rheumatoid arthritis. Arthritis Rheum 14:650-665, 1971.

135. Farr M, Scott DL, Constable TJ, et al: Thrombocytosis of active rheumatoid disease. Ann Rheum Dis 42:545-549, 1983.

136. Bowman SJ, Sivakumaran M, Snowden N, et al: The large granular lymphocyte syndrome with rheumatoid arthritis: immunogenetic evidence for a broader definition of Felty's syndrome. Arthritis Rheum 37:1326-1330, 1994.

137. Combe B, Andary M, Caraux J, et al: Characterization of an expanded subpopulation of large granular lymphocytes in a patient with rheumatoid arthritis. Arthritis Rheum 29:672-679, 1986.

138. Loughran TP Jr: Clonal diseases of large granular lymphocytes. Blood 82:1-14, 1993.

139. Kelly C, Baird G, Foster H, et al: Prognostic significance of paraproteinaemia in rheumatoid arthritis. Ann Rheum Dis 50:290, 1991.

140. Voskuyl AE, Zwinderman AH, Westedt ML, et al: Factors associated with the development of vasculitis in rheumatoid arthritis: results of a case-control study. Ann Rheum Dis 55:190, 1996.

141. Fischer M, Mielke H, Glaefke S, et al: Generalized vasculopathy and finger blood flow abnormalities in rheumatoid arthritis. J Rheumatol 11:33-37, 1984.

142. Soter NA, Mihm MC Jr., Gigli I, et al: Two distinct cellular patterns in cutaneous necrotizing angiitis. J Invest Dermatol 66:344-350, 1976.

143. Mongan ES, Cass RM, Jacox RF, et al: A study of the relation of seronegative and seropositive rheumatoid arthritis to each other and to necrotizing vasculitis. Am J Med 47:23-25, 1969.

144. Weinstein A, Peters K, Brown D, et al: Metabolism of the third component of complement (C3) in patients with rheumatoid arthritis. Arthritis Rheum 15:49-56, 1972.

145. Conn DL, McDuffie FC, Dyck PJ: Immunopathologic study of sural nerves in rheumatoid arthritis. Arthritis Rheum 15:135-143, 1972.

146. Schmid FR, Cooper NS, Ziff M, et al: Arteritis in rheumatoid arthritis. Am J Med 30:56, 1961.

147. Markenson JA, McDougal JS, Tsairis P, et al: Rheumatoid meningitis: a localized immune process. Ann Intern Med 119:359, 1967.

148. Siomopoulus V, Shah N: Acute organic brain syndrome associated with rheumatoid arthritis. J Clin Psychol 40:46, 1979.

149. Geirsson AJ, Sturfelt G, Truedsson L: Clinical and serological features of severe vasculitis in rheumatoid arthritis: prognostic implications. Ann Rheum Dis 46:727-733, 1987.

150. Voskkuyl AE, Zwinderman AH, Westedt ML, et al: The mortality of rheumatoid vasculitis compared with rheumatoid arthritis. Arthritis Rheum 39:266, 1996.

151. Dodson WH, Hollingsworth JW: Pleural effusion in rheumatoid arthritis: impaired transport of glucose. N Engl J Med 275:1337-1342, 1966.

152. Frank ST, Weg JG, Harkleroad LE, et al: Pulmonary dysfunction in rheumatoid disease. Chest 63:27-34, 1973.

153. Tishler M, Grief J, Fireman E, et al: Bronchoalveolar lavage: a sensitive tool for early diagnosis of pulmonary involvement in rheumatoid arthritis. J Rheumatol 13:547-550, 1986.

154. Constantopoulos SH, Tsianos EV, Moutsopoulos HM: Pulmonary and gastrointestinal manifestations of Sjögren's syndrome. Rheum Dis Clin North Am 18:617-635, 1992.

155. Caplan A: Certain unusual radiographic appearances in the chest of coal miners suffering from RA. Thorax 8:29, 1953.

156. Shenberger KN, Schned AR, Taylor TH: Rheumatoid disease and bronchogenic carcinoma: case report and review of the literature. J Rheumatol 11:226-228, 1984.

157. Dawson JK, Goodson NG, Graham DR, et al: Raised pulmonary artery pressures measured with Doppler echocardiography in rheumatoid arthritis patients. Rheumatology 39:1320-1325, 2000.

158. Radoux V, Menard HA, Begin R, et al: Airways disease in rheumatoid arthritis patients: one element of a general exocrine dysfunction. Arthritis Rheum 30:249-259, 1987.

159. Sassoon CS, McAlpine SW, Tashkin DP, et al: Small airways function in non-smokers with rheumatoid arthritis. Arthritis Rheum 27:1218-1226, 1984.

160. Wislowska M, Sypula S, Kowalik I: Echocardiographic findings and 24-hour electrocardiographic Holter monitoring in patients with nodular and non-nodular rheumatoid arthritis. Rheumatol Int 18:163-169, 1999.

161. MacDonald WJ Jr., Crawford MH, Klippel JH, et al: Echocardiographic assessment of cardiac structure and function in patients with rheumatoid arthritis. Am J Med 63:890-896, 1977.

162. McRorie ER, Wright RA, Errington ML, et al: Rheumatoid constrictive pericarditis. Br J Rheumatol 36:100, 1997.

163. Iveson JM, Thadani U, Ionescu M, et al: Aortic valve incompetence and replacement in rheumatoid arthritis. Ann Rheum Dis 34:312-320, 1975.

164. Ahern M, Lever JV, Cosh J: Complete heart block in rheumatoid arthritis. Ann Rheum Dis 42:389-397, 1983.

165. Camilleri JP, Douglas-Jones AG, Pritchard MH: Rapidly progressive aortic valve incompetence in a patient with rheumatoid arthritis. Br J Rheumatol 30:379-381, 1991.

166. Saraux A, Berthelot JM, Gérald C, et al: Ability of the American College of Rheumatology 1987 criteria to predict rheumatoid arthritis in patients with early arthritis and classification of these patients two years later. Arthritis Rheum 44:2485-2491, 2001.

167. Visser H, le Cessie S, Vos K, et al: How to diagnose rheumatoid arthritis early: a prediction model for persistent (erosive) arthritis. Arthritis Rheum 46:357-365, 2002.

168. Hoffman GS: Polyarthritis: The differential diagnosis of rheumatoid arthritis. Semin Arthritis Rheum 8:115-141, 1978.

169. Pinals RS: Polyarthritis and fever. N Engl J Med 330:769-774, 1994.

170. Davies PG, Fordham JN: Arthritis and angioimmunoblastic lymphadenopathy. Ann Rheum Dis 42:516-518, 1983.

171. Fallet GH, Mason M, Berry H, et al: Rheumatoid arthritis and ankylosing spondylitis occurring together. BMJ 1:804-807, 1976.

172. Chamot AM, Benhamou CL, Kahn MF, et al: Le syndrome acne pustulose hyperostose osteite (SAPHO): —85 observations. Rev Rhum Mal Osteoartic 54:187-196, 1987.

173. McEwen C, Lingg C, Kirsner JB: Arthritis accompanying ulcerative colitis. Am J Med 33:923, 1962.

174. Zizic TM, Stevens MB: The arthropathy of Behçet's disease. Johns Hopkins Med J 136:243-250, 1975.

175. Ahvonen P, Sievers K, Ano K: Arthritis associated with *Yersinia enterocolitica* infection. Acta Rheumatol Scand 15:232-253, 1969.

176. Bland JH, Frymoyer JW: Rheumatic syndromes of myxedema. N Engl J Med 282:1171-1174, 1970.

177. Churchill MD Jr., Geraci JE, Hunder GG: Musculoskeletal manifestations of bacterial endocarditis. Ann Intern Med 87:754-759, 1977.

178. Utsinger PD, Zvaifler NJ, Resnick D: Calcium pyrophosphate dihydrate deposition disease without chondrocalcinosis. J Rheumatol 2:258-264, 1975.

179. Halla JT, Hardin JG: Clinical features of the arthritis of mixed connective tissue disease. Arthritis Rheum 21:497-503, 1978.

180. Martin JR, Huang SN, Lacson A, et al: Congenital contractural deformities of the fingers and arthropathy. Ann Rheum Dis 44:826-830, 1985.

181. Wolfe F, Cathey MA, Kleinkeksel SM, et al: Psychological status in primary fibrositis and fibrositis associated with rheumatoid arthritis. J Rheumatol 11:500-506, 1984.

182. Talbott JH, Altman RD, Yu TF: Gouty arthritis masquerading as rheumatoid arthritis or vice versa. Semin Arthritis Rheum 8: 77-114, 1978.

183. Kozin F, McCarty DJ: Rheumatoid factor in the serum of gouty patients. Arthritis Rheum 20:1559-1560, 1977.

184. McDonnell SM, Preston BL, Jewell SA, et al: A survey of 2851 patients with hemochromatosis: symptoms and response to treatment. Am J Med 106:621, 1999.

185. Schumacher HR, Dorwart BB, Bond J, et al: Chronic synovitis with early cartilage destruction in sickle cell disease. Ann Rheum Dis 36:413-419, 1977.

186. DeCeulaer K, Forbes M, Roper D, et al: Non-gouty arthritis in sickle cell disease: report of 37 consecutive cases. Ann Rheum Dis 43:599-603, 1984.

187. Calabrese LH: Human immunodeficiency virus infection and arthritis. Rheum Dis Clin North Am 19:477-488, 1993.

188. Solomon G, Brancato L, Winchester R: An approach to the human immunodeficiency virus-positive patient with a spondyloarthropathic disease. Rheum Dis Clin North Am 17:43-58, 1991.

189. Schumacher HR, Gall EP: Arthritis in acute hepatitis and chronic active hepatitis: pathology of the synovial membrane with evidence for the presence of Australia antigen in synovial membranes. Am J Med 57:655-664, 1974.

190. Lee YH, Ji JD, Yeon JE, et al: Cryoglobulinaemia and rheumatic manifestations in patients with hepatitis C virus infection. Ann Rheum Dis 57:728, 1998.

191. Kremer JM, Alarcon GS, Lightfoot RWJ, et al: Methotrexate for rheumatoid arthritis: suggested guidelines for monitoring liver toxicity. Arthritis Rheum 37:316, 1994.

192. Hasunuma T, Tadanobu M, Hoa TTM, et al: Tenosynovial nodulosis in a patient infected with human T cell lymphotropic virus I. Arthritis Rheum 40:578, 1997.

193. Von Kempis J, Kohler G, Herbst EW, et al: Intravascular lymphoma presenting as symmetric polyarthritis. Arthritis Rheum 41:1126, 1998.

194. Gold RH, Metzger AL, Mirra JM, et al: Multicentric reticulohistiocytosis (lipoid dermato-arthritis): an erosive polyarthritis with distinctive clinical, roentgenographic and pathological features. Am J Roentgenol 124:610-624, 1975.

195. Ordenstein L: Sur la Paralysie Agitante et la Sclérose en Plaques Generalisée. Paris, Imprimerie de E Martinet, 1864.

196. Ginsburg WW, Cohen MD, Hall SB, et al: Seronegative polyarthritis in giant cell arteritis. Arthritis Rheum 28:1362-1366, 1985.

197. Bywaters EGL: Relation between heart and joint disease including "rheumatoid heart disease" and chronic post-rheumatic arthritis (type Jaccoud). Br Heart J 12:101, 1950.

198. Poncet A: Address to the Congress Français de Chirurgie, 1897. Bull Acad Med Paris 46:194, 1901.

199. Relman DA, Schmidt TM, MacDermott RP, et al: Identification of the uncultured bacillus of Whipple's disease. N Engl J Med 372:293, 1992.

200. Knight SM, Symmons DPM: A man with intermittent fever and arthralgia. Ann Rheum Dis 57:711, 1998.

201. Valkenburg HA: Pattern of rheumatoid disease in society: change or disappearance? Scand J Rheumatol 5(Suppl 12):89-95, 1975.

202. Pinals RS, Masi AT, Larsen RA: Preliminary criteria for clinical remission in rheumatoid arthritis. Arthritis Rheum 24:1308-1315, 1981.

203. Bukhari M, Harrison B, Lunt M: Time to first occurrence of erosions in inflammatory polyarthritis. Arthritis Rheum 44: 1248-1253, 2001.

204. Bukhari M, Lunt M, Harrison BJ, et al: Rheumatoid factor is the major predictor of increasing severity of radiographic erosions in rheumatoid arthritis. Arthritis Rheum 46:906-912, 2002.

205. Cranney A, Goldstein R, Pham B, et al: A measure of limited joint motion and deformity correlates with HLA-DRB1 and DQB1 alleles in patients with rheumatoid arthritis. Ann Rheum Dis 58:703-708, 1999.

206. Orces CH, del Rincón I, Abel M, et al: The number of deformed joints as a surrogate measure of damage in rheumatoid arthritis. Arthritis Care Res 47:67-72, 2002.

207. Pincus T: Why should rheumatologists collect patient self-report questionnaires in routine rheumatologic care? Rheum Dis Clin North America 21:271-319, 1995.

208. Kraan MC, Reece RJ, Smeets TJM, et al: Comparison of synovial tissues from the knee joints and the small joints of rheumatoid arthritis patients. Arthritis Rheum 48:2034-2038, 1995.

209. Drossaers-Bakker KW, Zwinderman AH, Vlieland TPMV: Long-term outcome in rheumatoid arthritis: a simple algorithm of baseline parameters can predict radiographic damage, disability, and disease course at 12-year followup. Arthritis Care Res 47:383-390, 2002.

210. Pinals RS: Survival in rheumatoid arthritis. Arthritis Rheum 30:473-475, 1987.

211. Vandenbroucke JP, Hazevoet HM, Cats A: Survival and cause of death in rheumatoid arthritis: a 25-year prospective followup. J Rheumatol 11:158-161, 1984.

212. Reilly PA, Cosh JA, Maddison PJ, et al: Mortality and survival in rheumatoid arthritis: a 25-year prospective study of 100 patients. Ann Rheum Dis 49:363-369, 1990.

213. Sherrer YS, Block DA, Mitchell DM, et al: The development of disability in rheumatoid arthritis. Arthritis Rheum 29:494-500, 1986.

214. Kirwan JR: The relationship between synovitis and erosions in rheumatoid arthritis. Br J Rheumatol 36:225, 1997.

215. Goodson NJ, Wiles NJ, Lunt M, et al: Mortality in early inflammatory polyarthritis: cardiovascular mortality is increased in seropositive patients. Arthritis Rheum 46:2010-1019, 2002.

216. del Rincón I, Williams R, Stern MP, et al: High incidence of cardiovascular events in a rheumatoid arthritis cohort not explained by traditional cardiac risk factors. Arthritis Rheum 44:2737-2745, 2001.

217. Kumeda Y, Inaba M, Goto H, et al: Increased thickness of the arterial intima-media detected by ultrasonography in patients with rheumatoid arthritis. Arthritis Rheum 46:1489-1497, 2002.

218. Knijff-Dutmen EAJ, Koerts J, Nieuwland R, et al: Elevated levels of platelet microparticles are associated with disease activity in rheumatoid arthritis. Arthritis Rheum 46:1498-1503, 2002.

219. Van Doornum S, McColl G, Wicks IP: Accelerated atherosclerosis: an extraarticular feature of rheumatoid arthritis? Arthritis Rheum 46:862-873, 2002.

220. Mitchell DM, Spitz PW, Young DY, et al: Survival, prognosis, and causes of death in rheumatoid arthritis. Arthritis Rheum 29: 706-714, 1986.

221. Erhardt CC, Mumford PA, Venables PJ, et al: Factors predicting a poor life prognosis in rheumatoid arthritis: an eight-year prospective study. Ann Rheum Dis 48:7-13, 1989.

222. Pincus T, Callahan LF, Sale WG, et al: Severe functional declines, work disability, and increased mortality in seventy-five rheumatoid arthritis patients studied over nine years. Arthritis Rheum 27:864-872, 1984.

223. Escalante A, del Rincon I: How much disability in rheumatoid arthritis is explained by rheumatoid arthritis? Arthritis Rheum 42:1712-1721, 1999.

224. Kellgren JH, O'Brien WM: On the natural history of rheumatoid arthritis in relation to the sheep cell agglutination test (SCAT). Arthritis Rheum 5:115, 1962.

225. Masi AT, Maldonado-Cocco JA, Kaplan SB, et al: Prospective study of the early course of rheumatoid arthritis in young adults: comparison of patients with and without rheumatoid factor positivity at entry and identification of variables correlating with outcome. Semin Arthritis Rheum 4:299-326, 1976.

226. Withrington RH, Teitsson I, Valdimarsson H, et al: Prospective study of early rheumatoid arthritis. II. Association of rheumatoid factor isotypes with fluctuations in disease activity. Ann Rheum Dis 43:679-685, 1984.

227. Sharp JT, Calkins E, Cohen AS, et al: Observations on the clinical, chemical, and serological manifestations of rheumatoid arthritis, based on the course of 154 cases. Medicine 43:41, 1964.

228. Geborek P, Saxne T, Pettersson H, et al: Synovial fluid acidosis correlates with radiological joint destruction in rheumatoid arthritis knee joints. J Rheumatol 16:468-472, 1989.

229. Edworthy SM, Bloch DA, Brant RF, et al: Detecting treatment effects in patients with rheumatoid arthritis: the advantage of longitudinal data. J Rheumatol 20:40, 1993.

230. Pincus T, Callahan LF, Brooks RH, et al: Self-report questionnaire scores in rheumatoid arthritis compared with traditional physical, radiographic, and laboratory measures. Ann Intern Med 110:259, 1989.

231. Thompson PW, Silman A, Kirwan JR, et al: Articular indices of joint inflammation in rheumatoid arthritis. Arthritis Rheum 30: 618-625, 1987.

232. Felson DT, Anderson JJ, Boers M, et al: The American College of Rheumatology preliminary core set of disease activity measures for rheumatoid arthritis clinical trials. Arthritis Rheum 36:729, 1993.

67

Treatment of Rheumatoid Arthritis

MARK C. GENOVESE · EDWARD D. HARRIS, JR.

Since the mid 1990's have been major changes in the treatment and management of rheumatoid arthritis (RA). In general, approaches have been aimed at earlier identification of the disease, earlier intervention with disease-modifying antirheumatic drugs (DMARDs), aggressive dosing of existing medications, combination therapy, and the introduction of anticytokine therapies. This has resulted in the prospect of patients having their symptoms suppressed, their joints preserved from destruction, and their function improved. These prospects all come with the possibly of fewer side effects than were seen with older treatment regimens.

The evolution of the changes in the approach to treatment is based on the great progress investigators in many laboratories have made in understanding basic mechanisms that underlie the development of RA and its perpetuation within joints. In addition, sound epidemiologic studies have provided useful information on the factors that amplify disease in those who have it, and well-planned double-blind, placebo-controlled clinical trials have added the crucial ingredient of evidence-based therapy to physicians' strategies of care. Underlying better treatment regimens has been an awareness that in patients with established disease, loss of function and destruction of joints begin relatively early after the onset of synovitis.

The case for early intervention has been made using several lines of evidence:

1. Functional health status declines early, with mild functional loss as early as 1 year and moderate to severe functional losses by 6 years.[1] Subsequently, work disability also occurs, especially early in disease, with work disability estimated to occur in 25 percent of RA patients at 6.4 years and 50 percent at 20.9 years after disease onset.[2]
2. Mortality rates are increased in patients with RA. Mortality rate has been shown to rise over 5 to 20 years, with as high as 35 percent mortality by 20 years.[3] Morbidity and mortality rates in RA are predicted by, and are directly proportional to, clinical status. More severe and active disease has a poorer outcome.[4]
3. Radiographic changes develop early in disease.[5-7] Erosions of bone and narrowing of joint spaces develop within the first 2 years of disease in most patients and are progressive afterward over several decades.[8] The rate of progression of radiographic scores is rapid early in disease and appears to continue along a similar trajectory for the duration of the disease if left untreated. Once the proliferative

synovium has begun to invade and destroy articular cartilage, joints are at risk for irreversible destruction, even when disease activity decreases (Fig.67–1).
4. In terms of economic impact, early disease activity predicts long-term costs. Data suggest that long-term

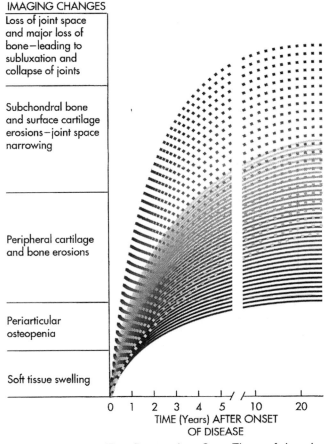

IMAGING CHANGES

Loss of joint space and major loss of bone—leading to subluxation and collapse of joints

Subchondral bone and surface cartilage erosions—joint space narrowing

Peripheral cartilage and bone erosions

Periarticular osteopenia

Soft tissue swelling

0 1 2 3 4 5 // 10 20
TIME (Years) AFTER ONSET OF DISEASE

FIGURE 67–1 · The Progression Over Time of Imaging Changes of Rheumatoid Joints. This figure emphasizes two major points about rheumatoid arthritis. One is that there is great variation in the degree of joint destruction among patients. Some (*solid black lines*) never develop more than periarticular osteopenia. Others, with sustained and aggressive disease, go on to destruction of cartilage, bone, and tendon (*dotted lines*). Others (*dotted/solid mix*) have erosions without complete joint destruction. The other point made by this figure is that the rate of destruction is greater in the first 2 years of disease than in later years. For this reason, it is essential that effective therapy be instituted early in hopes of altering the slope of the curves. Measurable determinants of the rate of progression include the mean erythrocyte sedimentation rate, joint count, Health Assessment Questionnaire results, pain, and a positive rheumatoid factor test. (Modified from Wolfe F, Sharp JT: Long term radiographic outcome of patients seen in the course of rheumatoid arthritis [Abstract No. 1056]. Arthritis Rheum 38 [Suppl 9]: 1995; used by permission.)

medical costs and outcomes are significantly associated with early changes in disabilty.[9] Further data would support the fact that persons with very poor function may experience direct medical costs 2.55 to 6.97 times as high as patients with relatively good function, with the majority of those costs coming from hospitalization.[10]

5. An interval of time may exist in which the introduction of DMARD therapy can result in a change in the natural course of disease—not just for a transient to short-lived time frame, but more fundamentally in the scope of the progression of the disease for a lifetime.[11] Data supporting this view have come from a number of trials looking at intervention in early RA. In the hydroxychloroquine in early RA (HERA) trial,[12] patients with RA were randomized to receive either hydroxychloroquine sulfate (HCQ) or placebo over a period of 36 weeks. At the conclusion of the study it was not surprising that those patients who had received HCQ had improvements in joint findings, pain, and physical function superior to what was seen in the placebo group. Of more interest, however, were the results seen after 3 years of follow-up of the original cohorts. Those patients who had therapy instituted early in the disease (the HCQ arm) versus those who had DMARD therapy delayed for 9 months (the placebo arm) continued to have significantly less pain and disability. These results could not be explained based on differences in glucocorticoid, DMARD, or nonsteroidal anti-inflammatory drug (NSAID) use subsequent to the trial and were attributed to the delay in the introduction of therapy.[13] However, the strongest support for this line of thinking stems from data from the COBRA Trial.[14] Patients were initially randomized to receive monotherapy with sulfasalasine or combination therapy in a step-down approach with sulfasalasine, methotrexate (MTX), and high-dose glucocorticoids. At the end of 28 weeks there appeared to be a significant advantage for the use of combination therapy based on clinical response, and at 1 year there was also less radiographic progression on the combination group. Of the greatest interest, however, is the 4-year follow-up data from this cohort. Those patients who had been treated with the initial 6-month cycle of intensive combination treatment had a sustained suppression of the rate of radiographic progression independent of subsequent antirheumatic therapy. Those patients initially treated with monotherapy had a change in Sharp score of 8.6 units/year, whereas those on the combination regimen progressed at only 5.6 units/year.[15] Thus, an interval of time may exist for intervention whereupon the outcome is a long-term change in the nature of the disease, irrespective of what type of therapy or intervention is used in the future.

Another element in the evolving optimism about treatment of RA has been the use of multiple agents in combination therapy, many of which are aimed at a different segment of the pathophysiologic processes within the synovium. Beginning with uncontrolled, but encouraging, results using combination therapy in the early 1980s,[16] it has been demonstrated more recently[17-21] that a combination of disease-modifying drugs provides additive, perhaps synergistic, benefit to patients without increasing toxicity.

The addition of newer therapeutic agents generated by recombinant or monoclonal antibody biotechnology has enhanced the concept and practice of combination therapy and has effectively exploited the promise of treatments that target certain inflammatory mediators believed to play an important role in both initiation and amplification of proliferative synovitis. As a class, the most effective of these to date has been the tumor necrosis factor (TNF) antagonists (e.g., adalimumab, etanercept, and infliximab). In refractory disease, the addition of adalimumab, etanercept, or infliximab to MTX treatment provides additional benefit to patients with persistent active disease.[19,20,22] With all three of the available TNF inhibitors, trials have demonstrated that more than 50 to 70 percent of the patients had at least a 20-percent response, and more than 40 percent of patients had a 50-percent improvement, as measured by the American College of Rheumatology (ACR) criteria.[23] Although each of the cohorts studied in these trials was slightly different, no significant side effects were apparent in the combination arms above and beyond what was seen in the MTX-only arms of the studies, suggesting a relatively good safety profile and strong benefit-to-risk ratio when put into perspective with the relative severity of the disease.

These studies have confirmed the rationale of using recombinant engineering to target crucial steps that have been identified by laboratory research in the pathogenesis of disease. In addition, they have raised the bar that defines efficacy in therapy. One caveat that must be applied to this class of agents is the relative cost of this approach (Table 67–1). At more than $15,000 per year, access to this type of therapy may be prohibitive for many patients and clearly affects prescribing patterns. The challenge to industry is clear: Develop drugs that are as safe and effective as the TNF inhibitors but less expensive.

This growing body of data lends credence to the belief that early identification and initiation of therapy in RA is appropriate and necessary to maximize the short- and long-term benefits to the patient. And although a unique opportunity for intervention may exist early in the course of disease, it is believed that DMARDs should be introduced at all stages of disease for long-term disease modification; whether that should occur as single therapy or as combination therapy is yet to be resolved. What has also become fundamentally clear is that even in later stages of disease, the use of DMARDs can reduce symptoms and signs, as well as improve function.[19,20,22]

In the years ahead, it will be increasingly important for both rheumatologists and primary care physicians treating patients with RA to demand rigorous confirmation of efficacy and safety by double-blind placebo-controlled studies of all new products. Physicians must be armed with data, because their patients will be coming at them armed with testimonies from the Internet

TABLE 67–1 • AVERAGE WHOLESALE PRICES OF THERAPY*

Medication	Cost Per Unit
Nonsteroidal Anti-inflammatory Drugs (NSAIDs)	
Rofecoxib	
12.5-mg tab	$2.64
25-mg tab	$2.64
50-mg tab	$3.85
Celecoxib	
100-mg tab	$1.57
200-mg tab	$2.64
Generic ibuprofen	
800-mg tab	$0.10
Disease-Modifying Antirheumatoid Drugs (DMARDs)	
Methotrexate	
2.5-mg tab	$1.26
Leflunomide	
10-mg tab	$9.08
20-mg tab	$9.08
Etanercept	
25-mg vial	$155.70
Adalimumab	
40-mg syringe	$653.30
Infliximab	
100-mg vial	$691.61
Anakinra	
100 mg syringe	$41.25

*Based on the average wholesale price in 2002 Redbook.

and convincing ads from television, newspapers, and magazines for many diverse drugs. Another issue will be finding suitable patients to enroll in studies of the most promising medications that are ready to move into phase II trials. Rheumatologists must take a leading role in making sure their patients have the chance to participate in studies of the most promising drugs and devices.

Readers of this chapter are encouraged to be familiar with material in previous chapters (see Chapters 56 to 66), which give thorough details of individual drugs, combination therapy, specific clinical trials, epidemiologic studies, clinical course and complications, indications for drug use, and toxicity. Additionally, the very helpful adjunctive therapy of surgery by experienced orthopedic surgeons, hand surgeons, and foot surgeons is discussed in detail in Chapters 115 and 116. In this chapter, emphasis will be placed on determining prognosis in individual patients and thereby arriving at the best treatment plan for individual patients.

Estimating Prognosis and Choosing Appropriate Therapy

The challenge for the physician is to form an appreciation for the severity of a patient's disease and formulate a treatment plan accordingly. As demonstrated in Figure 67–1, patients with the same diagnosis may have variable courses, ranging from those who progress rela-

tively rapidly to complete destruction of joints if left untreated to those who, with few pharmacologic interventions, smolder along with minimal disease that leaves cartilage functional and activities of daily living unchanged from the premorbid state.

As a general guideline, it can be said that the rate of progression toward joint destruction and disability in RA is proportional to the intensity of inflammatory and proliferative reactions within the joints and to the persistence of this disease over time. In other words, a patient who has low-grade attacks of synovitis that are separated in time from each other will be much less likely to advance to joint deformity than the patient who has continuous, highly active synovitis. The measurable parameters that affect intensity will be discussed in sections that follow.

One factor in prognosis that is virtually impossible for the physician to enter into calculations is how an individual patient responds to pain. Some individuals develop the "arthritis robustus" form of the disease, being aware of little discomfort in their joints (see Chapter 66). They continue to work hard and play hard. Radiographs may reveal substantial erosions and loss of joint space, but their joint function remains good as long as tendon function is maintained and bone structure is intact. At the other end of the scale, there are patients with a low tolerance for pain. Their activities of daily living and quality of life are diminished considerably by disease that often produces relatively little apparent damage to joints. This impression that pain can be dissociated from severity of RA is fortified by data demonstrating that, in 149 patients with early RA (symptoms present for less than 1 year), in contrast to joint swelling, no significant correlation was found for joint pain either with the acute-phase response or radiologic progression,[24] both of which are well-established markers for the progression of joint disease in RA.

THE ROLE OF THE RHEUMATOLOGIST IN MANAGEMENT

Increasing complexity of management options, combination therapies, and possible toxicities of therapy have all but necessitated that the rheumatologist be involved in the management decisions of patients suffering from RA. Data indicate that continuing care by a rheumatologist (mean of 8.6 visits per year) results in a crude rate of progression of functional disability that is significantly less (p 0.001) than for those who receive only intermittent, sporadic care by a rheumatologist.[25] Analysis of the data has supported the interpretation that worsening disability was not the reason for intermittent care, but rather a consequence of it.

In another series of 561 patients with definite RA followed over 20 years, the patients seen by a rheumatologist during the first 2 years of disease improved significantly when compared to others.[26] This favorable outcome could be related to an early start with relatively aggressive therapy. It is probable that the best care is given by a team of a rheumatologist and a primary care physician working closely with each patient, plus adequate consultation from physical and occupational therapists and orthopedic surgeons. Additional evidence supporting this demonstrated that patients who had access to a specialist (rheumatologist) had higher performance scores than patients who saw only a general practitioner. Importantly, access to both primary and specialist care resulted in significant improvements in arthritis care, comorbid illness, and health care maintenance overall beyond seeing a primary care doctor alone.[27]

It is important to note that among rheumatologists there is a wide variation of frequency with which follow-up visits are scheduled, even though clinical outcome for patients varies little.[28] With the increasing restraints of managed care on medical care, all physicians must struggle to give adequate time to each patient.

PARAMETERS OF PROGNOSIS

It is important to identify measures for estimating a prognosis that can be determined quickly in physicians' offices and with minimal laboratory expense. Measures identified vary widely with the individual studies, the end points used, and the types of therapy implemented. An instructive study was carried out on 142 consecutive patients with early RA (median duration of disease was 7 months) treated actively with disease-modifying drugs and followed prospectively for an average of 6.2 years. Functional outcome and radiographic damage were the end points. The significant prognostic factors at 1 year were high clinical disease activity at baseline, including morning stiffness, pain, grip strength, joint count, hemoglobin, and erythrocyte sedimentation rate (ESR), and a positive test for rheumatoid factor.[29] The functional outcome itself (measured by a modified health assessment,[30] age, and comorbid conditions) predicted 5-year mortality rate more effectively than radiographic or laboratory data.[31] The implication of this study is that measures of inflammatory activity may underestimate severity in RA.

Yet another indication of how function may predict outcome comes from an extensive study of the predictors for total joint replacement in 1600 patients seen during a period of observation that extended 23 years was reported in 1998. Patients with highly abnormal values on the health assessment questionnaire (HAQ), global severity of disease, and the ESR had a three- to sixfold increased risk of having a joint replacement.[32]

MARKERS FOR PROGNOSIS

In general, the markers discussed previously, including severe or aggressive baseline disease, poor function, the presence of rheumatoid factor, and elevation of acute phase markers, all suggest a worse prognosis.[33] Beyond this, the presence of erosions and joint-space narrowing early in the disease may also be predictive. It is possible to predict progression in individual patients by estimating yearly progression. This is based on evidence of radiographic damage and assumes no change in either disease or treatment. The estimate is obtained by dividing individual composite radiographic scores by the reported disease duration, thus providing an estimated yearly progression.

Additional markers of prognosis can include genetic predispositions, such as the presence of certain genetic loci (e.g., HLA-DR alleles that are associated with RA). Whereas some studies have yielded conflicting results, it is generally believed that the HLA-DRB1 locus can increase the likelihood of developing RA as well as the severity. There have already been attempts to use HLA-DRB1 typing in RA to predict responses to specific treatments.[34] In one study, the patients previously had been followed carefully in a study of combination therapy (hydroxychloroquine/sulfasalazine (SSZ)/MTX, hydroxychloroquine/SSZ, or MTX alone).[17] Patients were classified, in simplest terms, as "successes" or "failures" in achieving 50-percent improvement. DR4 subtyping was detected by hybridization of the patients' DNA with allele-specific oligonucleotide probes specific for the shared epitope region that enhances susceptibility to RA and is associated with greater severity of disease. Seventy-four percent of the patients were positive for at least one shared epitope allele, and 29 percent were positive for two. Although simplified, it can be concluded that patients who had one or two of the shared epitopes in their DRB1 chains were less likely to respond to MTX alone than to all three drugs, whereas those who had no shared epitopes in DRB1 chains did equally well on MTX alone and with all three drugs. For example, among patients positive for the shared epitope, 94 percent were "successes" if treated with triple therapy, but only 32 percent were "successes" if treated with MTX alone. These data are consistent with observations that patients positive for the shared epitope are at greatest risk for progressively active erosive disease (Fig. 67–2) and will need more-aggressive therapy earlier. Genetic analyses like these could lead to the choice of early effective therapy custom-designed for each patient. In future years, it may be possible—using relatively inexpensive microchip technology—to obtain a detailed printout that records the genetic predisposition to develop RA of each patient, as well as those genes governing autoantibody formation and the B cell repertoire, T cell receptor sequences, cytokine and adhesion molecule production, receptor density for inflammatory ligands, and susceptibility to both good and toxic effects of drugs.[35]

Biomarkers (surrogate markers found in the blood, urine, or other specimens) offer the promise of identifying patients with a poor prognosis or potentially identifying those who may benefit from specific therapies. Investigators found that patients in the COBRA trial[14] (mentioned earlier in the chapter) with high baseline levels of urinary C-terminal cross-linking telopeptide of type I (CTX-I) and type II (CTX-II) collagen were at the highest risk for radiographic progression.[36] Although this biomarker will need additional validation by other investigators, it demonstrates the point that over the next decade, large strides in diagnosis, prognosis, and patient-specific therapies may be viable based on advances in the field of biomarkers (see Chapter 50).

Refined imaging techniques can help in the staging of disease as well as in following effects of therapy. Magnetic resonance imaging (MRI) (see Chapter 51), although not yet justified as a cost-effective measure of

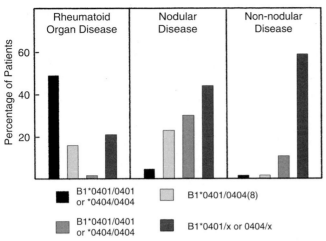

FIGURE 67–2 · Correlation of Allelic Combinations at the HLA-DRB1 Locus with Disease Severity in Rheumatoid Arthritis. A total of 102 patients with rheumatoid arthritis were grouped into subset according to their extra-articular disease manifestations. Thirty-seven patients had erosive disease without extra-articular manifestations; most of these patients combined an HLA-DRB1 *04 variant with a disease-nonassociated HLA-DRB1 allele. Patients with nodular disease but no major organ involvement (n = 43) were frequently homozygous for the disease-associated sequence polymorphism, by combining either two HLA-DRB1 *0 variants or one HLA-DRB1 *04 variant with HLA-DRB1 *0101. Patients with major organ involvement were predominantly homozygous for an HLA-DRB1 *04 allele. (From Weyland CM, Goronzy JJ: Functional domains on HLA-DR molecules: Implications for the linkage of HLA-DR genes to different autoimmune diseases. Clin Immunol Immunopathol 70: 94, 1994; used by permission.)

synovitis, can nevertheless provide a good estimate of synovial volume within joints. In a study using gadopentetate dimeglumine (Gd-DTPA)–enhanced MRI,[37] it was found that the rate of erosive progression on MRI was highly correlated with the values of synovial membrane volume, but not with local or global clinical or laboratory parameters. Erosions of bone seen on MRI grew into radiographically visible erosions, but with a delay of up to 1 year. Ultrasound is also proving potentially useful for diagnosing active disease at an early stage. When compared to clinical examination, MRI, three-phase bone scan, and conventional radiology in a study of 60 patients with various types of arthritis, ultrasound proved to be a sensitive tool. When looking specifically at 32 of the 60 patients without radiographic erosions, bone scan identified 58 percent of the joints as abnormal, ultrasound identified 54 percent as abnormal, and MRI demonstrated erosions in 20 percent of the joints and enhancement in 41 percent.[38] As imaging modalities hopefully decrease in cost, increase in availability, and grow in sophistication, it is possible they will have increased utility in the future for both diagnosic and prognositic purposes in patients with inflammatory arthritis.

▌ Undifferentiated Polyarthritis

Even without a clear diagnosis of RA, it is important for physicians to realize that effective treatment can be instituted for patients before a definite diagnosis is established. The patient who very recently has developed pain, stiffness, and swelling of hands, wrists, and feet, for example, may have one of many chronic diseases, or even self-limited ones. The differential diagnosis includes many possibilities, many of which are outlined in chapters 35 and 66. In cohorts of patients presenting to physicians in outpatient clinics with arthralgias, swelling of several joints, and a perception of partial disability, more than half are likely to have complete resolution of symptoms, and fewer than 20 percent go on to be diagnosed with RA.[39]

The mean time to diagnosis of RA from the onset of symptoms in one study of patients in a Massachusetts HMO in 1994 was 36 weeks.[25,40] This delay seems long, but it is related to reluctance of patients to seek help for a symptom complex that begins perniciously, as well as to a reluctance of physicians to make a diagnosis of a chronic disease when the patient presents with no acute manifestations. On the other hand, it is important to emphasize to patients that the longer they can go without a specific diagnosis of a symptom complex involving joints (assuming they are being cared for appropriately), the better their prognosis.

The point for emphasis is that much can be done for patients with undifferentiated polyarthritis, regardless of whether it represents the beginning of RA or another process. Education, pain control, a balance of rest and exercise, and drug therapy all can be instituted. Table 67–2 offers a useful tabulation of principles of rehabilitation for RA patients, but it is useful in all patients with polyarthritis.

EDUCATION

The point has been made that a "low formal educational level is a composite/surrogate variable [that] identifies behavioral risk factors predisposing to the etiology and poor outcomes in most chronic diseases."[41] In studies of RA, morbidity and mortality rates over a 9-year period in one series were inversely proportional to the formal educational level and could not be explained by age, duration of disease, joint count, functional measures, or medications.[42] Although the reasons behind this link of formal education to outcome are obscure, the corollary is that teaching patients about how arthritis affects people, how they can be involved in helping themselves, and what doctors use to treat arthritis leads to better outcomes.[43] Use of the Arthritis Self-Management Program (ASMP) has been rigorously shown to enable pain reduction, decrease visits to physicians, and save money.[44] Participation of spouses in educational group sessions for patients leads to additional beneficial effects.[45] Psychologic counseling, a form of education, is also useful for patients with arthritis. Stress-management training can be particularly effective, leading to statistically significant improvements in measures of helplessness, self efficacy, coping, pain, and health status.[46]

A more in-depth discussion of education and its role in arthritis can be found in Chapter 52; however, in general, patients need to feel they have some control over

TABLE 67–2 · PRINCIPLES AND APHORISMS FOR REHABILITATIVE THERAPIES IN RHEUMATOID ARTHRITIS

1. *Pain control* is the first consideration in any rehabilitative regimen.
2. *The treatment regimen* should be as brief and as simple as possible to be consistent with its goal (e.g., if 3 stretches of the shoulder one time daily will maintain the range of motion prescribed, 3 one-time daily and not 3 three-times daily, nor 30, etc., should be prescribed).
3. *Adherence* (compliance) to a treatment regimen at the very least requires sufficient patient instruction to achieve an understanding of its specifics and to motivate its ongoing implementation. The motivation also requires understanding the patient and his or her style, fears, beliefs, and goals.
4. *Rest* and restriction of skeletal motion can reduce inflammation but can also promote weakness and contractures. Rest must be balanced with appropriate movement whenever feasible.
5. *Joint protection principles:*
   (a) Joints protected by splints, rest, or during activities should be positioned to avoid deformities.
   (b) Transferring skills (e.g., ability to arise from a chair or get into a car) must be taught to provide optimal independence, joint protection, safety, and energy conservation.
   (c) The strongest joints should be used insofar as possible during activities (e.g., shoulder strap versus a handle on a purse).
   (d) Planning and pacing of activities should minimize prolonged or excessive joint use and conserve energy.
6. *Exercise therapy* has many objectives, and typically only one objective is achieved optimally by any specific exercise:
   (a) Preserve motion
   (b) Restore lost motion
   (c) Increase strength and static endurance
   (d) Increase dynamic (kinetic) endurance
   (e) Enhance a feeling of well-being
   (f) Provide cardiovascular conditioning
   (g) Provide active recreation

Adapted from Swezey RL. Rheumatoid arthritis: The role of the kinder and gentler therapies. J Rheumatol 17(Suppl 25):8, 1990; used by permission.

their illnesses—a capacity to do something for themselves that will have a positive effect. They do not want to be bystanders, watching a contest between a disease they did nothing to bring on and physicians whose words and strategies they insufficiently understand. Education can make a big difference, enabling patients to form a therapeutic contract with their physicians and making it more likely that they will not turn, out of frustration, to alternative therapies that may do more harm than good.

PAIN CONTROL

Pain can be the factor that limits effectiveness of physical and occupational therapy, and as pointed out during a special workshop sponsored by the National Advisory Board for Arthritis and Musculoskeletal and Skin Diseases, it is frequently undertreated in patients with arthritis.[47] In addition to inhibiting function, pain is a major cause of depression in patients with polyarthritis. To maximize therapy in patients with early RA or undifferentiated polyarthritis, pain must be controlled without altering consciousness or generating addiction. In general, treatment strategies favoring education, rest, exercise, and disease-modifying therapies are favored as an approach to pain control in arthritis, and strategies reliant on narcotic derivatives alone are discouraged. In most medical centers, experts in the management of pain are available for consultation by rheumatologists and primary care physicians.

REST, EXERCISE, AND ACTIVITIES OF DAILY LIVING

Education and supervision of a patient by trained professionals on the importance of finding the best balance of rest and exercise for inflamed joints is essential. Again,

this component of therapy can be started well before a definitive diagnosis is made. No matter what the cause, finding this balance should ensure that a patient will develop, or retain, sufficient strength to support joint function without exacerbating inflammation.

Details of physical and occupational therapy are outlined in Chapter 55. The patient with acutely and severely inflamed joints may need application of resting splints to immobilize the joint until anti-inflammatory medication takes effect. Even the most painful joints, when splinted, must be moved passively through a full range of motion each day to prevent flexion contractures, particularly in children. For moderately inflamed joints, isometric exercise with muscles contracted in a fixed position (the resting length of the muscle) provides adequate muscle tone without exacerbating joint inflammation and pain. Maximal contractions, held for 6 seconds and repeated 5 to 10 times, performed several times each day, can prevent further loss of muscle mass around arthritic joints.

Patients with inactive or well-controlled arthritis can profit from variable-resistance programs or even high-intensity strength training, which has been shown to provide significant improvements in strength, pain, and fatigue. Elderly patients with RA can benefit from progressive resistance exercises, as can younger patients. In a study of older patients given closely regulated workouts on pneumatic resistance equipment, maximal strength of all major exercised muscle groups was increased up to 75 percent without exacerbation of clinical disease activity.[48] Not only does prescribed sustained exercise increase muscle strength, it also helps the ability of patients to perform daily routines, improves global assessments and moods, and can decrease pain.[49]

Every patient with RA deserves one or more sessions with a licensed occupational therapist to learn how to preserve joint function and alignment while carrying out both the necessary and enjoyable activities of daily living. The basic concept is to avoid excessive force applied across non–weight-bearing joints and to avoid unnecessary impact loading on weight-bearing joints. The Arthritis Society Home Service in Toronto, Canada participated in a prospective and controlled trial demonstrating that home therapy by occupational therapists produced a statistically significant and clinically important improvement in function in rheumatoid patients.[50]

DRUG THERAPY

Patients with polyarthritis need relief of pain generated by the inflammation in their joints. Analgesics, NSAIDs, and glucocorticoids are the classes of compounds that do this effectively. For RA, these therapies must be considered adjunctive therapy, rather than primary therapy (disease-modifying drugs). Adjunctive therapy may be useful in the short term, and in some cases it will be sufficient for management, particularly in cases of polyarthritis that do not become chronically imbedded in joints and defined as RA. The goal of therapy should be to make these adjunctive drugs unnecessary and redundant through control of the disease. The reasons for this are their toxicities, which are varied, additive, and substantial. The NSAIDs are covered in detail in Chapter 56, and glucocorticoids are discussed in depth in Chapter 57. The goal in this chapter will be to suggest strategies for using these and other compounds to treat RA.

ANALGESICS

Acetaminophen is a very useful drug and can prove a useful adjunct in the treatment of arthritis. In patients without evidence of liver disease, it can be taken in doses up to 3 g or more per day without generating significant side effects. Combination of acetaminophen with codeine or other narcotic derivatives produces a powerful and potentially addictive combination. Their use alone in polyarthritis for more than 6 weeks (i.e., the minimum period for acceptably classifying a polyarthritis as RA) should be discouraged and reserved only for those patients who have severe and persistent disease despite all attempts to bring the disease under better control through the use of DMARDs.

NONSTEROIDAL ANTI-INFLAMMATORY DRUGS

More than 70 million prescriptions for NSAIDs are written each year in the United States, and more than 30 billion over-the-counter tablets are sold annually. As a class, NSAIDs are the most-often used and perhaps the most effective adjunctive therapy in RA, providing both analgesic and anti-inflammatory benefits. Chapter 56 provides a comprehensive review of these compounds, with details of their molecular activity as well as toxicity. The introduction of the potentially safer cyclooxygenase-2 (COX-2) selective agents has further fueled debate as to safety, toxicity, and costs of NSAID therapy. Given that the majority of patients with RA will be treated with NSAID therapy, physicians must carefully evaluate the individual patient to assess chronicity of use, risk factors for NSAID toxicity, risk factors for heart disease, and the ability of the patient or the insurance plan to cover the costs of the agent prescribed. Risk factors for use of NSAIDs (including aspirin) have been identified and include the following[51]:

- Advanced age
- History of peptic ulcer (with or without a known infection with *Helicobacter pylori*)
- Concomitant use of glucocorticoids or anticoagulants
- Thrombocytopenia or platelet dysfunction
- Pregnancy
- Moderate or severe congestive heart failure, cirrhosis, or renal insufficiency
- Aspirin intolerance, asthma, and nasal polyposis

Which NSAID should be prescribed first is perhaps the most frequently encountered and possibly the most difficult question. In a relatively young patient without any of the aforementioned risk factors, salicylates should not be excluded automatically from use. Aspirin, for example, has the advantages of being relatively inexpensive (even in enteric-coated preparations), having an inexpensive test for blood levels, having toxicity directly related to dose, and having a biologic manifestation of excessive blood levels (i.e., tinnitus).

Nonacetylated salicylates (e.g., salsalate, choline salicylate) also deserve consideration. They are moderately effective, have a relatively good safety profile, and are inexpensive. They have only a weak and reversible effect on COX. This finding has led to studies demonstrating that, at concentrations below those needed to inhibit either COX-1 or COX-2, salicylates interrupt signal transduction across cell membranes in such a way that activation of inflammatory pathways in cells such as the neutrophil is inhibited.[52] If a clinician chooses to use an NSAID other than a salicylate, the only major differences, other than those afforded by the selective COX-2 inhibitors, are in frequency of dosing and in subtle differences in side effect profiles.

The selective COX-2 inhibitors have been described in detail in Chapter 56. They clearly are a product of clever chemistry based on sound basic research. The fundamental difference between COX-1 and COX-2 is that COX-1 is a constitutively expressed enzyme synthesized at a relatively constant rate by the tissues that produce it, whereas COX-2 is induced in monocytes or macrophages, endothelial cells, chondrocytes, synovial cells, and osteoblasts by cytokines and other products generated during inflammation.

The selective COX-2 inhibitors (e.g., celecoxib, rofecoxib, and valdecoxib) all appear to be more effective than placebo in the treatment of arthritis and appear as effective as moderate doses of standard nonselective NSAIDs. The utility of the selective agents comes from potential safety advantages, including a lower risk of the development of gastrointestinal bleeding.[53,54] The selective agents also have no significant effects on platelets.

They do not, however, confer any advantage to the kidney, and risks of increasing hypertension or renal insufficiency because of their use must be recognized. As well, there is some evidence to suggest that selective COX-2 inhibition may, in an at-risk individual, increase risks for cardiovascular events.[55] This controversy is further outlined in Chapter 56.

Early Rheumatoid Arthritis

For patients with a symmetric polyarthritis in three or more joint areas (see Chapters 35 and 66) involving the hands, feet, or both for at least 6 weeks, more aggressive treatment is warranted, as it would be if a diagnosis of RA were definite. Even though tests for rheumatoid factor (RF) may be negative, laboratory tests and clinical examination (including a detailed family history, review of systems, and medication exposure) have for the most part ruled out early forms of systemic lupus erythematosus (SLE), scleroderma, vasculitis, and polymyositis. Although seronegative spondyloarthropathies cannot be ruled out completely at this stage, the approach to therapy for these diseases would be quite similar. Many with early disease will have benefited from NSAIDs, but many or most still have morning stiffness, some tenderness, and definite swelling of joints. Patients are generally apprehensive and concerned about developing a chronic, debilitating disease. Anxiety, depression, loss of self esteem, inability to work, and an inability to develop new coping behaviors may be evolving. This "learned helplessness" must be combated by education, reassurance, counseling, and the confident attitude of the physician.

Most important is the initiation of a program to downregulate activity of the synovitis with the goal of inducing a remission, or at least marked improvement, in the disease. Disease-modifying therapy is clearly indicated at this point (see previous DMARD therapy section); however, some other forms of adjunctive therapy may be appropriate.

GLUCOCORTICOID THERAPY

Although it is arbitrary to place a discussion of glucocorticoid therapy in this section on treatment of early RA because the place and role of these steroids are constantly being debated, it is clear that steroids in short courses and at low doses can clearly result in a reduction of symptoms and signs of disease, as well as improve patient function. It is hoped that in future years their use can be minimized. Except for intra-articular or other forms of parenteral administration, prednisone is the glucocorticoid preparation most often used by rheumatologists.

Although not universally practiced, some rheumatologists have used intramuscular injections of depot preparations of methylprednisolone (80 mg) intermittently in patients with active polyarthritis. The rationale is that this route and quantity of glucocorticoids will give a sustained, gradually declining therapeutic effect that will not induce "dependence" to the drug that so often happens when even low doses are prescribed in pill form.

The same dose can be given again in 6 weeks or more if disease-modifying drugs have not yet brought the synovitis under control. Use of higher doses of glucocorticoids along with other DMARDs as early therapy in combination will be discussed in a following paragraph.

The following list identifies the different indications for glucocorticoid use in RA. The last item (daily therapy) has the greatest potential for harmful effects, and these drugs are prescribed for an estimated 20 to 30 percent of all RA patients.

- These drugs are prescribed in short, high-dose courses for drug toxicity (e.g., the thrombocytopenia that rarely occurs with parenteral gold therapy).
- They may also be prescribed for vasculitis presenting as skin ulcers, mononeuritis multiplex, rapidly progressive pulmonary interstitial disease, coronary arteritis, ischemic bowel syndromes, or severe systemic toxicity with fever and intense pain.
- Intra-articular injections using a long-acting compound such a triamcinolone hexacetonide can be particularly useful when only a few joints are involved in a flare of arthritis.
- These drugs can be used as principal therapy, when needed, during pregnancy.
- They can be used as low-dose, daily therapy for moderately active disease.

The last point, daily use of glucocorticoids, has caused the most problems with long-term toxicity. Although the benefits of low-dose therapy (less than 7.5 mg/day given as one dose in the morning) have been shown, many data suggest that the cumulative effects on bone produce osteoporosis and other deleterious effects associated with significant morbidity. There are multiple actions of glucocorticoids on bone, including a recognized decreased production of osteoclasts and both decreased production and apoptosis of osteoblasts resulting in decreased bone formation and trabecular width.[56]

The arguments supporting use of low-dose, daily prednisone are as follows:

1. The rheumatoid process diminishes bone formation in patients compared with control populations.[57] Physical impairment is the major determinant of both spinal and femoral bone-mass deficiency in RA patients and if the clinical activity of arthritis is factored into equations, the effect of low-dose glucocorticoid therapy on bone loss in these patients is minimal,[58] particularly if the glucocorticoid encourages more physical activity by relieving inflammation. Metabolic-marker studies have indicated that generalized bone turnover is increased in RA.[59]

2. Evidence also has been presented that low-dose daily glucocorticoids reduce the rate of radiographically detected progression of disease.[60] This work was done with 128 adults with active RA of less than 2 years' duration. Patients were randomly assigned to receive 7.5 mg prednisone per day in addition to other medications, and others received placebo. Most patients in both groups did not develop positive radiologic scores, but those who did were principally in the placebo group, and the erosions (using the Larsen

scale) progressed more rapidly over the next 2 years. In a more-recent 2-year, double-blind, placebo-controlled trial, the benefits and risks of 10 mg of prednisone per day were evaluated. Investigators found that, particularly in the first 6 months, patients receiving prednisone had more clinical improvement, and there was significantly less radiographic progression than seen in the placebo group.[61]

Counter to these data, however, are side-effect data showing that prednisone has higher cumulative toxicity over many years than nearly all other agents used to treat RA,[62] as well as a twofold increase in standardized mortality rates.[63] Although most emphasis has been placed on osteoporosis, there is a definite association of low-dose glucocorticoid use on a daily basis with cataracts, glaucoma, impaired glucose tolerance, hirsutism, and skin atrophy. And although side effects may be limited by alternate-day regimens, alternate-day administration of glucocorticoids in asthmatic patients did not produce less bone loss than daily regimens.[64]

The American College of Rheumatology task force on osteoporosis guidelines[65] has published recommendations for the following subsets of patients:

- Patients receiving long-term glucocorticoid treatment who develop a nontraumatic osteoporotic fracture
- Patients receiving long-term glucocorticoid treatment who do not have fractures
- Patients beginning long-term glucocorticoid treatment

Those in the first group, who have developed a fracture (usually a compression fracture of the spine), are often at great risk for a higher mortality rate not only from the fracture but from other side effects of the glucocorticoids. These individuals need not only pharmacologic intervention, but lifestyle changes as well.

Patients in the second group, who are receiving long-term glucocorticoid treatment and do not have fractures, should have the baseline laboratory tests and a DEXA determination of bone mineral density. Physical therapy and exercise should be started, along with calcium and vitamin D supplementation. If appropriate, additional pharmacologic therapy should be considered to prevent glucocorticoid-induced osteoporosis. The importance of yearly measurements of bone mineral density using the same equipment in these patients will enable the physician to determine the rate of bone loss and to institute therapy appropriately.

Patients in the third group, who have RA and are beginning glucocorticoid therapy, should be evaluated carefully for associated diseases other than RA that affect bone metabolism. Women who are postmenopausal should be evaluated for the consideration of hormone replacement therapy. Other risk factors should be removed, when possible, and exercise, supplemental calcium, and vitamin D should be prescribed. A baseline bone mineral density determination is appropriate.

Most importantly, the potential toxicity of the glucocorticoids, if taken for long periods, must be communicated to the patient, and both the patient and physician

must have as their goal to control the disease within 6 months to the point that glucocorticoids are no longer deemed necessary and can be slowly tapered. Additional discussion and therapeutic options for the treatment of osteoporosis can be found in Chapter 90.

MINOCYCLINE

Tetracycline derivatives have a capacity to inhibit biosynthesis and activity of matrix metalloproteinases (MMPs) that have a principal role in degrading articular cartilage in RA. The presumed mechanism is through their chelating capacity for calcium and zinc molecules that alter molecular conformation of the proenzymes sufficiently to inactive them.[66,67] Minocycline, used in trials of RA, has mild but definite inhibitory effects on synovial T cell proliferation and cytokine production. Given in a dose of 100 mg daily, moderate improvement in clinical parameters of disease activity was found in those treated with minocycline more often than in those given placebo.[68,69]

A study of 46 patients with early RA who had not received systemic glucocorticoids or second-line drugs reported 65 percent of patients meeting 50-percent improvement in tender and swollen joints, duration of morning stiffness, and the ESR,[70] whereas only 13 percent of the placebo recipients improved similarly over a 6-month period.

In 2001, the results of a 2-year trial comparing minocycline with hydroxychloroquine were published.[71] In this small study of patients with early RA, those patients treated with minocycline were more likely to achieve a 50% improvement than those treated with hydroxychloroquine (60% vs. 33%). This study reconfirms the potential utility of minocycline, particularly in early disease.

Although the doses used in the previously described studies do not differ from those for patients given tetracyclines for acne, some bothersome side effects have been noted, including light-headed feelings, vertigo, and, rarely, liver toxicity. More worrisome have been reports of patients who are taking tetracycline derivatives who develop lupus-like syndromes, complete with autoantibodies. "Minocycline-induced autoimmune syndrome" is characterized by reversible polyarthralgia or arthritis, morning stiffness, fever, frequent skin involvement, occasional chronic active hepatitis, positive tests for antinuclear antibodies, and increased titers of p-ANCA.[72] With proper warning to patients and careful monitoring, however, minocycline seems to be an appropriate drug for use in patients with early synovitis.

COMPLEMENTARY THERAPY AND DIET

Patients given a definite diagnosis of RA often will want to be personally involved in attempts to control the disease. Along with direct advertising about the latest COX-2 selective inhibitor, they will be saturated with information about complementary therapy and diets for RA.

It is important to inform patients of the risk of taking herbal medicines that can be toxic and to let them know that there are no data to support the claims that copper bracelets, glucosamine and chondroitin sulfate, wheat germ, or tomato-free diets will benefit RA. Those interested in trying dietary modification should be informed about addition of omega-3 or omega-6 fatty acids to the diet. Eicosapentaenoic acid (EPA), in doses of 54 mg/kg/day, and docosahexaenoic acid (DHA), in doses of 36 mg/kg/day, added to the diet have been demonstrated in double-blind, randomized, placebo-controlled studies to improve joint counts in a 30-week trial.[73] Another study proved the benefit of these fish oils over 12 months when compared to olive oil supplementation.[74]

Manipulation of the omega-6 pathway of metabolism of fatty acids has been achieved by giving 1.4 g/day of gamma-linolenic acid (GLA) to RA patients in a double-blind placebo-controlled study of 24 weeks' duration.[75] Joint tenderness improved significantly in the treated group.

Giving omega-3 fatty acids (EPA and DHA) diminishes PGE2 and leukotriene B4 (LTB4) biosynthesis and increases production of PGE3 and LTB5, both of which are less inflammatory than the usual products. Addition of GLA to diets increases PGE1 (an anti-inflammatory prostaglandin) production, and PGE2 and LTB4 levels do not change.

These added oils in the diet can leave a fishy taste in the mouth and generate oily, foul-smelling stools. Some patients will not tolerate these effects, but most can. Most important, the fish-oil supplements do no apparent harm.

No other diets have been useful besides those associated with enhancing weight loss. Excess weight is a liability for RA patients, and weight control is an important component of a good therapeutic plan. "Starvation diets," despite the fact that they may suppress the immune response, should be discouraged.

DISEASE-MODIFICATION THERAPY

Initiating DMARD therapy is paramount in the treatment of RA. However, the decision of which DMARD to start is less clear. In any given patient, any of the DMARDs can be efficacious and well tolerated. However, no one DMARD is efficacious and safe in every patient. In fact, few patients experience remission on any DMARDs, and most experience some sort of side effect from the medications prescribed to treat the disease. An algorithmic approach to the use of DMARDs has been put forward by the American College of Rheumatology[76] (Fig. 67–3). This provides a general guideline and considerations when starting, changing, or adding DMARDs to the treatment of a patient with active disease.

In general, DMARD therapy begins with the initiation of therapy with the traditional small molecules such as MTX, hydroxychloroquine, or SSZ. These agents are of proven benefit, are generally well tolerated with a well known side effect profiles, and can be prescribed at a reasonable cost. Of these three therapies, MTX is the most commonly prescribed DMARD. After consideration has been given to the use of these traditional small-molecule therapies, the practitioner must take stock of the growing efficacy and safety data in the support of the newer-generation DMARDs and

biologic-response modifiers, such as leflunomide, adalimumab, anakinra, etanercept, and infliximab. These agents have been well studied in clinical trials demonstrating efficacy alone or in combination with traditional therapies. The ability of these agents to slow radiographic progression of disease and restore function appears to be at least equal to, and in some cases greater than, that seen with traditional therapies. In general there is little debate that as a class, the inhibitors of TNF-α have been the most-effective therapies available to date for the treatment of RA.

The question of when to initiate or to add these therapies into the treatment regimen is a difficult one, and in many cases it can be a matter of individual style. However, in some cases it can be a socioeconomic decision based on the higher costs of these therapies (see Table 67–1). In some situations, utilization of the biologic agents may be limited by third-party payors, and in most circumstances they are allowed only after failure of one or more of the standard agents. For the most part, this is a prudent, cost-effective approach to the introduction of the new agents. There are considerable data suggesting that many therapies can be used in combination both safely and efficaciously. Growing numbers of patients are finding themselves on combination therapy in an attempt to achieve better control over the disease process. In most cases, MTX has served as the building block on which combination therapy is based.[77,78] Drugs that have demonstrated benefit when combined with MTX include hydroxychloroquine, SSZ, cyclosporine, leflunomide, anakinra, adalimumab, etanercept, and infliximab, to name a few.

An important cornerstone in the approach to combination therapy is data that "triple therapy," MTX, SSZ, and hydroxychloroquine, has been found to be more effective than MTX alone.[17] In a well-done trial, 77 percent of patients with active RA had a significant improvement on triple therapy, compared to 33 percent of patients started on MTX alone over a 2-year time frame.[17] A follow-up study to this one demonstrated that the combination of all three agents was superior to MTX plus SSZ or MTX plus PLQ.[79] Additional studies, including the COBRA trial,[14] and the FIN-RACO trial, demonstrated utility if not superiority with combinations of traditional DMARD therapy.[80] In the COBRA trial, patients were initially randomized to receive monotherapy with sulfasalasine or combination therapy in a step-down approach with sulfasalasine, MTX, and high-dose glucocorticoids. At the end of 28 weeks, there appeared to be a significant advantage for the use of combination therapy based on clinical response, and at 1 year, there was also less radiographic progression in the combination group.[14] In the FIN-RACO trial, patients with early RA treated with combination therapy (SSZ, MTX, PLQ, prednisone) had better responses, more remissions, and no more side effects then those treated with monotherapy (SSZ or MTX).[80,81]

In the past few years, increasing emphasis has been placed on the use of biologic agents (such as TNF inhibitors) in combination with small-molecule agents such as MTX. These combinations have proven very effective in the treatment of patients with severe or long-standing disease and have proven their ability to slow

ACR TREATMENT ALGORITHM

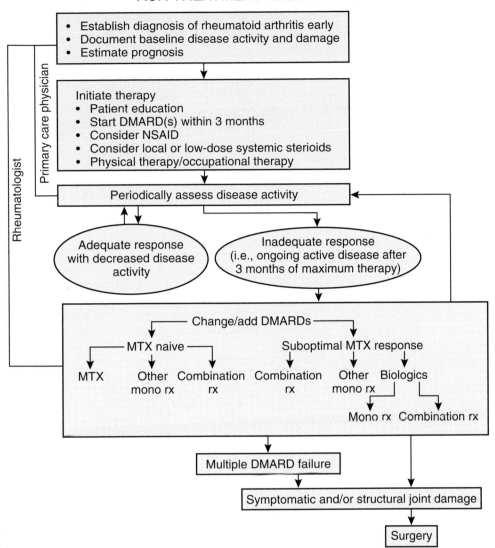

FIGURE 67–3 · Guidelines for the Management of Rheumatoid Arthritis. *Arthritis Rheum.* 2002;46: 328-346.

further radiographic progression of disease.[19,20,123] These combination approaches will be used with increasing frequency in the future as patients derive inadequate responses to monotherapies or as practitioners implement even more-aggressive therapy earlier in the disease course. Combination therapy in the treatment of RA is more completely described in Chapter 59 on MTX, leflunomide, and combination therapies in RA and Chapter 61 on anticytokine therapies.

In the past, considerable attention was given to the use of gold salts and penicillamine in the treatment of RA. Although not unreasonable therapy for an individual patient, their use has diminished in the past several years as combination therapies and new agents are used with increasing frequency in the treatment of RA.

Figure 67–3 presents a general guide for the physician after making a diagnosis of RA. The general theme of this guideline is adding multiple drugs to basic general care until the disease has been brought under control. There are so many options for drug therapy now that toxicity or lack of efficacy of one drug need not lead to

therapeutic nihilism or discouragement for either the patient or physician. Although MTX has become the mainstay of therapy in RA, a number of drugs (outlined in Chapters 58 and 60), now rarely used in RA, are options if toxicities prevent use of others.

HYDROXYCHLOROQUINE

Hydroxychloroquine is a logical consideration as an agent to add to NSAIDs and other components of general care very early in the disease process or in particularly mild disease. There are few side effects, and approximately 40 percent of patients will receive measurable benefit. In the United States, it is used more often than its cousin, chloroquine. When employing dosing schedules not exceeding 400 mg of hydroxychloroquine each day, fewer than 20 cases of true retinopathy causing visual loss have been reported,[82] which should reassure clinicians about its safety. It has been hypothesized that these antimalarial agents inhibit antigen processing and presentation, leading to downregulation of the CD4+

response in sites of immune damage.[83] Hydroxychloroquine (HCQ), has been found to have equal efficacy to SSZ[84] and was no less effective than the combination of SSZ and hydroxychloroquine. Some of the strong evidence supporting its utililty in early and in mild disease comes from the HERA trial[12] in which patients with RA were randomized to receive either HCQ or placebo over a period of 36 weeks. At the conclusion of the study, patients who had received HCQ had improvements in joint findings, pain, and physical function superior to what was seen in the placebo group. After 3 years of follow-up of the original cohorts, those patients who had previously been treated in the HCQ arm of the study continued to have significantly less pain and disability compared to those that had DMARD therapy delayed for 9 months (the placebo arm). These results could not be explained based on differences in glucocorticoid, DMARD, or NSAID use subsequent to the trial and were attributed to a delay in the introduction of therapy.[13] However, to date there are no convincing data on the ability of hydroxychloroquine to slow radiographic progression, and for those patients with active, progressing disease hydroxychloroquine will be inadequate as monotherapy In general, the mild benefits and the relative lack of toxicity make this a reasonable agent in early or mild disease, or as an adjunct to combination therapy.

SULFASALAZINE

SSZ is another DMARD alternative in the treatment of RA (see Chapter 58). Svartz reported, in uncontrolled studies, the benefits of this drug, which she synthesized from salicylic acid and a sulfonamide in 1942.[85] The drug was first used by gastroenterologists for treatment of inflammatory bowel disease. The drug is generally thought to be efficacious in doses of 2000 to 3000 mg/day. Although allergic reactions and rashes can occur, it is the gastrointestinal (GI) complaints that tend to be more common; these can potentially be lessened through the use of enteric-coated preparations.

Several studies have established the efficacy of SSZ in RA.[86-88] In early RA, investigators demonstrated that SSZ was superior to placebo in reducing both inflammation and clinical disease activity.[86] In a double-blind, randomized trial of 60 patients with RA who had not previously been treated with DMARDs, investigators demonstrated that patients randomized to receive SSZ had significantly less evidence of radiographic progression than did patients treated with hydroxychloroquine. This difference became apparent as early as 24 weeks in even this relatively small study, which suggested the possible superiority of this agent to hydroxychloroquine as a DMARD.[87]

A more recent study comparing SSZ to leflunomide demonstrated the clear utility of SSZ in the treatment of RA.[88] In this double-blind, placebo-controlled study, patients were treated with leflunomide, SSZ, or placebo, and ACR 20-percent response rates were seen at 24 weeks in 49, 45, and 29 percent of patients on each of the medications, respectively. Both leflunomide and SSZ were statistically better than placebo in reducing symptoms and signs of disease. As well, both leflunomide and

SSZ were significantly better than placebo at slowing radiographic progression of disease. In this study SSZ faired well both against placebo and the active comparator, leflunomide, helping solidify its role as a useful DMARD.

Beyond its role early in disease, or in the treatment of mild to moderate disease, is the potential role of SSZ in combination therapy. As previously discussed, this therapy clearly appears to be efficacious and well tolerated in combination with MTX and hydroxychloroquine.[14,17,80]

GOLD SALTS, D-PENICILLAMINE, AND AZATHIOPRINE

Three other secondary choices, some of which can be used in some combinations with primary choices in active synovitis, are intramuscular or oral gold, D-penicillamine, and azathioprine. These agents would generally not be favored in early disease and, in fact, have now been relegated to a role as agents used when other therapies have failed for either lack of efficacy or side effects. There is ample published evidence (see Chapter 58) that intramuscular gold therapy is beneficial for RA. Early use of gold-salt injections may retard progression of joint erosions.[89] There is also ample evidence that the two available compounds, gold sodium thiomalate and gold sodium thioglucose, are being used less and less by rheumatologists because of the need for meticulous monitoring for serious toxicity (e.g., cytopenias, proteinuria) and the costs of administration and monitoring (reviewed in Chapter 58).

It can be considered as a precursor of individual genetic analyses for potential therapeutic efficacy and toxicity that HLA-DR3 is found in more patients who develop either thrombocytopenia or nephropathy while taking gold injections.[90] These data must be balanced against the evidence that HLA-DR3 may be associated with a better response to gold therapy.

Auranofin, the triethylphosphine gold compound taken by mouth, has been available since the mid-1980s and continues to search for its niche in treatment strategies. Several issues are clear: Auranofin has different and less-severe toxicity than the intramuscular preparations. Cytopenia and proteinuria do not occur, but a bothersome mild enterocolitis that generates diarrhea leads to treatment failure in a number of cases. Auranofin is less efficacious than MTX, injectable gold, D-penicillamine, or SSZ.[91] The efficacy of auranofin, although less than the more-potent drugs, has been demonstrated, however[92]; and there is justification for combining it with hydroxychloroquine, SSZ, or even MTX in treating early stages of active synovitis.

Azathioprine, in doses of 1.5 to 2.5 mg/kg/day, has been used alone and in combination in RA, often as a "steroid-sparing agent." Neutropenia is the most common complication. One factor that leads to early toxicity from azathioprine is heterozygosity for mutant thiopurine methyltransferase alleles. Patients who have this defect (perhaps 10 percent of the population at risk) metabolize the drug poorly and are forced to discontinue azathioprine therapy within 1 month because of hematologic side effects.[93] Although not proved, this subset of patients could be those who, when azathioprine was added to a stable MTX regimen, developed an acute febrile toxic reaction characterized by fever, leukocytosis, and a cutaneous leukocytoclastic vasculitis.[94]

The story of D-penicillamine and RA is chronicled in Chapter 58. Initially used with apparent success, it was found to cause a selective decrease in CD4+ helper/inducer T cells. Although the "go low, go slow" sequence of starting with 125 or 250 mg/day and keeping doses no higher than 750 mg/day has resulted in diminished toxicity, yet there have been sufficient and worrisome side effects in many patients to discourage its routine use. Perhaps because of genetic differences among patients, the drug has been used with more apparent success and definite enthusiasm in the United Kingdom and Europe. In one study, 5 years in duration, 53 percent of patients remained on D-penicillamine, whereas only 34 percent continued taking gold salts, 31 percent remained on auranofin, and 30 percent remained on hydroxychloroquine.[95]

▮ Use of Methotrexate

As of the year 2004, the question for rheumatologists was not whether to use MTX, but rather, in a given patient with sustained synovitis beyond 2 to 3 months, whether there are any reasons not to use it.

Beginning with uncontrolled trials in the 1970s, and borrowed by rheumatologists from the dermatologists who were using it for psoriasis and psoriatic arthritis, there has been a gradual increase in enthusiastic acceptance of MTX as the preferred in the treatment of RA (see Chapter 59). A number of factors, now well documented, support this strategy:

• More patients are likely to be taking MTX than any other nonbiologic therapy 2 to 5 years after it is first prescribed.[96]
• MTX acts relatively quickly after being started, often within several weeks of the once-weekly dosing schedule.
• Doses can be escalated over time, from the initial levels of approximately 7.5 mg once weekly to more than 25 mg weekly (often given subcutaneously), to achieve efficacy without parallel increases in toxicity.
• MTX is relatively inexpensive, and the monitoring necessary for toxicity is less expensive than for gold, D-penicillamine, other immunosuppressive agents, or cytotoxic drugs.
• MTX can suppress disease activity in a significant proportion of patients with long-standing RA in whom other therapies have failed.[97]
• In addition to providing efficacy in clinical parameters, MTX appears to retard appearance of new erosions within involved joints.[98-101]
• Using MTX as a building block or the cornerstone of combination therapy has resulted in enhanced efficacy over MTX alone, without added increases in side effects.[17,19-21]
• There have been minimal unexpected side effects after more than 20 years of surveillance.

Most impressive is the documented evidence that MTX can reduce the radiographic evidence of joint destruction. In patients with early RA, it has been documented that MTX is effective at slowing progression. At 24 months of continued use in early RA patients, MTX is almost as effective as etanercept.[100,101] For patients with longer-standing disease, MTX appeared equally as effective as leflunomide in head-to-head studies.[102,103]

As a practical matter, it appears that the dose of MTX can be rapidly escalated. In the etanercept early-RA trial, patients were randomized to receive either etanercept or MTX. Those receiving MTX received a rapid dose escalation from 7.5 mg/week to 20 mg/week orally over a period of 8 weeks. This rapid dose escalation was well tolerated and led to rapid and sustained benefits in patients receiving MTX.[100,101] Patients on MTX with persistent disease should have their dose titrated higher (either rapidly or in the more traditional 2.5-mg increments) until they improve, develop side effects, or reach the 20- to 25-mg threshold. For patients unable to tolerate oral MTX, it is reasonable to consider changing to a subcutaneous or intramuscular injection once per week to limit some of the GI side effects. Another alternative would be to use folic acid daily or folinic acid weekly as a means to reduce some of the side effects of the medication.

Many studies, including one meta-analysis,[104] have reinforced the evidence that folic acid and folinic acid reduce the nausea and mucous-membrane ulcerations that are bothersome side effects of the drug; administration of 5 mg of folic acid once weekly appears to be sufficient, although many physicians prescribe 1 mg daily. Another reason to use folic acid in MTX-treated patients is for its effectiveness in reducing plasma homocysteine levels[105]; hyperhomocysteinemia is an independent risk factor for coronary artery disease, presumably mediated by a toxic effect on the endothelium.

Concerns by rheumatologists about liver toxicity of long-term MTX therapy have gradually diminished. Although the ACR guidelines for MTX use[106] are appropriate to follow, the general gestalt is that in patients with normal liver function, minimal use of alcohol, and negative serologies for hepatitis B and C, liver function tests are necessary only once every 4 to 8 weeks and should be measured 1 or a few days before the next dose. Routine biopsies of the liver, even after many years of continuous therapy, are not required. On the other hand, if liver-function tests do show hepatocellular disease and a decreasing serum albumin despite improvement in the clinical activity of disease, biopsies should be considered if the drug is to be continued.

There is definite conflict, without obvious resolution, between rheumatologists, who rarely have their patients' livers biopsied, and dermatologists, who recommend that their patients being treated with MTX for psoriasis have a liver biopsy performed after a cumulative dose of 1.5 g, and thereafter at 1.0- to 1.5-g intervals.[107] This may be related to as-yet-unknown genetic differences between psoriatic and rheumatoid patients, with the former having increased susceptibility to liver dysfunction in response to drugs, including alcohol.

The other organ threatened by MTX, more in an idiosyncratic or hypersensitivity pattern than liver toxicity, has been the lungs.[108] Reasonable criteria for the diagnosis of MTX-associated pneumonitis are summarized in Chapter 59. The pathology shows interstitial pneumonitis and bronchiolitis. Initial symptoms are often vague and nonspecific: a cough, or sometimes fever and dyspnea. While anticipating such a complication, the physician also must be concerned about and rule out infection with *Pneumocystis carinii* or, less commonly, cytomegalovirus-associated pneumonitis. Patients started on MTX must be told and reminded to report any upper respiratory symptoms to the physician.

It is also important to acknowledge that patients with RA are at increased risk for the development of malignancy. Although rare, lymphomas have been associated with the use of MTX particularly in association with Epstein-Barr virus infection. This is further discussed in Chapter 111, Musculosketal Syndromes and Malignancy.

CYCLOSPORINE

Cyclosporine, used by transplantation immunologists for many years to reduce solid organ allograft rejection, inhibits the activation of CD4+ helper-inducer T lymphocytes by blocking interleukin-2 (IL-2) and other T helper type 1 (Th1) cytokine production[109] and by inhibiting CD40 ligand expression in T lymphocytes.[110] The latter effect prevents T cells from delivering CD40L-dependent signals to B cells. Newer microemulsion forms of cyclosporine are absorbed better and more consistently than older oil-based formulations.

The drug was first used in Europe in doses (such as 10 mg/kg/day) that caused unacceptable reductions in renal function. Adding lower doses (2.5 to 5 mg/kg/day) to a stable dose of MTX and decreasing the cyclosporine if the patient's creatinine level rises to more than 30 percent of initial values has been demonstrated to provide substantial additive benefit over MTX alone.[111] Thirty-six patients (48 percent) of the cyclosporine/MTX group and 12 patients (16 percent) of the MTX-alone group achieved 20 percent improvement according to the ACR criteria. No unacceptable toxicity was observed during an open-label extension of the study for a year,[112] and similar to several of the other recommended regimens, this therapy appeared to slow radiographic progression of erosions.[113]

There is little to be gained by using this drug as monotherapy early in disease, but in patients with RA who cannot tolerate hydroxychloroquine and NSAIDs and, therefore, need a second-line drug to combine withthese, cyclosporine is a reasonable alternative.

TACROLIMUS

Similar to cyclosporine, tacrolimus (FK506) has specific effects limited to inhibiting CD4+ T cell function. It is metabolized and disposed of via the gut and liver, and adverse effects are dose-related and similar to cyclosporine (see Chapter 61). FK506 is not absorbed as readily or consistently as is the microemulsion formulation of cyclosporine. It can be useful in patients for whom cyclosporine is inappropriate, but for whom T cell suppression is desired. Recent work has demonstrated that some patients who have failed with MTX treatment can respond to carefully dose-adjusted tacrolimus.[114]

LEFLUNOMIDE

The role of leflunomide in the treatment of RA is evolving over time. It appears very effective as a monotherapy as an alternative to MTX or safe and effective as an addition to MTX in combination therapy. Leflunomide suppresses the de novo synthesis of pyrimidine (uridine and cytidine) nucleotides by inhibiting dihydroorotate dehydrogenase. Both T and B lymphocytes have low amounts of this enzyme and no salvage pathways for pyrimidine nucleotide synthesis. Therefore, the action of leflunomide is relatively specific for lymphocytes[115] (see Chapter 59).

In what has been referred to often as the "pivotal" trial of leflunomide versus MTX versus placebo, the ACR "responder index" over the 52-week study was 52 percent with leflunomide, 46 percent with MTX, and 26 percent with placebo.[102] Progression of joint erosions were at a rate significantly slower for leflunomide and MTX than in the placebo group. Assays of quality of life, using several instruments such as the Health Assessment Questionnaire Disability Index (HAQ-DI), were slightly better for leflunomide than MTX, and both were substantially better than placebo. As for adverse events, diarrhea was more common in leflunomide-treated patients, but others were the same as for MTX, including sporadic elevations of parenchymal liver enzymes.

A second multicenter phase-III study compared leflunomide head to head with MTX.[103] In this study of 999 patients with RA, both agents demonstrated substantial abilities to improve the symptoms and signs of disease. However, the improvements seen with MTX at 52 weeks were significantly greater than those with leflunomide. Both drugs were well tolerated and both led to inhibition of radiographic progression as assessed by radiographs.

A third phase III, double-blind, randomized, multicenter trial of leflunomide, placebo, and SSZ in active RA (358 patients) showed that leflunomide was more effective than placebo in treatment but no more effective than SSZ.[88]

Clearly, leflunomide is effective as monotherapy and has the ability to slow the radiographic progression of RA.[116] However, it is appropriate to consider using leflunomide as an add-on to MTX for patients who have only a partial response to MTX. Starting with 10 mg of leflunomide daily after a loading dose smaller than usual (e.g., 100 mg for the first 2 days) is a reasonable strategy.[21] Based on the results of the 24-week, 263-patient multicenter study, the addition of leflunomide to MTX resulted in 46 percent of patients achieving an ACR-20 compared to only 24 percent who had placebo added to background MTX.[21] The rates of liver-function test abnormalities, diarrhea, rash, and alopecia were all similar to what had been seen in the prior phase III studies.

One of the most interesting aspects of this drug is its extended plasma half-life of 15 to 18 days, because it binds to plasma proteins. This has led to the recommendation that it be given as a loading dose (100 mg/day for 3 days), followed by doses of 20 mg/day. However, it also means that if a patient has an adverse GI event (e.g., nausea, diarrhea) during or after the loading schedule, it may take some time to for the symptoms to subside. Alternative dosage schedules have evolved with time and experience with the drug, including the attenuated loading regimen and daily therapy used in the combination trial (100 mg/day for 2 days then 10 mg/day).[21] Completely avoiding the loading dose may also decrease the likelihood of side effects in some patients but not necessary negatively impact the efficacy of the drug in the long term. In one of the first randomized, placebo-controlled (phase II) studies, leflunomide was more effective than was placebo, and it was almost as effective as a 10-mg daily dose as is was as a 25-mg daily dose.[117] The higher dose had disproportionately more skin rash/allergic reactions, GI symptoms, weight loss, and reversible alopecia than the 10-mg daily dose. Therefore, it is not unreasonable to think that the lower 10-mg daily dose can be tried initially, with subsequent escalation to a 20-mg dose after safety has been established or after the patient has failed to achieve adequate response. Maintenance therapy of 10 mg rather than 20 mg daily, or 20 mg every other day because of the long biologic half-life, can be beneficial for some patients. It has been recommended that if the serum aspartate transaminase (AST) or alanine transaminase (ALT) increases to twice the upper limits of normal, or if they are repeatedly mildly abnormal, that the leflunomide dose be reduced and discontinued if these abnormalities persist. In general it is prudent to consider following the same guidelines for monitoring leflunomide that are applied to MTX,[106] including warnings for patients regarding alcohol intake and screening for pre-existing hepatitis B and C.

The place in strategies for use of leflunomide should be alongside MTX; it can be given to patients instead of MTX when the latter drug is poorly tolerated or contraindicated. It can also be used in addition to MTX in resistant active arthritis.

INHIBITION BY TUMOR NECROSIS FACTORS

The pivotal roles for tumor necrosis factor-alpha (TNF-α) in initiation and perpetuation of the inflammatory and proliferative processes of rheumatoid synovitis are clearly outlined in Chapter 61 and are summarized in Figure 67–4. As a class, the TNF inhibitors (adalimumab, etanercept, and infliximab) appear to be the most effective means of improving symptoms and signs of disease, increasing function, and reducing radiographic evidence of progression of RA.

Etanercept was the first TNF-α inhibitor to be approved by the Food and Drug Administration (FDA) for use in RA. It is a fusion protein of the soluble portion of the human TNF p75 chain of the receptor and the fragment crystallizable (Fc) portion of human immunoglobulin G1 (IgG1). The receptor portion binds extracellular TNF-α, effectively neutralizing it, and the Fc moiety prolongs its circulating half-life. This drug is traditionally administered as a subcutaneous injection of 25 mg twice weekly. However, the development of a new formulation will now allow the delivery of a single 50-mg injection once a week.

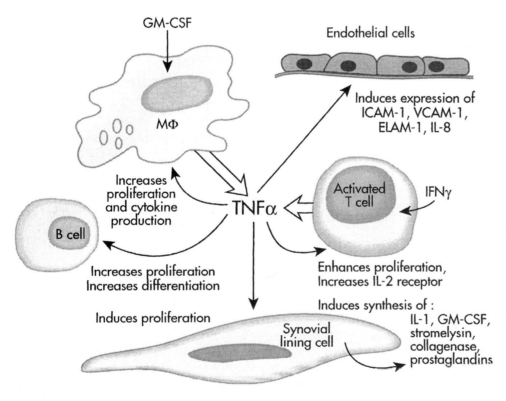

FIGURE 67–4 · TNF-α is a cytokine with multiple potentials for driving many engines of the inflammatory/proliferative processes in rheumatoid arthritis. It appears that both activated macrophages and T cells produce TNF-α, which in turn, can act back on these cells as well as on the synovial lining cells, endothelium, and B cells. All the major activity of TNF-α in model systems can be inferred to be proinflammatory. The fact that active TNF-α enhances IL-1 production by cells is additional evidence for its primacy in generating and sustaining rheumatoid synovitis.

Similar to other trials of newer agents, etanercept was tested in combination with MTX (stable dose of 15 to 25 mg/week) against MTX alone. The results set a new standard against which therapeutic agents for RA must be measured.[20] At 24 weeks, 71 percent of the patients receiving etanercept plus MTX and 27 percent of those receiving placebo plus MTX met the ACR-20 criteria (p < 0.001). Very important were the data that 39 percent of those receiving the combination and only 3 percent of those receiving MTX alone met the ACR-50 percent improvement criteria (p < 0.001), and 15 percent of the combination group met the ACR-70 criteria. The ACR-70 criteria have been proposed by the FDA as the criteria for a major clinical response.

A second important study involved patients in whom one to four second-line drugs had essentially failed (e.g., azathioprine, MTX, SSZ, penicillamine, hydroxychloroquine, or gold salts) and who were able to take NSAIDs and less than 10 mg prednisone each day.[118] They received etanercept or placebo. At 6 months, 59 percent of those receiving 25 mg of etanercept twice weekly and 11 percent of the placebo group had achieved a 20-percent ACR criteria response; 40 and 5 percent, respectively, achieved an ACR-50 response (p < 0.01). No patient developed signs or symptoms of another autoimmune disease.

A third important study looked at patients with early RA and compared the effects of MTX or etanercept on symptoms and signs, joint destruction, and function.[100,101] In this study, 632 patients with less than 3 years of disease and who were naïve to MTX and biologic agents were randomized to receive either aggressively dosed MTX (20 mg/wk) or one of two different doses of etanercept (10 mg subcutaneously twice a week or 25 mg subcutaneously twice a week). Patients treated with etanercept had a more rapid response than was seen with MTX. This led to significantly greater improvements at the ACR-20, -50, and -70 levels with etanercept compared to MTX for the first 4 months of the study. Interestingly, although there was still a numerical trend favoring the 25-mg dose of etanercept over MTX at 1 year, the statistical significance was lost. Both agents were very effective at reducing the symptoms and signs of RA in patients with early and aggressive disease. As part of this study, radiographs were also obtained, and there was good correlation between the clinical improvement and a lack of radiographic progression. There was a statistically significant advantage for etanercept at 6 months but, as with the clinical improvement, the radiographic assessments showed a trend but no statistical significance at 1 year.[100]

At 2 years the improvement in symptomatic benefits favored those patients who had been in the 25 mg of etanercept cohort. The ACR-20 response rate was 72 percent, versus 59 percent in the MTX arm. Etanercept appeared to be better tolerated with fewer side effects than seen in the MTX cohort. This was also reflected in the attrition seen in the study, with 74 percent of 25 mg etanercept patients remaining in the study after 2 years versus 59 percent of patients receiving MTX.[101]

Possibly the most interesting result of these studies, however, was the ability of etanercept to slow radiographic progression more than MTX. The mean change in the total Sharp score at 2 years was 1.3 in the 25 mg etanercept arm versus 3.2 in MTX group, demonstrating statistically meaningful differences in radiographic progression between the two arms. There was also a statistically significant difference seen between the number of patients with no evidence of radiographic progression at 2 years (63% etanercept versus 51% MTX). Patients also showed a significant improvement in function and a reduction in disability measured by the HAQ-DI; 55 percent of the etanercept patients achieved a 0.5 reduction in HAQ-DI, as did 37 percent of the MTX patients.

Infliximab is a chimeric anti-TNF monoclonal antibody. It was the second agent approved for use by the FDA in treatment of RA and had previously been approved for use in Crohn's disease. The majority of the antibody is human; however, a small portion of the Fab region is murine in origin. The antibody is given via intravenous infusions of 3 to 10 mg/kg. The recommended dosing regimen is 3 mg/kg with infusions at weeks 0, 2, and 6 and every 8 weeks thereafter. If patients fail to achieve a significant benefit, the dose can be increased or the dosing interval shortened. For pharmacokinetic and pharmacoeconomic reasons it may be more desirable to shorten the dosing interval rather than to increase the dose.[119] Concomitant administration of MTX gives more sustained benefit, may reduce the clearance of the drug and may possibly lead to less immunogenicity, reflected by a reduction in human antichimeric antibody (HACA) formation.[120,121] Whether concomitant use of other small molecules affords the same advantage is unknown, but plausible.

In the ATTRACT trial, a phase III study involving 428 patients, infliximab demonstrated significant benefit in patients with long-standing and refractory RA. Patients failing to respond to MTX were randomized to receive either placebo, infliximab (3 mg/kg every 4 weeks or every 8 weeks), or infliximab (10 mg/kg every 4 weeks or every 8 weeks). After 54 weeks there was a statistically significant advantage favoring all the infliximab/MTX arms when compared to the placebo/MTX arm. The ACR-20 response rate seen with placebo/MTX was 17 percent, compared to 42, 48, 59, and 59 percent, respectively, in the infliximab 3 mg/kg q 4 wks, 3 mg/kg q 8 wks, 10 mg/kg q 4 wks, and 10 mg/kg q 8 wks groups. ACR-50 responses were also significant and exceeded 34 percent in the three highest-dosed cohorts.[19]

Although infliximab demonstrated marked improvements in the symptoms and signs of disease, the most impressive results of this study were the ability of infliximab to slow the radiographic progression of RA. Each of the infliximab/MTX arms demonstrated a dramatic decrease in what would have been their predicted rate of radiographic progression, and statistical superiority to the placebo/MTX arm. Commensurate with the improvement in clinical manifestations was an improvement in function and a reduction in disability measured by the HAQ-DI and the short-form 36.[19]

Adalimumab (D2E7) is the latest of the biologic agents directed against TNF to be approved by the FDA for the treatment of RA. This is a fully human monoclonal antibody directed against TNF and is delivered as a subcutaneous injection once every other week or, in patients with insufficient response, it can be given once a week. Use of background MTX with this agent also appears to increase the duration of response, possibly by slowing the clearance of the drug. As was demonstrated with etanercept and infliximab, adalimumab showed significant benefits when combined with MTX.[22]

In the Anti-TNF Research Study Program of the Monoclonal Antibody D2E7 in Patients with Rheumatoid Arthritis (ARMADA) with adalimumab, patients with severe refractory RA were randomized to receive placebo or subcutaneous D2E7, at doses of 20, 40, or 80 mg every other week, in combination with MTX. The efficacy of adalimumab given subcutaneously every other week in combination with MTX was significantly better than MTX plus placebo, with ACR-20, -50, and -70 scores of 65, 53, and 26 percent, respectively, at the 40 mg every - other - week dose. In a second large study,[122] patients with active RA, after a 4-week DMARD washout period, were randomized to one of five groups: 20 mg of adalimumab every other week (EOW) or weekly, 40 mg of adalimumab EOW or weekly, or placebo. Patients who received 40 mg of adalimumab EOW showed substantial benefit, with an ACR-20 response of 46 percent, compared to placebo response of 19 percent. Those in the 40-mg group with weekly (QW) treatment did even better, with an ACR-20 response of 53.4 percent.

A 52-week, double-blind, placebo-controlled study[123] was carried out on patients with active RA who were receiving stable doses of MTX. Patients were randomly assigned to receive adalimumab, 20 mg subcutaneously QW; adalimumam, 40 mg EOW with placebo on the alternate weeks; or placebo QW. Substantial inhibition of radiographic progression was observed for both joint-space narrowing and erosions, particularly for the 40 mg EOW treatment group. The authors concluded that adalimumab given subcutaneously QW (20 mg) or EOW (40 mg) with concomitant MTX significantly inhibited progression of structural joint damage and improved signs and symptoms of RA in patients who previously were incomplete responders to MTX.

SAFETY OF TUMOR NECROSIS FACTOR INHIBITION

Tempering enthusiasm about the anti-TNF approaches to treatment is the reality that the beneficial effects are not permanent. Cessation of therapy is followed by a recrudescence of disease. The cytokine "rheostat" is not reset and the as-yet-unknown forces initiating the inflammatory and proliferative process are still at work.[124] Moreover, TNF inhibition does not work in all patients; exceptions are noted in the following list.

- *Serious infections (excluding tuberculosis).* When TNF inhibitors were first introduced in the late 1990s, there was concern that blocking TNF might impair the host defense system. Clinicians have since been reassured that, in general, there have not been significant problems with serious bacterial infections in patients treated with TNF inhibitors. Occasional

patients on etanercept, infliximab, or adalimumab have developed an opportunistic infection. Predicting which patients will develop an infection is almost impossible. Therefore, a degree of vigilance and the recognition that infections can occur should be part of all treatment initiation and monitoring efforts. In addition, it is apparent that in debilitated patients (those with infections such as skin ulcers or pneumonia or those with other illnesses that would increase the risk of infection or diminished immune surveillance) TNF inhibition is contraindicated.

- *Tuberculosis.* Reactivation of tuberculosis (TB) has been reported with all the TNF inhibitors. So far, there are more reports with infliximab than with etanercept or adalimumab. Researchers are not clear as to whether these differences are related to differing mechanism of action, pharmacokinetics, or the patient populations studied. Given the potential for reactivation of TB, appropriate screening should be done prior to the initiation of treatment with a TNF inhibitor.

- *Malignancies.* There has been no increase in the reported rate of malignancy among patients on TNF inhibitors. It is not known whether the rate of malignancy in these patients will increase over the expected number of cases in the general population as patients move beyond the current treatment-experience level of 6 years.

- *Demyelination.* Rare cases of multiple sclerosis, optic neuritis, and demyelination have been reported in patients taking TNF inhibitors.[125-128] These have been sporadic and appear in most cases to resolve when the TNF inhibitor is withdrawn. Because demyelination is a rare occurrence in the population at large, it is unclear whether these events are occurring more often than expected. It is recommended that TNF inhibition be avoided in patients with a history of demyelinating illness or who have features of unique neurologic problems.

TUMOR NECROSIS FACTOR INHIBITION AND THE TREATMENT OF RHEUMATOID ARTHRITIS

The TNF-inhibiting agents have demonstrated superior ability to reduce the signs and symptoms of RA, inhibit the progression of structural damage, and improve physical function in patients with this disease. Despite this, their role in the armamentarium remains debated. The debate focuses on several factors including the costs (Table 67–2), lack of long-term safety data, and the ability of traditional approaches to effectively treat a large number of patients.

In the previously mentioned etanercept early-RA trial, etanercept demonstrated statistically significant benefits over MTX. However, questions are raised as to whether this numerical/statistical advantage is clinically meaningful enough to warrant the difference in cost. For individual patients this can be a difficult issue, but given the cost differential and the lack of biomarkers or surrogates available to distinguish those likely to respond to therapy from those who will not, it is reasonable to suggest that the vast majority of patients should be treated with MTX prior to advancing to a TNF inhibitor. However, should a patient fail to achieve a significant response to MTX over a period of a few months, switching the patient to a TNF inhibitor as monotherapy or adding a TNF inhibitor and treating in combination with background DMARDs should be considered.

Without head-to-head studies, the question as to which agent affords the greatest efficacy cannot be answered. However, there is evidence that some patients may respond better to one TNF inhibitor than another. In fact, failure of one TNF inhibitor should not preclude switching to another. Based on a small series, there is reason to believe that more than 60 percent of patients who switch from etanercept to infliximab or from infliximab to etanercept are likely to experience significantly better results.[129] Deciding which agent to use for which patient is a difficult decision and is often influenced by a host of issues, including patient preference of injection or infusion, monotherapy or combination therapy, and most frequently, what agent insurance companies will reimburse.

INTERLEUKIN-1 RECEPTOR ANTAGONIST AND INTERLEUKIN-1 RECEPTOR

IL-1, like TNF-α has been implicated in the pathogenesis of RA. There is a circulating protein found in extracellular tissues, IL-1 receptor antagonist (IL-1Ra), which is a biologically important protein that functions as a naturally occurring antagonist to IL-1. It is produced by rheumatoid synovium and other tissues, predominantly by macrophages. A recombinant human form, anakinra, has been prepared for subcutaneous injection. In 2002, anakinra was approved by the FDA for the treatment of RA. It is given as a daily subcutaneous injection of 100 mg.

A 24-week double-blind, randomized, placebo-controlled, multicenter study of 472 patients reported that of the patients who received 150 mg/day of anakinra as monotherapy, 43 percent met the ACR-20 criteria for improvement, although 27 percent of the placebo group did as well.[130] A study of combination anakinra/MTX was done in 419 patients who had failed to achieve an adequate response to MTX alone.[131] At 24 weeks, the ACR-20 response rate in the anakinra 1.0-mg/kg (46%) and 2.0-mg/kg (38%) dose groups was significantly greater than in the placebo group (19%). Anakinra has also been demonstrated to be both safe and effective with a number of other DMARDs, including hydroxychloroquine, SSZ, and leflunomide.[132] However, two separate trials looking at combination use of anakinra with etanercept showed higher rates of infections and failed to demonstrate clinical benefits of the combination of these two anticytokine therapies.[133,134] In addition to the clinical benefits in signs and symptoms of disease, two studies have demonstrated that use of anakinra can reduce radiologic progression of RA.[135,136]

In general, anakinra has been demonstrated to be safe and well tolerated. The most frequent side effect has been injection-site reactions that occur in more than 50 percent of the patients who take this medication. Although mild and self limited, this problem can be a very uncomfortable one. In time it will become more clear about where in the armamentarium for treatment of RA anakinra will best fit. Currently, it is most often used in patients who have tried and failed a TNF inhibitor. This is in part related to its cost (see Table 67–2), the need for need for daily subcutaneous injections, and the perception of being less effective as a therapeutic biologic compound than are the TNF inhibitors. A number of biologic compounds and small molecules under development are based on good scientific rationale (see Chapter 62), and the role of inhibition of IL-1 will need to be constantly reevaluated in the face of new information.

PROTEIN A IMMUNOABSORPTION COLUMN

The FDA has approved as a device this staphylococcal protein that binds IgG and IgG-antigen complexes, removing them from the circulation of patients with severe RA that is not responsive to second-line therapy. The device has been effective in immune thrombocytopenic purpura and has been moderately more effective in RA than a "placebo" that provided sham immunoabsorption.[137] Its use is expensive, time-consuming for expert staff, and accompanied by many side effects. The trials in RA necessitated a column treatment once a week for 12 weeks; postmarketing trials will be essential to determine whether the treatment is effective in patients resistant to combinations of small molecules and biologic response modifiers. This remains an option only for patients who have failed treatment with traditional DMARDs as well as the newer anticytokine agents.

▌ Future Directions in Therapy of Rheumatoid Arthritis

The effectiveness of etanercept, infliximab, and adalimumab, drugs conceived of and developed from theoretic considerations born of basic research in pathophysiology, has bolstered enthusiasm that similar strategies will be effective as they focus on other arms of the process leading to a proliferative synovitis. The gradual addition and amplification of components linking together to produce RA in its mature form are outlined in Chapter 65. Some of the current strategies—whether well developed (addressed in this chapter and chapters 59 and 61) or only in concepts—(see Chapter 62) will clearly evolve in the coming years. Gone are the days of broad-based cytotoxic approaches, and we are well beyond the days when physicians had only rest, exercise, aspirin, and injectable gold to use. The new therapies will be targeted, specific, and additive. It is likely that synergism will be found among some of the future therapies and existing ones.

Several important caveats, however, must be emphasized. No matter how seductive the concept or clever the methodology in production of the product, any new therapy must be proven to have efficacy and minimal toxicity by randomized, double-blind, placebo-controlled trials.

On a practical note, evidence is mounting that early and aggressive therapy may afford a window of opportunity for substantive disease modification, which may lead to long-term protective benefits. In addition to the growing emphasis on early intervention, the rheumatology community is continually striving to improve overall response rates among current patients and expand intervention into untreated populations. There is also a strong desire to develop therapies that work in 90 to 100 percent of patients, not the 60 percent seen today. The long-term goal of treatment intervention should be to achieve remission. The remarkable efficacy and safety of biologic agents has been reassuring. However, monitoring for adverse events and for unforeseen occurrences must continue. Differences between agents also warrant considerable research. It may well be that different populations and disease states will be better suited to one or another agent either as monotherapy or in combination with other agents. More well-designed studies combining biologic agents and biologics with small-molecule DMARDs are needed. Rheumatologists must continually evaluate the pros and cons of mono-therapy and combination therapies and adjust treatment regimens in ways that lead to successful clinical outcomes.

REFERENCES

1. Wolfe F, Cathey MA: The assessment and prediction of functional disability in rheumatoid arthritis. J Rheumatol 18(9):1298-1306, 1999.
2. Wolfe F, Hawley DJ: The longterm outcomes of rheumatoid arthritis: Work disability; a prospective 18 year study of 823 patients. J Rheumatol 25(11):2108-2117, 1998.
3. Scott DL, Symmons DPM, Coulton BL, et al: Long-term outcome of treating rheumatoid arthritis: Results after 20 years. Lancet 1(8542):1108, 1987.
4. Pincus T, Callahan LF, Sale WG, et al: Severe functional declines, work disability, and increased mortality in seventy-five rheumatoid arthritis patients studied over nine years. Arthritis Rheum 27:864, 1984.
5. Wolfe F, Sharp JT: Radiographic outcome of recent-onset rheumatoid arthritis: a 19-year study of radiographic progression. Arthritis Rheum 41(9):1571-1582, 1998.
6. Pincus T, Callahan LF, Fuchs HA, et al: Quantitative analysis of hand radiographs in rheumatoid arthritis: time course of radiographic changes, relation to joint examination measures, and comparison of different scoring methods. J Rheumatol 22(10):1983-1989, 1995.
7. Pincus T, Fuchs HA, Callahan LF, et al: Early radiographic joint space narrowing and erosion and later malalignment in rheumatoid arthritis: a longitudinal analysis. J Rheumatol 25(4):636-640, 1998.
8. Fuchs HA, Kaye JJ, Callahan LF, et al: Evidence of significant radiographic damage in rheumatoid arthritis within the first two years of disease. J Rheumatol 16:585, 1989.
9. Singh G, Terry R, Ramey D, et al: Long-term medical costs and outcomes are significantly associated with early changes in disability in rheumatoid arthritis. Arthritis Rheum 39(9):S318, 1996.
10. Yelin E, Wanke LA: An assessment of the annual and long-term direct costs of rheumatoid arthritis: the impact of poor function and functional decline. Arthritis Rheum 42(6):1209-1218, 1999.
11. O'Dell JR: Treating rheumatoid arthritis early: a window of opportunity? Arthritis Rheum 46(2):283-285, 2002.
12. A randomized trial of hydroxychloroquine in early rheumatoid arthritis. The HERA Study. Am J Med 98(2):156-168, 1995.
13. Tsakonas E, Fitzgerald AA, Fitzcharles MA, et al: Consequences of delayed therapy with second-line agents in rheumatoid arthritis: a 3 year followup on the hydroxychloroquine in early rheumatoid arthritis (HERA) study. J Rheumatol 27(3):623-629, 2000.
14. Boers M, Verhoeven AC, Markusse HM, et al: Randomised comparison of combined step-down prednisolone, methotrexate and sulphasalazine with sulphasalazine alone in early rheumatoid arthritis. Lancet 350(9074):309-318, 1997.
15. Landewe RB, Boers M, Verhoeven AC, et al: COBRA combination therapy in patients with early rheumatoid arthritis: long-term structural benefits of a brief intervention. Arthritis Rheum 46(2):47-356, 2002.
16. McCarty DJ, Carrera GF: Treatment of intractable rheumatoid arthritis with combined cyclophosphamide, azathioprine and hydroxychloroquine. JAMA 255:2215, 1982.
17. O'Dell JR, Haire CE, Erikson N, et al: Treatment of rheumatoid arthritis with methotrexate alone, sulfasalazine and hydroxychloroquine, or a combination of all three medications. N Engl J Med 334:1287, 1996.
18. Mottonen T, Hannonen P, Leirisalo-Repo M, et al: Comparison of combination therapy with single-drug therapy in early rheumatoid arthritis: a randomised trial. Lancet 353:1568, 1999.
19. Lipsky PE, van der Heijde DM, St Clair EW, et al: Infliximab and methotrexate in the treatment of rheumatoid arthritis: Anti-tumor necrosis factor trial in rheumatoid arthritis with concomitant therapy study group. N Engl J Med 343(22):1594-1602, 2000.
20. Weinblatt ME, Kremer JM, Bankhurst AD, et al: A trial of etanercept, a recombinant tumor necrosis factor receptor: Fc fusion protein, in patients with rheumatoid arthritis receiving methotrexate. N Engl J Med 340:253-259, 1999.
21. Kremer JM, Genovese MC, Cannon GW, et al: Concomitant leflunomide therapy in patients with active rheumatoid arthritis despite stable doses of methotrexate: A randomized, double-blind, placebo-controlled trial. Ann Intern Med 137(9):726-733, 2002.
22. Weinblatt ME, Keystone EC, Furst DE, et al: Adalimumab, a fully human anti-tumor necrosis factor alpha monoclonal antibody, for the treatment of rheumatoid arthritis in patients taking concomitant methotrexate. The ARMADA trial. Arthritis Rheum 48(1):35-45, 2003.
23. Felson DT, Anderson JJ, Boers M, et al: American College of Rheumatology preliminary definition of improvement in rheumatoid arthritis. Arthritis Rheum 38:727, 1995.
24. van Leeuwen MA, van der Heijde DMFM, van Rijswijk MH, et al: Interrelationship of outcome measures and process variables in early rheumatoid arthritis: A comparison of radiologic damage, physical disability, joint counts, and acute phase reactants. J Rheumatol 21:3, 1994.
25. Ward MM, Leigh JP, Fries JF: Progression of functional disability in patients with rheumatoid arthritis. Arch Intern Med 153:2229, 1993.
26. Wolfe F, Hawley DJ, Cathey MA: Clinical and health status measures over time: Prognosis and outcome assessment in rheumatoid arthritis. J Rheumatol 18:1290, 1991.
27. MacLean CH, Louie R, Leake B, et al: Quality of care for patients with rheumatoid arthritis. JAMA 284(8):984-992, 2000.
28. Criswell LA, Such CL, Neuhaus JM, et al: Variation among rheumatologists in clinical outcomes and frequency of office visits for rheumatoid arthritis. J Rheumatol 24:7, 1997.
29. Mottonen T, Paimela L, Leirisalo-Repo M, et al: Only high disease activity and positive rheumatoid factor indicate poor prognosis in patients with early rheumatoid arthritis treated with "sawtooth" strategy. Ann Rheum Dis 57:533, 1998.
30. Callahan LF, Brooks RH, Summey JA, et al: Quantitative pain assessment for routine care of rheumatoid arthritis patents, using a pain scale based on activities of daily living and a visual analog pain scale. Arthritis Rheum 30:630, 1987.
31. Callahan LF, Pincus T, Huston JW III, et al: Measures of activity and damage in rheumatoid arthritis: Depiction of changes and prediction of mortality over five years. Arthritis Care Res 10:381, 1997.
32. Wolfe F, Zwillich SH: The long-term outcomes of rheumatoid arthritis: A 23-year prospective, longitudinal study of total joint replacement and its predictors in 1,600 patients with rheumatoid arthritis. Arthritis Rheum 41:1072, 1998.
33. Kim JM, Weisman MH: When does rheumatoid arthritis begin and why do we need to know? Arthritis Rheum 43(3):473-484, 2000.
34. O'Dell JR, Nepom BS, Haire C, et al: HLA-DRB1 typing in rheumatoid arthritis: Predicting response to specific treatments. Ann Rheum Dis 57:209, 1998.
35. Weyand C, Goronzy J: Prognosis in rheumatoid arthritis: Applying new technologies to old questions. J Rheumatol 20:11, 1993.

36. Garnero P, Landewe R, Boers M, et al: Association of baseline levels of markers of bone and cartilage degradation with long-term progression of joint damage in patients with early rheumatoid arthritis. Arthritis Rheum 46(11):2847-2856, 2002.

37. Ostergaard M, Hansen M, Stoltenberg M, et al: Magnetic resonance imaging–determined synovial membrane volume as a marker of disease activity and a predictor of progressive joint destruction in the wrists of patients with rheumatoid arthritis. Arthritis Rheum 42(5):918, 1999.

38. Backhaus M, Kamradt T, Sandrock D, et al: Arthritis of the finger joints: a comprehensive approach comparing conventional radiography, scintigraphy, ultrasound, and contrast-enhanced magnetic resonance imaging. Arthritis Rheum 42(6):1232-1245, 1999.

39. Wolfe F, Ross K, Hawley DJ, et al: The prognosis of rheumatoid arthritis and undifferentiated polyarthritis syndrome in the clinic: A study of 1141 patients. J Rheumatol 20:2005, 1993.

40. Chan KWA, Felson DT, Yood RA, et al: The lag time between onset of symptoms and diagnosis of rheumatoid arthritis. Arthritis Rheum 37:814, 1994.

41. Pincus T: Formal educational level: A marker for the importance of behavioral variables in the pathogenesis, morbidity, and mortality of most diseases? J Rheumatol 15:10, 1988.

42. Pincus T, Callahan LF: Formal education as a marker for increased mortality and morbidity in rheumatoid arthritis. J Chronic Dis 311:552, 1984.

43. Lorig K, Seleznick M, Lubeck D, et al: The beneficial outcomes of the arthritis self-management course are not adequately explained by behavioral change. Arthritis Rheum 32:91, 1989.

44. Lorig KR, Mazonson PD, Holman HR: Evidence suggesting that health education for self-management in patients with chronic arthritis has sustained health benefits while reducing health care costs. Arthritis Rheum 36:439, 1993.

45. Taal E, Rasker JJ, Wiegman O: Patient education and self-management in the rheumatic diseases: A self-efficacy approach. Arthritis Care Res 9:229, 1996.

46. Parker JC, Smarr KL, Buckelew SP, et al: Effects of stress management on clinical outcomes in rheumatoid arthritis. Arthritis Rheum 38:1807, 1995.

47. Bellamy N, Bradley L: Workshop on chronic pain, pain control, and patient outcomes in rheumatoid arthritis and osteoarthritis. Arthritis Rheum 39:357, 1996.

48. Rall LC, Meydani SN, Kehayias JJ, et al: The effect of progressive resistance training in rheumatoid arthritis. Arthritis Rheum 39:415, 1996.

49. Harcom TM, Lampan RM, Banwell BF, et al: Therapeutic value of graded aerobic exercise training in rheumatoid arthritis. Arthritis Rheum 28:32, 1985.

50. Helewa A, Goldsmith CH, Lee P, et al: Effects of occupational therapy home service on patients with rheumatoid arthritis. Lancet 337:1453, 1991.

51. Wolfe MM, Lichtenstein DR, Singh G: Gastrointestinal toxicity of nonsteroidal antiinflammatory drugs. N Engl J Med 340:1888, 1999.

52. Abramson S, Weissmann G: The mechanisms of action of nonsteroidal anti-inflammatory drugs. Arthritis Rheum 32:1, 1989.

53. Silverstein FE, Faich G, Goldstein JL, et al: Gastrointestinal toxicity with celecoxib vs nonsteroidal anti-inflammatory drugs for osteoarthritis and rheumatoid arthritis: the CLASS (Celecoxib Long-Term Arthritis Safety Study) study: A randomized controlled trial. JAMA 284(10):1247-1255, 2000.

54. Bombardier C, Laine L, Reicin A, et al: Comparison of upper gastrointestinal toxicity of rofecoxib and naproxen in patients with rheumatoid arthritis. VIGOR Study Group. N Engl J Med 343(21):1520-1528, 2000.

55. Strand V, Hochberg MC: The risk of cardiovascular thrombotic events with selective cyclooxygenase-2 inhibitors. Arthritis Rheum 47(4):349-355, 2002.

56. Weinstein RS, Jilka RL, Parfitt AM, et al: Inhibition of osteoblastogenesis and promotion of apoptosis of osteoblasts and osteocytes by glucocorticoids. J Clinical Invest 102:274, 1998.

57. Compton JE, Vedi S, Croucher PL, et al: Bone turnover in nonsteroid treated rheumatoid arthritis. Ann Rheum Dis 53:163, 1994.

58. Kröger H, Honkanen R, Saarikoski S, et al: Decreased axial bone mineral density in perimenopausal women with rheumatoid arthritis: A population based study. Ann Rheum Dis 53:18, 1994.

59. Dequeker J, Geisems P: Osteoporosis and arthritis. Ann Rheum Dis 49:276, 1990.

60. Kirwan JR: The effect of glucocorticoids on joint destruction in rheumatoid arthritis. N Engl J Med 333:142, 1995.

61. van Everdingen AA, Jacobs JW, Siewertsz Van Reesema DR, etal: Low-dose prednisone therapy for patients with early active rheumatoid arthritis: clinical efficacy, disease-modifying properties, and side effects: a randomized, double-blind, placebo-controlled clinical trial. Ann Intern Med 136(1):1-12, 2002.

62. Fries JF, Williams CA, Ramsey DR, Bloch DA: The relative toxicity of disease-modifying antirheumatic drugs. Arthritis Rheum 36:297, 1993.

63. Wolfe F, Mitchell DM, Sibley JT, et al: The mortality of rheumatoid arthritis. Arthritis Rheum 37:481, 1994.

64. Ruegsegger P, Medici TC, Anliker M: Corticosteroid-induced bone loss: A longitudinal study of alternate day therapy in patients with bronchial asthma using quantitative computed tomography. Eur J Clin Pharmacol 25:615, 1994.

65. Hochberg MC, Prashker MJ, Greenwald M, et al: Recommendations for the prevention and treatment of glucocorticoid-induced osteoporosis. Am Coll Rheum 39(11):1791, 1996.

66. Yu LP Jr., Smith GN, Hasty KA, et al: Doxycycline inhibits type XI collagenolytic activity of extracts from human osteoarthritis cartilage and of gelatinase. J Rheumatol 18:1450, 1991.

67. Smith GN Jr., Brandt KD, Hasty KA: Activation of recombinant human neutrophil procollagenase in the presence of doxycycline results in fragmentation of the enzyme and loss of enzyme activity. Arthritis Rheum 39:235, 1996.

68. Kloppenburg M, Breedveld FC, Terwiel JP, et al: Minocycline in active rheumatoid arthritis: a double-blind, placebo-controlled trial. Arthritis Rheum 37:629, 1994.

69. Tilley B, Alarcon G, Heyse S, et al: Minocycline in rheumatoid arthritis: A 48-week, double blind, placebo-controlled trial. Ann Intern Med 122:81, 1995.

70. Odell JR, Haire CE, Palmer W, et al: Treatment of early rheumatoid arthritis with minocycline or placebo: Results of a randomized, double-blind, placebo-controlled trial. Arthritis Rheum 40:842, 1997.

71. O'Dell JR, Blakely KW, Mallek JA, et al: Treatment of early seropositive rheumatoid arthritis: a two-year, double-blind comparison of minocycline and hydroxychloroquine. Arthritis Rheum 44(10):2235-2241, 2001.

72. Elkayam Ori, Levartovsky D, Brautbar C, et al: Clinical and immunological study of 7 patients with minocycline-induced autoimmune phenomena. Am J Med 105:484, 1998.

73. Kremer JM, Jubiz W, Michalek A, et al: Fish-oil fatty acid supplementation in active rheumatoid arthritis: A double-blinded, controlled, crossover study. Ann Intern Med 106:497, 1987.

74. Geusens P, Wouters C, Nijs J, et al: Long-term effect of omega-3 fatty acids of active rheumatoid arthritis. Arthritis Rheum 37:824, 1994.

75. Leventhal LJ, Boyce EG, Zurier RB: Treatment of rheumatoid arthritis with gamma-linolenic acid. Ann Intern Med 119:867, 1993.

76. Guidelines for the management of rheumatoid arthritis: 2002 Update. Arthritis Rheum 46(2):328-346, 2002.

77. Pincus T, O'Dell JR, Kremer JM: Combination therapy with multiple disease-modifying antirheumatic drugs in rheumatoid arthritis: a preventive strategy. Ann Intern Med 131(10):768-774, 1999.

78. Kremer JM: Rational use of new and existing disease-modifying agents in rheumatoid arthritis. Ann Intern Med 134(8):695-706, 2001.

79. O'Dell JR, Leff R, Paulsen G, et al: Treatment of rheumatoid arthritis with methotrexate and hydroxychloroquine, methotrexate and sulfasalazine, or a combination of the three medictions: results of a two-year, randomized, double-blind, placebo-controlled trial. Arthritis Rheum 46(5):1164-1170, 2002.

80. Mottonen T, Hannonen P, Leirisalo-Repo M, et al: Comparison of combination therapy with single-drug therapy in early rheumatoid arthritis: a randomised trial. FIN-RACo trial group. Lancet 353(9164):1568-1573, 1999.

81. Mottonen T, Hannonen P, Korpela M, et al: Delay to institution of therapy and induction of remission using single-drug or combination-disease modifying antirheumatic drug therapy in early rheumatoid arthritis. Arthritis Rheum 46(4):894-898, 2002.

82. Bernstein HN: Ocular safety of hydroxychloroquine. Ann Ophthalmol 23:292, 1991.

83. Fox RI, Kang H: Mechanism of action of antimalarial drugs: Inhibition of antigen processing and presentation. Lupus 2(Suppl 1):S9, 1993.

84. Faarvang KL, Egsmose C, Kryger P: Hydroxychloroquine and sulphasalazine alone and in combination in rheumatoid arthritis: A randomised double blind trial. Ann Rheum Dis 52:711, 1993.

85. Svartz N: A new sulfanilamide preparation. Acta Med Scand 110:577, 1942.

86. Hannonen P, Mottonen T, Hakola M, et al: Sulfasalazine in early rheumatoid arthritis: A 48-week double-blind, prospective, placebo-controlled study. Arthritis Rheum 36:1501, 1993.

87. van der Heijde DM, van Riel PL, Nuver-Zwart IH, et al: Effects of hydroxychloroquine and sulphasalazine on progression of joint damage in rheumatoid arthritis. Lancet 1(8646):1036-1038, 1989.

88. Smolen JS, Kalden JR, Scott DL: Efficacy and safety of leflunomide compared with placebo and sulfasalazine in active rheumatoid arthritis: A double-blind, randomised, multicentre trial. European leflunomide study group. Lancet 353(9149):259, 1999.

89. Buckland-Wright JC, Clarke GS, Chikanza IC, et al: Quantitative microfocal radiography detects changes in erosion area in patients with early rheumatoid arthritis treated with Myochrysine. J Rheumatol 20:243, 1993.

90. Sakkas LI, Chikanza IC, Vaughn RW, et al: Gold induced nephropathy in rheumatoid arthritis and HLA class II genes. Ann Rheum Dis 52:300, 1993.

91. Felson DT, Anderson JJ, Meenan RF: The comparative efficacy and toxicity of second-line drugs in rheumatoid arthritis: Results of second-line drugs in rheumatoid arthritis. Arthritis Rheum 33:1449, 1990.

92. Borg G, Allander E, Berg E: Auranofin treatment in early rheumatoid arthritis may postpone early retirement: Results from a 2-year double blind trial. J Rheumatol 18:1015, 1991.

93. Black AJ, McLeod HL, Capell HA: Thiopurine methyltransferase genotype predicts therapy limiting severe toxicity from azathioprine. Ann Intern Med 129:716, 1998.

94. Blanco R, Martinez-Taboada VM, Gonzalez-Gay MA: Acute febrile toxic reaction in patients with refractory rheumatoid arthritis who are receiving combined therapy with methotrexate and azathioprine. Arthritis Rheum 39:1016, 1996.

95. Jessop JD, O'Sullivan MM, Lewis PA, et al: A long term five-year randomized trial of hydroxychloroquine, sodium aurothiomalate, auranofin and penicillamine in the treatment of patients with rheumatoid arthritis. Br J Rheumatol 37:992, 1998.

96. Weinblatt ME, Maier AL: Longterm experience with low dose weekly methotrexate in rheumatoid arthritis. J Rheumatol 17(Suppl 22):33, 1990.

97. Rau R, Schleusser B, Herborn G, et al: Long term treatment of destructive rheumatoid arthritis with methotrexate. J Rheumatol 24:1881, 1997.

98. Rau R, Herborn G, Karger T, et al: Retardation of radiologic progression in rheumatoid arthritis with methotrexate therapy: A controlled study. Arthritis Rheum 34:1236, 1991.

99. Jeurissen MEC, Boerbooms AMT, van de Putte LBA, et al: Influence of methotrexate and azathioprine on radiologic progression in rheumatoid arthritis: A randomized, double-blind study. Ann Intern Med 114:999, 1991.

100. Bathon JM, Martin RW, Fleischmann RM, et al: A comparison of etanercept and methotrexate in patients with early rheumatoid arthritis. N Engl J Med 343(22):1586-1593, 2000.

101. Genovese MC, Bathon JM, Martin RW, et al: Etanercept versus methotrexate in patients with early rheumatoid arthritis: two-year radiographic and clinical outcomes. Arthritis Rheum 46(6):1443-1450, 2002.

102. Strand V, Cohen S, Schiff M, et al: Treatment of active rheumatoid arthritis with leflunomide compared with placebo and methotrexate. Leflunomide Rheumatoid Arthritis Investigators Group. Arch Intern Med 159(21):2542-2550, 1999.

103. Emery P, Breedveld FC, Lemmel EM, et al: A comparison of the efficacy and safety of leflunomide and methotrexate for the treatment of rheumatoid arthritis. Rheumatology (Oxford) 39(6):655-665, 2000.

104. Ortiz Z, Shea B, Suarez-Almazoe ME, et al: The efficacy of folic acid and folinic acid in reducing methotrexate gastrointestinal toxicity in rheumatoid arthritis: A meta-analysis of randomized controlled trials. J Rheumatol 25:36, 1998.

105. Morgan SL, Baggott JE, Lee JV, et al: Folic acid supplementation prevents deficient blood folate levels and hyperhomocystinemia during long-term, low dose methotrexate therapy for rheumatoid arthritis: Implications for cardiovascular disease prevention. J Rheumatol 25:441, 1998.

106. Kremer JM, Alacron GS, Lightfoot RW, et al: Methotrexate for rheumatoid arthritis: Suggested guidelines for monitoring liver toxicity. Arthritis Rheum 37:316, 1994.

107. Hassan W: Methotrexate and liver toxicity: Role of surveillance liver biopsy. Conflict between guidelines for rheumatologists and dermatologists. Ann Rheum Dis 55:273, 1996.

108. Barrera P, Laan RFJM, van Riel PLCM, et al: Methotrexate-related pulmonary complications in rheumatoid arthritis. Ann Rheum Dis 53:434, 1994.

109. Dronke M, Leonard WJ, Depper JM, et al: Cyclosporin A inhibits T-cell growth factor gene expression at the level of mRNA transcription. Proc Natl Acad Sci USA 81:5214, 1984.

110. Fuleihan R, Ramesh N, Horner A, et al: Cyclosporin A inhibits CD40 ligand expression in T lymphocytes. J Clin Invest 93:1315, 1994.

111. Tugwell P, Pincus T, Yocum D, et al: Combination therapy with cyclosporine and methotrexate in severe rheumatoid arthritis. N Engl J Med 333:137, 1995.

112. Stein CM, Pincus T, Yocum D, et al: Combination treatment of severe rheumatoid arthritis with cyclosporine and methotrexate for forty-eight weeks: An open-label extension study. The Methotrexate-Cyclosporine Combination Study Group. Arthritis Rheum 40:1843, 1997.

113. Tugwell P, Bombardier C, Gent M, et al: Low-dose cyclosporin versus placebo in patients with rheumatoid arthritis. Lancet 335:1051, 1990.

114. Furst DE, Saag K, Fleischmann MR, et al: Efficacy of tacrolimus in rheumatoid arthritis patients who have been treated unsuccessfully with methotrexate: a six-month, double-blind, randomized, dose-ranging study. Arthritis Rheum 46(8):2020-2028, 2002.

115. Fox RI: Mechanisms of action of leflunomide. J Rheumatol (Suppl 53):20, 1998.

116. Sharp JT, Strand V, Leung H, et al: Treatment with leflunomide slows radiographic progression of rheumatoid arthritis: results from three randomized controlled trials of leflunomide in patients with active rheumatoid arthritis. Leflunomide Rheumatoid Arthritis Investigators Group. Arthritis Rheum 43(3):495-505, 2000.

117. Mladenovic V, Domljan Z, Rozman B, et al: Safety and effectiveness of leflunomide in the treatment of patients with active rheumatoid arthritis. Arthritis Rheum 38(11):1595, 1995.

118. Moreland LW, Schiff MH, Baumgartner SW, et al: Etanercept therapy in rheumatoid arthritis. Ann Intern Med 130:478, 1999.

119. St Clair EW, Wagner CL, Fasanmade AA, et al: The relationship of serum infliximab concentrations to clinical improvement in rheumatoid arthritis: Results from ATTRACT, a multicenter, randomized, double-blind, placebo-controlled trial. Arthritis Rheum 46:1451-1459, 2002.

120. Maini RN, Breedveld FC, Kalden JR, et al: Therapeutic efficacy of multiple intravenous infusions of anti-tumor necrosis factor alpha monoclonal antibody combined with low-dose weekly methotrexate in rheumatoid arthritis. Arthritis Rheum 41(9):1552-1563, 1998.

121. Infliximab [package insert]. Malvern, Penn., Centocor, 2002.

122. Van de Putte LBA, Atkins C, Malaise M, et al: Adalimumab (D2E7) monotherapy in the treatment of patients with severely active rheumatoid arthritis [abstract]. Arthritis Rheum 45(Suppl):456, 2002.

123. Keystone E, Kavanaugh AF, Sharp J, et al: Adalimumab (D2E7), a fully human anti-TNF-α monoclonal antibody, inhibits the progression of structural joint damage in patients with active RA despite concomitant methotrexate therapy. Arthritis Rheum 46(Suppl):468, 2002.

124. Firestein GS, Zvaifler NJ: Anticytokine therapy in rheumatoid arthritis. N Engl J Med 337(3):195, 1997.

125. Robinson WH, Genovese MC, Moreland LW: Demyelinating and neurologic events reported in association with tumor necrosis factor alpha antagonism: by what mechanisms could tumor necrosis

factor alpha antagonists improve rheumatoid arthritis but exacerbate multiple sclerosis? Arthritis Rheum 44:1977-1983, 2001.

126. Sicotte NL, Voskuhl RR: Onset of multiple sclerosis associated with anti-TNF therapy. Neurology 57:1885-1888, 2001.

127. van Oosten BW, Barkhof F, Truyen L, et al: Increased MRI activity and immune activation in two multiple sclerosis patients treated with the monoclonal anti-tumor necrosis factor antibody cA2. Neurology 47:1531-1534, 1996.

128. Mohan N, Edwards ET, Cupps TR, et al: Demyelination occurring during anti-tumor necrosis factor alpha therapy for inflammatory arthritides. Arthritis Rheum 44(12):2862-2869, 2001.

129. van Vollenhoven R, Harju A, Brannemark S, et al: Switching between etanercept and infliximab: data from the Stockholm TNF-alpha antagonist registry (STURE) [abstract, EULAR]. Ann Rheum Dis 61(Suppl 1):Abstract OP0071, 2002.

130. Bresnihan B, Alvaro-Gracia JM, Cobby M, et al: Treatment of rheumatoid arthritis with recombinant human interleukin-1 receptor antagonist. Arthritis Rheum 41:196, 1998.

131. Cohen S, Hurd E, Cush J, et al: Treatment of rheumatoid arthritis with anakinra, a recombinant human interleukin-1 receptor antagonist, in combination with methotrexate: results of a twenty-four-week, multicenter, randomized, double-blind, placebo-controlled trial. Arthritis Rheum 46(3):614-624, 2002.

132. Fleischman R, Tesser J, Schechtman J, et al: A safety trial Of anakinra: recombinant interleukin-1 receptor antagonist (Il-1ra) in a large, placebo controlled heterogeneous population of patients with rheumatoid arthritis. Arthritis Rheum 45(9): Abstract #190, 2001.

133. Schiff MH, Bulpitt K, Weaver AA, et al: Safety of combination therapy with anakinra and etanercept in patients with rheumatoid arthritis. Arthritis Rheum 45(9):Abstract#157, 2001.

134. Genovese M, Cohen S, Moreland L, et al: A randomized double blind controlled study evaluating the safety and efficacy of etanercept vs etanercept plus anakinra in patients with rheumatoid arthritis despite treatment with MTX., in press.

135. Jiang Y, Genant HK, Watt I, et al: A multicenter, double-blind, dose-ranging, randomized, placebo-controlled study of recombinant human interleukin-1 receptor antagonist in patients with rheumatoid arthritis:radiologic progression and correlation of Genant and Larsen scores. Arthritis Rheum 43(5):1001-1009, 2000.

136. Shergy WJ, Cohen S, Greenwald M, et al: Anakinra inhibits the progression of radiographically measured joint destruction in rheumatoid arthritis. Arthritis Rheum 46(12):3420, 2002.

137. Wiesenhutter CW, Irish BL, Bertram JR: Treatment of patients with refractory rheumatoid arthritis with extracorporeal protein A immunoadsorption columns: A pilot trial. J Rheumatol 21:5, 1994.

68

Felty's Syndrome

ROBERT S. PINALS

In 1924, Felty described the triad of chronic arthritis, splenomegaly, and granulocytopenia. Felty's syndrome represents one of many systemic complications of seropositive rheumatoid arthritis (RA) occurring in patients with unusually severe extra-articular disease and immunologic abnormalities.[1] Persistent granulocytopenia ($<2000/mm^3$) must be present, but the complete triad is not required for a diagnosis of Felty's syndrome, because patients without splenomegaly resemble those with full-blown Felty's syndrome in terms of most clinical, serologic, and immunogenetic features.[1]

Epidemiology

The true prevalence of Felty's syndrome is unknown, but it may be as high as 3 percent in RA patients.[2] About two thirds of patients are women. HLA-DR4 is found in 95 percent of patients with Felty's syndrome.[1] This may account for the rarity of Felty's syndrome in blacks, who are known to have a low frequency of DR4. The condition is usually recognized in the fifth through seventh decades of life in patients who have had rRA for 10 years or more.[2] Splenomegaly and granulocytopenia may be present before symptoms or signs of arthritis in rare instances.[3]

Genetics

The familial occurrence of Felty's syndrome suggests that immunogenetic factors are operative.[4] HLA-DR4 is present more frequently than in other RA patients, and there also appears to be a DQ-linked susceptibility gene and a C4B-null allele that increase the risk of Felty's syndrome in HLA-DR4–positive RA patients.[1]

About one third of patients with Felty's syndrome have significant clonal expansions of CD3+CD8+ large granular lymphocytes in their peripheral blood (Fig. 68–1). When originally described, this group of patients with RA and large granular lymphocytosis (LGL) was considered to represent a separate syndrome. However, immunogenetic studies have demonstrated the same HLA-DR4 associations in LGL as in other Felty's syndrome patients. Furthermore, 19 to 35 percent of patients with Felty's syndrome have clonal expansion of LGL.[5] Additionally, there is an absence of distinguishing clinical or serologic features, suggesting that separation on the basis of peripheral blood lymphocyte morphology may be unjustified.[5,6] Large granular lymphocytes make up about 5 percent of the mononuclear cell population in normal human blood. Cells with natural-killer and antibody-dependent cell-mediated cytotoxic activity are found in this population. They usually lack surface immunoglobulin but frequently express certain surface phenotypes such as CD 3, 8, and 57. Among patients with an abnormal proliferation of these cells, neutropenia, splenomegaly, and susceptibility to infections are common. In some cases, there is a progressive course of malignant proliferation, but most cases are relatively benign and require no specific therapy. Up to a third of patients with LGL have inflammatory arthritis, and these patients have an immunogenetic pattern typical of Felty's syndrome. In contrast, the frequency of HLA-DR4 in patients without arthritis is not different from that in control subjects.

Pathogenesis

Mechanisms for the development of granulocytopenia include accelerated removal of granulocytes from the circulating pool and suppression of granulopoiesis. Ingestion and surface coating of immune complexes leads to impaired granulocyte function and facilitates their removal by the reticuloendothelial system. Specific antibodies directed against granulocyte cell surface antigens and complement activation may also be involved. Sequestration or margination of granulocytes in the spleen and venules in the lungs and elsewhere results in a diminished circulating pool. In some patients, the marrow does not respond appropriately to granulocytopenia because of humoral or T cell suppression of myelopoiesis.[7-9] There may be different subsets of Felty's syndrome, based on humoral and cell-mediated mechanisms, and more than one mechanism may account for neutropenia in an individual patient. Autoantibodies against granulocyte colony-stimulating factor (G-CSF) may play a role in some cases.[9] Elevated levels of serum G-CSF are usually present, irrespective of the presence or absence of autoantibodies, suggesting that the myeloid cells in Felty's syndrome are hyposensitive to the growth factor.

In LGL, an additional factor in the pathogenesis of neutropenia is the Fas ligand (FasL), a member of the tumor necrosis factor (TNF) family.[7,10] FasL is expressed on the surface of activated cytotoxic T cells, and elevated levels of soluble FasL are found in serum of most patients.[11] Serum from LGL patients has been shown to facilitate apoptosis of normal neutrophils in vitro.

The increased susceptibility to infection is probably related to several factors in addition to granulocytopenia.

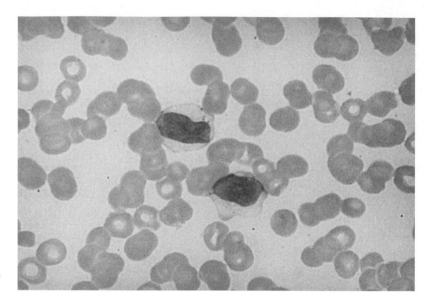

FIGURE 68–1 · Peripheral Blood Smear with Large Granular Lymphocytes.

Granulocyte reserves are diminished, and defective function of granulocytes in phagocytosis, chemotaxis, and superoxide production has been demonstrated.

Clinical Features

The articular disease is usually severe but not more so than in seropositive RA of comparable duration.[2] About one third of the patients have relatively inactive synovitis as judged by signs and symptoms, but even these patients continue to have an elevated erythrocyte sedimentation rate (ESR). In one large series, the mean ESR was 85 mm/hour.[12]

The spleen size is variable. In 5 to 10 percent of patients, it is not large enough to be palpable, but occasionally there is massive splenomegaly.[12] The median splenic weight in Felty's syndrome is about four times normal. There is no correlation between spleen size and the degree of granulocytopenia.[12]

Patients with Felty's syndrome tend to have more extra-articular manifestations than others with RA (Table 68–1). Weight loss may be striking and unexplained, often occurring for several months before the diagnosis of Felty's syndrome is made. Brown pigmentation over exposed surfaces of the extremities, especially over the tibia, may be related to stasis and to extravasation of red blood cells secondary to disease of small vessels.[12] Leg ulcers are frequently seen but do not seem to differ from those in other RA patients in terms of chronicity, recurrence, and presumed relationship to vasculitis.

Complications

Felty's syndrome patients have an increase in frequency of infections compared to matched RA control subjects.[1,13] The degree of granulocytopenia correlates poorly with the number and severity of infections until the granulo-cyte count falls below 1000/mm³. Other risk factors for infection include skin ulcers, corticosteroids, comorbid medical conditions, severity of the underlying rheumatoid process, and resulting disability.[13,14] Most of the infections are caused by common bacteria, such as staphylococcus, streptococcus, and gram-negative bacilli,[1,14] and involve common sites, particularly the skin and respiratory tract. In spite of the granulocytopenia, pus may accumulate in an appropriate fashion, suggesting that the site of infection is capable of competing successfully with the spleen for available granulocytes. The response to antibiotic therapy is usually adequate.[12,14]

Mild hepatomegaly is common in Felty's syndrome, and elevations of alkaline phosphatase and the transaminases are described in about a quarter of the patients.[1,12] An unusual type of liver involvement may be associated with Felty's syndrome but occurs rarely in other RA patients.[15] Histologically, the picture is described as nodular regenerative hyperplasia. Although there is mild portal fibrosis or infiltration with lymphocytes and plasma cells, the appearance is not characteristic of cirrhosis. Obliteration of portal venules may compromise

---

TABLE 68–1 · FREQUENCY OF EXTRA-ARTICULAR MANIFESTATIONS IN FELTY'S SYNDROME*

Manifestation	Frequency
Rheumatoid nodules	76%
Weight loss	68%
Sjögren's syndrome†	56%
Lymphadenopathy	34%
Leg ulcers	25%
Pleuritis	19%
Skin pigmentation	17%
Neuropathy	17%
Episcleritis	8%

*From a review of 10 reports since 1962.[12]
†Determined by positive Schirmer's test.

portal blood flow, leading to atrophy and regenerative nodule formation, portal hypertension, and gastrointestinal hemorrhage.

Patients with Felty's syndrome are at increased risk for the development of malignancies, particularly non-Hodgkin's lymphoma.[16]

Hematologic and Serologic Features

The leukopenia in Felty's syndrome is relative and absolute granulocytopenia, in contrast to systemic lupus erythematosus, in which lymphopenia is a more prominent feature. There is often considerable spontaneous variation in the granulocyte count. Patients with mild lowering may return to the normal range, but this is rarely seen when depression is severe. Thus, spontaneous remissions have been observed[1] but are uncommon.[12] During infections or other stressful episodes, the granulocyte count often returns to the normal range but is seldom elevated. This may conceal the diagnosis temporarily, because blood counts may be ordered mainly in the setting of an infection or other acute illness. The bone marrow may show no abnormality, but in most cases, there is a myeloid hyperplasia, with a relative excess of immature forms, often described as "maturation arrest." Although this might reflect an impaired myelopoietic response, early release of mature forms would result in the same appearance.[12] Rarely, the marrow suggests a depression in myeloid activity or shows an increased lymphocytic infiltration. A mild to moderate anemia is found in most patients, representing the anemia of chronic disease with an additional component of shortened red blood cell survival, which is corrected by splenectomy. Thrombocytopenia is seldom severe enough to cause purpura.

The alterations in immune response commonly found in RA are amplified in patients with Felty's syndrome. Rheumatoid factor is present in 98 percent of the patients, generally in high titer,[1,12] antinuclear antibodies are found in 62 to 80 percent,[1] and antineutrophil cytoplasmic antibodies in 77 percent. Most of the latter are reactive against lactoferrin.[17] Immunoglobulin levels are higher than in other RA patients, and complement levels are occasionally low, although most patients have levels within the normal range.[1,12] Immune complexes have been detected by various techniques in the majority of Felty's syndrome patients, always in much higher frequency than in RA control subjects.[1,12]

Differential Diagnosis

Patients with RA may also develop superimposed illnesses that result in splenomegaly or granulocytopenia. Drug reactions, myeloproliferative disorders, reticuloendothelial malignancies, hepatic cirrhosis, amyloidosis, sarcoidosis, tuberculosis, and other chronic infections must be considered and excluded with reasonable clinical certainty before the diagnosis of Felty's syndrome is accepted.

Management

There have been no controlled trials of any treatment for Felty's syndrome. Specific treatment for granulocytopenia is unnecessary except in patients who have experienced bacterial infections or those who are at high risk (granulocyte count below 1000/mm^3).

Frequently, granulocytopenia may improve during treatment with disease-modifying antirheumatic drugs (DMARDs).[12] Gold salt injections resulted in a complete hematologic response in 60 percent of patients and partial response in 20 percent in the largest reported series, but this and other older DMARDs have been displaced by newer drugs. Methotrexate is currently the most commonly used agent.[7,18] No controlled or comparative studies are available, but granulocytopenia usually improves with this treatment more rapidly than with gold, often within 2 months. Some patients have been followed for more than 1 year, without relapse or infection.[18] Low doses of corticosteroids do not produce consistent improvement in granulocytopenia and predispose to infection. There is limited experience with other drugs including leflunomide and cyclosporine A.[7] The mechanisms whereby second-line agents raise granulocyte counts are undetermined, as are their response rates and relative efficacy.

Treatment may be directed specifically at the granulocytopenia, using the granulopoietic growth factors. Several years of experience with the granulopoietic growth factors have confirmed their usefulness in increasing granulocyte counts within a short time and aiding in the resolution of infection.[19-22] However, continued therapy is necessary to maintain these benefits, and high costs may become an issue. Prolonged use has been reported in some patients,[21,22] but it may be more reasonable to utilize granulopoietic growth factors for a limited period, during which DMARD therapy is undertaken. G-CSF appears to have fewer adverse effects than granulocyte-macrophage colony-stimulating factor (GM-CSF). Significant adverse effects of these agents include exacerbation of arthritis, new onset of leukocytoclastic vasculitis, anemia, thrombocytopenia, and bone pain. To avoid or minimize these adverse effects, the initial use of low doses of G-CSF (3 μg/kg/day) and a short course of prednisone (20 to 30 mg/day) has been suggested.[7] A minority of patients are partially or completely unresponsive to G-CSF.

Because splenectomy usually reverses the hematologic abnormalities in Felty's syndrome, it has been advocated in the past as the treatment of choice.[12] However, currently it is reserved for patients who have not responded adequately to drug therapy. A prompt hematologic response is observed within minutes or hours after splenectomy, but granulocytopenia recurs and persists in about one quarter of these patients.[12] Continuing immune-mediated granulocyte sequestration may be responsible for these secondary failures. Recurrent or persistent infection was noted in only 26 percent of patients in one large series but in 60 percent in four others.[12] Patients who did not experience infection prior to splenectomy usually continued to be free of infection afterward, whereas those with the most severe infections had variable and inconsistent responses to splenectomy, suggesting that functional defects in granulocytes and disease severity variables may be as important as granulocytopenia in determining susceptibility to infection.[14]

Thrombocytopenia usually improves after splenectomy, as does anemia, to the extent that it is due to a hemolytic component. Although dramatic improvement in synovitis has been observed, it is often temporary and does not occur in most cases. Leg ulcers may also respond, even those that are not significantly infected, but the variability in etiology and natural course makes these reports difficult to interpret.[12]

Remission was induced in two patients with refractory Felty's syndrome by immunoablative high-dose cyclophosphamide without stem-cell rescue.[23] This approach is experimental, and long-term results are unknown.

The treatment of granulocytopenia in patients with LGL is generally similar to that in Felty's syndrome. Methotrexate[7,24] and G-CSF[20] have been used successfully. Cyclosporin may be indicated in refractory cases because it inhibits secretion of FasL.[7]

▌Prognosis

Patients with Felty's syndrome had a death rate similar to matched RA control subjects in a prospective study initiated in 1966. Despite a higher rate of infection, death due to sepsis (10 percent) was not more frequent in Felty's syndrome than in control subjects.[2] In another large series, 25 percent of deaths in Felty's syndrome were due to sepsis.[1] There is little information on survival and prognosis in the large granular lymphocyte syndrome, but no marked differences from Felty's syndrome have been reported.[6]

REFERENCES

1. Campion G, Maddison PJ, Goulding N, et al: The Felty syndrome: a case-matched study of clinical manifestations and outcome, serologic features, and immunogenetic association. Medicine 69:69, 1990.
2. Sibley JT, Haga M, Visram DA, et al: The clinical course of Felty's syndrome compared to matched controls. J Rheumatol 18:1163, 1991.
3. Bradley JD, Pinals RS: Felty's syndrome presenting without arthritis. Clin Exp Rheumatol 1:257, 1983.
4. Runge LA, Davey FR, Goldberg J, Boyd PR: The inheritance of Felty's syndrome in a family with several affected members. J Rheumatol 13:39, 1986.
5. Bowman SJ, Corrigall V, Panayi GS, et al: Hematologic and cytofluorographic analysis of patients with Felty's syndrome: a hypothesis that a discrete event leads to large granular lymphocyte expansions in this condition. Arthritis Rheum 38:1252, 1995.
6. Starkebaum G, Loughran TP Jr, Gaur LK, et al: Immunogenetic similarities between patients with Felty's syndrome and those with clonal expansions of large granular lymphocytes in rheumatoid arthritis. Arthritis Rheum 40:62, 1997.
7. Starkebaum G: Chronic neutropenia associated with autoimmune disease. Semin Hematol 39:121, 2002.
8. Ditzel HJ, Masaki Y, Nielsen H, et al: Cloning and expression of a novel human antibody-antigen pair associated with Felty's syndrome. Proc Natl Acad Sci U S A 97:9234, 2000.
9. Hellmich B, Csernok E, Schatz H, et al: Autoantibodies against granulocyte colony-stimulating factor in Felty's syndrome and neutropenic systemic lupus erythematosus. Arthritis Rheum 46:2384, 2002.
10. Perzova R, Loughran TP: Constitutive expression of Fas ligand in large granular lymphocyte leukemia. Br J Haematol 97:123, 1997.
11. Liu JH, Wei S, Lamy T, et al: Chronic neutropenia mediated by fas ligand. Blood 95:3219, 2000.
12. Goldberg J, Pinals RS: Felty syndrome. Semin Arthritis Rheum 10:52, 1980.
13. Doran MF, Crowson CS, Pond GR, et al: Predictors of infection in rheumatoid arthritis. Arthritis Rheum 46:2294, 2002.
14. Breedveld FC, Fibbe WE, Hermans J, et al: Factors influencing the incidence of infections in Felty's syndrome. Arch Intern Med 147:915, 1987.
15. Thorne C, Urowitz MB, Wanless IR, et al: Liver disease in Felty's syndrome. Am J Med 73:35, 1982.
16. Gridley G, Klippel JH, Hoover RN, et al: Incidence of cancer among men with the Felty syndrome. Ann Intern Med 120:35, 1994.
17. Coremans IEM, Hagen EC, van der Voort EAM, et al: Autoantibodies to neutrophil cytoplasmic enzymes in Felty's syndrome. Clin Exp Rheumatol 11:255, 1993.
18. Wassenberg S, Herborn G, Rau R: Methotrexate treatment in Felty's syndrome. Br J Rheumatol 37:908, 1998.
19. Hellmich B, Schnabel A, Gross WL: Treatment of severe neutropenia due to Felty's syndrome or systemic lupus erythematosus with granulocyte colony-stimulating factor. Semin Arthritis Rheum 29:82, 1999.
20. Stanworth SJ, Bhavnani M, Chattopadhya C, et al: Treatment of Felty's syndrome with the haemopoietic growth factor granulocyte colony-stimulating factor (G-CSF). Q J Med 91:49, 1998.
21. Starkebaum G: Use of colony-stimulating factors in the treatment of neutropenia associated with collagen vascular disease. Curr Opin Hematol 4:196, 1997.
22. Graham KE, Coodley GO: A prolonged use of granulocyte colony stimulating factor in Felty's syndrome. J Rheumatol 22:174, 1995.
23. Brodsky RA, Petri M, Smith BD, et al: Immunoablative high-dose cyclophosphamide without stem-cell rescue for refractory, severe autoimmune disease. Ann Intern Med 129:1031, 1998.
24. Hamidou MA, Sadr FB, Lamy T, et al: Low-dose methotrexate for the treatment of patients with large granular lymphocyte leukemia associated with rheumatoid arthritis. Am J Med 108:730, 2000.

69

Sjögren's Syndrome

STEVE CARSONS

In 1933, Henrik Sjögren[1] described the association of filamentary keratitis with arthritis. Previously, in 1882, Leber[2] had described filamentary keratitis, and in 1888, Mikulicz[3] described a patient with bilateral lacrimal and parotid enlargement. Biopsy of these glands revealed extensive round-cell infiltration. In 1953, Morgan and Castleman[4] noted the commonality between the glandular enlargement described by Mikulicz and the keratitis described by Sjögren. Subsequently, these disorders were considered to be variants of the same process and the term *Sjögren's syndrome* (SS) became more widely used.[5] In 1980, Talal[6] introduced the term *autoimmune exocrinopathy*; subsequently, Skopouli and Moutsopoulos introduced the term *autoimmune epitheliitis*[7]; both emphasize the etiologic and systemic nature of the disease.

Definitions

The utilization of multiple terms in the literature to describe this condition, coupled with—until very recently—a lack of consensus in the investigative community regarding classification criteria, has led to confusion with respect to nomenclature. Primary SS is best defined as dry eyes and dry mouth secondary to autoimmune dysfunction of the exocrine glands. Secondary SS is defined as the former definition in the presence of another autoimmune connective tissue disorder. Until relatively recently (1980), the terms *sicca syndrome* and *sicca complex* were used interchangeably with SS in the literature, and their routine use in clinical settings persists today. Sicca is probably best used in its most literal sense, which is "dry" (lat.). Some clinicians use the term *sicca* to describe patients with dry eyes, dry mouth, or both, who do not fulfill accepted criteria for complete Sjögren's syndrome. The term *Sjögren's syndrome* is preferred for describing all patients who meet classification criteria for, or who are firmly diagnosed with, the disorder.

Epidemiology

SS is a common autoimmune disorder. Prevalence estimates range from approximately 0.5 to 5 percent. The incidence rate in Olmstead County, Minnesota has been estimated to be 3.9 cases per 100,000 population.[8] Approximately one half of all cases of SS are primary. Similar to most autoimmune disorders, the vast majority of cases (approximately 90%) occur in women.[8] The majority of cases occur in midlife; however, the disorder is also seen in children[9] and the elderly.[10] Remarkably little difference in clinical presentation is noted among populations that differ on the basis of age, gender, and geographic origin.[9,11-13] Prevalence rates stated in the literature vary depending on the identifying variable chosen for study. For instance, a postmortem survey of lachrymal pathology found that 7.8 percent of individuals lacking a premortem diagnosis of an autoimmune disorder had moderate-severe (grade III or IV) lymphocytic infiltration.[14] Of 2500 sera obtained from female blood donors between the ages of 20 and 50, 0.44 percent had antibodies to SS-A.[15] Schein and colleagues assessed 2481 elderly individuals residing in Salisbury, MD (Maryland, USA) for the presence of dry eye or mouth and found the prevalence of dryness (eye or mouth) to be 27 percent.[16] In populations in which the prevalence of keratoconjunctivitis sicca (KCS) and primary SS are measured simultaneously, the prevalence of KCS always exceeds that of complete primary SS.[10,17-23] Table 69–1 describes the prevalence of primary SS in several diverse populations in

TABLE 69–1 · PREVALENCE OF PRIMARY SJÖGREN'S SYNDROME REPORTED FROM DIFFERENT POPULATIONS

Author of Study	Year of Study	Population Studied	Criteria Used	Findings	Reference
Strickland	1987	103 Caucasian females	European	pSS – 2% prob. pSS – 12%	10
Drosos	1988	62 Greek nursing home residents	Greek	pSS – 6% prob. pSS – 12%	17
Jacobsson	1989	705 Swedish adults	Copenhagen	KCS – 14.9% pSS – 2.7%	18
Zhang	1995	2166 Chinese adults	Copenhagen	pSS – 0.77%	19
Bjerrum	1997	504 Danish adults (30 to 60 yrs old)	Prelim. European	KCS – 8% pSS – 0.6 – 2.1%	20
Dafni	1997	837 rural Greek females	Prelim. European	pSS – 0.6% prob. pSS – 2.99%	21
Thomas	1998	1000 British adults	Prelim. European	pSS – 3.3%	22
Tomsic	1999	332 Slovenian adults	Prelim. European	pSS – 0.6%	23

Abbreviations: KCS, Keratoconjunctivitis sicca; prob. pSS, probable primary Sjögren's syndrome; pSS, primary Sjögren's syndrome.

which investigators have applied classification criteria for diagnosis.

Etiology and Pathogenesis

Animal models of SS have provided some important insights regarding the immunopathogenesis of this disease: 1) SS has a strong immunogenetic component; 2) the inflammatory infiltrate is largely T cell driven; 3) autoimmune sialadenitis can be triggered by viral infection; 4) relatively specific autoantibodies are produced; and 5) genes regulating apoptosis influence the chronicity of lymphocytic infiltration and are candidates for therapeutic manipulation.

IMMUNOGENETICS

Direct clinical observation has provided evidence suggesting a genetic component to SS, such as the observation of primary SS and autoimmune hemolytic anemia in sisters,[24] and the identification of primary SS in Caucasian monozygotic twins and their mother.[25] Like many other autoimmune disorders, early HLA studies identified an association with serologically defined HLA-B8[26] and HLA-DR3.[27] Later studies demonstrated that the -DR2 and -DR3 associations were secondary to linkage disequilibrium with HLA-DQ alleles.[28] Genetically defined allelic markers have subsequently identified a large number of polymorphisms involving the HLA DRB1/DQA1/DQB1 haplotype, which adds to the complexity of the genetic background of SS. These polymorphisms have been shown to vary with ethnicity, clinical manifestations, and, importantly, with the autoantibody response.

In Caucasian individuals, the HLA DRB1*0301/DQA1*0501/DQB1*0201 haplotype has the strongest association with the production of SS-A and SS-B. Additional genes located in the major histocompatibility complex (MHC) region on chromosome 6, but not classically associated with class I or II alleles, have been linked to SS. These include transporters associated with antigen processing (TAPs), genes situated between the DP and DQ regions,[29,30] and the tumor necrosis factor (TNF) alleles (particularly TNF-α[10]) located in the central MHC, telomeric to the complement-synthesis genes.[31] Recently, two genes located on chromosome 1, the interleukin-10 (IL-10) promoter region[32] and glutathione S-transferase M1,[33] have been linked to susceptibility to SS.

IMMUNOLOGIC ALTERATIONS IN PERIPHERAL BLOOD

Similar to other autoimmune disorders, the peripheral blood of patients with SS demonstrates a relative T cell lymphopenia, normal ratios of CD4+ and CD8+ T cells, and increases in activated T cells as determined by coexpression of CD3, CD4, and CD8 antigens with HLA-DR, CD-25 (IL-2R), and very late antigen-1 (VLA-1) (CD49a).[34-36] Expression of natural killer (NK) antigens (CD16) is variable, ranging from normal to diminished.[34,37] However, killing of K562 cells by SS peripheral blood mononuclear cells is reduced compared to normal controls.[38]

In contrast to T cells, circulating B cells are increased in SS.[39] B cells from the majority of SS patients express enhanced levels of CD5 (also known as Ly-1 or B1),[40] a finding of interest considering the role played by CD5 B cells in B cell malignancies such as CLL.

In addition to displaying antibody to SS-A and SS-B in 75 and 40 percent of patients, respectively,[41] approximately two thirds of SS patients have serum antinuclear antibody and rheumatoid factor (RF) activity. Many SS patients have striking polyclonal hypergammagloubulinemia. In fact, immunoglobulin (Ig) levels in SS are often higher than seen in rheumatoid arthritis (RA), systemic lupus erythematosus (SLE), and other connective tissue disorders. Several studies have pointed to a role for IgA in the immunopathogenesis of this disorder, especially because it appears to be synthesized locally in inflamed glands (see following). IgA is frequently elevated in the serum of SS patients,[42] particularly as IgA-containing RF.[43]

AUTOIMMUNE SIALADENITIS: THE IMMUNOPATHOLOGIC LESION

The hallmark of autoimmune exocrinopathy is infiltration of tissue by mononuclear cells that form distinct aggregates termed *foci*[44]. Aggregates tend to occur in periductal and periacinar locations and may become confluent, resulting in the replacement of epithelial structure (Fig. 69–1). Remnants of glands surrounded by large numbers of infiltrating mononuclear cells are known as epimyoepithelial islands. Plasma cells are noted within foci and at the periphery of periductal and periacinar foci. Glands with significant mononuclear infiltration may also display germinal center formation.

PHENOTYPE OF THE INFILTRATING LYMPHOCYTES: THE T CELL COMPARTMENT

In 1982, Fox and coworkers[45] described the classic finding of the predominance of CD4+ T cells among lym-

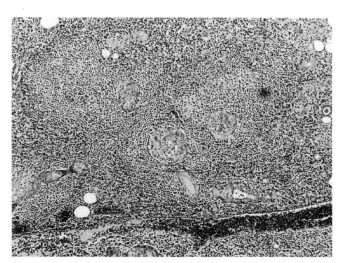

FIGURE 69–1 · Histopathologic Section of a Salivary Gland from a Patient with Sjögren's Syndrome. Normal glandular architecture is replaced by a sea of mononuclear cells. Remnants of acinar and ductal structures can be seen. Formation of a germinal center-like cluster can be noted. (Courtesy of Dr. John Fantasia, Long Island Jewish Medical Center.) (See color plate 35.)

phocytes infiltrating the minor salivary gland. In this study the CD4-to-CD8 ratio was 3:1. CD4+ predominance was also noted in peripheral blood. Although a minority, CD8+ T cells tend to localize around acinar epithelial cells.[46] B cells comprise a minority of the lymphocyte population in tissue, and a subset of B cells present in tissue is absent in peripheral blood.[47] Infiltrating lymphocytes are activated, expressing DR, DQ, and CD25, CD9, and CD10, but they are specifically distributed in the peripheral portion of the periductal foci. Bias in T cell receptor (TCR) gene utilization has been examined as a measure of response to putative autoantigen. Most studies do not support clonal T cell restriction, but relative expansion of certain TCR genes. Studies from Japan and Europe have identified expansion of Vβ2, Vβ8, and Vβ13 T cells.[48-50]

B CELL COMPARTMENT

Plasma cells expressing IgG, IgA, and IgM are found in SS salivary glands. IgA appears to be the predominant isotype; however, enrichment of IgM-positive cells to a level exceeding 10 percent seems specific for SS.[51] Clusters of IgA-positive cells have been localized adjacent to DR-expressing epithelium,[52] suggesting that the microenvironment of the activated glandular epithelium contributes to plasma cell differentiation and local IgA synthesis. Enhanced local synthesis of immunoglobulin is suggested by the finding of enrichment of anti–SS-B IgA in the saliva of SS patients.[53]

TRAFFICKING AND ADHESION OF INFLAMMATORY CELLS

The first step in inflammatory cell infiltration occurs at the glandular endothelium. Vessels in the inflamed gland express vascular cell adhesion molecule-1 (VCAM-1), intercellular adhesion molecules (ICAMs), and P- and E-selectins. Mononuclear cells surrounding blood vessels express lymphocyte function–associated antigen-1 (LFA-1), α4 and α5 integrins, and CD44.[54] Marked expression of ICAM and VCAM-1 can be observed in venules surrounded by CD4+CD45RO+ T cells.[55] High levels of the chemokine CXCL-13 has been found on endothelial cells and its counterreceptor, CXCR5, is observed on B cells organizing into germinal center-like structures.[56] Treatment of nonobese diabetic (NOD) mice with antibody to VCAM-1, α4 integrin, L-selectin, or LFA-1 almost completely inhibits lymphocyte ingress into inflamed glands.[57] Mononuclear cells utilize adhesion mechanisms to migrate to epithelial structures. Enhanced laminin expression is often found in the ductal epithelium of involved glands and is observed in areas yet unaffected by lymphocytic infiltrate,[58] leading to speculation that laminin expression is an early event in the disease process. ICAM-1 is expressed on ductal and acinar epithelial cells together with LFA-1, which is expressed on surrounding mononuclear cells.[54] In contrast to the marked expression of CXCL-13 seen on endothelium, CXCL-12 (SDF-1) is strongly expressed on ductal epithelium accompanied by only weak expression of CXCL-13. CXCR4, the counterreceptor for CXCL-12, localizes to periductal T cells.[56] CD8+ T cells surrounding acinar epithelium display the integrin αEβ7 and, thus, may utilize cadherin E to bind epithelial cells.[46] Importantly, acinar epithelial cells adjacent to αEβ7+ CD8+ T cells display apoptotic changes consistent with cytotoxic acinar cell destruction.

CYTOKINE PROFILE

Studies using immunohistochemical and in situ hybridization methodology demonstrate the uniform presence of the proinflammatory cytokines IL-1β, TNF-α IL-2, and IL-6 in SS minor salivary gland biopsies.[59-63] These cytokines localize to mononuclear cell infiltrates and epithelium. TNF-α and TNF-receptor (TNF-R) are present in the inflammatory infiltrate, vascular endothelium, and ductal epithelium, where they appear to be tightly coexpressed.[64] Acinar cells, however, do not express TNF-α or TNF-R-p75, but they do express TNF-R-p55, suggesting regional differences in susceptibility to apoptosis. Interestingly, CD4+ T cell clones originating from minor salivary gland (MSG) in organ culture produce levels of IL-10 that are 15-fold higher than those produced by similar clones derived from peripheral blood. In peripheral blood, B cells and monocytes produce approximately 90 percent of mononuclear-derived IL-10.[65] Perhaps factors present in MSG tissue in vivo inhibit IL-10 production.

MECHANISMS OF GLANDULAR DESTRUCTION

Role of Apoptosis

Mononuclear cells infiltrating affected tissue display elevated levels of apoptosis-related molecules Fas, FasL, and Bcl-2[66,67] and undergo apoptosis rarely (approximately 1%)[68]—a phenomenon referred to as "blocked apoptosis." Approximately 50 percent of infiltrating mononuclear cells express CD40 and CD40L. Bcl-2 expression colocalizes with that of CD40, suggesting that signaling through CD40 increases the expression of Bcl-2.[69] Interestingly, lymphocytes from patients with enlarged exocrine glands display reduced levels of Fas but enhanced sensitivity to steroids.[70] Despite a paucity of apoptosis in infiltrating mononuclear cells, apoptosis appears to play a role in glandular epithelial cell dysfunction. Enhanced expression of Fas and DNA strand breaks have been demonstrated on acinar epithelial cells.[66] DNA strand breaks occur even more frequently in ductal epithelium (68%) in SS, far exceeding the rate in controls (3%). This is accompanied by a significant reduction in Bcl-2 expression and enhancement of Bax expression in SS ductal epithelium.[67,71] Acinar epithelial cells adjacent to CD8+ T cells are apoptic.[46]

Role of Metalloproteinases

In addition to epithelial cell death, degradation of extracellular matrix contributes to destruction of glandular architecture. Metalloproteinase-2 (MMP-2), -3, and -9 are present in SS salivary glands, where they may degrade basement membrane collagen IV. Immunohis-tochemical studies reveal localization of MMPs to glandular cells, particularly acinar end-piece cells[72] and acinar cells adjacent to lymphocytic infiltrates.[73]

MULTIPLE AUTOANTIGENS MAY BE ETIOLOGIC FOR SJÖGREN'S SYNDROME

The existence of a strong autoantibody response and the presence of germinal center-like structures in the salivary glands of SS patients imply that the aberrant immune response is directed against one or multiple autoantigens. Molecular characterization of B cell Ig genes has provided considerable evidence for an antigen-driven response in SS. Analysis of heavy chain Ig rearrangements using RT-PCR on tissue obtained by biopsy of SS labial salivary gland and lymph node revealed that 92 of 94 V(H)-D-J(H) transcripts were modified by somatic mutation.[74] Analysis of rearranged V genes from B cells obtained by microdissection of germinal center-like clusters in SS labial salivary glands revealed a mixture of polyclonality containing some somatic mutation, along with dominant B cell clones expressing hypermutated V genes.[75]

Candidate Autoantigens

Epstein-Barr Virus

Case reports detailing the development of SS following acute mononucleosis[76,77] and evidence identifying salivary glands as sites for latent Epstein-Barr virus (EBV) infection have given credence to a role for EBV in the pathogenesis of SS. Some studies have demonstrated elevated antibody titers to EBV antigens in SS patients,[78] whereas others have not. EBV DNA has been detected by in situ hybridization and by PCR in SS glandular tissue, saliva, and tears.[79] These studies suggest that in certain patients, persistent glandular EBV infection may be associated with or result in immunoregulatory abnormalities, which lead to persistent inflammation and possibly lymphomagenesis (see following).

α-Fodrin is a 120-kD constituent of the epithelial cytoskeleton that was first observed to be a target of the autoimmune response in the NFS/sld mouse model of SS.[80] Serum IgG from affected mice recognized α-fodrin in immunoblots of salivary gland homogenates. Mouse IgG and human IgG isolated from SS patients also bind to a recombinant α-fodrin fusion protein. EBV activation of lymphoid cells results in the cleavage of α-fodrin to 120-kD fragments, which occurs concomitantly with cellular apoptosis and expression of ZEBRA protein, which is a marker for activation of the lytic cycle of EBV.[81] This cleavage can be blocked by caspase inhibitors. α-Fodrin is also cleaved into a unique 155-kD fragment by enzymes present in the granules of cytotoxic lymphocytes.[82] As demonstrated by these animal and in vitro experimental models, viruses such as EBV may, via intrinsic epithelial cell apoptosis and cytotoxic lymphocyte granule release, induce the formation of autoantigens linked to SS.

Antimuscarinic M3 Receptor

Thirty-five years ago, antibodies directed against salivary duct epithelium (ASDA) were reported[83] and were assumed to be a consequence of organ-specific autoimmunity in SS. Identification of specific glandular autoantigens was hampered by methodologic issues and perhaps by the intense interest in SS-A and SS-B, which were to be discovered shortly thereafter. Thirty years later, IgG present in the sera of SS patients was found to bind to and activate cholinergic receptors present on rat parotid gland.[84] Pharmacologic stimulation and inhibition studies pointed to a type M3 muscarinic receptor (M3R). Subsequently, it was demonstrated that serum and purified IgG from 11 of 15 patients with primary and secondary SS inhibited carbachol-induced contraction of isolated bladder strips, indicative of an inhibitory effect on parasympathetic neurotransmission.[85] Interestingly, M3R can be cleaved in vitro by granzyme B derived from cytotoxic granules,[82] consistent with the model of autoantigen production described previously.

SS-A and SS-B

SS-A and SS-B (Ro and La) represent the dominant humoral immune target to nuclear antigen in SS. Thus, these antigens have long been speculated to be of prime diagnostic and etiologic importance, especially because the antibody response to SS-A and SS-B has characteristics of an antigen-driven response.[86] A more detailed description and characterization of these antigens is found in Chapter 20. Evidence suggesting a local response to autoantigen is derived from studies demonstrating local antibody synthesis in salivary gland. All eight submucosal salivary gland biopsies studied from SS patients with circulating anti–SS-A demonstrated local production of anti–52-kD Ro.[87] In addition, the expression pattern of SS-B in acinar epithelial cells was found to be aberrant in SS patients, demonstrating cytoplasmic and nucleoplasmic staining in contrast to normal individuals in whom staining was restricted to the nucleolus.[88]

❚ Clinical Manifestations

OCULAR MANIFESTATIONS

Although the most prominent ocular manifestation of SS is the dry eye, patients often are not aware of dryness as a presenting symptom. Instead, patients may complain of a foreign body-type sensation as manifested by scratchiness, grittiness, or irritation from a "grain of sand." These symptoms may be interpreted by the patient and physician alike as atopic in nature. An early manifestation of the dry eye is the inability of the patient to tolerate contact lenses. Other common symptoms of dry eye include photophobia, redness, and ocular fatigue. Thick mucous strands may cause blurring of vision and the eyelids may be encrusted, especially upon awakening. If the condition persists and is untreated, symptoms may reflect complications of xeropthalmia including pain, intense photophobia indicative of corneal abrasion, and discharge possibly indicative of infection (Fig. 69–2). Infections threaten sight and are most often caused by gram-positive bacteria. Previous corneal surgery, topical corticosteroid therapy, and the use of contact lenses have been identi-

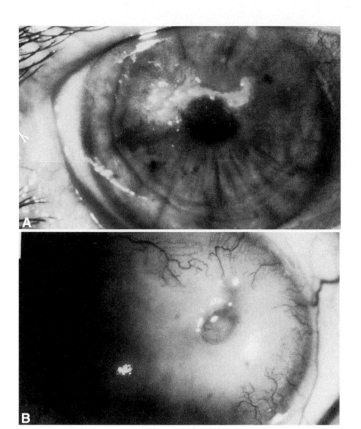

FIGURE 69-2 · Patient with moderate dry eye (A), in addition to surface staining, develop filamentary keratitis, in which the epithelium of the cornea sloughs off and becomes attached to the ocular surface along with mucin and debris. This causes significant foreign body sensation and discomfort. Patient with severe dry eye who did not receive adequate treatment (B) has developed corneal scarring. (Courtesy of Dr. Reza Dana, Harvard Medical School.)

fied as predisposing to infection.[89] Rarely, patients may present with an orbital mass representing a swollen lacrimal gland. Examination may reveal a paucity of tears in the conjunctival sac. The conjuctivae may appear injected. Specific maneuvers such as the Schirmer test and slit lamp examination may somewhat quantitate dryness and corneal disease, respectively. Corneal examination is aided by the installation of dye. Flourescein stains epithelial defects, whereas Rose Bengal binds devitalized cells and, thus, is more sensitive. Small punctate defects are often first observed at the inferior corneal margin.[90] Lissamine green is thought to be equally sensitive to Rose Bengal but less irritating.

ORAL MANIFESTATIONS

In contrast to dry eye, patients often directly complain of a dry mouth. Physicians caring for SS patients are accustomed to seeing SS patients carrying plastic water bottles. These patients require a constant supply of moisture to be comfortable. The dry-mouth patient will describe a parched feeling in the mouth, often extending to the throat. Eating is often difficult without supplemental liquids. Talal has popularized the "cracker sign" in which a patient is asked whether he or she can chew and swallow a saltine cracker without any exogenous liquid. The dry-mouth patient will often respond

with visible disgust or by demonstrating a choking sign by bringing his or her hand up to the neck. Patients also may describe a thickened saliva and may experience dysguesia. Many of the more severe symptoms associated with dry mouth are secondary to complications of chronic dryness.

Due to a reduction in salivary volume and the subsequent loss of the antibacterial properties of saliva in the dry mouth, tooth decay is accelerated. In fact, unexplained rampant dental caries may be the first sign of a dry mouth. Caries occurring in unusual places such as the incisal surfaces and at the gingival line are common in the dry mouth. Enamel at the junction of fillings and crowns is particularly susceptible to decay in the dry mouth. "Fillings falling out" may also be an early sign of a dry mouth. In a European Community study, 40 percent of a consecutive series of SS patients experienced early dental loss. In partially or completely edentulous patients, dental loss occurred an average of 9 years prior to the first symptom of xerostomia.[91] For the reasons stated previously, the dry mouth is also extremely susceptible to the development of intraoral candidiasis. In one study, more than 80 percent of all SS subjects were culture positive for *C. albicans* versus none of the controls.[92] Patients report a burning mouth and tongue. During the course of their illness, the majority of SS patients will experience swelling of the salivary glands. The parotids are most commonly involved; however, the sublingual and submandibular glands may also be affected. Swelling may be bilateral or unilateral and may fluctuate with time (Fig. 69–3). Of a series of patients with adult recurrent sialadenitis of the parotid glands followed prospectively, more than 50 percent developed SS.[93] These patients experienced parotid swelling a mean of 5 years prior to xerostomia. Patients may experience "glandular flares" manifested by periods of increased swelling accompanied by pain and tenderness. Thickened, inspissated saliva places SS patients at increased risk for formation of calculi, which may be incidentally found on imaging studies. Infectious parotitis or abscess presents as erythematous, painful swelling of the gland, often accompanied by fever, chills, and malaise. The presence of a dominant, hard mass should raise suspicion of lymphoma.

Examination of the oral cavity of the SS patient often reveals multiple caries in the distribution noted previously. Patients with more advanced disease may be edentulous or have complete dentures. The mouth appears dry, the mucosa is thin and parchment-like, and a tongue blade will adhere to the tongue and buccal surfaces in a "sticky" fashion. Centers specializing in SS or dry mouth will measure salivary flow rate quantitatively; however, by asking the patient to open the mouth and elevate the tongue for 1 minute, the clinician may estimate flow rate by observing infralingual salivary pooling. Massaging the parotid will yield little or no saliva from Stenson's duct. In the dry mouth, candidiasis is not manifested by thrush. Rather, there is extensive erythema of the oral mucosa and loss of filliform papillae from the dorsal surface of the tongue. Small amounts of thin, whitish exudate may be found on the tongue and buccal mucosa. Bilateral angular chelitis is often observed. Examination of the parotid glands often reveals some degree of swelling,

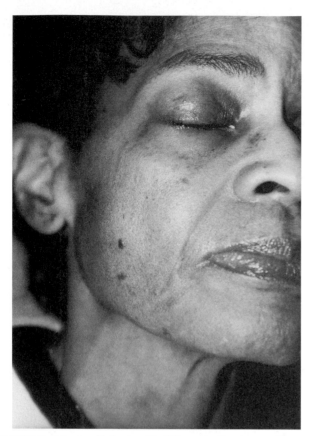

FIGURE 69-3 · Patient with Sjögren's Syndrome Demonstrating Moderate Parotid Swelling. In this patient, parotid enlargement fluctuates with time and is bilateral.

TABLE 69-2 · SYSTEMIC MANIFESTATIONS ASSOCIATED WITH SJÖGREN'S SYNDROME

Musculoskeletal
Arthralgias
Myalgias
Cutaneous
Dry skin
Hyperglobulinemic purpura
Vasculitis
Pulmonary
Xerotrachea
Pulmonary infiltrate
Gastrointestinal
Esophageal dysmotility
Pancreatitis
Hepatitis
Renal
Renal tubular acidosis
Interstitial nephritis
Neurologic
Peripheral neuropathy
Cranial neuropathy (especially 5th cranial nerve)
Central nervous system (CNS) disease
Hematologic
Leukopenia
Anemia
Lymphoma

often appreciated as a subtle, "grainy" enlargement. In severe cases, "chipmunk-like facies" indicative of massive bilateral glandular involvement is seen.

OTHER XEROSES

Dry nose is common and may lead to inflammation with subsequent congestion, crusting, and epistaxis. Xerotrachea may result in a chronic dry cough. Dry skin may lead to pruritus and excoriation. Rarely, secondary infection may occur. Vaginal dryness may lead to pruritus, irritation, and dyspareunia. Although the most common cutaneous manifestation of SS is dryness, little is known regarding the precise etiology and whether cutaneous dryness is truly part of the autoimmune exocrinopathy of SS. Sweat volume is reduced in SS patients,[94] and a skin biopsy has revealed lymphocytic infiltrates surrounding eccrine glands and ducts in one patient suffering from severe anhidrosis.[95] Dryness often leads to pruritus and excoriation and occasionally to superinfection.

▎ Systemic Manifestations

MUSCULOSKELETAL SYMPTOMS

Patients with primary SS often experience musculoskelatal symptoms, including arthralgias and transient sy-

novitis (Table 69–2). Prevalence estimates range from 54 to 84 percent.[96,97] Joint erosion is rare; however, mild joint-space narrowing appears to be common.[97,98] Muscle pain is common in SS; however, persistent and significant elevation in creatine phosphokinase (CPK) is extremely uncommon.[99] Nonetheless, two studies demonstrated abnormal muscle biopsy findings in a relatively high number (72 and 73%, respectively) of primary SS patients. These abnormalities consisted of inflammatory myositis, perivascular lymphocytic infiltrates, and inclusion bodies. Despite these findings, only 11 percent of the combined series had clinical evidence of polymyositis.[99,100] Muscle biopsy findings did not correlate with muscle pain; 27 percent of patients in one series met American College of Rheumatology (ACR) criteria for fibromyalgia.[99]

PULMONARY INVOLVEMENT

Clinical pulmonary involvement is relatively common in primary SS. Cough has been reported to occur in 40 to 50 percent of patients.[101,102] It is usually a symptom of xerotrachea, which, in turn, is strongly associated with impaired mucociliary clearance.[103,104] Morphometric analysis made at postmortem examination of SS patients' lungs reveals increases in the size of bronchial glands and goblet cells in central airways and in the mucus-occupying ratio in small airways; these are changes not dissimilar to those seen in chronic bronchitis.[105] Cough may also be secondary to bronchial hyperresponsiveness, which is found in 50 to 60 percent of primary SS patients when studied by methacholine challenge.[106] Additional pulmonary sympotmatology including dyspnea and chest pain (referable to pleural and parenchymal disease, respectively) has been estimated to occur in 9 to 43 percent of patients.[107,108] When abnormalities found on pulmonary function testing are included, approximately 75 percent of patients display evidence of pulmonary involvement.[109] Abnormal high resolution CT (HRCT) findings occur in 65 to 92 percent and primarily include ground-glass attenuation, bronchiectasis, septal thicking, micronodules, and parenchymal cysts.[110,111] HRCT abnormalities do not necessarily correlate with abnormal pulmonary function tests (PFTs).

Despite the absence of clinical symptoms and normal chest radiographs, primary SS patients may show evidence of subclinical lung inflammation on bronchioalveolar lavage (BAL).[112] A wide range of PFT abnormalities have been reported to occur in primary SS; however, the most common appear to be reduction in maximal expiratory flow (MEF), which is indicative of small airways disease, and reduced DLCO secondary to interstitial involvement.[101,102,108] Lung biopsy reveals a spectrum of inflammatory changes including bronchiolitis, lymphoid interstitial pneumonia, and fibrosis.[113] Immunohistochemical analysis demonstrates an increase in CD4+ T cells in the bronchial submucosa.[114] Taken together, the predominance of small airways disease, correlation with indicators of systemic inflammation, and CD4+ T cell infiltration of bronchial submucosa implies a significant role for autoimmune exocrinpoathy in SS lung disease.

RENAL INVOLVEMENT

The predominant form of renal disease seen in primary SS is a distal renal tubular acidosis syndrome resulting from tubulointerstitial lymphocytic infiltration. On rare occasions, the first presenting symptom of SS has been hypokalemic paralysis. In these cases the sicca component had been mild and previously unrecognized.[115] Overt renal disease of any form was seen in 4 percent of 471 patients followed for 10 years by Goules and colleagues.[116] More commonly, renal metabolic studies reveal mild disturbances in tubular function in the absence of clinical disease.[117] Proteinuria is not infrequently detected in primary SS (in approximately 20% of cases) and is mainly of tubular origin (β_2-microglobulin and α_1-microglobulin), suggesting a component of proximal tubular dysfunction. Filtration of increased amounts of proteins, such as Ig light chain and β_2-microglobulin (MHC class I–associated light chain), and local synthesis of these proteins by tubular lymphocytes may result in tubular damage. On renal biopsy, Talal and coworkers [118] noted lymphocytic infiltrates in all patients with tubular acidification defects. Similar to findings observed in exocrine glands, most infiltrating lymphocytes are CD4+ (CD4:CD8 = approximately 2:1); however, lymphocytes invading tubular epithelial cells are CD8+, suggesting a cytotoxic role.[119] Glomerular disease is rare but has been shown in 1 to 2 percent of cases by clinical and biopsy studies.[116] Patients with glomerulonephritis (GN) have been shown to have type II mixed cryoglobulins and low C4.[116]

GASTROINTESTINAL MANIFESTATIONS

Xerostomia is the most common upper alimentary abnormality in SS, and hyposalivation undoubtedly contributes to digestive abnormalities. Dysphagia has been reported in approximately 75 percent of patients,[120] and manometric evidence of esophageal dysmotility has been reported in at least one third.[121] More significant dysphagia may signify the presence of esophageal webs, which have been noted in 10 percent.[120] Gastric symptoms have been recorded in approximately half of patients with primary SS.[122] Endoscopic examination with biopsy reveals evidence of atrophic (usually antral) gastritis in 10 to 25 percent and superficial gastritis in approximately 80 percent.[122,123] Hypopepsinogenemia has been reported in up to two thirds[124]; however, parietal cell antibodies have only been detected in 10 percent.[122] Endoscopic surveillance may be required for persistent symptoms of epigastric discomfort, fullness, and early satiety, which could indicate the presence of severe atrophic gastritis or a MALT-associated lymphoma (see following).

HEPATIC INVOLVEMENT

Evidence of mild autoimmune hepatitis has been identified in approximately one quarter of primary SS patients,[125] with smooth muscle antibodies seen in 7 to 33 percent.[125,126] Antimitochondrial antibodies (AMA) have been reported in 7 to 13 percent of patients,[125-127] suggesting a close association of primary SS with primary biliary cirrhosis (PBC). In one series, more than 90 percent of AMA-positive SS patients revealed stage I PBC on liver biopsy.[127] Ninety-three percent of PBC patients display focal sialadenitis on salivary gland biopsy[128]; however, significant clinical evidence of SS has been reported in only 33 to 47 percent,[128] although some features of SS may be observed in up to three quarters of patients.[129]

Hepatitis C Virus and Sjögren's Syndrome

Within the past 10 years, an interesting relationship has emerged between hepatitis C infection and SS. Surveys of patients diagnosed with hepatitis C virus (HCV) infection reveal clinical and histologic abnormalities suggestive of SS in 57 to 77 percent.[130-132] Similarly, HCV was detected in 6 to 19 percent of patients with SS.[133-135] Not surprisingly, patients diagnosed with SS who are HCV positive have a much greater incidence of hepatic involvement (approximately 90% vs. approximately 10%).[133,136] HCV-positive SS patients also have a higher prevalence of cryoglobulinemia, hypocomplementemia, and neurologic involvement, but they are less often SS-A or SS-B positive (10 vs. 38%). Primary SS patients with cryoglobulinemia are sixfold more likely to have antibodies to HCV than those without cryoglobulins.[137] Histologically, the salivary lesion in HCV-positive SS patients is similar to HCV-negative SS patients, except for the severity of the infiltrate. HCV-positive patients have milder lesions and lower focus scores.[131] Immunohistochemically, the lesions are also similar, displaying a preponderance of T cells with a CD4:CD8 ratio of 2:1.[138] Of interest is a report describing the onset of SS after interferon-α (IFN-α) treatment for HCV.[139] HCV may be another viral agent that triggers autoimmune exocrinopathy in the appropriate genetic and immunologic background.

PANCREATIC INVOLVEMENT

Laboratory evidence of exocrine pancreatic functional abnormality is not infrequent in SS. Some abnormality in pancreatic function testing has been reported in one half to three quarters of patients.[140,141] The most frequent abnormality is elevation of immunoreactive trypsin in 30 to 40 percent.[140] Episodes of abdominal pain and steatorrhea occur in SS but are not always easily attributed to pancreatitis, in part due to difficulties in interpretation of serum amylase elevations. Approximately 30 percent of primary SS patients have elevations of P and S amylase.[142]

VASCULAR INVOLVEMENT

Vasculitis has been reported to occur in approximately 15 percent of SS patients. Subtypes range from hypersensitivity vasculitis to a necrotizing vasculitis resembling polyarteritis nodosa.[143] By far the majority of cases involve the skin and manifest as recurrent crops of purpura. The lesions range from micropetechiae to large purpura and may be noninflammatory, demonstrating only extravasated red blood cells (RBC), or may be vasculitic. Urticarial lesions also may occur. Immunopathologically, these purpura are caused by a combination of blood hyperviscosity and immune complex–mediated cutaneous vasculitis. Most biopsy specimens display immunofluorescent staining for immunoglobulin in the vessel wall.[144] Exacerbations of purpura occur secondary to increased hydrostatic pressure, such as that caused by prolonged standing and the wearing of constricting elastic stockings. Patients with long-standing purpura often display chronic older brawny lesions with superimposed showers of new petechiae-purpura (Fig. 69–4). Approximately 20 years ago, Alexander and colleagues[145] described the association of SS with cutaneous vasculitis, purpura, and adenopathy. Eighty-four percent of patients had antibodies to SS-A. It is important to rule out the presence of HCV in individuals presenting with cutaneous vasculitis, cryoglobulinemia, and sicca complaints. Regardless, the constellation of purpura, mixed cryoglobulinemia, and hypocomplementemia (C4) has recently been identified as a risk for lymphoproliferation in SS patients (see following).

Raynaud's phenomenon is not uncommon in SS, affecting 13 to 66 percent of patients.[146-149] It is often associated with nonerosive arthritis, frequently precedes the onset of xerostomia, and rarely results in digital ulceration. Nailfold capillary microscopic changes include increased loop dilatation and tortuosity and resemble changes seen in SLE.[150]

ASSOCIATION WITH AUTOIMMUNE THYROID DISEASE

A strong association between SS and thyroid disease has been documented. In patients with primary SS who are examined for thyroid disease, the prevalence of thyroid

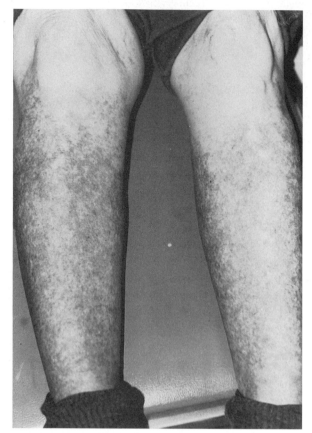

FIGURE 69–4 · Sjögren's Syndrome Patient Demonstrating Dermopathy Involving the Lower Extremities Secondary to Hyperglobulinemic Purpura. Recurrent showers of micropetechiae become chronic resulting in brawny hyperpigmentation.

abnormality has ranged from 35 to 45 percent,[151,152] and the prevalence autoimmune thyroiditis from 18 to 24 percent.[151,152] Autoimmune thyroid disease occurs much more frequently in patients with SS than RA.[153]

NEUROLOGIC DISORDERS

Neurologic disease is perhaps the most common significant extraglandular manifestation of SS and can involve the cranial nerves, peripheral nerves, and rarely the central nervous system (CNS). Clinical reports suggest that half of SS patients have some form of neurologic involvement, with estimates ranging from 22 to 76 percent.[154-160] Peripheral neuropathy has been found in approximately 20 percent of SS patients.[161,162] Peripheral neuropathy was symmetric in one third and the presenting symptom in approximately 10 percent.[161] A predominately sensory neuropathy may be observed and may present with ataxia.[163] Sural nerve biopsy in SS patients with sensorimotor polyneuropathy reveals perivascular inflammatory infiltrates and changes suggestive or diagnostic of vasculitis in the majority.[164,165] Progressive neuropathy, especially with motor involvement (i.e., foot drop), may indicate the presence of necrotizing vasculitis, particularly in the context of palpable purpura or cutaneous ulceration. Biopsies of SS patients with pure sensory neuropathy demonstrate dorsal root ganglionitis in addition to perivascular mononuclear cell infiltrates involving cutaneous nerves.[163] Approximately one quarter of patients with peripheral neuropathy will have a superimposed autonomic or cranial neuropathy.[165]

Cranial neuropathy, particularly trigeminal neuropathy, is the most distinctive type of neuropathy associated with pSS.[156,157,166] Sensorineural hearing loss, especially involving high frequencies, is noted in approximately one half of pSS patients upon audiometric testing.[167] Disturbances in autonomic nervous system function can be demonstrated by objective testing (e.g., tilt table, digital blood flow, deep breathing) in a significant number of pSS patients[168,169]; however, clinical symptoms are uncommon. Rarely, patients may develop significant postural hypotension. Adie's pupil has been described in several reports.[170,171]

The incidence of CNS disease in pSS ranges from 0 to 30 percent. Interpretation of these figures has been a subject of controversy due to several issues, including lack of a uniform description of the clinical syndrome of CNS Sjögren's, especially cases for which symptoms are restricted to mild cognitive or depressive features; inclusion of cases defined solely by electrophysiologic or imaging abnormalities; and the question of the strict exclusion of SLE, primary angiitis of the central nervous system (PACNS), antiphospholipid syndrome (APL), or other etiologies, including hepatitis C. In rheumatologic practice, significant CNS disease is rare, whereas peripheral and cranial neuropathies are common. The largest series of CNS Sjögren's cases reporting clinical, serologic, and pathologic characteristics has been published at Johns Hopkins by Alexander and colleagues. The patients in this study have an increased frequency of SS-A positivity and a strong association with peripheral inflammatory vascular disease most commonly expressed as cutaneous vasculitis (see previous discussion). There is also an association with peripheral neuropathy and inflammatory myopathy.[172,173] Postmortem examination of pSS patients from another center has revealed mixed inflammatory infiltrates in the leptomeninges and choroid plexus; only 5 of 11 patients had neurologic symptoms.[174] Seventy-five percent of SS patients from the Hopkins cohort with active neuropsychiatric disease had abnormalities on magnetic resonance imaging (MRI), particularly in the subcortical and periventricular white matter.[175] Twenty patients from this cohort were reported to have neurologic disease mimicking multiple sclerosis (MS).[176] Over the past several years, surveys of MS outpatient populations from whom evidence of SS was sought have been published.[177-184] Of 486 patients reported collectively, 3.3 percent met criteria for SS, and 8.4 percent had at least one feature of SS. Of 100 patients consecutively admitted to an inpatient neurology service, three had SS.[185] Thus, only a very small percentage of MS patients may have undetected SS. Additionally, the existence of an SS-MS overlap syndrome cannot be excluded. Myelopathy was a prominent component of the MS-like disease reported in the Hopkins series and has subsequently been reported on multiple occasions, as summarized by Williams.[186] The majority of patients demonstrate an acute or progressive transverse myelopathy. Good therapeutic outcomes have been reported with a combination of corticosteroid and cyclophosphamide. Several instances of optic neuropathy in pSS have been reported in the absence of MS.[187] pSS patients lacking clinical CNS disease have also been reported to have MRI abnormalities.[188] pSS patients who display no evidence of neurologic abnormality except cognitive dysfunction were found to have abnormal SPECT scans but normal MRI studies.[189] Extreme caution must be utilized when the diagnosis of "neuro-Sjögren's" is entertained in patients demonstrating mild cognitive or psychiatric symptoms and minor abnormalities on sensitive imaging techniques, particularly in the absence of objective focal and serologic findings.

LYMPHOPROLIFERATIVE DISEASE

One of the major concerns of internists and rheumatologists caring for SS patients is the potential for the development of lymphoma. Kassan's original study[190] estimated that a primary SS patient has an approximately 40-fold enhanced risk of developing non-Hodgkin's lymphoma (NHL) compared to age-matched controls. Subsequent studies have confirmed this risk but at a somewhat lower magnitude. This may, in part, be secondary to population differences. Table 69–3 summarizes studies examining the risk of lymphoma in primary SS.[191-199] Younger SS patients may be at somewhat higher risk than older patients.[200] A survey of 113 patients with NHL revealed that 12 percent had SS.[201]

SS-associated NHLs are largely B cell in origin[202] and may display a monocytoid phenotype.[203] They frequently involve MALT near the marginal zone.[204] Extranodal sites are often involved and include the salivary glands themselves (50%),[204] the gastrointestinal (GI) tract (see previous discussion), the lung, skin, thymus, and thyroid gland.[205-207] These NHL are often indolent but may transform into large-cell NHL.[208] Waldenström's macroglobulinemia may be heralded by the onset of the hyperviscosity syndrome accompanied by lower extremity purpura. The clinician should be aware of signs suggestive of lymphoproliferation, including a significant increase in the size of the salivary

TABLE 69–3 • RISK OF LYMPHOPROLIFERATION IN SJÖGREN'S SYNDROME

Number in Study	Region	Method	Risk	Reference
110	Finland	SIR	13	191
676	Finland	SIR	8.7	192
136	USA	RR	44	190
62	France	PP	6.4	193
331	Italy	RR	33	194
55	France	PP	9	195
30	Netherlands	PP	10	196
261	Greece	IR	12.2	197
723	Greece	PP	3.9	198
138	USA	PP	6.0	199

Abbreviations: IR, incidence ratio per 1000 person-years; PP, point prevalence (%); RR, relative risk; SIR, standardized incidence ratio.

glands, especially when accompanied by dominant masses, lymphadenopathy, splenomegaly, and pulmonary infiltrates. Longitudinal monitoring of laboratory parameters is appropriate. Development of a monoclonal protein, new-onset leukopenia and anemia, and a loss of previously present specific autoantibodies (i.e., ANA, SS-A, SS-B) have all been associated with the development of lymphoma. More recently, a study of 261 Greek patients revealed that the presence of a low C4 and cryoglobulins conferred an approximates six- to eightfold increase in risk for the development of lymphoma.[197] On occasion, a patient presents with significant increases in glandular swelling and lymphadenopathy suggestive of lymphoma. Tissue biopsy, however, is inconclusive, revealing lymphoid architecture that is atypical but not diagnostic of malignancy. This condition is referred to as "pseudolymphoma" and may represent an intermediate step in lymphomagenesis.[209]

Secondary Sjögren's Syndrome

Although secondary SS is defined as xerostomia and xeropthalmia in the presence of an autoimmune connective tissue disease, it is important to note that secondary SS is not monolithic. In other words, characteristics of SS that occur among the various connective tissue disorders may differ. Additionally, SS is a common accompaniment of autoimmune disorders not generally considered to be "connective tissue diseases," such as thyroiditis, primary biliary cirrhosis, and MS. Thus, signs of SS should not be overlooked in these contexts. Finally, because of clinical, immunogenetic, and serologic overlap, many investigators and clinicians consider SS and SLE to be more intimately related than other contexts in which secondary SS is observed.

Clinical signs suggestive of SS have been noted in 8 to 31 percent of patients with SLE,[210,211] whereas lymphocytic infiltration of minor salivary glands has been reported in 50 percent of unselected SLE patients.[212] SLE patients who have more severe grades of lymphocytic infiltration appear to have less renal disease but more adenopathy, circulating RF, positivity to SS-A and SS-B, and erosive arthritis,[210-212] in addition to overt xeropthalmia and parotid enlargement. SLE patients with renal tubular acidosis and interstitial nephritis have been described as having concomitant primary SS.[213] In several reported series, primary SS has been observed to transition into SLE at intervals ranging from 1 to 10 years after the diagnosis of pSS.[214-218]

Clinical SS affects approximately 20 percent of patients with RA. Thirty-one percent have positive MSG biopsies.[219] SS-A antibodies have been found in 4 to 23 percent of RA patients.[219-221] These patients have more common and severe sicca complaints, positive MSG biopsies, and are less likely to display HLA-DR4–related antigens. Interestingly, focal sialadenitis was found to be common among an early synovitis cohort, 70 percent of whom had been diagnosed with RA 1 year later.[222]

Between 17 and 20 percent of scleroderma patients have been diagnosed with SS.[223,224] On histopathologic examinaton, salivary glands from some patients with scleroderma display fibrosis alone, whereas others demonstrate typical lymphocytic sialadenitis and fibrosis. Despite similarities in the prevalence of SS in scleroderma and RA, individuals with scleroderma are more frequently symptomatic, perhaps due to the high prevalence of fibrosis.[223] SS is well known to complicate limited scleroderma.[225] An overlap among SS-CREST and primary biliary cirrhosis (PBC) is known to occur. Among a cohort of patients with MCTD, one third had antibodies to SS-A, and 42 percent had sicca symptoms.[226] Approximately 15 percent of pSS patients have cardiolipin antibodies.[227] When sought, β2-glycoprotein I antibodies were not detected, and clinical evidence of antiphospholipid syndrome was absent.

Clinical Outcomes

When followed over a 10-year period, approximately one third of patients with sicca complaints eventually fulfill criteria for SS.[228,229] Development of disease and severity of sicca symptoms correlate with the presence of autoantibodies, particularly ANA and SS-A, and the level of serum IgG.[228,230] More advanced sialographic findings are also seen in patients who are SS-A positive.[231] Glandular SS appears to progress very slowly. Once established, diminished salivary flow remains relatively constant for several years, despite increases in focus score upon rebiopsy.[228,229,232] The most prevalent extraglandular manifestations developing during 9 years of follow-up were arthralgias, arthritis, Raynaud's phenomenon, dry skin, skin rash, and leucopenia.[233] The severity of extraglandular disease has been correlated to the severity of exocrine surface disease and to the presence of SS-A.[234,235] SS-A positivity has also been linked to the development of other rheumatologic diagnoses, including SLE, RA, and scleroderma.[236] Overall, there does not appear to be excess mortality in patients with pSS.[237] The risk of and mortality associated with lymphoma has been discussed previously. Using the short form-36 (SF-36), it was found that women with pSS had a diminished quality of life (QOL) on all SF-36 scales. Although the psychologic-subdimension scales were similar to women with RA and fibromyalgia, the physical function QOL was better in women with pSS.[238]

Differential Diagnosis

Many common conditions cause dryness. Human immunodeficiency virus (HIV) causes a syndrome known as diffuse infiltrative lymphocytosis syndrome (DILS) in approximately 3 to 8 percent of patients.[239,240] These patients display nearly an exact replica of SS symptoms including dry eyes, dry mouth, salivary swelling, and a propensity to develop lymphomas.[241] They are more commonly male, however, and lack specific SS-A and SS-B antibodies, although approximately 10 percent may exhibit ANA and RF. In cases in which it may be particularly difficult to distinguish SS from DILS, immunohistochemical study of minor salivary glands may be useful revealing a CD4+:CD8+ ratio of approximately 0.66 in DILS, in contrast to a ratio of more than 3.0 in SS.[239,240] In Japan, where HTLV-1 infection is endemic, a relationship between a Sjögren-like syndrome and HTLV-1 disease has been described. Clinical and serologic findings differ little between HTLV-1–positive and –negative SS patients,[242] although HTLV-1–positive SS patients may not possess characteristic sialographic findings.[243] Lymphocytic infiltration of salivary glands in graft-versus-host disease results in a syndrome that mimics SS[244] and appears within 12 weeks of bone marrow transplantation (BMT). Infiltration peaks between 26 and 52 weeks post BMT. Dry eye and mouth occurs between 12 and 24 months. Symptoms may abate after 2 years.[245,246] ANA and smooth muscle antibodies are frequently positive; however, SS-A and SS-B are not.[247] Infiltrate T cell CD4/CD8 is either lower than that found in SS or the inverse.[248] In these individuals, skin changes may mimic scleroderma. Patients with sarcoidosis may present with lacrimal and salivary swelling, hypergammaglobulinemia, bone, muscle and joint pain, and pulmonary infiltrates. In most cases, the characteristic features of sarcoidosis should pose little difficulty in diagnosis. MSG biopsy reveals noncaseating granulomas.[249] Amyloid infiltration may also result in salivary gland enlargement, tongue swelling, and dry mouth, in addition to joint pain and renal insufficiency. MSG biopsy demonstrates birefringence and immunochemical staining typical of amyloid.[250] Lymphoma may arise spontaneously in a salivary gland. The majority of tumors occur in the parotid gland and present as firm masses that are usually painless. Sicca symptoms are present in a minority (approximately 15%) of cases.[251] Other conditions causing sicca complaints are listed in Table 69–4.[252-260]

APPROACH TO THE WORKUP OF SJÖGREN'S SYNDROME

The modalities utilized for the workup of SS have formed the basis for most of the criteria sets proposed for the classification of SS. Thus, the evaluation of a patient with suspected SS often requires cooperation among the rheumatologist, ophthalmologist, and dental specialist. Figure 69–5 is a stepwise approach to the workup of SS based on the American-European Consensus Group modification of the European Community criteria shown in Table 69–5.[261] It is critical to ensure that clinical conditions listed as exclusions, including medications that cause dryness, are absent. It is also important to have an understanding of the performance characteristics of the testing components utilized. No individual test is absolutely specific for SS, including MSG biopsy. Among ophthalmologic tests, the Schirmer test, tear breakup time and Rose Bengal dye test are all sensitive; however, only the Rose Bengal is specific (approximately 95%).[262,263] The Schirmer test is not very reproducible, either in controls[264] or in SS patients.[265] The salivary scintigraphic time-activity pattern correlates well with salivary flow rate[266] but is diagnostically nonspecific; abnormalities could be caused by any infiltrative disorder. Sialography has the capacity to visualize the salivary ductal pattern, demonstrating abnormal aborization and ductal ectasia. Sialography appears to be as sensitive as biopsy and only slightly less specific,[267,268] but it is invasive, potentially causing flares of glandular pain and swelling. At focus scores greater than 3, scintigraphy, sialography, and biopsy display fairly good agreement.[269] Recently, parenchymal heterogeneity on ultrasonography and alterations in signal strength on MRI have been shown to be relatively specific for glandular involvement with SS.[270,271] The MSG biopsy is often used to confirm a diagnosis of SS. It is important to verify that the biopsy is read by a pathologist experienced in interpreting salivary gland pathology. Vivino and colleagues[272] have documented a revision in diagnosis in 53 percent of biopsy samples reexamined at a university center. Only samples demonstrating periductal lymphocytic infiltrates in the form of foci should be regarded as being consistent with SS. Biopsies revealing nonspecific scattered lymphocytic infiltrates, fibrosis, or fatty change should not. In patients assessed specifically for the ocular and oral components of SS, only focal sialadenitis correlated with KCS[273]; however, even biopsies with focus scores greater than 1 are not always specific for SS. Approximately 15 to 20 percent of specimens obtained from random postmortem samples and from healthy individuals have focus scores greater than 1.[274,275] Approximately 10 percent of samples from healthy elderly individuals[255] can be interpreted as positive. Focal lymphocyte sialadenitis (FLS) has been found on biopsy of a submandibular gland, despite repeatedly negative minor salivary gland (lip) biopsies.[276] Cigarette smoking appears to lower the focus score of MSG biopsies.[277] An MSG biopsy should always be performed if the clinician cannot rule out or suspects an alternative cause of salivary swelling (i.e., lymphoma or sarcoidosis). In cases in which SS is not reasonably suspected or in which the diagnosis is readily apparent from noninvasive testing, the biopsy adds little.[278] Serologies, particularly ANA and SS-A and-B, correlate with focus score on biopsy.[279] Serum IgG is the most specific predictor of a positive biopsy but has relatively low sensitivity.[280] Anti–SS-B may be useful in identifying pSS among patients presenting with xerostomia, xerophthalmia, and undifferentiated features of connective tissue disorder.[268]

TABLE 69–4 · SYSTEMIC CONDITIONS ASSOCIATED WITH SICCA SYMPTOMS

Viral : Mumps, EBV, HIV, HTLV-1	See text
GVHD	See text
Sarcoidosis	See text
Amyloidosis	See text
Lymphoma	See text
Radioiodine therapy	Reference 252
Fibromyalgia-like syndromes: Chronic fatigue syndrome; dry eye and mouth syndrome	References 253, 254
Aging	Reference 255
Dyslipoproteinemia	Reference 256
Hemochromatosis	Reference 257
Lipodystrophy	References 258, 259
Bulimia	Reference 260

Abbreviations: EBV, Epstein Barr virus; HIV, human immunodeficiency virus; HTLV-1, human T cell leukemia virus–1; GVHD, graft versus host decrease.

FIGURE 69–5 · An Approach to Utilizing the European-American Consensus Criteria for the Diagnosis of Sjögren's Syndrome.[261] The six criteria are: 1) symptoms of dry eye; 2) symptoms of dry mouth or salivary swelling; 3) evidence of dry eye (Schirmer test or abnormal corneal staining); 4) evidence of salivary dysfunction (abnormal salivary flow, scintigram, or sialogram); 5) presence of SS-A or SS-B; and 6) positive minor salivary gland biopsy. Patients must have four of the criteria, at least one of which must be either autoantibodies or positive biopsy. Major exclusions include other major connective tissue disorders (for primary Sjögren's), lymphoma, sarcoidosis, amyloidosis, human immunodeficiency virus (HIV), and treatment with anticholinergic medication. In the algorithm depicted in Figure 69-1, a patient may attain four criteria via a simple office history, physical examination, and laboratory testing. If required, patients should be referred to an ophthalmologist, oral surgeon, otolaryngologist, or nuclear medicine physician to complete the workup.

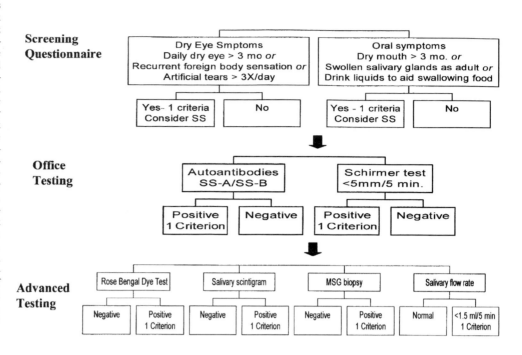

TABLE 69–5 · EUROPEAN-AMERICAN CONSENSUS GROUP MODIFICATION OF THE EUROPEAN COMMUNITY CRITERIA FOR SJÖGREN'S SYNDROME (SS)[261]

I. Symptoms of dry eye
Patients must have a positive response to at least one of the following:
Have you had daily, persistent, troublesome dry eyes for more than 3 months?
Do you have a recurrent sensation of sand or gravel in the eyes?
Do you use tear substitutes more than 3 times a day?

II. Oral symptoms
Patients must have a positive response to at least one of the following:
Have you had a daily feeling of dry mouth for more than 3 months?
Have you had recurrently or persistently swollen salivary glands as an adult?
Do you frequently drink liquids to aid in swallowing dry food?

III. Ocular signs
Patients must have objective evidence of ocular involvement, defined as a positive result from at least one of the following two tests:
1) Schirmer's test performed without anesthesia (5 mm in 5 min).
2) Rose Bengal score or other ocular dye score (4 according to van Bijsterveld's scoring system)

IV. Histopathology
This criterion is met if in patient's minor salivary glands (obtained through normal-appearing mucosa) focal lymphocytic sialadenitis is evaluated by an expert histopathologist with a focus score of 1. This score is defined as the number of lymphocytic foci adjacent to normal-appearing mucous acini and containing more than 50 lymphocytes per 4 mm^2 of glandular tissue.

V. Salivary gland involvement
Patient must have objective evidence of salivary gland involvement defined by a positive result for at least one of the following diagnostic tests:
1) Unstimulated whole salivary flow (1.5 ml in 15 min)
2) Parotid sialography showing the presence of diffuse sialectasis, punctuate, cavitary, or destructive pattern) without evidence of obstruction in the major ducts
3) Salivary scintigraphy showing delayed uptake, reduced concentration, delayed excretion of tracer, or some combination of these

VI. Autoantibodies
Patient must have presence in the serum of the following autoantibodies:
1) Antibodies to Ro(SS-A) or La (SS-B)
Definite SS requires the presence of four criteria, one of which must be either positive biopsy or autoantibodies.

Exclusions: Prior head and neck radiation; hepatitis C infection; human immunodeficiency virus (HIV) or acquired immunodeficiency syndrome (AIDS); preexisting lymphoma; sarcoidosis; graft-versus-host disease; use of anticholinergic drugs

Treatment

Therapy for SS can be viewed as having three phases. The first phase consists of external moisture replacement or capture. This approach can be applied to the oral cavity, eyes, nose, skin, and genital tract. The next phase consists of stimulation of endogenous secretions and has been proven effective mainly for xerostomia. This approach is currently under investigation for other xeroses including the eyes and skin. Finally, patients with systemic manifestations such as pulmonary disease, vasculitis, and pseudolymphoma may require corticosteriods, cytotoxic agents, or both.

OCULAR DISEASE

Therapy of xerophthalmia begins with moisture replacement. Patients should be encouraged to use tear substitutes often. Myriad over-the-counter (OTC) preparations exist. The rheumatologist should become familiar with one or two preparations from each of the following categories: (1) Standard artificial tears consist of polyvinyl alcohol or methylcellulose. (2) If irritation occurs with frequent use, preservative-free tears should be utilized. These preparations exist as sealed, sterile, individual units that must be refrigerated or discarded after single use. (3) A subset of tear preparations are of higher viscosity by virtue of inclusion of 0.1 percent dextran or 1 percent carboxymethylcellulose. These are useful for periods of increased symptomatology but may cause some blurring. (4) Lubricating ointments and hydroxypropyl cellulose inserts are generally longer lived; however, they leave residue, may cause significant blurring, and are often reserved for nocturnal use. Vivino and Orlin[281] have published an excellent detailed compendium of these agents. Existing tears may be retained in the eye by blocking their drainage or by inhibiting their evaporation. The former may be accomplished by occluding the punctae by inserting collagen or silicone plugs (temporary) or by electrocautery (permanent). The latter may be accomplished by wearing goggles or glasses with specially constructed side chambers. These devices are not well accepted by patients but are valuable in certain environmental conditions (i.e., wind). Inflammation of the meibobian glands (blepharitis) may complicate the dry eye and can be treated with warm compresses, cleansing of the lids, and a topical antibiotic when needed.

ORAL DISEASE

Surprisingly, replacement of saliva is not as successfully accomplished as tear supplementation. Artificial salivas are available[281]; however, they are generally felt to be short lived and unappetizing. A moisturizing gel (e.g., Oral Balance) is longer lived but must be applied intraorally. Most patients find it most suitable for nighttime application. Patients should be counseled with regard to general environmental measures designed to enhance moisture, such as the use of a humidifier and avoidance of forced-hot-air heating systems and excessive air conditioning. Emphasis should be given to fastidious dental care, including frequent examinations and office and home fluoride application. Patients should be advised to avoid retaining sugar-containing foods in the mouth for long periods of time. SS patients often chew gum or candy for the gustatory stimulus for salivation; only sugar-free products should be used. Some of the more severe symptoms encountered by the dry mouth patient are secondary to intraoral candidiasis.[282] Treatment should be initiated with mycostatin. The oral suspension (100,000U/5 ml QID for 10 days) is commonly used; however, it contains significant amounts of sucrose and could, therefore, be cariogenic. Mycostatin vaginal tablets dissolved orally offer an alternative. Cotrimazole troches (10-mg troche dissolved in the mouth five times per day for 14 days) also may be used. Dentures require removal and immersion in antifungal solutions to avoid recontamination. Oral candidiasis is recurrent and often requires retreatment. Systemic antifungals may be used, but they become ineffective as salivary flow diminishes. IFN-α lozenges appear to increase salivary flow and reduce symptoms.[283]

SECRETORY STIMULATION

Patients whose symptoms of dryness are not optimally controlled by moisture replacement should be considered for treatment with secretory stimulants (secretagogues).

Secretagogues stimulate muscarinic receptors in salivary glands and other organs, leading to enhanced secretion. Because there is a poor correlation between length of disease, biopsy findings, and response to these agents, and because M3R are upregulated in pSS labial salivary gland acini,[284] a trial of secretagogue therapy should be offered. Because secretagogues stimulate muscarinic activity in multiple organ systems, caution should be used in patients with asthma, narrow-angle glaucoma, acute iritis, severe cardiovascular disease, biliary disease, nephrolithiasis, diarrhea, and ulcer disease. There are two approved agents available for use as secretagogues in SS: pilocarpine (Salagen) and cevemiline (Evoxac). Both agents have been shown, in controlled clinical trials, to significantly increase salivary flow rate in SS.[285-287] Preliminary data suggests that other xeroses may be improved as well. Pilocarpine is administered as 5-mg tablets QID. Cevemiline is administered as 30-mg capsules TID. Table 69–6 compares the properties of these agents. Oral corticosteroid has not been convincingly shown to improve salivary flow.[288] Methotrexate (MTX) and oral cyclosporine A have been shown to improve subjective symptoms of dryness but not exocrine function.[289,290] Recently, a 14-week pilot study[291] with a subsequent 1-year follow-up[292] has demonstrated a potential use for infliximab in treating the ocular, oral, and systemic inflammatory manifestations of SS. Additional placebo-controlled studies will be required to demonstrate efficacy and safety, particularly with regard to lymphoproliferation.

TREATMENT OF SYSTEMIC DISEASE

Minor musculoskeletal symptoms usually respond to nonsteroidal anti-inflammatory drug (NSAID) therapy.

TABLE 69–6 • COMPARISON OF MUSCARINIC STIMULANTS FOR SJÖGREN'S SYNDROME

	Pilocarpine	Cevimeline
Brand name	Salagen	Evoxac
Dose form	Tablet	Capsule
Dose strength	5 mg	30 mg
Half-life	Approximately 1 hr	Approximately 5 hr
Peak onset of reaction	1 hr	1.5 to 2.0 hr
Major muscarinic side effects (%)	Diaphoresis (40) Nausea (10) Rhinitis (9) Diarrhea (9)	Diaphoresis (19) Nausea (14) Rhinitis (11) Diarrhea (10)

Because erosive joint disease is rare, therapy with disease-modifying antirheumatic drugs (DMARDs) is usually unnecessary; however, hydroxychloroquine (HCQ) at doses of 6 to 7 mg/kg/day has been used to treat fatigue, arthralgia, and myalgia in primary SS. HCQ has not been shown to improve dryness; however, HCQ administration does result in reduction of acute-phase proteins and elevated immunoglobulin levels in primary SS.[293] Rarely, short courses of low-dose corticosteroid (i.e., 5 to 10 mg/day of prednisolone may be necessary for very painful or disabling joint symptoms).

To combat cutaneous dryness, patients should be instructed never to dry completely after bathing but rather to gently blot the skin dry, leaving a slight amount of moisture, to be followed by application of a moisturizer. There is some data suggesting that secretagogues (such as pilocarpine), when taken at doses of 20 to 30 mg/day, ameliorate the symptoms of dry skin. Tight or constricting elastic clothing on the lower extremities may exacerbate hypergammaglobulinemic purpura. On the other hand, support hosiery may be helpful. Intermittent use of a mild corticosteroid cream may be useful to control pruritus. Mild cases of leukocytoclastic vasculitis may be treated expectantly as described previously. Severe cases manifested by necrotic or ulcerating lesions require more aggressive therapy.

Xerotrachea can be managed with humidification, secretagogues, and guaifenesin (1200 mg bid). Cough and dyspnea associated with pulmonary lymphocytic infiltration may be treated with moderate-dose corticosteroid, but may also require low-to-moderate-dose oral cyclophosphamide (50 to 150 mg/day). Frank lymphoma, when demonstrated by biopsy, requires standard chemotherapeutic intervention.

Treatment for mild to moderate renal tubular acidosis consists of supplementation with potassium chloride and alkalinization with potassium citrate. For cases resistant to replacement therapy or demonstrating evidence of renal insufficiency, consideration of corticosteroid therapy (0.5 to 1.0 mg/kg) should be given.

Manifestations of GERD are usually managed with antacids, H2 blockers, and PPIs. Intermittent endoscopic evaluation and intervention may be required. Sjögren's-associated hepatitis is often mild and may not require specific therapy. Persistent and progressive linear function test (LFT) elevation may require therapy with prednisone and azathioprine. Standard measures for the management of acute pancreatitis or pancreatic enzyme deficiency should be employed. Corticosteroid therapy has not been proven useful and may itself be associated with pancreatitis; it should be avoided unless abdominal vasculitis is suspected.

Cranial and peripheral neuropathy may be treated with low-dose tricyclic antidepressants or gabapentin (300 to 1800 mg/day). Symptomatic cases resistant to the previously mentioned therapies may be treated with intravenous gammaglobulin (0.4 g/kg/day for 5 days). When demonstrated by muscle and nerve biopsy, vasculitis should be treated with moderate-dose corticosteroid (approximately 1 mg/kg/day with subsequent tapering) and cyclophosphamide (50 to 150 mg PO daily). If felt to be due to primary SS, CNS manifestations should be treated aggressively with high-dose oral (1 to 2 mg/kg) or pulse intravenous (1 g/day for 3 days) corticosteroid and daily (50 to 150 mg/day) or monthly intravenous pulse (0.5 to 1 g/m²) cyclophosphamide.

REFERENCES

1. Sjögren H: Zur Kenntnis der keratoconjunctivitis sicca (keratitis filiformis bei hypofunktion der tranendrusen). Acta Ophthalmol (Kbh) 11(Suppl 2):1, 1933.
2. Leber: Uber die entstenhung der netzhautablosung. Klin Monatsbl Augenheilkd 20:165, 1882.
3. Mikulicz J: In discussion at Verein fur wissenschaftliche Heilkunde zu Konigsberg. Berl Klin Wochenschr 25:759,1888.
4. Morgan WS, Castleman B: A clinicopathologic study of Mikulicz's disease. Am J Pathol 29:471, 1953.
5. Mason AM, Gumpel JM, Golding PL: Sjögren's syndrome: A clinical review. Sem Arthritis Rheum 2:301, 1973.
6. Talal N: Recent developments in the immunology of Sjögren's syndrome (autoimmune exocrinopathy). Scand J Rheumatol Suppl 61:76, 1986.
7. Skopouli FN, Moutsopoulos HM: Autoimmune epitheliitis: Sjögren's syndrome. Clin Exp Rheumatol 12(Suppl 11):S9, 1994.
8. Pillemer SR, Matteson EL, Jacobsson LT, et al: Incidence of physician-diagnosed primary Sjögren's syndrome in residents of Olmsted County, Minnesota. Mayo Clin Proc 76:593, 2001.
9. Chudwin DS, Daniels TE, Wara DW, et al: Spectrum of Sjögren's syndrome in children. J Pediatr 98:213, 1981.
10. Strickland RW, Tesar JT, Berne BH, et al: The frequency of sicca syndrome in an elderly female population. J Rheumatol 14:766, 1987.
11. Molina R, Provost TT, Arnett FC, et al: Primary Sjögren's syndrome in men: Clinical, serologic and immunogenetic features. Am J Med 80:23, 1986.
12. Brennan MT, Fox PC: Sex differences in primary Sjögren's syndrome. J Rheumatol 26:2373, 1999.
13. Cervera R, Font J, Ramos-Casals M, et al: Primary Sjögren's syndrome in men: Clinical and immunological characteristics. Lupus 9:61, 2000.
14. Nasu M, Matsubara O, Yamamoto H: Postmortem prevalence of lymphocytic infiltration of the lacrimal gland: A comparative study in autoimmune and non-autoimmune diseases. J Pathol 143:11, 1984.
15. Fritzler MJ, Pauls JD, Kinsella TD, et al: Antinuclear, anticytoplasmic, and anti-Sjögren's syndrome antigen A (SS-A/Ro) antibodies in female blood donors. Clin Immunol Immunopathol 36:120, 1985.
16. Schein OD, Hochberg MC, Munoz B, et al: Dry eye and dry mouth in the elderly: A population-based assessment. Arch Intern Med 159:1359, 1999.

17. Drosos AA, Andonopoulos AP, Costopoulos JS, et al: Prevalence of primary Sjögren's syndrome in an elderly population. Br J Rheumatol 27:123, 1988.

18. Jacobsson LT, Axell TE, Hansen BU, et al: Dry eyes or mouth: An epidemiological study in Swedish adults, with special reference to primary Sjögren's syndrome. J Autoimmun 2:521, 1989.

19. Zhang NZ, Shi CS, Yao QP, et al: Prevalence of primary Sjögren's syndrome in China. J Rheumatol 22:659, 1995.

20. Bjerrum KB: Keratoconjunctivitis sicca and primary Sjögren's syndrome in a Danish population aged 30-60 years. Acta Ophthalmol Scand 75:281, 1997.

21. Dafni UG, Tzioufas AG, Staikos P, et al: Prevalence of Sjögren's syndrome in a closed rural community. Ann Rheum Dis 56:521, 1997.

22. Thomas E, Hay EM, Hajeer A, et al: Sjögren's syndrome: A community-based study of prevalence and impact. Br J Rheumatol 37:1069, 1998.

23. Tomsic M, Logar D, Grmek M, et al: Prevalence of Sjögren's syndrome in Slovenia. Rheumatology (Oxford) 38:164, 1999.

24. Boling EP, Wen J, Reveille JD, et al: Primary Sjögren's syndrome and autoimmune hemolytic anemia in sisters: A family study. Am J Med 74:1066, 1983.

25. Bolstad AI, Haga HJ, Wassmuth R, et al. Monozygotic twins with primary Sjögren's syndrome. J Rheumatol 2000 27:2264.

26. Fye KH, Terasaki PI, Moutsopoulos H, et al: Association of Sjögren's syndrome with HLA-B8. Arthritis Rheum 19:883, 1976.

27. Chused TM, Kassan SS, Opelz G, et al: Sjögren's syndrome association with HLA-Dw3. N Engl J Med 296:895, 1977.

28. Arnett FC, Bias WB, Reveille JD: Genetic studies in Sjögren's syndrome and systemic lupus erythematosus. J Autoimmun 2:403, 1989.

29. Kumagai S, Kanagawa S, Morinobu A, et al: Association of a new allele of the TAP2 gene, TAP2*Bky2 (Val577), with susceptibility to Sjögren's syndrome. Arthritis Rheum 40:1685, 1997.

30. Jean S, Quelvenec E, Alizadeh M, et al: DRB1*15 and DRB1*03 extended haplotype interaction in primary Sjögren's syndrome genetic susceptibility. Clin Exp Rheumatol 16:725, 1998.

31. Guggenbuhl P, Veillard E, Quelvenec E, et al: Analysis of TNF alpha microsatellites in 35 patients with primary Sjögren's syndrome. Joint Bone Spine 67:290, 2000.

32. Hulkkonen J, Pertovaara M, Antonen J, et al: Genetic association between interleukin-10 promoter region polymorphisms and primary Sjögren's syndrome. Arthritis Rheum 44:176, 2001.

33. Morinobu A, Kanagawa S, Koshiba M, et al: Association of the glutathione S-transferase M1 homozygous null genotype with susceptibility to Sjögren's syndrome in Japanese individuals. Arthritis Rheum 42:2612, 1999.

34. Ichikawa Y, Shimizu H, Takahashi K, et al: Lymphocyte subsets of the peripheral blood in Sjögren's syndrome and rheumatoid arthritis. Clin Exp Rheumatol 7:55, 1989.

35. Ichikawa Y, Shimizu H, Yoshida M, et al: Activation antigens expressed on T cells of the peripheral blood in Sjögren's syndrome and rheumatoid arthritis. Clin Exp Rheumatol 8:243, 1990.

36. Ichikawa Y, Shimizu H, Yoshida M, et al: Activation of T cell subsets in the peripheral blood of patients with Sjögren's syndrome: Multicolor flow cytometric analysis. Arthritis Rheum 33:1674, 1990.

37. Struyf NJ, Snoeck HW, Bridts CH, et al: Natural killer cell activity in Sjögren's syndrome and systemic lupus erythematosus: Stimulation with interferons and interleukin-2 and correlation with immune complexes. Ann Rheum Dis 49:690, 1990.

38. Miyasaka N, Seaman W, Bakhshi A, et al: Natural killing activity in Sjögren's syndrome: An analysis of defective mechanisms. Arthritis Rheum 26:954, 1983.

39. Bakhshi A, Miyasaka N, Kavathas P, et al: Lymphocyte subsets in Sjögren's syndrome: a quantitative analysis using monoclonal antibodies and the fluorescence-activated cell sorter. J Clin Lab Immunol 10:63, 1983.

40. Dauphinee M, Tovar Z, Talal N: B cells expressing CD5 are increased in Sjögren's syndrome. Arthritis Rheum 31:642, 1988.

41. Carsons SE: The medical workup of Sjögren's syndrome. In Carsons SE, Harris EK, (eds): The New Sjögren's Syndrome Handbook. New York: Oxford, Oxford University Press, 1998, pp 29-36.

42. Basset C, Durand V, Jamin C, et al: Increased N-linked glycosylation leading to oversialylation of monomeric immunoglobulin A1 from patients with Sjögren's syndrome. Scand J Immunol 51:300, 2000.

43. Atkinson JC, Fox PC, Travis WD, et al: IgA rheumatoid factor and IgA-containing immune complexes in primary Sjögren's syndrome. J Rheumatol 16:1205, 1989.

44. Daniels TE, Aufdermonte TB, Greenspan JS: Histopathology of Sjögren's syndrome. In Talal N, Moutsopolous HM, Kassan S (eds): Sjögren's Syndrome: Clinical and Immunological Aspects. Berlin, Springer Verlag, 1987, pp 41-54.

45. Fox RI, Carstens SA, Fong S, et al: Use of monoclonal antibodies to analyze peripheral blood and salivary gland lymphocyte subsets in Sjögren's syndrome. Arthritis Rheum 25:419, 1982.

46. Fujihara T, Fujita H, Tsubota K, et al: Preferential localization of CD8+alpha E beta 7+ T cells around acinar epithelial cells with apoptosis in patients with Sjögren's syndrome. J Immunol 163:2226, 1999.

47. Adamson TC III, Fox RI, Frisman DM, et al: Immunohistologic analysis of lymphoid infiltrates in primary Sjögren's syndrome using monoclonal antibodies. J Immunol 130:203, 1983.

48. Sumida T, Yonaha F, Maeda T, et al: T cell receptor repertoire of infiltrating T cells in lips of Sjögren's syndrome patients. J Clin Invest 89:681, 1992.

49. Smith MD, Lamour A, Boylston A, et al: Selective expression of V beta families by T cells in the blood and salivary gland infiltrate of patients with primary Sjögren's syndrome. J Rheumatol 21:1832, 1994.

50. Roncin S, Guillevin L, Beaugrand M, et al: Identification of the T cell antigen receptor V beta gene product in labial salivary glands from patients with primary Sjögren's syndrome. Ann Med Interne (Paris) 146:226, 1995.

51. Speight PM, Cruchley A, Williams DM: Quantification of plasma cells in labial salivary glands: increased expression of IgM in Sjögren's syndrome. J Oral Pathol Med 19.126, 1990.

52. Thrane PS, Sollid LM, Haanes HR, et al: Clustering of IgA-producing immunocytes related to HLA-DR-positive ducts in normal and inflamed salivary glands. Scand J Immunol 35:43, 1992.

53. Horsfall AC, Rose LM, Maini RN: Autoantibody synthesis in salivary glands of Sjögren's syndrome patients. J Autoimmun 2:559, 1989.

54. Aziz KE, McCluskey PJ, Wakefield D: Expression of selectins (CD62 E,L,P) and cellular adhesion molecules in primary Sjögren's syndrome: questions to immunoregulation. Clin Immunol Immunopathol 80:55, 1996.

55. Saito I, Terauchi K, Shimuta M, et al: Expression of cell adhesion molecules in the salivary and lacrimal glands of Sjögren's syndrome. J Clin Lab Anal 7:180, 1993.

56. Amft N, Curnow SJ, Scheel-Toellner D, et al: Ectopic expression of the B cell-attracting chemokine BCA-1 (CXCL13) on endothelial cells and within lymphoid follicles contributes to the establishment of germinal center-like structures in Sjögren's syndrome. Arthritis Rheum 44:2633, 2001.

57. Mikulowska-Mennis A, Xu B, Berberian JM, et al: Lymphocyte migration to inflamed lacrimal glands is mediated by vascular cell adhesion molecule-1/alpha(4)beta(1) integrin, peripheral node addressin/1-selectin, and lymphocyte function-associated antigen-1 adhesion pathways. Am J Pathol 159:671, 2001.

58. McArthur CP, Daniels PJ, Kragel P, et al: Sjögren's syndrome salivary gland immunopathology: increased laminin expression precedes lymphocytic infiltration. J Autoimmun 10:59, 1997.

59. Oxholm P, Daniels TE, Bendtzen K: Cytokine expression in labial salivary glands from patients with primary Sjögren's syndrome. Autoimmunity 12:185, 1992.

60. Boumba D, Skopouli FN, Moutsopoulos HM: Cytokine mRNA expression in the labial salivary gland tissues from patients with primary Sjögren's syndrome. Br J Rheumatol 34:326, 1995.

61. Cauli A, Yanni G, Pitzalis C, et al: Cytokine and adhesion molecule expression in the minor salivary glands of patients with Sjögren's syndrome and chronic sialoadenitis. Ann Rheum Dis 54:209, 1995.

62. Ohyama Y, Nakamura S, Matsuzaki G, et al: Cytokine messenger RNA expression in the labial salivary glands of patients with Sjögren's syndrome. Arthritis Rheum 39:1376, 1996.

63. Sun D, Emmert-Buck MR, Fox PC: Differential cytokine mRNA expression in human labial minor salivary glands in primary Sjögren's syndrome. Autoimmunity 28:125, 1998.

64. Koski H, Janin A, Humphreys-Beher MG, et al: Tumor necrosis factor-alpha and receptors for it in labial salivary glands in Sjögren's syndrome. Clin Exp Rheumatol 19:131, 2001.

65. Villarreal GM, Alcocer-Varela J, Llorente L: Differential interleukin IL-10 and IL-13 gene expression in vivo in salivary glands and peripheral blood mononuclear cells from patients with primary Sjögren's syndrome. Immunol Lett 49:105, 1996.

66. Kong L, Ogawa N, Nakabayashi T, et al: Fas and Fas ligand expression in the salivary glands of patients with primary Sjögren's syndrome. Arthritis Rheum 40:87, 1997.

67. Polihronis M, Tapinos NI, Theocharis SE, et al: Modes of epithelial cell death and repair in Sjögren's syndrome (SS). Clin Exp Immunol 114:485, 1998.

68. Ohlsson M, Skarstein K, Bolstad AI, et al: Fas-induced apoptosis is a rare event in Sjögren's syndrome. Lab Invest 81:95, 2001.

69. Nakamura H, Kawakami A, Tominaga M, et al: Expression of CD40/CD40 ligand and Bcl-2 family proteins in labial salivary glands of patients with Sjögren's syndrome. Lab Invest 79:261, 1999.

70. Tsubota K, Fujita H, Tadano K, et al: Abnormal expression and function of Fas ligand of lacrimal glands and peripheral blood in Sjögren's syndrome patients with enlarged exocrine glands. Clin Exp Immunol 129:177, 2002.

71. Manganelli P, Quaini F, Andreoli AM, et al: Quantitative analysis of apoptosis and Bcl-2 in Sjögren's syndrome. J Rheumatol 24:1552, 1997.

72. Konttinen YT, Halinen S, Hanemaaijer R, et al: Matrix metalloproteinase (MMP)-9 type IV collagenase/gelatinase implicated in the pathogenesis of Sjögren's syndrome. Matrix Biol 17:335, 1998.

73. Azuma M, Motegi K, Aota K, et al: Role of cytokines in the destruction of acinar structure in Sjögren's syndrome salivary glands. Lab Invest 77:269, 1997.

74. Gellrich S, Rutz S, Borkowski A, et al: Analysis of V(H)-D-J(H) gene transcripts in B cells infiltrating the salivary glands and lymph node tissues of patients with Sjögren's syndrome. Arthritis Rheum 42:240, 1999.

75. Stott DI, Hiepe F, Hummel M, et al: Antigen-driven proliferation of B cells within the target tissue of an autoimmune disease: The salivary glands of patients with Sjögren's syndrome. J Clin Invest 102:938, 1998.

76. Whittingham S, McNeilage J, Mackay IR: Primary Sjögren's syndrome after infectious mononucleosis. Ann Intern Med 102:490, 1985.

77. Gaston JS, Rowe M, Bacon P: Sjögren's syndrome after infection by Epstein-Barr virus. J Rheumatol 17:558, 1990.

78. Inoue N, Harada S, Miyasaka N, et al: Analysis of antibody titers to Epstein-Barr virus nuclear antigen in sera of patients with Sjögren's syndrome and with rheumatoid arthritis. J Infect Dis 164:22, 1991.

79. Fox RI, Pearson G, Vaughan JH: Detection of Epstein-Barr virus-associated antigens and DNA in salivary gland biopsies from patients with Sjögren's syndrome. J Immunol 137:3162, 1986.

80. Haneji N, Nakamura T, Takio K, et al: Identification of alpha-fodrin as a candidate autoantigen in primary Sjögren's syndrome. Science 276:604, 1997.

81. Inoue H, Tsubota K, Ono M, et al: Possible involvement of EBV-mediated alpha fodrin cleavage for organ-specific autoantigen in Sjögren's syndrome. J Immunol 166:5801, 2001.

82. Nagaraju K, Cox A, Casciola-Rosen L, et al: Novel fragments of the Sjögren's syndrome autoantigens alpha-fodrin and type 3 muscarinic acetylcholine receptor generated during cytotoxic lymphocyte granule-induced cell death. Arthritis Rheum 44:2376, 2001.

83. MacSween RN, Goudie RB, Anderson JR, et al: Occurrence of antibody to salivary duct epithelium in Sjögren's disease, rheumatoid arthritis, and other arthritides: A clinical and laboratory study. Ann Rheum Dis 26:402, 1967.

84. Bacman S, Sterin-Borda L, Camusso JJ, et al: Circulating antibodies against rat parotid gland M3 muscarinic receptors in primary Sjögren's syndrome. Clin Exp Immunol 104:454, 1996.

85. Waterman SA, Gordon TP, Rischmueller M: Inhibitory effects of muscarinic receptor autoantibodies on parasympathetic neurotransmission in Sjögren's syndrome. Arthritis Rheum 43:1647, 2000.

86. Lindstrom FD, Eriksson P, Tejle K, et al: IgG subclasses of anti-SS-A/Ro in patients with primary Sjögren's syndrome. Clin Immunol Immunopathol 73:358, 1994.

87. Tengner P, Halse AK, Haga HJ, et al: Detection of anti-Ro/SSA and anti-La/SSB autoantibody-producing cells in salivary glands from patients with Sjögren's syndrome. Arthritis Rheum 41:2238, 1998.

88. de Wilde PC, Kater L, Bodeutsch C, et al: Aberrant expression pattern of the SS-B/La antigen in the labial salivary glands of patients with Sjögren's syndrome. Arthritis Rheum 39:783, 1996.

89. Ormerod LD, Fong LP, Foster CS: Corneal infection in mucosal scarring disorders and Sjögren's syndrome. Am J Ophthalmol 105:512, 1988.

90. Friedlaender MH: Ocular manifestations of Sjögren's syndrome: Keratoconjunctivitis sicca. Rheum Dis Clin North Am 18:591, 1992.

91. Baudet-Pommel M, Albuisson E, Kemeny JL, et al: Early dental loss in Sjögren's syndrome: Histologic correlates—European Community Study Group on Diagnostic Criteria for Sjögren's Syndrome (EEC COMAC). Oral Surg Oral Med Oral Pathol 78:181, 1994.

92. Rhodus NL, Bloomquist C, Liljemark W, et al: Prevalence, density and manifestations of oral Candida albicans in patients with Sjögren's syndrome. J Otolaryngol 26:300, 1997.

93. Wang SL, Zou ZJ, Yu SF, et al: Recurrent swelling of parotid glands and Sjögren's syndrome. Int J Oral Maxillofac Surg 22:362, 1993.

94. Katayama I, Yokozeki H, Nishioka K: Impaired sweating as an exocrine manifestation in Sjögren's syndrome. Br J Dermatol 133:716, 1995.

95. Mitchell J, Greenspan J, Daniels T, et al: Anhidrosis (hypohidrosis) in Sjögren's syndrome. J Am Acad Dermatol 16:233, 1987.

96. Castro-Poltronieri A, Alarcon-Segovia D: Articular manifestations of primary Sjögren's syndrome. J Rheumatol 10:485, 1983.

97. Pease CT, Shattles W, Barrett NK, et al: The arthopathy of Sjögren's syndrome. Br J Rheumatol 32:609, 1993.

98. Tsampoulas CG, Skopouli FN, Sartoris DJ, et al: Hand radiographic changes in patients with primary and secondary Sjögren's syndrome. Scand J Rheumatol 15:333, 1986.

99. Lindvall B, Bengtsson A, Ernerudh J, et al: Subclinical myositis is common in primary Sjögren's syndrome and is not related to muscle pain. J Rheumatol 29:717, 2002.

100. Vrethem M, Lindvall B, Holmgren H, et al: Neuropathy and myopathy in primary Sjögren's syndrome: Neurophysiological, immunological and muscle biopsy results. Acta Neurol Scand 82:126, 1990.

101. Papiris SA, Maniata M, Constantopoulos SH, et al: Lung involvement in primary Sjögren's syndrome is mainly related to the small airway disease. Ann Rheum Dis 58:61, 1999.

102. Mialon P, Barthelemy L, Sebert P, et al: A longitudinal study of lung impairment in patients with primary Sjögren's syndrome. Clin Exp Rheumatol 15:349, 1997.

103. Fairfax AJ, Haslam PL, Pavia D, et al: Pulmonary disorders associated with Sjögren's syndrome. Q J Med 50:279, 1981.

104. Mathieu A, Cauli A, Pala R, et al: Tracheobronchial mucociliary clearance in patients with primary and secondary Sjögren's syndrome. Scand J Rheumatol 24:300, 1995.

105. Andoh Y, Shimura S, Sawai T, et al: Morphometric analysis of airways in Sjögren's syndrome. Am Rev Respir Dis 148:1358, 1993.

106. La Corte R, Potena A, Bajocchi G, et al: Increased bronchial responsiveness in primary Sjögren's syndrome: A sign of tracheobronchial involvement. Clin Exp Rheumatol 9:125, 1991.

107. Strimlan CV, Rosenow EC III, Divertie MB, et al: Pulmonary manifestations of Sjögren's syndrome. Chest 70:354, 1976.

108. Kelly C, Gardiner P, Pal B, et al: Lung function in primary Sjögren's syndrome: A cross sectional and longitudinal study. Thorax 46:180, 1991.

109. Constantopoulos SH, Papadimitriou CS, Moutsopoulos HM: Respiratory manifestations in primary Sjögren's syndrome: A clinical, functional, and histologic study. Chest 88:226, 1985.

110. Uffmann M, Kiener HP, Bankier AA, et al: Lung manifestation in asymptomatic patients with primary Sjögren's syndrome: Assessment with high resolution CT and pulmonary function tests. J Thorac Imaging 16:282, 2001.

111. Koyama M, Johkoh T, Honda O, et al: Pulmonary involvement in primary Sjögren's syndrome: Spectrum of pulmonary abnormalities and computed tomography findings in 60 patients. J Thorac Imaging 16:290, 2001.

112. Hatron PY, Wallaert B, Gosset D, et al: Subclinical lung inflammation in primary Sjögren's syndrome: Relationship between bronchoalveolar lavage cellular analysis findings and characteristics of the disease. Arthritis Rheum 30:1226, 1987.

113. Deheinzelin D, Capelozzi VL, Kairalla RA, et al: Interstitial lung disease in primary Sjögren's syndrome: Clinical pathological evaluation and response to treatment. Am J Respir Crit Care Med 154:794, 1996.

114. Papiris SA, Saetta M, Turato G, et al: CD-4 positive T-lymphocytes infiltrate the bronchial mucosa of patients with Sjögren's syndrome. Am J Respir Crit Care Med 156:637, 1997.

115. Raskin RJ, Tesar JT, Lawless OJ: Hypokalemic periodic paralysis in Sjögren's syndrome. Arch Intern Med 141:1671, 1981.

116. Goules A, Masouridi S, Tzioufas AG, et al: Clinically significant and biopsy-documented renal involvement in primary Sjögren's syndrome. Medicine 79:241, 2000.

117. Shiozawa S, Shiozawa K, Shimizu S, et al: Clinical studies of renal disease in Sjögren's syndrome. Ann Rheum Dis 46:768, 1987.

118. Talal N, Zisman E, Schur PH: Renal tubular acidosis, glomerulonephritis and immunologic factors in Sjögren's syndrome. Arthritis Rheum 11:774, 1968.

119. Matsumura R, Kondo Y, Sugiyama T, et al: Immunohistochemical identification of infiltrating mononuclear cells in tubulointerstitial nephritis associated with Sjögren's syndrome. Clin Nephrol 30:335, 1988.

120. Kjellen G, Fransson SG, Lindstrom F, et al: Esophageal function, radiography, and dysphagia in Sjögren's syndrome. Dig Dis Sci 1986 31:225.

121. Tsianos EB, Chiras CD, Drosos AA, et al: Oesophageal dysfunction in patients with primary Sjögren's syndrome. Ann Rheum Dis 44:610, 1985.

122. Ostuni PA, Germana B, DiMario F, et al: Gastric involvement in primary Sjögren's syndrome. Clin Exp Rheumatol 11:21, 1993.

123. Pokorny G, Karacsony G, Lonovics J, et al: Types of atrophic gastritis in patients with primary Sjögren's syndrome. Ann Rheum Dis 50:97, 1991.

124. Maury CP, Tornroth T, Teppo AM: Atrophic gastritis in Sjögren's syndrome: Morphologic, biochemical and immunologic findings. Arthritis Rheum 28:388, 1985.

125. Lindgren S, Manthorpe R, Eriksson S: Autoimmune liver disease in patients with primary Sjögren's syndrome. J Hepatol 20:354, 1994.

126. Manthorpe R, Permin H, Tage-Jensen U: Autoantibodies in Sjögren's syndrome, with special reference to liver-cell membrane antibody (LMA). Scan J Rheumatol 8:168, 1979.

127. Skopouli FN, Barbatis C, Moutsopoulos HM: Liver involvement in primary Sjögren's syndrome. Br J Rheumatol 33:745, 1994.

128. Hansen BU, Lindgren S, Eriksson S, et al: Clinical and immunological features of Sjögren's syndrome in patients with primary biliary cirrhosis with emphasis on focal sialadenitis. Acta Med Scand 224:611, 1988.

129. Uddenfeldt P, Danielsson A, Forssell A, et al: Features of Sjögren's syndrome in patients with primary biliary cirrhosis. J Intern Med 230:443, 1991.

130. Haddad J, Deny P, Munz-Gotheil C, et al: Lymphocyte sialadenitis of Sjögren's syndrome associated with chronic hepatitis C virus liver disease. Lancet 339:321, 1992.

131. Pirisi M, Scott C, Fabris C, et al: Mild sialoadenitis: A common finding in patients with hepatitis C virus infection. Scand J Gastroenterol 29:940, 1994.

132. Verbaan H, Carlson J, Eriksson S, et al: Extrahepatic manifestations of chronic hepatitis C infection and the interrelationship between primary Sjögren's syndrome and hepatitis C in Swedish patients. J Intern Med 245:127, 1999.

133. Jorgensen C, Legouffe MC, Perney P, et al: Sicca syndrome associated with hepatitis C virus infection. Arthritis Rheum 39:1166, 1996.

134. Garcia-Carrasco M, Ramos M, Cervera R, et al: Hepatitis C virus infection in "primary" Sjögren's syndrome: prevalence and clinical significance in a series of 90 patients. Ann Rheum Dis 56:173, 1997.

135. Szodoray P, Csepregi A, Hejjas M, et al: Study of hepatitis C virus infection in 213 Hungarian patients with Sjögren's syndrome. Rheumatol Int 21:6, 2001.

136. Ramos-Casals M, Garcia-Carrasco M, Cervera R, et al: Hepatitis C virus infection mimicking primary Sjögren's syndrome: A clinical and immunologic description of 35 cases. Medicine 80:1, 2001.

137. Ramos-Casals M, Cervera R, Yague J, et al: Cryoglobulinemia in primary Sjögren's syndrome: prevalence and clinical characteristics in a series of 115 patients. Semin Arthritis Rheum 28:200, 1998.

138. Coll J, Gambus G, Corominas J, et al: Immunohistochemistry of minor salivary gland biopsy specimen from patients with Sjögren's syndrome with and without hepatitis C virus infection. Ann Rheum Dis 56:390, 1997.

139. Unoki H, Moriyama A, Tabaru A, et al: Development of Sjögren's syndrome during treatment with recombinant human interferon-alpha-2b for chronic hepatitis C. J Gastroenterol 31:723, 1996.

140. Coll J, Navarro S, Tomas R, et al: Exocrine pancreatic function in Sjögren's syndrome. Arch Intern Med 149:848, 1989.

141. Nishimori I, Morita M, Kino J, et al: Pancreatic involvement in patients with Sjögren's syndrome and primary biliary cirrhosis. Int J Pancreatol 17:47, 1995.

142. Tsianos EB, Tzioufas AG, Kita MD, et al: Serum isoamylases in patients with autoimmune rheumatic diseases. Clin Exp Rheumatol 2:235, 1984.

143. Tsokos M, Lazarou SA, Moutsopoulos HM: Vasculitis in primary Sjögren's syndrome: Histologic classification and clinical presentation. Am J Clin Pathol 88:26, 1987.

144. Sugai S, Shimizu S, Tachibana J, et al: Hypergammaglobulinemic purpura in patients with Sjögren's syndrome: A report of nine cases and a review of the Japanese literature. Jpn J Med 28:148, 1989.

145. Alexander EL, Arnett FC, Provost TT, et al: Sjögren's syndrome: association of anti-Ro(SSA) antibodies with vasculitis, hematologic abnormalities, and serologic hyperreactivity. Ann Int Med 98:155, 1983.

146. Youinou P, Pennec YL, Katsikis P, et al: Raynaud's phenomenon in primary Sjögren's syndrome. Br J Rheumatol 29:205, 1990.

147. Skopouli FN, Talal A, Galanopoulou V, et al: Raynaud's phenomenon in primary Sjögren's syndrome. J Rheumatol 17:618, 1990.

148. Kraus A, Caballero-Uribe C, Jakez J, et al: Raynaud's phenomenon in primary Sjögren's syndrome: Association with other extraglandular manifestations. J Rheumatol 19:1572, 1992.

149. Garcia-Carrasco M, Siso A, Ramos Casals M, et al: Raynaud's phenomenon in primary Sjögren's syndrome: Prevalence and clinical characteristics in a series of 320 patients. J Rheumatol 29:726, 2002.

150. Ohtsuka T: Nailfold capillary abnormalities in patients with Sjögren's syndrome and systemic lupus erythematosus. Br J Rheumatol 136:94, 1997.

151. Ramos-Casals M, Garcia-Carrasco M, Cervera R, et al: Thyroid disease in primary Sjögren's syndrome: Study in a series of 160 patients. Medicine (Baltimore) 79:103, 2000.

152. Perez B, Kraus A, Lopez G, et al: Autoimmune thyroid disease in primary Sjögren's syndrome. Am J Med 99:480, 1995.

153. Youinou P, Mangold W, Jouquan J, et al: Organ-specific autoantibodies in non-organ-specific autoimmune diseases with special reference to rheumatoid arthritis. Rheumatol Int 7:123, 1987.

154. Andonopoulos AP, Lagos G, Drosos AA, et al: The spectrum of neurologic involvement in Sjögren's syndrome. Br J Rheumatol 29:21-23, 1990.

155. Hietaharju A, Yli-Kerttula U, Hakkinen V, et al: Nervous system manifestations in Sjögren's syndrome. Acta Neurol Scand 81:144, 1990.

156. Mauch E, Volk C, Kratzsch G, et al: Neurological and neuropsychiatric dysfunction in primary Sjögren's syndrome. Acta Neurol Scand 89:31, 1994.

157. Tajima Y, Mito Y, Owada Y, et al: Neurological manifestations of primary Sjögren's syndrome in Japanese patients. Intern Med 36:690, 1997.

158. Govoni M, Bajocchi G, Rizzo N, et al: Neurological involvement in primary Sjögren's syndrome: Clinical and instrumental evaluation in a cohort of Italian patients. Clin Rheumatol 18:299, 1999.

159. Lafitte C, Amoura Z, Cacoub P, et al: Neurological complications of primary Sjögren's syndrome. J Neurol 248:577, 2001.
160. Terenzi TJ, Dennis, KA, Carsons SE: Primary Sjögren's with systemic manifestations: Effects of classification utilizing the New European-American Consensus Criteria and the ACR Criteria for SLE. Arthritis Rheum 46:S367, 2002.
161. Gemignani F, Marbini A, Pavesi G, et al: Peripheral neuropathy associated with primary Sjögren's syndrome. J Neurol Neurosurg Psychiatry 57:983, 1994.
162. Barendregt PJ, van den Bent MJ, van Raaij-van den Aarssen VJ, et al: Involvement of the peripheral nervous system in primary Sjögren's syndrome. Ann Rheum Dis 60:876, 2001.
163. Griffin JW, Cornblath DR, Alexander E, et al: Ataxic sensory neuropathy and dorsal root ganglionitis associated with Sjögren's syndrome. Ann Neurol 27:304, 1990.
164. Malinow K, Yannakakis GD, Glusman SM, et al: Subacute sensory neuronopathy secondary to dorsal root ganglionitis in primary Sjögren's syndrome. Ann Neurol 20:535, 1986.
165. Mellgren SI, Conn DL, Stevens JC, et al: Peripheral neuropathy in primary Sjögren's syndrome. Neurology 39:390, 1989.
166. Kaltreider HB, Talal N: The neuropathy of Sjögren's syndrome: Trigeminal nerve involvement. Ann Intern Med 70:751, 1969.
167. Tumiati B, Casoli P, Parmeggiani A: Hearing loss in Sjögren's syndrome. Ann Intern Med 126:450, 1997.
168. Mandl T, Jacobsson L, Lilja B, et al: Disturbances of autonomic nervous function in primary Sjögren's syndrome. Scand J Rheumatol 26:401, 1997.
169. Andonopoulos AP, Christodoulou J, Ballas C, et al: Autonomic cardiovascular neuropathy in Sjögren's syndrome: A controlled study. J Rheumatol 25:2385, 1998.
170. Vetrugno R, Liguori R, Cevoli S, et al: Adie's tonic pupil as a manifestation of Sjögren's syndrome. Ital J Neurol Sci 18:293, 1997.
171. Bachmeyer C, Zuber M, Dupont S, et al: Adie syndrome as the initial sign of primary Sjögren's syndrome. Am J Ophthalmol 123:691, 1997.
172. Molina R, Provost TT, Alexander EL: Peripheral inflammatory vascular disease in Sjögren's syndrome: Association with nervous system complications. Arthritis Rheum 28:1341, 1985.
173. Alexander EL, Ranzenbach MR, Kumar AJ, et al: Anti-Ro(SS-A) autoantibodies in central nervous system disease associated with Sjögren's syndrome (CNS-SS): Clinical, neuroimaging, and angiographic correlates. Neurology 44:899, 1994.
174. de la Monte SM, Hutchins GM, Gupta PK: Polymorphous meningitis with atypical mononuclear cells in Sjögren's syndrome. Ann Neurol 14:455, 1983.
175. Alexander EL, Beall SS, Gordon B, et al: Magnetic resonance imaging of cerebral lesions in patients with Sjögren's syndrome. Ann Intern Med 108:815, 1988.
176. Alexander EL, Malinow K, Lejewski JE, et al: Primary Sjögren's syndrome with central nervous system disease mimicking multiple sclerosis. Ann Intern Med 104:323, 1986.
177. Noseworthy JH, Bass BH, Vandervoort MK, et al: The prevalence of primary Sjögren's syndrome in a multiple sclerosis population. Ann Neurol 25:95, 1989.
178. Montecucco C, Franciotta DM, Caporali R, et al: Sicca syndrome and anti-SSA/Ro antibodies in patients with suspected or definite multiple sclerosis. Scand J Rheum 18:407, 1989.
179. Metz LM, Seland TP, Fritzler MJ: An analysis of the frequency of Sjögren's syndrome in a population of multiple sclerosis patients. J Clin Lab Immunol 30:121, 1989.
180. Miro J, Pena-Sagredo JL, Berciano J, et al: Prevalence of primary Sjögren's syndrome in patients with multiple sclerosis. Ann Neurol 27:582, 1990.
181. Ellemann K, Krogh E, Arlien-Soeborg P, et al: Sjögren's syndrome in patients with multiple sclerosis. Acta Neuro Scand 84:68, 1991.
182. Sandberg-Wollheim M, Axell T, Hansen BU, et al: Primary Sjögren's syndrome in patients with multiple sclerosis. Neurology 42:845, 1992.
183. de Andres C, Guillem A, Rodriguez-Mahou M, et al: Frequency and significance of anti-Ro(SS-A) antibodies in multiple sclerosis patients. Acta Neurol Scand 104:83, 2001.
184. de Seze J, Devos D, Castelnovo G, et al: The prevalence of Sjögren's syndrome in patients with primary progressive multiple sclerosis. Neurology 57:1359, 2001.
185. Olsen ML, O'Connor S, Arnett FC, et al: Autoantibodies and rheumatic disorders in a neurology inpatient population: A prospective study. Am J Med 90:479, 1991.
186. Williams CS, Butler E, Roman GC: Treatment of myelopathy in Sjögren's syndrome with a combination of prednisone and cyclophosphamide. Arch Neurol 58:815, 2001.
187. Wise CM, Agudelo CA: Optic neuropathy as an initial manifestation of Sjögren's syndrome. J Rheumatol 15:799, 1988.
188. Pierot L, Suave C, Leger JM, et al: Asymptomatic cerebral involvement in Sjögren's syndrome: MRI findings of 15 cases. Neuroradiology 35:378, 1993.
189. Belin C, Moroni C, Caillat-Vigneron N, et al: Central nervous system involvement in Sjögren's syndrome: Evidence from neuropsychological testing and HMPAO-SPECT. Ann Med Interne (Paris) 150:598, 1999.
190. Kassan SS, Thomas TL, Moutsopoulos HM, et al: Increased risk of lymphoma in sicca syndrome. Ann Int Med 89:888, 1978.
191. Pertovaara M, Pukkala E, Laippala P, et al: A longitudinal cohort study of Finnish patients with primary Sjögren's syndrome: Clinical, immunological, and epidemiologic aspects. Ann Rheum Dis 60:467, 2001.
192. Kauppi M, Pukkala E, Isomaki H: Elevated incidence of hematologic malignancies in patients with Sjögren's syndrome compared with patients with rheumatoid arthritis (Finland). Cancer Causes Control 8:201, 1997.
193. Pariente D, Anaya JM, Combe B, et al: Non Hodgkin's lymphoma associated with primary Sjögren's syndrome. Eur J Med 1:337, 1992.
194. Valesini G, Priori R, Bavoillot D, et al: Differential risk of non-Hodgkin's lymphoma in Italian patients with primary Sjögren's syndrome. J Rheumatol 24:2376, 1997.
195. Zufferey P, Meyer OC, Grossin M, et al: Primary Sjögren's syndrome (SS) and malignant lymphoma: A retrospective cohort study of 55 patients with SS. Scand J Rheumatol 24:342, 1995.
196. Kruize AA, Hene RJ, van der Heide A, et al: Long-term follow-up of patients with Sjögren's syndrome. Arthritis Rheum 39:297, 1996.
197. Skopouli FN, Dafni U, Ioannidis JP, et al: Clinical evolution, and morbidity and mortality of primary Sjögren's syndrome. Semin Arthritis Rheum 29:296, 2000.
198. Ioannidis JP, Vassikiou VA, Moutsopoulos HM: Long-term risk of mortality and lymphoproliferative disease and predictive classification of primary Sjögren's syndrome. Arthritis Rheum 46:741, 2002.
199. McCurley T, Collins RD, Ball E, et al: Nodal and extranodal lymphoproliferative disorders in Sjögren's syndrome: A clinical and immunopathologic study. Hum Pathol 21:482, 1990.
200. Ramos-Casals M, Cervera R, Font J, et al: Young onset of primary Sjögren's syndrome: clinical and immunological characteristics. Lupus 7:202, 1998.
201. Janin A, Morel P, Quiquandon I, et al: Non-Hodgkin's lymphoma and Sjögren's syndrome: An immunopathological study of 113 patients. Clin Exp Rheumatol 10:565, 1992.
202. Zulman J, Jaffe R, Talal N: Evidence that the malignant lymphoma of Sjögren's syndrome is a monoclonal B-cell neoplasm. New Eng J Med 299:1215, 1978.
203. Sheibani K, Burke JS, Swartz WG, et al: Monocytoid B-cell lymphoma: clinicopathological study of 21 cases of a unique type of low-grade lymphoma. Cancer 62:1531, 1988.
204. Voulgarelis M, Dafni UG, Isenberg DA, et al: Malignant lymphoma in primary Sjögren's syndrome: A multicenter, retrospective, clinical study by the European Concerted Action on Sjögren's Syndrome. Arthritis Rheum 42:1765, 1999.
205. Isaacson P, Wright DH: Extranodal malignant lymphoma arising from mucosa-associated lymphoid tissue. Cancer 53:2515, 1984.
206. Hansen LA, Prakash UB, Colby TV: Pulmonary lymphoma in Sjögren's syndrome. May Clin Proc 64:920, 1989.
207. Royer B, Cazals-Hatem D, Sibilia J, et al: Lymphomas in patients with Sjögren's syndrome are marginal zone B cell neoplasms, arise in diverse extranodal and nodal site and are not associated with viruses. Blood 90:766, 1997.
208. Biasi D, Caramaschi P, Ambrosetti A, et al: Mucosa-associated lymphoid tissue lymphoma of the salivary glands occurring in patients affected by Sjögren's syndrome: Report of 6 cases. Acta Haematol 105:83, 2001.

209. Talal N, Aufdemorte TB, Kincaid WL, et al: Two patients illustrating lymphoma transition and response to therapy in Sjögren's syndrome. J Autoimmun 1:171, 1988.

210. Andonopoulos AP, Skopouli FN, Dimou GS, et al: Sjögren's syndrome in systemic lupus erythematosus. J Rheumatol 17:201, 1990.

211. Grennan DM, Ferguson M, Williamson J, et al: Sjögren's syndrome in SLE. Part 1. The frequency of the clinical and subclinical features of Sjögren's syndrome in patients with SLE. N Z Med J 86:374, 1977.

212. Skopouli F, Siouna-Fatourou H, Dimou GS, et al: Histologic lesion in labial salivary glands of patients with systemic lupus erythematosus. Oral Surg Oral Med Oral Pathol 72:208, 1991.

213. Graninger WB, Steinberg AD, Meron G, et al: Interstitial nephritis in patients with systemic lupus erythematosus: A manifestation of concomitant Sjögren's syndrome? Clin Exp Rheumatol 9:41, 1991.

214. Romero RW, Nesbitt LT Jr., Ichinose H: Mikulicz disease and subsequent lupus erythematosus development. JAMA 237:2507, 1977.

215. Provost TT, Talal N, Harley JB, et al: The relationship between anti-Ro(SS-A) antibody-positive Sjögren's syndrome and anti-Ro(SS-A) antibody-positive lupus erythematosus. Arch Dermatol 124:63, 1988.

216. Chevalier X, de Bandt M, Bourgeois P, et al: Primary Sjögren's syndrome preceding the presentation of systemic lupus erythematosus as a benign intracranial hypertension syndrome. Ann Rheum Dis 51:808, 1992.

217. Zufferey P, Meyer OC, Bourgeois P, et al: Primary systemic Sjögren's syndrome (SS) preceding systemic lupus erythematosus: a retrospective study of 4 cases in a cohort of 55 SS patients. Lupus 4:23, 1995.

218. Satoh M, Yamagata H, Watanabe F, et al: Development of anti-Sm and anti-DNA antibodies followed by clinical manifestation of systemic lupus erythematosus in an elderly woman with long-standing Sjögren's syndrome. Lupus 4:63, 1995.

219. Andonopoulos AP, Drosos AA, Skopouli FN, et al: Secondary Sjögren's syndrome in rheumatoid arthritis. J Rheumatol 14:1098, 1987.

220. Skopouli FN, Andonopoulos AP, Moutsopoulos HM: Clinical implications of the presence of anti-Ro(SSA) antibodies in patients with rheumatoid arthritis. J Autoimmun 1:381, 1988.

221. Boire G, Menard HA, Gendron M, et al: Rheumatoid arthritis: anti-Ro antibodies define a non-HLA-DR associated clinicoserological cluster. J Rheumatol 20:1654, 1993.

222. Brennan MT, Pillemer SR, Goldbach-Mansky R, et al: Focal sialadenitis in patients with early synovitis. Clin Exp Rheumatol 19:444, 2001.

223. Cipoletti JF, Buckingham RB, Barnes EL, et al: Sjögren's syndrome in progressive systemic sclerosis. Ann Intern Med 87:535, 1977.

224. Andonopoulos AP, Drosos AA, Skopouli FN, et al: Sjögren's syndrome in rheumatoid arthritis and progressive systemic sclerosis: A comparative study. Clin Exp Rheumatol 7:203, 1989.

225. Frayha RA, Tabbara KF, Geha RS: Familial CREST syndrome with sicca complex. J Rheumatol 4:53, 1977.

226. Setty YN, Pittman CB, Mahale AS, et al: Sicca symptoms and anti-SSA/Ro antibodies are common in mixed connective tissue disease. J Rheumatol 29:487, 2002.

227. Jedryka-Goral A, Jagiello P, D'Cruz DP, et al: Isotype profile and clinical relevance of anticardiolipin antibodies in Sjögren's syndrome. Ann Rheum Dis 51:889, 1992.

228. Pertovaara M, Korpela M, Uusitalo H, et al: Clinical follow-up study of 87 patients with sicca symptoms (dryness of eyes or mouth, or both). Ann Rheum Dis 58:423, 1999.

229. Kruize AA, van Bijsterveld OP, Hene RJ, et al: Long-term course of tear gland function in patients with keratoconjunctivitis sicca and Sjögren's syndrome. Br J Ophthalmol 81:435, 1997.

230. Haga HJ: Clinical and immunological factors associated with low lacrimal and salivary flow rate in patients with primary Sjögren's syndrome. J Rheumatol 29:305, 2002.

231. Miyachi K, Naito M, Maeno Y, et al: Sialographic study in patients with and without antibodies to Sjögren's syndrome A (Ro). J Rheumatol 10:387, 1983.

232. Jonsson R, Kroneld U, Backman K, et al: Progression of sialadenitis in Sjögren's syndrome. Br J Rheumatol 32:578, 1993.

233. Markusse HM, Oudkerk M, Vroom TM, et al: Primary Sjögren's syndrome: clinical spectrum and mode of presentation based on an analysis of 50 patients selected from a department of rheumatology. Neth J Med 40:125, 1992.

234. Asmussen K, Andersen V, Bendixen G, et al: Quantitative assessment of clinical disease status in primary Sjögren's syndrome: A cross-sectional study using a new classification model. Scand J Rheumatol 26:197, 1997.

235. Kelly CA, Foster H, Pal B, et al: Primary Sjögren's syndrome in northeast England-a longitudinal study. Br J Rheumatol 30:437, 1991.

236. Davidson BK, Kelly CA, Griffiths ID: Primary Sjögren's syndrome in the northeast of England: A long-term follow-up study. Rheumatology (Oxford) 38:245, 1999.

237. Martins PB, Pillemer SR, Jacobsson LT, et al: Survivorship in a population based cohort of patients with Sjögren's syndrome, 1976-1992. J Rheumatol 26:1296, 1999.

238. Strombeck B, Ekdahl C, Manthorpe R, et al: Health-related quality of life in primary Sjögren's syndrome, rheumatoid arthritis and fibromyalgia compared to normal population data using SF-36. Scand J Rheumatol 29:20, 2000.

239. Williams FM, Cohen PR, Jumshyd J, et al: Prevalence of the diffuse infiltrative lymphocytosis syndrome among human immunodeficiency virus-type 1-positive outpatients. Arthritis Rheum 41:863, 1998.

240. Kordossis T, Paikos S, Aroni K, et al: Prevalence of Sjögren's-like syndrome in a cohort of HIV-1-positive patients: Descriptive pathology and immunopathology. Br J Rheumatol 37:691, 1998.

241. Ulirsch RC, Jaffe ES: Sjögren's syndrome-like illness associated with the acquired immunodeficiency syndrome-related complex. Hum Pathol 18:1063, 1987.

242. Nakamura H, Kawakami A, Tominaga M, et al: Relationship between Sjögren's syndrome and human T-lymphotropic virus type 1 infection: Follow-up study of 83 patients. J Lab Clin Med 135:139, 2000.

243. Izumi M, Nakamura H, Nakamura T, et al: Sjögren's syndrome (SS) in patients with human T cell leukemia virus 1 associated myelopathy: Paradoxical features of the major salivary glands compared to classical SS. J Rheumatol 26:2609, 1999.

244. Gratwhol AA, Moutsopoulos HM, Chused TM, et al: Sjögren-type syndrome after allogeneic bone marrow transplantation. Ann Int Med 87:703, 1977.

245. Lindahl G, Lonnquist B, Hedfors E: Lymphocytic infiltration of lip salivary glands in bone marrow recipients: A model for the development of the histopathological changes in Sjögren's syndrome? J Autoimmun 2:579, 1989.

246. Janin-Mercier A, Devergie A, Arrago JP, et al: Systemic evaluation of Sjögren-like syndrome after bone marrow transplantation in man. Transplantation 43:677, 1987.

247. Rouquette-Gally AM, Boyeldieu D, Gluckman E, et al: Auto-immunity in 28 patients after allogeneic bone marrow transplantation: Comparison with Sjögren's syndrome and scleroderma. Br J Haematol 66:45, 1987.

248. Hiroki A, Nakamura S, Shinohara M, et al: A comparison of glandular involvement between chronic graft-versus-host disease and Sjögren's syndrome. Int J Oral Maxillofac Surg 25:298, 1996.

249. Drosos AA, Constantopoulos SH, Psychos D, et al: The forgotten cause of sicca complex: sarcoidosis. J Rheumatol 16:1548, 1989.

250. Gogel HK, Searles RP, Volpicelli NA, et al: Primary amyloidosis presenting as Sjögren's syndrome. Arch Intern Med 143:2325, 1983.

251. Nime FA, Cooper HS, Eggleston JC: Primary malignant lymphomas of the salivary glands. Cancer 37:906, 1976.

252. Solans R, Bosch JA, Galofre P, et al: Salivary and lacrimal gland dysfunciton (sicca syndrome) after radioiodine therapy. J Nuc Med 42:738, 2001.

253. Sirois DA, Natelson B: Clinicopathological findings consistent with primary Sjögren's syndrome in a subset of patients diagnosed with chronic fatigue syndrome: preliminary observations. J Rheumatol 28:126, 2001.

254. Price EJ, Venables PJ: Dry eyes and mouth syndrome: A subgroup of patients presenting with sicca symptoms. Rheumatology (Oxford) 41:416, 2002.

255. De Wilde PC, Baak JP, van Houwelingen JC, et al: Morphometric study of histological changes in sublabial salivary glands due to aging process. J Clin Pathol 39:406, 1986.

256. Goldman JA, Julian EH: Pseudo-Sjögren's syndrome with hyperlipoproteinemia. JAMA 237:1582, 1977.

257. Takeda Y, Ohya T: Sicca symptom in a patient with hemochromatosis: Minor salivary gland biopsy for differential diagnosis. Int J Oral Maxillofac Surg 16:745, 1987.

258. Alarcon-Segovia D, Ramos-Niembro F: Association of partial lipodystrophy and Sjögren's syndrome. Lett Ann Int Med 85:474, 1976.

259. Ipp MM, Howard NJ, Tervo RC, et al: Sicca syndrome and total lipodystrophy. Ann Int Med 85:443, 1976.

260. Levin PA, Falko JM, Dixon K, et al: Benign parotid enlargement in bulimia. Ann Int Med 93:827, 1980.

261. Vitali C, Bombardiere S, Jonsson R, et al: Classification criteria for Sjögren's syndrome: A revised version of the European criteria proposed by the American-European Consensus Group. Ann Rheum Dis 61:554, 2002.

262. Paschides CA, Kitsios G, Karakostas KX, et al: Evaluation of tear break-up time, Schirmer's-1 test and Rose Bengal staining as confirmatory tests for keratoconjunctivitis sicca. Clin Exp Rheumatol 7:155, 1989.

263. Kalk WW, Mansour K, Vissink A, et al: Oral and ocular manifestations in Sjögren's syndrome. J Rheumatol 29:924, 2002.

264. Clinch TE, Benedetto DA, Felberg NT, et al: Schirmer's test. Arch Ophthalmol 101:1383, 1983.

265. Haga HJ, Hulten B, Bolstad AI, et al: Reliability and sensitivity of the diagnostic tests for primary Sjögren's syndrome. J Rheumatol 26:604, 1999.

266. Saito T, Fukuda H, Horikawa M, et al: Salivary gland scintigraphy with 99mTc-pertechnetate in Sjögren's syndrome: Relationship to clinicopathologic features of salivary and lacrimal glands. J Oral Pathol Med 26:46, 1997.

267. Vitali C, Tavoni A, Simi U, et al: Parotid sialography and minor salivary gland biopsy in the diagnosis of Sjögren's syndrome: A comparative study of 84 patients. J Rheumatol 15:262, 1988.

268. Vitali C, Monti P, Giuiggioli C, et al: Parotid sialography and lip biopsy in the evaluation of oral component in Sjögren's syndrome. Clin Exp Rheumatol 7:131, 1989.

269. Lindvall AM, Jonsson R: The salivary gland component of Sjögren's syndrome: An evaluation of diagnostic methods. Oral Surg Oral Med Oral Pathol 62:32, 1986.

270. Niemela RK, Paakko E, Suramo I, et al: Magnetic resonance imaging and magnetic resonance sialography of parotid glands in primary Sjögren's syndrome. Arthritis Rheum 45:512, 2001.

271. Izumi M, Eguchi K, Ohki M, et al: MR imaging of the parotid gland in Sjögren's syndrome: A proposal for new diagnostic criteria. Am J Roentgenol 166:1483, 1996.

272. Vivino FB, Gala I, Hermann GA: Change in final diagnosis on second evaluation of labial minor salivary gland biopsies. J Rheumatol 29:938, 2002.

273. Daniels TE, Whitcher JP: Association of patterns of labial salivary gland inflammation with keratoconjunctivitis sicca: Analysis of 618 patients with suspected Sjögren's syndrome. Arthritis Rheum 37:869, 1994.

274. Segerberg-Konttinen M: A postmortem study of focal adenitis in salivary and lacrimal glands. J Autoimmun 2:553, 1989.

275. Radfar L, Kleiner DE, Fox PC, et al: Prevalence and clinical significance of lymphocytic foci in minor salivary glands of healthy volunteers. Arthritis Rheum 47:520, 2002.

276. Katz J, Yamase H, Parke A: A case of Sjögren's syndrome with repeatedly negative findings on lip biopsy. Arthritis Rheum 34:1325, 1991.

277. Manthorpe R, Benoni C, Jacobsson L, et al: Lower frequency of focal lip sialadenitis (focus score) in smoking patients: Can tobacco diminish the salivary gland involvement as judged by histological examination and anti-SSA/Ro and anti-SSB/La antibodies in Sjögren's syndrome? Ann Rheum Dis 59:54, 2000.

278. Lee M, Rutka JA, Slomovic AR, et al: Establishing guidelines for the role of minor salivary gland biopsy in clinical practice for Sjögren's syndrome. J Rheumatol 25:247, 1998.

279. Shah F, Rapini RP, Arnett FC, et al: Association of labial salivary gland histopathology with clinical and serologic features of connective tissue diseases. Arthritis Rheum 33:1682, 1990.

280. Brennan MT, Sankar V, Leakan RA, et al: Risk factors for positive minor salivary gland biopsy findings in Sjögren's syndrome and dry mouth patients. Arthritis Rheum 47:189, 2002.

281. Vivino FB, Orlin SE: Sjögren's syndrome: Giving dry mouth and dry eye the full treatment. J Musculoskel Med 17:350, 2000.

282. Hernandez YL, Daniels TE: Oral candidiasis in Sjögren's syndrome: prevalence, clinical correlations, and treatment. Oral Surg Oral Med Oral Pathol 68:324, 1989.

283. Shiozawa S, Tanaka Y, Shiozawa K: Single-blinded controlled trial of low-dose oral IFN-alpha for the treatment of xerostomia in patients with Sjögren's syndrome. J Interferon Cytokine Res 18:255, 1998.

284. Beroukas D, Goodfellow R, Hiscock J, et al: Up-regulation of M3-muscarinic receptors in labial salivary gland acini in primary Sjögren's syndrome. Lab Invest 82:203, 2002.

285. Fox PC, Atkinson JC, Macynski AA, et al: Pilocarpine treatment of salivary gland hypofunction and dry mouth (xerostomia). Arch Intern Med 151:1149, 1991.

286. Vivino FB, Al-Hashimi I, Khan Z, et al: Pilocarpine tablets for the treatment of dry mouth and dry eye symptoms in patients with Sjögren's syndrome: A randomized, placebo-controlled, fixed-dose, multicenter trial: P92-01 Study Group. Arch Intern Med 159:174, 1999.

287. Fife RS, Chase WF, Dore RK, et al: Cevimeline for the treatment of xerostomia in patients with Sjögren's syndrome: A randomized trial: Arch Intern Med 162:1293, 2002.

288. Fox PC, Datiles M, Atkinson JC, et al: Prednisone and piroxicam for treatment of primary Sjögren's syndrome. Clin Exp Rheumatol 11:149, 1993.

289. Skopouli FN, Jagiello P, Tsifetaki N, et al: Methotrexate in primary Sjögren's syndrome. Clin Exp Rheumatol 14:555, 1996.

290. Drosos AA, Skopouli FN, Costopoulos JS, et al: Cyclosporin A (CyA) in primary Sjögren's syndrome: A double-blind study. Ann Rheum Dis 45:732, 1986.

291. Steinfeld SD, Demols P, Salmon I, et al: Infliximab in patients with primary Sjögren's syndrome: A pilot study. Arthritis Rheum 44:2371, 2001.

292. Steinfeld SD, Demols P, Appelboom T: Infliximab in primary Sjögren's syndrome: One year follow-up. Arthritis Rheum 46:3301, 2002.

293. Fox RI, Chan E, Benton L, et al: Treatment of primary Sjögren's syndrome with hydroxychloroquine. Am J Med 85:62, 1988.

Spondyloarthropathies

70 · Ankylosing Spondylitis

SJEF VAN DER LINDEN · DÉSIRÉE VAN DER HEIJDE · JUERGEN BRAUN

Ankylosing spondylitis (AS) is a human leucocyte antigen (HLA)-B27–associated chronic inflammatory disease of unknown etiology. Usually it affects the sacroiliac joints at early stages and may involve the axial skeleton at later stages of the disease. Peripheral joint involvement may also be an important feature. The disease can be accompanied by extraskeletal manifestations, such as acute anterior uveitis, aortic incompetence, cardiac conduction defects, fibrosis of the upper lobes of the lungs, neurologic involvement, or renal (secondary) amyloidosis.

AS belongs to the group of spondyloarthropathies. This group of disorders constitutes a family of related but heterogeneous conditions rather than a single disease with different clinical manifestations[1] (Tables 70–1 and 70–2).

Historical Aspects

In 1850, Brodie described the clinical features of a 31-year-old man who had developed an ankylosed spine and who "occasionally [was] suffering severe inflammation of the eye." In 1884, Struempell from Germany described two patients who showed complete ankylosis of the spine and hip joints.[2] This report was soon followed by descriptions of the disease by von Bechterew from St. Petersburg, Russia, and Pierre Marie from France.[3,4] Roentgen had developed the radiographic technique by 1896, but it was not until 1930 that sacroiliac disease, now considered the radiographic hallmark of AS, was fully recognized.

Nomenclature

The term *ankylosing spondylitis* is derived from the Greek roots ankylos ("bent"), although now it usually implies fusion or adhesions, and spondylos ("vertebral disk"). Because ankylosis of the spine tends to appear in late stages of the disease and does not occur in many patients with mild disease, it has been suggested that it would be better to rename the disease spondylitis or spondylitic disease.[5]

Classification

CLASSIFICATION CRITERIA FOR SPONDYLOARTHROPATHIES

The spectrum of spondyloarthropathies is wider than the sum of the disorders mentioned in Table 70–1. To also encompass patients with seronegative oligoarthritis, dactylitis, or polyarthritis of the lower extremities; heel pain due to enthesitis; and other undifferentiated spondyloarthropathies; classification criteria for the whole group of spondyloarthropathies have been developed[1] (Table 70–3). The European Spondyloarthropathy Study Group (ESSG) criteria resulted in a sensitivity of 86 percent and a specificity of 87 percent. In the subgroup of early cases (i.e., those in whom signs and symptoms had developed within the last year), the sensitivity declined to 68 percent, although the specificity increased to 93 percent. These criteria, although clearly not intended for diagnostic purposes, might be useful for identification of atypical and undifferentiated forms of spondyloarthropathies. This set of criteria performed quite well in patients with different sociocultural and geographic characteristics.[6]

CLASSIFICATION CRITERIA FOR ANKYLOSING SPONDYLITIS

The diagnosis of AS is based on clinical features. The disease is "primary" or "idiopathic" if no associated disorder

---

TABLE 70–1 · DISEASES BELONGING TO THE SPONDYLOARTHROPATHIES

Ankylosing spondylitis
Reiter's syndrome or reactive arthritis
Arthropathy of inflammatory bowel disease (Crohn's disease, ulcerative colitis)
Psoriatic arthritis
Undifferentiated spondyloarthropathies
Juvenile chronic arthritis and juvenile-onset ankylosing spondylitis

TABLE 70–2 · CLINICAL CHARACTERISTICS OF SPONDYLOARTHROPATHIES

Typical pattern of peripheral arthritis: predominantly of lower limb, asymmetric
Tendency to radiographic sacroiliitis
Absence of rheumatoid factor (RF)
Absence of subcutaneous nodules and other extra-articular features of rheumatoid arthritis (RA)
Overlapping extra-articular features characteristic of the group (e.g., anterior uveitis)
Significant familial aggregation
Association with HLA-B27

TABLE 70–3 · EUROPEAN SPONDYLOARTHROPATHY STUDY GROUP (ESSG) CLASSIFICATION CRITERIA

Inflammatory spinal pain
  OR
Synovitis (asymmetric, predominantly in lower limbs)
  AND
any one of the following:
  Positive family history
  Psoriasis
  Inflammatory bowel disease
  Alternate buttock pain
  Enthesopathy
Sensitivity, 77%; specificity, 89%
Adding:
  Sacroiliitis
Sensitivity, 86%; specificity, 87%

From Dougados M, van der Linden S, Juhlin R, et al: The European Spondylarthropathy Study Group preliminary criteria for the classification of spondylarthropathy. Arthritis Rheum 34:1218, 1991.

is present, and "secondary" if the disease is associated with psoriasis or chronic inflammatory bowel disease.

In daily practice, a presumptive clinical diagnosis of AS is usually supported by radiologic evidence of sacroiliitis. Indeed, many think of AS as "symptomatic sacroiliitis." However, the presence of sacroiliitis per se does not necessarily mean the presence of AS. Moreover, although radiographic sacroiliitis is very frequent in AS, it is by no means an early or obligate manifestation of the disease.[7] Lack of either sensitivity or specificity in previous classifications led to a modification of the New York criteria for AS[8] (Table 70–4). The criteria of "limitation of motion of the lumbar spine" and "limitation of chest expansion" appear to reflect disease duration; they are usually not present in early disease.[9] Indeed, it should be stressed that classification criteria are usually not well suited for early diagnosis of disease.

▌ Epidemiology

PREVALENCE

The prevalence of AS closely parallels the frequency of HLA-B27. This holds for those B27 subtypes that are associated with the disease but not for populations in which certain subtypes that lack association with AS occur rather frequently such as in the Indonesian population.[10-12]

TABLE 70–4 · CRITERIA FOR ANKYLOSING SPONDYLITIS

Rome, 1961

Clinical Criteria

1. Low back pain and stiffness for more than 3 months, not relieved by rest
2. Pain and stiffness in the thoracic region
3. Limited motion in the lumbar spine
4. Limited chest expansion
5. History or evidence of iritis or its sequelae

Radiologic Criterion

6. Roentgenogram showing bilateral sacroiliac changes characteristic of ankylosing spondylitis (this would exclude bilateral osteoarthritis of the sacroiliac joints)

Definite ankylosing spondylitis if:
1. Grade 3 or 4 bilateral sacroiliitis with at least one clinical criterion
2. At least four clinical criteria

New York, 1966

Diagnosis

1. Limitation of motion of the lumbar spine in all three planes: anterior flexion, lateral flexion, and extension
2. Pain at the dorsolumbar junction or in the lumbar spine
3. Limitation of chest expansion to 2.5 cm or less measured at the level of the fourth intercostal space

Grading of Radiographs

Normal, 0; suspicious, 1; minimal sacroiliitis, 2; moderate sacroiliitis, 3; ankylosis, 4

Definite ankylosing spondylitis if:
1. Grade 3 or 4 bilateral sacroiliitis with at least one clinical criterion
2. Grade 3 or 4 unilateral or grade 2 bilateral sacroiliitis with clinical criterion 1 or with both clinical criteria 2 and 3
Probable ankylosing spondylitis:
Grade 3 or 4 bilateral sacroiliitis with no clinical criteria

Modified New York, 1984

Criteria

1. Low back pain of at least 3 months' duration improved by exercise and not relieved by rest
2. Limitation of lumbar spine in sagittal and frontal planes
3. Chest expansion decreased relative to normal values for age and sex
4. Bilateral sacroiliitis grade 2 to 4
5. Unilateral sacroiliitis grade 3 or 4
Definite ankylosing spondylitis or unilateral grade 3 or 4, or bilateral grade 2 to 4 sacroiliitis and any clinical criterion

Data from van der Linden, Valkenburg, Cats: Evalution of diagnostic criteria for ankylosing spondylitis: a proposal for modification of the New York criteria. Arthritis Rheum 27:361, 1984.

Among whites, the estimated prevalence rate of AS as defined by the (modified) New York criteria ranges from 67.7 per 100,000 population older than 20 years of age in the Netherlands to 197 per 100,000 in the United States.[13,14] The prevalence of clinically significant AS in Finland was within this range, with a figure of 0.15 percent.[15]

However, in Central Europe, higher prevalence rates have been reported. An epidemiologic study from Berlin reports a prevalence figure of 0.86 percent.[16] In the general population, AS is likely to develop in about

1 to 2 percent of HLA-B27–positive adults who have a disease-associated B27 subtype, although there may still be regional or geographic differences.

For example, in northern Norway AS may develop in 6.7 percent of HLA-B27–positive people.[17] The disease is much more common among HLA-B27–positive first-degree relatives of HLA-B27–positive AS patients, because roughly 10 to 30 percent of them have signs or symptoms of AS.[13] In fact, a positive family history of AS is a strong risk factor for the disease.

INCIDENCE

There is no adequate evidence that the incidence has really changed within the last decades. Clinical features, age of onset, and survival time have remained stable.[18] One study revealed an overall age and gender-adjusted incidence of 7.3 per 100,000 person-years. This U.S. figure compares quite well with the Finnish study, which revealed an incidence of 8.9 per 100,000 people aged 16 or older.[15]

RACIAL DISTRIBUTION

AS occurs in all parts of the world, but there are race-related differences in the prevalence. This might reflect differences in the distribution of HLA-B27 among races (Table 70–5). Approximately 90 percent of white patients with AS possess HLA-B27, but AS and HLA-B27 (prevalence of B27 below 1 percent) are nearly absent in African blacks and Japanese. In African Americans, owing to racial admixture with whites, 2 percent possess B27, but only about 50 percent of black patients with AS possess B27. Correspondingly, African Americans are affected far less frequently than American whites.

▌ Etiology and Genetics

HYPOTHESES

The precise etiology of AS is still unclear. The disease has a well-known genetic component. The strong association with most subtypes of HLA-B27 supports the view that the disease is due to a genetically determined immune response to environmental factors in susceptible individuals. The genetic marker HLA-B27 is present in 80 to 98 percent of white patients, in contrast to only about 8 percent of the general population. HLA-B27 accounts for only 16 percent of the total genetic risk for the disease, whereas the major histocompatibility complex (MHC), located on chromosome 6, as a whole accounts for about half of the genetic variability for AS.[19] The role of *Klebsiella pneumoniae* polysaccharides is a matter of continuing debate, as levels of immunoglobulin (Ig) G and IgA antibodies against these bacteria were increased in patients with AS compared to those in healthy controls, but also in patients with inflammatory bowel disease.[20]

The arthritogenic peptide hypothesis postulates that AS results when external antigenic challenge activates autoreactive T cells that recognize endogenous peptides presented by HLA-B27. In normal situations, the HLA-B27 molecule on the surface of the antigen-presenting cells presents endogenously derived peptides to cell determinant (CD)8+ T cells. These peptides, which are usually nine amino acids long and have arginine in position 2, are mostly self derived, but they may also be of viral or bacterial origin.

Figure 70–1 shows the B27 antigen-binding cleft and the important amino acid residues of the binding cleft.

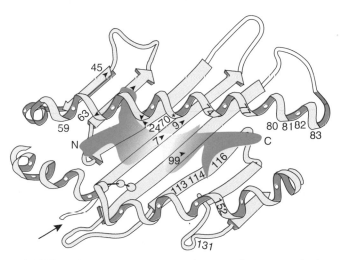

FIGURE 70–1 · A Schematic Ribbon Diagram of the Antigen-Binding Cleft of the HLA-B* 2705 Molecule Containing a Nonameric (Nine Amino Acids Long) Antigenic Peptide, as Seen from the Viewpoint of a T cell Receptor. The letters N and C indicate the amino acid carboxytermini of the bound peptide, and the *arrow* indicates the aminoterminus of the heavy (α) chain of the HLA-B27 molecule. The floor of the antigen-binding cleft is formed by the β strands, which are shown as *broad arrows* pointing away from the amino-terminus. The margins of the cleft are formed by α-helices shown as helical ribbons. The top α-helix and the four β strands to the left are from the α₁ domain of the α-chain, whereas the bottom α-helix and the four β strands to the right are from the α₂ domain. The disulfide bond is shown as two connecting spheres. The polymorphic residues of the eight subtypes of HLA-B27 are shown; these subtypes differ from each other at residues 59, 74, 77, 80, 81, 82, 83, 97, 113, 114, 116, 131, and 152. Location of the B27 family-specific residues (Lys) at position 70 is marked by an *asterisk*. The amino acids that form pocket B are at positions 7, 9, 24, 34, 45, 63, 67, and 99 (*black arrowheads*). Tyr7, Val34, and Glu63 are conserved in all HLA class I molecules. Thus, the prime residues that determine the size and chemical nature of pocket B of all of the HLA-B27 subtypes are His9, Thr24, Glu45, Cys67, and Tyr99. This side chain of the second residue (Arg) of the bound peptide is shown anchored into pocket B of the HLA-B27 molecule. (From Khan MA: Spondyloarthropathies. Editorial overview. Curr Opin Rheumatol 6:351, 1994. Copyright Rapid Science Publishers.)

TABLE 70–5 · HLA-B27 PREVALENCE IN WHITE POPULATIONS

Population Subgroups	HLA-B27 Phenotype Frequency (%)
UrgoFinnish	12-18
Northern Scandinavians	10-16
Slavic	7-14
Western Europeans	6-9
Southern Europeans	2-6
Basques	9-14
Gypsies (Spain)	16-18
Arabs, Jews, Armenians, Iranians	3-5
Pakistanis	6-8
Indians	2-6

HLA-B27–positive individuals with differing subtypes may also differ in their ability to present peptides to autoreactive cytotoxic T cells. This could possibly also result from inherited differences in HLA-linked proteasome genes, which influence an individual's risk for the disease.[21] Also, tumor necrosis factor-α (TNF-α) promoter allele variability might contribute to genetic susceptibility to the development of AS. The idea that, among other factors, HLA-B27 itself is involved in disease pathogenesis is supported by the spontaneous development of spondyloarthropathy in HLA-B27 transgenic rats, as has been known for about a decade.[22] These animals get colitis and arthritis, two major features of AS. The model requires T cells, gut bacteria, and high expression of B27 in bone marrow–derived cells. Control rats with HLA-B7 remain healthy. Rats with a mutant B27 bearing a Cys67→Ser substitution resemble wild-type B27 transgenics, but with a lower prevalence of arthritis. Disease-prone lewis rats, but not controls, develop high serum-IgA levels. Arthritis is associated with high levels of interleukin-6 (IL-6). The model is intriguing, but it seems unlikely that it will allow much deeper insights into the pathogenesis of AS.[22]

SUBTYPES OF HLA-B27

HLA-B27 itself is a serologic specificity that encompasses 25 subtypes (HLA-B*2701 to B*2725) that are products (proteins) of 27 different alleles related by nucleotide sequence homology.[23] At the protein-sequence level, only 24 different mature protein products are observed. In fact, three alleles (B*27052, B*27053, and B*27054) differ only by silent mutations, whereas B*2713 differs only in the leader segment of the gene, which is not part of the expressed product. Therefore, at the cell surface, the HLA-B27 molecules encoded by these two alleles are identical.[23] Among HLA-B27–positive people, B*2705 is the predominant subtype in most populations, especially among northern Europeans, people from Siberia, and North Americans, whereas HLA-B*2704 is the most prevalent Asian subtype.[23] HLA-B*2706 has been reported as not associated with AS. However, there is now some evidence that it is in fact HLA-B*2722, previously mistyped as B*2706, that is reduced in Thai HLA-B27–positive patients as compared to controls.[24,25] HLA-B*2709, a rare subtype primarily restricted to people from Sardinia, Italy, is the only other HLA-B27 subtype that seems not to be associated with the disease. It differs from the disease-associated subtype B*2705 by having histidine at amino acid position 116.

OTHER GENETIC FACTORS

In most white populations only 1 to 3 percent (sometimes, as in northern Norway, up to 6 percent) of HLA-B27–positive persons develop AS, in contrast to some 20 percent of HLA-B27–positive first-degree relatives of white AS patients (although there are no differences between the HLA-B27 molecules from relatives and HLA-B27–positive individuals in these populations). A positive family history for AS is, therefore, a very strong risk factor for the disease. The overall sibling recurrence rate of about 10 percent is markedly in excess of the general population prevalence of this disease. Family studies strongly support the view that, apart from HLA-B27 or its subtypes, there are additional genetic factors (including non-HLA genes) that contribute to the development of AS. For example, studies of AS in twins have shown that concordance in monozygotic twins is 63 percent, whereas concordance in dizygotic twins is 12.5 percent, although it rises to 23 percent in HLA-B27–positive dizygotic twins[19] (Table 70–6). This large difference between monozygotic and HLA-B27–positive dizygotic twins suggests the existence of considerable non–HLA-B27 genetic susceptibility to AS. It has been proposed that there is polygenic inheritance of a genetic component to the disease that accounts for more than 90 percent of the population variance, whereas as much as 69 percent of the genetic effect may arise from outside the HLA region.[19] Therefore, the predisposition to AS is not entirely determined by genes. The nongenetic factors might correspond to an environmental effect such as a specific microbial infection, as implicated in reactive arthritis, or it might correspond to random or stochastic events in development, such as the emergence of specific immune cells. Only a small number of random events (such as infections, exposure to toxins, or somatic genetic mutations) need to occur in predisposed people to allow the emergence of rheumatic diseases such as AS.[26] Other HLA types might contribute to the genetic susceptibility to AS. HLA-B60 has been demonstrated to be associated with a three- to sixfold increase in susceptibility to AS, both in HLA-B27–positive and HLA-B27–negative individuals.[19,27] A large genetic study of 129 families with 181 affected sibling pairs with AS support a role for HLA-DRB1*0101 and 1501, but not for HLA-B60 (B4001).[28] However, still other HLA factors (B7-Creg, B38, B39, DR1, DR8) and non-HLA factors (possibly Crohn's disease locus on chromosome 16 or psoriasis genes on chromosome 17) should be considered as candidates.[19] Recently, an association between AS and B14 (mainly the B*1403 subtype) was found in a West African population. HLA-B27 was nearly absent,

TABLE 70–6 • POOLED DATA ON CONCORDANCE IN TWINS

Category	1997 UK Study	All Twins Reported
MZ		
Both affected	6	17
Total	8	27 (42-81)
% (95% CI)	75	63 (42-81)
DZ		
Both affected	4	7
Total	32	56
% (95% CI)	12.5	12.5 (5-24)
B27 + DZ		
Both affected	4	7
Total	15	30
% (95% CI)	27	23 (10-42)

Abbreviations: CI, Confidence interval; DZ, dizygotic; MZ, monozygotic.
Modified from Brown MA, Kennedy LG, MacGregor A, et al: Genetic susceptibility to ankylosing spondylitis in twins: the role of genes, HLA, and the environment. Arthritis Rheum 40:1823, 1997.

being observed in only one of eight Togolese patients (B*2703).[29]

Possibly less than 10 percent of the population variance is due to environmental effects.[19] The apparent decreasing north to south gradient in the prevalence of AS might be due to geographic differences in the occurrence of such environmental factors.

Pathology

An important pathologic site in AS is the enthesis, or the insertion of tendons or ligament capsules into bone. Changes due to enthesitis explain the typical findings in AS: syndesmophyte formation, squaring of vertebral bodies, vertebral end-plate destruction, and Achilles tendinitis (Fig. 70–2).

There is definitely a role for T cells in AS. As shown in an immunohistologic study with probes obtained by computed tomography (CT)-guided sacroiliac biopsies, CD4+, CD8+ T cells, and macrophages are present in inflamed sacroiliac joints. Abundant mRNA of TNF-α was seen near the characteristic myxoid infiltrates, whereas mRNA of transforming growth factor-β (TGF-β) was found near areas of new bone formation.[30]

Clinical Manifestations

SKELETAL MANIFESTATIONS

Low Back Pain and Stiffness

Back pain is an extremely common symptom, occurring in up to 80 percent of the general population. Therefore, it is important to note that back pain in AS has special features that differentiate it from mechanic back pain[31] (Table 70–7).

The pain is initially felt primarily deep in the gluteal region, is dull in character, is difficult to localize, and is

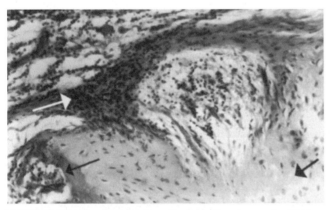

FIGURE 70–2 · Postmortem Autopsy Specimen of a 51-Year-Old Human Leukocyte Antigen (HLA)-B27–Positive Ankylosing Spondylitis Patient Who Died from Amyloidosis After at Least 2 Decades of Disease. Growing front of a syndesmophyte (*thin black arrow*) on the right side of the distal end plate of vertebra Th 12, next to granulation tissue with numerous inflammatory cells (*white arrow*) in proximity to the bone marrow (above) and chondroid metaplasia (*heavy black arrow*) (Courtesy of Dr. R. Francois, Brussels, Belgium.) (From Francois RJ: Lerachis dans la spondylarthrite ankylosante. Edis Arscia, Brussels, Belgium, 1976.)

TABLE 70–7 · DIAGNOSTIC FEATURES OF ANKYLOSING SPONDYLITIS

Consider a Diagnosis of Ankylosing Spondylitis if There Is:
Inflammatory spinal pain
Onset before age 40
Insidious onset
Persistence for at least 3 months
Morning stiffness
Improvement with exercise
Chest pain
Alternate buttock pain
Acute anterior uveitis
Synovitis (predominantly of lower limbs, asymmetric)
Enthesitis (heel, plantar)
Radiographic sacroiliitis
Positive family history for
Ankylosing spondylitis
Chronic inflammatory bowel disease
Psoriasis

insidious in onset. The pain can be severe at this early phase of the disease; it localizes in sacroiliac joints but is occasionally referred toward the iliac crest or greater trochanteric region or down the dorsal thigh. Radiation of buttock pain may suggest root compression of the ischiatic nerve. The buttock pain may typically alternate from side to side. Coughing, sneezing, or other maneuvers that cause a sudden twist of the back may accentuate pain. Although the pain is often unilateral or intermittent at first, within a few months it usually becomes persistent and bilateral and the lower lumbar area becomes stiff and painful. The pain is associated with a feeling of low back stiffness that is worse in the morning and that may awaken the patient from sleep. Many patients do not differentiate between low back pain and stiffness. The morning stiffness may last up to 3 hours. Both the stiffness and the pain tend to be eased by a hot shower, an exercise program, or physical activity. Fatigue as a result of chronic back pain and stiffness may be an important problem and can be accentuated by sleep disturbances due to these symptoms.

Chest Pain

With subsequent involvement of the thoracic spine (including costovertebral and costotransverse joints) and occurrence of enthesopathy at costosternal and manubriosternal joints, patients may experience chest pain accentuated on coughing or sneezing, which sometimes is characterized as "pleuritic." The chest pain may often be associated with tenderness over sternocostal or costosternal junctions. Mild to moderate reduction of chest expansion is often detectable in an early stage of AS. Chest pain occurs relatively often in HLA-B27–positive relatives, even in the absence of radiographic evidence of sacroiliitis.[32]

Tenderness

Extra-articular tenderness at certain loci is a prominent complaint in some patients. These lesions are due to enthesitis, an inflammatory reaction at the insertion of a tendon in the bone. Prevailing tender sites are the costosternal junctions, spinous processes, iliac crests, greater trochanters, ischial tuberosities, tibial tubercles, or heels (Achilles tendinitis or plantar fasciitis). Radiologically, bone spurs may develop at these sites.

Joints

The girdle or "root" joints (hips and shoulders) are the most frequently involved extra-axial joints in AS, and pain in these areas may be the presenting symptom in up to 15 percent of patients. Shoulder involvement, but especially hip involvement, may cause considerable physical disability. Coexisting disease in the lumbar spine often contributes significantly to disability of the lower extremities. Hips and shoulders are involved at some stage of disease in up to 35 percent of the patients. Hip disease is more often seen in Algeria, India, and Mexico. It is relatively more common as a presenting manifestation if the disease starts in childhood (juvenile AS). In boys 8 to 10 years of age, hip disease as a manifestation of juvenile AS is the most frequent type of chronic arthritis. These children with hip disease are mostly HLA-B27–positive, but they are serologically negative for antinuclear antibodies.

The knee joint may also be affected in AS, frequently as an intermittent effusion. Temporomandibular joint involvement occurs in about 10 percent of patients.

EXTRASKELETAL MANIFESTATIONS

General Symptoms

Constitutional symptoms, such as fatigue, loss of weight, and low-grade fever, occur frequently. Other extraskeletal manifestations are more localized.

Eye Disease

Acute anterior uveitis or iridocyclitis is the most common extra-articular manifestation of AS, occurring in 25 to 30 percent of patients at some time in the course of the disease. There is no clear relationship between activity of the articular disease and this extra-articular manifestation. The onset of the eye inflammation is usually acute and typically unilateral, but the attacks may alternate. The eye is red and painful, with visual impairment. Photophobia and increased lacrimation may be present. If the eye remains untreated or if treatment is delayed, posterior synechiae and glaucoma may develop. Most attacks subside in 4 to 8 weeks without sequelae if treatment is provided at an early stage. Acute anterior uveitis is more common in B27-positive than B27-negative patients with AS.[33] Relatives who have acute anterior uveitis seem at higher risk for AS themselves. The calculated incidence of acute anterior uveitis in a Swiss family study was 89 attacks per 1000 patient-years for AS patients but only 8 per 1000 person-years among healthy B27-positive relatives.[34]

Cardiovascular Disease

Cardiac involvement may be clinically silent or may cause considerable problems for the patient. Manifestations of cardiac involvement include ascending aortitis, aortic valve incompetence, conduction abnormalities, cardiomegaly, and pericarditis. In rare situations, aortitis may precede other features of AS. Aortic incompetence was noted in 3.5 percent of patients who had the disease for 15 years and in 10 percent after 30 years.[35] Cardiac conduction disturbances are seen with increasing frequency with the passage of time, occurring in 2.7 percent of those with disease of 15 years' duration and in 8.5 percent after 30 years.[35] Both aortic incompetence and cardiac conduction defects occur twice as often in patients with peripheral joint involvement.

Pulmonary Disease

Lung involvement is a rare and late manifestation of AS. It is characterized by slowly progressive fibrosis of the upper lobes of the lungs, appearing, on average, two decades after the onset of AS. The lesions eventually become cystic; the cavities may subsequently be colonized by *Aspergillus*, with the formation of mycetoma. Patients may complain of cough, dyspnea, and sometimes hemoptysis.[36]

High-resolution CT may be helpful in detecting interstitial lung disease in patients with respiratory symptoms who have normal results on plain radiographs of the chest.[37]

Pulmonary ventilation is usually well maintained; an increased diaphragmatic contribution helps to compensate for chest wall rigidity, which is due to involvement of the thoracic joints in the inflammatory process. Vital capacity and total lung capacity may be moderately reduced as a consequence of the restricted chest wall movement, whereas residual volume and functional residual capacity are usually increased.

Neurologic Involvement

Neurologic complications of AS can be caused by fracture, instability, compression, or inflammation. Traffic accidents or minor trauma can cause spinal fractures. The C5-C6 or C6-C7 level is the most commonly involved site.

As in rheumatoid arthritis (RA), atlantoaxial joint subluxation, atlanto-occipital subluxation, and upward subluxation of the axis may occur in AS as a consequence of instability resulting from the inflammatory process. Spontaneous anterior atlantoaxial subluxation is a well-recognized complication in about 2 percent of patients and manifests with or without signs of spinal cord compression. It is observed more commonly in patients with spondylitis and peripheral arthritis than in those with exclusively axial involvement.[38]

Causes of neurologic complications due to compression include ossification of the posterior longitudinal ligament (which may lead to compressive myelopathy), destructive intervertebral disk lesions, and spinal stenosis.

The cauda equina syndrome is a rare but serious complication of long-standing AS. The syndrome affects lumbosacral nerve roots. This gives rise to pain and sensory loss, but frequently there are also urinary and bowel symptoms. There is a gradual onset of urinary and fecal incontinence, impotence, saddle anesthesia, and occasionally loss of ankle jerks. Motor symptoms, if present, are usually mild. Newer imaging techniques, such as CT and magnetic resonance imaging (MRI), allow accurate noninvasive diagnosis of this complication of AS.[39] There are no compressive lesions. Arachnoiditis and arachnoid adhesions may be important in the pathogenesis.

Renal Involvement

IgA nephropathy has been reported in many patients with AS. These patients with IgA nephropathy often have an elevated IgA level (93 percent) and renal impairment (27 percent) at presentation.[40] Microscopic hematuria and proteinuria may occur in up to 35 percent of patients. The significance of these findings for subsequent deterioration of renal function is unclear.[41] Amyloidosis (secondary type) is a rare complication. Amyloid deposits detected through abdominal subcutaneous fat aspiration are not invariably associated with a poor renal prognosis.[42]

Osteoporosis

Osteopenia is already seen in early stages of AS.[43] In patients with this disease, osteoporotic deformities of the thoracic vertebrae occur and, together with wedging of the thoracic disks, contribute significantly to fixed hyperkyphosis of the spine.[44] The prevalence of symptomatic osteoporotic spinal fractures is increased.[45] Neurologic complications occur rather frequently, even after minor trauma.[46] Proper assessment of bone density in the spine is difficult in the presence of syndesmophytes, because they may give rise to falsely high values. This measurement error can be avoided by using quantitative CT. Bone density and the true fracture risk and complication rate need to be assessed further in early and late disease and to be related to disease activity. Currently, it is unclear whether any specific preventive therapy is warranted.

▉ Physical Findings

SPINAL MOBILITY

To arrive at an early diagnosis, the physician must perform a thorough physical examination. On spine examination, there is usually some limitation of motion of the lumbar spine as elicited by forward flexion, hyperextension, or lateral flexion. Early loss of the normal lumbar lordosis is easily assessed on inspection.

The Schober test (or its modifications) is useful for detecting limitation of forward flexion and hyperextension of the lumbar spine. The patient stands erect; one mark is placed with a pen on the skin overlying the fifth lumbar spinous process (usually at the level of the posterosuperior iliac spine or the "dimple of Venus"), and the other mark is placed 10 cm above in the midline. The patient is then asked to bend forward maximally without bending the knees. In healthy people, the distance between the two marks on the skin should increase as the skin stretches. If the distance between both marks does not reach 15 cm, reduced lumbar spine mobility is indicated. Lateral flexion may also be diminished, and spinal rotation may cause pain.

CHEST EXPANSION

Mild to moderate reduction of chest expansion is often detectable in an early stage of AS. Normal values are age dependent and sex dependent, and there is a lot of overlap between normal values and values obtained from AS patients. Reduction below 5 cm in young persons with insidious onset of chronic, inflammatory low back pain should strongly suggest AS. Chest expansion should be measured on maximal inspiration after forced maximal expiration at the level of the fourth intercostal space in males and just below the breasts in females.

ENTHESITIS

Examining the ischial tuberosities, greater trochanters, spinous processes, costochondral and manubriosternal junctions, and iliac crests can assess the presence of enthesitis. In addition, Achilles tendinitis and plantar fasciitis are manifestations of enthesitis.

SACROILIITIS

Direct pressure over the sacroiliac joints may elicit pain, as may special maneuvers, although these tests lack specificity. These signs may also be negative in early disease or may become negative in late stages, as inflammation is replaced by fibrosis or bony ankylosis.

POSTURE

In the course of the disease, the patient may lose normal posture. Involvement of the cervical spine is manifested by pain and limitation of neck movements. The patient may develop a forward slope of the neck that can be detected by having the patient stand against a wall and try to touch his or her occiput to it.

After many years of disease progression in patients with severe disease, the entire spine may become increasingly stiff, with loss of normal posture from gradual loss of lumbar lordosis and the development of thoracic kyphosis. The abdomen becomes protuberant; breathing is primarily by diaphragmatic action. These typical deformities usually evolve after disease duration of 10 years or more.

▉ Laboratory Tests

Generally, routine blood tests are not helpful. A normal erythrocyte sedimentation rate (ESR) or normal

C-reactive protein (CRP) levels do not exclude active disease. An elevated ESR or CRP is reported in up to 75 percent of patients, but it may show lack of correlation with clinical disease activity.[47] In an unselected patient population, an elevated ESR or CRP, respectively, was present in 45 percent and 38 percent of the patients with spinal disease only, compared to 62 percent and 61 percent, respectively, in patients with peripheral arthritis with or without inflammatory bowel disease. Neither is superior in assessing disease activity.[48] A mild normochromic anemia may be present in 15 percent of patients. Elevation of serum alkaline phosphatase (primarily derived from bone) is seen in some patients, but it is unrelated to the activity or duration of the disease. Some elevation of serum IgA is frequent in AS. Its level correlates with acute-phase reactants.

∎ Radiography and Imaging

CONVENTIONAL RADIOGRAPHY

The typical radiographic changes of AS are seen primarily in the axial skeleton, especially in the sacroiliac, diskovertebral, apophyseal, costovertebral, and costotransverse joints. They evolve over many years, and the earliest, most consistent, and most characteristic findings are seen in the sacroiliac joints. However, otherwise typical AS has been described in the absence of radiographic evidence of sacroiliitis.[13] The roentgenographic findings of sacroiliitis are usually symmetric and consist of blurring of the subchondral bone plate, followed by erosions and sclerosis of the adjacent bone. The changes in the synovial portion of the joint (i.e., the lower two thirds of the joint) result from inflammatory chondritis and osteitis of the adjacent subchondral bone.[49] The cartilage covering the iliac side of the joint is much thinner than that covering the sacral side. Therefore, the erosions and subchondral sclerosis are typically seen first and tend to be more prominent on the iliac side.

In the upper one third of the sacroiliac joint, where strong intra-articular ligaments hold the bones together, the inflammatory process may lead to similar roentgenographic abnormalities. Progression of the subchondral bone erosions can lead to "pseudowidening" of the sacroiliac joint space. With time, gradual fibrosis, calcification, interosseous bridging, and ossification occur. Erosions become less obvious, but the subchondral sclerosis persists, becoming the most prominent radiologic feature.

Ultimately, usually after several years, there may be complete bony ankylosis of the sacroiliac joints, with resolution of bony sclerosis. It is practical to grade radiographic sacroiliitis according to the New York criteria (grades 0 to 4) (Table 70–8).

Bony erosions and osteitis ("whiskering") at sites of osseous attachment of tendons and ligaments are frequently seen, particularly at the calcaneus, ischial tuberosities, iliac crest, femoral trochanters, and spinous processes of the vertebrae. In the early stages of the evolution of syndesmophytes, there is inflammation of the superficial layers of the annulus fibrosis, with subsequent reactive sclerosis and erosions of the adjacent corners of the vertebral bodies. This combination of destructive osteitis and repair leads to "squaring" of the vertebral bodies. This squaring is associated with gradual ossification of the annulus fibrosis and eventual "bridging" between vertebrae by syndesmophytes.[50] There are often concomitant inflammatory changes, ankylosis in the apophyseal joints, and ossification of the adjacent ligaments. In a number of patients this may ultimately result in a virtually complete fusion of the vertebral column ("bamboo spine").

Hip or shoulder joint involvement may lead to symmetric, concentric joint-space narrowing, irregularity of the subchondral bone with subchondral sclerosis, osteophyte formation at the outer margin of the articular surface, and, ultimately, bony ankylosis.

COMPUTED TOMOGRAPHY AND MAGNETIC RESONANCE IMAGING

The conventional plain pelvic radiograph is still the initial tool for evaluation of sacroiliac joints for patients with inflammatory low back pain. This technique, how-

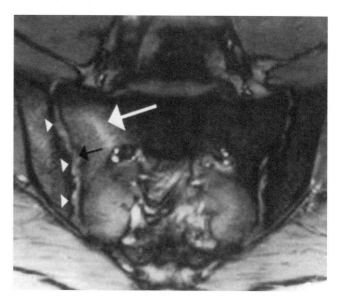

FIGURE 70–3 · T1-Weighted opposed phase gradient echo sequence 3 minutes after intravenous injection of gadolinium-DTPA (dynamic MR image), showing acute sacroiliitis demonstrated by the strong contrast enhancement of the right sacroiliac joint (*arrowheads*), with impressive bone marrow edema (*white arrow*) and erosions (*black arrow*). Enhancement factor 150%, graded 3B right, 1× left, in a male 23-year-old ankylosing spondylitis patient with severe inflammatory back pain localized mainly to the right side, 3 years' disease duration.

TABLE 70–8 · GRADING OF SACROILIITIS ACCORDING TO THE NEW YORK CRITERIA

Grade
0, Normal
1, Suspicious
2, Minimal sacroiliitis
3, Moderate sacroiliitis
4, Ankylosis

ever, lacks sensitivity in the early stages of sacroiliac inflammation. In such cases dynamic MRI with a T1-weighted sequence after intravenous injection of gadolinium diethylenetriaminepentaacetic acid is able to demonstrate early stages of sacroiliitis[51,52] (Fig. 70–3). Fat-saturating techniques such as short tau inversion recovery (STIR) sequences are very sensitive in the detection of bone marrow edema, which is a frequent finding in AS-related inflammatory states of the musculoskeletal system.[53] STIR imaging is cheaper than Gd-DTPA sequences and almost as good. Thus, active early sacroiliitis can best be searched for by STIR or contrast-based sequences.

Similarly, spinal inflammation is first assessed by conventional radiography. Square vertebrae, shiny corners (Romanus lesion), spondylodiscitis (Anderson lesion), and syndesmophytes with partial and complete fusion are typical radiographic features of AS. Early spinal inflammation cannot be well assessed by conventional radiography, but can be visualized better by MRI.[16] For the detection of bone changes, such as erosions and ankylosis, CT is usually considered superior to MRI, but MRI is better in the imaging of cartilage and provides the possibility of dynamic measurements.[51,54,55] CT is definitely not indicated in the routine evaluation of the sacroiliac joint. CT scanning may be useful in the diagnosis of spinal fractures, spinal stenosis, or thecal diverticula. Also MRI has been helpful in visualizing arachnoid diverticula associated with the cauda equina syndrome.[39,56]

Diagnosis

Clinical manifestations of AS usually begin in late adolescence or early adulthood and only rarely start after age 40.[13] The diagnosis of AS at an early stage of disease depends primarily on a careful history and physical examination. Two features of the history are critically important: 1) the presence of inflammatory low back pain and stiffness and 2) a positive family history for AS.

Low back pain is very common in the general population and is frequently due to noninflammatory, nonspecific mechanic causes. However, the low back pain in AS has typical "inflammatory" features (see Table 70–7). A history of inflammatory low back pain can be used as a diagnostic tool. Inflammatory back pain was reported to have a sensitivity of 95 percent and a specificity of 85 to 90 percent when at least four of the inflammatory spinal pain items in Table 70–7 were present.[31,57]

Because the prevalence of AS in many white population is as low as approximately 0.1 percent, applying the clinical history as a screening test for the disease in such a low-probability setting provides a positive predictive value of only 1 percent. However, a positive family history increases the pretest probability of AS from 0.1 percent for a person belonging to the general population to about 10 percent for any first-degree relative of an AS proband.[13] The probability of having AS for a first-degree relative with a positive family history of AS increases from a probability of 10 percent to a probability of nearly 50 percent if this relative has inflammatory low back pain. In contrast, the likelihood of having AS increases from 0.1 percent to only 1.0 percent for a person who has inflammatory back pain but gives a negative family history for AS. A definite diagnosis of AS is usually established by radiographic evidence of bilateral sacroiliitis. The plain anteroposterior view of the pelvis is usually adequate for diagnostic purposes. There is, however, considerable intra- and interobserver variation in the radiographic diagnosis of sacroiliitis for both conventional pelvic films and CT of the sacroiliac joints. Training in reading these films has limited value. Improvement in sensitivity tends to be associated with decrease in specificity.[58]

In most adult patients, AS can be diagnosed clinically without the HLA-B27 test. This assessment has no value in established disease or as screening and should not be regarded as diagnostic or confirmatory in patients with low back pain.[59] However, in (young) patients with inflammatory chronic back pain, a positive HLA-B27 test increases the likelihood of having AS, in particular if imaging of the sacroiliac joints does not provide conclusive results.

Problems in Diagnosis

Physicians are reluctant to make the diagnosis of AS when radiologic evidence of sacroiliitis is not present. In particular, relatives of AS patients may have signs and symptoms of AS, including inflammatory back pain, but sometimes persistently do not show radiographic sacroiliitis even after lengthy follow-up.[7] Radiographic sacroiliitis is frequent in AS but is by no means an early or obligate manifestation of the disease. In patients with a clinical diagnosis of possible AS, radiographic sacroiliitis may become manifest only after appropriate follow-up.

Patients with symptomatic spondylitic disease often have associated thoracic pain and stiffness. Sometimes individuals may have just recurrent thoracic pain and stiffness without radiographic evidence of sacroiliitis or even without inflammatory lumbar back pain.[7] The chest pain may be accentuated on coughing or sneezing (because of involvement of costovertebral joints), and it may be characterized as "pleuritic" pain.

AS rarely develops after age 40. However, late-onset AS does occur. There may then initially be little or no clinical involvement of the axial skeleton, but patients may show moderate oligoarthritis with low cell counts in the synovial fluid and pitting edema of the lower limbs.[60]

At the lower end of the age scale, juvenile-onset AS is not uncommon among patients with spondyloarthropathies. Such patients tend to have enthesopathy and peripheral arthritis that may be severe and disabling.

Both the seronegative enthesopathy and arthropathy syndrome and juvenile AS are conditions that occur predominantly in HLA-B27–positive boys in late childhood. In one study, after 5 years, 75 percent of the 20 patients with the seronegative enthesopathy and arthropathy syndrome had definite AS.[61]

Spondylitis in Males and Females

Clinically, AS is more commonly seen in males; the reported male-to-female ratio is about 2:1 to 3:1. However, extrapolation of studies employing the genetic marker HLA-B27 suggests that based on radiographs of the sacroiliac joints, prevalence rates are about equal in both sexes.[13]

Disease expression has been considered different in males and females. A case-control study comparing 35 female patients to 70 male patients as controls showed no differences regarding spinal symptoms, chest expansion, peripheral arthritis, extra-articular manifestations, or functional outcome. The males with AS more often had radiologic spinal changes and hip joint involvement than their female counterparts. There is still some controversy, but overall, there are no significant clinical or radiographic differences between women and men with AS. However, on average, the disease seems more severe in men.[62,63]

Prognosis

The course of AS is highly variable. Characterized by spontaneous remissions and exacerbations, its prognosis has generally been considered rather favorable. The disease may run a relatively mild or self-limiting course.

However, the disease may also remain active over many years. Life expectancy is somewhat reduced, in particular after 10 years of disease.[64] A study from Finland indicates that the risk of dying for patients with AS is increased by 50 percent compared to controls matched for age and gender. Causes of death include complications of the disease such as amyloidosis and spinal fractures, but also cardiovascular, gastrointestinal, and renal disease.[65] There is no convincing evidence that the natural history of the disease has essentially changed.[66,67] No differences exist between familial and sporadic AS regarding age at onset of disease, age at diagnosis, or the prevalence of peripheral arthritis and acute anterior uveitis.[68]

Functional limitations increase with duration of disease. Structural damage seen on radiographs is not directly related to physical function and spinal mobility. Even with normal spinal radiographs there might be a major reduction in spinal mobility, and patients with severe abnormalities on the radiographs might function quite well in every day tasks.

Recent data show that the functional prognosis of AS is less favorable than thought for many years. Withdrawal from work in those with a paid job varies from 10 percent after 20 years of disease duration to 30 percent after 10 years, depending on characteristics of patients included and social security system considered[69-72] (Table 70–9). Age- and sex-adjusted withdrawal rate from labor force participation was 3.1 times higher among Dutch patients as compared to the general population.[72] Older age at disease onset, manual work, a lower educational level, and coping strategies characterized by limiting and pacing activities were associated with a higher risk for work disability.[70-72] Vocational counseling, job training, easy access to the workplace, and support of colleagues and management may reduce the probability of withdrawal from work.[69,73] Sick leave in those with a paid job was linked to disease activity and presence of extraspinal disease manifestations.[69,74,75] Patients with peripheral joint involvement are more likely to experience sick leaves than AS patients with axial manifestations only.

Apart from the impact on labor force participation, patients have an important health care and non–health care resource utilization, resulting in yearly mean total costs (direct and productivity) per patient of about $6700 to $9500 when applying the human capital approach to calculate the productivity costs.[74,76,77]

Overall, the first 10 years of disease is particularly important with respect to subsequent outcome. Most of the loss of function among patients with AS occurs within this period and is associated with the presence of peripheral arthritis, spinal radiographic changes, and development of a so-called "bamboo spine."[78] In a retrospective study of patients with spondyloarthropathies, including AS, who had a disease duration of at least 10 years, seven variables were associated with disease severity if these factors occurred within the first 2 years of follow-up. These patients regularly attended one university department of rheumatology. These factors, expressed as an odds ratio together with its 95-percent confidence interval, are as follows: arthritis of hip joints (22.9; 4.4 to 118); ESR more than 30 mm/hr (7; 4.8 to 9.5); poor efficacy of nonsteroidal anti-inflammatory drugs (NSAIDs) (8.3; 2.6 to 27.1); limitation of lumbar spine (7; 2 to 25); sausage-like digits (8.5; 1.5 to 9.0); oligoarthritis (4.3; 1.4 to 13.1); onset before age 16 years (3.5; 1.1 to 12.8).[79]

The long-term results of total hip replacement in AS are satisfactory. The outcome of 138 total hip replacements and 12 revisions was good or very good in 86 percent, and 63 percent of patients had no pain. Mobility

TABLE 70–9 • WITHDRAWAL FROM LABOR FORCE DUE TO WORK DISABILITY AMONG PATIENTS WITH ANKYLOSING SPONDYLITIS (AS) WHO HAVE A PAID JOB AT ONSET OF DISEASE

	Withdrawal Rate	Comments
Mexico (103 patients)	3% per year	
France (182 patients)	36% after 20 years	
Netherlands (529 patients)	30% after 20 years	RR compared to the general population: 3.1 (95% CI: 2.5 to 3.7)
USA (234 patients)	10% after 20 and 30 years	Highly educated patients; IBD excluded

Abbreviations: IBD, inflammatory bowel disease; RR, relative risk; CL, confidence interval.

was good or very good in 44 percent. The mean follow-up was 7.5 years (range 1 to 34 years). Altogether, 69 percent of the male hip recipients younger than 60 years were at work at the time of the survey.[80]

Assessment and Monitoring

Signs and symptoms such as spinal pain and limitation of motion might be due to disease activity or to damage as a result of prolonged periods of active disease. A plethora of tools aim at assessment of the same dimensions. For example, there are many ways to measure limitation of motion of the lumbar spine. New instruments have been developed to assess various aspects of the disease, including the Bath Ankylosing Spondylitis Metrology Index, Bath Ankylosing Spondylitis Global, Bath Ankylosing Spondylitis Radiology Index, Bath Ankylosing Spondylitis Disease Activity Index, and Dougados functional index.[81-84] However, standardization and validation of many of the instruments has been lacking or incomplete. An international Assessment in Ankylosing Spondylitis (ASAS) working group was formed with the aims of selecting, proposing, and testing core sets of measures for different settings.[85] It was felt that a certain set of variables should be targeted to a specific task. For example, in the assessment of efficacy of physical therapy, it would not be realistic to include measures aiming to demonstrate radiographic changes of the spine. Clearly, a set of measures that show disease-modifying capabilities of a drug will differ from a core set that show analgetic effectiveness only. Four settings have been defined: 1) disease-controlling antirheumatic therapy (DCART); 2) symptom-modifying antirheumatic drugs (SMARDs) such as NSAIDs; 3) phys-

ical therapy; and 4) clinical record keeping in daily practice.[85] Recently, there has been an update of the core sets. The results for the four settings of the updated core sets are presented in Table 70–10. These core sets are now known as the World Health Organization/International League of Associations for Rheumatology (WHO/ILAR) core set for the assessment of AS. Also, criteria to assess response of individual patients (in contrast to the just-mentioned core sets intended to assess improvement at the group level) to NSAIDs have been developed and validated. They are now known as the ASAS-20 improvement criteria. Recently, criteria to define partial remission have also been defined. Both the improvement and partial remission criteria are presented in Table 70–11.[86]

Assessment of outcomes and process variables of patients with AS can be done in a homogenous and reliable way across centers. The smallest detectable difference of current measures among stable patients varies mostly between 10 percent (enthesis index) and 40 percent (spinal pain at night).[87] For each variable, only changes larger than the smallest detectable difference for that specific instrument can confidently be regarded as real change due to a particular therapeutic intervention or due to an alteration in the natural course of the disease. A well accepted and easy to perform needs-based quality of life instrument (ASQoL) specific for AS for assessing the impact of interventions has shown good scaling and psychometric properties.[88]

Management

For most patients, AS is a relatively mild disease with a good functional prognosis. Most do not experience sig-

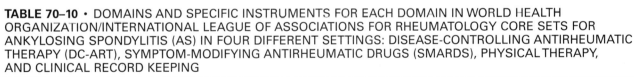

TABLE 70–10 · DOMAINS AND SPECIFIC INSTRUMENTS FOR EACH DOMAIN IN WORLD HEALTH ORGANIZATION/INTERNATIONAL LEAGUE OF ASSOCIATIONS FOR RHEUMATOLOGY CORE SETS FOR ANKYLOSING SPONDYLITIS (AS) IN FOUR DIFFERENT SETTINGS: DISEASE-CONTROLLING ANTIRHEUMATIC THERAPY (DC-ART), SYMPTOM-MODIFYING ANTIRHEUMATIC DRUGS (SMARDS), PHYSICAL THERAPY, AND CLINICAL RECORD KEEPING

Domain	Instrument
1. Function	BASFI or Functional Index Dougados
2. Pain	VAS: last week, spine-at-night, due to AS and VAS: last week, spine, due to AS
3. Spinal mobility	Chest expansion and modified Schober and occiput to wall distance and (lateral spinal flection or BASMI)
4. Patient global assessment	VAS: last week
5. Stiffness	Duration of morning stiffness, spine, last week
6. Peripheral joints and entheses	Number of swollen joints (44 joint count); validated enthesis index
7. Acute-phase reactants	Erythrocyte sedimentation rate (ESR)
8. Spine radiographs	Anteroposterior and lateral view of lumbar spine, lateral view of cervical spine, and pelvic radiograph including sacroiliac joints and hip
9. Hip radiographs	Pelvic radiograph including sacroiliac joints and hips
10. Fatigue	VAS on fatigue from BASDAI

Abbreviations: BASFI, Bath Ankylosing Spondylitis Functional Index; VAS, visual analogue scale.
DC-ART domains: 1, 2, 3, 4, 5, 6, 7, 8, 9, 10
SMARD: domains: 1, 2, 3, 4, 5, 10
Physical therapy: domains: 1, 2, 3, 4, 5, 10
Clinical record keeping: domains: 1, 2, 3, 4, 5, 6, 7
From van der Heijde D, Calin A, Dougados M, et al: Selection of instruments in the core set for DC-ART, SMARD, physical therapy, and clinical record keeping in ankylosing spondylitis: progress report of ASAS Working Group—Assessments in ankylosing spondylitis. J Rheumatol 26:951, 1999.

TABLE 70–11 • ASSESSMENT IN ANKYLOSING SPONDYLITIS INTERNATIONAL WORKING GROUP (ASAS) IMPROVEMENT CRITERIA (ASAS-20) AND ASAS PARTIAL REMISSION CRITERIA

ASAS-20 Improvement Criteria
At least 20-percent improvement AND 10 units improvement in three out of the four following domains, without worsening of 20 percent or more AND 10 units in the remaining domain: -Bath Ankylosing Spondylitis Functional Index (BASFI) -Morning stiffness -Patient global assessment -Pain

ASAS Partial Remission Criteria
A value below 20 units in all four domains

nificant extraskeletal manifestations, except for acute anterior uveitis, which occurs in about 30 percent of patients. Usually, this eye disease can be well managed with eye drops containing corticosteroids to reduce inflammation and with pupil-dilating, atropine-like agents to prevent or diminish synechiae. At the outset, patients should be warned about the possibility of the occurrence of acute anterior uveitis at any time during the course of their disease.

The objectives for treatment of AS are to relieve pain, stiffness, and fatigue and to maintain good posture and good physical and psychosocial functioning.[89] The principles of management are summarized in Table 70–12. No drug is currently available that has been shown to significantly influence the course of spinal disease and retard the process of ossification in particular. Similarly, evidence is lacking to suggest that any of the conventional disease-modifying antirheumatic drugs (DMARDs), including sulfasalazine and methotrexate (MTX), may alter or inhibit the inflammation seen in the spine and entheses in AS.

A full explanation of the disease, its course, possible complications such as acute anterior uveitis, and its prognosis is essential to achieve appropriate compli-

TABLE 70–12 • PRINCIPLES OF MANAGEMENT OF ANKYLOSING SPONDYLITIS (AS)

1. No cure, but most patients can be well managed
2. Early diagnosis very important
3. Education of patient to increase compliance
4. Appropriate use of antirheumatic drugs, primarily nonsteroidal, anti-inflammatory drugs (NSAIDs)
5. Continuity of care
6. Daily exercises very important (e.g., swimming)
7. Sleep on firm mattress
8. Appropriate sports and recreation
9. Supportive measures and counseling
10. Avoidance of smoking
11. Avoidance of trauma (osteoporosis of the spine)
12. Patient support groups
13. Family counseling

Adapted from Khan MA, Skosey JL: Ankylosing spondylitis and related spondyloarthropathies. In Samter M (ed): Immunological Diseases. Boston, Little, Brown & Co, 1988, pp 1509-1538.

ance by the patient. Self-help groups provide important information and social support. In addition, patient organizations often provide access to hydrotherapy and group physiotherapy. Exercises are the mainstay of treatment. Preferably, they should be started after a hot shower or a hot bath. Swimming and extension-promoting exercises or sporting activities, such as volleyball or, wherever possible, wintertime cross-country skiing, are appropriate. These activities counteract the kyphotic effects of pain and fatigue on posture and reduce stiffness.

The patient should avoid vigorous or contact sports if the spine has become fused or osteoporotic because such a spine is susceptible to fracture.

Appliances such as driving mirrors may improve comfort and safety for the patient and society, especially if there is considerable involvement of the cervical spine. In that case, appropriate neck support is also required to reduce the risk of fracturing the vulnerable osteoporotic cervical spine as a consequence of road traffic accidents. For the same reason, automobile air bags should be strongly recommended.

PHYSIOTHERAPY

There is now ample evidence that physiotherapy provided as exercises is effective, at least in the short term (up to 1 year), in particular to groups of patients with AS. Scientific evidence for long-term effectiveness is not yet available.[90-92]

In a randomized controlled trial, a program of supervised physiotherapy in groups was found to be superior to individualized programs in improving thoracolumbar mobility and fitness. The program, which consisted of hydrotherapy, exercises, and sporting activities twice weekly for 3 hours per session, resulted in improved overall health, as reported by the patient, whereas stiffness was also reduced.[91] An intensive 3-week spa-exercise therapy program showed marked improvement in both subjective and objective assessments that lasted for up to 9 months. Health resource utilization, in particular NSAID usage and sick leave, decreased in the 9-month follow-up period after spa-exercise therapy. Clinical benefits of such treatments can be reached at acceptable costs.[93,94]

Lying prone for 15 to 30 minutes once or several times a day is useful to reverse the tendency toward kyphosis, which is aggravated by pain and fatigue, and flexion contractures of the hip joints. The patient should preferably sleep fully supine on a firm mattress with only a small neck-support pillow.

MEDICATION

Nonsteroidal Anti-inflammatory Drugs

The efficacy and effectiveness of NSAID therapy have been well established. Phenylbutazone (100 mg three or four times daily) is very effective, but it is now used only in severe cases under close monitoring of the full blood count. Many NSAIDs are effective in patients with AS. No NSAID has documented superiority in terms of efficacy.

Selective cyclooxygenase-2 (COX-2) inhibitors showed similar efficacy to conventional NSAIDs. Although not tested directly in clinical trials in AS, better gastrointestinal safety is expected with the usage of COX-2 inhibitors, similar to that in other rheumatic conditions.[95] Once-daily drug prescription regimens may improve patient compliance. It is not well known whether continuous treatment with NSAIDs has long-term advantages over intermittent therapy in terms of functional ability and prevention of structural damage.

Second-Line Drugs

The rationale for the use of sulphasalazine in AS is the common association between inflammatory bowel disease and spondyloarthropathies, as well as the description of inflammatory lesions in the ileum of patients with spondyloarthropathies.[96]

Corticosteroids may be effective for local intra-articular treatment in AS including the sacroiliac joints. Systemically, steroids work less well than in RA. A small subgroup of AS patients seems to respond, in particular those with peripheral arthritis or associated inflammatory bowel disease.[97,98]

Sulphasalazine has been used in AS since 1984. A meta-analysis showed sulphasalazine to be superior to placebo for three clinical variables (duration of morning stiffness, severity of morning stiffness, and severity of pain) and one laboratory parameter (IgG level).[99] Since that publication, however, new evidence for the effectiveness of this drug in the treatment of AS is less convincing, at least for patients who have axial involvement only. Sulfasalazine proved to be more efficacious than placebo in patients with spondyloarthropathies (including AS).[100] However, subgroup analysis showed that patients with (peripheral) polyarthritis, mostly those with psoriatic arthritis but including patients with AS with peripheral joint involvement, had the best response. Therefore, sulfasalazine was effective in reducing synovitis in patients with peripheral polyarticular involvement but had no results on axial involvement. A study from the United States has confirmed that there was no evidence of effect on axial disease given the results of a large subgroup of 187 patients with AS who had axial involvement only.[101]

A small uncontrolled trial suggests that MTX may be effective in treating AS that is unresponsive to NSAIDs and sulfasalazine, but better-designed studies are required to confirm these preliminary findings, in particular for patients with isolated axial involvement.[102] Currently, there is no convincing evidence that MTX works in AS. Leflunomide showed little efficacy in an open trial.[103]

NEWER TREATMENT MODALITIES

Treatment with intravenously administered bisphosphonates has provided conflicting results. The drug has been shown to be efficacious in AS for spinal pain, functioning, and global assessment; the higher dosage of pamidronate (60 mg intravenously) was superior to a low dosage of 10 mg intravenously.[104]

Thalidomide, a sleeping pill with definite toxicity in pregnancy, administered orally has now been used in AS. In a small, 6-month open trial, 5 of the 12 patients dropped out before completion of the study due to side effects. The most prominent effects were reduction of ESR and CRP levels.[105] In another open 1-year study in China with 30 male patients with severe and refractory disease, 80 percent of 26 completers achieved 20-percent improvement in four of seven predefined clinical measures including pain and patient global assessment.[106]

The usage of anti–TNF-α in the treatment of AS can be regarded as a definite advantage in the therapy of this disease. Currently approved anti–TNF-α agents include infliximab, a chimeric monoclonal anti–TNF-α antibody (3 to 5 mg/kg every 6 to 8 weeks after an initial saturation phase), and etanercept, a 75-kD TNF-α receptor fusion protein (25 mg subcutaneously two times each week), have been shown to improve the signs and symptoms of active AS patients.[98,107] The number of patients who must be treated to achieve one patient who will experience at least 50-percent improvement in disease activity with this expensive therapy is just two (the 95-percent confidence limits range from 1 to 6 patients).

Continuous treatment with these compounds is necessary in most patients. More than two thirds of the patients stay on therapy after 1 year. It is now well known that CRP levels normalize during treatment with anti–TNF-α therapy. It is not yet known whether patients with low CRP respond to the same degree as those with high CRP levels.

Guidelines for the use of anti–TNF-α–directed therapies have recently been developed[108,109] (Table 10–13) (see also http://www.ASAS-group.org). The new therapeutic modalities identify important clinical questions to be answered by further research. Clearly, infliximab and etanercept have disease-modifying properties, but their long-term safety and disease-controlling effects in terms of improvement or maintaining of function, as well as the prevention of structural damage, still has to be demonstrated. A major challenge is to try to understand which patients will develop functional limitations and how these relate to proliferative and other structural spinal changes. Given the efficacy and possible side effects of the new and expensive treatments, better prediction of outcome with and without such interventions at the level of individual patients with AS is clearly of paramount importance.

▌ Other Treatments

SURGERY

Involvement of the hip joint may cause serious disability. Ectopic bone formation may occur, but generally the outcome of total hip replacement is favorable.[80]

Vertebral osteotomy may be required in selected cases to correct marked flexion deformity when forward vision is severely impaired. Diaphragmatic herniation may result from the procedure.

TABLE 70–13 • ASAS RECOMMENDATION FOR THE INITIATION OF TREATMENT WITH BIOLOGICS IN PATIENTS WITH ANKYLOSING SPONDYLITIS (AS)

	Specification (Definition of the Terms)
Which patients?	

Diagnosis	Patients normally fulfilling modified New York Criteria for definite AS
	Modified New York criteria
	  Radiologic criterion
	    Sacroiliitis, grade ≥ II bilaterally or grade III to IV unilaterally
	  Clinical criteria
	    Low back pain and stiffness for more than 3 months that improves with exercise but is not relieved by rest
	    Limitation of motion of the lumbar spine in both the sagittal and frontal planes
	    Limitation of chest expansion relative to normal values correlated for age and sex

Active disease	For at least 4 weeks BASDAI ≥4 (0-10) AND Expert's* Opinion† (Initiation yes/no)
Treatment failure	All patients must have had adequate therapeutic trials of at least two NSAIDs An adequate therapeutic trial would be defined by: Treatment for at least 3 months at maximal recommended or tolerated anti-inflammatory dose unless contraindicated Treatment for <3 months where treatment was withdrawn because of intolerance or toxicity or contraindicated Patients with symptomatic peripheral arthritis (normally having or failing local steroid injection for those with oligoarticular involvement) must have had adequate therapeutic trial of NSAIDs and at least salazopyrine‡ Patients with symptomatic enthesitis must have adequate therapeutic trial of at least two local steroid injections unless contraindicated.

Contraindication	Women who are pregnant or breast feeding; effective contraception must be practiced
	Active infection
	Patients at high risk of infection including:
	  Chronic leg ulcer
	  Previous tuberculosis (note: please follow local recommendations for prevention or treatment)
	  Septic arthritis of a native joint within the last 12 months
	  Sepsis of a prosthetic joint within the last 12 months, or indefinitely if the joint remains in situ
	  Persistent or recurrent chest infections
	  Indwelling urinary catheter
	  Multiple sclerosis
	  Malignancy or premalignancy states excluding:
	  Basal cell carcinoma
	  Malignancies diagnosed and treated more than 10 years previously (where the probability of total cure is very high)

	How to Assess the Disease?
ASAS core set for daily practice	Physical function (BASFI or Dougados functional index) Pain (VAS, last week, spine at night, due to AS AND VAS, last week, spine due to AS) Spinal mobility (chest expansion AND modified Schober AND occiput to wall distance) Patient's global assessment (VAS, last week) Stiffness (duration of morning stiffness, spine, last week) Peripheral joints and entheses (number of swollen joints, enthesitis score such as developed in Maastricht, Berlin, or San Francisco) Acute-phase reactants (ESR OR CRP) Fatigue (VAS)
BASDAI	VAS (or Likert scale) overall level of fatigue/tiredness past week VAS (or Likert scale) overall level of AS neck, back, or hip pain past week VAS (or Likert scale) overall level of pain/swelling in joints other than neck, back, or hips past week VAS (or Likert scale) overall discomfort from any areas tender to touch or pressure past week VAS (or Likert scale) overall level of morning stiffness from time of awakening past week Duration and intensity (VAS or Likert scale) of morning stiffness from time of awakening (up to 120 minutes)
	How to Assess a Response?
Responder criteria **Time of evaluation**	(BASDAI: 50% relative change OR absolute change of 20 mm) *AND* expert's opinion: Continuation yes/no Between 6 and 12 weeks

Abbreviations: BASDAI, Bath Ankylosing Spondylitis Disease Activity Index; NSAIDs, nonsteroidal anti-inflammatory drugs; BASFI, bath ankylosing spondylitis functional index.

*The expert is a physician, normally a rheumatologist, with expertise in inflammatory back pain and the use of biologics. Expert should be locally defined.
†Expert's opinion comprises clinical features, and the physician would normally have available clinical features (history and examination) or acute-phase response or imaging modalities, such as radiographs demonstrating rapid progression and magnetic resonance imaging (MRI) indicating inflammation.
‡Sulfasalazine treatment for at least 4 months at standard target dose or maximally tolerated dose unless contraindicated or not tolerated. Treatment for less than 4 months, where treatment was withdrawn because of intolerance or toxicity or contraindicated.

◼ Summary

Although our understanding of the genetics of AS has improved greatly, our knowledge about the etiology and pathogenesis is still far from complete. A lot has been accomplished regarding classification and assessment of the disease. Treatment with biologics such as anti–TNF-α therapy is very effective and may be the first therapy that really can control the disease. The challenge now is to find out how to predict and improve outcome at the level of individual patients.

REFERENCES

1. Dougados M, van der Linden S, Juhlin R, et al: The European Spondylarthropathy Study Group: preliminary criteria for the classification of spondylarthropathy. Arthritis Rheum 34:1218, 1991.
2. Struempell A: Lehrbuch der speziellen Pathologie und Therapie der inneren Krankheiten. Leipzig, Vogel, 1884, Band 2, Teil 2, pp 152-153.
3. von Bechterew W: Steifheit der Wirbelsaeule und ihre Verkruemmung als besondere Erkrankungsform. Neurologisches Zentralbl 12:426, 1893.
4. Marie P: Sur la spondylose rhizomélique. Revue Médicale 18:285, 1889.
5. Arnett F: Seronegative spondylarthropathies. Bull Rheum Dis 37:1, 1987.
6. Cury SE, Vilar MJP, Ciconelli RM, et al: Evaluation of the European Spondyloarthropathy Study Group (ESSG) preliminary classification criteria in Brazilian patients. Clin Exp Rheumatol 15:79, 1997.
7. Khan MA, van der Linden SM, Kushner I, et al: Spondylitic disease without radiologic evidence of sacroiliitis in relatives of HLA-B27 positive ankylosing spondylitis patients. Arthritis Rheum 28:40, 1985.
8. Van der Linden SM, Valkenburg HA, Cats A: Evaluation of diagnostic criteria for ankylosing spondylitis: a proposal for modification of the New York criteria. Arthritis Rheum 27:361, 1984.
9. Goethé HS, Steven MM, van der Linden S, et al: Evaluation of diagnostic criteria for ankylosing spondylitis: a comparison of the Rome, New York and modified New York criteria in patients with a positive clinical history screening test for ankylosing spondylitis. Br J Rheumatol 24:242, 1985.
10. D'Amato M, Fiorillo MT, Carcassi C, et al: Relevance of residue 116 of HLA-B27 in determining susceptibility to ankylosing spondylitis. Eur J Immunol 25:3199, 1995.
11. Lopez-Larrea C, Sujirachato K, Mehra NK, et al: HLA-B27 subtypes in Asian patients with ankylosing spondylitis. Tissue Antigens 45:169, 1995.
12. Nasution AR, Marjuadi A, Kunmartini S, et al: HLA-B27 subtypes positively and negatively associated with spondylarthropathy. J Rheumatol 24:1111, 1997.
13. Van der Linden SM, Valkenburg HA, de Jongh BM, et al: The risk of developing ankylosing spondylitis in HLA-B27 positive individuals: a comparison of relatives of spondylitis patients with the general population. Arthritis Rheum 27:241, 1984.
14. Ahearn JM, Hochberg MC: Epidemiology and genetics of ankylosing spondylitis. J Rheumatol 16(Suppl):22, 1988.
15. Kaipiainen-Seppanen O, Aho K, Heliovaara M: Incidence and prevalence of ankylosing spondylitis in Finland. J Rheumatol 24:496, 1997.
16. Braun J, Bollow M, Remlinger G, et al: Prevalence of spondylarthropathies in HLA-B27 positive and negative blood donors. Arthritis Rheum 41: 58, 1998.
17. Gran JT, Husby G: Ankylosing spondylitis: a comparative study of patients in an epidemiological survey, and those admitted to a department of rheumatology. J Rheumatol 11:788, 1984.
18. Carbone LD, Cooper C, Michet CJ, et al: Ankylosing spondylitis in Rochester, Minnesota, 1935-1989. Arthritis Rheum 35:1476, 1992.
19. Brown MA, Kennedy LG, MacGregor AJ, et al: Susceptibility to ankylosing spondylitis in twins: the role of genes, HLA, and the environment. Arthritis Rheum 40:1823, 1997.
20. Ahmadi K, Wilson C, Tiwana H, et al: Antibodies to *Klebsiella pneumoniae* lipopolysaccharide in patients with ankylosing spondylitis. Br J Rheumatol 37:1330, 1998.
21. Fraile A, Nieto A, Vinasco J, et al: Association of large molecular weight proteasome 7 gene polymorphism with ankylosing spondylitis. Arthritis Rheum 41:560, 1998.
22. Taurog JD, Maika SD, Satumtira N, et al: Inflammatory disease in HLA-B27 transgenic rats. Immunol Rev 169:209, 1999.
23. Ball E, Khan MA: HLA-B27 polymorphism. Bone Joint Spine 68:378, 2001.
24. Lopez-Larrea C, Sujirachato K, Mehra NK, et al: HLA-B27 subtypes in Asian patients with ankylosing spondylitis: evidence for new associations. Tissue Antigens 45:169, 1995.
25. Garcia-Fernandez S, Gonzales S, Blanco Am, et al: New insights regarding HLA-B27 diversity in the Asian population. Tissue Antigens 58:259, 2001.
26. Roberts-Thomson PJ, Jones ME. Walker JG, et al: Stochastic processes in the causation of rheumatic diseases. J Rheumatol 29:2628, 2002.
27. Robinson WP, van der Linden S, Khan MA, et al: HLA-Bw60 increases susceptibility to ankylosing spondylitis in HLA-B27+ patients. Arthritis Rheum 32:1135, 1989.
28. Khan MA, Akey J, BruckelJ, et al: HLA-DRB1*0101 and DRB1*1504, but not HLA-B60 (B*4001) contribute to susceptibility to ankylosing spondylitis. Arthritis Rheum 46:S435, 2002.
29. Lopez-Larrea C, Mijiyawa M, Gonzales S, et al: Association of ankylosing spondylitis with HLA-B*1403 in a West African population. Arthritis Rheum 46:2968, 2002.
30. Braun J, Bollow M, Neure L, et al: Use of immunohistologic and in situ hybridization techniques in the examination of sacroiliac joint biopsy specimens from patients with ankylosing spondylitis. Arthritis Rheum 38:499, 1995.
31. Calin A, Porta J, Fries JF, Schurman DJ: Clinical history as a screening test for ankylosing spondylitis. JAMA 237:2613, 1977.
32. Van der Linden S, Khan MA, Rentsch HU, et al: Chest pain without radiographic sacroiliitis in relatives of patients with ankylosing spondylitis. J Rheumatol 15:836, 1988.
33. Khan MA, Kushner I, Braun WE: Comparison of clinical features in HLA-B27 positive and negative patients with ankylosing spondylitis. Arthritis Rheum 20:909, 1977.
34. Van der Linden S, Rentsch HU, Gerber N, et al: The association between ankylosing spondylitis, acute anterior uveitis and HLA-B27: the results of a Swiss family study. Br J Rheumatol 27(Suppl 2):39, 1988.
35. Graham DC, Smythe HA: The carditis and aortitis of ankylosing spondylitis. Bull Rheum Dis 9:171, 1958.
36. Strobel ES, Fritschka E: Case report and review of the literature: fatal pulmonary complications in ankylosing spondylitis. Clin Rheumatol 16:617, 1997.
37. Casserly IP, Fenlon HM, Breatnach E, et al: Lung findings on high-resolution computed tomography in idiopathic ankylosing spondylitis B correlation with clinical findings, pulmonary function testing and plain radiography. Br J Rheumatol 36:677, 1997.
38. Ramos-Remus G, Gomez-Vargas A, Hernandez-Chavez A, et al: Two year follow-up of anterior and vertical atlantoaxial subluxation in ankylosing spondylitis. J Rheumatol 24:507, 1997.
39. Tyrrell PNM, Davies AM, Evans N: Neurological disturbances in ankylosing spondylitis. Ann Rheum Dis 53:714, 1994.
40. Lai KN, Li PKT, Hawkins B, et al: IgA nephropathy associated with ankylosing spondylitis: occurrence in women as well as in men. Ann Rheum Dis 48:435, 1989.
41. Vilar MJP, Cury SE, Ferraz MB, et al: Renal abnormalities in ankylosing spondylitis. Scand J Rheumatol 26:19, 1997.
42. Gratacos J, Orellana C, Sanmarti R, et al: Secondary amyloidosis in ankylosing spondylitis: a systematic review of 137 patients using abdominal fat aspiration. J Rheumatol 24:912, 1997.
43. Lee YSL, Schlotzhauer T, Ott SM et al: Skeletal status of men with early and late ankylosing spondylitis. Am J Med 103:233, 1997.
44. Geusens P, Vosse D, van der Heijde D, et al: High prevalence of thoracic vertebral deformities and discal wedging in ankylosing

spondylitis patients with hyperkyphosis. J Rheumatol 28:1856, 2001.

45. Cooper C, Carbone L, Michet CJ, et al: Fracture risk in patients with ankylosing spondylitis: a population based study. J Rheumatol 21:1877, 1994.

46. Graham B, van Peteghem PK: Fractures of the spine in ankylosing spondylitis: diagnosis, treatment, and complications. Spine 14:803, 1989.

47. Khan MA, Kushner I: Diagnosis of ankylosing spondylitis. In Cohen AS (ed): Progress in Clinical Rheumatology. Vol 1. Orlando, Fla., Grune and Stratton, 1984, pp 145-178.

48. Spoorenberg A, van der Heijde D, de Klerk E, et al: Relative value of erythrocyte sedimentation rate and C-reactive protein in assessment of disease activity in ankylosing spondylitis. J Rheumatol 26: 980, 1999.

49. Schichikawa K, Tsujimoto M, Nishioka J, et al: Histopathology of early sacroiliitis and enthesitis in ankylosing spondylitis. In Ziff M, Cohen SB (eds): The Spondyloarthropathies: Advances in Inflammation Research. Vol 9. New York, Raven Press, 1985.

50. Aufdermaur M: Pathogenesis of square bodies in ankylosing spondylitis. Ann Rheum Dis 48:628, 1989.

51. Braun J, Bollow M, Eggens U, et al: Use of dynamic magnetic resonance imaging with fast imaging in the detection of early and advanced sacroiliitis in spondylarthropathy patients. Arthritis Rheum 37:1039, 1994.

52. Braun J, Bollow M, Remlinger G, et al: Prevalence of spondyloarthropathies in HLA-B27 positive and negative blood donors. Arthritis Rheum 41:58, 1998.

53. McGonagle D, Gibbon W, O'Connor P, et al: Characteristic magnetic resonance imaging entheseal changes of knee synovitis in spondylarthropathy. Arthritis Rheum 41:694, 1998.

54. Wittram C, Whitehouse GH, Williams JW, et al: A comparison of MR and CT in suspected sacroiliitis. J Comput Assist Tomogr 20:68, 1996.

55. Geijer M, Sihlbom H, Gothlin JH, et al: The role of CT in the diagnosis of sacroiliitis. Acta Radiol 39:265, 1998.

56. Rubenstein DJ, Alvarez O, Ghelman B, et al: Cauda equina syndrome complicating spondylitis: MR features. J Comput Assist Tomogr 13:511, 1989.

57. Van der Linden SM, Fahrer H: Occurrence of spinal pain syndromes in a group of apparently healthy and physically fit sportsmen (orienteers). Scand J Rheumatol 17:475, 1988.

58. van Tubergen A, Heuft-Dorenbosch L, Schulpen G, et al: Radiographic assessment of sacroiliitis by radiologists and rheumatologists: does training improve quality? Ann Rheum Dis 62:519, 2003.

59. Khan MA, Khan MK: Diagnostic value of HLA-B27 testing in ankylosing spondylitis and Reiter's syndrome. Ann Intern Med 96:70, 1982.

60. Dubost JJ, Sauvezie B: Late onset peripheral spondylarthropathy. J Rheumatol 16:1214, 1989.

61. Burgos-Vargas R, Clark P: Axial involvement in the seronegative enthesopathy and arthropathy syndrome and its progression to AS. J Rheumatol 16:192, 1989.

62. Kidd B, Mullee M, Frank A, et al: Disease expression of ankylosing spondylitis in males and females. J Rheumatol 15:1407, 1988.

63. Jimenez-Balderas FJ, Mintz G: AS: Clinical course in women and men. J Rheumatol 20:2062, 1993.

64. Khan MA, Khan MK, Kushner I: Survival among patients with ankylosing spondylitis: a lifetable analysis. J Rheumatol 8:86, 1981.

65. Lehtinen K: Mortality and causes of death in 398 patients admitted to hospital with ankylosing spondylitis. Ann Rheum Dis 52:174, 1993.

66. Calin A, Elswood J, Rigg S, et al: Ankylosing spondylitis: an analytical review of 1500 patients—the changing pattern of disease. J Rheumatol 15:1234, 1988.

67. Fries JF, Singh G, Bloch DA, et al: The natural history of ankylosing spondylitis: Is the disease really changing? [Editorial]. J Rheumatol 16:860, 1989.

68. Van de Paardt M, Dijkmans B, Giltay E, van de Horst-Bruinsma I: Dutch patients with familial and sporadic ankylosing spondylitis do not differ in disease phenotype. J Rheumatol 29:2583, 2002.

69. Guillemin F, Briancon S, Pourel J, Gaucher A: Long-term disability and prolonged sick leaves as outcome measurements in ankylosing spondylitis: possible predictive factors. Arthritis Rheum 33:1001, 1990.

70. Ramos-Remus C, Prieto-Parra RE, Michel-Diaz J, et al: A five-year cumulative analysis of labor-status and lost working days in patients with ankylosing spondylitis (AS). Arthritis Rheum 41(Suppl):1136, 1998.

71. Ward M, Kuzis S: Risk factors for work disability in patients with ankylosing spondylitis. J Rheumatol 28:315, 2001.

72. Boonen A, Chorus A, Miedema H, et al: Withdrawal from labour force due to work disability in patients with ankylosing spondylitis. Ann Rheum Dis 60:1033, 2001.

73. Chorus AMJ, Boonen A, Miedema HS, van der Linden S: Employment perspectives of patients with ankylosing spondylitis. Ann Rheum Dis 61:693, 2002.

74. Boonen A, van der Heijde D, Landewe R, et al: Work status and productivity costs due to ankylosing spondylitis: comparison of three European countries. Ann Rheum Dis 61:429, 2002.

75. Boonen A, Chorus A, Miedema H, et al: Employment, work disability, and work days lost in patients with ankylosing spondylitis: a cross sectional study of Dutch patients. Ann Rheum Dis 60:353, 2001.

76. Boonen A, van der Heijde D, Landewé R, et al: Direct costs of ankylosing spondylitis and its determinants: an analysis among three European countries. Ann Rheum Dis 62:732, 2003.

77. Ward MM: Functional, disability predicts total costs in patients with ankylosing spondylitis. Arthritis Rheum 46:223, 2002.

78. Gran JT, Skomsvolly JF: The outcome of ankylosing spondylitis: A study of 100 patients. Brh J Rheumatol 36:766, 1997.

79. Amor B, Silva-Santos R, Nahal R, et al: Predictive factors for the long-term outcome of spondylarthropathies. J Rheumatol 21:1883, 1994.

80. Calin A, Elswood J: The outcome of 138 total hip replacements and 12 revisions in ankylosing spondylitis: high success rate after a mean followup of 7.5 years. J Rheumatol 16:955, 1989.

81. Calin A, Garrett S, Whitelock H, et al: A new approach to defining functional ability in ankylosing spondylitis: the development of the Bath Ankylosing Spondylitis Functional Index (BASFI). J Rheumatol 21:2281, 1994.

82. Dougados M, Gueguen A, Nakache JP, et al: Evaluation of a functional index and an articular index in ankylosing spondylitis. J Rheumatol 15:302, 1988.

83. Garrett S, Jenkinson T, Whitelock H, et al: A new approach to defining disease status in AS: The Bath Ankylosing Spondylitis Disease Activity Index (BASDAI). J Rheumatol 21:2286, 1994.

84. Jenkinson TR, Mallorie PA, Whitelock H, et al: Defining spinal mobility in ankylosing spondylitis (AS): The Bath AS Metrology Index (BASMI). J Rheumatol 21:1694, 1994.

85. Van der Heijde D, Calin A, Dougados M, et al: Selection of specific instruments for each domain in core set for DC-ART, SM-ARD, physical therapy and clinical record keeping in ankylosing spondylitis: progress report of ASAS working group. J Rheumatol 26:951, 1999.

86. Anderson JJ, Baron G, van der Heijde D, et al: Ankylosing spondylitis assessment group preliminary definition of short-term improvement in ankylosing spondylitis. Arthritis Rheum 44:1876, 2001.

87. Auleley GR, Benbouazza K, Spoorenberg A, et al: Evaluation of the smallest detectable difference in outcome or process variables in ankylosing spondylitis. Arthritis Rheum 47:582, 2002.

88. Doward LC, Spoorenberg A, Cook SA, et al: Development of the ASQoL: a quality of life instrument specific to ankylosing spondylitis. Ann Rheum Dis 62:20, 2003.

89. Khan MA, Skosey JL: Ankylosing spondylitis and related spondylarthropathies. In Samter M (ed): Immunological Diseases. Boston, Little, Brown & Co, 1988, pp 1509-1538.

90. Band DA, Jones SD, Kennedy LG, et al: Which patients with ankylosing spondylitis derive most benefit from inpatient management program? J Rheumatol 24:2381, 1997.

91. Hidding A, van der Linden S, Boers M, et al: Is group physical therapy superior to individualized therapy in ankylosing spondylitis? A randomized controlled trial. Arthritis Care Res 6:117, 1993.

92. Dagfinder H, Hagen K: Physiotherapy interventions for ankylosing spondylitis (Cochrane review). In The Cochrane Library, Oxford: Oxford: update software, 2001.

93. van Tubergen A, Landewé R, van der Heijde D, et al: Combined spa-exercise therapy is effective in patients with ankylosing spondylitis: a randomized controlled trial. Arthritis Rheum 45:430, 2001.

94. van Tubergen A, Boonen A, Landewé R, et al: Cost-effectiveness of combined spa-exercise therapy in ankylosing spondylitis: a randomized controlled trial. Arthritis Rheum 47:459, 2002.

95. Dougados M, Behier JM, Jolchine I, et al: Efficacy of celecoxib, a cyclooxygenase 2-specific inhibitor, in the treatment of ankylosing spondylitis: a six-week controlled study with comparison against placebo and against a conventional nonsteroidal antiinflammatory drug. Arthritis Rheum 44:180, 2001.

96. Mielants H, Veys EM: Inflammation of the ileum in patients with B27 positive reactive arthritis. Lancet 1:288, 1984.

97. Maugars Y, Mathis C, Berthelot JM, et al: Assessment of the efficacy of sacroiliac corticosteroid injections in spondylarthropathies: a double-blind study. Br J Rheumatol 35:76, 1996.

98. Braun J, Sieper J: Therapy of ankylosing spondylitis and other spondyloarthritides: established medical treatment, anti-TNF-alpha therapy and other novel approaches. Arthritis Res 4:307, 2002.

99. Ferraż MB, Tugwell P, Goldsmith CH, et al: Meta-analysis of sulphasalazine in ankylosing spondylitis. J Rheumatol 17:1481, 1990.

100. Dougados M, van der Linden S, Juhlin R, et al: Sulphasalazine in spondylarthropathy: a randomized, multicenter, double-blind, placebo-controlled study. Arthritis Rheum 38:618, 1995.

101. Clegg DO, Reda DJ, Weisman MH, et al: Comparison of sulfasalazine and placebo in the treatment of ankylosing spondyli-tis: a Department of Veterans Affairs cooperative study. Arthritis Rheum 39:2004, 1996.

102. Creemers MCW, Franssen MJAM, van de Putte LBA, et al: Methotrexate in severe ankylosing spondylitis: an open study. J Rheumatol 22:1104, 1995.

103. Haibel H, Rudwaleit M, Braun J, Sieper J: Therapy of active ankylosing spondylitis with leflunomide. Ann Rheum Dis 6(Suppl 1):301, 2002.

104. Maksymowych WP, Fitzgerald A, LeClercq S, et al: A 6 month randomized double-blinded dose response comparison of i.v. pamidronate (60 mg vs 10 mg) in the treatment of NSAID-refractory ankylosing spondylitis (AS). Arthritis Rheum 46:766, 2002.

105. Breban M, Gombert B, Amor B, Dougados M: Efficacy of thalidomide in the treatment of refractory ankylosing spondyli-tis. Arthritis Rheum 42:580, 1999.

106. Huang F, Gu J, Zhao W, et al: One-year open-label trial of thalidomide in ankylosing spondylitis. Arthritis Rheum 47:249, 2002.

107. Gorman JD, Sack KE, Davis JC Jr.: Treatment of ankylosing spondylitis by inhibition of tumor necrosis factor alpha. N Engl J Med 346:1349, 2002.

108. Maksymowych W, Inman RD, Gladman D, et al: Spondylarthritis research consortium of Canada: Canadian rheumatology association consensus on the use of anti-TNF-alpha-directed therapies in the treatment of spondyloarthritis. J Rheumatol 30:1356, 2003.

109. Braun J, Pham T, Sieper J, et al for the ASAS working group: International ASAS consensus statement for the use of biologic agents inpatients with ankylosing spondylitis. Ann Rheum Dis 62:817, 2003.

71 Reiter's Syndrome, Undifferentiated Spondyloarthropathy, and Reactive Arthritis

DAVID TAK YAN YU · PENG THIM FAN

In recent years, the introduction of biologic modifiers to the treatment of the spondyloarthropathies has ushered in a new era. Never before has the response of spondyloarthropathy patients to treatment been so rapid and so profound. With effective treatment it has become even more important for practicing clinicians to understand why the diverse conditions are grouped together, to understand their natural course, and to diagnose individual members accurately.

Definition and Classification Criteria

Reiter's syndrome, undifferentiated spondyloarthropathy, and reactive arthritis belong to the family of spondyloarthropathies, a group that also includes ankylosing spondylitis (AS), psoriatic arthritis, and arthritis associated with inflammatory bowel disease. Until recently, these diseases were grouped together only by convention because of the cardinal clinical features they share. The Amor criteria, published in 1990, were the first set of classification criteria based on case-controlled examination of the entire spondyloarthropathy family.[1] The European Spondyloarthropathy Study Group (ESSG) criteria, published in 1991, were the second set.[2] These criteria provide a uniform standard for the inclusion of patients in studies.

The Amor criteria require the separate evaluation of 12 features, which are listed in Table 71–1. Each feature carries a preassigned probability point count of 1, 2, or 3. A patient is considered to have a spondyloarthropathy if the sum of the point counts is 6 or more.

In contrast to the Amor criteria, the ESSG criteria use only two entry parameters. According to this classification, patients should be evaluated if they have one of the following:

1. Inflammatory spinal pain
2. Synovitis that is asymmetric or predominantly of the lower limbs

A patient is considered to have spondyloarthropathy if one of the above is present, plus any one of the following features:

1. Positive family history, which is defined as presence in first-degree or second-degree relatives of any of the following: AS, psoriasis, acute uveitis, reactive arthritis, or inflammatory bowel diseases
2. Psoriasis diagnosed by a physician

3. Inflammatory bowel disease (either Crohn's disease or ulcerative colitis) diagnosed by a physician and confirmed by radiographic examination or endoscopy
4. Nongonococcal urethritis or cervicitis, or acute diarrhea within 1 month before arthritis
5. Buttock pain alternating between right and left gluteal areas
6. Enthesopathy, defined as spontaneous pain or tenderness at the site of insertion of the Achilles tendon or plantar fascia

TABLE 71–1 · PARAMETERS IN THE AMOR CRITERIA FOR DIAGNOSING SPONDYLOARTHOPATHY

Criterion	Points
A. Clinical Symptoms or Past History	
1. Lumbar or dorsal pain during the night, or morning stiffness of lumbar or dorsal spine	1
2. Asymmetric Diagnosing Spondyloarthopathy oligoarthritis	2
3. Buttock pain	1
if affecting alternately the right or the left buttock	2
4. Sausage-like toe or digit	2
5. Heel pain	2
6. Iritis	2
7. Nongonococcal urethritis or cervicitis accompanying, or within 1 month before, the onset of arthritis	1
8. Acute diarrhea accompanying, or within 1 month before, the onset of arthritis	1
9. Presence or history of psoriasis, balanitis, or inflammatory bowel disease (ulcerative colitis or Crohn's disease)	2
B. Radiologic Finding	
10. Sacroiliitis (grade >2 if bilateral; grade >3 if unilateral)	3
C. Genetic Background	
11. Presence of HLA-B27, or familial history of ankylosing spondylitis (AS), Reiter's syndrome, uveitis, psoriasis, or chronic enterocolopathies	2
D. Response to Treatment	
12. Clear-cut improvement of rheumatic complaints with nonsteroidal anti-inflammatory drugs (NSAIDs) in less than 48 hours, or relapse of the pain in less than 48 hours if NSAIDs discontinued	2

7. Radiographic evidence of sacroiliitis by plain films
8. Spinal pain has to be "inflammatory" to qualify as an entry parameter; inflammatory spinal pain has at least four of the following five features:

At least 3 months' duration
Onset before 45 years of age
Insidious onset
Improved by exercise
Associated with morning stiffness

Both the Amor and the ESSG criteria represent a consensus opinion among multiple experts. To create the criteria, each individual expert evaluated a number of patients and assigned the diagnosis of spondyloarthropathy based on his or her own clinical judgment, rather than any set of validated criteria. These individual expert opinions form the "gold standard of diagnosis" in these studies. The final criteria represent a statistical compilation of all the opinions. Because of this, there may be disagreements when one particular opinion is measured against the consensus criteria. In the ESSG criteria, for example, the sensitivity and specificity are 78.5 percent and 89.6 percent, respectively. The positive and negative predictive values are 60.3 percent and 99.2 percent, respectively. The ESSG criteria work less well in patients with onset of arthritis of less than 1 year. The sensitivity decreases to 67.9 percent. However, the criteria are still highly specific at 92.8 percent. The two sets of classification criteria have been validated in several countries and are generally considered by academicians to be useful as diagnostic adjuncts. When evaluated by a Spanish multicenter group, for example, the sensitivities of the Amor and ESSG criteria were 90.8 percent and 83.5 percent, respectively, and their were specificities 96.2 percent and 95.2 percent, respectively.[3]

Once a patient is classified as having a spondyloarthropathy, other clinical features may allow further subclassification into psoriatic arthritis, arthritis related to inflammatory bowel disease, reactive arthritis, or AS. However, there remains a large number of patients who fulfill the criteria for spondyloarthropathy but cannot be allocated into one of those subcategories. They are then designated as having "undifferentiated spondyloarthropathy." In addition to one of the two ESSG entry parameters, these patients have one or more of the following: positive family history, alternating buttock pain, enthesopathy, or sacroiliitis. This is an important diagnostic designation because undifferentiated spondyloarthropathy is one of the two most common members of the family, the other being AS. The ESSG criteria are currently the best tools we have to secure the diagnosis of undifferentiated spondyloarthropathy.

The name "Reiter's syndrome" is the most restrictive and least useful designation. It originated in a 1916 report by Hans Reiter of a single patient showing the clinical triad of arthritis, urethritis, and conjunctivitis.[4] In 1981, the American Rheumatism Association (ARA) widened the scope by defining the syndrome as a peripheral arthritis lasting longer than 1 month associated with urethritis, cervicitis, or diarrhea.[5] Since then, Reiter's syndrome has become synonymous with *reactive arthritis*, a term introduced by Ahvonen in 1969.[6] In the

last decade, the ARA criteria have become obsolete. As a result, the term *Reiter's syndrome* has been superceded by the Amor and the ESSG classification criteria for spondyloarthropathies, as well as the definitions of reactive arthritis to be described in the next section.

The concept of "reactive arthritis" has evolved through several changes. Originally, it was defined as "an arthritis induced by bacterial infections in which live bacteria could not be detected in the affected joints."[6] Over the years, many clinical settings involving a variety of pathogens satisfied this definition, leading to a lack of uniformity in the clinical features. "Poststreptococcal reactive arthritis," for instance, is clinically distinct from the spondyloarthropathies, but it has nevertheless been classified as a reactive arthritis.[7] Currently most experts in this field would limit the term *reactive arthritis* strictly to arthritis induced by the following bacteria: *Chlamydia, Salmonella, Shigella, Yersinia,* and *Campylobacter.* Only these forms of postinfection arthritis share the same clinical features of the spondyloarthropathy family. Investigators have also changed the definition of reactive arthritis by omitting the requirement for lack of infectious organisms in the joints. As we improve our ability to detect bacteria in the joints, it becomes clear that they can be found in other types of arthritis and even in normal individuals.

There are no validated criteria for the classification or diagnosis of reactive arthritis. The following working definition was adapted from the 3rd International Workshop on Reactive Arthritis in 1996.[8] Two features are considered to be critical requirements:

1. An acute inflammatory arthritis, inflammatory low back pain, or enthesitis
2. Evidence of an infection preceding this condition by 4 to 8 weeks

Evidence of preceding infection can be clinical, such as diarrhea or nongonococcal urethritis. It can also be based on laboratory tests, such as positive bacterial culture in stools or urogenital swabs, identification of *Chlamydia trachomatis* from urine, or elevated serum antibodies to the pathogens. According to this working definition, a diagnosis of reactive arthritis can be made if a patient has a history of a preceding infection without laboratory evidence to support it. Conversely, a patient has reactive arthritis if there is laboratory evidence of a recent infection even though the infection may be symptomatically silent.

▌ Epidemiology

There have been very few population surveys on the prevalence of the entire spondyloarthropathy family. The most recent assessment was a telephone survey conducted in Brittany, France. The prevalence of spondyloarthropathy and rheumatoid arthritis was found to be 0.47 and 0.62 percent, respectively.[9] This value is not very different from a 1998 assessment of blood donors in Berlin using the ESSG criteria. There, as in previous studies, the prevalence of spondyloarthropathy was highly linked to that of the HLA-B27 antigen.[10] Prevalence is

13.6 percent among HLA-B27–positive subjects and 0.8 percent among HLA-B27–negative subjects. The frequency of HLA-B27 in white Western European subjects is 9.3 percent. Hence, the overall prevalence of spondyloarthropathy in Berlin is 1.9 percent. Twenty spondyloarthropathy patients are identified among the Berlin blood donors: 45 percent have AS, whereas 35 percent have undifferentiated spondyloarthropathy. These percentages support the impression that in clinical practice, undifferentiated spondyloarthropathy is as common as AS. Because the frequency of HLA-B27 varies with ethnicity, parallel differences in prevalence are observed with the spondyloarthropathy.[11] For example, the 1.9-percent prevalence of spondyloarthropathy in a white population is less than the 2.5 percent among Alaskan Eskimos,[12] partly owing to the higher frequency of HLA-B27 among the Eskimos, which is 25 to 40 percent. An additional feature of Eskimos is that both undifferentiated spondyloarthropathy (1.3%) and reactive arthritis (1.0%) are more common than AS (0.4%). A similarly high prevalence of reactive arthritis is reported among Native American Navajo Indians, Greenland Inuit Eskimos, Alaskan Inupiat Eskimos, and Alaskan Yupik Eskimos. This observation is attributed to their higher frequency of HLA-B27, as well as enteric or sexually transmitted diseases.

The frequency of reactive arthritis has been assessed in several ways: the prevalence or incidence in the general population, the frequency following endemic infections, or the frequency following outbreaks of infections. As to the general prevalence, little data are available. It has been commonly regarded as 1 per 10,000, which is about one tenth those of AS and undifferentiated spondyloarthropathy. The second type of assessment is incidence, for which more information is available. From 1950 to 1980, the incidence of Reiter's syndrome in Olmsted County, Rochester, MN was 3.5 per 100,000 population per year in men, and there were no female cases.[13] In an Hispanic population, the incidence rates between 1975 and 1989 were 2.66 and 0.65 per 100,000 for men and women, respectively.[14] A higher number of cases (43.6 per 100,000 inhabitants) was reported in Finland, published in 1978.[15] In general, there has been a gradual decline in cases of reactive arthritis over the years. A decade later in Norway, between 1988 and 1990, the incidence was only one tenth that of the Finnish study: 4.6 cases per 100,000 for arthritis induced by *Chlamydia* and 5 cases per 100,000 for arthritis induced by enteric bacteria.[16] A study in the Greek army also showed this decline with 27 cases from 1980 to1983 and only 4 from 1989 to1992.[17] This decrease to range of 1 to 10 cases per 100,000 population is probably caused by a decline in the rate of arthritis-inducing infections.

Another way to study the frequency of reactive arthritis is to enumerate the frequency of patients with rheumatologic sequelae after endemic infections by individual species of bacteria. There are very few such studies. In 1995, 271 patients (almost all black) attending a sexually transmitted disease clinic in Alabama were evaluated for the presence of *Chlamydia*-induced arthritis. Among those with genital infections, 4.1 percent had reactive arthritis.[18] None of the patients was positive for HLA-B27, but this population had a low prevalence of HLA-B27. Regarding enteric infections, at least two surveys have been reported, both based on Finnish National Health Department reports. In one study, investigators recruited 198 subjects who were culture positive for *Salmonella* during the period of 1 year, starting in May 1998.[19] Several serotypes of *Salmonella* were involved. Only 4 percent were diagnosed as having reactive arthritis when reviewed by rheumatologists. HLA-B27 probably contributed to the severity and duration of joint symptoms, because 75 percent of the confirmed cases of *Salmonella*-induced reactive arthritis were HLA-B27 positive. The second study focused on 609 people infected with *Campylobacter*.[20] Almost all the *Campylobacter* infections were by *C. jejuni*. Seven percent fulfilled their criteria for reactive arthritis, and 1 percent for reactive tendinitis. None of these was observed in a control group of 771 individuals. In summary, the incidence of reactive arthritis following endemic infections is 1 to 5 percent.

A final way to evaluate the frequency of reactive arthritis is to study the number of arthritis patients discovered following epidemics of enteric infections. The rate is not very different from those observed following endemic infections, varying from 1 to 2 percent, except for *Salmonella*, which can be higher.[21]

Lastly, the incidence of reactive arthritis might depend on unique host factors. Musculoskeletal symptoms are common among human immunodeficiency virus (HIV)-infected patients and are often caused by a spondyloarthropathy.[22] Thus, a higher frequency of spondyloarthropathy among patients infected with HIV has been suggested, but this might depend on the population.

■ Pathogenesis of Spondyloarthropathy

The pathogenesis of AS is almost entirely genetic. Some of the AS genes probably also contribute to other members of the spondyloarthropathy family. Details of the genes contributing to AS are provided in Chapter 70. In the other spondyloarthropathies, HLA-B27 is currently the only gene identified with certainty. In those patients who possess HLA-B27, it is believed that the gene is a pivotal factor. However, unlike AS, a considerable proportion of spondyloarthropathy patients are HLA-B27 negative. Environmental factors play very minor roles in AS. How much they contribute to the other members of the spondyloarthropathy family is not clear. In the case of reactive arthritis, the initial bacterial infection is, by definition, an essential factor. In the case of undifferentiated spondyloarthropathy, a considerable proportion of patients have clinically silent infections by pathogens known to cause reactive arthritis. The pathogenesis in these patients may actually be the same as reactive arthritis.

Among the members of the spondyloarthropathy family, the pathogenesis of reactive arthritis has been the most extensively studied.[23] This is because the pathogens that cause reactive arthritis are known and readily available for experimental analysis. These pathogens share certain characteristics. They primarily infect mucosal surfaces and are then conveyed to the joint compartment by monocytes.[24] On arrival at the joint, the pathogens will remain, perhaps indefinitely, either as bacterial fragments or intact with nucleotides.[25] Such homing of bacteria to joints is not restricted to reactive-arthritis pathogens. Many strains of bacteria have been detected by polymerase chain reactions, (PCR) in joints of various arthritis conditions, and also in apparently healthy individuals. In some arthritic joints, more than one species of bacteria are found. The *Chlamydia* species represents a prototype of how arthritis-causing bacterial strains have evolved to become persistent in the host. In a persistent *Chlamydial* infection, the bacteria change the composition of their major outer membrane proteins and their pathways of energy utilization. In defense from host attack, they develop mechanisms to inhibit apoptosis of the host cells in which they reside, induce apoptosis of host T lymphocytes, and downregulate the expression of antigen-presenting molecules of host antigen-presenting cells. Antibiotics are ineffective against bacteria during the persistent infective state and may contribute to their conversion into such a persistent state. This poses great difficulty to the physician.[23]

The host, on the other hand, also mounts multiple responses against the bacteria. Some of these reactions may contribute to the inflammatory process in the joints. Two types of anti-*Chlamydial* T lymphocyte responses are observed: cell determinant (CD)4+ and CD8+. The following *Chlamydial* proteins are antigenic for synovial CD4+ T lymphocytes: Hcl, hsp60, omp-2, enolase, pmpD, and CT579.[26] In the past, the major focus of research has been on CD8+ T lymphocytes, because the only known HLA-B27–specific immune reactivity was with the T cell receptors (TCR) of CD8+ T lymphocytes. This specificity is directed against a complex of HLA-B27 and the peptides they carry. Early efforts tried to identify peptides derived from candidate bacterial proteins, such as the stress proteins.[27] Subsequent attempts at peptide identification have been carried to the extreme by screening for the entire genome of *Chlamydia trachomatis*. Eleven *Chlamydial* peptides have been identified. However, only 1 of the 11 peptides is reactive with 3 of 3 patients tested. This peptide is derived from clp protease-adenosine triphosphatase (ATPase), and carries the sequence: NRAKQVIKL.[28] These studies leave no doubt that there is an active T lymphocyte response against bacterial peptides in the joints of patients with reactive arthritis. Further validation comes from an analysis of TCR showing that, in the acute stage of reactive arthritis, the T lymphocyte response is oligoclonal, indicating that only a small number of dominant bacterial antigens are involved.[29] It is highly likely that these interactions are partly responsible for the arthritis process. Whether the reactivity in the acute stage is subsequently perpetuated by a cross-reactive autoantigen remains to be demonstrated. Proteins such as HLA-B27 itself, aggrecans, or versicans of the proteoglycan family are potential candidates for autoantigens that may perpetuate the process.[30]

This emphasis on CD8+ T lymphocytes is based on the premise that an HLA-B27 molecule exists as complexes of heavy chain, light chain, and peptide.[31] This trimolecular structure was reported more than a decade ago. Since 1996, alternative structures of HLA-B27 have been reported, ushering in new theories on how HLA-B27 mediates arthritis. The major new observation is that HLA-B27 can exist free of the β2-microglobulin light chain. These free heavy chains have been observed in cell lines, transgenic mice, and monocytes of patients with AS.[32] There are at least two conceivable ways the generation of free heavy chains of HLA-B27 could lead to arthritis. One, the free heavy chains could provide ligands for receptors on immune cells such as natural killer (NK) receptors.[33] Another equally appealing hypothesis is that these free heavy chains are generated because HLA-B27 matures more slowly inside cells, compared to other HLA class I alleles. This delay in maturation may generate signaling responses designated as endoplasmic "unfolded protein response" and "overloading response."[34] The latter activates nuclear factor kappa B (NFκB), which is the transcription factor for pivotal proinflammatory cytokines. This hypothesis is supported by other conceptually independent experiments demonstrating that expression of HLA-B27 on cell lines modifies the signaling response of the cells to enable invasion by arthritis-causing bacteria.[35] It is of course quite unlikely that all responses occur simultaneously in all the cells of an HLA-B27 host. Using microarray, preliminary experiments suggest that such processes take place in the macrophages of the synovial compartment.[36] The macrophages must play a central role in the inflammatory response in spondyloarthropathies because they secrete tumor necrosis factor-α (TNF-α), the major mediator of inflammation in these diseases.

In summary, multiple factors contribute to the pathogenesis of spondyloarthropathy. Even HLA-B27 plays several different roles. A most important observation is that treatment of the spondyloarthropathies with TNF-inhibitors leads to a profound suppression of all the features of inflammation. This factor suggests that, irrespective of the many potential pathways of activation listed previously, the ultimate number of mediators might be very limited. It would appear that additional therapeutic success will depend on identifying more downstream mediators, rather than on discovering the initiating pathogenic mechanisms.

Diagnostic Strategy for the Spondyloarthropathies

How should a practicing clinician or an academician diagnose spondyloarthropathy? There are no diagnostic criteria. Most practicing rheumatologists accomplish it intuitively. This is not sufficient for an academic rheumatologist. An academician would address three questions: How useful are the classification criteria as diagnostic tools? What are the essential items in the history and physical examination? And, what is a simple scheme a rheumatologist could use to increase the accuracy of diagnosis beyond individual intuitive judgment? For the asymmetry of this inflammatory disease and characteristic "sausage" digits, see Figures 71–1 and 71–2.

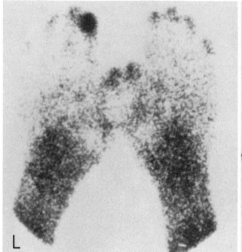
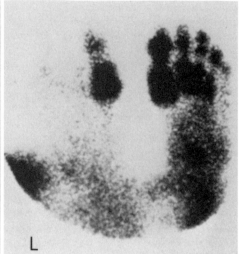

FIGURE 71–1 · Scintiscan in undifferentiated spondyloarthropathy demonstrating asymmetry of the inflammatory disease involving the distal digit of the left index finger and several "sausage" toes, especially on the right. (Courtesy of Dr. Rodney Bluestone.)

USEFULNESS OF THE CLASSIFICATION CRITERIA FOR DIAGNOSIS

Even though the ESSG and Amor criteria are classification criteria, academicians have recommended them as aids to diagnosis. For that purpose, a major shortcoming is that they were based only on a single evaluation of each patient, with no follow-up studies to substantiate their accuracy. However, follow-up studies were subsequently carried out by the Spanish Spondy-loarthropathy Study Group. Based on his or her own judgment, each rheumatologist in the Spanish group classified patients at entry into three categories: definite, possible, or absence of spondyloarthropathy. This approach closely simulates that of most practicing rheu-matologists. Fifty-two patients were followed prospectively for 5 years. The Group's conclusion was that the Amor criteria have a positive predictive value of 76 percent and a negative predictive value of 89 percent. The ESSG criteria have positive predictive value of 46 percent and negative predictive value of 82 percent. Hence, both classification criteria offer substantial diagnostic help, at least in eliminating the diagnosis of spondyloarthropathy. The Amor criteria, being more complex, are more accurate than the ESSG criteria. Inclusion of HLA-B27 and response to nonsteroidal anti-inflammatory drugs (NSAIDs) may have contributed to the higher sensitivity of the Amor criteria in this study.[37] Another important observation of the study is that patients suspected of having a spondyloarthropathy, but not satisfying the criteria, may go on to develop a definite spondyloarthropathy within several years. For this reason, an initial diagnosis of probable spondyloarthropathy is a practically useful one. The Spanish Group also found that the potential usefulness of the ESSG criteria varies with the prevalence of spondyloarthropathy in a rheumatology practice. Not surprisingly, the ESSG criteria are more accurate in an area of higher prevalence than one with a lower prevalence.[3] Therefore, a rheumatologist with a major interest in spondyloarthropathy will find the criteria more useful. Table 71–2 outlines a simple strategy for practicing rheumatologists.

WHAT BASIC CLINICAL FEATURES SHOULD A RHEUMATOLOGIST USE TO DIAGNOSE SPONDYLOARTHROPATHY?

The spondyloarthropathy family is a group of diseases with both shared and unique clinical findings. In the past, textbooks have listed the individual clinical features and their frequencies. It is probably more useful for diagnostic purposes to define the individual sensitivity and specificity of each clinical feature. The ESSG study group has listed 25 independent candidate variables according to their sensitivity and specificity in classifying a patient as having spondyloarthropathy. All variables were found to have high specificity. Because of that, practicing physicians are encouraged to evaluate these components in the history and physical examination (see Table 71–3).

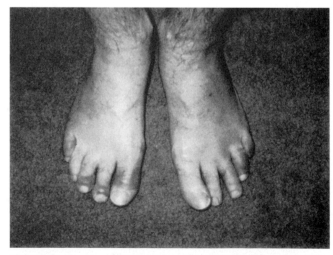

FIGURE 71–2 · Asymmetric Inflammatory Disease of the Feet. Especially specific for spondyloarthropathy are the "sausage" toes with severe swelling of the phalangeal shafts. Note also swelling of the tarsus.

TABLE 71–2 · DIAGNOSTIC STRATEGY FOR SPONDYLOARTHROPATHY

Features	Probability
Inflammatory low back pain or oligoarthritis of lower extremity PLUS	14%
Additional features from Amor or European Spondyloarthopathy Study Group, (O) criteria PLUS	30 to 70%
HLA-B27, sacroiliitis, or both	95%

Diagnostic Strategy for Reactive Arthritis

This varies according to whether the patient is being seen in a specialty rheumatology clinic or in a general practice clinic. From an analysis of the numerous reports from specialty clinics, it appears that the two entry parameters of the ESSG criteria—inflammatory spinal pain and asymmetric synovitis involving the lower limbs—are also the most important for a correct diagnosis of reactive arthritis. Clinical or laboratory evidence of recent infection completes the entry criteria for reactive arthritis. The role of serologic tests in securing evidence of infection varies according to the locale and the organism involved. HLA-B27 positivity greatly enhances the accuracy of the diagnosis.[38] A diagnostic strategy is provided in Table 71–4.

This diagnostic approach is based on data derived from patients attending rheumatology clinics. In the general population, many patients with reactive arthritis do not have severe enough symptoms to attend specialty clinics. Their spectrum of clinical features is somewhat different. No statistical compilation of such patients has been carried out. In a community study of *Salmonella*-induced arthritis, the majority had lower-limb involvement, with the knees being the most frequently affected. Tendon symptoms of enthesopathy affected 4.5 percent of patients.[19] In a study of *Campylobacter*-induced arthritis, 20 percent of the reactive-arthritis patients had inflammatory low back pain without peripheral arthritis. Fifty percent of patients with peripheral arthritis had polyarticular distribution, which is quite different from those seen in specialty clinics. The most frequently affected joint was the knee, although small joints were also affected. Almost all cases were mild. The percent of HLA-B27 in *Campylobacter*-

TABLE 71–3 · PARAMETERS USEFUL FOR DIAGNOSING SPONDYLOAROPATHIES

Essential Elements in the History

Information from History	% Sensitivity	% Specificity
Spinal pain	85	29
Inflammatory spinal pain	7	83)
Synovitis, predominantly in the lower limbs	35	89
Asymmetric synovitis	41	87
Mono- or oligo-versus polyarticular involvement	14	75)
Buttock pain	53	74
Buttock pain, alternating between right and left	20	97
Buttock pain, unilateral, without radiation below the knee	13	93
Anterior chest wall pain	44	86
Heel pain	37	89
Conjunctivitis	17	88
Uveitis (acute anterior)	22	97
Psoriasis	23	95
Mucosal ulceration	6	97
Acute diarrhea (1 month before arthritis)	12	98
Inflammatory bowel disease	10	97
Nongonococcal urethritis or cervicitis (I month before arthritis)	7	97
Family history (see text)	32	95
Positive effect of NSAIDs	65	49

Essential Elements in the Physical Examination

Feature	% Sensitivity	% Specificity
Detection of synovitis, predominantly in the lower limbs	35	89
Synovitis being asymmetric	41	87
Synovitis being mono- or oligo- and not polyarthritis	14	75
Dactylitis	18	96
Reduction in spinal mobility*	37	90
Chest expansion <2.5 cm	15	96
Psoriasis	23	96

*For spinal mobility, the cervical and lumbar spines should be evaluated separately. Ranges of movement of the spine are defined as being "restricted" only if the reduction is in more than one plane. Degree of flexion deformity of the cervical spine is measured by the occiput (or tragus) to wall distance. Range of forward flexion of the lumbar spine is measured by the Schober test.

Abbreviations: NSAIDs, nonsteroidal anti-inflammatory drugs.

TABLE 71–4 · DIAGNOSTIC STRATEGY IN REACTIVE ARTHRITIS

Features	Probability
Inflammatory low back pain or oligoarthritis of lower extremity PLUS	
Symptoms of preceding acute symptomatic urethritis, cervicitis, or enteritis PLUS	30 to 50%
Positive bacterial recognition test PLUS	70 to 80%
Positive HLA-B27	>80%

induced arthritis was strikingly no different than that of the control population.[20]

In summary, taking all these factors into consideration, the most reliable indicator of reactive arthritis is the presence of an infection by an arthritis-causing pathogen within 1 to 2 months preceding the onset of arthritis. The clinical features of the arthritis and presence of HLA-B27 are helpful when patients are seen in specialty clinics but not necessarily so in general practice.

SPECIFIC FEATURES

Mucous Membrane and Skin

Small, shallow, painless ulcers of the glans penis and urethral meatus, termed *balanitis circinata*, have been described, and they may precede the symptoms of arthritis. In uncircumcised patients the lesions are moist and are asymptomatic unless secondarily infected. The foreskin has to be retracted during the physical examination to detect these lesions. On the circumcised penis the lesions harden to a crust, which may scar and cause pain (Fig. 71–3).

Keratoderma blenorrhagica is a hyperkeratotic skin lesion that is seen in 12 to 14 percent of patients (Fig. 71–4). It begins as clear vesicles on erythematous bases and progresses to macules, papules, and nodules. The lesions are frequently found on the soles of the feet, and they may also involve the toes, scrotum, penis, palms, trunk, and scalp. The lesions cannot be distinguished either clinically or microscopically from pustular psoriasis, although it has been claimed that a superficial leukocytoclastic vasculitis is seen in keratoderma blenorrhagica but not in pustular psoriasis.[39] These lesions do not correlate with the course of the disease. The nails can become thickened and ridged. Keratotic material accumulates under the nail and lifts it from the nail bed (Fig. 71–5). Superficial oral ulcers are an early and transient feature of the disease. They begin as vesicles and progress to small, shallow, sometimes confluent, ulcers. Because they are often painless, they may go unnoticed by the patient. Erythema nodosum is unique to post-*Yersinia* reactive arthritis.

Eye

Conjunctivitis is the most common complication of reactive arthritis. Patients experience redness, smarting, and tearing, and a few have photophobia, chemosis, and swelling of the lids. The mucopurulent discharge is typically sterile, although, rarely, *Chlamydia* organisms have been cultured from the eye during bouts of inclusion conjunctivitis.[40] Symptoms commonly subside within a week, but they may persist for 7 months.

Uveitis probably occurs as an independent, asynchronous event due to the shared genetic susceptibility of HLA-B27 positivity.[41] It does not occur in undifferentiated spondyloarthropathy in the absence of HLA-B27. The initial attack is always acute and unilateral, but recurrent episodes often affect the other eye. The inflammation is anterior (iritis) and tends to spare the choroid and retina. Patients with iritis complain of photophobia, redness, and pain, and occasionally reduced vision and increased tearing. The inflammation tends to resolve completely within 2 to 4 months.

Spondyloarthropathy Associated with Human Immunodeficiency Virus Infection

Spondyloarthropathy, including undifferentiated spondyloarthropathy, Reiter's syndrome, reactive arthritis, and psoriatic arthritis, are seemingly common rheumatic

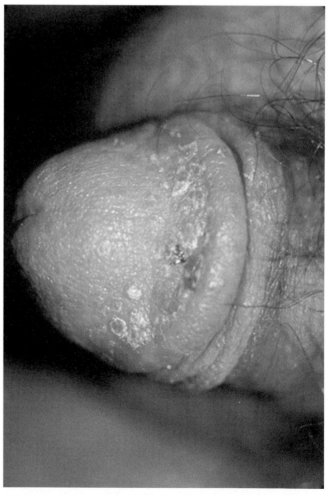

FIGURE 71–3 · Balanitis Circinata in an Uncircumcised Penis. Moist, painless, shallow ulcers are seen at the corona when the foreskin is retracted. (Courtesy of Dr. Kenneth Landow.)

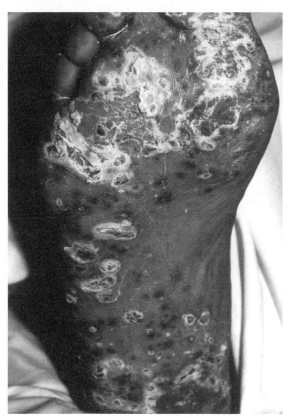

FIGURE 71–4 · Keratoderma Blennorrhagica. Hyperkeratotic vesicles, papules, and plaques on the sole of the foot. (Courtesy of Dr. Kenneth Landow.)

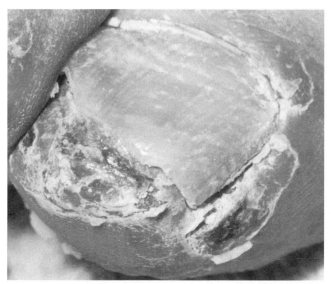

FIGURE 71–5 · The Toenail is Thickened and Ridged. Part of the nail is trimmed to reveal keratotic deposits, which are lifting the nail from the nail bed. (Courtesy of Dr. Kenneth Landow.)

complaints in patients with HIV infection. Extra-articular manifestations include enthesitis, nail involvement with subungual hyperkeratosis, circinate balanitis, keratoderma blenorrhagica, oral ulcers, and uveitis. In Caucasian patients, there is an association with HLA-

B27. The prevalence of HIV-related spondyloarthropathy in Western countries seems to have declined to become the same as in the general population.[42] This is not the case in Africa, where aggressive treatment of HIV infection is not available. In Zambia, for example, the prevalence of spondyloarthropathy in HIV-positive individuals is 180 per 100,000. This is more than 10-fold the prevalence in HIV-negative individuals. In those populations, HIV infection is a predisposing factor to spondyloarthropathy.[43]

Juvenile-Onset Spondyloarthropathy

Juvenile-onset spondyloarthropathy is common in Mexican Mestizos, Chinese, Indians, and North Africans. Unlike adult-onset spondyloarthropathy, axial symptoms are uncommon at onset. Instead, the patients present with peripheral arthritis and enthesitis predominantly of the lower extremities. Among Chinese patients, for example, 82 percent of juvenile patients present as peripheral arthritis at onset versus 47 percent in adult patients. Only 11 percent of juvenile patients present as low back pain at onset versus 45 percent of adult patients. The course is variable. It can be self-limiting, intermittent, or persistent. Unlike adult-onset spondyloarthropathy, the joints may develop contracture and ultimately ankylosis. Foot enthesitis is especially disabling. Some patients develop AS after a number of years.[44]

LABORATORY EVALUATION

The most useful laboratory tests are those that prove the presence of an arthritis-causing bacterium in the urogenital tract or bowel. When positive, they support a diagnosis of reactive arthritis and are useful even in the absence of overt signs and symptoms of infection. Together with typical clinical rheumatologic features, they provide a diagnostic probability of greater than 50 percent.[38] Laboratory testing is particularly important in *Chlamydia*-induced arthritis because a considerable proportion of patients are clinically silent. The clinical course of "silent" *Chlamydia*-induced arthritis is the same as those with symptomatic urethritis.[45] Bacterial studies are also helpful with undifferentiated spondyloarthropathy. One study of 74 patients with undifferentiated oligoarthritis identified triggering infections in 47 percent of patients, including *Yersinia*, *Salmonella*, and *Chlamydia*.[46]

To identify *Chlamydia* infections, urine samples or genital swabs should be submitted for culture or for assessment of nucleotide hybridization.[47] Stool cultures are necessary for securing the diagnosis of enteric infections. However, a negative culture does not rule out reactive arthritis, because the stool cultures can become negative by the time the arthritis appears. The significance of a positive serologic test for any organism depends on the prevalence of such antibodies in that community. Many papers have been published on the detection of bacteria in the joint compartments. It is generally agreed that identification of infectious pathogens of reactive arthritis in synovium and synovial fluid is of little diagnostic value because these tests are frequently positive in patients with other established forms of arthritis. This is the case regardless of the method being used.

The second group of laboratory tests reflects the presence of inflammation. A moderate neutrophilic leukocytosis, elevated erythrocyte sedimentation rate (ESR), and elevated C-reactive protein level are common during the acute illness. Chronic cases show a mild normocytic anemia. These laboratory tests, however, are very poor substitute for clinical assessment. In AS, the gold standard for assessment of disease activity is a set of clinical parameters tabulated as the Bath Ankylosing Spondylitis Disease Activity Index BASDAI. This has been modified recently by the Assessment in Ankylosing Spondylitis ASAS working group (see Chapter 70). Laboratory tests by themselves have poor predictive value of disease activity in the spondyloarthropathies. Studies are underway to see if laboratory studies combined with the results of imaging are more accurate, and validated recommendations should be available in the near future.

Synovial fluid may be mildly to severely inflammatory, and synovial biopsies show inflammatory changes. Efforts are underway to identify spondyloarthropathy-specific features in these tissues.[48] Both synovial fluid and biopsies are certainly useful when it appears necessary to exclude diagnoses of septic arthritis and mycobacterial infections.

HLA-B27 typing is helpful but, by itself, lacks diagnostic specificity. It carries a positive point in the Amor criteria, and a positive test strengthens the diagnosis of both spondyloarthropathy and reactive arthritis. It is also of minor help in assessing prognosis and development of axial disease,[21] carditis, and uveitis.

DIAGNOSTIC IMAGING

The two diagnostic features of spondyloarthropathy are enthesopathy (Fig. 71–6) and sacroiliitis. They can be detected by ultrasound, magnetic resonance imaging (MRI), computed tomography (CT) scan, and plain radiographs. These are described in Chapter 70. Plain radiograph of the sacroiliitis should always be carried out in patients suspected of spondyloarthropathy. Positive sacroiliitis carries a specificity of more than 90 percent.

▌ Management

With the advent of anti–TNF-α therapy, effective treatment of inflammation of both peripheral joints and the axial skeleton is now possible. Nevertheless, first line treatment for all patients should still be NSAIDs. With the wide array of conventional NSAIDs and including cycloxygenase-2 (COX-2) inhibitor (COX-2) inhibitors available, selection will depend on personal preference, susceptibility to side effects, and other factors. Studies are showing that COX-2 inhibitors are similar, but not superior, in efficacy to other NSAIDs. Celecoxib, for example, is effective in AS.[49] Whether they should be used in sustained dosage or only on demand is an important question. Several studies show that when used continuously, NSAIDs provide maximum suppression of pain and inflammation within 2 weeks. After that, there is no information on whether there is a therapeutic difference between sustained use versus intermittent use as symptoms demand. When assessing their effect, the control of pain and stiffness is a good guide. For a patient to stay on a particular NSAID, a minimum of 20 percent improvement is expected; however, ESR and C-reactive protein may stay elevated. Narcotic analgesics are useful adjuncts, and concern over dependency is unjustified. The rate of opioid dependency in patients with AS is low, even when one to seven tablets equivalent of 30 mg of codeine have been prescribed daily for several years.[50]

Local injections of corticosteroids are useful for areas of localized inflammation. Swollen joints will respond to aspiration and injection. Heel pain can be relieved by injections into the plantar fascia. However, direct injection into the Achilles tendon should be avoided as it may cause tendon rupture. The sacroiliac joints respond well to direct corticosteroid injection (see

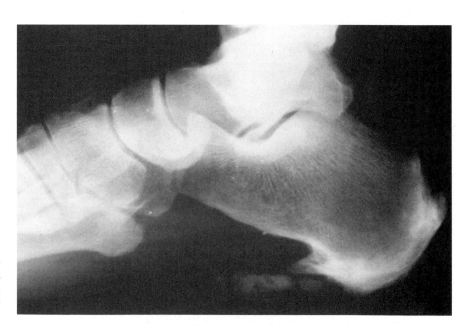

FIGURE 71–6 · Calcaneal Spurs at the Plantar Fascial Insertion, with Sclerosis and Fluffy Periosteal New Bone. Note ossification of the plantar fascia and normal ankle and talonavicular joints.

Chapter 70). When symptoms permit, range-of-motion and isometric strengthening exercises are probably helpful. Formal studies on the effect of joint resting and splinting have not been performed. Short-term exercise does not improve most parameters of spinal mobility.[51] There are no good studies on the effect of diet or other modalities of alternative medicine.

Because reactive arthritis is induced by a preceding bacterial infection, multiple trials of antibiotics for varying periods have been carried out. It is quite clear that the selection, dose, and length of use of antibiotics should be tailored only to treat any acute infection, if needed. As for extension beyond the acute phase, a combination of 10 separate studies shows that it will not result in a significant improvement in the long-term outcome of reactive arthritis.[52]

Topical corticosteroids and keratolytic agents are useful for keratoderma blenorrhagica. Circinate balanitis should be treated with weak topical corticosteroids such as hydro-cortisone valerate cream. More resistant skin lesions usually respond to methotrexate (MTX) or retinoids, such as etretinate. Phototherapy, especially Psoralen with exposure to ultraviolet A light PUVA, is reserved for the more resistant skin lesions, but there is a risk for late-onset genital cancer and melanoma. *Chlamydia* infection of the conjunctivae requires antibiotic treatment. Anterior uveitis should be promptly treated with frequent applications of topical corticosteroids, mydriatics, and cycloplegics.

If a patient fails on NSAID treatment, then a disease-modifying antirheumatic drug (DMARD) rather than systemic corticosteroids should be employed, because systemic corticosteroids are rarely beneficial, even at moderate doses of 20 to 40 mg/day. Sulfasalazine is the only nonbiologic DMARD that has been tested in double-blind controlled studies.[53,54] It has a modest effect on peripheral arthritis but does not improve axial disease. It is still indicated in localities where more effective DMARDs are unavailable or unaffordable. Sulfasalazine is started at 500 mg/day, with gradual weekly increase to 1 g twice a day. If there is still no response in 3 to 4 weeks, it can be increased to a maximum of 3 g/day. The enteric-coated form of sulfasalazine is preferred. If an improvement appears, the drug can be decreased gradually after 6 months and then stopped completely. If the drug is ineffective after 4 months at maximum tolerable dose, it should be discontinued. Most of the side effects are nausea, flatulence, and headache. Anemia, leucopenia, and hepatotoxicity can occur. In populations with glucose-6-phosphate dehydrogenase deficiency, a screening test is required. For monitoring, complete blood counts and liver chemistry are recommended every 2 weeks for the first 3 months, and subsequently every 3 months. If a skin rash develops, the drug should be discontinued. Oligospermia may cause infertility in men, but it may be reversed by stopping the drug for 6 months. There is no study to indicate how long it should be used. Because undifferentiated spondyloarthropathy and reactive arthritis are potentially self-remitting diseases, clinicians can consider stopping treatment after 6 months or remission.

There are no double-blind control studies on the use of other DMARDs, such as MTX, in treatment of reactive arthritis and undifferentiated spondyloarthropathy.

Their efficacy in most patients is not dramatic and rather doubtful. If the drug is not effective within 6 months, it should be discontinued.

The most effective treatment currently is with a TNF-α inhibitor: etanercept or infliximab. Etanercevt has been approved by the Food and Drug Administration (FDA) for treatment of AS. Additional TNF-α inhibitors such as/adalimumab might also become available for spondyloarthropathy. Although a consensus statement among experts on their use in AS will be available shortly, there are no published guidelines for undifferentiated spondyloarthropathy indicating when these agents should be used. The decision should be made individually with each patient, or based on the response to a 1 to 2 month trial. There is no doubt that both biologics are extremely useful in patients with AS. At least 80 percent of AS patients will respond to these agents, with 50 percent showing at least 50-percent improvement. This response is very similar to that seen in a 12-week, double-blind, placebo-controlled trial of 40 spondyloarthropathy patients, which included undifferentiated spondyloarthropathy.[55] These patients received intravenous infusions of 5 mg/kg of infliximab at 0, 2, and 6 weeks. Seventeen of 18 patients who completed the trial experienced dramatic improvement in disease activity with significant improvement noted as early as week 2. The same investigators carried out an open-label pilot study with similar beneficial results.[56] There was no loss of efficacy when the open trial was extended to 1 year.[57] Synovial histology of the knee in responsive patients showed reduced synovial lining thickness, vascularity, and infiltration with neutrophils and macrophages.[58] A small open-label study of six patients with undifferentiated spondyloarthropathy suggests that the effect of 3 mg/kg is less than that of 5 mg/kg.[59] For practical purposes, it is reasonable to start treatment with 3 mg/kg at weeks 0, 2, 6, and then continue treatment every 8 weeks. The dose can be increased and the infusion intervals shortened according to clinical response. Most patients will require increases in dose as well as frequency of infusions. There are no controlled studies on the effect of etanercept in spondyloarthropathy patients other than AS. An open study indicates that the effect is also dramatic and rapid.[60] Anecdotal reports suggest that these biologics are also effective in patients with reactive arthritis without reactivating the initiating infections. Open studies indicate that they are also useful in juvenile spondyloarthropathy.[44]

For both infliximab and etanercept, the spectrum of side effects resembles that seen in patients treated for rheumatoid arthritis (RA). As in RA, disseminated tuberculosis is a possible side effect of infliximab therapy, and one case was reported in the placebo-controlled trial.[55] Anti–TNF-α therapy is, of course, contraindicated with patients with HIV infections. It will take several more years to discover whether these biologics will actually arrest the progression of spondyloarthropathy. Judging by the long-term beneficial response in RA and the case reports of resolution of calcaneal enthesitis[61] and axial enthesitis by scintigraphy[62] during infliximab treatment, there is considerable hope that disease progression can be halted. In the etanercept study, more than 80 percent of MRI-positive active entheseal lesions either improved or regressed with treatment[60] (Box 71–1).

Box 71-1

Treatment Plan in Spondyloarthropathy

1. Eradicate acute bacterial infection with an antibiotic
2. Use nonsteroidal anti-inflammatory drug (NSAID) to relieve pain and inflammation
3. Add an opioid if necessary
4. Inject swollen joints and tendons with glucocorticoid
5. For painful sacroiliac joint, inject under computed tomography (CT) guidance
6. Add disease-modifying antirheumatic drug (DMARD) if the disease is still active and progressive; use sulfasalazine if biologics are unavailable
7. Infliximab and etanercept will lead to rapid and dramatic improvement in the majority of patients with severe disease

---

Course and Prognosis Prior to the Availability of Biologics

The introduction of TNF-α inhibitor therapy promises to drastically improve the course and prognosis of the spondyloarthropathies. The following data describe patients before this new era. This information is important to assist a clinician in deciding whether a particular patient with undifferentiated spondyloarthropathy should be placed on a biologic. At least five studies of 2 to 10 years follow-up have been published.[63] Thirteen to 34 percent of patients in the studies became asymptomatic, and 12 to 59 percent developed into a definite form of spondyloarthropathy, mostly AS. The others remained categorized as undifferentiated or probable spondyloarthropathy, typically in the form of recurrent oligoarthritis (Table 71-5). When first seen, there are no clinical or laboratory features that can predict an outcome for an individual patient. It is possible that the development of more sensitive imaging techniques for sacroiliitis may provide prognostic help, but this remains to be tested.

For reactive arthritis, the course and prognosis vary with the pathogen and the particular patient. Table 71–6 shows the outcome of reactive arthritis induced by three enteric pathogens and by *Chlamydia*. The number of patients studied for *Campylobacter*-induced arthritis is too small for meaningful comparison. As for those who evolve into chronic arthritis, two features contribute to a severe form: *Chlamydia* as the infective agent and HLA-B27 positivity.

The effect of treatment by biologics on the course of these spondyloarthropathies will require many years of follow-up to become clear. The improvement of inflammation observed by MRI is very encouraging.

Future Directions

The current status of understanding of spondyloarthropathy is not unlike that of RA. The basic arthritis-causing mechanisms are postulated to be either an antigen-driven lymphocyte response or cellular processes independent of the immune responses. Like RA, it is now certain that spondyloarthropathy is mediated by multiple genes of

TABLE 71–5 • OUTCOME OF UNDIFFERENTIATED SPONDYLOARTHROPATHY AFTER 2 TO 10 YEARS OF FOLLOW-UP

Authors	Patients	% HLA-B27	Follow-up	% Progression
Sany et al[64]	23	100	2.3 years	Definite SpA: 30
Schattenkirchner et al[65]	119	100	2 to 6 years	Definite SpA: 25 Recurrent oligoarthritis: 26 Asymptomatic: 34
Mau et al[66]	54	76	10 years	Definite SpA: 59 Unchanged: 19
Sampaio-Barros et al[63]	68	54	2 years	Definite SpA: 12 Unchanged: 75 Remission: 13

TABLE 71–6 • OUTCOME OF REACTIVE ARTHRITIS

	Yersinia		Salmonella		Shigella		Chlamydia
Years of follow-up	4 to 5	10	1.5 to 2	5	2	20	10 to 20
Number of patients	58	111	17	27	6	100	
% recovered	19	45	5/6*	33	1/6*	20	30
% arthralgia	32	20	0/6*	NA	3/6*	NA	68
% recurrent arthritis	3	6	8/17*	37	3/6*	18	38
% chronic arthritis	8	2	NA	52	2/6*	18	16
Ankylosing spondylitis	7	15	NA	NA	NA	14	26

*These values are absolute numbers and not percentages.

Abbreviations: NA, not available.

which the MHC play a critical but only partial role. Identifying the yet unknown arthritis-causing genes or the biologic processes they mediate is very important. This will allow a more rational approach to classification, diagnosis, treatment, and prevention of these diseases.

REFERENCES

1. Amor B, Dougados M, Mijiyawa M: Criteres de classification des spondyloarthropathies. Reve Rhum 57:85, 1990.
2. Dougados M, van der Linden S, Juhlin R, et al: The European spondyloarthropathy study group preliminary criteria for the classification of spondyloarthropathy. Arthritis Rheum 34:1218, 1991.
3. Gomariz E, del Mazo A, Guijo V, et al: The potential of European Spondyloarthropathy Study Group Spondyloarthropathy classification criteria as diagnostic aid in rheumatic practice. J Rheumatol 29:326, 2002.
4. Reiter H: Ueber eine bister unerkannte Spirochateninfektion (Spirochaetosis arthritica). Dtsch Med Wschr 42:1535, 1916.
5. Wilkens R, Arnett F, Bitter T, et al: Reiter's syndrome: Evaluation of preliminary criteria for definite disease. Arthritis Rheum 24:844, 1981.
6. Ahvonen P, Sievers K, Aho K: Arthritis associated with *Yersinia enterocolitica* infection. Acta Rheum Scand 15:232, 1969.
7. Sibilia J, Limbach F-X: Reactive arthritis or chronic infectious arthritis? Ann Rheum Dis 61:580, 2002.
8. Braun J, Kingsley G, D v. d. H, Sieper J: On the difficulties of establishing a consensus on the definition of and diagnostic investigations for reactive arthritis: Results and discussion of a questionnaire prepared for the 4th International Workshop on Reactive Arthritis, Berlin, Germany, July 3-6, 1999. J Rheumatol 27:2185, 2000.
9. Saraux A, Guedes C, Allain J, et al: Prevalence of rheumatoid arthritis and spondyloarthropathy in Brittany, France, Societe de Rhumatologie de l'Quest. J Rheumatol 26:2622, 1999.
10. Braun J, Bollow M, Remlinger G, et al: Prevalence of spondyloarthropathies in HLA-B27 positive and negative donors. Arthritis Rheum 41:58, 1988.
11. Lau C, Burgos-Vargas R, Louthrenoo W, et al: Features of spondyloarthropathies around the world. Rheum Dis Clin North Am 24:753, 1998.
12. Boyer G, Templin D, Cornoni-Huntley J, et al: Prevalence of spondyloarthropathies in Alaskan Eskimos. J Rheumatol 21:2292, 1994.
13. Michet C, Machado E, Ballard D, McKenna C: Epidemiology of Reiter's syndrome in Rochester, Minnesota. Arthritis Rheum 31:428, 1988.
14. Silman A. *In*: M. C. H., Alan J Silman (eds): Epidemiology of the Rheumatic Diseases. New York, 2001.
15. Isomaki H, Raunio J, von Essen R, et al: Incidence of rheumatic diseases in Finland. Scand J Rheumatol 7:188, 1979.
16. Kvien T, Glennas A, Melby K, et al: Reactive arthritis: Incidence, triggering agents and clinical presentation. J Rheumatol 21:115, 1994.
17. Iliopoulos A, Karras D, Ioakimidis D, et al: Changes in the epidemiology of Reiter's syndrome (reactive arthritis) in the post-AIDS era? An analysis of cases appearing in the Greek army. J Rheumatol 22:252, 1995.
18. Rich E, Hook ER, Alarcon G, Moreland L: Reactive arthritis in patients attending an urban sexually transmitted diseases clinic. Arthritis Rheum 39:1172, 1996.
19. Ekman P, Kirveskari J, Granfors K: Modification of disease outcome in Salmonella-infected patients by HLA-B27. Arthritis Rheum 43:1527, 2000.
20. Hannu T, Mattila L, Rautelin H, et al: Campylobacter-triggered reactive arthritis: a population-based study. Rheumatology 41:312, 2002.
21. Leirisalo-Repo M: Enteric infections and arthritis: clinical aspects. *In* C A, T JD (eds): The Spondylarthritides. Oxford, 1998, p 59.
22. Luthrenoo W: Musculoskeletal manifestation of HIV infection in Thailand: An analysis of 100 cases. J Clin Rheumatol 3:258, 1997.
23. Yu D, Kuipers J: Role of bacteria and HLA-B27 in the pathogenesis of reactive arthritis. Rheum Dis Clin North Am 29:1, 2003.

24. Kuipers JG, Jurgens-Saathoff B, Bialowons A, et al: Detection of *Chlamydia trachomatis* in peripheral blood leukocytes of reactive arthritis patients by polymerase chain reaction. Arthritis Rheum 41:1894, 1998.
25. Gerard HC, Branigan PJ, Schumacher HR Jr., Hudson AP: Synovial *Chlamydia trachomatis* in patients with reactive arthritis/Reiter's syndrome are viable but show aberrant gene expression. J Rheumatol 25:734, 1998.
26. Goodall J, Yeo G, Huang M, et al: Identification of *Chlamydia trachomatis* antigens recognized by human CD4+ T lymphocytes by screening an expression library. Euro J Immunol 31:1513, 2001.
27. Marker-Hermann E, Hohler T: Pathogenesis of human leukocyte antigen-positive arthritis. Rheum Dis Clin North Am 24:865, 1998.
28. Kuon W, Holzhutter HG, Appel H, et al: Identification of HLA-B27-restricted peptides from the *Chlamydia trachomatis* proteome with possible relevance to HLA-B27-associated diseases. J Immunol 167:4738, 2001.
29. Dulphy N, Peyrat MA, Tieng V, et al: Common intra-articular T cell expansions in patients with reactive arthritis: identical beta-chain junctional sequences and cytotoxicity toward HLA-B27. J Immunol 162:3830, 1999.
30. Ramos M, De Castro J: HLA-B27 and the pathogenesis of spondyloarthritis. Tissue Antigens 60:191, 2002.
31. Madden DR, Gorga JC, Strominger JL, Wiley DC: The structure of HLA-B27 reveals nonamer self-peptides bound in an extended conformation. Nature 353:321, 1991.
32. Tsai W, Chen C, Yen J, et al: Free HLA class I heavy chain-carrying monocytes: a potential role in the pathogenesis of spondyloarthropathies. J Rheumatol 966, 2002.
33. Allen R, Bowness P, McMichael A: The role of HLA-B27 in spondyloarthritis. Immunogenetics 50:220, 1999.
34. Colbert RA: HLA-B27 misfolding: a solution to the spondyloarthropathy conundrum? Molec Med Today 6:224, 2000.
35. Ikawa T, Ikeda M, Yamaguchi A, et al: Expression of arthritis-causing HLA-B27 on Hela cells promotes induction of c-fos in response to in vitro invasion by Salmonella typhimurium. J Clin Invest 101:263, 1998.
36. Gu J, Rihl M, Marker-Hermann E, et al: Clues to the pathogenesis of spondyloarthropathy derived from synovial-fluid-mononuclear-cell gene expression profiles. J Rheumatol 2159, 2002.
37. Collantes E, Veroz R, Escudero A, et al: Can some cases of "possible" spondyloarthropathy be classified as "definite" or "undifferentiated" spondyloarthropathy? Value of criteria for spondyloarthropathies. Joint Bone Spine 67:516, 2000.
38. Sieper J, Rudwaleit M, Braun J, van der Heijde D: Diagnosing reactive arthritis: Role of clinical setting in the value of serologic and microbiologic assays. Arthritis Rheum 2002:319, 2001.
39. Magro C, Crowson A, Peeling R: Vasculitis as the basis of cutaneous lesions in Reiter's disease. Hum Pathol 26:633, 1995.
40. Keat A: Reiter's syndrome and reactive arthritis in perspective. N Engl J Med 309:1606, 1983.
41. Arnett F: Seronegative spondyloarthropathies. Bull Rheum Dis 37:1, 1987.
42. Cuellar M, Espinoza L: Rheumatic manifestations of HIV-AIDS. Bailliere's Clin Rheumatol 14:579, 2000.
43. Njobvu P, McGill P, Kerr H, et al: Spondyloarthropathy and human immunodeficiency virus infection in Zambia. J Rheumatol 25:1553, 1998.
44. Huang F, Zhang J, Zhu J, Yang C: Juvenile spondyloarthropathies: The Chinese experience. Rheum Dis Clin North Am, in press.
45. Wollenhaupt J, Kolbus F, Weissbrodt H, et al: Manifestations of Chlamydia induced arthritis in patients with silent versus symptomatic urogenital chlamydial infection. Clin Exper Rheumatol 13:453, 1995.
46. Fendler C, Laitko S, Sorensen H, et al: Frequency of triggering bacteria in patients with reactive arthritis and undifferentiated oligoarthritis and the relative importance of tests used for diagnsosis. Ann Rheum Dis 60:337, 2001.
47. Johnson R, Newhall W, Papp J, et al: Screening tests to detect *Chlamydia trachomatis* and *Neiseeria gonorrhoeae* infections - 2002. MMWR Recomm Rep 51(RR-15):1, 2002.
48. Baeten D, Demeter P, Cuvelier C, et al: Comparative study of the synovial histology in rheumatoid arthritis, spondyloarthropathy, and osteoarthritis: influence of disease duration and activity. Ann Rheum Dis 59:945, 2000.

49. Dougados M, Behier J, Jolchine I, et al: Efficacy of celecoxib, a cyclooxygenase 2-specific inhibitor, in the treatment of ankylosing spondylitis: a six-week controlled study with comparison against placebo and against a conventional nonsteriodal antiinflammatory drug. Arthritis Rheum 44:180, 2001.

50. Ytterberg S, Mahowald M, Woods S: Codeine and oxycodone use in patients with chronic rheumatic disease pain. Arthritis Rheum 42:830, 1999.

51. Heikkila S, Viitanen J, Kautiainen H, Kauppi M: Sensitivity to change of mobility tests: effect of short term intensive physiotherapy and exercise on spinal, hip, and shoulder measurements in spondyloarthropathy. J Rheumatol 27:1251, 2000.

52. Leirisalo-Repo M: Prognosis, course of disease, and treatment of the spondyloarthropathies. Rheum Dis Clin North Am 24:737, 1998.

53. Dougados M, van der Linden S, Leirisalo-Repo M, et al: Sulfasalazine in the treatment of spondyloarthropathy: A randomized, double blind, placebo controlled study. Arthritis Rheum 38:618, 1995.

54. Clegg D, Reda D, Weisman M, et al: Comparison of sulfasalazine and placebo in the treatment of reactive arthritis (Reiter's syndrome). A Department of Veterans Affairs Cooperative Study. Arthritis Rheum 39:2021, 1996.

55. Van den Bosch F, Kruithof E, Baeten D: Randomized double-blind comparison of chimeric monoclonal antibody to tumor necrosis factor a (infliximab) versus placebo in active spondyloarthropathy. Arthritis Rheum 46:755, 2002.

56. Van den Bosch F, Kruithof E, Baeten D, et al: Effects of a loading dose regimen of three infusions of chimeric monoclonal antibody to tumour necrosis factor alpha (infliximab) in spondyloarthropathy: an open pilot study. Ann Rheum Dis 59:428, 2000.

57. Kruithof E, Van den Bosch F, Baeten D, et al: Repeated infusions of infliximab, a chimeric anti-TNF alpha monoclonal antibody, in patients with active spondyloarthropathy: one year follow up. Ann Rheum Dis 61:207, 2002.

58. Baeten D, Kruithof K, Van den Bosch F: Immunomodulatory effects of anti-tumor necrosis factor a therapy on synovium in spondyloarthropathy. Arthritis Rheum 44:186, 2001.

59. Brandt J, Haibel H, Reddig J, et al: Successful short term treatment of severe undifferentiated spondyloarthroapthy with anti-tumor necrosis factor-alpha monoclonal antibody infliximab. J Rheumatol 29:118, 2002.

60. Marzo-Ortega H, McGonagle D, O'Connor P, Emery P: Efficacy of etanercept in the treatment of the entheseal pathology in resistant spondyloarthropathy: a clinical and magnetic resonance imaging study. Arthritis Rheum 44:2112, 2001.

61. D'Agostino M, Breban M, Said-Nahal R: Refractory inflammatory heel pain in spondyloarthropathy: a significant response to infliximab documented by ultrasound. Arthritis Rheum 46:840, 2002.

62. Haidi A, Hicking P, Brown M: Scintigraphic evidence of effect of infliximab on disease activity in ankylosing spondylitis. Rheumatology 41:114, 2002.

63. Sampaio-Barros P, Bertolo M, Kraemer M, et al: Undifferentiated spondyloarthropathies: a 2-year follow-up study. Clin Rheumatol 20:201, 2001.

64. Sany J, Ronsenberg F, Panis G, Serre H: Unclassified HLA-B27 inflammatory rheumatic diseases: follow-up of 23 patients. Arthritis Rheum 23:258, 1980.

65. Schattenkirchner M, Kruger K: Natural course and prognosis of HLA-B27 oligoarthritis. Clin Rheumatol 6(Suppl 2):83, 1987.

66. Mau W, Zeidler H, Mau R, et al: Clinical features and prognosis of patients with possible ankylosing spondylitis: results of a 10-year followup. J Rheumatol 15:1109, 1988.

72

Psoriatic Arthritis

DAFNA D. GLADMAN

Psoriatic arthritis (PsA) is an inflammatory arthritis associated with psoriasis. It was initially considered a variant of rheumatoid arthritis (RA) but was distinguished from it when it was found that the majority of patients with PsA were seronegative for rheumatoid factor (RF). Although most patients with PsA have a benign course, a subset of patients has a severe, unrelenting, and sometimes mutilating form of arthritis.

Epidemiology

The first description of arthritis in a patient with psoriasis was published in 1818, but the notion of a specific form of arthritis associated with psoriasis was first cultivated by Wright.[1] There is still debate as to whether PsA is a distinct entity.[2] It is argued that both psoriasis and arthritis are common conditions, and, thus, their occurrence in the same patient is expected. Extensive epidemiologic evidence, however, supports the concept of PsA as a distinct entity.

Whereas the prevalence of arthritis in the general population is estimated at 2 to 3 percent, in psoriatic patients, it varies from 7 to 42 percent.[2] Conversely, the prevalence of psoriasis in persons with arthritis is 2.6 to 7.0 percent, whereas it is 0.1 to 2.8 percent in the general population.[2-4] Moreover, the descriptions of the arthritis associated with psoriasis suggest that it is a distinct entity. Unlike osteoarthritis (OA), PsA is inflammatory in nature and affects both proximal and distal joints. It differs from RA by the lack of gender preference, the frequent involvement of distal interphalangeal (DIP) joints, the tendency to asymmetry, the absence of rheumatoid factor (RF), the presence of spondyloarthropathy, the association with HLA-B27, and the presence of extra-articular features common to the spondyloarthropathies. Therefore, PsA is considered an inflammatory arthritis associated with psoriasis and usually seronegative for RF. It is classified among the seronegative, HLA-B27-associated spondyloarthropathies.

The exact prevalence of PsA is unknown, and estimates have varied from 0.04 to 1.4 percent. A recent survey of the National Psoriasis Foundation[5] identified a prevalence of 1.5 percent.

Pathogenesis

The exact etiology of PsA is unclear. Genetic, immunologic, and environmental elements are thought to play a role in the perpetuation of the inflammatory process.[6,7]

GENETIC FACTORS

Psoriasis and PsA have a familial clustering. Specific family investigations have shown that the disease is much more likely to occur in first-degree relatives of affected individuals than in the general population or in spouses.[8] Twin studies in psoriasis have also demonstrated the genetic predisposition to the disease, with a high rate of concordance in monozygotic twins.[9] Population studies have shown that psoriasis is associated with the HLA antigens B13, B16 (particularly its B39 split), B17, B27, B37, B38, Cw6, DR4, and DR7.[10] HLA-B7 and HLA-B27 identify patients with psoriasis destined for the development of arthritis. HLA-DR7a has been found in high frequency among patients with psoriasis and PsA.[9] HLA-Cw*0602 is increased in both psoriasis and PsA and is associated with an earlier age of onset of psoriasis.[11] Whereas T cell receptor gene expression has not been found to be biased in PsA, Southern blot analysis using DNA probes for the immunoglobulin H (IgH) gene region (immunoglobulin heavy chain gene on chromosome 14q32) suggests that the gene may confer susceptibility to arthritis in patients with psoriasis.[9] Another set of genes that may be important in the etiopathogenesis of PsA include the killer immunoglobulin-like receptor (KIR) genes. These genes are located on chromosome 19q13.4. KIRs are present on natural killer (NK) cells and participate in the normal function of innate immunity (see Chapter 8). There are both inhibitory and activating KIRs. KIRs recognize HLA molecules as their ligands, particularly those encoded by the B and C loci. A recent study found that KIR2DS1/2DS2, in the absence of their corresponding ligands, are independent susceptibility genes for PsA.[12]

In psoriasis, whole-genome scans have demonstrated linkage with loci on chromosomes 17q, 4q, and 6p.[13] The strongest evidence for linkage is on chromosome 6p. However, none of the linkage studies in psoriasis have attempted to identify the susceptibility genes related to PsA. A recent study identified a locus for PsA on chromosome 16q.[14] PsA is a clinically heterogeneous disorder, and it is likely, therefore, that a number of different genes with low-to-moderate penetrance play a role in susceptibility. One aspect of such genetic heterogeneity is a "parent of origin" effect in which there is heterogeneity of linkage of paternal and maternal meiosis. Recent studies in psoriasis and PsA have demonstrated a differential expression of disease depending on the gender of the disease-transmitting parent. For both these disorders, an excess paternal transmission pattern has been noted.[15,16]

IMMUNOLOGIC FACTORS

The pathology of skin and joint lesions in PsA is that of an inflammatory reaction, and there is evidence for autoimmunity as well, perhaps mediated by complement activation.[17] The inflammatory nature of the skin and joint lesions in PsA is demonstrated by synovial lining cell hyperplasia and mononuclear infiltration, resembling the histopathologic changes in RA.[18] However, there is less synovial lining hyperplasia, fewer macrophages, and greater vascularity in PsA compared to RA synovium. The cytokine profile in PsA reflects a complex interplay between T cells and monocytes or macrophages. The presence of T helper type 1 (Th1) cytokines (i.e., tumor necrosis factor-α [TNF-α], interleukin [IL]-1β and IL-10) in PsA was higher than in a group of RA patients, suggesting that these two disorders may result from different underlying mechanisms.[19]

Antinuclear antibodies have been demonstrated in the sera of patients with PsA and have been thought to react with stratum corneum antigens. Antiepidermal keratin and anti-cytokeratin18 (CK18) antibodies have also been found in the sera of patients with psoriasis and PsA.[17,20]

Several studies have shown a significant reduction in the number and percentage of cell determinant (CD)4+ T cells in the peripheral blood, although they are found throughout the skin lesions and synovium.[17] Dendritic cells have been found in the synovial fluid of patients with PsA and are reactive in the mixed-leukocyte reaction[21]; the inference is that the dendritic cells present an unknown antigen to CD4+ cells within the joints and skin of patients with PsA, leading to T cell activation.[17,22] Fibroblasts from the skin and synovia of patients with PsA have an increased proliferative activity and the capability to secrete increased amounts of IL-1, IL-6, and platelet-derived growth factors (PDGFs).[23,24] Several studies suggest that cytokines secreted from activated T cells and other mononuclear proinflammatory cells induce proliferation and activation of synovial and epidermal fibroblasts. T lymphocytes, particularly CD8+ cells, are thought to play an important role in the pathogenesis of both the skin and joint manifestations.[17,20,22,25] Moreover, common clonal expansions of the T cell antigen receptor beta chain variable (TCRβV) gene repertoires in both skin and synovium were documented, suggesting both manifestations may be triggered by a common antigen.[26] Injection of activated T cells from individuals affected with psoriasis into a severe combined immunodeficiency (SCID) mouse previously engrafted with unaffected human skin lead to the development of psoriasis in the graft and surrounding skin.[27] These activated T cells likely contribute to the enhanced production of cytokines noted both in the synovial fluid and synovial cultures from patients with PsA.[19] Monocytes may also play an important role in the pathogenesis of PsA.[28] Monocytes are responsible for the production of metalloproteinase-2 (MMP-2) and MMP-9, which have been demonstrated to be increased in PsA and to correlate with higher vascularity.[29,30] These cytokines are thought to mediate cartilage erosion in inflammatory arthritides. More recently, Ritchlin and colleagues[31] described an expanded population of osteoclast precursors in the peripheral blood of patients with PsA, as well as enhanced osteoclastogenesis by supernatant released by peripheral blood mononuclear cells from these patients. They suggest that this enhanced osteoclastogenesis may explain the erosive nature of the disease. The fact that anti-TNF therapy led to a reduction in the number of these precursor cells lends credence to this theory.

Psoriatic plaques in skin have increased levels of leukotriene B_4.[32] Injections of leukotriene B_4 cause intraepidermal microabscesses, suggesting a role for this compound in the development of psoriasis.[33]

ENVIRONMENTAL FACTORS

Infections

The temporal relationship between certain viral or bacterial infections and the development or exacerbation of psoriasis or PsA suggests a pathogenetic role for these organisms.[6] The response to streptococcal antigens by cells from patients with PsA, however, was no different from that of cells from patients with RA,[34] making the role of *Streptococcus* in PsA doubtful. Psoriasis and PsA have also been reported to be associated with human immunodeficiency virus (HIV) infection.[35] Although the prevalence of psoriasis in patients infected with HIV is similar to that in the general population, patients with HIV usually have more extensive erythrodermic psoriasis, and patients with psoriasis may present with exacerbation of their skin disease after being infected with HIV.

Trauma

A few studies have reported the occurrence of arthritis and acroosteolysis following physical trauma in patients with psoriasis. A retrospective search of medical records revealed that 12 (9 percent) of 138 patients with PsA, and only 2 (1 percent) of 138 RA patients experienced acute illness or trauma before the onset of their arthritis.[36] Clinical and laboratory findings of 25 post-traumatic PsA patients was similar to 275 PsA patients without a history of trauma, except for erythrocyte sedimentation rate (ESR) and C-reactive protein (CRP) at disease onset (first 6 months). These differences in acute-phase responses were not sustained in follow-up of these patients.[37] It has been suggested that trauma-induced arthritis represents a deep Koebner phenomenon,[38] perhaps related to peripheral nerve release of substance P.[39]

▮ Clinical Features

PsA is a systemic inflammatory disease with articular and extra-articular features.[4,40-50] The onset of arthritis is usually insidious, but it can occur acutely. There are five general patterns of PsA[4]:

1. Arthritis of the DIP joints (Fig. 72–1)
2. Destructive (mutilans) arthritis (Fig. 72–2)

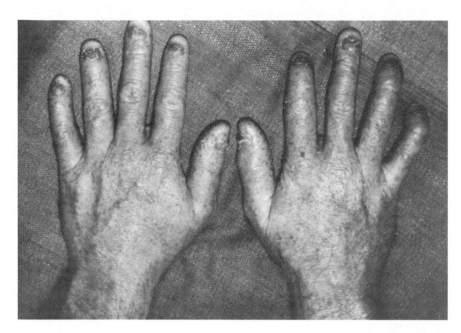

FIGURE 72–1 · Arthritis of the Distal Interphalangeal Joints (DIP) in a Patient with Psoriatic Arthritis (PsA).

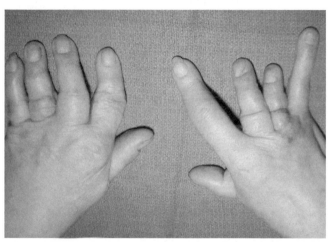

FIGURE 72–2 · Destructive Arthritis (arthritis mutilans) Involving all Digits, some with Shortening, others with Ankylosis. (See color plate 36.)

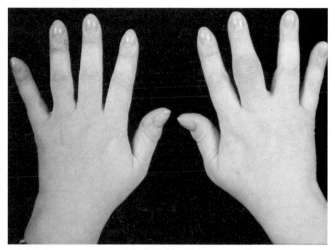

FIGURE 72–4 · Asymmetric Oligoarthritis Involving the Third Proximal Interphalangeal Joint; the Other Hand is Normal. (See color plate 38.)

3. Symmetric polyarthritis indistinguishable from RA (Fig. 72–3)
4. Asymmetric oligoarthritis (Fig. 72–4)
5. Spondyloarthropathy (Figs. 72–5 and 72–6)

Variability in definition of symmetry, symmetric oligoarthritis, and peripheral and axial overlap pattern has led to differences in the reported frequency of the subsets of PsA among different studies[40-50] (Table 72–1). Most patients with PsA present with polyarthritis. All peripheral joints may be involved in PsA. Spondyloarthropathy alone occurs in only 2 to 4 percent of the patients. Moreover, it is clear that patterns of PsA are not permanent: More than 60 percent change from their initial pattern.[47,51] A patient may begin with an oligoarticular pattern that evolves into polyarthritis; another patient presenting with polyarticular disease may end up with only a few involved joints. The arthritis is inflammatory in nature, presenting with

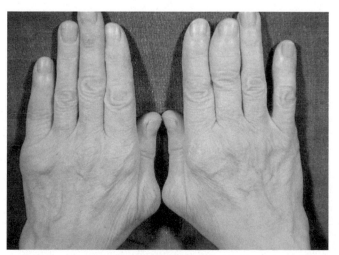

FIGURE 72–3 · Symmetric Polyarthritis Indistinguishable from Rheumatoid Arthritis (RA). (See color plate 37.)

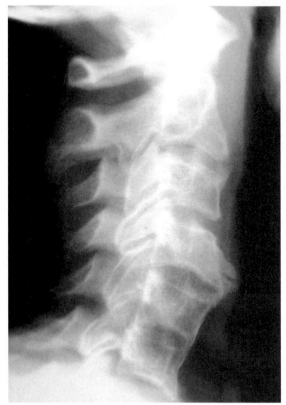

FIGURE 72-5 · Both Classic (C5-6) and Paramarginal (C4-5) Syndesmophytes in the Cervical Spine of a Patient with Psoriatic Arthritis (PsA).

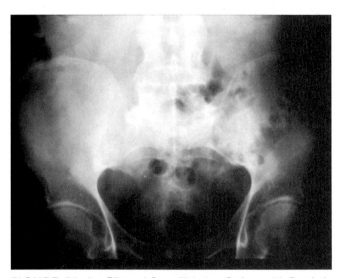

FIGURE 72-6 · Bilateral Sacroiliitis in a Patient with Psoriatic Arthritis (PsA). Note syndesmophytes in the lower lumbar vertebrae.

pain and swelling in the affected joints. The joints may be erythematous. Patients with PsA have been found to be less tender than patients with RA, a fact that may explain why it had been thought to be a mild disease.[51] Although PsA tends to have a more asymmetric distribution than RA, 53 percent of patients with polyarticular disease demonstrate symmetry.[43] Whether the presenting or subsequent pattern is of prognostic value has not been resolved.

Spondyloarthropathy develops in 20 to 40 percent of the patients, but rarely is it detected at the onset of PsA.[52] The spondyloarthropathy tends to affect men and older patients and tends to begin later in the course of the disease.[51–54] In many patients, the spondyloarthropathy was diagnosed only after radiography at first visit to the PsA clinic.[51,53] The clinical features of the spondyloarthropathy include sacroiliitis, which is often asymmetric; and spinal disease similar to ankylosing spondylitis (AS) associated with pain and stiffness of the cervical, thoracic, and lumbar spine. Sixty-five percent of psoriatic patients with spondyloarthropathy reported inflammatory neck or back pain or back stiffness, and 17 percent had clinical sacroiliitis (based on eliciting pain in the sacroiliac region by Gaenslen or flexion abduction external rotation [FABER] maneuvers).[53] In one study,[54] there was radiologic evidence for cervical spine involvement in 40 (70 percent) of 57 patients with PsA, only 40 percent of whom had symptoms of inflammatory neck disease. In another study,[55] sacroiliitis was detected radiographically in 71 percent of the patients. Patients with AS have more severe spinal disease,[56] as evidenced by the presence of syndesmophytes and grade 4 sacroiliitis, whereas patients with PsA more commonly have peripheral arthritis. In both psoriatic spondyloarthropathy and AS, men have a more severe disease than women.[56]

Other clinical features of PsA include dactylitis, tenosynovitis, and enthesitis.[1,2,4,40-54] Dactylitis (Fig. 72–7) occurs in more than 30 percent of patients and is characterized by a diffuse swelling of the entire digit along with arthritis of the DIP, proximal interphalangeal, and metacarpophalangeal or metatarsophalangeal joints. Whether dactylitis reflects a severe inflammatory process in all of these joints, extensive tenosynovitis of a digit, or both, is unclear. Studies using ultrasound and magnetic resonance imaging (MRI) revealed effusions in the affected joints and within tendon sheaths.[57] Heel pain, a manifestation of enthesitis, can be severe and disabling (Fig. 72–8). Diffuse swelling of the upper limb in patients with PsA has also been described.[58]

ASSOCIATED EXTRA-ARTICULAR FEATURES

Most patients with PsA have the classic psoriasis vulgaris pattern of skin lesions. Association with pustular psoriasis and erythroderma have been reported as well.[59] There is no direct relation between the severity of skin lesions and the degree of joint inflammation in PsA.[50] Only 35 percent of the patients recognize a link between the joint and skin disease.[43] Indeed, in every study, 15 to 20 percent of the patients have joint disease that preceded the skin manifestations (see Table 72–1). Nail lesions, including pitting, ridging, and onycholysis, are the only clinical feature of skin psoriasis significantly associated with the development of PsA. Nail lesions occur in 90 percent of patients with PsA and in only 41 percent of those with psoriasis uncomplicated by arthritis.[60]

Ocular involvement, either conjunctivitis or iritis, occurs in 7 to 33 percent of patients.[43,60,61] Aortic incompetence was reported in less than 4 percent of patients with psoriatic arthropathy and usually develops late in the course of the disease.[4]

TABLE 72–1 · CLINICAL FEATURES OF PSORIATIC ARTHRITIS (PSA) IN REPORTED SERIES

Feature	Roberts (1976)	Kammer (1979)	Scarpa (1984)	Gladman (1987)	Helliwell (1991)	Torre-Alonse (1991)	Veale (1994)	Jones (1994)	Trobace (1994)	Marsal (1999)	Cohen (1999)
No. of Patients	168	100	62	220	50	180	100	100	58	73	221
Male / Female	67/101	47/53	29/33	104/116	32/18	99/81	59/41	43/57	35/33	37/36	169/51
Age of Onset (yr)	36-45	33-45	40-60	37	39	39	34	37.6	42	42	37
Oligoarthritis(%)	53	54	16	14	14	37	43	26	50	7	?
Polyarthritis (%)	54	25	39	40	78	35	33	63	40	88	?
Distal (%)	17	?	7.5	12	0	0	16	1	?	4	?
Back (%)	5	21	21	2	6	7	4	6	?	1	?
Mutilans (%)	5	?	2.3	16	2	4	2	4	?	14	?
Sacroiliitis (%)	?	?	16	27	36	20	15	6	43	14	74
Joints Before Skin (%)	16	30	?	17	?	15	?	18	?	?	13.7

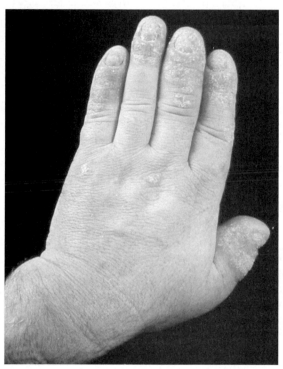

FIGURE 72–7 · Dactylitis in the Third Digit and Thumb in a Patient with Psoriatic Arthritis (PsA). (See color plate 39.)

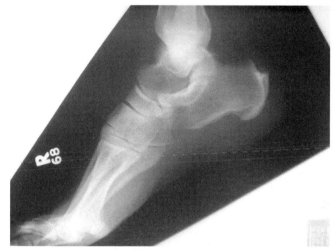

FIGURE 72–8 · Achilles Insertion Spur.

Laboratory Features

There is no diagnostic laboratory test for PsA. The ESR is elevated in 40 to 60 percent of the patients, particularly in those with the polyarticular form.[34] It may reflect the severity of the skin disease. In the past, the lack of RF activity was considered as the most distinctive laboratory feature of PsA.[1] Recent studies have indicated, however, that low titers of RF are detected in 5 to 16 percent of patients and that antinuclear autoantibodies are present in 2 to 16 percent of patients.[4,40-50,60] Hypergammaglobulinemia, particularly elevated IgA levels, and increased complement activity are also found.[43] Elevated uric acid levels in patients with PsA led to an erroneous diagnosis of gout in a patient presenting with acute monoarthritis.

It is, therefore, important to look for crystals in patients with PsA who present with an acutely inflamed joint, particularly in the presence of hyperuricemia. Hyperuricemia does not reflect the extent of skin involvement and is associated with other metabolic abnormalities in patients with PsA.[62]

RADIOGRAPHIC FEATURES

The radiographic features characteristic of PsA include asymmetric distribution, involvement of DIP joints, sacroiliitis and spondylitis, bone erosions with new bone formation, bony ankylosis, and resorption of the distal phalanges[63] (Fig. 72–9). The typical change in the peripheral joint is the "pencil-in-cup" picture of marked lysis of the distal end of a phalanx with remodeling of the proximal end of the more distal phalanx. Involvement of temporomandibular, sternoclavicular, and manubriosternal joints is common in PsA. The detection of abnormalities of these joints, however, requires special radiologic techniques, including computed tomography (CT) scan.[64] The presence of spurs and the periosteal reaction are also characteristic of the enthesopathy of PsA. In the spine, both typical

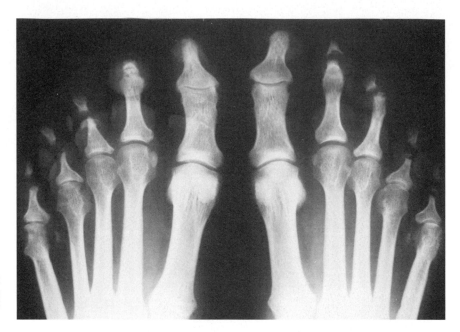

FIGURE 72–9 · Bone Resorption in Feet with "Pencil-in-cup" changes, as well as Resorption of Distal Tuft in Left First Distal Phalanx.

marginal syndesmophytes and paramarginal syndesmophytes are seen (see Fig. 72–6). The latter may be difficult to distinguish from the coarse paraspinal ossification seen in patients with diffuse idiopathic skeletal hyperostosis (DISH). The ossification of PsA is thick and fluffy, however, and patients with DISH have ossification primarily on the right side of the thoracic spine with normal sacroiliac joints.[53,54] The radiologic features of PsA may be as severe as those of RA.[65]

Diagnosis

There are no diagnostic or classification criteria for PsA.[2] The diagnosis is made when a patient with psoriasis presents with features of an inflammatory arthritis. The diagnosis is easier if RF is negative. If RF is positive, the clinician must try to rule out the possibility that the patient has a coexistence of both psoriasis and RA. A patient with psoriasis who presents only with DIP joint disease may also pose a diagnostic dilemma, because psoriasis and osteoarthritis can coexist; the presence of inflammatory features and the radiologic appearance may help to identify the correct diagnosis. It is more difficult to make the diagnosis of PsA in a patient not known to have psoriasis; clinical and radiographic features, including the pattern of the arthritis, the distribution and joints involved, and the presence of a spondyloarthropathy, may facilitate the diagnosis. It is, therefore, crucial to perform a careful history and physical examination, looking for hidden psoriatic lesions, particularly in the ears, the hairline, the umbilical area, the anal cleft, and the nails.

Clinical Course and Outcome

The course of PsA is usually characterized by flares and remissions. Arthritis mutilans was recognized as a typi-

cal form of PsA, and earlier studies suggested that PsA results in joint destruction and severe disability in a large proportion of the patients.[4] Destructive arthritis developed in 25 percent of patients with oligoarticular arthritis and 64 percent of the patients with polyarticular arthritis. Studies in earlier years have indicated that PsA is a mild disease and that only a minority of patients (less than 5 percent) experience erosive and deforming arthritis.[40,42] Of a large group of 220 patients with PsA, of whom 67 percent had at least one erosion, 37 (17 percent) had erosions in five or more joints.[43] Joint damage progresses despite control of the inflammatory process of the disease, and in 5 years of follow-up, the number of patients with five or more damaged joints more than doubles.[51] In one group of patients,[44] 57 percent had erosive arthritis and 19 percent had American Rheumatism Association (ARA) class III or IV functional impairment. A younger age at the onset of the arthritis, female gender, and acute onset of arthritis were more common in patients with severe arthritis.[51] Remission occurred in 17.6 percent of patients with PsA followed in a longitudinal clinic.[66] One study found that although death is no more common in patients hospitalized with PsA than in the general population, many patients have restricted functional ability.

A long-term follow-up study of patients with psoriatic spondyloarthropathy revealed a significant increase in the number of patients with syndesmophyte formation and sacroiliitis, although clinically these patients continued to have excellent spinal mobility, suggesting that spondyloarthropathy has a favorable prognosis.[53] A logistic regression analysis indicated that more advanced spondyloarthropathy occurs in men.[56]

A group of 305 patients who entered a PsA clinic with fewer than 10 deformed joints were observed prospectively.[67] The presence of five or more swollen joints and the use of advanced therapeutic modalities at first visit to the PsA clinic were associated with progression of deformities over the follow-up period. An ESR of less than 15 was "protective." There was no effect of disease duration on these findings. A further analysis of 276 patients who underwent HLA typing revealed that the HLA antigens HLA-B27, in the presence of HLA-DR7, and DQw3, in the absence of HLA-DR7, were predictors of progression through all states of damage, whereas B39 was associated with disease progression in early disease.[68] A further analysis of the addition of all HLA antigens noted among these patients to the previously mentioned model suggested that the presence of HLA-B22 was protective for progression of clinical damage.[69] A further study in the same clinic found that actively inflamed joints at each visit predict progression of damage in a subsequent visit.[70] A recent study from another center also identified the presence of polyarthritis as an indicator of disease progression.[71] Thus, it is important to monitor patients with PsA for active inflammation and treat them appropriately to prevent further joint damage.

Seven percent of patients followed in a large outpatient PsA clinic required musculoskeletal surgery.[72] The average disease duration prior to the first surgery was 13 years. The number of actively inflamed joints and the extent of radiologic damage at first assessment were highly predictive of subsequent surgery.

The mortality of PsA patients followed in a large outpatient clinic was noted to be significantly higher than that of the general population. Twelve percent of patients (53 patients) had died. The standard mortality ratio (SMR) for the female cohort was 1.59 and for the men was 1.65.[73] Overall, a 62-percent increased mortality risk was noted. Thirty-six percent of the deaths were attributed to disease of the circulatory system, 21 percent to respiratory system disease, 17 percent to malignant neoplasm, and 14.9 percent to injury or poisonings. A multivariate analysis revealed that ESR of more than 15 mm/hour, a high level of medication use prior to initial visit, radiologic damage, and absence of nail lesions were associated with an increased overall mortality.[74]

OUTCOME MEASURES IN PSORIATIC ARTHRITIS

Traditional methods of monitoring patients with rheumatic conditions include clinical assessment for joint inflammation and damage, as well as radiographic evaluations.[2] The methods used to evaluate patients with PsA are also those used to assess patients with RA. The American College of Rheumatology (ACR) joint count was found reliable in patients with PsA,[75] and the Ritchie articular index has also been used.[76] Clegg and colleagues[77] developed a new outcome measure for their clinical trial of sulfasalazine in PsA: the Psoriatic Arthritis Response Criteria (PsARC). The measure includes four items: tender joint count (which must be reduced by at least 30% for response), swollen joint count (must be reduced by 30% for response), physician global assessment (decreased by one point), and patient global assessment (decreased by one point for response) on a visual analogue scale. To count as a responder, a patient must demonstrate an improvement in at least two of the four items, one of which

must be either the tender or a swollen joint count. In addition, a patient must not demonstrate worsening in any of the items. Although the PsARC was not validated for face or construct validity prior to the study, it did show a modest response in the sulfasalazine trial and has since been used in other trials (see upcoming section on treatment) and appears to function well. Other features of PsA, such as dactylitis, tendinitis, and enthesitis, as well as the spondyloarthropathy, have not been adequately measured in PsA.

The radiologic scoring methods evaluating peripheral joints in PsA were all developed for patients with RA. A recent study validated the original Steinbrocker's, a modified Steinbrocker's, and Larsen's method for assessment of radiographs in patients with PsA.[78] The modified Steinbrocker's and Larsen's method were noted to be more responsive to change than the original Steinbrocker's. A radiologic method that includes both destruction and bony proliferation was recently developed and validated in a small group of patients with PsA.[79] These methods can now be used to assess disease progression in PsA.

Health status instruments are increasingly being used to assess outcome in rheumatologic diseases. The Health Assessment Questionnaire (HAQ), as well as its modification for spondyloarthropathy (HAQ-S), the Arthritis Impact Measurement Scales (AIMS/AIMS2), and a generic instrument known as the Medical Outcomes Study 36-item Short Form Health Survey (SF-36) have all been validated in PsA.[80] Based on these instruments, patients with PsA have reduced function and quality of life and fare as poorly as patients with RA.[81,82] The choice of the health status index used may partially depend on the dimension of most interest to the patient or physician. The HAQ, AIMS2, and SF-36 are responsive to changes in general health and to a lesser degree inflammatory disease activity. However, no instrument has demonstrated responsiveness to disease progression. Therefore, it may be prudent to use range of outcome measures to monitor patients with PsA.

▌ Treatment

The treatment of PsA is directed at controlling the inflammatory process. Although there is no clear correlation between the skin and joint inflammation in every patient, the skin and joint aspects of the disease need to be treated simultaneously. Initial treatment is nonsteroidal anti-inflammatory drugs (NSAIDs) for joint disease and topical therapies for the skin.[5,83,84] In many patients, this approach is sufficient to control disease manifestations, although some patients have a worsening of psoriasis with NSAIDs. In these cases, a drug belonging to a different family of NSAIDs should be used.

In individuals whose arthritis is persistent, disease-modifying antirheumatic drugs (DMARDs) should be used. If the skin disease is well controlled with topical medication, the joint disease can be treated with a variety of second-line or cytotoxic drugs. These include gold salts, antimalarials, D-penicillamine, and azathioprine. Intramuscular gold is more effective than oral gold.[85] Antimalarials have been useful in uncontrolled trials and have not caused more skin flares in a case-controlled study.[86]

In patients with severe skin inflammation, medications such as methotrexate (MTX),[87,88] retinoic acid derivatives,[89] or psoralen plus ultraviolet light (PUVA)[90,91] should be considered. These medications have been shown to work for both skin and joint manifestations.[5,83]

Sulfasalazine was tested in randomized controlled trials in PsA.[77,92] In the largest randomized controlled trial to date, sulfasalazine, at a dose of 2000 mg/day, was shown to be more effective than placebo in the treatment of PsA.[77] However, the effect size was small. Although sulfasalazine was well tolerated in the randomized controlled trials, this has not been the experience in clinical practice, where up to 44 percent of patients are not able to tolerate sulfasalazine due to side effects.[93] Sulfasalazine may also be of some help for the treatment of psoriasis in these patients. Cyclosporin A appears to be an effective agent for the treatment of psoriasis and PsA.[94] The major concern with cyclosporin A is its toxicity, especially nephrotoxicity and hypertension. However, of the 170 patients reviewed from 16 studies of cyclosporin A in PsA, 9.4 percent discontinued the drug because of side effects (6% with nephrotoxicity and 2% with hypertension).[83]

Several other modalities have been tried in PsA, including vitamin D_3, bromocriptine, peptide T, and fish oils, but their effect remains to be proved.[83,84]

Although the second-line cytotoxic drugs may control the acute inflammation in PsA, they have not been helpful in arresting the progression of clinical and radiologic damage.[93,95-97] Thus, either the disease needs to be treated earlier, or better drugs are necessary to prevent the damage that may ensue as a result of PsA.

There has been a recent interest in studying new drugs in PsA. The treatment with leflunomide in psoriatic arthritis (TOPAS) study, using leflunomide, an agent that affects activated lymphocytes by inhibition of de novo pyrimidine synthesis and reduction of pyrimidines, demonstrated its efficacy for both skin and joint manifestations in PsA.[98] The primary outcome measure of the TOPAS study was the PsARC. In a double-blind, randomized, placebo-controlled study that included 188 patients, the PsARC response was achieved by 59 percent of the leflunomide-treated patients compared to 29.7 percent of the placebo-treated patients (p < 0.0001). The ACR-20 response was achieved by only 36.3 percent of the leflunomide-treated patients and 20 percent of the placebo-treated patients (p = 0.014). The psoriasis area severity index (PASI) score was reduced by 24 percent in the leflunomide group and did not change at all in the placebo-treated group (p = 0.003); however, the target lesion demonstrated a 48.4-percent response in the leflunomide-treated patients and 25.6 percent in the placebo-treated group (p = 0.0048).

Based on the major role of TNF in the inflammation of both skin and joint lesions of PsA, several studies using anti-TNF agents were recently carried out. In a phase 2 trial of etanercept, a soluble TNF receptor, in 60 patients with PsA, 30 were randomized to etanercept and 30 to placebo.[99] Half of the patients in each group were receiving concomitant MTX therapy. The end points were the proportion of patients who met the PsARC and those who met the ACR-20 response criteria for RA. At 3 months, 87 percent of the etanercept-treated patients achieved the PsARC response and 73 percent achieved the ACR-20 response, compared to 23 and 13 percent of the placebo-treated patients, respectively. This medication was effective against skin psoriasis as measured by reduction in the PASI score by 46 percent in the etanercept-treated group and by 9 percent in the placebo-treated group. Target lesions demonstrated improvement in 50 percent of the etanercept patients and in none of the placebo patients. A phase 3, randomized, placebo-controlled trial of etanercept in 205 patients with PsA demonstrated a 72 percent PsARC response at 3 months and a 70 percent response at 6 months, with the corresponding placebo responses of 31 and 24 percent, respectively (p < 0.001).[100] The ACR-20 response in the larger trial was 59 percent at 3 months and 50 percent at 6 months with corresponding placebo responses of 15 and 13 percent, respectively (p < 0.001). The PASI scores were decreased by 46 percent in the etanercept group and did not change in the placebo group (p < 0.001). Similar responses were noted among patients who were concomitantly treated with MTX and those who were MTX naïve.

The chimeric monoclonal anti-TNF antibody infliximab was studied in a double-blind, randomized, controlled fashion in 100 patients with PsA.[101] The PsARC response at 16 weeks was 76.5 percent in infliximab-treated patients and 18 percent in placebo-treated patients (p < 0.0001). The ACR-20 response was 69 percent in infliximab patients and 8 percent in the placebo group (p < 0.0001). There was a remarkable improvement in the PASI score, with a reduction of 81 percent in the infliximab group compared to an increase of 35 percent in the placebo group (p < 0.001). These studies suggest that anti-TNF agents have an important role in the management of patients with PsA. There are now several other biologic agents in various stages of clinical trials for PsA.

REFERENCES

1. Wright V: Psoriasis and arthritis. Ann Rheum Dis 15:348, 1956.
2. Gladman DD: Criteria for psoriatic arthritis. Baillières Clin Rheumatol 9:319, 1995.
3. O'Neill T, Silman AJ: Historical background and epidemiology. Baillières Clin Rheumatol 8:245, 1994.
4. Wright V, Moll JMH: Psoriatic arthritis. Seronegative Polyarthritis. Amsterdam, North Holland, 1976, p 169.
5. http://www.psoriasis.org
6. Gladman DD: Psoriatic arthritis: Recent advances in pathogenesis and treatment. Rheum Dis Clin North Am 18:247, 1992.
7. Abu-Shakra M, Gladman DD: Aetiopathogenesis of psoriatic arthritis. Rheumatol Rev 3:1, 1994.
8. Moll JMH, Wright V: Familial occurrence of psoriatic arthritis. Ann Rheum Dis 32:181, 1973.
9. Farber EM, Noll ML: Genetics of psoriasis: Twin studies. In Farber EM, Cox AJ (eds): Psoriasis: Proceedings of the International Symposium. Stanford, Calif., Stanford University Press, 1971, p 7.
10. Eastmond CJ: Genetics and HLA antigens. Baillières Clin Rheumatol 8:263, 1994.
11. Gladman DD, Cheung C, Ng CM, Wade JA: HLA C-locus alleles in psoriatic arthritis. Human Immunol 60:259-261, 1999.
12. Martin MP, Nelson G, Lee J-H, et al: Susceptibility to Psoriatic Arthritis: Influence of activating *Killer Immunoglobulin-like Receptor*

genes in the absence of their corresponding HLA ligands. J Immunol 169:2818-2822, 2002.

13. Elder JT, Nair RP, Henseler T, et al: The genetics of psoriasis 2001: The odyssey continues. Arch Dermatol 137:1447-1454, 2001.

14. Karason A, Gudjonsson JE, Upmanyu R, et al: A susceptibility gene for psoriatic arthritis maps to chromosome 16q: Evidence for imprinting. Am J Hum Genet 72:125-131, 2003.

15. Morrison IM, Reeve AE: A catalogue of imprinted genes and parent of origin effect in humans and animals. Hum Mol Genet 7(10):1599, 1998.

16. Rahman P, Gladman DD, Schentag CT, Petronis A: Excess paternal transmission in PsA. Arthritis Rheum 41:1228-1231, 1999.

17. Gladman DD: Toward unravelling the mystery of psoriatic arthritis. Arthritis Rheum 36:881, 1993.

18. Veale D, Yanni G, Rogers S, et al: Reduced synovial membrane macrophage numbers, ELAM1 expression, and lining layer hyperplasia in psoriatic arthritis as compared with rheumatoid arthritis. Arthritis Rheum 36:893, 1993.

19. Ritchlin C, Haas-Smith SA, Hicks D: Patterns of cytokine production in psoriatic synovium. J Rheumatol 25:8:1544, 1998.

20. Panayi G: Immunology of psoriasis and psoriatic arthritis. Baillières Clin Rheumatol 8:419, 1994.

21. Stagg AJ, Harding B, Hughes RA, et al: The distribution and functional properties of dendritic cells in patients with seronegative arthritis. Clin Exp Immunol 84:66, 1991.

22. Veale DJ, Barnes L, Rogers S, FitzGerald O: Immunohistochemical markers for arthritis in psoriasis. Ann Rheum Dis 53:450, 1994.

23. Espinoza LR, Aguilar JL, Espinoza CG, et al: Fibroblast function in psoriatic arthritis. I. Alteration of cell kinetics and growth factor responses. J Rheumatol 21:1502, 1994.

24. Espinoza LR, Aguilar JL, Espinoza CG, et al: Fibroblast function in psoriatic arthritis. II. Increased expression of PDGF receptors and increased production of GF and cytokines. J Rheumatol 21:1507, 1994.

25. Costello P, Bresnihan B, O'Farrell C, Fitzgerald O: Predominance of CD8+ T lymphocytes in psoriatic arthritis. J Rheumatol 26:1117-24, 1999.

26. Tassiulas I, Duncan SR, Centola M, et al: Clonal characteristics of T cell infiltrates in skin and synovium of patients with psoriatic arthritis. Human Immunol 60:479-491, 1999.

27. Wrone-Smith T, Nickoloff BJ: Dermal injection of immunocytes induces psoriasis. J Clin Invest 98:1878-1887, 1996.

28. Neumüller J, Dunky A, Burtscher H, et al: Interaction of monocytes from patients with psoriatic arthritis with cultured microvascular endothelial cells. Clin Immunol 98:143-152, 2001.

29. Fraser A, Fearon U, Reece R, et al: Matrix metalloproteinase 9, apoptosis, and vascular morphology in early arthritis. Arthritis Rheum 44:2024-2028, 2001.

30. Hitchon CA, Danning CL, Illei GG, et al: Gelatinase expression and activity in the synovium and skin of patients with erosive psoriatic arthritis. J Rheumatol 29:107-117, 2002.

31. Ritchlin C, Haas-Smith SA, Schwartz E: Osteoclast precursors are markedly increased in the peripheral blood of psoriatic arthritis patients. Arthritis Rheum 44(suppl 9):S325, 2001.

32. Voorhees JJ: Leukotrienes and other lipoxygenase products in the pathogenesis and therapy of psoriasis and other dermatoses. Arch Dermatol 119:541, 1983.

33. Brain S, Camp R, Dowd P, et al: The release of leukotriene B4—like material in biologically active amounts from lesional skin of patients with psoriasis. J Invest Dermatol 83:70, 1984.

34. Grilington FM, Skinner MA, Birchall NM, Tan PLI: Gamma delta positive T cells from patients with psoriatic and rheumatoid arthritis respond to streptococcal antigen. J Rheumatol 20:983, 1993.

35. Espinoza LR, Jara LJ, Espinoza CG, et al: There is an association between human immunodeficiency virus infection and spondyloarthropathies. Rheum Dis Clin North Am 18:257, 1992.

36. Scarpa R, Del Puente A, di Girolamo C, et al: Interplay between environmental factors, articular involvement, and HLA B27 in patients with psoriatic arthritis. Ann Rheum Dis 51:78, 1992.

37. Punzi L, Pianon M, Bertazzolo N, et al: Clinical, laboratory and immunogenetic aspects of post-traumatic psoriatic arthritis: A study of 25 patients. Clin Exp Rheumatol 16:277, 1998.

38. Vasey FB: Etiology and pathogenesis of psoriatic arthritis. In Gerber LH, Espinoza LR (eds): Psoriatic Arthritis. Orlando, Fla., Grune & Stratton, 1985, p 45.

39. Lotz M, Carson DA, Vaughan JH: Substance P activation of rheumatoid synoviocytes: Neural pathway in pathogenesis of arthritis. Science 335:893, 1987.

40. Roberts MET, Wright V, Hill AGS, et al: Psoriatic arthritis: Followup study. Ann Rheum Dis 35:206, 1976.

41. Kammer GM, Soter NA, Gibson DJ, et al: Psoriatic arthritis: Clinical, immunologic and HLA study of 100 patients. Semin Arthritis Rheum 9:75, 1979.

42. Scarpa R, Oriente P, Pulino A, et al: Psoriatic arthritis in psoriatic patients. Br J Rheumatol 23:246, 1984.

43. Gladman DD, Shuckett R, Russell ML, et al: Psoriatic arthritis: Clinical and laboratory analysis of 220 patients. Q J Med 62:127, 1987.

44. Torre Alonso JC, Perez AR, Castrillo JMA, et al: Psoriatic arthritis (PA): A clinical, immunological and radiological study of 180 patients. Br J Rheumatol 30:245, 1991.

45. Helliwell P, Marchesoni A, Peters M, et al: A reevaluation of the osteoarticular manifestations of psoriasis. Br J Rheumatol 30:339, 1991.

46. Veale D, Rogers S, Fitzgerald O: Classification of clinical subsets in psoriatic arthritis. Br J Rheumatol 33:133, 1994.

47. Jones SM, Armas JB, Cohen MG, et al: Psoriatic arthritis: Outcome of disease subsets and relationship of joint disease to nail and skin disease. Br J Rheumatol 33:834, 1994.

48. Trabace S, Cappellacci S, Ciccarone P, et al: Psoriatic arthritis: a clinical, radiological and genetic study of 58 Italian patients. Acta DermVenereol Suppl (Stockh) 106:69-70, 1994.

49. Marsal S, Armadans-Gil L, Martinez M, et al: Clinical, radiographic and HLA associations as markers for different patterns of psoriatic arthritis. Rheumatology (Oxford) 38:332-337, 1999.

50. Cohen MR, Reda DJ, Clegg DO: Baseline relationship between psoriasis and psoriatic arthritis: Analysis of 221 patients with active psoriatic arthritis: J Rheumatol 26:1752-1756, 1999.

51. Gladman DD: Natural history of psoriatic arthritis. Baillières Clin Rheumatol 8:379, 1994.

52. Lambert JB, Wright V: Psoriatic spondylitis: A clinical and radiological description of the spine in psoriatic arthritis. Q J Med 46:411, 1977.

53. Hanly J, Russell ML, Gladman DD: Psoriatic spondyloarthropathy: A long term prospective study. Ann Rheum Dis 47:386, 1988.

54. Salvarani C, Macchioni P, Cromones T, et al: The cervical spine in patients with psoriatic arthritis: A clinical, radiological and immunogenetic study. Ann Rheum Dis 51:73, 1992.

55. Ballistone MJ, Manaster BJ, Reda DJ, Clegg DO: The prevlance of sacroiliitis in psoriatic arthritis: New perspectives from a large, multicenter cohort. Skeletal Radiology 28:196-201, 1999.

56. Gladman DD: Psoriatic arthritis: Spondyloarthropathies. Rheum Dis Clin North Am 24:829, 1998.

57. Lehtinen A, Traavisainen M, Leirisalo Repo M: Sonographic analysis of enthesopathy in the lower extremities of patients with spondyloarthropathy. Clin Exp Rheumatol 12:143, 1994.

58. Mulherin DM, FitzGerald O, Bresnihan B: Lymphedema of the upper limb in patients with psoriatic arthritis. Semin Arthritis Rheum 22:350, 1993.

59. Wright V, Roberts MC, Hill AGS: Dermatological manifestations in psoriatic arthritis: A followup study. Acta Dermatovenereol 59:235, 1979.

60. Gladman DD, Anhorn KB, Schachter RK, et al: HLA antigens in psoriatic arthritis. J Rheumatol 13:586, 1986.

61. Queiro R, Torre JC, Belzunegui J, et al: Clinical features and predictive factors in psoriatic arthritis-related uveitis. Semin Arthritis Rheum 31:264-270, 2002.

62. Bruce IN, Schentag C, Gladman DD: Hyperuricemia in psoriatic arthritis (PsA) does not reflect the extent of skin involvement. J Clin Rheumatol 6:6-9, 2000.

63. Avila R, Pugh DG, Slocumb CH, et al: Psoriatic arthritis: A roentgenologic study. Radiology 75:691, 1960.

64. Taccari E, Spedarr A, Ricieri V, et al: Sternoclavicular joint disease in psoriatic arthritis. Ann Rheum Dis 51:372, 1992.

65. Rahman P, Gladman DD, Cook RJ, et al: Radiological assessment in psoriatic arthritis. Br J Rheumatol 37:760-765, 1998.

66. Gladman DD, Ng Tung Hing E, Schentag CT, Cook R: Remission in psoriatic arthritis. J Rheumatol 28:1045-1048, 2001.

67. Gladman DD, Farewell VT, Nadeau C: Clinical indicators of progression in psoriatic arthritis (PSA): Multivariate relative risk model. J Rheumatol 22:675, 1995.

68. Gladman DD, Farewell VT: The role of HLA antigens as indicators of disease progression in psoriatic arthritis (PSA): Multivariate relative risk model psoriatic arthritis. Arthritis Rheum 38:845, 1995.

69. Gladman DD, Farewell VT, Kopciuk K, Cook RJ: HLA antigens and progression in psoriatic arthritis. J Rheumatol 25:730, 1998.

70. Gladman DD, Farewell VT: Progression in psoriatic arthritis: Role of time varying clinical indicators. J Rheumatol 26:2409-2413, 1999.

71. Queiro-Silva R, Torre-Alonso JC, Tinture-Eguren T, Lopez-Lagunas I: A polyarticular onset predicts erosive and deforming disease in psoriatic arthritis. Ann Rheum Dis 62:68-70, 2003.

72. Zangger P, Gladman DD, Bogoch ER: Musculoskeletal surgery in psoriatic arthritis: J Rheumatol 25:725, 1998.

73. Wong K, Gladman DD, Husted J, et al: Mortality studies in psoriatic arthritis. Results from a single outpatient clinic. I. Causes and Risk of Death. Arthritis Rheum 40:1868, 1997.

74. Gladman DD, Farewell VT, Wong K, Husted J: Mortality studies in psoriatic arthritis: Results for a single outpatient center. II. Prognostic indicators for death. Arthritis Rheum 41:1103, 1998.

75. Gladman DD, Farewell V, Buskila D, et al: Reliability of measurements of active and damaged joints in psoriatic arthritis. J Rheumatol 17:62-64, 1990.

76. Daunt AON, Cox MJ, Robertson JC, Cawley MJD: Indices of disease activity in psoriatic arthritis. J Roy Soc Med 80:556-558, 1987.

77. Clegg DO, Rea DJ, Mejias E, et al: Comparison of sulfasalazine and placebo in the treatment of psoriatic arthritis. 39:2013, 1996.

78. Rahman P, Gladman DD, Cook RJ, et al: Radiological assessment in psoriatic arthritis. Br J Rheumatol 37:760, 1998.

79. Wassenberg S, Fischer O, Kahle V, et al: A method to score radiographic change in psoriatic arthritis. Z Rheumatol 60:156-166, 2001.

80. Husted J, Gladman DD, Cook RJ, Farewell VT: Responsiveness of health status instruments to changes in articular status and perceived health in patients with psoriatic arthritis. J Rheumatol 25:11:2146, 1998.

81. Husted JA, Gladman DD, Farewell VT, Cook R: Health-related quality of life of patients with psoriatic arthritis: A comparison with patients with rheumatoid arthritis. Arthritis Care Res 45:151-158, 2001.

82. Sokoll KB, Helliwell PS: Comparison of disability and quality of life in rheumatoid and psoriatic arthritis. J Rheumatol 28:1842-1846, 2001.

83. Bruce I, Gladman DD: Psoriatic arthritis: Recognition and management. BioDrugs 9:271,1998.

84. Brockbank J, Gladman DD: Diagnosis and management of psoriatic arthritis. BioDrugs 62:2447-2457, 2002.

85. Palit J, Hill J, Capell HA, et al: A multicentre doubleblind comparison of auranofin, intramuscular gold thiomalate and placebo in patients with psoriatic arthritis. Br J Rheumatol 29:280, 1990.

86. Gladman DD, Blake R, Brubacher B, Farewell VT: Chloroquine therapy in psoriatic arthritis. J Rheumatol 19:1724, 1992.

87. Willkens RF, Williams HJ, Ward JR, et al: Randomized, double-blind, placebo-controlled trial of low dose pulse methotrexate in psoriatic arthritis. Arthritis Rheum 27:376, 1984.

88. Espinoza LR, Zakraoni L, Espinoza CG, et al: Psoriatic arthritis: Clinical response and side effects of methotrexate therapy. J Rheumatol 19:872, 1992.

89. Klinkhoff AV, Gertner E, Chalmers A, et al: Pilot study of etretinate in psoriatic arthritis. J Rheumatol 16:789, 1989.

90. Perlman SG, Gerber LH, Roberts M, et al: Photochemotherapy and psoriatic arthritis: A prospective study. Ann Intern Med 91:717, 1979.

91. de Misa RF, Azafia JM, Harto A, et al: Psoriatic arthritis: One year of treatment with extracorporeal photochemotherapy. J Am Acad Dermatol 30:1037, 1994.

92. Dougados M, van der Linden S, Leirisalo-Repo M: Sulfasalazine in the treatment of spondyloarthropathy: A randomized, multicenter, double-blind, placebo controlled study. Arthritis Rheum 38:618, 1995.

93. Rahman P, Gladman DD, Cook RJ, et al: The use of sulfasalazine in psoriatic arthritis: A clinic experience J Rheumatol 25:1957, 1998.

94. Gupta AK, Matteson EI, Ellis CN, et al: Cyclosporin in the treatment of psoriatic arthritis. Arch Dermatol 125:507, 1989.

95. Mader R, Gladman DD, Long J, et al: Does injectable gold retard radiologic evidence of joint damage in psoriatic arthritis. Clin Invest Med 18:139-143, 1995.

96. Abu-Shakra M, Gladman DD, Thorne JC, et al: Longterm methotrexate therapy in psoriatic arthritis: Clinical and radiologic outcome. J Rheumatol 22:241-245, 1995.

97. Lee JCT, Gladman DD, Schentag CT, Cook RJ: The long-term use of azathioprine in patients with psoriatic arthritis. J Clin Rheumatol 7:160-165, 2001.

98. Kaltwasser P, Nash P, Gladman D, et al: A double blind placebo controlled trial of the efficacy and safety of leflunomide in the treatment of psoriatic arthritis: Results from the TOPAS trial. Presented at the American College of Rheumatology Annual Meeting. New Orleans, October 29, 2002.

99. Mease PJ, Goffe BS, Metz J, et al: Etanercept in the treatment of psoriatic arthritis and psoriasis: A randomised trial. Lancet 356:385-390, 2000.

100. Mease P, Kivitz A, Burch F,et al: Improvement in disease activity in patients with psoriatic arthritis receiving etanercept (Enbrel®): Results of a phase 3 multicenter clinical trial [Abstract]. Arthritis Rheum 44(suppl 9):S90, 2001.

101. Antoni C, Kavanaugh A, Kikham B, et al: The Infliximab Multinational Psoriatic Arthritis Controlled Trial (IMPACT). Arthritis Rheum 46(suppl 9):S381, 2002.

73

Enteropathic Arthritis

FRANK A. WOLLHEIM

The definition of enteropathic arthritis is a pragmatic rather than a scientific one and is based on clinical observations—made over the centuries—that gastrointestinal disturbances such as dysentery often are followed by arthritis. The gut mucosa is a first line of defense against ingested environmental noxious factors, and gut permeability is obviously an important variable to investigate. Even the healthy intestine allows the transmission of large molecules, such as cow-milk allergen. In a nursing mother, these can, after absorption, reach her breast milk in amounts sufficient to cause symptoms of cow-milk allergy in the infant.

We should realize that most microorganisms and antigens do not cause immune reactions in the gut, but rather induce tolerance. The specialized gut-associated immune system (GALT) is still not completely understood. Cell trafficking between the gut and joints is an important pathogenetic event.[1] Disease susceptibility and severity is often under genetic control and carriage of human leukocyte antigen (HLA)-B27 could contribute to susceptibility through nonimmunologic mechanisms.

Relevant Gut Biology

The gut in healthy adults has an estimated mucous surface of 400 m^2, which is more than 200 times that of the skin. Absorption, secretion, and exclusion of foreign materials are delicately regulated. Molecules smaller than 5000 D can pass through the epithelial membranes of the microvilli, whereas larger molecules can enter Peyer's patches by endocytosis. Altered gut permeability can be observed in several diseases; the causes are in part genetic but are triggered by exogenous factors such as drugs and microorganisms.[2] Oral feeding of lactalbumin, lactoglobulin, polyethylene glycol particles, ^{51}Cr-labeled ethylene diamine tetraacetic acid (EDTA), and sugars such as lactulose and mannitol followed by urine analysis is used to quantify pathologic changes. In addition, intestinal permeability and function may be studied by regional perfusion with help of endoscopic techniques that close off segments of the gut with inflatable balloons.[3] Ethnic differences in gut permeability have been described.[4]

GALT is a highly specialized tissue constituting 25 percent of the mucosa. The gut has been called "the most misunderstood and under-appreciated lymphoid organ in the body."[5] The epithelial glycoprotein, now called secretory component or polymeric immunoglobulin receptor (pIgR), is a 100-kD transmembrane receptor for polymeric immunoglobulin (Ig), that is, J chain–containing IgA and IgM. It is abundantly present in Peyer's patches in the distal ileum. It forms complexes, secretory immunoglobulin A (sIgA) and to some extent secretary immunoglobin M (sIgM), that are secreted into the lumen and constitute a non-inflammatory, non–complement-binding first line of defense. It is estimated that a healthy adult secretes 3 to 5 g sIgA daily into the gut. From the Peyer's patches, primed B lymphocytes disseminate throughout the body's mucous membranes, notably to other parts of the alimentary tract. Primed T lymphocytes also disseminate into the circulation and lymph nodes and home into target organs such as salivary gland in Sjögren's disease, lungs, and synovium.[6] The mechanisms are still incompletely worked out, but vascular adhesion protein-1 expressed on synovial epithelial cells is involved in lymphocyte homing, and P-selectin is a part of macrophage recruitment.[7] Most T lymphocytes in the mucosal lamina propria are cell determinant (CD)4+, whereas intraepithelial T cells are mostly CD8+. Gut-associated lymphocytes preferentially express the integrins $\alpha_4\beta_7$ or $\alpha_E\beta_7$.[6] A scheme of the human mucosal immune system is depicted in Figure 73–1.

A chain of events in the pathogenesis of enteropathic arthritis can involve gastrointestinal infection with the appropriate microorganism in the genetically predisposed patient. This causes a local inflammation in the gut mucosa, formation of sIgA, increased permeability, absorption of foreign material, and triggering of T lymphocytes. Circulating immune complexes and memory T cells localize to joints and cause synovitis (Fig. 73–2).

Spondyloarthropathies

Seronegative spondyloarthropathy is presently an accepted designation for a group of diseases fulfilling some common characteristics and showing overlapping features. These are both genetic and clinical[8] and include, among other conditions, reactive arthritis, arthritis with inflammatory bowel disease (IBD), and a syndrome termed *undifferentiated spondyloarthropathy*. The gut is a putative or proven port of entry for microbial agents, and the joint disease is characterized by sacroiliitis, spinal involvement, enthesopathy, or peripheral oligoarthritis with dominant localization to the lower extremities. Systemic manifestations from the eyes, skin, heart, and urogenital tract are also common.

Mucosal inductive sites

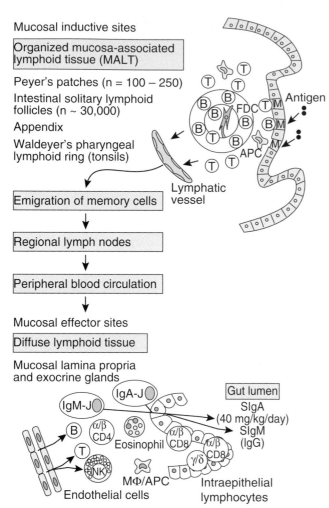

FIGURE 73–1 · The Human Mucosal Immune System. (From Brandtzaeg P, Berstad AE, Farstad IN, et al: Mucosal immunity: A major adaptive defence mechanism. Behring Inst Mitt 98:1, 1997.)

Inflammatory Bowel Disease

Crohn's disease and ulcerative colitis are distinct entities with different pathogenesis (Table 73–1). Both are familial, but hereditary factors are more important in Crohn's disease, according to twin studies.[9] Recent evidence implicates involvement of genes outside the HLA region on chromosome 6. Concurrence in the same family of the two diseases has been described but is rare. Interestingly, a tumor necrosis factor-α (TNF-α) microsatellite gene factor is associated with Crohn's disease but not with ulcerative colitis.[10] Although the entire gut wall is involved in a patchy way in Crohn's disease, diffuse, mainly mucosal pathology is typical of ulcerative colitis. T lymphocyte proliferation and cytokine generation is also different. In Crohn's disease, a T helper type 1 (Th1) response dominates,[11,12] but no such dominance has been documented for ulcerative colitis. Increased amounts of so-called proinflammatory cytokines—TNF-α, interleukin (IL)-1β, IL-6, and IL-8—are released locally in both diseases.[13] Despite the differences at bedside and in the laboratory, the tradition of dealing with the two diseases is retained on the basis of the remarkable similarities with regard to joint involvement. The prevalence of Crohn's disease and ulcerative colitis is about equal and ranges between 50 and 100 cases per 100,000.[14]

AXIAL INVOLVEMENT

Table 73–2 shows that spinal involvement occurs in 10 to 20 percent of cases. It is symptomatic or silent and may precede the onset of IBD or appear later.[14] In contrast to ankylosing spondylitis (AS), there is no sex difference. In general, the involvement is similar or identical to that in classic AS. In a retrospective study designed to identify differences,[15] it was observed that

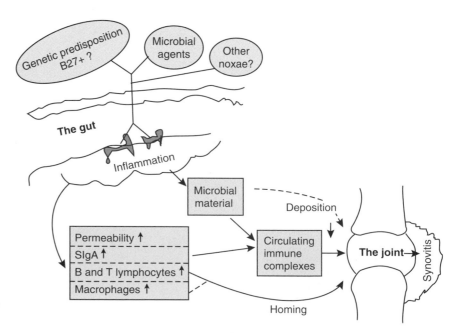

FIGURE 73–2 · Pathogenesis of Enteropathic Arthritis.

TABLE 73–1 • DISTINCTIVE FEATURES OF INFLAMMATORY BOWEL DISEASE (IBD)

	Crohn's Disease	Ulcerative Colitis
Genetic base	Strong, recessive	Weaker, dominant
Non-HLA genes	TNF-α	?
Gut permeability sensitive to ASA on genetic base	Yes	?
T lymphocyte response in gut	Th1 (IFN-$\gamma\uparrow$)	No Th1 or Th2 imbalance
Fas ligand expression	No	Yes
Effect of smoking	None (?)	Protective
Correlation gut activity to arthritis symptoms	No	Yes
ICAM-1 antisense rx	Beneficial	No response (?)
Infliximab rx	Dramatically effective	Not effective (?)

Abbreviations: ASA, acetylsalicylic acid; ICAM-1, intercellular adhesion molecule; IFN-γ, interferon-γ; rx,therapy; Th1, T helper type 1; Th2, T helper type 2.

TABLE 73–2 • EXTRAINTESTINAL MANIFESTATIONS OF INFLAMMATORY BOWEL DISEASE (IBD)

	Crohn's Disease	Ulcerative Colitis
Peripheral arthritis	$\cong$15%	$\cong$10%
Axial or sacroiliac arthritis	$\cong$15-20%	$\cong$10-15%
Septic arthritis	Rare	Not reported
Skin: Erythema nodosum	9% or less	?
Erythema multiforme	Rare	?
Pyoderma gangrenosum	0.5%	0.3-0.4% (in severe disease)
Aphtous ulcers	Rare	8%
Nephrolithiasis (oxalate)	<15%	?
Amyloidosis	Very rare	?
Liver disease	3-5%	7%
Uveitis	13%	4%
Vasculitis	Takayasu's	<5%
Clubbing of fingers	4-13%	1-5%

changes in enteropathic disease tended to be milder, squaring of vertebrae was more prevalent, and Romanus lesions occurred only in isolated AS. The majority of radiologic features were not different. The symptoms of spinal involvement, when present, do not vary with intestinal disease activity. The issue is complicated by the well-established association of AS with silent Crohn's disease, diagnosed by biopsy.[16] Isolated sacroiliitis is often silent and not associated with HLA-B27. In full-blown IBD-related AS, the prevalence of B27 is between 50 and 70 percent.[14]

PERIPHERAL JOINT INVOLVEMENT

Between 5 and 15 percent of patients in most studies develop peripheral arthritis, slightly more often in Crohn's disease than in ulcerative colitis (see Table 73–2). It is commonly nondestructive and reversible, but erosive changes may also occur. Only limited information on the histopathologic appearance is available, and it indicates presence of granulomas in cases with Crohn's disease and unspecific synovitis in ulcerative colitis.[14] In Crohn's disease, septic arthritis has been reported in the hip, which rapidly destroys the joint and requires aggressive therapy. The symptoms tend to coincide with gut activity in ulcerative colitis but not in Crohn's disease. Total colectomy is associated with remission of arthritis in half of the patients with ulcerative colitis, but paradoxically, the arthritis may begin after surgery,[17] perhaps representing a form of bypass arthritis related to altered gut microbiology. Based on examination of approximately 1500 patients with ulcerative colitis and Crohn's disease, a distinction was made between two forms of peripheral arthritis: oligoarthritis of type 1 (less than five joints) and polyarthritis of type 2 (more than five joints). The highest prevalence was found in metacarpophalangeal, proximal interphalangeal, knee, and ankle joints. Shoulder involvement was more common in ulcerative colitis, but joint involvement was otherwise strikingly similar. Importantly, the majority of type 1 cases were acute and resolved within 6 weeks, whereas the type 2 cases persisted[18] (Fig. 73–3). Type 1 arthritis was 12 times more prevalent in carriers of the rare HLA-DRB1*0103 allele.[19] This represents a newly recognized example of genetic influence on disease phenotype and may be a clue to different pathogenesis[19] (Table 73–3).

OTHER MANIFESTATIONS

As seen in Table 73–2, clubbing of fingers, uveitis, and skin manifestations are also observed in IBD, with higher frequency in Crohn's disease. The pathogenesis of these lesions is unclear, but immunologic mechanisms are likely. Pyoderma gangrenosum is a painful, ulcerating skin reaction, frequently associated with a systemic disease (Fig. 73–4). In a series of 86 patients seen at the Mayo Clinic between 1970 and 1983, 31 had

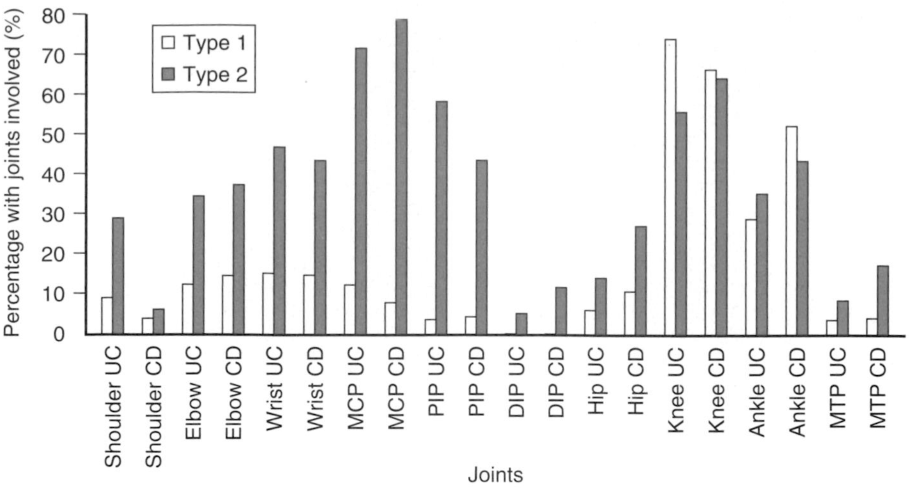

FIGURE 73-3 · Articular Distribution of Peripheral Arthropathies in Inflammatory Bowel Disease (IBD). UC, ulcerative colitis; CD, Crohn's disease; type 1, oligoarthritis; type 2, polyarthritis. (From Orchard TR, Wordsworth BP, Jewell DP: Peripheral arthropathies in inflammatory bowel disease: their articular distribution and natural history. Gut 42:387, 1998.)

TABLE 73-3 · PERIPHERAL JOINT DISEASE AND INFLAMMATORY BOWEL DISEASE (IBD)

	Type 1 (<5 joints)	Type 2 (>5 joints)
Prevalence in UC/CD	3.3%/6.0%	2.5%/4.6%
Clinical course	Self-limiting arthritis	Persistent arthritis
Type of IBD	Relapsing in < 85%	Relapsing in 30-40%
Major histocompatibility complex (MHC) association	HLA-B27, -B35, -DRB1*0103	HLA-B44

Abbreviations: CD, Crohn's disease; IBD, inflammatory bowel disease; UC, ulcerative colitis.

Data from Orchard TR, Wordsworth BP, Jewell DP: Peripheral arthropathies in inflammatory bowel disease: Their articular distribution and natural history. Gut 42:387, 1998; and Orchard TR, Thiyagaraja S, Welsh KI, et al: Clinical phenotype is related to HLA genotype in the peripheral arthropathies of inflammatory bowel disease. Gastroenterology 118:274, 2000.

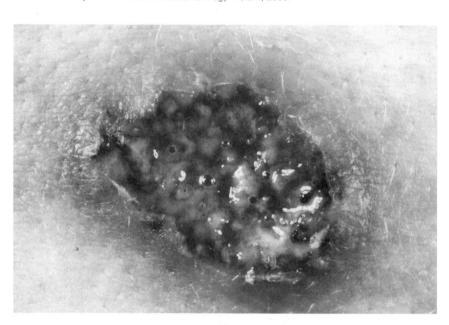

FIGURE 73-4 · Pyoderma Gangrenosum in a Patient with Ulcerative Colitis. (Courtesy of Professor H. Rorsman, Lund, Sweden.)

IBD[14]; a similar proportion, 14 of 44, was observed in a more recent report.[20] Erythema nodosum, uveitis, and peripheral arthritis commonly occur together in IBD and have been linked to HLA DRB1*0103 and TNF-α gene polymorphism.[21] Uveitis is also a feature of other spondyloarthropathies, such as AS and reactive arthritis. In IBD, however, uveitis is more often bilateral, and the tendency toward chronicity is more pronounced.

Response to topical therapy with glucocorticoids may also be less prompt.[22]

PATHOGENESIS

Genetic factors are important for susceptibility, but it is not known by what mechanism. Experimental work with transgenic animals transfected with human

HLA-B27 and β_2-microglobulin has shown that certain strains of conventional mice and rats develop spondyloarthropathies, whereas identical animals in a germ-free environment are protected.[23,24] In human disease, HLA-B27 is clearly one predisposing factor, but only in the minority of cases with spinal joint involvement. The microbial contribution is still largely unclear, and animal work indicates that parts of the normal gut flora may be involved.[25] In jejunal juice from patients with AS and rheumatoid arthritis (RA) collected with the closed-segment endoscopic technique,[3] antibodies were found against *Klebsiella pneumoniae*, *Escherichia coli*, and *Proteus mirabilis*.[26] Disturbed and augmented local immune response in parts of the gut against a variety of microorganisms is emerging as a prevalent feature of several chronic joint diseases.

Gene manipulation in mice indicates that IL-2, IL-10, and transforming growth factor-β (TGF-β) may be protective factors and that HLA-B27 may influence cytokine expression.[27] Altered cytokine balance in the gut mucosa may, thus, be an important pathogenic factor.

Increased gut permeability has already been alluded to as an important factor in pathogenesis.[3,4] Bacteria recovered from the gut lumen in IBD are covered by IgG antibodies in addition to sIgA and sIgM.[28] Increased leakage from the inflamed mucosa thus allows egress of complement-binding IgG, which can contribute to inflammation, which in turn further augments permeability. The increased and altered immune response to bacteria differs between Crohn's disease and ulcerative colitis.[29] The pathogenetic significance of such differences remains uncertain. Increased gut permeability in IBD has been known for a number of years. In part, this may be under genetic influence. A study showed that although basal permeability was normal in relatives of patients with Crohn's disease, gut permeability was abnormally increased after ingestion of acetylsalicylic acid.[30] Environmental influences on permeability could be partly mediated by bacterial endotoxin. An in vitro perfusion study on rat gut showed serosal rather than mucosal application to impair the barrier.[31] Absorbed bacterial material could, thus, add to the already damaged barrier.

MANAGEMENT

A general rule in managing arthritis complicating IBD can be formulated as "what is good for the gut is also helpful for the joints." Thus, sulfasalazine is of proven value in long-term management. This drug has been shown to inhibit the function of nuclear factor kappa B (NFκB) and may thereby favorably influence the expression of proinflammatory cytokines. Azathioprine, glucocorticoids, and methotrexate (MTX) are also widely used. There is a striking paucity of controlled trials of the effects of these agents on joint symptoms, partly because they also affect the intestinal disease, which often is the main indication for their use.[32]

TNF inhibition with infliximab (but not with etanercept) results in remission of gastrointestinal manifesta-

tions in close to 60 percent of patients with Crohn's disease.[33] Infliximab is also effective in AS, but only anecdotal evidence supports its effect on the associated arthritis.[34] Alicaforsen (ISIS2302), an antisense inhibitor of intercellular adhesion molecule-1 (ICAM-1), is in development for the treatment of Crohn's.[35] No information on effects on the arthritis have been published.

Pain control with nonsteroidal anti-inflammatory drugs (NSAIDs) is a problem; it has been convincingly shown that they increase gut permeability and thereby may exacerbate gut inflammation. Paradoxically, they are in wide clinical use and are often well tolerated.[14,36]

■ Enteric Reactive Arthritis

Postdysentery arthritis was recognized by several physicians in the 19th century. Because of a confusing case report in 1916, the eponym Reiter's has been used to designate a syndrome of arthritis, urethritis, and conjunctivitis, which, for good reasons, should be replaced by Fiessinger-Leroy syndrome if an eponym is to be used.[37,38] *Yersinia* was identified as a human pathogen in the 1960s and as a trigger of reactive arthritis in 1959.[14]

CLINICAL FEATURES

Reactive arthritis can be identified with considerable accuracy as a condition with acute onset of asymmetric oligoarthritis with dominant localization to lower extremities, often affecting large joints. Enthesopathy, manifested by heel pain, for example, is common. Glomerulonephritis and myocarditis are not unusual.[14] It is said that postenteric reactive arthritis is less likely to be chronic and to recur than is posturethritic reactive arthritis.[39] However, several follow-up studies have documented some chronicity in two thirds of patients.[14,40] The initiating and triggering enteritis is often mild or even asymptomatic, indicating that a vigorous inflammatory response in the gut is protective against triggered arthritis. Rheumatoid factor (RF) is not present in these patients. Fever and acute-phase reaction may be low grade or intense. Spinal disease eventually develops in approximately 20 percent of patients.[14]

TRIGGERING AGENTS

The triggering agents are usually gram-negative obligate or facultative intracellular organisms. Table 73–4 shows the selective agents that are mostly implicated as triggers. No organism can be identified in one quarter of most series of patients.[14]

Two publications claim group A streptococci as triggers of reactive arthritis. In one pediatric center in Florida, 25 children were identified.[41] Only 11 had a history of sore throat, and only 5 of 7 cultures were positive, but all had significant anti–streptococcal antibody titers. The arthritis was not migratory, lasted on average 60 days, and was often axial; thus, it was not similar to rheumatic fever. HLA-B27 was not increased. Four adult patients, all with positive throat cultures,

TABLE 73–4 · ETIOLOGIC AGENTS IN POSTENTERIC REACTIVE ARTHRITIS

Common	Uncommon
Shigella flexneri	Shigella sonnei
Salmonella typhimurium	Shigella dysenteriae
Salmonella enteritidis	Salmonella paratyphi B
Yersinia enterocolitica 03	Salmonella paratyphi C
Yersinia enterocolitica 09	Yersinia enterocolitica 08
Yersinia pseudotuberculosis	Giardia lamblia
Campylobacter jejuni	Group A streptococci (?)

developed nonmigratory oligoarthritis.[42] *Giardia lamblia* has been implicated in occasional cases.[14] It is likely that other triggers will be identified in time, yet it can be said that only a minority of organisms have the potency to trigger reactive arthritis. It is not clear which features determine arthritogenicity.[14]

Brucellosis is rare in North America and in most western countries, but it is still enedemic in Peru, northern Spain, and the Middle East, where sheep, goats, and camels are vectors. Nonpasteurized milk is the major source of infection. Arthralgias, asymmetric peripheral arthritis, unilateral sacroiliitis, and spondylitis are frequent. Joint effusions are often culture negative, and the diagnosis then rests on serologic tests. The recommended therapy is 6 weeks administration of doxycyclineand rifampicin.[43] Brucellosis may be a cause of spinal compression.[44] Brucella arthritis has been suspected of sometimes being reactive, based on failure to grow microorganisms from joint fluid and poor response to antibiotic therapy, but this needs confirmation.

PATHOGENESIS

After three decades, the mechanism by which HLA-B27 mediates susceptibility to postenteric reactive arthritis remains unclear (see Fig. 73–2). Reactive arthritis invites mechanism studies: Obviously, eliciting antigens should be present in the etiologic agent. Persistence of microbial antigen in the joint has been convincingly proved not only for *Chlamydia* and *Salmonella*[14] but also for *Yersinia enterocolitica*.[45] These investigators found evidence of bacterial lipopolysaccharide and heat-shock protein (HSP) in joint tissue up to 4 years after the acute episode. Carriage of HLA B27 does not influence the duration of fecal presence of bacteria in salmonellosis, and joint involvement does not correlate with this either.[46] New roles of HLA-B27 are indicated by elegant transfection experiments in which human HLA-B27 expression enhanced and prolonged upregulation of NFκB upon LPS stimulation[47] and facilitated cell penetration of arthritogenic salmonella but not yersinia organisms.[48] Attempts to implicate molecular mimicry have, however, not met with success.[14,39] Another approach has been to isolate and propagate synovial cytotoxic T lymphocytes from B27-positive patients with *Yersinia* arthritis and expose them to nonapeptides from *Yersinia* HSP. This allowed identification of a single peptide that was immunogenic for the T cell lines.[49] This complicated but intriguing work needs confirmation.

TREATMENT

Symptomatic therapy with analgesics or NSAIDs is commonly practiced; although, for reasons related to permeability discussed previously, their use should be restricted. Local injections with glucocorticoids are possibly less effective than in RA, but formal studies have not been performed. Large multicenter trials with antibiotics such as sulfasalazine have shown marginal effects at best. The problem with these studies is that they involve mixed groups of patients, some of whom may respond better than others. Reactive arthritis, in the majority of cases, is self limiting. Even when they are given at the onset of diarrhea in *Salmonella* epidemics, antibiotics are not effective in preventing or modifying arthritis[50]; although, in theory, they should prevent reinfection and thereby be beneficial. Furthermore, tetracyclines are protease inhibitors, and sulfasalazine inhibits NFκB. Therefore, efficacy in treatment does not necessarily mean an antimicrobial mechanism. Because widespread use of antibiotics has negative general health consequences, they have no place in the treatment of enteric reactive arthritis. A paper from Finland claiming that a 3 month treatement with eiprofloxacin in the acute stage prevents later HLA-B27–associated morbidity is methodologically unconvincing and needs confirmation.[50a]

▌ Bypass Arthritis-Dermatitis Syndrome

Surgical treatment of overweight patients by creation of a blind loop is no longer in use. It was often complicated by incapacitating joint and skin symptoms. The syndrome is of interest because it is a human model disease for distant complications of bacterial overgrowth in the gut. The main features were an intensely painful oligoarthritis of large and small joints and spine without structural changes, recurrent papulopustular rash (Fig. 73–5), and complement-binding circulating immune complexes that contained components of gut microorganisms. Surgical elimination of the blind loop as well as antibiotic therapy cured the arthritis but did little for the rash.[14] A similar syndrome has been observed in some patients with IBD after colorectal surgery.[17] This involves ileoanal anastomosis, creating a so-called ileal pouch, which may become inflamed. A case report describes a case of arthritis that responded to surgery.[51] An intriguing report describes delayed occurrence of asymmetric oligoarthritis combined with a necrotizing vasculitic skin lesion. This happened 18 years after bypass surgery and 6 weeks after laparoscopic division of adhesions. The condition cleared after treatment with doxycycline.[52]

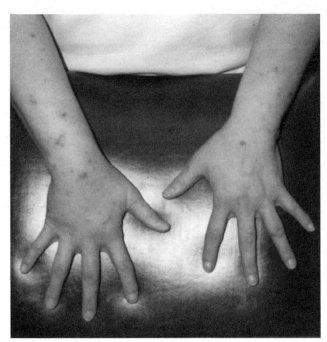

FIGURE 73-5 · Papulopustular rash in a case with Bypass Arthritis-dermatitis. The rash remained a recurrent problem even after the joint symptoms subsided.

Arthritis and Celiac Disease

Celiac disease is strongly associated with HLA-DQ2, and concordance in monozygotic twins is 70 percent. It is probably a Th1-driven disease in which wheat gliadins are the implicated antigens. Villous atrophy and altered gut permeability for β-lactalbumin are associated with this pathologic process. Deamidation of gliadin seems to be of key importance for DQ2 binding and T cell recognition.[53] Arthritis is a recognized complication in children and adults.[14] Arthritis was present in 52 of 200 adults with celiac disease.[54] There was no definite clinical difference between patients with and without arthritis, although body mass index was slightly lower in the arthritic patients. The arthritis ranges from mono- to oligo- or polyarthritis, and axial involvement is not uncommon. The arthritis is usually nondestructive.[55] Gluten-free diet is helpful in at least half of the cases, and arthritis is less prevalent among patients observing a gluten-free diet.[54]

Whipple's Disease

Whipple's disease, or intestinal lipodystrophy, as it was called by its originator in 1907,[14] is an intestinal infection with a unique microorganism called *Tropheryma whippelii*, belonging to the actinomycete family. It was identified in the rod-shaped material from periodic acid– and Schiff-positive gut lesions by polymerase chain reaction (PCR) analysis with use of broad-range primers searching for bacterial 16S ribosomal RNA.[14] This now allows specific diagnosis with a PCR tech-

nique, although it still has not been possible to propagate the organism in culture. PCR-positive material has been identified in paraffin-embedded gut biopsy specimens, diskitis material, synovial fluid, vitreous fluid, blood, and cerebrospinal fluid.[56]

Despite the advent of this improved diagnostic tool, Whipple's disease is still a rare condition. A retrospective French study identified 52 patients, 73 percent of whom were men.[57] Articular symptoms were the presenting features in 67 percent, and intestinal ones in only 15 percent. Later, 83 percent developed diarrhea and abdominal pain. Neurologic and ophthalmic symptoms are also sometimes present. The arthralgias and arthritis are most commonly seen in knee joints but can localize in any peripheral joint and also in spinal joints and disks. The source of infection is still unknown, and there is no evidence of person-to-person transmission. The time of the infectious event is also unclear. In some individuals, joint symptoms have been present for more than 10 years before diagnosis. *T. whippelii* was found in wastewater from sewage treatment plants in an unconfirmed German study. Antibiotic therapy is mandatory. The recommended regimen is daily parenteral administration of benzylpenicillin and streptomycin for 2 weeks, followed by trimethoprim and sulfamethoxazole for 1 to 2 years.[58]

Collagenous Colitis and Lymphocytic Colitis

Collagenous colitis was described in 1976 by Lindström, who found a characteristic thickening of the collagen layer under the gut epithelium. This is normally 3 μm, but it is more than 10 μm in collagenous colitis and may reach 50 to 100 μm (Fig. 73-6). Lymphocytic colitis or microscopic colitis is a distinct entity characterized by lymphocyte infiltration of the upper colon.[59]

Collagenous colitis is nine times more common in women and occurs with a prevalence of 15 cases and an incidence of 1.8 cases per 100,000.[14,60] The peak incidence is between 70 and 80 years of age. The

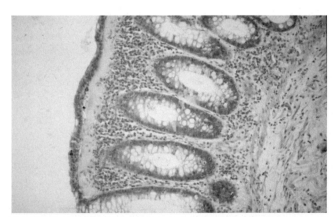

FIGURE 73-6 · Biopsy Specimen of Colon in a case of Collagenous Colitis (H+E). Arrow points at layer of abnormal collagen deposition. (Courtesy of Dr. C. Lindström, Malmö, Sweden.)

epidemiology of lymphocytic colitis is less well defined, but the gender distribution in this condition is even.[60] The intestinal symptoms consist of painful, watery stools of chronic-intermittent or sometimes chronic-persistent character, weight loss, and fatigue. Although unrelated, these syndromes are of rheumatologic interest because both are associated with autoimmune thyroid disease, positive antinuclear antibodies, and joint symptoms in 40 to 60 percent of cases. The best studied entity, collagenous colitis, is associated with a variety of joint syndromes, including Sjögren's syndrome, nondestructive oligoarthritis, migratory arthralgias, sacroiliitis, and RA. A recent survey of 63 consecutive cases in one Swedish center identified eight cases of RA and three cases of AS, clearly suggesting a correlation between the colitis and chronic joint diseases.[61] Celiac disease has also been described.[14]

Therapy consists of antidiarrheal measures, sulfasalazine, and antibiotics such as metronidazole, as well as glucocorticoids. In a few resistant cases, partial colonic resection has been performed. A pathogenic role has been discussed but seems unlikely. Unexpectedly, some cases respond favorably to NSAID therapy.

◾ Poncet's Disease and *Bacille Calmette-Gueorin*–Induced Reactive Arthritis

Tuberculous arthritis or Poncet's disease is a rare aseptic form of insidious fever, weakness, and arthritis described mostly in young adults suffering from extrapulmonary tuberculosis.[14] It is said to respond slowly to antituberculous therapy, and in the absence of pulmonary changes, the intestine is assumed to be the port of entry. The attenuated *Mycobacterium* bacille Calmette-Guerin (BCG) strain is used intradermally as an adjuvant in cancer therapy to stimulate T cell–mediated immunity. It is also instilled into the urinary bladder to treat superficial cancer. Aseptic arthritis occurs in 0.4 to 0.8 percent of these patients, and anecdotal evidence indicates an increased prevalence of HLA-B27 among these.[62] This was associated with sacroiliitis in some 20 percent and with oligoarthritis with predominant localization to the lower limbs, and it occurred more often in men. In cases of reactive arthritis occurring after intradermal administration of BCG, on the other hand, 6 of 10 patients were women, and symmetric hand arthritis dominated. The prognosis was good in these cases; symptoms cleared within 3 months.

Mycobacterium HSP (HSP65) has been incriminated in both these sterile forms of arthritis, as well as in other forms of arthritis.[63] Mycobacterial and human HSPs are 50 percent homologous, and one hypothesis is that both therapeutic efficacy and arthritis complication could be caused by cross-reactive T lymphocytes. HSP also has homologies with proteoglycan and HLA-DR. The pathogenesis of arthritis after intravesical instillation could be different and related to antigen persistence, setting the stage for a kind of reactive arthritis.

◾ Summary

The concept of enteropathic arthritis has gained importance from advances in knowledge regarding gut immunology and function and cell trafficking. It is a safe prediction that expanding knowledge in the field of host–microbe interactions will shed better light on pathogenic mechanisms of the diseases dealt with in this chapter, other diseases in the spondylarthritis family, and RA.

REFERENCES

1. Wollheim FA: Enteropathic arthritis: How do the joints talk with the gut? Curr Opin Rheumatol 13:305, 2001.
2. Unno N, Fink MP: Intestinal hyperpermeability: Mechanisms and relevance to disease. Gastroenterol Clin North Am 27:289, 1998.
3. Lennernas H: Human intestinal permeability. J Pharm Sci 87:403, 1998.
4. Iqbal TH, Lewis KO, Gearty JC, Cooper BT: Small intestinal permeability to mannitol and lactulose in the three ethnic groups resident in west Birmingham. Gut 39:199, 1996.
5. Mestecky J, Russel MW, Elson CO: Intestinal IgA: Novel views on its function in the defence of the largest mucosal surface. Gut 44:2, 1999.
6. Brandtzaeg P: Review article: Homing of mucosal immune cells—a possible connection between intestinal and articular inflammation. Aliment Pharmacol Ther 11(Suppl 3):24, 1997.
7. Salmi M, Rajala P, Jalkanen S: Homing of mucosal leukocytes to joints: Distinct endothelial ligands in synovium mediate leukocyte-subtype specific adhesion. J Clin Invest 99:2165, 1997.
8. Taurog JD: HLA-B27 subtypes, disease susceptibility, and peptide binding specificity. In Calin A, Taurog JD (eds): The Spondylarthritides. Oxford, Oxford University Press, 1998, p 257.
9. Tysk C, Lindberg E, Jarnerot G, Floderus-Myrhed B: Ulcerative colitis and Crohn's disease in an unselected population of monozygotic and dizygotic twins. A study of heritability and the influence of smoking. Gut 29:990, 1988.
10. Plevy SE, Targan SR, Yang H, et al: Tumor necrosis factor microsatellites define a Crohn's disease–associated haplotype on chromosome 6. Gastroenterology 110:1053, 1996.
11. Fuss IJ, Neurath M, Boirivant M, et al: Disparate CD4⁺ lamina propria (LP) lymphokine secretion profiles in inflammatory bowel disease: Crohn's disease LP cells manifest increased secretion of IFN-γ, whereas ulcerative colitis LP cells manifest increased secretion of IL-5. J Immunol 157:1261, 1996.
12. Camoglio L, Te Velde AA, Tigges AJ, et al: Altered expression of interferon-γ and interleukin-4 in inflammatory bowel disease. Inflamm Bowel Dis 4:285, 1998.
13. Guimbaud R, Bertrand V, Chauvelot-Moachon L, et al: Network of inflammatory cytokines and correlation with disease activity in ulcerative colitis. Am J Gastroenterol 93:2397, 1998.
14. Wollheim FA: Enteropathic arthritis. In Kelley WN, Harris ED Jr, Ruddy S, Sledge CB (eds): Textbook of Rheumatology, 5th ed. Philadelphia, WB Saunders, 1997, p 1006.
15. Helliwell PS, Hickling P, Wright V: Do the radiological changes of classical ankylosing spondylitis differ from the changes found in the spondylitis associated with inflammatory bowel disease, psoriasis, and reactive arthritis? Ann Rheum Dis 57:135, 1998.
16. Mielants H, Veys EM, Goemaere S, et al: A prospective study of patients with spondylarthropathy with special reference to HLA-B27 and to gut histology. J Rheumatol 20:1353, 1993.
17. Andreyev HJ, Kamm MA, Forbes A, Nicholls RJ: Joint symptoms after restorative proctocolectomy in ulcerative colitis and familial polyposis coli. J Clin Gastroenterol 23:35, 1996.
18. Orchard TR, Wordsworth BP, Jewell DP: Peripheral arthropathies in inflammatory bowel disease: Their articular distribution and natural history. Gut 42:387, 1998.
19. Orchard TR, Thiyagaraja S, Welsh KI, et al: Clinical phenotype is related to HLA genotype in the peripheral arthropathies of inflammatory bowel disease. Gastroenterology 118:274, 2000.

20. von den Driesch P: Pyoderma gangrenosum: A report of 44 cases with follow-up. Br J Dermatol 137:1000, 1997.

21. Orchard TR, Chua CN, Ahmad T, et al: Uveitis and erythema nodosum in inflammatory bowel disease: Clinical features and the role of HLA genes. Gastroenterology 123:714, 2002.

22. Banares A, Hernandez-Garcia C, Fernandez-Guitiérrez B, Jover JA: Eye involvement in the spondyloarthropathies. Rheum Dis Clin North Am 24:771, 1998.

23. Hammer RE, Maika SD, Richardson JA, et al: Spontaneous inflammatory disease in transgenic rats expressing HLA-B27 and human β_2m: An animal model of HLA-B27–associated human disorders. Cell 63:1099, 1990.

24. Taurog JD, Richardson JA, Croft JT, et al: The germfree state prevents development of gut and joint inflammatory disease in HLA-B27 transgenic rats. J Exp Med 180:2359, 1994.

25. Rath HC, Herfarth HH, Ikeda JS, et al: Normal luminal bacteria, especially *Bacteroides* species, mediate chronic colitis, gastritis, and arthritis in HLA-B27/human β_2-microglobulin transgenic rats. J Clin Invest 98:945, 1996.

26. Gaston JS: Pathogenic role of gut inflammation in the spondyloarthropathies. Curr Opin Rheumatol 9:302, 1997.

27. Maki-Ikola O, Hallgren R, Kanerud L, et al: Enhanced jejunal production of antibodies to *Klebsiella* and other Enterobacteria in patients with ankylosing spondylitis and rheumatoid arthritis. Ann Rheum Dis 56:421, 1997.

28. Macpherson A, Khoo UY, Forgacs I, et al: Mucosal antibodies in inflammatory bowel disease are directed against intestinal bacteria. Gut 38:365, 1996.

29. Tiwana H, Walmsley RS, Wilson C, et al: Characterization of the humoral immune response to *Klebsiella* species in inflammatory bowel disease and ankylosing spondylitis. Br J Rheumatol 37:525, 1998.

30. Söderholm JD, Olaison G, Lindberg E, et al: Different intestinal permeability patterns in relatives and spouses of patients with Crohn's disease: An inherited defect in mucosal defence? Gut 44:96, 1999.

31. Osman NE, Wastrom B, Karlsson B: Serosal but not mucosal endotoxin exposure increases intestinal permeability in vitro in the rat. Scand J Gastroenterol 33:1170, 1998.

32. Rutgeerts P: Medical therapy of inflammatory bowel disease. Digestion 59:433, 1998.

33. Hanauer SB, Feagan BG, Lichtenstein GR, et al: Maintenance infliximab for Crohn's disease: the ACCENT I randomised trial. Lancet 359:9317, 2002.

34. Van den Bosch F, Kruithof E, De Vos M, et al: Crohn's disease associated with spondyloarthropathy: effect of TNF-alpha blockade with infliximab on articular symptoms. Lancet. 356(9244):1821, 2000.

35. Yacyshyn BR, Chey WY, Goff J, et al: Double blind, placebo controlled trial of the remission inducing and steroid sparing properties of an ICAM-1 antisense oligodeoxynucleotide, alicaforsen (ISIS 2302), in active steroid dependent Crohn's disease. Gut 51:30, 2002.

36. Sigthorsson G, Tibble J, Hayllar J, et al: Intestinal permeability and inflammation in patients on NSAIDs. Gut 43:506, 1998.

37. Wallace DJ, Weisman M: Should a war criminal be rewarded with eponymous distinction? The double life of Hans Reiter (1881–1969). J Clin Rheumatol 6:49, 2000.

38. Fiessinger M, Leroy B: Contribution à l'étude d'une épidemie de dysenterie dans la Somme. Bull Soc Med Hop Paris 40:2030, 1916.

39. Schumacher HR Jr: Reactive arthritis. Rheum Dis Clin North Am 24:261, 1998.

40. Thomson DGT, DeRubeis DA, Hodge MA, et al: Post-salmonella reactive arthritis: Late clinical sequelae in a point source cohort. Am J Med 98:13, 1995.

41. Ahmed S, Ayoub EM, Scornik JC, et al: Poststreptococcal reactive arthritis: Clinical characteristics and association with HLA-DR alleles. Arthritis Rheum 41:1096, 1998.

42. Jansen TL, Janssen M, de Jong AJ: Reactive arthritis associated with group C and group G β-hemolytic streptococci. J Rheumatol 25:1126, 1998.

43. Rajapakse CN: Bacterial infections: osteoarticular brucellosis. Baillieres Clin Rheumatol 9:161, 1995.

44. Ibero I, Vela P, Pascual E: Arthritis of shoulder and spinal cord compression due to *Brucella* disc infection. Br J Rheumatol 36:377, 1997.

45. Granfors K, Merilahti-Palo R, Luukkainen R, et al: Persistence of *Yersinia* antigens in peripheral blood cells from patients with *Yersinia enterocolitica* O:3 infection with or without reactive arthritis. Arthritis Rheum 41:855, 1998.

46. Ekman P, Kirveskari J, Granfors K: Modification of disease outcome in *Salmonella*-infected patients by HLA-B27. Arthritis Rheum 43:1527, 2000.

47. Penttinen MA, Holmberg CI, Sistonen L, Granfors K: HLA-B27 modulates nuclear factor kappaB activation in human monocytic cells exposed to lipopolysaccharide. Arthritis Rheum 46:2172, 2002.

48. Saarinen M, Ekman P, Ikeda M, et al: Invasion of *Salmonella* into human intestinal epithelial cells is modulated by HLA-B27. Rheumatology (Oxford) 41:651, 2002.

49. Ugrinovic S, Mertz A, Wu P, et al: A single nonamer from the *Yersinia* 60-kDa heat shock protein is the target of HLA-B27–restricted CTL response in *Yersinia*-induced reactive arthritis. J Immunol 159:5715, 1997.

50. Sieper J, Braun J: Treatment of reactive arthritis with antibiotics. Br J Rheumatol 37:717, 1998.

50a.Yli-Kerttula T, Luukkainen R, Yli-Kerttula U, et al: Effect of a three month course of ciprofloxacin on the late prognosis of reactive orthritis. Ann Rheum Dis 62:880, 2003.

51. ter Borg EJ, Nadorp JH, Elbers JR: Ileal pouch arthritis: A case report. Eur J Gastroenterol Hepatol 8:957, 1996.

52. Fisch C, Schiller P, Harr T, Maclachlan D: First presentation of intestinal bypass syndrome 18 yr after initial surgery. Rheumatology (Oxford) 40:351, 2001.

53. Sjöström H, Lundin KE, Molberg O, et al: Identification of a gliadin T-cell epitope in coeliac disease: General importance of gliadin deamidation for intestinal T-cell recognition. Scand J Immunol 48:111, 1998.

54. Lubrano E, Ciacci C, Ames PR, et al: The arthritis of coeliac disease: Prevalence and pattern in 200 adult patients. Br J Rheumatol 35:1314, 1996.

55. Slot O, Locht H: Arthritis as presenting symptom in adult coeliac disease: Two cases and review of the literature. Scand J Rheumatol 29:260, 2000.

56. Louie JS, Liebling MR: The polymerase chain reaction in infectious and post-infectious arthritis. Rheum Dis Clin North Am 24:227, 1998.

57. Durand DV, Lecomte C, Cathebras P, et al: Whipple disease: Clinical review of 52 cases—The SNFMI research group on Whipple disease. Societé Nationale Francaise de Medecine Interne. Medicine (Baltimore) 76:170, 1997.

58. Singer R: Diagnosis and treatment of Whipple's disease. Drugs 55:669, 1998.

59. Giardiello FM, Lazenby AJ, Bayless TM, et al: Lymphocytic (microscopic) colitis: Clinicopathologic study of 18 patients and comparison to collagenous colitis. Dig Dis Sci 34:1730, 1989.

60. Bohr J, Tysk C, Eriksson S, Jarnerot G: Collagenous colitis in Orebro, Sweden, an epidemiological study 1984–1993. Gut 37:394, 1995.

61. Domargård A, Skogh T, Bohr J, et al: Collagenous colitis and rheumatoid arthritis: Is there a relation? Ann Rheum Dis 61(suppl 1):78, 2002.

62. Buchs N, Chevrel G, Miossec P: Bacillus Calmette-Gueorin induced aseptic arthritis: An experimental model of reactive arthritis. J Rheumatol 25:1662, 1998.

63. Iwata H, Kinoshita M, Sumiya M, et al: Emergence of erosive polyarthritis coincident with *Mycobacterium kansasii* pulmonary infection in a patient with systemic sclerosis-rheumatoid arthritis overlap syndrome. Clin Exp Rheumatol 17:757, 1999.

Systemic Lupus Erythematosus and Related Syndromes

74

Pathogenesis of Systemic Lupus Erythematosus

BEVRA HANNAHS HAHN · GEORGE A. KARPOUZAS · BETTY P. TSAO

The pathogenesis of systemic lupus erythematosus (SLE) is complex, as shown in Figure 74–1 and reviewed elsewhere.[1] Target tissue damage is caused primarily by pathogenic autoantibodies and immune complexes. The abnormal immune response that permits persistence of pathogenic B and T cells has multiple components that include processing of increased quantities of self antigens by antigen-presenting cells, hyperactivation of T and B cells, and failure of multiple regulatory networks to interrupt this process. The immunologic abnormalities occur in a framework of interactions between multiple susceptibility genes (and insufficient protective genes)[2,3] and environmental stimuli, at least one of which (ultraviolet light) can induce apoptosis in dermal cells that results in presentation of RNA protein, DNA protein, and phospholipid self antigens to the immune system.[4]

The Effectors of Systemic Lupus Erythematosus

PATHOGENIC AUTOANTIBODIES

All individuals produce numerous antibodies that react with self molecules. The characteristics of the background antiself normal repertoire include the following: Most of the antibodies are immunoglobulin (Ig) M; they have weak avidity for self antigens; and they are widely cross-reactive with multiple antigens. Pathogenic autoantibodies are different (Table 74–1). They are usually IgG, have high avidity for self antigens, and have restricted specificity.[5,6] High-avidity antiself antibodies can be constructed from many different immunoglobulin genes, but they tend to derive from a few "preferred" families of genes, suggesting derivation from an initial, antigen-activated "mother" B cell.[7,8] Pathogenic Ig molecules are often highly mutated, particularly in

the hypervariable (complementarity determining) regions of their heavy and light chains.[5-10]

Several features of autoantibodies influence their pathogenic potential, including what antigens they bind, avidity for those antigens, the net charge of the Ig molecule and the immune complex it forms with antigen, the presence in the Ig molecule of charged amino acids that interact with opposite charges on cell membranes or DNA, presence in the Ig molecules of sequences recognized by helper T cells, and ability to fix and activate complement.[10] Even though we understand many of these principles, it is difficult to predict that a given monoclonal antiself antibody will be a pathogen. For example, two high-avidity, IgG2a, complement-fixing murine monoclonal anti-DNA antibodies were administered to normal mice; one caused nephritis on transfer to normal BALB/c mice; the other did not.[11] Among monoclonal human antibodies to DNA, some caused proteinuria upon transfer to severe combined immunodeficiency (SCID) mice, whereas others did not.[12]

In terms of antigens bound, it is convenient to think of the autoantibodies of SLE as belonging to one of several groups directed against DNA/protein complexes, RNA/protein complexes, cell membrane structures, and intracellular molecules that reach cell surfaces during cell activation. The antibodies considered to be the hallmark of SLE are IgG antibodies to double-stranded (ds)-DNA. These antibodies probably develop from antibodies to histone proteins on nucleosomes (antinucleosomal antibodies). Nucleosomes are presented to the immune system in surface membrane blebs of cells undergoing apoptosis and are released from cells undergoing programmed cell death.[4,13] Studies in mice suggest that the initial antibodies to DNA/protein are directed against nucleosomes.[14] As those antibodies mature and gain somatic mutations, some daughter cells bind single-stranded DNA (ss-DNA), and then ultimately both anti–ss-DNA and anti–ds-DNA. In support of this "antinucleosome-to-anti–ds-DNA hyporthesis"

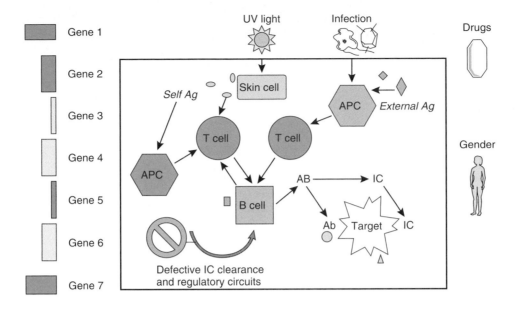

FIGURE 74–1 · Overview of the Pathogenesis of SLE. The immune abnormalities that characterize SLE are pictured inside the framework of susceptibility (and preventive) genes and possible environmental stimuli that trigger the immune responses. External antigens are pictured as diamonds; self antigens are pictured as ovals, circles, triangles, and squares. External factors introduce their own antigens to be processed by antigen-presenting cells, and they cause apoptosis, activation, or death of host cells, thus releasing self antigen (e.g., nucleosomes, U1 RNP, and Ro/SS-A), which can in turn be processed by antigen-presenting cells and B cells. These processed peptides stimulate T cells and bind to antigen receptors on B cells, thus driving the production of harmful antibodies, which can in turn combine with antigen to form harmful immune complexes. The target cells (glomeruli, endothelial cells, platelets) then release more self antigen to perpetuate the process. Meanwhile, the multiple regulatory circuits that are supposed to alter this response to self so that it is harmless are not working effectively. It is likely that multiple genes control each of these responses—including genes for T and B cell hyperactive responses, characteristics of the target cells, and inability to mount regulation, like immune complex clearance and regulatory T cells.

TABLE 74–1 · CHARACTERISTICS OF PATHOGENIC AUTOANTIBODIES

- Many different V-, D-, and J-region genes of the immunoglobulin (Ig) heavy chain and V- and J-region genes of the light chain, used to assemble protective antibodies against external antigens, can also be used to assemble pathogenic autoantibodies.
- There is probably some restriction in the Ig genes used to assemble autoantibodies, because they tend to derive from a few families, suggesting that many cells are daughters of cells initially activated by antigen.
- Many pathogenic autoantibodies are mutated in variable regions (and often in framework regions), suggesting modification by specific antigenic stimulation.
- General characteristics that favor ability of an autoantibody to be pathogenic are as follows:
  Ability to bind directly to target tissues, such as erythrocytes, lymphocytes, and platelet membranes, or to glomerular antigens
  Ability to activate complement
  Cationic charge favoring adherence to polyanionic regions of membranes
  High avidity for the autoantigen present in target tissue
  Presence of amino acids in antigen-contacting region of the Ig molecule that favor charge-charge or hydrogen-bonding interactions with molecules in the antigen; this contributes to high avidity for antigen

are observations that both mice and humans with SLE have T cells activated by nucleosomes and nucleosomal peptides: Such cells can help B cell synthesis of IgG anti–ds-DNA.[15-17] It is likely that at least some pathogenic anti-DNA antibodies bind directly or in complexes to DNA deposited in basement membranes and to other renal structures, including heparan sulfate, histone, laminin, alpha-actinin, and collagen in glomerular basement membranes.[10,11,18-22] Sera from patients with lupus nephritis contain antibodies that bind to glomeruli; some bind DNA, and others do not.[23,24] Non–DNA-binding autoantibodies that probably can cause nephritis include antibodies to C1q,[25,26] nucleosomes,[11] and Ro/SS-A.[27]

Another autoantibody highly specific for SLE is anti-Smith (anti-Sm). High-affinity anti-Sm antibodies have a prevalence of 5 to 25 percent in SLE patients. They are usually of IgG subclass, suggesting T cell dependence. T cell immunity against Sm peptides has been described in peripheral blood mononuclear cells (PBMCs) and lymphoid tissues of both SLE patients and mice.[28] Sm-reactive T cells demonstrate highly restricted T cell receptor (TCR) usage, which is characteristic of an antigen-driven response. SmD1 appears to be the most frequently recognized peptide in the molecule. It is remarkably conserved and bears a 99-percent homology with the mouse D1 protein. The epitope SmD1$_{83-119}$ appears to be recognized with remarkable sensitivity and specificity by human SLE sera (70 percent in SLE vs. 8.3 percent in healthy controls and other autoimmune diseases), possibly due to its highly positive charge and its conformation.[29,30] In murine systems SmD1$_{83-119}$ is very effective both as an immunogen (accelerating disease) and as a tolerogen (preventing or delaying disease) in lupus-prone mice.[31]

Other autoantibodies that directly cause disease include those that coat platelets or erythrocytes. Interestingly, antibodies against platelets in lupus patients with thrombocytopenia recognize a wider variety of antigens than do antibodies in patients with idiopathic thrombocytopenic purpura. In both diseases, antibodies are directed against surface glycoprotein II and III antigens on intact platelets; but in SLE, there are additional antibodies against cytoplasmic antigens, which come to the surface of activated platelets, and against phospholipids, suggesting that activated, damaged cells and cells undergoing apoptosis (in which antigenic portions of phospholipids in cell membranes are directed outward rather than inward) are important in stimulating pathogenic responses in SLE.[32]

Antibodies against proteins associated with the Ro/La particle are probably also direct pathogens, particularly in congenital heart block.[33-37] IgG anti-Ro crosses the placenta, can bind to certain areas of fetal heart conduction system tissue, alter myosin-actin function, and probably cause heart block. The syndrome has been essentially reproduced in fetal mice; infusion of IgG anti-Ro from mothers with fetuses with congenital heart block induces electrocardiographic abnormalities in the fetal mouse heart compatible with heart block.[34] Furthermore, once a woman has produced a fetus with congenital heart block, the chances of subsequent fetuses having the same problem are greatly increased. Most babies with congenital heart block have mothers with anti-Ro (or rarely anti-ribonucleoprotein [RNP] or anti-La); many of those mothers are healthy at the time of this occurrence, but some develop SLE or lupus-like syndromes later.[35]

Antibodies against phospholipids (either anticardiolipin or the lupus anticoagulant) increase the risk for venous or arterial thrombosis, for fetal loss, and for thrombocytopenia.[38] They are likely to be involved directly in induction or maintenance of blood clots. Antibodies to ribosomal P have been associated with depression and psychosis in SLE patients in some studies and with hepatitis and nephritis in others.[39-41] The mechanism by which they cause disease is unclear but may be related to the fact that they, like some antibodies to DNA and RNP, can penetrate membranes of living cells, bind cytoplasmic or nuclear structures, and alter cell function.[42]

PATHOGENIC IMMUNE COMPLEXES

Like autoreactive antibodies, some immune complexes are pathogenic and others are not. The characteristics of pathogenic immune complexes are summarized in Table 74–2 and reviewed elsewhere.[43] Size of the immune complex is important; large immune complexes are cleared by the mononuclear phagocytic cell

---

TABLE 74–2 • FACTORS FAVORING TISSUE DEPOSITION AND PATHOGENICITY OF IMMUNE COMPLEXES

- Excessive quantities of immune complexes, which overwhelm clearance mechanisms
- "Correct" size (large complexes are bound by the mononuclear phagocytic system and cleared rapidly; small complexes are excreted in urine; intermediate size complexes are most likely to escape these mechanisms and to be tissue bound)
- Tissue tropism of immune complexes (cationic charge of complexes allows binding to anions in tissue; antibody may recognize components of tissues)
- Decreased immune-complex clearance and catabolism (relates to acquired and genetically determined low levels of surface complement receptors, genetic acquisition of fragment crystallizable (Fcγ receptors that are inefficient binders of immunoglobulin (Ig) in immune complexes, decreased solubilization of immune complexes by complement as complement levels fall or are genetically low)

---

system on their first "pass" through the circulation; small immune complexes are more likely to deposit in tissue. Excessive quantities of immune complexes overwhelm the mechanisms used to clear them, as discussed before. Finally, some immune complexes are "tissue tropic" and prone to bind to tissues because they have a net cationic charge or because the antibodies they contain are directed against tissue components. It is well accepted that immune complexes that fix complement are responsible for much of the tissue damage that characterizes SLE. In mammals, immune complexes are transported bound to complement receptor 1 (CR1) receptors, predominantly on erythrocytes. If surface CR1 molecule numbers are low, either because of genetic factors or because they have been stripped from the cell surfaces by an overload of activated complement, pathogenic immune complexes may persist long enough to cause tissue damage.[44,45]

Genetics of Systemic Lupus Erythematosus

As with other autoimmune diseases, susceptibility to SLE depends on multiple genes.[2,3] Susceptibility genes are defined as genes that increase the relative risk for a disease, even though most individuals with that gene are healthy. The number of genes a person must inherit to develop clinical SLE is unknown; it is likely to be several, with full gene effect depending partly on other modifying or protective genes in the same individual, gender, and the strength of environmental stimuli that can trigger disease (e.g., a severe sunburn in a person with susceptibility genes). Evidence for genetic predisposition in humans includes the following:

1. An approximately 10-fold increase in clinical disease in monozygotic compared to dizygotic twins[46-48]
2. An 8-fold or greater relative risk for SLE in first-degree relatives, with 10 to 16 percent of

patients with SLE having an affected first- or second-degree relative[49-50]

3. Association and linkage studies associating disease with particular gene variants and haplotypes[2,3,51]
4. Scans of the human genome linking disease with several regions on multiple chromosomes[52-54]

Because the highest reported concordance rate in monozygotic twins is 58 percent,[48] it is likely that environmental factors are also required.

The evidence for genetic control of disease is even more compelling in mice. Several strains are predisposed to SLE, with almost all individuals (gender dependent in some strains) developing the disease as they age. Major histocompatibility complex (MHC) class II genes on chromosome 6 (similar to human leukocyte antigen [HLA]-D on chromosome 17) and regions on several other chromosomes contribute to susceptibility in these strains.[55-63] Some locations on mouse chromosomes have potential homologues in the human genome. Mice predisposed to lupus that also inherit the *lpr* or *gld* genes have accelerated disease based on mutations in the genes encoding Fas (in *lpr*) and Fas ligand (in *gld*) that impair apoptosis[64-66] and permit autoreactive T and B cells to persist for abnormally long periods. Bx satin beige (BXSB) male mice spontaneously develop severe systemic autoimmunity due to the presence of the *yaa* gene in the Y chromosome, which accelerates a lupus-like disease mediated by interactions with several genes in the BXSB genome.[66a]

Human Genetic Studies

Multiple ethnic populations have been analyzed for susceptibility genes. Three principles have emerged:

1. For most ethnic populations, some of the susceptibility genes differ from those of other populations.
2. There are individual genes that predispose to disease across multiple ethnic groups.
3. Genetic predisposition may be linked to autoantibody repertoires and to clinical subsets of disease.

The currently known genes and gene regions associated with murine and human SLE are shown in Table 74–3. Table 74–4 shows the putative susceptibility loci significantly linked to SLE by genome scanning. Some genes associated with SLE in humans are located on chromosome 6, in the region that encodes HLA genes, especially class II (DR, DQ, DP) and class III (C2, C4).[2,3,53] Other chromosomes contain susceptibility genes, with general agreement that those linked to SLE include two regions on chromosome 1, and chromosomes 2, 4, and 16.[51-54,67]

Extended haplotypes predispose to disease in certain ethnic groups. As shown in Table 74–3, several investigators have reported an association between HLA class I-B8 and SLE in whites of Western and Northern European ancestry.[3,68-72] There is linkage disequilibrium between class I-B8 and class II-DR3. DR3 and DR2 are linked to SLE in different haplotypes and predispose to different

clinical subsets of disease.[68,69,72-86] For example, HLA-B8/DR3/DQw2/C4AQO is a haplotype associated with a deletion of class III genes-*C4A* and a neighboring *CYP21A* gene[73-77] and predisposes to SLE in whites. In nonwhite SLE populations, a defective *C4A* gene is also frequent but usually results from mechanisms other than deletion.[78-83] The extended haplotype HLA-A10/B18/C4A4/C4B2/BFS is in disequilibrium with class III complement C2 deficiency[2]; homozygous deficiency for C2 occurs in 1 in 10,000 individuals,[87-90] many of whom have SLE or similar disease. The SLE is clinically distinct; patients have primarily joint and skin disease and are often antinuclear antibody negative. A recent study using a large cohort (334 families containing 576 SLE patients) identifies three distinct SLE-associated haplotypes containing DRB1*1501/DQB1*0602, DRB1*0801/DQB1*0402, and DRB1*0301/DQB1*0201 alleles, respectively.[91] By defining ancestral recombinants, the DRB1*1501 (formerly known as DR2) risk haplotype contains both the DRB1 and DQB1 genes, but excludes the class I and class III regions including tumor necrosis factor-α (TNF-α). The DRB1*0301 haplotype corresponds to the HLA A1-B8-DR3 haplotype of the Northern European origin that has been associated with several other autoimmune diseases, including type 1 diabetes, Graves' disease, and myasthenia gravis.[92] The extensive linkage disequilibrium of the DRB1*0301 haplotype makes ancestral recombinants within this region rather rare and difficult to narrow the SLE-associated region beyond the 1-megabase (1-Mb) interval containing most class III and class II genes.[91] The DRB1*0801 (DR8) haplotype is less common in this cohort, and ancestral recombinants narrows the risk region to approximately 500 kb containing both the DRB1 and DQB1 genes.[91] These three SLE class II risk haplotypes are highly enriched in white families; among the 254 families carrying at least one risk haplotype, 229 (90%) are white or have known white admixture. Analysis of haplotype frequencies in 280 female SLE cases from the family collection and 174 female white controls reveals an approximately twofold increase in frequencies of risk haplotypes of SLE patients compared to controls and a doubling of risk for homozygotes compared to heterozygotes.[91] The disease-associated HLA genotypes appear to be not-as-strong contributors for risks to develop SLE compared to other autoimmune diseases such as ankylosing spondilitis (AS), type 1 diabetes, or rheumatoid arthritis (RA).

Individual Human Leukocyte Antigen Genes Predisposing to Systemic Lupus Erythematosus

High risk for SLE is conferred by homozygous deficiencies of early complement components or their inhibitors, including C2 and C4 within the HLA gene complex and non-HLA C1q, C1r, and C1-INH.[87-90] Individuals with nearly total absence of these proteins are rare and account for less than 5 percent of those with SLE. However, most people with homozygous deficiencies have SLE or SLE-like diseases. Although null alleles for C4 are genes predisposing to SLE in multiple ethnic groups (see Table 74–3), complete deficiency of C4 is rare, because four alleles (two at *C4A* and two at

TABLE 74–3 • THE GENETIC BASIS OF SYSTEMIC LUPUS ERYTHEMATOSUS (SLE)

Genes Involved in Murine Lupus

Major histocompatibility complex (MHC) (chromosome 17): *H2z* of NZW mouse permits production of pathogenic immunoglobulin G (IgG) antibodies to DNA
lpr (chromosome 19): Contains mutation in Fas that accelerates SLE on permissive genetic backgrounds, such as MRL/lpr
gld (chromosome 1): Contains mutation in Fas ligand that accelerates SLE on permissive genetic backgrounds
yaa (chromosome Y): Accelerates SLE in males of genetically predisposed strains (BXSB)
Multiple regions on different chromosomes protect NZW mice from developing SLE although they possess several predisposing genes.

In Mice with Combined New Zealand Black (NZB) and New Zealand White (NZW) Backgrounds

Chromosome 1: Contains at least two regions that predispose to SLE
Nba2: Associated with break in tolerance to DNA-containing molecules; a candidate susceptibility gene for the *Nba2* locus has recently been identified—*Ifi202* (chromosome 1)—a NZB-derived interferon-inducible gene
Sle1: Promotes loss of tolerance to nucleosomes and permits development of histone-specific T cells; ANA develops along with minimal nephritis; this chromosomal region contains four separate susceptibility loci—*Sle1a, Sle1b, Sle1c,* and *Sle1d*—the NZM2410/NZW-derived complement receptor 2 gene, *Cr2*, has been implicated as a candidate susceptibility gene for the *Sle1c* locus
Chromosome 4: *Sle2* permits hyperactivation of B cells with high levels of IgM, no nephritis
Chromosome 7: *Sle3* permits hyperactivation of T cells, increased numbers of CD4+ T cells with delayed apoptosis, increased IgG antibodies to nucleosomal antigens, moderate nephritis
Combination of *Sle1* and *Sle3* permits severe SLE with IgG antibodies to DNA and lethal, early nephritis
Sle1 suppressor in MHC regimen reduces percentage of mice with lethal nephritis in Sle1 + Sle2 + Sle1s

Genes Involved in Human Lupus

Histocompatibilty (HLA) Genes

Extended haplotypes predispose to lupus in some ethnic groups:
  HLA-B8/DRB1*0301/DQB1*0201/C4AQO (anti-Ro)
  HLA-DRB1*1501/DQB1*0602 (nephritis, low levels of tumor necrosis factor-α [TNF-α])
  HLA-DRB1*0801/DQB1*0402
  HLA-A10/B18/C4A4/C4B2/BFS (associated with C2 deficiency)
  DR2 (increases relative risk two- to threefold)
  DR3 (increases relative risk two- to threefold)
  DR2/DQw1 (anti-Ro)
  DR3/DQw2 (anti-Ro plus anti-La)
  DR2 or DR3 with DQB1*0201, 0602, 0302 (anti-DNA)
  DR4 with DQw5, w8 and others (anti-U1 RNP)
  DR2 with DQw6 or w7 and others (anti-Sm)
  DR4, DR7 with DQw7, w8, w6 and others (lupus anticoagulant)
Homozygous deficiencies of early complement components (C2, C4)

Nonhistocompatibility Genes

C1q (chromosome 1)
FcγRIIA receptor allele (chromosome 1)
FcγRIIIA receptor allele (chromosome 1)
Promoter polymorphisms of interleukin (IL)-10 (chromosome 1)
PDCD1 polymorphisms (chromosome 2)
Mannose-binding ligand polymorphisms (chromosome 10)

TABLE 74–4 • PUTATIVE SUSCEPTIBILITY LOCI SIGNIFICANTLY LINKED TO SYSTEMIC LUPUS ERYTHEMATOSUS (SLE) BY GENOME SCANNING

Locus	LOD Scores	Candidate Genes	Syntenic Murine Susceptibility Loci
1q22-24	3.4	*FCGR2A, FCGR3A*	*Sle1a, Sle1b*
1q41-43	3.3, 3.5	*PARP*	*Sle1d, Bxs3*
2q35-37	4.2	*PDCD1*	
4p16-15	3.8		
6p11-22	4.2	*DR, DQ*	*Lbw1, Sle1s*
16q12-13	3.8	*NOD2*	

Abbreviations: LOD scores, logarithm of the odds that the two loci are linked PARP, poly(ADP-rivase) polymerase; PDCD1, programmed cell death 1 gene.

C4B) contribute to synthesis of the protein. In affected populations, about 50 percent of SLE patients have a C4 gene abnormality, compared to 15 percent or less in healthy, ethnically matched control subjects.

DR3 and DR2 are individual genes that predispose to SLE in multiple ethnic groups, but the relative risk conferred by those genes alone is 2 to 3.[2,68,69,84-86,93] As described previously, DR3 is a part of an extended HLA haplotype in linkage disequilibrium with the promoter polymorphism of the TNF-α gene (−308A *TNFA*).[94] The −308A *TNFA* allele has been shown to confer higher transcriptional activity than the −308G *TNFA* allele.[95] The high-activity allele has been associated with SLE in multiple studies and may be an independent risk factor or a part of the HLA risk haplotype.[96-100] However, neither the disease association nor the elevated activity has been consistently demonstrated in similar studies.[101]

Human Leukocyte Antigen Genes and Autoantibody Production

A strong association exists between certain HLA genes, particularly amino acid sequences in the DR and DQα and DQβ regions, and the ability to make certain autoantibodies.[3,102-108] Anti-Ro/SS-A and La/SS-B are examples.[104,105] They are genetically linked antibodies specific for proteins associated with small nuclear RNP; they are associated clinically with sicca complex, neonatal lupus, and subacute cutaneous lupus. Anti-Ro without anti-La is associated with DR2/DQw1; anti-Ro plus anti-La is associated with DR3/DQw2 and exhibits a gene-dose effect. That is, patients heterozygous for DQw1/DQw2 have high quantities of anti-Ro,[104] which strengthens the evidence linking the genes and the autoantibodies. In fact, most patients who have anti-Ro plus anti-La have three or four of the relevant DR/DQ alleles, and none has less than two.[2] All of the DQα alleles associated with anti-Ro share a Glu in position 34; all the DQβ alleles have Leu in position 26. These amino acids are found in those positions in the I-A molecules of MRL/lpr mice, the only murine lupus model that makes large quantities of anti-Ro and anti-La.[2,105]

Genetic associations with autoantibodies have been reported for anti-DNA,[102] anti–U1 RNP,[106] the 70-kD polypeptide of U1 RNP,[106,107] the lupus anticoagulant,[108] and autoantibodies to nucleosomes[67] and C1q.[103] Many of these autoantibodies are associated with certain clinical manifestations of SLE. Thus, the genetic background may control the autoantibody pattern, which, in turn, helps, determine the clinical subset.

Nonhuman Leukocyte Antigen Genes Predisposing to Systemic Lupus Erythematosus

Non-HLA gene/genomic regions linked to or associated with SLE are listed in Table 74–3. A strong association between the rare disorder of complement C1q deficiency and SLE reveals the importance of C1q in preventing the development of SLE. Among the 32 patients identified to have homozygous deficiency of C1q, more than 90 percent (30 individuals) have developed SLE.[109,110] Mice lacking C1q are defective in removal of apoptotic bodies, and many develop lupus-like glomerulonephritis on a permissive genetic background.[111] Structurally similar to C1q, mannose binding ligand (MBL) activates both classic and alternative pathways of the complement cascade and opsonizes bacteria. Polymorphisms in the *MBL* promoter and exon 1, which result in lower levels of MBL, are more prevalent in SLE patients than in ethnically matched controls from several different populations.[112-115] Human leukocytes express surface receptors that bind the fragment crystallizable (Fc) portions of Ig, including Ig in immune complexes. Certain polymorphisms of the genes encoding FcγIIA and FcγIIIA receptors (*FCGR2A* and *FCGR3A*) predispose to SLE. *FCGR2A*, located on human chromosome 1q23, has two codominant alleles differing at amino acids in position 131 of the molecule, H131 and R131. H131 is associated with stronger binding and more efficient phagocytosis of IgG2 and IgG3 than is R131. Among African Americans, Dutch, South Koreans, and

Hispanics with SLE, particularly those with lupus nephritis, there is less inheritance of H131 (or more inheritance of R131) than in healthy control subjects from the same populations.[116-119] In whites, there may be no correlation between this gene polymorphism and disease susceptibility,[120-124] but it may relate to severity, because homozygotes for R131 have earlier disease and more proteinuria.[125] Similarly, polymorphisms in the extracellular portion of the FcγIIIA receptor (mapped to the 1q23 region) predispose to SLE; patients with SLE, especially nephritis, are likely to inherit the polymorphism that binds IgG1 and IgG3 weakly compared with the allele encoding a high-binding molecule.[119,123,126,127] Using a large, multiethnic cohort of SLE patients, the low-binding allele of *FCGR3A* associates with whites but not with nonwhites (i.e., Hispanics, Asian/Pacific Islanders, blacks).[119] A possible consequence of inheriting Fcγ receptors that bind Ig weakly is impaired ability to clear immune complexes, which would be likely to predispose an individual to nephritis or other sequelae of circulating immune complexes. Interleukin-10 (IL-10), an immunoregulatory cytokine, can inhibit monocyte and dendritic cell function, but it stimulates B cell activation, proliferation, differentiation, and Ig secretion.[128] Increased serum levels of IL-10 in SLE patients compared to normals have been shown consistently.[128] The molecular basis of high IL-10 levels in SLE has been associated with several promoter polymorphisms (including two CA-repeat microsatellites, and 10 single nucleotide polymorphisms [SNPs]). One microsatellite, IL-10.G, has been associated with susceptibility to SLE in Scottish, Mexican-American, and Italian populations,[121,129,130] but not in Mexican, Swedish, or Taiwanese.[131-133] Although no association between the three SNP haplotypes (−1082 G/A,−819 C/T, and −592 C/A) and SLE has been established in five studies, significant association with various SLE manifestation has been reported.[134-138] The remaining seven promoter SNPs were identified more recently and led to the definiton of eight SNP haplotypes.[139] These haplotypes correlated with IL-10 production in normals and were significantly associated with SLE in African Americans.[139] These studies suggested a genetic basis for elevated levels of IL-10 contributing in the pathogenesis of SLE.

Linkage analysis in complex diseases (such as SLE) usually leads to the identification of large genomic intervals of approximately 20 centimorgan (cM) (approximately 20 million base pairs; Mb) that are likely to contain disease-susceptibility genes. This method uses DNA samples from families with multiple affected members to assess cosegregation of the test genetic marker allele with a phenotype of interest (e.g., SLE). As shown in Table 74–3, genome scanning of genetic markers from several groups using different collections of multiplex pedigree materials shows significant linkage of the 1q22-24,[140] 1q41-42,[51,140,141] 2q37,[142] 4p16-15,[143] 6p21-11,[144,145] and 16q12-13[144,145] chromosomal regions to SLE (the threshold for significant linkage is defined as a logarithm of odds [LOD] scores ≥3.3 or 3.6 depending on linkage methods).[146] Remarkably, confirmation of significant linkage in an independent cohort has been established for all six loci, providing strong evidence for the presence of SLE susceptibility gene(s) in each putative locus.[141,143,145,147-149] Because linkage analysis identifies large genomic intervals that are likely to harbor disease-susceptibility genes, efforts to fine-map and assess positional candidate genes (candidate genes mapped within the linked region) are in progress. To this end, a positional candidate gene for the 2q37 locus,[142,150] the programmed cell death 1 gene (PDCD1, also called PD-1), has recently been associated with SLE.[151] It is a strong candidate because mice deficient in PDCD1 are defective in peripheral tolerance of T and B cells and develop lupus-like arthritis and glomerulonephritis.[152,153] An intronic SNP in PDCD1 is associated with susceptibility to SLE in Europeans and Mexicans with relative risks of 2.6 and 3.5, respectively.[151] This SLE-associated SNP located in an intronic enhancer abolishes binding to the RUNX1 transcription factor, which could lead to aberrant regulation of PDCD1 contributing to breakdown of immune tolerance and the development of SLE. The 1q41-42 linked region contains polyadenosine diphosphate [ADP]-ribose polymerase, an enzyme that participates in DNA repair triggered by apoptosis and that has been associated with SLE by one group of investigators,[51] but not confirmed by others.[154-156] The 1q22-24–linked region contains FCGR2A and FCGR3A, which have been associated with SLE susceptibility in many studies as described previously. These two genes may be in linkage disequilibrium because of their physical proximity, which complicates the assessment of the relative role of each gene in susceptibility to SLE. A recent study provides strong genetic evidence (linkage and both family-based and population-based association) to support a role of FCGR3A in susceptibility to SLE.[157] Thus far no positional candidate genes within the 4p16-15 region have been associated with SLE. The 6p21-11–linked region contains the approximately 3.6-Mb HLA region that contains several class II risk haplotypes of SLE. NOD2, encoding a protein involved in bacterial recognition by monocytes, is the positional candidate gene within the 16q12-13 region linked to SLE. The functional role of NOD2 in innate immunity makes its genetic variants candidate genetic factors for autoimmune diseases. It is generally accepted that multiple polymorphisms of NOD2 contribute to susceptibility to Crohn's disease.[158-160] Interaction between genetic risk factors may impact susceptibility; data supporting linkage and genetic interaction of 1q23 and 16q12 have been observed in a multiethnic cohort containing 145 SLE-affected sibling pairs.[149]

The highly heterogeneous nature of manifestations among SLE patients may represent genetic heterogeneity that confounds the identification of lupus-susceptibility genes. One approach to reduce heterogeneity is to stratify pedigrees for the presence of a single manifestation and to reevaluate the genome-wide scanning data for linkage evidence for the particular manifestation-associated SLE locus. This strategy has lead to the identification of 1) a vitiligo-related SLE locus, SLEV1, at chromosome 17p13[161]; 2) a SLE susceptibility locus, SLEH1, at 11q14 in African-American (AA) SLE pedigrees stratified by hemolytic anemia (maximum LOD [MLOD] = 4.5 at D11S2002)[162] and a nucleolar antibody pattern (MLOD = 5.62 at D11S2002)[163]; 3) a SLEB3 locus at 4p16 in 23 European-American (EA) SLE pedigrees stratified by neuropsychiatric manifestations (MLOD = 5.19 at D4S2366)[164]; 4) a SLED1 locus at 19p13.2 (MLOD = 4.93 at D19S714) and another SLED2 at 18q21.1 (MLOD = 3.40 at D18S858) in 37 EA and 29 AA pedigrees, respectively, containing at least one affected with a positive anti–ds-DNA[165]; 5) SLEN1 at 10q22.3 (MLOD = 3.16 at D10S2470), SLEN2 at 2q34-35 (MLOD = 2.15 at D2S2972) in 31 EA pedigrees and SLEN3 at 11p15.6 (MLOD = 3.34 at D11S1984) in 20 AA pedigrees with two or more patients with SLE and renal disease, when stratified by renal disease.[166] The advantage of this approach is the improved evidence for linkage revealed by pedigree stratification based on select clinical manifestations compared to the disease status of SLE. However, these results from testing each manifestation separately increase the possibility of false-positive results using a smaller subset of family materials. These results could be strengthened by replications in independent samples.

Murine Lupus Genetic Studies

Several inbred mouse strains are genetically "programmed" to develop SLE.[167,168] New Zealand Bielchowsky/Black (NZB/Bl) mice develop IgG1 antibodies to erythrocytes, IgM antibodies to single-stranded DNA, and mild lymphoprolifcration; most die of hemolytic anemia, with disease earlier in females than in males. NZB/NZW and NZB/SWR F1 hybrids develop IgG2a and IgG2b anti–double-stranded DNA; females die of glomerulonephritis mediated primarily by anti-DNA; males develop slowly progressive disease at a later age. NZB/NZW F1 hybrid brother-sister matings have generated substrains of mice designated NZM mice that vary widely in prevalence and severity of nephritis, serum levels of IgG and IgM, and antibodies to nucleosomes and DNA. MRL/lpr mice develop lymphoproliferation; high levels of IgM and IgG; and antibodies to ss-DNA, ds-DNA, Ro and La, and rheumatoid factors (RFs). Clinically, they develop mild (histologic) polyarthritis, marked lymphadenopathy, salivary gland lymphocytic infiltration, and lethal glomerulonephritis. Males are affected almost as early as females are. Their disease is markedly accelerated by the lpr (for lymphoproliferation) gene added to an MRL/lpr; genetic background.[169,170] BXSB mice develop IgG anti–ds-DNA, with lethal nephritis affecting males, who have an accelerating gene (Yaa) on the Y chromosome.[66a] Other strains with lupus-like disease have been reported, such as Palmerston North and mice with the gld accelerating gene.[171] Extensive genetic studies in several of these strains have established the following principles:

1. SLE is a multigenic disease.
2. No single gene can account for all of the manifestations of disease.
3. Many susceptibility genes confer a change in immune responses that contribute to disease

when they are mixed with other susceptibility genes.

4. Modifying and protective genes exist that protect some mouse strains from developing SLE even though they inherit multiple susceptibility genes.

5. Lupus susceptibility loci appear to colocalize with susceptibility loci of other autoimmune diseases.

Genes influencing autoimmunity have been studied extensively in MRL/, MRL/lpr, NZB/Bl, NZB/ NZW F1, NZB/NZW F1 × NZW backcross, NZM, BXSB, and SWR mice. Recent analyses have employed microsatellite DNA technology, which allows examination of an entire genome and identification of regions of chromosomes that segregate with qualitative or quantitative clinical characteristics. In parallel with the genetics of human SLE, MHC class II genes (located on mouse chromosome 17) have been linked to lupus nephritis in strains with an NZW background.[55-58] In addition, the importance of the lpr gene (on chromosome 19), which encodes a defective Fas receptor, has been elucidated.[64-66,170,171] This defect probably accounts for acceleration of autoimmunity in mice bearing the lpr gene because MRL/lpr mice transgenic for the normal gene encoding Fas do not exhibit accelerated lupus.[170] The gld gene, another accelerator of autoimmunity, encodes a defective Fas ligand.[171] Therefore, the inability to eliminate autoreactive lymphocytes by apoptosis mediated through Fas–Fas ligand interactions promotes autoimmunity.

Linkage studies of the entire mouse genome in NZB, NZW, NZB/NZW F1, NZM, BXSB, SWR, and MRL/lpr mice have identified one or more regions on chromosomes 1, 3, 4, 5, 6, 7, 9, 10, 11, 12, 13, 14, 16, 17, 18, and 19 that are likely to contain genes conferring lupus susceptibility or resistance.[58,63,172-174] Although more than 30 chromosomal intervals thus far have been identified, each analyzed strain has three or more intervals linked to disease susceptibility, suggesting that murine lupus is oligogenic and mediated by combinations of several genes. Of note, specific regions of chromosomes 1, 4, 7, and 17 (containing the MHC region) have been independently mapped in multiple strains. The importance of DNA regions on chromosomes 1, 4, 7, and 17 of the New Zealand genetic background has been elucidated by detailed phenotypic characterization and successive backcrosses into another normal mouse strain (C57BL/6 or B6) to analyze the locations and component phenotypes of individual susceptibility gene. Heterozygosity at the H2 locus on chromosome 17 (particularly containing H2z from NZW) has been identified as important in conferring certain autoantibodies and nephritis.[55-58,175] The regions of interest on chromosomes 1 and 4 contain DNA contributed by both NZB and NZW parents. One NZB-derived locus on chromosome 1, Nba2, may contribute to loss of tolerance to DNA-containing self antigens.[55] The Nba2 lupus susceptibility locus was further characterized by developing congenic mice via repeatedly backcrossing mice containing the NZB chromosomal 1 interval into the normal B6 genetic background and then intercrossing siblings to generate B6.Nba2 congenic mice homozygous for the Nba2 locus. Comparisons

of 11,000 gene microarrays revealed only two differentially expressed genes of spleen cells from B6.Nba2 and B6 mice: interferon (IFN)-inducible Ifi202 and Ifi203.[176] Ifi202 has been implicated as a candidate susceptibility gene supported by studies of strain distribution of expression, the promoter polymorphisms, and the effects on cell proliferation and apoptosis. A similar approach has produced multiple congenic strains of mice, each carrying a single susceptibility locus from the NZM2410 genome.[177] For example, the region designated Sle1 on chromosome 1 (close to Nba2), when expressed in B and T cells of a normal B6 background (B6.NZMc1), promotes development of IgG antibodies to nucleosome and generates histone-specific T cells.[58-60,63,178] Although the mice lose tolerance to nucleosome and develop antinuclear antibodies induced by the exposed portion of chromatin (H2A/H2B/DNA)—antibodies thought to precede pathogenic anti-DNA—these antibodies do not evolve, and animals develop minimal nephritis. Subsequent studies reveal that the potent autoimmunity conferred by the genomic interval of Sle1 reflects the combined effects of a cluster of four independent, but functionally related, susceptibility genes: Sle1a, Sle1b, Sle1c, and Sle1d.[179] Congenic strains for each of these four subintervals have been generated, in which Sle1b is the strongest contributor of the observed Sle1 phenotype. Within the genomic interval of Sle1b locus, the immune receptor cell determinant (CD)2/SLAM family of genes is a good candidate as a susceptibility gene. The congenic interval of Sle1c contains the gene Cr2 (encoding complement receptors 1 and 2 by alternative splicing of a common transcript) that has been implicated as a candidate susceptibility gene.[174] A single nucleotide polymorphism of the NZM2410/NZW Cr2, creating a novel glycosylation site within the C3d binding domain, may interfere with receptor dimerization, reduce receptor-mediated signaling, and consequently lower the threshold for negative selection of autoreactive B cells.[180] Cr2-deficient mice have impaired humoral immunity. Studies of Cr2-deficient mice with or without a concomitant Fas mutation in the B6 genetic background demonstrate a role of Cr2 in modulating serum levels of antinuclear antibodies (ANA) and anti–ds-DNA autoantibodies.[181] Mice congenic for the region on chromosome 4 (B6.NZMc4 expressing the Sle2 region) show hyperactivation of B cells with hypersecretion of IgM but develop no nephritis.[61,63] Mice congenic for the chromosome 7 region (B6.NZMc7 containing the Sle3 region) have hyperactivation of T cells, increased numbers of CD4+ helper T cells, reduced apoptosis, and increased levels of IgG antibodies to multiple nucleosomal antigens; they develop moderate nephritis.[63] When mice are bred to express Sle1 and Sle3, they develop severe disease, with IgG antibodies to DNA and other self antigens, and lethal, early glomerulonephritis—confirming the hypothesis that multiple genes conferring multiple abnormalities in immune tolerance and B and T cell function are required for an individual to develop severe lupus.[63] Finally, studies of this type have shown that several chromosome regions in NZW mice (a strain that inherits multiple susceptibility genes, including H2z, Sle1, and Sle3) are linked to protection from disease.[63]

One of these, Sle1 suppressor (Sle1s), when bred into mice with Sle1 plus Sle3, reduces the incidence of severe nephritis by half.[182] Sle1s is located in the MHC/TNF-α region. Thus, both modifying and protective genes are critical in determining exactly how "predisposed" an individual is to this autoimmune disease.

Environmental Factors, Apoptosis, and Systemic Lupus Erythematosus

As mentioned in the discussion of genetics, the fact that most monozygotic twins are discordant for clinical SLE suggests that environmental factors play a role in disease pathogenesis.[2,46-48] These factors are summarized in Table 74–5. Two are clearly important: ultraviolet (UV) light and gender. As many as 70 percent of SLE patients have disease flared by exposure to UV light.[183] The B spectrum may be more important than the A spectrum in activating disease in humans. Although patients might be wise to avoid intense exposure to both UVA and UVB spectra, some data suggest that exposure to UVA might benefit SLE.[184] Several experiments have suggested mechanisms by which exposure to UV light might accelerate disease. For example, exposure of DNA to UV light increases thymine dimers, which ren-

TABLE 74–5 • ENVIRONMENTAL FACTORS THAT MAY PLAY A ROLE IN THE PATHOGENESIS OF SYSTEMIC LUPUS ERYTHEMATOSUS (SLE)

Definite
Ultraviolet B light

Probable
Sex hormones: In humans, female-to-male ratio is 9:1 between menarche and menopause, 3:1 in young and old

Possible
Dietary factors
Alfalfa sprouts and related sprouting foods containing L-canavanine
Pristane and similar substances
High intake of saturated fats
Infectious agents
Bacterial DNA
Human retroviruses
Endotoxins, bacterial lipopolysaccharides
Exposure to certain medications*
Hydralazine
Procainamide
Isoniazid
Hydantoins
Chlorpromazine
Methyldopa
D-Penicillamine
Minocycline
Antibodies to tumor necrosis factor-α (TNF-α)
Interferon-α (IFN-α)

*Although each of the drugs listed, and many others, can induce lupus-like symptoms in predisposed individuals, there is little evidence that they can induce true SLE or even activate disease in individuals with established SLE. Therefore, if the clinical care of a patient with SLE would benefit from use of one of these drugs, the drug should not be withheld.

ders the DNA more immunogenic.[185] Of great interest are recent observations that exposure of keratinocytes to UV light induces apoptosis.[4,186] During apoptosis, three events occur that might expose self molecules to the immune system or render them immunogenic: 1) movement of nuclear and cytoplasmic DNA-protein and RNA-protein antigens to the surface of cells in membrane-encased blebs (nucleosomes, Ro/SS-A, and U1 RNP antigens, for example);[4,186] 2) flipping of the membrane inside-out so that antigenic portions of membrane phospholipids are exposed on the cell surface; and 3) modification of intracellular proteins that might render them antigenic.[187] Each of these changes presents nucleoprotein and cytoplasmic and phospholipid self antigens to the immune system. This might be the major stimulus that allows the few lymphocytes that escape self-tolerance mechanisms to become self reactive. In addition, damage to cells induced by UV light increases release of heat-shock proteins (HSP), which participate in activation of autoreactive T cells.[188]

Gender is obviously of great importance in susceptibility to SLE, which is predominantly a disease of women, particularly during their reproductive years.[189] The basis of this sex predisposition is not understood. It seems unlikely that the X chromosome is involved, because the disease does not follow a sex-linked genetic pattern. A recent idea is that women who have been pregnant may have fetal cells that persist for decades in their circulation or tissues, where the fetal cells induce chronic graft-versus-host disease, which resembles SLE.[190] Abnormalities in sex-hormone metabolism might contribute to gender differences in susceptibility to SLE. Men and women with SLE have accelerated metabolism of testosterone.[191] Estrone is preferentially hydroxylated at the C-16 position in men and women with SLE and in their first-degree relatives, resulting in the accumulation of 16-hydroxylated metabolites,[192] which have sustained high estrogenic activity.[193] Thus, men and women with SLE might have too much estrogenic and too little androgenic hormone, shifting their immune system toward increased responses. Menopausal nurses treated with hormone replacement therapy have an increased risk for development of SLE compared to nurses who do not receive hormone replacement therapy,[194] and women exposed to estrogen-containing oral contraceptives also have increased risk for SLE,[195] adding to the evidence that female sex hormones are permissive for development of SLE. Prolactin levels are elevated in some individuals with SLE and may increase disease activity.[196]

An additional factor that may promote development of disease in genetically predisposed individuals is diet. Some macaque monkeys fed alfalfa sprouts developed SLE; sprouting vegetables contain an aromatic amino acid, L-canavanine, that is immunostimulatory.[197] Mice with SLE are protected from disease if they have severely restricted calorie intake, restricted fat intake, or high intake of omega-3 unsaturated fat such as eicosapentaenoic acid (fish oil).[198-201] A study in human SLE suggested that 20 g of fish oil daily may be steroid sparing.[201] The role of these dietary observations in human disease is uncertain, but we recommend that patients with SLE minimize their dietary intake of sprouts, excessive calories, and saturated fat. Reports suggesting that exposure of women to hair dye, permanent-wave solutions, and lipstick increased their risk for SLE were not confirmed in subsequent studies.[202,203]

Many searches have been made for infectious agents that cause lupus; results have been largely unconvincing. However, infections may play a role in expanding undesirable immune responses. For example, administration of bacterial lipopolysaccharides to mice with SLE accelerates disease.[204] One study[205] detected antibodies to the retroviral gag protein p24 from human immunodeficiency virus (HIV)-1 in one third of SLE patients compared to 1 of 120 control subjects. Type C oncornavirus has been implicated in the nephritis of NZB/Bl mice and related strains.[206] One group has found persistent BK polyoma virus more frequently in patients with SLE than in control subjects,[207] and a study of children showed that those with SLE were significantly more likely to have evidence of infection with Epstein-Barr virus than were matched non-SLE control children from the same population.[208] Investigators in one laboratory have implicated human retrovirus-5 in the synovitis of SLE and RA.[209] All these observations require confirmation by other groups. It seems likely that infectious agents (and their products, such as superantigens and lipopolysaccharides) that can activate the innate immune system monocytes, B cells, and T cells could worsen SLE, possibly by a burst of proinflammatory cytokines, or even induce the disease in an individual with the appropriate predisposing genes.

Drugs appear on the list of environmental exposures that might induce SLE-like disease. The drugs listed in Table 74–4 are relatively frequently implicated in drug-induced lupus.[210] This disease is probably different from true SLE. The clinical manifestations of drug-induced lupus are predominantly arthritis, serositis, fatigue, malaise, and low-grade fever; nephritis and central nervous system disease are rare. These manifestations disappear in most patients within a few weeks of discontinuation of the offending drug, never to reappear unless reexposure occurs. Although antinuclear antibodies appear in all patients, it is unusual for high titers of anti–ds-DNA or profound hypocomplementemia to develop. Antibodies to histones are common with some of the inducing drugs; these antibodies are also found in SLE. In drug-induced lupus and SLE, the response is probably directed primarily against chromatin nucleosomes, with different histones dominating the response in the two diseases.[210] Antibodies to lymphocytes, platelets, erythrocytes, and phospholipids occur in drug-induced lupus and SLE. It is possible that an individual predisposed to SLE might have the disease triggered by exposure to one of these drugs. However, experience has suggested that such an event is rare. Therefore, if a patient with established, true SLE needs one of these drugs (hydantoin or isoniazid, for example), the drug should not be withheld. On the other hand, if one drug has probably induced lupus, the patient should not be rechallenged with that agent. Specificity of autoantibodies to DNA-protein or RNA-protein may spread over time to involve other self antigens in individuals with the correct permissive genes.

Of note to rheumatologists is the recent implication of minocycline[211] and antibodies to TNF-α[212] as potential inducers of SLE-like reactions.

In summary, then, what are the antigens that induce SLE? Are the stimulating antigens foreign (cross-reacting or mimicking "self"), or are they normal or altered self molecules that induce responses that overwhelm tolerance? The role of DNA has been a particular mystery, because mammalian DNA (in contrast to bacterial DNA) is weakly immunogenic,[213,214] and yet the IgG anti–ds-DNA response correlates with disease activity and nephritis in some patients with SLE, and antibodies to DNA clearly cause nephritis in mice.[11] Immunogenic DNA could originate from certain bacteria after infection,[215] but it is likely that mammalian DNA-protein complexes, particularly those in nucleosomes, are the initial stimulators of this response.[216] Early responses in mice are directed against nucleosomes and "spread" to involve ss-DNA and ds-DNA over time.[217] Helper T cells that support anti-DNA production are activated by nucleosomes,[217] and some nephritogenic monoclonal antibodies to DNA bind DNA-histone complexes; the anti-DNA/DNA-histone complex can then bind to heparan sulfate in glomerular basement membranes.[11] Some antibodies of this type can penetrate cells and bind to cytoplasmic and nuclear structures, probably altering cell function and contributing to disease by mechanisms other than classic complement-mediated tissue injury.[42,218] The stimulatory role of the Ro molecules is probably similar in that RNA-protein globular complexes induce an immune response in B cells.[219] As discussed before, cells undergoing apoptosis are capable of presenting nucleosomes, Ro, U1 RNP, and antigenic portions of membrane phospholipids to immune systems and may be critical in inducing autoreactivity or permitting it to persist. The same is true for infectious agents. In humans, defects in Fas are associated with lymphoproliferative disease and autoimmunity, particularly hemolytic anemia and thrombocytopenia—the Canale-Smith syndrome[220] (see Chapter 21). On the other hand, apoptosis that is too rapid might allow quantitative increases in presentation of self antigens. Apoptosis in human SLE is defective; levels of the Bcl-2 protein that protects from apoptosis are high in human SLE T cells,[221] but levels of Fas ligand are also high, and in vitro apoptosis of lymphocytes is increased.[220-222] Another potential mechanism promoting SLE through altered apoptosis involves deficiencies of C1q. It is likely that C1q is involved in clearance of cells undergoing apoptosis[223]; perhaps failure to clear such cells is important in individuals with homozygous deficiencies of C1q, almost all of whom develop SLE.[87] Mice homozygous for C1q deficiency are also predisposed to lupus nephritis.[224]

■ Abnormal Immune Responses Characteristic of Systemic Lupus Erythematosus

The result of interactions between susceptibility genes and triggering environmental factors is development of these pathogenic autoantibodies and immune complexes that characterize SLE. This requires hyperactivity of B and T cells and failure of multiple immunoregulatory circuits to downregulate those responses. The most prominent of these abnormalities are listed in Table 74–6.

Characteristics of Lupus B Cells

Recent evidence suggests a broad role of B cells in the development of immune responses and autoimmunity. Along with their traditional functions as antigen-presenting cells (APC) and precursors of antibody producing plasma cell (PCs), B cells regulate APC and T cell functions, produce cytokines, and express receptor-ligand pairs (i.e., CD154-CD40) previously thought to be restricted to other cell types.[225]

Several abnormalities of the SLE B cell have been described over the years in both human and murine systems:

1. Aberrant recruitment and survival of polyreactive autoantibody-producing cells in the functional repertoire of SLE patients, which normally die in the healthy host

2. Enhanced B cell activation, increased signaling responses to ligation of surface receptors, diminished activity of inhibitory signaling pathways, and a decreased tendency for apoptosis[226]

3. Enhanced production and response to several cytokines

It was recently demonstrated that B cell–B cell interactions mediated by CD154-CD40 are essential for differentiation of germinal center (GC) B cells into memory cells, as well as for the formation of secondary GC structures that allow reactivated memory B cells to differentiate into PCs secreting high-affinity antibodies.[227,228] In murine lupus models, CD154-expressing B cells stimulate autoantibody production by such B cell–B cell interactions.[225] Freshly isolated B cells from the periphery of patients with active SLE constitutively express CD154, as assessed by flow cytometry and mRNA analysis, and are enriched in cells with a GC phenotype, in contrast to cells from normal healthy controls or inactive SLE patients, which do not. Treatment of SLE nephritis patients with an antibody to CD154 (h5c8, BG9588) has resulted in the disappearance of such B

TABLE 74–6 · CHARACTERISTICS OF THE ABNORMAL IMMUNE RESPONSE IN PATIENTS WITH SYSTEMIC LUPUS ERYTHEMATOSUS (SLE)

Hyperactivated B Cells

- The number of B cells secreting immunoglobulin is increased in peripheral blood (up to 50-fold).
- Total numbers of B cells in all stages of maturation are increased.
- B cell abnormalities can precede the development of SLE.
- Much of the immunoglobulin (Ig) produced is autoreactive against multiple self antigens; some antibodies are pathogenic.
- SLE B cells may be intrinsically easy to activate polyclonally. Polyclonal activation may precede autoantigen-specific activation.
- Some SLE B cells are activated by specific antigens. The B cell repertoire in each patient may be skewed toward a limited number of autoantibodies, probably depending on that person's susceptibility genes.
- Elevated levels of certain cytokines may promote B cell hyperfunction, such as interleukin (IL)-10 and IL-6.
- B cell responses to activating signals are abnormal, with increased intracellular calcium flux.

Hyperactivated T Cells

- The total number of T cells is decreased in most patients with active SLE, but the function of the remaining cells is skewed toward help. Cells with cell determinant (CD)4+ CD8–, CD4– CD8+, CD4– CD8–, αβ or γδ surface phenotypes can give help for autoantibody production, suggesting persistence of autoreactive helper T cells and lack of maturation or appearance of appropriate downregulating T cells.
- Antibodies to T cell subsets are present in most patients with active disease.
- Early activation events, including calcium responses, protein kinase A activation, and generation of cyclic adenosine monophosphate, are abnormal.
- Increased numbers of T cells in peripheral blood express activation markers (IL-2R, DR, DP, Fas).
- Serum levels of IL-2, sIL-2R, and interferon-γ (IFN-γ) are increased.
- Circulating T cells in patients with active disease are "exhausted," which means they produce little IL-2 and are programmed for activation-induced cell death (AICD), or apoptosis.
- Autoantibodies are processed into peptides that are presented in B cell and other antigen-presenting cell major histocompatibility complex (MHC) class II molecules and activate T cell help for additional autoantibody production.
- SLE T cells cannot drive natural killer (NK) cells to produce active transforming growth factor-β (TGF-β), which in turn helps maturation of CD8+ T cells to regulate B cells.

Abnormalities of Monocytes and Macrophages

- Phagocytic cells of several types cannot bind or process immune complexes efficiently.
- Large quantities of IFN-γ are released from monocytes and macrophages during periods of disease activity.

Abnormalities of Immunoregulation

- Mechanisms of immune tolerance may be defective.
- Clearing of immune complexes is inadequate because of low levels of complement and poorly functioning fragment crystallizable (Fc)γ receptors on cell surfaces.
- Downregulation of activated T and B cell networks by suppressor T cells and interacting NK cells is inadequate.
- Idiotypic circuits in B and T cell networks, which in health downregulate antibody production and T cell activation, are inadequate.

cells from the circulation.[225] Enhanced spontaneous proliferation and Ig secretion by highly purified B cells was also inhibited.[229] Likewise, spontaneous in vitro proliferation, survival, and Ig secretion of B cells from BXSB and BWF1 mice was inhibited by an anti-CD154 antibody.[230] In healthy controls, mature B cells are free to recirculate into secondary lymphoid tissues, and to form, enter, and participate in GC reactions,[231] whereas immature polyreactive and autoreactive B cells are generally excluded, resulting in anergy or apoptosis. In SLE, such polyreactive autoantibody-producing B cells may be redirected into T cell–dependent GC reactions and lead to differentiation into PCs secreting pathogenic autoantibodies.[225] Evidence from studies in MRL/lpr[232] and (NZB/NZW) F1 mice[233] suggests that autoreactive B cells are able to form or enter splenic follicles, but are retained outside follicles in the T cell zone of non–autoimmune control mice. By contrast, anti-DNA–producing B cells were localized within the follicles of lupus-prone mice.[234] Several factors contribute to the aberrant recruitment of these autoreactive B cells in the functional repertoire of patients with SLE:

1. Decreased phagocytic function in SLE provides sufficient quantities of autoantigen for the surface Ig engagement necessary to positively select autoreactive B cells that would otherwise become anergic or die.
2. SLE B cells may have a lower threshold for positive selection, as evidenced by enhanced activity of tyrosine kinases and increased Ca^{2+} release compared to normal controls.[226]
3. Altered signaling through surface Ig or enhanced expression of costimulatory molecules such as CD154 may rescue SLE autoreactive B cells from anergy or deletion that normally follows autoantigen binding in healthy controls.[225]

Beyond their aberrant recruitment in the functional repertoire of lupus patients, autoreactive B cells display impaired apoptosis, thus perpetuating high-affinity autoantibody production and autoimmunity. As discussed elsewhere in this chapter, defects in the induction or regulation of B cell apoptosis have been well characterized in both human and murine systems of SLE:

1. Mutations of Fas or Fas-L genes are associated with both quantitative and qualitative apoptotic defects in lpr and gld mice, respectively,[235] and linked to lymphoproliferation and systemic autoimmunity. Sporadic cases of humans with Fas and Fas-L mutations have been reported who also develop lupus-like disease.[236] Moreover, there are recent reports for aberrant expression of Fas-L on anti-DNA secreting B cells in patients with SLE, killing Fas+ immunoregulatory T cells and thus facilitating escape of autoreactive B cells from the immune tolerance system.[237]
2. Mice congenitally deficient for the preapoptotic protein Bim (Bim −/−)[238] or transgenic for the antiapoptotic protein Bcl-2[239] develop a lupus-like disorder.
3. Mice transgenic for BlyS (a new member of the TNF superfamily) develop lymphoproliferation and a lupus-like disorder associated with inhibition of B cell apoptosis mediated by Bcl-2 upregulation.[240] In

addition, lupus-prone NZB/NZW F1 mice have elevated levels of circulating Blys,[241] and SLE patients exhibit elevated serum levels of this protein.[242]
4. As described elsewhere, the altered selection of naïve B cells and their rescue from tolerance induction and persistence in the periphery, as a result of hormonal treatment with estradiol[243] or prolactin,[244] is associated with an upregulation of Bcl-2 expression and impaired apoptosis in these cells.

Several functional studies incriminate an intrinsically deranged B cell in the initiation and propagation of lupus autoimmunity in murine systems of SLE:

1. MRL/lpr mice congenitally deficient in TCR α/β T cells are still able to produce anti-DNA antibodies and manifest immune complex–mediated glomerulonephritis.[245]
2. MRL/lpr mice genetically manipulated to express B cells bearing surface Ig b cell receptor (BCR) but unable to secrete any antibody also develop nephritis, verifying the importance of B cells in the expression of disease.[246]
3. Adoptive transfer of pre-B cells from embryonic liver of NZB/NZW F1 mice into SCID mice resulted in production of anti-DNA antibodies and sustained a lupus-like disease.[247]

B cell activation is clearly abnormal in individuals with SLE, both human and murine.[248,249] In fact, in some mouse models, hyperactivated B cells can be demonstrated in fetal life.[250] In people with SLE, there is often a marked increase in the number of plasma cells in the peripheral blood that are secreting Ig and in numbers of B cells at all stages of activation.[248,251] Studies of twins and family members have shown that such increased numbers can precede clinical disease.[252] Stimulation of freshly isolated B cells from SLE patients through their BCR results in abnormally high Ca^{2+} responses, increased generation of inositol triphosphate, and increased production of tyrosine phosphorylated proteins as compared to B cell responses from normal or control subjects.[226] These signaling abnormalities are disease specific and activity independent, suggesting a potentially intrinsic lupus B cell defect.[253] In lupus mice, polyclonal activation of B cells precedes the high-avidity, single autoantigen–specific B cell activation that characterizes well-developed disease. This suggests that B cells in SLE are subject to increased polyclonal activation and antigen-specific activation.[248,254] Either type of stimulation induces altered intracellular events that result in increased B cell function. Because patients have autoantibody repertoires that differ among individuals (e.g., almost all have antinuclear antibodies but only some anti–ds-DNA, anti-Ro, anti-RNP, or anti-platelet antibodies), it is likely that many B cells are activated by specific antigens. After autoantibody responses are initiated, B cells and helper T cells develop that recognize additional antigens—a process known as epitope spreading. Thus, a lupus-predisposed individual may make an antibody to immunogenic portions of nucleosome, Sm peptides, or Ig-derived peptides, and a few months later, B cells can be detected that make antinucleosome or anti-Sm, anti–ds-DNA, and antinuclear antibodies.[255-257] Whether spreading is more common in SLE than in normal individuals may depend on these intrinsic abnormalities of B and T cells, the failure to regulate the initial response, the presence of an antigen that mimics these DNA-protein or RNA-protein complexes, or all three.

Inhibitory signaling pathways are impaired in SLE B cells. In that regard, the coreceptors that negatively regulate surface Ig-signaling, CD22 and CD45, as well as a downstream signal transduction molecule (SH2-containing phosphatase 1 [SHP]), have all been shown to be downregulated in SLE B cells[258-260] and to be present in human SLE susceptibility loci.[261-264]

There are recent reports of abnormally enhanced production and response to cytokines such as IL-6 and IL-10 by SLE B cells. SLE B cells are more easily driven to differentiate by IL-6 than are normal B cells.[265] SLE patients have increased numbers of IL-6–secreting cells,[266] and SLE B cells constitutively express surface receptors for IL-6, in contrast to B cells from normal controls.[267] IL-6 increases in vitro production by B cells of both IgG and anti-DNA–IgG, whereas addition of anti–IL-6 inhibits those effects.[267] Furthermore, administration of IL-6 to mice accelerates lupus.[268] IL-10 has both immunostimulatory and immunosuppressive effects. SLE patients display increased serum concentrations of IL-10[265] and increased numbers of IL-10–secreting cells[269] during active disease. Administration of anti–IL-10 to SLE-predisposed mice is effective in preventing disease, probably by permitting transforming growth factor-β (TGF-β)–mediated suppression of T and B cell functions.[270] In patients with SLE, anti–IL-10 mAb suppressed the in vitro production of auto-Ab from B cells, whereas recombinant IL-10 promoted it.[271] More recent evidence, however, has demonstrated an immunoprotective role of IL-10 in lupus-prone MRL/lpr mice; mice made deficient in IL-10 (MRL/lpr/IL-10$^{-/-}$) developed severe lupus with earlier skin lesions, increased lymphadenopathy, and more severe glomerulonephritis than IL-10–sufficient mice. The protective effect of IL-10 was mediated through downregulation of pathogenic T helper type 1 (Th1) responses.[272] The standing hypothesis reconciling the previous contrasting observations is that during the initial phase of SLE, in which IFN-γ and its induced IgG2a promote disease, IL-10 is needed to suppress the pathogenic Th1 responses. By contrast, at later phases of disease, excessive IL-10 production may lead to enhanced autoantibody production and subsequent formation of pathogenic immune complexes.

CHARACTERISTICS OF LUPUS T CELLS

Abnormalities in T cell function are probably critical to both murine and human SLE. In all the strains of lupus mice that have been tested, elimination or inactivation of CD4+ helper T cells protects from disease,[273,274] and athymic mice do not develop SLE.[275,276] Quantitative variations in T cells and their subsets may be important. In human SLE, the total number of T cells is usually reduced, probably due to the effects of antilymphocyte antibodies (ALAs).[277,278] Decreased CD4+ T cell numbers correlate well with ALAs specifically reactive against CD4+, and there is strong correlation among high ALA titers, lymphopenia, and disease activity.[279,280] Data vary as to which T cell subset is most frequently reduced, and the characteristics of cells in peripheral blood may not be as important as cells in target organs. Early reports in humans have indicated a relative decrease of CD8+ cells in SLE.[281,282] Later reports showed considerable variation in the numbers and ratios of peripheral blood CD4+ and CD8+ T cells in SLE patients. Patients with high CD4-to-CD8 ratios demonstrated low numbers of CD8+ cells and defective CD8+ suppressor and effectors, whereas patients with low CD4-to-CD8 ratios had either low CD4+ numbers or defective CD4+ suppressor and inducers.[283] Another T cell subset, natural killer (NK) T cells may also be decreased in numbers in peripheral blood of patients with SLE.[284,285] NK T cells respond to glycolipid antigens presented by nonpolymorphic MHC molecules such CD1. These cells lack expression of CD4 or CD8 double negative (DN) and are CD3+, CD56+, TCRαβ+, or γδ+, and can provide help for autoantibody production in SLE.[286,287] In addition, certain subsets of DN cells possess potent suppressive activity. Such a subset (bearing the invariant Va24JaQ TCR) was decreased in peripheral blood of Japanese SLE patients[288] and in the affected sibling of identical twins discordant for autoimmune diabetes.[289] CD1-restricted CD4–CD8– T cells were increased in peripheral blood of U.S. patients with active SLE, and could help fetal B cells switch from IgM to IgG production (similar cells from healthy individuals did not function as helpers in this system).[285] In general, subsets of all these populations of human SLE peripheral blood T cells (CD4+CD8–, CD4–CD8+, CD4–CD8–) can give help for autoantibody production, whereas only CD4+CD8– cells have this capacity in healthy individuals.

Several functional abnormalities have been reported in SLE T cells in terms of proliferation, activation, expression of costimulatory or effector surface molecules, intracellular signaling pathways, and helper or cytolytic activity. Accessory cell–dependent TCR/CD3-mediated proliferation in unfractionated peripheral blood mononuclear, cell (PBMC) cultures from SLE patients is significantly decreased compared to normal controls,[290] whereas CD3/TCR-mediated proliferation of purified SLE T cells ranges from normal to enhanced.[291] Decreased proliferative responses have been reported in some patients in response to mitogenic lectins (PHA, ConA, PWM), anti-CD2, and both allogeneic and autologous mixed lymphocyte reactions.[277,292] There is considerable evidence for the presence of in vivo polyclonal T cell activation in SLE. Increased numbers of circulating T cells demonstrate spontaneous proliferation[293] and express proliferating cell nuclear antigen.[294] There is increased expression of MHC class II molecules[293] on T cell surfaces, as well as increased release of soluble IL-2 receptors,[295] TNF receptors,[296] and CD40-L into the serum.[297]

A pan–T cell dysfunction appears to exist in SLE, which is characterized by exaggerated CD4+ and diminished CD8+ T cell activities. Moreover, NK cell functions are defective.[298] Due in part to loss of effective CD8[+] T and NK cell negative feedback on B cells,[299] forbidden B cell clones produce autoantibodies against an array of intra- and extracellular autoantigens (see the preceding section for discussion of intrinsic abnormalities in SLE B cells). The ability of T cells to help antibody production, and their inability to suppress it, are probably the T cell functions most pertinent to clinical SLE. Because many of the pathogenic autoantibodies in patients with SLE are IgG, T cell help is necessary for their production and maintenance. As mentioned previously, in human SLE, T cells with many different surface phenotypes give help for autoantibody production,[287-287,300] including classic helper cells (CD4+CD8– αβ TCR) and also CD4–CD8+ αβ TCR, CD4–CD8– αβ, or γδ TCR cells, and CD1-restricted DN T cells.[301] Whether this unusual situation of cells of many phenotypes driving disease represents intrinsic defects in the cells, failure of effector CD8+ cell precursors to mature into suppressive cells, or absence of other downregulating networks is unknown. Furthermore, the presence of excess help in human SLE PBL T cells is not always found: In some in vitro studies, helper activity stimulated by PWM or specific antigen was either decreased[302] or normal.[303]

CD8+ T cell function is impaired in peripheral blood T cells from patients with SLE. For example, impaired generation of CD8+ cytolytic T cells against allogeneic targets[304] and of cytolytic activity induced by anti-CD3 stimulation have been reported.[305] Moreover, CD8+ cells from some lupus patients sustain, rather than suppress, spontaneous polyclonal IgG production; they synergize with CD4+ T cells to support autoantibody synthesis.[306] CD8+ suppressive activity for autoantibody production is also defective in several murine models of SLE.[307-309]

Inquiries into the mechanisms causing the aforementioned T cell dysfunctions have led to identification of several new defects of signal transduction and have begun to reveal their molecular basis. In contrast to T cells from the peripheral blood of normal individuals or patients with nonlupus rheumatic diseases, peripheral blood T cells from SLE patients show diminished TCR ζ-chain expression.[310] This may be associated with decreased elaboration of IFN-γ in response to TCR-initiated cell signals[311] and can account for both the decreased activation-induced cell death (AICD) and the diminished NK cell activity in SLE.[311] An enhanced and prolonged rise in intracellular Ca^{2+} concentration ($[Ca^{2+}]_i$) following TCR-mediated cell activation has been identified in human primary SLE T cells, T cell lines, and antigen-specific T cell clones,[311] which is unrelated to disease activity or specific organ involvement. Ca^{2+} as a second messenger mediates calcineurin-catalyzed dephosphorylation of nuclear factor of activated T cell (NF-AT), its nuclear translocation and overexpression of CD154, Fas-L, and c-myc in SLE T cells.[312,313] There are reports of defective cyclic adenosine monophosphate (camp)-dependent protein phosphorylation in peripheral blood T cells from SLE patients. This defect may be attributed to deficient activities of type I and type II isoenzymes of protein kinase A (PKA).[314,315] Among SLE patients, the preva-

lences of deficient PKA-I and PKA-II activities are approximately 80 and 40 percent, respectively.[315] These deficiencies are persistent over time and are independent of clinical disease activity. The molecular basis of the deficient enzyme activity is under investigation.

Regulation of apoptosis in both human and murine SLE T cells is impaired, as described elsewhere in this chapter. Although mutations in the apoptosis-mediating Fas receptor or the Fas-L in the lpr and gld mouse backgrounds, respectively, are associated with impaired lymphocyte apoptosis and lupus-like disease, the Fas-mediated signaling pathway appears normal in human SLE.[316] However, SLE T cells in many patients demonstrate defective AICD. This could be due to abnormalities in a second major pathway leading to AICD, which involves signaling between members of the TNF-α surface receptor family and their ligands. For example, T cells from peripheral blood of some SLE patients show decreased intracellular synthesis of TNF-α, which could result in undesirable survival of autoreactive cells.[317] In contrast, increased spontaneous apoptosis has been also observed in SLE.[318] Such accelerated apoptosis is likely to provide more autoantigens to stimulate the immune system. Therefore, apoptosis must be in perfect balance for avoidance of autoreactivity—if autoreactive lymphocytes persist too long, as in MRL/lpr mice, or are increased in quantity with cell survival too brief, as in some people with active SLE, autoimmunity results. Disruption of the mitochondrial transmembrane potential ($\Delta\Psi_m$ with mitochondrial hyperpolarization has been proposed as the point of no return in apoptotic signaling. This phenomenon precedes caspase activation and phosphatidylserine externalization in the early phase of Fas-, p53-, and H_2O_2-induced apoptosis.[319-321] Recently, deviations in key mitochondrial checkpoints associated with abnormal T cell apoptosis in SLE have been identified[322]: 1) deficient elevation of $\Delta\Psi_m$; 2) diminished CD3/ CD28-induced reactive oxygen intermediates (ROI) and H_2O_2 production; and 3) reduced H_2O_2-induced apoptosis.

One of the cardinal biochemical abnormalities in SLE T cells is a global decrease in genomic deoxymethylcytosine (d[m]C) content.[323] Because methylation of deoxycytosine in regulatory sequences can suppress transcription of the associated gene,[324] abnormal hypomethylation could contribute to overexpression of some genes in SLE T cells. More importantly, T cells treated with methylation inhibitors, including procainamide and hydralazine, become autoreactive as a result of surface lymphocyte function antigen-1 (LFA-1; CD11a) overexpression, leading to a lupus-like disease in murine models.[325] LFA-1 overexpression lowers the threshold for T cell activation, allowing the cells to respond to self–class II MHC molecules presenting inappropriate antigens.[326] In particular, it appears to overstabilize the normally low-affinity interaction between the TCR and class II MHC molecules lacking the relevant antigenic peptide, thus allowing the signaling apparatus to assemble and transmit its signal.[327] Defective signaling via the extracellular regulating kinase (ERK) pathway in active SLE T cells has been associated with DNA hypomethylation.

Disease activity in some patients with SLE has been associated with anergy to recall antigens by skin testing. This anergy may reflect peripheral T cell anergy secondary to impaired IL-2 secretion. Mechanisms likely to contribute to deficient IL-2 production by SLE T cells are the absence of the p65/p50 nuclear factor kappa B (NFκB) heterodimer and reduced AP-1 activity.[328] Another alternative is the inhibition of IL-2 enhancer/promoter of transcriptional activation. c-AMP-responsive element modulator (CREM) is a transcriptional repressor that binds to cAMP response elements and downregulates the expression of genes having this binding site.[329] It was recently shown that p-CREM binds to the IL-2 enhancer/promoter and contributes to T cell energy.[330]

Altered cytokine homeostasis characterizes active SLE. Increased levels of IL-10 in the serum and increased numbers of lL-10–secreting cells are observed. IL-10 inhibits some T cell functions and can lead to downregulation of IL-2, TNF-α, and IFN-γ,[331] each of which plays a cardinal role in the generation of cytotoxic and suppressive T cells. The exact role of Th1 cytokines (see Chapter 8) in SLE is unclear. During periods of disease activity, peripheral blood cells secrete low levels of IL-2 and IFN-γ in some patients with SLE.[265] However, murine lupus seems to depend strongly on increased levels of IFN-γ, because mice that are congenitally deficient for the IFN-γ receptor (IFN-γ–/–) are partially protected from developing SLE,[332] and treatment with soluble IFN-γ receptor prevents disease.[333] Perhaps the cells isolated from patients with active disease are exhausted, and the cytokine profile they produce does not reflect the initiation of disease or flares.

Recent observations in murine lupus suggest that autoantibodies can activate their own T cell help; that is, B cells process their surface Ig and present Ig-derived peptides in their surface MHC class II molecules to nearby helper T cells, which are then activated to help the synthesis of additional autoantibody.[255,334] This may be an important mechanism for sustaining the production of pathogenic autoantibodies in SLE. The V regions of anti-DNA antibodies contain determinants that can drive the autoimmune response in SLE. V_H-derived peptides accelerate the disease process in lupus-prone NZB/NZW F1 mice and elicit lupus-like inflammatory changes in normal control strains. V_H-Reactive T cells spontaneously arise during disease and assist production of both anti-peptide antibodies and anti-DNA antibodies that deposit in glomeruli.[335] Peripheral blood T cells from many patients with SLE recognize V_H-determinants of human anti-DNA. Therefore V-region reactive T cells are not deleted in the periphery of healthy individuals. Used as a tolerogen, an artificial V_H-peptide (pCONSENSUS) inhibits responses to V_H and other autoantigens, but it leaves the murine immune system intact and able to generate responses to external antigens.[335] Similarly, patients with SLE have circulating T cells that recognize peptides from nucleosomes, and it is likely that these cells also upregulate anti-DNA antibody production.[287]

The role of T cells in directly causing tissue damage in SLE has not been emphasized, but it is probably important. Most evidence suggests that polymyositis, whether it occurs alone or with another connective tissue disease such as SLE, depends on cytotoxic T cells destroying muscle cells.[336] Because 50 percent of individuals with subacute cutaneous lupus and anti-Ro/SS-A do not have Ig and complement deposited at the dermal-epidermal junction, dermatitis in those individuals may be caused by T cells sensitized to Ro.[337] Finally, although the classic explanation for vasculitis is deposition of immune complexes in vessel walls, some T cells, probably sensitized to endothelial cell antigens, can cause vasculitis.[338] Kidney infiltrating T cells in SLE patients demonstrate a relatively restricted TCR Vbeta repertoire. TCR Vbeta8 and Vbeta20 were preferentially expressed in 50 and 40 percent of kidney biopsies, respectively, in one study,[339] and junctional sequences of complementary DNA encoding the TCR Vbeta8 and Vbeta20 genes in intrarenal T cells showed oligoclonal expansion, indicating antigen-driven stimulation.

Where are the suppressor/regulatory T cells that should eliminate these pathogenic, hyperactive T and B cells? Recent work has suggested abnormalities in interactions between CD4+ T cells that are required for maturation of cytotoxic CD8+ regulatory cells and the NK cells that participate in nonspecific regulation. This might result from the inability of NK cells from SLE patients to secrete adequate quantities of activated TGF-β[340] It is likely that CD4+ T cells stimulate the NK cells to secrete active TGF-β under normal circumstances, but not when SLE is active. In the chronic graft-versus-host mouse model of lupus-like disease, autoantibody formation and nephritis are delayed by administration of T cells preincubated with TGF-β, suggesting that this cytokine may partially restore suppression/regulation in individuals with autoimmunity.[341]

In summary, T lymphocytes are quantitatively and qualitatively abnormal in human lupus and in murine models of the disease. Qualitative abnormalities include increased responsiveness to surface activating signals, which results in increased calcium flux that may depend on defects in PKA I and II isoenzymes. Hypomethylation of DNA may be one outcome, or it may be an independent abnormality. For unknown reasons, T cells with many different surface phenotypes, such as CD4–CD8+, and DN T cells promote help of autoantibody production instead of suppression. Quantitative abnormalities in several cytokines, such as IL-2, IFN-γ, IL-10, and TGF-β are important in aberrant cell function, but it is not clear whether these are primary or secondary. There are several adverse outcomes of all these abnormalities, including resistance to apoptosis in some autoreactive cells, accelerated apoptosis in other lymphocytes that release autoantigens, and defective regulation of the skewing of many different subsets to provide help. Finally, the direct role of cytotoxic, activated, poorly regulated T cells in tissue damage must be important in disease pathogenesis.

▮ Abnormalities in Immunoregulation

The ability to make pathogenic subsets of autoantibodies and immune complexes must be accompanied by inability to downregulate them if disease is to be sustained. In murine lupus, once autoantibodies appear, they increase steadily until organ damage occurs, and death follows. In humans, SLE is more frequently characterized by fluctuating levels of autoantibodies with clinical exacerbations and periods of improvement; although, if patients were not treated, many might assume an inexorable downhill course. Nevertheless, virtually every mechanism of regulating antibodies that has been studied in human SLE is abnormal.

IMMUNE TOLERANCE

Highly autoreactive B and T lymphocytes are removed in healthy individuals by processes of immune tolerance. Two major mechanisms occur in both B and T cells: deletion and anergy.[342,343]

For T cells, interaction with MHC class I and class II molecules on thymic epithelial cells may deliver one or two signals to the cells: 1) cross-linking of antigen receptors, possibly followed by 2) engagement of second surface receptors after activation of T cell help. If two signals are received, apoptosis results; the cells are deleted. A few that "leak" into the periphery can be deleted there. Cells that receive only one activation signal are anergized; they cannot be activated when they reach the periphery, and they may eventually undergo apoptosis. B cells undergo the same processes, with the bone marrow and peripheral lymphoid organs as sites of deleting and anergizing signals. In addition, B cells can undergo receptor editing—a process in which an autoreactive surface Ig molecule is changed by different combinations of heavy and light chains. The resultant Ig molecule is no longer highly autoreactive; the edited "safe" B cells are selected for expansion.[344-346] T cell functions can be altered by shifts in the cytokines they release; deviation from Th1 to Th2 patterns protects from some T cell–induced autoimmune diseases in animals, such as experimental allergic encephalitis and diabetes.[347]

INADEQUATE CLEARING OF IMMUNE COMPLEXES

Several defects contribute to inadequate clearing of soluble and insoluble immune complexes.[43] Immune complexes are transported by complement receptors, primarily on erythrocytes in humans. The numbers of complement receptors on cell surfaces are reduced in patients with active SLE[90] so that immune complexes are not transported adequately to the mononuclear phagocytic cell system that clears them, leaving the immune complexes to deposit in tissues. In some individuals, the low numbers of complement receptors may be genetically determined; in most, they are probably low because they have been stripped away by large quantities of immune complex.[90] Phagocytosis of immune complexes occurs after binding to Fcγ receptors of several types on monocytes, macrophages, and neutrophils. Binding and internalization of Ig in immune complexes may be less than normal in some SLE patients with certain alleles of FcγRIIA and FcγRIIIA.[116,117,120,126] In many SLE patients, immune complexes are not phagocytosed

properly, and this also permits persistence of harmful immune complexes in the circulation.[90,348] In an earlier section, we discussed impaired clearing of apoptotic bodies in patients with SLE; persistence of these bodies probably permits sustained exposure of the immune system to autoantigens contained in them and contributes to autoantibody production.

INADEQUATE DOWNREGULATION BY T CELLS

Autoimmune disease is prevented by mechanisms of central and peripheral immune tolerance, among which a cardinal role is played by regulatory/inhibitory cells.[349-351] These cells belong to the CD4+, CD8+, or NK T cell compartments and exert an array of complex functions on diverse cell subsets. Several functional abnormalities have been described for each of these T cell subsets in both human and murine SLE.

In the CD8+ compartment, two distinct subsets of suppressor cells have been identified in mice and humans that share the CD8+CD28– surface phenotype, are not cytotoxic, and do not induce apoptosis. The first CD8+ suppressor subset induces antigen-specific immune suppression through cell-to-cell contact with APC presenting antigen.[352-354] The second subset mediates an antigen nonspecific suppression of T cell proliferation via soluble factors such as IFN-γ and IL-6.[355,356] This subset is functionally impaired in relapses of multiple sclerosis (MS)[355] and SLE,[356] suggesting involvement in disease pathogenesis. Earlier reports emphasized the loss of suppressor T cell functions in both murine and human SLE. Krakauer and Waldmann showed loss of suppressor T cells in adult female BWF1 mice using PWM-driven IgM biosynthesis as a detection system.[357] ConA-pulsed splenocytes (or supernatants) from adult BWF1 females (in contrast to cells from normal mice or young BWF1 mice) added into PWM-driven splenocytes of normal mice, failed to suppress IgM production. Ly2+ (CD8+) cells from older BWF1 mice fail to decrease IgG anti-DNA in cocultures of B with L3T4+ (CD4+) cells, in contrast to cells from young mice.[358] Similarly, in a chronic graft-versus-host disease murine lupus-like model,[359] resistance to induction of lupus-like disease by CD4+ T cells depends on the presence of adequate numbers and intact function of CD8+ cytotoxic cells. In human SLE there is impaired generation of CD8+ cytolytic T cells against allogeneic targets[360] and depressed anti-CD3–dependent cytolytic activity.[361] Moreover, CD8+ lymphocytes from lupus patients sustain, rather than suppress, spontaneous polyclonal IgG production; they synergize with CD4+ T cells to support autoantibody synthesis.[362]

In addition to loss of function, numbers of CD8+ cells may also decline as autoimmune disease appears. Studies in mice and dogs have shown that CD8+ cells fall in numbers or do not expand at the rapid rate occurring in CD4+ T cells and B cells as the animals develop SLE.[363] In patients with SLE, there is considerable variation in numbers of CD8+ cells;[364] in some individuals they are lower than normal.[365,366] How do suppressor T cells evolve? In mice and humans, interactions between CD4+ and CD8+ cell subsets are required to induce suppression of Ig production in antigen, PWM, or autologous mixed lymphocyte response (AMLR) systems.[367,368] Similarly, differentiation of cytotoxic CD8+ precursors into cytotoxic CD8+ effectors requires the presence of CD4+ cells.[368] Several years ago, a group reported that anti-2H4 antibody (anti-CD45R) identified a suppressor/inducer (CD4+2H4+) cell subset. Although not directly suppressive, this subset induced CD8+ cells to become suppressor/effectors.[369] Another group reported that patients with SLE demonstrate a selective relative reduction in that subset during active phases and reconstitution during remissions.[370] We are not aware of more recent data describing characteristics of suppressor/inducer CD4+ cells in SLE.

Studies in mice and humans with lupus have indicated that generation of CD8+ suppressor/effectors requires interactions between CD4+ and CD8+ cell subsets, and humoral factors such as IL-2 and TGF-β.[371-373] Many of them have reported decreased IL-2 secretion by T cells.[371-379] Although untreated CD8+ T cells from peripheral blood of patients with SLE enhanced Ig production by B cells, exposure of CD8+ cells to IL-2 plus TGF-β prevented this "helper" effect and decreased polyclonal IgG and antinucleoprotein antibody production.[380] Addition of anti–TGF-β blocked the interference with T cell help, so it is likely that CD8+ inhibitory cells (Ti) depend in part on that cytokine. CD8+ T cells activated in the presence of TGF-β suppress antibody production.[380]

Unmanipulated adult BWF1 mice cannot generate Ti capable of suppressing autoantibody production.[381] That could result from defects in generation of Ti, inadequate functional capacities of Ti, or presence of downregulating cells such as regulatory CD4+ T cells. Studies in normal humans[369] and rodents[382,383] have demonstrated that CD4+ suppressor/inducer cells, through cell-to-cell contact or production of humoral factors, and in the presence of IL-2 and TGF-β, mediate the generation of CD8+ suppressor/effector cells from CD8+ suppressor precursors. Absence of such cells results in inability to generate CD8+ suppressor/effectors. Dendritic cells may also participate in generation of Ti. Generation of cytotoxic CD8+ cells requires help from a CD4+ helper cell through CD40-CD40L interactions with the surface of a dendritic cell.[384-386] However, other studies have reported that if CD8+ cytotoxic precursor frequencies are high, priming of CD8+ T cell responses may not require CD4+ T cell help.[387] Once generated, the CD8+ suppressor/effector can subsequently act directly on the CD4+ T helper cell and abrogate its ability to provide help. Alternatively, it can act on an APC via cell-to-cell contact and render it tolerogenic through induction of surface expression of inhibitory receptors, such as ILT-3 and ILT-4, and downregulation of surface expression of CD80 and CD86.[388] Such a "tolerogenic" APC, upon subsequent contact with a CD4+ T helper, will render it anergic. From a regulatory standpoint, the functional abilities of normally generated CD8+ suppressor cells may be inhibited by regulatory CD4+ cells, whereas their proliferative capacity and survival remain intact.[389] Based on this model, failure to generate CD8+ Ti in BWF1 mice could result from abnormalities in dendritic cells or in CD4+ T cell suppressor/inducers. It is also possible that the Ti are generated but cannot function well enough to oppose activated T helper and B cells. Interestingly, the multiple defects described in the CD8+ T cells can be overcome. There is recent evidence suggesting that, in the BWF1 model of lupus, CD8+ inhibitory cells may still be present and may be induced to protect against the development of systemic autoimmunity in young BWF1 mice: Vaccination of BWF1 mice with plasmid DNA vectors encoding Ig VH-derived MHC class I–binding epitopes activates cytotoxic T cells that ablate autoantibody-producing B cells and inhibit the development of lupus nephritis.[390] This observation, in the context of the previously mentioned model, leads us to hypothesize that the CD8+ Ti cells in the old BWF1 mouse are not absent. It is more likely that the pathways leading to the generation of functionally competent CD8+ suppressor/effector T cells are deficient. These may include a deficiency of IL-2 and TGF-β in the microenvironment, or the absence or defective function of a CD4+ suppressor/inducer cell.

As described in the T cell section, certain subsets of DN cells possess potent suppressive activity. Such a subset (bearing the invariant Va24JaQ TCR) was reported to be decreased in peripheral blood of Japanese SLE patients,[288] and in the affected sibling of identical twins discordant for autoimmune diabetes.[289] NK T cells may also be decreased in numbers in peripheral blood of patients with SLE.[284,285] Furthermore, spontaneous and induced production of TGF-β by NK cells from patients with active SLE is reduced compared to normal controls.[299]

Another subset of regulatory or suppressor cells is a thymus-derived CD4+ subset constitutively expressing the IL-2 receptor α-chain (CD25); these cells protect the host from spontaneous organ-specific autoimmune disease. CD4+CD25+ cells have been called "professional" suppressor cells and have a contact-dependent mechanism of action in vitro.[391] In mice, CD4+CD25+ T cells appear in the peripheral immune system on day three of life and are preceded by CD4+CD25- T cells that can be detected from birth. A murine model of day thymectomy (D3Tx) has been extensively used for the study of regulatory cells in vivo.[392-395] This intervention creates a repertoire depleted of regulatory CD4+CD25+ T cells and enriched for autoreactive CD4+CD25- T cells. Upon stimulation by endogenous antigens, they then cause severe and progressive organ-specific autoimmune disease.[393,394] Little is known, however, about the role of CD4+CD25+ T cells in murine systemic autoimmunity. It was recently reported that day thymectomized SNF1 mice were protected from lupus-like glomerulonephritis; however, they developed organ-specific autoimmune responses including prostatitis, orchitis, and oophoritis.[396] Data on human systemic autoimmunity have not been published to date

In summary, several sets of regulatory/suppressor T cells, including CD8+CD28-, CD4+CD25+, and NK T cells protect from autoimmunity in normal mice, and probably in healthy humans. It is likely that abnormalities affecting any of these subsets contribute to the imbalance between autoantibody synthesis and regulation that is characteristic of SLE.

INADEQUATE IDIOTYPIC CIRCUITS CONTROLLING PATHOGENIC B AND T CELLS

In SLE, both human and murine, a substantial proportion of autoantibodies express a restricted number of public idiotypes (Ids).[397,398] Ids are sequences within the heavy and light chains of Ig molecules that are themselves antigenic; they induce anti-Id responses. Normally, those anti-Ids can suppress Ids and, therefore, downregulate production of Id+ antibodies. Some Ids (e.g., 16/6, O-81, and IdGN2) dominate tissue lesions in human SLE.[397-399] In murine lupus, treating mice with anti-Ids directed against the public Ids dominating their anti–ds-DNA antibodies can prevent or suppress disease, at least temporarily.[398] T cells have a similar idiotypic regulatory system; the Ids reside in the TCR molecules and the anti-Ids on TCR of regulatory T cells that are expected to suppress the Id+ T cells. It is unclear why this idiotypic B and T cell process is not operating normally to suppress disease in either human or murine SLE.

▌Summary

As shown in Table 74–7, many of the clinical manifestations of SLE are probably caused by or are associated with the pathogenic autoantibodies, immune complexes, and T cells that have been described. Certain immune complexes, selected antibodies to DNA or Ro/SS-A, and antibodies that bind glomerular structures can cause nephritis. Antibodies that bind to the fetal conduction system or cell membranes (lymphocytes, erythrocytes, platelets, neurons) or enter cells and alter cell functions also have the potential to cause disease. Immune complexes, antibodies to endothelial cells, antineutrophil cytoplasmic antibodies, and T cells may participate in vasculitis and in endothelial cell damage that promotes accelerated atherosclerosis—onto which may be added the prothrombotic effects of antibodies to phospholipids. A person's ability to manufacture pathogenic Ig and sustain its production depends on intrinsic abnormalities of B and T lymphocytes, and those, in turn, depend on inheriting an appropriate number of susceptibility genes, lacking protective genes, and encountering an environmental stimulus that sets the whole process into action. Understanding of this complex process is evolving rapidly, making the study of the pathogenesis of SLE one of the most fascinating areas in modern medicine.

TABLE 74–7 • CORRELATION AMONG CLINICAL MANIFESTATIONS OF SYSTEMIC LUPUS ERYTHEMATOSUS (SLE) AND AUTOANTIBODIES, IMMUNE COMPLEXES, AND T CELLS

Manifestation	Autoantibodies	Immune Complexes	T cells
Nephritis	Anti–double-stranded (ds)-DNA Anti-Ro Anti-Ciq Ids 16/6 and GN2	+	+
Arthritis	?	+	+
Dermatitis	Anti-Ro Anti–ds-DNA Id 16/6		+
Vasculitis	Anti-Ro?	+	+
Central nervous system	Anti-ribosomal P Antineuronal?	+	
Hematologic			
Lymphopenia	Antilymphocyte		
Hemolysis	Antierythrocyte		
Thrombocytopenia	Antiplatelet	+	
Clotting	Antiphospholipid		
Fetal loss	Antiphospholipid		
Neonatal lupus	Anti-Ro		
Sicca syndrome	Anti-Ro		+
Mild disease	Anti-RNP without other Autoantibody except ANA		

REFERENCES

1. Oelke K, Richardson B: Pathogenesis of lupus. Arthritis Rheum 47(3):343-345, 2002.
2. Tsao BP: An update on genetic studies of systemic lupus erythematosus. Curr Rheumatol Rep 4(4):359-367, 2002.
3. Harley JB, Moser KL, Gaffney PM, et al: The genetics of human systemic lupus erythematosus. Curr Opin Immunol 10:690, 1998.
4. Casciola-Rosen L, Rosen A: Ultraviolet light–induced keratinocyte apoptosis: A potential mechanism for the induction of skin lesions and autoantibody production in LE. Lupus 6:175, 1997.
5. Peeva E, Diamond B, Putterman C: Immunoglobulins and autoantibodies. *In* Wallace DR, Hahn BH (eds): Dubois' Lupus Erythematosus, 6th ed. Philadelphia, Lippincott, Williams and Wilkens, 2002, pp 391-415.
6. Katz JB, Limpanasithikul W, Diamond B: Mutational analysis of an autoantibody: Differential binding and pathogenicity. J Exp Med 180:925, 1994.
7. Shlomchik M, Mascelli M, Shan H, et al: Anti-DNA antibodies from autoimmune mice arise by clonal expansion and somatic mutation. J Exp Med 171:265, 1990.
8. Tilman DM, Jou N-T, Marion TN: Both IgM and IgG anti-DNA antibody are the products of clonally selective B cell stimulation in (NZB × NZW)/F1 mice. J Exp Med 176:361, 1992.
9. VanEs JH, Gmelig-Meyling FJH, van de Akker WRM, et al: Somatic mutations in the variable regions of a human IgG anti–double-stranded DNA autoantibody suggest a role for antigen in the induction of SLE. J Exp Med 173:461, 1991.
10. Hahn BH: Antibodies to DNA. N Engl J Med 338(19):1359-1368, 1998.
11. Ohnishi K, Ebling FM, Mitchell B, et al: Comparison of pathogenic and nonpathogenic murine antibodies to DNA: Antigen binding and structural characteristics. Int Immunol 6:817, 1994.
12. Ehrenstein MR, Katz DR, Griffiths MH, et al: Human IgG anti-DNA antibodies deposit in kidneys and induce proteinuria in SCID mice. Kidney Int 48:705, 1995.
13. Mevorach D: The immune response to apoptotic cells. Ann N Y Acad Sci 887:191-198, 1999.

14. Burlingame RW, Rubin RL: Autoantibody to the nucleosome subunit (H2A-H2B)-DNA is an early and ubiquitous feature of lupus-like conditions. Mol Biol Rep 23(3-4):159-166, 1996.

15. Kaliyaperumal A, Michaels MA, Datta SK: Naturally processed chromatin peptides reveal a major autoepitope that primes pathogenic T and B cells of lupus. J Immunol 168(5):2530-2537, 2002.

16. Bruns A, Blass S, Hausdorf G, et al: Nucleosomes are major T and B cell autoantigens in systemic lupus erythematosus. Arthritis Rheum 43(10):2307-2315, 2000.

17. Lu L, Kaliyaperumal A, Boumpas DT, Datta SK: Major peptide autoepitopes for nucleosome-specific T cells of human lupus. J Clin Invest 104(3):345-355, 1999.

18. Raz E, Brezis M, Roenmann E, et al: Anti-DNA antibodies bind directly to renal antigens and induce kidney dysfunction in the isolated perfused rat kidney. J Immunol 142:3076, 1989.

19. Madaio MP, Carlson J, Cataldo J, et al: Murine monoclonal anti-DNA antibodies bind directly to glomerular antigens and form immune deposits. J Immunol 138:2883, 1987.

20. Mostoslavsky G, Fischel R, Yachimovich N, et al: Lupus anti-DNA autoantibodies cross-react with a glomerular structural protein: A case for tissue injury by molecular mimicry. Eur J Immunol 31(4):1221-1227, 2001.

21. Deocharan B, Qing X, Lichauco J, Putterman C: Alpha-actinin is a cross-reactive renal target for pathogenic anti-DNA antibodies. J Immunol 168(6):3072-3078, 2002.

22. Chan TM, Leung JK, Ho SK, Yung S: Mesangial cell-binding anti-DNA antibodies in patients with systemic lupus erythematosus. J Am Soc Nephrol 13(5):1219-1229, 2002.

23. Lefkowith JB, Kiehl M, Rubenstein J, et al: Heterogeneity and clinical significance of glomerular-binding antibodies in systemic lupus erythematosus. J Clin Invest 98(6):1373-1380, 1996.

24. Gilkeson GS: Glomerular binding antibodies in systemic lupus erythematosus. In Kammer GM, Tsokos GC (eds): Lupus: Molecular and Cellular Pathogenesis. Totowa, NJ, Humana Press, 1999, p 448.

25. Siegert CE, Daha MR, Tseng CM, et al: Predictive value of IgG autoantibodies against C1q for nephritis in systemic lupus erythematosus. Ann Rheum Dis 52:851, 1993.

26. Horvath L, Czirjak L, Fekete B, et al: High levels of antibodies against C1q are associated with disease activity and nephritis but not with other organ manifestations in SLE patients. Clin Exp Rheumatol 19(6):667-672, 2001.

27. Maddison PJ, Reichlin M: Deposition of antibodies to a soluble cytoplasmic antigen in the kidneys of patients with systemic lupus erythematosus. Arthritis Rheum 22:553, 1979.

28. Riemekasten G, Kawald A, Weiss C, et al: Strong acceleration of murine lupus by injection of the SmD1(83-119) peptide. Arthritis Rheum 44(10):2435-2445, 2001.

29. Riemekasten G, Weiss C, Schneider S, et al: T cell reactivity against the SmD1(83-119) C terminal peptide in patients with systemic lupus erythematosus. Ann Rheum Dis 61(9):779-785, 2002.

30. Riemekasten G, Marell J, Trebeljahr G, et al: A novel epitope on the C-terminus of SmD1 is recognized by the majority of sera from patients with systemic lupus erythematosus. J Clin Invest 102(4):754-763, 1998.

31. Riemekasten G, Langnickel D, Ebling FM, et al: Identification and characterization of SmD183-119-reactive T cells that provide T cell help for pathogenic anti-double-stranded DNA antibodies. Arthritis Rheum 48(2):475-485, 2003.

32. Rioux JD, Zdarsky E, Newkirk MM, et al: Anti-DNA and anti-platelet specificities of SLE-derived autoantibodies: Evidence for CDR2H mutations and CDR3H motifs. Mol Immunol 32:683,1995.

33. Reichlin M, Brucato A, Frank MB, et al: Concentration of autoantibodies to native 60-kd Ro/SS-A and denatured 52-kd Ro/SS-A in eluates from the heart of a child who died with congenital complete heart block. Arthritis Rheum 37:1698, 1994.

34. Mazel JA, El-Sherif N, Buyon J, et al: Electrocardiographic abnormalities in a murine model injected with IgG from mothers of children with congenital heart block. Circulation 99(14): 1914-1918, 1999.

35. Buyon JP: Autoimmune-associated congenital heart block. In Kammer GM, Tsokos GC (eds): Lupus: Molecular and Cellular Pathogenesis. Totowa, NJ, Humana Press, 1999, p 492.

36. Tran HB, Ohlsson M, Beroukas D, et al: A serologic marker for fetal risk of congenital heart block. Arthritis Rheum 46(5): 1233-1241, 2002.

37. Salomonsson S, Dorner T, Theander E, et al: Subcellular redistribution of la/SSB autoantigen during physiologic apoptosis in the fetal mouse heart and conduction system: a clue to the pathogenesis of congenital heart block. Arthritis Rheum 46(1):202-208, 2002.

38. McCarty GA: The lupus anticoagulant and antiphospholipid antibodies. In Wallace DR, Hahn BH (eds): Dubois' Lupus Erythematosus, 6th ed. Philadelphia, Lippincott, Williams and Willkins, 2002, pp 495-508.

39. Bonfa E, Golombek SJ, Kaufman LD, et al: Association between lupus psychosis and anti-ribosomal P protein antibodies. N Engl J Med 317:265, 1986.

40. Schneebaum AB, Singleton JD, West SG, et al: Association of psychiatric manifestations with antibodies to ribosomal P proteins in SLE. Am J Med 90:54, 1992.

41. Hulsey M, Goldstein R, Scully L, et al: Anti-ribosomal P antibodies in SLE: A case control study correlating hepatic and renal disease. Clin Immunol Immunopathol 74:252, 1995.

42. Reichlin MN: Autoantibodies to intracellular antigens in SLE that bind and penetrate cells. In Kammer GM, Tsokos GC (eds): Lupus: Molecular and Cellular Pathogenesis. Totowa, NJ, Humana Press, 1999, p 389.

43. Salmon JE: Abnormalities in immune complex clearance and Fcγ receptor function. In Wallace DJ, Hahn BH (eds): Dubois' Lupus Erythematosus, 6th ed. Phildelphia, Lippincott, Williams and Wilkens, 2002, pp 219-242.

44. Walport MJ, Lachmann PJ: Erythrocyte complement receptor type 1, immmune complexes, and the rheumatic diseases. Arthritis Rheum 31:153, 1988.

45. Carroll MC: The Role of complement in B cell activation and tolerance. Adv Immunol 74:61-88, 2000.

46. Jarvinen P, Kaprio J, Makitalo R, et al: Systemic lupus erythematosus and related systemic diseases in a nationwide twin cohort: An increased prevalence of disease in MZ twins and concordance of disease features. J Intern Med 231:67, 1992.

47. Deapen D, Escalante A, Weinrib L, et al: A revised estimate of twin concordance in SLE. Arthritis Rheum 35:311, 1992.

48. Block SR, Lockshin MD, Winfield JB, et al: Studies of twins with systemic lupus erythematosus: A review of the literature and presentation of 12 additional sets. Am J Med 59:533, 1975.

49. Hochberg MC, Florsheim F, Scott J, et al: Familial aggregation of SLE. Am J Epidemiol 122:526, 1985.

50. Lawrence JS, Martins CL, Drake GL: A family survey of lupus erythematosus: Heritability. J Rheumatol 14:913, 1987.

51. Tsao BP, Cantor RM, Grossman JN, et al: PARP alleles within the linked chromosomal region are associated with systemic lupus erythematosus. J Clin Invest 103:1135, 1999.

52. Moser KL, Neas BR, Salmon JE, et al: Genome scan of human systemic lupus erythematosus: Evidence for linkage on chromosome 1q in African-American pedigrees. Proc Natl Acad Sci USA 95:14869, 1998.

53. Gaffney PM, Kearns GM, Shark KB, et al: A genome-wide search for susceptibility genes in human systemic lupus erythematosus sib-pair families. Proc Natl Acad Sci U S A 95:14875, 1998.

54. Shai R, Quismorio FP Jr, Li L, et al: Genome-wide screen for systemic lupus erythematosus susceptibility genes in multiplex families. Human Mol Gen 8:639, 1999.

55. Vyse TJ, Rozzo SJ, Drake CG, et al: Control of multiple autoantibodies linked with a lupus nephritis susceptibility locus in New Zealand black mice. J Immunol 158:5566, 1997.

56. Vyse TJ, Rozzo SJ, Drake CG, et al: Contributions of Ea(z) and Eb(z) MHC genes to lupus susceptibility in New Zealand mice. J Immunol 160:2757, 1998.

57. Rozzo SJ, Vyse TJ, David CS, et al: Analysis of MHC class II genes in the susceptibility to lupus in New Zealand mice. J Immunol 162:2623, 1999.

58. Morel L, Wakeland EK: Susceptibility to lupus nephritis in the NZB/W model system. Curr Opin Immunol 10:718, 1998.

59. Sobel ES, Mohan C, Morel L, et al: Genetic dissection of SLE pathogenesis: Adoptive transfer of Sle1 mediates the loss of tolerance by bone marrow–derived B cells. J Immunol 162:2415, 1999.

60. Mohan C, Alas E, Morel L, et al: Genetic dissection of SLE pathogenesis: Sle1 on murine chromosome 1 leads to a selective loss of tolerance to H2A/H2B/DNA subnucleosomes. J Clin Invest 191:1362, 1998.

61. Mohan C, Morel L, Yang P, et al: Genetic dissection of systemic lupus erythematosus pathogenesis: Sle2 on murine chromosome 4 leads to B cell hyperactivity. J Immunol 159:454, 1997.
62. Morel L, Mohan C, Yu Y, et al: Functional dissection of systemic lupus erythematosus using congenic mouse strains. J Immunol 158:6019, 1997.
63. Mohan C, Morel L, Wakeland EK: Genetic insights into murine lupus. In Kammer GM, Tsokos GC (eds): Lupus: Molecular and Cellular Pathogenesis. Totowa, NJ, Humana Press, 1999, p 124.
64. Watson ML, Rao JK, Gilkeson GS, et al: Genetic analysis of MRL/lpr mice: Relationship of the Fas apoptosis gene to disease manifestations and renal disease–modifying loci. J Exp Med 176:1645, 1992.
65. Russell JH, Rush B, Weaver C, et al: Mature T cells of autoimmune lpr/lpr mice have a defect in antigen-stimulated suicide. Proc Natl Acad Sci U S A 90:4409, 1993.
66. Cohen PL, Eisenberg RA: Lpr and gld: Single gene models of systemic autoimmunity and lymphoproliferative disease. Annu Rev Immunol 9:243, 1991.
66a. Amano H, Amano E, Moll T, et al: The yaa mutation promoting murine lupus causes defective development of marginal zone B cells. J Immunol 170(5):2293-2301, 2003.
67. Tsao BP, Cantor RM, Kalunian KC, et al: Evidence for linkage of a candidate chromosome 1 region to human systemic lupus erythematosus. J Clin Invest 99:725, 1997.
68. Schur PH, Marcus-Bagley D, Awdeh Z, et al: The effect of ethnicity on major histocompatibility complex complement allotypes and extended haplotypes in patients with SLE. Arthritis Rheum 33:985, 1990.
69. Bell DA, Rigsby R, Stiller CR, et al: HLA antigens in SLE: Relationship to disease severity, age at onset, and sex. J Rheumatol 11:475, 1984.
70. Gibofsky AM, Winchester RJ, Patarroyo M, et al: Disease association of the Ia-like human alloantigens: Contrasting patterns in rheumatoid arthritis and SLE. J Exp Med 148:1728, 1978.
71. Stasny P: HLA-D and Ia antigens in rheumatoid arthritis and SLE. Arthritis Rheum 21:1728, 1978.
72. So AK, Fiedler AH, Warner CA, et al: DNA polymorphisms of MHC class II and class III genes in SLE. Tissue Antigens 35:133, 1990.
73. Carroll MC, Palsdottir A, Belt KT, et al: Deletion of complement C4 and 21-OH hydroxylase genes in the HLA class II region. EMBO J 4:2567, 1985.
74. Kemp ME, Atkinson JP, Skanes VM, et al: Deletion of C4A genes in patients with SLE. Arthritis Rheum 30:1015, 1987.
75. Sturfelt G, Truedsson L, Johansen P, et al: Homozygous C4A deficiency in SLE: Analysis of patients from a defined population. Clin Genet 38:271, 1993.
76. Fielder AH, Walport MJ, Batchelor JR, et al: Family study of the major histocompatibility complex in patients with SLE: Importance of null alleles of C4A and C4B in determining disease susceptibility. BMJ 286:425, 1983.
77. Howard PF, Hochberg M, Bias WB, et al: Relationship between C4 null genes, HLA-D region antigens and genetic susceptibility to SLE in Caucasians and black Americans. Am J Med 81:187, 1989.
78. Wilson WA, Perez MC, Ramantis PE: Partial C4A deficiency is associated with susceptibility to SLE in black Americans. Arthritis Rheum 31:1171, 1988.
79. Dunckley H, Gatenby PA, Hawkins RB, et al: Deficiency of C4A is a genetic determinant of SLE in three ethnic groups. J Immunogenet 14:209, 1987.
80. Christiansen FG, Zhang WJ, Griffiths M, et al: Major histocompatibility complex: C4 deficiency explains some but not all of the influence of the MHC. J Rheumatol 18:1350, 1991.
81. Hawkins BR, Wong KL, Wong RW, et al: Strong associations between the MHC and SLE in southern Chinese. J Rheumatol 14:1128, 1987.
82. Tokunaga K, Omoto K, Akaza T, et al: Haplotype study on C4 polymorphism in Japanese: Associations with MHC alleles, complotypes, and HLA-complement haplotypes. Immunogenetics 22:539, 1985.
83. deJuan E, Martin-Villa JM, Gomez-Reino JJ, et al: Differential contributions of C4 and HLA-DQ genes to SLE susceptibility. Genetics 91:579, 1993.
84. Kaschru RB, Sequeira W, Mitta KK, et al: A significant increase of HLA-DR3 and DR2 in SLE among blacks. J Rheumatol 11:471, 1984.
85. Gladman DD, Terasaki PI, Park MS, et al: Increased frequency of HLA-DRw2 in SLE. Lancet 2:902, 1972.
86. Reveille JC, Schrohenloher RE, Acton RT, et al: DNA analysis of HLA-DR and DQ genes in American blacks with SLE. Arthritis Rheum 32:1243, 1989.
87. Walport MJ, Davies KA, Morley BJ, et al: Complement deficiency and autoimmunity. Ann N Y Acad Sci 815:267, 1997.
88. Agnello V: Lupus diseases associated with hereditary and acquired deficiencies of complement. Springer Semin Immunopathol 9:161, 1986.
89. Bowness P, Davies KA, Norsworthy PJ, et al: Hereditary C1q deficiency and systemic lupus erythematosus. QJM 87:455, 1994.
90. Atkinson JP, Schifferli JA: Complement system and systemic lupus erythematosus. In Kammer GM, Tsokos GC (eds): Lupus: Molecular and Cellular Pathogenesis. Totowa, NJ, Humana Press, 1999, p 529.
91. Graham RR, Ortmann WA, Langefeld CD, et al: Visualizing human leukocyte antigen class II risk haplotypes in human systemic lupus erythematosus. Am J Hum Genet 71:543-553, 2002.
92. Erlich HA, Nepom GT, Tyan DB: Autoimmunity: genetics and immunological mechanisms. In Rimoin DL, Connor JM, Pyeritz RE, Korf BR (eds): Principles and Practice of Medical Genetics. London, UK, Harcourt Publishers Limited, 2002, pp 1997-2011.
93. Hochberg MC, Boyd RE, Ahearn JM, et al: A review of clinico-laboratory features and immunogenetic markers in 150 patients with emphasis on demographic subsets. Medicine (Baltimore) 64:285, 1985.
94. Wilson AG, de Vries N, Pociot F, et al: An allelic polymorphism within the human tumor necrosis factor alpha promoter region is strongly associated with HLA A1, B8, and DR3 alleles. J Exp Med 177:557-560, 1993.
95. Wilson AG, Symons JA, McDowell TL, et al: Effects of a polymorphism in the human tumor necrosis factor alpha promoter on transcriptional activation. Proc Natl Acad Sci USA 94: 3195-3199, 1997.
96. Lu L-Y, Ding W-Z, Fici D, et al: Molecular analysis of major histocompatibility complex allelic associations with systemic lupus erythematosus in Taiwan. Arthritis Rheum 40:1138-1145, 1997.
97. Rood MJ, Keijsers V, van der Linden MW, et al: Neuropsychiatric systemic lupus erythematosus is associated with imbalance in interleukin 10 promoter haplotypes. Ann Rheum Dis 58:85-89, 1999.
98. Rudwaleit M, Tikly M, Khamashta M, et al: Interethnic differences in the association of tumor necrosis factor promoter polymorphisms with systemic lupus erythematosus. J Rheumatol 23:1725-1728, 1996.
99. Sullivan KE, Wooten C, Schmeckpeper BJ, et al: A promoter polymorphism of tumor necrosis factor a associated with systemic lupus erythematosus in African-Americans. Arthritis Rheum 40:2207-2211, 1997.
100. Wilson AG, Gordon C, di Giovine FS, et al: A genetic association between systemic lupus erythematosus and tumour necrosis factor-alpha. Euro J Immunol 24:191-195, 1994.
101. Bidwell J, Keen L, Gallagher G, et al: Review: Cytokine gene polymorphism in human disease: On-line databases. Genes Immunity 1:3-19, 1999.
102. Fronek Z, Timmerman LA, Alper CA, et al: MHC genes and susceptibility to SLE. Arthritis Rheum 33:1542, 1990.
103. Haseley LA, Wisnieski JJ, Denburg MR, et al: Antibodies to C1q in systemic lupus erythematosus: Characteristics and relation to FcγRIIA alleles. Kidney Int 52:1375, 1997.
104. Hamilton RG, Harley JB, Bias WB, et al: Two Ro (SS-A) responses in SLE: Correlation of HLA-DR/DQ specificities with quantitative expression of Ro (SS-A) autoantibody. Arthritis Rheum 31:496, 1988.
105. Reveille JD, MacLeod MJ, Whittington K, et al: Specific amino acid residues in the second hypervariable region of HLA-DQA1 and DQB1 chains promote the Ro (SS-A)/La (SS-B) autoantibody responses. J Immunol 146:3871, 1991.
106. Hoffman RW, Rettenmaier LJ, Takeda Y, et al: Human autoantibodies against the 70-kd peptide of U1 small nuclear RNP are associated with HLA-D4 among connective tissue disease patients. Arthritis Rheum 33:666, 1990.

107. Kaneoka H, Hsu K-C, Takeda Y, et al: Molecular genetic analysis of HLA-DR and HLA-DQ genes among anti–U1-70-kd autoantibody positive connective tissue disease patients. Arthritis Rheum 35:83, 1992.

108. Arnett FC Jr., Olsen ML, Anderson KL, et al: Molecular analysis of major histocompatibility complex alleles associated with the lupus anticoagulant. J Clin Invest 87:1490, 1991.

109. Walport MJ: The Roche Rheumatology Prize Lecture: Complement deficiency and disease. Br J Rheumatol 32:269-273, 1993.

110. Slingsby JH, Norsworthy P, Pearce G, et al: Homozgous hereditary C1q deficiency and systemic lupus erythematosus: a new family and the molecular basis of C1q deficiency in three families. Arthritis Rheum 39:663-670, 1995.

111. Botto M, Dell'Agnola C, Bygrave AE, et al: Homozygous C1q deficiency causes glomerulonephritis associated with multiple apoptotic bodies. Nat Genet 19:56-59, 1998.

112. Davies EJ, Snowden N, Hillarby MC, et al: Mannose-binding protein gene polymorphism in systemic lupus erythematosus. Arthritis Rheum 38:110, 1995.

113. Sullivan KE, Wooten C, Goldman D, et al: Mannose-binding gene protein polymorphisms in black patients with systemic lupus erythematosus. Arthritis Rheum 39:2046, 1996.

114. Ip WK, Chan SY, Lau CS, Lau YL: Association of systemic lupus erythematosus with promoter polymorphisms of the mannose-binding lectin gene. Arthritis Rheum 41:1663-1668, 1998.

115. Lau YL, Lau CS, Chan SY, et al: Mannose-binding protein in Chinese patients with systemic lupus erythematosus. Arthritis Rheum 39:706-708, 1996.

116. Salmon JE, Millard S, Schachter LA, et al: FcγRIIA alleles are heritable risk factors for lupus nephritis in African Americans. J Clin Invest 97:1348, 1996.

117. Song YW, Han CW, Kang SW, et al: Abnormal distribution of Fcγ receptor type IIa polymorphisms in Korean patients with systemic lupus erythematosus. Arthritis Rheum 41:421, 1998.

118. Duits AJ, Bootsma H, Derksen RHWM, et al: Skewed distribution of IgG Fc receptor IIa (CD32) polymorphism is associated with renal disease in systemic lupus erythematosus patients. Arthritis Rheum 39:1832-1836, 1995.

119. Zuniga R, Ng S, Peterson MG, et al: Low-binding alleles of Fcgamma receptor types IIA and IIIA are inherited independently and are associated with systemic lupus erythematosus in Hispanic patients. Arthritis Rheum 44:361-367, 2001.

120. Botto M, Theodoridis E, Thompson EM, et al: FcγRIIa polymorphism in systemic lupus erythematosus (SLE): No association with disease. Clin Exper Immunol 104:264-268, 1996.

121. D'Alfonso S, Rampi M, Bocchio D, et al: Systemic lupus erythematosus candidate genes in the Italian population: Evidence for a significant association with interleukin-10 [published erratum appears in Arthritis Rheum 43(7):1442, 2000]. Arthritis Rheum 43:120-128, 2000.

122. Dijstelbloem HM, Bijl M, Fijnheer R, et al: Fcgamma receptor polymorphisms in systemic lupus erythematosus: Association with disease and in vivo clearance of immune complexes. Arthritis Rheum 43:2793-2800, 2000.

123. Koene HR, Kleijer M, Swaak AJ, et al: The Fc gammaRIIIa-158F allele is a risk factor for systemic lupus erythematosus. Arthritis Rheum 41:1813-1818, 1998.

124. Manger K, Repp R, Spriewald BM, et al: Fcγ receptor IIa polymorphism in Caucasian patients with systemic lupus erythematosus: Association with clinical symptoms. Arthritis Rheum 41:1181-1189, 1998.

125. Manger K, Repp R, Spriewald BM, et al: Fcγ receptor IIA polymorphism in Caucasian patients with systemic lupus erythematosus: Association with clinical symptoms. Arthritis Rheum 41:1181, 1998.

126. Wu J, Edberg JC, Redecha PB, et al: A novel polymorphism of FcγRIIIa (CD16) alters receptor function and predisposes to autoimmune diseases. J Clin Invest 100:1059, 1997.

127. Salmon JE, Ng S, Yoo DH, et al: Altered distribution of Fcgamma receptor IIIA alleles in a cohort of Korean patients with lupus nephritis. Arthritis Rheum 42:818-819, 1999.

128. Beebe A, Cua D, de Waal MR: The role of interleukin-10 in autoimmune disease: systemic lupus erythematosus (SLE) and multiple sclerosis (MS). Cytokine Growth Factor Rev 13:403, 2002.

129. Eskdale J, Wordsworth P, Bowman S, et al: Association between polymorphisms at the human IL-10 locus and systemic lupus erythematosus [published erratum appears in Tissue Antigens 50(6):699, 1997]. Tissue Antigens 49:635-639, 1997.

130. Mehrian R, Quismorio FPJ, Strassmann G, et al: Synergistic effect between IL-10 and bcl-2 genotypes in determining susceptibility to systemic lupus erythematosus. Arthritis Rheum 41:596-602, 1998.

131. Alarcon-Riquelme ME, Lindqvist AK, Jonasson I, et al: Genetic analysis of the contribution of IL10 to systemic lupus erythematosus. J Rheumatol 26:2148-2152, 1999.

132. Ou TT, Tsai WC, Chen CJ, et al: Genetic analysis of interleukin-10 promoter region in patients with systemic lupus erythematosus in Taiwan. Kaohsiung J Med Sci 14:599-606, 1998.

133. Johansson C, Castillejo-Lopez C, Johanneson B, et al: Association analysis with microsatellite and SNP markers does not support the involvement of BCL-2 in systemic lupus erythematosus in Mexican and Swedish patients and their families. Genes Immun 1:380-385, 2000.

134. Lazarus M, Hajeer AH, Turner D, et al: Genetic variation in the interleukin 10 gene promoter and systemic lupus erythematosus [See comments]. J Rheumatol 24:2314-2317, 1997.

135. Mok CC, Lanchbury JS, Chan DW, Lau CS: Interleukin-10 promoter polymorphisms in Southern Chinese patients with systemic lupus erythematosus [See comments]. Arthritis Rheum 41:1090-1095, 1998.

136. Rood MJ, Keijsers V, van der Linden MW, et al: Neuropsychiatric systemic lupus erythematosus is associated with imbalance in interleukin 10 promoter haplotypes.

137. van der Linden MW, Westendorp RG, Sturk A, et al: High interleukin-10 production in first-degree relatives of patients with generalized but not cutaneous lupus erythematosus. J Investig Med 48:327-334, 2000.

138. Crawley E, Woo P, Isenberg DA: Single nucleotide polymorphic haplotypes of the interleukin-10 5′ flanking region are not associated with renal disease or serology in Caucasian patients with systemic lupus erythematosus. Arthritis Rheum 42:2017-2018, 1999.

139. Gibson AW, Edberg JC, Wu J, et al: Novel single nucleotide polymorphisms in the distal IL-10 promoter affect IL-10 production and enhance the risk of systemic lupus erythematosus. J Immunol 166:3915-3922, 2001.

140. Moser KL, Neas BR, Salmon JE, et al: Genome scan of human systemic lupus erythematosus: Evidence for linkage on chromosome 1q in African-American pedigrees. Proc Natl Acad Sci USA 95:14869-14874, 1998.

141. Graham RR, Langefeld CD, Gaffney PM, et al: Genetic linkage and transmission disequilibrium of marker haplotypes at chromosome 1q41 in human systemic lupus erythematosus. Arthritis Res 3:299-305, 2001.

142. Lindqvist AK, Steinsson K, Johanneson B, et al: A susceptibility locus for human systemic lupus erythematosus (hSLE1) on chromosome 2q. J Autoimmun 14:169-178, 2000.

143. Gray-McGuire C, Moser KL, Gaffney PM, et al: Genome scan of human systemic lupus erythematosus by regression modeling: evidence of linkage and epistasis at 4p16-15.2. Am J Hum Genet 67:1460-1469, 2000.

144. Gaffney PM, Kearns GM, Shark KB, et al: A genome-wide search for susceptibility genes in human systemic lupus erythematosus sib-pair families. Proc Natl Acad Sci USA 95:14875-14879, 1998.

145. Gaffney PM, Ortmann WA, Selby SA, et al: Genome screening in human systemic lupus erythematosus: Results from a second Minnesota cohort and combined analyses of 187 sib-pair families. Am J Hum Genet 66:547-556, 2000.

146. Lander ES, Kruglyak L: Genetic dissection of complex traits: guidelines for interpreting and reporting linkage results. Nat Genet 11:241-247, 1995.

147. Moser KL, Gray-McGuire C, Kelly J, et al: Confirmation of genetic linkage between human systemic lupus erythematosus and chromosome 1q41. Arthritis Rheum 42:1902-1907, 1999.

148. Shai R, Quismorio FP Jr., Li L, et al: Genome-wide screen for systemic lupus erythematosus susceptibility genes in multiplex families. Hum Mol Genet 8:639-644, 1999.

149. Tsao BP, Cantor RM, Grossman JM, et al: Linkage and interaction of loci on 1q23 and 16q12 may contribute to susceptibility

to systemic lupus erythematosus. Arthritis Rheum 46:2928-2936, 2002.

150. Magnusson V, Lindqvist AK, Castillejo-Lopez C, et al: Fine mapping of the SLEB2 locus involved in susceptibility to systemic lupus erythematosus. Genomics 70:307-314, 2000.

151. Prokunina L, Castillejo-Lopez C, Oberg F, et al: A regulatory polymorphism in PDCD1 is associated with susceptibility to systemic lupus erythematosus in humans. Nat Genet 32:666-669, 2002.

152. Nishimura H, Nose M, Hiai H, et al: Development of lupus-like autoimmune diseases by disruption of the PD-1 gene encoding an ITIM motif-carrying immunoreceptor. Immunity 11:141-151, 1999.

153. Nishimura H, Honjo T: PD-1: an inhibitory immunoreceptor involved in peripheral tolerance. Trends Immunol 22:265-268, 2001.

154. Boorboor P, Drescher BE, Hartung K, et al: Poly(ADP-ribose) polymerase polymorphisms are not a genetic risk factor for systemic lupus erythematosus in German Caucasians [Letter] [In Process Citation]. J Rheumatol 27:2061, 2000.

155. Criswell LA, Moser KL, Gaffney PM, et al: PARP alleles and SLE: failure to confirm association with disease susceptibility [Letter; comment] [See comments]. J Clin Invest 105:1501-1502, 2000.

156. Delrieu O, Michel M, Frances C, et al: Poly(ADP-ribose) polymerase alleles in French Caucasians are associated neither with lupus nor with primary antiphospholipid syndrome: GRAID Research Group—Group for Research on Auto-Immune Disorders [See comments]. Arthritis Rheum 42:2194-2197, 1999.

157. Edberg JC, Langefeld CD, Wu J, et al: Genetic linkage and association of Fcgamma receptor IIIA (CD16A) on chromosome 1q23 with human systemic lupus erythematosus. Arthritis Rheum 46:2132-2140, 2002.

158. Hugot JP, Chamaillard M, Zouali H, et al: Association of NOD2 leucine-rich repeat variants with susceptibility to Crohn's disease. Nature 411:599-603, 2001.

159. Lesage S, Zouali H, Cezard JP, et al: CARD15/NOD2 mutational analysis and genotype-phenotype correlation in 612 patients with inflammatory bowel disease. Am J Hum Genet 70:845-857, 2002.

160. Ogura Y, Bonen DK, Inohara N, et al: A frameshift mutation in NOD2 associated with susceptibility to Crohn's disease. Nature 411:603-606, 2001.

161. Nath SK, Kelly JA, Namjou B, et al: Evidence for a susceptibility gene, SLEV1, on chromosome 17p13 in families with vitiligo-related systemic lupus erythematosus. Am J Hum Genet 69:1401-1406, 2001.

162. Kelly JA, Thompson K, Kilpatrick J, et al: Evidence for a susceptibility gene (SLEH1) on chromosome 11q14 for systemic lupus erythematosus (SLE) families with hemolytic anemia. Proc Natl Acad Sci U S A 99:11766-11771, 2002.

163. Sawalha AH, Namjou B, Nath SK, et al: Genetic linkage of systemic lupus erythematosus with chromosome 11q14 (SLEH1) in African-American families stratified by a nucleolar antinuclear antibody pattern. Genes Immun 3(Suppl 1):S31-S34, 2002.

164. Nath SK, Kelly JA, Reid J, et al: SLEB3 in systemic lupus erythematosus (SLE) is strongly related to SLE families ascertained through neuropsychiatric manifestations. Hum Genet 111:54-58, 2002.

165. Namjou B, Nath SK, Kilpatrick J, et al: Genome scan stratified by the presence of anti-double-stranded DNA (dsDNA) autoantibody in pedigrees multiplex for systemic lupus erythematosus (SLE) establishes linkages at 19p13.2 (SLED1) and 18q21.1 (SLED2). Genes Immun 3(Suppl 1):S35-S41, 2002.

166. Quintero-Del-Rio AI, Kelly JA, Kilpatrick J, et al: The genetics of systemic lupus erythematosus stratified by renal disease: Linkage at 10q22.3 (SLEN1), 2q34-35 (SLEN2), and 11p15.6 (SLEN3). Genes Immun 3(Suppl 1):S57-S62, 2002.

167. Andrews BS, Eisenberg RA, Theofilopoulos AN, et al: Spontaneous murine lupus-like syndrome: Clinical and immunopathological manifestations in several strains. J Exp Med 148:1198, 1978.

168. Hahn BH: Animal models of systemic lupus erythematosus. In Wallace DJ, Hahn BH (eds): Dubois' Lupus Erythematosus, 5th ed. Baltimore, Williams & Wilkins, 1997, p 339.

169. Watanabe-Fukunaga R, Brannan CI, Clopeland NG, et al: Lymphoproliferation disorder in mice explained by defects in Fas antigen that mediates apoptosis. Nature 356:314, 1992.

170. Wu J, Zhou T, Zhang J, et al: Correction of accelerated autoimmune disease by early replacement of the mutated *lpr* gene with the normal Fas apoptosis gene in the T cells of transgenic MRL-lpr/lpr mice. Proc Natl Acad Sci U S A 91:2344, 1994.

171. Takahashi T, Tanaka M, Brannan CI, et al: Generalized lymphoproliferative disease in mice, caused by a point mutation in the Fas ligand. Cell 76:969, 1994.

172. Vidal S, Kono DH, Theofilopoulos AN: Loci predisposing to autoimmunity in MRL-Fas lpr and C57Bl/6-Fas lpr mice. J Clin Invest 101:696, 1998.

173. Wakeland EK, Liu K, Graham RR, Behrens TW: Delineating the genetic basis of systemic lupus erythematosus. Immunity 15:397-408, 2001.

174. Xie S, Chang S, Yang P, et al: Genetic contributions of nonautoimmune SWR mice toward lupus nephritis. J Immunol 167:7141-7149, 2001.

175. Morel L, Tian XH, Croker BP, Wakeland EK: Epistatic modifiers of autoimmunity in a murine model of lupus nephritis. Immunity 11:131-139, 1999.

176. Rozzo SJ, Allard JD, Choubey D, et al: Evidence for an interferon-inducible gene, Ifi202, in the susceptibility to systemic lupus. Immunity 15:435-443, 2001.

177. Morel L, Yu Y, Blenman KR, et al: Production of congenic mouse strains carrying genomic intervals containing SLE-susceptibility genes derived from the SLE-prone NZM24 D10 strain. Mamm Genome 7:335, 1996.

178. Sobel ES, Satoh M, Chen Y, et al: The major murine systemic lupus erythematosus susceptibility locus Sle1 results in abnormal functions of both B and T cells. J Immunol 169:2694-2700, 2002.

179. Morel L, Blenman KR, Croker BP, Wakeland EK: The major murine systemic lupus erythematosus susceptibility locus, Sle1, is a cluster of functionally related genes. Proc Natl Acad Sci USA 98:1787-1792, 2001.

180. Boackle SA, Holers VM, Chen X, et al: Cr2, a candidate gene in the murine Sle1c lupus susceptibility locus, encodes a dysfunctional protein. Immunity 15:775-785, 2001.

181. Wu X, Jiang N, Deppong C, et al: A role for the Cr2 gene in modifying autoantibody production in systemic lupus erythematosus. J Immunol 169:1587-1592, 2002.

182. Morel L, Tian HH, Croker BP, et al: Epistatic modifiers of autoimmunity in a murine model of lupus nephritis. Immunity 11:131, 1999.

183. Wysenbeck AJ, Block DA, Fries JF: Prevalence and expression of photosensitivity in SLE. Rheum Dis 48:461, 1989.

184. McGrath H Jr: Ultraviolet-A1 irradiation decreases clinical disease activity and autoantibodies in patients with SLE. Clin Exp Rheumatol 12:129, 1994.

185. Natali PG, Tan EM: Experimental skin lesions in mice resembling SLE. Arthritis Rheum 16:579, 1973.

186. Casciola-Rosen LA, Anhalt G, Rosen A: Autoantigens targeted in systemic lupus erythematosus are clustered in two populations of surface structures on apoptotic keratinocytes. J Exp Med 179:1317, 1994.

187. Casiano CA, Ochs RL, Tan EM: Distinct cleavage products of nuclear proteins in apoptosis and necrosis revealed by autoantibody probes. Cell Death Differ 5:183, 1998.

188. Schultz DR, Arnold PI: Heat shock (stress) proteins and autoimmunity in rheumatic diseases. Semin Arthritis Rheum 22:357, 1993.

189. Lahita RG: Sex hormones and systemic lupus erythematosus. Rheum Dis Clin North Am 26(4):951-968, 2000.

190. Nelson JL: Microchimerism and autoimmune disease [Editorial; comment]. N Engl J Med 338:1224, 1998.

191. Lahita RG, Kunkel HG, Bradlow HL: Increased oxidation of testosterone in SLE. Arthritis Rheum 26:1517, 1983.

192. Lahita RG, Bradlow L, Fishman J, et al: Estrogen metabolism in systemic lupus erythematosus: Patients and family members. Arthritis Rheum 25:843, 1982.

193. Fishman J, Martucci C: Biological properties of 16α-hydroxyestrone: Implications in estrogen physiology and pathophysiology. J Clin Endocrinol Metab 51:611, 1980.

194. Sanchez-Guerrero J, Liang MH, Karlson EW, et al: Post-menopausal estrogen therapy and the risk for developing systemic lupus erythematosus. Ann Intern Med 122:430, 1995.

195. Sanchez-Guerrero J, Karlson EW, Liang MH, et al: Past use of oral contraceptives and the risk of developing systemic lupus erythematosus. Arthritis Rheum 40:804, 1997.

196. Walker SE, McMurray RW, Houri JM, et al: Effects of prolactin in stimulating disease activity in systemic lupus erythematosus. Ann N Y Acad Sci 840:762, 1998.

197. Manilow MR, Bardana EJ Jr, Pirofsky B, et al: Systemic lupus erythematosus–like syndrome in monkeys fed alfalfa sprouts: Role of a nonprotein amino acid. Science 216:1500, 1978.

198. Jolly CA, Muthukumar A, Avula CP, et al: Life span is prolonged in food-restricted autoimmune-prone (NZB × NZW)F(1) mice fed a diet enriched with (n-3) fatty acids. J Nutr 131(10): 2753-2760, 2001.

199. Jolly CA, Muthukumar A, Reddy Avula CP, Fernandes G: Maintenance of NF-kappaB activation in T-lymphocytes and a naive T-cell population in autoimmune-prone (NZB/NZW)F(1) mice by feeding a food-restricted diet enriched with n-3 fatty acids. Cell Immunol 213(2):122-133, 2001.

200. Kelley VE, Ferreti A, Izui S, et al: A fish oil diet rich in eicosapentaenoic acid reduces cyclooxygenase metabolites and suppresses lupus in MRL/lpr mice. J Immunol 134:1914, 1985.

201. Walton AJE, Snaith ML, Locniskar M, et al: Dietary fish oil and the severity of symptoms in patients with SLE. Ann Rheum Dis 50:463, 1991.

202. Freni-Titulauer LWJ, Kelley DB, Grow AG, et al: Connective tissue disease in southeastern Georgia: A case control study of etiologic factors. Am J Epidemiol 130:404, 1989.

203. Sanchez-Guerrero J, Karlson EW, Colditz G, et al: Hair dye use and the risk of developing systemic lupus erythematosus. Arthritis Rheum 39:657, 1996.

204. Cavallo T, Granholm NA: Bacterial lipopolysaccharide transforms mesangial into proliferative lupus nephritis without interfering with processing of pathogenic immune complexes in NZB/W mice. Am J Pathol 137:971, 1990.

205. Talal N, Garry RF, Schur PH, et al: A conserved idiotype and antibodies to retroviral proteins in SLE. J Clin Invest 85:1866, 1990.

206. Erausquin C, Merino R, Izui S, et al: Therapeutic effect of early thymic irradiation in (NZB × NZW)F1 mice, associated with a selective decrease in the levels of IgG3 and gp70–anti-gp70 immune complexes. Cell Immunol 161:207, 1995.

207. Sundsfjord A, Osei A, Rosenqvist H, et al: BK and JC viruses in patients with systemic lupus erythematosus: Prevalent and persistent BK viruria, sequence stability of the viral regulatory regions, and nondetectable viremia. J Infect Dis 180:1, 1999.

208. Harley JB, James JA: Epstein-Barr virus infection may be an environmental risk factor for systemic lupus erythematosus in children and teenagers [Letter]. Arthritis Rheum 42:1782, 1999.

209. Griffiths DJ, Cooke SP, Herve C, et al: Detection of human retrovirus 5 in patients with arthritis and systemic lupus erythematosus. Arthritis Rheum 42:448, 1999.

210. Rubin RL: Drug-induced lupus. In Wallace DJ, Hahn BH (eds): Dubois' Lupus Erythematosus, 5th ed. Baltimore, Williams & Wilkins, 1997, p 871.

211. Elkayam O, Yaron M, Caspi D: Minocycline-induced autoimmune syndromes: An overview. Semin Arthritis Rheum 28:392, 1999.

212. Sandborn WJ, Hanauer SB: Antitumor necrosis factor therapy for inflammatory bowel disease: A review of agents, pharmacology, clinical results, and safety. Inflamm Bowel Dis 5:119, 1999.

213. Gilkeson GS, Grudier JP, Karounos DG, et al: Induction of anti–double-stranded DNA antibodies in normal mice by immunization with bacterial DNA. J Immunol 142:1482, 1989.

214. Schwartz RS, Stollar BD: The origins of anti-DNA antibodies. J Clin Invest 75:321, 1985.

215. Neujahr DC, Reich CF, Pisetsky DS: Immunostimulatory properties of genomic DNA from different bacterial species. Immunobiology 200:106, 1999.

216. Datta SK, Kaliyaperumal A: Nucleosome-driven autoimmune response in lupus: Pathogenic T helper cell epitopes and costimulatory signals. Ann N Y Acad Sci 815:155, 1997.

217. Burlingame R, Boey ML, Starkebaum G, et al: The central role of chromatin in autoimmune responses to histones and DNA in SLE. J Clin Invest 94:184, 1994.

218. Reichlin M: Cellular dysfunction induced by penetration of autoantibodies into living cells: Cellular damage and dysfunction mediated by antibodies to dsDNA and ribosomal P proteins. J Autoimmun 11:557, 1998.

219. McCluskey J, Farris AD, Keech CL, et al: Determinant spreading: Lessons from animal models and human disease. Immunol Rev 164:209, 1998.

220. Vaishnaw AK, McNally JD, Elkon KB: Apoptosis in the rheumatic diseases. Arthritis Rheum 40:1917, 1997.

221. Lorenz HM, Grunke M, Hieronymus T, et al: In vitro apoptosis and expression of apoptosis-related molecules in lymphocytes from patients with systemic lupus erythematosus and other autoimmune diseases. Arthritis Rheum 40:306, 1997.

222. Georgescu L, Vakkalanka RK, Elkon KB, et al: Interleukin-10 promotes activation-induced cell death of SLE lymphocytes mediated by Fas ligand. J Clin Invest 100:2622, 1997.

223. Korb LC, Ahearn JM: C1q binds directly and specifically to surface blebs of apoptotic human keratinocytes: Complement deficiency and systemic lupus erythematosus revisited. J Immunol 158:4525, 1997.

224. Mitchell DA, Taylor PR, Cook HT, et al: Cutting edge: C1q protects against the development of glomerulonephritis independently of C3 activation. J Immunol 162:5676, 1999.

225. Grammer AC, Lipsky PE: CD154-CD40 interactions mediate differentiation to plasma cells in healthy individuals and persons with systemic lupus erythematosus. Arthritis Rheum 46(6): 1417-1429, 2002.

226. Tsokos GC, Wong HK, Enyedy EJ, Nambiar MP: Immune cell signaling in lupus. Curr Opin Rheumatol 12(5):355-363, 2000.

227. Shakhov AN, Nedospasov SA: Expression profiling in knockout mice: Lymphotoxin versus tumor necrosis factor in the maintenance of splenic microarchitecture. Cytokine Growth Factor Rev 12(1):107-119, 2001.

228. Matsumoto M: Role of TNF ligand and receptor family in the lymphoid organogenesis defined by gene targeting. J Med Invest 46(3-4):141-150, 1999.

229. Grammer AC, McFarland RD, Heaney J, et al: Expression, regulation, and function of B cell-expressed CD154 in germinal centers. J Immunol 163(8):4150-4159, 1999.

230. Lettesjo H, Burd GP, Mageed RA: CD4+ T lymphocytes with constitutive CD40 ligand in preautoimmune (NZB × NZW)F1 lupus-prone mice: Phenotype and possible role in autoreactivity. J Immunol 165(7):4095-4104, 2000.

231. Calame KL: Plasma cells: finding new light at the end of B cell development. Nat Immunol 2(12):1103-1108, 2001.

232. Mandik-Nayak L, Bui A, Noorchashm H, et al: Regulation of anti-double-stranded DNA B cells in nonautoimmune mice: Localization to the T-B interface of the splenic follicle. J Exp Med 186(8):1257-1267, 1997.

233. Wellmann U, Werner A, Winkler TH: Altered selection processes of B lymphocytes in autoimmune NZB/W mice, despite intact central tolerance against DNA. Eur J Immunol 31(9):2800-2810, 2001.

234. Jacobson BA, Rothstein TL, Marshak-Rothstein A: Unique site of IgG2a and rheumatoid factor production in MRL/lpr mice. Immunol Rev 156:103-110, 1997.

235. Cohen PL, Eisenberg RA: Lpr and gld: Single gene models of systemic autoimmunity and lymphoproliferative disease. Annu Rev Immunol 9:243-269, 1991.

236. Vaishnaw AK, Toubi E, Ohsako S, et al: The spectrum of apoptotic defects and clinical manifestations, including systemic lupus erythematosus, in humans with CD95 (Fas/APO-1) mutations. Arthritis Rheum 42(9):1833-1842, 1999.

237. Nagafuchi H, Wakisaka S, Takeba Y, et al: Aberrant expression of Fas ligand on anti-DNA autoantibody secreting B lymphocytes in patients with systemic lupus erythematosus: "Immune privilege"-like state of the autoreactive B cells. Clin Exp Rheumatol 20(5):625-631, 2002.

238. Bouillet P, Metcalf D, Huang DC, et al: Proapoptotic Bcl-2 relative Bim required for certain apoptotic responses, leukocyte homeostasis, and to preclude autoimmunity. Science 286(5445):1735-1738, 1999.

239. Strasser A, Whittingham S, Vaux DL, et al: Enforced BCL2 expression in B-lymphoid cells prolongs antibody responses and elicits autoimmune disease. Proc Natl Acad Sci USA 88(19):8661-8665, 1991.

240. Khare SD, Sarosi I, Xia XZ, et al: Severe B cell hyperplasia and autoimmune disease in TALL-1 transgenic mice. Proc Natl Acad Sci U S A 97(7):3370-3375, 2000.

241. Gross JA, Johnston J, Mudri S, et al: TACI and BCMA are receptors for a TNF homologue implicated in B-cell autoimmune disease. Nature 404(6781):995-999, 2000.

242. Cheema GS, Roschke V, Hilbert DM, Stohl W: Elevated serum B lymphocyte stimulator levels in patients with systemic immune-based rheumatic diseases. Arthritis Rheum 44(6): 1313-1319, 2001.

243. Bynoe MS, Grimaldi CM, Diamond B: Estrogen up-regulates Bcl-2 and blocks tolerance induction of naive B cells. Proc Natl Acad Sci USA 97(6):2703-2708, 2000.

244. Peeva E, Michael D, Cleary J, et al: Prolactin modulates the naive B cell repertoire. J Clin Invest 111(2):275-283, 2003.

245. Peng SL, Madaio MP, Hughes DP, et al: Murine lupus in the absence of alpha beta T cells. J Immunol 156(10):4041-4049, 1996.

246. Chan OT, Hannum LG, Haberman AM, et al: A novel mouse with B cells but lacking serum antibody reveals an antibody-independent role for B cells in murine lupus. J Exp Med 189(10):1639-1648, 1999.

247. Reininger L, Radaszkiewicz T, Kosco M, et al: Development of autoimmune disease in SCID mice populated with long-term "in vitro" proliferating (NZB × NZW)F1 pre-B cells. J Exp Med 176(5):1343-1353, 1992.

248. Klinman DM: B-cell abnormalities characteristic of systemic lupus erythematosus. In Wallace DJ, Hahn BH (eds): Dubois' Lupus Erythematosus, 5th ed. Baltimore, Williams & Wilkins, 1997, p 195.

249. Reininger L, Radaszkiewicz T, Kosco M, et al: Development of autoimmune disease in SCID mice populated with long-term "in vitro" proliferating (NZB × NZW)F1 pre-B cells. J Exp Med 176:1343, 1992.

250. Moutsopoulos HM, Boehm-Truitt M, Kassan SS, et al: Demonstration of activatin of B lymphocytes in New Zeland black mice at birth by an immunoradiometric assay for murine IgM. J Immunol 119:1639, 1977.

251. Klinman DM, Shirai A, Ishigatsubo Y, et al: Quantitation of IgM- and IgG-secreting B cells in the peripheral blood of patients with SLE. Arthritis Rheum 34:11, 1991.

252. Fauci AS, Moutsopoulos HM: Polyclonally triggered B cells in the peripheral blood and bone marrow of normal individuals and in patients with SLE and Sjögren's syndrome. Arthritis Rheum 24:577, 1983.

253. Liossis SN, Kovacs B, Dennis G, et al: B cells from patients with systemic lupus erythematosus display abnormal antigen receptor-mediated early signal transduction events. J Clin Invest 98(11):2549-2557, 1996.

254. Dziarski R: Autoimmunity: Polyclonal activation of antigen induction? Immunol Today 9:340, 1988.

255. Singh RR, Hahn BH, Tsao BP, et al: Evidence for multiple mechanisms of polyclonal T cell activation in murine lupus. J Clin Invest 102:1841, 1998.

256. James JA, Harley JB: B-cell epitope spreading in autoimmunity. Immunol Rev 164:185, 1998.

257. Craft J, Fatenejad S: Self antigens and epitope spreading in systemic autoimmunity. Arthritis Rheum 40:1374, 1998.

258. Majeti R, Xu Z, Parslow TG, et al: An inactivating point mutation in the inhibitory wedge of CD45 causes lymphoproliferation and autoimmunity. Cell 103(7):1059-1070, 2000.

259. Huck S, Le Corre R, Youinou P, Zouali M: Expression of B cell receptor-associated signaling molecules in human lupus. Autoimmunity 33(3):213-224, 2001.

260. Mary C, Laporte C, Parzy D, et al: Dysregulated expression of the Cd22 gene as a result of a short interspersed nucleotide element insertion in Cd22a lupus-prone mice. J Immunol 165(6):2987-2996, 2000.

261. Shai R, Quismorio FP Jr, Li L, et al: Genome-wide screen for systemic lupus erythematosus susceptibility genes in multiplex families. Hum Mol Genet 8(4):639-644, 1999.

262. Gray-McGuire C, Moser KL, Gaffney PM, et al: Genome scan of human systemic lupus erythematosus by regression modeling: evidence of linkage and epistasis at 4p16-15.2. Am J Hum Genet 67(6):1460-1469, 2000.

263. Gaffney PM, Kearns GM, Shark KB, et al: A genome-wide search for susceptibility genes in human systemic lupus erythematosus sib-pair families. Proc Natl Acad Sci USA 95(25):14875-14879, 1998.

264. Moser KL, Neas BR, Salmon JE, et al: Genome scan of human systemic lupus erythematosus: Evidence for linkage on chromosome 1q in African-American pedigrees. Proc Natl Acad Sci USA 95(25):14869-14874, 1998.

265. Honda M, Linker-Israeli M: Cytokine gene expression in human systemic lupus erythematosus. In Kammer GM, Tsokos GC (eds): Lupus: Molecular and Cellular Pathogenesis. Totowa, NJ, Humana Press, 1999, p 341.

266. Hagiwara E, Gourley MF, Lee S, Klinman DK: Disease severity in patients with systemic lupus erythematosus correlates with an increased ratio of interleukin-10:interferon-gamma-secreting cells in the peripheral blood. Arthritis Rheum 39(3):379-385, 1996.

267. Nagafuchi H, Suzuki N, Mizushima Y, Sakane T: Constitutive expression of IL-6 receptors and their role in the excessive B cell function in patients with systemic lupus erythematosus. J Immunol 151(11):6525-6534, 1993.

268. Fink BK, Chan B, Wofsy DM: IL-6 promotes murine lupus in NZB/NZW F1 mice. J Clin Invest 94:585, 1995.

269. Hagiwara E, Gourley MF, Lee S, et al: Disease severity in patients with systemic lupus erythematosus correlates with an increased ratio of interleukin-10:interferon-γ-secreting cells in the peripheral blood. Arthritis Rheum 39:379, 1996.

270. Ishida H, Muchamuel T, Sakaguchi S, et al: Continuous administration of anti–interleukin 10 antibodies delays onset of autoimmunity in NZB/NZW F1 mice. J Exp Med 179:305, 1994.

271. Llorente L, Zou W, Levy Y, et al: Role of interleukin 10 in the B lymphocyte hyperactivity and autoantibody production of human systemic lupus erythematosus. J Exp Med 181(3):839-844, 1995.

272. Yin Z, Bahtiyar G, Zhang N, et al: IL-10 regulates murine lupus. J Immunol 169(4):2148-2155, 2002.

273. Wofsy D, Seaman WE: Successful treatment of autoimmunity in NZB/NZW F1 mice with monoclonal antibody to L3T4. J Exp Med 161:378, 1985.

274. Wofsy D: Administration of monoclonal anti–T cell antibodies retards murine lupus in BXSB mice. J Immunol 136:4554, 1986.

275. Mihara M, Ohsugi Y, Saito K, et al: Immunologic abnormality in NZB/NZW F1 mice: Thymus-independent occurrence of B cell abnormality and requirement for T cells in the development of autoimmune disease, as evidenced by an analysis of the athymic nude individuals. J Immunol 141(1):85-90, 1988.

276. Shoenfeld Y, Mozes E:. Pathogenic idiotypes of autoantibodies in autoimmunity: Lessons from new experimental models of SLE. FASEB J 4(9):2646-2651, 1990.

277. Horwitz D: The role of T lymphocytes in SLE. In Wallace DJ, Hahn BH (eds): Dubois' Lupus Erythematosus, 5th ed. Baltimore, Williams & Wilkins, 1997, p 155.

278. Winfield JB: Antilymphocyte autoantibodies. In Wallace DJ, Hahn BH (eds): Dubois' Lupus Erythematosus, 5th ed. Baltimore, Williams & Wilkins, 1997, p 505.

279. Yamada A, Winfield JB: Inhibition of soluble antigen-induced T cell proliferation by warm-reactive antibodies to activated T cells in systemic lupus erythematosus. J Clin Invest 74(6):1948-1960, 1984.

280. Butler WT, Sharp JT, Rossen RD, et al: Relationship of the clinical course of systemic lupus erythematosus to the presence of circulating lymphocytotoxic antibodies. Arthritis Rheum 15(3):251-258, 1972.

281. Morimoto C, Reinherz EL, Schlossman SF, et al: Alterations in immunoregulatory T cell subsets in active systemic lupus erythematosus. J Clin Invest 66:1171, 1980.

282. Tsokos GC, Balow JE: Phenotypes of T lymphocytes in systemic lupus erythematosus: Decreased cytotoxic/suppressor subpopulation is associated with deficient allogeneic cytotoxic responses rather than with concanavalin A-induced suppressor cells. Clin Immunol Immunopathol 26:267, 1983.

283. Koide J, Takano M, Takeuchi T, et al: Direct demonstration of immunoregulatory T-cell defects in patients with systemic lupus erythematosus. Scand J Immunol 23:449, 1986.

284. Devi BS, Van Noordin S, Krausz T, Davies KA: Peripheral blood lymphocytes in SLE–hyperexpression of CD154 on T and B

lymphocytes and increased number of double negative T cells. J Autoimmun 11(5):471-475, 1998.

285. Sieling PA, Porcelli SA, Duong BT, et al: Human double-negative T cells in systemic lupus erythematosus provide help for IgG and are restricted by CD1c. J Immunol 165(9):5338-5344, 2000.

286. Rajagopalan S, Zordan T, Tsokos GC, Datta SK: Pathogenic anti-DNA autoantibody-inducing T helper cell lines from patients with active lupus nephritis: isolation of CD4-8-T helper cell lines that express the gamma delta T-cell antigen receptor. Proc Natl Acad Sci U S A 87(18):7020-7024, 1990.

287. Shivakumar S, Tsokos GC, Datta SK: T cell receptor alpha/beta expressing double-negative (CD4-/CD8-) and CD4+ T helper cells in humans augment the production of pathogenic anti-DNA autoantibodies associated with lupus nephritis. J Immunol 143(1):103-112, 1989.

288. Oishi Y, Sumida T, Sakamoto A, et al: Selective reduction and recovery of invariant Valpha24JalphaQ T cell receptor T cells in correlation with disease activity in patients with systemic lupus erythematosus. J Rheumatol 28(2):275-283, 2001.

289. Wilson SB, Kent SC, Horton HF, et al: Multiple differences in gene expression in regulatory Valpha 24Jalpha Q T cells from identical twins discordant for type I diabetes. Proc Natl Acad Sci U S A 97(13):7411-7416, 2000.

290. Kaneoka H, Morito F, Yamaguchi M: Low responsiveness to the anti Leu 4 antibody by T cells from patients with active systemic lupus erythematosus. J Clin Lab Immunol 28(1):15-26, 1989.

291. Stohl W: Impaired generation of polyclonal T cell-mediated cytolytic activity despite normal polyclonal T cell proliferation in systemic lupus erythematosus. Clin Immunol Immunopathol 63(2):163-172, 1992.

292. Tsokos GC, Liossis SN: Lymphocytes, cytokines, inflammation, and immune trafficking. Curr Opin Rheumatol 10:417, 1998.

293. Raziuddin S, Nur MA, al-Wabel AA: Increased circulating HLA-DR+ CD4+ T cells in systemic lupus erythematosus: Alterations associated with prednisolone therapy. Scand J Immunol 31(2):139-145, 1990.

294. Horwitz DA, Stastny P, Ziff M: Circulating deoxyribonucleic acid–synthesizing mononuclear leukocytes. I. Increased numbers of proliferating mononuclear leukocytes in inflammatory disease. J Lab Clin Med 76(3):391-402, 1970.

295. Manoussakis MN, Papadopoulos GK, Drosos AA, Moutsopoulos HM: Soluble interleukin 2 receptor molecules in the serum of patients with autoimmune diseases. Clin Immunol Immunopathol 50(3):321-332, 1989.

296. Davas EM, Tsirogianni A, Kappou I, et al: Serum IL-6, TNFalpha, p55 srTNFalpha, p75srTNFalpha, srIL-2alpha levels and disease activity in systemic lupus erythematosus. Clin Rheumatol 18(1):17-22, 1999.

297. Kato K, Santana-Sahagun E, Rassenti LZ, et al: The soluble CD40 ligand sCD154 in systemic lupus erythematosus. J Clin Invest 104(7):947-955, 1999.

298. Stohl W, Elliott JE, Hamilton AS, et al: Impaired recovery and cytolytic function of CD56+ T and non-T cells in systemic lupus erythematosus following in vitro polyclonal T cell stimulation: Studies in unselected patients and monozygotic disease-discordant twins. Arthritis Rheum 39(11):1840-1851, 1996.

299. Horwitz DA, Gray JD, Ohtsuka K, et al: The immunoregulatory effects of NK cells: The role of TGF-beta and implications for autoimmunity. Immunol Today 18(11):538-542, 1997.

300. Datta SK, Patel H, Berry D: Induction of cationic shift in IgG anti-DNA autoantibodies: Role of T helper cells with classical and novel phenotypes in three models of lupus nephritis. J Exp Med 165:1252, 1987.

301. Zeng D, Dick M, Cheng L, et al: Subsets of transgenic T cells that recognize CD1 induce or prevent murine lupus: Role of cytokines. J Exp Med 187:525, 1998.

302. Tan P, Pang G, Wilson JD: Immunoglobulin production in vitro by peripheral blood lymphocytes in systemic lupus erythematosus: Helper T cell defect and B cell hyperreactivity. Clin Exp Immunol 44(3):548-554, 1981.

303. Fauci AS, Moutsopoulos HM: Polyclonally triggered B cells in the peripheral blood and bone marrow of normal individuals and in patients with systemic lupus erythematosus and primary Sjögren's syndrome. Arthritis Rheum 24(4):577-583, 1981.

304. Tsokos GC, Smith PL, Christian CB, et al: Interleukin-2 restores the depressed allogeneic cell-mediated lympholysis and natural killer cell activity in patients with systemic lupus erythematosus. Clin Immunol Immunopathol 34:379, 1985.

305. Stohl W: Impaired polyclonal T cell cytolytic activity: A possible risk factor for systemic lupus erythematosus. Arthritis Rheum 38:506, 1995.

306. Linker-Israeli M, Quismorio FP Jr, Horwitz DA: CD8+ lymphocytes from patients with systemic lupus erythematosus sustain, rather than suppress, spontaneous polyclonal IgG production and synergize with CD4+ cells to support autoantibody synthesis. Arthritis Rheum 33:1216, 1990.

307. Gray D, Hirokawa M, Ohtsuka K, Horwitz DA: Generation of an inhibitory circuit involving CD8+ T cells, IL-2, and NK cell-derived TGF-beta: Contrasting effects of anti-CD2 and anti-CD3. J Immunol 160:2248, 1998.

308. Sekigawa I, Okada T, Noguchi K, et al: Class-specific regulation of anti-DNA antibody synthesis and the age-associated changes in (NZB × NZW) F1 hybrid mice. J Immunol 138:2890, 1987.

309. Via CS, Sharrow SO, Shearer GM: Role of cytotoxic T lymphocytes in the prevention of lupus-like disease occurring in a murine model of graft-vs-host disease. J Immunol 139:1840, 1987.

310. Liossis SN, Ding XZ, Dennis GJ, Tsokos GC: Altered pattern of TCR/CD3-mediated protein-tyrosyl phosphorylation in T cells from patients with systemic lupus erythematosus: Deficient expression of the T cell receptor zeta chain. J Clin Invest 101(7):1448-1457, 1998.

311. Tsokos GC, Liossis SN: Immune cell signaling defects in lupus: activation, anergy and death. Immunol Today 20(3):119-124, 1999.

312. Koshy M, Berger D, Crow MK: Increased expression of CD40 ligand on systemic lupus erythematosus lymphocytes. J Clin Invest 98(3):826-837, 1996.

313. Kovacs B, Liossis SN, Dennis GJ, Tsokos GC: Increased expression of functional Fas-ligand in activated T cells from patients with systemic lupus erythematosus. Autoimmunity 25(4):213-221, 1997.

314. Kammer GM, Khan IU, Malemud CJ: Deficient type I protein kinase A isozyme activity in systemic lupus erythematosus T lymphocytes. J Clin Invest 94(1):422-430, 1994.

315. Mishra N, Khan IU, Tsokos GC, Kammer GM: Association of deficient type II protein kinase A activity with aberrant nuclear translocation of the RII beta subunit in systemic lupus erythematosus T lymphocytes. J Immunol 165(5):2830-2840, 2000.

316. Mysler E, Bini P, Drappa J, et al: The apoptosis-1/Fas protein in human systemic lupus erythematosus. J Clin Invest 93(3):1029-1034, 1994.

317. Kovacs B, Vassilopoulos D, Vogelgesang SA, Tsokos GC: Defective CD3-mediated cell death in activated T cells from patients with systemic lupus erythematosus: Role of decreased intracellular TNF-alpha. Clin Immunol Immunopathol 81(3):293-302, 1996.

318. Emlen W, Niebur J, Kadera R: Accelerated in vitro apoptosis of lymphocytes from patients with systemic lupus erythematosus. J Immunol 152(7):3685-3692, 1994.

319. Banki K, Hutter E, Gonchoroff NJ, Perl A: Elevation of mitochondrial transmembrane potential and reactive oxygen intermediate levels are early events and occur independently from activation of caspases in Fas signaling. J Immunol 162(3):1466-1479, 1999.

320. Li PF, Dietz R, von Harsdorf R: p53 regulates mitochondrial membrane potential through reactive oxygen species and induces cytochrome c-independent apoptosis blocked by Bcl-2. EMBO J 18(21):6027-6036, 1999.

321. Puskas F, Gergely P Jr, Banki K, Perl A: Stimulation of the pentose phosphate pathway and glutathione levels by dehydroascorbate, the oxidized form of vitamin C. FASEB J 14(10):1352-1361, 2000.

322. Gergely P Jr, Grossman C, Niland B, et al: Mitochondrial hyperpolarization and ATP depletion in patients with systemic lupus erythematosus. Arthritis Rheum 46(1):175-190, 2002.

323. Richardson B, Scheinbart L, Strahler J, et al: Evidence for impaired T cell DNA methylation in systemic lupus erythematosus and rheumatoid arthritis. Arthritis Rheum 33(11):1665-1673, 1990.

324. Bird AP, Wolffe AP: Methylation-induced repression—belts, braces, and chromatin. Cell 99(5):451-454, 1999.

325. Kammer GM, Perl A, Richardson BC, Tsokos GC: Abnormal T cell signal transduction in systemic lupus erythematosus. Arthritis Rheum 46(5):1139-1154, 2002.

326. Yung R, Powers D, Johnson K, et al: Mechanisms of drug-induced lupus. II. T cells overexpressing lymphocyte function-associated antigen 1 become autoreactive and cause a lupuslike disease in syngeneic mice. J Clin Invest 97(12):2866-2871, 1996.

327. Kaplan MJ, Beretta L, Yung RL, Richardson BC: LFA-1 overexpression and T cell autoreactivity: Mechanisms. Immunol Invest 29(4):427-442, 2000.

328. Wong HK, Kammer GM, Dennis G, Tsokos GC: Abnormal NF-kappa B activity in T lymphocytes from patients with systemic lupus erythematosus is associated with decreased p65-RelA protein expression. J Immunol 163(3):1682-1689, 1999.

329. Sassone-Corsi P:. Coupling gene expression to cAMP signalling: role of CREB and CREM. Int J Biochem Cell Biol 30(1):27-38, 1998.

330. Powell JD, Lerner CG, Ewoldt GR, Schwartz RH: The-180 site of the IL-2 promoter is the target of CREB/CREM binding in T cell anergy. J Immunol 163(12):6631-6639, 1999.

331. Mosmann TR: Properties and functions of interleukin-10. Adv Immunol 56:1-26, 1994.

332. Schwarting A, Wada T, Kinoshita K, et al: IFN-γ receptor signaling is essential for the initiation, acceleration, and destruction of autoimmune kidney disease in MRL-Fas(lpr) mice. J Immunol 161:494, 1998.

333. Ozmen L, Roman D, Fountoulakis M, et al: Experimental therapy of systemic lupus erythematosus: The treatment of NZB/W mice with mouse soluble interferon-γ receptor inhibits the onset of glomerulonephritis. Eur J Immunol 25:6, 1995.

334. Singh RR, Ebling FM, Sercarz EE, et al: Immune tolerance to autoantibody-derived peptides delays development of autoimmunity in murine lupus. J Clin Invest 96:2990, 1995.

335. Hahn BH, Singh RR, Wong WK, et al: Treatment with a consensus peptide based on amino acid sequences in autoantibodies prevents T cell activation by autoantigens and delays disease onset in murine lupus. Arthritis Rheum 44(2):432-441, 2001.

336. O'Hanlon TP, Dalakas MC, Plotz PH, et al: Predominant TCR αβ variable and joining gene expression by muscle-infiltrating lymphocytes in the idiopathic inflammatory myopathies. J Immunol 152:2569, 1994.

337. Werth VP, Dutz JP, Sontheimer RD: Pathogenetic mechanisms and treatment of cutaneous lupus erythematosus. Curr Opin Rheumatol 9:400, 1997.

338. Danning CL, Illei GG, Boumpas DT: Vasculitis associated with primary rheumatologic diseases. Curr Opin Rheumatol 10:58, 1998.

339. Murata H, Matsumura R, Koyama A, et al: T cell receptor repertoire of T cells in the kidneys of patients with lupus nephritis. Arthritis Rheum 46(8):2141-2147, 2002.

340. Radic MZ, Erikson J, Litwin S, et al: B lymphocytes may escape tolerance by revising their antigen receptors. J Exp Med 177:1165, 1993.

341. Horwitz DA, Gray JD, Zheng SG: The potential of human regulatory T cells generated ex vivo as a treatment for lupus and other chronic inflammatory diseases. Arthritis Res 4(4):241-246, 2002.

342. Walker LS, Abbas AK: The enemy within: keeping self-reactive T cells at bay in the periphery. Nat Rev Immunol 2(1):11-19, 2002.

343. Healy JI, Goodnow CC: Positive versus negative signaling by lymphocyte antigen receptors. Annu Rev Immunol 16:645, 1998.

344. Chen C, Radic MZ, Erikson J, et al: Deletion and editing of B cells that express antibodies to DNA. J Immunol 152:1970, 1994.

345. Radic MZ, Erikson J, Litwin S, et al: B lymphocytes may escape tolerance by revising their antigen receptors. J Exp Med 177:1165, 1993.

346. Tiegs SL, Russell DM, Nemazee D: Receptor editing in self-reactive bone marrow B cells. J Exp Med 177:1009, 1993.

347. Kumar V, Sercarz E: Induction or protection from experimental autoimmune encephalomyelitis depends on the cytokine secretion profile of TCR peptide-specific regulatory CD4 T cells. J Immunol 161:6585, 1998.

348. Salmon JE: Abnormalities in immune complex clearance and in Fcγ-receptor function. In Wallace DJ, Hahn BH (eds): Dubois' Lupus Erythematosus, 5th ed. Baltimore, Williams & Wilkins, 1997, p 221.

349. Sakaguchi S, Sakaguchi N, Shimizu J, et al: Immunologic tolerance maintained by CD25+ CD4+ regulatory T cells: Their common role in controlling autoimmunity, tumor immunity, and transplantation tolerance. Immunol Rev 182:18-32, 2001.

350. Shevach EM: Regulatory T cells in autoimmmunity. Annu Rev Immunol 18:423-449, 2000.

351. Mason D: T-cell-mediated control of autoimmunity. Arthritis Res 3(3):133-135, 2001.

352. Liu Z, Tugulea S, Cortesini R, Suciu-Foca N: Specific suppression of T helper alloreactivity by allo-MHC class I-restricted CD8+CD28-T cells. Int Immunol 10(6):775-783, 1998.

353. Ciubotariu R, Liu Z, Colovai AI, et al: Persistent allopeptide reactivity and epitope spreading in chronic rejection of organ allografts. J Clin Invest 101(2):398-405, 1998.

354. Chang CC, Ciubotariu R, Manavalan JS, et al: Tolerization of dendritic cells by T(S) cells: The crucial role of inhibitory receptors ILT3 and ILT4. Nat Immunol 3(3):237-243, 2002.

355. Balashov KE, Khoury SJ, Hafler DA, Weiner HL: Inhibition of T cell responses by activated human CD8+ T cells is mediated by interferon-gamma and is defective in chronic progressive multiple sclerosis. J Clin Invest 95(6):2711-2719, 1995.

356. Filaci G, Bacilieri S, Fravega M, et al: Impairment of CD8+ T suppressor cell function in patients with active systemic lupus erythematosus. J Immunol 166(10):6452-6457, 2001.

357. Krakauer RS, Waldmann TA, Strober W: Loss of suppressor T cells in adult NZB/NZW mice. J Exp Med 144:663, 1976.

358. Sekigawa I, Okada T, Noguchi K, et al: Class-specific regulation of anti-DNA antibody synthesis and the age-associated changes in (NZB × NZW) F1 hybrid mice. J Immunol 138:2890, 1987.

359. Via CS, Sharrow SO, Shearer GM: Role of cytotoxic T lymphocytes in the prevention of lupus-like disease occurring in a murine model of graft-vs-host disease. J Immunol 139:1840, 1987.

360. Tsokos GC, Smith PL, Christian CB, et al: Interleukin-2 restores the depressed allogeneic cell-mediated lympholysis and natural killer cell activity in patients with systemic lupus erythematosus. Clin Immunol Immunopathol 34:379, 1985.

361. Stohl W: Impaired polyclonal T cell cytolytic activity: A possible risk factor for systemic lupus erythematosus. Arthritis Rheum 38:506, 1995.

362. Linker-Israeli M, Quismorio FP Jr, Horwitz DA:. CD8+ lymphocytes from patients with systemic lupus erythematosus sustain, rather than suppress, spontaneous polyclonal IgG production and synergize with CD4+ cells to support autoantibody synthesis. Arthritis Rheum 33:1216, 1990.

363. Karpouzas GA, Singh RR, Ebling FM, et al: Defects in CD8+ T cell function characterize lupus-prone (NZB × NZW) F1 mice. Arthritis Rheum 48:5198-5199, 2003.

364. Koide J, Takano M, Takeuchi T, et al: Direct demonstration of immunoregulatory T-cell defects in patients with systemic lupus erythematosus. Scand J Immunol 23:449, 1986.

365. Morimoto C, Reinherz EL, Schlossman SF, et al: Alterations in immunoregulatory T cell subsets in active systemic lupus erythematosus. J Clin Invest 66:1171, 1980.

366. Tsokos GC, Balow JE: Phenotypes of T lymphocytes in systemic lupus erythematosus: decreased cytotoxic/suppressor subpopulation is associated with deficient allogeneic cytotoxic responses rather than with concanavalin A-induced suppressor cells. Clin Immunol Immunopathol 26: 267, 1983.

367. Morimoto C, Distaso JA, Borel Y, et al: Communicative interactions between subpopulations of human T lymphocytes required for generation of suppressor effector function in a primary antibody response. J Immunol 128:1645, 1982.

368. Gatenby PA, Kotzin BL, Kansas GS, Engleman EG: Immunoglobulin secretion in the human autologous mixed leukocyte reaction: Definition of a suppressor-amplifier circuit using monoclonal antibodies. J Exp Med 156:55, 1982.

369. Tanaka S, Matsuyama T, Steinberg AD, et al: Antilymphocyte antibodies against CD4+2H4+ cell populations in patients with systemic lupus erythematosus. Arthritis Rheum 32:398, 1989.

370. Raziuddin S, Nur MA, Alwabel AA: Selective loss of the CD4+ inducers of suppressor T cell subsets (2H4+) in active systemic lupus erythematosus. J Rheumatol 16:1315, 1989.

371. Theofilopoulos A, Dixon FJ: Etiopathogenesis of murine SLE. Immunol Rev 55:179, 1981.

372. Lin LC, Chen YC, Chou CC, et al: Dysregulation of T helper cell cytokines in autoimmune prone NZB × NZW F1 mice. Scand J Immunol 42:466, 1995.

373. Sato MN, Minoprio P, Avrameas S, Ternynck T: Defects in the regulation of anti-DNA antibody production in aged lupus-prone (NZB × NZW) F1 mice: Analysis of T-cell lymphokine synthesis. Immunology 85:26, 1995.

374. Alcocer-Varela J, Alarcon-Segovia D: Decreased production of and response to interleukin-2 by cultured lymphocytes from patients with systemic lupus erythematosus. J Clin Invest 69:1388, 1982.

375. Linker-Israeli M, Bakke AC, Kitridou RC, et al: Defective production of interleukin 1 and interleukin 2 in patients with systemic lupus erythematosus (SLE). J Immunol 130:2651, 1983.

376. Murakawa Y, Takada S, Ueda Y, et al: Characterization of T lymphocyte subpopulations responsible for deficient interleukin 2 activity in patients with systemic lupus erythematosus. J Immunol 134:187, 1985.

377. De Faucal P, Godard A, Peyrat MA, et al: Impaired IL2 production by lymphocytes of patients with systemic lupus erythematosus. Ann Immunol (Paris) 135D:161, 1984.

378. Takada S, Ueda Y, Suzuki N, et al: Abnormalities in autologous mixed lymphocyte reaction-activated immunologic processes in systemic lupus erythematosus and their possible correction by interleukin 2. Eur J Immunol 15:262, 1985.

379. Hagiwara E, Gourley MF, Lee S, Klinman DK: Disease severity in patients with systemic lupus erythematosus correlates with an increased ratio of interleukin-10: interferon-gamma-secreting cells in the peripheral blood. Arthritis Rheum 39:379, 1996.

380. Gray JD, Hirokawa M, Horwitz DA: The role of transforming growth factor beta in the generation of suppression: an interaction between CD8+ T and NK cells. J Exp Med 180:1937, 1994.

381. Singh RR, Ebling FM, Albuquerque DA, et al: Induction of autoantibody production is limited in nonautoimmune mice. J Immunol 169(1):587-594, 2002.

382. Frankel AH, Sayegh MH, Rothstein DM, et al: Requirements for the induction of allospecific CD8+ suppressor T cells in the rat primary mixed lymphocyte response. CD4+, CD45R+ T cells, or supernatant factor. Transplantation 48:639, 1989.

383. Hall BM, Pearce NW, Gurley KE, Dorsch SE: Specific unresponsiveness in rats with prolonged cardiac allograft survival after treatment with cyclosporine. III. Further characterization of the CD4+ suppressor cell and its mechanisms of action. J Exp Med 171:141, 1990.

384. Ridge JP, Di Rosa F, Matzinger P: A conditioned dendritic cell can be a temporal bridge between a CD4+ T-helper and a T-killer cell. Nature 393:474, 1998.

385. Bennett SR, Carbone FR, Karamalis F, et al: Help for cytotoxic-T-cell responses is mediated by CD40 signalling. Nature 393:478, 1998.

386. Schoenberger SP, Toes RE, van der Voort EI, et al: T-cell help for cytotoxic T lymphocytes is mediated by CD40-CD40L interactions. Nature 393:480, 1998.

387. Mintern JD, Davey GM, Belz GT, et al: Cutting edge: precursor frequency affects the helper dependence of cytotoxic T cells. J Immunol 168:977, 2002.

388. Feinberg MB, Silvestri G: T (S) cells and immune tolerance induction: a regulatory renaissance? Nat Immunol 3:215, 2002.

389. Lin CY, Graca L, Cobbold SP, Waldmann H: Dominant transplantation tolerance impairs CD8+ T cell function but not expansion. Nat Immunol 3:1208, 2002.

390. Fan GC, Singh RR: Vaccination with minigenes encoding V (H)-derived major histocompatibility complex class I-binding epitopes activates cytotoxic T cells that ablate autoantibody-producing B cells and inhibit lupus. J Exp Med 196:731, 2002.

391. Shevach EM: Certified professionals: CD4(+)CD25(+) suppressor T cells. J Exp Med 193(11):F41-46, 2001.

392. Sakaguchi S, Takahashi T, Nishizuka Y: Study on cellular events in post-thymectomy autoimmune oophoritis in mice. II. Requirement of Lyt-1 cells in normal female mice for the prevention of oophoritis. J Exp Med 156(6):1577-1586, 1982.

393. Suri-Payer E, Amar AZ, McHugh R, et al: Post-thymectomy autoimmune gastritis: fine specificity and pathogenicity of anti-H/K ATPase-reactive T cells. Eur J Immunol 29(2):669-677, 1999.

394. Alard P, Thompson C, Agersborg SS, et al: Endogenous oocyte antigens are required for rapid induction and progression of autoimmune ovarian disease following day-3 thymectomy. J Immunol 166(7):4363-4369, 2001.

395. Itoh M, Takahashi T, Sakaguchi N, et al: Thymus and autoimmunity: production of CD25+CD4+ naturally anergic and suppressive T cells as a key function of the thymus in maintaining immunologic self-tolerance. J Immunol 162(9):5317-5326, 1999.

396. Bagavant H, Thompson C, Ohno K, et al: Differential effect of neonatal thymectomy on systemic; and organ-specific autoimmune disease. Int Immunol 14(12):1397-1406, 2002.

397. Shoenfeld Y, Isenberg DA: DNA antibody idiotypes: A review of their genetic, clinical and immunopathological features. Semin Arthritis Rheum 16:215, 1987.

398. Hahn BH, Ebling FM: Idiotypes and idiotype networks. In Wallace DJ, Hahn BH (eds): Dubois' Lupus Erythematosus, 5th ed. Baltimore, Williams & Wilkins, 1997, p 291.

399. Kalunian KC, Panosian-Sahakian N, Ebling FM, et al: Idiotypic characteristics of immunoglobulins associated with human SLE: Studies of antibodies deposited in glomeruli. Arthritis Rheum 32:513, 1989.

75

Clinical Manifestations of Systemic Lupus Erythematosus

STEVEN M. EDWORTHY

This chapter reviews the clinical manifestations of lupus. It begins by examining the question: What is systemic lupus erythematosus (SLE)?[1] A broad conceptual framework is illustrated in Figure 75–1 to encompass the many considerations clinicians deal with in caring for lupus patients. A historical perspective is provided, along with reflections on the diversity of lupus manifestations. The critical differences between diagnosis and classification are revisited so that clinicians will reconsider how criteria are to be applied.[2] The incidence and prevalence of the disease are reviewed, and then data on disease activity, outcomes, and prognostic factors are provided. The role of the Internet is discussed in the context of the expanding knowledge base about lupus. Finally, a few complex problems facing clinicians are highlighted before concluding remarks are presented on the role the clinician can play in improving the current understanding of SLE.

Chapter 74 reviews the biologic data that have been gathered on the etiopathogenesis of SLE, particularly with respect to the mouse models used as surrogates for the human experience. Genetic, as well as humoral and cell-mediated, immune factors are discussed in detail. Although the dominant pathophysiologic process appears to be driven by antinuclear autoantibodies, this does not explain the entire range of clinical findings of SLE. Imbalance of cytokines, excess activity of helper T cells, effects of hormonal changes, abnormalities of C1q receptors, abnormal neurovascular response to temperature, excess release of adhesion molecules, and antibodies against phospholipid moieties of the cell membrane are all thought to have a potential ancillary pathologic role. The discovery that lupus-like syndromes in murine models (*1pr* mice and transgenic *bcl2* mice) are associated with dysregulation of molecules that control lymphocyte survival (apoptosis), along with observations on human keratinocytes, suggests that this more generalized defect in tolerance underlies the multiple disease manifestations of lupus.[3-5]

■ What Is Systemic Lupus Erythematosus?

SLE lacks a single, unifying pathognomonic marker. It is a disease with a complex set of immunologic abnormalities that appear to involve multiple mechanisms of dysregulation and that may be linked to more than 20 different genetic determinants. Early in the disease course, the signs may be subtle or may be suggestive of

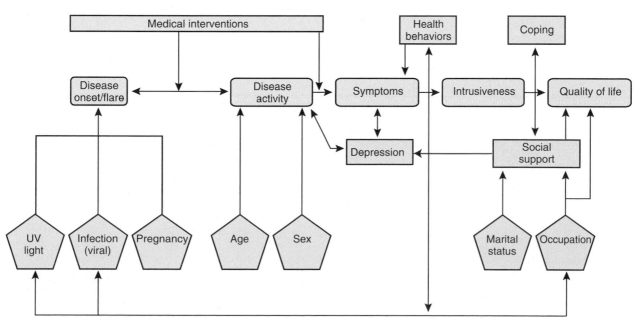

FIGURE 75–1 · Conceptual Framework of Systemic Lupus Erythematosus.

other entities, such as rheumatoid arthritis (RA), palindromic rheumatism, antiphospholipid syndrome, polymorphous light eruptions, Still's disease, rheumatic fever, sarcoidosis, Lyme disease, multiple sclerosis (MS), thrombotic thrombocytopenic purpura, cryoglobulinemia, Weber-Christian disease, viral illnesses, vasculitis, or even fibromyalgia.

Nevertheless, there are definitions of SLE that have been embedded in the foundations of our scientific literature. For example, the National Library of Medicine scope for the medical subject heading (MeSH) "Lupus Erythematosus, Systemic," under which most medical literature on the subject is indexed, reads as follows:

> Scope: A chronic, relapsing, inflammatory, and often febrile multisystemic disorder of connective tissue, characterized principally by involvement of the skin, joints, kidneys, and serosal membranes. It is of unknown etiology, but is thought to represent a failure of the regulatory mechanisms of the autoimmune system. The disease is marked by a wide range of system dysfunctions, an elevated erythrocyte sedimentation rate, and the formation of LE cells in the blood or bone marrow.
>
> Used For:
> Libman-Sacks disease
> Lupus erythematosus disseminatus
> NOTE: if not specified as "systemic" it is still probably correct to index here, not also discoid; LUPUS NEPHRITIS is also available; See Related: ANTIPHOSPHOLIPID SYNDROME LUPUS COAGULATION INHIBITOR

This indexing term (i.e., the MeSH term) used to guide the referencing of the world literature, reflects its historical roots when it refers to the LE cell but not autoantibodies. It highlights the multisystemic nature of the condition and uses the term *connective tissue* to indicate where the effect is found. The scope statement does not shed light on how discoid lupus should be considered, except that it is "still probably correct to index" it under SLE, along with Libman-Sacks disease and lupus erythematosus disseminatus. The index points out that, when searching the literature, researchers should also look at the terms *antiphospholipid syndrome* and *lupus coagulation inhibitor*.[6]

Another perspective on how SLE is defined can be gained by examining the coding system of the *International Statistical Classification of Diseases and Related Health Problems* (ICD), which has gone through 10 iterations since its inception in the 1890s. These codes are used by many payors in North America, Australia, and Europe as a method of keeping track of the resource utilization and costs of this resource; thus, these codes represent a relevant factor in the proper deployment of health care delivery. The World Health Organization (WHO), which maintains the nomenclature of ICD, places SLE among the "710" group of diseases of the connective tissues in ICD-9 (edition 9), the most commonly used ICD in North America. These codes reflect the consideration that SLE has similarities to scleroderma, dermatomyositis, and eosinophilic fasciitis. ICD-10, the latest version, uses a series of letters and numbers to designate diseases and, as such, has proposed M32.1 for SLE.

■ Historical Perspective

The history of lupus has been divided into the classic period of cutaneous description, the neoclassic period that recognized the systemic nature of the disease, and the modern period heralded by the finding of the LE cell.[7] We are now in the "postmodern" lupus period, using techniques of molecular and cellular biology to find underlying themes of immunologic intolerance. Currently, more than 80 percent of the American public has become aware of SLE as an immunologic disease.[8]

Sir William Osler coined the term *systemic lupus erythematosus*, which included the observations of cutaneous manifestations of lupus first made by Cazenave in 1851, and subsequently by Kaposi in 1872, as well as his own recognition of cardiac, pulmonary, and renal problems in some patients. The notion that lupus is a collagen disease was put forward by Klemperer in 1942; however, he emphasized in his original paper that other elements of connective tissue were involved and that collagen was simply the unusual component identified in his histologic findings.[9] Perhaps Klinge had expressed a more correct view in the German literature of the early 1930s when he called lupus a connective tissue disease.[9] Clinically, we often see changes in the connective tissue elements of the body accumulated around the basement membrane of the skin, the glomerulus, and the lung parenchyma. These changes are associated with immunologic markers such as complement or antibodies, with the end result being scar formation involving connective tissue cells and their products. However, other effects not directly related to autoantibody deposition are also seen. These include the altered sensorium in central nervous system (CNS) lupus; the vasospastic phenomenon of Raynaud's phenomenon; thromboembolic problems of the antiphospholipid syndrome; peripheral neuropathies associated with vasculitis; and systemic symptoms of fever, malaise, and profound fatigue.

From 1956 to 1965, the observed prevalence of SLE rose from 41.4 to 134.4 per million in New York City. It was noted that this was "coincident in time with the development of serological techniques for detecting antinuclear and DNA antibodies."[10] In 1957, Holman and Kunkel were among the first to describe autoantibodies directed against nuclear particles by use of an immunofluorescent technique.[11] Their observations were made in 32 patients who had LE cells. Holman and Kunkel linked antibodies to DNA near the time when Watson and Crick were discovering the double helix of DNA. Lupus and double-stranded (ds)-DNA have been inextricably linked since then.[12-15]

Thomas Kuhn wrote that science can be stymied in its progress by an overwhelming belief system that prevents creative breakthroughs from occurring, such as happened in the pre-Copernican era of astronomy. In 1994, Holman,[16] reflecting on this observation, pointed out that medical science had not made quantum leaps in its understanding of rheumatic disease in general, and lupus in particular, in the preceding 40 years. He thought this was due to 1) mistaken notions about the causation of chronic rheumatic disease, 2) the dominance of the acute disease model, and 3) the strategy of reductionism in scientific investigation. He implied that laboratory models that reduce lupus to a few immunologic factors would not provide a far-reaching understanding of the disease. To understand lupus, we need to approach it with an appreciation of the diversity of clinical presentation, as well as an awareness of its ability to vary over time within a given patient. Perhaps breakthroughs such as the link with abnormal apoptosis[17-19] will provide the quantum leap necessary to explain the diversity seen in lupus.[5] Since 1957, there have been more than 30 nuclear antigens against which lupus patients' sera have been found to react.[20,21]

In 1976, Marion Ropes[9] used an "activity index" to describe patients seen for an extended time, from before to after the corticosteroid period. This represented a critical transition in the description of lupus manifestations, preparing the way for our current understanding of disease management. Subsequently, several activity measures have been validated and found to be reliable.[22-24] Proceedings from the Outcome Measures in Rheumatoid Arthritis Clinical Trials (OMERACT) convention recommended including activity measures in both clinical trials and longitudinal cohort studies.[25]

What we now know is that SLE is not just a collagen-vascular disease, nor is it confined to the connective tissues. It is a disease of fluctuating immune dysfunction, having strong association with antinuclear antibodies, and it has enormous potential for variation both within a single patient over time and across populations of patients. In the course of 100 years, we have gone from assessment of patients without any reliance on laboratory markers to a sophisticated repertoire of autoantibody tests to help make the diagnosis. Measuring disease activity, along with the prediction of the activity, underpins the advances that will be made with the introduction of postmodern therapeutic agents.

▌ Epidemiology and Management

Except for the obvious association with female gender and hormonal status (or lack of predilection for men), finding the etiopathogenesis of lupus through traditional epidemiologic studies is hampered by the difficulty of tracing the initial symptoms back to an originating event that triggers the immune system in a susceptible individual. Also, the potential of a lagged response to environmental factors, such as a virus or ultraviolet light exposure, makes analysis of events more complex than tracing an outbreak of *Salmonella* infection, for example. As well, it may take some time for sufficient symptoms and signs to manifest themselves for identification of a case using the currently accepted classification scheme. Therefore, it is difficult to arrive at accurate estimates of the incidence of this disease. Nevertheless, attempts have been made with use of case-finding methods in defined populations.

Although it is commonly understood that lupus has a higher incidence in young women,[26] this may not be true. A study from Sweden, using well-defined populations (1981-1986) and reliable case-finding methodology, identified a female incidence of 5.4 cases per 100,000 populaion per year and a male incidence of 1 per 100,000 per year. The highest incidence was found in the age-group 55 to 74 years at approximately 7.5 per 100,000 per year; the lowest adult incidence, in the 15- to 24-year-old age-group, was 1.2 per 100,000 per year.[27]

A population study using capture-recapture methodology to find cases in Allegheny County, Pennsylvania, identified 191 definite cases and 78 probable cases between January 1, 1985, and December 31, 1990. This yielded a crude incidence for definite SLE of 3.5 per 100,000 per year for white women and 9.2 per 100,000 per year for black women. The overall rate for both genders and ethnicities was 2.4 per 100,000 per year (95-percent confidence interval [CI] 2.1 to 2.8). A rate of 1.0 per 100,000 per year (95-percent CI 0.8 to 1.3) was found for probable cases of SLE.[28]

Prevalence rates rely on identifying all cases, according to an accepted definition, within a sample that is representative of the entire population. Populations defined by a particular health maintenance organization or enrolled members of an insurance plan may have subtle selection bias frelated to employee status, cost of enrollment, or perception of wellness by the individual. Samples drawn from specific geographic areas may have distinct age distributions because of varying life expectancies, infant birth and mortality rates, or age-related immigration and emigration patterns. In addition, physicians in certain regions may not identify or record cases when they occur.[29] Ethnic origin may also vary considerably and will affect the disease prevalence estimates. Estimates of prevalence range from 40 per 100,000 women (Mayo Clinic) to 565 per 100,000 women.[8,30] Ascertainment techniques and the nature of the population from which the lupus patients are identified account for a large amount of the variation. Nevertheless, within the United States, during periods of relatively stable population dynamics in San Francisco in the late 1960s, prevalence of lupus for white women was found to be 90.5 per 100,000 (Kaiser Permanente, 1965 to 1973).[31] The prevalence among black women in the San Francisco study was estimated at 280 per 100,000 individuals. A more recent estimate from the United States used random-digit dialing to 16,607 households and from this derived a sample of 4034 women older than 18 years. Cases that were reported and validated through medical chart review provide a prevalence estimate of 124 per 100,000 adult women (95-percent CI 40 to 289).[32] A third method of estimating prevalence was undertaken by the Lupus Foundation of America. Self report from a mailed survey suggested that there might be as many as 565 lupus patients per 100,000 population. However, this study did not validate the diagnostic formulation, and it was considered a considerable overestimation of the actual rate.[8]

SLE occurs 10 times more commonly in women than in men. Therefore, in interpreting prevalence figures, a correction for gender should be undertaken. For example, because approximately 50 percent of the world's population of 6 billion people is female and the overall prevalence of SLE in women is approximately 100 per 100,000 (considering the world racial distribution and varying life expectancy), there are approximately 3 million women and 300,000 men affected worldwide. Of course, more accurate estimates would take into account the age distribution and life expectancy in different continents as well as the prevalence rates for different ethnicities. North America, in particular, has a population bulge of individuals in the 50- to 60-year-old age-group, whereas India has a much younger population. The number of "definite" lupus patients in a modern urban region of 5 million people would be 2500 to 3000, assuming 75 percent of individuals are older than 18 years, a survival rate after diagnosis of 80 percent at 10 years, and an average age at onset of 30 years. There would likely be another 1000 to 1500 "possible" lupus patients who would require investigation and observation.

Classification and Diagnosis

CLASSIFICATION CRITERIA

In 1971, criteria were developed to deal with a growing concern that epidemiologic studies and clinical trials involving lupus patients would be difficult to compare with one another if there was no documented consensus on what constituted the findings of systemic lupus.[33,34] The revised American College of Rheumatology (ACR) classification criteria were published 11 years later,[35] before the demonstration of the antiphospholipid syndrome[36] and also before the plethora of studies on new autoantigens was reported. One of the driving forces of the revised criteria was to incorporate the antinuclear antibody (ANA) tests that had become widely available and that had essentially replaced the LE cell preparation for detecting the characteristic laboratory finding of lupus. Another factor was to rely less heavily on invasive diagnostic procedures, such as the kidney biopsy. A third consideration was to remove elements such as Raynaud's phenomenon and alopecia because the low specificity of these criteria, combined with the low prevalence of SLE in the population, could cause a high false-positive rate of classification.[2,37]

More recently, changes have been recommended to two of the criteria. In 1997, the antiphospholipid component of item 10, immunologic factors, was revisited. The work of Drs. Graham Hughes and Donato Alarcon-Segovia, and other investigators who explained the relevance of antiphospholipid antibodies, was cited. At the recommendation of Dr. Eng Tan, who had been chairman of the 1971 criteria committee, Dr. Marc Hochberg called for the deletion of the LE cell preparation criteria and established the accepted methods for identifying antiphospholipid antibodies based on anticardiolipin antibodies, lupus anticoagulant testing, or a false-positive serologic test for syphilis. In 1999, Dr. Matt Liang and the committee on neuropsychiatric lupus suggested that the case definitions for 19 different neuropsychiatric (NP) conditions be used instead of the existing neurologic criteria of seizure disorder

and psychosis. This ratification has not been formally accepted but is worth considering, given the detailed operational definitions and investigative procedures the committee provided. The caveat that has been raised is that some of the findings—such as headache, cognitive dysfunction, and mood disorders—are common in the general public and lack specificity, whereas some of the other criteria—such as the movement disorder of chorea and cranial nerve involvement—are so rare that they contribute very little to sensitivity. Nevertheless, this demonstrates that the criteria are an evolving set and that the SLE community of investigators continues to revisit the concept of the systemic nature of lupus from a phenomenonologic perspective.

The operational approach to using the criteria will be familiar to rheumatologists, but perhaps not to students and residents. The fundamental rule is that a patient must have four or more of the 11 criteria to qualify for the classification category of SLE (see Classification of Systemic Lupus Erythematosus). Learning and remembering 11 criteria may seem a daunting task for the individual who is also learning the anatomy and physiology of all the joints, muscles, and tendons in the body. Instead of considering 11 separate criteria, it may be useful to think through six logical clinical groupings: joints, skin, serosal surfaces, kidneys, hematologic elements, neuropsychiatric elements, and then finally the system that links these all together: immunologic abnormalities. Granted, each of these six clinical areas has further subgroupings that need to be recalled; however, if one pictures an "archtypical" lupus patient who has arthritis, photosensitive rash, pleurisy, proteinuria, thrombocytopenia, and seizures when considering the diagnosis, the criteria will naturally follow.

DIAGNOSTIC CERTAINTY

Once you have become familiar with the classification criteria and can use them fluently on the wards, it will be worthwhile to think more deeply about the difference between classification and diagnosis. The process of deriving criteria from diagnosed cases is inherently circular, because criteria are based on diagnosed cases of SLE.[1] Hence, it is critical to improve the understanding of diagnosis. Rarely can the diagnosis of SLE be made with absolute certainty at the first onset of symptoms. To accommodate this it has been common for rheumatologists to refer to cases as probable, definite, or classic.[38] An operational definition of this, derived from the 1982 criteria,[39,40] is included here to provide a clinical framework of certainty[41] (Fig. 75–2).

Antibodies to ds-DNA, particularly when found with renal abnormalities, are closely associated with systemic lupus. When these are found in the presence of a positive ANA test result, the certainty of diagnosis approaches 90 percent, and further scrutiny of the patient's course will increase certainty to 100 percent if the disease is present. Malar rash is also a strong indicator that the underlying disease process is that of systemic lupus. However, clinicians must be careful that the appropriate inflammatory components are present and that the changes of the malar region are not due to

CLASSIFICATION OF SYSTEMIC LUPUS ERYTHEMATOSUS

Criterion	Definition
1) Malar rash	Fixed erythema, flat or raised, over the malar eminences, tending to spare the nasolabial folds
2) Discoid rash	Erythematous raised patches with adherent keratotic scaling and follicular plugging; atrophic scarring may occur in older lesions
3) Photosensitivity	Skin rash as a result of unusual reaction to sunlight, by patient history or physician observation
4) Oral Ulcers	Oral or nasopharyngeal ulceration, usually painless, observed by a physician
5) Arthritis	Nonerosive arthritis involving two or more peripheral joints, characterized by tenderness, swelling, or effusion
6) Serositis	a) Pleuritis: convincing history of pleuritic pain or rub heard by a physician or evidence of pleural effusion OR b) Pericarditis: documented by ECG, rub, or evidence of pericardial effusion
7) Renal disorder	a) Persistent proteinuria greater than 0.5 g per day or greater than 3+ if quantitation not performed OR b) Cellular casts, which may be red cell, hemoglobin, granular, tubular, or mixed
8) Neurologic disorder	a) Seizures: in the absence of offending drugs or known metabolic derangements (e.g., uremia, ketoacidosis, or electrolyte imbalance) OR b) Psychosis: in the absence of offending drugs or known metabolic derangements (e.g., uremia, ketoacidosis, or electrolyte imbalance)
9) Hematologic disorder	a) Hemolytic anemia, with reticulocytosis OR b) Leukopenia: less than 4000/mm^3 total on two or more occasions OR c) Lymphopenia: less than 1500/mm^3 on two or more occasions d) Thrombocytopenia: less than 100,000/mm^3 in the absence of offending drugs
10) Immunologic disorder	a) Anti-DNA: antibody to native DNA in abnormal titer OR b) Anti-Sm: presence of antibody to Sm nuclear antigen OR c) Positive finding of antiphospholipid antibodies based on 1) an abnormal serum level of IgG or IgM anti-cardiolipin antibodies, 2) a positive test result for lupus anticoagulant using a standard method, or 3) a false-positive serologic test for syphilis known to be positive for at least 6 months and confirmed by *Treponema pallidum* immobilization or fluorescent treponemal antibody absorption test
11) Antinuclear antibody	An abnormal titer of antinuclear antibody (ANA) by immunofluorescence or an equivalent assay at any point in time and in the absence of drugs known to be associated with "drug-induced lupus" syndrome

a polymorphous light eruption, acne rosacea, a drug reaction, or simply weathered skin. The presence of convincing serositis in the absence of an infectious etiology and in the presence of a highly positive ANA response should make SLE probable. Discoid rash, which is so striking when it is present, can evolve into a systemic process. However, this may take many years to occur and will be picked up only by looking for hematologic, renal, central nervous system (CNS), or musculoskeletal involvement on an annual basis. A doctor's clinical acumen is tested when patients have less obvious or less specific features of lupus, such as myalgias, low-grade fevers, fatigue, Raynaud's phenomenon, and alopecia.[42] In these instances, the type of ANA present, the levels of complement (C3 and C4), and the profile of white blood cells (WBCs), platelets, and hemoglobin, along with historic features of photosensitivity, recurrent miscarriages, or fluctuating mental state, might cause consideration of SLE at the possible (50 percent) level. However, if only a positive ANA response

and myalgia consistent with fibromyalgia are present, it is likely a disservice to the patient and the health care system to label the patient with lupus (Table 75–1).

◾ Autoantibodies

Currently, the sine qua non of established lupus is the ANA test; however, the results of current laboratory testing for ANAs may vary considerably.[43] With the widespread availability of ANA tests and the general knowledge that nonspecific symptoms may be associated with connective tissue diseases, it has become common practice for general practitioners to order ANA tests in a broad range of patients. This testing is ordered to rule out the diagnosis when the results are negative, rather than as a confirmatory test.[44] A positive ANA response points toward a connective tissue disease, among which SLE is the most common, but it may also represent a nonspecific finding.

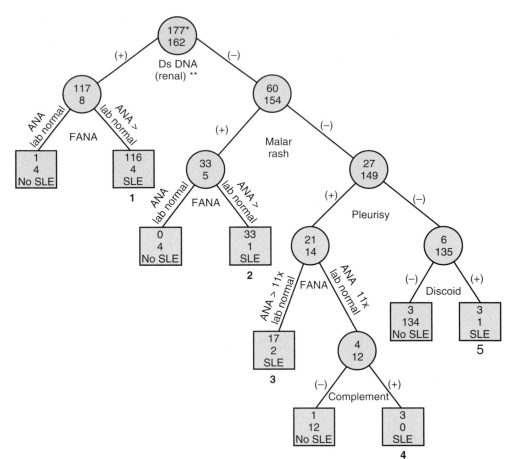

FIGURE 75–2 · Classification Tree for Systemic Lupus Erythematosus (SLE). *Upper number = SLE; lower number = control. **Surrogate. Sensitivity, 97 percent; specificity, 95 percent.

TABLE 75–1 · DIAGNOSTIC CERTAINTY

	Certainty*	Antinuclear Antibodies†	Immunology Laboratory‡	Clinical Signs§
Definite	90%	≥1:80	ds-DNA or Sm	Proteinuria
	80%	≥1:160		Malar rash
	80%	≥1:160	Low complement	Serositis‖
Probable	70%	≥1:160	Low complement	Discoid rash
Possible	60%	≥1:160	RNP, SS-A, SS-B, antiphospholipid antibody	Lymphocytopenia (<1000), thrombocytopenia, or Coombs-positive anemia
	50%¶	≥1:160	No abnormalities	Nonspecific skin findings; urticaria, unwitnessed photosensitivity, or malar rash**
Unlikely	25%	≥1:160	No abnormalities	Severe fatigue, arthralgias, and myalgias††

*Certainty scale is anchored at five points: 0 = not possible, 25 = conceivable but unlikely, 50 = possible, 75 = probable, 100 = absolutely.

†Antinuclear antibody testing should not include cytoplasmic staining except when mitochondria, Golgi, or centriole antibodies are positively identified. Age older than 50 years, medications, or malignant neoplasms may elevate antinuclear antibodies nonspecifically.

‡Immunology laboratory items include extractable nuclear antigens such as Sm, ds-DNA, SS-A, SS-B, and RNP as well as low complement levels by reliable methods.

§Signs are interpreted findings by examination or laboratory analysis that are witnessed by a certified specialist.

‖Serositis for diagnostic purposes requires a convincing history with evidence on examination or historical evidence on radiography (chest), electrocardiography and echocardiography (cardiac), or examination (mesenteric).

¶Borderline lupus, when the diagnosis is uncertain, has been described as latent, incipient, incomplete[42] or probable.[28]

**Symptoms of rashes that are not witnessed by a certified specialist or accompanied by reliable photographs should be considered unwitnessed.

††Fibromyalgia may reduce certainty of painful symptoms such as arthralgias, particularly when certainty is in the 50 percent range.

Although highly specific, depending on the test methods employed, anti–ds-DNA is not necessarily highly sensitive for lupus, nor is it always predictive of disease activity.[45-49] It has been strongly associated with immune complex disease, particularly of the kidney. Within an individual patient, it may be possible to find patterns of antibody expression that are predictive; however, there is sufficient biologic variability within the antibody types that this cannot be used to predict outcomes in populations. In addition to ds-DNA, a number of specific epitopes within the nucleus have been shown to give rise to positive test results in lupus patients.[21] These include small nuclear ribonucleoproteins (Sm and RNP), SS-A/Ro, SS-B/La, single-stranded (ss)-DNA, the nuclear matrix, the nucleolar organizing region, the chromosomal coat protein, and histones.[12,50,51] Other epitopes that are targeted by antibodies in the sera of SLE patients are the phospholipid moieties on platelets and other tissue,[52-55] lymphocyte markers, and red blood cell (RBC) antigens. Although thought to be more specific for scleroderma, both the centromere and topoisomerase antibodies can be found in lupus patients. In addition, two new antigenic determinants, ASE-1 and HsEG5, which are associated with the nucleolar organizing region, have been found more commonly in SLE patients.[44] Of considerable interest has been the finding that many of these epitopes from the nucleus are expressed within blebs on the surface of apoptotic cells.[54] This has led to the consideration that the finding of ANAs may be an epiphenomenon of cell death. Although of some pathologic significance in certain instances, they are also markers of an immune system that has become disrupted (Table 75–2).

▊ Clinical Findings

SKIN

The skin provides one of the best windows through which to view the activity of lupus, both from the patient's perspective in recalling specific features and from the clinician's in establishing the diagnosis or assessing disease activity. Examination of the skin should include inspection for malar rash, discoid rash, Raynaud's phenomenon, acral cyanosis, periungual erythema, livedo reticularis, and maculopapular rashes of the trunk or extremity. Of these, the most strongly associated with SLE is malar rash[39,56,57] (Fig. 75–3). The annular lesions of subacute cutaneous lupus are associated with less-severe disease.[58] Alopecia, particularly when it is associated with inflammatory changes in the scalp, is a sign of lupus. Hair thinning often occurs when patients have suffered a flare of lupus and may also be associated with immunosuppressant drugs. The relative contribution to hair thinning of the flare or its treatment with steroids, azathioprine, or cyclophosphamide is difficult to differentiate. Hairs at the anterior margin of the scalp may have a stiff, spike appearance (lupus hairs) and allow the clinician to evaluate the patient's claims of hair problems. Clinicians should always consider photosensitivity[59,60] and the effect that ultraviolet light can have on the epidermal and dermal elements, which may include increased apoptosis,[19] increased release of adhesion molecules, and possibly greater reactivity of lymphocytes in the region.[19,61] Ultraviolet light in the 300- to 320-nm range (UVB) induces the greatest erythemal response in human skin and has increasing effect as the ozone layer thins or the light intensity increases with seasonal changes. The degree of melanin production associated with race may have an ameliorating effect on ultraviolet light absorption. Of interest is the role that diet and drugs might play in increasing photosensitivity response. Such foods as celery and parsley can act as natural psoralens that increase the likelihood of inciting a photosensitive reaction.[62]

Features such as sclerodactyly and telangiectasia may occasionally be found in individuals with lupus and may signify an evolution to different disease types, such as scleroderma.[63] This can create a diagnostic and management dilemma because it may signify that the process of fibrosis and collagen abnormalities associated with scleroderma will occur in organs other than the skin. Previous formulations of a mixed connective tissue disease[64,65] have been challenged,[66,67] and the clinician must carefully observe the patient over time before applying diagnostic labels with great certainty in these settings.

Although not life-threatening, discoid lupus can have severe effects on the emotional well-being of the patient. When the condition persists in the face of adequate treatment, it is critical to review all medications and sources of provocation for the disease. Discoid disease

---

▊ **TABLE 75–2 · AUTOANTIBODY PREVALENCE IN DIFFERENT DIAGNOSTIC GROUPS**

Epitope Specificity	Comments
double-stranded (ds) DNA	Associated with more severe lupus; kidney disease association is diffuse proliferative glomerulonephritis; central nervous system, cardiac, and pulmonary also associated
Smith (sm)	Associated with membranous nephropathy
RNP	Generally associated with Raynaud's phenomenon and may indicate pulmonary or muscle involvement
SS-A	Cutaneous manifestations, sicca complex, and neonatal lupus syndrome to be watched for (52-kD more ominous)
SS-B	When present, increases the concerns about neonatal lupus
Phospholipid	Increasing pathophysiologic significance
Centromere	Can occur in SLE patients without signs of CREST syndrome other than Raynaud's
SCL-70 (topoisomerase)	May indicate a changing disease presentation toward scleroderma

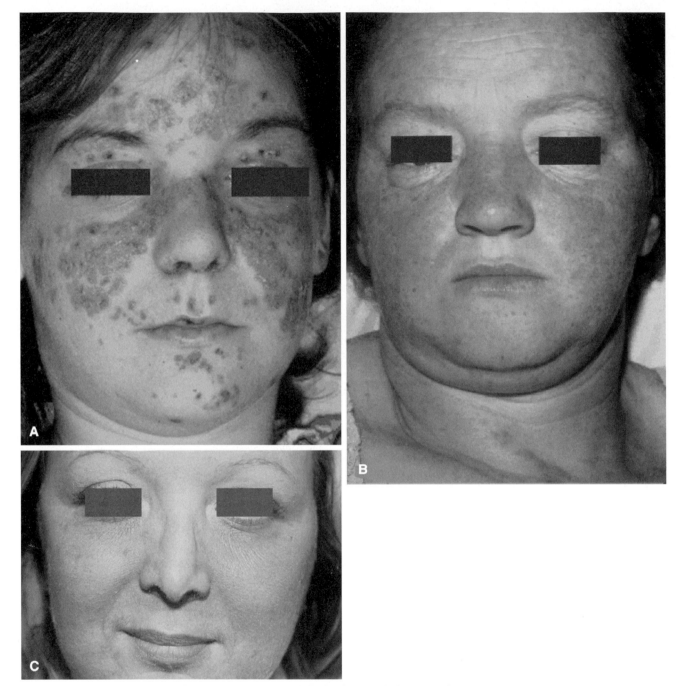

FIGURE 75–3 · *A–C,* Rash of systemic lupus erythematosus.

can have the worst impact on skin, much more so than subacute cutaneous lesions, malar rashes, or telangiectatic changes.

In severe, life-threatening flares of lupus, there may be evidence of Janeway lesions and Osler's nodes in the hands or feet. These may be caused by immune complex deposition and must be distinguished from septic emboli from a source such as the mitral or aortic valve. Blood cultures, echocardiograms, and careful observation of the patient are required,[68] although distinguishing Libman-Sacks endocardial lesions from bacterial endocarditis remains a problem.[69,70] There is increasing evidence that SLE patients with antiphospholipid antibodies are at increased risk of having valvular problems along with associated thromboembolic manifestations of the disease.[71-73]

MUSCULOSKELETAL INVOLVEMENT

Whereas skin manifestations provide a window through which to view lupus activity, the musculoskeletal examination can reveal the impact of the disease on a patient's activities of daily living. Arthritis is the most common sign patients exhibit over time, although there may be an age-dependent distribution of the symptom,[74] which affects the prevalence of the finding at disease onset as well as over the course of the disease. Arthritis that progresses to erosions and deformity is rare.[65,75] The nonerosive deforming arthropathy found in SLE, which carries the eponym Jaccoud's arthropathy, involves the same distribution as RA, including the metacarpophalangeal joints, wrists, and metatarsophalangeal joints. More common is the finding of arthralgia in these joints that migrates during a 24- to 48-hour period across several joint regions, including both the large and small joints of the appendicular skeleton. On occasion, warmth can be felt in these joints, but typically there is little evidence of inflammation aside from some mild soft tissue swelling around the joints. This degree of inflammation is typically not debilitating. In fact, it is usually the associated fatigue that patients complain of as the most debilitating symptom. Synovial fluid, when it is possible to aspirate it, is clear or straw colored, and on microscopic analysis has a type II cell quantity and distribution. In addition, it is common for patients to experience other musculoskeletal problems, such as tenosynovitis and bursitis. Nodules may form on tendons, particularly the flexor tendons of the hand. Fibromyalgia is a common problem for lupus patients, as with other rheumatic conditions, and it probably contributes to the overall fatigue of which patients complain.[76-78] Myositis is less common, although still possible as a feature of SLE.[79,80]

HEMATOLOGIC INVOLVEMENT

Hematologic processes are generally identified when laboratory investigations are prompted by other disease manifestations. Rarely is anemia, leukopenia, or thrombocytopenia the presenting feature of SLE without concomitant problems of the skin, joints, CNS, or cardiopulmonary systems. Once SLE has been identified and routine monitoring of patients is undertaken, it is common to find anemia, often with low mean corpuscular volume, of chronic inflammatory processes that inhibit iron transfer. Coombs-positive anemia, indicating an antibody-mediated process, is relatively uncommon when patients are observed longitudinally.[81,82]

Leukopenia is common, primarily owing to decreased numbers of lymphocytes. The disease or its treatment may cause lymphopenia. If the patient is not receiving steroids or immunosuppressive agents, this is an indication of ongoing immunologic activity. Lymphocyte populations are dynamic, and yet it is well known now that the balance of lymphocyte subpopulations is critical for stable immunologic status. The investigation of these subtypes is not fruitful in terms of identifying prognosticators or relevant markers for treatment schedules, in large part owing to the lack of reliable and available laboratory testing. Combinations of findings, including the lymphocyte levels and complement levels or blood pressure, for example, may be more important than the refined subtype assessments for predicting the progression of disease.[83]

Thrombocytopenia is often documented, and although it is of some concern with respect to bleeding propensity, if levels drop below 30,000, the association with antiphospholipid syndrome and the sequelae of thromboembolic disease is of greatest concern.[84-86] Fulminant thrombotic thrombocytopenic purpura can occur, although rarely.[84] There is occasionally need for splenectomy in situations of prolonged, unresponsive, severe thrombocytopenia.[87] However, splenectomized patients may have more problems with cutaneous vasculitis and infections in the postsplenectomy period without obvious benefits over those treated medically.[88] A strong association with the antiphospholipid syndrome has been documented, and it is speculated that the phospholipid moiety exposed by activation of the platelet membrane may explain the association.[89,90]

Circulating neutropenia is a rare condition that does not necessarily reflect severe lupus involvement. Patients may go for years without significant problems associated with this condition. Certainly, infection is not found commonly in these settings, and when infection occurs, it is not necessarily causally related to the neutropenia.[81]

KIDNEY

Renal involvement is always to be considered and can often be found, sometimes even in the absence of urinary or serum evidence.[91] The huge capillary bed, along with the negatively charged basement membrane and the intricate functional capacity of the cells embedded in the glomerular apparatus and the conducting tubules, creates an environment that is highly susceptible to inflammatory insults caused by autoantibodies. Even though renal biopsy is readily performed in tertiary care settings, examination of urine for proteinuria, cells, and casts and serum analysis for azotemia remain the most effective methods for monitoring patients at routine visits. With these simple measures, clinicians can handle most therapeutic decisions as well as provide prognostic information for the patient. Clinical findings such as hypertension, low complement levels, and lymphopenia may provide a clearer indication of the likelihood of progression to worse states of renal function.[83]

Transitions between better and worse states of renal involvement have been quantified with respect to the likelihood that they would progress or improve (Table 75–3). Individuals who exhibit normal kidney function are likely to retain normal function during the coming year if they have serum albumin levels greater than 40 mg/liter and normal systolic blood pressure at their annual checkup. However, if serum albumin is low and lymphocyte counts are less than 1000, the likelihood of progression is at least 50 percent. Approximately 25 percent of patients found to have proteinuria, but without evidence of azotemia, will progress to azotemia during the next 10 to 12 months, particularly those with a combination of excess RBCs on urinalysis and either low WBC count or low complement levels. Once kidney function has decreased sufficiently to produce a serum creatinine level of more than 400 mg/liter, it is most likely patients will require dialysis or kidney transplantation within a year. Some studies have suggested that patients who progress to renal failure will have far less immunologic disease activity subsequently. However, exceptions to this rule have been noted, and it is important to continue to monitor patients for other organ involvement that may be immunologically mediated.

Along with these parameters, the levels of serum albumin and serum cholesterol will provide markers for the nephrotic syndrome as well as for the severity of the proteinuria. Worsened proteinuria is an indicator of

TABLE 75–3 • TRANSITION OF SYSTEMIC LUPUS ERYTHEMATOSUS PATIENTS BETWEEN STATES OF RENAL FUNCTION

State at Entry	No. Before Transition	Follow-up	Subsequent State During Follow-up Period*			
			Normal	Proteinuria Alone	Moderate Filtration Dysfunction	Severe Azotemia Deterioration
Normal	172	300 days	113 (65)	34 (20)	24 (14)	1 (.5)
Proteinuria alone	113	300 days	28 (25)	54 (48)	28 (25)	3 (2)
Moderate filtration dysfunction	103	100 days	23 (22)	34 (33)	41 (40)	5 (5)
Severe azotemia	21	300 days Improvement	0 (0)	0 (0)	0 (0)	21 (100)

*The numbers on the diagonal (113, 54, 41, 21) show how many patients did not change from initial state.

poor outcomes with respect to renal function.[92] Nephrologists, rheumatologists, and pathologists have debated the utility of kidney biopsy for almost 30 years.[93] Studies suggest that it may be helpful in establishing the diagnosis before the institution of immunosuppressive therapy, such as cyclophosphamide[94,95]; however, questions have been raised regarding the added value of biopsies over the impression of a clinician after review of disease duration, involvement, and activity.[96] Some advocate that biopsies be performed to ensure that there is adequate renal tissue to be benefited by aggressive therapy, using the degree of sclerosis and interstitial fibrosis to indicate damage that is no longer amenable to intervention.[97,98]

The WHO classification of lupus nephritis is based on biopsy findings. These pathologic classifications have been correlated with clinical and laboratory findings and are often used to suggest renal prognosis in individual patients. In general, class I (normal findings on biopsy) is thought to have an excellent prognosis. Individuals designated class II (mesangial hypertrophy and mesangial immune deposits) generally have a good prognosis. Those designated class III (mesangial and endothelial proliferation with immune deposits along capillaries, but less than 50 percent of glomeruli involved) have a moderate prognosis. Class IV (diffuse proliferative glomerulonephritis with greater than 50% of glomeruli involved and cell proliferation resulting in crescent formation) indicates a poor prognosis but may be amenable to aggressive immunosuppressive therapy. Class V (membranous glomerulonephritis with subepithelial granular immune deposits) designation is associated with nephrotic-range proteinuria in two thirds of patients, but patients often maintain normal creatinine clearance. Finally, class VI (sclerosing changes with fibrous crescents and vascular sclerosis) designation is an ominous sign that there are few reversible elements to the kidney involvement and that progression to renal failure is likely. The clinical and laboratory associations with class II through class V are provided in Table 75–4.

There is a strong association of diffuse proliferative glomerulonephritis with ds-DNA antibodies[99] and of

TABLE 75–4 • CORRELATIONS BETWEEN CLINICAL AND LABORATORY FINDINGS AND PATHOLOGIC CLASSIFICATIONS IN LUPUS NEPHRITIS PATIENTS

	Mesangial		Focal Proliferative	Diffuse Proliferative	Membranous	Tubulo-interstitial	Infection	Drug-Induced
	IIA	IIB	III	IV	V			
Symptoms	None	None	None	Renal failure Nephrotic syndrome	Nephrotic syndrome	None	Dysuria	Renal failure (rare)
Hypertension	None	None	±	Common	Late-onset	Late-onset	Late-onset	None
Proteinuria (g/day)	None	<1	<2	1-20	3.5-20	±	±	±
Hematuria (RBCs/hpf)	None	5-15	5-15	Many	None	±	±	None
Pyuria (WBCs/hpf)	None	5-15	5-15	Many	None	±	Many	None
Casts	None	±	±	None	None	None	None	None
GFR (ml/min)	NI	NI	60-80	<60	NI	NI	NI	NI or ↓
CH$_{50}$	NI	± ↓	↓	↓ ↓	NI	NI	NI	NI
C3	NI	± ↓	↓	↓ ↓	NI	NI	NI	NI
Anti-DNA	NI	± ↑	↑	↑ ↑	NI	NI	NI	NI
Immune complexes	NI	± ↑	↑	↑ ↑	NI	NI	NI	NI

Abbreviations: C3, Complement 3; CH$_{50}$, total serum hemolytic complement (expressed in 50% hemolytic units); GFR, glomerular filtration rate; hpf, high-power field; NI, normal; RBC, red blood cell; WBC, white blood cell; ±, occasional, small amounts; ↑, somewhat increased; ↓, somewhat decreased; ↑ ↑, greatly increased; ↓ ↓, greatly decreased.

membranous glomerulopathy with Sm antibodies.[100-102] Renal involvement can be seen in the presence of other autoantibodies, and there is a veno-occlusive phenomenon that can be seen with antiphospholipid antibodies.

CARDIOPULMONARY INVOLVEMENT

Lupus can affect both the heart and lungs in a variety of ways. In addition to the inflammatory process caused by immune complex disease and the resulting fibrosis, the lung can suffer acute insult from pulmonary embolus, capillary leak, or serositis.[103-105] The lung also exhibits an unusual "shrinking" phenomenon in some patients, which could be due to either a weakened or fibrotic diaphragmatic muscle or involvement of the phrenic nerve.[106] Cardiac involvement may occur in any component, including the valves, the myocardium, the conducting system, or the pericardium. The Libman-Sacks lesion of the mitral and aortic valves has been recognized more frequently in sites where echocardiograms can routinely be performed. There is an emerging recognition of the association between antiphospholipid syndrome and Libman-Sacks disease.[72,107,108]

A clue to pulmonary involvement may be cough or chest pain on breathing; however, neither has a high positive predictive value. Chest pain occurs in approximately 50 percent of patients, but this can often be demonstrated to be chest wall pain involving musculoskeletal elements. This is commonly associated with fibromyalgia but may also represent costochondritis or Tietze's syndrome. The patient can be reassured that this does not represent lung involvement. Cough is most often associated with upper respiratory infection of a viral etiology. Nevertheless, pulmonary involvement in lupus must be carefully assessed to ensure that acute lupus pneumonitis, characterized by pleurisy, dyspnea, cough, and fever with radiologic findings of pulmonary infiltrates, is not present. Once infection has been ruled out, it is imperative that immunosuppressant therapy and supportive respiratory care be given. Prognosis is poor (50% mortality), and a sequela for survivors is severe restrictive lung disease.

Pericardial effusions may develop rapidly in lupus patients in association with symptoms of pericarditis and general lupus activity. These effusions are often responsive to high-dose steroids, unlike the effusions found in patients with RA, which are more insidious in onset and are found to have fibrinous adhesions. A pericardial window is occasionally required to be placed surgically to maintain cardiac function in the setting of extensive pericardial effusions impinging on the filling phase of the cardiac cycle.

More emphasis has been placed on the premature occurrence of coronary artery disease in recent years. It has been shown that women in their thirties and forties may be at more than 50 times the risk of age- and gender-matched control subjects, particularly if hypercholesterolemia, prednisone use, hypertension, early ovarian failure, and obesity are present.[109-112]

THROMBOEMBOLIC COMPLICATIONS

The association of SLE and the antiphospholipid antibodies can be traced to the initial finding of false-positive serologic test results for syphilis before 1950 and then to their inclusion in the classification criteria as one of the immunologic criteria along with antibodies to ds-DNA, Sm, and the LE cell.[35] In 1997, an amendment was made to the ACR criteria in favor of adding the antiphospholipid antibody tests and removing the LE cell preparation.[36] There were significant advances in understanding the phenomenon of thromboembolism during the 1980s.[113-116] The full spectrum of disease association may not be complete yet; however, most of the problems associated with SLE have been identified.[53-55,90,117] The antiphospholipid syndrome is covered in detail in Chapter 77.

Subtle findings on magnetic resonance imaging (MRI) of the brain or massive life-threatening events in the lungs, as well as many clinical situations between these extremes, have been noted in association with the antiphospholipid syndrome.[52,84,85,118,119] Transverse myelitis, optic neuropathy, and epilepsy are associated, suggesting a role for early anticoagulation when these entities are encountered.[120,121] Antiphospholipid antibodies are likely to have a pathophysiologic role in recurrent miscarriages, early pregnancy loss, and poor outcomes of pregnancy.[122-125] The degree to which platelet aggregation, prostaglandin changes, plasminogen activation and inhibition, and fibrinolysis play a role in causing thrombotic and thromboembolic problems is not known.[126] However, it is clear that ischemia of vulnerable tissues such as brain, spinal cord, lung, placenta, and bowel is a major problem for lupus patients. The first sign of an embolic event may be acute and associated with dysfunction of the imperiled organ system. Sudden pain in the gut associated with postprandial pain or chest pain with shortness of breath could indicate thromboembolic disease. It is occasionally impossible to distinguish inflammatory processes from the effects of a clot, and the two processes may actually coincide. The clinician may be required to treat both possibilities, using anticoagulation as well as immunosuppression, to avoid a fatal occurrence or irreversible damage.

NEUROPSYCHIATRIC INVOLVEMENT

The human brain, arguably our most complex end-organ, and one of the products of millions of years of mammalian evolution, can be affected by disease in a multitude of ways. Being warm-blooded creatures, with a high metabolic rate and rich blood supply to the CNS, infarctions from either thrombotic or embolic processes can cause havoc. Inflammation of neural tissue adjacent to blood vessels can also disrupt normal function. Hypothetically, immune-mediated effects on neuronal cells could cause dysfunction. Demyelination of axons leading to a situation not unlike MS has been cited as one example of such a process. Transverse myelitis is another example. The finding of elevated levels of immunoglobulin G (IgG) anticardiolipin antibodies in cerebrospinal fluid (CSF), greater than expected from a vascular supply alone, suggests there may be a central production of this potentially pathologic element. Metabolic abnormalities, as a consequence of other organ dysfunction, could play a role in changing the metabolic capability of neurons and their component parts of axons, dendrites, and synapses. It is also possible that the subtle balance of neurotransmitters in the hindbrain, such as serotonin, could be altered by effects of lupus or its treatment. Irrespective of the mechanisms, it is recognized that a great many patients with lupus have cognitive dysfunction and other neuropsychiatric problems.[128-130]

Neuropsychiatric lupus (NPSLE) is now the accepted term for the presentation of psychologic, CNS, or peripheral nervous system abnormalities. NPSLE has replaced CNS lupus, neurolupus, CNS vasculitis, cerebral vasculitis, or organic brain syndrome, as the general term to be used. The 1999 ACR Nomenclature Committee, an international panel (including United States, Canada, Mexico, United Kingdom, and Germany) with experts from neurology, rheumatology, psychiatry, psychology, and hematology identified 19 different NP conditions that are part of the lupus complex. Twelve are associated with the CNS and seven with the peripheral nervous system. This marks a step forward in the understanding of a very difficult aspect of lupus. A number of key points are made in their recommendations. One of these is that this new set of 19 NP definitions could be used to expand the neuropsychiatric criteria of the ACR classification criteria of SLE from just seizures and psychosis. As noted previously, this has not yet been ratified by the classification criteria committee of the ACR. These NP criteria are not to replace clinical judgment or to interfere with the clinical diagnosis given to patients.

To establish meaningful, reproducible terms, the committee developed case definitions that are published on the ACR Web site (*www.rheumatology.org/ ar/ar.html*). These definitions follow a rigorous outline that not only spells out the definition, but also indicates the diagnostic criteria, exclusionary conditions, associated conditions, and methods for ascertainment, as well as the findings that should be recorded for comparison or research purposes. It has been noted that patients may have more than one NP manifestation at the same time, or accumulated over time, and that the diagnosis may change from the time of presentation to the time of final diagnosis as treatment unfolds.

An example of one of these case definitions, cerebrovascular disease, is shown in the box on the following page. Strokes, transient ischemic attacks (TIAs), multi-infarct processes, hemorrhages, and thromboses are accepted if infection, hypoglycemia, tumor, trauma, or vascular malformation can be excluded. Potential associated conditions such as hypertension, atrial fibrillation, antiphospholipid antibodies, and others should be noted, because it may be impossible to determine whether the conditions are causal. Acceptable diagnostic maneuvers are identified, and finally, the concomitant disease elements relevant to the ongoing record are indicated.

Headache, one of the more nonspecific and common NP categories listed, is described as "discomfort in the region of the cranial vault" and is divided into five categories: migraine, cluster, tension, benign intracranial hypertension, and "intractable headache." Controlled studies using normal populations indicate that these categories may be equally common in the general public as they are in SLE; however, it is still considered reasonable to use this classification of headaches to describe the experience many patients report. The case definitions point out that aseptic meningitis (including drug-induced), pseudotumor cerebri caused by oral contraceptives, sulfonamides, trimethoprim, and others, CNS infection, tumors, trauma, caffeine withdrawal, and intracranial hemorrhage or vascular occlusions must be excluded as the cause.

Cognitive dysfunction is widely recognized as one of the most common NP conditions, after headache, from which SLE patients suffer. It has been described in up to 80 percent of patients in some studies. Even after acknowledging the potential impact of treatment with steroids, cytotoxics, and other medications, as well as the negative effects of depression or dysphoria, there still remains a component of cognitive dysfunction that is specific to SLE. The actual cognitive processes typically measured in psychologic tests include intelligence, attention, reasoning, learning, recall, fluency, language, and perceptual-motor capacity. An appropriate set of tests is outlined in the NP committee's recommendations. Of these, the very essential human element of learning is most commonly disrupted. The distinction is made that patients can recall information appropriately, but their ability to encode information accurately or completely is lacking. Hence, some have postulated that attention to both auditory and visual tasks are affected by pathophysiologic mechanisms of lupus. Hippocampal regions of the brain are associated with new learning, and it is possible that SLE patients have brain abnormalities in these structures. This may be the meaning behind the very commonly cited problem of "poor memory" that patients report in the clinic. Interesting work by Gladman and Urowitz on patients with inactive SLE reveals that a high degree of disease activity at onset, a history of vasculitis, or both will predict cognitive dysfunction, whereas the presence of fibromyalgia, previous evidence of renal disease or damage, previous evidence of NP lupus, steroid use, atherosclerosis, or cytotoxic drug use will not.

Less common, but still present often enough to cause concern, are mood disorders, including anxiety. It is recommended that the DSM-IV classification of psychiatric conditions be used to describe these. SLE patients may be understandably anxious about their situation, given the effect of steroids on their physical features, cytotoxics on their reproductive capacity, and the general ominous nature of the condition relative to what their healthy peers have experienced. Nevertheless, some patients are more intensely anxious than seems warranted, and many express severe depressive features out of keeping with the situation they are in. Without an immunopathophysiologic explanation for either anxiety or depression, it is difficult to impute a causal relationship to SLE; however, it is recommended that these symptoms be noted as part of the NP lupus complex.

CASE DEFINITION—CEREBROVASCULAR DISEASE

Cerebrovascular Disease

Cerebrovascular disease is defined as neurologic deficits due to arterial insufficiency or occlusion, veno-occlusive disease, or hemorrhage. These are mainly focal deficits but may be multifocal in recurrent disease.

Diagnostic criteria:

One of the following and supporting radioimaging study:

1. *Stroke syndrome:* Acute focal neurologic deficit persisting more than 24 hours (or lasting less than 24 hours with computed tomography [CT] or magnetic resonance imaging [MRI] abnormality consistent with physical findings and symptoms
2. *Transient ischemic attack:* Acute, focal neurologic deficit with clinical resolution within 24 hours (without corresponding lesion on CT or MRI)
3. *Chronic multifocal disease:* Recurrent or progressive neurologic deterioration attributable to cerebrovascular disease
4. *Subarachnoid and intracranial hemorrhage:* Bleeding documented by cerebrospinal fluid (CSF) findings and MRI or CT
5. *Sinus thrombosis:* Acute, focal neurologic deficit in the presence of increased intracranial pressure

NB: The finding of unidentified bright objects on MRI without clinical manifestations is not classified at the present time.

Exclusions:

Infection with space occupying lesions in the brain, intracranial tumor, trauma, vascular malformation, hypoglycemia

Associations:

Diabetes mellitus, dyslipidemia, atherosclerotic vascular disease, atrial fibrillation, valvular heart disease, atrial septal defect, hypercoagulability state, antiphospholipid antibody syndrome, hypertension, smoking, cocaine or amphetamine abuse

Ascertainment:

History and physical examination
CT or MRI
Angiogram as indicated
Antiphospholipid antibodies
Lumbar puncture as indicated
ECG for suspected cardiac arrhythmias
ECG for suspected Libman-Sacks, valvular disease, or atrial septal defect
Duplex ultrasound of carotid arteries for suspected carotid artery disease

Record:

Basic descriptors of demographics, systemic lupus erythematosus (SLE) criteria and duration, laboratory, medications
Associated findings, chronology, SLE activity, change with management, severity
Type of cerebrovascular pathology (e.g., infarct, hemorrhage)
Antiphospholipid antibodies
Other coagulation studies obtained

Acute confusional state is diagnosed when there is a disturbance of consciousness, or level of arousal, with reduced ability to focus, maintain, or shift attention. Typically the condition develops over a short period of time (hours to days) and tends to fluctuate during the course of the day. Often, cognitive dysfunction is present during the "acute confusional state"; however, if present alone without the acute confusion, then the patient should only be classified as having "cognitive dysfunction." Both acute or subacute cognitive changes and sudden mood or behavioral changes are recognized as part of this state. For example, patients may exhibit reversal of the sleep-wake cycle or severe irritability mixed with anxiety and even paranoia. On the other hand, they may exhibit severe obtundation and even appear to be entering a comatose state. The "acute confusional state" is equivalent in the DSM-IV and ICD-9 classification of "delirium," which is often the term used by psychiatrists. Neurologists, on the other hand, refer to this as "encephalopathy," which refers to a diffuse cerebral dysfunction thought to be due to a pathophysiologic process usually seen in metabolic disorders. Therefore, overt metabolic abnormalities of glucose, electrolytes, fluids, or osmolarity should be ruled out, as well as other primary mental and neurologic disorders unrelated to SLE such as tumors or infection. Of note, it is no longer recommended to use the term *organic brain syndrome.* This term has lost its meaning in the face of the more precise definitions currently used.

Another acute CNS condition is psychosis, which is defined as a severe disturbance in the perception of reality characterized by delusions, hallucinations, or both. The patient experiences impairment in social or occupational roles, not exclusively during a period of hallucination. Other explanations such as schizophrenia, use of street or prescribed drugs, and a psychologically induced process from stress need to be ruled out. It is often difficult to separate the effects of high-dose steroids from NP psychosis until changes in the steroid regimen have been undertaken and the patient's situation observed. Some patients note adverse changes in their symptoms at doses of 20 mg or more.

Seizure disorder, one of the disease classification criteria for SLE, is relatively uncommon when compared to cognitive dysfunction, headaches, or mood and anxiety disorders. It is an abnormal paroxysmal neuronal discharge in the brain, which causes abnormal function. About 3 percent of the population has epilepsy, which must be distinguished from isolated seizures associated with SLE. Alcohol, narcotic, or barbiturate withdrawal, exposure to toxic compounds, high fevers with or without infection, tumors, and severe sleep deprivation are some of the causes of seizures that need to be ruled out in the patient with SLE. Additionally, vasovagal or cardiac syncope, narcolepsy and cataplexy, panic attacks, conversion disorder, or occasionally malingering need to be considered in some patients who present with unusual acute CNS events.

The diagnosis of seizure disorder could have a profound effect on the patient's functioning in society, particularly with respect to driving. Clearly, the condition must be correctly diagnosed and treated to ensure the safe use of moving vehicles and other equipment. It is worthwhile to elicit a careful history of credible witnesses regarding the type of seizure because electroencephalogram (EEG) may not be diagnostic during the interictal state. The seizure may be "primary generalized," as in a tonic/clonic, atonic, or petit mal type; or, they may be partial (also called focal and referred to as Jacksonian, temporal lobe, or psychomotor seizure), in which the seizure begins locally and is simple, without impairment of consciousness; or complex, which refers to partial impairment of consciousness. The symptoms may be motor, sensory, aphasic, cognitive, affective, dysmnesic, illusional, olfactory, or psychologic. It likely will require the expert assistance of a neurologist to correctly identify the seizure features once you suspect they are occurring in your patient. The response to therapy, diagnostic imaging interpretation (MRI or CAT scan), and EEG findings will all be needed to correctly manage the patient with a suspected seizure disorder.

Other abnormalities of the CNS include aseptic meningitis, demyelinating syndrome, movement disorders such as choreiform movements, and central myelopathy. Each of these requires close attention to history taking and appropriate examination of the patient. Signs of meningeal irritation with a stiff, painful neck will raise the possibility of meningitis, whereas rapid onset of band-like sensory changes in the trunk associated with gait disturbance may tip the clinician off to transverse myelitis. The demyelinating syndrome associated with SLE is very difficult to distinguish from MS and may actually be the chance occurrence of two diseases. MRI is particularly useful in these settings, particularly if the diagnostician can provide a correlation between symptoms and findings. Rapid treatment is paramount, particularly with transverse myelitis. At times, the clinician is forced to treat the condition as both a potential inflammatory lesion, as well as a thrombotic event, when the antiphospholipid antibody

syndrome is found in association, or is suspected. There are insufficient trials, and insufficient experience in most locations, with the detailed interpretation of diagnostic images to safely distinguish between these alternative mechanisms.

The peripheral nervous system can be involved in many ways. Some patients with SLE will present with a Guillain-Barré picture with an inflammatory demyelinating process. Myasthenia gravis can also occur in the setting of SLE. The other processes involving the peripheral nervous system may occur in isolated nerves including the motor, sensory, or autonomic components either singly or in combination. The cranial nerves can also be affected. It is relevant to record any associated elements or diagnoses, such as stroke or TIA, migraine, TTP, or metabolic dysregulation, such as hypoglycemia, hypoxemia, or uremia, with each of these manifestations of peripheral nervous system involvement.

In summary, the neuropsychiatric manifestations of SLE are both protean and complex. Invariably, clinicians are left with a sense of inadequacy in determining the cause and effect of the disease, its treatment, and the complications thereof. Very often, it is only the long-term knowledge of individual patients that allows a decision to be made regarding the introduction of new therapy or withdrawal of medications. Support and understanding of patients regarding their concerns about cognitive dysfunction, their dysphoria and anxiety, or the debilitating effects of a cerebrovascular accident should always be considered a key element of therapy.

INFECTION AND OTHER COMPLICATING FACTORS

Activity of disease is often difficult to differentiate from infection. A patient with lupus receiving low doses of steroids and possibly an immunosuppressive agent such as azathioprine is at higher risk of infection. If the patient presents with fever and malaise, this could represent further activation of the disease process or, alternatively, an infection that has developed during the immunosuppressive process. Unusual organisms such as *Pneumocystis carinii*, *Candida*, and *Mycobacterium* may be present. Measures of acute-phase reactants, such as the erythrocyte sedimentation rate (or C-reactive protein), may confirm the inflammatory state but fail to differentiate infection from disease activity. Examination for bands (immature polymorphonuclear leukocytes) could point toward an acute bacterial infection, but the result is often equivocal. The finding of lowered complement levels, with both C3 and C4 depressed, when it is known that the SLE patient does not have the C4-null allele, could point to an immune complex–mediated process rather than infection.

Close attention should be paid to the lungs, heart, and gastrointestinal tract. Chest radiograph examination is useful for ruling out pulmonary involvement; however, if radiologic changes are found, it may be difficult to distinguish pneumonia from other lupus-related problems, such as pneumonitis, intra-alveolar hemorrhage, vasculitis, congestive heart failure, acute respiratory distress syndrome, and even the effects of pulmonary embolus. Biopsy of the lung parenchyma is occasionally required in the rapidly failing individual. Nail bed infarcts, Osler's nodes, and Janeway lesions in the extremities are probably the peripheral findings of immune complex disease, but they demand careful auscultation of the cardiac valves along with an echocardiogram, if it is available, to rule out bacterial endocarditis as a source of fever. Blood cultures in both pulmonary and cardiac settings will help with decision making as the clinician considers whether to use strong immunosuppressive medications or antibiotic therapy. It is usually not difficult to identify infection of the urinary tract; often the patient has localized symptoms. However, urine culture may be required in the patient who is thought to have occult infection. Any suggestion of CNS involvement complicates the diagnostic process considerably. Viral or bacterial meningitis, viral encephalopathy, and even septic emboli should be considered in a patient with seizures, delirium, or altered sensorium. Of course, through all this investigation, the clinician must always consider that both lupus activity and infection may be contributing factors.

Another consideration is to differentiate disease activity from allergic reactions to medications or alternative therapies. Care providers prescribe lupus patients a wide variety of medications and agents. Sulfonamides may be used for symptoms of urinary tract infection by the naïve care provider and thereby provoke an activation of the immune system. The patient could purchase ibuprofen for symptomatic relief of muscle or joint pain and then have CNS disease activation. Antihypertensive agents such as thiazide diuretics can cause photosensitivity reactions, mimicking or perhaps provoking a lupus skin condition. Certain antiepileptic compounds, such as phenytoin, have been associated with rashes, including malar rash, which can fool even the most astute clinician. Cardiac medications associated with drug-induced lupus may also cause symptoms in the SLE patient that appear to be activation of the disease but necessitate removal of the cardiac compound to return the patient to a quiescent state. Hormone replacement therapy, often used in the setting of premature ovarian failure secondary to cyclophosphamide therapy or in the setting of long-term steroid use with consequent osteoporosis, is suspected of inducing flares in some individuals.[124,131-133]

Disease Activity

Remission of all lupus activity is unusual.[86,134] Control of activity with medications such as corticosteroids, immunosuppressants, and antimalarials can be achieved with some risk of iatrogenesis. Decisions regarding therapy are rooted in an estimation of the degree of damage that may result from untreated disease activity. Therefore, determining activity in a systematic fashion is a prerequisite to optimal clinical care. This section discusses the current approaches to quantifying disease activity, identifying flares, and predicting flares. This is followed by a discussion of damage that results from the disease activity or its treatment.

QUANTIFYING ACTIVITY

At least five formal measures of disease activity are currently considered acceptable. All five correlate with each other better than they do with the clinician's "gestalt" of a patient's activity (Table 75–5). It may be that the experienced clinician weights each sign of activity in a different fashion, or that different elements of activity are brought into the clinical summation. Alternatively, clinicians may not be consistent in their determination of activity between different patients, and, therefore, reduced correlation of their findings with the activity indices occurs. However, both approaches—standardized scoring and clinical judgment—have merit and provide useful information.[24,135,136]

Four of the five indices measure activity on the basis of clinical findings alone, without incorporating intent to treat. Each one provides a score related to the extent of inflammation involved. The British Isles Lupus Assessment Group Score, developed in the United Kingdom, incorporates treatment decisions into the assessment.[142] There is inherent logic to this approach, given the premise that providing therapy is an indication of the clinician's overall impression of activity.[22,137,138]

The weights assigned to each variable do not always correspond to the degree of inflammation present; instead, they may relate to the seriousness of the organ

TABLE 75–5 • DISEASE ACTIVITY INDICES*

	SLAM	SLEDAI	SIS	BILAG	ECLAM	Physician
SLAM	1.0	0.827	0.884	0.786	0.755	0.614
SLEDAI		1.0	0.800	0.762	0.785	0.656
SIS			1.0	0.762	0.754	0.535
BILAG				1.0	0.725	0.629
ECLAM					1.0	0.686

*SLAM, Systemic Lupus Activity Measure[138-140]; SLEDAI, SLE Disease Activity Index[138-141]; SIS, SLE Index Score[138]; BILAG, British Isles Lupus Assessment Group[142]; ECLAM, European Consensus Lupus Activity Measurement.[22]

involvement according to the life-threatening nature or threat to the functional capacity of the individual. For example, the weights given by the SLE Disease Activity Index are much greater for CNS involvement than they are for cutaneous involvement. Thus, retinal hemorrhage or optic neuritis may have less actual immunologic activity than a discoid patch; the former are given eight points, whereas skin involvement is given two. The SLE Disease Activity Index is scored (present or absent) on 24 items observed during the preceding 10 days. The six neurologic elements, each scoring eight points, include seizure, psychosis, organic brain syndrome, visual changes with retinal involvement, cranial nerve involvement, and new cerebrovascular accident. Vasculitis also scores eight points. Renal involvement with new-onset proteinuria, casts, hematuria, and pyuria would accumulate 16 points of activity, allowing four points for each item. Arthritis and myositis score four points each. Pleurisy, pericarditis, and mucosal membrane ulcerations each receive two points, as do the onset of a new rash and the occurrence of alopecia. Low complement level and abnormal ds-DNA add two points each; fever, thrombocytopenia, and leukopenia add one point each. Thus, a patient who has developed a new rash, arthritis, and pleurisy while demonstrating thrombocytopenia and low complement levels would score nine points. Alternatively, a patient with new-onset proteinuria with hematuria (not due to infection) who has abnormal complement and ds-DNA would score 12 points. If that person also has vasculitis as evidenced by periungual infarction and splinter hemorrhage, the score will be 20.

Another index, the Systemic Lupus Activity Measure, has a rating scale (0 to 3) on 31 items, and the total score can range from 0 to 84. The SLE Disease Activity Index has been used retrospectively, apparently with reliable effect when complete data are available on the charts. Assessment of activity from chart review using the Systemic Lupus Activity Measure demonstrates correlation with concurrent assessments; however, the authors caution against its use for retrospective review.[136]

DEFINING A "FLARE"

Flares of disease activity occur in patients in a variety of ways. In fact, variety seems to be the rule, even within a given patient. Sometimes a flare will begin with overwhelming fatigue. At other times, it will begin with subtle neurologic findings. Most commonly, it begins with pain in the joints, accompanied by some changes in the skin. Lymphadenopathy, particularly in the cervical area, is often found coincident with other signs of a flare. Definitions of flares usually rely on an increase of activity from a lower state to a higher state. However, a flare may in fact persist for a relatively long time, and, thus, it is not entirely correct to refer to a flare as an increase in activity alone. Determining the range of activity, or the change in activity, that constitutes a flare is a current challenge for clinician scientists. Several attempts have been made to operationalize the concept

of a flare with a uniform approach. However, this area is still under investigation, and a consistent method has not been adopted.[143-146]

PREDICTING A "FLARE"

Conflicting results have been published regarding the ability of particular findings to predict flares. Some authors report excellent predictability of ds-DNA antibodies in selected patients,[147] whereas others have found virtually no predictive capability of such measures as autoantibody formation or complement activation. Complement split products may have more predictive value.[148] Timing of the antecedent measures is another critical difference among the studies reported. Esdaile and colleagues[49,144] were unable to find predictive elements when 3-, 6-, and 9-month laboratory information was used to predict changes in activity scores of 6 or more on the SLE Disease Activity Index. TerBorg and associates,[149] using serial weekly measures, detected rises in autoantibody titers before clinical flares.

▌ End-Organ Damage

DISEASE PROCESS

End-organ damage begins with the formation of scar tissue in response to inflammation and ischemia. Some tissues, such as the skin, may heal well without leaving irreparable damage. However, the kidneys, heart, brain, and lungs are not so readily repaired without leaving a dysfunctional organ. In particular, the damage that results can be seen in a permanently altered filtration function of the kidney, seizure disorder in the brain, and damaged parenchyma or myocardium.

TREATMENT EFFECTS

The treatments that are effective in dealing with active lupus have their own attendant risks. Corticosteroids can cause a great deal of damage, ranging from severe osteoporosis to increased atherosclerosis and cataracts. Less severe, but intrusive nevertheless, is the effect on weight and on skin thickness. Immunosuppressive medications, including cyclophosphamide and azathioprine, primarily, are linked to premature ovarian failure.

QUANTIFYING DAMAGE

A consensus has been reached about how to tabulate these effects: each of the areas is scored according to whether irreparable damage has occurred. The Systemic Lupus Index of the Consensus Committee has quantified damage caused by either disease or its treatment. The scale has been shown to have good reliability and has validity at face value as well as through convergence with other approaches of quantifying damage.[150,151]

ILLNESS INTRUSIVENESS INTO PSYCHOSOCIAL WELLBEING

SLE is stressful, both psychologically and physiologically. For many people, the disease contributes to emotional distress in the form of anxiety, frustration, and depressed mood. A number of psychosocial stressors and adaptive challenges may underlie these difficulties.

Organ involvement is unpredictable in SLE because disease activity may affect one or more systems over time, including the kidney, lungs, joints, liver, hematologic, and central nervous systems. The unpredictable nature of the disease and widespread potential for harm leads to anxiety. Shortened life expectancy raises concerns about mortality and this, in turn, can compromise effective coping. Treatment may have severe repercussions at many different levels. Body image can be threatened, for example, by cushingoid facial changes resulting from prednisone therapy. Important life goals can be undermined when immunosuppression agents exert toxic effects on reproductive capacity. Economic resources can be strained when physicians prescribe medications that are not reimbursed by drug plans. Because SLE is a rare disease, with a prevalence of less than 1 per 1000 in many population studies, patients often feel isolated, unsupported, and misunderstood by their doctors, family members, and friends.

SLE affects women predominantly, often during the reproductive years when they are establishing families and careers. Family and social relationships are especially salient for women. Because SLE affects them at a life stage when they would otherwise have expected to begin and raise a family, women may experience the condition as especially stressful. We introduced the concept of *illness intrusiveness* to summarize the extent to which chronic conditions, such as SLE, and their treatments interfere with psychologically meaningful activities.[151a] Many of the psychosocial challenges faced by women with SLE are subsumed by the concept of illness intrusiveness.

Illness intrusiveness involves illness-induced disruptions to lifestyles, activities, and interests and compromises quality of life in chronic disease.[151b] It intervenes between the objective circumstances of disease (e.g., pain, shortness of breath, weakness, memory loss) and treatment (e.g., negative side effects, costs of medications, time for provider visits), on the one hand, and subjective well-being and emotional distress on the other. Illness intrusiveness is a stressor that threatens quality of life. It is not a facet of quality of life itself. Different variables correlate with illness intrusiveness as compared to emotional distress and subjective well-being. Considerable evidence substantiates the illness intrusiveness theoretical framework across chronic conditions, including SLE.[151c] The Illness Intrusiveness Ratings Scale (IIRS) taps illness intrusiveness as it relates to three separate life domains: relationships and personal development, intimacy, and instrumental life domains. Stress-process research shows that women are more sensitive than men when stressors arise in the context of interpersonal relationships. In terms of the IIRS, such effects might be more evident when examining illness intrusiveness into intimacy or relationships and personal development as compared to instrumental life domains. Adjunctive psychosocial interventions, such as brief supportive-expressive group psychotherapy, focus on minimizing illness-induced difficulties in relationships and intimacy. Their psychosocial benefits may, therefore, be evident in reduced illness intrusiveness into intimacy or relationships and personal development (e.g., as compared to instrumental life domains, such as work and finances).[151d]

▌ Prognosis

DEFINING PROGNOSIS

Prognostication is the prediction of outcomes. Outcomes may be the results of disease activity or of disease treatment. A primary outcome of interest has been mortality, or quantity of life.[90,152-154] Emphasis has also been placed on quality of life.[155-159] With lupus, there are also the intermediate outcomes related to failures of certain critical systems, such as the kidneys, heart, brain, and lungs.[26,92,94,96,151,160-166] The OMERACT group has developed a consensus on which parameters should be considered imperative in the reporting of outcomes in randomized clinical trials and in longitudinal observational studies.[24] The key measures identified for both randomized clinical trials and longitudinal observational studies are disease activity, health-related quality of life, damage indices, and toxicity or adverse events (including death). Of these, disease-activity measures are considered the most important for both types of investigative effort.

Mortality rates have changed over the years in North America.[90,153,154] Results from the 1950s give worst-case estimates, based on cohorts of patients who have severe disease to begin with and who do not have the benefit of adequate therapy for serious consequences, such as renal failure. These would apply to patients who live in areas where only severe disease is recognized and patients are without access to renal dialysis or for whom management of acute cardiorespiratory problems with intensive care support is not available. In these situations, the 5-year life expectancy is approximately 50 percent. However, under optimal conditions of diagnosis and treatment, with good social support, life expectancy can be 90 percent at 10 years.[167]

CHALLENGING SITUATIONS

Socioeconomic Isolation

Socioeconomic factors are becoming increasingly evident as determinants of the outcomes of people with lupus. Results from South America indicate that the poorer socioeconomic mestizos have twice the rate of severe outcomes, including renal failure and death, than do whites who are better educated, have higher social status, and have better medical coverage.[168] This mirrors what has been found in other populations in which there is a distinct difference in socioeconomic class.[169-171] Such elements as access to laboratory testing, ability to obtain medications, proximity of tertiary care facilities, and ability to deal with intensive care patients or renal dialysis patients are considered critical for successful management of lupus patients.

Pregnancy

The likelihood of poor outcome for fetus or mother can be determined best through an assessment of existing disease activity, assessment of previous pregnancy outcomes, and knowledge of antiphospholipid and SS-A/SS-B antibody status. An ominous sign of poor outcome for both the mother and the fetus is renal or CNS activity immediately before pregnancy. Thrombocytopenia, although not an absolute contraindication, presents considerable management problems. The presence of antiphospholipid syndrome should raise red flags, particularly regarding the likelihood of fetal wastage, whereas the presence of SS-A (or SS-B) is an indication for closer monitoring of the fetus for cardiac or neurologic problems. If a second pregnancy is anticipated, the first pregnancy will have strong predictive power. There may be as high as an 80 percent likelihood of poor fetal outcome if a miscarriage occurred in the 14th to 20th week of the first pregnancy.[172]

Observation of outcomes suggests that up to 40 percent of pregnancies may result in either miscarriages (38 percent) or stillbirths (2 percent),[173] which is higher than for age-matched individuals without chronic disease. Deliveries are more likely to be premature, and intrauterine growth retardation occurs in about 10 percent of pregnancies. Neonatal lupus is closely associated with the presence of maternal SS-A or SS-B antibodies and occurs in about 3 percent of pregnancies.[174,175] Myocardial involvement in utero, when detected, is best treated with fluorinated steroids, which can cross the placenta without deactivation.[176]

The presence of antiphospholipid antibodies is predictive of poor outcomes, but the negative results can be ameliorated by the use of low-molecular-weight heparin and aspirin.[177,178] Low-dose prednisone has also been used, although well-controlled studies are lacking.[179] Other laboratory parameters may need special interpretation during pregnancy. Complement levels are increased in normal pregnancies and, thus, may not be sensitive indicators of complement activation, whereas the split products of complement activation could be if they are available from the laboratory.[180]

There is still controversy about whether pregnancy induces flares.[181-184] It has been noted that if flares of lupus activity in the mother occur, they are often relatively mild, involving the skin and joints. It is possible to treat patients with low-dose prednisone or hydroxychloroquine.[182,183,185,186] Treatment of flares, using a multidisciplinary approach, improves the outcome for the fetus dramatically.[123] Immunosuppressive agents have been used during pregnancies without evidence of teratogenic effects being observed.[183,187] Few studies have been done on the development of children born to mothers with lupus. However, retrospective assessments suggest that male offspring may have a higher rate of hyperactivity and attention deficit than their peers born to mothers without lupus.[188]

■ Information on the Internet

A new challenge has arisen for clinicians, particularly in North America. The widespread use of computers and the spread of information on the Internet has increased tremendously during the past 5 years, and now millions of individuals have ready access to an increasing number of Web sites that deal directly with health issues. In a disease such as SLE, in which there is great variability in clinical manifestations and some potential for controversy over treatment alternatives, confusion can arise. Patients and their care providers may find themselves at odds with respect to appropriate management. Matching the right information to the individual patient is the art of medicine. In some instances, information on the Internet may be accurate but not appropriate for all clinical presentations. Patients and their families may find discrepancies between the information obtained from the Internet and that obtained from their treating care providers. For this reason, a listing of stable Web sites that demonstrate a sensible approach to SLE has been developed (Table 75-6). Although it is expected that these sites may change during the next 5 years, they will provide an initial point of departure for clinicians who are interested in the new class of "Internet patients."

■ Concluding Remarks

GLOBAL IMPACT

SLE is an uncommon disease. However, at a prevalence of 1 per 1000 women, 3 million families worldwide are touched by this disease. For most of the world, diagnosis and treatment require laboratory tests and medications beyond the capabilities of their current health budget. The detailed knowledge that rheumatologists have for managing the disease is not available to most of the physicians who will encounter patients. North America and Europe dedicate the greatest amount of resources for health care services from their existing gross domestic product. However, even they have difficulty providing sufficient resources to manage the difficult health problems associated with lupus, particularly for people who live outside urban centers or who have insufficient health care insurance to pay for services. Strategies to effectively deal with the disease burden by decreasing the rate of renal failure[189]; reducing the incidence of stroke; lowering the cardiovascular risk factors; and improving the general well-being of patients affected by rash, arthritis, and fatigue requires a coordinated effort by several sectors of the health care system. The first step is to accurately diagnose cases and then to provide access for these individuals to providers with appro-

TABLE 75–6 · SYSTEMIC LUPUS ERYTHEMATOSUS SITES ON THE INTERNET

Organization	Universal Resource Locator (URL)	Comments
Hamline University, St. Paul, Minnesota	http://www.hamline.edu/lupus/index.html	This site fosters a mailing list and a newsgroup on lupus as well as occasional chats open to participants, lupus patients, supporters, and health care providers.
Canadian Rheumatology Association (CRA)	http://www.cra-scr.ca	Password-protected site for rheumatologists to share case studies in a secure environment.
American College of Rheumatology (ACR)	http://www.rheumatology.org	General information on lupus with links to many journals.
International League of Associations for Rheumatology (ILAR)	http://www.ilar.org	Links to PANLAR, EULAR, AFLAR, and APLAR*.
Lupus HealthNet	http://www.lupus.org	Patient-focused information on lupus and its management, including how to participate in research projects.
Lupus Foundation of America (LFA)	http://www.lupus.org	Extensive source of information on lupus links to LFA chapters for the local states organizations in the United States.
Lupus Canada	http://www.lupuscanada.org	Information on lupus links to provincial lupus organizations in Canada.
European Lupus Erythematosus Federation (ELEF)	http://www.elef.rheumanet.org	Formed by members of ELEF, lupus organizations in 15 European countries with links to each country member organization; online ELEF newsletter.
Lupus Multiplex Registry and Repository	http://omrf.ouhsc.edu/lupus/	Homepage for the NIH- and OMRF-sponsored repository to recruit and store multiplex family DNA for current and future studies on lupus. Its purpose is to inform as well as to recruit families for the repository.
Lupus Association (Singapore)	http://home1.pacific.net.sg/~lupusas	Information on lupus site is in English, but also available in Chinese.
	http://www.mtio.com/lupus/seclin.htm	Links to non-English sites for lupus organizations around the world.
Lupus	http://www.arnoldpublishers.com/journals/pages/lupus	Online sample available.
The Journal of Rheumatology	http://www.jrheum.com/	Table of contents for the most recent issue, an archive of articles, and author indices printed since January 1996.
Arthritis and Rheumatism	http://www.rheumatology.org/ar/ar.html	Official journal of the American College of Rheumatology; index of articles and abstracts available since 1995.

*PANLAR, Pan American League Against Rheumatism; EULAR, European League Against Rheumatism; AFLAR, African League Against Rheumatism; APLAR, Asia Pacific League of Associations for Rheumatology; NIH, National Institutes of Health; OMRF, Oklahoma Medical Research Foundation.

priate knowledge and skills to deal with a complex, multisystem chronic illness.

SPREAD OF KNOWLEDGE

A phenomenon of knowledge dissemination is occurring that provides a partial solution to this problem. The Internet can connect the most geographically remote physician to the urban specialist. As we explore this potential for communication, we find a great number of opportunities to provide individualized advice on specific issues, along with means of disseminating more general knowledge. Issues of security, reimbursement, and authentication of knowledge must be addressed. Training of health care providers in the use of e-mail and Web services is required. However, the momentum of Internet use in the general public is creating the rising tide of ability that will push health care providers to expand their electronic skills. There are already a number of excellent Web sites available for accessing knowledge on the subject. Sites have also been established to assist with genetic studies, with attempts to identify a broad group of patients, some of whom have familial involvement. Support networks have also been developed, with chat groups and news groups providing new information on therapies and investigations.

CLINICAL PRACTICE

Clinical acumen is being supplemented by more sophisticated laboratory and imaging tests than ever before. A greater appreciation of the role that socioeconomic factors play in the health of individuals with chronic disease is leading to more comprehensive management plans. New immunosuppressive strategies that take into account subtle effects of cytokine imbalance or inappropriate T cell receptors and their ligands are now being considered. With all this, there is greater opportunity than ever before to reduce the intrusiveness of SLE on the lives of affected individuals and their families.

The clinician should remain open to any and all manifestations that can give clues to early diagnosis, accurate assessment of activity, and awareness of the damage that can occur from the disease and its treatment. Most important, the quality of life of individuals with SLE must be kept in mind while developing a management strategy for lupus patients.

REFERENCES

1. Lockshin MD: What is SLE [Editorial]. J Rheumatol 16:419, 1989.
2. Fries JF: Methodology of validation of criteria for SLE. Scand J Rheumatol Suppl 65:25, 1987.
3. Casciola-Rosen LA, Anhalt G, Rosen A: Autoantigens targeted in systemic lupus erythematosus are clustered in two populations of surface structures on apoptotic keratinocytes. J Exp Med 179:1317, 1994.
4. Vaishnaw AK, McNally JD, Elkon KB: Apoptosis in the rheumatic diseases. Arthritis Rheum 40:1917, 1997.
5. Elkon KB: Apoptosis and SLE [editorial]. Lupus 3:1, 1994.
6. National Library of Medicine and National Institutes of Health: Medical Subject Headings, Annotated Alphabetic List. Bethesda, Maryland, The Library, 1998.
7. Hochberg MC: The history of lupus erythematosus. Md Med J 40:871, 1991.
8. Lahita RG: Special report: Adjusted lupus prevalence—Results of a marketing study by the Lupus Foundation of America. Lupus 4:450, 1995.
9. Ropes MW: Systemic Lupus Erythematosus. Cambridge, Mass., Harvard University Press, 1976.
10. Siegel M, Holley HL, Lee SL: Epidemiologic studies on systemic lupus erythematosus: Comparative data for New York City and Jefferson County, Alabama, 1956–1965. Arthritis Rheum 13:802, 1970.
11. Robbins WC, Holman HR, Deicher H, Kunkel HG: Complement Fixation with Cell Nuclei and DNA in Lupus Erythematosus. New York, Society for Experimental Biology and Medicine, 1957, pp 575-579.
12. Hahn BH: Antibodies to DNA [Review]. N Engl J Med 338:1359, 1998.
13. Hahn BH, Singh RR, Ebling FM: Self Ig peptides that help anti-DNA antibody production: Importance of charged residues [see comments]. Lupus 7:307, 1998.
14. Pauls JD, Gohill J, Fritzler MJ: Antibodies from patients with systemic lupus erythematosus and drug-induced lupus bind determinants on histone 5 (H5). Mol Immunol 27:701, 1990.
15. Ebling FM, Hahn BH: Pathogenic subsets of antibodies to DNA (Review). Int Rev Immunol 5:79, 1989.
16. Holman HR: Thought barriers to understanding rheumatic diseases. Arthritis Rheum 37:1565, 1994.
17. Rose LM, Latchman DS, Isenberg DA: Bcl-2 and Fas, molecules which influence apoptosis: A possible role in systemic lupus erythematosus? [Review]. Autoimmunity 17:271, 1994.
18. Rose LM, Latchman DS, Isenberg DA: Apoptosis in peripheral lymphocytes in systemic lupus erythematosus: A review. Br J Rheumatol 36:158, 1997.
19. Sontheimer RD: Photoimmunology of lupus erythematosus and dermatomyositis: A speculative review. Photochem Photobiol 63:583, 1996.
20. Fritzler MJ: Antinuclear antibodies in the investigation of rheumatic diseases. Bull Rheum Dis 35:1, 1985.
21. Sontheimer RD, McCauliffe DP, Zappi E, Targoff I: Antinuclear antibodies: Clinical correlations and biologic significance [review]. Adv Dermatol 7:3, discussion 53, 1992.
22. Gladman DD: Indicators of disease activity, prognosis, and treatment of systemic lupus erythematosus [Review]. Curr Opin Rheumatol 6:487, 1994.
23. Gladman DD, Goldsmith CH, Urowitz MB, et al: Sensitivity to change of 3 systemic lupus erythematosus disease activity indices: International validation. J Rheumatol 21:1468, 1994.
24. Fortin PR, Abrahamowicz M, Danoff D: Small changes in outpatients' lupus activity are better detected by clinical instruments than by laboratory tests. J Rheumatol 22:2078, 1995.
25. Smolen JS, Strand V, Cardiel M, et al: Randomized clinical trials and longitudinal observational studies in systemic lupus erythematosus: Consensus on a preliminary core set of outcome domains. J Rheumatol 26:504, 1999.
26. Klippel JH: Systemic lupus erythematosus: Demographics, prognosis, and outcome [Review]. J Rheumatol 48(Suppl):67, 1997.
27. Jonsson H, Nived O, Sturfelt G, Silman A: Estimating the incidence of systemic lupus erythematosus in a defined population using multiple sources of retrieval [See comments]. Br J Rheumatol 29:185, 1990.
28. McCarty DJ, Manzi S, Medsger TA Jr., et al: Incidence of systemic lupus erythematosus: Race and gender differences. Arthritis Rheum 38:1260, 1995.
29. Hochberg MC: Prevalence of systemic lupus erythematosus in England and Wales, 1981–2. Ann Rheum Dis 46:664, 1987.
30. Lawrence RC, Hochberg MC, Kelsey JL, et al: Estimates of the prevalence of selected arthritic and musculoskeletal diseases in the United States. J Rheumatol 16:427, 1989.
31. Fessel WJ: Systemic lupus erythematosus in the community. Arch Intern Med 134:1027, 1974.
32. Hochberg MC, Perlmutter DL, Medsger TA, et al: Prevalence of self-reported physician-diagnosed systemic lupus erythematosus in the USA. Lupus 4:454, 1995.
33. Cohen AS, Canoso JJ: Criteria for the classification of systemic lupus erythematosus: status 1972. Arthritis Rheum 15:540, 1972.
34. Canoso JJ, Cohen AS: A review of the use, evaluations, and criticisms of the preliminary criteria for the classification of systemic lupus erythematosus. Arthritis Rheum 22:917, 1979.
35. Tan EM, Cohen AS, Fries JF, et al: The 1982 revised criteria for the classification of systemic lupus erythematosus. Arthritis Rheum 25:1271, 1982.
36. Hochberg MC: Updating the American College of Rheumatology revised criteria for the classification of systemic lupus erythematosus [Letter; see comments]. Arthritis Rheum 40:1725, 1997.
37. Edworthy SM: Classification criteria: What value do they serve? J Rheumatol 19:192, 1992.
38. Schur PH: Clinical features of SLE. In Kelly WN, Harris ED, Ruddy S, Sledge CB (eds): Textbook of Rheumatology. Philadelphia, WB Saunders, 1989, pp 1101-1129.
39. Edworthy SM, Zatarain E, McShane DJ, Bloch DA: Analysis of the 1982 ARA lupus criteria data set by recursive partitioning methodology: New insights into the relative merit of individual criteria [See comments]. J Rheumatol 15:1493, 1988.
40. Perez-Gutthann S, Petri M, Hochberg MC: Comparison of different methods of classifying patients with systemic lupus erythematosus. J Rheumatol 18:1176, 1991.
41. Edworthy SM: A database for systemic lupus erythematosus and systemic connective tissue disorders [Review]. Rheum Dis Clin North Am 21:501, 1995.
42. Panush SR, Greer JM, Morshedian KK: What is lupus? What is not lupus? [Abstract]. Controversies Clin Rheumatol 19:223, 1993.
43. Tan EM, Feltkamp TE, Smolen JS, et al: Range of antinuclear antibodies in "healthy" individuals [See comments]. Arthritis Rheum 40:1601, 1997.
44. Suarez-Almazor ME, Gonzales-Lopez J, Gamez-Nava I, et al: Utilization and predictive value of laboratory tests in patients referred to rheumatologists by primary care physicians. J Rheumatol 25:1980, 1998.
45. Isenberg DA, Dudeney C, Williams W, et al: Measurement of anti-DNA antibodies: A reappraisal using five different methods. Ann Rheum Dis 46:448, 1987.
46. Villarreal GM, Drenkard C, Villa AR, et al: Prevalence of 13 autoantibodies and of the 16/6 and related pathogenic idiotypes in 465 patients with systemic lupus erythematosus and their relationship with disease activity. Lupus 6:425, 1997.
47. Ravirajan CT, Rahman MA, Papadaki L, et al: Genetic, structural and functional properties of an IgG DNA-binding monoclonal

antibody from a lupus patient with nephritis. Eur J Immunol 28:339, 1998.

48. Williams WM, Isenberg DA: A cross-sectional study of anti-DNA antibodies in the serum and IgG and IgM fraction of healthy individuals, patients with systemic lupus erythematosus and their relatives. Lupus 5:576, 1996.

49. Esdaile JM, Joseph L, Abrahamowicz M, et al: Routine immunologic tests in systemic lupus erythematosus: Is there a need for more studies? [See comments]. J Rheumatol 23:1891, 1996.

50. Isenberg DA, Garton M, Reichlin MW, Reichlin M: Long-term follow-up of autoantibody profiles in black female lupus patients and clinical comparison with Caucasian and Asian patients. Br J Rheumatol 36:229, 1997.

51. Cabral AR, Alarcon-Segovia D: Autoantibodies in systemic lupus erythematosus [Review]. Curr Opin Rheumatol 9:387, 1997.

52. Alarcon-Segovia D, Estanol B, Garcia-Ramos G, Villa AR: Antiphospholipid antibodies and the antiphospholipid syndrome: Clinical relevance in neuropsychiatric systemic lupus erythematosus. Ann N Y Acad Sci 823:279, 1997.

53. Alarcon-Segovia D, Mestanza M, Cabiedes J, Cabral AR: The antiphospholipid/cofactor syndromes. II. A variant in patients with systemic lupus erythematosus with antibodies to β_2-glycoprotein I but no antibodies detectable in standard antiphospholipid assays. J Rheumatol 24:1545, 1997.

54. Casciola-Rosen L, Rosen A, Petri M, Schlissel M: Surface blebs on apoptotic cells are sites of enhanced procoagulant activity: Implications for coagulation events and antigenic spread in systemic lupus erythematosus. Proc Natl Acad Sci USA 93:1624, 1996.

55. Mujic F, Cuadrado MJ, Lloyd M, et al: Primary antiphospholipid syndrome evolving into systemic lupus erythematosus. J Rheumatol 22:1589, 1995.

56. Werth VP, Dutz JP, Sontheimer RD: Pathogenetic mechanisms and treatment of cutaneous lupus erythematosus [Review]. Curr Opin Rheumatol 9:400, 1997.

57. McCauliffe DP, Sontheimer RD: Dermatologic manifestations of rheumatic disorders (Review). Prim Care 20:925, 1993.

58. Sontheimer RD, Maddison PJ, Reichlin M, et al: Serologic and HLA associations in subacute cutaneous lupus erythenmatosus, a clinical subset of lupus erythematosus. Ann Intern Med 97:664, 1982.

59. Wysenbeek AJ, Block DA, Fries JF: Prevalence and expression of photosensitivity in systemic lupus erythematosus. Ann Rheum Dis 48:461, 1989.

60. Cohen MR, Isenberg DA: Ultraviolet irradiation in systemic lupus erythematosus: Friend or foe? [Review]. Br J Rheumatol, 35:1002, 1996.

61. Del Papa N, Conforti G, Gambini D, et al: Characterization of the endothelial surface proteins recognized by anti-endothelial antibodies in primary and secondary autoimmune vasculitis. Clin Immunol Immunopathol 70:211, 1994.

62. Sontheimer RD: Fluorescent light photosensitivity in patients with systemic lupus erythematosus: Comment on the article by Rihner and McGrath [Letter; comment]. Arthritis Rheum 36:428, 1993.

63. Asherson RA, Angus H, Mathews JA, et al: The progressive systemic sclerosis/systemic lupus overlap: An unusual clinical progression. Ann Rheum Dis 50:323, 1991.

64. Alarcon-Segovia D: Mixed connective tissue disease: A decade of growing pains. J Rheumatol 8:535, 1981.

65. Grennan DM, Bunn C, Hughes GR, et al: Frequency and clinical significance of antibodies to ribonucleoprotein in SLE and other connective tissue disease subgroups. Ann Rheum Dis 36:442, 1977.

66. Black C, Isenberg DA: Mixed connective tissue disease: Goodbye to all that [Review; see comments]. Br J Rheumatol 31:695, 1992.

67. Alarcon-Segovia D, Cardiel MH: Comparison between 3 diagnostic criteria for mixed connective tissue disease: Study of 593 patients. J Rheumatol 16:328, 1989.

68. Martin L, Edworthy SM, Ryan JP, Fritzler MJ: Upper airway disease in systemic lupus erythematosus: A report of 4 cases and a review of the literature [Review]. J Rheumatol 19:1186, 1992.

69. Cervera R, Font J, Pare C, et al: Cardiac disease in systemic lupus erythematosus: Prospective study of 70 patients. Ann Rheum Dis 51:156, 1992.

70. Ames DE, Asherson RA, Coltart JD, et al: Systemic lupus erythematosus complicated by tricuspid stenosis and regurgitation: Successful treatment by valve transplantation. Ann Rheum Dis 51:120, 1992.

71. Chartash EK, Lans DM, Paget SA, et al: Aortic insufficiency and mitral regurgitation in patients with systemic lupus erythematosus and the antiphospholipid syndrome. Am J Med 86:407, 1989.

72. Khamashta MA, Cervera R, Asherson RA, et al: Association of antibodies against phospholipids with heart valve disease in systemic lupus erythematosus [see comments]. Lancet 335: 1541, 1990.

73. Asherson RA, Gibson DG, Evans DW, et al: Diagnostic and therapeutic problems in two patients with antiphospholipid antibodies, heart valve lesions, and transient ischemic attacks. Ann Rheum Dis 47:947, 1988.

74. Cervera R, Khamashta MA, Font J, et al: Systemic lupus erythematosus: Clinical and immunologic patterns of disease expression in a cohort of 1,000 patients—The European Working Party on Systemic Lupus Erythematosus. Medicine (Baltimore) 72:113, 1993.

75. Richter Cohen M, Steiner G, Smolen JS, Isenberg DA: Erosive arthritis in systemic lupus erythematosus: Analysis of a distinct clinical and serological subset. Br J Rheumatol 37:421, 1998.

76. Wang B, Gladman DD, Urowitz MB: Fatigue in lupus is not correlated with disease activity. J Rheumatol 25:892, 1998.

77. Gladman DD, Urowitz MB, Gough J, MacKinnon A: Fibromyalgia is a major contributor to quality of life in lupus. J Rheumatol 24:2145, 1997.

78. Petri M: Clinical features of systemic lupus erythematosus [Review]. Curr Opin Rheumatol 7:395, 1995.

79. Garton MJ, Isenberg DA: Clinical features of lupus myositis versus idiopathic myositis: A review of 30 cases. Br J Rheumatol 36:1067, 1997.

80. Gertner E. Goodman R, Gladman DD: Successive unfolding of two different collagen vascular diseases in the same patient. J Rheumatol 16:126, 1989.

81. Keeling DM, Isenberg DA: Haematological manifestations of systemic lupus erythematosus [Review]. Blood Rev 7:199, 1993.

82. Deleze M, Alarcon-Segovia D, Oria CV, et al: Hemocytopenia in systemic lupus erythematosus: Relationship to antiphospholipid antibodies [published erratum appears in J Rheumatol 16:1523, 1989]. J Rheumatol 16:926, 1989.

83. Edworthy SM, Bloch DA, McShane DJ, et al: A "state model" of renal function in systemic lupus erythematosus: Its value in the prediction of outcome in 292 patients. J Rheumatol 16:29, 1989.

84. Jorfen M, Callejas JL, Formiga F, et al: Fulminant thrombotic thrombocytopenic purpura in systemic lupus erythematosus. Scand J Rheumatol 27:76, 1998.

85. McDonagh JE, Khamashta MA, Menon S, et al: A young woman with SLE: Diagnostic and therapeutic challenges. Lupus 6:633, 1997.

86. Drenkard C, Villa AR, Garcia-Padilla C, et al: Remission of systemic lupus erythematosus. Medicine (Baltimore) 75:88, 1996.

87. Hakim AJ, Machin SJ, Isenberg DA: Autoimmune thrombocytopenia in primary antiphospholipid syndrome and sytemic lupus erythematosus: The response to splenectomy. Semin Arthritis Rheum 28:20, 1998.

88. Rivero SJ, Alger M, Alarcon-Segovia D: Splenectomy for hemocytopenia in systemic lupus erythematosus: A controlled appraisal. Arch Intern Med 139:773, 1979.

89. Hughes GR, Khamashta MA: The antiphospholipid syndrome [Review]. J R Coll Physicians Lond 28:301, 1994.

90. Drenkard C, Villa AR, Alarcon-Segovia D, Perez-Vazquez ME: Influence of the antiphospholipid syndrome in the survival of patients with systemic lupus erythematosus. J Rheumatol 21:1067, 1994.

91. Font J, Torras A, Cervera R, et al: Silent renal disease in systemic lupus erythematosus. Clin Nephrol 27:283, 1987.

92. Fraenkel L, MacKenzie T, Joseph L, et al: Response to treatment as a predictor of longterm outcome in patients with lupus nephritis. J Rheumatol 21:2052, 1994.

93. Fries JF, Porta J, Liang MH: Marginal benefit of renal biopsy in systemic lupus erythematosus. Arch Intern Med 138:1386, 1978.

94. McLaughlin JR, Bombardier C, Farewell VT, et al: Kidney biopsy in systemic lupus erythematosus. III. Survival analysis

controlling for clinical and laboratory variables. Arthritis Rheum 37:559, 1994.

95. Gladman DD, Urowitz MB, Cole E, et al: Kidney biopsy in SLE. I. A clinical-morphologic evaluation. Q J Med 73:1125, 1989.

96. Esdaile JM, MacKenzie T, Barre P, et al: Can experienced clinicians predict the outcome of lupus nephritis? Lupus 1:205, 1992.

97. Balow JE, Austin HA III, Muenz LR, et al: Effect of treatment on the evolution of renal abnormalities in lupus nephritis. N Engl J Med 311:491, 1984.

98. Austin HA III, Muenz LR, Joyce KM, et al: Prognostic factors in lupus nephritis. Contribution of renal histologic data. Am J Med 75:382, 1983.

99. Houssiau FA, D'Cruz D, Vianna J, Hughes GR: Lupus nephritis: The significance of serological tests at the time of biopsy. Clin Exp Rheumatol 9:345, 1991.

100. Fries JF: The clinical aspects of systemic lupus erythematosus. Med Clin North Am 61:229, 1977.

101. Fritzler MJ, O'Brien MD: The purification, characterization and amino acid analysis of nuclear ribonuclear protein and Sm antigens reacting with human autoimmune sera. Clin Invest Med 6:61, 1983.

102. Bunn CC, Gharavi AE, Hughes GR: Antibodies to extractable nuclear antigens in 173 patients with DNA-binding positive SLE: An association between antibodies to ribonucleoprotein and Sm antigens observed by counterimmunoelectrophoresis. J Clin Lab Immunol 8:13, 1982.

103. Karsh J, Klippel JH, Balow JE, Decker JL: Mortality in lupus nephritis. Arthritis Rheum 22:764, 1979.

104. Merrill JT, Lahita RG: The antiphospholipid syndrome and SLE: Is there a clue in the link between complement and coagulation? [review]. Lupus 5:6, 1996.

105. Asherson RA, Cervera R: Review: Antiphospholipid antibodies and the lung. J Rheumatol 22:62, 1995.

106. Rubin LA, Urowitz MB: Shrinking lung syndrome in SLE—a clinical pathologic study. J Rheumatol 10:973, 1983.

107. Asherson RA, Hughes GR: The expanding spectrum of Libman Sacks endocarditis: The role of antiphospholipid antibodies [Review]. Clin Exp Rheumatol 7:225, 1989.

108. Mont MA, Glueck CJ, Pacheco IH, et al: Risk factors for osteonecrosis in systemic lupus erythematosus [See comments]. J Rheumatol 24:654, 1997.

109. Bruce IN, Gladman DD, Urowitz MB: Detection and modification of risk factors for coronary artery disease in patients with systemic lupus erythematosus: A quality improvement study. Clin Exp Rheumatol 16:435, 1998.

110. Dinu AR, Merrill JT, Shen C, et al: Frequency of antibodies to the cholesterol transport protein apolipoprotein A1 in patients with SLE. Lupus 7:355, 1998.

111. Manzi S, Meilahn EN, Rairie JE, et al: Age-specific incidence rates of myocardial infarction and angina in women with systemic lupus erythematosus: Comparison with the Framingham Study. Am J Epidemiol 145:408, 1997.

112. Petri M, Perez-Gutthann S, Spence D, Hochberg MC: Risk factors for coronary artery disease in patients with systemic lupus erythematosus. Am J Med 93:513, 1992.

113. Boey ML, Colaco CB, Gharavi AE, et al: Thrombosis in systemic lupus erythematosus: Striking association with the presence of circulating lupus anticoagulant. Br Med J Clin Res Ed 287:1021, 1983.

114. Hughes GR, Mackworth-Young C, Harris EN, Gharavi AE: Venoocclusive disease in systemic lupus erythematosus: Possible association with anticardiolipin antibodies? [Letter]. Arthritis Rheum 27:1071, 1984.

115. Harris EN, Gharavi AE, Hughes GR: Anti-phospholipid antibodies [Review]. Clin Rheum Dis 11:591, 1985.

116. Harris EN, Hughes GR, Gharavi AE: Antiphospholipid antibodies: An elderly statesman dons new garments. J Rheumatol 14(Suppl)13:208, 1987.

117. Lawrie AS, Lloyd ME, Mohamed F, et al: Assay of protein S in systemic lupus erythematosus. Blood Coagul Fibrinolysis 6:322, 1995.

118. Tishler M, Alosachie I, Chapman Y, et al: Anti-neuronal antibodies in antiphospholipid syndrome with central nervous system envolvement: The difference from systemic lupus erythematosus. Lupus 4:145, 1995.

119. Cervera R, Khamashta MA, Font J, et al: Anti-endothelial cell antibodies in systemic lupus erythematosus: Association with vascular and renal lesions [in Spanish]. Med Clin (Barc) 99:605, 1992.

120. Cordeiro MF, Lloyd ME, Spalton DJ, Hughes GR: Ischaemic optic neuropathy, transverse myelitis, and epilepsy in an antiphospholipid positive patient with systemic lupus erythematosus [Letter]. J Neurol Neurosurg Psychiatry 57:1142, 1994.

121. Lavalle C, Pizarro S, Drenkard C, et al: Transverse myelitis: A manifestation of systemic lupus erythematosus strongly associated with antiphospholipid antibodies [See comments]. J Rheumatol 17:34, 1990.

122. Martinez-Rueda JO, Arce-Salinas CA, Kraus A, et al: Factors associated with fetal losses in severe systemic lupus erythematosus. Lupus 5:113, 1996.

123. Lima F, Buchanan NM, Khamashta MA, et al: Obstetric outcome in systemic lupus erythematosus (Review). Semin Arthritis Rheum 25:184, 1995.

124. Boumpas DT, Fessler BJ, Austin HA III, et al: Systemic lupus erythematosus: Emerging concepts. II.: Dermatologic and joint disease, the antiphospholipid antibody syndrome, pregnancy and hormonal therapy, morbidity and mortality, and pathogenesis [Review]. Ann Intern Med 123:42, 1995.

125. Petri M: Systemic lupus erythematosus and pregnancy [Review]. Rheum Dis Clin North Am 20:87, 1994.

126. Lockshin MD: Why do patients with antiphospholipid antibody clot? [Editorial; comment]. Lupus 6:351, 1997.

127. Chinn RJ, Wilkinson ID, Hall-Craggs MA, et al: Magnetic resonance imaging of the brain and cerebral proton spectroscopy in patients with systemic lupus erythematosus. Arthritis Rheum 40:36, 1997.

128. Hanly JG, Liang MH: Cognitive disorders in systemic lupus erythematosus. Epidemiologic and clinical issues [Review]. Ann N Y Acad Sci 823:60, 1997.

129. Ginsburg KS, Wright EA, Larson MG, et al: A controlled study of the prevalence of cognitive dysfunction in randomly selected patients with systemic lupus erythematosus. Arthritis Rheum 35:776, 1992.

130. Khamashta MA, Cervera R, Hughes GR: The central nervous system in systemic lupus erythematosus [Review]. Rheumatol Int 11:117, 1991.

131. Mok CC, Lau CS, Ho CT, et al: Safety of hormonal replacement therapy in postmenopausal patients with systemic lupus erythematosus. Scand J Rheumatol 27:342, 1998.

132. Kreidstein S, Urowitz MB, Gladman DD, Gough J: Hormone replacement therapy in systemic lupus erythematosus. J Rheumatol 24:2149, 1997.

133. Mok CC, Wong RW, Lau CS: Ovarian failure and flares of systemic lupus erythematosus. Arthritis Rheum 42:1274, 1999.

134. LeBlanc BA, Urowitz MB, Gladman OD: Serologically active, clinically quiescent systemic lupus erythematosus: Longterm followup [Letter]. J Rheumatol 21:174, 1994.

135. Abrahamowicz M, Fortin PR, du Berger R, et al: The relationship between disease activity and expert physician's decision to start major treatment in active systemic lupus erythematosus: A decision aid for development of entry criteria for clinical trials. J Rheumatol 25:277, 1998.

136. Wluka AE, Liang MH, Partridge AJ, et al: Assessment of systemic lupus erythematosus disease activity by medical record review compared with direct standardized evaluation. Arthritis Rheum 40:57, 1997.

137. Vitali C, Bencivelli W, Isenberg DA, et al: Disease activity in systemic lupus erythematosus: Report of the Consensus Study Group of the European Workshop for Rheumatology Research. II. Identification of the variables indicative of disease activity and their use in the development of an activity score: The European Consensus Study Group for Disease Activity in SLE [Review]. Clin Exp Rheumatol 10:541, 1992.

138. Liang MH, Socher SA, Larson MG, Schur PH: Reliability and validity of six systems for the clinical assessment of disease activity in systemic lupus erythematosus. Arthritis Rheum 32:1107, 1989.

139. Isenberg D: Comparison of lupus activity indices. Clin Exp Rheumatol 8(Suppl 5):37, 1990.

140. Liang MH, Fortin PR, Isenberg DA, Snaith L: Quantitative clinical assessment of disease activity in systemic lupus erythemato-

sus: Progress report and research agenda. Rheumatol Int 11:133, 1991.

141. Bombardier C, Gladman DD, Urowitz MB, et al: Derivation of the SLEDAI: A disease activity index for lupus patients. The Committee on Prognosis Studies in SLE. Arthritis Rheum 35:630, 1992.

142. Hay EM, Bacon PA, Gordon C, et al: The BILAG index: A reliable and valid instrument for measuring clinical disease activity in systemic lupus erythematosus. Q J Med 86:447, 1993.

143. Liang MH, Fortin PR: Response criteria for clinical trials in systemic lupus erythematosus [published erratum appears in Lupus 6:619, 1997]. Lupus 4:336, 1995.

144. Esdaile JM, Abrahamowicz M, Joseph L, et al: Laboratory tests as predictors of disease exacerbations in systemic lupus erythematosus: Why some tests fail [See comments]. Arthritis Rheum 39:370, 1996.

145. Ehrenstein MR, Conroy SE, Heath J, et al: The occurrence, nature and distribution of flares in a cohort of patients with systemic lupus erythematosus: A rheumatological view [See comments]. Br J Rheumatol 34:257, 1995.

146. Petri M, Genovese M, Engle E, Hochberg M: Definition, incidence, and clinical description of flare in systemic lupus erythematosus. A prospective cohort study. Arthritis Rheum 34:937, 1991.

147. Cabral AR, Alarcon-Segovia D: Anti–β_2-glycoprotein I antibody testing in patients with antiphospholipid syndrome [Letter; comment]. Br J Rheumatol 36:1235, 1997.

148. Buyon JP, Tamerius J, Belmont HM, Abramson SB: Assessment of disease activity and impending flare in patients with systemic lupus erythematosus: Comparison of the use of complement split products and conventional measurements of complement. Arthritis Rheum 35:1028, 1992.

149. Ter Borg EJ, Horst G, Hummel EJ, et al: Measurement of increases in anti–double-stranded DNA antibody levels as a predictor of the disease exacerbation in systemic lupus erythematosus: A long-term, prospective study. Arthritis Rheum 33:634, 1990.

150. Ruiz-Arguelles A, Angles-Cano E, Perez-Romano B, et al: Serum antibodies to distinct epitopes of the tissue-type plasminogen activator (t-PA) in patients with systemic lupus erythematosus. Am J Hematol 49:109, 1995.

151. Stoll T, Seifert B, Isenberg DA: SLICC/ACR Damage Index is valid, and renal and pulmonary organ scores are predictors of severe outcome in patients with systemic lupus erythematosus. Br J Rheumatol 35:248, 1996.

151a. Devins GM, Edworthy SM, Paul LC, et al: Restless sleep, illness intrusiveness, and depressive symptoms in three chronic illness conditions: Rheumatoid arthritis, end-stage renal disease, and multiple sclerosis. J Psychosom Res 37(2):163-70, 1993.

151b. Devins GM, Edworthy SM: Illness intrusiveness explains race-related quality-of-life differences among women with systemic lupus erythematosus. Lupus 9(7):534-41, 2000.

151c. Devins GM, Dion R, Pelletier LG, et al: Structure of lifestyle disruptions in chronic disease: A confirmatory factor analysis of the Illness Intrusiveness Ratings Scale. Med Care 39(10):1097-104, 2001.

151d. Edworthy SM, Dobkin PL, Clarke AE, et al: Group psychotherapy reduces illness intrusiveness in systemic lupus erythematosus. J Rheumatol 30(5):1011-6, 2003.

152. Gladman DD: Prognosis and treatment of systemic lupus erythematosus [Review]. Curr Opin Rheumatol 7:402, 1995.

153. Abu-Shakra M, Urowitz MB, Gladman DD, Gough J: Mortality studies in systemic lupus erythematosus: Results from a single center. II. Predictor variables for mortality. J Rheumatol 22:1265, 1995.

154. Abu-Shakra M, Urowitz MB, Gladman DD, Gough J: Mortality studies in systemic lupus erythematosus: Results from a single center. I. Causes of death. J Rheumatol 22:1259, 1995.

155. Stoll T, Gordon C, Seifert B, et al: Consistency and validity of patient administered assessment of quality of life by the MOS SF-36; its association with disease activity and damage in patients with systemic lupus erythematosus. J Rheumatol 24:1608, 1997.

156. Gladman DD, Urowitz MB, Ong A, et al: Lack of correlation among the 3 outcomes describing SLE: Disease activity, damage and quality of life. Clin Exp Rheumatol 14:305, 1996.

157. Gladman DD, Urowitz MB, Ong A, et al: A comparison of five health status instruments in patients with systemic lupus erythematosus (SLE). Lupus 5:190, 1996.

158. Shortall E, Isenberg D, Newman SP: Factors associated with mood and mood disorders in SLE. Lupus 4:272, 1995.

159. Peterson MG, Horton R, Engelhard E, et al: Effect of counselor training on skills development and psychosocial status of volunteers with systemic lupus erythematosus. Arthritis Care Res 6:38, 1993.

160. Gladman DD: Prognosis and treatment of systemic lupus erythematosus [Review]. Curr Opin Rheumatol 8:430, 1996.

161. Molina JF, Drenkard C, Molina J, et al: Systemic lupus erythematosus in males. A study of 107 Latin American patients [Review]. Medicine (Baltimore) 75:124, 1996.

162. Simmons-O'Brien E, Chen S, Watson R, et al: One hundred anti-Ro (SS-A) antibody positive patients: A 10-year follow-up. Medicine (Baltimore) 74:109, 1995.

163. Esdaile JM: Prognosis in systemic lupus erythematosus [Review]. Springer Semin Immunopathol 16:337, 1994.

164. Esdaile JM, Joseph L, MacKenzie T, et al: The benefit of early treatment with immunosuppressive agents in lupus nephritis [see comments]. J Rheumatol 21:2046, 1994.

165. Esdaile JM, Joseph L, MacKenzie T: The pathogenesis and prognosis of lupus nephritis: Information from repeat renal biopsy. Semin Arthritis Rheum 23:135, 1993.

166. Seleznick MJ, Fries JF: Variables associated with decreased survival in systemic lupus erythematosus. Semin Arthritis Rheum 21:73, 1991.

167. Urowitz MB, Gladman DD, Abu-Shakra M, Farewell VT: Mortality studies in systemic lupus erythematosus: Results from a single center. III. Improved survival over 24 years. J Rheumatol 24:1061, 1997.

168. Pons-Estel R: Lupus Around the World Workshops. CW-2: Lupus in Latin Americans. In Hughes G (ed): Programs and Abstracts from the Fifth International Conference on SLE, Cancun, Mexico, April 20-25, 1998. Lupus 7(suppl 1):9, 1998.

169. Karlson EW, Daltroy LH, Lew RA, et al: The relationship of socioeconomic status, race, and modifiable risk factors to outcomes in patients with systemic lupus erythematosus. Arthritis Rheum 40:47, 1997.

170. Liang MH, Partridge AJ, Daltroy LH, et al: Strategies for reducing excess morbidity and mortality in blacks with systemic lupus erythematosus [Review]. Arthritis Rheum 34:1187, 1991.

171. Callahan LF, Pincus T: Associations between clinical status questionnaire scores and formal education level in persons with systemic lupus erythematosus. Arthritis Rheum 33:407, 1990.

172. Ramsey-Goldman R, Kutzer JE, Kuller LH, et al: Previous pregnancy outcome is an important determinant of subsequent pregnancy outcome in women with systemic lupus erythematosus. Am J Reprod Immunol 28:195, 1992.

173. Rahman P, Gladman DD, Urowitz MB: Clinical predictors of fetal outcome in systemic lupus erythematosus. J Rheumatol 25:1526, 1998.

174. Brucato A, Franceshini F, Buyon JP: Neonatal lupus: Long-term outcomes of mothers and children and recurrence rate [Review]. Clin Exp Rheumatol 15:467, 1997.

175. Silverman ED, Buyon J, Laxer RM, et al: Autoantibody response to the Ro/La particle may predict outcome in neonatal lupus erythematosus. Clin Exp Immunol 100:499, 1995.

176. Khamashta MA, Hughes GR: Pregnancy in systemic lupus erythematosus [Review]. Curr Opin Rheumatol 8:424, 1996.

177. Magid MS, Kaplan C, Sammaritano LR, et al: Placental pathology in systemic lupus erythematosus: A prospective study. Am J Obstet Gynecol 179:226, 1998.

178. Buchanan NM, Khamashta MA, Morton KE, et al: A study of 100 high risk lupus pregnancies [Review]. Am J Reprod Immunol 28:192, 1992.

179. Harris EN, Asherson RA, Hughes GR: Antiphospholipid antibodies: Autoantibodies with a difference [Review]. Annu Rev Med 39:261, 1988.

180. Abramson SB, Buyon JP: Activation of the complement pathway: Comparison of normal pregnancy, preeclampsia, and systemic lupus erythematosus during pregnancy [Review]. Am J Reprod Immunol 28:183, 1992.

181. Ruiz-Irastorza G, Khamashta M, Hughes GR: Does SLE flare during pregnancy? [Review]. Scand J Rheumatol Suppl 107:76, 1998.

182. Khamashta MA, Ruiz-Irastorza G, Hughes GR: Systemic lupus erythematosus flares during pregnancy [Review]. Rheum Dis Clin North Am 23:15, 1997.

183. Ruiz-Irastorza G, Lima F, Alves J, et al: Increased rate of lupus flare during pregnancy and the puerperium: A prospective study of 78 pregnancies. Br J Rheumatol 35:133, 1996.

184. Lockshin MD: Does lupus flare during pregnancy? [Editorial]. Lupus 2:1, 1993.

185. Buchanan NM, Toubi E, Khamashta MA, et al: Hydroxychloroquine and lupus pregnancy: Review of a series of 36 cases. Ann Rheum Dis 55:486, 1996.

186. Gladman DD, Urowitz MB, Senecal JL, et al: Aspects of use of antimalarials in systemic lupus erythematosus. J Rheumatol 25:983, 1998.

187. Ramsey-Goldman R, Mientus JM, Kutzer JE, et al: Pregnancy outcome in women with systemic lupus erythematosus treated with immunosuppresive drugs. J Rheumatol 20:1152, 1993.

188. McAllister DL, Kaplan BJ, Edworthy SM, et al: The influence of systemic lupus erythematosus on fetal development: Cognitive, behavioral, and health trends. J Int Neuropsychol Soc 3:370, 1997.

189. McInnes PM, Schuttinga J, Sanslone WR, et al: The economic impact of treatment of severe lupus nephritis with prednisone and intravenous cyclophosphamide. Arthritis Rheum 37:1000, 1994.

76

Management of Systemic Lupus Erythematosus

BEVRA HANNAHS HAHN

Management of systemic lupus erythematosus (SLE) is a challenge because no interventions can result in cure, exacerbations of disease can occur after months of stable maintenance treatment, and undesirable side effects of the therapies can be as troublesome as the disease. Careful and frequent monitoring of patients is important in selecting management plans, monitoring efficacy, and changing treatments.

Initial Therapeutic Decisions

Because most therapeutic interventions in patients with SLE are associated with significant undesirable side effects, the physician must first decide whether a patient needs treatment and, if so, whether conservative management is sufficient or aggressive immunosuppression is necessary. Figure 76–1 presents an algorithm for this decision making.

In general, patients with manifestations of SLE that are not life threatening and are unlikely to be associated with organ damage should be treated conservatively. If quality of life is mildly impaired, education and careful follow-up may be adequate. If quality of life is impaired, it is appropriate to initiate strategies listed in Figure 76–1 as conservative measures. On the other hand, if the disease is life threatening or if major organ systems are at high risk for irreversible damage, aggressive intervention is mandatory. Aggressive therapy usually consists of immunosuppression. A few clinical subsets of SLE have been recognized, however, for which immunosuppression is either not effective or alternative therapies may be preferable. The best example of this is patients who have recurring thrombosis as the major manifestation of SLE. In the subsequent sections, conservative therapies, the approach to patients with life-threatening SLE, and therapies effective in different clinical subsets are reviewed.

The pharmacology, mechanisms of action, benefits, and side effects of most of the drugs used in the management of SLE are reviewed in Section VII of this book. This chapter discusses the use of these agents in SLE.

Conservative Management

ARTHRITIS, ARTHRALGIA, AND MYALGIA

Arthritis, arthralgia, and myalgia are the most common manifestations of SLE. Severity ranges from mild to disabling. For patients with mild symptoms, administration of analgesics, nonsteroidal anti-inflammatory drugs (NSAIDs), or salicylates may provide adequate relief, although none of these is as effective as glucocorticoids.[1-3]

Nonacetylated salicylates are useful because they inhibit prostaglandin synthesis less than acetylated salicylates and NSAIDs and, therefore, are associated with a relatively low incidence of gastrointestinal symptoms and bleeding. They usually do not impair platelet function. Therapeutic range (approximately 150 to 200 mg/dl) can be assessed by measuring serum salicylate levels.

The use of standard NSAIDs that inhibit both cyclooxygenase-1 and -2 (COX-1 and -2), or NSAIDs that are more specific inhibitors of COX-2, requires special caution in patients with SLE. Several agents (ibuprofen, tolmetin, sulindac, rofecoxib) can cause aseptic meningitis.[4,5] Through their effects on renal prostaglandins, all NSAIDs can reduce glomerular filtration rates and renal blood flow, especially in patients who have clinical or subclinical nephritis, who are taking diuretics, or who have congestive heart failure or cirrhosis. Although sulindac is least likely to have this effect, it does occur; serum creatinine levels should be monitored after introduction of any salicylate or NSAID. Hyperkalemia and interstitial nephritis are uncommon side effects of NSAIDs. Salt retention secondary to NSAID use may elevate blood pressure and cause pedal edema; NSAIDs may reduce the efficacy of furosemide and thiazide diuretics. Gastrointestinal toxicity with ulcer symptoms, perforation, or bleeding can develop at any time during therapy. Protection from gastrointestinal adverse events has not been studied in patients with SLE, but the prevalence of this problem is lower in individuals treated with NSAIDs that inhibit COX-2 more than COX-1, at least for the first year of therapy.[4,6] Finally, patients with SLE have a higher incidence of hepatotoxicity than other patients taking standard NSAIDs[4]; hepatotoxicity is usually manifested as transaminitis without permanent hepatic damage. In summary, SLE patients treated with NSAIDs should be monitored regularly for renal, gastrointestinal, and hepatic side effects.

Concomitant use of glucocorticoids and NSAIDs that strongly inhibit COX-1 substantially increases the risk of gastrointestinal bleeding. Use of such NSAIDs with or without glucocorticoids may require addition of gastroprotective therapies—either proton pump inhibitors such as omeprazole or the prostaglandin analogue misoprostol.[7] Glucocorticoids also increase clearance of salicylates; lowering glucocorticoid doses may be accompanied by increases in serum salicylate levels.

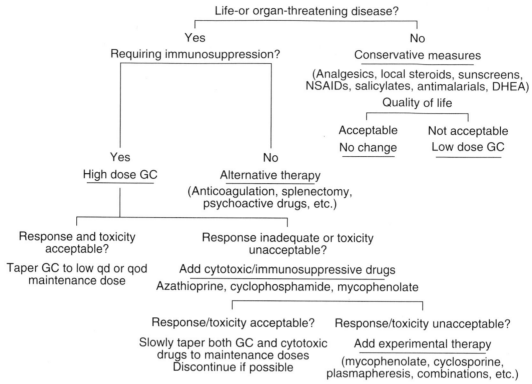

FIGURE 76–1 · An Algorithm for Selecting Management of Patients with Systemic Lupus Erythematosus (SLE).

In many SLE patients, musculoskeletal symptoms are not well controlled by salicylate or NSAID therapy. A trial of antimalarial drugs may be useful in such individuals, or as initial therapy in patients with prominent arthralgia or arthritis.[8,9] Antimalarials are discussed later with the treatment of cutaneous manifestations. Hydroxychloroquine is the preferred antimalarial agent in the United States (chloroquine may be more effective but has a higher incidence of retinal toxicity; quinacrine is often effective but, rarely, can cause aplastic anemia). The usual dose of hydroxychloroquine for SLE patients with arthritis is 400 mg daily. If response does not occur within 6 months, the patient can be considered a nonresponder and the drug stopped. If hydroxychloroquine is used for more than 6 months or chloroquine is used for more than 3 months, regular examination by an ophthalmologist for retinal damage is mandatory. If antimalarials are effective, the maintenance dose should be reduced periodically if possible, or the drug should be withdrawn when a patient is doing well, because the retinal toxicity is cumulative.

Some patients with arthritis or arthralgia do not benefit from NSAIDs or salicylates, with or without antimalarials. Administration of dihydroandrosterone (DHEA), 100 to 200 mg daily, lowers activity of SLE in some patients, including arthritis and arthralgias.[10] A recent study has suggested that 200 mg/day is more effective than lower doses.[11] Acne is a side effect in 10 to 30 percent of patients; the potential adverse effects of elevated serum levels of testosterone, which occurs in all women treated with DHEA in these doses, is unknown.

Methotrexate (MTX) in weekly oral or parenteral doses of 10 to 20 mg may also be considered, because there are reports of its efficacy in lupus arthritis.[12] Recent uncontrolled studies of leflunomide treatment in patients with SLE have suggested that disease activity, including arthritis, is reduced.[13] However, none of these interventions is as reliable as glucocorticoid therapy in suppressing lupus arthritis and arthralgia. If quality of life is seriously impaired by joint pain, the physician should consider institution of low-dose glucocorticoids, not to exceed 15 mg each morning. Rare patients require high-dose glucocorticoids or even cytotoxic drugs. Such interventions should be avoided if possible. In fact, if arthritis is the major manifestation of disease that compels the physician to choose high-dose immunosuppressive treatments, it may be preferable to use around-the-clock non-narcotic or narcotic analgesics to control pain, rather than risk the life-threatening side effects of immunosuppression.

Pain that persists in one or two joints may be due to ischemic necrosis of bone or, rarely, to septic arthritis. Ischemic necrosis of bone can be associated with warmth and swelling in contiguous joints; it should be ruled out in patients with a small number of persistently inflamed or painful joints (especially knees, hips, shoulders, wrists, or ankles) who do not have additional evidence of active SLE before these patients are treated for lupus arthritis.

CUTANEOUS LUPUS

As many as 70 percent of patients with SLE are photosensitive.[14] Flares of SLE can be caused by ultraviolet

(UV) light, infrared light, heat, or rarely, fluorescent light. Some patients are sensitive to UVB (290 to 320 nm), some to UVA (320 to 400 nm), and some to both. Photosensitive patients should minimize their exposure by wearing protective clothing, using tinted glass in car windows, avoiding direct sun exposure, and applying sunscreens. Most topical sunscreens are creams, oils, lotions, or gels that physically block or scatter UVB light; contain UV light–blocking chemicals such as para-aminobenzoic acid (PABA) and its esters, benzophenones, salicylates, anthranilates, and cinnamates; or both.[15] All absorb UVB light; UVA is absorbed partially by benzophenones and anthranilates. The sun protection factor (SPF) is the ratio of the time required for UVB to produce erythema when sunscreen is worn compared to the time required to produce the same degree of erythema in unprotected skin. SPFs range from 2 to 50; lupus patients should use preparations with an SPF of 15 or higher. The agents should be reapplied after toweling or sweating.

Table 76–1 lists some available high-protection sunscreens that are free of PABA; there is a relatively high prevalence of contact dermatitis to PABS. Patients should begin with preparations that block UVA and UVB. Sunscreens can be locally irritating (especially those that contain PABA); patients may need to try several preparations to find one that is not irritating, drying, or staining and that stays on well. Cosmetic preparations of concealing makeup that cover disfiguring lesions and also contain products that block UV light are also listed in Table 76–1. Local glucocorticoids, including topical creams and ointments and injections into severe skin lesions, are also helpful in lupus dermatitis.[15,16] Patients with disfiguring (discoid) or extensive lesions should be seen by a dermatologist, because management of severe lupus dermatitis can be difficult. Because topical steroids, especially fluorinated preparations, can cause skin atrophy, depigmentation, telangiectasia, and fragility, care

should be taken to choose the correct preparations for the involved area. Facial lesions should be treated with low- to medium-potency nonfluorinated preparations (hydrocortisone, desonide); trunk and arm lesions with medium-potency fluorinated preparations (betamethasone valerate, triamcinolone acetonide); and scalp lesions with medium-potency preparations administered as lotions. Hypertrophic lesions elsewhere and disabling lesions on the palms and soles should be treated with high-potency topical glucocorticoids (betamethasone dipropionate, clobetasol).[15,16] Continuous use of high-potency creams should be limited to 2 weeks, if possible, after which time less-potent preparations should be substituted for a brief time, or topical steroid therapy could be stopped altogether. Because skin lesions often worsen when topical therapies are discontinued, additional strategies may be required.

An alternative to topical steroids is topical tacrolimus, which is FDA-approved for contact dermatitis. Tacrolimus inhibits T cell activation locally. Use of 0.1% cream on lesions twice a day for 3 weeks has been repeated in open trials as effective in some patients for molar SLE rash, discoid lupus, and subacute cutaneous lupus.[16,16a]

Antimalarial agents are useful in many patients with lupus dermatitis, whether the lesions are those of SLE, subacute cutaneous lupus, or discoid lupus.[8,16-19] Antimalarials have multiple sunblocking, anti-inflammatory, and immunosuppressive effects. They may be immunosuppressive as a result of binding to lysosomal cell membranes, where they alter pH with subsequent impairment of protein processing to peptides, assembly of the α- and β-chains of HLA class II molecules, and of transport of mature class II molecules containing peptides to the surfaces of antigen-presenting cells (APC). Thus, T cell activation is impaired. In addition, antimalarials reduce the release of interleukin 1 (IL-1), IL-6, and tumor necrosis factor-α (TNF-α) from monocytes

TABLE 76–1 · SUNSCREEN PREPARATIONS WITH SUN PROTECTION FACTOR (SPF) OF 15 OR GREATER

Product	SPF	Contents	Comments
Physical sunscreens Dermablend, Covermark, Clinique, AFil Shiseido	15 15	Zinc oxide (has been improved to finer particles to permit transparent products; recent silicone coating improved absorption of reflected light), titanium dioxide, talc, petrolatum	Advantage: Can hide lesions Disadvantages: Some preparations are messy, sandy; recently products have improved
Chemical sunscreens (UVA plus UVB blockers)		Aminobenzoates (e.g., PABA), benzophenones, cinnamates, dibenzoylmethones, salicylates, avobenzone	May be mixed with physical sunscreens
Bain de Soleil*	15, 30		
Photoplex	15		
Shade UVAGuard	15		
Total Eclipse	15		
PreSun*	15		
Coppertone Sunscreen	15		
Ti Screen	15, 30		
Sundown Sunblock*	15		
Presun	30, 39		
Neutragena oil-free sunblock	30		
Bull Frog	36		

*Contains PABA, which can occasionally sensitize skin, as can most ingredients listed.

Abbreviations: PABA, Para-aminobenzoic acid; UVA, ultraviolet A; UVB, ultraviolet B.

and macrophages, and of IL-2 and interferon-γ (IFN-γ) from T cells. They also bind melanin and serve as sunscreens, and they have antiplatelet and cholesterol-lowering effects. All these properties may be beneficial to patients with SLE.

A controlled trial of hydroxychloroquine in patients with stable lupus showed that replacement of the anti-malarial agent with placebo resulted in a significant increase in flare-ups, some of which were serious.[9] In addition, multiple open studies of hundreds of patients with discoid lupus erythematosus (LE), SLE, or suba-cute cutaneous LE have reported that 60 to 90 percent of patients with cutaneous lupus have good to excellent responses to antimalarials.[8,16] Higher doses of each agent give earlier responses, and a larger proportion of patients improve. (Higher doses are more toxic.) Responses to chloroquine and quinacrine are usually demonstrable within 1 to 3 months; responses to hydrox-ychloroquine may require 3 to 6 months. Antimalarials may be steroid sparing. Recommended initial doses of antimalarials are as follows: hydroxychloroquine, 400 mg daily; chloroquine phosphate, 500 mg daily; and quinacrine, 100 mg daily. Higher doses can be given for brief periods (2 to 4 weeks). After disease is well controlled, the drugs can be slowly tapered. Daily doses can be reduced, or the drug can be given less frequently (e.g., a few days each week). The combina-tion of hydroxychloroquine (or chloroquine) and quinacrine is probably synergistic and can be used in patients refractory to single-drug therapy.

Toxicities of these agents are important but infrequent in comparison with other agents used to treat SLE.[8] Retinal damage is the most important; it can occur in up to 10 percent of patients receiving chronic chloroquine therapy but in less than 5 percent of those receiving hydroxychloroquine. Regular ophthalmologic examina-tions with appropriate special testing can identify retinal changes early. If changes occur, antimalarial therapy should be stopped or the daily dose decreased. This strat-egy substantially lowers the incidence of clinically impor-tant retinal toxicity. Other significant adverse events associated with all the antimalarials include gastrointesti-nal disturbances (nausea, diarrhea, weight loss), rashes, peripheral neuropathies, and myopathies of skeletal and cardiac muscles. Quinacrine is associated with aplas-tic anemia, especially in patients who experience an antecedent lichen planus–like rash.[8] Pigment changes are common with quinacrine (usually a yellow discoloration of skin). They occur less frequently with chloroquine and hydroxychloroquine, which can cause depigmenta-tion, hyperpigmentation, and blue-black discoloration of skin, nails, and mucous membranes. If neuropathies or myopathies develop, antimalarials should be discontin-ued; skin changes are usually tolerated by patients (in the case of quinacrine, any dermatitis other than pig-ment changes or lupus dermatitis should cause the physi-cian to discontinue treatment). The use of antimala-rials during pregnancy is controversial, with conflicting reports of fetal damage and of good outcomes; most reports indicate no adverse effects on the fetus.[18] Use of antimalarial agents in lupus is reviewed in Table 76–2.

For individuals with lupus rash resistant to antimalari-als and other conservative strategies, systemic therapy with retinoids such as isotretinoin or topical therapy with tretinoin have been beneficial.[16,17] Initial doses of 1 mg/kg divided into two daily doses are recommended; within a few weeks response occurs and the dose should be tapered. Discontinuing the therapy is often followed by flare of skin lesions. Systemic retinoids are teratogenic, cause cheilitis in most patients, and elevate cholesterol

TABLE 76–2 • USE OF ANTIMALARIALS AND EXPERIMENTAL REGIMENS TO TREAT CUTANEOUS LUPUS

Agent	Initial Dose	Maintenance Dose	Response	Toxicities
Hydroxychloroquine	400-600 mg/day	100-400 mg/day	Dermatitis (SLE, DLE, SCLE), arthralgia, arthritis, oral ulcers, fatigue	Retinal damage, corneal deposit, skin pigmentation, rashes, alopecia, peripheral neuropathy, peripheral myopathy, cardiomyopathy, nausea, anorexia, diarrhea, psychosis
Chloroquine	500mg/day for one week	250 mg daily or every other day (*do not exceed 4mg/kg)	As for hydroxychloroquine; probably most effective for arthritis	As for hydroxychloroquine; probably most toxic for the retina
Quinacrine	100 mg/day	50-100 mg/day	Probably most effective for fatigue	Aplastic anemia (often preceded by lichen planus rash); little or no retinal damage; yellow pigmentation of skin
Hydroxychloroquine or chloroquine plus quinacrine	As indicated above	As indicated above	Effects probably additive for dermatitis	Toxicities probably not additive
Experimental dapsone	25 mg twice daily	25 mg/day	Dermatitis (especially DLE and bullous LE)	Methemoglobinemia, sulfhemoglobinemia, hemolytic anemia, gastrointestinal intolerance
Etretinate	1 mg/kg/day in 2 divided doses	0.25-0.5 mg/kg/day	Dermatitis (especially DLE and SCLE)	Hyperlipidemia, cheilitis, fetal abnormalities

Abbreviations: DLE, Disseminated lupus erythematosus; LE, lupus erythematosus; SCLE, subacute cutaneous lupus erythematosus; SLE, systemic lupus erythematosus.

and triglyceride levels in some. Patients resistant to anti-malarials and retinoids may require systemic glucocorti-coids, which improve lupus skin lesions of any type.

Additional treatments, which should be considered experimental for dermatologic lupus because there are no controlled prospective trials, include dapsone, thalidomide, and tacrolimus (FK506).[16,19-22] Dapsone has been used in discoid lupus, urticarial vasculitis, and bullous LE lesions with some success. The recommended initial dose is 50 mg daily; that can be increased to 100 mg daily for a few weeks if needed. Dapsone has significant hematologic toxicities (including methemoglobinemia, sulfhemoglobinemia, hemolytic anemia, and aplastic anemia) as well as exfoliative dermatitis, acute tubular necrosis, peripheral neuropathy, and hepatotoxicity. It can occasionally worsen the rashes of LE. Many experts have reported success with thalidomide therapy in approximately 50 percent of individuals with refractory skin lesions of SLE or subacute cutaneous lupus (as well as for other manifestations of active lupus including refractory aphthous-type mouth ulcers).[20,21] Low doses (e.g., 50 mg twice a day) may be effective and are reported to be substantially less toxic than higher doses. Adverse effects include, most importantly, teratogenesis, so use of thalidomide in the United States is severely restricted and is provided only after contact with and screening by the manufacturer. Fertility control must be maintained. Other side effects may include peripheral neuropathy, neutropenia, hypertension, bradycardia, and seizures, along with drowsiness, dizziness, diarrhea, and fever. Topical tacrolimus (FK506) interferes with cutaneous T cell function: The preparation is approved in the United States for treatment of atopic dermatitis, at 0.03 or 0.1 percent concentrations applied twice a day. There are a few reports of efficacy in refractory cutaneous lupus.[22]

Some steroid-resistant cases of lupus dermatitis have improved when treated with cytotoxic drugs such as asazathioprine or MTX.[16,17] I have found MTX particularly useful in this situation; I begin doses of 10 mg/week and escalate the dose every few weeks if needed (as for management of patients with rheumatoid arthritis [RA]), then taper slowly if efficacious. Folic acid supplementation is recommended. Side effects of these cytotoxic drugs include bone marrow suppression (particularly leukopenia), hepatotoxicity, increased infections (including herpes zoster), nausea and diarrhea, and aphthous stomatitis.

FATIGUE AND SYSTEMIC COMPLAINTS

Fatigue is common in patients with SLE and may be the major disabling complaint. It reflects multiple problems, including depression, sleep deprivation, and fibromyalgia, as well as disease activity.[23,24] Some patients are improved by treatment of any of these aspects, with glucocorticoids and antimalarials sometimes suppressing this manifestation, at least in part. Complaints of fatigue should be approached sympathetically, with recommendations for increased rest periods and flexibility in working hours when possible. Fever and weight loss, if mild, can be managed with the conservative approaches out-

lined in the preceding paragraphs. When severe, systemic glucocorticoid therapy is necessary.

SEROSITIS

Episodes of chest and abdominal pain may be secondary to lupus serositis. In some patients, complaints respond to salicylates, NSAIDs (indomethacin may be best), antimalarial therapies, or to low doses of systemic glucocorticoids, such as 15 mg/day.[1] In others, systemic glucocorticoids must be given in high doses to achieve disease control.

Aggressive Therapy

INDICATIONS

Institution of aggressive therapy, beginning with high-dose glucocorticoids, should be used whenever a patient has life-threatening SLE that is likely to respond to steroids. The serious manifestations of lupus that usually improve with glucocorticoid therapy are listed in Table 76–3. Some manifestations may not be steroid responsive (e.g., pure membranous glomerulonephritis, vascular occlusions). Other manifestations respond to therapy but may be mild enough that high doses of glucocorticoids are not necessary, such as hemolytic anemia with hematocrit values of 30 to 34 percent and no symptoms, thrombocytopenia of 50,000 to 120,000 cells/mm^3 without bleeding, mesangial glomerulonephritis, and mild cognitive dysfunction.

TABLE 76–3 • SERIOUS AND LIFE-THREATENING MANIFESTATIONS OF SYSTEMIC LUPUS ERYTHEMATOSUS (SLE): RESPONSES TO GLUCOCORTICOIDS

Manifestations usually responsive to high-dose glucocorticoids
  Vasculitis
  Severe dermatitis of subacute cutaneous lupus
    erythematosus or SLE
  Polyarthritis
  Polyserositis—pericarditis, pleurisy, peritonitis
  Myocarditis
  Lupus pneumonitis*
  Glomerulonephritis—proliferative forms
  Hemolytic anemia
  Thrombocytopenia
  Diffuse central nervous system syndrome*—acute
    confusional state, demyelinating syndromes,
    intractable headache
  Serious cognitive defects
  Myelopathies
  Peripheral neuropathies
  Lupus crisis*—high fever and prostration
Manifestations not often responsive to glucocorticoids
  Thrombosis—includes strokes
  Glomerulonephritis—scarred end-stage renal disease,
    pure membranous glomerulonephritis
  Resistant thrombocytopenia or hemolytic anemia—occurs
    in a minority of patients; consider splenectomy, cytotoxics,
    danazol, or cyclosporine/neoral therapies
  Psychosis related to conditions other than SLE, such as
    glucocorticoid therapy

*Special care should be taken to rule out infectious processes before immunosuppressive therapies are instituted.

Infectious causes of the manifestations interpreted as lupus must be carefully excluded before instituting or increasing glucocorticoid therapy, especially in the presence of pulmonary infiltrates, confusion states, hematuria with pyuria, and fever. Finally, the physician must consider the presence of comorbid conditions that increase the risk of glucocorticoid therapy, such as infection, hypertension, diabetes mellitus, obesity, osteoporosis, and psychiatric disorders. When all factors are carefully analyzed and the decision is made to institute aggressive therapy, institution of high-dose glucocorticoids is the appropriate first step, sometimes with addition of cytotoxic drugs.

CLASSIFICATION OF LUPUS NEPHRITIS

Table 76–4 lists the current World Health Organization (WHO) morphologic classification of lupus nephritis, as modified. Most of the prospective controlled trials in patients with SLE have been conducted in patients with proliferative forms of glomerulonephritis (classes IIIA or B, IV, or VB). Others have included patients with clinical evidence of active nephritis, such as worsening proteinuria, microscopic hematuria, or rising levels of serum creatinine, whether or not the patients have had a renal biopsy. In general, aggressive immunosuppression is recommended in patients with proliferative forms of lupus nephritis with a high histologic score for active lesions and a low score for chronic lesions.

GLUCOCORTICOID THERAPY

Efficacy of Daily High-Dose Therapy

Most of the randomized, prospective, controlled trials of glucocorticoid therapy in SLE have been conducted in patients with life-threatening forms of lupus nephritis, with comparisons made between the efficacy of steroids and that of other interventions, which usually consist of steroids plus a cytotoxic drug. Therefore, guidelines for management of all serious disease come primarily from studies of patients with nephritis.

The most convincing evidence that high-dose glucocorticoids can be lifesaving was provided by Pollak and colleagues[25,26] in retrospective studies of patients with diffuse proliferative glomerulonephritis (DPGN). Figure 76–2 illustrates their outcomes. Their original data antedate the availability of dialysis and renal transplantation. Two years after renal biopsy, patients with DPGN treated with less than 40 mg of prednisone a day had a survival rate of 0 percent; patients treated with 40 to 60 mg of prednisone for 4 to 6 months had a survival rate of 55 percent. The average doses were, in the low-dose group, 10 to 15 mg/day and, in the high-dose group, 47.5 mg/day for 6 months. These studies form the basis of current practice,[2,3] although the use of 40 to 60 mg of prednisone daily is rarely continued for more than 4 to 12 weeks. Standard practice for treatment with single-drug therapy in patients with severe forms of lupus nephritis is to begin 1 mg/kg per day (usually 40 to 60 mg of prednisone daily) for 4 to 6 weeks. Thereafter, the dose should be tapered as rapidly as disease activity permits. Alternatively, patients who have severe, active SLE may be treated with high doses of intravenous (IV) methylprednisolone (10 to 20 mg/kg, usually 500 to 1000 mg total) daily for 1 to 3 days to "induce" response, followed by daily glucocorticoid treatment. The advantages of this approach are discussed in the section on IV methylprednisolone.

Monitoring Responses

Several problems arise when these guidelines for glucocorticoid therapy are followed[1-3]:

1. Some patients do not respond.
2. Some patients respond initially but relapse when the dose is tapered.
3. Toxic side effects of glucocorticoids are virtually universal.

To minimize these problems, the physician should establish what constitutes acceptable clinical responses and set time limits to achieve those responses.

The criteria for response should include both clinical and laboratory parameters, when the laboratory parameters provide good measures of the clinical problem being addressed. For example, in patients with nephritis, serum levels of creatinine, complement, and blood urea nitrogen should improve within 2 to 10 weeks of institution of therapy. Quantities of antibodies to DNA should fall during the same period. Proteinuria should diminish and renal function should improve after 2 to 10 weeks of daily high-dose prednisone. In some unusual patients, clinical improvement occurs without changes in autoantibody titers or serum complement levels. In contrast to nephritis, hemolysis and thrombocytopenia usually begin to improve within 5 to 15 days after glucocorticoid therapy is instituted. Manifestations of central nervous system (CNS) lupus, such as acute confusional states, severe headache, and diffuse demyelination syndromes, often improve within days; other manifestations such as psychosis, movement disorders, and cognitive changes may require several weeks to improve. If the desired effect is not obtained within the appropriate time frame, the next decision is whether to change the glucocorticoid dose, to introduce additional therapy, or to stop immunosuppression. Patients with several months of renal insufficiency (e.g., serum creatinine levels above 2 mg/dl) and high chronicity indices on renal biopsy are unlikely to improve. It is appropriate to plan for dialysis or renal transplantation in such patients. (See the discussion later in this chapter in the section on outcomes in patients with SLE.)

Intravenous Pulse Therapy and Alternate-Day Regimens

In an effort to increase response rates and the rapidity of responses, and to decrease side effects of daily high-dose glucocorticoid therapy, several experts have studied the efficacy of administering methylprednisolone (10 to 30 mg/kg, 500 to 1000 mg/dose), in single high IV doses for three to six doses, then maintaining responses with

TABLE 76-4 · USE OF GLUCOCORTICOIDS IN SYSTEMIC LUPUS ERYTHEMATOSUS (SLE)

Severe, Active SLE

Preparations	Dose	Advantages	Toxicities
REGIMEN 1: Daily oral short-acting (prednisone, prednisolone, methylprednisolone)	1–2 mg/kg daily; begin in divided doses	Controls disease rapidly; 5–10 days for hematologic or central nervous system disease, serositis, or vasculitis; 2–10 wks for glomerulonephritis	High—infections, sleeplessness, mood swings, hyperglycemia, psychosis, hypertension, weight gain, hypokalemia, fragile skin, bruising, osteoporosis, ischemic necrosis of bone, irregular menses, muscle cramps, sweats, acne, hirsutism, cataracts
REGIMEN 2: Intravenous methylprednisolone	500–1000 mg every day for 3–5 days. Then, 1–1.5 mg/kg/day of oral glucocorticoid	Controls disease rapidly: may achieve results more rapidly than daily oral therapy; a few nonresponders to regimen 1 respond to regimen 2	High—same as for daily except more rapid taper of daily maintenance steroid dose may be possible, leading to lower cumulative doses
REGIMEN 3: Combine regimen 1 or 2 with a cytotoxic or other immunosuppressive drug (see Table 76–5)			

SLE Well Controlled by Therapy (Maintenance Regimens)

REGIMEN 1: Continue daily oral glucocorticoid. Consolidate to a single morning dose. Then, begin a slow taper of single daily dose: reduce by 5 to 15% every week if tolerated. When a dose of 30 mg/day is reached, reduce by 2.5-mg increments. When a dose of 10–15 mg/day is reached, reduce by 1-mg increments. If disease flares, increase to most recent effective dose and hold there for a few weeks.

REGIMEN 2: Begin to taper to an alternate-day glucocorticoid regimen. Consolidate to single-dose daily therapy, then begin taper on alternate-day regimen. For example, 60 mg/day tapers to 60 mg alternating with 50 mg. Work down to 60 mg every other day, then taper by 5–15% increments every 1–2 weeks.

REGIMEN 3: To regimen 1 or 2, add additional therapies that optimize glucocorticoid taper, such as antimalarials for dermatitis or arthritis or nonsteroidal anti-inflammatory drugs (NSAIDs) for fever, arthritis, and serositis.

If tapering to 15 mg daily, 30 mg every other day, or less is achieved without disease flare, consider managing the disease with glucocorticoids alone. If maintenance doses are higher, consider adding a cytotoxic drug (see Table 76–5).

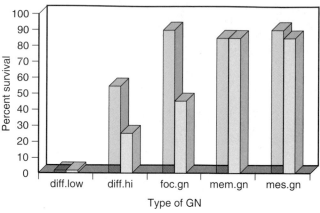

FIGURE 76-2 · Survival in Patients with Systemic Lupus Erythematosus (SLE). Percentage of patients surviving in each group defined by renal biopsy histology is shown for 2 years (black bars) and 5 years (gray bars). Survival was calculated by life table analysis from the time at which the renal biopsy was performed. Note that high-dose prednisone improved survival in patients with diffuse proliferative glomerulonephritis (DPGN), that 100 percent with that lesion and insignificant immunosuppressive therapy died (data precede the era of dialysis and renal transplantation), and that histologic diagnoses other than DPGN are associated with a better prognosis, particularly if there are no proliferative changes outside the mesangium. Diff.low, patients with DPGN (class IV) who received no prednisone or low-dose prednisone (less than 40 mg/day); diff.hi, patients with DPGN who received 40 to 60 mg/day of prednisone for 4 to 6 months; foc.gn, patients with focal proliferative (class III) nephritis, therapy unspecified; mem.gn, patients with purely membranous nephritis, therapy unspecified; mes.gn, patients with minimal changes confined to mild proliferation in mesangial areas only, therapy not specified. (Based on data from Pollak VE, Dosekun AK: Evaluation of treatment in lupus nephritis: Effects of prednisone. Am J Kidney Dis 2(Suppl 2):170, 1982.)

high doses of daily oral prednisone (40 to 60 mg), which are rapidly tapered.[1] Uncontrolled trials[1,27,28] suggest that 75 percent or more of lupus patients with severe active nephritis, CNS disease, pneumonitis, polyserositis, vasculitis, or thrombocytopenia improve within a few days.

Some patients who fail to improve on 40 to 60 mg of prednisone daily respond to high-dose pulse therapy.[1,27,28] Patients who have active disease with rapid increases in proteinuria and rapid increases in serum creatinine level are most likely to respond. In a prospective, randomized controlled trial,[29] initial pulses followed by daily oral prednisone therapy improved renal function a mean of 12 weeks earlier than standard daily therapy; the final renal function (measured as inulin clearances) was similar in both groups. Another controlled trial in a small number of patients[30] compared 12 months of repeated pulses of IV methylprednisolone (given three sequential days each month and followed by high-dose daily prednisone, then tapered) to daily high-dose prednisone (then tapered) in SLE patients with DPGN. After 1 year, renal function was significantly better and maintenance prednisone requirement was significantly lower in the group that received IV steroid pulses. Therefore, use of pulse glucocorticoids followed by daily oral glucocorticoids, compared to daily oral glucocorticoids alone, has the benefit of earlier response, but probably not better response.

With regard to the comparison of pulse glucocorticoids followed by oral daily glucocorticoids to pulse cyclophosphamide with oral daily glucocorticoids, most

data suggest that the cyclophosphamide regimen is superior. In three recent studies,[31,33,34] renal function was preserved better in patients randomized to cyclophosphamide groups, provided that cyclophosphamide was given for at least 6 months (results were even better in patients treated with IV cyclophosphamide for 30 months). In one of these studies,[34] the cohort was followed for a mean of 11 years. In a study[32] that concluded the two regimens did not differ in influence on outcomes, the IV cyclophoshamide versus methylprednisolone regimens were administered for only 4 months.

To address the question of whether combinations of cyclophosphamide plus IV pulses of methylprednisolone might be superior to regimens containing only one of these therapies, one study[33] compared pulse cyclophosphamide (0.5 to 1.0 g/m^2 body surface area), pulse methylprednisolone (1 g/m^2 body surface area once a month for at least 1 year), and combined therapies in SLE patients with nephritis. Renal remission rates over a 5-year period were 85 percent in the combination group, 62 percent in the cyclophosphamide group, and 29 percent in the methylprednisolone group. Although differences between combination therapy and cyclophosphamide did not reach statistical significance, both groups receiving cyclophosphamide did better than the methylprednisolone group, and there was a trend for combination therapy to be better than cyclophosphamide alone. Amenorrhea, cervical dysplasia, at least one important infection, and herpes zoster were all more common in the groups receiving cyclophosphamide; ischemic necrosis of bone was found somewhat more frequently in the pulse methylprednisolone group.

Overall, the incidence of adverse side effects is probably not increased when high-dose pulse therapy with glucocorticoids is compared with high-dose daily therapy. However, steroid withdrawal syndromes, acute psychosis, rapid increases in blood pressure, seizures, arrhythmias, and sudden death have been reported.[1]

In summary, many patients with severe, active SLE respond within days or a few weeks to IV pulses of methylprednisolone followed by daily oral glucocorticoids. Response of renal disease occurs earlier if pulse steroids are added to daily glucocorticoids. The physician can administer methylprednisolone therapy for 3 days, then start 1 mg/kg (40 to 60 mg) of prednisone daily, then rapidly taper the dose to low levels of daily or alternate-day oral glucocorticoid maintenance therapy. The author uses pulse glucocorticoid regimens in patients with severe SLE who are experiencing rapid clinical deterioration. Repeating pulse glucocorticoid therapy monthly (1 to 3 days a month) is an acceptable alternative to addition of cytotoxic drugs. However, long-term results (5 years or more) suggest that addition of cyclophosphamide to glucocorticoid regimens improves renal outcomes, and that pulses of cyclophosphamide are more effective in controlling nephritis than pulses of methylprednisolone. However, in patients refractory to standard daily glucocorticoid therapy plus IV cyclophosphamide, regular IV pulses of methylprednisolone may offer better disease control.

With regard to treatment regimens that use alternate-day glucocorticoids, one study[35] reported good responses in five of seven patients with lupus nephritis treated initially with prednisone (100 to 120 mg every other day); however, I have had little success with alternate-day therapy in patients with severe active disease and cannot recommend it. It is desirable to initiate daily glucocorticoid therapy, then taper to maintenance regimens of a short-acting glucocorticoid (e.g., prednisone, prednisolone, methylprednisolone) given in the morning once every 48 hours. Such regimens, compared with daily glucocorticoid administration, are associated with significantly less suppression of the hypothalamic-pituitary axis, as well as less potassium and nitrogen wasting, hypertension, cushingoid changes, and infection.[36] Disease must be well suppressed before such regimens are appropriate.

Summary of Glucocorticoid Use in Severe Systemic Lupus Erythematosus

Glucocorticoid regimens and their side effects are reviewed in Table 76–5. Most patients with severe active SLE improve substantially on glucocorticoid regimens.

Initial therapy should be either high-dose daily glucocorticoids (40 to 100 mg prednisone daily, or 1 to 1.5 mg/kg) given in divided doses, or high-dose IV methylpredniso-lone pulses followed by 40 to 60 mg prednisone (or equivalent short-acting glucocorticoid) daily. Some manifestations may respond as early as 1 to 5 days, others require 2 to 10 weeks (especially nephritis). If the desired response is obtained within an appropriate time, tapering of daily glucocorticoid doses is initiated. Daily doses may be decreased by 5 to 15 percent weekly if flares do not occur. A substantial proportion of patients experience steroid withdrawal during tapering (e.g., fever, nausea, joint pain, malaise, frank arthritis); such reactions should not last more than 3 days. There should be an attempt to reach a maintenance low daily or alternate-day glucocorticoid dose. In most cases, the disease flares during the tapers; when this occurs, the dose should be increased and held at the level necessary to control severe disease. If the maintenance requirement is unacceptable because of side effects, institution of an additional agent is recommended.

TABLE 76–5 • USE OF CYTOTOXIC DRUGS IN SYSTEMIC LUPUS ERYTHEMATOSUS (SLE) IN ADDITION TO GLUCOCORTICOIDS

Drug	Initial Dose	Maintenance Dose	Advantages	Adverse Side Effects	Incidence (%)
Azathioprine; requires 6–12 months to work well	1–3 mg/kg/day	1–2 mg/kg/day	Probably reduces flares, reduces renal scarring, reduces glucocorticoid dose requirement	Bone marrow suppression	<5
				Leukopenia	15
				Infections (including herpes zoster)	40–70
				Malignancies	<5
				Infertility	15
				Early menopause	10
				Hepatic damage	<5
				Nausea	15
Cyclophosphamide; requires 2–16 weeks to work well	1–3 mg/kg/day orally or 8–20 mg/kg intravenously once a month plus mesna	0.5–2 mg/kg/day orally or 8–20 mg/kg intravenously every 4–12 wks plus mesna	As for azathioprine, probably effective in higher proportion of patients	Bone marrow suppression	<5
				Leukopenia	30
				Infections	30
				Malignancies	<5
				Cystitis*	15
				Infertility	50
				Menopause	50
				Nausea	20
				Alopecia	20
Mycophenolate mofetil	Initial Dose 500 mg bid, increase over a few weeks to 1500 mg bid	Unknown	Improves nephritis, better tolerated than cyclophosphamide	Diarrhea Nausea, W, GIsx	17 / 23
				Infection	30–42
				Neutropenia	<5
				Thrombocytopenia	<5
Combination therapy: Azathioprine plus	1.5–2.5 mg/kg/day orally	1–2 mg/kg/day orally	Possibly more effective than one drug	Infections	40
Cyclophosphamide	1.5–2.5 mg/kg/day orally	1–2 mg/kg/day orally		Cystitis*	15

*Hemorrhagic cystitis, urinary bladder sclerosis, and carcinoma of the urinary bladder are infrequent if cyclophosphamide is given intravenously, especially with mesna.

CYTOTOXIC DRUGS

Life-Threatening Lupus and Severe Forms of Lupus Nephritis

Two groups of cytotoxic drugs have been used in large numbers of patients with severe SLE—purine antagonists and alkylating agents. There is increasing use of MTX and of the T cell–specific immunosuppressive agent mycophenolate mofetil, and new cytotoxic drugs are being studied. The first cytotoxic agent used in SLE was nitrogen mustard.[37] The two drugs used most frequently are azathioprine (Imuran) and cyclophosphamide (Cytoxan); of the two, cyclophosphamide is more effective and more toxic. Cyclophosphamide suppresses both humoral and cellular immune responses more effectively than azathioprine, and in contrast to azathioprine is not cell cycle–dependent. Mycophenolate mofetil is coming into wide usage. Doses of these drugs, their side effects, and guidelines to combination therapies are reviewed in Table 76–6.

Azathioprine

With regard to azathioprine in doses of 2 to 3 mg/kg/day, short-term studies (1 to 2 years in duration) have failed to show a better outcome in patients with severe SLE treated with glucocorticoids plus azathioprine compared with those treated with glucocorticoids alone.[38] In studies that follow patients for 5 to 15 years, however, individuals who receive combination therapy have fewer chronic changes on renal biopsy, better renal function, fewer severe disease flares, and lower glucocorticoid requirements.[39-41] Significant adverse side effects of chronic azathioprine therapy include increased rates of infection with opportunistic organisms (especially herpes zoster), ovarian failure, bone marrow suppression (especially leukopenia), hepatic damage, and increased susceptibility to malignancies.[41-43] For patients with severe SLE, some experts use daily or pulse glucocorticoid regimens and a cytotoxic drug (azathioprine in slowly progressive disease; cyclophosphamide or mycophenolate mofetil in rapidly progressive disease).

In general, the physician should allow 6 to 12 months for azathioprine to be effective. After disease is well controlled and glucocorticoid doses are tapered to the lowest possible maintenance levels, doses of azathioprine should be slowly tapered and discontinued if disease is well controlled for a year or more.

Cyclophosphamide

The benefits of cyclophosphamide therapy have been somewhat controversial due to conflicting reports regarding its efficacy in severe SLE and its numerous undesirable side effects. Some authorities have suggested that it is effective over the short term in only a small proportion of patients with severe lupus nephritis[44,45] and that it does not change long-term outcome. Furthermore, many patients prefer azathioprine because it less toxic, even when informed that cyclophosphamide may be more efficacious.[46] Other data[31,33,34,39-41] suggest that cyclophosphamide is effective in most patients with

TABLE 76–6 • STRATEGIES TO MINIMIZE THE ADVERSE EFFECTS OF TREATMENT WITH GLUCOCORTICOIDS OR CYTOTOXIC DRUGS IN PATIENTS WITH SYSTEMIC LUPUS ERYTHEMATOSUS (SLE)

I. Methods of using drugs
  A. Initiate use only in patients with life-threatening disease or severely impaired quality of life.
  B. Monitor at frequent intervals.
    1. Glucocorticoids—electrolytes, CBC count, glucose levels, evidence of infection, blood pressure, intraocular pressure, formation of cataracts, evidence for osteoporosis
    2. Cytotoxic drugs—CBC count, platelet count, liver function tests, evidence of infection, urinalysis for microscopic hematuria (with oral cyclophosphamide), signs of malignancy
  C. Reduce drug doses as frequently as possible.
II. Treatment and prevention of infections
  A. Be aware of the high incidence of infections, both ordinary and opportunistic. The most frequent organisms are herpes zoster, urinary tract infections with gram-negative bacteria, and infections with *Staphylococcus*, *Candida* (including sepsis), *Pneumocystis carinii*. Mycobacteria, fungi, and viruses such as CMV are not unusual. Monitor carefully for evidence of these.
  B. If infection is suspected, treat for the most likely organisms. Therapy can be discontinued or changed after culture information is available.
  C. Immunize to prevent infections. Annual influenza vaccination and one immunization with pneumococcal vaccine (Pneumovax 23) are recommended for all patients.
  D. Some recurring infections can be prevented, or their frequency diminished, by use of prophylactic antibiotics. Examples include acyclovir for herpes, trimethoprim-sulfamethoxazole (Bactrim) for urinary tract infections with susceptible organisms, trimethoprim-sulfamethoxazole for *Pneumocystis* infection.
III. Correct manifestations of glucocorticoid toxicity
  A. Control hypertension
  B. Control hypokalemia
  C. Control symptomatic hyperglycemia
IV. Encourage exercise to counter the weight gain and myopathy of glucocorticoid therapy
V. Minimize the osteoporosis associated with glucocorticoid therapy
  A. Advise adequate daily calcium intake (1000 mg for premenopausal women and for men; 1500 mg for postmenopausal women).
  B. If 24-hour urinary calcium excretion is less than 120 mg, add vitamin D, 50,000 units 1–3 times weekly (or calcitriol, 0.5 µg daily), to maintain urinary calcium levels at 150–200 mg. Monitor serum and urinary calcium levels every 3–4 months if this is instituted.
  C. When women become menopausal, consider hormone replacement therapy if not contraindicated and SLE is stable.
  D. If risk for osteoporosis is high or if fractures occur, add bisphosphonate, calcitonin, or teriparatide.

Abbreviations: CBC, Complete blood cell; CMV, cytomegalovirus.

severe lupus nephritis over both the short and the long term; many experts believe that it should be included in initial therapeutic regimens in most SLE patients with severe nephritis (or other life-threatening, rapidly progressive organ involvement). Most experts agree that a high rate of relapse of nephritis (in patients with diffuse proliferative nephritis) occurs during the 5 to 10 years after initiation of combined glucocorticoid and cytotoxic regimens. In one recent long-term study,[47] the cumulative risk of renal flare in patients treated with IV cyclophosphamide was 45 percent at 10 years, and 27 percent of patients progressed to renal failure. This is similar to long-term outcomes reported previously.[48,49] I have reviewed this work and formed the following opinions. When cyclophosphamide is given intravenously once a month for 6 months and then discontinued, 50 to 80 percent of patients can be expected to improve. That improvement is lost in more than half during the subsequent 6 to 24 months.[31,33,47-49] In contrast, if IV cyclophosphamide is given monthly for 6 months, then at longer intervals for an additional 12 to 24 months, numbers of disease flares and preservation of renal function are better than in groups treated with glucocorticoids alone.[31] After cyclophosphamide is discontinued, about 25 percent of patients experience flares of SLE within 5 years, and about 50 percent within 10 years.[47,49]

Adverse reactions to cyclophosphamide are more common, however, with longer duration of therapy. For example, irreversible ovarian failure occurs in a much higher proportion of women on a 30-month regimen of IV cyclophosphamide (39 percent) than on a 6-month regimen (12 percent). In fact, 100 percent of women over the age of 30 years had ovarian failure in one study.[50] Some data[51] suggest that serious infections are more frequent in patients receiving both cyclophosphamide and steroids (49 percent) compared to steroids alone (29 percent), particularly if the nadir of total leukocyte count after cyclophosphamide doses is below 3000 cells/dl. In my experience, introducing granulocyte colony-stimulating factor (G-CSF) treatments at the time of this nadir, particularly if an infection is present, will prevent infection or enhance antibiotic therapies without activating disease. Others have reported that administration of G-CSF to patients with SLE is relatively safe: There is a small chance of aggravating a disease flare.[52] In many patients, lupus nephritis is a process that progresses over a period of many years. Acute changes can be reversed by aggressive immunosuppression with glucocorticoids or glucocorticoids plus cytotoxics. Scarring may progress inexorably in some individuals, however, and that process probably occurs more rapidly in patients treated with steroids alone, but it does occur in those with combination therapy as well. It may be useful and more acceptable to patients to induce improvement with glucocorticoid plus cyclophosphamide than to maintain the improvement with a safer regimen, such as low-dose daily or alternate-day steroids plus daily azathioprine, mycophenolate mofetil, or IV cyclophosphamide at long intervals (every 2 or 3 months). Data supporting this approach are appearing in the literature, and a prospective controlled trial comparing continuation of therapy (after administration of monthly IV cyclophosphamide) with azathioprine versus quarterly IV cyclophosphamide is in progress.[53-55] Recent studies have challenged the current community standard for treatment of severe lupus nephritis with cyclophosphamide among rheumatologists in the United States. Neither route of administration nor dose are known to be ideal. The six monthly IV cyclosphosphamide doses usually used (0.5 to 1 g/m^2 body surface area, beginning at the lower end and escalating until leukopenia occurs),

followed by two quarterly pulses, was compared to lower doses in a recent prospective randomized study conducted in Europe.[53] The comparison group received a fixed dose of 500 mg of cyclophosphamide intravenously once every 2 weeks for six doses. Both groups, after conclusion of cyclophosphamide, were maintained on azathioprine. At the beginning of the trial all patients in both groups received IV pulses of methylprednisolone, followed by 0.5 mg/kg of prednisolone daily. After a median follow-up of 41 months, the two groups had similar rates of renal remission (71 percent in the low-dose group and 54 percent in the high-dose group), and renal flares occurred in 27 percent of the low-dose and 29 percent of the high-dose groups. Severe infections were twice as frequent in the high-dose group, but differences did not reach statistical significance. These data suggested that we can administer lower doses of cyclophosphamide than are standard, for shorter periods of time, with lower glucocorticoid doses. One cautionary note should be added: The vast majority of patients were Caucasian; data cannot be compared directly to most trials in SLE patients conducted in the United States.

IV cyclophosphamide is effective in some patients with serious extrarenal manifestations of SLE, including diffuse CNS disease, thrombocytopenia, and interstitial pulmonary inflammation.[56,57] If in the initial suppression of severe lupus, intermittent IV cyclophosphamide and daily glucocorticoids are not effective, alternative strategies (added to daily glucocorticoids) include the following: 1) monthly IV pulses of methylprednisolone (Solu-Medrol, discussed earlier); 2) daily doses of oral cyclophosphamide; 3) daily oral doses of both cyclophosphamide and azathioprine; 4) mycophenolate mofetil; 5) cyclosporine; and 6) the experimental therapies plasmapheresis or immunoablative doses of cyclophosphamide, with or without stem cell infusion.

Several regimens combine daily oral cytotoxic drugs and glucocorticoids. Combination therapies studied in patients with lupus nephritis include glucocorticoids plus 1) daily oral cyclophosphamide, 2 to 3 mg/kg/day; 2) daily oral cyclophosphamide, 1.5 to 2.5 mg/kg/day, plus daily oral azathioprine, 1.5 to 2.5 mg/kg/day[39-41,48]; and 3) daily oral mycophenolate mofetil.[55-55b] The oral regimens have the advantages of convenience and daily immunosuppression of severe disease. Oral administration of cyclophosphamide, however, carries a substantial risk of urinary bladder toxicity (hemorrhagic cystitis, sclerosing chronic cystitis, and carcinoma of the bladder). That risk is much lower with IV administration, especially if cyclophosphamide doses are accompanied by administration of mesna, which inactivates the oxazaphosphorine metabolite of cyclophosphamide that irritates the bladder.[58] (I give 1 mg of IV mesna for every 1 mg of IV cyclophosphamide, half of the mesna just before and half 2 hours after the cyclophosphamide infusion.) IV pulse cyclophosphamide is effective in most patients with severe disease. In my experience, daily oral administration may be more effective than intermittent high-dose pulses (and more toxic) in some patients, and combination therapy of oral daily glucocorticoids plus azathioprine plus cyclophosphamide is effective in some patients who fail standard glucocorticoids-plus-pulse-cyclophosphamide regimens. There are no prospective controlled studies in human SLE that support these views. Addition of mycophenolate can also be effective, and there are increasing published data supporting this approach.[55-55b]

Several questions about therapy with IV or oral cyclophosphamide remain unanswered. The minimal effective dose is unknown and probably varies from patient to patient. Some authorities recommend that the dose be increased until the leukocyte nadir 10 to 14 days later is below 3500 cells/mm; there is no evidence that such a nadir is required for clinical response. Another problem is when and how to stop this therapy, as discussed earlier. My approach is to give monthly doses of the highest cyclophosphamide dose tolerated until response is achieved, then either continue IV cyclophosphamide at longer intervals (every 2 months instead of every 1 month, then, if response is sustained, every 3 months), or to add azathioprine or mycophenolate mofetil, continuing the treatments for a total of 2 years. The methods of using cytotoxic drugs are reviewed in Table 76–6.

Most patients treated with cyclophosphamide experience adverse side effects.[39,42-44,50,51,53-55] The most important adverse side effect is disabling or life-threatening infections. The most common infections are herpes zoster and staphylococcal, gram-negative bacterial, *Candida*, and *Pneumocystis carinii* infections. These infections must be carefully sought if appropriate symptoms are present, because, (with the exception of herpes zoster) they are often fatal. Other toxicities include bone marrow suppression (especially leukopenia) and increased malignancies. Infertility is common in both men and women (banking of sperm should be considered before cyclophosphamide regimens are instituted in men) and may be reversible if detected early in young patients so the drug can be stopped. Loss of ovarian function may also contribute to osteopenia and to accelerated atherosclerotic disease in women receiving chronic glucocorticoid therapy. Hair loss is common, as are gastrointestinal side effects, including nausea, diarrhea, and dyspepsia. Some patients experience malaise and fatigue, which improve after cytotoxic drugs are discontinued (see Table 76–6 for a review of adverse effects).

Methotrexate

MTX is reported to be effective in SLE arthritis, myositis, vasculitis, rash, serositis, and nephritis in some patients.[59-61] Most studies of MTX therapy in SLE have evaluated mainly cutaneous and joint involvement. The most recent prospective, randomized, placebo-controlled trial[60] showed lower pain scores, lower numbers of cutaneous lesions, higher complement levels, lower systemic lupus erythematosus disease activity index (SLEDAI) scores of disease activity and lower prednisone doses in the patients receiving MTX compared to the placebo control group. Two studies evaluating response of lupus nephritis reached different conclusions regarding efficacy. Currently, MTX has a place in the treatment of patients with relatively mild disease, particularly cutaneous and articular, who have not achieved adequate responses to NSAIDs, antimalarials, and low-dose glucocorticoids.

Mycophenolate Mofetil

Mycophenolate mofetil, widely used to prevent rejection of allografts, has been successful in treatment of murine lupus.[62] Small open trials and two recent prospective controlled trial in patients have suggested that many individuals respond.[55-55b,62-64] This drug is a selective, noncompetitive reversible inhibitor of inosine monophosphate dehydrogenase, which blocks de novo guanosine nucleotide incorporation into DNA. T and B lymphocytes depend on de novo synthesis of purines and lack salvage pathways present in other cell types. Therefore, mycophenolate is relatively specific for lymphocytes; therapy should spare ovarian and testicular function (not proven). Mycophenolate suppresses antibody formation and glycosylation of adhesion molecules. Adverse side effects are similar to those of azathioprine, with a higher incidence of nausea and diarrhea and a rare association with gastrointestinal ulceration and perforation. Infection (including herpes zoster), leukopenia, lymphoma, and nonmelanoma carcinoma are more common than with placebo[64] (similar to azathioprine).

At a dose of 2 to 3 g/day, mycophenolate is superior to azathioprine (1 to 2 mg/kg/day) in preventing graft rejection. A prospective, randomized trial[55] comparing daily oral cyclophoshamide given for 6 months (followed by daily azathioprine) to daily oral mycophenolate mofetil given for 12 months in patients with diffuse proliferative glomerulonephritis showed complete or partial remission in 90 percent of the cyclophophamide group and 95 percent of the mycophenolate group over a 12-month period. The rate of infections was higher in the cyclophosphamide group, as were amenorrhea, alopecia, leukopenia, and death. Rates of relapse did not differ in the first 12 months (11 to 15% in the two groups). However, at 24 months, the flare rate was higher in the mycophenolate group.[63] All patients in the study were Chinese, and the severity of nephritis was probably less than that of patients included in the National Institute of Health (NIH) studies of cyclophosphamide. Ethnic and disease-severity differences might account for the high response rate in this group. Much data supports the fact that outcomes of nephritis are worse and responses to therapy less in patients with lupus nephritis who are African American.[66,67] Thus, interpretation of the results of clinical trials must consider the ethnic composition of patients studied as well as different criteria for inclusion in the study, different therapeutic regimens, and different definitions of the outcomes measured. A recent prospective trial in the United States[55a,55b] compared treatment of severe lupus nephritis with IV cyclophosphamide versus mycophenolate mofetil 2 to 3 g a day. At 6 months, complete or partial remissions occurred in 49% of mycophenolate and 26% of cyclophosphamide—a statistically significant difference favoring mycophenolate. Side effects were less in the mycophenolate group. The durability of the responses and the acquisition of more responses beyond 6 months of therapy are not known. To administer mycophenolate mofetil, I begin 250 mg twice daily and gradually increase the dose over a few weeks to a total of 2 to 3 g daily. In my experience, response occurs more rapidly to mycophenolate than to azathioprine. In addition, I concur with the opinion of other experts that some patients refractory to high-dose glucocorticoids and cyclophosphamide respond to mycophenolate.[64]

OTHER IMMUNOSUPPRESSIVE APPROACHES USED IN SYSTEMIC LUPUS ERYTHEMATOSUS

Several other cytotoxic drugs have been used in uncontrolled studies of patients with SLE, including nitrogen mustard, chlorambucil, cyclosporine, and leflunomide. I have used nitrogen mustard or chlorambucil (with some success) in patients who are unresponsive to azathioprine and in whom bladder toxicity from cyclophosphamide has developed. Cyclosporine can be used as a second agent added to glucocorticoids; reports of the utility of cyclosporine in SLE give mixed results. One open randomized study compared cyclosporine (5 mg/kg/day) to prednisolone plus cyclophosphamide (2 mg/kg/day) for 1 year in children with lupus DPGN: Both groups showed a reduction of urine protein and maintenance of renal function, with better growth in the neoral group.[68] An open trial (unblinded) assigned patients with moderately severe active SLE to pulse methylprednisolone plus daily glucocorticoids plus cyclosporine (less than 5 mg/kg/day) or to steroids alone; the cyclosporine group had a significantly lower 12-month mean cumulative dose of prednisone and few disease flares.[69] In contrast, a retrospective review suggested that cyclosporin is useful primarily in management of lupus thrombocytopenia and that side effects or failure to control disease activity led to withdrawal of the therapy in most patients.[70] In uncontrolled trials of cyclosporine in adults with lupus nephritis,[71] some of whom have failed steroid-plus-cytotoxic therapies, at least half show diminished disease activity scores, reduced proteinuria, and stable or improved renal function. Deterioration in renal function is a frequent side effect of cyclosporine; other side effects include hypertension, hypertrichosis, gingival hyperplasia, paresthesias, tremor, and gastrointestinal symptoms. Nevertheless, these drugs are acceptable alternatives in patients doing poorly on standard, proven regimens who have normal or close-to-normal renal function and good control of blood pressure.

Leflunomide, a new agent released for treatment of RA, which is immunosuppressive by impairing lymphocyte function, has also been used in patients with SLE. One retrospective analysis of a small number of patients treated with 100-mg loading doses daily for 3 days, then maintenance daily doses of 20 mg, reported improvement in 10 of 14 patients.[72] The major adverse effects of leflunomide include nausea, diarrhea, infections, allergic reactions, and hepatotoxicity. It is not yet clear that this agent has an important role in the management of SLE.

Finally, in patients with life-threatening disease who are refractory or intolerant to all these "standard" strategies, maximal "immunoablative" cytotoxic or immunosuppressive therapy can be considered with or without infusion of autologous stem cells.[73-76] These procedures are discussed in this chapter in a later section on experimental therapies.

Summary

In treatment of acute, severe SLE, combination therapy with glucocorticoids and cytotoxic drugs is probably superior to glucocorticoids alone in controlling active disease, preventing irreversible tissue damage, minimizing maintenance glucocorticoid requirements, and prolonging survival. Progressive organ damage may occur over several years despite good short-term responses to these interventions. Cyclophosphamide is more effective than azathioprine but is also more toxic. Longer duration of therapy with cyclophosphamide is associated with fewer disease flares but higher toxicities, and the ideal duration of immunosuppressive therapy varies from patient to patient. Cyclophosphamide may be used in intermittent IV regimens in doses ranging from 7 to 20 mg/kg, or in daily oral doses from 1 to 2.5 mg/kg. Triple therapy with glucocorticoids, azathioprine, and cyclophosphamide is probably useful but accompanied by a high incidence of adverse side effects. In patients who fail to improve or do not tolerate cyclophosphamide or azathioprine, use of repeated monthly pulses of methylprednisolone, mycophenolate mofetil, or cyclosporine may be considered. There is recent evidence that mycophenolate mofetil may be useful to induce improvement as the initial cytotoxic drug in severe lupus nephritis. MTX is probably not beneficial in severe disease. Leflunomide has potential but current data are inadequate to recommend it. Immunoablation with autologous stem cell rescue is available at a few centers for patients with life-threatening disease refractory to all standard therapies. All these therapies, whether glucocorticoids alone or glucocorticoids plus cytotoxics, require close patient follow-up with frequent monitoring for adverse side effects.

Maximizing Disease Control

The most important criteria for disease control are clinical outcomes. In most patients, equilibrium is reached between mild, non–life-threatening disease activity and acceptable side effects of maintenance therapies. Complete long-term disease suppression usually is not possible, especially in the absence of side effects. Acceptable clinical outcomes include stable renal function (even though proteinuria is present), safe platelet and erythrocyte levels, arthralgias without arthritis, and mild skin lesions. The efficacy of treating to normalize serum levels of complement, antibodies to DNA (or other autoantibodies), and erythrocyte sedimentation rates (ESR) is controversial.[77-81] Although disease flares are usually fewer in patients with serum complement levels and antibodies to DNA kept in the normal range, particularly in patients with nephritis,[77,78,81] a few patients with persistently low complement levels and high anti-DNA have good outcomes,[79,80] and disease activity in some patients does not correlate with serum levels of any autoantibodies or of complement.[79] It is useful to establish in each individual patient what changes in laboratory tests herald a disease flare; these tests can then be used to help guide therapy. One study

TABLE 76–7 • MANIFESTATIONS OF SYSTEMIC LUPUS ERYTHEMATOSUS (SLE) THAT CAN BE MANAGED WITH STRATEGIES OTHER THAN, OR IN ADDITION TO, IMMUNOSUPPRESSION

Manifestation	Intervention
Thrombosis	Anticoagulation
Recurrent fetal loss with antiphospholipid	Heparin in low dose or low-molecular-weight heparin with or without aspirin; if heparin ineffective or not tolerated, use low-dose aspirin alone; glucocorticoids plus aspirin in moderate to high dose may be used but is controversial
Thrombocytopenia or hemolytic anemia	Intravenous gamma globulin, splenectomy, danazol, cyclosporine, cytotoxic drugs
Seizures without other serious manifestations	Anticonvulsants
Behavior disorders or psychosis without other serious manifestations	Psychoactive drugs, neuroleptics
Pure membranous glomerulonephritis	Limited trials of immunosuppressives or no specific treatment

shows that altering treatment in response to changes in laboratory tests significantly lowers the occurrence of disease flares.[81]

Minimizing Adverse Outcomes of Therapies and Long-Term Disease

Several strategies are useful for minimizing adverse outcomes related to glucocorticoid and cytotoxic therapies[41,82-85] as summarized in Table 76–7. Patients should be monitored frequently for signs of infection, and appropriate antimicrobial agents should be prescribed as soon as infection is suspected, then changed or discontinued as results of cultures become available. Infections with opportunistic organisms are common in immunosuppressed patients with SLE[42,43]; special procedures may be required to identify these organisms. For example, diagnosis of *Pneumocystis* infection, invasive *Candida* infection, aspergillosis, mycobacterial disease, and viruses such as cytomegalovirus may require biopsy of the affected organs. Immunization of SLE patients with influenza and pneumococcal vaccines (and probably with most other vaccines) is safe and usually effective,[82] although patients who receive high doses of immunosuppressive drugs may make inadequate protective-antibody responses.

Careful attention to blood pressure control and correction of hypokalemia and symptomatic hyperglycemia are recommended for patients receiving glucocorticoids. Frequent monitoring for adverse effects on bone marrow, liver, and lung are recommended for patients receiving cytotoxic drugs.

Osteoporosis can be a serious problem (overall prevalence of approximately 15 percent in SLE patients) in glucocorticoid-treated patients, especially in individuals who are Caucasian, postmenopausal, older than 50 years, and those with a high cumulative dose of glucocorticoids.[83-86] Several strategies help maintain bone mass in such individuals.[83,84] These strategies include calcium supplementation to achieve a total daily intake of 1000 to 1500 mg, plus 50,000 units vitamin D one to three times a week, or daily calcitriol in patients with low urinary calcium (below 120 mg in 24 hours). In addition, estrogen replacement therapy in menopausal women, progesterone, androgens, calcitonin, and bisphosphonates have all been shown to stabilize bone mass in patients on glucocorticoid therapy. Administration of estrogen to patients with SLE is controversial for several reasons. First, there is a possibility that disease might be aggravated by female sex hormones. Studies of a large cohort of nurses showed a higher incidence of SLE in women who had ever received oral contraceptives or estrogen replacement therapy compared to women without such therapies.[87,88] A prospective, randomized controlled trial addressing the safety of estrogen therapies in women with SLE has been completed[88a] and shows a higher rate of mild but not severe disease flares in women on hormone replacement therapy (estrogen plus progesterone) compared to placebo. Secondly, recent studies have shown that administration of estrogen/progesterone combinations to healthy postmenopausal women increases the risk for myocardial infarction and stroke, as well as previously known increases in venous thromboses and breast cancer.[89] Because morbidity and mortality from atherosclerosis, including myocardial infarcts and strokes, are increased in women with SLE, particularly after a decade of disease, hormone replacement therapy that includes estrogen and progesterone may do harm in some. Virtually all data support the benefit of estrogen replacement for preventing osteoporosis, so the physician must decide which risk is greater. To prevent osteoporosis, use of calcium, adequate vitamin D, and bisphosphonates seems the safest choice at the time of this writing.

Atherosclerosis is accelerated in some patients with SLE: The overall risk for symptomatic atherosclerosis may be increased as much as 50-fold in women with SLE between the ages of 35 and 44.[90,91] In women with SLE older than 40, the relative risk for myocardial infarction is approximately 10.[91-91b] Predisposing factors include hypertension, increasing age, increasing disease duration, and hyperlipidemia.[91,92] One study[91a] showed that SLE patients with carotid plaque compared to those without had lower mean daily doses of prednisone and less use of cytotoxics, suggesting that more aggressive control of SLE disease activity might decrease the acceleration of atherosclerosis. Therefore, the physician must pay close attention to control of all treatable risk factors predisposing to this complication. There is interest in considering statin therapies in SLE,[93,94] not only for their abilities to decrease risk for myocardial infarction and to lower levels of total cholesterol and low-density lipoproteins, but also because they may have anti-inflammatory effects. Data are available showing that postmenopausal women with preexisting heart disease, receiving estrogen and progesterone, are protected from increased risk for myocardial infarction if they are receiving statin therapies.[93] There are no prospective data published as yet in patients with SLE; such a study is in progress.

TABLE 76–8 · OUTCOME OF PREGNANCIES IN WOMEN WITH ANTIPHOSPHOLIPID ANTIBODIES TREATED WITH DIFFERENT INTERVENTIONS

Treatment	Successful Births with No Interventions (%)	Successful Births with Interventions (%)
Review of Literature as of 1992:		
Aspirin alone	12-15	57-80
Aspirin + prednisone	7-30	36-100
Low-dose heparin + prednisone	4	64
Low-dose heparin + aspirin	19	64
High-dose heparin	5-6	93-100
Literature after 1992:		
Direct Comparison Trials 1. Heparin + ASA: 80% vs. ASA alone: 44% 2. High-dose heparin: 80% vs. low dose: 76%		

Review as of 1992 adapted from Many A, Pauzner R, Carp H, et al: Treatment of patients with antiphospholipid antibodies during pregnancy. Am J Reprod Immunol 28:216, 1992. Literature after 1992 adapted from Kutteh WH, Ermel LD: A clinical trial for the treatment of antiphospholipid antibody-associated recurrent pregnancy loss with lower dose heparin and aspirin. Am J Reprod Immunol 35:402, 1996; Kutteh WH: Antiphospholipid antibody-associated recurrent pregnancy loss: Treatment with heparin and low-dose aspirin is superior to low-dose aspirin alone. Am J Obstet Gynecol 174:1584, 1996.

Treatment with Strategies Other Than Immunosuppression

Some patients have disease manifestations that require management with interventions other than immunosuppression. They are discussed here and are reviewed in Table 76–7.

THROMBOSIS

Among those with SLE who experience recurrent thrombosis as their sole or major disease manifestation (predominantly patients with antiphospholipid antibodies), anticoagulation is probably the therapy of choice. There are no controlled studies to support this view, but most experts recommend it[95-97] based on failure of immunosuppressive interventions to prevent clotting and generally favorable experiences with anticoagulation. In fact, retrospective studies suggest that the only intervention that significantly lowers the incidence of reclotting (which is approximately 50 percent in 2 years after the initial clot) is aggressive anticoagulation with warfarin, keeping the international normalization ratio (INR) at 3.0 to 3.5.[95-97] This is particularly important in patients with clotting that affects branches of the internal carotid arteries, who have a greater than 80 percent recurrence.[97] The major adverse event related to such therapy is bleeding. A recent British study showed that in patients with anti-phospholipid

syndrome (APS) anticoagulated with a target INR of 3.5, the rate of major bleeding was six cases per 100 patient-years (intracranial bleeds were 1.5 per 100 patient-years), whereas recurrence of thrombosis rate was 9.1 cases per 100 patient-years.[98] Thus, benefit outweighs risk for most patients. The lupus anticoagulant is usually steroid responsive and diminishes if high-dose glucocorticoid therapy is begun. Antibodies to cardiolipin are more resistant; they may not be decreased by either glucocorticoids or cytotoxic drugs. Although high levels of immunoglobulin G (IgG) anticardiolipin antibodies confer a higher risk for clotting than other Ig subsets or lower quantities, it is not clear that it is useful to reduce titers of these antibodies. Immunosuppression has limited utility in these patients and is not recommended—unless other manifestations of SLE require it. Some patients show a combination of vasculitis and clotting and require both immunosuppression and anticoagulation.[99] These issues are addressed in more detail in Chapter 77.

PREGNANCY AND LUPUS: TREATMENT PROBLEMS

Patients with Recurrent Fetal Loss

The most important cause of fetal loss in mothers with SLE is the presence of active disease during pregnancy.[100] It is essential to suppress disease during this period, and many experts recommend administration of glucocorticoids (using preparations such as prednisone or prednisolone that do not cross the placenta in active forms, while avoiding hydrocortisone, betamethasone, and dexamethasone, which do cross the placenta in active forms and, thus, expose the fetus[101]) in doses required to maintain suppression of serious disease activity. There is debate regarding whether or not betamethasone or dexamethsone given antenatally are associated with low birth weights, reduced brain weights, and later maturational abnormalities of brain development in human fetuses;[102] these become issues when the goal is to treat the fetus with neonatal lupus myocarditis or prematurity. In general, systemic treatment with fluorinated glucocorticoids such as betamethasone and dexamethasone should be avoided in treatment of pregnant women with SLE. Some women (with or without SLE) experience fetal loss in the presence of antiphospholipid antibodies, especially if the antibodies are high-titer IgG anticardiolipin or the lupus anticoagulant. There are several therapeutic choices in these women. First, if there have been no previous fetal losses, the physician can choose not to intervene; many pregnancies go well. The higher the number of previous fetal losses (especially if there are no live births), the lower the chance that subsequent pregnancies will have a good outcome.[103]

Several studies have addressed the benefits of different interventions. The administration of aspirin alone has had mixed results, with some studies suggesting a higher birth rate of live infants, and others suggesting no positive effects.[103-105] Similarly, the use of glucocorticoids along with aspirin has had advocates, but the majority of data suggest that moderate to high doses of glucocorticoids do not improve fetal survival and are associated with considerable maternal toxicity, including hypertension and diabetes.[105-107] There is general agreement that anticoagulation with heparin or low-molecular-weight heparin are effective in improving live birth rates.[103,104,106] Both treatments probably are associated with loss of maternal bone mass, sometimes leading to vertebral fractures. A recent clinical trial showed that 5000 units of heparin daily was not better than aspirin alone[108]; studies using 5000 units of heparin twice daily have shown benefits, and that is the dose I recommend. Dicumarol (Coumadin) is teratogenic when administered in the first trimester and should be avoided during that time. In general, with use of heparin (usually given with aspirin) or low-molecular-weight heparin, the rate of live births is 70 to 90 percent.[103-106] Frequent fetal and maternal monitoring is critical to good outcomes with any of these interventions: These high-risk pregnancies often require early delivery in response to clinical evidence of fetal distress.

Neonatal Lupus

Several lupus syndromes can occur in neonates,[109-112] usually associated with maternal antibodies to Ro. Manifestations can include rash (the most frequent), congenital heart block, cardiomyopathy, hepatobiliary disease, and thrombocytopenia (the last of which is more strongly associated with maternal thrombocytopenia than anti-Ro). The rash consists of plaques of slightly raised erythema that clear spontaneously over several weeks as maternal IgG is metabolized. Congenital heart block can be fatal; in children who survive neonatal cardiac lupus, subsequent cardiomyopathy or total heart block are common.[111] Therefore, patients with SLE who are pregnant should be screened for anti-Ro, and fetal heart rates should be closely monitored in women with anti-Ro so that early delivery and cardiac pacing can be offered if heart block occurs. Treatment of antibody-positive women with prior fetuses with congenital heart block, or evidence of cardiac distress in a current fetus, has been reported. Glucocortoids (dexamethasone or betamethasone), IV gamma globulin, or plasmapheresis have been administered in an attempt to prevent congenital heart block.[109-112] It is likely that the therapies are effective in suppressing fetal myocarditis as well as fetal pleural effusions, ascites, and hydrops, but chances of reversing heart block, once established, are probably poor.[111,112]

Thrombocytopenia can occur in newborns, probably from maternal antiplatelet antibodies crossing the placenta. The mother may or may not have thrombocytopenia. It is short-lived in the newborn but may be associated with bleeding. Treatment of maternal thrombocytopenia with glucocorticoids is recommended.

Influence of Pregnancy on Systemic Lupus Erythematosus in the Mother

Although a minority of patients experience severe disease flares or worsening during pregnancy, most women do well[100] (see Chapter 74). Patients at high risk for adverse effects include those with active renal, cardiac, pulmonary, or CNS lupus. Patients should be examined at frequent intervals during pregnancy. Signs of increasing disease activity or impending preeclampsia include rising liver enzymes (preeclampsia or HELLP [hemolysis, elevated liver enzymes, low platelets] syndrome), hypertension (either SLE or preeclampsia), new or increasing proteinuria (either SLE or preeclampsia), thrombocytopenia (lupus), and falling levels of serum complement (lupus). These signs indicate a need for aggressive intervention to treat both mother and fetus.

SEVERE CYTOPENIAS

Patients with the thrombocytopenia of SLE may benefit from several therapies in addition to immunosuppression. Most authorities recommend high-dose glucocorticoids (60 to 100 mg prednisone daily) as the initial intervention in adults. Platelet counts begin to rise 3 to 10 days after introduction of glucocorticoids; the increase is usually sustained. Administration of IV gamma globulin (0.4 g/kg on each of 2 to 5 days) for 4 to 7 days is usually followed by rapid increase in platelet counts, which is usually transient. A study that compared prednisone alone to IV gamma globulin alone to combination therapy in idiopathic immune thrombocytopenia showed response appearing in a median of 5 days for each single-drug therapy and in 3 days for combination therapy.[113] Relapse rates and the percentage of patients that required subsequent splenectomy were similar in the three groups.

Splenectomy[114,115] should be considered whenever glucocorticoid or IV gamma globulin therapy is ineffective, either initially or when tapered or discontinued. The objective of therapy is to maintain adequate levels of platelets ($50,000/mm^3$ or higher). The efficacy of splenectomy in lupus cytopenias is somewhat controversial. If the criterion of permanently sustained normal counts in the absence of any maintenance therapies is used, the response rate may be as low as 15 percent.[116] If the criterion of adequate platelet counts with or without requirement for additional maintenance therapies is used, about 90 percent of patients have good initial responses and 65 to 70 percent have good sustained responses.[114,115] Asplenic patients are at increased risk for infection with encapsulated microorganisms, particularly *Pneumococcus*; patients should receive pneumococcal vaccine before splenectomy if possible.

Danazol, an anabolic steroid, may be useful in some cases of SLE thrombocytopenia.[117,118] Administration of danazol, 400 to 800 mg daily, may increase platelet counts to acceptable levels over 2 to 12 weeks. Danazol has been effective in some patients who failed on glucocorticoid therapy, splenectomy, and cytotoxic drugs. Side effects of danazol include weight gain, lethargy, myalgia, mild virilization, menopausal symptoms, rash, pruritus, hepatic tumors, hepatitis, and pancreatitis.[117-119]

Cyclosporine (Neoral) is also useful in some patients with thrombocytopenia.[70,71] Doses of 3 to 5 mg/kg/day should be initiated; platelet counts usually increase in 2 to 3 weeks, and the dose can be slowly tapered to maintain the response. Use of cyclosporine has been discussed previously.

Cytotoxic drugs, including cyclophosphamide (daily or intermittent IV pulses), azathioprine, and vinca alkaloids are sometimes effective in patients with thrombocytopenia who are steroid and splenectomy resistant.

See previous discussion for dosage and administration recommendations.

A recent French retrospective review of patients with SLE and "severe" thrombocytopenia (defined as platelet counts less than 50×10^9 per liter)[114] concluded that glucocorticoids plus another intervention result in better long-term control than glucocorticoids alone. Initial response to glucocorticoid therapy (1 mg/kg per day) resulted in improvement in 80 percent, but the improvement was sustained in only 22 percent. In contrast, combinations of prednisone and hydroxychloroquine or danazol or splenectomy increased long-term responses to 50 to 65 percent. Responses to glucocorticoids plus cytotoxic agents were not sustained as well; however, the numbers of patients in each of the subgroups studied was too small to be confident that these data are applicable to all SLE patients. Because some patients have only one major episode of severe thrombocytopenia, I recommend beginning with glucocorticoids alone. Additional strategies can be introduced if the problem recurs. In most patients with stable platelet counts at or above 40,000/liter, I do not recommend treatment unless the counts are steadily falling, bleeding is or has occurred during episodes of moderate thrombocytopenia, there is additional risk for bleeding, or some other manifestation of SLE requires intervention. Hemolytic anemia of SLE, if severe, should also be treated initially with high-dose glucocorticoids. Splenectomy, danazol, cyclosporine, and cytotoxic drugs are useful in some steroid-resistant individuals.

The leukopenia (usually lymphopenia) of SLE is rarely associated with important clinical sequelae. Rare patients with granulocytopenia, however, experience recurrent bacterial infections that may resolve after the granulocyte count is increased by treatment with glucocorticoid therapy, cyclosporine, splenectomy, or G-CSF. Treatment with G-CSF has been successful in lupus granulocytopenia if doses are kept at the minimum required to maintain absolute neutrophil counts above 1000/mm³.[120] High doses run the risk of activating SLE.[120,121] Use of G-CSF to manage granulocytopenia secondary to cyclophosphamide or other cytotoxic therapies in patients with SLE is reasonable, provided the risk of infection is greater than the risk of flaring the SLE.

CENTRAL NERVOUS SYSTEM LUPUS

The diagnosis and management of CNS lupus have been reviewed recently.[122] New classifications of the neurologic syndromes of SLE have been published and are intended to increase the uniformity of diagnosis so that results of interventions can be assessed accurately.[123] It is useful to divide patients with CNS lupus into two large groups to select appropriate therapies: those with vascular occlusions and those with more diffuse CNS disease.

Patients with strokes are likely to have hypercoagulability syndromes. It may be useful to consider anticoagulation rather than immunosuppression if strokes are the only CNS manifestations of lupus, especially if antibodies to phospholipids or vegetations of Libman-Sachs endocarditis are present. On the other hand, if there are signs of diffuse brain disease, especially with peripheral vasculitis, immunosuppression should be instituted. In patients with nonthrombotic diffuse CNS abnormalities, the nature of the manifestations may determine the best therapeutic choices. For example, seizures of various types are frequent in patients with SLE. If SLE is not active in other organ systems, treatment with anticonvulsants may be adequate therapy. Similarly, behavior disorders and psychosis may be manifestation of SLE or may be unrelated. Psychoactive drugs may be a safer initial intervention than immunosuppression. If patients improve, immunosuppression can be avoided.

I usually do not treat mild cognitive disorders with glucocorticoids, because their side effects are so great. However, one study suggested that cognitive defects may be improved significantly by the administration of 30 mg prednisone daily for a few weeks, and improvement can be maintained in some patients after the dose is tapered or withdrawn.[124] More extensive CNS disease, such as acute confusional states, diffuse demyelinating disease, and myelopathies, require immediate and aggressive intervention with high-dose glucocorticoids with or without cytotoxic drugs.

PURE MEMBRANOUS NEPHRITIS

Treatment of pure membranous lupus glomerulonephritis may be different from treatment of proliferative glomerulonephritis. A recent review discusses histology, diagnosis, clinical manifestations, and therapy.[125] Renal biopsy is necessary to establish the diagnosis, because most SLE patients with membranous changes in glomeruli also have some inflammatory proliferative changes. Patients with pure membranous lupus glomerulonephritis usually present with nephrotic syndrome; renal failure occurs but is less frequent and later than renal failure in proliferative glomerulonephritis.[125,126] This disease may not improve during glucocorticoid or cytotoxic therapies, using 24-hour protein excretion as the measure of response. I usually treat this patient subset with high-dose daily or alternate-day glucocorticoids for 6 to 12 weeks. If proteinuria does not diminish, the therapy is discontinued. It is possible that long-term benefit would be obtained from 6- to 12-month administration of alternate-day glucocorticoids or glucocorticoids plus cytotoxics, or cyclosporine, as in non–lupus idiopathic membranous glomerulonephritis; no prospective controlled trials are available in patients with SLE, because only 10 to 20 percent of patients with lupus nephritis have this histologic type. Addition of angiotensin-converting enzyme (ACE) inhibitors may reduce proteinuria in this and other SLE nephropathies; inadequate data are available in SLE patients to prove this.

THROMBOTIC THROMBOCYTOPENIA PURPURA

A small proportion of SLE patients develop episodes of thrombotic thrombocytopenia purpura (TTP) with the typical presentation of CNS symptoms, renal disease, and thrombocytopenia. Peripheral blood smears show schistocytes, and serum levels of LDH are usually very high. Clinicians must be alert to the possibility of this diagnosis, because initial symptoms mimic SLE flares. Treatment with plasmapheresis or plasma exchange is often lifesaving; the syndrome usually does not respond to glucocorticoid or other immunosuppressive therapies.[127] Recurrences are common.

Experimental Therapies

APHERESIS

Plasmapheresis, leukoplasmapheresis, and cryopheresis have all been used to treat patients with SLE. Although some dramatic benefits have been reported with a combination of glucocorticoids, IV cyclophosphamide, and plasmapheresis,[128] controlled trials in lupus nephritis have shown no benefit of plasmapheresis when added to standard therapies.[129] Theoretically, because apheresis removes serum IgG and reduces levels of autoantibodies and immune complexes, rapid disease control should result. There may still be a place for this therapy in patients with life-threatening manifestations of SLE that are not controlled with standard therapies. High levels of antibodies serve as negative feedback for B cells; a few days after autoantibody levels fall, they usually rebound in high quantities. Therefore, initiation of apheresis requires administration of a cytotoxic drug (usually IV cyclophosphamide) between days 5 to 10 of the treatment. Apheresis is expensive and requires vascular access. Clotting factors are removed along with immunoglobulin; the plasma removed can be replaced initially with plasma substitutes, but substances (usually fresh frozen plasma) that contain clotting factors have to be provided, thus introducing risks of transmission of hepatitis viruses and human immunodeficiency virus (HIV).

MANIPULATION OF SEX HORMONE LEVELS

Because estrogenic hormones have been implicated in the pathogenesis of SLE, several investigators have studied the efficacy of administering androgenic hormones or luteinizing hormone–blocking agents. Danazol is useful in some patients,[117,118] especially those with thrombocytopenia (see previous discussion). There has been recent interest in DHEA, which reduced the activity of SLE and was steroid-sparing in an open trial and in a controlled prospective trial.[10,11] These agents are not effective in severe SLE; however, they probably have steroid-sparing properties in some individuals with mild disease. Doses of DHEA from 50 to 200 mg daily can be used to reduce SLE activity and steroid requirements in patients with relatively mild disease; the major side effect of this intervention is acne, which occurs in 10 to 30 percent of patients.

REGULATION OF T CELL AND B CELL INTERACTIONS

Biologic interventions that suppress B cell activation—either by direct effects on B cell receptors or on helper T cells—have been effective in mouse models of lupus. These interventions include interrupting idiotypic circuits, binding B cell receptors with nucleotides on a framework that prevents binding to fragment crystallizable (Fc) receptors with activation of second signals, interrupting expansion of B cells with a fusion protein that binds Blys growth factor, inactivating helper T cells through antibody blockade of surface molecules cell determinant (CD)4 or CD3, inactivating second-signal molecules on T cells such as CD40L and CTLA4, blocking recognition of antigen presented in class II major histocompatibility complex (MHC) gene products on surfaces of APCs, inhibiting cytokines that, among other functions, increase B cell maturation and secretion of autoantibodies, including IL-6 and IL-10, and replacing bone marrow of lupus mice with allogeneic marrow from mice resistant to lupus.[130-141] Activation of T cells requires two signals delivered by APCs: one antigen-specific signal via the T cell receptor and a second nonspecific signal by linking of additional surface molecules. For T cell activation, linkage between CD28 on T cells and B7.1 or B7.2 (CD80 and CD86) on APC is required. There is at least one additional signal, between CTLA4 on T cells and CD80 and CD86 on APC, that may in some cases give a negative signal that stops T cell activation. The interaction between CD28 and its ligands, B7.1 and B7.2, can be interrupted by administration of the experimental fusion protein CTLA4-Ig.[135-137] For T cell activation that leads to B cell activation, the second signal requires links between CD40L (CD154) on T cells and CD40 on B cells. This interaction can be interrupted by administration of the experimental monoclonal antibody, anti-CD154.[136] Blys is a surface molecule with increased expression on activated T cells; interaction between soluble Blys and its receptor on B cells expands activated B cells and increases autoantibody production.[133,134]

Most of these biologics have been studied in phase I or phase II studies in patients with SLE, but development is not far enough along to recommend their use in patients at this time. There is also interest in treatment with a monoclonal antibody to CD20, which eliminates most mature B cells for several months.[142] A promising biologic in the treatment of human SLE is La Jolla Pharmaceuticals 394 (LJP 394, "Riquent") a "tolerogen" consisting of four small nucleotides held in an "X" configuration by a tetrameric scaffold.[143,144] The idea is to bind anti-DNA B cell receptors, but not Fc gamma receptors, so that second signals are not activated. Administration of LJP 394 intravenously to SLE patients with high antibodies to DNA reduces the quantities of those antibodies. One phase II prospective, randomized, placebo-controlled study of patients with recent flares of lupus nephritis but stable disease at the time of treatment suggested reduction of renal flares in the treatment group.[145a]

A small series of SLE patients with diffuse membranoproliferative nephritis resistant to treatment with glucocorticoids and cytotoxics was treated with total lymph node irradiation, which inactivates both B and T lymphocytes over the short term, and some T cells for many months.[146] After 10 years of follow-up, approximately 20 percent of patients had good renal function without immunosuppressive therapies. This therapy is not popular currently, but it might be considered for individuals who have not responded to the many alternative therapies now available.

INTRAVENOUS GAMMA GLOBULIN

Administration of IV gamma globulin may have favorable effects on active SLE.[147] Such treatment may solubilize immune complexes and provide anti-idiotypic downregulation of autoantibody production, thus interfering with T cell and B cell signaling. In addition to the utility of this treatment in the management of lupus-induced thrombocytopenia,[113] there are reports of improvement (and of worsening) of dermatitis and nephritis.[144,147]

IMMUNOABLATION WITH OR WITHOUT AUTOLOGOUS STEM CELL TRANSPLANTATION

The idea of these therapies is to induce disease remission in patients with SLE. Thus, the increased short-term danger of infections and bleeding during periods of inadequate numbers of leukocytes and platelets is offset by the possibility that over the long-term patients will not require chronic immunosuppressive therapies, including glucocorticoids. There is at least one report studying administration of immunoablative doses of cyclophosphamide (200 mg/kg divided into four daily IV doses) without subsequent transfer of stem cells.[76] The majority of patients showed excellent improvement in the disease activity of SLE, and over a period of 2 years the flare rate approximated 30 percent. The advantage of this approach is the avoidance of the manipulations required to mobilize stem cells into the peripheral blood (usually done by administration of cyclophosphamide and G-CSF); this mobilization process is associated with increased risk for infections, bleeding, and death. On the other hand, many experts suggest that providing autologous stem cells after immunoablation is safer than not doing so. In this experimental procedure stem cells are induced in the peripheral blood, then harvested and cultured.[73-75] Therapies that completely ablate bone marrow and much of the immune system are administered (usually consisting of very-high-dose cyclophosphamide, and total body irradiation or antithymocyte globulin), stem cells are reinfused, and stem cell growth factor is administered. Peripheral leukocytes are repopulated in an average of 10 days, with platelets reaching safe levels by a mean of 14 days. The advantage of this approach is that, ultimately, post-treatment immunosuppression is not required: The disadvantage is the well-known dangers of immunoablation during the harvest period, then of immunoablation during the period around the administration of the stem cells, as well as the risk of flaring SLE with administration of G-CSF. Several patients with SLE have been treated with this approach in Europe and in the United States.[73-75a] To date, short-term follow-up (approximately 3 years) has suggested that the great majority of patients with autologous stem cell therapy respond with greatly diminished disease activity; 50 to 75 percent achieve "remission" requiring no immunosuppression, or therapy with only antimalarials or low-dose prednisone (10 mg or less), and 25 to 35 percent flare by 3 years. Flares may be easier to control than the severe disease that led the patient to be a candidate for stem cell

transplantation. Mortality rates (including deaths during the induction period) are reported as 3 to 8 percent. The ultimate utility of this therapy, particularly its ability to induce long-standing remissions, is being studied.

Outcome in Patients with Systemic Lupus Erythematosus

In some patients with lupus nephritis, planning for dialysis or renal transplantation, rather than immunosuppression, is appropriate. Patients who present with serum creatinine levels over 2.4 mg/dl, in whom the creatinine has slowly risen over a period of a few years, often have irreversible kidney lesions.[126,148-151] Black race and hematocrit levels below 26 percent also predict a high risk for end-stage renal disease.[66,67,150] The irreversibility of lesions can be confirmed by high chronicity scores and low activity scores on renal biopsy specimens.[126] The 2-year survival rate in SLE patients with renal transplants is approximately 85 percent, with renal graft survival rates at 1 and 5 years of 68 and 54 percent, respectively.[152,153] Recent data suggest that patients with SLE have about twice the risk of renal transplant failure than patients with other types of renal disease.[153] SLE recurs in approximately 10 percent of transplanted kidneys, and standard laboratory measures of lupus activity may or may not predict this recurrence.[154] With regard to extrarenal SLE, a decrease in disease activity scores and numbers of disease flares usually occur after initiation of dialysis or transplantation.

Death is caused most frequently by infection or severe nephritis; other manifestations of active SLE and atherosclerotic thrombotic events also account for a substantial proportion of deaths.[148-152] Extrarenal manifestations of SLE that are frequently fatal include carditis, pneumonitis,

TABLE 76–9 · SURVIVAL RATES IN SYSTEMIC LUPUS ERYTHEMATOSUS (SLE)

Years After Diagnosis (%)	Survival Rates
1*	95-97
5	85-91
10	73-80
15	63-64

*Certain disease subsets and ethnic groups have worse outcomes, on the lower end of those shown here. Those subsets include individuals of black race, those presenting with serum Cr >2.4 or hematocrit values <26% or with renal histologic features showing high activity and chronicity indices. Austin HA III, Boumpas DT, Vaughan EM, et al: High-risk features of lupus nephritis: Importance of race and clinical and histological factors in 166 patients. Nephrol Dialysis Transplant 10:1620, 1995.

Data derived from Ginzler E, Diamond HS, Weiner M, et al: A multicenter study of outcome in systemic lupus erythematosus. Arthritis Rheum 25:605, 1982; Ward MM, Pyun E, Studenski S: Long-term survival in systemic lupus erythematosus: Patient characteristics associated with poorer outcomes. Arthritis Rheum 38:274, 1995; Jacobsen S, Petersen J, Ullman S, et al: A multicentre study of 513 Danish patients with systemic lupus erythematosus. II. Disease mortality and clinical factors of prognostic value. Clin Rheumatol 17:478, 1998; Boumpas DT, Fessler BJ, Austin HA III, et al: Systemic lupus erythematosus: Emerging Concepts. II. Ann Intern Med 123:42, 1995.

pulmonary hypertension, diffuse brain disease, stroke, myocardial infarction, intestinal perforations in areas of vasculitis, and extracranial arterial thromboses.

The prognosis of patients with SLE has improved considerably in the past four decades. Current survival rates are shown in Table 76–9. Older age, male gender, African-American race, lower income without medical insurance, and nephritis are associated with the highest mortality rates.[148-151] Fortunately, the mortality rate in SLE patients has declined steadily over the past 30 years.[155] Nevertheless, current survival rates are not good enough—a fact that demands more effective approaches to the treatment of SLE.

REFERENCES

1. Wallace DJ: Principles of therapy and local measures. *In* Wallace DJ, Hahn BH (eds): Dubois' Lupus Erythematosus, 6th ed. Philadelphia, Lippincott Williams & Wilkins, 2002, p 1131.
2. Kirou KA, Boumpas DT: Systemic glucocorticoid therapy in systemic lupus erythematosus. *In* Wallace DJ, Hahn BH (eds): Dubois' Lupus Erythematosus, 6th ed. Philadelphia. Lippincott Williams & Wilkins, 2002, p 1173.
3. Chatham WW, Kimberly RP: Treatment of lupus with corticosteroids. Lupus 10(3):140-147, 2001.
4. Ostensen M, Villiger PM: Nonsteroidal anti-inflammatory drugs in systemic lupus erythematosus. Lupus 10(3):135-139, 2001.
5. Bonnel RA, Villalba ML, Karwoski CB, Beitz J: Aseptic meningitis associated with rofecoxib. Arch Intern Med 162(6):713-715, 2002.
6. Langman MJ, Jensen DM, Watson DJ, et al: Adverse upper gastrointestinal effects of rofecoxib compared with NSAIDs. JAMA 282:1929, 1999.
7. Hawkey CJ: Progress in prophylaxis against nonsteroidal anti-inflammatory drug-associated ulcers and erosions: Omeprazole NSAID Steering Committee. Am J Med 104(3A):67S, 1998.
8. Wallace DJ: Antimalarial therapies. *In* Wallace DJ, Hahn BH (eds): Dubois' Lupus Erythematosus, 6th ed. Philadelphia, Lippincott, Williams & Wilkins, 2002, p 1149.
9. Canadian Hydroxychloroquine Study Group: A randomized study of the effect of withdrawing hydroxychloroquine sulfate in systemic lupus erythematosus. N Engl J Med 324:150, 1991.
10. van Vollenhoven RF, Morabito LM, Engleman EG, et al: Treatment of systemic lupus erythematosus with dehydroepiandrosterone: 50 patients treated up to 12 months. J Rheumatol 25:285, 1998.
11. Petri, MA, Lahita RG, Van Vollenhoven RF, et al: Effects of prasterone on corticosteroid requirements of women with systemic lupus erythematosus: A double-blind, randomized, placebo-controlled trial. Arthritis Rheum 46(7):1820-1829, 2002.
12. Sato EI: Methotrexate therapy in systemic lupus erythematosus. Lupus 10(3):162-164, 2001.
13. Remer CF, Weisman MH, Wallace DJ: Benefits of leflunomide in systemic lupus erythematosus: A pilot observational study. Lupus 10(7):480-483, 2001.
14. Wysenbeek AJ, Block DA, Fries JF: Prevalence and expression of photosensitivity in systemic lupus erythematosus. Ann Rheum Dis 48:461, 1989.
15. Ting WW, Sontheimer RD: Local therapy for cutaneous and systemic lupus erythematosus: Practical and theoretical considerations. Lupus 10(3):171-184, 2001.
16. Callen JP: Management of skin disease in patients with lupus erythematosus. Best Pract Res Clin Rheumatol 16(2):245-264, 2002.
16a. Walker SL, Kinby B, Chalmers RJ: The effect of topical tacrolimus on severe recalcitrant chronic discoid lupus erythematosus. Br J Dermatol 147:405-406, 2002.
17. Duna GF, Cash JM: Treatment of refractory cutaneous lupus erythematosus. Rheum Dis Clin North Am 21:99, 1995.
18. Al-Herz A, Schulzer M, Esdaile JM: Survey of antimalarial use in lupus pregnancy and lactation. J Rheumatol 29(4):700-706, 2002.
19. Boumpas DT, Fessler BJ, Austin HA III, et al: Systemic lupus erythematosus: Emerging concepts. II. Dermatologic and joint disease, the antiphospholipid antibody syndrome, pregnancy and hormonal therapy, morbidity and mortality, and pathogenesis. Ann Intern Med 123:42, 1995.
20. Thomson KF, Goodfield MJ: Low-dose thalidomide is an effective second-line treatment in cutaneous lupus erythematosus. J Dermatolog Treat 12(3):145-147, 2001.
21. Karim MY, Ruiz-Irastorza G, Khamashta MA, Hughes GR: Update on therapy: Thalidomide in the treatment of lupus. Lupus 10(3):188-192, 2001.
22. Toshimasu T, Ohtani T, Sakamoto T, et al: Topical FK506 (tacrolimus) therapy for facial erythematous lesions of cutaneous lupus erythematousus and dermatomyositis. Eur J Dermatol 12:50-52, 2002.
23. McKinley PS, Ouellette SC, Winkel GH: The contributions of disease activity, sleep patterns and depression to fatigue in systemic lupus erythematosus: A proposed model. Arthritis Rheum 38:826, 1995.
24. Wang B, Gladmann DD, Urowitz MB: Fatigue in lupus is not correlated with disease activity. J Rheumatol 25:892, 1998.
25. Pollak VE, Pirani CL, Kark RM: Effect of large doses of prednisone on the renal lesions and life span of patients with lupus glomerulonephritis. J Lab Clin Med 57:495, 1961.
26. Pollak VE, Dosekun AK: Evaluation of treatment in lupus nephritis: Effects of prednisone. Am J Kidney Dis 2(Suppl 2):170, 1982.
27. Cathcart ES, Scheinberg MA, Idelson BA, et al: Beneficial effects of methylprednisolone "pulse" therapy in diffuse proliferative lupus nephritis. Lancet 1:163, 1976.
28. Isenberg DA, Morrow WJW, Snaith ML: Methylprednisolone pulse therapy in the treatment of systemic lupus erythematosus. Ann Rheum Dis 41:347, 1982.
29. Barron KS, Person DA, Brewer EJ Jr, et al: Pulse methylprednisolone therapy in diffuse proliferative lupus nephritis. J Pediatr 101:137, 1982.
30. Liebling MR, McLaughlin K, Boonsue S, et al: Monthly pulses of methylprednisolone in SLE nephritis. J Rheumatol 9:543, 1982.
31. Boumpas DR, Austin HA III, Vaughn EM, et al: Controlled trial of pulse methylprednisolone versus two regimens of pulse cyclophosphamide in severe lupus nephritis. Lancet 340:741, 1992.
32. Sesso R, Monteiro M, Sato E, et al: A controlled trial of pulse cyclophosphamide versus pulse methylprednisolone in severe lupus nephritis. Lupus 3:107, 1994.
33. Gourley MF, Austin HA III, Scott D, et al: Methylprednisolone and cyclophosphamide, alone or in combination, in patients with lupus nephritis. Ann Intern Med 125:549, 1996.
34. Illei GG, Austin HA, Crane M, et al: Combination therapy with pulse cyclophosphamide plus pulse methylprednisolone improves long-term renal outcome wtihout adding toxicity in patients with lupus nephritis. Ann Intern Med 135:248-257, 2001.
35. Ackerman GL: Alternate-day steroid therapy in lupus nephritis. Ann Intern Med 72:511, 1970.
36. Fauci AS: Alternate day corticosteroid therapy. Am J Med 64:729, 1978.
37. Dubois EL: Nitrogen mustard in treatment of systemic lupus erythematosus. Arch Intern Med 93:667, 1954.
38. Hahn BH, Kantor OS, Osterland CK: Azathioprine plus prednisone compared with prednisone alone in the treatment of systemic lupus erythematosus: Report of a prospective controlled trial in 24 patients. Ann Intern Med 85:597, 1975.
39. Bansal VK, Beto JA: Treatment of lupus nephritis: A meta-analysis of clinical trials. Am J Kidney Dis 29:193, 1997.
40. Balow JE, Austin HA III, Tsokos GC, et al: Lupus nephritis. Ann Intern Med 106:79, 1987.
41. Ginzler EM, Bollet AJ, Friedman EA: The natural history and response to therapy of lupus nephritis. Annu Rev Med 31:463, 1980.
42. Hellmann DB, Petri M, Whiting O'Keefe Q: Fatal infections in systemic lupus erythematosus: The role of opportunistic organisms. Medicine 66:341, 1987.
43. Klippel JH: Systemic lupus erythematosus: Treatment related complications superimposed on chronic disease. JAMA 263:1812, 1990.
44. Donadio JV Jr, Glassock RJ: Immunosuppressive drug therapy in lupus nephritis [Review]. Am J Kidney Dis 21:239, 1993.
45. Lewis EJ: The treatment of lupus nephritis: Revisiting Galen. Ann Intern Med 21:296-298, 2001.

46. Fraenkel L, Bogardus S, Concato J: Patient preferences for treatment of lupus nephritis. Arthritis Rheum 47:421-428, 2002.
47. Illei GG, Takada K, Psarkin D, et al: Renal flares are common in patients with severe proliferative lupus nephritis treated with pulse immunosuppressive therapy: Long-term follow-up of a cohort of 145 patients participating in randomized controlled studies. Arthritis Rheum 46:995-1002, 2002.
48. Steinberg AD, Steinberg SC: Longterm preservation of renal function in patients with lupus nephritis receiving treatment that includes cyclophosphamide versus those treated with prednisone only. Arthritis Rheum 34:945, 1991.
49. Ciruelo E, de la Cruz J, Lopez I, et al: Cumulative rate of relapse of lupus nephritis after successful treatment with cyclophosphamide. Arthritis Rheum 39:2028, 1996.
50. Boumpas DT, Austin HA III, Vaughan EM, et al: Risk for sustained amenorrhea in patients with systemic lupus erythematosus receiving intermittent pulse cyclophosphamide therapy. Ann Intern Med 119:366, 1993.
51. Pryor BD, Bologna SG, Kahl LE: Risk factors for serious infection during treatment with cyclophosphamide and high-dose corticosteroids for systemic lupus erythematosus. Arthritis Rheum 39:1475, 1996.
52. Hellmich B, Schnabel A, Gross WL: Treatment of severe neutropenia due to Felty's syndrome or systemic lupus erythematosus with granulocyte colony-stimulating factor. Semin Arthritis Rheum 29:82-99, 1999.
53. Houssiau FA, Vasconcelos C, D'Cruz D, et al: Immunosuppressive therapy in lupus nephritis: the Euro-Lupus Nephritis Trial, a randomized trial of low-dose versus high-dose intravenous cyclophosphamide. Arthritis Rheum 46:2121-2131, 2002.
54. Mok CC, Ho CT, Chan KW, et al: Outcome and prognostic indicators of diffuse proliferative lupus glomerulonephritis treated with sequential oral cyclophosphamide and azathioprine. Arthritis Rheum 46:1003-1013, 2002.
55. Chan TM, Li FK, Tang CS, et al: Efficacy of mycophenolate mofetil in patients with diffuse proliferative lupus nephritis. Hong Kong-Guangzhou Nephrology Study Group. N Engl J Med 343:1156-1162, 2000.
55a.Ginzler EM, Aranow C, Merrill JT, et al: Toxicity and tolerability of mycophenolate mofetil vs. intravenous cyclophosphamide in a multicenter trial as induction therapy for lupus nephritis [Abstract]. Arthritis Rheum 48:S586, 2003.
55b.Ginzler EM, Aranow C, Buyon J, et al: A multicenter study of mycophenolate mofetil vs. intravenous cyclophosphamide as induction therapy for severe lupus nephritis: Preliminary results [Abstract]. Arthritis Rheum 48:S647, 2003.
56. Eiser ER, Shanies HM: Treatment of lupus interstitial lung disease with intravenous cyclophosphamide. Arthritis Rheum 37:428, 1994.
57. Boumpas DT, Barez S, Klippel JH, et al: Intermittent cyclophosphamide for the treatment of autoimmune thrombocytopenia in systemic lupus erythematosus. Ann Intern Med 112:674, 1990.
58. deVries CR, Freiha FS: Hemorrhagic cystitis: A review. J Urol 143:1, 1990.
59. Walz LeBlanc BA, Dagenais P, Urowitz MB, et al: Methotrexate in systemic lupus erythematosus. J Rheumatol 21:836, 1994.
60. Carneiro JR, Sato EI: Double blind, randomized, placebo controlled clinical trial of methotrexate in systemic lupus erythematosus. J Rheumatol 26(6).1275-1279, 1999.
61. Sato EI: Methotrexate therapy in systemic lupus erythematosus. Lupus 10:162-164, 2001.
62. McMurray RW, Elbourne KB, Lagoo A, et al: Mycophenolate mofetil suppresses autoimmunity and mortality in the female NZB/NZW F1 mouse model of systemic lupus erythematosus. J Rheumatol 25:2364, 1998.
63. Chan TM, Wong WS, Lau CS, et al: Prolonged followup of patients with diffuse proliferative lupus nephritis treated with prednisone and mycophenolate mofetil [Abstract]. J Am Soc Nephrol 12:195A, 2001.
64. Karim MY, Alba P, Cuadrado MJ, et al: Mycophenolate mofetil for systemic lupus erythematosus refractory to other immunosuppressive agents. Rheumatology 41:876-882, 2002.
65. Roche Laboratories: Cellcept (mycophenolate mofetil capsules). In Physician's Desk Reference, 52nd ed. Medical Economics, Montvale, New Jersey, 1998, p 2265.
66. Dooley MA, Hogan S, Jennette C, et al: Cyclophosphamide therapy for lupus nephritis: Poor renal survival in black Americans. Kidney Int 51;1188-1195, 1997.
67. Lea JP: Lupus nephritis in African Americans. Am J Med Sci 323:85-89, 2002.
68. Fu LW, Yang LY, Chen WP, et al: Clinical efficacy of cyclosporin as neoral in the treatment of paediatric lupus nephritis with heavy proteinuria. Br J Rheumatol 37:217, 1998.
69. Dammacco F, Della Casa Alberighi O, Ferraccioli G, et al: Cyclosporine-A plus steroid versus steroids alone in the 12-month treatment of systemic lupus erythematosus. Int J Clin Lab Res 30:67-73, 2000.
70. Morton SJ, Powell RJ: An audit of cyclosporin for systemic lupus erythematosus and related overlap syndromes: Limitations of its use. Ann Rheum Dis 59:487-489, 2000.
71. Caccavo D, Lagana B, Mitterhofer AP, et al: Long-term treatment of systemic lupus erythematosus with cyclosporin A. Arthritis Rheum 40:27, 1997.
72. Remer CF, Weisman MH, Wallace DJ: Benefits of leflunomide in systemic lupus erythematosus: A pilot observational study. Lupus 10:480-483, 2001.
73. Traynor AE, Schroeder J, Rosa RM, et al: Treatment of severe systemic lupus erythematosus with high-dose chemotherapy and haemopoietic stem-cell transplantation: A phase I study. Lancet 356:701-707, 2000.
74. Furst DE: Stem cell transplantation for autoimmune disease: progress and problems. Curr Opin Rheumatol 14:220-224, 2002.
75. Tyndall A, Passweg J, Gratwohl A: Haemopoietic stem cell transplantation in the treatment of severe autoimmune diseases. Ann Rheum Dis 60:702-707, 2001.
75a.Trayner AE, Barr WG, Rosa RM, et al: Hematopoietic stem cell transplantation for severe and refractory lupus. Analysis after 5 years and 15 patients. Arthritis Rheum 46:2917-2923, 2002.
76. Brodsky RA, Petri M, Smith BD, et al: Immunoablative high-dose cyclophosphamide without stem-cell rescue for refractory, severe autoimmune disease. Ann Intern Med 129:1031, 1998.
77. Hahn BH: Antibodies to DNA. N Engl J Med 338:1359, 1998.
78. terBorg EJ, Horst G, Hummel EJ, et al: Measurement of increases in anti-double-stranded DNA antibody levels as a predictor of disease exacerbation in systemic lupus erythematosus: A long-term, prospective study. Arthritis Rheum 33:634, 1990.
79. Esdaile JM, Abrahamowicz M, Joseph L, et al: Laboratory tests as predictors of disease exacerbations in systemic lupus erythematosus: Why some tests fail. Arthritis Rheum 39:370, 1996.
80. Gladman DD, Urowitz MB, Keystone EC: Serologically active clinically quiescent systemic lupus erythematosus: A discordance between clinical and serologic features. Am J Med 66:210, 1979.
81. Bootsma H, Spronk P, Derksen R, et al: Prevention of relapses in systemic lupus erythematosus. Lancet 345:1595, 1995.
82. Battafarano DF, Battafarano NJ, Larsen L, et al: Antigen-specific antibody responses in lupus patients following immunization. Arthritis Rheum 41:1828, 1998.
83. Recommendations for the prevention and treatment of glucocorticoid-induced osteoporosis: American College of Rheumatology Task Force on Osteoporosis Guidelines. Arthritis Rheum 39:1791, 1996.
84. Cunnane G, Lane NE: Steroid-induced osteoporosis in systemic lupus erythematosus. Rheum Dis Clin North Am 26(2):311-329, 2000.
85. Zonana-Nacach A, Barr SG, Magder LS, Petri M: Damage in systemic lupus erythematosus and its association with corticosteroids. Arthritis Rheum 43(8):1801-1808, 2000.
86. Ramsey-Goldman R, Manzi S: Association of osteoporosis and cardiovascular disease in women with systemic lupus erythematosus. Arthritis Rheum 44(10):2338-2341, 2001.
87. Sanchez-Guerrero J, Liang MH, Karlson EW, et al: Postmenopausal estrogen therapy and the risk for developing systemic lupus erythematosus. Ann Intern Med 122:430, 1995.
88. Sanchez-Guerrero J, Karlson EW, Liang MH, et al: Past use of oral contraceptives and the risk of developing systemic lupus erythematosus. Arthritis Rheum 40:804, 1997.
88a.Buyon JP, Petri M, Kim M, et al: Estrogen/cyclic progesterone replacement is associated with an increased rate of mild/moderate but not severe flares in SLE patients in the SELENA trial. Presented at ACR as late-breaking abstract, 2003. http://www.abstractsonline.com
89. Writing Group for the Women's Health Initiative Investigators: Risks and benefits of estrogen plus progestin in healthy postmenopausal women: Principal results from the Women's Health Initiative randomized controlled trial. JAMA 17:321-323, 2002.

90. Manzi S, Selzer F, Sutton-Tyrrell K, et al: Prevalence and risk factors of carotid plaque in women with systemic lupus erythematosus. Arthritis Rheum 42(1):51-60, 1999.

91. Manzi S, Meilahn EN, Rairie JE, et al: Age-specific incidence rates of myocardial infarction and angina in women with systemic lupus erythematosus: Comparison with the Framingham Study. Am J Epidemiol 145:408-415, 1997.

91a. Roman MJ, Shanker BA, Davis A, et al: Prevalence and correlates of accelerated atherosclerosis in systemic lupus erythematosus. N Eng J Med 349:2399–2406, 2003.

91b. Asanuma Y, Oeser A, Shintani AK, et al: Premature coronary artery atherosclerosis in SLE. N Eng J Med 349:2407–2415, 2003.

92. Petri M: Detection of coronary artery disease and the role of traditional risk factors in the Hopkins Lupus Cohort. Lupus 9(3):170-175, 2000.

93. Schrott HG, Blumenthal RS, Levy R: HERS Study Group: Statin therapy, cardiovascular events, and total mortality in the heath and Estrogen/Progestin Replacement Study (HERS). Circulation 105:2962-2967, 2002.

94. Wierzbicki AS: Lipid-lowering drugs in lupus: An unexplored therapeutic intervention. Lupus 10(3):233-236, 2001.

95. Petri M: Clinical and management aspects of the antiphospholipid syndrome. In Wallace DJ, Hahn BH (eds): Dubois' Lupus Erythematosus, 6th ed. Baltimore, Lippincott, Williams & Wilkins, 2002, p 1093.

96. Khamashta MA, Cuadrado MJ, Mujic F, et al: The management of thrombosis in the antiphospholipid-antibody syndrome. N Engl J Med 332:993, 1995.

97. Rosove MH, Brewer PMC: Antiphospholipid thrombosis: Clinical course after the first thrombotic event in 70 patients. Ann Intern Med 117:303, 1992.

98. Ruiz-Irastorza G, Khamashta MA, Hunt BJ, et al: Bleeding and recurrent thrombosis in definite antiphospholipid syndrome: Analysis of a series of 66 patients treated with oral anticoagulation to a target international normalized ratio of 3.5. Arch Intern Med 162:1164-1169, 2002.

99. Rocca PV, Siegel LB, Cupps TR: The concomitant expression of vasculitis and coagulopathy: Synergy for marked tissue ischemia. J Rheumatol 21:556, 1994.

100. Kitridou RC: The mother in systemic lupus erythematosus. The fetus in systemic lupus erythematosus. In Wallace DJ, Hahn BH (eds): Dubois' Lupus Erythematosus, 6th ed. Baltimore, Lippincott, Williams & Wilkins, 2002, pp 985, 1023.

101. Moore LE, Martin JN Jr: When betamethasone and dexamethasone are unavailable: Hydrocortisone. J Perinatol 21(7):456-458, 2001.

102. O'Shea TM, Doyle LW: Perinatal glucocorticoid therapy and neurodevelopmental outcome: An epidemiologic perspective. Semin Neonatol 6(4):293-307, 2001.

103. Empson M, Lassere M, Craig JC, Scott JR: Recurrent pregnancy loss with antiphospholipid antibody: A systematic review of therapeutic trials. Obstet Gynecol 99(1):135-144, 2002.

104. Rai R, Cohen H, Dave M, et al: Randomised controlled trial of aspirin and aspirin plus heparin in pregnant women with recurrent miscarriage associated with phospholipid antibodies. Br Med J 25:314, 1997.

105. Laskin CA, Bombardier C, Hannah ME, et al: Prednisone and aspirin in women with autoantibodies and unexplained recurrent fetal loss. N Engl J Med 337:148, 1997.

106. Cowchock FS, Reece EA, Balaban D, et al: Repeated fetal losses associated with antiphospholipid antibodies: A collaborative randomized trial comparing prednisone with low-dose heparin treatment. Am J Obstet Gynecol 166:1318, 1992.

107. Lockshin MD, Druzin ML, Qamar MA: Prednisone does not prevent recurrent fetal death in women with antiphospholipid antibody. Am J Obstet Gynecol 169:439, 1989.

108. Farquharson RG, Quenby S, Greaves M: Antiphospholipid syndrome in pregnancy: A randomized, controlled trial of treatment. Obstet Gynecol 100(3):408-413, 2002.

109. Lee LA: Neonatal lupus: Clinical features, therapy, and pathogenesis. Curr Rheumatol Rep 3(5):391-395, 2001.

110. Tseng CE, Buyon JP: Neonatal lupus syndromes. Rheum Dis Clin North Am 23:31, 1997.

111. Moak JP, Barron KS, Hougen TJ, et al: Congenital heart block: development of late-onset cardiomyopathy, a previously underappreciated sequela. J Am Coll Cardiol 37(1):238-242, 2001.

112. Saleeb S, Copel J, Friedman D, Buyon JP: Comparison of treatment with fluorinated glucocorticoids to the natural history of autantibody-associated congenital heart block: Retrospective review of the research registry for neonatal lupus. Arthritis Rheum 42:2335-2345, 1999.

113. Jacobs P, Wood L: The comparison of gamma globulin to steroids in treating adult immune thrombocytopenia: An interim analysis. Blut 59:92, 1989.

114. Arnal C, Piette JC, Leone J, et al: Treatment of severe immune thrombocytopenia associated with systemic lupus erythematosus: 59 cases. J Rheumatol 29(1):75-83, 2002.

115. Hakim AJ, Machin SJ, Isenberg DA: Autoimmune thrombocytopenia in primary antiphospholipid syndrome and systemic lupus erythematosus: The response to splenectomy. Semin Arthritis Rheum 28:20, 1998.

116. Hall S, McCormick JL Jr, Greipp PR, et al: Splenectomy does not cure the thrombocytopenia of systemic lupus erythematosus. Ann Intern Med 102:325, 1985.

117. West SG, Johnson SC: Danazol for the treatment of refractory autoimmune thrombocytopenia in systemic lupus erythematosus. Ann Intern Med 108:703, 1988.

118. Blanco R, Martinez-Taboada VM, Rodriguez-Valverde V, et al: Successful therapy with danazol in refractory autoimmune thrombocytopenia associated with rheumatic diseases. Br J Rheumatol 36:1095, 1997.

119. Weill BJ, Menkes CJ, Cormier C, et al: Hepatocellular carcinoma after danazol therapy. J Rheumatol 15:1447, 1988.

120. Hellmich B, Schnabel A, Gross WL: Treatment of severe neutropenia due to Felty's syndrome or systemic lupus erythematosus with granulocyte colony-stimulating factor. Semin Arthritis Rheum 29(2):82-99, 1999.

121. Burt RK, Fassas A, Snowden J, et al: Collection of hematopoietic stem cells from patients with autoimmune diseases. Bone Marrow Transplant 28(1):1-12, 2001.

122. Hermosillo-Romo D, Brey RL: Neuropsychiatric involvement in systemic lupus erythematosus. Curr Rheumatol Rep 4(4):337-344, 2002.

123. ACR Ad Hoc Committee on Neuropsychiatric Lupus Nomenclature: The American College of Rheumatology nomenclature and case definitions for neuropsychiatric lupus syndromes. Arthritis Rheum 42:599, 1999. For definitions, see Internet site www.rheumatology.org, click on Arthritis Rheum, click on Appendix A: Case definitions for neuropsychiatric syndromes in SLE.

124. Denburg SD, Carbotte RM, Denburg JA: Corticosteroids and neuropsychological functioning in patients with SLE. Arthritis Rheum 37:1311, 1994.

125. Kolasinski SL, Chung JB, Albert DA: What do we know about lupus membranous nephropathy? An analytic review. Arthritis Rheum 47(4):450-455, 2002.

126. Austin HA III, Boumpas DT, Vaughan EM, et al: Predicting renal outcomes in severe lupus nephritis: Contributions of clinical and histologic data. Kidney Int 45:544, 1994.

127. Musio F, Bohen EM, Yuan CM, et al: Review of thrombotic thrombocytopenic purpura in the setting of systemic lupus erythematosus. Semin Arthritis Rheum 28:1, 1998.

128. Eular HH, Schroeder JO, Harten P, et al: Treatment-free remission in severe systemic lupus erythematosus following synchronization of plasmapheresis with subsequent pulse cyclophosphamide. Arthritis Rheum 37:1784, 1994.

129. Lewis DJ, Hunsicker LG, Lan SP, et al for the Lupus Nephritis Collaborative Study Group: A controlled trial of plasmapheresis therapy in severe lupus nephritis. N Engl J Med 326:1373, 1992.

130. Wofsy D, Seaman WE: Reversal of advanced murine lupus in NZB/NZW F1 mice by in vivo treatment with anti-L3T4. J Immunol 138:2089, 1987.

131. Hahn BH, Ebling FM: Suppression of murine lupus nephritis by administration of an antiidiotypic antibody to antiDNA. J Immunol 132:187, 1984.

132. Uner AH, Knupp CJ, Tatum AH, et al: Treatment with antibody reactive with the nephritogenic idiotype, IdLNF1, suppresses its

production and leads to prolonged survival of NZB(SWR)F1 mice. J Autoimmun 7:27, 1994.

133. Gross JA, Johnston J, Mudri S, et al: TACI and BCMA are receptors for a TNF homologue implicated in B-cell autoimmune disease. Nature 404(6781):995-999, 2000.

134. Dorner T, Putterman C: B cells, BAFF/zTNF4, TACI, and systemic lupus erythematosus. Arthritis Res 3(4):197-199, 2001.

135. Finck BK, Linsley PS, Wofsy D: Treatment of murine lupus with CTLA4Ig. Science 265:1225, 1994.

136. Daikh DI, Finck BK, Linsley PS, et al: Long-term inhibition of murine lupus by brief simultaneous blockade of the B7/CD28 and CD40/p39 costimulation pathways. J Immunol 159:3104, 1997.

137. Daikh DI, Wofsy D: Cutting edge: Reversal of murine lupus nephritis with CTLA4Ig and cyclophosphamide. J Immunol 166:2913-2916, 2001.

138. Hahn BH, Singh RR, Wong WK, et al: Treatment with a consensus peptide based on amino acid sequences in autoantibodies prevents T cell activation by autoantigens and delays disease onset in murine lupus. Arthritis Rheum 44(2):432-441, 2001.

139. Ishida H, Muchamuel T, Sakaguchi S, et al: Continuous administration of anti-interleukin 10 antibodies delays onset of autoimmunity in NZB/W F1 mice. J Exp Med 179:305, 1994.

140. Kiberd BA: Interleukin-6 receptor blockage ameliorates murine lupus nephritis. J Am Soc Nephrol 4:58, 1993.

141. Wang B, Yamamoto Y, El-Badri NS, Good RA: Effective treatment of autoimmune disease and progressive renal disease by mixed bone-marrow transplantation that establishes a stable mixed chimerism in BXSB recipient mice. Proc Natl Acad Sci USA 96(6):3012-3016, 1999.

142. Leandro MJ, Edwards JC, Cambridge G, et al: An open study of B lymphocyte depletion in systemic lupus erythematosus. Arthritis Rheum 46(10):2673-2677, 2002.

143. Lorenz HM: Abetimus (La Jolla pharmaceuticals). Curr Opin Investig Drugs 3(2):234-239, 2002.

144. Wallace DJ: Management of lupus erythematosus: recent insights. Curr Opin Rheumatol 14(3):212-219, 2002.

145. Furie RA, Cash JM, Cronin ME, et al: Treatment of systemic lupus erythematosus with LJP 394. J Rheumatol 28(2):257-266, 2001.

145a.Alarcon-Segovia D, Tumlin JA, Furie RA, et al: CJP 394 for the prevention of renal flare in patients with SLE: Results from a randomized, double-blind placebo controlled study. Arthritis Rheum 48:442–454, 2003.

146. Genovese MC, Uhrin Z, Bloch DA, et al: Long-term followup of patients treated with total lymphoid irradiation for lupus nephritis. Arthritis Rheum 46(4):1014-1018, 2002.

147. Sany J: Intravenous immunoglobulin therapy for rheumatic diseases [Review]. Curr Opin Rheumatol 6:305, 1994.

148. Ginzler E, Diamond HS, Weiner M, et al: A multicenter study of outcome in systemic lupus erythematosus. Arthritis Rheum 25:605, 1982.

149. Ginzler EM, Schorn K: Outcome and prognosis in systemic lupus erythematosus. Rheum Dis Clin North Am 14:67, 1988.

150. Ward MM, Pyun E, Studenski S: Long-term survival in systemic lupus erythematosus: Patient characteristics associated with poorer outcomes. Arthritis Rheum 38:274, 1995.

151. Jacobsen S, Petersen J, Ullman S, et al: A multicentre study of 513 Danish patients with SLE. II. Disease mortality and clinical factors of prognostic value. Clin Rheumatol 17:478, 1998.

152. Nossent HC, Swaak TJG, Berden JHM, et al: Systemic lupus erythematosus after renal transplantation: Patient and graft survival and disease activity. Ann Intern Med 114:183, 1991.

153. Stone JH, Amend WJ, Criswell LA: Outcome of renal transplantation in 97 cyclosporin-era patients with systemic lupus erythematosus and matched controls. Arthritis Rheum 41:438, 1998.

154. Stone JH, Millward CL, Olson JL, et al: Frequency of recurrent lupus nephritis among 97 renal transplant patients during the cyclosporine era. Arthritis Rheum 41:678, 1998.

155. Urowitz MB, Gladman DD, Abu-Shakra M, et al: Mortality studies in SLE: Results from a single center. III. Improved survival over 24 years. J Rheumatol 24:1061, 1997.

77

Antiphospholipid Antibody Syndrome

MICHAEL D. LOCKSHIN

▐ Definition and Classification

DEFINITION OF THE ANTIPHOSPHOLIPID ANTIBODY SYNDROME

Synonyms for the antiphospholipid antibody syndrome (APS) are anticardiolipin antibody, lupus anticoagulant, and Hughes' syndrome. Diagnosis requires that a patient have both a clinical event (thrombosis or pregnancy loss) and an antiphospholipid antibody (aPL) documented by a solid-phase serum assay (anticardiolipin), an inhibitor of phospholipid-dependent clotting (lupus anticoagulant), or both. A false-positive test for syphilis does not fulfill the laboratory criterion. Preliminary 1999 classification criteria for APS are listed in Table 77–1.[1] New data indicate that elements not included as criteria also identify patients with APS: immunoglobulin A (IgA) aPL antibody, valvular heart disease, thrombocytopenia, preeclampsia, and livedo reticularis, but not intrauterine growth restriction[2] (Table 77–2). Antibody to the phospholipid-binding protein β_2 glycoprotein I (β_2GPI) will likely be a future diagnostic criterion (see following).

APS can occur as an isolated diagnosis, known as primary antiphospholipid antibody syndrome (PAPS), or it can be associated with systemic lupus erythematosus (SLE) or another rheumatic disease and known as secondary APS (sAPS). aPL, but not the syndrome, can be induced by drugs and by infections.[3] Positive tests for aPL may precede symptoms for many years.[4] The probability that an asymptomatic person incidentally found to have aPL will eventually develop the syndrome is unknown, but it is likely low.

DIAGNOSTIC AUTOANTIBODIES

The antigen to which aPL binds is β_2GPI (apolipoprotein H). β_2GPI is normally present at a concentration of 200 μg/ml, is a member of the complement control protein family, and has five repeating domains and several alleles. An octapeptide in the fifth domain and critical cysteine bonds are necessary for both phospholipid-binding and antigenicity; a first-domain site is also critical for pathogenicity.[5] In vivo, β_2GPI binds to phosphatidylserine on activated or apoptotic cell membranes, including those of trophoblast, platelets, and endothelial cells. This binding may also initiate cell activation or apoptosis and may initiate coagulation. Other phospholipid binding proteins, such as prothrombin, may substitute for β_2GPI in some patients with this disorder.

Although the widely available enzyme-linked immunosorbent assay (ELISA) for anticardiolipin antibody is standardized, considerable variability exists among commercial laboratories that perform the test.[6] Normal persons have IgG and IgA antibody less than 16 GPL or APL (G = IgG; A = IgA; PL = phospholipid) units/ml and IgM less than 5 MPL (M = IgM) units/ml. The low-positive range is 17 to 40 GPL, MPL, or APL units, and high-positive values are above 80 GPL or 40 MPL or APL units. The anticardiolipin ELISA is sensitive but not specific for the diagnosis of APS.[7]

Documentation of a lupus anticoagulant requires the four-step process outlined in Table 77–1. Most patients with APS defined by a lupus anticoagulant have highly abnormal activated partial thromboplastin time (aPTT) or Russell viper venom time (RVVT). Low-level aPTT or RVVT abnormalities are not clearly linked to the APS. Approximately 80 percent of patients with lupus anticoagulant have anticardiolipin antibody, and 20 percent of patients positive for anticardiolipin antibody have lupus anticoagulant.

Autoimmune aPLs bind β_2GPI or other phospholipid-binding proteins, which in turn bind negatively charged phospholipids (β_2GPI-dependent aPL). Infection-induced aPLs are β_2GPI-independent; they bind phospholipid directly and are induced by infections such as syphilitic and nonsyphilitic *Treponema*, *Borrelia burgdorferi*, human immunodeficiency virus (HIV), *Leptospira*, and parasites.[8] β_2GPI-independent aPLs are not associated with thrombosis or with pregnancy loss.

Negative predictive value is high for β_2GPI-dependent anticardiolipin, lupus anticoagulant, and anti-β_2GPI tests, but positive predictive value is not. The clinical tests for antibody to phosphatidylserine and phosphatidyl-ethanolamine are neither standardized nor widely accepted as predictors of clinical illness. Antibodies to prothrombin (factor II), thrombomodulin, and other coagulation proteins sometimes accompany aPLs directed against β_2GPI.[9] Antiprothrombin may cause hemorrhage by depleting prothrombin. Some APS patients also have antibody to endothelial cell antigens.[10,11]

▐ Epidemiology and Genetics

Low-titer anticardiolipin antibody occurs in 2 to 7 percent of normal blood donors and moderate- to high-titer anticardiolipin antibody or lupus anticoagulant in 0.2 percent. The prevalence of positive tests increases with age. From 60 to 80 percent of patients with PAPS are women. Familial disease is frequent, but HLA typing of patients has not revealed a single consistent profile. Patients of

TABLE 77–1 • PRELIMINARY CLASSIFICATION CRITERIA FOR ANTIPHOSPHOLIPID ANTIBODY SYNDROME (APS)

Type	Criteria
Clinical	
Vascular thrombosis	One or more episodes of: Arterial thrombosis, *or* Venous thrombosis, *or* Small vessel thrombosis, in any tissue or organ, confirmed by imaging or Doppler studies or histopathologic studies. For histopathologic confirmation, thrombosis should be present without significant evidence of inflammation in the vessel wall.
Pregnancy morbidity	One or more: Unexplained deaths of a morphologically normal fetus at or after the 10th week of gestation with fetal morphology documented by ultrasound or by direct examination of the fetus, *or* Premature birth of a morphologically normal neonate at or before the 34th week of gestation because of severe preeclampsia, eclampsia, or severe placental insufficiency, *or* Three or more unexplained consecutive miscarriages with anatomic, genetic, or hormonal causes excluded.
Laboratory	
Anticardiolipin antibody (aCL)	Immunoglobulin G (IgG) and/or IgM isotype present in medium or high titer on two or more occasions, 6 weeks or more apart, *and* Measured by a standardized ELISA for β_2 glycoprotein I–dependent anticardiolipin antibody Abnormality present in plasma on two or more occasions, 6 weeks or more apart, *and* Detected according to the guidelines of the International Society on Thrombosis and Hemostasis Scientific Subcommittee on Lupus Anticoagulants/phospholipid-dependent antibodies in the following steps: 1. Demonstration of a prolonged phospholipid-dependent coagulation screening test (e.g., activated partial thromboplastin time, kaolin clotting time, dilute Russell viper venom time, dilute prothrombin time) 2. Failure to correct the prolonged screening test by mixing with normal platelet poor plasma 3. Shortening or correction of the prolonged screening test by the addition of excess phospholipid 4. Exclusion of other coagulopathies as clinically indicated (e.g., factor VIII inhibitor, heparin)

Adapted from Wilson WA, Gharavi AE, Koike T, et al: International consensus statement on preliminary classification criteria for antiphospholipid syndrome: Report of an international workshop. Arthritis Rheum 42:1309, 1999.

African ancestry may be more likely than are those of European ancestry to have IgA isotype antibody.[12]

TABLE 77–2 • NONDEFINING CLINICAL AND LABORATORY FEATURES OF THE ANTIPHOSPHOLIPID ANTIBODY SYNDROME*

Type	Features
Clinical	Livedo reticularis* Thrombocytopenia (usually 50,000 to 100,000 platelets/mm³)* Autoimmune hemolytic anemia Cardiac valve disease (late finding)* Multiple sclerosis–like syndrome and other myelopathy Nonfocal neurologic symptoms Chorea Catastrophic vascular occlusion syndrome* Pulmonary hypertension Systemic hypertension Renal failure
Laboratory	Immunoglobulin A (IgA) anticardiolipin antibody* Antibodies to phosphatidylserine, phosphatidylinositol, phosphatidylglycerol, phosphatidylethanolamine Antibody to β_2 glycoprotein I* Proteinuria False-positive test for syphilis* Hyperintense lesions on T2-weighted brain magnetic resonance imaging (MRI)

*Components identified with an asterisk have been shown in formal studies to be statistically associated with the syndrome subsequent to publication of the Sapporo Criteria (see Table 77–1).

According to a study of normal male physicians followed prospectively for 3 years, those with moderate to high titers of IgG anticardiolipin antibody have a risk for thrombophlebitis or pulmonary embolus eight times higher than do men with negative tests.[13] Approximately 10 percent of first-stroke victims have aPL,[14] especially those who are young,[15] as do up to 21 percent of women who have suffered three or more consecutive fetal losses.[16] In a retrospective study, 60 percent of women identified to have aPL after an abnormal pregnancy suffered a thrombotic event in the subsequent 10 years.[17]

β_2GPI polymorphisms influence the generation of aPL in individuals, but they have only a weak relationship to occurrence of APS.[18] Both persons congenitally lacking β_2GPI and β_2GPI knockout mice appear normal.[19]

Etiology

In experimental animal models, passive or active immunization with viral peptides,[20] bacterial peptides,[21] and heterologous β_2GPI[22] induce polyclonal aPL, lupus anticoagulant, and clinical events associated with APS. These data suggest that pathologic aPL is induced in humans by infection; direct proof of this hypothesis is lacking.

Pathogenesis and Pathophysiology

Because high-titer antibody may persist for years in asymptomatic persons, it is likely that vascular injury.

FIGURE 77–1 • Proposed Mechanism of Thrombosis and Placental Injury. The negatively charged phospholipid, phosphatidylserine (PS, orange circles), migrates from the inner to the outer cell membrane during activation or apoptosis of platelets and endothelial cells, and it is normally present on trophoblasts. (The neutral phospholipid, phosphatidylcholine [PC, green circles], is the major constituent of the outer layer of unactivated cells.) Dimeric β_2 glycoprotein I (β_2GPI) then binds to PS and antiphospholipid antibody (aPL) binds to β_2GPI, activating complement and triggering several signals, leading to expression of adhesion molecules (e.g., ICAM-1) and tissue factor (TF), platelet aggregation, and thrombosis. Placental effects of aPL are indicated in red. Placental anticoagulant protein I (PAP-1, annexin V) normally provides a shield on trophoblast PS, protecting the fetus against activation of maternal prothrombotic processes. This shield is broken by β_2GPI-APS complex. It is likely that complement activation, recruiting and stimulating inflammatory cells, is a critical downstream element of fetal injury. APLs also downregulate expression of trophoblast signal transducer and activator of transcription 5 (STAT-5), reducing endometrial stromal cell production of prolactin (PRL) and insulin growth factor binding protein-1 (IGFBP-1). (Adapted from Rai R, Roubey R, Rand J, et al. Presented at the 10th International Antiphospholipid Antibody Conference, Taormina, Sicily, October, 2002). (See color plate 40.)

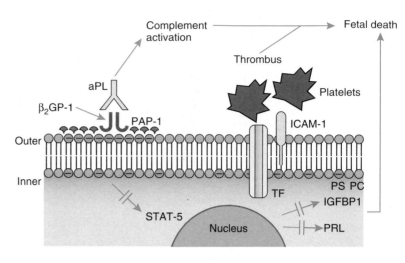

endothelial cell activation, or both immediately precede the occurrence of thrombosis in persons bearing the antibody. A proposed pathogenesis is illustrated in Figure 77–1. The process begins with activation or apoptosis of platelets, endothelial cells, or trophoblasts, during which the negatively charged phospholipid phosphatidylserine migrates from the inner to the normally electrically neutral outer cell membrane. Circulating β_2GPI then binds to phosphatidylserine. APL then binds to a β_2GPI dimer,[23] initiating a signaling cascade that induces cell surface tissue factor expression and adhesion molecules, causing platelets to aggregate and initiate thrombosis.[24] In the placenta, aPL competes for phosphatidylserine with the natural anticoagulant placental anticoagulant protein I (annexin V),[25,26] interrupting a shield that is thought to protect the fetus from maternal prothrombotic mechanisms.[27] Through downregulation of signal transducer and activator of transcription 5 (Stat5) aPLs also inhibit production of placental prolactin, insulin growth factor β-1,[28] and they adversely affect formation of a trophoblast syncytium, placental apoptosis, and trophoblast invasion—all processes required for normal establishment of placental function. In vitro, pathogenic aPLs induce adhesion molecules and enhance adherence of leukocytes to endothelium.[29,30] In experimental animal models, aPL causes fetal resorption and increases size and duration of trauma-induced venous and arterial thrombi.[31,32] Inhibiting complement activation prevents experimental aPL-induced fetal death, and C5 knockout mice carry pregnancies normally despite aPL,[33] implying that a complement-mediated effector mechanism is an absolute requirement for fetal death to occur.

Low-level aPL is present in normal people; under physiologic conditions, β_2GPI may function in the elimination of apoptotic cells.[34]

Independent coagulopathies (heritable deficiencies of protein C, protein S, or antithrombin III; mutations of factor V [A506G, factor V_{Leiden}], prothrombin [G20210A], or methylene tetrahydrofolate reductase [MTHFR C677T, hyperhomocysteinemia]) may further increase thrombotic risk of patients with aPL. aPL binds to oxidized low-density lipoprotein, possibly contributing to the development of atherosclerosis.[35] A function of normal aPL may be to participate in the physiologic removal of oxidized lipids.

Diagnosis

CLINICAL MANIFESTATIONS

Vascular Occlusion and Miscellaneous Manifestations

APS occurs as a multisystem disease affecting all organ systems. Its principal manifestations are recurrent venous or arterial thromboses, recurrent pregnancy loss, and catastrophic vascular occlusion. Many patients have livedo reticularis (Figure 77–2). Except for its severity, the youth of affected patients, and unusual anatomic locations (Budd-Chiari syndrome and sagittal sinus and upper extremity thromboses), venous thromboses in APS do not clinically differ from thromboses attributable to other causes. Similarly, arterial thromboses differ from those not associated with aPL only because of their recurrent nature, unusual locations, and occurrence in young patients. Glomerular capillary endothelial cell injury or thrombosis of renal vessels causes proteinuria without celluria or hypocomplementemia and may lead to severe hypertension, renal failure, or both.[36] Table 77–2 lists additional nondefining clinical and laboratory features that commonly occur in APS.

Valvular heart disease, a late manifestation, may necessitate valve replacement. Its pathogenesis in APS is unknown. Some patients develop nonfocal neurologic symptoms such as lack of concentration, forgetfulness, and dizzy spells. Multiple small, hyperintense

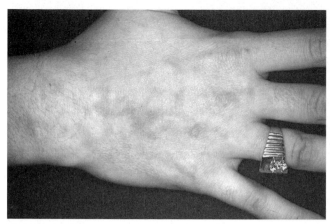

FIGURE 77–2 · Livedo reticularis in a patient with the primary antiphospholipid antibody syndrome (APS).

lesions seen on magnetic resonance imaging (MRI), primarily in the periventricular white matter, do not correlate well with clinical symptoms.

Pregnancy Loss

Pregnancy losses in patients with aPL typically occur after 10 weeks' gestation, but early losses also occur.[37] However, early pregnancy losses are more commonly due to chromosomal and other genetic defects. An APS pregnancy is often normal until the second trimester, when fetal growth slows and amniotic fluid volume decreases. APS patients may develop severe, early preeclampsia and HELLP (*h*emolysis, *e*levated *l*iver enzymes, *l*ow *p*latelets) syndrome. Placental infarction is a cause of fetal growth restriction or death; nonthrombotic mechanisms of placental dysfunction also occur.[26-28] Prior pregnancy losses predict future losses independent of aPL titer.

Catastrophic Vascular Occlusion Syndrome

The catastrophic vascular occlusion syndrome is a rare, abrupt, life-threatening complication of APS. It consists of multiple thromboses of medium and small arteries occurring (despite apparently adequate anticoagulation) over a period of days, causing stroke, cardiac, hepatic, adrenal, renal, and intestinal infarction and peripheral gangrene.[38] Proposed formal criteria for this syndrome are shown in Table 77–3.[39]

Acute adrenal failure may be the initial clinical event. Patients often have moderate thrombocytopenia, erythrocytes are less fragmented than in the hemolytic-uremic syndrome or thrombotic thrombocytopenic purpura, and fibrin split products are not strikingly elevated. Renal failure and pulmonary hemorrhage may occur. Tissue biopsies show noninflammatory vascular occlusion.[40]

LABORATORY TESTS

Blood

Patients with APS have persistent, moderate- or high-titer IgG or IgM anticardiolipin antibody (rarely IgA only), lupus anticoagulant, or both. (Tests for antibody to β_2GPI and other phospholipid-binding proteins will likely supplant anticardiolipin as a defining antibody.) Because commercial laboratories vary in their consistency of measurement, tests should be repeated for verification. High antibody titer, IgG isotype, and IgG_2 subclass impart poor prognoses.[41] Lupus anticoagulant is a more specific but less sensitive predictor of thromboses than is anticardiolipin. Low-titer, transient, or IgD and IgE antibody, and antibody to noncardiolipin (phosphatidylserine, phosphatidylethanolamine) phospholipids do not have a proven relationship to APS.

Antinuclear and anti-DNA antibodies occur in approximately 45 percent of patients clinically diagnosed as having PAPS[42]; they do not mandate the additional diagnosis of SLE if the patient has no clinical indicators of SLE. Thrombocytopenia in APS is usually modest (more than 50,000/mm^3); proteinuria and renal insufficiency occur in patients with thrombotic microangiopathy. Pathologic examination demonstrates small artery and glomerular thrombi and recanalization (Fig. 77–3). Hypocomple-

TABLE 77–3 · PRELIMINARY CRITERIA FOR THE CLASSIFICATION OF CATASTROPHIC ANTIPHOSPHOLIPID SYNDROME (APS)

1. Evidence of involvement of three or more organs, systems, or tissues[*]
2. Development of manifestations simultaneously or in less than 1 week
3. Confirmation by histopathology of small vessel occlusion in at least one organ or tissue[†]
4. Laboratory confirmation of the presence of antiphospholipid antibody (aPL) (LA or aCL or anti-β_2–glycoprotein antibodies)[‡]

Definite catastrophic APS
  All four criteria
Probable catastrophic APS
  Criteria 2 through 4 and two organs, systems, or tissues involved
  Criteria 1 through 3, except no confirmations 6 weeks apart due to early death of patient not tested before catastrophic episode
  Criteria 1, 2, 4
  Criteria 1, 3, 4 and development of a third event more than 1 week but less than 1 month after first despite anticoagulation

[*]Usually, clinical evidence of vessel occlusions, confirmed by imaging techniques when appropriate. Renal involvement is defined by a 50-percent rise in serum creatinine, severe systemic hypertension, proteinuria, or some combination of these.

[†]For histopathologic confirmation, significant evidence of thrombosis must be present, although vasculitis may coexist occasionally.

[‡]If the patient had not been previously diagnosed as having APS, laboratory confirmation requires that presence of aPL be detected on two or more occasions at least 6 weeks apart (not necessarily at the time of the event), according to the proposed preliminary criteria for the classification of APS.

Adapted from Asherson RA, Cervera R, de Goot PG, et al: Catastrophic antiphospholipid syndrome: International consensus statement on classification criteria and treatment guidelines. Lupus 12:530, 2003.

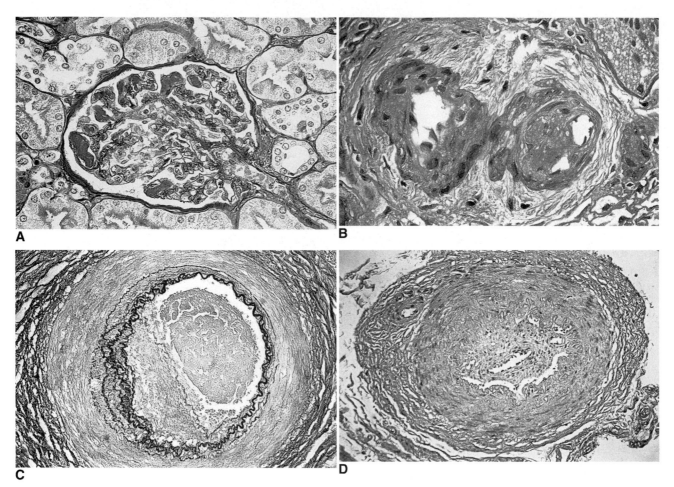

FIGURE 77–3 • Thrombotic Microangiopathy in the Antiphospholipid Antibody Syndrome (APS). *A*, Kidney biopsy from a 35-year-old woman with primary antiphospholipid syndrome (PAPS), microhematuria, and non-nephrotic proteinuria. Note the glomerulus containing microthrombi occluding capillary lumina, with endothelial swelling. *B*, Same patient's small renal artery containing organized thrombus with recanalization and arteriosclerosis (periodic acid–Schiff, ×100). *C*, Autopsy specimen from a 45-year-old man with PAPS. Note the thrombus in various stages of organization, intact elastic lamina with focal reduplication, and medial thickening (elastic Verhoff's stain, ×100). *D*, Same patient's medium-sized peripheral artery. Note the organized thrombus with recanalization, severe fibrointimal thickening, medial hypertrophy, and extreme stenosis of lumen (H&E, ×75). (Slides and caption provided by Dr. Surya V. Seshan.) (See color plate 41).

mentemia, erythrocyte casts, and pyuria are not characteristic of thrombotic microangiopathy and imply lupus glomerulonephritis. Erythrocyte sedimentation rate (ESR), hemoglobin, and leukocyte count are usually normal in patients with uncomplicated PAPS, except during acute thrombosis. Prothrombin fragment 1 plus 2 and other markers of coagulation activation do not predict impending thrombosis.

Serologic Tests

Initial diagnosis requires testing for anticardiolipin by ELISA or lupus anticoagulant with an aPTT or a dilute RVVT, confirming an abnormal clotting test with a formal test of lupus anticoagulant (see Table 77–1). At least one of these tests must be abnormal in moderate to high titer. Positive results require a repeat test after several weeks to exclude a transient, clinically unimportant antibody. Patients repeatedly normal in both tests who are still suspected of having APS should be tested for anti-

body to β_2GPI. Whether to test persons with venous occlusive disease simultaneously for protein C, protein S, and antithrombin III deficiency or for the factor V Leiden or prothrombin mutations is a matter of economics and clinical likelihood; all genetic thrombophilias likely cause recurrent fetal loss. Such testing is advisable when feasible. It is useful to test persons with arterial occlusive disease for hyperhomocystinemia.

Patients positive for aPL should also be tested for platelet count, antinuclear antibody (ANA), urinalysis, and ESR, with further evaluation for lupus if abnormalities are found. (Patients tested as part of pregnancy counseling should also be tested for anti-Ro/SSA and anti-La/SSB antibodies, because the risk of neonatal lupus occurs in the same patient population.)

IMAGING STUDIES

MRI studies show vascular occlusion and infarction consistent with clinical symptoms, without special characteristics, except that multiple otherwise unexplained cerebral infarctions in a young person suggest the syndrome. Multiple small, hyperintense white-matter lesions are common and do not unequivocally imply brain infarction. Occlusions usually occur in vessels below the resolution limits of angiography; hence, angiography or magnetic resonance angiography is not indicated unless clinical findings suggest medium- or large-vessel disease. Echocardiography or cardiac MRI may show severe Libman-Sacks endocarditis and intracardiac thrombi.[43]

PATHOLOGY

Skin, renal, and other tissues show noninflammatory occlusion of all caliber arteries and veins, acute and chronic endothelial injury and its sequelae, and recanalization in late lesions. The finding of inflammatory necrotizing vasculitis suggests concomitant lupus or other connective tissue disease. There are no other diagnostic immunofluorescence or electron microscopic findings.

Differential Diagnosis

POSITIVE ANTIPHOSPHOLIPID ANTIBODY TESTS

Nonautoimmune causes for a positive aPL test are outlined in Table 77–4. High-titer β_9GPI-dependent aPL, repeatedly demonstrable over several months, in a patient with appropriate symptoms, confirms a diagnosis of APS. Infection-induced antibody is usually transient and is more commonly IgM than IgG.[44] Transient and low-titer antibodies are inconclusive for diagnosis. Research laboratories can distinguish autoimmune from infection-induced aPL by determination of the antibody's β_9GPI dependence. In a patient who has lupus or lupus-like disease, livedo reticularis, or long-standing thrombocytopenia, and who has a strongly positive aPL test, it is usually unnecessary to exclude other diagnoses.

PREGNANCY

Five to 21 percent of women with recurrent pregnancy losses, and 0.5 to 2 percent of normal pregnant women, have aPL. Heritable deficiency of protein C, protein S, and antithrombin III and presence of the factor V Leiden, prothrombin, and methylene tetrahydrofolate reductase (MTHFR) mutations are other, less common

causes of fetal loss.[45,46] Attribution of pregnancy loss to APS is most certain when there is no coexisting plausible alternative, when the loss occurs after the demonstration of fetal heart beat (10 weeks), when high-titer aPL is repeatedly positive before and after pregnancy, and when the placenta shows vasculopathy and infarction. A single pregnancy loss before 10 weeks' gestation in a patient with a low-positive aPL test is more likely to be attributable to fetal chromosomal abnormalities, infection, or maternal hormonal or anatomic abnormalities.

THROMBOSIS

Fourteen percent of patients with recurrent venous thromboembolic disease have aPL.[47] Nephrotic syndrome; venous insufficiency; immobility; venous obstruction; thromboplastin-releasing tumors; factor V Leiden; prothrombin 20210; and protein C, protein S, and antithrombin III deficiency are alternative causes of venous thromboembolic disease. Arterial occlusion occurs in patients with thrombotic thrombocytopenic purpura, infected or sterile emboli of cardiac or vascular origin, septicemia, hyperhomocystinemia, myxoma, Takayasu's arteritis, polyarteritis nodosa, and severe Raynaud's disease. The relationship of Sneddon syndrome (stroke and livedo reticularis, with or without aPL) to APS is uncertain.

CATASTROPHIC VASCULAR OCCLUSION

This disastrous syndrome has few mimics. Among them are polyarteritis nodosa and disseminated embolization from myxoma, atrial thrombus, or atherosclerotic plaque. Small vessel occlusions occurring in rapid succession suggest disseminated intravascular coagulation. Severe cerebral and renal disease suggest thrombotic thrombocytopenic purpura; renal failure and hemolysis suggest hemolytic-uremic syndrome. APL is rarely present in patients with the alternative diagnoses. Acute adrenal insufficiency is characteristic only of APS and Waterhouse-Friderichsen syndrome.

Treatment

GENERAL PRINCIPLES

Anticoagulation is the treatment for APS. Warfarin, heparin, and low-molecular-weight heparin, often in

TABLE 77–4 · NONAUTOIMMUNE CAUSES FOR POSITIVE ANTIPHOSPHOLIPID ANTIBODY TESTS

Assay Type	Antibody Type	Causes
ELISA	β_2-Glycoprotein independent	Infection: syphilis, Lyme disease, leptospirosis, pinta, human immunodeficiency virus (HIV)
	β_2-Glycoprotein dependent	Advanced age
		Medications
	Either	Lymphoproliferative disease
		Hyperimmunoglobulin M
Lupus anticoagulant	None	Infection: HIV, drugs

association with low-dose aspirin, are all used. Anti-coagulation is indicated for seropositive patients with thrombosis and at the diagnosis of pregnancy in a seropositive woman who has had prior pregnancy losses attributable to APS. Anticoagulation is not indicated for prophylactic treatment of asymptomatic seropositive persons. Because warfarin is teratogenic, only unfrac-tionated or low-molecular-weight heparin is used for treatment of affected pregnancies in the United States; in other countries, converting to warfarin after the first trimester is considered acceptable.[48,49]

Anticoagulation for thrombosis is initiated in a stan-dard manner with heparin, followed by long-term maintenance with warfarin, usually at international normalized ratio (INR) of 2.5.[50,51] Some patients require larger than expected doses of both heparin and warfarin to achieve therapeutic anticoagulation. Although most physicians with special interest in this field now use low-molecular-weight heparin for pregnant patients and for patients unable or unwilling to take warfarin, no clinical trial has compared low-molecular-weight heparin to unfractionated heparin or warfarin. Many physicians add low-dose (81 to 325 mg/day) aspirin, hydroxychloro-quine, or both to heparin or warfarin; the justification for this practice rests primarily on retrospective data and association studies. Cortico-steroids have no established role in the treatment of PAPS but are used for rheumatic symptoms in sAPS. However, high doses of cortico-steroids are usually empirically given to patients with severe thrombocytopenia, hemolytic anemia, and the catastrophic syndrome.

In some patients, lupus anticoagulants cause the INR to be unreliable.[52] Such patients may be treated with war-farin, monitored by special assays, or with unfractionated or low-molecular-weight heparin monitored by measure-ment of antifactor Xa activity or other appropriate assay. For well-anticoagulated patients who continue to have thromboses, aspirin, hydroxychloroquine, a statin drug, intravenous Ig, and plasmapheresis have theoretical bases for efficacy and have all been used. No published experi-ence in APS patients exists for clopidogrel, pentoxifylline, Aggrenox, argatroban, hirudins, and other new anticoag-ulant agents. Clinical experience suggests that throm-bolytic agents for acute thrombosis are unhelpful, because reocclusion rapidly occurs. Treatment recom-mendations are summarized in Table 77–5.

POSITIVE, ASYMPTOMATIC PERSONS

Asymptomatic persons serendipitously found to have a weakly or transiently positive aPL test need no prophylac-tic therapy. For those with moderate- to high-titer, persist-ent aPL, education about the meaning of the abnormal test is appropriate, as is a discussion of warning signs to report. Persistence of aPL for decades without clinical events is well documented. Ongoing prospective clinical trials will determine whether asymptomatic persons with high-titer aPL should be treated prophylactically. Pregnant women with low-titer antibody should be closely monitored and retested during pregnancy, because the titer of the aPL may increase during pregnancy, and prog-nosis is related to the highest titer documented.

TABLE 77–5 • TREATMENT RECOMMENDATIONS

Antibody Titer	Clinical Circumstance	Recommendation
Moderate or high positive	Asymptomatic	No treatment*
	Equivocal thrombosis	Aspirin, 81 mg/day
	Recurrent venous thrombosis	Warfarin INR 2.5 indefinitely
	Arterial thrombosis	Warfarin INR 2.5 indefinitely
	First pregnancy	No treatment*
	Single pregnancy loss at less than 10 weeks	No treatment*
	Recurrent fetal loss or loss after 10 weeks, no thrombosis	Low-dose heparin (5000 U bid) or low-molecular-weight heparin throughout pregnancy, discontinue 6 to 12 weeks postpartum
	Recurrent fetal loss or loss after 10 weeks, thrombosis	Therapeutic heparin or low-molecular-weight heparin throughout pregnancy, warfarin postpartum
	Livedo reticularis	No treatment†
	Leg ulcers	Warfarin, INR 2.5
	Valve nodules or deformity	No known effective treatment; full anticoagulation if emboli or intracardiac thrombi demonstrated
	Thrombocytopenia of more than 50,000/mm³	No treatment
	Thrombocytopenia *less than or equal to* 50,000/mm³	Prednisone up to 60 mg/day
Absent or low-positive	Recurrent venous thrombosis	Evaluate for protein C, protein S, or antithrombin III deficiency, factor V Leiden; warfarin, INR 2.0 to 3.0 indefinitely
	Arterial thrombosis	Evaluate for homocystinemia, atherosclerosis, vasculitis; warfarin 2.5 indefinitely
	Recurrent pregnancy loss	Evaluate for other coagulopathies, other causes of pregnancy loss; consider heparin, 5000 U bid or low-molecular-weight heparin throughout pregnancy; discontinue 6 to 12 weeks postpartum

*Aspirin (81 mg/day) may be given.
†Anticoagulation may be considered.

POSITIVE PATIENTS WITH AN AMBIGUOUS CLINICAL EVENT

Some patients with positive aPL tests have clinical events of ambiguous meaning (dizzy or confusional episodes, nonspecific visual disturbance, very early pregnancy loss). There is no consensus for the treatment of such persons. Because full anticoagulation carries high risk, many physicians prescribe low-dose (81 mg) aspirin, hydroxychloroquine, or both daily. No published data support or repudiate this recommendation.

VENOUS THROMBOSIS

Retrospective studies advocate warfarin anticoagulation to very high INRs, but recent prospective studies indicate that an anticoagulation target INR of 2.5 is sufficient for uncomplicated patients with either venous or arterial thrombosis.[51] Venous thrombosis APS patients have high recurrence rates if anticoagulation is discontinued. Lifelong anticoagulation of patients is appropriate.[53,54]

ARTERIAL THROMBOSIS

Patients with arterial thrombosis should receive high-dose anticoagulation indefinitely, even though the risk of hemorrhage is high.[55] Normalization of the lupus anticoagulant or anticardiolipin antibody tests is *not* an indication to discontinue anticoagulation, because patients remain at risk for new thrombosis regardless of change in titer.

PREGNANCY

Prior Fetal Losses Later Than 10 Gestational Weeks

Subcutaneous heparin, 5000 units twice daily, with low-dose aspirin, increases the fetal survival rate from 50 to 80 percent among women who have had at least two fetal losses and who have unequivocally positive tests for aPL.[56] Most experts in the field now use low-molecular-weight heparin, such as enoxaparin, 40 mg/day until 12 weeks then 40 mg q 12 h thereafter. Treatment begins after confirmation of pregnancy, continues until 48 hours before anticipated delivery (to allow epidural anesthesia), and resumes for 12 weeks postpartum. Corticosteroid therapy is not useful for patients who do not have concomitant SLE. Some physicians recommend initiation of heparin prior to conception; no clinical trial supports this recommendation, and the risk of longer duration of heparin therapy is considerable. Patients in most published series received low-dose aspirin as well as heparin, but the benefit of adding aspirin is unknown.

No Prior Fetal Losses or Fetal Losses Before 10 Gestational Weeks

No studies unequivocally justify treatment of women with aPL during a first pregnancy, women with only very early losses, or women whose aPL titers are low or transient. Nonetheless, it is common to offer such patients low-dose aspirin.

Prior Thrombosis in Pregnancy

Women who have had prior thromboses must be fully anticoagulated throughout pregnancy because the risk of new thrombosis markedly increases both during pregnancy and postpartum. In these women, warfarin is changed to heparin or low-molecular-weight heparin prior to conception if possible. Clopidogrel and newer antithrombotic agents are not cleared for use in pregnancy, but, together with intravenous Ig and hydroxychloroquine, may be considered in patients unable to use heparin.

Postpartum Therapy

Because of the risk of thrombosis, it is prudent to continue anticoagulation for 6 to 12 weeks postpartum and to discontinue it thereafter by tapering doses. If desired, conversion from heparin to warfarin may be accomplished after the first or second postpartum week. Breast feeding is permissible with both heparin and warfarin.

CATASTROPHIC VASCULAR OCCLUSION

Onset of the catastrophic vascular occlusion syndrome is usually sudden, diagnostically confusing, and immediately life threatening. There are no systematic studies of treatment for this syndrome. Detailed reviews conclude that the most effective treatment combines full-dose anticoagulation, high-dose corticosteroid, plasmapheresis, and intravenous Ig.[38-40]

NEGATIVE ANTIPHOSPHOLIPID ANTIBODY TEST AND A CLINICAL EVENT

In patients clinically suspected of having APS but having normal anticardiolipin, lupus anticoagulant, and anti-β_2GPI tests, alternative causes of clotting must be sought. Even among patients with concomitant rheumatic disease, APS may not be the cause of recurrent thromboembolism or pregnancy loss. Patients with SLE develop emboli from SLE-related cardiac valvular disease, vasculitis, or atheromata. Other patients have factor V Leiden or other procoagulant mutation. Recurrent pregnancy losses may be caused by chromosomal abnormalities, uterine infection, diabetes, hypertension, or non–aPL coagulopathy. The concept of "seronegative" APS is not recognized.

SPECIAL SITUATIONS

Effects of Aging

Because the prevalence of positive ELISA aPL tests increases with age, and because the differential diagnosis of vascular occlusion is broader than it is in young adults, particular care is necessary in diagnosing PAPS in patients older than 60 years. Sustained high-titer IgG antibody, livedo reticularis, thrombocytopenia, coexisting rheumatic disease, and absence of alternative causes support a diagnosis of APS.

Lupus-Inducing Drugs

Although drugs that induce lupus (hydralazine, phenytoin) may also induce aPL, if alternatives are not available, they may be prescribed for patients with aPL. Drugs that promote thrombosis (estrogen and estrogen-containing oral contraceptives) are not currently deemed safe, even for asymptomatic women serendipitously known to bear high-titer antibody. This advice does not translate to a recommendation to test all normal women prior to prescription of such medications, but it does suggest special attention to and further evaluation of those with family histories or clinical suggestions of rheumatic disease, livedo reticularis, biologic false-positive tests for syphilis, or borderline thrombocytopenia. There is no reliable information regarding the safety of progestin-only contraception, "morning after" contraception, or use of raloxifene, bromocriptine, or leuprolide in APS patients. A small retrospective review of women undergoing artificial reproductive technology (in vitro fertilization ["IVF"]) procedures demonstrated no thrombotic events.[57]

Other Conditions

Based on presumed pathogenesis, some physicians prescribe anticoagulation for patients with livedo reticularis, thrombocytopenia, leg ulcers, thrombotic microangiopathy, or valvulopathy. The efficacy of anticoagulation is unknown in these conditions.

▌ Complications and Prognosis

The absolute risk to an asymptomatic person serendipitously found to have the antibody is unknown. A biologic false-positive test for syphilis, in the absence of aPL, does not predict pregnancy loss.[58] A single strongly positive ELISA predicts an increased risk of thrombophlebitis or pulmonary embolus,[13] but the absolute risk is low. In normal primiparas, aPL doubles to quadruples the risk of pregnancy loss,[59] but most antibody-positive women have normal pregnancies. In separate studies of obstetric APS patients without thrombosis, half developed thromboses during 3 to 10 years of follow-up and 10 percent developed SLE.[17,60,61] The studied populations were highly selected referral populations that may have been biased toward severe disease, but follow-up studies of obstetric patients with autoantibodies show similar results.[62]

Even with treatment, prematurity and fetal growth restriction still occur. Long-term outcomes of children born of APS pregnancies are not known. In many patients with long-standing APS, development of severe cardiac valvular disease necessitates valve replacement. Atherosclerosis also occurs, as does progressive multi-infarct dementia. Recent studies suggest that APS does not add to the risk of atherosclerosis imparted by SLE.[63,64]

REFERENCES

1. Wilson WA, Gharavi AE, Koike T, et al: International consensus statement on preliminary classification criteria for antiphospholipid syndrome: Report of an international workshop. Arthritis Rheum 42:1309, 1999.
2. Petri M, Branch DW, Brey R, et al: Evidence-based classification criteria for antiphospholipid antibody syndrome. Lupus, in press.
3. Gharavi AE, Sammaritano LR, Wen J, et al: Characteristics of human immunodeficiency virus and chlorpromazine-induced antiphospholipid antibodies: Effect of beta 2 glycoprotein I on binding to phospholipid. J Rheumatol 21:94, 1994.
4. Arbuckle MR, James JA, Kohlhase KF, et al: Development of anti-dsDNA autoantibodies prior to clinical diagnosis of systemic lupus erythematosus. Scand J Immunol 54:211, 2001.
5. Reddel SW, Wang YX, Sheng YH, et al: Epitope studies with anti-beta 2-glycoprotein I antibodies from autoantibody and immunized sources. J Autoimmun 15:91, 2000.
6. Tincani A, Allegri F, Sanmarco M, et al: Anticardiolipin antibody assay: a methodological analysis for a better consensus in routine determination—a cooperative project of the European Anti-phospholipid Forum. Thromb Haemost 86:575, 2001.
7. Day HM, Thiagarajan P, Ahn C, et al: Autoantibodies to ß2-glyco-protein I in systemic lupus erythematosus and primary antiphospholipid syndrome: Clinical correlations in comparison with other antiphospholipid antibody tests. J Rheumatol 25:667, 1998.
8. Arvieux J, Renaudineau Y, Mane I, et al: Distinguishing features of anti-beta2 glycoprotein I antibodies between patients with leprosy and the antiphospholipid syndrome. Thromb Haemost 87:599, 2002.
9. Horbach DA, Vanoort E, Derksen RHWM, et al: The contribution of anti-prothrombin-antibodies to lupus anticoagulant activity: Discrimination between functional and non-functional anti-prothrombin antibodies. Thromb Haemost 79:790, 1998.
10. Atsumi T, Khamashta MA, Haworth RS, et al: Arterial disease and thrombosis in the antiphospholipid syndrome: A pathogenic role for endothelin 1. Arthritis Rheum 41:800, 1998.
11. Delpapa N, Sheng YH, Raschi E, et al: Human ß2-glycoprotein I binds to endothelial cells through a cluster of lysine residues that are critical for anionic phospholipid binding and offers epitopes for anti-ß2-glycoprotein I antibodies. J Immunol 160:5572, 1998.
12. Diri E, Cucurull E, Gharavi AE, et al: Antiphospholipid (Hughes') syndrome in African-Americans: IgA aCL and beta2 glycoprotein-I is the most frequent isotype. Lupus 8:263, 1999.
13. Ginsburg JS, Liang MH, Newcomer L, et al: Anticardiolipin antibodies and the risk for ischemic stroke and venous thrombosis. Ann Intern Med 117:997, 1992.
14. The Antiphospholipid Antibody Stroke Study (APASS) Group: Anticardiolipin antibodies are an independent risk factor for first ischemic stroke. Neurology 43:2069, 1993.
15. Levine SR, Brey RL, Sawaya KL, et al: Recurrent stroke and thrombo-occlusive events in the antiphospholipid syndrome. Ann Neurol 38:119, 1995.
16. Stephenson MD: Frequency of factors associated with habitual abortion in 197 couples. Fertil Steril 66:24, 1996.
17. Erkan D, Merrill JT, Yazici Y, et al: High thrombosis rate after fetal loss in antiphospholipid syndrome: Effective prophylaxis with aspirin. Arthritis Rheum 44:1466, 2001.
18. Kamboh MI, Manzi S, Mehdi H, et al: Genetic variation in apolipoprotein H (beta2-glycoprotein I) affects the occurrence of antiphospholipid antibodies and apolipoprotein H concentrations in systemic lupus erythematosus. Lupus 8:742, 1999.
19. Sheng Y, Reddel SW, Herzog H, et al: Impaired thrombin generation in beta 2-glycoprotein I null mice. J Biol Chem 276:13817, 2001.
20. Gharavi AE, Pierangeli SS, Harris EN: Origin of antiphospholipid antibodies. Rheum Dis Clin North Am 27:551, 2001.
21. Blank M, Krause I, Fridkin M, et al: Bacterial induction of autoantibodies to beta2-glycoprotein-I accounts for the infectious etiology of antiphospholipid syndrome. J Clin Invest 109:797, 2002.
22. Gharavi AE, Sammaritano LR, Wen J, et al: Induction of antiphospholipid antibodies by immunization with beta 2 glyco-protein I (apolipoprotein H). J Clin Invest 90:1105, 1992.

23. Lutters BC, Derksen RH, Tekelenburg WL, et al: Dimers of beta 2-glycoprotein 1 increase platelet deposition to collagen via interaction with phospholipids and the apolipoprotein E receptor 2′.

24. Bordron A, Dueymes MY, Levy Y, et al: Anti-endothelial cell antibody binding makes negatively charged phospholipids accessible to antiphospholipid antibodies. Arthritis Rheum 41:1738, 1998.

25. Sammaritano LR, Gharavi AE, Soberano C, et al: Phospholipid binding of antiphospholipid antibodies and placental anticoagulant protein. J Clin Immunol 12:27, 1992.

26. Rand JH, Wu X, Andree HAM, et al: Pregnancy loss in the antiphospholipid-antibody syndrome: A possible thrombogenic mechanism. N Engl J Med 337:154, 1997.

27. Rand JH: Molecular pathogenesis of the antiphospholipid syndrome. Circ Res 90:29, 2002.

28. Mak IYH, Brosens JJ, Christian M, et al: Regulated expression of signal transducer and activator of transcription, Stat5, and its enhancement of PRL expression in human endometrial stromal cells in vitro. J Clin Endocrinol Metab 87:2581, 2002.

29. Simantov R, LaSala J, Lo SK, et al: Activation of cultured vascular endothelial cells by antiphospholipid antibodies. J Clin Invest 96:2211, 1996.

30. Font J, Espinosa G, Tassies D, et al: Effects of b_2-glycoprotein I and monoclonal anticardiolipin antibodies in platelet interaction with subendothelium under flow conditions. Arthritis Rheum 46:3283, 2002.

31. Pierangeli SS, Liu XW, Barker JH, et al: Induction of thrombosis in a mouse model by IgG, IgM, and IgA immunoglobulins from patients with the antiphospholipid syndrome. Thromb Haemost 74:1361, 1995.

32. Jankowski M, Vreys I, Wittevrongel C, et al: Thrombogenicity of ß2-glycoprotein I-dependent antiphospholipid antibodies in a photochemically-induced thrombosis model in the hamster. Blood 101:157, 2003.

33. Girardi G, Berman J, Spruce L, et al: A critical role for complement c5 in antiphospholipid antibody-induced pregnancy loss [Abstract]. Arthritis Rheum 46:S219, 2002.

34. Casciola-Rosen L, Rosen A, Petri M, et al: Surface blebs on apoptotic cells are sites of enhanced procoagulant activity: Implications for coagulation events and antigenic spread in systemic lupus erythematosus. Proc Natl Acad Sci USA 93:1624, 1996.

35. Horkko S, Olee T, Mo L, et al: Anticardiolipin antibodies from patients with the antiphospholipid antibody syndrome recognize epitopes in both beta(2)-glycoprotein 1 and oxidized low-density lipoprotein. Circulation 103:941, 2001.

36. Bhandari S, Harnden P, Brownjohn AM, et al: Association of anticardiolipin antibodies with intraglomerular thrombi and renal dysfunction in lupus nephritis. QJM 91:401, 1998.

37. Oshiro BT, Silver RM, Scott JR, et al: Antiphospholipid antibody and fetal death. Obstet Gynecol 87:489, 1996.

38. Asherson RA, Cervera R, Piette J-C, et al: "CAPS Registry": A review of 150 cases from the international registry of patients with catastrophic antiphospholipid syndrome (CAPS) [Abstract]. Arthritis Rheum 46:S218, 2002.

39. Asherson RA, Cervera R, de Groot PG, et al: Catastrophic antiphospholipid syndrome: International consensus statement on classification criteria and treatment guidelines. Lupus, 12:530, 2003.

40. Asherson RA, Cervera R, Piette JC, et al: Catastrophic antiphospholipid syndrome: Clues to the pathogenesis from a series of 80 patients. Medicine (Baltimore) 80:355, 2001.

41. Sammaritano LR, Ng S, Sobel R, et al: Anticardiolipin IgG subclasses: Association of IgG2 with arterial and/or venous thrombosis. Arthritis Rheum 40:1998, 1997.

42. Lockshin MD, Sammaritano LR, Schwartzman S: Brief report: Validation of the Sapporo Criteria for antiphospholipid antibody syndrome. Arthritis Rheum 43:440, 2000.

43. Erel H, Erkan D, Lehman TJ, et al: Diagnostic usefulness of 3 dimensional gadolinium enhanced magnetic resonance venography in antiphospholipid syndrome. J Rheumatol 29:1338, 2002.

44. Levy RA, Gharavi AE, Sammaritano LR, et al: Characteristics of IgG antiphospholipid antibodies in patients with systemic lupus erythematosus and syphilis. J Rheum 17:1036, 1990.

45. Kupferminc MJ, Eldo A, Steinman N, et al: Increased frequency of genetic thrombophilia in women with complications of pregnancy. N Engl J Med 340:9, 1999.

46. Spitzer KA, Clark CA, Laskin AS, et al: Prevalence of inherited thrombophilias in women with unexplained recurrent pregnancy loss [Abstract]. Arthritis Rheum 46:S231, 2002.

47. Ginsberg JS, Wells PS, Brill-Edwards P, et al: Antiphospholipid antibodies and venous thromboembolism. Blood 86:3685, 1995.

48. Pauzner R, Dulitzki M, Langevitz P, et al: Low molecular weight heparin and warfarin in the treatment of patients with antiphospholipid syndrome during pregnancy. Thromb Haemost 86:1379, 2001.

49. Vilela VS, de Jesus NR, Levy RA: Prevention of thrombosis during pregnancy. Isr Med Assoc J 4:794, 2002.

50. Khamashta MA, Cuadrado MJ, Mujic F, et al: The management of thrombosis in the antiphospholipid antibody syndrome. N Engl J Med 332:993, 1995.

51. Crowther MA, Ginsberg JS, Julian J, et al: A comparison of two intensities of warfarin for prevention of recurrent thrombosis in patients with the antiphospholipid antibody syndrome. N Engl J Med 349:1133, 2003.

52. Ortel TL, Moll S: Monitoring warfarin therapy in patients with lupus anticoagulants. Ann Intern Med 127:177, 1997.

53. McCrae KR: Antiphospholipid antibody associated thrombosis: Consensus for treatment. Lupus 5:560, 1996.

54. Brunner HI, Chan WS, Ginsberg JS, et al: Long term anticoagulation is preferable for patients with antiphospholipid antibody syndrome. result of a decision analysis. J Rheumatol 29:490, 2002.

55. Petty GW, Brown RD, Whisnant JP, et al: Frequency of major complications of aspirin, warfarin, and intravenous heparin for secondary stroke prevention: A population-based study. Ann Intern Med 130:14, 1999.

56. Balasch J, Cervera R: Reflections on the management of reproductive failure in the antiphospholipid syndrome—the clinician's perspective. Lupus 11:467, 2002.

57. Guballa N, Sammaritano L, Schwartzman S, et al: Ovulation induction and in vitro fertilization in systemic lupus erythematosus and antiphospholipid syndrome. Arthritis Rheum 43:550, 2000.

58. Koskela P, Vaarala O, Makitalo R, et al: Significance of false positive syphilis reactions and anticardiolipin antibodies in a nationwide series of pregnant women. J Rheumatol 15:70, 1998.

59. Lynch A, Marler R, Murphy J, et al: Antiphospholipid antibodies in predicting adverse pregnancy outcome: A prospective study. Ann Intern Med 120:470, 1994.

60. Shah NM, Khamashta MA, Atsumi T, et al: Outcome of patients with anticardiolipin antibodies: A 10 year follow-up of 52 patients. Lupus 7:3, 1998.

61. Silver RM, Draper ML, Scott JR, et al: Clinical consequences of antiphospholipid antibodies: An historic cohort study. Obstet Gynecol 83:372, 1994.

62. Clark CA, Spitzer KA, Goldberg AS, et al: Long-term Follow-up of women with autoantibodies and recurrent pregnancy loss (RPL) [Abstract]. Arthritis Rheum 46:S45, 2002.

63. Roman MJ, Shankar BA, Davis A, et al: Prevalence and correlates of accelerated atherosclerosis in systemic lupus erythematosus. N Engl J Med 349:2399, 2003.

64. Maksimowicz K, Petri M, Magder L: Predictors of carotid atherosclerosis in systemic lupus erythematosus [Abstract]. Arthritis Rheum 46:S54, 2002.

Mixed Connective Tissue Disease, Scleroderma, and Inflammatory Myopathies

78 | Mixed Connective Tissue Disease and Other Overlap Syndromes

ROBERT M. BENNETT

The clustering of symptoms and signs into readily recognizable groupings has an important historic precedence in the classification of disease. With the progress of knowledge, such groupings may become more precisely defined in terms of distinctive pathology or specific laboratory findings. According to current nosology, there are five diffuse connective tissue diseases (DCTDs):

- systemic lupus erythematosus (SLE)
- scleroderma (Scl)
- polymyositis (PM)
- dermatomyositis (DM)
- rheumatoid arthritis (RA)

Each of these may be associated with Sjögren's syndrome, which in its primary form may be the most common of the connective tissue diseases.[1] All five classic DCTDs are descriptive syndromes, and none has a "gold standard" for diagnosis. They all exhibit a considerable heterogeneity in their clinical expression. The diagnosis of a well-differentiated DCTD is usually readily apparent without recourse to extensive investigations. However, in the early stages, there are often common features such as Raynaud's phenomenon, arthralgias, myalgias, esophageal dysfunction, and positive tests for antinuclear antibodies (ANAs). In such cases, the diagnosis often is not obvious, and these patients may be referred to as having undifferentiated connective tissue disease (UCTD).[2] About 25 percent of such patients have clinical overlap syndromes, whereas most differentiate into a clinical picture consistent with the traditional description of a DCTD. In some instances, one DCTD evolves into another DCTD over time.

The propensity for differentiation into a classic DCTD or the maintenance of an overlap state is often associated with distinctive serologic profiles and major histocompatibility complex (MHC) linkages. Although most rheumatologists generally feel more comfortable thinking in terms of the classic DCTD paradigms, a case can be advanced for using serologic profiles and human leukocyte antigen (HLA) typing to better understand the clinical features and prognoses. In this respect, a careful analysis of the overlap syndromes and their serologic associations has provided insights for understanding the clinical heterogeneity of the DCTDs.[3] Numerous clinical correlations of autoantibodies have been reported and are summarized in Table 78–1.

Autoimmunity in Overlap Syndromes

There is compelling evidence that autoimmunity is often antigen driven by components of subcellular particles—in particular spliceosomes, nucleosomes, and proteasomes.[4]

AUTOIMMUNITY TO SPLICEOSOMAL COMPONENTS

Certain components of the spliceosome are common targets of autoimmunity in the DCTDs.[5,6] Furthermore it appears that post-translational modifications of these molecules, as occurs during apoptosis, often are associated with increased immunogenicity.[7] Spliceosomes are complex nuclear particles involved in the processing of premessenger RNA into mature "spliced RNA"[8] (Fig. 78–1). There are two major spliceosomal subunits that are antigenic targets in autoimmunity: 1) small nuclear ribonucleoprotein protein particles (snRNP) and 2) heterogeneous nuclear RNP particles (hnRNP).[1] The snRNPs contain small RNA species ranging in size from 80 to 350 nucleotides that are complexed with proteins. These RNAs contain a high content of uridine and are therefore called U-RNAs; five different U-RNAs were defined on the basis of immunoprecipitation (U1, U2, U4, U5, and U6).[9] Autoantibodies to these complexes are mainly directed to the protein components. Anti-Sm antibodies precipitate five proteins with molecular weights of 28,000 (B'B), 16,000 (D), 13,000 (E), 12,000 (F) and 11,000 (G); five of these polypeptides are com-

TABLE 78-1 · CORRELATION OF AUTOANTIBODIES WITH CLINICAL FEATURES

Autoantigen	Clinical Associations
Nucleosome	SLE, Scl, MCTD
Proteasome	SLE, PM/DM, Sjögren's syndrome, multiple sclerosis
ds-DNA	SLE, glomerulonephritis, vasculitis
Histones H1, H2A, H2B,H3, H4	SLE, DILE, UCTD, RA, PBC, generalized morphea Scl with renal and cardiac involvement
RF	RA, erosive arthritis, cryoglobulinemia
Sm snRNP	SLE
U1 snRNP	MCTD, SLE, PM
68-kD peptide of U1-RNP	MCTD, Raynaud's, pulmonary hypertension
Centromere	Limited Scl, CREST, Raynaud's, pulmonary hypertension, PBC
Topoisomerase 1 (Scl-70)	Diffuse Scl with prominent organ involvement
B2-glycoprotein	Thrombosis, thrombocytopenia, miscarriages
Anticardiolipin, which is B2-glycoprotein independent	MCTD
Ro/La	Sjögren's syndrome, SCLE, congenital heart block, photosensitivity, PBC
Ribosomal P	SLE psychosis
Proteinase 3	Wegener's, pulmonary capillaritis
Myeloperoxidase	Churg Straus, pauci-immune GN
hnRNP-A2 (2nd RNA binding region domain)	RA, SLE, erosive arthritis in SLE and Scl
hnRNP-A2 (both RNA binding domains)	MCTD
hnRNP-I	Scl (early diffuse and limited)
RNA polymerase 1	Scl (diffuse with renovascular hypertension)
PM / Scl	PM/SCL overlap, arthritis, skin lesions, mechanic's hands
Ku	SLE, PM/Scl overlap, primary pulmonary hypertension, Grave's disease
Signal recognition particle (SRP)	PM (severe course with cardiac disease and high mortality)
Histidyl t-RNA synthetase (Jo1)	PM with arthritis and interstitial lung disease
Th/To	Limited form of Scl
Ro 52	PM/Scl overlap
Mi 2	Dermatomyositis
U5 snRNP	PM/Scl overlap
U3 snRNP	Limited Scl
Fibrillarin	Severe generalized Scl
Endothelial cell	Pulmonary hypertension, severe digital gangrene

Abbreviations: ds, double stranded; RE, rheumatoid factor; RNP, ribonucleoprotein; PM/ScL, palymiositis/Scleruderma; SN, small nuclear; HN, heterogenous nuclear; RNA, ribonucleic acid; DNA, deoxyribonucleic acid.

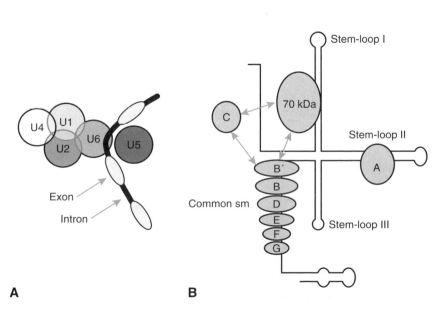

A   **B**

FIGURE 78-1 · *A.* The spliceosome is made up of five small nuclear RNAs (snRNAs) complexed with proteins to form a small nuclear ribonucleoprotein particle (snRNP). This subcellular structure is responsible for splicing introns from pre-mRNA to form mRNA. Antibodies to various spliceosomal constituents are a common feature of autoimmune rheumatic disorders with a tendency to associate with different clinical profiles (see Table 78-1). *B.* The U1 small nuclear RNP (U1 snRNP) particle of the spliceosome is composed of U1 RNA, RNP proteins (70 kD, A, and C), and common Sm proteins (B'B, D, E, F, and G). The structure of U1 RNA consists of single-stranded RNA and double-stranded RNA called stem-loops I, II, III, and IV. The 70-kD protein can bind directly to stem-loop I of U1 RNA, and the A protein can bind directly to stem-loop II of U1 RNA through an RNA-binding domain known as the RNP-80 motif. The common Smith (Sm) proteins bind as a complex to single-stranded RNA at the position shown. Because C protein does not have an RNA-binding domain, it cannot bind directly to U1 RNA. However, it does have a zinc-finger domain that facilitates its joining U1 snRNP through protein-protein interactions (*arrows*) of its zinc-finger domain with the 70-kD and common Sm proteins. (Item B from: Hoffman RW, Greidinger EL: Mixed connective tissue disease. Curr Opin Rheum 12:386-390, 2000.)

mon to the U1, U2, U4, U5, and U6 RNAs. Anti-RNP antibodies precipitate three proteins with molecular weights of 68,000 (70K), 33,000 (A'), and 22,000 (C); these polypeptides are uniquely associated with U1 RNA (see Fig. 78–1). The clinical correlates considered to be distinctive of mixed connective tissue disease (MCTD) are associated with the 70-kD specificity[10,11] with an immunodominant epitope embracing amino acid residue 125 flanked by important conformational residues at positions 119 to 126.[12] On the other hand, SLE is associated with anti-Sm antibodies.[3,13] Further definition of clinical syndromes is afforded by measuring multiple antibodies. In one study, the combination of antibodies against 70 kD, A, and C was exclusively observed in MCTD patients, whereas the combination against 70 kD, A, C, Sm-B'B, and Sm-D was restricted to patients with SLE.[14] There has been recent recognition of other U1 RNP reactive autoantibodies in that some anti–U1 RNP–positive sera specifically recognize a conformational structure generated by the binding of the 70-kD protein to U1 RNA[15] and SR proteins.[16]

(2) The hnRNP particles contain pre-mRNA associated with about 30 small proteins that are all structurally related and have molecular weights of 33 to 43 kD.[17] Nine hnRNP core proteins have been designated A1, A2, B1a, B1b, B1c, B2, C1, C2, and C3.[18] An antibody termed anti-RA33, which targets the 33-kD hnRNP-A2, is particularly interesting because it is found in sera from about one third of patients with RA, SLE, or MCTD[19] (Fig. 78–2). Furthermore, it has associations with patient subsets of erosive arthritis in SLE, scleroderma, and MCTD[20-22] and predicts the eventual development of RA

in patients with early polyarthritis.[23] Importantly, this association with anti-RA33 is not seen in scleroderma (sine erosions), PM, or overlaps of PM/Scl or PM/DM.[19] The antigenic epitopes of hnRNP-A2 contain two RNA-binding regions at the N-terminal end and a glycine-rich C-terminal region. Certain disease subsets target these two RNA binding regions differently. For instance RA and SLE sera preferentially react with the complete second RNA binding domain, whereas MCTD sera target an epitope that spans both RNA binding domains.[24]

AUTOIMMUNITY TO NUCLEOSOMAL COMPONENTS

Nucleosomes are the compact building blocks of chromatin and consist of an octamer of two copies of histones H2A, H2B, H3, and H4, around wrapped approximately 146 base pairs of DNA (Fig. 78–3). During apoptosis endonucleases cleave chromatin with the liberation of nucleosomal particles. Normally these particles are phagocytosed by macrophages. In animal models of lupus, antinucleosome antibodies emerge before the occurrence of anti–double-stranded (ds)-DNA and antihistone antibodies[25] and is linked to defective phagocytosis of apoptotically released constituents.[26,27] Nucleosomal antibodies are directed to antigenic determinants on the intact nucleosome rather than its individual components, DNA and histones.[28] In a study of 496 patients with 13 different DCTD and 100 patients with hepatitis C, antinucleosome antibodies were found only in the sera of patients with SLE (71.7%), Scl

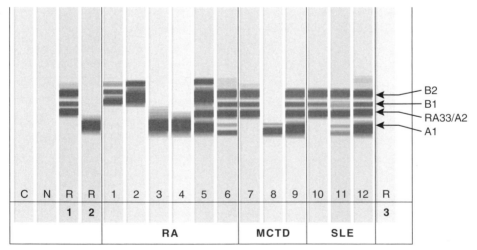

AUTOIMMUNITY TO SPLICEOSOMAL hnRNP PROTEINS

FIGURE 78–2 · Spliceosomal heterogeneous nuclear ribonucleoprotein particle (hnRNP) proteins are targets for autoantibodies in rheumatoid arthritis (RA), mixed connective tissue disease (MCTD), and systemic lupus erythematosus (SLE). This is demonstrated on this Western blot of the partially purified hnRNP proteins A1, which have been resolved by sodium dodecyl sulfate-polyacrylamide gel electrophoresis. Autoantibody reactivities to RA33 and A2, B1, and B2 are found in sera from patients with RA (lanes 1 to 6), MCTD (lanes 7 to 9), and SLE (lanes 10 to 12). The RA33 and A2 band is seen in lanes 1, 2, 5 to 7, and 9 to 12; the A1 double band is seen in lanes 3 to 6, 8, 9, 11, and 12. The double band above the RA33 and A2 band corresponds to hnRNP proteins B1 and B2 and is visible in all sera with RA33 and A2 reactivity. Other experiments have shown that MCTD sera react with a different epitope on RA33 and A2 compared with SLE and RA sera. C, control (no serum); N, normal human serum; R1, reference serum positive for anti-RA33; 1A2, B1, B2, R2, reference serum positive for anti-A1; R3, reference serum positive for anti-UI small nuclear ribonucleoprotein particles, Sm. (Adapted from Hassfeld W, Steiner G, Studnicka-Benke A, et al: Arthritis Rheum 38:777-785, 1995.)

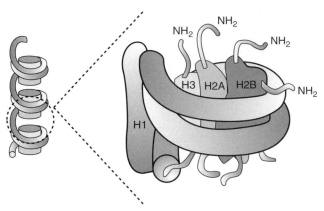

FIGURE 78-3 · The nucleosome is the fundamental repeating unit of chromatin. The central part of the nucleosome is composed of a tetramer composed of two molecules of histones H3 and H4, flanked by two dimers of histones H2A and H2B. This central core is surrounded by two superhelical turns, consisting of 146 base pairs of histone-free DNA. Histone H1 is located at the point where DNA enters and exits the nucleosome. Antibodies to the nucleosome arise early in the evolution of SLE—before anti-DNA and antihistone antibodies. Thus, the nucleosome is thought to be an important early autoantigen in the development of epitope spreading. Nucleosome antibodies are also found in scleroderma and mixed connective tissue disease (MCTD). (From Zahir Amoura Koutouzov S, Piette C, et al: The role of nucleosomes in lupus. Curr Opin Rheumatol 12:369-373, 2000.)

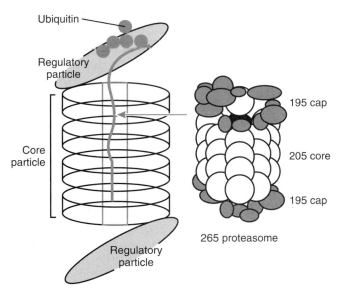

FIGURE 78–4 · Most proteins in the cytosol and nucleus are degraded via the proteasome-ubiquitin pathway. The 26S proteasome is a huge complex of 2.5 mega-datton, (MD), made up of approximately 35 different subunits. It contains a protolytic core complex, the 20S proteasome, and one or two 19S regulatory complexes that associate with the termini of the barrel-shaped 20S core. The function of proteasomes is two-fold: 1) to degrade intracellular proteins that have been tagged with ubiquitin, and 2) to generate antigenic peptides for presentation by the MHC class I molecules. Antibodies to proteasomal subunits have been reported in several autoimmune diseases (especially systemic lupus erythematosus [SLE] and polymyostis/dermatomyositis, (PM/DM) and elevated levels of proteasomes have been correlated with disease activity.

(45.9%), and MCTD (45.0%). Antinucleosome antibodies of the immunoglobulin G3 (IgG3) subclass were found only in the sera of patients with active SLE, and their levels showed a positive correlation with SLE disease activity.[29] Some 90 percent of SLE sera are positive for antinucleosome antibodies; it is claimed that they are a more sensitive marker of both active and inactive SLE than any other antibody system.[25]

AUTOIMMUNITY TO PROTEOSOMAL COMPONENTS

The 26S proteasome is a large subcellular particle involved in the degradation of proteins that have been tagged with ubiquitin and the generation peptides for presentation by the MHC class I molecules[30] (Fig. 78–4). There is increasing evidence that it maybe the target of an autoimmune response in DCTD.[31] Antibodies to proteasomal subunits have been reported in patients with autoimmune myositis, SLE, and primary Sjogren's syndrome.[32-34] Furthermore, increased levels of proteasome subunits have been detected in the sera of patients with autoimmune myositis, SLE, primary Sjögren's syndrome, RA, and autoimmune hepatitis; they are correlated with disease activity.[35] It is claimed that circulating proteasomal subunits are sensitive markers of the autoimmune inflammatory processes and reflect the magnitude of cellular damage.

▋ Generation of Autoimmunity

The antibody response to just one component of an intracellular structure, such as a spliceosome, will result in the uptake of the entire particle by antigen-processing cells (APC). Thus, all the proteins making up the particle will be subject to antigen processing with potential peptide presentation linked to their affinity to class II HLA antigens. Depending on the polymorphisms of the individual's HLA molecules, there will be a diversification of the antibody response to include some of these other antigens. This process is called "epitope spreading" and is considered pivotal in the development of the linked antibody responses observed in different DCTDs.[36,37] For instance, it has been shown that the induction of an immune response to one component of a U-RNP complex can induce a diversified autoantibody response to other components of the complex[38] (Fig. 78–5). In this way, an immune response becomes modified over time, and this change has been associated with changes in the clinical picture.[39,40]

The interaction of T cell receptors (TCR) and peptides presented by HLA molecules are a critical event in the generation of autoimmunity. The 70-kD anti–U1 RNP antibody response is associated with the HLA DR4 and DR2 phenotype.[41,42] DNA sequencing of HLA-DB genes has revealed that DR2- and DR4-positive patients share a common set of amino acids in the beta chain at positions 26, 28, 30, 31, 32, 70, and 73.[43] Such amino acids form a pocket for antigen binding (Fig. 78–6). It is hypothesized that these two HLA subtypes represent a critical genetic specificity for the presentation of antigenic peptides to their cognate TCRs. The shared epitope on HLA-DR4 and -DR2 that is associated with an anti–U1 RNP response is different from the shared epitope associated with HLA-DR4 and -DR1 in RA patients.[44] The 68-kD polypeptide has several different epitopes, the most consistent sequence being KDK DRD RKR RSS RSR.[45] This region is preferentially targeted by MCTD sera, but not by SLE sera.[46] Reactivities to

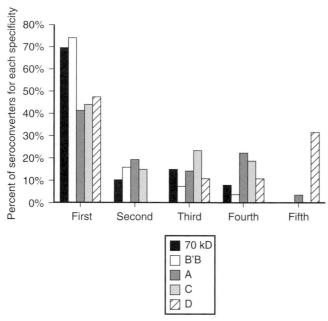

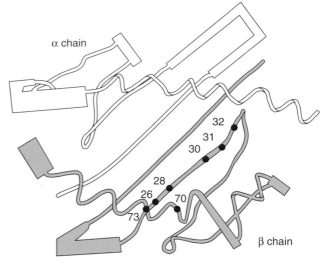

FIGURE 78-6 · DR2- and DR4-positive patients with mixed connective tissue disease (MCTD) share a common set of amino acids in the β chain of both class II HLA molecules at positions 26, 28, 30, 31, 32, 70, and 73. These amino acids form a pocket for antigen binding and are thought to present a restricted set of processed peptides to cognate T cells. (From Kallenberg CG: Overlapping syndromes, undifferentiated connective tissue disease, and other fibrosing conditions. Curr Opin Rheumatol 4:837-842, 1992.)

FIGURE 78-5 · One hundred sixty-three patients with serial serum samples from 1989 to 1999 were identified from the University of Missouri Antibody Testing Laboratory. All sera tested were initially negative for U1 RNP peptide antibodies, but over the ensuing years, they developed antibodies to at least one U1 RNP peptide. The order in which seroconversion occurred was ranked from first through fifth for 70 kD, B′B, A, C, and D. For each individual peptide, the number of patients in each rank group divided by the total number of seroconverters for that peptide is shown. The first RNP antibodies to appear were most often directed against the 70 kD and B′B peptides. Antibodies to the A and C peptides usually developed after other RNP peptide antibodies, and antibodies to D often emerged only after immunity to multiple other U1 RNP proteins had appeared. Thus, there appears to be an orderly pattern of emergence of U1 RNP peptide antibodies, with the 70-kD and B′B molecules being important early immunogens in the development of human RNP immunity. (From Hoffman RW, Greidinger EL: The appearance of U1 RNP antibody specificities in sequential autoimmune human antisera follows a characteristic order that implicates the U1–70 kd and B9/B proteins as predominant U1 RNP immunogens. Arthritis Rheum 44([2]):368-375, 2001.)

spliceosomal proteins are seldom seen in connective tissue disorders other than SLE, MCTD, and RA. The autoimmune response to the spliceosome in these three disorders is characterized by differential degrees of epitope spreading. The widest range of antibodies, to both snRNP and hnRNP, is seen in SLE, a more restricted antispliceosomal antibody repertoire to snRNP and hnRNP is seen in MCTD, and in RA, the antispliceosomal antibody repertoire is restricted to hnRNP.[19]

In general the autoimmune rheumatic diseases are characterized by the production of autoantibodies that recognize evolutionarily conserved molecules. The mechanisms whereby these "hidden" intracellular molecules become autoantigens remains an area of intensive research. The two main theories are apoptotic modification[47] and molecular mimicry.[48]

APOPTOTIC MODIFICATION

The biochemical hallmark of apoptosis is the cleavage of DNA into oligonucleotides that produce characteris-

tic "DNA ladders" when separated on agarose gels. Interestingly, similar DNA ladders are found in the serum of lupus patients.[49] Although rheumatic disease autoantigens are not unified by common structure or function, they have the common feature of becoming clustered and concentrated in the surface blebs of apoptotic cells (Fig. 78–7). A population of smaller blebs contain fragmented endoplasmic reticulum and ribosomes, as well as the ribonucleoprotein, Ro. Larger blebs (apoptotic bodies) contain nucleosomal DNA, Ro, La, and the snRNAs.[50] Apoptosis also generates modified proteins, through cleavage with a class of enzymes called capsases. Many potentially autoantigenic fragments result from cleavage with a capsase called granzyme B.[51] During the process of apoptosis several enzyme systems are upregulated, producing posttranslational modifications of the cleaved proteins.[52] It is thought that these modifications, which include citrullination, phosphorylation, dephosphorylation, transglutimination, and conjugation to ubiquitin, render the molecules more antigenic. For instance, the U1-70K protein is specifically cleaved by the enzyme caspase-3, converting it into a C-terminally truncated 40-kD fragment, which is still associated with the complete U1-snRNP complex. Similar modifications have *not* been found with any of the other U1 snRNPs.[53] At least one "death-associated" modification affects every major autoantigen that has been identified to date.[52] Over time it is envisaged that this immune response is modified by epitope spreading, with the resulting generation of the distinctive clinical features of the classic DCTDs such as SLE and MCTD.[54,55] It is hypothesized that the cell surface translocation of snRNPs facilitates the exposure of apoptotically modified antigens to the immune system. Whether such apoptotic cleavage fragments

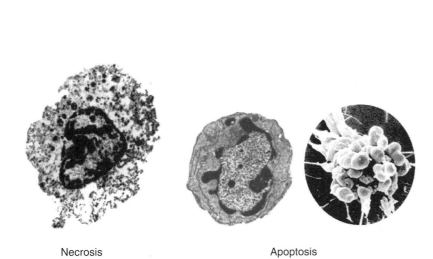

Necrosis   Apoptosis

FIGURE 78–7 · Cells either die in an unregulated distension and protein denaturation (necrosis) or in a tightly programmed series of events (apoptosis). In necrosis, the cell swells up due to the cessation of the energy dependent sodium and calcium pumps, resulting in water influx. Proteins begin to denature, turning white as in heated egg white. Necrotic cells enlarge in the process of dying, whereas in apoptosis the cell shrinks to about half its original size. In apoptosis, the cell membrane softens forming surface blebs and the cell's nucleus shrinks prior to disintegrating. The surface blebs are readily seen in the scanning electron micrograph on the right. Eventually the cells break into large fragments, which are engulfed by macrophages. Enzymes called caspases trigger programmed cell death. Autoantigens, which have been chemically modified during apoptosis, are clustered within the blebs at the surface of apoptotic cells. Smaller blebs contain fragmented endoplasmic reticulum, ribosomes, and Ro. The larger blebs contain nucleosomal DNA, Ro, La, and the small nuclear ribonucleoproteins. It is hypothesized that modified nucleoprotein complexes, which escape phagocytosis, present neoepitopes that drive an autoimmune response in genetically vulnerable individuals.

induce an autoimmune response is probably dependent on both genetic susceptibility and delayed clearance or repeated exposure.[26] It has been estimated that in vivo scavenger mechanisms have 12 hours to remove apoptotic material from the circulation.[56] The normal ratio of apoptotic cells to healthy cells is less than 1 percent, and this may be increased in diverse conditions such as complement deficiencies and infections.[26]

MOLECULAR MIMICRY

The initial stimulus for a first antibody response may be a nonself protein possessing a peptide region that mimics a self epitope—so called "molecular mimicry."[57] The most likely environmental triggers are infectious agents that display molecular mimicry. This theory postulates that the development of autoimmunity depends on the chance association of an environmental agent in a host with a permissive genetic background.[58] A critical limitation to molecular mimicry is the necessity for the antigenic sequence to undergo TCR recognition.[59] Helper T lymphocytes (cell determinant [CD]4+) usually recognize peptides of 12 to 16 amino acids in the context of HLA class II molecules. However, in some instances smaller peptides may be recognized, and in some instances these are *more* immunostimulatory than the parent ligand.[60] Such observations indicate that antigen recognition by T cells is highly degenerate and expands the potential for molecular mimicry; the universe of molecules containing a pentapeptide, for example, is many-fold greater than for a 12–amino residue peptide. If a virus has a stretch of amino acids identical to such an immunostimulatory peptide, an autoimmune response may result.[61] Once an immune response to one component of an infectious agent has been elicited, other proteins or epitopes may become antigenic by the same process of epitope spreading. Despite this wealth of basic research, there is not one human autoimmune disease that has definitively been linked to the mechanism of molecular mimicry.[62]

▋ Scleroderma Overlaps

There is a widespread heterogeneity of disease expression in Scl ranging from a diffuse cutaneous disease, with a poor prognosis, to a limited cutaneous involvement, with generally a good prognosis (see Chapter 79). Furthermore, some patients with Scl have a prominent overlap with other connective tissue diseases.[63] In many cases, these overlaps occur in those patients who do not have prominent skin involvement (*sine* scleroderma) or with the limited form of the disease, known as CREST (calcinosis, Raynaud's phenomenon, esophageal dysmotility, sclerodactyly, and telangiectasia) or incomplete CREST. Approximately 90 percent of patients with Scl have a positive ANA. Scl-related antibodies include topoisomerase 1 (Scl-70), anticentromere, hnPNP-I, RA33, p23, p25, RNA polymerase I (RNAP-1), RNA polymerase III, U1-RNP, PM/Scl, fibrillarin, histone, Ku, endothelial cell, and Th/To[63-70] (see Table 78–1). Specific antibody profiles are associated with distinctive patterns of morbidity and mortality. Patients possessing anticentromere, anti–U3 snRNP and anti-Th/To antibodies tend to have the limited form of Scl. Patients with anti-RNAP antibodies have a poor prognosis (less than a 50% 5-year survival rate) and are at greater risk for cardiac or renal involvement—in particular a Scl hypertensive crisis. About 60 percent of patients with Scl have obvious synovitis, and 35 percent are positive for rheumatoid factor (RF).[71] Erosive arthritis is uncommon, but an RA/Scl overlap has been reported.[72-74] Erosive arthritis in Scl has an association with anti-RA33; the Scl component in such overlap patients is often an incomplete form of CREST.[22]

The limited form of Scl has a well-documented overlap with primary biliary cirrhosis (PBC); this is often referred to as Reynold's syndrome after the lead author of a 1970 paper describing this association.[75] The distinctive antibody association of Scl with PBC is antimitochondrial antibodies.[76] Conversely, anticentromere antibodies have been found in 10 to 29 percent of patients with PBC; approximately half developed some features of the CREST syndrome.[77] Hence, a serologic overlap between the two syndromes is more prevalent than the clinical overlap. Patients with this overlap commonly have Sjögren's syndrome and Hashimoto's thyroiditis. Autoimmune hepatitis (AIH) has also been associated with Scl,[78] and PBC and AIH may coexist.[79]

The characteristic vessel pathology in Scl is a bland intimal proliferation. A necrotizing vasculitis is rare, but it has been described in association with a CREST/Sjögren's syndrome overlap; such patients are often anti-Ro positive.[80]

Low-grade muscle involvement is not uncommon in Scl and is described in 50 to 80 percent of patients.[81] A European review of 114 Scl overlap patients reported a 95-percent PM-Scl antibody positivity,[82] with 80 percent having an inflammatory myositis. This "scleromyositis" differed from MCTD by coexistent features of dermatomyositis (myalgia, myositis, Gottron sign, heliotrope rash, calcinosis), but no features of SLE—as is characteristic of classic MCTD. Many of these patients had a deforming arthritis of the hands. In general, they had a chronic benign course and most were steroid responsive.

Scl/lupus overlaps are less common. However, Scl patients often have ANAs other than anticentomere and Scl-70. Antihistone antibodies maybe seen in association with anticentromere antibodies; patients with this combination have an increased prevalence of SLE features, especially lung, kidney, and heart involvement.[83] In one report, anti–Scl-70 antibodies were found in 25 percent of SLE patients.[84] Their presence correlated with the disease activity score systemic lupus activity measure (SLAM) and anti–ds-DNA antibodies. SLE patients with anti–Scl-70 were at greater risk for pulmonary hypertension and renal involvement. SLE patients who develop Raynaud's phenomenon often have U1-RNP antibodies and nailfold capillaroscopic findings that are typical of Scl.[85]

▪ Polymyositis Overlaps

Polymyositis has the most specific "end organ" response of all the classic DCTDs. Yet the same clinical picture and investigational findings may be found in patients with SLE, Scl, MCTD, and Sjögren's syndrome. When clinical overlaps emerge, they are most commonly associated with three specific autoantibodies, namely anti–PM-Scl, anti-Ku, and anti–U1 RNP.[86-88] The major autoantigens that are recognized by anti-PM/Scl autoantibodies are PM/Scl-100 and PM/Scl-75. These autoantigens associate in a large complex consisting of 11 to 16 proteins that play a pivotal role in ribosome synthesis.[89] The PM/Scl complex is the human counterpart of the yeast exosome—an RNA-processing complex consisting of 11 3′ → 5′ exoribonucleases.[89]

The following clinical features have been described in North American patients with anti–PM-Scl antibodies[88]:

Raynaud's phenomenon (100%)
Sclerodactyly (96%)

Arthritis or arthralgia (96%; 28% of these had an Erosive arthritis)
Myositis (88%)
Restrictive lung disease (78%)
Calcinosis (47%)
Sicca symptoms (34%)

Antibodies to the Ku nuclear antigen, reported in about 10 percent of myositis patients,[90] have also been associated with a PM/Scl overlap syndrome[91] and primary pulmonary hypertension.[92] Some patients with polymyositis develop an unusual but distinctive syndrome of Raynaud's phenomenon, inflammatory arthritis, and interstitial lung disease. The arthropathy associated with polymyositis is characterized by deforming subluxations (particularly of the DIPs and thumbs) with only minor erosive changes.[93] Another myositis overlap syndrome is seen in patients with anti–amino-acyl trRNA synthetase antibodies. This is a family of enzymes that catalyze the transfer of a specific amino acid to its cognate transfer RNA[94]—the most common association is with anti–Jo 1 (histidine-trRNA synthetase). The clinical syndromes associated with antisynthetase antibodies are similar.[95] There is usually a subacute onset with remissions and exacerbations characterized by inflammatory myositis, fever (80%), Raynaud's, and skin problems (e.g., mechanic's hands in 70%). Arthropathy is seen in 50 to 90 percent and interstitial lung disease in 50 to 80 percent of patients.[96] A distinctive feature of the inflammatory myopathies is the presence of MHC class I antigens on the surface of muscle cells. Transgenic mice that overexpress MHC class I in skeletal muscle develop an inflammatory myopathy that is often accompanied by autoantibodies to histidyl-tRNA synthetase.[97] It has been suggested that autoimmune inflammatory myopathies arise as a consequence of a nonspecific environmental event that causes sustained upregulation of MHC class in skeletal muscle.

The association of myositis in patients with anti–U1-RNP antibodies is usually seen in the context of MCTD. However, some patients with an inflammatory myositis, without Raynaud's, have anti–U1-RNP antibodies in association with interstitial lung disease, arthritis, and neurologic symptoms.[98]

PMS1 is a DNA mismatch repair enzyme that appears to be fairly specific for inflammatory myositis; it occurs in 7.5 percent of PM patients, but not in the sera of patients with other autoimmune disorders.[99] Interestingly sera recognizing PMS1 also recognized several other proteins involved in DNA repair and remodeling, all of which are efficiently cleaved by granzyme B during apoptosis. This has led to the notion that an immune response to granzyme B substrates is a characteristic feature of a myositis-specific phenotype.

Antibodies to the signal-recognition particle (SRP) have been reported in 4 percent of 265 patients with Scl/PM overlap.[100] Anti-SRP–positive patients have a severe, rapidly progressive myositis in the absence of Raynaud's phenomenon, pulmonary fibrosis, or arthritis.[101] Muscle biopsies show minimal inflammation, muscle fiber necrosis, regeneration with prominent endomysial fibrosis, and deposits of the terminal components of complement (C5b-9) in endomysial capillaries.[101]

Mixed Connective Tissue Disease

MCTD was described by Sharp and his colleagues in a 1972 paper reporting an overlap of SLE, Scl, and PM.[102] This was the first overlap syndrome defined in terms of a specific antibody—namely antibodies directed against a ribonuclease-sensitive extractable nuclear antigen (ENA). Over the last 30 years, many studies have explored the clinical correlates of this antibody system (now called U1 RNP).

SEROLOGIC FEATURES

The basic premise of MCTD is that the presence of high-titer anti–U1 RNP antibodies modifies the expression of a DCTD in ways that are relevant to prognosis and treatment. The first clue to diagnosing MCTD is usually a positive ANA with a high-titer, speckled pattern. The titer is often greater than 1:1000 and sometimes greater than 1:10,000. This finding should prompt the measurement of antibodies to U1 RNP, Sm, Ro, and La. It is also pertinent to note whether the serum contains antibodies to ds-DNA and histones, as patients destined to follow a course most consistent with MCTD have sera with predominant U1-RNP reactivity. Antibodies to ds-DNA, Sm, and Ro are occasionally seen as a transient phenomenon in patients with MCTD. But when they are found consistently as the predominant antibody system, the clinical picture is usually more consistent with classic SLE. Antibodies to the 70-kD antigen are most closely associated with the clinical correlates of MCTD.[42,103,104]

CLINICAL FEATURES

Diagnosis

The central premise of MCTD is that of an overlap syndrome embracing features of SLE, Scl, and PM/DM.[105] These overlap features of MCTD seldom occur concurrently; it usually takes several years before enough overlapping features have appeared to be confident that MCTD is the most appropriate diagnosis.[106] The most common clinical associations with U1 RNP antibodies in the early phase of the disease are hand edema, arthritis, Raynaud's phenomenon, inflammatory muscle disease, and sclerodactyly.[106,107] There are four diagnostic criteria sets that have been used for defining MCTD patients.[108-111] A comparative study indicated that two criteria sets, those of Alarcon-Segovia and Kahn, had the best sensitivity and specificity (62.5 and 86.2%, respectively)[112] (Table 78–2). The sensitivity could be improved to 81.3 percent if the term *myalgia* was substituted for *myositis*.[113] Some patients initially diagnosed as having MCTD will evolve into a clinical picture most consistent with SLE or RA; in one long-term follow-up, more than half of the subjects continued to satisfy criteria for MCTD.[114] A comparison of the clinical and serologic features of MCTD with SLE, RA, Scl, and PM/DM is given in Table 78–3.

General Features and Epidemiology

The prevalence of MCTD in Caucasians is not known. An epidemiologic study in Japan suggested a prevalence of

TABLE 78–2 · TWO DIAGNOSTIC CRITERIA FOR MIXED CONNECTIVE TISSUE DISEASE (MCTD)

Alarcón-Segovia's Criteria[110]	Kahn's Criteria[109]
Serologic criteria Anti-RNP at hemagglutination	A. Serologic criteria High-titer anti-RNP corresponding titer of ≥1:1600 to a speckled antinuclear antibodies (ANA) of ≥1:1200 titer
B. Clinical criteria Swollen hands Synovitis Myositis (biologically proven) Raynaud's phenomenon Acrosclerosis	Clinical criteria Swollen fingers Synovitis Myositis Raynaud's phenomenon
Mixed connective tissue disorder (MCTD) present if: Criterion A is accompanied by 3 or more clinical criteria, one of which must include synovitis or myositis	Mixed connective tissue disorder (MCTD) present if: Criterion A is accompanied by Raynaud's phenomenon and two or more the three emaining rclinical criteria

2.7 percent for MCTD compared to 20.9 percent for SLE, 5.7 percent for Scl, and 4.9 percent for PM/DM.[115] The female-to-male ratio in this study was 16:1. The age of onset in MCTD is similar to the other DCTDs, with most cases presenting in the second or third decades. The syndrome of MCTD usually occurs as an isolated finding, but there are reports of a familial occurrence.[116,117] Unlike SLE, precipitation by sun exposure has not been described in patients with MCTD. Likewise, drug exposure has not been related to the onset of MCTD, although a transient appearance of anti-RNP antibodies has been noted at the initiation of procainamide therapy.[118] Vinyl chloride[119] and silica[120] are the only environmental agents that have so far been associated with MCTD.

Early Symptoms

In the early stages, most patients destined to develop MCTD cannot be differentiated from the other classic DCTDs. The assumption that a diagnosis of MCTD implies a simultaneous presence of features usually seen in SLE, Scl, and PM is erroneous. It is unusual to see such an overlap during the early course of MCTD, but with the progress of time, the overlapping features usually occur sequentially. Early in the course of the disease most patients complain of easy fatigability, poorly defined myalgias, arthralgias, and Raynaud's phenomenon; at this point in time a diagnosis of RA, SLE, or UCTD seems most appropriate.[121,122] If such a patient is found to have swollen hands, puffy fingers, or both in association with a high-titer, speckled ANA, they should be carefully followed for the evolution of overlap features. A high titer of anti-RNP antibodies in a patient with UCTD is a powerful predictor for later evolution into MCTD[123]; this highlights the importance of anti-RNP antibodies as a serologic marker for MCTD.[124] Less commonly, there is an acute onset of MCTD that gives little clue to the subsequent course; such presentations have included

TABLE 78–3 • DIFFERENTIAL FEATURES OF THE MAJOR DCTDS

Clinical Feature	SLE	RA	Scl	PM	MCTD
Pleurisy or pericarditis	++++	+	+	–	+++
Erosive joint disease	±	++++	+	±	+
Raynaud's phenomenon	++	–	++++	+	++++
Inflammatory myositis	+	+	+	++++	+++
Sclerodactyly	±	–	++++	–	++
Nonacral skin thickening	–	–	+++	–	–
Interstitial pulmonary fibrosis	+	+	+++	++	+
Pulmonary hypertension	++	±	+	+	+++
Butterfly rash	++++	–	–	–	++
Oral ulcers	+++	–	–	–	++
Seizures or psychosis	+++	–	–	–	–
Trigeminal neuropathy	+	–	++	–	+++
Peripheral neuropathy	++	++	±	–	++
Transverse myelopathy	+++	+	–	–	++
Aseptic meningitis	+++	+	–	–	+++
Diffuse proliferative glomerulonephritis	++++	–	–	–	+
Membranous glomerulonephritis	+++	–	–	–	++
Renovascular hypertension	+	–	++++	–	+++
Inflammatory vasculitis	++	++	+	+	+
Noninflammatory vasculopathy	–	–	++++	–	+++
Esophageal dysmotility	+	±	++++	+	+++

polymyositis, acute arthritis, aseptic meningitis, digital gangrene, high fever, acute abdomen, and trigeminal neuropathy.

Fever

Fever may be a prominent feature of MCTD in the absence of an obvious cause.[106] Fever of unknown origin has been the initial presentation of MCTD; after careful evaluation, fever in MCTD can usually be traced to a coexistent myositis, aseptic meningitis, serositis, lymph adenopathy, or intercurrent infection.

Joints

Joint pain and stiffness is an early symptom in nearly all patients who develop MCTD syndrome. Over the past two decades, it has become increasingly apparent that joint involvement in MCTD is more common and more severe than in classic SLE. About 60 percent of patients eventually develop an obvious arthritis, often with deformities commonly seen in RA such as ulnar deviation, swan neck, and boutonniére changes.[107] Radiographs usually show a characteristic absence of severe erosive changes; they often resemble Jaccoud's arthropathy. However, a destructive arthritis, including an arthritis mutilans, is a well-established association[107,125,126] (Fig. 78–8). Occasionally, an acute inflammatory destructive arthritis may be the presenting feature.[127] Small marginal erosions, often with a well-demarcated edge, are the most characteristic radiologic feature in patients with severe joint disease.[128,129] Rib erosions may rarely be seen.[130] Some patients develop a flexor tenosynovitis, which is an additional cause for hand deformities.[131]

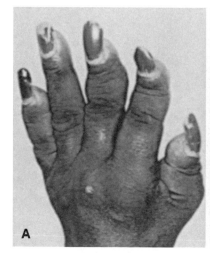
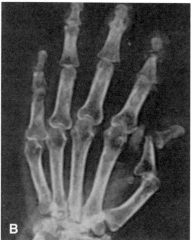

FIGURE 78–8 • *A*, In a few patients with mixed connective tissue disease (MCTD), a severe destructive form of arthritis (arthritis mutilans) develops. *B*, The radiograph shows almost complete osteolysis of the carpal bones with focal osteolytic changes in several digits and bony fusion of the third distal interphalangeal joint. (From Bennett RM, O'Connell DJ: Mixed connective tissue disease: A clinicopathological study of 20 cases. Semin Arthritis Rheum 10:25, 1980.)

A positive RF is found in 50 to 70 percent of patients with MCTD; indeed, patients may be diagnosed as having RA and fulfill American College of Rheumatology (ACR) criteria for RA.[106,123] Joint histology in MCTD reveals a hyperplastic synovium with surface fibrinoid necrosis, increased vascularity, interstitial edema, and infiltration of macrophages, lymphocytes, neutrophils, and multinucleated giant cells,[132] indistinguishable from that found in RA.

Skin and Mucous Membranes

Most patients with MCTD develop mucocutaneous changes sometime during the course of the syndrome. Raynaud's phenomenon is the most common problem and one of the earliest manifestations of MCTD.[40,105,106,133] It may be accompanied by puffy, swollen digits and sometimes total hand edema.,[105] In some patients, skin changes commonly associated with classic SLE are prominent findings, particularly malar rash and discoid plaques.[134] Mucous membrane lesions have included buccal ulceration,[106] sicca complex,[135] orogenital ulceration,[136] livedo vasculitis,[137] and nasal septal perforation.[138] Peritendinous and subcutaneous nodules may occur over the flexors of forearms, the extensors of the hands and feet, and the Achilles tendons.[126,139]

Muscle

Myalgia is a common symptom in patients with the MCTD syndrome.[105,106] Sometimes an inflammatory myositis is seen in patients with anti–U1-RNP who do not have the characteristic features of MCTD.[98,140] Most patients have no demonstrable weakness, electromyography (EMG) abnormalities, or muscle-enzyme changes. It is often unclear whether the symptom represents a low-grade myositis, physical deconditioning, or an associated fibromyalgia syndrome. The inflammatory myopathy associated with MCTD is identical clinically and histologically to classic PM.[141] In most patients myositis occurs as an acute flare against a background of general disease activity. Such patients usually respond well to a short course of high-dose corticosteroid therapy. Another scenario is that of a low-grade inflammatory myopathy, which is often insidious in its onset; these patients often have a poor therapeutic response to corticosteroids. Some patients with polymyositis associated with MCTD develop an impressive fever[106]; other patients may give a history of febrile myalgias that have been diagnosed as "flu."

Heart

All three layers of the heart may be involved in MCTD. An abnormal electrocardiogram (ECG) is noted in about 20 percent of patients.[142] The most common ECG changes are right ventricular hypertrophy, right atrial enlargement, and interventricular conduction defects. Pericarditis is the most common clinical manifestation of cardiac involvement; it is reported in 10 to 30 percent of patients[143,144]; pericardial tamponade is rare.[145] Involvement of the myocardium is increasingly recognized.[146,147] In some patients, myocardial involvement is secondary to pulmonary hypertension; this is often asymptomatic in its early stages.[148] The early detection of pulmonary hypertension is important for initiating early therapy. Clinical criteria for diagnosis of pulmonary hypertension were derived from a study of 555 Japanese patients with MCTD, of whom 83 had pulmonary hypertension.[149] Four or more of the following six criteria had a diagnostic sensitivity of 92 percent and specificity of 100 percent:

1. exertional dyspnea
2. systolic pulsation of the left sternal border
3. accentuated second pulmonary sound
4. dilatation of the pulmonary artery on chest radiograph
5. right ventricular hypertrophy on ECG
6. right ventricular enlargement on ECHO

Lung

The majority of MCTD patients have some evidence of pulmonary involvement; in the early stages this is asymptomatic.[148] A review of 81 adult patients with MCTD noted pleuropulmonary involvement in 25 percent of patients.[150] Symptoms were dyspnea (16%), chest pain (7%), and cough (5%). Chest radiographs showed interstitial changes (19%), pleural effusions (6%,), pneumonic infiltrates (4%), and pleural thickening (2%); the most discriminatory lung-function test in this series was the single breath diffusing capacity for carbon monoxide. Pleuritic chest pain is common. Interstitial lung disease is usually progressive; in a 6-year follow-up study there was a decrease in vital capacity of 35 percent and a reduction in diffusing capacity of lungs for carbon monoxide, (DLCO) of 43 percent. In rare cases, pulmonary insufficiency may result from diaphragmatic dysfunction.[151]

High-resolution computed tomography (CT) scan is the most sensitive test to determine the presence of interstitial lung disease in MCTD (Fig. 78–9). A review of 35 patients came to the conclusion that CT findings in MCTD were a combination of those seen in other connective tissue disorders.[152] The most common CT finding was septal thickening, whereas ground-glass opacity was lower than in other connective tissue disorders; honeycombing was less frequent than in Scl but higher than in PM/DM. Another high-resolution CT study of 41 MCTD patients reported that the most characteristic pulmonary involvements are a ground-glass attenuation, nonseptal linear opacities, and peripheral/lower lobe predominance.[153] An acute interstitial pneumonia is an occasional event.[154] Pulmonary hemorrhage has occasionally been reported.[155,156] The major cause of death in MCTD is pulmonary hypertension.[40,157,158] Unlike Scl, in which pulmonary hypertension is usually secondary to an interstitial pulmonary fibrosis, pulmonary hypertension in MCTD is usually caused by a bland intimal proliferation and medial hypertrophy of pulmonary arterioles[159,160] (Fig. 78–10). A comparison of the autopsy findings in MCTD patients with and without pulmonary hypertension found intimal proliferation, fibrosis, and thrombi in both groups. Progression to severe pulmonary hypertension was associ-

FIGURE 78–9 · Computed tomography (CT) scans of a patient with mixed connective tissue disease (MCTD) and pulmonary hypertension (A, upper zones; B, lower zones). There are bilateral pleural effusions and enlarged bilateral mediastinal lymph nodes in the right paratracheal region and left prevascular areas. The pulmonary artery has a diameter greater than that of the ascending aorta—consistent with the diagnosis of pulmonary hypertension. Both hilar pulmonary arteries are also enlarged. A fairly large pericardial effusion is present. The lung windows show evidence of a diffuse abnormality with linear opacities and some areas of ground-glass attenuation in the upper zones. At the lung bases there are more confluent opacities, both reticular and ground glass, and some air-space consolidation. No honeycombing is identified, and there is no distortion of the lung architecture. (From Yasuharu Saito Terada M, Ishida T, et al: Pulmonary involvement in mixed connective tissue disease: comparison with other collagen vascular diseases using high resolution CT. J Comput Assist Tomog 26([3]:349-357, 2002.)

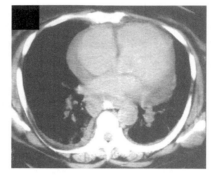
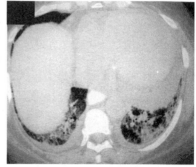

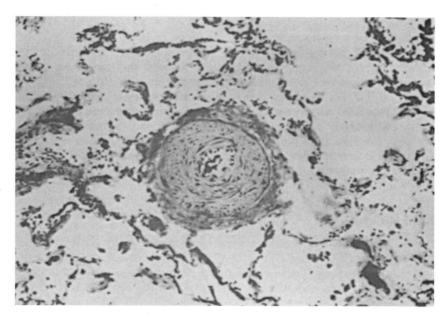

FIGURE 78–10 · Intimal hyperplasia and smooth muscle hypertrophy without accompanying inflammation are the characteristic features of the vasculopathy of mixed connective tissue disease (MCTD). When it occurs in the lung, as shown here, it may give rise to severe pulmonary hypertension. (Note absence of pulmonary fibrosis.) (From Alpert MA, Goldberg SH, Singsen BH, et al: Cardiovascular manifestations of mixed connective tissue disease in adults. Circulation 6:1182, 1983. By permission of the American Heart Association, Inc.)

ated with endothelial damage, microthrombi, proliferation of intimal myocytes, and diffuse involvement of pulmonary arterioles more than 200 microns in diameter.[161] The development of pulmonary hypertension has been correlated with a nailfold capillary pattern similar to that seen in Scl,[148] anti–endothelial cell antibodies,[162-164] anticardiolipin antibodies,[40,165,166] and anti–U1-RNP antibodies.[165] There is now evidence that all forms of pulmonary hypertension are linked by defects in the signaling pathway involving angiopoietin-1, a protein involved in the recruitment of smooth-muscle cells around blood vessels; TIE2, the endothelial-specific receptor for angiopoietin-1; and bone morphogenetic protein receptor type 1A (BMP-R1A) and BMP-R2.[167] These are potential molecular targets for therapeutic intervention.

Kidney

In the initial description of MCTD, renal involvement was considered to be rare.[105] After some three decades of observations, it is now evident that renal involvement

occurs in about 25 percent of patients.[121,168,169] However high titers of anti–U1 RNP antibodies are relatively protective against the development of diffuse proliferative glomerulonephritis, irrespective of whether they occur in a setting of classic SLE or MCTD.[85,170,171] When patients with MCTD do develop renal changes, they usually take the form of a membranous glomerulonephritis.[168,169,172] This is often asymptomatic but may sometimes cause an overt nephrotic syndrome.[169] The development of diffuse proliferative glomerulonephritis or parenchymal interstitial disease has been rarely recorded in MCTD.[169,173] There is increasing recognition that MCTD patients are at risk of developing a renovascular hypertensive crisis similar to the Scl kidney.[174,175]

Gastrointestinal

Gastrointestinal involvement is a major feature of the overlap with Scl, occurring in about 60 to 80 percent of patients.[176] The most common abdominal problem in MCTD is disordered motility in the upper gastrointestinal tract.[176,177] There have been case reports of hemoperitoneum,[178] hematobilia,[179] duodenal bleeding,[180] megacolon,[181] ascites,[182] protein-losing enteropathy,[183,184] PBC,[185] portal hypertension,[186,187] pneumatosis intestinalis,[188-191] splenic vasculitis,[192] and autoimmune hepatitis.[185,193,194] Abdominal pain in MCTD may result from bowel hypomotility, serositis, mesenteric vasculitis, colonic perforation, and pancreatitis. One patient with mesenteric vasculitis died from hemorrhage involving the small and large bowel.[195] Malabsorption syndrome can occur secondary to small bowel dilation with bacterial overgrowth.[191,196] Liver involvement in the form of chronic active hepatitis and Budd-Chiari syndrome has been described.[181,197] There are occasional reports of secretory diarrhea[198] and pancreatitis.[199] Pseudodiverticulae, identical to those seen in SCL, may be seen along the antimesenteric border of the colon.[192] Examples of these features are shown in Figure 78–11.

Central Nervous System

In keeping with Sharp's original description, central nervous system (CNS) involvement has not been a conspicuous clinical feature of MCTD. There is a general agreement that the most common problem is a trigeminal neuropathy.[200-202] This is of some heuristic interest as it is also the most frequent CNS manifestation of Scl.[203,204] In a review of 81 cases of trigeminal neuropathy seen in a neurologic clinic, the most frequently associated connective tissue diseases were UCTD (47%), MCTD (26%), and Scl (19%).[205] In a few instances, trigeminal neuropathy has been the presenting feature of MCTD.[206,207] In contrast to CNS involvement in classic SLE, frank psychosis and convulsions have rarely been reported in MCTD.[200,201] Headaches are a relatively common symptom in MCTD; in the majority of patients they are probably vascular in origin with many of the components of classic migraines.[208] Some patients experience headaches accompanied by fever and sometimes myalgia, somewhat reminiscent of a viral syndrome.[200] In a subset of these patients, signs of meningeal irritation develop, and examination of the cerebral spinal fluid reveals the changes of aseptic meningitis.[200,209,210] Aseptic meningitis in MCTD has also been described as a hypersensitivity reaction to nonsteroidal anti-inflammatory drugs (NSAIDs), in

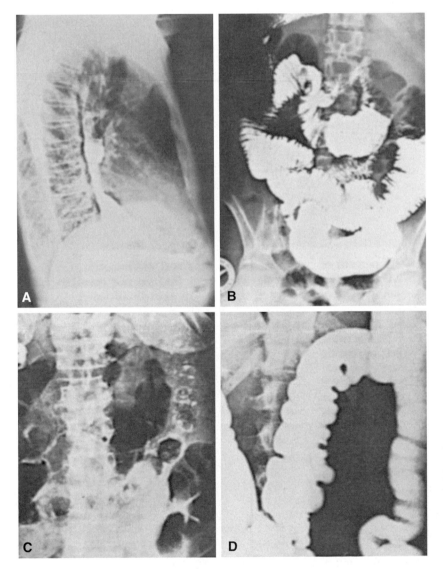

FIGURE 78–11 · Four examples of gastrointestinal changes in patients with mixed connective tissue disease (MCTD) that resemble those seen in scleroderma. A, Reduced peristalsis in the lower two thirds of the esophagus. B, Dilatation of the duodenal loop and proximal small bowel. C, Pneumatosis cystoides intestinalis of the small bowel (arrows). D, Wide-mouthed pseudodiverticula in the antimesenteric border of the colon. (From Bennett RM, O'Connell DJ: Mixed connective tissue disease: A clinicopathological study of 20 cases. Semin Arthritis Rheum 10:25, 1980, and Br J Radiol 50:620, 1977.)

particular sulindac[211] and ibuprofen.[212] A new but rare CNS correlation with anti–U1 RNP antibodies is cerebral hemorrhage; this was described in patients with U1 RNP–associated Scl[65] and in two juvenile MCTD patients.[213] There are several reports of transverse myelitis[214-216] and cauda equina syndrome,[217] and isolated reports of tongue atrophy,[218] retinal vasculitis,[219] optic neuropathy,[220,221] progressive multifocal leukoencephalopathy,[222] cold-induced brain ischemia,[223] myasthenia gravis,[224] polyradiculopathy,[225] berry aneurysms,[226] demyelinating disorder,[227] and peripheral neuropathy.[201,202]

Blood Vessels

A bland, intimal proliferation and medial hypertrophy affecting medium and small vessels is the characteristic vascular lesion of MCTD.[160,199,228,229] When this vessel pathology is widespread in the lung or kidney, there is an association with pulmonary hypertension and renovascular crises.[40] This vascular lesion differs from the usual changes encountered in SLE, in which a perivascular inflammatory infiltrate and fibrinoid necrosis are more characteristic. An angiographic study reported a high prevalence of medium-size vessel occlusions[230] (Fig. 78–12). Fingernail capillaroscopy is abnormal in most MCTD patients, with the same pattern of capillary dilatation and drop out reported in Scl.[230] In one study, all MCTD patients had Scl-like capillaroscopy pattern, and a "bushy organization" was noted in 73 percent; this finding was reputed to have an 87-percent predictive value.[231] It would appear that an Scl pattern on nailfold capillaroscopy is a distinctive feature of MCTD that is not seen in classic SLE.[232] As nailfold capillaroscopy can be readily performed in the office or at the bedside, it may provide useful clinical information in distinguishing patients destined to develop an MCTD syndrome. Anti–endothelial cell antibodies have been reported in 45 percent of patients with MCTD; the presence of these antibodies tends to correlate with pulmonary changes and spontaneous abortion.[163,164] Further support for

endothelial cell injury in MCTD is provided by elevated serum levels of factor VIII Rag[233] and elevated plasma levels of endothelin-1.[162] Anti–U1-RNP antibodies may have a pathologic role in the small-vessel pathology of MCTD as anti–U1-RNP antibodies induce the release of proinflammatory cytokines from cultured endothelial cells.[234]

Blood

Hematologic abnormalities are a common finding in MCTD. Anemia is found in 75 percent of patients; the usual profile is most consistent with the anemia of chronic inflammation.[85,106] A positive Coombs test is seen in about 60 percent of patients, but an overt hemolytic anemia is uncommon.[105,106,235] As in SLE, a leukopenia affecting mainly the lymphocyte series is seen in about 7 percent of patients and tends to correlate with disease activity.[105,106,170] Less-common associations have been thrombocytopenia,[106,235] thrombotic thrombocytopenia purpura,[236-238] and red cell aplasia.[239] Hypocomplementemia has been described in several studies;[105,106,240] it is not as prevalent as in classic SLE and has not been correlated with any particular clinical situation. Positive tests for RF have been found in about 50 percent of patients.[85,106,171] The presence of RF is associated with more severe degrees of arthritis,[241,242] especially if anti-A2 or -RA33 are also present.[19] A false-positive VDRL has been noted in about 10 percent of patients.[105,106] Anticardiolipin antibodies, lupus anticoagulants, or both have also been reported.[166,243] Unlike the anticardiolipin antibodies found in SLE, they are β2-glycoprotein independent[244] and tend to be associated with thrombocytopenia[245] rather than thrombotic events.[243]

Pregnancy

In a comparison study of patients with MCTD and SLE, the fertility rates in both were unaltered, whereas the parity and fetal wastage was increased in both.[246] Forty

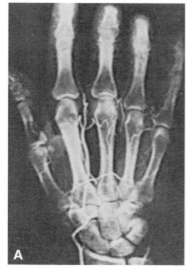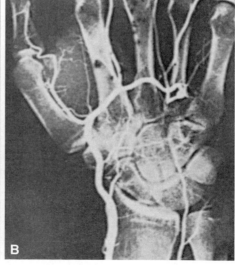

FIGURE 78–12 • *A*, Digital angiogram showing multiple arterial occlusions with collateral formation. *B*, Digital angiogram showing ulnar artery occlusions. (From Peller JS, Gabor GT, Porter JM, Bennett RM: Angiographic findings in mixed connective tissue disease: Correlation with fingernail capillary photomicroscopy and digital photoplethysmography findings. Arthritis Rheum 28:768, 1985. Reprinted with permission of the American College of Rheumatology.)

percent of patients exhibited an exacerbation of MCTD during pregnancy. In contradistinction, other studies have not reported exacerbations of maternal disease or postpartum flares.[106,247,248] Lundberg noted a tendency to low birth weights in MCTD,[249] as has been found in other conditions associated with Raynaud's phenomenon.[250] The mechanism for pregnancy complications is probably an autoimmune reaction against placental tissues, as immunostaining studies show deposits of fibrinogen, IgG, IgM, IgA, and complement 3 (C3) localized to the trophoblast basement membrane. These deposits are associated with intervillous fibrin deposition and infarction.[251] Furthermore, there is an association of antiendothelial antibodies with spontaneous abortion in MCTD.[163]

Juvenile MCTD

MCTD may first become apparent in childhood (see Chapter 97). From the reports to date, it would seem that juvenile MCTD is associated with more morbidity than the disease in adults. Significant myocarditis, glomerulonephritis, thrombocytopenia, seizures, and aseptic meningitis have been described.[252] Grab reported on two children with severe CNS problems; one had a hemiparesis and aphasia secondary to occlusion of the left internal carotid artery but recovered after treatment with prednisone and cytoxan. The other child died due to an intracranial hemorrhage; an autopsy showed small vessel fibrinoid necrosis.[213] Another death was reported in a 15-year-old girl with MCTD who developed an accelerated hypertension with a hemolytic-uremic syndrome and pancreatitis; on autopsy, a widespread vasculopathy was found with bland, intimal proliferation.[199] Other studies have reported a more benign course.[253,254] A metanalysis of 224 patients reported a 7.6-percent mortality rate due to sepsis or infection,[7] cerebral complications,[3] heart failure,[2] pulmonary hypertension,[2] renal failure,[2] or gastrointestinal bleeding.[1] This was a similar mortality rate to juvenile SLE, DM, and Scl.[255]

PROGNOSIS

The original description of MCTD stressed two points, namely: "... a relatively good prognosis and an excellent response to corticosteroids."[105] With the benefit of two decades of hindsight, it is now apparent that both of these claims need to be qualified. There is now unequivocal evidence that patients with high-titer U1 RNP antibodies have a low prevalence of serious renal disease and life-threatening neurologic problems; in this sense, MCTD can be favorably compared to classic SLE. However, not all patients with MCTD have a favorable prognosis, and death may occur from progressive pulmonary hypertension and its cardiac sequelae.[40] Pulmonary hypertension sometimes follows a rapidly accelerated course, which leads to death in a few weeks.[106] Rare causes of death are myocarditis,[146] renovascular hypertension, and cerebral hemorrhage.[65,213] In contrast to SLE, in which the major cause of death is often related to secondary infections, nosocomial infections have rarely been described in

patients with MCTD.[40] A 29-year follow-up of 47 MCTD patients from Sharp's group at the University of Missouri reported a favorable course in 62 percent and continuing active disease in 38 percent. Eleven (23%) patients had a fatal outcome; to pulmonary hypertension, in 9 patients, and two deaths unrelated to MCTD.[40] In a Japanese study of 45 MCTD patients, the survival rate at 5 years was 90.5 percent and 82.1 percent at 10 years[256]; patients with predominant Scl-PM overlap had a worse prognosis, with a 33 percent 10-year survival. It is evident that the course of MCTD is unpredictable; many patients do follow a relatively benign course, but it is major organ involvement that ultimately dictates the morbidity and mortality of the disease.

MANAGEMENT

There is no cure for MCTD. The rational management of MCTD is confounded by the absence of controlled trials. Recommendations for management are based on conventional treatments for SLE, PM/DM, RA, and Scl.

Pulmonary hypertension is the main cause of death in MCTD, and patients should be evaluated at regular intervals for the development of this complication. This diagnosis should be suspected in patients with increasing exertional dyspnea. Two-dimensional echocardiography with Doppler flow studies is the most useful screening test,[257] with a definitive diagnosis requiring cardiac catheterization showing a mean resting pulmonary artery pressure greater than 25 mmHg at rest.[258] Recent advances in the treatment of pulmonary hypertension have led to reduced morbidity and mortality.[259] Overall effective management requires anticoagulation and vasodilator therapy, such as calcium channel blockers or prostacyclin analogues. Long-term treatment with intravenous epoprostenol or prostacyclin improves exercise capacity, hemodynamics, and survival in most patients,[258] as does therapy with inhaled iloprost.[260] Bosentan, an oral endothelium-1 antagonist, appears to be another useful addition to the armamentarium.[261]

Many of the problems causing morbidity tend to be intermittent and responsive to glucocorticoids (e.g., aseptic meningitis, myositis, pleurisy, pericarditis, and myocarditis). On the other hand, nephrotic syndrome, Raynaud's phenomenon, deforming arthropathy, acrosclerosis, and peripheral neuropathies are usually steroid resistant. Many of the Scl-like gastrointestinal problems can be managed according to the usual practice in Scl, such as management of renal crisis with ACE inhibitors, Raynaud's phenomenon with calcium channel blockers, and gastrointestinal reflux disease with proton pump inhibitors.[262]

As in SLE, it is worthwhile to consider the use of intravenous gammaglobulin[263,264] or danazol[265] in patients with steroid-resistant thrombocytopenia, refractory myosis, or hemolytic anemia.

Successful autologous peripheral blood stem cell transplantation has been reported in a patient with refractory mysositis and MCTD.[266]

General guidelines for treating specific features of the MCTD spectrum are given in Table 78–4. Over the long term, concern usually mounts over the total glucocorti-

TABLE 78–4 • GUIDELINES FOR MANAGING MIXED CONNECTIVE TISSUE DISORDER (MCTD)

Problems	Treatments
Fatigue, arthralgias, myalgias	NSAIDs, antimalarials, low-dose prednisone (less than 10 mg/day)
Arthritis	NSAIDs, antimalarials, gold,* methotrexate, ? TNF inhibition
Pleurisy	Indomethacin, short course of prednisone: about 20 mg/day
Aseptic meningitis	Discontinue NSAIDs;† short course of high-dose prednisone: about 60 mg/day
Myositis	Acute onset/severe: prednisone, 60 to 100 mg/day
	Chronic/low-grade: prednisone, 10 to 30 mg/day‡
	Consider methotrexate and IVIG
Membranous glomerulonephropathy	Mild: no treatment required
	Progressive proteinuria: trial of angiotensin-converting enzyme inhibitor; trial of low-dose aspirin combined with dipyridamole
	Severe: trial of prednisone (15 to 60 mg/day) plus monthly pulse cyclophosphamide or daily chlorambucil
Nephrotic syndrome	Steroids seldom effective; low-dose aspirin combined with dipyridamole to prevent thrombotic complications; trial of prednisone (15 to 60 mg/day) plus monthly pulse cyclophosphamide or daily chlorambucil; may require dialysis/transplantation
Raynaud's phenomenon	Keep warm, avoid finger trauma, stop smoking; nifedipine as tolerated; pentoxifylline in severe cases with ischemic eschars
Acute-onset digital gangrene	Intra-arterial prostacyclin, local nitroglycerin ointment; consider endothelin receptor antagonist such as bosentan (Tracleer)
Myocarditis	Trial of steroids and cyclophosphamide; avoid digoxin§
Incomplete heart block	Avoid chloroquine¶
Asymptomatic pulmonary hypertension	Trial of steroids and cyclophosphamide, low-dose aspirin and angiotensin-converting enzyme inhibitors; consider endothelin receptor antagonist (oral bosentan)
Symptomatic pulmonary hypertension	Intravenous prostacyclin, angiotensin-converting enzyme inhibitors, anticoagulation; endothelin receptor antagonist (oral bosentan); sildenafil trial; heart-lung transplantation
Vascular headache	Trial of propranolol or alternate-day aspirin (350 mg); symptomatic use of sumatriptin
Dysphagia	Mild: no treatment
	With reflux: proton pump inhibitor; consider Nissen fundoplication
	Severe: calcium channel antagonist, alone or in combination with an anticholinergic agent
Intestinal dysmotility	Prokinetic agents such as metoclopramide, domperidone, octreotide, and erythromycin
	Small bowel bacterial overgrowth: tetracycline, erythromycin
Osteoporosis	Calcium and vitamin D supplements, estrogen replacement or raloxifene; biphosphonates; nasal calcitonin; carboxyl truncated PTH analogues such as hPTH-(1-34)
Heartburn	Raise head of bed, discontinue smoking and avoid caffeine; H2 antagonists, H+ proton blockers; metoclopramide trial pump
Trigeminal neuropathy	None

*Has been associated with frequent hypersensitivity reactions.
†Sulindac and ibuprofen have been associated with a hypersensitivity aseptic meningitis.
‡Remain alert for steroid myopathy, aseptic necrosis of bone, and accelerated osteoporosis.
§Predisposes to ventricular arrhythmias.
¶Predisposes to complete heart block.
¶Cannot be used if esophagus is more than mildly involved.

coid burden and the possibility of inducing an iatrogenic steroid myopathy, nosocomial infection, aseptic necrosis of bone, or accelerated osteoporosis. Routine evaluation of bone mineral density is warranted to detect early, presymptomatic osteoporosis and initiate therapy with antiresorptive agents. Unless contraindicated, all patients should take supplementary calcium and vitamin D. Postmenopausal patients should be offered estrogen orprogesterone replacement therapy, or raloxifene, unless there are specific contraindications; anecdotally, estrogen therapy has not been associated with flares of MCTD. In patients requiring long-term glucocorticoids it would seem reasonable to use antimalarials[267,268] or methotrexate[269] in an attempt to minimize the cumulative steroid burden. Digitalis is relatively contraindicated in patients with myocarditis due to the risk of inducing ventricular arrhythmias. Antimalarials should be used with caution in patients with a fascicular or bundle branch block due to the risk of causing a complete heart

block.[270] Patients with severe hand deformities may be helped by soft tissue release operations and selected joint fusions. There is often a tendency to assume that all patients with MCTD should be on long-term steroids; this mistake is compounded by the assumption that all medical problems in these patients are related to their underlying MCTD. For instance, apparent flares of discomfort and pain in MCTD may be due to myofascial pain syndrome or fibromyalgia and are, thus, unresponsive to corticosteroids.[271,272] Likewise the feeling of malaise and easy fatigability may be related to a reactive depression or the fact that the patient has become deconditioned. There is an increasing appreciation that the ability of any one individual to deal effectively with a chronic rheumatic disease is a result of multiple variables such as level of education, level of aerobic fitness, associated depression, maintenance of a strong locus of internal control, and an adequate social support framework. It is now evident that the initial claim of the disease's "being characterized by an excellent response to corticosteroid therapy"[105] has a ring of truth but needs to be qualified. The management of patients with MCTD requires continuing reassessment of an ever-changing pattern of clinical problems and a constant alertness to the iatrogenic disease. As with any disease of unknown etiology, effective management of patients with the MCTD syndrome presents a constant and ever-evolving challenge.

REFERENCES

1. Thomas E, Hay EM, Hajeer A, Silman AJ: Sjogren's syndrome: a community-based study of prevalence and impact. Br J Rheumatol. 37(10):1069-1076, 1998.
2. Fiori G, Pignone A, Cerinic MM: Overlap syndromes. Reumatizam 49(2):12-15, 2002.
3. Jury EC, D'Cruz D, Morrow WJ: Autoantibodies and overlap syndromes in autoimmune rheumatic disease. J Clin Pathol. 54(5):340-347, 2001.
4. Fritzler MJ: Autoantibodies: diagnostic fingerprints and etiologic perplexities. Clin Invest Med. 20(1):50-66, 1997.
5. Bruns A, Blass S, Hausdorf G, et al: Nucleosomes are major T and B cell autoantigens in systemic lupus erythematosus. Arthritis Rheum 43(10):2307-2315, 2000.
6. McClain MT, Ramsland PA, Kaufman KM, et al: Anti-sm autoantibodies in systemic lupus target highly basic surface structures of complexed spliceosomal autoantigens. J Immunol 168(4):2054-2062, 2002.
7. Utz PJ, Anderson P: Posttranslational protein modifications, apoptosis, and the bypass of tolerance to autoantigens. Arthritis Rheum 41(7):1152-1160, 1998.
8. Newman A: RNA splicing: Activity in the spliceosome. Curr Biol. 4(5):462-464, 1994.
9. Lerner MR, Boyle JA, Hardin JA, et al: Two novel classes of small ribonucleoproteins detected by antibodies associated with lupus erythematosus. Science 211:400, 1981.
10. Hoffman RW, Greidinger EL: Mixed connective tissue disease. Curr Opin Rheumatol. 12(5):386-390, 2000.
11. Fenning S, Wolff-Vorbeck G, Hackl W, et al: T cell lines recognizing the 70-kD protein of U1 small nuclear ribonucleoprotein (U1snRNP). Clin Exp Immunol 101(3):408-413, 1995.
12. Welin HE, Wahren-Herlenius M, Lundberg I, et al: Key residues revealed in a major conformational epitope of the U1-70K protein. Proc Natl Acad Sci U S A 96(25):14487-14492, 1999.
13. Yokota S: Mixed connective tissue disease in childhood. Acta Paediatr Jpn 35(5):472-479, 1993.
14. Gaubitz M, Wegmann C, Schotte H, et al: Differentiation of RNP- and SM-antibody subsets in SLE and MCTD patients by a new ELISA using recombinant antigens. Cell Mol Biol 48(3):317-321, 2002.
15. Murakami A, Kojima K, Ohya K, et al: A new conformational epitope generated by the binding of recombinant 70-kd protein and U1 RNA to anti-U1 RNP autoantibodies in sera from patients with mixed connective tissue disease. Arthritis Rheum 46(12):3273-3282, 2002.
16. Neugebauer KM, Merrill JT, Wener MH, et al: SR proteins are autoantigens in patients with systemic lupus erythematosus: Importance of phosphoepitopes. Arthritis Rheum 43(8):1768-1778, 2000.
17. Gorlach M, Burd CG, Portman DS, et al: The hnRNP proteins. Mol Biol Rep 18(2):73-78, 1993.
18. Wilk HE, Werr H, Friedrich D, et al: The core proteins of 35S hnRNP complexes: Characterization of nine different species. Eur J Biochem. 146(1):71-81, 1985.
19. Hassfeld W, Steiner G, Studnicka-Benke A, et al: Autoimmune response to the spliceosome: An immunologic link between rheumatoid arthritis, mixed connective tissue disease, and systemic lupus erythematosus. Arthritis Rheum 38(6):777-785, 1995.
20. Isenberg DA, Steiner G, Smolen JS: Clinical utility and serological connections of anti-RA33 antibodies in systemic lupus erythematosus. J Rheumatol 21(7):1260-1263, 1994.
21. Richter CM, Steiner G, Smolen JS, et al: Erosive arthritis in systemic lupus erythematosus: analysis of a distinct clinical and serological subset. Br J Rheumatol 37(4):421-424, 1998.
22. Zimmermann C, Steiner G, Skriner K, et al: The concurrence of rheumatoid arthritis and limited systemic sclerosis: clinical and serologic characteristics of an overlap syndrome. Arthritis Rheum 41(11):1938-1945, 1998.
23. Hassfeld W, Steiner G, Graninger W, et al: Autoantibody to the nuclear antigen RA33: a marker for early rheumatoid arthritis. Br J Rheumatol 32(3):199-203, 1993.
24. Skriner K, Sommergruber WH, Tremmel V, et al: Anti-A2/RA33 autoantibodies are directed to the RNA binding region of the A2 protein of the heterogeneous nuclear ribonucleoprotein complex: Differential epitope recognition in rheumatoid arthritis, systemic lupus erythematosus, and mixed connective tissue disease. J Clin Invest 100(1):127-135, 1997.
25. Amoura Z, Chabre H, Koutouzov S, et al: Nucleosome-restricted antibodies are detected before anti-dsDNA and/or antihistone antibodies in serum of MRL-Mp lpr/lpr and +/+ mice, and are present in kidney eluates of lupus mice with proteinuria. Arthritis Rheum 37(11):1684-1688, 1994.
26. Navratil JS, Ahearn JM: Apoptosis, clearance mechanisms, and the development of systemic lupus erythematosus. Curr Rheumatol Rep 3(3):191-198, 2001.
27. Cohen PL, Caricchio R, Abraham V, et al: Delayed apoptotic cell clearance and lupus-like autoimmunity in mice lacking the c-mer membrane tyrosine kinase. J Exp Med 196(1):135-140, 2002.
28. Amoura Z, Koutouzov S, Piette JC: The role of nucleosomes in lupus. Curr Opin Rheumatol 12(5):369-373, 2000.
29. Amoura Z, Koutouzov S, Chabre H, et al: Presence of antinucleosome autoantibodies in a restricted set of connective tissue diseases: antinucleosome antibodies of the IgG3 subclass are markers of renal pathogenicity in systemic lupus erythematosus. Arthritis Rheum 43(1):76-84, 2000.
30. Zwickl P, Voges D, Baumeister W: The proteasome: a macromolecular assembly designed for controlled proteolysis. Philos Trans R Soc Lond B Biol Sci 354(1389):1501-1511, 1999.
31. Mountz JD: Significance of increased circulating proteasome in autoimmune disease. J Rheumatol 29(10):2027-2030, 2002.
32. Feist E, Dorner T, Kuckelkorn U, et al: Diagnostic importance of anti-proteasome antibodies. Int Arch Allergy Immunol 123(1):92-97, 2000.
33. Feist E, Kuckelkorn U, Dorner T, et al: Autoantibodies in primary Sjögren's syndrome are directed against proteasomal subunits of the alpha and beta type. Arthritis Rheum 42(4):697-702, 1999.
34. Feist E, Dorner T, Kuckelkorn U, et al: Proteasome alpha-type subunit C9 is a primary target of autoantibodies in sera of patients with myositis and systemic lupus erythematosus. J Exp Med 184(4):1313-1318, 1996.
35. Egerer K, Kuckelkorn U, Rudolph PE, et al: Circulating proteasomes are markers of cell damage and immunologic activity in autoimmune diseases. J Rheumatol 29(10):2045-2052, 2002.
36. Vanderlugt CL, Miller SD: Epitope spreading in immune-mediated diseases: implications for immunotherapy. Nat Rev Immunol 2(2):85-95, 2002.
37. Tuohy VK, Kinkel RP: Epitope spreading: a mechanism for progression of autoimmune disease. Arch Immunol Ther Exp (Warsz) 48(5):347-351, 2000.
38. Fatenejad S, Mamula MJ, Craft J: Role of intermolecular/intrastructural B- and T-cell determinants in the diversification of autoantibodies to ribonucleoprotein particles. Proc Natl Acad Sci U S A 90:12010-12014, 1993.
39. Orth T, Mayet WJ, Deister H, et al: Analysis of epitope spreading over an eleven-year period in a patient with systemic lupus erythematosus. Scand J Rheumatol 27(6):461-464, 1998.
40. Burdt MA, Hoffman RW, Deutscher SL, et al: Long-term outcome in mixed connective tissue disease: longitudinal clinical and serologic findings. Arthritis Rheum 42(5):899-909, 1999.
41. Genth E, Zarnowski H, Mierau R, et al: HLA-DR4 and Gm(1,3,5,21) are associated with U1-nRNP antibody positive connective tissue disease. Ann Rheum Dis 46:189-196, 1987.
42. Hoffman RW, Rettenmaier LJ, Takeda Y, et al: Human autoantibodies against the 70-kd polypeptide of U1 small nuclear RNP are associated with HLA-DR4 among connective tissue disease patients. Arthritis Rheum 33:666-673, 1990.

43. Kaneoka H, Hsu KC, Takeda Y, et al: Molecular genetic analysis of HLA-DR and HLA-DQ genes among anti-U1-70-kd autoantibody positive connective tissue disease patients. Arthritis Rheum 35:83-94, 1992.

44. Merryman PF, Crapper RM, Lee S, et al: Class II major histocompatibility complex gene sequences in rheumatoid arthritis: the third diversity region of both DR beta 1 and DR beta 2 genes in two DR1, DRw10-positive individuals specify the same inferred amino acid sequence as the DR beta 1 and DR beta 2 genes of a DR4(Dw14) haplotype. Arthritis Rheum 32:251-258, 1989.

45. James JA, Scofield RH, Harley JB: Basic amino acids predominate in the sequential autoantigenic determinants of the small nuclear 70K ribonucleoprotein. Scand J Immunol 39:557-566, 1994.

46. Barakat S, Briand JP, Abuaf N, et al: Mapping of epitopes on U1 snRNP polypeptide A with synthetic peptides and autoimmune sera. Clin Exp Immunol 86:71-78, 1991.

47. Eguchi K: Apoptosis in autoimmune diseases. Intern Med 40(4):275-284, 2001.

48. Karlsen AE, Dyrberg T: Molecular mimicry between non-self, modified self and self in autoimmunity. Semin Immunol 10(1): 25-34, 1998.

49. Rumore PM, Steinman CR: Endogenous circulating DNA in systemic lupus erythematosus: Occurrence as multimeric complexes bound to histone. J Clin Invest 86(1):69-74, 1990.

50. Casciola-Rosen LA, Anhalt G, Rosen A: Autoantigens targeted in systemic lupus erythematosus are clustered in two populations of surface structures on apoptotic keratinocytes. J Exp Med 179(4):1317-1330, 1994.

51. Casciola-Rosen L, Andrade F, Ulanet D, et al: Cleavage by granzyme B is strongly predictive of autoantigen status: implications for initiation of autoimmunity. J Exp Med 190(6):815-826, 1999.

52. Utz PJ, Gensler TJ, Anderson P: Death, autoantigen modifications, and tolerance. Arthritis Res 2(2):101-114, 2000.

53. Greidinger EL, Foecking MF, Ranatunga S, Hoffman RW: Apoptotic U1-70 kd is antigenically distinct from the intact form of the U1-70-kd molecule. Arthritis Rheum 46(5):1264-1269, 2002.

54. Deshmukh US, Kannapell CC, Fu SM: Immune responses to small nuclear ribonucleoproteins: antigen-dependent distinct B cell epitope spreading patterns in mice immunized with recombinant polypeptides of small nuclear ribonucleoproteins. J Immunol 168(10):5326-5332, 2002.

55. Monneaux F, Muller S: Epitope spreading in systemic lupus erythematosus: identification of triggering peptide sequences. Arthritis Rheum 46(6):1430-1438, 2002.

56. Van Nieuwenhuijze AE, Van Lopik T, Smeenk RJ, Aarden LA: Time between onset of apoptosis and release of nucleosomes from apoptotic cells: putative implications for systemic lupus erythematosus. Ann Rheum Dis 62(1):10-14, 2003.

57. Davies JM: Introduction: Epitope mimicry as a component cause of autoimmune disease. Cell Mol Life Sci 57(4):523-526, 2000.

58. Francioni C, Galeazzi M, Fioravanti A, et al: Long-term i.v. Ig treatment in systemic lupus erythematosus. Clin Exp Rheumatol 12:163-168, 1994.

59. Wucherpfennig KW: Structural basis of molecular mimicry. J Autoimmun 16(3):293-302, 2001.

60. Hemmer B, Kondo T, Gran B, et al: Minimal peptide length requirements for CD4(+) T cell clones–implications for molecular mimicry and T cell survival. Int Immunol 12(3):375-383, 2000.

61. Mamula MJ: Epitope spreading: the role of self peptides and autoantigen processing by B lymphocytes. Immunol Rev 164: 231-239, 1998.

62. Rose NR, Mackay IR: Molecular mimicry: a critical look at exemplary instances in human diseases. Cell Mol Life Sci 57(4): 542-551, 2000.

63. Pope JE: Scleroderma overlap syndromes. Curr Opin Rheumatol 14(6):704-710, 2002.

64. Kuwana M, Kimura K, Hirakata M, et al: Differences in autoantibody response to Th/To between systemic sclerosis and other autoimmune diseases. Ann Rheum Dis 61(9):842-846, 2002.

65. Kuwana M, Kaburaki J, Okano Y, et al: Clinical and prognostic associations based on serum antinuclear antibodies in Japanese patients with systemic sclerosis. Arthritis Rheum 37:75-83, 1994.

66. Phan TG, Cass A, Gillin A, et al: Anti-RNA polymerase III antibodies in the diagnosis of scleroderma renal crisis sine scleroderma. J Rheumatol 26(11):2489-2492, 1999.

67. Negi VS, Tripathy NK, Misra R, Nityanand S: Antiendothelial cell antibodies in scleroderma correlate with severe digital ischemia and pulmonary arterial hypertension. J Rheumatol 25(3): 462-466, 1998.

68. Arnett FC, Reveille JD, Goldstein R, et al: Autoantibodies to fibrillarin in systemic sclerosis (scleroderma): An immunogenetic, serologic, and clinical analysis. Arthritis Rheum 39(7):1151-1160, 1996.

69. Pope JE, Thompson A: The frequency and significance of anticardiolipin antibodies in scleroderma. J Rheumatol 27(6): 1450-1452, 2000.

70. Yamane K, Ihn H, Kubo M, et al: Antibodies to Th/To ribonucleoprotein in patients with localized scleroderma. Rheumatology (Oxford) 40(6):683-686, 2001.

71. Clark JA, Winkelman RK, McDuffie FC, Ward LE: Synovial tissue changes and rheumatoid factor in scleroderma. Mayo Clin Proc 46:97-103, 1971.

72. Misra R, Darton K, Jewkes RF, et al: Arthritis in scleroderma. Br J Rheumatol 34(9):831-837, 1995.

73. Armstrong RD, Gibson T: Scleroderma and erosive polyarthritis: a disease entity. Ann Rheum Dis 41:141-146, 1982.

74. Catoggio LJ, Evison G, Harkness JA, Maddison PJ: The arthropathy of systemic sclerosis (scleroderma), comparison with mixed connective tissue disease. Clin Exp Rheumatol 1(2):101-112, 1983.

75. Leclech C, Friedel J, Jeandel C, et al: Reynolds' syndrome: the combination of scleroderma of CREST syndrome type and primary biliary cirrhosis. Ann Dermatol Venereol 114(6-7):857-859, 1987.

76. Akimoto S, Ishikawa O, Muro Y, et al: Clinical and immunological characterization of patients with systemic sclerosis overlapping primary biliary cirrhosis: a comparison with patients with systemic sclerosis alone. J Dermatol 26(1):18-22, 1999.

77. Makinen D, Fritzler M, Davis P, Sherlock S: Anticentromere antibodies in primary cirrhosis. Arthritis Rheum 26:914-917, 1983.

78. Marie I, Levesque H, Tranvouez JL, et al: Autoimmune hepatitis and systemic sclerosis: a new overlap syndrome? Rheumatology (Oxford) 40(1):102-106, 2001.

79. Chazouilleres O, Wendum D, Serfaty L, et al: Primary biliary cirrhosis-autoimmune hepatitis overlap syndrome: clinical features and response to therapy. Hepatology 2(82):296-301, 1998.

80. Oddis CV, Eisenbeis CH, Reidbord HE, et al: Vasculitis in systemic sclerosis: association with Sjögren's syndrome and the CREST syndrome variant. J Rheumatol 14:942-948, 1987.

81. Clements PJ, Furst DE, Campion DS, et al: Muscle disease in progressive systemic sclerosis: diagnostic and therapeutic considerations. Arthritis Rheum 21:62-71, 1978.

82. Jablonska S, Blaszczyk M: Scleroderma overlap syndromes. Adv Exp Med Biol. 455:85-92, 1999.

83. Parodi A, Drosera M, Barbieri L, Rebora A: Scleroderma subsets are best detected by the simultaneous analysis of the autoantibody profile using commercial ELISA. Dermatology 204(1):29-32, 2002.

84. Gussin HA, Ignat GP, Varga J, Teodorescu M: Anti-topoisomerase I (anti-Scl-70) antibodies in patients with systemic lupus erythematosus. Arthritis Rheum 44(2):376-383, 2001.

85. Sharp GC, Irvin WS, May CM, et al: Association of antibodies to ribonucleoprotein and Sm antigens with mixed connective-tissue disease, systematic lupus erythematosus and other rheumatic diseases. N Engl J Med 295(21):1149-1154, 1976.

86. Venables PJ, Mumford PA, Maini RN: Antibodies to nuclear antigens in polymyositis: relationship to autoimmune 'overlap syndromes' and carcinoma. Ann Rheum Dis 40(3):217-223, 1981.

87. Mimori T: Scleroderma-polymyositis overlap syndrome. Int J Dermatol 26:419-425, 1987.

88. Marguerie C, Bunn CC, Copier J, et al: The clinical and immunogenetic features of patients with autoantibodies to the nucleolar antigen PM-Scl. Medicine (Baltimore) 71:327-336, 1992.

89. Brouwer R, Pruijn GJ, Van Venrooij WJ: The human exosome: an autoantigenic complex of exoribonucleases in myositis and scleroderma. Arthritis Res 3(2):102-106, 2001.

90. Mimori T, Suwa A, Hama N: Clinical significance of anti-Ku antibodies. Nippon Rinsho 48(Suppl):535-538, 1990.

91. Yamanishi Y, Maeda H, Katayama S, et al: Scleroderma-polymyositis overlap syndrome associated with anti-Ku antibody and rimmed vacuole formation. J Rheumatol 23(11):1991-1994, 1996.

92. Isern RA, Yaneva M, Weiner E, et al: Autoantibodies in patients with primary pulmonary hypertension: association with anti-Ku. Am J Med 93(3):307-312, 1992.

93. Oddis CV, Medsger TA, Cooperstein LA: A subluxing arthropathy associated with the anti-Jo-1 antibody in polymyositis/dermatomyositis. Arthritis Rheum 33:1640-1645, 1990.

94. Mathews MB, Bernstein RM: Myositis autoantibody inhibits histidyl-tRNA synthetase: a model for autoimmunity. Nature 304:177-179, 1983.

95. Marguerie C, Bunn CC, Beynon HL, et al: Polymyositis, pulmonary fibrosis and autoantibodies to aminoacyl-tRNA synthetase enzymes. Q J Med 77(282):1019-1038, 1990.

96. Hirakata M, Nagai S: Interstitial lung disease in polymyositis and dermatomyositis. Curr Opin Rheumatol 12(6):501-508, 2000.

97. Nagaraju K, Raben N, Loeffler L, et al: Conditional up-regulation of MHC class I in skeletal muscle leads to self-sustaining autoimmune myositis and myositis-specific autoantibodies. Proc Natl Acad Sci U S A 97(16):9209-9214, 2000.

98. Coppo P, Clauvel JP, Bengoufa D, et al: Inflammatory myositis associated with anti-U1-small nuclear ribonucleoprotein antibodies: a subset of myositis associated with a favourable outcome. Rheumatology (Oxford) 41(9):1040-1046, 2002.

99. Casciola-Rosen LA, Pluta AF, Plotz PH, et al: The DNA mismatch repair enzyme PMS1 is a myositis-specific autoantigen. Arthritis Rheum 44(2):389-396, 2001.

100. Targoff IN, Johnson AE, Miller FW: Antibody to signal recognition particle in polymyositis. Arthritis Rheum 33:1361-1370, 1990.

101. Miller T, Al Lozi MT, Lopate G, Pestronk A: Myopathy with antibodies to the signal recognition particle: clinical and pathological features. J Neurol Neurosurg Psychiatry 73(4):420-428, 2002.

102. Sharp GC, Irvin WS, LaRoque RL, et al: Association of autoantibodies to different nuclear antigens with clinical patterns of rheumatic disease and responsiveness to therapy. J Clin Invest 50:350-359, 1971.

103. Hoffman RW, Cassidy JT, Takeda Y, et al: U1-70-kd autoantibody-positive mixed connective tissue disease in children: A longitudinal clinical and serologic analysis. Arthritis Rheum 36(11):1599-1602, 1993.

104. McHugh N, James I, Maddison P: Clinical significance of antibodies to a 68 kDa U1RNP polypeptide in connective tissue disease. J Rheumatol 17:1320-1328, 1990.

105. Sharp GC, Irvin WS, Tan EM, et al: Mixed connective tissue disease: an apparently distinct rheumatic disease syndrome associated with a specific antibody to an extractable nuclear antigen. Am J Med. 52:148-159, 1972

106. Bennett RM, O'Connell DJ. Mixed connective tisssue disease: a clinicopathologic study of 20 cases. Semin Arthritis Rheum 10(1):25-51, 1980.

107. Bennett RM, O'Connell DJ: The arthritis of mixed connective tissue disease. Ann Rheum Dis 37(5):397-403, 1978.

108. Sharp GC: Diagnostic criteria for classification of MCTD. In Kasukawa R, Sharp G (eds): Mixed Connective Tissue Disease and Antinuclear Antibodies. Amsterdam, Elsevier, 1987, pp 23-32.

109. Kahn MF, Appelboom T: Syndrom de Sharp. In Kahn MF, Peltier AP, Meyer O, Piette JC (eds): Les Maladies Systemiques. Paris, Flammarion, 1991, pp 545-556.

110. Alarcon-Segovia D, Villareal M: Classification and diagnostic criteria for mixed connective tissue disease. In Kasukawa R, Sharp G (eds): Mixed Connective Tissue Disease and Antinuclear Antibodies. Amsterdam, Elsevier, 1987, pp 33-40.

111. Salden MH, van Eekelen CA, Habets WJ, et al: Anti-nuclear matrix antibodies in mixed connective tissue disease. Eur J Immunol 12(9):783-786, 1982.

112. Alarcon-Segovia D, Cardiel MH: Comparison between 3 diagnostic criteria for mixed connective tissue disease. Study of 593 patients. J Rheumatol 16(3):328-334, 1989.

113. Amigues JM, Cantagrel A, Abbal M, Mazieres B: Comparative study of 4 diagnosis criteria sets for mixed connective tissue disease in patients with anti-RNP antibodies. Autoimmunity Group of the Hospitals of Toulouse. J Rheumatol 23(12):2055-2062, 1996.

114. van den Hoogen FH, Spronk PE, Boerbooms AM, et al: Long-term follow-up of 46 patients with anti-(U1)snRNP antibodies. Br J Rheumatol 33:1117-1120, 1994.

115. Nakae K, Furusawa F, Kasukawa R, et al: A nationwide epidemiological survey on diffuse collagen diseases: Estimation of prevalence rate in Japan. In Kasukawa R, Sharp G (eds): Mixed Connective Tissue Disease and Antinuclear Antibodies. Amsterdam, Excerpta Medica, 1987, pp 9-13.

116. Ramos-Niembro F, Alarcon-Segovia D: Familial aspects of mixed connective tissue disease (MCTD). I. Occurrence of systemic lupus erythematosus in another member in two families and aggregation of MCTD in another family. J Rheumatol 5(4):433-440, 1978.

117. Horn JR, Kapur JJ, Walker SE: Mixed connective tissue disease in siblings. Arthritis Rheum 21(6):709-714, 1978.

118. Winfield JB, Koffler D, Kunkel HG: Development of antibodies to ribonucleoprotein following short term therapy with procainamide. Arthritis Rheum 18:531, 1975.

119. Kahn MF, Bourgeois P, Aeschlimann A, et al: Mixed connective tissue disease after exposure to polyvinyl chloride. J Rheumatol 16(4):533-535, 1989.

120. Sanchez-Roman J, Wichmann I, Salaberri J, et al: Multiple clinical and biological autoimmune manifestations in 50 workers after occupational exposure to silica. Ann Rheum Dis 52:534-538, 1993.

121. Kashiwazaki S, Kondo H, Fukui T: Clinical features of anti-nRNP antibody positive patients. In Kasukawa R, Sharp G (eds): Mixed Connective Tissue Disease and Antinuclear Antibodies. Amsterdam, Excerpta Medica, 1987, pp 261-266.

122. LeRoy EC, Maricq H, Kahaleh M: Undifferentiated connective tissue syndrome. Arthritis Rheum 23:341-343, 1980.

123. Piirainen HI, Kurki PT: Clinical and serological follow-up of patients with polyarthritis, Raynaud's phenomenon, and circulating RNP antibodies. Scand J Rheumatol 19:51-56, 1990.

124. Sharp GC, Hoffman RW: Clinical, immunologic, and immunogenetic evidence that mixed connective tissue disease is a distinct entity: comment on the article by Smolen and Steiner. Arthritis Rheum 42(1):190-191, 1999.

125. Halla JT, Hardin JG: Clinical features of the arthritis of mixed connective tissue disease. Arthritis Rheum 21:497-503, 1978.

126. Ramos-Niembro F, Alarcon-Segovia D, Hernandez-Ortiz J: Articular manifestations of mixed connective tissue disease. Arthritis Rheum 22(1):43-51, 1979.

127. Krishnamoorthy L, O'Toole G, Jaffe W, et al: Mixed connective tissue disease presenting to the acute hand service. Ann Plast Surg 41(1):86-88, 1998.

128. O'Connell DJ, Bennett RM: Mixed connective tissue disease: clinical and radiological aspects of 20 cases. Br J Radiol 50(597):620-625, 1977.

129. Udoff EJ, Genant HK, Kozin F, et al: Mixed connective tissue disease: the spectrum of radiographic manifestations. Radiology 124(3):613-618, 1977.

130. Martinez-Cordero E, Lopez-Zepeda J: Resorptive arthropathy and rib erosions in mixed connective tissue disease. J Rheumatol 17:719-722, 1990.

131. Lewis RA, Adams JP, Gerber NL, et al: The hand in mixed connective tissue disease. J Hand Surg 3(3):217-222, 1978.

132. Fujinami M, Saito K, Okawa-Takatsuji M, et al: Histological evaluation of destructive monoarthropathy in mixed connective tissue disease. Scand J Rheumatol 26(5):395-398, 1997.

133. Nedumaran K, Rajendran CP, Porkodi R, et al: Mixed connective tissue disease: clinical and immunological profile. J Assoc Physicians India 49:412-414, 2001.

134. Gilliam JN, Prystowsky SD: Conversion of discoid lupus erythematosus to mixed connective tissue disease. J Rheumatol 4(2):165-169, 1977.

135. Konttinen YT, Tuominen TS, Piirainen HI, et al: Signs and symptoms in the masticatory system in ten patients with mixed connective tissue disease. Scand J Rheumatol 19(5):363-373, 1990.

136. Hamza M: Orogenital ulcerations in mixed connective tissue disease. J Rheumatol 12:643-644, 1985.

137. Oh YB, Jun JB, Kim CK, et al: Mixed connective tissue disease associated with skin defects of livedoid vasculitis. Clin Rheumatol 19(5):381-384, 2000.

138. Willkens RF, Roth GJ, Novak A, et al: Perforation of nasal septum in rheumatic diseases. Arthritis Rheum 19:119-121, 1976.

139. Lazaro MA, Maldonado Cocco JA, et al: Clinical and serologic characteristics of patients with overlap syndrome: is mixed connective tissue disease a distinct clinical entity? Medicine (Baltimore) 68(1):58-65, 1989.

140. Targoff IN: Idiopathic inflammatory myopathy: autoantibody update. Curr Rheumatol Rep 4(5):434-441, 2002.

141. Oxenhandler R, Hart M, Corman L, et al: Pathology of skeletal muscle in mixed connective tissue disease. Arthritis Rheum 20(4):985-988, 1977.

142. Rebollar-Gonzalez V, Torre-Delgadillo A, Orea-Tejeda A, et al: Cardiac conduction disturbances in mixed connective tissue disease. Rev Invest Clin 53(4):330-334, 2001.

143. Alpert MA, Goldberg SH, Singsen BH, et al: Cardiovascular manifestations of mixed connective tissue disease in adults. Circulation 68(6):1182-1193, 1983.

144. Oetgen WJ, Mutter ML, Lawless OJ, et al: Cardiac abnormalities in mixed connective tissue disease. Chest 83(2):185-188, 1983.

145. Nunoda S, Mifune J, Ono S, et al: An adult case of mixed connective tissue disease associated with perimyocarditis and massive pericardial effusion. Jpn Heart J 27(1):129-135, 1986.

146. Whitlow PL, Gilliam JN, Chubick A, et al: Myocarditis in mixed connective tissue disease: Association of myocarditis with antibody to nuclear ribonucleoprotein. Arthritis Rheum 23(7):808-815, 1980.

147. Lash AD, Wittman AL, Quismorio FP Jr: Myocarditis in mixed connective tissue disease: clinical and pathologic study of three cases and review of the literature. Semin Arthritis Rheum 15(4):288-296, 1986.

148. Sullivan WD, Hurst DJ, Harmon CE, et al: A prospective evaluation emphasizing pulmonary involvement in patients with mixed connective tissue disease. Medicine (Baltimore) 63(2):92-107, 1984.

149. Ueda N, Mimura K, Maeda H, et al: Mixed connective tissue disease with fatal pulmonary hypertension and a review of literature. Virchows Arch A Pathol Anat Histopathol 404(4):335-340, 1984.

150. Udaya BS, Prakash MD: Intrathoracic manifestations in mixed connective tissue disease. Mayo Clin Proc 60:813-821, 1985.

151. Martens J, Demedts M: Diaphragm dysfunction in mixed connective tissue disease: A case report. Scand J Rheumatol 11(3):165-167, 1982.

152. Saito Y, Terada M, Takada T, et al: Pulmonary involvement in mixed connective tissue disease: comparison with other collagen vascular diseases using high resolution CT. J Comput Assist Tomogr 26(3):349-357, 2002.

153. Kozuka T, Johkoh T, Honda O, et al: Pulmonary involvement in mixed connective tissue disease: high-resolution CT findings in 41 patients. J Thorac Imaging 16(2):94-98, 2001.

154. Suzuki M, Shimizu K, Sakamoto K, et al: Interstitial pneumonia associated with mixed connective tissue disease–marked improvement with azathioprine. Nihon Kyobu Shikkan Gakkai Zasshi 34(1):101-105, 1996.

155. Sanchez-Guerrero J, Cesarman G, Alarcon-Segovia D: Massive pulmonary hemorrhage in mixed connective tissue diseases. J Rheumatol 16:1132-1134, 1989.

156. Germain MJ, Davidman M: Pulmonary hemorrhage and acute renal failure in a patient with mixed connective tissue disease. Am J Kid Dis 3:420-424, 1984.

157. Miyasaka N: Pulmonary hypertension complicating mixed connective tissue disease. Intern Med 37(4):347-348, 1998.

158. Jones MB, Osterholm RK, Wilson RB, et al: Fatal pulmonary hypertension and resolving immune-complex glomerulonephritis in mixed connective tissue disease: A case report and review of the literature. Am J Med 65(5):855-863, 1978.

159. Manthorpe R, Elling H, van der Meulen JT, et al: Two fatal cases of mixed connective tissue disease: Description of case histories terminating as progressive systemic sclerosis. Scand J Rheumatol 9(1):7-10, 1980.

160. Singsen BH, Swanson VL, Bernstein BH, et al: A histologic evaluation of mixed connective tissue disease in childhood. Am J Med 68:710, 1980.

161. Mikami Y, Sawai T: Pulmonary hypertension in autopsy cases of mixed connective tissue disease. Ryumachi 33(2):117-124, 1993.

162. Filep JG, Bodolay E, Sipka S, et al: Plasma endothelin correlates with antiendothelial antibodies in patients with mixed connective tissue disease. Circulation 92(10):2969-2974, 1995.

163. Bodolay E, Bojan F, Szegedi G, et al: Cytotoxic endothelial cell antibodies in mixed connective tissue disease. Immunol Lett 20(2):163-167, 1989.

164. Watanabe H, Kaise S, Takeda I, et al: Anti-endothelial cell antibodies in the sera of patients with mixed connective tissue disease: the clinical significance. Fukushima J Med Sci 43(1):13-28, 1997.

165. Nishimaki T, Aotsuka S, Kondo H, et al: Immunological analysis of pulmonary hypertension in connective tissue diseases. J Rheumatol 26(11):2357-2362, 1999.

166. Hainaut P, Lavenne E, Magy JM, et al: Circulating lupus type anticoagulant and pulmonary hypertension associated with mixed connective tissue disease. Clin Rheumatol 5(1):96-101, 1986.

167. Du L, Sullivan CC, Chu D, et al: Signaling molecules in nonfamilial pulmonary hypertension. N Engl J Med 348(6):500-509, 2003.

168. Bennett RM, Spargo BH: Immune complex nephropathy in mixed connective tissue disease. Am J Med 63(4):534-541, 1977.

169. Kitridou RC, Akmal M, Turkel SB, et al: Renal involvement in mixed connective tissue disease: a longitudinal clinicopathologic study. Semin Arthritis Rheum 16(2):135-145, 1986.

170. Maddison PJ, Mogovero H, Reichlin M: Patterns of clinical disease associated with antibodies to nuclear ribonucleoprotein. J Rheumatol 5:407, 1978.

171. Lemmer JP, Curry NH, Mallory JH, et al: Clinical characteristics and course in patients with high titer anti-RNP antibodies. J Rheumatol 9:536, 1982.

172. Kobayashi S, Nagase M, Kimura M, et al: Renal involvement in mixed connective tissue disease: Report of 5 cases. Am J Nephrol 5(4):282-289, 1985.

173. Suzuki T, Shibata T: Clinical and microscopical study on renal involvement of patients with mixed connective tissue disease. *In* Kasukawa R, Sharp G (eds): Mixed Connective Tissue Disease and Antinuclear Antibodies. Amsterdam, Excerpta Medica, 1987, pp 303-308.

174. Selva OA, Labrador HM, Vilardell TM: Case 26-2001: scleroderma renal crisis and polymyositis. N Engl J Med 346(24):1916-1918, 2002.

175. Szigeti N, Fabian G, Czirjak L: Fatal scleroderma renal crisis caused by gastrointestinal bleeding in a patient with scleroderma, Sjögren's syndrome and primary biliary cirrhosis overlap. J Eur Acad Dermatol Venereol 16(3):276-279, 2001.

176. Marshall JB, Kretschmar JM, Gerhardt DC, et al: Gastrointestinal manifestations of mixed connective tissue disease. Gastroenterology 98(5 Pt 1):1232-1238, 1990.

177. Weston S, Thumshirn M, Wiste J, et al: Clinical and upper gastrointestinal motility features in systemic sclerosis and related disorders. Am J Gastroenterol 93(7):1085-1089, 1998.

178. Ohtomo Y, Higasi Y: A case of MCTD patient with recurrent hemoperitoneum receiving CAPD who had a successful recovery with an increase in steroids. Nippon Jinzo Gakkai Shi 34(3):325-329, 1992.

179. Kuipers EJ, van Leeuwen MA, Nikkels PG, et al: Hemobilia due to vasculitis of the gall bladder in a patient with mixed connective tissue disease. J Rheumatol 18(4):617-618, 1991.

180. Hirose W, Nakane H, Misumi J, et al: Duodenal hemorrhage and dermal vasculitis associated with mixed connective tissue disease. J Rheumatol 20(1):151-154, 1993.

181. Rolny P, Goobar J, Zettergren L: HBsAg-negative chronic active hepatitis and mixed connective tissue disease syndrome: An unusual association observed in two patients. Acta Med Scand 215(4):391-395, 1984.

182. Linana Santafe JJ, Calvo CJ, Hortelano ME, et al: Acute ascites as the onset of mixed connective tissue disease. An Med Interna 10(10):504-506, 1993.

183. Nosho K, Takahashi H, Ikeda Y, et al: A case of protein-losing gastroenteropathy in association with mixed connective tissue disease which was successfully treated with cyclophosphamide pulse therapy. Ryumachi 38(6):818-824, 1998.

184. Terren P: Protein-losing enteropathy and mixed connective-tissue disease. Med J Aust 149(10):558-559, 1988.

185. Matsumoto T, Kobayashi S, Shimizu H, et al: The liver in collagen diseases: pathologic study of 160 cases with particular reference to hepatic arteritis, primary biliary cirrhosis, autoimmune hepatitis and nodular regenerative hyperplasia of the liver. Liver 20(5):366-373, 2000.

186. Sekiguchi Y, Amano K, Takano Y, et al: Portal and pulmonary hypertension in a patient with MCTD. Ryumachi 39(4):657-663, 1999.

187. Hirasaki S, Koide N, Ogawa H, et al: Mixed connective tissue disease associated with idiopathic portal hypertension and chronic thyroiditis. J Gastroenterol 32(6):808-811, 1997.

188. Gessner C, Kaltenhauser S, Borte G, et al: Pneumatosis cystoides intestinalis, a rare complication of mixed connective tissue disease. Dtsch Med Wochenschr 126(40):1099-1102, 2001.

189. Lynn JT, Gossen G, Miller A, et al: Pneumatosis intestinalis in mixed connective tissue disease: Two case reports and literature review. Arthritis Rheum 27:1186-1189, 1984.

190. Pun YL, Russell DM, Taggart GJ, et al: Pneumatosis intestinalis and pneumoperitoneum complicating mixed connective tissue disease. Br J Rheumatol 30(2):146-149, 1991.

191. Wakamatsu M, Inada K, Tsutsumi Y: Mixed connective tissue disease complicated by pneumatosis cystoides intestinalis and malabsorption syndrome: case report and literature review. Pathol Int 45(11):875-878, 1995.

192. Iguchi Y, Ohmoto K, Shibata K, et al: A case of esophageal intramural pseudodiverticulosis complicated with primary biliary cirrhosis and mixed connective tissue disease. Nippon Shokakibyo Gakkai Zasshi 94(3):180-185, 1997.

193. Aoki S, Tada Y, Ohta A, et al: Autoimmune hepatitis associated with mixed connective tissue disease: Report of a case and a review of the literature. Nihon Rinsho Meneki Gakkai Kaishi 24(2):75-80, 2001.

194. Min JK, Han NI, Kim JA, et al: A case of cholestatic autoimmune hepatitis and acute liver failure: An unusual hepatic manifestation of mixed connective tissue disease and Sjögren's syndrome. J Korean Med Sci 16(4):512-515, 2001.

195. De Coo IF, Renier WO, Ruitenbeck W, et al: A 4-base pair deletion in the mitochondrial cytochrome b gene associated with parkinsonism/MELAS overlap syndrome. Ann Neurol 45(1):130-133, 1999.

196. Zaoui A, Galian A, Rioche M, et al: Selective immune deficiency in IgA. Intestinal malabsorption syndrome and mixed connective tissue disease. Rev Med Interne 8(3):320-323, 1987.

197. Cosnes J, Robert A, Levy VG, et al: Budd-Chiari syndrome in a patient with mixed connective-tissue disease. Dig Dis Sci 25(6):467-469, 1980.

198. Thiele DL, Krejs GJ: Secretory diarrhea in mixed connective tissue disease. Am J Gastroenterol 80(2):107-110, 1985.

199. Braun J, Sieper J, Schwarz A, et al: Widespread vasculopathy with hemolytic uremic syndrome, perimyocarditis and cystic pancreatitis in a young woman with mixed connective tissue disease: Case report and review of the literature. Rheumatol Int 13(1):31-36, 1993.

200. Bennett RM, Bong DM, Spargo BH: Neuropsychiatric problems in mixed connective tissue disease. Am J Med 65(6):955-962, 1978.

201. Nadeau SE: Neurologic manifestations of connective tissue disease. Neurol Clin 20(1):151-178, 2002.

202. Nitsche A, Leiguarda RC, Maldonado Cocco JA, et al: Neurological features in overlap syndrome. Clin Rheumatol 10(1):5-9, 1991.

203. Lee P, Bruni J, Sukenik S: Neurological manifestations in systemic sclerosis (scleroderma). J Rheumatol 11(4):480-483, 1984.

204. Teasdall RD, Frayha RA, Shulman LE: Cranial nerve involvement in systemic sclerosis (scleroderma): A report of 10 cases. Medicine (Baltimore) 59(2):149-159, 1980.

205. Hagen NA, Stevens JC, Michet CJ Jr: Trigeminal sensory neuropathy associated with connective tissue diseases. Neurology 40(6):891-896, 1990.

206. Vincent FM, Van Houzen RN: Trigeminal sensory neuropathy and bilateral carpal tunnel syndrome: The initial manifestation of mixed connective tissue disease. J Neurol Neurosurg Psychiatry 43(5):458-460, 1980.

207. Searles RP, Mladinich EK, Messner RP: Isolated trigeminal sensory neuropathy: Early manifestation of mixed connective tissue disease. Neurology 28(12):1286-1289, 1978.

208. Bronshvas MM, Prystowsky SD, Traviesa DC: Vascular headaches in mixed connective tissue disease. Headache 18:154, 1978.

209. Harris GJ, Franson TR, Ryan LM: Recurrent aseptic meningitis as a manifestation of mixed connective tissue disease (MCTD). Wis Med J 86:31-33, 1987.

210. Fujimoto M, Kira J, Murai H, et al: Hypertrophic cranial pachymeningitis associated with mixed connective tissue disease, a comparison with idiopathic and infectious pachymeningitis. Intern Med 32(6):510-512, 1993.

211. Yasuda Y, Akiguchi I, Kameyama M: Sulindac-induced aseptic meningitis in mixed connective tissue disease. Clin Neurol Neurosurg 91(3):257-260, 1989.

212. Hoffman M, Gray RG: Ibuprofen-induced meningitis in mixed connective tissue disease. Clin Rheumatol 1(2):128-130, 1982.

213. Graf WD, Milstein JM, Sherry DD: Stroke and mixed connective tissue disease. J Child Neurol 8(3):256-259, 1993.

214. Mok CC, Lau CS: Transverse myelopathy complicating mixed connective tissue disease. Clin Neurol Neurosurg 97(3):259-260, 1995.

215. Obara K, Tanaka K: A case of mixed connective tissue disease (MCTD) associated with transverse myelitis responding to pulse therapy. Rinsho Shinkeigaku 31(11):1197-1201, 1991.

216. Pedersen C, Bonen H, Boesen F: Transverse myelitis in mixed connective tissue disease. Clin Rheumatol 6(2):290-292, 1987.

217. Kappes J, Bennett RM: Cauda equina syndrome in a patient with high titer anti-RNP antibodies. Arthritis Rheum 25:349-352, 1982.

218. Gibson J, Lamey PJ, Zoma A, et al: Tongue atrophy in mixed connective tissue disease. Oral Surg Oral Med Oral Pathol 71(3):294-296, 1991.

219. Kraus A, Cervantes G, Barojas E, et al. Retinal vasculitis in mixed connective tissue disease: A fluoroangiographic study. J Rheumatol 12(6):1122-1124, 1985.

220. Flechtner KM, Baum K: Mixed connective tissue disease: recurrent episodes of optic neuropathy and transverse myelopathy: Successful treatment with plasmapheresis. J Neurol Sci 126(2):146-148, 1994.

221. Gressel MG, Tomsak RL: Recurrent bilateral optic neuropathy in mixed connective tissue disease. J Clin Neuroophthalmol 3(2):101-104, 1983.

222. Schneider F: Progressive multifocal leukoencephalopathy as a cause of neurologic symptoms in Sharp syndrome. Z Rheumatol 50:222-224, 1991.

223. Yoshihara S, Fukuma N, Masago R: Cold-induced reversible brain ischemia in mixed connective tissue disease, a case report. Nihon Rinsho Meneki Gakkai Kaishi 22(3):158-163, 1999.

224. Yasuda M, Loo M, Shiokawa S, et al: Mixed connective tissue disease presenting myasthenia gravis. Intern Med 32(8):633-637, 1993.

225. Katada E, Ojika K, Uemura M, et al: Mixed connective tissue disease associated with acute polyradiculoneuropathy. Intern Med. 36(2):118-124, 1997.

226. Masuzawa T, Nakahara N, Kobayashi S: Intracranial multiple berry aneurysms associated with fibromuscular dysplasia and mixed connective tissue disease: case report. Neurol Med Chir (Tokyo) 27:42-50, 1987.

227. Luostarinen L, Himanen SL, Pirttila T, et al: Mixed connective tissue disease associated with chronic inflammatory demyelinating polyneuropathy. Scand J Rheumatol 28(5):328-330, 1999.

228. Yamaguchi T, Ohshima S, Tanaka T, et al: Renal crisis due to intimal hyperplasia in a patient with mixed connective tissue disease (MCTD) accompanied by pulmonary hypertension. Intern Med 40(12):1250-1253, 2001.

229. Suzuki M, Hamada M, Sekiya M, et al: Fatal pulmonary hypertension in a patient with mixed connective tissue disease: report of an autopsy case. Intern Med 31(1):74-77, 1992.

230. Peller JS, Gabor GT, Porter JM, et al: Angiographic findings in mixed connective tissue disease: Correlation with fingernail capillary photomicroscopy and digital photoplethysmography findings. Arthritis Rheum 28(7):768-774, 1985.

231. Granier F, Vayssairat M, Priollet P, et al: Nailfold capillary microscopy in mixed connective tissue disease. Comparison with systemic sclerosis and systemic lupus erythematosus. Arthritis Rheum 29(2):189-195, 1986.

232. Maricq HR, LeRoy EC, D'Angelo WA, et al: Diagnostic potential of in vivo capillary microscopy in scleroderma and related disorders. Arthritis Rheum 23:183, 1980.

233. James JP, Stevens TR, Hall ND, et al: Factor VIII related antigen in connective tissue disease patients and relatives. Br J Rheumatol 29:6-9, 1990.

234. Okawa-Takatsuji M, Aotsuka S, Uwatoko S, et al: Increase of cytokine production by pulmonary artery endothelial cells induced by supernatants from monocytes stimulated with autoantibodies against U1-ribonucleoprotein. Clin Exp Rheumatol 17(6):705-712, 1999.

235. Segond P, Yeni P, Jacquot JM, Massias P: Severe autoimmune anemia and thrombopenia in mixed connective tissue disease. Arthritis Rheum 21:995, 1978.

236. ter Borg EJ, Houtman PM, Kallenberg CG, et al: Thrombocytopenia and hemolytic anemia in a patient with mixed connective tissue disease due to thrombotic thrombocytopenic purpura. J Rheumatol 15(7):1174-1177, 1988.

237. Paice EW, Snaith ML: Thrombotic thrombocytopenia purpura occurring in a patient with mixed connective tissue disease. Rheumatol Int 4:141-142, 1984.

238. Kato A, Suzuki Y, Fujigaki Y, et al: Thrombotic thrombocytopenic purpura associated with mixed connective tissue disease. Rheumatol Int 22(3):122-125, 2002.

239. Julkunen H, Jantti J, Pettersson T: Pure red cell aplasia in mixed connective tissue disease. J Rheumatol 16(10):1385-1386, 1989.

240. Paller AS: Juvenile dermatomyositis and overlap syndromes. Adv Dermatol 10:309-326; discussion 327:309-326, 1995.

241. Ginsburg WW, Conn DL, Bunch TW, McDuffie FC: Comparison of clinical and serologic markers in systemic lupus erythematosus and overlap syndrome: a review of 247 patients. J Rheumatol 10(2):235-241, 1983.

242. Radwan L, Maszczyk Z, Koziorowski A, et al: Control of breathing in obstructive sleep apnoea and in patients with the overlap syndrome. Eur Respir J 8(4):542-545, 1995.

243. Komatireddy GR, Wang GS, Sharp GC, Hoffman RW: Antiphospholipid antibodies among anti-U1-70 kDa autoantibody positive patients with mixed connective tissue disease. J Rheumatol 24(2):319-322, 1997.

244. Mendonca LL, Amengual O, Atsumi T, et al: Most anticardiolipin antibodies in mixed connective tissue disease are beta2-glycoprotein independent . J Rheumatol 25(1):189-190, 1998.

245. Doria A, Ruffatti A, Calligaro A, et al: Antiphospholipid antibodies in mixed connective tissue disease. Clin Rheumatol 11(1):48-50, 1992.

246. Kaufman RL, Kitridou RC: Pregnancy in mixed connective tissue disease: comparison with systemic lupus erythematosus. J Rheumatol 9(4):549-555, 1982.

247. Bodolay E, Bacsko G, Bezsilla E, Szegedi G: Pregnancy in mixed connective tissue disease. Orv Hetil 132(12):619-622, 1991.

248. Kari JA: Pregnancy outcome in connective tissue diseases. Saudi Med J 22(7):590-594, 2001.

249. Lundberg I, Hedfors E: Pregnancy outcome in patients with high titer anti-RNP antibodies: A retrospective study of 40 pregnancies. J Rheumatol 18:359-362, 1991.

250. Kahl LE, Blair C, Ramsey-Goldman R, et al: Pregnancy outcomes in women with primary Raynaud's phenomenon. Arthritis Rheum 33:1249-1255, 1990.

251. Ackerman J, Gonzalez EF, Gilbert-Barness E: Immunological studies of the placenta in maternal connective tissue disease. Pediatr Dev Pathol 2(1):19-24, 1999.

252. Yokota S, Imagawa T, Katakura S, et al: Mixed connective tissue disease in childhood: a nationwide retrospective study in Japan. Acta Paediatr Jpn 39(2):273-276, 1997.

253. Peskett SA, Ansell BM, Fizzman P, et al: Mixed connective tissue disease in children. Rheumatol Rehabil 17(4):245-248, 1978.

254. Tiddens HA, van der Net JJ, Graeff-Meeder ER, et al: Juvenile-onset mixed connective tissue disease: longitudinal follow-up. J Pediatr 122(2):191-197, 1993.

255. Michels H: Course of mixed connective tissue disease in children. Ann Med 29(5):359-364, 1997.

256. Miyawaki S, Onodera H: Clinical course and prognosis of patients with mixed connective tissue disease. In Kasukawa R, Sharp G (eds): Mixed Connective Tissue Disease and Antinuclear Antibodies. Amsterdam, Excerpta Medica, 1987, pp 331-336.

257. McGoon MD: The assessment of pulmonary hypertension. Clin Chest Med 22(3):493-508, 2001.

258. Chemla D, Castelain V, Herve P, et al: Haemodynamic evaluation of pulmonary hypertension. Eur Respir J 20(5):1314-1331, 2002.

259. McLaughlin VV: Medical management of primary pulmonary hypertension. Expert Opin Pharmacother 3(2):159-165, 2002.

260. Olschewski H, Simonneau G, Galie N, et al: Inhaled iloprost for severe pulmonary hypertension. N Engl J Med 347(5):322-329, 2002.

261. Rubin LJ, Badesch DB, Barst RJ, et al: Bosentan therapy for pulmonary arterial hypertension. N Engl J Med 346(12):896-903, 2002.

262. Sapadin AN, Fleischmajer R: Treatment of scleroderma. Arch Dermatol 138(1):99-105, 2002.

263. Godeau B, Chevret S, Varet B, et al: Intravenous immunoglobulin or high-dose methylprednisolone, with or without oral prednisone, for adults with untreated severe autoimmune thrombocytopenic purpura: a randomised, multicentre trial. Lancet 359(9300):23-29, 2002.

264. Cherin P, Pelletier S, Teixeira A, et al: Results and long-term followup of intravenous immunoglobulin infusions in chronic, refractory polymyositis: an open study with thirty-five adult patients. Arthritis Rheum 46(2):467-474, 2002.

265. Blanco R, Martinez-Taboada VM, Rodriguez-Valverde V, et al: Successful therapy with danazol in refractory autoimmune thrombocytopenia associated with rheumatic diseases. Br J Rheumatol 36(10):1095-1099, 1997.

266. Myllykangas-Luosujarvi R, Jantunen E, Kaipiainen-Seppanen O, et al: Autologous peripheral blood stem cell transplantation in a patient with severe mixed connective tissue disease. Scand J Rheumatol 29(5):326-327, 2000.

267. Wallace DJ: Antimalarials: the 'real' advance in lupus. Lupus 10(6):385-387, 2001.

268. D'Cruz D: Antimalarial therapy: a panacea for mild lupus? Lupus 10(3):148-151, 2001.

269. Sato EI: Methotrexate therapy in systemic lupus erythematosus. Lupus 10(3):162-164, 2001.

270. Nolan RJ, Shulman ST, Victorica BE: Congenital complete heart block associated with maternal mixed connective tissue disease. J Pediatr 95(3):420-422, 1979.

271. Middleton GD, McFarlin JE, Lipsky PE: The prevalence and clinical impact of fibromyalgia in systemic lupus erythematosus. Arthritis Rheum 37:1181-1188, 1994.

272. Bennett R: The concurrence of lupus and fibromyalgia: implications for diagnosis and management. Lupus 6(6):494-499, 1997.

79 Scleroderma

JAMES R. SEIBOLD

Systemic sclerosis (scleroderma) is a generalized disorder of connective tissue characterized clinically by thickening and fibrosis of the skin (scleroderma) and by distinctive forms of involvement of internal organs, notably the heart, lungs, kidneys, and gastrointestinal tract. The etiology and pathogenesis are unknown. Any unifying hypothesis concerning the pathogenesis must explain the following: 1) the remarkable heterogeneity of patterns of the extent and progression of disease and of internal organ involvement, 2) the accelerated rate of accumulation of extracellular matrix in both skin and internal organs, 3) the frequent and somewhat characteristic immunologic abnormalities, 4) the variable contributions of acute and chronic inflammatory change, and 5) the ubiquitous and characteristic abnormalities of vascular function and structure.

Systemic sclerosis is often of tragic consequence to the patient. Morbidity and mortality are substantial and are directly related to the extent and severity of visceral involvement. Although much is available for the supportive care of the individual with systemic sclerosis, there are no therapies known to modify the natural history of disease. This is in part due to the dearth of appropriately designed clinical studies of potentially effective agents.

Definition and Classification

The term *scleroderma* (Greek *skleros* ["hard"] + *derma* ["skin"]) is a descriptive construct that includes a number of clinical disorders otherwise minimally related or unrelated to systemic sclerosis (Table 79–1). A multicenter study by the American College of Rheumatology (ACR) proposed preliminary criteria for the classification of systemic sclerosis based on clinical and laboratory assessments of nearly 800 patients with early-diagnosed connective tissue disease, including systemic sclerosis, systemic lupus erythematosus (SLE), inflammatory muscle disease, and isolated Raynaud's phenomenon.[1] Sclerodermatous skin change in any location proximal to the metacarpophalangeal joints was the single major criterion for classification of systemic sclerosis, with a sensitivity of 91 percent and specificity greater than 99 percent. The presence of two or more of the following features contributed further as minor criteria: sclerodactyly, digital pitting scars on fingertips or loss of digital finger pad substance, and bibasilar pulmonary fibrosis.[1] It is recognized that many patients with confident diagnoses of systemic sclerosis do not fulfill these criteria.[2] Furthermore, proximal skin thickening is an intrinsic clinical feature of many of the disorders listed in Table

TABLE 79–1 • DIFFERENTIAL DIAGNOSIS OF SCLERODERMA AND SYSTEMIC SCLEROSIS

Systemic sclerosis
  See Table 83–2
Disorders characterized by or associated with skin
  thickening on the fingers and hands
  Bleomycin-induced scleroderma
  Digital sclerosis of diabetes mellitus
  Chronic reflex sympathetic dystrophy
  Mycosis fungoides
  Vinyl chloride disease
  Amyloidosis
  Acrodermatitis chronica atrophicans
  Adult celiac disease
  Vibration disease
Disorders characterized by or associated with generalized
  skin thickening, but typically sparing the fingers and hands
  Scleroderma adultorum of Buschke
  Scleromyxedema
  Eosinophilic fasciitis
  Eosinophilic-myalgia syndrome
  Generalized subcutaneous morphea
  Pentazocine-induced scleroderma
  Human graft-versus-host disease
  Porphyria cutanea tarda
  Amyloidosis
Disorders characterized by asymmetric skin change
  Morphea
  Linear scleroderma
  Coup de sabre
Disorders characterized by similar internal organ involvement
  Primary pulmonary hypertension
  Primary biliary cirrhosis
  Intestinal pseudo-obstruction
  Collagenous colitis
  Infiltrative cardiomyopathy
  Idiopathic pulmonary fibrosis
Disorders characterized by Raynaud's phenomenon
  See Table 83–4

79–1. Thus, although the ACR criteria are useful in ensuring uniformity in clinical research, they are without value in clinical differential diagnosis.[3]

Within the diagnosis of systemic sclerosis, most observers recognize subgroups of clinical and prognostic importance[4,5] that are not discriminated by the classification criteria[1] and that are the subject of terminologic controversy.[3] A consensus proposal on nomenclature has been developed to permit the separation of systemic sclerosis by clinical features alone, with the extent of skin involvement serving as a principal guide[6] (Table 79–2). Some think patients with skin thickening that is proximal to the fingers yet spares the trunk (acrosclerosis) represent an intermediate group between those with diffuse cutaneous scleroderma and those with finger involvement

TABLE 79–2 • CLASSIFICATION OF SYSTEMIC SCLEROSIS

With diffuse cutaneous scleroderma

Skin thickening present on the trunk in addition to face, proximal and distal extremities

With limited cutaneous scleroderma

Skin thickening limited to sites distal to the elbow and knee but also involving the face and neck
   Synonym: CREST syndrome (C, calcinosis; R, Raynaud's phenomenon; E, esophageal dysmotility; S, sclerodactyly; T, telangiectases)

Sine scleroderma

Characteristic internal organ manifestations, vascular and serologic abnormalities but without clinically detectable skin change

In overlap

Any of the three previous classifications occurring concomitantly with a diagnosis of systemic lupus erythematosus (SLE), inflammatory muscle disease, or rheumatoid arthritis (RA). Synonyms: Mixed connective tissue disease, lupoderma, sclerodermatomyositis (see Chapters 74 and 84)

Undifferentiated connective tissue disease

Raynaud's phenomenon with clinical features, serologic features, or both, of systemic sclerosis (digital ulceration, abnormal nail fold capillary loops, serum anticentromere antibody, finger edema) but without skin thickening and without internal organ abnormalities of systemic sclerosis

only (sclerodactyly).[5] It should be recognized that virtually all the proposed stratifications of systemic sclerosis are somewhat arbitrary and are likely subject to clinical ascertainment bias. The majority of the clinical and laboratory information on which classification is based has been derived from cross-sectional or point-prevalence surveys or retrospective study of some specific feature of illness.[3,6,7]

Incidence and Epidemiology

The incidence of systemic sclerosis, derived from modern, well-designed studies, is between 18 and 20 individuals per million population per year[8,9] and appears to be stable. A study of Raynaud's phenomenon in South Carolina has found evidence of substantial numbers of previously undiagnosed individuals.[10] Data suggest that true prevalence may be more than fourfold higher than previously recognized. Coupled with studies of mortality demonstrating 7-year survival rates of 81 percent for limited scleroderma and 72 percent for diffuse scleroderma,[11] these figures suggest that there are 75,000 to 100,000 cases of systemic sclerosis in the United States. It remains likely that many cases are unrecognized or are misdiagnosed as Raynaud's phenomenon only or as having a related connective tissue disease.[10]

Systemic sclerosis is found in all geographic areas and all racial groups, although blacks may be at moderately increased risk.[11,12] Although all age-groups may

be affected, the onset of disease is highest between the ages of 30 and 50 years.[8,911,12] Systemic sclerosis is three to four times more common in women than in men,[11,12] with women of childbearing age at peak risk.[11] The majority of cases occur sporadically without reference to season, geography, occupation, and socioeconomic status.[12] Case reports and series linking the occurrence of systemic sclerosis to organic solvent exposure have not been supported by a focused epidemiologic survey.[13,14] Occupational silica or metal dust exposure has been linked with the occurrence of systemic sclerosis.[15] Although the disease is clinically indistinguishable from idiopathic systemic sclerosis, genomic differences in both class II HLA and tumor necrosis factor (TNF) alleles suggest a difference in the mechanism of disease.[15] Anecdotal reports have linked the occurrence of systemic sclerosis with silicone augmentative mammoplasty,[16-18] but large epidemiologic studies have failed to confirm any association.[19,20]

Although reports of the familial occurrence of systemic sclerosis are rare, it is more common than would be expected by chance alone.[14] The concordance of scleroderma in identical twins is 5.9 percent,[21] roughly 300-fold that of chance alone. A genetic contribution to disease is considered likely. Studies of HLA phenotypes by serologic techniques have suggested linkages of disease with the HLA-A1, -B8, and -DR3 haplotype or with DR3/DR52.[22,23] Major histocompatibility complex (MHC) analysis at the DNA level has revealed strong associations with C4AQ0 and DQA2.[24] Furthermore, there are strong associations of class II MHC alleles with serologically and clinically defined subsets of disease.[24] Detailed study of a well-defined case cluster of scleroderma in Choctaws in southeastern Oklahoma has linked the expression of disease with a unique Amerindian HLA haplotype (B35, Cw4, DRB1*1602 [DR2], DQA1*0501, and DQB1*0301 [DQ7]).[25] A multilocus 2-cM haplotype on chromosome 15q homologous to the murine *tsk1* region has also been linked to systemic sclerosis in the Choctaw.[26] First-degree relatives of patients with systemic sclerosis are more likely to have serum antinuclear antibody.[27] There is not an increased familial occurrence of more specific serologic features such as serum anticentromere antibody.[28]

Initial Presentations

RAYNAUD'S PHENOMENON AND SYSTEMIC SCLEROSIS

Raynaud's phenomenon is the initial complaint in approximately 70 percent of patients with systemic sclerosis and in virtually all patients whose disease is destined to evolve into systemic sclerosis with limited scleroderma (formerly known as CREST syndrome: *c*alcinosis, *R*aynaud's phenomenon, *e*sophageal dysmotility, *s*clerodactyly, *t*elangiectases)[29] (see Table 79–2). Individuals with diffuse scleroderma are more likely to present with finger and hand swelling, complaints of arthritis, evidence of specific internal organ involvement, or skin thickening. In diffuse scleroderma, any of these features may occur either contemporaneously or within 1 to 2 years of the development of Raynaud's phenomenon.

The small subgroup of patients who never develop Raynaud's phenomenon are more frequently male, are at high risk for developing renal and myocardial involvement, and have poor survival.

The exact incidence of Raynaud's phenomenon is not known. However, it is viewed as an important index characteristic for epidemiologic study of systemic sclerosis.[10] Population surveys have suggested a prevalence of 5 to 10 percent in nonsmokers[10,30] and up to 30 percent in premenopausal females.[30] Reconciliation of the prevalence of Raynaud's phenomenon with the relative rarity of systemic sclerosis is difficult. The experiences of academic centers are likely subject to a referral bias that selects for cases of relative clinical severity, thereby skewing the case mix toward secondary forms of this syndrome.

Advances in techniques of laboratory diagnosis permit the dismissal of older, clinically based studies of the natural history of Raynaud's phenomenon and its potential to evolve into systemic sclerosis. In any modern study of Raynaud's phenomenon, few patients have been encountered who at initial assessment were free of clinical and laboratory abnormality and at some later time were noted to develop features of systemic sclerosis. Support for this view derives from studies of architectural abnormalities of the nail fold capillary bed[31]; serologic abnormalities including antinuclear and anticentromere antibodies[32,33]; physiologic assessments of digital perfusion[34]; and measures of in vivo platelet activation[35]. To term patients with systemic sclerosis at the stage of Raynaud's phenomenon only as "transitional" from primary Raynaud's describes a biologic and clinical sequence that is virtually never encountered. Terming such patients "undifferentiated connective tissue disease" allows for diverse subsequent clinical outcomes, including systemic sclerosis[36] (Fig. 79–1).

EDEMATOUS CHANGE

An intrinsic feature of undifferentiated connective tissue disease is the painless swelling of the fingers and hands known as early "puffy" or edematous scleroderma. Similar presentations are described in rheumatoid arthritis (RA) and SLE and as the most typical early sign of overlap syndromes.[37] From the clinical standpoint, the longer an individual patient remains at this stage, the more favorable the long-term prognosis. Symptoms of morning stiffness and arthralgia are typical, and median nerve compression is a frequent occurrence. Pitting edema of the fingers and dorsum of the hands is easily elicited on physical examination. The edema is also typically present in unexpected locations such as the upper arms, face, and trunk, even in patients with clear diagnoses of limited scleroderma. The extent and severity of skin edema are unrelated to either the duration or the classification of disease.

The edema is in part due to the deposition of hydrophilic glycosaminoglycan in the dermis but may also reflect local inflammation, hydrostatic effects, and microvascular disruption.[38] It is not known what causes the edema to regress; in fact, some data suggest that it does not. The percentage contribution of tissue water to weight in trimmed punch-skin biopsies is remarkably consistent (about 70 percent) in all patients, irrespective of their clinical classification, duration of disease, or degree of clinical skin thickness and edema at the site of biopsy.[39] It is possible that the edema does not resolve but the clinical ability to detect such changes becomes more limited as the dermis becomes more fibrotic.

▌ Skin Involvement

CLINICAL FINDINGS

The skin thickening of systemic sclerosis begins on the fingers and hands in nearly all cases. The skin initially appears shiny and taut and may be erythematous at early stages (Fig. 79–2). Superficial landmarks such as transverse digital skin creases are obscured, and hair growth is sparse. The skin of the face and neck is usually next involved and is associated with an immobile and pinched

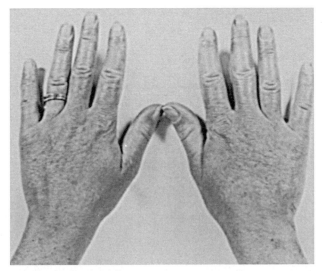

FIGURE 79–1 · The Hands of a Young Woman with Undifferentiated Connective Tissue Disease. The fingers are swollen, with mild pitting edema, and there is digital tip cyanosis. The skin is not yet thickened.

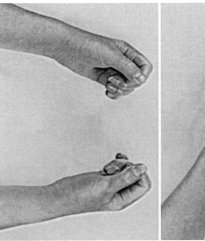
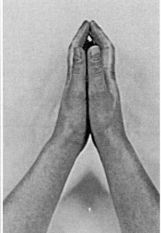

FIGURE 79–2 · The Hands of a Young Woman After Several Months of Rapidly Progressive Scleroderma. The skin is taut and indurated, and there is limitation of both fist closure and finger extension.

facies (Fig. 79–3). The lips become thin and pursed, and radial furrowing may develop about the mouth (Fig. 79–4). Skin tightening and thickening may limit the oral aperture, impairing effective dental hygiene. The skin change may stay restricted to fingers, hands, and face and may remain relatively mild. Extension to the forearms is followed by a spontaneous arrest of progression (limited scleroderma) or by rapid centripetal spread to the upper arms, shoulders, anterior chest, back, abdomen, and legs (diffuse scleroderma). Impressive areas of hyper- and hypopigmentation may develop (Fig. 79–5), or there may be generalized deepening of skin tone.

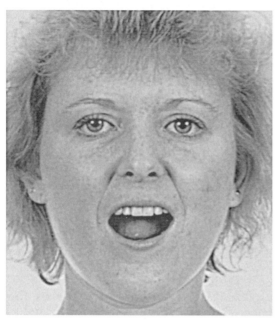

FIGURE 79-3 · The Face of a Young Woman with Several Months of Rapidly Progressive Scleroderma. The facial skin is taut with an immobile facies and limitation of the oral aperture.

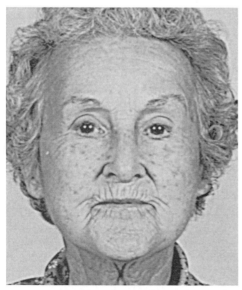

FIGURE 79-4 · The Face of a Woman with Long-standing Diffuse Scleroderma Exhibiting Multiple Telangiectasias and Exaggerated Radial Furrowing about the Lips.

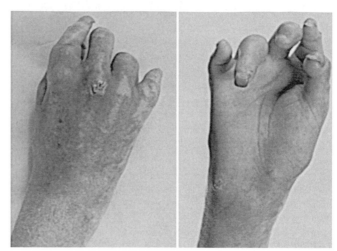

FIGURE 79-5 · Advanced Changes of Scleroderma in the Hand of a Woman with Long-Standing Disease. The skin is taut and thickened, with irregular pigmentary change and palmar telangiectasias. Ulcerations are present over bony prominences and the fingers reveal extensive trophic abnormalities.

In diffuse scleroderma, the pace of extension of skin change is somewhat variable, ranging from the development of total body skin thickening within a few months to more insidious progression over several years. Whereas some patients mimic the relapsing patterns of SLE with intermittent periods of rapidly progressive skin involvement interspersed with periods of clinical quiescence, the typical pattern is of unremitting progression. Some data suggest that untreated diffuse scleroderma is uniphasic, with peaking of skin involvement in both extent and severity within 3 years of the onset of disease[39,40] (Fig. 79–6). In contrast, patients with limited

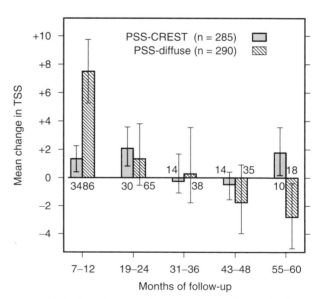

FIGURE 79-6 · The natural history of scleroderma skin involvement as assessed by the total skin score (TSS) in a large number of patients followed for periods as long as 5 years. Individuals with diffuse scleroderma worsen in extent and severity for the first 2 to 3 years of disease but thereafter improve spontaneously. Limited scleroderma (formerly known as CREST syndrome) is typified by slow but continual worsening. (From Medsger TA Jr.: Progressive systemic sclerosis. Clin Rheum Dis 9: 655, 1983.)

scleroderma inexorably worsen with time without periods of spontaneous improvement or arrest. However, these patients may enjoy so slow a rate of progression of skin change as to be clinically unchanged from year to year.

At later stages of disease, atrophy develops, leading to fragility and laxity of the superficial dermis, although tethering to deeper tissues may still be appreciated. The clinical observation of improving skin change in late diffuse scleroderma[39,40] may reflect this atrophic phase. This renders interpretation of clinical trials difficult.

ASSESSMENT AND CLASSIFICATION

The diagnosis of systemic sclerosis is usually clinically obvious once skin thickening has developed, and skin biopsies are rarely necessary. However, virtually all the proposed classification schemes[3-6] are based on clinical determinations of the extent of sclerodermatous skin change (see Table 79–2). As discussed in detail in subsequent sections, there are important relations between classification and prognosis. A useful aphorism is that the relative risk of acquiring new internal organ involvement closely parallels the pace, progression, and extent of skin involvement. Because internal organ involvement is the principal determinant of morbidity and mortality, the clinical ability to accurately recognize the extent of skin change is paramount. Similarly, the clinical ability to recognize serial changes in the extent and severity of skin thickening is necessary for monitoring the stage and "activity" of systemic sclerosis and in assessing the response to therapy.

The most widely accepted method for monitoring skin changes in systemic sclerosis is by simple clinical palpation. The modified Rodnan skin score[41,42] employs a qualitative rating scale (0, normal skin; 1, mild; 2, moderate; 3, severe thickening) of findings on clinical palpation of 17 body areas and, thus, permits a semiquantitative tool for clinical research as well as a measure of clinical progress in the individual patient (Fig. 79–7). Other proposed systems estimate both skin thickening and tethering.[43] Skin thickness ratings of experienced clinical investigators by clinical palpation correlate closely with skin core biopsy weights.[38] Total skin scoring is used increasingly as the primary outcome measure in clinical research trials. The measurement is considered accessible and sensitive to change.[44,45] Studies have confirmed a high degree of reproducibility (intraobserver error) and accuracy (interobserver error) of skin-scoring techniques.[41,42]

HISTOPATHOLOGIC FINDINGS

The tightening and thickening of the skin in systemic sclerosis is due to the accumulation of excess collagen and other extracellular matrix constituents including glycosaminoglycan and fibronectin. Skin biopsies from early stages of illness disclose an increase in compact hyalinized collagen fibers in the lower dermis and upper subcutaneum in association with perivascular and interstitial lymphocyte and histiocyte infiltrates[46-49]

Right		Left
Total skin score by palpation		
Right		Left
0 1 2 (3) 4	Fingers	0 1 2 (3) 4
0 1 2 (3) 4	Hands	0 1 2 (3) 4
0 1 (2) 3 4	Forearms	0 1 (2) 3 4
0 1 (2) 3 4	Arms	0 1 (2) 3 4
0 (1) 2 3 4	Shoulders	0 (1) 2 3 4
0 (1) 2 3 4	Neck	
0 1 (2) 3 4	Face	
0 1 (2) 3 4	Chest	
0 (1) 2 3 4	Breasts	0 (1) 2 3 4
0 (1) 2 3 4	Abdomen	
0 (1) 2 3 4	Upper back	
(0) 1 2 3 4	Lower back	
(0) 1 2 3 4	Thighs	(0) 1 2 3 4
(0) 1 2 3 4	Legs	(0) 1 2 3 4
0 (1) 2 3 4	Feet	0 (1) 2 3 4
0 1 2 (3) 4	Toes	0 1 2 (3) 4
	Total 37	

FIGURE 79–7 · An example of the total skin score (TSS) technique (Rodnan) of assessing scleroderma skin thickening by clinical palpation. The presence of skin change on the trunk permits classification of this patient as systemic sclerosis with diffuse scleroderma. Serial examinations are used to follow the clinical course and to assess the response to therapy.

(Fig. 79–8). Direct skin immunofluorescence is minimal,[48] and electron microscopy reveals an increase in fine collagen fibrils of 10 to 20 nm in diameter, and in ground substance.[46,49] At later stages, atrophic change is noted, including thinning of the epidermis with a loss of rete pegs and of dermal appendages.[46]

ABNORMALITIES OF EXTRACELLULAR MATRIX

Collagen accumulation by cultured fibroblasts derived from the skin of patients with systemic sclerosis is increased.[50] The relative proportion of the two major skin procollagens, types I and III, is that of normal skin, and this, along with some forms of keloid, separates systemic sclerosis as unique among fibrosing disorders. There is some evidence of disproportionately increased synthesis of basement membrane collagen, as well as of fibronectin and glycosaminoglycan.[50] The collagen is biochemically normal. Studies with complementary DNA probes for pro-$\alpha 1$(I), $\alpha 2$(I), and α(I)IV collagens have failed to reveal a disease-associated genomic polymorphism.[51] The increased synthesis of types I and III collagen is associated with a coordinate increase in messenger RNA (mRNA) levels.[50,51]

Collagen degradation in systemic sclerosis is normal. The activity of intracellular enzymes responsible for post-translational modification of collagen, prolylhydroxylase, and lysylhydroxylase, is increased,[52] and the response of scleroderma fibroblasts to feedback regulation by the aminopropeptide of collagen is normal.[53]

The fundamental basis for the hyperproliferative and hypersecretory "scleroderma fibroblast phenotype" has

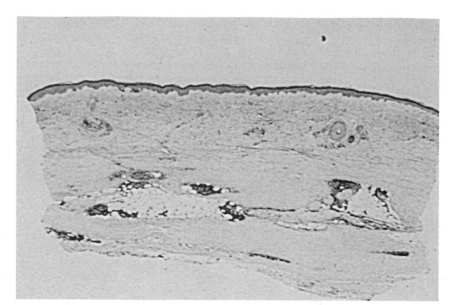

FIGURE 79–8 · Photomicrograph of a Punch Skin Biopsy Obtained from a Patient with early Diffuse Scleroderma. The epidermis is thinned and shows loss of appendages. The lower dermis and subcutis are markedly thickened from an increase in compact hyalinized collagen. Lymphocyte infiltrates (typically T helper phenotype) are readily apparent in the lower dermis and at the dermal-subcuticular interface.

not been determined. Clonal selection of a hyperproliferative fibroblast subpopulation is supported by much data. Both normal and scleroderma fibroblasts are heterogeneous in their level of collagen synthesis, and high-collagen–producing cells are overrepresented in scleroderma.[54] Scleroderma skin contains a higher percentage of fibroblasts resistant to anti-Fas–mediated killing, suggesting a defect in apoptosis.[55] The defect in fibroblast regulation may be autocrine or paracrine effects of immigrant immune cells[56] or endothelium.[57] Scleroderma fibroblasts both are more responsive to transforming growth factor-β (TGF-β)[50,58] and express increased levels of TGF-β receptor.[58]

INFLUENCES ON MATRIX METABOLISM

To assume that the fibrosis of systemic sclerosis is a secondary event casts focus on potential primary signals of connective tissue activation (Table 79–3). A diverse array of cytokines and growth factors are capable of inducing or modulating the scleroderma fibroblast phenotype (enhanced proliferation and synthetic function).[50] The microenvironment of the scleroderma tissue lesion contains a variety of cellular populations capable of local release of cytokines.

TABLE 79–3 · CYTOKINES IMPLICATED IN THE FIBROBLAST BIOLOGY OF SYSTEMIC SCLEROSIS

Inhibition of Growth or Proliferation or Matrix Synthesis	Inhibition of Growth or Synthesis
Transforming growth factor-β	Interferon-γ
Leukotriene B$_4$	Tumor necrosis factor-α
Interleukin-1	Fibroblast growth factor
Interleukin-4	Endothelial growth factor
Interleukin-6	Interleukin-8

Mast cell infiltration[59,60] and degranulation[60] have been demonstrated in scleroderma skin preceding clinically apparent fibrosis. Similar findings are noted in murine models of scleroderma including the tight skin (Tsk) mouse[61] and chronic graft-versus-host disease,[62] as well as in a variety of other fibrosing conditions.

Mast cell or monocyte release of TNF might be implicated in this process. TNF-α and lymphotoxin (TNF-β) are mitogenic for fibroblasts, inhibitory to endothelium, and pleotropic for matrix synthesis[63] and may represent the prime mitogenic signal released by monocytes. Their effects are augmented by interferon-γ (IFN-γ). Rosenbloom and colleagues[64] have demonstrated in studies of systemic sclerosis that recombinant IFN-γ causes potent inhibition of fibroblast collagen production and an associated coordinate decrease in types I and III procollagen mRNA levels. This effect is noted at very low concentrations of IFN-γ[64] and has been shown to persist through serial passages of cultured scleroderma fibroblasts.[65]

Antigen- and mitogen-stimulated T lymphocytes release factors that are both chemotactic for fibroblasts[66] and stimulatory to both fibroblast proliferation and collagen accumulation.[67] Soluble mediators derived from concanavalin A–incubated normal human mononuclear cells have been shown to induce systemic sclerosis-like fibroblast growth and glycosaminoglycan synthesis,[68] and phytohemagglutinin-stimulated monocytes from systemic sclerosis enhance collagen accumulation.[69]

Platelet-derived growth factors (PDGFs) have been implicated,[63] and, perhaps most important, TGF-β has been implicated; it stimulates fibroblast proliferation and matrix synthesis,[50] in part by stimulation of the autocrine release of PDGF and also by being inhibitory to endothelium. When injected subcutaneously, TGF-β causes intense mononuclear cell infiltrate, neoangiogenesis, and fibrosis.[50] Continued investigation of these various influences on connective tissue metabolism in systemic sclerosis may lead to effective approaches to therapeutic manipulation.[63]

▌ Vascular and Microvascular Abnormalities

A vascular hypothesis for the pathogenesis of systemic sclerosis is supported by a variety of clinical and laboratory observations. Characteristic structural alterations of the small artery and microvasculature are present at the earliest recognizable stages of illness, and clinical manifestations reflecting the vascular derangement dominate aspects of the disease course in all forms of the disorder.

RAYNAUD'S PHENOMENON

Raynaud's phenomenon is the most typical presenting manifestation of systemic sclerosis. The digital arteries of patients with systemic sclerosis exhibit marked intimal hyperplasia consisting predominantly of collagen and to a lesser degree of ground substance[29] (Fig. 79–9). Medial changes are relatively inconspicuous, but adventitial fibrosis is seen in 40 percent of cases.[29] Severe narrowing (more than 75 percent) of the arterial lumen results, which may in itself be of sufficient severity to account for Raynaud's phenomenon. A normal vasoconstrictor response to cold or emotional stimuli, superimposed on the anatomic obstruction, could cause complete or near-complete occlusion of the arterial lumen.[29] Similar histopathologic changes are evident in the small arteries and arterioles of affected internal organs[70,71] (Fig. 79–10). Certain important clinical syndromes such as scleroderma renal crisis[72] and pulmonary hypertension[73] are due principally to the presence of this fibrotic arteriosclerotic lesion.

MECHANISMS OF RAYNAUD'S PHENOMENON

Perfusion to the skin is ordinarily 10- to 20-fold that required for nutrition and oxygenation. Alterations in skin blood flow are thus a principal mechanism of body thermoregulation. Peripheral vasoconstriction in response to cold is physiologic, and vasoconstriction sufficient to produce digital pallor or cyanosis may occur in healthy persons, given a prolonged or severe-enough cold exposure. Individuals with Raynaud's phenomenon, irrespective of the cause, have undue intolerance to environmental cold. No single pathophysiologic mechanism adequately explains cold-induced vasospasm in all forms of the syndrome, and, in fact, there is no single form of Raynaud's phenomenon for which the pathophysiology is entirely understood.[74] Sufficient information is available to classify Raynaud's phenomenon according to reasonable estimations regarding the predominant pathophysiologic abnormality (Table 79–4).

Although structural features perforce govern consideration of the mechanism of Raynaud's phenomenon in systemic sclerosis, other factors doubtless are participatory. Platelet activation in vivo[35] is associated with the local release of substances that exert powerful local effects on vascular smooth muscle tone. Potentially important are unstable products of arachidonic acid metabolism, such as thromboxane A_2, and stable constituents of the platelet dense granule, principally serotonin. Whereas unaggregated platelets do not cause contraction of human digital artery muscle strips, the addition of platelets after induced aggregation causes brisk contraction of these preparations.[75] Of probable relevance is the observation that cooling to 24°C augments the platelet-induced vasoconstrictive response.[76] The status of the endothelium is felt to have important influences on arterial smooth muscle responses to serotonin and thromboxane. Endothelial release of prostacyclin and endothelial monoamine oxidase activity in the catabolism of serotonin represent the opposing vasodilatory influences. Ketanserin, an experimental S_2-serotonergic antagonist, improves digital artery perfusion across a broad range of temperatures in both short-term oral and intravenous usage in patients with systemic sclerosis,[77] suggesting a continual level of in vivo

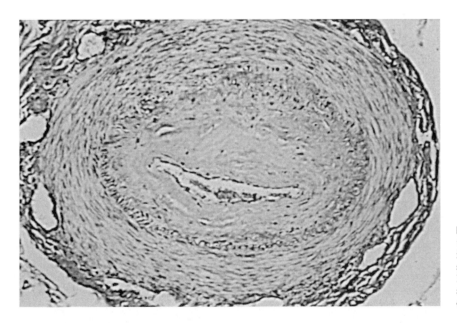

FIGURE 79–9 · Photomicrograph of a digital artery in cross-section obtained post mortem from a patient with long-standing systemic sclerosis. The intima shows dramatic collagenous hyperplasia with a 90-percent reduction of the arterial lumen. Medial changes are inconspicuous, but the adventitia is mildly fibrosed.

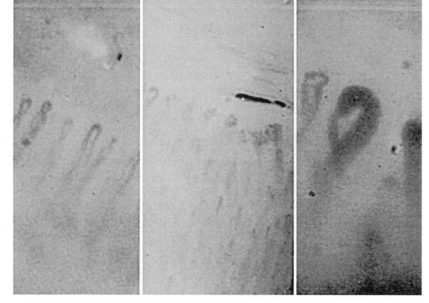

FIGURE 79–10 · Nail Fold Capillary Loop Photography. On the left are the delicate and symmetric hairpin loops of normal nail fold circulation. The center photograph reveals tortuosity and redundancy of multiple capillary loops and might be encountered in both systemic sclerosis and other connective tissue disorders. The right photograph reveals change and disease-specific changes of systemic sclerosis, including a paucity of capillary loops and a single loop with gross dilatation of both the venular and arteriolar limbs. (Reproduced from Dieppe PA, et al: Scleroderma, dermatomyositis and polymyositis. Slide Atlas of Rheumatology. London, Gower Medical, 1986.)

TABLE 79–4 · MECHANISTIC CLASSIFICATION OF RAYNAUD'S PHENOMENON

Vasospastic
Primary Raynaud's phenomenon (Raynaud's disease)
Drug induced
  Ergot
  Methysergide
  β-Adrenergic blockers
Pheochromocytoma
Carcinoid syndrome
Primary with other vasospastic syndromes (migraine, variant angina)
Structural
Large and medium arteries
  Thoracic outlet syndrome
  Crutch pressure
  Brachiocephalic trunk disease (Takayasu's, atherosclerosis)
Small artery and arteriolar
  Vibration disease
  Arteriosclerosis and thromboangiitis obliterans
  Cold injury (frostbite, pernio)
  Polyvinyl chloride disease
  Chemotherapy (bleomycin, vinblastine)
  Connective tissue disease
    Systemic sclerosis
    Systemic lupus erythematosus (SLE)
    Inflammatory myopathy (dermatomyositis → polymyositis)
    Overlap syndromes
Hemorrheologic
Cryoglobulinemia
Cryofibrinogenemia
Paraproteinemia and hyperviscosity syndromes
Cold agglutinin disease
Polycythemia (essential thrombocythemia, polycythemia vera)

serotonergic tone. The antiplatelet effects of calcium channel blockers such as nifedipine may be partially responsible for their favorable effects in the treatment of Raynaud's phenomenon complicating systemic sclerosis. Iloprost, an experimental stable prostacyclin, has been shown to improve cold tolerance, lessen Raynaud's phenomenon, and facilitate the healing of ischemic digital ulcers in patients with systemic sclerosis.[78] Individuals with primary Raynaud's phenomenon do not have evidence of in vivo platelet activation.[35]

Adrenergic influences in the Raynaud's phenomenon of systemic sclerosis may be of fundamental importance.[79] The α-adrenergic receptor response is a key clinical determinant of perfusion in primary Raynaud's phenomenon.[80] Ex vivo responsiveness to α_2-receptor agonists by skin arterioles from patients with scleroderma is increased.[81] There is histopathologic evidence of destructive changes in the peripheral sympathetic ganglia, and physiologic evidence of reduced electric resistance of skin in systemic sclerosis.[74] Dysautonomia and peripheral nerve dysfunction are frequent in scleroderma.[79]

INTERNAL ORGANS IN RAYNAUD'S PHENOMENON

Fibrotic arteriosclerotic changes of the small artery and arteriole are present in the internal organs of patients with systemic sclerosis[71,72] and have clinical and functional significance. This has been long suspected from clinical observations such as the increased incidence of scleroderma renal crisis during cold weather months and is now supported by a variety of modern clinical physiologic investigations (Table 79–5).

Myocardial involvement from systemic sclerosis has been particularly well studied in this regard. Intermittent ischemia is suggested by histopathologic study, revealing myocardial contraction band necrosis.[82] Clinical physiologic studies have supported this notion, including the demonstrations of a high prevalence of both fixed and reversible thallium perfusion abnormalities in individuals with diffuse scleroderma[83] and a comparable prevalence of fixed perfusion defects in patients with limited skin involvement.[84] Thallium perfusion abnormalities have been demonstrated to improve in response to nifedipine therapy, as has myocardial perfusion and

TABLE 79–5 · EVIDENCE OF REVERSIBLE COLD-INDUCED PERFUSION CHANGES IN THE INTERNAL ORGANS IN SYSTEMIC SCLEROSIS

Myocardial

Fixed and reversible thallium perfusion defects in diffuse scleroderma
Fixed thallium perfusion defects in limited scleroderma (formerly known as CREST syndrome)
Reversible thallium perfusion defects with nifedipine and dipyridamole
Transient regional wall motion abnormalities by echocardiography
Transient left ventricular dysfunction by gated ventriculoscintigraphy

Pulmonary

Transient perfusion changes by [81]M krypton scanning
Attenuated rise in diffusing capacity during cold challenge
Transient elevation in pulmonary artery pressure

Renal

Transient elevation of plasma renin activity
Transient reduction in renal cortical perfusion by xenon washout

Abbreviations: CREST syndrome, C, calcinosis; R, Raynaud's phenomenon; E, esophageal dysmotility; S, sclerodactyly; T, telangiectases.

metabolic function by positron-emission tomography.[85] Transient regional wall motion abnormalities have been demonstrated to occur during cold challenge by both echocardiographic[86] and scintigraphic[87] techniques, suggesting a Raynaud-like reactivity of the coronary microvasculature.

It is perhaps not entirely correct to term these transient changes in visceral perfusion Raynaud's phenomenon, because the phases of cyanosis and of reactive erythema have not been successfully demonstrated. In fact, some of the "cold-induced" perfusion abnormalities of systemic sclerosis may simply reflect the behavior of hypocompliant, structurally fixed vasculature. For example, the increase in pulmonary diffusing capacity seen in healthy persons during cold exposure is lacking in patients with systemic sclerosis. However, similar findings are noted with the assumption of a recumbent posture (another maneuver that increases central venous volume and an elevation of the diffusing capacity), suggesting an inability of a fibrosed pulmonary vasculature to accommodate increased venous return rather than cold-induced vasospasm. However, other sensitive techniques such as [81]M krypton lung scanning have demonstrated transient cold-induced perfusion decreases in approximately half of patients.[88]

MICROVASCULAR ABNORMALITIES

Concomitant with, and possibly antedating, the arteriolar abnormalities are characteristic architectural abnormalities of the microvasculature[10] (see Fig. 79–10) that are easily appreciated by wide-field microscopy of the nail fold capillary bed.[89] The changes of systemic sclerosis include enlargement and tortuosity of individual capillary loops, interspersed with areas of capillary loop

dropout.[89] The mechanism of the capillary loop injury remains unresolved. Tissue pressure in the proximal digit is known to exceed that of the capillary bed; thus, it is possible that hydrostatic effects contribute to capillary "varicosity."

Ultrastructural study has demonstrated a loss of endothelium and associated basement membrane thickening and reduplication in systemic sclerosis.[71,90] The finding of increased plasma von Willebrand's factor activity, factor VIII–von Willebrand's factor antigen,[91] tissue plasminogen activator, and endothelin-1[92] in patients with systemic sclerosis suggests that in vivo endothelial cell injury is ongoing. The factor or factors responsible for the initiation and perpetuation of endothelial injury are unknown. Circulating immune complexes are present in many patients,[93] but immunohistologic evidence for tissue deposition of these is lacking. Sparse deposits of antibody have been noted in areas of serum protein exudate in biopsies of the nail fold capillary bed.[94]

The initial lesion of vascular injury, by whatever mechanism, can be seen as perpetuating a variety of local tissue responses important among which is platelet activation and the attendant release of PDGF[85,86] and vasoconstrictive substances. Exposure of subendothelial matrix constituents may induce an "amplification loop" of immunologically mediated vascular injury, including the development of circulating antibodies to type IV collagen[95] and antibody-dependent endothelial injury.[96] T lymphoctyes from patients with systemic sclerosis both proliferate[97] and express interleukin-2 (IL-2) receptor (CD25 positivity)[98] on exposure to subendothelial laminin. Adhesion molecule expression is increased, as well as endothelial pleiotropic chemokines[79,99]

Immunologic Features

Systemic sclerosis is known to occur in overlap with other connective tissue disorders, most commonly SLE and polymyositis, but also RA, Sjögren's syndrome, and organ-specific autoimmune disorders such as Hashimoto's thyroiditis and primary biliary cirrhosis. More frequently, patients with systemic sclerosis present with clinical features and laboratory abnormalities reminiscent of a specific concomitant disorder but insufficient to sustain a second diagnosis.

NONSPECIFIC SEROLOGIC ABNORMALITIES

Antinuclear antibodies are present in the sera of more than 90 percent of patients with systemic sclerosis and most typically include patterns of homogeneous, speckled, and nucleolar immunofluorescent staining when sought on fixed-tissue substrates. With few exceptions, these antinuclear antibodies are not complement fixing and persist after antigen denaturation with ribonuclease and deoxyribonuclease. Similarly, by direct testing, antibody to native DNA is either lacking or present in extremely low titer. As a rule, patients with systemic sclerosis lack anti-Sm antibody,[100] and only about 20 percent have antibody directed against nuclear ribonucleoprotein (anti-nRNP).[101] There are no consistent clinical associations of any of these serologic features. Around 30 percent of patients have serum rheumatoid factor (RF), and serum cryoglobulins are detectable in low concentration in as many as 50 percent. Anticardiolipin antibodies are either lacking (immunoglobulin G [IgG]) or present in low titer (IgM).

Serum immune complexes have been found in systemic sclerosis. Although their significance remains speculative, the presence of immune complexes has been correlated with cardiopulmonary involvement,[88,102] the overall severity of disease, and other evidence of serologic abnormality.[102] Additional laboratory features include polyclonal hypergammaglobulinemia and other evidence of acute-phase response.

ANTICENTROMERE ANTIBODIES

When tissue culture substrates for indirect immunofluorescent study, most notably the human laryngeal carcinoma cell line HEp-2, are used, anticentromere antibodies give rise to coarse, speckled patterns on interphase nuclei and appear as centromeric clustering on metaphase nuclei. The original reports suggested that between 50 and 96 percent of patients with limited systemic sclerosis had detectable serum anticentromere antibody.[32,103] In contrast, anticentromere antibody is found in less than 10 percent of individuals with diffuse scleroderma and is infrequent in other nonsystemic sclerosis connective tissue diseases. Inasmuch as its presence parallels that of limited systemic sclerosis, serum anticentromere antibody confers a favorable prognosis[103,104] and is a useful tool in the assessment and classification of patients with early systemic sclerosis. In comparisons of patients with clinical diagnoses of limited scleroderma, those with serum anticentromere antibody were more likely to have telangiectasias and calcinosis and less likely to have restrictive lung disease than those lacking anticentromere antibody.[105] Retrospective analysis of banked sera suggests that anticentromere titers do not change with time or the course of disease. The presence of serum anticentromere antibody is of great value in the recognition of limited scleroderma at the stage of Raynaud's phenomenon only.[32,106] The origin and biologic role of anticentromere antibody remains unclear.

ANTI–DNA TOPOISOMERASE I

Between 20 and 40 percent of patients classified as having systemic sclerosis have serum antibody reactive with an extractable nuclear antigen of 70 kD termed Scl-70.[107] The antigen has been definitely characterized as DNA topoisomerase I, an intracellular enzyme involved in the initial uncoiling of supercoiled DNA before transcription and present at both centromeric and other intracellular locations.[108] Anti–topoisomerase I antibodies inhibit the function of the enzyme and may modulate collagen production in systemic sclerosis.[109] There are data to suggest that Scl-70 is a fragment of protease degradation of a 96-kD topoisomerase[110] and similarly of an 86-kD antigen,[111] both of which have kinetochore localization and DNA topoisomerase function.

Antigenicity to DNA topoisomerase I has been isolated to an 11–amino acid sequence that contains six sequential amino acids similar to a sequence present in the group-specific p30^{gag} of mammalian retrovirus.[112] Serum antibody to retroviral p24^{gag} is present in 25 percent of patients with diffuse scleroderma but is unrelated to the presence of anti–DNA topoisomerase I.[113] Others have identified at least two independent antigenic epitopes of DNA topoisomerase I unrelated to the region of retroviral homology.[114] It remains possible that antibody elicited by previous or persistent retrovirus infection cross-reacts with intracellular topoisomerase. A retroviral cause of disease would be consistent with the sporadic occurrence, variable latency, and broad spectrum of disease expression that typifies systemic sclerosis.

Those patients with diffuse scleroderma who lack anti–topoisomerase antibody reactivity frequently have antibody to either RNA polymerase I or RNA polymerase III.[115]

The specific autoantibodies of systemic sclerosis are mutually exclusive.[116] Cell injury in conditions of hypoxemia reperfusion leads to selective release of scleroderma-specific antigen.[117]

ABNORMALITIES OF CELLULAR IMMUNITY

Lymphocyte infiltration of the lower dermis occurs early in systemic sclerosis (see Fig. 79–8) and consists largely of T lymphocytes, typically expressing surface markers of helper T cell phenotype.[47,118] Mononuclear cell infiltration has been correlated with the severity of local skin thickening[118] and is most frequent at the early stages of disease. Because a variety of studies have suggested that lymphokines and monokines may stimulate collagen accumulation by fibroblasts[50] (see Table 79–1), it is likely that these immigrant inflammatory cells are important participants in the evolution of disease.

Although total peripheral lymphocyte counts are typically normal or slightly reduced in untreated systemic sclerosis, analysis of T lymphocyte subpopulations has noted a relatively increased proportion of cell determinant (CD)4+ (helper T) cells due mainly to an absolute reduction in CD8+ (suppressor T) cells.[98,119,120] Within the CD4+ subpopulation, the percentage of CD4/4B4+ cells (inducers of help) is lowered, whereas the CD4/2H4+ cells (inducers of suppression) are increased.[98] Soluble plasma levels of the CD8 molecule are elevated, suggesting increased turnover or activation of the CD8+ population.[98]

Serum or plasma levels of soluble IL-2 receptors are increased in patients with systemic sclerosis[121,122] and correlate with the severity, progression of, and mortality from the disease. The proportion of T lymphocytes expressing IL-2 receptors (CD25+) is slightly increased in systemic sclerosis.[98] Exposure to mitogen (phytohemagglutinin and concanavalin A) stimulates CD25+ expression comparable to that of lymphocytes from healthy persons.[98]

IL-1 production by peripheral blood mononuclear cells is diminished in systemic sclerosis.[123,124] Elevated levels of serum IL-2, by both immunoreactive and biologic assay, have been reported and are correlated with the extent of skin involvement and disease activity.[125] There are reports of inconsistent elevations of IL-4, IL-6, and TNF levels.[126]

Preliminary studies reveal the use of a restricted T cell receptor repertoire in the advancing skin lesion of patients with systemic sclerosis.[127] These findings are similar to those of the involved skin of the Tsk-2 murine model of scleroderma.[128] Studies of CD8+ lymphocytes obtained by bronchoalveolar lavage from patients with alveolitis reveal oligoclonal dominance within each subject.[129]

There is, thus, ample evidence of T lymphocyte activation and turnover from early stages of systemic sclerosis. Whether this process is antigen driven or is attributable to a specific cytokine effect or to an unidentified cytokine inhibitor is unclear. Although the macrophage-activating effects of IFN-γ have been discussed previously, additional information links platelet-derived autacoids, including serotonin, via the S_2-serotonergic receptor to macrophage activation in scleroderma[130] or via the effects of TGF-β.[50,63] Clinically, patients with systemic sclerosis are not prone to opportunistic or even an increased incidence of infection, and cutaneous delayed hypersensitivity is normal.

A Theory of Pathogenesis

EXPERIMENTAL MODELS

Convincing animal models of systemic sclerosis have been lacking. The Tsk mouse develops thickened and adherent skin due to collagen and glycosaminoglycan accumulation in the dermis.[131,132] Elegant experiments have identified the fibrillin gene as the mutant locus of the disease.[132] Chronic graft-versus-host disease in BALB/c mice,[62] another animal model, is characterized by dermal fibrosis in the setting of mononuclear cell infiltrate.[133] The predictability of these models of dermal fibrosis is seen as providing a mechanism for the screening of potential therapies of systemic sclerosis.

The "scleroderma chicken" phenotype is an inherited fibrotic disorder of White Leghorn chickens characterized by dermal and esophageal fibrosis and diffuse occlusive change of small- and medium-sized arteries.[134] Although the blood vessel changes are largely in the media as opposed to the intimal disruption of human systemic sclerosis, in the presence of diverse autoantibody formation and evidence of T cell infiltration in affected tissues,[134,135] the arthritis, peripheral vascular insufficiency (digital and comb necrosis), and extensive visceral involvement offer many parallels with human disease.

HUMAN MODELS—FETAL MICROCHIMERISM

Although uncommon, human graft-versus-host disease is associated with scleroderma-like skin thickening, sicca syndrome, and interstitial lung disease.[136] A "graft-versus-host" mechanism for idiopathic scleroderma has been proposed. Individuals with systemic sclerosis are more likely to have evidence of persistent fetal cells in their peripheral circulation,[137] as well as higher numbers of such cells than controls.[138] Evidence of fetal microchimerism extends to the demonstration of persistent fetal cells in the involved skin of patients with systemic sclerosis.[139]

PATHOGENIC INTERRELATIONSHIPS

In general, hypotheses about the pathogenesis of systemic sclerosis can be segregated by their emphasis on vascular, immunologic, and collagen abnormalities. As discussed earlier, virtually all the available evidence suggests that the accumulation of collagen and other matrix constituents is a secondary process. The principal research questions posed revolve around the determination of which of the various cytokines and growth factors have biologic relevance in systemic sclerosis and by what mechanism they operate. It is fair to emphasize that the dermal fibrosis from which the disorder is named is the least consistent clinical feature of disease. Sclerodermatous skin change is limited in approximately half of patients to the fingers, hands, and face and is either absent or trivial in systemic sclerosis sine scleroderma and in undifferentiated connective tissue disease. Furthermore, the fibrotic change of visceral tissues is inconsistent, and in many cases its contribution to organ dysfunction is difficult to differentiate from that of vascular and inflammatory change. Last, there is evidence that even in diffuse scleroderma, progressive fibrosis of skin is typical only of the early stages of disease.

As an intellectual strategy in a disease so complex as systemic sclerosis, it would seem appropriate to address the abnormalities present at the first recognizable stages of illness, and this typically directs attention to the clinical presentation of Raynaud's phenomenon. However, clinical investigations of such patients have revealed that immunologic features,[32] abnormalities of microvascular architecture and endothelial integrity,[10,31,33,35] and abnormalities of arteriolar structure and function are well established at this earliest stage of disease. The issues of pathogenesis become paradigms of "the chicken versus the egg" and would include the inability to elucidate whether platelet activation in systemic sclerosis is a primary or secondary event to vascular injury and the inability to recognize whether the specific immunologic features are fundamental to pathogenesis or merely epiphenomena of chronic tissue injury. The demonstration of specific scleroderma-associated antigen release in conditions of hypoxemia or reperfusion hints that the initial injury is vascular.[117] There is no known "prescleroderma" clinical syndrome, and the absence of convincing kindreds of scleroderma has made the investigation of potential host factors difficult. If there is a principal exogenous agent that triggers the disease in the susceptible individual, the absence of geographic and seasonal clusters of case outbreaks has rendered its identification problematic.

Figure 79–11 illustrates one attempt to link the various descriptive abnormalities of systemic sclerosis.

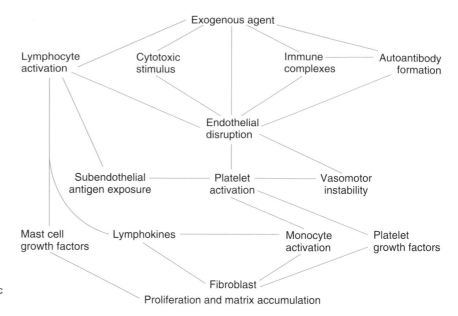

FIGURE 79-11 · Potential Pathogenic Interrelationships in Systemic Sclerosis.

Although there is reason or evidence, or both, to implicate each and all of these various possibilities in the development and expression of disease, their relative importance and order of occurrence remain entirely speculative. For the clinician and researcher considering the heterogeneity of patterns of disease, prioritization of pathogenic influences becomes even more problematic. The differences in diffuse versus limited classifications of systemic sclerosis could be seen as a feature of the magnitude and duration of tissue insult and response; they could represent entirely different causes of disease with a common response; or they could represent the same cause with host factors influencing the presence and degree of any particular aspect of response.

▉ Clinical Features

The individual with systemic sclerosis is confronted with a wide array of symptoms and difficulties, ranging from complaints attributable to specific internal organ involvement to the protean manifestations of chronic catabolic illness. Fever, even low grade, is uncommon in systemic sclerosis and should prompt a search for an alternative cause. Malaise and ease of fatigue are virtually universal complaints, as is weight loss, even in the absence of gastrointestinal involvement. Many patients suffer waxing and waning of systemic symptoms in a pattern reminiscent of that of SLE or RA. Reactive depression is common, and diminished self esteem and concern over cosmetic features of scleroderma can dominate the patient's sense of well-being. Systemic sclerosis is uncommon enough that many patients have neither met another with the illness nor heard of the disease until diagnosed. The burden on the psyche is made greater by the lack of understanding of cause and by the absence of consistently effective treatments.

MUSCULOSKELETAL FEATURES

Generalized arthralgia and morning stiffness are typical symptoms of systemic sclerosis and may be confused with early RA. Clinically appreciable joint inflammation is uncommon, although erosive arthropathy has been demonstrated to occur in some series in as many as 29 percent of patients.[140] An inexorable loss of hand function is the rule as skin thickening worsens and the underlying joints become tethered and restricted in motion. Inflammatory and fibrinous involvement of tendon sheaths may mimic arthritis. Leathery tendon friction rubs are appreciated by palpation during active or passive motion of involved areas and on rare occasions are audible. Although most typically manifest over the wrists, ankles, and knees, an occurrence in the subscapular bursae may mimic the auscultatory findings of pleural friction rubs, and deep involvement surrounding the hip girdle may cause anterior thigh pain on weight-bearing and suggest possible aseptic necrosis of the hip.

Insidious muscle weakness, both proximal and distal, occurs in many patients with systemic sclerosis secondary to disuse atrophy. In other patients, there is also ample evidence of a primary myopathy characterized by mild proximal muscle weakness and mild elevations of levels of serum muscle enzymes, including aldolase and creatine phosphokinase.[141,142] Electromyographic abnormalities are typical and include increased polyphasic potentials of normal and decreased amplitude and duration but without the insertional irritability and fibrillation that are hallmarks of polymyositis and dermatomyositis. Muscle biopsy reveals interstitial fibrosis and fiber atrophy with less conspicuous evidence of inflammatory cell infiltration and muscle fiber degeneration.[141,142] An indolent clinical course characterized by waxing and waning of symptoms and laboratory features, generally unresponsive to glucocorticoid therapy, serves further to differentiate the simple myopathy of systemic sclerosis from inflammatory myositis occurring in overlap.

Although seldom a source of clinical complaints, osteopenia is common in systemic sclerosis and is related to impaired intestinal absorptive function, disuse, and diminished perfusion. Resorption and dissolution of the digital tufts (acro-osteolysis) (Fig. 79–12) occurs in long-standing disease and is best explained by chronic digital ischemia.

Subcutaneous calcinosis occurs in approximately 40 percent of patients with long-standing limited scleroderma and less frequently in diffuse disease. The most characteristic locations include the fingers (see Fig. 79–12), preolecranon area, olecranon and prepatellar bursae, and the anterior compartment of the lower extremity. Widespread involvement of tendon sheaths may occur, as well as involvement of bizarre and strategically troublesome locations such as the ischial tuberosities, lateral malleoli, and thoracic outlet. These deposits are intermittently inflamed and a source of discomfort, and spontaneous extrusion through the skin with complicating superinfection is a frequent problem. Protein rich in γ-carboxyglutamic acid is increased locally[143] in both the calcinosis of dermatomyositis and that of systemic sclerosis.

GASTROINTESTINAL INVOLVEMENT

Involvement of the gastrointestinal tract is the third most common manifestation of systemic sclerosis, following only sclerodermal skin change and Raynaud's phenomenon. Particularly with reference to esophageal dysmotility, there is no significant difference in prevalence or severity between individuals with generalized and limited scleroderma, and esophageal involvement is a principal feature of systemic sclerosis sine scleroderma.

Impaired function of the lower esophageal sphincter is associated with symptoms of intermittent heartburn, typically described as a retrosternal burning pain, but with frequent radiation into the pharynx and associated with a sour or bitter regurgitation. Disordered peristalsis of the lower two thirds of the esophagus presents as dysphagia and odynophagia for solid foods. Patients frequently complain of a "sticking" sensation of extraordinary reproducibility in location and severity. Although the passage of food can be improved by thorough mastication of smaller quantities taken with liquids, many patients tend to subtly reduce their dietary intake in an attempt to minimize symptoms. The lower esophageal dysmotility also exacerbates the symptoms of reflux by allowing pooling of acid in the esophagus.[144]

Histopathologic study at the late stages of illness has emphasized smooth muscle atrophy with fibrous replacement of the muscularis, fibrosis of the submucosa and lamina propria, and varied degrees of mucosal thinning and erosion.[70] Motility studies of early esophageal involvement have suggested that disordered cholinergic neural function is present in the nutritive vasculature,[145] and capillary alterations of endothelial swelling and basement membrane lamination are typical.[146] It seems likely that impaired perfusion and microvascular disruption contribute to the pathogenesis, first as disordered myoelectric function and later as influences on muscle atrophy and fibrosis.

Esophageal function may be assessed by a variety of techniques including manometrics,[144] thin-barium recumbent cine-esophagraphy (Fig. 79–13), radionuclide transit studies, and esophagoscopy. Although the sensitivities of these modalities of assessment appear comparable, the choice of a functional test should be

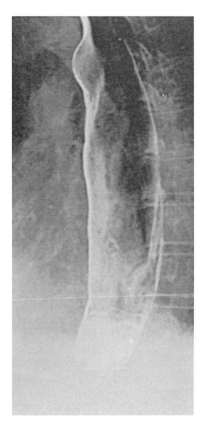

FIGURE 79–13 · Barium esophagram demonstrating dilatation and aperistalsis of the distal esophagus and a patulent lower esophageal sphincter.

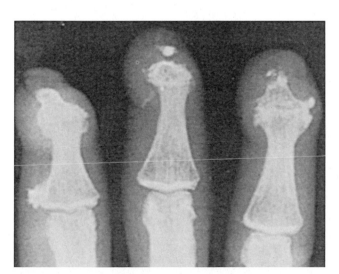

FIGURE 79–12 · Roentgenogram of the fingers revealing resorption and dissolution of the phalangeal tufts and multiple areas of punctate subcutaneous calcinosis.

guided by the specificity of information needed for clinical management. The abnormalities of esophageal function are not unique to systemic sclerosis. It is also clear that there are patients within the spectrum of idiopathic intestinal hypomotility syndromes who share immunologic features of systemic sclerosis, such as serum antinuclear antibody, but in whom a confident diagnosis cannot be sustained.

Complications of chronic esophageal reflux include erosive esophagitis with bleeding, Barrett's esophagus, and lower esophageal stricture,[144,147] which when present further contributes to solid food dysphagia. The presence of lower esophageal dysmotility is the principal influence on the development of erosive esophagitis, which may be present in surprising degree even in the asymptomatic patient. Upper esophageal dysmotility and impaired deglutition occur rarely. In contrast to the situation in polymyositis, aspiration is uncommon in systemic sclerosis[148] but should be suspected if patients present with productive cough or pulmonary infiltrates.

Involvement of the stomach occurs in systemic sclerosis and presents clinically as ease of satiety and on occasion as either functional gastric outlet obstruction or acute gastric dilatation. Gastric antral venous ectasia ("watermelon stomach") is increasingly recognized as a cause of upper gastrointestinal bleeding in scleroderma.[149] Telangiectases of the gastrointestinal tract may rarely be the cause of both upper and lower intestinal bleeding.

Small bowel involvement is one of the most vexing complications of systemic sclerosis and is more likely encountered in patients with long-standing limited scleroderma. Symptoms include intermittent bloating with abdominal cramps, intermittent or chronic diarrhea, and presentations suggestive of intestinal obstruction. Malabsorption occurs in a minority and is most readily detected as impaired D-xylose absorption or as increased quantitative fecal fat elimination. The basic mechanism of small bowel dysfunction is similar to that of the esophagus, where fibrosis and smooth muscle atrophy are noted in either a patchy or a diffuse distribution.[145,147] Bacterial overgrowth in areas of intestinal stasis occurs frequently and is often responsive to empirical courses of broad-spectrum oral antibiotics such as tetracycline, vancomycin, or metronidazole.[147] Jejunal cultures and the bile acid breath test are useful in diagnosis. Pneumatosis cystoides intestinalis may occur and is an ominous clinical sign. Volvulus and perforation are reported rare complications.

Colonic involvement is present in the majority of patients with systemic sclerosis but is infrequently a prominent cause of clinical symptoms. Constipation, obstipation, and pseudo-obstruction may occur and are related to abnormal colonic motility.[147] Wide-mouthed diverticula along the antimesenteric border of the colon occur but are seldom the site of bleeding or of diverticular abscess. Rectal prolapse and fecal incontinence reflect sclerodermal involvement of the anal sphincter.

Primary biliary cirrhosis is well described as occurring in overlap with systemic sclerosis, principally in individuals with long-standing limited disease. In one series, 17 percent of patients whose disease was classified as "primary" biliary cirrhosis had clinical evidence of systemic sclerosis,[150] and anticentromere antibody was detected in 10 of 110 consecutive patients, all of whom had clinical features of systemic sclerosis.[151] The antimitochondrial antibodies of systemic sclerosis most typically react with a DNAse-sensitive antigen rather than the mitochondrial adenosine triphosphatase (ATPase) typical of primary biliary cirrhosis.[152] Hepatic and biliary tract fibrosis are distinctly uncommon.

PULMONARY MANIFESTATIONS

As the ability to manage other complications of systemic sclerosis has improved, pulmonary involvement has emerged as the leading cause of mortality and a principal source of morbidity. No organ illustrates the diversity of pathologic processes operative in scleroderma as much as the lung, in which combinations of vascular obliteration, fibrosis, and inflammation may be present. The clinical onset is frequently insidious, perhaps because of the relative physical inactivity of many patients with systemic sclerosis. Progressive dyspnea on exertion, limited effort tolerance, and a nonproductive cough are typical, whereas chest pain, pleuritic symptoms, and increased sputum are less likely. Physical findings include fine early inspiratory crackling rales in the case of interstitial fibrotic disease or may instead reflect signs of pulmonary hypertension, including an audibly increased and palpable pulmonic component of the second heart sound, right ventricular gallops, murmurs of pulmonic and tricuspid insufficiency, jugular venous distention, hepatojugular reflux, and pedal edema.[73,153]

As a general rule, patients with diffuse scleroderma are at risk for progressive interstitial fibrotic lung disease. Histologic changes of diffuse fibrosis and variable degrees of inflammatory infiltrate are seen in alveoli, interstitium, and the peribronchiolar tissues (Fig. 79–14). Individuals with limited systemic sclerosis may develop interstitial disease but are also at risk for progressive pulmonary hypertension in the absence of interstitial change, a complication most typical of long-standing disease.[73] Autopsy studies have defined the presence of intimal proliferation and medial myxomatous change in the small- to medium-sized pulmonary arteries in 29 to 47 percent of these patients[70,71] (Fig. 79–15). In a prospective clinical study of 49 patients with systemic sclerosis, pulmonary arterial hypertension was detected by right-sided heart catheterization in 33 percent of all patients and in five of the 10 with limited scleroderma.[154]

Chest radiography reveals increased interstitial markings most prominently at the bases but is a relatively insensitive screening test. High-resolution computerized tomography (CT) is a more sensitive test and permits discrimination of fibrosis from interstitial inflammation.[155,156] Pulmonary function testing remains the mainstay of clinical diagnosis and serial functional assessment. Evidence of restriction including reduced vital capacity, diminished compliance, and increased ratios of forced expiratory volume to vital capacity is typical.[157,158] A reduction of diffusing capacity is the most sensitive abnormality and if isolated or dispropor-

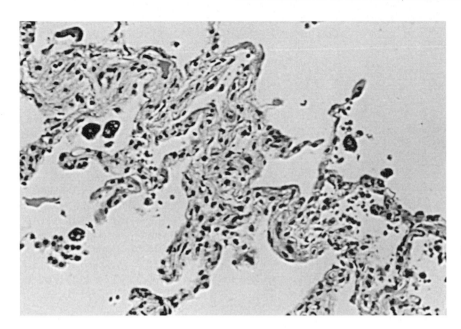

FIGURE 79-14 · Photomicrograph of lung tissue obtained post mortem from a patient with interstitial pulmonary involvement from systemic sclerosis. There is interstitial thickening and fibrosis and continuing evidence of interstitial inflammation.

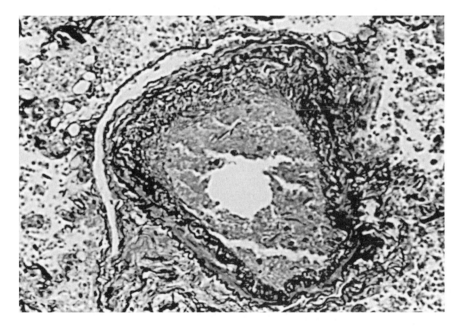

FIGURE 79-15 · Intimal proliferation with reduplication of the internal elastic lamella and medial myxomatous change are seen in this photomicrograph of a pulmonary arteriole obtained post mortem from a patient with long-standing limited scleroderma and severe pulmonary hypertension. The surrounding interstitium is thickened, reveals a mild inflammatory infiltrate, and emphasizes the heterogeneity of pathologic processes operative in scleroderma lung (Verhoeff-van Gieson stain for elastin).

tionately decreased should suggest pulmonary vascular involvement.[159] Most of the studies to date have suggested that pulmonary involvement, once established, is continually progressive and that prevalence increases in parallel with the duration of systemic sclerosis.[157] Occasional patients improve either their measures of volume or their diffusing capacity,[157] although variability in testing or difficulties in the performance of pulmonary function testing such as a diminished oral aperture might be contributory. Isolated reduction in diffusing capacity confers a poor prognosis.[159] Obstructive disease is usually attributed to cigarette smoking. Complications typical of interstitial lung disease, such as spontaneous pneumothorax secondary to cicatricial emphysema, occur only rarely.

Gallium lung scanning has been advocated in the assessment of the inflammatory component but is generally less sensitive than in idiopathic interstitial fibrosis. Bronchoalveolar lavage reveals elevated proportions of neutrophils, lymphocytes, and occasionally eosinophils in the majority of patients,[160] as well as selectively increased concentrations of immune complexes and fibronectin.[161] A consensus has developed that identification of alveolitis or inflammation should guide subsequent therapy.[162]

MYOCARDIAL INVOLVEMENT

Pathologic series have noted patchy myocardial fibrosis in as many as 81 percent of patients with systemic sclerosis.[70] As have large retrospective clinical analyses,[163] these studies have suggested that myocardial involvement is a principal determinant of survival in systemic sclerosis. Clinically, however, myocardial involvement is less confidently detected, and principal presentations are frequently attributed to concomitant lung, pericardial, or renal disease.

As discussed earlier (see Table 79–5), the fibrosis seems inseparable from and may be due to intermittent microvascular ischemia of the myocardium, perhaps mediated by myocardial mast cell infiltrates.[164] Physical findings are nonspecific and include ventricular gallops, sinus tachycardia, signs of congestive heart failure, and occasional pericardial friction rubs. Echocardiography reveals evidence of pericardial thickening or fluid, or both, in about half the patients, but clinical presentations of pericarditis and of tamponade are infrequent.

Resting electrocardiographic abnormalities, including atrial and ventricular arrhythmias and conduction disturbances, are encountered in nearly 50 percent of patients.[165] Ambulatory electrocardiographic features include a high prevalence of both supraventricular and ventricular tachyarrhythmias,[166] with the latter associated strongly with both overall mortality and the syndrome of sudden death.[166] Of the plethora of available techniques of cardiovascular assessment, Holter monitor studies both are sensitive and yield information of potential therapeutic benefit. Patients with limited systemic sclerosis are at only slightly decreased risk of myocardial involvement.[167] Discrimination of the relative roles of heart and lung involvement in the clinical complaints of the individual patient is often difficult.[166,167]

RENAL INVOLVEMENT

The sudden onset of accelerated to malignant hypertension, rapidly progressive renal insufficiency, hyperreninemia, and evidence of microangiopathic hemolysis describes the syndrome of "scleroderma renal crisis."[72,168] The clinical setting is usually an individual with diffuse scleroderma whose disease is at an early stage in which there is rapid progression of skin involvement.[168] The onset is most typically in cold weather months,[168] although exceptions to all these statements are frequent. The predominance of patients with early, diffuse scleroderma contributes substantially to the shortened survival of patients with this classification of disease.

Histopathologic study reveals the typical intimal proliferative lesion of systemic sclerosis (Fig. 79–16) with accompanying evidence of fibrinoid necrosis of the media,[70,72] the latter a nonspecific finding of malignant hypertension. Changes are most conspicuous in the interlobular and arcuate arteries and are in anatomic relation to areas of renal cortical necrosis. Sparse deposits of complement and immunoglobulin are noted in vessel walls, but vasculitis is uncommon.

Patients at risk for the development of scleroderma renal disease cannot be identified by elevations of plasma renin activity,[168] and pathologic evidence of renal vascular disease is present in many patients without clinical renal disease.[70-72] Transient elevations of plasma renin activity and diminished cortical perfusion may be evoked with cold challenge but do not reliably identify impending renal disease. Nonetheless, markedly elevated plasma renin activity is encountered in virtually all patients at the onset of hypertension.[168] Functional vasospasm superimposed on the intimal proliferative lesion is hypothesized to result in sufficient renal cortical hypoperfusion to trigger the release of renin.[169] Ultimately, the vasoconstrictive effects of angiotensin II perpetuate the renal cortical ischemia, and the accelerated hypertension contributes the element of injury to the media, resulting in a fixed and irreversible deprivation of cortical blood flow and necrosis. Diffuse extrarenal vascular injury occurs as well with intimal disruption, fibrin deposition, and microangiopathic hemolysis. Although renal "Raynaud's" is doubtless participatory in many cases, other factors may evoke scleroderma renal crisis

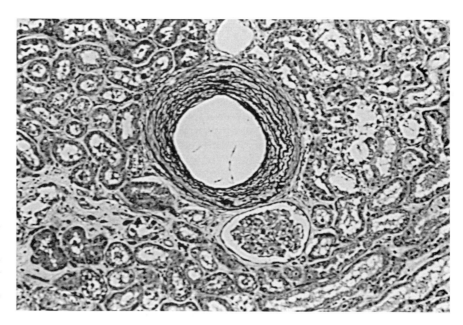

FIGURE 79–16 • Photomicrograph of a small renal artery obtained from a patient with a successfully aborted scleroderma renal crisis. The intimal proliferative changes with reduplication of the internal elastic lamella are characteristic and highly reminiscent of the digital artery changes shown in Figure 79–9 (Verhoeff-van Gieson stain for elastin).

including sudden depletion of intravascular fluid. Normotensive renal failure related to arteriolar thrombosis is associated with previous glucocorticoid therapy.[170]

Profound decreases in the amount of hemoglobin may occur as well as thrombocytopenia. Peripheral blood smears demonstrating fragmented red blood cells can be key to an early diagnosis. Serum fibrinogen levels are usually normal, although frequently decreased from previous values, and fibrin degradation products can be detected. Urinary sediment typically reveals modest amounts of protein and red blood cells, but casts and nephrosis are unusual. Progression to anuric renal failure is the expected outcome if the diagnosis is not promptly established and hypertension controlled.

ENDOCRINE FEATURES

Histologic evidence of thyroid gland fibrosis was found in 14 percent of a series of autopsied patients with scleroderma.[171] Evidence of hypothyroidism, frequently occult, is noted in as many as one fourth of patients and is best detected by abnormal responses to thyrotropin-releasing hormone. Serum antithyroid antibodies, lymphocytic infiltration of the gland, and clinical presentations of acute autoimmune thyroiditis are uncommon. Impotence is described as an early feature of scleroderma[172] and is felt to represent an abnormality of penile vascular function.[173]

EXOCRINE FEATURES

Sicca syndrome occurs in 20 to 30 percent of patients with systemic sclerosis. Fibrosis in the absence of mononuclear cell infiltration is noted on minor salivary gland biopsy.[174] Antibodies to the Sjögren's precipitins (SS-A and SS-B) occur in approximately one half of patients.[175] Clinical presentations include dry eyes and dry mouth, but salivary gland enlargement is uncommon. Dry mouth coupled with the mechanical problems of limited oral aperture and impaired hand function make adequate dental hygiene a formidable task. Pancreatic insufficiency has been reported, but pathologic evidence of pancreatic fibrosis is lacking. Vaginal dryness is a bothersome and common complication.

PREGNANCY

There is little known concerning the effects of scleroderma on pregnancy and vice versa. Irregular menses and amenorrhea occur in severely ill patients, and women with scleroderma frequently have difficulty with conception. Intrauterine growth retardation and low birth weights have been reported.[176] In general, pregnancy does not worsen the scleroderma,[176] although the course of pregnancy is typified by worsened symptoms of reflux esophagitis and by exacerbation of cardiopulmonary symptoms.

NEUROLOGIC MANIFESTATIONS

Systemic sclerosis spares the central nervous system. Entrapment neuropathies that include carpal tunnel syndrome, meralgia paresthetica, trigeminal neuropathy, and facial nerve palsies are well known. Subclinical autonomic dysfunction has been demonstrated,[79,177] and physiologic study has suggested that both gastrointestinal cholinergic and peripheral adrenergic nervous function are impaired. Peripheral sensory deficits are best attributed to concomitant diseases or to adverse effects of therapy.

SCLERODERMA AND MALIGNANCY

The coincidence of malignancy and scleroderma has been described, including the occurrence of lung carcinoma superimposed on long-standing interstitial pulmonary disease.[178] In one series, the relative risk of lung cancer in systemic sclerosis was 16.5.[178] In contrast, a detailed epidemiologic comparison comprising more than 1000 patient-years and an expected seven to eight malignancies found 14 malignancies, mainly pulmonary, and a relative risk of 1.81.[179] Although there was no increase in breast carcinoma, a biologic relationship was suggested by its occurrence in close temporal relationship to the onset of scleroderma.[179] Esophageal carcinoma is so rare that regular surveillance is not thought to be cost effective.

▌ Therapy for Systemic Sclerosis

IMPACT OF CLASSIFICATION AND DURATION

Individuals at the early stages of diffuse scleroderma are most likely to manifest an increasing extent and severity of sclerodermal skin thickening and are at the highest risk of developing new internal organ involvement.[39,40,168] At later stages of diffuse disease, slowly improving skin change is typical.[40,44] Spontaneous regression to clinical features of limited disease occurs, but complete remission is exceedingly rare.[180] In later disease, the risk of developing new visceral involvement is much reduced, although still present, and it should be emphasized that spontaneous improvement in established internal organ dysfunction is most uncommon.

Limited scleroderma is typified by insidious progression of skin involvement; often the skin is unrecognizably changed from year to year. Internal organ involvement including the heart and lungs is known to occur with frequencies close to those of diffuse disease, but the onset of involvement and dysfunction is typically delayed for years. Other than the association of renal disease with diffuse scleroderma and pulmonary hypertension with limited scleroderma, there is little difference between these subgroups at very late stages of disease. Patients with chronic diffuse and limited scleroderma who are matched for sex, age, and disease duration differ only in terms of the frequency of skeletal muscle involvement and, by definition, extent of scleroderma.[181]

Although vast gaps remain in our understanding of the natural history of systemic sclerosis, it would seem apparent that the syndrome is clinically divergent at early stages and clinically convergent late in the disease course. Assuming that truly remittive or effective drug therapy were available, the goals of treatment in any given subgroup would be somewhat different. For example, an agent of potential effectiveness in the prevention of new skin involvement would be most appropriately employed and most easily assessed in patients with early diffuse disease.[44] Given the slowness of collagen turnover, improvement from the baseline might not be detected for 1 to 3 years. However, the benefit over that of a placebo in attenuating new skin involvement would be more easily demonstrated. It should also be emphasized that the clinical progression of skin involvement in early diffuse disease is somewhat variable. Many patients can have prolonged periods of months or more in which skin thickening appears unchanged. Others can seem to improve rapidly, although this likely represents waxing and waning of skin edema rather than changes in dermal collagen accumulation. In later years of diffuse disease, placebo-treated patients would be predicted to somewhat improve in the extent and severity of skin involvement. Thus, the potential therapeutic effect of a drug would be obscured and a larger number of patients would need be studied and for prolonged periods of time. Agents chosen to affect skin involvement would not be applicable to patients with limited scleroderma.

Parallel arguments apply to a consideration of therapeutic agents for visceral involvement. Individuals with early diffuse disease could be seen as the subgroup in which a therapeutic benefit would be most easily demonstrable if the goal of therapy were the prevention of new internal organ involvement. A study of therapies directed toward the reversal of preexisting internal organ dysfunction would require the unlikely effect of visceral tissue remodeling. Irrespective of which elements of pathogenesis were approached and with which modality, including antifibrotic agents, immunomodulators, or therapies directed against vascular features of systemic sclerosis, a clinical benefit would be difficult to prove.

Therapeutic studies of systemic sclerosis can easily be criticized for a lack of controls matched for the duration, severity, and classification of disease; inappropriate choices of the duration of the study; unclear therapeutic end points; and a lack of standardization of the measures of outcome. The paradox of adequately designed therapeutic studies of systemic sclerosis is that any trial of less than 1 year's duration is likely to risk a false-negative outcome, whereas any trial of longer than 3 years risks false-positive results.

IMPACT OF DISEASE PROCESS

Systemic sclerosis encompasses a diverse array of pathologic insults, including obliterative vasculopathy, fibrosis, immunologic and inflammatory changes, and "irreversible" tissue atrophy. Table 79–6 outlines principal clinical features of systemic sclerosis according to the dominant pathologic process. Absent some fundamental breakthrough in our understanding of the etiology and pathogenesis of this disease, rational approaches to therapy can be constructed in this context. An immunosuppressant therapy could slow fibrosis in the lung. An

TABLE 79–6 • CLINICAL FEATURES OF SYSTEMIC SCLEROSIS SEGREGATED BY FEATURES OF DISEASE PROCESS

Development and clinical choice of "disease-modifying" therapy requires attention to both the process and the potential outcome

Vascular features	Fibrotic features
Raynaud's phenomenon	Sclerodermal skin thickening
Renal crisis	Interstitial pulmonary disease
Pulmonary hypertension	*Atrophic features*
Inflammatory features	Gastrointestinal involvement
Alveolitis	Ischemic ulcerations
Myositis	Exocrinopathy
Arthritis	Peripheral neuropathy
Tendinitis	

antifibrotic therapy could reduce skin involvement and perhaps stabilize lung function. We currently lack any reasonable therapy to slow or reverse vascular injury, yet organs affected dominantly by scleroderma vasculopathy can be effectively managed; examples of relevant conditions are scleroderma renal crisis and pulmonary hypertension (see later). No therapy should be expected to reverse atrophic features such as a loss of gastrointestinal smooth muscle.[44]

DISEASE-MODIFYING THERAPIES

A truly "disease-modifying" therapy for systemic sclerosis should enhance survival, reduce disability and comorbidity from the disease, or both.[182] Goals of treatment in addition to improved survival might include 1) the prevention of internal organ involvement, 2) the arrest or slowing of deterioration of function in previously involved organs, 3) improvement in the function of previously involved organs (including the skin), or 4) all three of these. Against this definition, there are *no* drug therapies of proven value in the management of systemic sclerosis.[183] Controlled and prospective clinical trials have been performed but with disappointingly uniformly negative results. A variety of trials of one or more agents have claimed to demonstrate clinical benefit but have been, by and large, of inadequate design.[183] This would include retrospective analyses, uncontrolled observational series, and prospective studies that include multiple end points.

Glucocorticoids have no efficacy in slowing the progress of systemic sclerosis. Their usefulness is limited to the management of inflammatory myositis, occurring in overlap with systemic sclerosis, and potentially in inflammatory stages of interstitial lung disease.[160] Short courses of low-dose glucocorticoids have had palliative benefit in the arthralgias and myalgias of early edematous scleroderma and in the management of painful tendinous involvement. High-dose glucocorticoids (30 mg or more of prednisone per day) are linked to the syndrome of normotensive renal failure[170] and other vaso-occlusive complications of this disease. Unconfirmed reports have shown that tamoxifen, the estrogen inhibitor, also binds to TGF-β

receptors and may inhibit the fibrinogenic activity of this cytokine in scleroderma.

Immunosuppressive agents have been relatively well studied. A 3-year controlled trial of chlorambucil that incorporated detailed laboratory assessments of internal organ involvement found no benefit of the drug over a placebo.[184] Azathioprine employed for periods up to 23 months was similarly inefficacious.[185] A 6-month study of 5-fluorouracil failed to demonstrate clinically important change.[186] A pilot study of cyclosporine suggested usefulness for skin involvement although dose-limiting adverse reactions, especially nephrotoxicity, were frequent.[187] In view of the prominent abnormalities of cellular and humoral immune dysfunction present at early stages of systemic sclerosis, immunosuppressive therapy would seem a rational approach to management but one that is unsupported by the published results of trials.

Ketotifen, an antihistamine claimed to also inhibit mast cell degranulation, produced no benefit in skin involvement, pulmonary function, or other clinical parameters in a 6-month controlled trial.[188]

Recombinant IFN-γ has been the subject of three open-label trials in early diffuse disease,[189,190] with data supportive of an effect on skin involvement. Further development of this agent is limited by its apparently deleterious effect on vascular features of scleroderma, including the provocation of renal crisis and worsening of Raynaud's phenomenon.[190]

Photopheresis employs extracorporeal ultraviolet A irradiation to activate 8-methoxypsoralen[191] and is an approved therapy for cutaneous T cell lymphoma. A short-term comparison with D-penicillamine treatment suggested minor benefits, including an improved sense of well-being in pheresed subjects, but an inconsistent and poorly quantified effect on skin involvement. A sham-controlled prospective trial of this cumbersome and expensive therapy was carried out, but not published and did not replicate this effect.

There have been a number of well-designed and well-performed studies directed at the vascular aspects of systemic sclerosis, including the chronic in vivo platelet activation. Vasodilators, including captopril,[192] the S_2-serotonergic antagonist ketanserin,[193] and aspirin with dipyridamole, in a controlled study[194] were not associated with clinical benefit.

A variety of therapies of less-apparent rationale have been attempted, including dimethylsulfoxide, colchicine, N-acetylcysteine, anabolic steroids, griseofulvin, potassium aminobenzoate, minocycline, and others.[183]

Since the 1970s, the most commonly employed agent in systemic sclerosis has been D-penicillamine. In a large retrospective analysis, D-penicillamine, given at high dosage and for prolonged periods was reported to improve skin involvement and to be associated with a lesser incidence of new visceral involvement, notably renal, and improved survival in comparison to a matched group of patients receiving other therapies.[40] Similar outcomes were reported in an uncontrolled prospective study.[195] There are also two retrospective experiences suggesting modest efficacy in established interstitial lung disease.[196,197] Adverse effects occur in approximately 30 percent of patients,[198] and there is

no evidence that D-penicillamine therapy improves vascular and immunologic features of systemic sclerosis. A randomized, controlled prospective trial has been completed comparing 1000 mg/day to 125 mg every other day.[199] No benefit of D-penicillamine could be shown with regard to survival, the behavior of visceral involvement, skin thickening, the quality of life, or the functional status of the patient.[199] D-penicillamine therapy should be abandoned.

Although there are obvious benefits to controlled and prospective trials in systemic sclerosis, the reader should be aware that such trials are expensive, particularly if they incorporate laboratory measures of internal organ status, and the number of patients required is substantial.[44] The relative rarity of systemic sclerosis has not traditionally accorded this disorder a position of priority in privately sponsored therapeutic research.

In spite of these impediments, randomized controlled trials are increasingly the case in scleroderma research. Not-yet-published trials include prospective controlled studies of IFN-α and oral methotrexate, neither of which had benefit. Recombinant human relaxin, a pregnancy-related hormone with antifibrotic effects, has been reported to reduce skin thickening, stabilize pulmonary involvement, and improve patient function in comparison to placebo.[200,201] A large-scale study is in progress. Immunoablation with autologous stem cell transplantation[202] and thalidomide are the subjects of ongoing pilot trials.

Pulmonary arterial hypertension (PAH) is now recognized to be the most important cause of late disease morbidity and mortality in scleroderma. PAH develops as isolated pulmonary vasculopathy in later years in approximately 20 percent of patients with limited scleroderma but also as a contributory component to interstitial lung injury in approximately 20 percent of patients with diffuse scleroderma.[203] Pulmonary hypertension is defined as a mean pulmonary artery pressure (PAP) of more than 25 mmHg at rest or more than 30 mmHg during exercise in patients with no concurrent evidence for left ventricular failure.[204]

The pathophysiology of PAH includes reduced prostacyclin production and increased synthesis of endothelin-1 both as secondary effects of endothelial injury. Endothelin is profibrotic and proinflammatory as well as vasoconstrictive.[205] Therapies with chronic prostacyclin replacement (epoprostenol, treprostinil) are associated with improvement in vascular smooth muscle proliferation.[204,206]

The diagnosis of PAH is not easy. Exertional dyspnea or fatigue is the principal symptom. Noninvasive testing including electrocardiography, echocardiography with Doppler, ventilation/perfusion lung scanning, pulmonary function testing and high resolution CT are the basic screening tests. Right heart catheterization is necessary to confirm the diagnosis[207] (Fig. 79–17).

As for the management of PAH, the largest current killer of patients with scleroderma, there are a substantial number of pharmacologic treatment options. Currently, there are three drugs approved in the United States for the treatment of PAH: continuous intravenous epoprostenol infusion; the prostacyclin analogue treprostinil

PULMONARY DIAGNOSTIC ALGORITHM FOR PATIENTS WITH SCLERODERMA

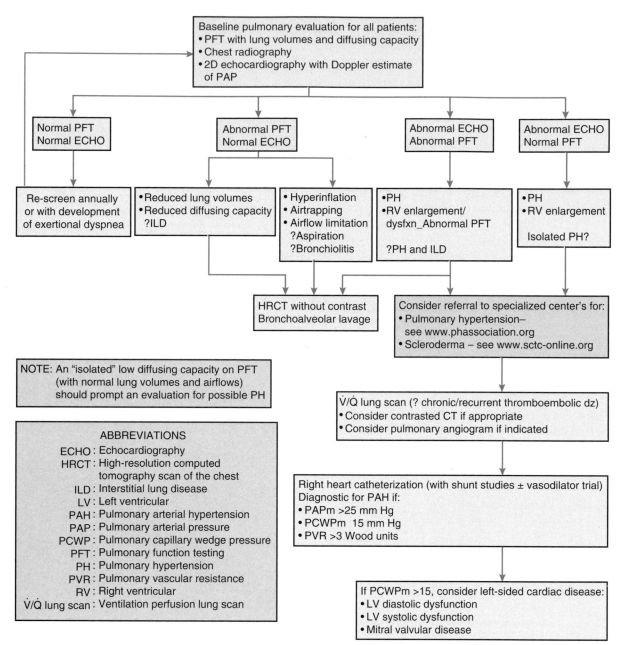

FIGURE 79–17 · Pulmonary Diagnostic Algorithm for Patients with Scleroderma.

administered via continuous subcutaneous infusion; and the orally active, nonpeptide bosentan. Continuous infusion of epoprostenol improves exercise capacity, functional class, hemodynamics, and survival in PAH patients, and there is some evidence that sildenafil can offer additional benefit. It is approved for class III/IV patients, who are those severely limited by their disease. Bosentan (Tracleer), the endothelin receptor (both A and B receptors) antagonist is approved for the same subset of patients. It has liver toxicity, but has proved useful and may be the best avenue of approach for this component of the disease. In a trial that expands the possible efficacy and indications for this drug, a double-blind, randomized, placebo-controlled multicenter study to assess the efficacy,

safety, and tolerability of bosentan in patients with active interstitial lung disease associated with systemic sclerosis (125 mg/placebo bid) is underway.

SUPPORTIVE MEASURES

Much is available in the supportive therapy of the individual patient with systemic sclerosis. Proper clinical management mandates an awareness of the multiplicity of symptoms and the palliative potential of the modern therapeutic armamentarium. All patients benefit from education about their condition. Although the clinician may feel somewhat frustrated by the lack of disease-modifying therapeutic options, attentive and individualized monitoring can help many patients to lead full and productive lives. The management of Raynaud's phenomenon should focus on reduction of both the frequency and the severity of episodes of cold-induced vasospasm and on prevention of digital tip ischemic ulcerations. All patients benefit from cessation of smoking and common-sense lifestyle changes. Dress can be important and, in addition to mittens and warm footwear, should include hats and layered clothing on the trunk so as to minimize the contribution of reflex responses to central body cold stimuli. The choice of drug therapy is a complicated issue in systemic sclerosis, and the response is dominated by the degree of fixed obstructive change in the digital vasculature. Calcium channel blockers including nifedipine, isradipine, amlodipine, diltiazem, and nicardipine are subjectively efficacious in many patients, although the physiologic benefit is less consistently demonstrable.[79,81] The availability of sustained-release preparations of both nifedipine and diltiazem has increased their usefulness by permitting higher dosages with improved tolerance. These agents cause vascular smooth muscle relaxation by interference with the trans-sarcolemmal influx of calcium through membrane channels termed *slow channels*[208] and likely function as antivasoconstrictors rather than as vasodilators. Their clinical use is somewhat limited by their potential to interfere with esophageal motility, and they may, in some patients, actually worsen peripheral vascular resistance by increasing perfusion of the fixed distal vasculature. Prazosin, an orally active selective antagonist of α_1-adrenoceptors, is of occasional benefit.[209] Other therapies, including sympatholytics, biofeedback, and Pavlovian conditioning, are more useful in primary Raynaud's phenomenon. An occasional patient may benefit from sympathectomy and can be chosen by monitoring the short-term response to sympathetic ganglion instillation of bupivacaine.

Digital ischemic ulcerations (Fig. 79–18) require attention to the role of superinfection and consideration of the possible contribution of underlying calcinosis. In addition to agents for peripheral vasodilation, aspirin and dipyridamole are theoretically helpful, although of dubious clinical efficacy, and pentoxifylline may be added for the enhancement of microvascular perfusion. The S_2-serotonergic receptor antagonist ketanserin is unavailable in the United States.[77] Iloprost, an intravenously administered stable prostacyclin analogue, remains investigational but appears efficacious for both the control of Raynaud's phenomenon and the healing of digital tip ulcerations.[78] An orally bioavailable analogue was demonstrated to be ineffective.[210] The ischemically compromised digit is an indication for angiography, which permits localization of the site of vascular occlusion, recognition of embolus, and assessment of the component of reversible vasoconstriction.

Nonsteroidal anti-inflammatory drugs (NSAIDs) are generally useful in the management of arthralgias and myalgia, although occasional patients require low-dosage oral glucocorticoids. Control of musculoskeletal discomfort facilitates effective physical and occupational therapy, which is appropriate for most patients. Although few patients maintain normal hand function,

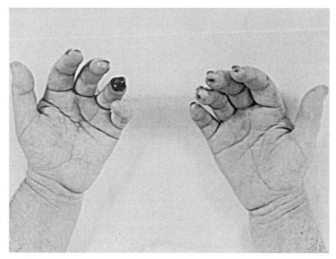

FIGURE 79–18 · Multiple ischemic digital tip ulcerations and a single digit with sharply demarcated dry gangrene in the hands of a woman with long-standing limited scleroderma.

the early institution of a vigorous and sustained physical therapy program can attenuate the effects of the inexorably progressive tethering and atrophy responsible for the loss of function.

Skin care is important and should include moisturizing agents and the prompt treatment of infected ulcerations. There are no current effective therapies for subcutaneous calcinosis. Surgical débridement of strategically located deposits is often necessary, although recurrence is common.

Symptoms of reflux esophagitis are typical of systemic sclerosis but generally amenable to therapy.[147] Patients should be encouraged to avoid large meals and tight clothing so as to minimize increased gastric pressure. Reflux can be minimized by the avoidance of postprandial recumbency and by elevation of the head of the bed. Type 2 histamine receptor blockade with cimetidine, ranitidine, famotidine, or nizatidine supplemented with antacid is generally useful, as is mucosal protection with sucralfate administered postprandially. Omeprazole and lansoprazole, inhibitors of gastric acid secretion due to inhibition of the H^+,K^+-ATPase proton pump of the parietal cell, are remarkably effective in palliation of pyrosis but are limited by expense. Long-term safety and efficacy have been demonstrated.[211] Dysphagia can be minimized by careful mastication of small quantities of food. Occasional patients benefit clinically from the esophageal motility–enhancing effects of metoclopramide or cisapride.[147,212] Refractory dysphagia should suggest lower esophageal stricture and the need for mechanic dilation. Symptoms of small bowel involvement may respond to broad-spectrum antibiotics and occasionally to dietary lactose restriction. Constipation is best managed with agents that soften and increase the bulk of stool.

Although myocardial perfusion abnormalities have been demonstrated to improve in response to nifedipine and dipyridamole, evidence of clinical efficacy is lacking.[84,85] Symptomatic pericarditis responds to both NSAIDs and glucocorticoids. Although cardiac dysrhythmias are felt to have important prognostic value, studies demonstrating enhanced survival by treatment of the arrhythmias are lacking.

Pulmonary involvement has been considered not consistently amenable to therapy. A patient in whom there was evidence of pulmonary interstitial inflammation might be treated with glucocorticoids and immunosuppressive agents in the hope of arresting the development of interstitial fibrosis.[162] Two trials of oral cyclophosphamide in both active disease of moderate severity[213] and in earlier, milder disease[214] have suggested effectiveness in either halting progression, reversing pulmonary function abnormalities, or both. Cyclosporine[187] therapy was associated with stable pulmonary functions over 48 weeks, as was methotrexate in an open pilot trial.[215] Interstitial fibrosis has been treated with D-penicillamine,[196,197] although substantial questions concerning its efficacy remain unanswered.[199]

Pulmonary hypertension has emerged as a principal cause of morbidity and mortality in late systemic sclerosis. Vasodilator therapy with calcium channel blockers[216] is of uncertain clinical benefit and may on occasion lead to paradoxical worsening of pulmonary artery pressure and pulmonary vascular resistance.[153] Centrally infused prostacyclin (epoprostenol) improves both short- and long-term hemodynamics, as well as the quality of life and survival.[217,218] Supplemental oxygen and careful attention to fluid balance are the mainstays of symptomatic management. Selected patients have received single lung transplants as definitive management.

The key to management of scleroderma renal involvement is prompt recognition of the diagnosis and aggressive treatment of the accompanying accelerated hypertension. Patients at high risk, namely, early generalized scleroderma, should be taught ambulatory self-monitoring of blood pressure. Previously refractory to all but the most desperate therapies, such as bilateral nephrectomy, a variety of modern and effective antihypertensive agents have revolutionized the clinical management. Angiotensin-converting enzyme inhibitors such as captopril and enalapril are mechanistically suited to the hyperreninemic hypertension of scleroderma renal crisis and are the treatment of choice.[168,169,193] Successful control of hypertension and arrest of progressive renal insufficiency have also been reported with minoxidil, α-methyldopa, and other agents. If blood pressure is controlled before the serum creatinine level rises to 4 mg/dl, arrest of renal insufficiency and occasional improvement of renal function result.[219] Peritoneal dialysis is the modality of choice for the management of uremia and facilitates the option for renal transplantation. Although there are reports of regression of sclerodermal skin thickening after successful medical management of sclerodermal renal crisis, this is uncommon and in part likely due to the spontaneous improvement typical of later stages of diffuse scleroderma.

▌ Localized Scleroderma

Localized scleroderma is the term employed to describe a variety of conditions of clinical and histopathologic similarity to the skin manifestations of systemic sclerosis but in which the characteristic internal organ and vascular features are lacking.[220]

LINEAR SCLERODERMA

Linear scleroderma is an uncommon disorder of unknown cause characterized by a band of sclerotic induration and hyperpigmentation occurring on a single extremity or on the face. Although the onset may occur at any age, linear scleroderma is most typically encountered in children and young adults. Women are affected approximately three times as often as men, and the condition is uncommon in blacks. The onset is heralded by a frequently asymptomatic band of erythema followed by rapid evolution of induration and thickening of skin with tethering to deeper tissues. The original lesion frequently extends insidiously to involve the entire length of the affected extremity, and satellite lesions of morphea (see later) are common. Irregular atrophy of underlying subcutaneous fat is typical, and extension to underlying muscle and bone (melorheostosis) may occur. In the adult, the principal functional impact is contracture of underlying joints. Involvement of the face (coup de sabre) in children (Fig. 79–19) is associated with asymmetric growth and progressive facial disfigurement. Linear scleroderma of an extremity in childhood leads to substantial muscle atrophy and progressive leg length discrepancy (Fig. 79–20).

Peripheral blood eosinophilia and polyclonal hypergammaglobulinemia are present in many patients at clinically active stages of disease,[221] as are antinuclear and anti–single-stranded DNA antibodies. Biopsy of affected skin reveals lower dermal and subcutaneous fibrosis and infiltration with lymphocytes and plasma cells and is essentially indistinguishable from the changes of systemic sclerosis. Augmented accumulation of collagen and glycosaminoglycan is noted in studies of cultured dermal fibroblasts derived from patients with linear scleroderma.

The typical patient has active disease for 2 to 3 years.[222] Involutional atrophic change dominates the later stages

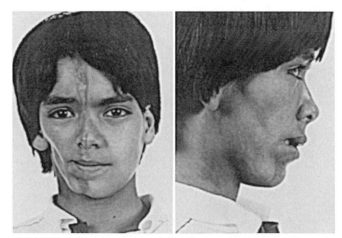

FIGURE 79–19 • Linear Scleroderma of the Face (Coup de Sabre) in a 13-Year-Old Boy with 8 Years of Disease. Atrophy of the subcutaneum and of the mandible are apparent, as is an isolated depression of bone over the forehead. Progressive facial distortion has occurred along with the ongoing asymmetric growth. Reconstructive surgery is planned for early adulthood.

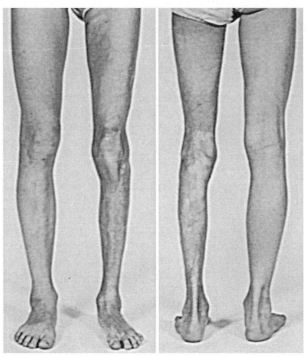

FIGURE 79-20 · Linear Scleroderma of the Left Leg in an 11-year-Old Girl. Diffuse muscle atrophy is apparent. As this patient enters puberty, progressive leg length discrepancy is expected.

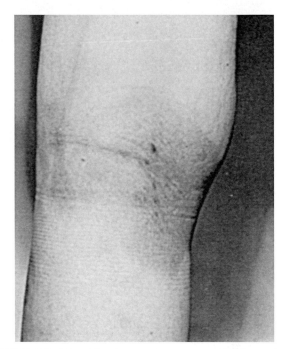

FIGURE 79-21 · Morphea en plaque present for 4 years is seen in the popliteal fossa of this 55-year-old woman. The recent course has been marked by progressive softening of this and other lesions.

of disease. Physical therapy of affected joint groups is useful. D-penicillamine, topical and systemic glucocorticoids, and hydroxychloroquine have been advocated, but convincing evidence of their effectiveness is lacking.[222]

MORPHEA

This variety of localized scleroderma may occur at any site and at any age and is characterized by either small discrete spots (guttate morphea) or by larger patches (morphea en plaque) (Fig. 79-21) of sclerodermatous skin induration. Slowly expanding "target" lesions with an erythematosus or violaceous border and with central hypopigmentation, tethering, and thickening may occur in many locations either simultaneously or as evolving continually over several months or years. Involutional atrophy with persistent pigmentary change, spontaneous improvement, and even total clinical resolution of morphea are typical after periods of several months to several years.[222] The clinical consequences of morphea are principally cosmetic, although contracture of underlying joint groups may occur. Biopsies at early stages of illness reveal an inflammatory infiltrate, felt by some observers to be more intense than that of systemic sclerosis, and fibrosis with the changes principally noted in the lower dermis and upper subcutaneous tissue.

On occasion, morphea can manifest in an extensively generalized distribution and with protean manifestations of catabolic illness including fatigue, weight loss, and inanition. Generalized subcutaneous morphea is a rare entity in which inflammation and fibrosis are centered in the subcutaneous tissue with apparent extension to the lower dermis and occasionally to the subtending fascia.[222] In one well-described series of 16 patients, many had features suggestive of systemic sclerosis including interstitial pulmonary disease, esophageal dysmotility, joint complaints, and serum antinuclear antibodies.[223]

RELATIONSHIP TO SYSTEMIC SCLEROSIS

Individuals with otherwise typical systemic sclerosis may on occasion manifest morphea and linear scleroderma-like skin changes,[222] as may rare patients with SLE and overlap syndromes. As a general rule, the converse occurs so rarely as to confirm a lack of association. The similarities of localized scleroderma to systemic sclerosis are limited to the histopathologic features, the serologic abnormalities, and the shared prevalence in young women.

SCLEREDEMA AND SCLEROMYXEDEMA

Scleredema (scleredema adultorum of Buschke) and scleromyxedema (papular mucinosis, lichen myxedematosus) are clinically similar, but distinct, connective tissue disorders characterized by widespread induration and thickening of the skin resulting from the accumulation of collagen and proteoglycan in the dermis. The skin involvement on the face and neck, which progresses acrally, and the sparing of the fingers and hands, as well as the absence of Raynaud's phenomenon and of visceral involvement, permit clinical differentiation from systemic sclerosis. Histopathologically, both scleredema and scleromyxedema show minimal epidermal changes, whereas the dermis is markedly thickened with variable degrees of proteoglycan, hyaluronic acid, and collagen deposits.[224,225]

The cause and pathogenesis of both diseases are obscure. Around half of adult scleredema patients have diabetes mellitus, and both conditions are associated with underlying plasma cell dyscrasia including multiple myeloma.[226] Sera from patients with scleromyxedema have been shown to stimulate DNA synthesis and cell proliferation of normal human skin fibroblasts in culture, and sera from patients with scleredema stimulate collagen and proteoglycan accumulation by autologous and homologous dermal fibroblast lines.[226] Serologic, internal organ, and vascular features of systemic sclerosis are conspicuously absent, and there are no known effective therapies.

EOSINOPHILIC FASCIITIS

Eosinophilic fasciitis is a scleroderma-like disorder characterized by inflammation and thickening of the deep fascia. Since the original description by Shulman in 1975, several hundred cases have been reported,[222,227,228] and the clinical description is still evolving. Extension to subjacent skeletal muscle may occur, and extension to overlying subcutaneum and lower dermis is common. The onset frequently follows periods of unusual physical exertion and trauma, particularly in males, and the condition has been reported to occur in children and elderly persons, although it is most frequent in young adults. The rapid onset of pain and swelling of the extremities is soon followed by progressive induration of the skin and subcutaneous tissues of the forearms, legs, and, on occasion, hands, feet, and trunk. In many cases, exaggerated deep grooving or "furrowing" of the subcutis surrounding superficial veins is noted (Fig. 79–22) and may be enhanced by an antidependent posture. The overlying skin is typically shiny and erythematous with a coarse "orange peel" appearance. Carpal tunnel syndrome is frequent, and contractures of underlying joints develop early in the course of illness.[228]

Raynaud's phenomenon and internal organ features of systemic sclerosis are absent, although peripheral vascular entrapment syndromes may occur. Several cases of accompanying hematologic disorders, including aplastic anemia and myeloproliferative syndromes, have been reported.[222,229]

Laboratory abnormalities at early stages of illness include peripheral eosinophilia, elevated erythrocyte sedimentation rates (ESR), polyclonal hypergammaglobulinemia, and elevated levels of circulating immune complexes.

Diagnosis is best established by a full-thickness (skin-to-skeletal muscle) wedge biopsy. Early in the course of the illness, the deep fascia and subcutis are edematous and infiltrated with lymphocytes, plasma cells, histiocytes, eosinophils,[228,230] and mast cells. As the disease progresses, these structures, and often the dermis as well, become thickened and fibrotic (Fig. 79–23).

Glucocorticoids in small doses (10 to 20 mg/day of prednisone) are useful in the palliation of limb discomfort and readily suppress the peripheral and tissue eosinophilia. Glucocorticoids have not been demonstrated to hasten the resolution of fibrosis nor to modify the long-term course of the disease. Their usage is reserved for individuals with early disease and actively inflamed biopsy lesions and as adjuncts in the management of carpal tunnel syndrome and flexion contracture. NSAIDs are useful for symptomatic relief as well. There is anecdotal evidence of the usefulness of hydroxychloroquine, methotrexate, and D-penicillamine.

The natural history of eosinophilic fasciitis remains to be resolved. Many patients improve spontaneously or while on glucocorticoids over periods of 2 to 5 years, although histopathologic evidence of fascial fibrosis may persist.[222,231] Other patients experience a course of

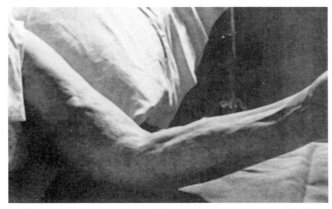

FIGURE 79–22 · The Arm of a 59-Year-Old Woman with 4 Months of Eosinophilic Fasciitis. The superficial skin is not thickened but is irregularly tethered to deeper tissues that have a woody induration. There is a coarse, orange peel appearance and patchy erythema. The exaggerated furrow over the course of superficial veins in the volar forearm is pathognomonic of idiopathic eosinophilic fasciitis and of the fasciitis secondary to the eosinophilia myalgia syndrome.

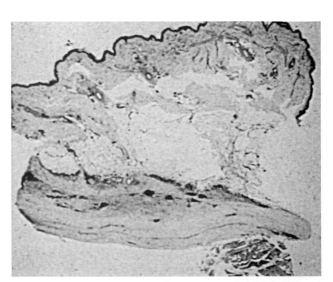

FIGURE 79–23 · Photomicrograph of a Full-Thickness Biopsy from the Forearm of a Patient with Eosinophilic Fasciitis. The epidermis and upper dermis are unremarkable. The fascia is several-fold thickened with dense fibrosis and persistent inflammatory infiltrate. Inflammation and patchy fibrosis extend into the subcutaneous fat and to the lower dermis. Although eosinophils were readily apparent on higher magnification in this case, they are inconsistently demonstrated and easily suppressed by glucocorticoid.

recurrent relapse and remission, and a minority have protracted clinical activity. Later disease can be dominated by painful symmetric joint complaints.

EOSINOPHILIA-MYALGIA SYNDROME

An epidemic of now more than 1500 cases of abrupt onset of myalgia, fatigue, and peripheral eosinophilia was identified in 1989 and rapidly linked to the use of L-tryptophan dietary supplement for insomnia, premenstrual symptoms, and depression.[228,232] A contaminant traced to a single Japanese manufacturer of L-tryptophan has been identified as the precipitating agent and attributed to both the use of a new strain of *Bacillus amyloliquefaciens* in the fermentation process and reduced use of powdered carbon in a purification step.[233]

The clinical spectrum of eosinophilia-myalgia syndrome includes rapid evolution of dermal and fascial induration of the extremities (lower more than upper), virtually indistinguishable from eosinophilic fasciitis.[228] In fact, retrospective analysis of patients previously diagnosed with eosinophilic fasciitis has identified a surprisingly prevalent prior use of L-tryptophan. Additional features include dyspnea, dry cough, and mild hypoxemia occasionally with a Löffler syndrome–like pneumonitis or with apparent pulmonary microvascular disruption, peripheral neuritis, and mild hepatitis. Muscle pain is frequently disabling. Although serum creatine kinase levels are usually normal, elevations of serum aldolase levels suggest myositis. Although some individuals seem to improve after cessation of L-tryptophan ingestion, the typical course is of progression to chronic and severe eosinophilic fasciitis. Glucocorticoids are useful in palliation of early symptoms but apparently do not alter the progression of the disease. Little is known about the usefulness of cytotoxic agents.

Histopathologic changes of tissue edema and perivascular accumulation of lymphocytes, plasma cells, and eosinophils are found at early stages. The evolution of hyaline sclerodermoid changes with mucinosis typify later disease.

OTHER SYNDROMES

An epidemic of acute pneumonitis followed by a chronic stage of scleroderma-like skin thickening, neuromyopathy, and sicca syndrome affected thousands of individuals in Spain in 1981.[228,234] A tainted rapeseed oil was implicated epidemiologically, although the precise chemical offending substance was not identified and the mechanism of the toxic oil syndrome remains unknown.[228,235]

Intramuscular pentazocine is associated with a local inflammatory fibrosing tissue reaction that, on occasion, may become more generalized,[236] and bleomycin therapy may induce both scleroderma-like fibrosis of skin and lungs.[237]

The syndromes of localized scleroderma should be considered if not accompanied by Raynaud's phenomenon or if the distribution of skin involvement is atypical for systemic sclerosis. Dermal fibrosis, frequently linked to inflammatory processes of diverse causes, suggests common pathogenic influences in the spectrum of the scleroderma disorders.

REFERENCES

1. Subcommittee for Scleroderma Criteria of the American Rheumatism Association Diagnostic and Therapeutic Criteria Committee: Preliminary criteria for the classification of systemic sclerosis (scleroderma). Arthritis Rheum 23:581, 1980.
2. Medsger TA, Steen VD: Classification, prognosis. *In* Clements PJ, Furst DE (eds): Systemic Sclerosis, 1st ed. Baltimore, Williams & Wilkins, 1996, pp 51-64.
3. Jablonska S, Blaszczyk M: Differential diagnosis of scleroderma-like disorders. *In* Clements PJ, Furst DE (eds): Systemic Sclerosis, 1st ed. Baltimore, Williams & Wilkins, 1996, pp 99-120.
4. Rodnan GP, Jablonska S, Medsger TA: Classification and nomenclature of progressive systemic sclerosis (scleroderma). Clin Rheum Dis 5:5, 1979.
5. Barnett AF: Scleroderma (progressive systemic sclerosis): Progress and course based on a personal series of 118 cases. Med J Aust 2:129, 1978.
6. LeRoy EC, Black C, Fleischmajer R, et al: Scleroderma (systemic sclerosis): Classification, subsets and pathogenesis. J Rheumatol 15:202, 1988.
7. Giordano M, Valentini G, Migliaresi S, et al: Different antibody patterns and different prognoses in patients with scleroderma with various extents of skin sclerosis. J Rheumatol 13:911, 1986.
8. Steen VD, Oddis CV, Conte CG, et al: Incidence of systemic sclerosis in Allegheny County, Pennsylvania: A twenty-year study of hospital-diagnosed cases, 1963-1982. Arthritis Rheum 40:441, 1997.
9. Mayes MD, Laing TJ, Gillespie BW, et al: Prevalence, incidence and survival rates of systemic sclerosis in the Detroit metropolitan area. Arthritis Rheum 39:S150, 1996.
10. Maricq HR, Weinrich MC, Keil JE, et al: Prevalence of scleroderma spectrum disorders in the general population of South Carolina. Arthritis Rheum 32:998, 1989.
11. Laing TJ, Gillespie BW, Toth MB, et al: Racial differences in scleroderma among women in Michigan. Arthritis Rheum 40:734, 1997.
12. Mayes MD: Epidemiology of systemic sclerosis and related diseases. Curr Opin Rheumatol 9:557, 1997.
13. Nietert PJ, Sutherland S, Silver RM, et al: Is occupational solvent exposure a risk factor for scleroderma? Arthritis Rheum 41:1111, 1998.
14. Lacey JV, Garabrant DH, Laing TW, et al: Petroleum distillate solvents as risk factors for undifferentiated connective tissue disease (UCTD). Am J Epidemiol 149:761, 1999.
15. Frank K-H, Fussel M, Conrad K, et al: Differential distribution of HLA class II and tumor necrosis factor alleles (TNF 308.2, TNFα2 microsatellite) in anti-topoisomerase I responders among scleroderma patients with and without exposure to quartz/metal dust. Arthritis Rheum 41:1306, 1998.
16. Varga J, Schumacher HR, Jimenez SA: Systemic sclerosis after augmentation mammoplasty with silicone implants. Ann Intern Med 111:377, 1989.
17. Spiera H: Scleroderma after silicone augmentation mammoplasty. JAMA 260:236, 1988.
18. Sanchez-Guerrero J, Schur PH, Sergent JS, Liang MH: Silicone breast implants and rheumatic disease: Clinical, immunologic, and epidemiologic studies. Arthritis Rheum 37:158, 1994.
19. Gabriel SE, O'Fallon WM, Kurland LT, et al: Risk of connective-tissue diseases and other disorders after breast implantation. N Engl J Med 330:1697, 1994.
20. Sanchez-Guerrero J, Colditz GA, Karlson EW, et al: Silicone breast implants and the risk of connective-tissue diseases and symptoms. N Engl J Med 332:1666, 1995.
21. Feghali CA, Wright TM: Epidemiologic and clinical study of twins with scleroderma. Arthritis Rheum 38:S308, 1995.
22. Whiteside TL, Medsger TA, Rodnan GP: Studies of the HLA antigens in progressive systemic sclerosis. *In* Black CM, Myers AR (eds): Systemic Sclerosis (Scleroderma), 1st ed. New York, Gower Medical, 1985, pp 89-96.
23. Lynch CJ, Singh G, Whiteside TL, et al: Histocompatibility antigens in progressive systemic sclerosis (scleroderma). J Clin Immunol 2:314, 1982.
24. Briggs D, Stephens C, Vaughan R, et al: A molecular and serologic analysis of the major histocompatibility complex and com-

plement component C4 in systemic sclerosis. Arthritis Rheum 36:943, 1993.

25. Arnett FC, Howard RF, Ta F, et al: Increased prevalence of systemic sclerosis in a Native American tribe in Oklahoma: Association with an Amerindian HLA haplotype. Arthritis Rheum 39:1362, 1996.

26. Tan FK, Stivers DN, Foster MW, et al: Association of microsatellite markers near the fibrillin 1 gene of human chromosome 15q with scleroderma in a Native American population. Arthritis Rheum 41:1729, 1998.

27. Rothfield NF, Rodnan, GP: Serum antinuclear antibodies in progressive systemic sclerosis (scleroderma). Arthritis Rheum 11:607, 1968.

28. Maddison PJ, Skinner RP, Pereira RS, et al: Antinuclear antibodies in the relatives and spouses of patients with systemic sclerosis. Ann Rheum Dis 45:793, 1986.

29. Rodnan GP, Myerowitz RL, Justh GO: Morphologic changes in the digital arteries of patients with progressive systemic sclerosis (scleroderma) and Raynaud phenomenon. Medicine 59:393, 1980.

30. Silman AJ, Black CM, Welsh KI: Epidemiology, demographics, genetics. In Clements PJ, Furst DE (eds): Systemic Sclerosis, 1st ed. Baltimore, Williams & Wilkins, 1996, pp 23-49.

31. Harper FE, Maricq HR, Turner RE, et al: A prospective study of Raynaud phenomenon and early connective tissue disease: A five-year report. Am J Med 72:883, 1982.

32. Kallenberg CGM, Pastoor GW, Wouda AA, et al: Antinuclear antibodies in patients with Raynaud's phenomenon: Clinical significance of anticentromere antibodies. Ann Rheum Dis 41:382, 1982.

33. Gerbracht DD, Steen VD, Ziegler GL, et al: Evolution of primary Raynaud's phenomenon (Raynaud's disease) to connective tissue disease. Arthritis Rheum 28:87, 1985.

34. Engelhart M, Seibold JR: The effect of local temperature versus sympathetic tone on digital perfusion in Raynaud's phenomenon. Angiology 41:715, 1990.

35. Seibold JR, Harris JN: Plasma beta-thromboglobulin in the differential diagnosis of Raynaud's phenomenon. J Rheumatol 12:99, 1985.

36. LeRoy EC, Maricq HR, Kahaleh MB: Undifferentiated connective tissue syndromes. Arthritis Rheum 23:341, 1980.

37. Buckingham RB, Prince RK, Rodnan GP: Progressive systemic sclerosis (PSS, scleroderma) dermal fibroblasts synthesize increased amounts of glycosaminoglycans. J Lab Clin Med 101:659, 1983.

38. Furst DE, Seibold JR, Steen VD, et al: The modified Rodnan skin score is an accurate reflection of skin thickness in systemic sclerosis. J Rheumatol 25:84, 1998.

39. Seibold JR, Furst DE, Clements PJ: Why everything (or nothing) seems to work in the treatment of scleroderma. J Rheumatol 19:673, 1992.

40. Steen VD, Medsger TA, Rodnan GP: D-Penicillamine therapy in progressive systemic sclerosis (scleroderma): A retrospective analysis. Ann Intern Med 97:652, 1982.

41. Clements PJ, Lachenbruch P, Seibold J, et al: Inter- and intraobserver variability of total skin thickness score (modified Rodnan TSS) in systemic sclerosis. J Rheumatol 22:1281, 1995.

42. Clements PJ, Lachenbruch P, Seibold JR, et al: Skin score: An assessment of inter-observer variability in three independent studies. J Rheumatol 20:1892, 1993.

43. Clements PJ, Lachenbruch PA, Ng SC, et al: Skin score: A semiquantitative measure of cutaneous involvement that improves prediction of prognosis in systemic sclerosis. Arthritis Rheum 33:1256, 1990.

44. Clements PJ, Furst DE, Seibold JR, Lachenbruch PA: Controlled trials: Trial design issues. In Clements PJ, Furst DE (eds): Systemic Sclerosis, 1st ed. Baltimore, Williams & Wilkins, 1996, pp 515-533.

45. Seibold JR, McCloskey DA: Skin involvement as a relevant outcome measure in clinical trials of systemic sclerosis. Curr Opin Rheumatol 9:571, 1997.

46. Fleischmajer R, Damiano V, Nedwich A: Alteration of subcutaneous tissue in systemic scleroderma. Arch Dermatol 105:59, 1972.

47. Fleischmajer R, Perlish JS, Reeves IRT: Cellular infiltrates in scleroderma skin. Arthritis Rheum 20:975, 1977.

48. Haynes DC, Gershwin ME: The immunopathology of progressive systemic sclerosis (PSS). Semin Arthritis Rheum 11:331, 1982.

49. Fleischmajer R, Prunieras M: II. Electron microscopy of collagen, cells, and the subcutaneous tissue. Arch Dermatol 106:515, 1972.

50. Varga J, Jimenez SA: Pathogenesis of scleroderma: Cellular aspects. In Clements PJ, Furst DE. (eds): Systemic Sclerosis, 1st ed. Baltimore, Williams & Wilkins, 1996, pp 123-152.

51. Jimenez SA, Feldman G, Bashey RI, et al: Co-ordinate increase in the expression of type I and type III collagen genes in progressive systemic sclerosis. Biochem J 237:837, 1986.

52. Peltonen L, Palotie A, Myllyla R, et al: Collagen biosynthesis in systemic scleroderma: Regulation of posttranslational modifications and synthesis of procollagen in cultured fibroblasts. J Invest Dermatol 84:14, 1985.

53. Krieg T, Horlein D, Wiestner M, et al: Aminoterminal extension peptides from type I procollagen normalize excessive collagen synthesis of scleroderma fibroblasts. Arch Dermatol Res 263:171, 1978.

54. Jelaska A, Arakawa M, Broketa G, Korn JH: Heterogeneity of collagen synthesis in normal and systemic sclerosis skin fibroblasts: Increased proportion of high collagen-producing cells in systemic sclerosis fibroblasts. Arthritis Rheum 39:1338, 1996.

55. Jelaska A, Korn JH: Apoptosis as a selection factor in the pathogenesis of scleroderma. Arthritis Rheum 40:S200, 1997.

56. Denton CP, Xu S, Black CM, et al: Scleroderma fibroblasts show increased responsiveness to endothelial cell-derived IL-1 and βFGF. J Invest Dermatol 108:269, 1997.

57. Serpier H, Gillery P, Salmon-Ehr V, et al: Antagonistic effects of interferon gamma and interleukin-4 on fibroblast cultures. J Invest Dermatol 109:158, 1997.

58. Kawakami T, Ihn H, Xu W, et al: Increased expression of TGF-beta receptors by scleroderma fibroblasts: Evidence for contribution of autocrine TGF-beta signaling to scleroderma phenotype. J Invest Dermatol 110:47, 1998.

59. Seibold JR, Giorno RC, Claman HN: Dermal mast cell degranulation in systemic sclerosis. Arthritis Rheum 33:1702, 1990.

60. Hawkins RA, Claman HN, Clark RAF, et al: Increased dermal mast cell populations in progressive systemic sclerosis: A link in chronic fibrosis? Ann Intern Med 102:182, 1985.

61. Walker M, Harley R, Maize J, et al: Mast cells and their degranulation in the Tsk mouse model of scleroderma. Proc Soc Exp Biol Med 180:323, 1985.

62. Lee Choi K, Giorno R, Claman HN: Cutaneous mast cell depletion and recovery in murine graft-vs-host disease. J Immunol 138:4093, 1987.

63. LeRoy EC, Smith EA, Kahaleh MB, et al: A strategy for determining the pathogenesis of systemic sclerosis: Is transforming growth factor beta the answer? Arthritis Rheum 32:817, 1989.

64. Rosenbloom J, Feldman G, Freundlich B, et al: Inhibition of excessive scleroderma fibroblast collagen production by recombinant gamma-interferon. Arthritis Rheum 29:851, 1986.

65. Duncan MR, Berman B: Persistence of a reduced-collagen-producing phenotype in cultured scleroderma fibroblasts after short-term exposure to interferons. J Clin Invest 79:1318, 1987.

66. Postlethwaite AE, Snyderman R, Kang AH: The chemotactic attraction of human fibroblasts to a lymphocyte-derived factor. J Exp Med 144:1188, 1976.

67. Wahl SM, Wahl LM, McCarthy JB: Lymphocyte-mediated activation of fibroblast proliferation and collagen production. J Immunol 121:942, 1978.

68. Worrall JG, Whiteside TL, Prince RK, et al: Persistence of scleroderma-like phenotype in normal fibroblasts after prolonged exposure to soluble mediators from mononuclear cells. Arthritis Rheum 29:54, 1986.

69. Perlish JS, Fleischmajer R: Effect of mitogen-stimulated scleroderma mononuclear cells on collagen synthesis by normal fibroblasts. In Black CM, Myers AR (eds): Systemic Sclerosis (Scleroderma), 1st ed. New York, Gower Medical, 1985.

70. D'Angelo WA, Fries JF, Masi AT, et al: Pathologic observations in systemic sclerosis (scleroderma): A study of fifty-eight autopsy cases and fifty-eight matched controls. Am J Med 46:428, 1969.

71. Norton WL, Nardo JM: Vascular disease in progressive systemic sclerosis (scleroderma). Ann Intern Med 73:317, 1970.

72. Cannon PJ, Hassar M, Cararella WJ, et al: The relationship of hypertension and renal failure in scleroderma (progressive systemic sclerosis) to structural and functional abnormalities of the renal cortical circulation. Medicine (Baltimore) 53:1, 1974.

73. Salerni R, Rodnan GP, Leon DF, et al: Pulmonary hypertension in the CREST syndrome variant of progressive systemic sclerosis (scleroderma). Ann Intern Med 86:394, 1977.

74. Seibold JR: Serotonin and Raynaud's phenomenon. In Vanhoutte PM (ed): Serotonin and the Cardiovascular System, 1st ed. New York, Raven Press, 1985.

75. Moulds RFW, Iwanov V, Medcalf RL: The effects of platelet-derived contractile agents on human digital arteries. Clin Sci 66:443, 1984.

76. Lindblad LE, Shepherd JT, Vanhoutte PM: Cooling augments platelet-induced contraction of peripheral arteries of the dog. Proc Soc Exp Biol Med 176:119, 1984.

77. Seibold JR, Jageneau AHM: Treatment of Raynaud's phenomenon with ketanserin, a selective antagonist of the serotonin$_2$ (5-HT$_2$) receptor. Arthritis Rheum 27:139, 1984.

78. Wigley FM, Wise RA, Seibold JR, et al: Intravenous iloprost infusion in patients with Raynaud phenomenon secondary to systemic sclerosis: A multicenter, placebo-controlled, double-blind study. Ann Intern Med 120:199, 1994.

79. Matucci Cerinic M, Generini S, Pignone A: New approaches to the treatment of Raynaud's phenomenon. Curr Opin Rheumatol 9:544, 1997.

80. Freedman RR, Baer RP, Mayes MD: Blockade of vasospastic attacks by alpha-2 adrenergic but not alpha-1 adrenergic antagonists in idiopathic Raynaud's disease. Circulation 92:1448, 1995.

81. Wigley FM, Flavahan NA: Raynaud's phenomenon. Rheum Dis Clin North Am 22:765, 1996.

82. Bulkley BH, Ridolfi RL, Salyer WR, et al: Myocardial lesions of progressive systemic sclerosis: A cause of cardiac dysfunction. Circulation 53:483, 1976.

83. Follansbee WP, Curtiss EI, Medsger TA, et al: Physiologic abnormalities of cardiac function in progressive systemic sclerosis with diffuse scleroderma. N Engl J Med 310:142, 1984.

84. Follansbee WP, Curtiss EI, Medsger TA, et al: Myocardial function and perfusion in the CREST syndrome variant of progressive systemic sclerosis: Exercise radionuclide evaluation and comparison with diffuse scleroderma. Am J Med 77:489, 1984.

85. Duboc D, Kahan A, Maziere B, et al: The effect of nifedipine on myocardial perfusion and metabolism in systemic sclerosis: A positron emission tomographic study. Arthritis Rheum 34:198, 1991.

86. Alexander EL, Firestein GS, Weiss JL, et al: Reversible cold-induced abnormalities in myocardial perfusion and function in systemic sclerosis. Ann Intern Med 105:661, 1986.

87. Ellis WW, Baer AN, Robertson RM, et al: Left ventricular dysfunction induced by cold exposure in patients with systemic sclerosis. Am J Med 80:385, 1986.

88. Furst DE, Davis JA, Clements PJ, et al: Abnormalities of pulmonary vascular dynamics and inflammation in early progressive systemic sclerosis. Arthritis Rheum 24:1403, 1981.

89. Maricq HR: Widefield capillary microscopy. Technique and rating scale for abnormalities seen in scleroderma and related disorders. Arthritis Rheum 24:1159, 1981.

90. Fleischmajer R, Perlish J, Shaw KV, et al: Skin capillary changes in early systemic scleroderma: Electron microscopy and "in vitro" autoradiography with tritiated thymidine. Arch Dermatol 112:1553, 1976.

91. Kahaleh MB, Osborn I, LeRoy EC: Increased factor VIII/von Willebrand factor antigen and von Willebrand factor activity in scleroderma and in Raynaud's phenomenon. Ann Intern Med 94:482, 1981.

92. Yamane K, Kashiwagi H, Suzuki N, et al: Elevated plasma levels of endothelin-1 in systemic sclerosis. Arthritis Rheum 34:243, 1991.

93. Seibold JR, Medsger TA, Winkelstein A, et al: Immune complexes in progressive systemic sclerosis (scleroderma). Arthritis Rheum 25:1167, 1982.

94. Thompson RP, Harper FE, Maize JC, et al: Nailfold biopsy in scleroderma and related disorders: Correlation of histologic, capillaroscopic, and clinical data. Arthritis Rheum 27:97, 1984.

95. Mackel AM, DeLustro F, Harper FE, et al: Antibodies to collagen in scleroderma. Arthritis Rheum 25:522, 1982.

96. Penning CA, Cunningham J, French MAH, et al: Antibody-dependent cellular cytotoxicity of human vascular endothelium in systemic sclerosis. Clin Exp Immunol 58:548, 1984.

97. Huffstutter JE, DeLustro FA, LeRoy EC: Cellular immunity to collagen and laminin in scleroderma. Arthritis Rheum 28:775, 1985.

98. Degiannis D, Seibold JR, Czarnecki M, et al: Soluble and cellular markers of immune activation in patients with systemic sclerosis. Clin Immunol Immunopathol 56:259, 1990.

99. Sato S: Abnormalities of adhesion molecules and chemokines in scleroderma. Curr Opin Rheumatol 11:490, 1999.

100. Munves EF, Schur PH: Antibodies to Sm and RNP: Prognosticators of disease involvement. Arthritis Rheum 26:848, 1983.

101. Ginsburg WW, Conn DL, Bunch TW, et al: Comparison of clinical and serologic markers in systemic lupus erythematosus and overlap syndrome: A review of 247 patients. J Rheumatol 10:235, 1983.

102. Seibold JR, Medsger TA, Winkelstein A, et al: Immune complexes in progressive systemic sclerosis (scleroderma). Arthritis Rheum 25:1167, 1982.

103. Fritzler MJ, Kinsella TD, Garbutt E: The CREST syndrome: A distinct serologic entity with anticentromere antibodies. Am J Med 69:520, 1980.

104. McCarty GA, Rice JR, Bembe ML, et al: Anticentromere antibody: Clinical correlations and association with favorable prognosis in patients with scleroderma variants. Arthritis Rheum 26:1, 1983.

105. Steen VD, Ziegler GL, Rodnan GP, et al: Clinical and laboratory associations of anticentromere antibody in patients with progressive systemic sclerosis. Arthritis Rheum 27:125, 1984.

106. Weiner ES, Hildebrandt S, Senecal J-L, et al: Prognostic significance of anticentromere antibodies and anti-topoisomerase I antibodies in Raynaud's disease. Arthritis Rheum 34:68, 1991.

107. Tan EM, Rodnan GP, Garcia I, et al: Diversity of antinuclear antibodies in progressive systemic sclerosis: Anti-centromere antibody and its relationship to CREST syndrome. Arthritis Rheum 23:617, 1980.

108. Maul GG, French BT, van Venrooij WJ, et al: Topoisomerase I identified by scleroderma 70 antisera: Enrichment of topoisomerase I at the centromere in mouse mitotic cells before anaphase. Proc Nat Acad Sci USA 83:5145, 1986.

109. Douvas A: Does Scl-70 modulate collagen production in systemic sclerosis? Lancet 2:475, 1988.

110. Guldner H-H, Szostecki C, Vosberg H-P, et al: Scl 70 autoantibodies from scleroderma patients recognize a 95 kDa protein identified as DNA topoisomerase I. Chromosoma 94:132, 1986.

111. Van Venrooij WJ, Stapel SO, Houben H, et al: Scl-86, a marker antigen for diffuse scleroderma. J Clin Invest 75:1053, 1985.

112. Maul GG, Jimenez SA, Riggs E, et al: Determination of an epitope of the diffuse systemic sclerosis marker antigen DNA topoisomerase-I: Sequence similarity with retroviral p^{30} gag protein suggests a possible cause for autoimmunity in systemic sclerosis. Proc Natl Acad Sci USA 86:8492, 1989.

113. Dang H, Garry RF, Seibold JR, Medsger TA: Antibodies to retroviral GAG proteins in progressive systemic sclerosis. Arthritis Rheum 34:1336, 1991.

114. D'Arpa P, White-Cooper H, Cleveland DW, et al: Use of molecular cloning methods to map the distribution of epitopes on topoisomerase I (Scl-70) recognized by sera of scleroderma patients. Arthritis Rheum 33:1501, 1990.

115. Okano Y, Steen VD, Medsger TA: Autoantibody reactive with RNA polymerase III in systemic sclerosis. Ann Intern Med 119:1005, 1993.

116. Douvas A: Pathogenesis: serologic correlates. In Clements PJ, Furst DE (eds): Systemic Sclerosis, 1st ed. Baltimore, Williams & Wilkins, 1996, pp 175-202.

117. Casciola-Rosen L, Wigley F, Rosen A: Scleroderma autoantigens are uniquely fragmented by metal-catalyzed oxidation reactions: Implications for pathogenesis. J Exp Med 185:71, 1997

118. Roumm AD, Whiteside TL, Medsger TA, et al: Lymphocytes in the skin of patients with progressive systemic sclerosis: Quantification, subtyping, and clinical correlations. Arthritis Rheum 27:645, 1984.

119. Whiteside TL, Kumagai Y, Roumm AD, et al: Suppressor cell function and T lymphocyte subpopulations in peripheral blood of patients with progressive systemic sclerosis. Arthritis Rheum 26:841, 1983.

120. Keystone EC, Lau C, Gladman CC, et al: Immunoregulatory T cell subpopulations in patients with scleroderma using monoclonal antibodies. Clin Exp Immunol 48:443, 1982.

121. Degiannis D, Seibold JR, Czarnecki M, et al: Soluble interleukin-2 receptors in patients with systemic sclerosis: Clinical and laboratory correlations. Arthritis Rheum 33:375, 1990.

122. Clements PJ, Peter JB, Agopian MS, et al: Elevated serum levels of soluble interleukin 2 receptor, interleukin 2 and neopterin in diffuse and limited scleroderma: Effect of chlorambucil. J Rheumatol 17:908, 1990.

123. Sandborg CI, Berman MA, Andrews BS, et al: Interleukin-1 production by mononuclear cells from patients with scleroderma. Clin Exp Immunol 60:294, 1985.

124. Whicher JT, Gilbert AM, Westacott C, et al: Defective production of leucocytic endogenous mediator (interleukin 1) by peripheral blood leucocytes of patients with systemic sclerosis, systemic lupus erythematosus, rheumatoid arthritis and mixed connective tissue disease. Clin Exp Immunol 65:80, 1986.

125. Kahaleh MB, LeRoy EC: Interleukin-2 in scleroderma: Correlation of serum level with extent of skin involvement and disease duration. Ann Intern Med 110:446, 1989.

126. Needleman BW, Wigley FM, Stair RW: Interleukin-1, interleukin-2, interleukin-4, interleukin-6, tumor necrosis factor and interferon levels in sera from patients with scleroderma. Arthritis Rheum 53:67, 1992.

127. Toth R, Allegretta M, Kim Y, Amento A: T cells derived from the skin of patients with systemic scleroderma preferentially utilize the T cell receptor VB3. Arthritis Rheum 38:S252, 1995.

128. Wooley PH, Sud S, Langendorfer A, et al: T cells infiltrating the skin of Tsk-2 scleroderma-like mice exhibit T cell receptor bias. Arthritis Rheum 38:S253, 1995.

129. Yurovsky VV, Wigley FM, Wise RA, White B: T cell repertoire in the lungs of patients with systemic sclerosis. Arthritis Rheum 38:S253, 1995.

130. Sternberg EM: Pathogenesis of scleroderma: The interrelationship of the immune and vascular hypotheses. Surv Immunol Res 4:69, 1985.

131. Jimenez SA, Gershwin ME: Animal models of systemic sclerosis. In Clements PJ, Furst DE (eds): Systemic Sclerosis, 1st ed. Baltimore, Williams & Wilkins, 1996, pp 251-273.

132. Bona CA, Murai C, Casares S, et al: Structure of the mutant fibrillin-1 gene in the tight skin (TSK) mouse. DNA Res 4:267, 1997.

133. Jaffee BD, Claman HN: Chronic graft-vs-host disease as a model for scleroderma. I. Description of model systems. Cell Immunol 77:1, 1983.

134. Van de Water J, Gershwin ME: Avian scleroderma: An inherited fibrotic disease of white leghorn chickens resembling progressive systemic sclerosis. Am J Pathol 120:478, 1985.

135. Van de Water J, Haapanen L, Boyd R, et al: Identification of T cells in early dermal lymphocytic infiltrates in avian scleroderma. Arthritis Rheum 32:1031, 1989.

136. Furst DE, Clements PJ, Graze P, et al: A syndrome resembling progressive systemic sclerosis after bone marrow transplantation. A model for scleroderma? Arthritis Rheum 22:904, 1979.

137. Nelson JL: Maternal-fetal immunology and autoimmune disease: Is some autoimmune disease auto-alloimmune or allo-autoimmune? Arthritis Rheum 39:191, 1996.

138. Nelson JL, Furst DE, Maloney S, et al: Microchimerism and HLA-compatible relationships of pregnancy in SSc. Lancet 351:559, 1998.

139. Artlett CM, Smith JB, Jimenez SA: Identification of fetal DNA and cells from skin lesions from women with systemic sclerosis. N Engl J Med 338:1186, 1998.

140. Blocka KLN, Bassett LW, Furst DE, et al: The arthropathy of advanced progressive systemic sclerosis: A radiographic survey. Arthritis Rheum 24:874, 1981.

141. Medsger TA, Rodnan GP, Moossy J, et al: Skeletal muscle involvement in progressive systemic sclerosis (scleroderma). Arthritis Rheum 11:554, 1968.

142. Clements PJ, Furst DE, Campion DS, et al: Muscle disease in progressive systemic sclerosis: Diagnostic and therapeutic considerations. Arthritis Rheum 21:62, 1978.

143. Lian JB, Pachman LM, Gundberg CM, et al: Gamma-carboxyglutamate excretion and calcinosis in juvenile dermatomyositis. Arthritis Rheum 25:1094, 1982.

144. Zamost BJ, Hirschberg J, Ippoliti AF, et al: Esophagitis in scleroderma: Prevalence and risk factors. Gastroenterology 92:421, 1987.

145. Cohen S, Laufer I, Snape WJ, et al: The gastrointestinal manifestations of scleroderma: Pathogenesis and management. Gastroenterology 79:155, 1980.

146. Russell ML, Friesen D, Henderson RD, et al: Ultrastructure of the esophagus in scleroderma. Arthritis Rheum 25:1117, 1982.

147. Sjogren RW: Gastrointestinal motility disorders in scleroderma. Arthritis Rheum 37:1265, 1994.

148. Troshinsky MB, Kane GC, Varga J, et al: Pulmonary function and gastroesophageal reflux in systemic sclerosis. Ann Intern Med 121:6, 1994.

149. Jabarri M, Cherry R, Lough JO, et al: Gastric antral venous ectasia: The watermelon stomach. Gastroenterology 87:1165, 1984.

150. Clarke AK, Galbraith RM, Hamilton EBD, et al: Rheumatic disorders in primary biliary cirrhosis. Ann Rheum Dis 37:42, 1978.

151. Bernstein RM, Callender ME, Neuberger JM, et al: Anticentromere antibody in primary biliary cirrhosis. Ann Rheum Dis 41:612, 1982.

152. Gupta RC, Seibold JR, Krishnan MR, et al: Precipitating autoantibodies to mitochondrial proteins in progressive systemic sclerosis. Clin Exp Immunol 58:68, 1984.

153. Seibold JR, Molony RR, Turkevich D, et al: Acute hemodynamic effects of ketanserin in pulmonary hypertension secondary to systemic sclerosis. J Rheumatol 14:519, 1987.

154. Ungerer RG, Tashkin DP, Furst D, et al: Prevalence and clinical correlates of pulmonary arterial hypertension in progressive systemic sclerosis. Am J Med 75:65, 1983.

155. Orens JB, Kazerooni EA, Martiniez FJ, et al: The sensitivity of high-resolution CT in detecting idiopathic pulmonary fibrosis proved by open lung biopsy: A prospective study. Chest 108:109, 1995.

156. Remy-Jardin M, Remy J, Wallaert B, et al: Pulmonary involvement in progressive systemic sclerosis: Sequential evaluation with CT, pulmonary function tests and bronchoalveolar lavage. Radiology 188:499, 1993.

157. Greenwald GI, Tashkin DP, Gong H, et al: Longitudinal changes in lung function and respiratory symptoms in progressive systemic sclerosis. Prospective study. Am J Med 83:83, 1987.

158. Owens GR, Fino GJ, Herbert DL, et al: Pulmonary function in progressive systemic sclerosis: Comparison of CREST syndrome variant with diffuse scleroderma. Chest 84:546, 1983.

159. Steen VD, Graham G, Conte C, et al: Isolated diffusing capacity reduction in systemic sclerosis. Arthritis Rheum 35:765, 1992.

160. Silver RM, Miller KS, Kinsella MB, et al: Evaluation and management of scleroderma lung disease using bronchoalveolar lavage. Am J Med 88:470, 1990.

161. Kinsella MB, Smith EA, Miller KS, et al: Spontaneous production of fibronectin by alveolar macrophages in patients with scleroderma. Arthritis Rheum 32:577, 1989.

162. Bolster MB, Silver RM: Assessment and management of scleroderma lung disease. Curr Opin Rheumatol 11:543, 1999.

163. Medsger TA, Masi AT, Rodnan GP, et al: Survival with systemic sclerosis (scleroderma): A life-table analysis of clinical and demographic factors in 309 patients. Ann Intern Med 75:369, 1971.

164. Lichtbroun AS, Sandhaus LM, Giorno RC, et al: Myocardial mast cells in systemic sclerosis: A report of three fatal cases. Am J Med 89:372, 1990.

165. Follansbee WP, Curtiss EI, Rahko PS, et al: The electrocardiogram in systemic sclerosis (scleroderma): Study of 102 consecutive cases with functional correlations and review of the literature. Am J Med 79:183, 1985.

166. Kostis JB, Seibold JR, Turkevich D, et al: Prognostic importance of cardiac arrhythmias in systemic sclerosis. Am J Med 84:1007, 1988.

167. Follansbee WP: The cardiovascular manifestations of systemic sclerosis (scleroderma). Curr Probl Cardiol 11(5):242, 1986.

168. Steen VD, Medsger TA, Osial TA, et al: Factors predicting development of renal involvement in progressive systemic sclerosis. Am J Med 76:779, 1984.

169. Whitman HH, Case DB, Laragh JH, et al: Variable response to oral angiotensin-converting-enzyme blockade in hypertensive scleroderma patients. Arthritis Rheum 25:241, 1982.

170. Helfrich DJ, Banner B, Steen VD, et al: Normotensive renal failure in systemic sclerosis. Arthritis Rheum 32:1128, 1989.

171. Gordon MB, Klein I, Dekker A, et al: Thyroid disease in progressive systemic sclerosis: Increased frequency of glandular fibrosis and hypothyroidism. Ann Intern Med 95:431, 1981.

172. Lally EV, Jimenez SA: Impotence in progressive systemic sclerosis. Ann Intern Med 95:150, 1981.

173. Nowlin NS, Brick JE, Weaver DJ, et al: Impotence in scleroderma. Ann Intern Med 104:794, 1986.

174. Cipoletti JF, Buckingham RB, Barnes EL, et al: Sjögren's syndrome in progressive systemic sclerosis. Ann Intern Med 87:535, 1977.

175. Osial TA, Whiteside TL, Buckingham RB, et al: Clinical and serologic study of Sjögren's syndrome in patients with progressive systemic sclerosis. Arthritis Rheum 26:500, 1983.

176. Steen VD, Conte C, Day N, et al: Pregnancy in women with systemic sclerosis. Arthritis Rheum 32:151, 1989.

177. Sonnex C, Paice E, White AG: Autonomic neuropathy in systemic sclerosis: A case report and evaluation of six patients. Ann Rheum Dis 45:957, 1986.

178. Peters-Golden M, Wise RA, Hochberg M, et al: Incidence of lung cancer in systemic sclerosis. J Rheumatol 12:1136, 1985.

179. Roumm AD, Medsger TA: Cancer and systemic sclerosis: An epidemiologic study. Arthritis Rheum 28:1336, 1985.

180. Black C, Dieppe P, Huskisson T, et al: Regressive systemic sclerosis. Ann Rheum Dis 45:384, 1986.

181. Furst DE, Clements PJ, Saab M, et al: Clinical and serological comparison of 17 chronic progressive systemic sclerosis (PSS) and 17 CREST syndrome patients matched for sex, age, and disease duration. Ann Rheum Dis 43:794, 1984.

182. White B, Bauer EA, Goldsmith LA, et al: Guidelines for clinical trials in systemic sclerosis (scleroderma). I. Disease-modifying interventions. Arthritis Rheum 38:351, 1995.

183. Seibold JR, Furst DE, Clements PJ: Treatment of systemic sclerosis by disease modifying agents. In Clements PJ, Furst DE (eds): Systemic Sclerosis, 1st ed. Baltimore, Williams & Wilkins, 1996, pp 535-548.

184. Furst DE, Clements PJ, Hillis S, et al: Immunosuppression with chlorambucil, versus placebo, for scleroderma: Results of a three-year, parallel, randomized, double-blind study. Arthritis Rheum 32:584, 1989.

185. Jansen GT, Barraza DF, Ballard JL, et al: Generalized scleroderma—Treatment with an immunosuppressive agent. Arch Dermatol 97:690, 1968.

186. Casas JA, Saway PA, Villarreal I, et al: 5-Fluorouracil in the treatment of scleroderma: A randomised, double blind, placebo controlled international collaborative study. Ann Rheum Dis 49:926, 1990.

187. Clements PJ, Lachenbruch PA, Sterz M, et al: Cyclosporine in systemic sclerosis: Results of a forty-eight week open safety study in ten patients. Arthritis Rheum 36:75, 1993.

188. Gruber BL, Kaufman LD: A double-blind randomized controlled trial of ketotifen versus placebo in early diffuse scleroderma. Arthritis Rheum 34:362, 1991.

189. Kahan A, Amor B, Menkes CJ, Strauch G: Recombinant interferon-gamma in the treatment of systemic sclerosis. Am J Med 87:273, 1989.

190. Freundlich B, Jimenez SA, Steen VD, et al: Treatment of systemic sclerosis with recombinant interferon-gamma: A Phase I/II clinical trial. Arthritis Rheum 35:1134, 1992.

191. Rook AH, Freundlich B, Jegasothy BV, et al: Treatment of systemic sclerosis with extracorporeal photochemotherapy: Results of a multicenter trial. Arch Dermatol 128:1517, 1992.

192. Beckett VL, Donadio JV, Brennan LA, et al: Use of captopril as early therapy for renal scleroderma: A prospective study. Mayo Clin Proc 60:763, 1985.

193. Seibold JR, Clements PJ, Lachenbruch PA, et al: Prospective, controlled trial of ketanserin vs placebo in systemic sclerosis. Arthritis Rheum 38:S335, 1995.

194. Beckett VL, Conn DL, Fuster V, et al: Trial of platelet-inhibiting drugs in scleroderma: Double-blind study with dipyridamole and aspirin. Arthritis Rheum 27:1137, 1984.

195. Jimenez SA, Sigal SH: A 15-year prospective study of treatment of rapidly progressive systemic sclerosis with D-penicillamine. J Rheumatol 18:1496, 1991.

196. Steen VD, Owens GR, Redmond C, et al: The effect of D-penicillamine on pulmonary findings in systemic sclerosis. Arthritis Rheum 28:882, 1985.

197. De Clerck LS, Dequeker J, Francx L, et al: D-Penicillamine therapy and interstitial lung disease in scleroderma: A long-term followup study. Arthritis Rheum 30:643, 1987.

198. Steen VD, Blair S, Medsger TA: The toxicity of D-penicillamine in systemic sclerosis. Ann Intern Med 104:699, 1986.

199. Clements PJ, Furst DE, Wong W-K, et al: High-dose versus low-dose D-penicillamine in early diffuse systemic sclerosis. Arthritis Rheum 42:1194, 1999.

200. Seibold JR, Clements PJ, Furst DE, et al: Safety and pharmacokinetics of recombinant human relaxin in systemic sclerosis. J Rheumatol 25:302, 1998.

201. Seibold JR, Korn JH, Simms R, et al: Recombinant human relaxin in the treatment of scleroderma: A randomized, double-blind, placebo-controlled multicenter trial. Ann Intern Med 132:871-879, 2000.

202. Clements PJ, Furst DE: Choosing appropriate patients with SSc for treatment by autologous stem cell transplantation. J Rheumatol 24(Suppl 48):85, 1997.

203. Chang B, Wigley FM, White B, Wise RA: Scleroderma patients with combined pulmonary hypertension and interstitial lung disease. J Rheumatol 30:2398-2405, 2003.

204. Sitbon O, Humbert M, Simonneau G: Primary pulmonary hypertension: current therapy. Prog Cardiovasc Dis 45:115-128, 2002.

205. Mayes MD: Endothelin and endothelin receptor antagonists in systemic rheumatic disease. Arthritis Rheum 48:1190-1199, 2003.

206. Tuder RM, Cool CD, Geraci MW, et al: Prostacyclin synthase expression is decreased in lungs from patients with severe pulmonary hypertension. Am J Resp Crit Care Med 159: 1925-1932, 1999.

207. Barst RJ, Seibold JR: Pulmonary arterial hypertension related to systemic sclerosis: A primer for the rheumatologist. Scleroderma Care Res 1:12-20, 2003.

208. Snyder SH, Reynolds IJ: Calcium-antagonist drugs: Receptor interactions that clarify therapeutic effects. N Engl Med 313:995, 1985.

209. Russell IJ, Lessard JA: Prazosin treatment of Raynaud's phenomenon: A double-blind single crossover study. J Rheumatol 12:94, 1985.

210. Wigley FM, Korn JH, Csuka ME, et al: Oral iloprost in patients with Raynaud phenomenon secondary to systemic sclerosis: A multicenter, placebo-controlled, double-blind study. Arthritis Rheum 41:670, 1998.

211. Klinkenberg-Knol EC, Festen HPM, Jansen JBM, et al: Long-term treatment with omeprazole for refractory reflux esophagitis: Efficacy and safety. Ann Intern Med 121:161, 1994.

212. DeVault KR, Castell DO: Current diagnosis and treatment of gastroesophageal reflux disease. Mayo Clin Proc 69:867, 1994.

213. Silver RH, Warrick JH, Kinsella MB, et al: Cyclophosphamide and low-dose prednisone therapy in patients with systemic sclerosis (scleroderma) with interstitial lung disease. J Rheumatol 20:838, 1993.

214. Akesson A, Scheja A, Ludin A, Wollheim FA: Improved pulmonary function in systemic sclerosis after treatment with cyclophosphamide. Arthritis Rheum 37:729, 1994.

215. Seibold JR, McCloskey DA, Furst DE: Pilot trial of methotrexate in treatment of early diffuse scleroderma. Arthritis Rheum 37:S262, 1994.

216. Rich S, Kaufmann E, Levy PS: The effect of high doses of calcium-channel blockers on survival in primary pulmonary hypertension. N Engl J Med 327:76, 1992.

217. Barst RJ, Rubin LJ, McGoon MD, et al: Survival in primary pulmonary hypertension with long-term continuous intravenous prostacyclin. Ann Intern Med 121:409, 1994.

218. Barst RJ, Rubin LJ, Long WA, et al: A comparison of continuous intravenous epoprostenol (prostacyclin) with conventional therapy for primary pulmonary hypertension. N Engl J Med 334:296, 1996.

219. Steen VD: Organ involvement: Renal. In Clements PJ, Furst DE (eds): Systemic Sclerosis. Baltimore, Williams & Wilkins, 1996, pp 425-439.

220. Rodnan GP: When is scleroderma not scleroderma? The differential diagnosis of progressive systemic sclerosis. Bull Rheum Dis 31:7, 1981.

221. Falanga V, Medsger TA, Reichlin M, et al: Linear scleroderma: Clinical spectrum, prognosis, and laboratory abnormalities. Ann Intern Med 104:849, 1986.

222. Peterson LS, Nelson AM, Su WPD: Classification of morphea (localized scleroderma). Mayo Clin Proc 70:1068, 1995.

223. Person JR, Su WPD: Subcutaneous morphea: A clinical study of sixteen cases. Br J Dermatol 100:371, 1979.

224. Venencie PY, Powell FC, Su WPD, et al: Scleredema: A review of thirty-three cases. J Am Acad Dermatol 11:128, 1984.

225. Feldman P, Shapiro L, Pick AI, et al: Scleromyxedema. Arch Dermatol 99:51, 1969.

226. Ohta A, Uitto J, Oikarinen AI, et al: Paraproteinemia in patients with scleredema: Clinical findings and serum effects on skin fibroblasts in vitro. J Am Acad Dermatol 16:96, 1987.

227. Shulman LE: Diffuse fasciitis with eosinophilia: A new syndrome? Trans Assoc Am Phys 88:70, 1975.

228. Varga J, Kahari V-M: Eosinophilia-myalgia syndrome, eosinophilic fasciitis, and related fibrosing syndromes. Curr Opin Rheumatol 9:562, 1997.

229. Hoffman R, Dainiak N, Sibrack L, et al: Antibody-mediated aplastic anemia and diffuse fasciitis. N Engl J Med 300:718, 1979.

230. Barnes L, Rodnan GP, Medsger TA, et al: Eosinophilic fasciitis: A pathologic study of twenty cases. Am J Pathol 96:493, 1979.

231. Moutsopoulos HM, Webber BL, Pavlidis NA, et al: Diffuse fasciitis with eosinophilia: A clinicopathologic study. Am J Med 68:710, 1980.

232. Martin RW, Duffy J, Engel AG, et al: The clinical spectrum of the eosinophilia-myalgia syndrome associated with L-tryptophan ingestion: Clinical features in 20 patients and aspects of pathophysiology. Ann Intern Med 113:124, 1990.

233. Belongia EA, Hedberg CW, Gleich GJ, et al: An investigation of the cause of the eosinophilia-myalgia syndrome associated with tryptophan use. N Engl J Med 323:357, 1990.

234. Tabuenca JM: Toxic-allergic syndrome caused by ingestion of rapeseed oil denatured with aniline. Lancet 2:567, 1981.

235. Mateo IM, Fernandez-Dapica MP, Izquierdo M, et al: Toxic epidemic syndrome: Musculoskeletal manifestations. J Rheumatol 11:333, 1984.

236. Palestine RF, Millens JL, Sligel GT: Skin manifestations of pentazocine abuse. J Am Acad Dermatol 2:47, 1980.

237. Finch WR, Rodnan GP, Buckingham RB, et al: Bleomycin-induced scleroderma. J Rheumatol 7:651, 1980.

80 Inflammatory Diseases of Muscle and Other Myopathies

ROBERT L. WORTMANN

The inflammatory diseases of muscle are a heterogeneous group of conditions characterized by proximal muscle weakness and nonsuppurative inflammation of skeletal muscle. Traditionally, the terms *polymyositis* and *polymyositis-dermatomyositis syndrome* (or *complex*) have been used to represent a variety of diagnoses, including adult and childhood forms of polymyositis and dermatomyositis, myositis associated with other defined collagen-vascular diseases, myositis associated with malignancy, inclusion body myositis, and other rare conditions. The imprecision of these groupings reflect a lack of understanding of the precise nature and causes of these diseases. Because of this limited understanding, it is perhaps more appropriate to use the term *idiopathic inflammatory myopathy* to represent the entire group and reserve the terms *polymyositis* and *dermatomyositis* for more specific conditions or subsets of patients. This allows differentiation from the inflammatory myopathies related to known infectious or toxic causes (Table 80–1).

Classifications of Inflammatory Diseases of Muscle

Although polymyositis (PM) and dermatomyositis (DM) were recognized as clinical entities more than 100 years ago, it was not until 1975 that generally accepted criteria for the diagnosis of these conditions were proposed by Bohan and Peter[1] (Table 80–2). Their work allowed, for the first time, a more systematic approach to the study of the inflammatory myopathies. According to these criteria, patients with polymyositis manifest 1) proximal muscle weakness, 2) elevated serum levels of enzymes derived from skeletal muscle, 3) myopathic changes demonstrated by electromyography (EMG), and 4) muscle biopsy evidence of inflammation. The addition of a skin rash (criterion 5) affords the diagnosis of DM. Patients are assigned to other categories based on their age and the coexistence of another disease. Bohan and Peter divided the idiopathic inflammatory myopathies among five groups: 1) primary idiopathic PM, 2) primary idiopathic DM, 3) DM or PM associated with neoplasia, 4) childhood DM (or PM) associated with vasculitis, and 5) PM or DM with associated collagen-vascular disease.

Additional classification schemes have been proposed based on newer studies of patients with idiopathic inflammatory myopathy.[2-4] The group of inclusion body myositis (IBM) emerged from studies of patients who fulfilled criteria for PM but were generally resistant to therapy. Criteria for the diagnosis of IBM have been proposed and employed for investigation of this diagnostic group[5] (Table 80–3). The application of criteria for the diagnosis of PM, DM, and IBM has proved quite useful, but these criteria have not been validated in a fashion similar to that proposed by the American College of Rheumatology for the diagnosis of rheumatoid arthritis (RA) or systemic lupus erythematosus (SLE).

More recently, circulating myositis-specific autoantibodies (MSAs) have been identified in some patients with idiopathic inflammatory myopathy[6] (Table 80–4). It appears that the presence of these may define relatively homogeneous groups with regard to disease manifestations and prognosis[2,6,7] (Table 80–5) Although promising, the clinical usefulness of a classification scheme based on MSAs is limited because studies to date have been on small and select populations, and the availability of testing for them is limited.

Despite these schemes, it is frequently difficult to classify some patients with idiopathic inflammatory myopathies (Fig. 80–1). This inability results from the lack of specificity provided by the various classification schemes. This is, in part, a reflection of the lack of specificity of each individual criterion, as well as the result of incomplete or atypical presentations. For example, a patient may have a biopsy characteristic of PM but also have a skin rash. This state will persist until more specific disease definitions can be developed, and this is unlikely to occur until there is a better

TABLE 80–1 · CLASSIFICATION OF INFLAMMATORY DISEASES OF MUSCLE

Idiopathic inflammatory myopathies
Polymyositis (PM)
Dermatomyositis (DM)
Juvenile (childhood) DM
Myositis associated with collagen vascular disease
Myositis associated with malignancy
Inclusion body myositis
Other forms of inflammatory myopathy
Myositis associated with eosinophilia
Myositis ossificans
Localized or focal myositis
Giant-cell myositis
Myopathies caused by infection
Myopathies caused by drugs and toxins

TABLE 80–2 • CRITERIA TO DEFINE POLYMYOSITIS (PM) AND DERMATOMYOSITIS (DM) PROPOSED BY BOHAN AND PETER

1. Symmetric weakness of limb girdle muscles and anterior neck flexors, progressing over weeks to months, with or without dysphagia or respiratory muscle involvement.
2. Skeletal muscle histologic examination showing evidence of necrosis of types I and II muscle fibers, phagocytosis, regeneration with basophilia, large sarcolemmal nuclei and prominent nucleoli, atrophy in a perifascicular distribution, variation in fiber size, and an inflammatory exudate.
3. Elevation of levels of serum skeletal muscle enzymes (CK, aldolase, ALT, AST, and LDH).
4. Electromyographic (EMG) triad of short, small polyphasic motor units; fibrillations, positive waves, and insertional irritability; and bizarre high-frequency discharges.
5. Dermatologic features including a lilac (heliotrope) discoloration of the eyelids with periorbital edema; a scaly, erythematous dermatitis over the dorsa of the hands, especially over the metacarpophalangeal and proximal interphalangeal joints (Gottron's sign); and involvement of the knees, elbows, medial malleoli, face, neck, and upper torso.

Abbreviations: ALT, alanine aminotransferase; AST, aspartate aminotransferase; CK, creatine kinase; LDH, lactate dehydrogenase.

Data from Bohan A, Peter JB: Polymyositis and dermatomyositis (first of two parts). N Engl J Med 292:344, 1975.

understanding of the underlying pathophysiologies and etiologies.

Epidemiology

The idiopathic inflammatory myopathies are relatively rare diseases. Estimates of prevalence range from 0.5 to 9.3 cases per million.[8,9] The incidence appears to be increasing, although this may simply reflect increased awareness and more accurate diagnosis.

Racial differences are apparent. In adults in the United States, the lowest rates are reported in those of Japanese descent and the highest in blacks. The incidence of childhood DM is significantly higher in Asians and Africans than in Europeans and Americans, and the incidence in blacks in the United States is twice that in whites.[9] In Europe, there is a significant latitude gradient of relative prevalence of DM and PM with the latter more common in the north.

Overall, the age at onset of the idiopathic inflammatory myopathies has a bimodal distribution, with peaks between ages 10 and 15 years in children and between 45 and 60 years in adults. However, the mean ages for specific groups differ. The age at onset of myositis associated with another collagen vascular disease is similar to that of

TABLE 80–3 • INCLUSION BODY MYOSITIS (IBM) DIAGNOSTIC CRITERIA

I. Diagnostic Classification
   A. *Definite* IBM
      Patients must exhibit all muscle biopsy including invasion of non-necrotic fibers by mononuclear cells, vacuolated muscle fibers, and intracellular (within muscle fibers) amyloid deposits or 15- to 18-nm tubulofilaments. None of the other clinical or laboratory features are mandatory if muscle biopsy features are diagnostic.
   B. *Probable* IBM
      If the muscle shows inflammation (invasion of non-necrotic muscle fibers by mononuclear cells) and vacuolated muscle fibers but without other pathologic features, a diagnosis of IBM can be given if the patient exhibits the characteristic clinical and laboratory features (see next sections of table).
II. Characteristic Features
   A. Clinical features
      Duration of illness
      Age of onset older than 30 years of age
      Muscle weakness
      Affects proximal and distal muscles of arms and leg
      and
      Patient must exhibit at least one of the following features:
      Finger flexor weakness
      Wrist flexor or wrist extensor weakness
      Quadriceps muscle weakness (Medical Research Council [MRC] grade 4)
   B. Laboratory features
      Serum creatine kinase less than 12 times upper limit as normal
      Muscle biopsy
      Inflammatory myopathy characterized by mononuclear cell invasion of non-necrotic muscle fibers
      Vacuolated muscle fibers
      Either:
         (i) Intracellular amyloid deposits (must use fluorescent method of identification before excluding the presence of amyloid)
         or
         (ii) 15 to 18 nm of tubulofilaments by electron microscopy
III. Electromyography must be consistent with features of an inflammatory myopathy (however, long-duration potentials are commonly observed and do not exclude diagnosis of sporadic IBM).

From Peng A, Koffman BM, Malley JD, et al: Disease progression in sporadic inclusion body myositis: observations in 78 patients. Neurology 55:296, 2000.

TABLE 80–4 · MYOSITIS-RELATED AUTOANTIBODIES

Name	Antigen	MW (kD)	HLA
Mytosis Specific			
Jo1	Histidyl-tRNA synthetase	50	D3;DRw52 DRB1*0501
PL7	Threonyl-tRNA synthetase	80	DRw52
PL12	Alanyl-tRNA synthetase	110	DRw52
EJ	Glycyl-tRNA synthetase	75	DRw52
OJ	Isoleucyl-tRNA synthetase	150	DRw52
KS	Asparaginyl-tRNA synthetase	65	
SRP	Signal recognition particle	54, 60, 72	DR5;DRw52 7SLRNA
Mi-2	CHO3 and CHO4 helicase components of histone acetylase complexes	240	DR7;DRw53
Mytosis Associated			
56kd	Component of ribonucleoprotein particle	56	none
Fer	Elongation factor-1α	48	none
Mas	tRNA^ser^-related antigen		DR4;DRw53
KJ	Unidentified translocation factor	120	DW52
PM-Sci	Unidentified	100	DR3
Ku	DNA-binding proteins	70, 80	
MJ	Unidentified	135	

Abbreviations: HLA, human leukocyte antigen; MW, molecular weight.

Adapted from Targoff IN: Autoantibodies. *In* Wortmann RL (ed): Clinical Disorders of Skeletal Muscle. Philadelphia, Lippincott, Williams & Wilkins, 2000, pp 268-269.

TABLE 80–5 · ADULT AND CHILDHOOD SYNDROMES ASSOCIATED WITH MYOSITIS-SPECIFIC AUTOANTIBODIES

Autoantibody	Clinical Features	Treatment Response
Anti–Jo-1 (and other antisynthetase)	Polymyositis or dermatomyositis with relatively acute onset Interstitial lung disease Fever Arthritis Raynaud's phenomenon "Mechanic's" hands	Moderate with disease persistence
Anti-SRP (signal recognition particle)	Polymyositis with very acute onset often in autumn Severe weakness Palpitations	Poor
Anti–Mi-2	Dermatomyositis with V sign and shawl sign Cuticular overgrowth	Good

the associated condition. Both myositis associated with malignancy and IBM are more common after the age of 50 years. Women are affected more frequently than men by a 2:1 ratio, with the exception of IBM, in which the ratio is reversed. Female predominance is especially great between the ages of 15 and 44 years, in myositis associated with other collagen-vascular diseases, and in blacks.

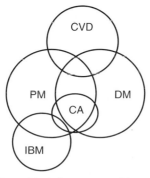

FIGURE 80–1 · Idiopathic Inflammatory Myopathies. Some individuals have clearly defined disease, whereas others have an overlap and a presentation more difficult to classify. CA, cancer associated myositis; CV, myositis with an associated collagen-vascular disease; DM, dermatomyositis; IBM, inclusion body myositis; PM, polymyositis.

Clinical Features

The dominant clinical feature of the idiopathic inflammatory myopathies is symmetric proximal muscle weakness.[10-14] Although strength may be essentially normal at the time of presentation, virtually all patients develop significant muscle weakness during the course of their illness. The weakness can be accompanied by myalgias and tenderness and eventually atrophy and fibrosis. Laboratory investigation reveals elevated serum enzyme levels of skeletal muscle origin, EMG demonstrates changes consistent with inflammation, and histologic examination of skeletal muscle shows changes characteristic of inflammation. These manifestations can occur in a variety of combinations or patterns. No single feature is specific or diagnostic.

Thus, the presence of any one feature should suggest the diagnosis of inflammatory myopathy, but the diagnosis is made by ruling out other causes for the abnormalities observed.

POLYMYOSITIS IN THE ADULT

Typically, adult-onset PM begins insidiously over 3 to 6 months with no identifiable precipitating event. Only rarely is the onset abrupt and associated with clinically evident rhabdomyolysis and myoglobinuria. The weakness initially affects the muscles of the shoulder and pelvic girdle, with the latter being slightly more common. Distal weakness is uncommon initially but can develop over time in severe cases. Weakness of neck muscles, particularly the flexors, occurs in about half the patients. Ocular muscles are virtually never involved. Facial and bulbar muscle weakness is rare, but dysphagia may develop secondary to esophageal dysfunction, cricopharyngeal obstruction, or macroglossia from tongue myositis.[15] Pharyngeal muscle weakness may cause dysphonia and difficulty in swallowing. In severe cases, attempts to swallow fluids may result in liquid coming out the nose or in aspiration.

PM is a systemic disease, and patients may develop morning stiffness, fatigue, anorexia, weight loss, and fever. Arthralgias are not uncommon, but frank synovitis is less usual. Raynaud's phenomenon is sometimes present. Muscle pain and tenderness are present in about half the patients. Periorbital edema may occur. The neurologic portion of the physical examination is normal except for motor function.

Pulmonary and cardiac manifestations may occur at any time during the course of the disease.[16,17] "Velcro"-like crackles may be heard on chest auscultation, and changes indicative of interstitial fibrosis may be seen on chest radiographs.[16,18] Interstitial pneumonitis may cause dyspnea, a nonproductive cough, hypoxemia, and fatal respiratory failure. Aspiration pneumonia may complicate the disease course in patients with esophageal dysmotility, swallowing difficulties, or dysphonia. Cardiac involvement is usually absent or is restricted to electrocardiographic abnormalities. However, heart block, supraventricular arrhythmia, or cardiomyopathy may develop, causing syncope, palpitations, or congestive heart failure.[19,20]

The creatine kinase (CK) level is elevated in almost every patient with PM at some time during the course of the disease. Normal levels of CK may be found in patients who present very early in the course of their disease, in advanced cases with significant muscle atrophy late in the course, or as a result of circulating inhibitors of CK activity that may be present during active disease and can lower serum levels to within the normal range.[21] However, in most patients, elevation of the serum CK level is a helpful indicator of the severity of the disease.[22] Although the range of CK elevations observed is great, levels peak at 10 times normal in the average case. Levels of other muscle enzymes (aldolase, aspartate aminotransferase [AST], alanine aminotransferase [ALT], and lactate dehydrogenase) are also found to be elevated in most cases, if the appropriate enzymes are measured repeatedly throughout the course of the disease. The finding of an elevated CK-MB isoenzyme does not necessarily signify cardiac involvement, although it can. A rising ratio of the MB fraction to the total CK or the presence of cardiac troponin I are more indicative of cardiac involvement.

EMG evaluation of patients with PM classically reveals the triad of 1) increased insertional activity, fibrillations, and sharp positive waves; 2) spontaneous, bizarre high-frequency discharges; and 3) polyphasic motor unit potentials of low amplitude and short duration. In larger series, the complete triad is found in approximately 40 percent of patients.[11,23] In contrast, 10 to 15 percent of patients may have completely normal studies. EMG abnormalities are limited to the paraspinal muscles in a small number of patients, even in the presence of widespread weakness.

Although the histopathologic changes of PM are well described, no specific change is pathognomonic. Wide variations in pathologic change can be observed within the tissue of an individual patient, as well as from individual to individual (Fig. 80–2). In the typical case, muscle fibers are found to be in varied stages of necrosis and regeneration. The inflammatory cell infiltrate is predominantly focal and endomysial, although perivascular accumulations may also occur. In some cases, T lymphocytes, especially T8+ cytotoxic cells, accompanied by a smaller number of macrophages are found surrounding and invading initially non-necrotic fibers.[24,25] In other cases, degeneration is seen in the absence of inflammatory cells in the immediate area. Using hematoxylin and eosin (H&E) staining, regenerating cells are identified by basophilic staining, large centrally located nuclei, and prominent nucleoli. Intact fibers may vary in size. Destroyed fibers are replaced by fibrous connective tissue and fat. However, in some cases, no fiber necrosis is observed, and the only recognized change is type II fiber atrophy (Fig. 80–3).

DERMATOMYOSITIS IN THE ADULT

The clinical features of DM include all those described for PM plus cutaneous manifestations.[26] Rash is often the presenting complaint and may antedate the onset of myopathic symptoms by more than a year. The skin involvement varies widely from patient to patient. In some, the severity of the rash and muscle weakness coincides. In other patients, the activity of the skin disease and muscle weakness are unrelated. The rash may change from one type to another during the course of the disease.

A variety of skin changes can be observed. Changes considered pathognomonic are termed *Gottron's papules* or *Gottron's sign*. These are symmetric, lacy, pink to violaceous, raised or macular areas typically found on the dorsal aspect of interphalangeal joints, elbows, patellae, and medial malleoli. Characteristic changes include heliotrope (violaceous) discoloration of the eyelids, often with associated periorbital edema; macular erythema of the posterior shoulders and neck (shawl sign), anterior neck and upper chest (V sign), face, and forehead; and dystrophic cuticles. Periungual

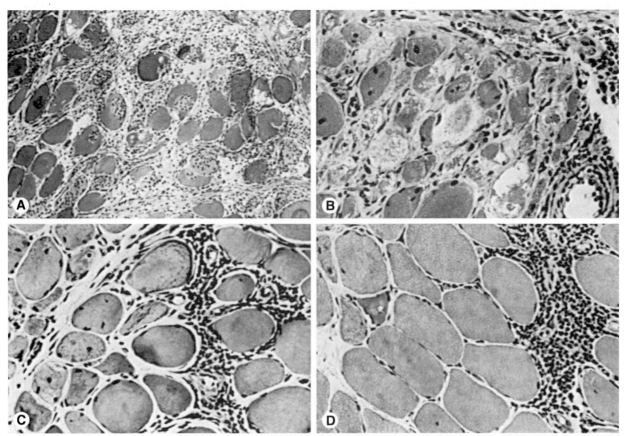

FIGURE 80–2 · Pathologic Changes in Idiopathic Inflammatory Myopathies. Classic changes in polymyositis (PM) show fiber necrosis and regeneration with endomysial mononuclear cell infiltration. Typical infiltrates in dermatomyositis (DM) are perimysial. It is not uncommon to find elements of each on an individual biopsy specimen. *A,* Extensive endomysial infiltration of inflammatory cells, with fiber invasion and necrosis. *B,* Necrotic fibers, regenerating fibers, and perivascular mononuclear cell infiltration. *C,* Variation in fiber size with endomysial infiltration. *D,* Primarily perimysial inflammatory infiltrate.

telangiectasias and nailfold capillary changes similar to those observed in patients with scleroderma or SLE and Raynaud's phenomenon can be seen. Darkened or dirty-appearing horizontal lines may be noted across the lateral and palmar aspects of the fingers. These

changes are termed *mechanic's hands* because of the similarity to changes noted in the hands of people who do manual labor. Cutaneous vasculitis can occur with livedo reticularis, digital infarcts, or palpable, white-centered petechiae. Less-specific skin changes include

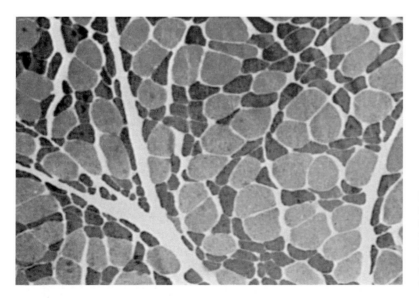

FIGURE 80–3 · Histochemical staining of muscle for adenosine triphosphatase (ATPase) activity; pH 9.4 allows differentiation between type II fibers (darker) and type I fibers (lighter). Type II fiber atrophy, shown here, is a nonspecific change that may occur in inflammatory muscle disease, steroid myopathy, cachectic states, upper motor neuron deficit, peripheral nerve disease, myasthenia gravis, and hyperparathyroidism.

poikiloderma, calcinosis cutis, erythema multiforme, subepidermal bullae, and photosensitivity.

The muscle biopsy histopathologic appearance of adult DM may be identical to that of PM but more often has its own characteristic pattern. Fiber invasion by T lymphocytes is rare, and a perivascular distribution of inflammatory cells, composed of higher percentages of B lymphocytes and helper T4+ lymphocytes, is the rule.[25,27] Biopsies reveal decreased capillary density perifascicular atrophy[28] (Fig. 80–4). Histopathologic skin lesions vary according to the stage of the disease and the type of lesion. Epidermal thickening; prominent dermal blood vessels; infiltration of lymphocytes (mostly CD4+), plasma cells, and histiocytes; and edema of the superficial layers of the dermis are seen in the earlier erythematous edematous regions.[29] Epidermal thinning, inflammatory cell infiltrates in the dermis, and increased connective tissue are seen in thickened, pigmented areas.

Some patients with biopsy-confirmed classic cutaneous findings of DM have no clinical laboratory evidence of muscle disease. The terms *amyopathic dermatomyositis* and *dermatomyositis sine myositis* have been used to describe patients with these findings.[30] These patients may constitute 10 percent of all patients with DM in some referral centers.[31] Today, the diagnosis of amyopathic DM is applied to patients who have Gottron's papules or sign; another cutaneous manifestation of DM; a skin biopsy histologic appearance compatible with DM; and no enzymatic or clinical evidence of myopathy. Pruritus and photosensitivity are common. In making the diagnosis of amyopathic DM, the clinician must exclude other causes of similar-appearing cutaneous conditions and recognize that the patient may be in an early or "skin disease only" phase of disease or have subclinical myositis.

It appears that perhaps one third to one half of such patients will retain the diagnosis over time, with some attaining partial or complete remission. The remainder progress and develop muscle involvement and weakness. Malignancy has developed in some cases.[32]

Changes in muscle enzymes and in EMG, magnetic resonance imaging (MRI), and ^{31}P (phosphorous) magnetic resonance spectroscopy results may precede the onset of clinical weakness.[33] Rarely, trichinosis infection, allergic contact dermatitis, and drugs (Table 80–6) can cause cutaneous changes that mimic DM.[34]

JUVENILE (CHILDHOOD) DERMATOMYOSITIS

The usual inflammatory myopathic process observed in children has a highly characteristic pattern, although a disease similar to adult PM is occasionally encountered in the pediatric age-group.[10,35] Juvenile DM differs from that of the adult form in many patients because of the coexistence of vasculitis, ectopic calcification, and lipodystrophy.[36-38] Classically, children develop cutaneous manifestations followed by muscle weakness. The rash is typically erythematous and is found on the malar region as well as the extensor surfaces of the elbows, knuckles, and knees. Involved muscles are often found

TABLE 80–6 · DRUGS AND DERMATOMYOSITIS (DM)

Induce DM
Antazoline
Bacille Calmette-Guérin (BCG) vaccine
Chlorpromazine
Clemizole
D-Penicillamine
Isoniazide
Penicillins
Pravastatin
Simistatin
Sulfonamides
Tamoxifen
Induce DM-like syndrome
Acetylsalicylic acid
Diclofenae
Hydroxyurea
Kava-kava
D-Penicillamine

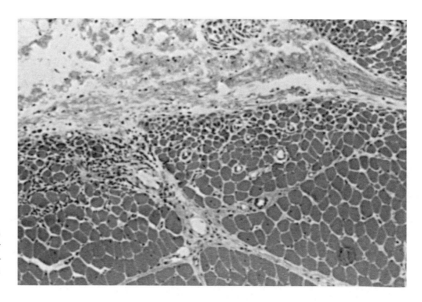

FIGURE 80–4 · Hematoxylin and Eosin (H&E) Stain of Skeletal Muscle Revealing Perifascicular Atrophy. The change is characteristic of juvenile dermatomyositis (DM) but may also be seen in adults with DM and other inflammatory myopathies.

to be tender and swollen on palpation. Amyopathic dermamyositis can also occur in children.[39] Juvenile DM is discussed more fully in Chapter 97.

MYOSITIS AND OTHER COLLAGEN-VASCULAR DISEASES

Muscle weakness is a frequent finding in patients with rheumatic diseases (Table 80–7). In some cases, the weakness may result from the systemic effects of cytokines (e.g., interleukin-1 [IL-1], IL-6, tumor necrosis factors [TNFs]) or side effects of therapies (e.g., glucocorticoids, D-Penicillamine, hydroxychloroquine). The features of idiopathic inflammatory myopathy (see Table 80–2) may dominate the clinical picture in some patients with scleroderma, SLE, mixed connective tissue disease, and Sjögren's syndrome.[40-45] In other cases, weakness may be accompanied by normal enzyme levels and an absence of abnormalities on EMG examination. The full picture of PM is less common but can occur in RA, adult Still's disease, Wegener's granulomatosis, and polyarteritis nodosa.[46,47] In vasculitic syndromes, muscle weakness is more commonly related to arteritis and nerve involvement than to nonsuppurative inflammatory changes of muscles. The histologic appearance of muscle in patients with myositis secondary to another connective tissue disease may be identical to that of patients with PM. In some patients, however, differences more representative of the associated condition are recognized.

MYOSITIS AND MALIGNANCY

The first association of myositis and malignancy was reported in 1916. Subsequent observations promoted the concept that patients with PM and DM had an increased risk of malignancy. Although this issue has been reinvestigated many times, questions still remain concerning the frequency of malignancy in patients with myositis and whether the risk is higher for those with DM.[48,49]

In studies reported after 1976, the frequency of malignancy associated with myositis is about 20 percent (with a range from 6 to 60 percent). Although this seems quite high, it is not different from the frequency of malignancy for the general population when appropriate control groups are analyzed. Some studies show that malignancy is more commonly associated with DM than with PM, but others demonstrate no difference

---

TABLE 80–7 · COLLAGEN-VASCULAR DISEASES THAT MAY BE ASSOCIATED WITH MYOPATHY

Adult Still's disease	Polymyalgia rheumatica
Allergic granulomatosis	Rheumatoid arthritis
Giant-cell arteritis	Scleroderma
Hypersensitivity vasculitis	Sjögren's syndrome
Leukocytoclastic vasculitis	Systemic lupus erythematosus
Mixed connective tissue disease	Wegener's granulomatosis
Polyarteritis nodosum	

---

between the two subsets.[48-50] Malignancies have developed in patients of all ages, as well as in those who present with amyopathic DM.[32]

Malignancy can develop before, at the same time as, or after the diagnosis of myositis. Occasionally, both conditions seem to follow a parallel course, but more commonly, the two seem to have only a temporal relationship, having developed within 1 year of each other. CK levels are elevated in most but not all patients with myositis with malignancy. Finding normal CK levels on repeated testing in patients with other features of myositis indicates an increased likelihood of malignancy.

Some evidence supports the premise that myositis and malignancy are associated more commonly in elderly persons. However, the two conditions are also well reported to coexist in adults younger than 40 years, as well as rarely in children. Malignancy has also been reported in IBM. It appears that the sites or types of malignancy that occur in patients with myositis are those expected for the age-group and sex of the individual, with the exception that ovarian cancer may be overrepresented in women with DM.[51]

INCLUSION BODY MYOSITIS

IBM is the most recently identified subset of inflammatory myopathies[5] (see Table 80–3). Some reports indicate that this diagnosis makes up 15 to 28 percent of all inflammatory myopathies.[59] It exists in sporadic and familial forms (see following regarding the familial cases). Although small numbers of cases of IBM have been diagnosed in patients younger than 40 years and rarely in childhood, this disease affects primarily older individuals.[52-54] The onset of symptoms is typically insidious, and progression is slow.[55] Symptoms may have been present for 5 or 6 years before a diagnosis. The clinical picture in some patients differs from that of typical PM in that it may include focal, distal, or asymmetric weakness.[56] Myalgias and muscle tenderness are rare. Dysphagia, noted in more than 20 percent of patients, tends to be a late occurrence but occasionally is a significant presenting symptom. Facial weakness is rare, and no cases with ptosis or ophthalmoplegia have been reported. The cardiovascular features are similar to those observed in PM. As the muscle weakness becomes severe, it is accompanied by atrophy and diminished deep tendon reflexes. In some patients, the disease continues a slow, steady progression. In others, it seems to plateau, leaving the individual with fixed weakness and atrophy of the involved musculature.

Serum CK levels are only slightly elevated in most patients with IBM and are normal in 25 percent. No correlation exists between the level of CK and the acuteness or severity of the disease. Elevated erythrocyte sedimentation rates (ESR) or positive tests for antinuclear antibodies (ANAs) are present in less than 20 percent of patients. Most patients have myopathic changes on EMG, with approximately half of the patients having EMG features consistent with neurogenic or mixed neurogenic and myopathic changes.[56]

The diagnosis is defined primarily by the pathologic findings. Histologic changes include necrosis and inflammation consistent with PM, although perivascular exudates are rare, and "ragged red" fibers and angulated atrophic fibers may be seen. The characteristic change is the presence of intracellular lined vacuoles (Fig. 80–5). On paraffin sections, the vacuoles appear lined with eosinophilic material, but on frozen preparations, they appear lined with basophilic granules. Lined vacuoles are not specific for IBM, as similar vacuoles have been described in other diseases (Table 80–8). Electron microscopy reveals either intracytoplasmic or intranuclear tubular or filamentous inclusions (Fig. 80–6). These structures are straight and rigid, appearing with periodic striations and resembling paramyxovirus nucleocapsid. Myelin figures, which are also called *myeloid bodies,* are membranous whorls that are common in, but not specific for, IBM.

TABLE 80–8 • MYOPATHIES ASSOCIATED WITH VACUOLES

Inflammatory	Adult dermatomyositis
	Inclusion body myositis
Dystrophic	Duchenne's muscular dystrophy (acute lesions)
	Oculopharyngeal muscular dystrophy
Toxic	Alcohol
	Chloroquine
	Colchicine
	Glycyrrhizin
	Zidovudine (AZT)
Metabolic	Acid maltase deficiency
	Other glycogen storage diseases
	Carnitine deficiency
Infectious	Echovirus
Miscellaneous	Distal myopathy
	Lafora's disease
	Periodic paralysis

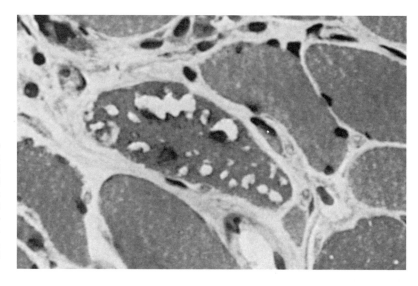

FIGURE 80–5 · Hematoxylin and eosin (H&E)–stained section of muscle from a patient with inclusion body myositis showing degenerating fibers with lined vacuoles, atrophic and angulated fibers, increased endomysium, and scattered mononuclear cells. (From Cohen MR, Sulaiman AR, Garancis JC, Wortmann RL: Clinical heterogeneity and treatment response in inclusion body myositis. Arthritis Rheum 32:734, 1989. Reprinted from Arthritis and Rheumatism Journal, Copyright 1989. Used with permission of the American College of Rheumatology.)

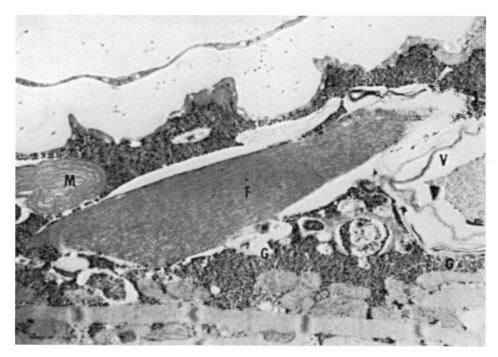

FIGURE 80–6 · Electron micrograph of muscle tissue from a patient with inclusion body myositis. Note the cytoplasmic inclusion (F) beneath the sarcolemma, a myelin figure (M), a vacuole (V), and pools of cytoplasmic glycogen (G). (From Cohen MR, Sulaiman AR, Garancis JC, Wortmann RL: Clinical heterogeneity and treatment response in inclusion myositis. Arthritis Rheum 32:734, 1989. Reprinted from Arthritis and Rheumatism Journal, Copyright 1989. Used with permission of the American College of Rheumatology.)

MYOSITIS AND EOSINOPHILS

Eosinophilic myositis is a rare disorder characterized by the subacute onset of proximal weakness, myalgias, elevated serum levels of muscle enzymes, myopathic EMG findings, and an eosinophilic inflammatory infiltrate in skeletal muscle.[57] Eosinophilic myositis can also be a focal disorder, relapsing or remitting spontaneously.[58] It can be associated with a predominant overlying eosinophilic fasciitis (Shulman's disease) or may represent one manifestation of a generalized hypereosinophilic syndrome.[59] Chronic eosinophilic perimyositis is a rare cause of persistent myalgia.[60] The majority of patients with eosinophilic myositis respond to prednisone.

The term *eosinophilia myalgia syndrome* is used for a neuromuscular condition caused by the ingestion of L-tryptophan that was contaminated during production. This syndrome reached epidemic status during the autumn of 1989. Only rarely has this syndrome been encountered since contaminated L-tryptophan was removed from sale and the toxicity resulting from its use was publicized. The syndrome typically caused myalgias, weakness, and profound peripheral blood hypereosinophilia (more than 1000 eosinophils/mm^3). Other features included arthralgias, alopecia, fever, weight loss, and pulmonary problems. Discontinuation of the L-tryptophan led to the resolution of symptoms in some patients, and glucocorticoid therapy was helpful in others. However, some patients continue to have persistent myalgias and paresthesias, and others have died, primarily from progressive pulmonary complications.[61]

MYOSITIS OSSIFICANS

Myositis ossificans can be divided into two types, localized and widespread. Localized myositis ossificans invariably follows trauma, although the trauma may have seemed trivial or may even have been forgotten. Initially, a warm, tender swelling of a doughy consistency is noted in the muscle.[62] When the swelling is close to a joint, the picture may simulate that of an acute monarticular arthritis. Soon thereafter, the area takes on the consistency of a mass and becomes firm and hard. At about 1 month, calcifications are seen on radiographs or with computed tomography (CT) scanning. Surgical excision is often necessary and leads to a good outcome. Lesions have a characteristic histologic appearance (Fig. 80–7).

The widespread, progressive form is termed *myositis ossificans progressiva* and is inherited in the autosomal dominant pattern.[63] Warm, tender swelling in many muscles is typically first noted during childhood. The lesions gradually shrink, become hard, and may disappear, only to recur, especially in the muscles of the spine, abdominal wall, chest, and extremities. Most patients also have some congenital skeletal defects, including microdactyly of the great toe and thumb, exostosis, and an absence of the two upper incisors, as well as hypogenitalism, an absence of the ear lobules, and deafness. Treatment with ethane-1-hydroxy-1, 1-diphosphonate has been effective in halting the progression of the disease in some patients.

LOCALIZED OR FOCAL MYOSITIS

Histologic changes identical to those observed in PM occasionally are present in biopsies of focal nodules from patients with only one muscle or one extremity involved. Characteristically, the nodules are painful, tender, and enlarge over a period of weeks.[64,65] This disorder may remit spontaneously, remain focal and confined to one limb for several years, or represent an unusual presentation of PM and progress to a more typical distribution after a few days or weeks.[66] Focal myositis can present with isolated nerve palsies. These lesions must be differentiated from a skeletal muscle tumor.

Orbital or ocular myositis is a focal myositis limited to extraocular muscles. Patients usually present with orbital or periorbital pain, diplopia, abnormal extraocular motion, and proptosis.[67] It can be seen alone or in association with PM, Lyme disease, or Crohn's disease.

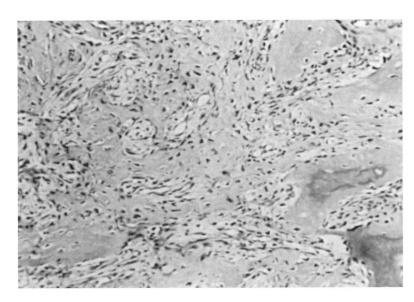

FIGURE 80–7 · Hematoxylin and Eosin (H&E)–Stained Section of Muscle from Localized Area of Myositis Ossificans. (From Siegert JJ, Wortmann RL: Myositis ossificans simulating acute monoarticular arthritis. J Rheumatol 13:652, 1986.)

CT and MRI are helpful in distinguishing orbital myositis from orbital pseudotumor, cellulitis, cavernous sinus thrombosis, or Graves' ophthalmopathy.

GIANT-CELL MYOSITIS

Multinucleated giant cells may occur in skeletal muscle as an isolated condition termed *giant-cell (granulomatous) myositis* or in association with a variety of conditions, including foreign body reactions, tuberculosis, inflammatory bowel disease, and sarcoidosis.[68,69] Regenerating muscle cells are multinucleated and may closely resemble giant cells. Therefore, the histopathologic appearance and overall clinical status of the patient should be reviewed carefully whenever giant cells are found in skeletal muscle.

MACROPHAGIC MYOFASCIITIS

First reported on 1993, macrophagic myofasciitis is characterized by unique pathologic pattern of focal infiltration of the epimysium, perimysium, and perifascicular endomysium by sheets of large, nonepithelial macrophages; occasional CD8+ T cells intermingled with macrophages or surrounding microvessels; and inconspicuous muscle fiber damage.[70] Affected patients generally report a syndrome of diffuse myalgia, anthralgia, marked asthenia, and, less frequently, muscle weakness and fever. Slight elevations of CK can occur in some patients, as well as elevated ESR and myopathic EMG changes. Gallium-67 scintigraphy may be useful in making the diagnosis.[71] The majority of cases have been identified in France, but the disease has also been seen in other parts of Europe and the United States. Steroids are generally effective treatment.

▌ Pathogenesis

The idiopathic inflammatory myopathies are believed to be immune-mediated processes possibly triggered by environmental factors in genetically susceptible individuals. This hypothesis is based on the recognized association with other autoimmune and collagen-vascular diseases, the prevalence and type of circulating autoantibodies, animal models, immunogenetic observations, specifics of the inflammatory changes in muscle, and the treatment response to immunosuppressive agents.

Two observations have provided strong support for the hypothesis that the idiopathic inflammatory myopathies are disorders of autoimmunity. First is the recognized association with other autoimmune diseases, including Hashimoto's thyroiditis, Graves' disease, myasthenia gravis, type I diabetes mellitus, primary biliary cirrhosis, inflammatory bowel disease, hepatitis C infection, dermatitis herpetiformis, primary vitiligo, and the collagen-vascular diseases. Second is the high prevalence of circulating autoantibodies.[2,6] The autoantibodies associated with PM and DM include the MSAs found almost exclusively in these diseases, autoantibodies that occur more commonly in myositis but are not specific, and those found in patients with overlap syndrome (see Table 80–5).

The MSAs can be categorized as to those directed at aminoacyl–transfer RNA (tRNA) synthetases, nonsynthetase cytoplasmic antigens, and nuclear antigens. The antisynthetases are the most commonly recognized MSAs, and anti–histidyl-tRNA synthetase, termed *anti–Jo-1*, is the most common of these. The antisynthetases show immunochemical properties, including the immunoprecipitation of tRNA, inhibition of enzyme function, and reaction with conformational epitopes. These properties are characteristic of autoantibodies. The antisynthetases do not cross-react. With extremely rare exceptions, an individual patient has only one antisynthetase.

The combination of the clinical observation that an individual can have only one MSA and the demonstration of strong immunogenetic associations indicates that the presence of an MSA defines a clinical syndrome (see Table 80–6). Individuals with anti–Jo-1 or another antisynthetase have PM or DM with an increased prevalence of interstitial lung disease, arthritis, Raynaud's phenomenon, fever, and mechanic's hands. In fact, perhaps 80 percent of patients with myositis and interstitial lung disease have circulating antisynthetase antibodies. In contrast, individuals with anti–signal recognition particle (SRP) antibodies have PM and are refractory to therapy; those with anti–Mi-2 have typical DM with a very good prognosis.

The cause, or triggering event, of the idiopathic inflammatory myopathies is unknown, but viruses have been strongly implicated. The seasonal variation in the onset of disease among different MSA subsets (first half of the year for antisynthetase syndrome and latter half for anti-SRP) is indirect evidence that infectious agents may play a role. Interestingly, certain picornaviruses can serve as a substrate for aminoacyl-tRNA synthetase activity and can be charged with the respective amino acid. Furthermore, some homology exists among amino acid sequences near the active site of *Escherichia coli* histidyl-tRNA synthetase (Jo-1), muscle proteins, and a capsid protein of encephalomyocarditis virus, which is a picornavirus that induces a model of myositis in mice. Although no homology exists between human and *E. coli* histidyl-tRNA synthetase, antibodies initially directed against a virus or a virus-enzyme complex could react with homologous areas of host proteins, resulting in autoantibody production by the process of molecular mimicry.

Although evidence suggests that viruses could cause autoantibody production, more compelling evidence supports the hypothesis that the idiopathic inflammatory myopathies are actually caused by viruses. Clearly, some viruses such as coxsackievirus A9, which has been cultured from muscle, can cause myositis. Elevated titers to coxsackievirus have been found in some children with juvenile DM; mumps virus antigen has been identified in inclusions in muscle from some patients with IBM; and enteroviral genomes have been identified in muscle from some patients with PM and DM.[70,71] Furthermore, human immunodeficiency virus (HIV) and human T lymphotropic virus type-1 induce a myositis in humans that is immunopathologically indistinguishable from idiopathic PM.[72]

The most striking evidence of a viral cause for the idiopathic inflammatory myopathies is found in animal models, in which chronic myositis develops after infection with a picornavirus and persists long after virus can no longer be detected in the tissue.[73] The best-described models are produced by injecting coxsackievirus B1 into neonatal Swiss mice or by infecting adult BALB/c mice with encephalomyocarditis virus 221A. A model of inflammatory myopathy induced by *Trypanosoma cruzi* infection of CBA/J mice provides evidence that other infectious agents might serve as environmental triggers for this disease.[74]

GENETIC MARKERS

Genetic factors are also important with regard to the inflammatory myopathies. Familial cases of idiopathic inflammatory myopathies are reported in monozygotic twins, siblings, parent-child pairs, and first-degree relatives of patients. These familial occurrences indicate an immunogenetic relationship in some cases. Although no direct relationships have been established between an inflammatory myopathy and a specific genetic marker, several observations support the premise that different pathogenetic mechanisms are involved in different diagnostic groups. The strongest associations exist for human leukocyte antigen (HLA)-B8, HLA-DR3, and DRW52 phenotypes in both children and adults with PM and DM.[2,27] In one study, white patients had a 48-percent prevalence of HLA-DR3 with a 96-percent linkage to B8, whereas black patients had no increase in HLA-DR3 but a 50 percent linkage to HLA-B8. The frequency of HLA-B8 and HLA-DR3 is especially high in the subset of white patients with anti-Jo-1 antibodies. The overall incidence of DRW52 is 75 percent, with more than 90 percent of patients with anti-Jo-1 antibodies carrying this marker.[6] Other studies have shown a greater frequency of HLA-B14 in whites and HLA-B7 and DRW6 in blacks with PM but not with DM. HLA-DRB1*0301, the linked allele DQA1 *0501, and DRB1 alleles sharing the first hypervariable region motif9 EYSTS13 are major genetic risk factors for the development of myositis in whites.[75,76] Both *0501 and *0401 are observed in blacks. These associations are stronger among patients with circulating antisynthetase antibodies. In contrast, no HLA-DRB1, nor DQA1 allele or motif, has been identified as a risk factor in Korean patients with myositis. This finding, and other data, indicate that the development of an idiopathic inflammatory myopathy is modulated by difficult genes and perhaps different environmental factors in different populations around the world.

Among the white patients with PM and DM with DQA1*0501 and in white patients with PM and DM,[76,77] there is a greater prevalence of TNF-α–308A allele (an A for G substitution at the-308 position of the TNF promoter region).[78] Children with TNF-α–308A allele tend to have disease course of longer duration.

The strongest genetic association for sporadic IBM is with HLA-DR3. In many cases there is a further association with an extended haplotype marked by HLA-DR3/B8.[79] A potential site for the susceptibility gene is the region between HLADR and C4.[80] Furthermore, phylogenetic analysis of the D-loop region of mitochondrial DNA has disclosed a common polymorphism, 16311C, in many patients with sporadic IBM.[81] The most common types of hereditary IBM are autosomal recessive. The abnormality is linked to chromosome 9p1-q1 and may be allelic.[82,83] A Swedish autosomal dominant form is linked to chromosome 17p13 and results from a missense mutation in the myosin heavy chain IIA gene.[84]

IMMUNOPATHOLOGY

The pathologic changes in muscle provide the strongest evidence that these diseases have an immune-mediated pathogenesis.[85,86] The changes in PM and IBM appear to result from cell-mediated antigen-specific cytotoxicity.[7,24,27] Non-necrotic muscle fibers are seen surrounded and invaded by CD8+ mononuclear cells, with cytotoxic cells outnumbering suppressor cells by a ratio of 3:1 in the CD8+ population. The activation marker HLA-DR is present in one third of all lymphocytes found in muscle and 50 percent of those invading muscle fibers. B cells and natural killer (NK) cells do not appear to play a significant role in PM or IBM.

CD8+ T cells do participate in antigen-directed cytotoxicity. To carry out this function, CD8+ T cells must recognize HLA class I molecules on the target, and class I molecules are upregulated in muscle fibers in PM and IBM. In addition, the muscle fibers in these diseases express the adhesive molecule intercellular adhesion molecule-1 (ICAM-1), and CD8+ T cells express the complementary adhesion molecule lymphocyte function–associated antigen-1, involving the cytotoxic lymphocytes to form their attack on muscle fibers.[86-88]

This does appear to be an antigen-driven process. The lymphocytes in muscle express the surface marker CD45R0, a marker indicating that they are antigen-primed T cells. In addition, the T cell antigen markers on the infiltrating and invading cells are oligoclonal, a finding implicating a cytotoxic process driven by defined antigens.[55,57] Finally, approximately 10 percent of the infiltrating lymphocytes bear the Ki-67 nuclear antigen. This finding suggests that a portion of the T cells in muscle have proliferated in situ. Reports of finding restricted expression of T cell receptor (TCR) gene families among the autoinvasive T cells persisting during the course of disease indicates that the same antigen drives the immune response throughout.[89]

When electron microscopy is used, the CD8+ cells are found to adhere to the fibers, sending spider-like projections through a seemingly intact membrane, indicating that these cells are attached to specific antigens on the sarcolemma. The mechanism causing cell death is uncertain. Possibilities include osmotic lysis as a result of perforin-created pores or apoptosis. Perforin and granzymes have been identified in the CD8+ cells infiltrating muscle, and these granules are oriented to the surface in contact with the muscle fibers. In addition, the elements necessary for apoptotic cell death,

Fas ligand on T cells, and Fas expression on muscle fibers, are present.[90] However, the pore-like structures suggestive of the effect of perforin have not been demonstrated, nor has any evidence of apoptosis been identified.[91] It appears that the expression of Fas antigen on diseased muscle fibers is related to an unknown biologic function in the process of fiber injury and not to apoptosis.

Although the previously mentioned features are observed in PM and IBM, the two conditions differ in other ways.[54] In IBM, the inflammatory infiltrate lessens over time, rimmed vacuoles are present on histologic examination, atrophic and angulated fibers (changes suggesting denervation) are observed, filamentous structures are found with electron microscopy, and amyloid (β-amyloid, β-amyloid precursor protein, hyperphosphorylated tau, and prion protein) deposits are present in all biopsies and in 70 percent of vacuolated fibers.[82,92] These amyloid proteins appear to accumulate before vacuolization and are similar to those found in Alzheimer's disease. Amyloid proteins are present in postsynaptic neuromuscular junctions in normal muscle. It is speculated that genetic control of amyloid accumulation is lost and the process spreads to nonjunctional sites. In experimental molecules, overproduction of amyloid is accompanied by the formation of small filaments, tubulofilaments, amorphous deposits, and small congophilic deposits similar to those seen in tissue from patients with IBM.[93] In addition, there is evidence of overexpression of αB-crystallin, a heat-shock protein. Upregulation of this protein in IBM muscle fibers indicates a tissue response to a stressor yet to be identified.[94]

In contrast to their role in PM and IBM, humoral immune mechanisms appear to play a greater role in DM.[7,27] The cellular infiltrates are predominantly perivascular and composed of B cells and CD4+ T cells. CD8+ cells, activated T cells, and perforin granules are rare. Major histocompatibility complex (MHC) class II molecules are expressed on muscle fibers. The vasculopathy that is so prominent in juvenile DM is also present in the adult form of the disease.

The findings suggest that DM is the result of antigen-driven CD4+ and T cells providing help to B cells that generate antibodies that participate with complement, damaging the microvasculature. Capillary damage may be the earliest lesion in DM[28] and lead to perifascicular atrophy (see Fig. 80–4). The vessels show upregulation of the adhesion molecule ICAM-1 and expression of vascular cell adhesion molecule-1 (VCAM-1)[87]; are the site of inflammatory cell clustering; and contain deposits of immunoglobulins (Igs) and the terminal (C5 to C9) membrane attack complex (MAC) of complement. The finding of decreased CD59 expression along with the MAC deposition on the sarcolemma and muscle vessels of patients with DM supports a role for complement in the pathway in the pathogenesis of this disease.[95]

Despite characteristic differences in the clinical features, histopathology, and immunohistochemistry among PM, DM, and IBM, interleukin 1α(1L-1α) is expressed in the muscle blood vessels in each and MCH class, I and II molecules are expressed on muscle fiber membranes in PM and dermamyositis.[96-98] These changes are present on vessels and fibers independent of adjacent inflammatory infiltration.[98,99] In addition, functional defects in muscle appear to be more related to 1L-1α expression in capillaries than to the presence of inflammatory cells. Finally, improvement of muscle function in patients with PM and DM correlates not only with a disappearance of T cells, but also with decreased expression of 1L-1α, ICAM-1, VCAM-1, leukocyte-associated function antigen-1 (LFA-1) in vessels and MHC class I antigens and fibers.[100]

CAUSES OF WEAKNESS

The muscle weakness that occurs in an inflammatory myopathy may result directly from the loss of muscle fibers destroyed by that immune response and subsequent fibrosis. On the other hand, additional mechanisms must come into play, at least in part, because weakness occurs in some individuals with muscle histologic examinations showing no inflammatory cells or evidence of fiber necrosis. These observations suggest that abnormalities of the contractile process or membrane defects may underlie the symptoms of muscle weakness. TNF-α, a cytokine found in some myositic muscle, is known to inhibit contractile function of skeletal muscle.[101]

Both muscle contraction and the maintenance of membrane integrity are energy (adenosine triphosphate [ATP])-dependent processes. It is also possible, therefore, that disordered energy metabolism in skeletal muscle fibers is responsible for at least some of the muscle weakness in the idiopathic inflammatory myopathies. The hypothesis that inflammatory myopathies are associated with altered muscle-cell energetics is supported by studies of animals and human disease.[27,102,103] Studies using magnetic resonance spectroscopy, a noninvasive method of measuring high-energy phosphate compounds in tissue, have shown that patients with PM and DM deplete ATP pools more rapidly and take longer to restore baseline levels than do healthy control subjects.[33,103] In addition, these parameters improve with effective therapy.

▌ Differential Diagnosis

Although the idiopathic inflammatory myopathies are relatively rare diseases, the list of diseases that cause myopathic symptoms for which patients seek medical attention is long (Table 80–9). Myopathic symptoms include fixed muscle weakness, or the inability to perform specific tasks, such as climbing stairs or raising the hands above the head; early or premature fatigue; and cramping or myalgia after muscular activity. The symptoms of myopathic diseases can range from chronic and mild to acute and fulminate. Some symptoms allow individuals to live comfortably, provided that they sufficiently limit their physical activity; others are severe and associated with profound disability or rhabdomyolysis, myoglobinuria, and renal failure.

TABLE 80–9 • CATEGORIES OF DISEASES AND DISORDERS THAT CAN CAUSE MYOPATHIC SYMPTOMS

Neuropathic Diseases
  Muscular dystrophies
  Denervating conditions
  Neuromuscular junction disorders
  Proximal neuropathies
  Myotonic diseases
Neoplasms
Drug-Related Conditions
Infections
Metabolic
  Primary
  Secondary
    Storage Diseases and Inborn Errors of Metabolism
    Mitochondrial myopathies
Nutritional Toxic
Endocrine disorders
Rhabdomyolysis
Miscellaneous Causes
  Amyloidosis
  Sarcoidosis
  Atherosclerotic emboli
  Behçet's disease
  Fibromyalgia
  Psychosomatic

NEUROLOGIC DISEASES

Neurologic diseases (Table 80–10) generally can be differentiated from PM because of the occurrence of asymmetric weakness, distal extremity involvement, altered sensorium, or abnormal cranial nerve function.[104] Generally, myopathies cause only proximal and symmetric weakness. Exceptions include some cases of mitochondrial myopathies, IBM, and myositis associated with anti-SRP antibodies, which may have "neuropathic" features.

The muscular dystrophies often have a positive family history. The limb-girdle dystrophy syndromes are perhaps most easily confused with inflammatory muscle disease. Upper and lower extremity proximal muscle weakness may begin in the first through third decades of life and is eventually accompanied by muscle wasting. Shoulder and pelvic girdle muscles are also most commonly affected in Duchenne's muscular dystrophy and Becker's muscular dystrophy. The onset of Duchenne's muscular dystrophy is usually by the age of 5 years. In addition to muscle weakness and wasting, individuals develop winging of the scapulae, a hyperlordotic gait, and pseudohypertrophy of the calf muscles. Patients usually cannot walk after the age of 11 years and die of respiratory failure by the age of 20 years. Becker's muscular dystrophy is similar but generally milder, with patients able to walk beyond the age of 16 years. Facioscapulohumeral muscular dystrophy is an autosomal dominant disorder with a better prognosis. Weakness characteristically begins in the facial muscles. Medical attention is usually sought after shoulder weakness develops.

The spinal muscle atrophies are generally autosomal recessive disorders that cause degeneration of the spinal anterior horn cells. The onset may occur at any age. The distribution of muscles involved is dependent on the specific cord segments affected, and accordingly, the weakness tends to be localized rather than diffuse. Amyotrophic lateral sclerosis is associated with lower motor neuron denervation, upper motor neuron signs, and bulbar or pseudobulbar palsy.

Although proximal muscle weakness, especially of the upper extremities, may be the dominant clinical feature of myasthenia gravis, extraocular and bulbar muscle involvement and marked fatigability help differentiate it from PM. Eaton-Lambert syndrome also causes proximal muscle weakness. Although approximately two thirds of individuals with Eaton-Lambert syndrome have an associated neoplastic disease, it can occur in the absence of cancer, especially when it develops before the age of 40 years.[105]

Conditions considered under the classification of proximal neuropathies can cause myopathic symptoms and are occasionally confused with PM. These include diabetic amyotrophy and plexopathy, Guillain-Barré syndrome, and acute intermittent porphyria.

NEOPLASIA

Cancer must be considered in the evaluation of patients with myopathic symptoms. The association between myositis and malignancy was discussed earlier. The weakness and fatigue that develop in the progress of a neoplastic disease may result from the systemic effects of cytokines released by the tumor cells or by virtue of the immune response to the malignancy. In addition, prominent neuromuscular changes can develop as features of paraneoplastic syndrome.[105] Eaton-Lambert syndrome is an example of this. These individuals have excessive fatigability on exertion and weakness that may be profound and exclusively proximal in distribution. Patients report that their strength is reduced at rest but may increase at the first of repetitive movements, only to decrease with continued exercise. EMG readily differentiates this diagnosis from myasthenia gravis and PM. The proximal myopathy that develops in patients with carcinoid syndrome is probably the result of compounds produced by the cancer cells.

TABLE 80–10 • NEUROLOGIC DISEASES MOST OFTEN CONFUSED WITH INFLAMMATORY MUSCLE DISEASE

Muscular Dystrophies	**Neuromuscular Junction**
Duchenne's muscular	**Disorders**
dystrophy	Myasthenia gravis
Becker's muscular dystrophy	Eaton-Lambert syndrome
Facioscapulohumeral muscular	**Proximal Neuropathies**
dystrophy	Diabetic amyotrophy
Limb-girdle muscular dystrophy	Guillain-Barré syndrome
Myotonic dystrophy	Autoimmune
Denervating Conditions	polyneuropathies
Spinal muscular atrophies	Acute intermittent
Amyotrophic lateral sclerosis	porphyria

DRUG-RELATED CONDITIONS

A long list of drugs can cause myopathic changes[106] (see Tables 80–6 and 80–11). The list includes some drugs commonly used in a rheumatology practice. Glucocorticoid use causes proximal muscle weakness and wasting. EMG changes are minimal and, if present, nonspecific. Biopsy of muscle shows only type II fiber atrophy. This condition may be difficult to diagnose when it develops in patients being treated for inflammatory muscle disease. In addition, glucocorticoid use is strongly implicated in the etiology of critical illness myopathy.[107,108]

Colchicine, chloroquine, and hydroxychloroquine can cause an axonal neuromyopathy with vacuoles on biopsy. This toxicity is invariably associated with high CK levels. Withdrawal of the drug should rapidly lead to clinical improvement and normalization of the CK level. Some patients receiving D-Penicillamine develop autoimmune syndromes, including PM and myasthenia gravis.

The exact mechanism by which many drugs cause myopathy is uncertain. Some myopathies, such as those caused by D-Penicillamine, hydralazine, and procainamide, are immune mediated. Some, such as those caused by alcohol, result from direct toxic effects. Still other drugs may cause metabolic or electrolyte abnormalities. For example, statins, fibrates and niacin may alter muscle fiber energetics, although statin use has also been associated with the development of PM.[109,110]

INFECTIONS

Numerous infections can cause a myopathy (Table 80–12), and many may be confused with PM.[111] For example, patients, especially children, with influenza A

TABLE 80–11 • DRUGS THAT CAN CAUSE MYOPATHIC SYMPTOMS OR SYNDROMES*

Amiodarone	Hydralazine
Aspirin	Hydroxychloroquine
Bezafibrate	Ipecac
Chloroquine	Ketoconazole
Cimetidine	Labetalol
Clofibrate	Levodopa
Cocaine	Lovastatin
Colchicine	Nicotinic acid
Cyclosporine	Nalidixic acid
D,L-Carnitine	Penicillin
Danazol	D-Penicillamine
Enalapril	Phenytoin
Epsilon aminocaproic acid	Pivampicillin
Etofibrate	Pravastatin
Fenofibrate	Ranitidine
Flecainide	Rifampin
Fluvastatin	Simvastatin
Gemfibrozil	Sulfonamides
Glucocorticoids	L-Tryptophan
Glycyrrhiza	Valproic acid
Gold salts	Vincristine
Heroin	Zidovudine (AZT)

*In addition, any drug or hormone that can raise or lower serum concentrations of sodium, potassium, calcium, phosphorus, or magnesium can induce myopathic symptoms.

TABLE 80–12 • INFECTIOUS CAUSES OF MYOSITIS

Viral
Adenoviruses 2, 21
Coxsackieviruses A9, B1, B2, B3, B4, B5
Cytomegalovirus
Echovirus A9
Epstein-Barr virus
Hepatitis B virus
Human immunodeficiency virus (HIV)
Human T cell lymphotrophic virus type 1
Influenza A and B viruses
Mumps virus
Rubella virus
Varicella-zoster virus
Fungal
Candida
Cryptococcus
Bacterial
Borrelia burgdorferi (Lyme spirochete)
Clostridium perfringens
Mycobacterium leprae
Tuberculosis
Mycoplasma pneumoniae
Rickettsia
Staphylococcus
Streptococcus
Parasitic
Microsporidia
Schistosoma
Toxoplasma gondii
Trypanosoma cruzi
Helminthic
Echinococcus
Trichinella

and B viral infections can experience severe myalgias associated with very high (up to 15 times normal) CK levels and nonspecific myopathic changes, including fiber necrosis and inflammatory cell infiltration on muscle biopsy. A subacute myositis has also been described after rubella infection and after immunization with live-attenuated rubella virus.

Acquired immune deficiency syndrome (AIDS) represents a very complicated situation.[112,113] Weakness is a common finding in patients suffering from AIDS. The possible causes include the generalized debilitated, cachectic state; central or peripheral nervous system diseases; PM emerging as a consequence of the altered immune function; infections with HIV, cytomegalovirus, Mycobacterium avium-intracellulare, Cryptococcus, Trichinella, or Toxoplasma; pyomyositis; and the toxic effects of zidovudine (AZT). Biopsies of muscle from patients with AIDS and the AIDS-related complex who have not received AZT therapy are abnormal in 70 to 96 percent of cases.[114] Among the changes noted are "moth-eaten" fibers (76 percent), type II fiber atrophy (58 percent), endomysial or perimysial or perivascular mononuclear cell infiltrates, or all of these (36 percent), and vasculitis with perifascicular atrophy (4 percent). AZT use can cause mitochondrial myopathy.

Bacterial causes of myositis are important to recognize because the diagnosis allows effective treatment with the appropriate antibiotics. Pyomyositis is a focal suppurative process.[115,116] Typically, abscesses, most often caused by streptococcal infection, are found in one or more proximal muscles, usually in the lower extremities. Myositis can also be associated with Lyme borreliosis.[117] Among the parasites that cause myositis, *Toxoplasma* is the most common in the United States. Toxoplasmosis can cause an acute or subacute illness resembling PM.[118]

METABOLIC MYOPATHIES

The term *metabolic myopathy* represents a heterogeneous group of conditions (Table 80–13) that have in common abnormalities in muscle energy metabolism that result in skeletal muscle dysfunction.[119] Some metabolic myopathies should be considered primary and are associated with known or postulated biochemical defects that affect the ability of the muscle fibers to maintain adequate levels of ATP.[120] The prevalence of

---

TABLE 80–13 • METABOLIC MYOPATHIES

Disordered Glycogen Metabolism
Myophosphorylase deficiency (McArdle's disease)
Phosphorylase *b* kinase deficiency
Phosphofructokinase deficiency
Debrancher enzyme deficiency
Brancher enzyme deficiency
Phosphoglycerate kinase deficiency
Phosphoglycerate mutase deficiency
Lactate dehydrogenase deficiency
Acid maltase deficiency
Endocrine
Acromegaly
Hypothyroidism
Hyperthyroidism
Hyperparathyroidism
Cushing's disease
Addison's disease
Hyperaldosteronism
Carcinoid syndrome
Diabetes mellitus
Myoadenylate Deaminase Deficiency
Mitochondrial Myopathies
Disordered Lipid Metabolism
Carnitine deficiency
Inherited
Acquired
Carnitine palmitoyltransferase deficiency
Fatty acid acyl-CoA dehydrogenase deficiency
Coenzyme Q$_{10}$ deficiency
Metabolic Nutritional
Uremia
Hepatic failure
Malabsorption
Periodic paralysis
Vitamin D deficiency
Vitamin E deficiency
Electrolyte Disorders
Hypernatremia
Hyponatremia
Hyperkalemia
Hypokalemia
Hypercalcemia
Hypocalcemia
Hypophosphatemia
Hypomagnesemia

---

these disorders appears to be greater than previously appreciated. Other metabolic myopathies may be considered secondary and attributed to various endocrine or electrolyte abnormalities.

Primary Metabolic Myopathies

Disorders of Glycogen Metabolism

Eleven diseases have been identified that have in common an underlying defect in glycogen synthesis, glycogenolysis, or glycolysis.[121] They are often referred to as the *glycogen storage diseases* (GSDs) because each defect results in the abnormal deposition and accumulation of glycogen in skeletal muscle. Many of these can present in children and adults in a fashion that is difficult to differentiate from an inflammatory myopathy.[122]

The classic clinical manifestation of a GSD is exercise intolerance, which may be attributed to pain, fatigue, stiffness, weakness, or intense cramping. Most afflicted persons are well at rest and can function without difficulty at low levels of activity and during periods when lipids provide the major source of muscle energy. Symptoms develop after activities of high intensity and short duration or of less intensive effort for longer intervals—times when the majority of energy for muscular work is derived from carbohydrate. Some patients experience a "second wind" phenomenon. Although they must stop an activity because of exercise-induced symptoms, they are often able to resume the exercise after a brief rest. Most patients develop some symptoms during childhood, but significant problems such as severe cramping or exercise-induced rhabdomyolysis and myoglobinuria with renal failure may not develop until the teenage years. A subset of patients, however, complain only of easy fatigability, whereas others develop the gradual onset of proximal muscle weakness. The latter presentation, which often occurs in adulthood (the oldest patient reported was diagnosed at the age of 78 years), may be difficult to differentiate from PM.

Confusion of GSD with inflammatory muscle disease results because serum CK levels are commonly elevated and EMG shows increased insertional irritability, increased numbers of polyphasic motor unit potentials, fibrillations, and positive waves. Each of these is a nonspecific abnormality that can be seen in inflammatory myopathies. On muscle biopsy, fiber necrosis and phagocytosis may be noted.

The diagnosis of GSDs may be suggested by finding the classic changes of glycogen deposition on muscle biopsy. The finding of excessive glycogen deposition is not specific and can be seen in IBM, mitochondrial myopathies, and other diseases. However, these changes may be missed in patients with a GSD in the presence of significant rhabdomyolysis. In other patients, the changes may be inapparent with the use of only light microscopy and may require electron microscopy to be appreciated. The forearm ischemic exercise test is a useful method of screening for a GSD. Individuals with GSD, except those with acid maltase deficiency, fail to generate lactate during ischemic exercise. The putative diagnosis should always be confirmed by specific enzyme analysis of muscle tissue whenever it is suspected, by either histologic examination or ischemic exercise testing.

Inherited deficiency of acid maltase presents in infantile, childhood, and adult forms. The last typically manifests as proximal muscle weakness beginning after the age of 20 years and may be misdiagnosed as PM or limb-girdle muscular dystrophy. Diaphragmatic involvement and respiratory failure develop in one third of patients. Acid maltase activity is localized to lysosomes and does not affect cytosolic glycogen metabolism. Therefore, a deficiency will not affect the results of ischemic exercise testing. The diagnosis of adult acid maltase deficiency should usually be suspected because of the characteristic EMG changes of intense electric irritability and myotonic discharges in the absence of clinical myotonia and can be established finding deficient α-glucosidase activity in muscle or leukocytes.

Disorders of Lipid Metabolism

The recognized disorders of lipid metabolism that cause myopathic problems are due to abnormalities in the transport and processing of fatty acids for energy. Carnitine palmitoyltransferase activities are necessary for the transport of long-chain fatty acid into mitochondria. Carnitine palmitoyltransferase deficiency is an autosomal recessive disorder that invariably causes attacks of severe myalgia and myoglobinuria.[120,123] These are typically associated with vigorous physical activity but may occur with fasting, infection, or cold exposure. The initiation of ibuprofen therapy has been implicated in one case. Serum CK levels, EMGs, and muscle histologic examinations are normal except during episodes of rhabdomyolysis. The diagnosis is made by assaying muscle tissue for enzyme activity, which reveals a partial deficiency.

Carnitine is an essential intermediate that acts as a carrier of long-chain fatty acids into mitochondria, where they can undergo β-oxidation. Carnitine deficiency causes abnormal lipid deposition in skeletal muscle and can result from inherited or acquired causes. Primary carnitine deficiencies can be divided into *systemic* and *muscle* types. Symptoms of *systemic carnitine deficiency* develop early in life, with episodes of coma and hypoketotic hypoglycemia similar to Reye's syndrome. This may be associated with deficiency of short-, medium-, or long-chain acyl-CoA dehydrogenase activities or a defect in cellular uptake of carnitine. Patients with *muscle carnitine deficiency* present in later childhood or during the early adult years with chronic muscle weakness. The process affects mainly proximal muscles but may also involve facial and pharyngeal musculature. Acquired carnitine deficiencies have been reported with pregnancy, renal failure requiring long-term hemodialysis, end-stage cirrhosis, myxedema, adrenal insufficiency, and therapy with valproate or pivampicillin.

Carnitine deficiency may be confused with PM because serum CK levels are elevated in more than half the patients and EMG often reveals polyphasic motor unit potentials (MUPs) of small amplitude and short duration. The diagnosis should be considered when abnormal deposits of lipid are identified by histochemical analysis of muscle tissue. Only 50 percent of patients with carnitine deficiency respond to dietary supplementation with L-carnitine. Treatment with dietary manipulation, prednisone, or propranolol has provided success in a few patients refractory to L-carnitine treatment.

Deficiencies of the three fatty acid acyl-CoA dehydrogenase activities have been reported in a 38-year-old man who presented with a 2-year history of proximal muscle weakness, neck pain, high CK levels, myopathic changes on EMG, and abnormal lipid accumulation in muscle tissue. Riboflavin therapy resulted in normalization of the histologic appearance of muscle and in improved strength. Riboflavin therapy was considered because the acyl-CoA dehydrogenases are flavin-containing proteins.

Muscle coenzyme Q10 deficiency has been described in two teenaged sisters who had abnormal fatigability and slowly progressive weakness of proximal limb and trunk muscles that began in childhood. Subsequently, each developed tremor, ataxia, and dysarthria. Coenzyme Q10 is an obligatory receptor of electrons derived from oxidation of fatty acids. Histologic examination of muscle revealed marked lipid accumulation, and all type I fibers were ragged andred. Oral coenzyme Q10 therapy improved muscle strength and other symptoms.

Myoadenylate Deaminase Deficiency

Myoadenylate deaminase deficiency exists in primary and secondary forms.[124] The primary form is inherited in an autosomal recessive pattern and is common, being found in up to 2 percent of muscle biopsy specimens. In the cast majority of individuals, the primary deficiency is due to a nonsense mutation at codon 12 of the adenosine monophosphate (AMP) deaminase-1 gene.[125] This mutation has also been identified in 22 percent of normal individuals and individuals with other recognized neuromuscular diseases, causing most to doubt the clinical significance of the deficiency state. Indeed, almost all patients with myoadenylate deaminase deficiency are asymptomatic. Symptomatic patients generally report weakness or cramping after exercise. Patients with primary myoadenylate deaminase deficiency have normal, or minimally elevated, serum CK levels, normal EMGs, and a normal histologic appearance of muscle. The forearm ischemic exercise test is, however, abnormal. Myoadenylate deaminase–deficient persons can release lactate into the circulation after ischemic exercise but fail to generate ammonia.

The secondary forms appear to be acquired in the course of a variety of neuromuscular diseases, including PM, DM, scleroderma, and SLE. The molecular basis for the secondary deficiencies appears to differ. In PM, the deficiency is correlated with diminishing amounts of otherwise normal AMP deaminase mRNA.

Mitochondrial Myopathies

The term *mitochondrial myopathy* refers to a clinically heterogeneous group of disorders that have in common morphologic abnormalities in the number, size, or structure of mitochondria.[126] The metabolic abnormalities described in these conditions are numerous and can be attributed to defects in nutrient transport; processing of pyruvate and acetyl coenzyme A; oxidative phosphorylation; the respiratory (electron transport) chain; or energy conservation. It appears that many mitochondrial myopathies are inherited through maternal transmission and are caused by defects in mitochondrial DNA. The clinical spectrum of these conditions is quite diverse and includes progressive muscular weakness, external ophthalmoplegia with or without proximal myopathy, progressive exercise intolerance, and multisystem disease. More than 25 specific enzyme abnormalities have been described, of which at least six may present with exercise intolerance or progressive muscular weakness in adults. In addition, mitochondrial myopathy may develop in patients who have received long-term AZT therapy.[114]

Secondary Metabolic Myopathies

A host of endocrine and metabolic disorders may lead to myopathic symptoms (see Table 80–13). Proximal muscle weakness is a major feature of Cushing's syndrome. Both hypothyroidism and hyperthyroidism can produce proximal muscle weakness and elevated serum CK values. Hyperparathyroidism may cause proximal weakness, high CK levels, and myopathic EMG changes. The basis for the weakness in these disorders is related, in part, to hormonal or toxic effects on muscle contractility. Electrolyte disorders must also play a crucial role. In fact, virtually any electrolyte disturbance may result in myopathic symptoms (Table 80–14). Finally, skeletal muscle infarction can occur in diabetes mellitus.[127]

Rhabdomyolysis

Rhabdomyolysis is not a disease. Rather, it is the consequence of any cause of extensive muscle necrosis. Although rhabdomyolysis is most commonly associated with severe muscle injury, it may be caused by a variety of conditions[128] (Table 80–15). The clinical result of rhabdomyolysis is intense myalgia associated with muscle tenderness and swelling. Serum CK values may reach levels 2000 times normal. If the cause or offending agent is corrected or removed, the muscle can heal remarkably quickly, with few or no residual effects. Permanent weakness and atrophy are rare unless significant infarction has occurred or the rhabdomyolysis has developed in relation to myositis or another myopathy.

Potential complications of massive muscle necrosis include hypocalcemia, hyperuricemia, myoglobinuria, and hyperkalemia. Hypocalcemia results from the sequestration of calcium by necrotic muscle. The risk of hypocalcemia decreases within the first days after the onset. Serum urate concentrations increase as a result of the accelerated breakdown of ATP associated with damaged muscle plus a block in uric acid excretion due to a concomitant acidosis or renal failure.

The most threatening complication of rhabdomyolysis is acute tubular necrosis. The risk of renal failure increases directly with the height of the serum CK, potassium, and phosphorus levels; with urine myoglobin levels higher than 1 μg/ml; inversely with serum albumin levels; and in the presence of dehydration or sepsis as the underlying cause. It is characterized by oliguria, myoglobinuria, urine containing pigmented granular casts, and a high serum creatinine level. Acute uric acid nephropathy may also complicate the picture. Treatment is essentially supportive. When myoglobinuria is identified, a diuresis should be established in hopes of preventing renal failure. An alkalinization of

TABLE 80–14 • MYOPATHIC SYMPTOMS RESULTING FROM ELECTROLYTE ABNORMALITIES

Ion	Abnormality	Weakness	Myalgia	Cramps
Calcium	Hypercalcemia	+	+	−
	Hypocalcemia	+	+	+
Magnesium	Hypomagnesemia	+	+	+
Phosphorus	Hypophosphatemia	+	+	+
Potassium	Hyperkalemia	+	−	−
	Hypokalemia	+	+	+
Sodium	Hypernatremia	+	+	+
	Hyponatremia	+	−	+

TABLE 80–15 • CAUSES OF RHABDOMYOLYSIS

Trauma
Crush injury (with or without coma)
Excessive exercise (marathon running, military training)
Electric shock (lightning, high-voltage injury, electroshock therapy)
Muscle activity (status epilepticus, delirium tremens)
High temperature (malignant hyperthermia, heat stroke, malignant neuroleptic syndrome, infection)
Ischemic injury (thromboembolism, sickle cell trait)
Drugs and Toxins
Recreational (alcohol, barbiturates, heroin, cocaine)
Lipid lowering (clofibrate, bezafibrate, gemfibrozil, lovastatin, pravastatin, simvastatin) high-dose niacin
Venoms (rattlesnake, sea snake, hornet, red spider)
Infections
Viral (influenza virus, coxsackievirus, herpesvirus, echovirus, adenovirus, HIV-1)
Bacterial (*Staphylococcus*, typhoid, *Legionella*, *Clostridium*)
Metabolic Causes
Genetic (glycogen storage diseases, CPT deficiency, mitochondrial myopathies)
Electrolyte imbalance (hypocalcemia, hypernatremia, hypophosphatemia, hyperosmolar nonketotic states, acidosis)
Collagen Vascular Causes
Polymyositis
Dermatomyositis
Unknown Causes

Abbreviations: CPT, Carnitine palmitoyltransferase, HIV-1, human immunodeficiency virus-1.

the urine is also recommended, but this has not been proved to alter outcomes unless uric acid nephropathy is a component. The patient should also be monitored for hyperkalemia.

Testing for Muscle Disease

PHYSICAL EXAMINATION

The findings on physical examination of patients with an inflammatory disease of skeletal muscle are typical of those of most myopathic processes. Abnormalities are generally limited to the motor component of the examination, with weakness in a proximal and symmetric distribution. An objective determination of strength proves very useful in assessing the severity of disease as well as the effectiveness of therapy. The most frequently used system for assessing individual muscle groups is that of the Medical Research Council, which grades strength on a scale of zero (no contraction) to 5 (normal) (Table 80–16). This method is relatively insensitive. A useful method for following the progress of the disease is the timed-stands test.[129] This test involves counting the time needed to stand 10 times from a chair. The time required to perform this activity is quite reproducible in healthy individuals but does increase with age (Fig. 80–8). Other techniques are available.[130] Of them, serial measurement of isometric muscle strength with a hand-held pull gauge may be among the more useful.

LABORATORY TESTING

Chemistries

Elevation of levels of serum enzymes derived from skeletal muscle including CK, aldolase, AST, ALT, and lactate dehydrogenase helps confirm the presence of a myopathic process. High levels of these enzymes are found in the inflammatory diseases of muscle but are not specific for those diagnoses.[131] The CK is generally considered to be the most sensitive indication of an inflammatory myopathy. However, these are cases in which the CK is normal but another muscle enzyme is elevated.

CK is a dimer and exists in the serum in three isoforms: MM, MB, and BB. The MM form predominates

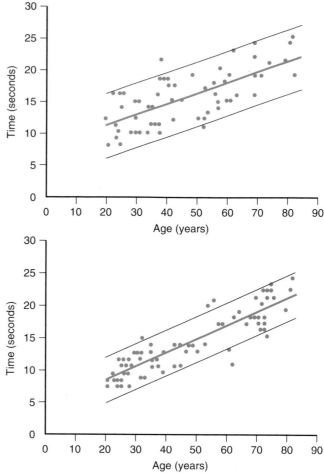

FIGURE 80–8 · Timed-stands Test as a Function of Age in 62 Healthy Women *(top)* and in 77 Healthy Men *(bottom)*. The mean and limits of normal (90% prediction region) are shown. (From Csuka M, McCarty DJ: A simple method for measurement of lower extremity muscle strength. Am J Med 78:77, 1985.)

in skeletal and cardiac muscle. MB constitutes about 25 percent of the total CK activity in cardiac tissue. MB is a very minor component in skeletal muscle but is present in that tissue in greater amounts in embryonal and regenerating fibers. BB is the major isoenzyme in brain and smooth muscle. It is important to determine the tissue source of CK whenever elevated levels are encountered.

The amount of CK in the serum is the result of that released from tissues minus that which is removed from the circulation. Most elevated serum CK levels result from muscle necrosis or leaking membranes. Accordingly, most elevations are of the MM isoform. However, the MB isoform can occur in myositis with no cardiac involvement and in healthy young women after submaximal eccentric exercise. Inflammatory or hypoxic injury, blunt trauma, and sharp trauma (intramuscular injections, EMG needle insertion, muscle biopsy) are well-recognized causes of high CK levels. Both isometric and aerobic exercise can also produce elevated CK levels, especially in poorly conditioned individuals. Furthermore, morphine, benzodiazepine derivatives, and barbiturate use may elevate the serum

TABLE 80–16 · SYSTEM FOR OBJECTIVE (SEMIQUANTITATIVE) GRADING OF MUSCLE STRENGTH

5	Normal power resistance
4	Power decreased but muscle contraction possible against resistance
3	Muscle contraction against gravity only
2	Muscle contraction possible only when gravity is eliminated
1	Contraction without motion
0	No contraction

CK levels by retarding the elimination of the enzyme from the circulation. CK elevations caused by cocaine use can be sustained even after months of abstinence. Circulating macro CK isoenzyme BB can cause misleading results.

Occasionally, elevated CK levels are observed in asymptomatic individuals. Racial differences in normal CK levels must be considered in this context. Healthy asymptomatic black males have higher total CK levels than those of whites or Hispanics, with the majority of values judged to be abnormal using the usual laboratory values. Men generally have higher values than women. Many of these asymptomatic elevations can be accounted for by exercise, medications, or hemolysis. Some indicate a carrier state for muscular dystrophy, and others are signs of early or mild myopathies. Some of these asymptomatic elevations, however, remain idiopathic. The terms asymptomatic (or benign) hyper-CK-emia are now being applied to individuals who have persistently elevated CK levels, but no evidence of disease.[132,133]

Myoglobin, the oxygen-binding heme protein, is released from injured skeletal and cardiac muscles and cleared in the urine. The serum myoglobin concentration is a sensitive indicator of muscle fiber integrity. Hypermyoglobinemia can result from any factor or disease that would raise serum CK levels. In some patients with myositis, the serum myoglobin level is occasionally elevated when CK levels are normal. Myoglobin may be detected in serum even when it goes undetected in urine. Myoglobinuria may occur in the absence of visible pigmenturia. The finding of positive tests for hemoglobin in the urine in the absence of red blood cells is indirect evidence of myoglobinuria.

The average man excretes 60 to 100 mg of creatine in the urine per 24 hours. Women excrete approximately twice those amounts. Increased excretion can occur with any cause of muscle atrophy.

Autoantibodies

Circulating autoantibodies can be detected in the sera in a large number of patients with inflammatory myopathies.[6,134] ANA testing may be positive at low titers in some patients with PM, 60 percent of children with childhood DM, and the majority of patients with an associated collagen-vascular disease or overlap syndrome. In the latter cases, patients may also have autoantibodies more specific for those diseases or syndromes (Table 80–17). Some patients with PM or DM have autoantibodies that are found almost exclusively in those conditions (see Table 80–5). These antibodies, termed *myositis-specific autoantibodies,* tend to be present in genetically restricted groups of patients, bind evolutionarily conserved epitopes, and identify relatively homogeneous groups of patients (see Table 80–6).

Electromyography

EMG is a valuable technique for determining the classification, distribution, and severity of diseases affecting skeletal muscle.[135] Although the changes identified are

TABLE 80–17 • AUTOANTIBODIES IN INFLAMMATORY MYOPATHIES ASSOCIATED WITH OTHER COLLAGEN-VASCULAR DISEASES OR OVERLAP SYNDROMES

Autoantibody	Disease Association
Anti-Sm	SLE
Anti-RNP	SLE, MCTD
Anti–Ro-SSA	Sjögren's syndrome
Anti-Ku	SLE, scleroderma
Anticentromere	CREST syndrome
ANCA	Wegener's granulomatosis
Anti–Scl-70	Scleroderma
Anti–PM-Scl	Scleroderma
Anti–U1-RNP	SLE, scleroderma

Abbreviations: SLE, systemic lupus erythematosus; MCTD, mixed connective tissue disease; CREST, calcinosis, Raynaud's phenomenon, esophageal motility disorders, sclerodactyly, and telangiectasia.

not specific, this technique should allow differentiation between myopathic and neuropathic conditions and, in the latter, localize the site of the abnormality to the central nervous system, spinal cord anterior horn cell, peripheral nerves, or neuromuscular junction. In addition, knowledge of the distribution and severity of abnormalities can guide selection of the most appropriate site for biopsy. Both spontaneous and voluntary activity can be affected by temperature, caffeine, and epinephrine, as well as the age of the patient.

Normal muscle is electrically silent at rest, with spontaneous activity noted only when the needle electrode passes through the muscle, mechanically stimulating or damaging the fibers. This is termed *insertional activity* and is characterized by a burst of spikes of varied amplitudes. Insertional activity may be increased with conditions causing irritability of fiber membranes or may be decreased if muscle fibers have been replaced by fat or fibrous tissue.

After insertional activity subsides, no potentials are generated in normal muscle unless the electrode is moved or the muscle is contracted. Abnormal spontaneous activity, however, may occur in a variety of disease states. Of the different forms of abnormal spontaneous activity, fibrillation potentials have the most diagnostic importance. These are generated by fibers that have lost their innervation. Most commonly, fibrillation potentials are the result of a loss of or damage to some part of a lower motor neuron; however, diseases of the neuromuscular junction and primary myopathies associated with fiber membrane damage also produce them. The term *positive waves* is used for fibrillation potentials with a characteristic form that are produced by fibers that have been damaged and have lost innervation. Myotonic discharges are another form of spontaneous activity. These differ from fibrillation in the rate and pattern of firing and are attributed to alterations in ion channels within the muscle fiber membrane. Myotonic discharges are not specific for any single disease or even for myopathic conditions. A third form of spontaneous activity is termed *complex repetitive discharges.* Also known as *bizarre high-frequency discharges* or *bizarre repetitive potentials*, these forms generally, but not invariably, indicate muscle disease and are more commonly observed in chronic disorders.

Additional information is provided from examination of potentials evoked by electric stimulation or those generated by a voluntary muscle contraction. Both methods cause the fibers within a motor unit to fire in a synchronous fashion, producing MUPs. The size and shape of an MUP depend on the number, density, size, conduction velocity, and synchrony of firing of muscle fibers within the recording area, as well as any intervening inactive fat or connective tissue. Normal MUPs are triphasic, ranging from 100 µV to 5 mV in amplitude and from 3 to 15 msec in duration. In general, the amplitude reflects the potential close to the electrode. During voluntary muscle contraction, the number of units activated increases with the force of contraction. The activation of additional motor units is termed *recruitment*.

Diseases can affect both the appearance of individual MUPs and recruitment. Typically, in diseases of muscle, MUPs have reduced amplitude and shortened duration. Although this pattern is often referred to as myopathic, these changes are not specific and also can be seen in neuropathic conditions such as anterior horn cell disease, diseases of peripheral nerves, and disturbances of neuromuscular transmission. An MUP is termed *polyphasic* if it contains more than four phases, or baseline crossings. Polyphasic MUPs occur when fibers within the unit fire asynchronously. This may result from degeneration and regeneration of fibers (as occurs in many myopathies), segmental fiber destruction, or longitudinal fiber splitting. Myopathies commonly cause altered recruitment, as do other diseases that reduce the number of motor units.

PATTERNS OF MYOPATHIC DISORDERS

The characteristic findings in myopathic disorders include individual MUPs of decreased duration and smaller amplitude; increased numbers of polyphasic potentials; a full recruitment pattern generated with full effort despite clinical weakness; and decreased amplitude and increased density of the complex interference pattern. Inflammatory myopathies cause changes that tend to be scattered in distribution and variable in character but are most marked in the proximal muscles and paraspinal muscles. Earlier in the disease, low-amplitude MUPs of short duration and spontaneous fibrillation potentials are observed. The spontaneous fibrillations often fire at a slower rate than those seen in neuropathic disorders. Over time, MUPs tend to become more polyphasic, and more positive waves are present within the fibrillation potentials.

The prominent spontaneous activity, which may also include scattered myotonic discharges and complex repetitive discharges, is characteristic of most inflammatory myopathies and distinguishes them from other myopathies. However, similar patterns of abnormalities can be seen with myasthenia gravis, GSDs, carnitine deficiency, congenital myopathies, botulism, Duchenne's muscular dystrophy, hyperkalemic periodic paralysis, rhabdomyolysis, and trauma.

The EMG pattern changes as the disease progresses and the myositic process becomes chronic. MUPs of longer duration and higher-than-normal amplitude appear as regenerated fibers are reinnervated. Recruitment is reduced in proportion to the number of motor units damaged or replaced. Insertional activity is diminished with increased fibrosis. Thus, it may be difficult to distinguish chronic myositis from chronic neurogenic atrophy.

The EMG features of primary metabolic myopathies are quite variable. Many patients may, in fact, have relatively normal studies. Myophosphorylase deficiency and carnitine deficiency may have so-called myopathic MUPs and some fibrillations, occasionally limited to the paraspinal muscles. The EMG features of acid maltase deficiency are, in contrast, pronounced, with prominent polyphasic MUPs in proximal muscles and striking fibrillation potentials, myotonic discharges, and complex repetitive discharges.

DISORDERS OF NEUROMUSCULAR TRANSMISSION

The findings in diseases that disturb neuromuscular transmission are among the most characteristic of EMG abnormalities. In myasthenia gravis, a standard EMG study may reveal small, short MUPs and fibrillations. The classic finding, however, is a decremental response to repetitive stimulation. Evoked potentials are initially normal but slowly and progressively decreased with successive stimuli. In contrast, repetitive stimulation of motor units in patients with Eaton-Lambert syndrome results in minimal responses initially, followed by progressive increases in amplitude.

NEUROPATHIC DISORDERS

Neuropathic disorders are characterized by denervation and reinnervation. These processes result in spontaneous activity, including a fibrillation potential and positive waves; polyphasic MUPs that are of large amplitude and long duration, particularly in areas of denervation; and an incomplete interference pattern. Biphasic MUPs of large amplitude and small duration are produced by denervated motor units, whereas polyphasic MUPs of long duration result from asynchronous firing of scattered reinnervated fibers. The fallout of motor units in neuropathic conditions results in an incomplete interference pattern with full-effort contraction.

MUSCLE BIOPSY AND HISTOLOGIC FINDINGS

This information is invaluable in assessing myopathic conditions and is essential for establishing the diagnosis of an inflammatory myopathy. Unfortunately, only in the case of an enzyme-deficient state can the examination of muscle tissue provide a specific diagnosis. Too often, the changes observed are simply too nonspecific.

Four types of evaluation can be performed on skeletal muscle: histologic studies, histochemical analysis, electron microscopy, and assays of enzyme activities or other constituents. The technique for the biopsy depends on which tests are to be done. If only histologic examination is required, a percutaneous needle biopsy may prove satisfactory.[136] On the other hand, if all four evaluations are desired, an open technique may be preferred.

The site of the biopsy should be selected carefully. A proximal muscle is preferred for the evaluation of myopathic problems. Ideally, the area selected should be actively involved with the process, but the most severely involved area should be avoided. Severely damaged muscle is often too necrotic or scarred for meaningful interpretation. Traditionally, an EMG is the most helpful technique used to localize the site for biopsy. MRI may also be used in this regard[137] (Fig. 80–9). EMG needles can traumatize the muscle. Because the distribution of most myopathies is symmetric, it is recommended to perform the study on one side of the body and take the biopsy specimen from the identified site on the opposite side when EMG is being used.

Infiltration of the muscle with a local anesthetic must also be avoided. Tissue for histologic examination is fixed in formalin and embedded in paraffin for sectioning. Specimens for histochemical analysis are rapidly frozen in liquid nitrogen and sectioned in a cryostat. H&E and modified Gomori's trichrome stains are used for most histologic examinations. A wide variety of stains are used for histochemical analysis, including adenosine triphosphatase (ATPase), which stains the enzyme of the myofibrils; the reduced form of nicotinamide adenine dinucleotide and succinic dehydrogenases, both oxidative enzymes in the mitochondria; myophosphorylase, which catalyzes the initiation of glycogenolysis; myoadenylate deaminase, the first enzyme in the purine nucleotide cycle; acid phosphatase and nonspecific esterase, which stain lysosomes and macrophages; periodic acid–Schiff, which stains glycogen; and oil red O for lipid. Staining for ATPase and enzymes of other metabolic systems is useful in determining the fiber type, size, and distribution (see Table 80–3).

This combination of histologic and histochemical analysis is generally useful in differentiating myopathic from neuropathic processes. Myopathic changes include rounding and increased random variation of fiber size, internal nuclei, fibrosis, and fatty replacement. Myopathic processes may also cause necrosis associated with phagocytosis. Inflammatory myopathies are associated with fiber atrophy, degeneration, and regeneration, plus inflammatory cell infiltrates in both endomysial and perimysial locations. Fiber necrosis, phagocytosis, and regeneration are also typically seen in muscular dystrophy.

Neuropathic conditions that cause denervation, such as disorders of the spinal cord and peripheral nerves, produce small, atrophic angular fibers. Target fibers can also result from denervation. Target fibers are seen using the ATPase stain and are generally type I cells. Each fiber has a central clear area surrounded by a zone of increased intensity of staining, with normal staining at the periphery. Reinnervation causes fiber type grouping, that is, aggregation of fibers all of the same type.

Histochemistry is also useful in identifying other neuromuscular diseases. Applying Gomori's trichrome

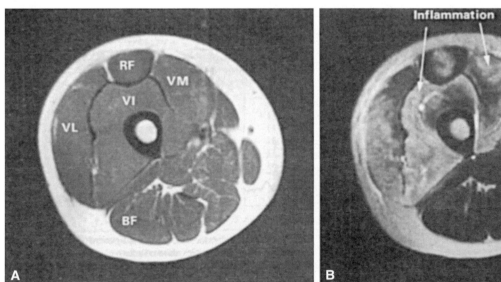
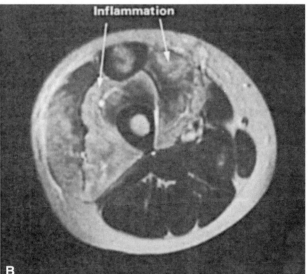

FIGURE 80–9 · A, T2-weighted image of upper leg muscle from a normal individual. B, T2-weighted image of upper leg muscle from a patient with dermatomyositis (DM). (From Park JH, Vital TL, Ryder NM, et al: Magnetic resonance imaging and P31 magnetic resonance spectroscopy provide unique quantitative data useful in the longitudinal management of patients with dermatomyositis. Arthritis Rheum 37:738, 1994. Reprinted from Arthritis and Rheumatism Journal, Copyright 1994. Used with permission of the American College of Rheumatology.)

stain to frozen sections identifies nemaline rod and some mitochondrial myopathies. The ragged, red fiber, characteristic of mitochondrial myopathies, is evident with the trichrome stain. Central core disease is apparent when the central portion of each fiber does not stain for mitochondrial enzymes. Abnormal accumulation of glycogen or lipid suggests either a GSD or a lipid-storage disease, respectively. Enzyme-deficient states may be identified with appropriate histochemical stains but are best diagnosed by subjecting the tissue protein to assays for the specific enzyme activity. Ultrastructural analysis will show characteristic changes in cases of IBM, increased numbers of mitochondria with altered morphology in mitochondrial myopathies, and abnormal glycogen or lipid deposition.

FOREARM ISCHEMIC EXERCISE TESTING

During vigorous ischemic exercise, skeletal muscle functions anaerobically, generating lactate and ammonia. Lactate is the product of the glycolytic metabolism of glycogen and glucose. Ammonia is generated through the conversion of AMP to inosine monophosphate (IMP) by the activity of myoadenylate deaminase. The forearm ischemic exercise test takes advantage of this physiology and has been standardized for use in screening for various metabolic myopathies, including most recognized GSDs (exceptions are acid maltase deficiency, brancher enzyme deficiency and, phosphorylase b kinase deficiency) and myoadenylate deaminase deficiency.[131]

The forearm ischemic exercise test is performed after drawing a venous blood sample for lactate and ammonia, preferably from the nondominant arm at rest and without the use of a tourniquet. Next, a sphygmomanometer is placed around the upper arm of the dominant side and inflated to 20 to 30 mmHg above systolic pressure. The patient then vigorously exercises that extremity by repeatedly squeezing a ball or grip strength testing device (one grip every 2 seconds). The exercise is continued, and the cuff inflated, for a total of 2 minutes (many healthy people can exercise for only 90 seconds under these conditions if they give maximal effort). This may cause some discomfort, which is immediately relieved when the cuff is deflated. Blood samples for levels of lactate and ammonia are drawn from the dominant arm after the cuff is deflated. Most research studies have drawn samples at intervals over 10 minutes. However, one sample obtained 2 minutes after the tourniquet is removed has proved useful in clinical practice. The normal response to forearm ischemic exercise is at least a threefold rise over baseline for each metabolite. In individuals with a GSD, the ammonia level increases normally, but lactate levels remain at baseline. In contrast, in myoadenylate deaminase deficiency, lactate levels increase but ammonia levels do not. The forearm ischemic exercise test is an effective screening test, provided that the patient exercises vigorously. A submaximal exercise effort, whether due to pain, weakness, or malingering, can cause a false-positive result. Therefore, failure to generate lactate or ammonia after ischemic exercise does not

ensure the diagnosis of the particular enzyme deficiency. Any abnormal result should be confirmed with the appropriate enzyme analysis.

IMAGING TECHNIQUES

Neither radiography nor radionuclide imaging has proved particularly useful in patients with muscle diseases. However, computer-based image analysis using ultrasonography, CT, and MRI techniques has provided useful images.[138,140] Each of these techniques can be used in selecting a site for muscle biopsy. With the use of B mode or real-time ultrasound techniques, normal muscle appears as a homogeneous echogenic matrix separated internally by a hyperechoic fascial plane. This procedure is most useful in identifying dystrophic muscle, abscess formation, and changes secondary to acute denervation. It can also be used to quantify muscle atrophy.[141] Although image resolution with ultrasonography is poor compared with that of CT or MRI, this technique has the advantage of no radiation exposure and is easily repeated.

CT can readily differentiate normal from diseased muscle. Consequently, it can be used to determine the distribution of disease, often revealing disease in muscles apparently uninvolved by clinical examination. This technique clearly delineates fat from other tissues. Muscular dystrophies generally cause the most striking abnormalities. Changes can also be seen in myositis and, to lesser extent, in neurogenic disorders. CT has an overall diagnostic accuracy of 85 percent compared to histologic examination of muscle tissue obtained by needle biopsy. Use of this technique is somewhat limited because it cannot distinguish connective tissue from muscle, and it exposes the patient to radiation.

Of available techniques, MRI offers the best view of soft tissue and internal muscle detail (see Fig. 80–9). It can detect early or subtle disease changes and show patchy muscle involvement. MRI can be used to semiquantitatively grade muscle involvement in muscular dystrophy, map patterns of motor unit loss after peripheral nerve trauma, and diagnose and follow the response to therapy in inflammatory muscle disease.[138,142]

Magnetic resonance spectroscopy can measure intramuscular pH and levels of ATP, creatine phosphate, and inorganic phosphorus. This technique has been used to demonstrate biochemical consequences of myophosphorylase deficiency (a lack of acidification of muscle during anaerobic exercise) and has proved useful in the longitudinal management of individuals with DM.

Treatment of Idiopathic Inflammatory Myopathies

To date, only four blinded, controlled therapeutic trials for the treatment of PM or DM have been published, and only recently have consensus-derived measures of disease activity and outcomes been described.[143-146] Consequently, the treatment of the inflammatory myopathics is largely empirical.[149] Before initiating treatment with any medication, it is important to ensure an accurate diagnosis. Because there is no specific diagnostic test for the idiopathic inflammatory myopathies, these diagnoses must be arrived at by excluding other possible causes. Unfortunately, it is difficult to determine the actual effects of therapy in some patients because some fail to respond to any treatment and others have only partial resolution of their weakness. It is, therefore, essential to evaluate the patient's clinical status as objectively as possible. Pretreatment testing of the strength of individual muscle groups and a timed-stands test provide valuable information. These baseline measures can be compared to those obtained after therapy is initiated. Blood pressure, chest examination, chest radiography, and pulmonary function studies are indicated. Fluoroscopic swallowing studies with contrast material may be important if the patient has difficulty swallowing, dysphagia, or dysphonia. Precautions that could prevent aspiration must be emphasized for patients at risk. Such precautions include education about swallowing, elevating the head of the bed on blocks, and the use of antacids or H_2 blockers to neutralize gastric secretions.

Levels of muscle enzymes including CK, aldolase, ALT, AST, and lactate dehydrogenase should be measured, although only the most abnormal value or values need to be tested routinely. In addition, blood cell counts; levels of electrolytes, creatinine, and glucose; and other values that might be affected by therapy should be quantified at baseline. The recognized association between the inflammatory myopathies and malignancy has led some physicians to perform extensive evaluations for an occult neoplasm whenever they encounter a patient with myositis. This, however, is not warranted unless some indication is provided by the history, physical examination, or routine testing. Cancer screening tests indicated by the patient's age and sex should not be overlooked, especially pelvic examinations in women.

Physical therapists can prove invaluable in the treatment of the patient with myositis. Not only are they well trained in testing muscle group strength, but also they can instruct and assist the patient in an exercise program. Exercise programs that take into account the amount of inflammatory activity may be critical for a good outcome. Bed rest is important, and an active range-of-motion activity is to be avoided during intervals of severe inflammation. Passive motion activities are encouraged during these intervals in an effort to maintain the range of motion and prevent contractures. As the individual improves, this program should include active assisted and then active exercises.[150,151] A soft cervical collar may greatly benefit patients with weakness of the neck flexor muscles.

Glucocorticoids are the standard first-line medication for patients with idiopathic inflammatory myopathy. Initially, prednisone is given in a single dose of 1 to 2 mg/kg (with an arbitrary maximum of 100 mg) per day. However, some individuals advocate dividing the daily dose or substitute daily doses of intravenous methylprednisolone.[152] Once instituted, daily high-dose prednisone therapy is continued until strength improves. Clinical improvement may be noted in the first weeks or gradually over 3 to 6 months. This variability is related, at least in part, to the timing of the treatment. The earlier in the course of the illness the prednisone is given, the faster and more effectively it works.

Regular evaluations of muscle strength and serum enzymes should be performed during treatment. Ideally, the initial steroid dosage is maintained until strength and CK values have returned to normal and have remained normal for 4 to 8 weeks. Although CK levels are a useful monitor, muscle strength is more important. Objective testing of strength is necessary to make certain that the patient's reported improvement is not simply due to a euphoric or "energizing" side effect of the steroids. Lowered CK values can be observed despite no improvement in strength because of circulating inhibitors present in active disease or as a nonspecific consequence of the effect of the glucocorticoids. On the other hand, CK values may remain high after complete normalization of muscle strength, presumably because the disease process has resulted in "leaky" cell membranes.

Once remission is apparent, the prednisone dosage can be tapered gradually by reducing the daily dose by about 10 mg/month. As the taper continues, therapy may be changed to an alternate-day schedule. Although alternate-day steroid therapy will cause fewer side effects, if initiated too soon it may well be accompanied by a flare of the disease. To control a flare encountered at any point during a taper will probably require that the dosage be returned to the level that initially brought about the remission.

During the course of treatment, some patients who have had a partial, if not a gratifying, response to glucocorticoid therapy, again develop weakness. The clinician is then faced with the dilemma of whether the decline in muscle strength is caused by a flare of the inflammatory disease process or by steroid myopathy. Unfortunately, no specific test will provide the answer. Even a muscle biopsy is of little value. An active inflammatory change can be observed even when steroid myopathy is contributing to the weakness. A provocative challenge with higher doses of glucocorticoids or rapidly tapering the dose is the only way of determining the cause of the clinical decline.

Exactly how many patients will benefit or will be cured by glucocorticoid therapy is not certain. As many as 90 percent of patients will improve at least partially with glucocorticoid therapy, with 50 to 75 percent of those achieving a complete remission.[12] Many glucocorticoid failures can be attributed to early discontinuation of prednisone therapy without appropriate low-dose maintenance therapy, early development of side effects necessitating taper, or an inaccurate diagnosis.[149]

If a patient fails to respond to glucocorticoid therapy after 6 weeks or if a patient has had some improvement but the level of strength has reached a plateau, serious consideration should be given to adding another agent. The choice of additional therapy is between the immunosuppressive agents azathioprine and methotrexate (MTX).

Beneficial results have been reported with MTX. This agent is usually given on a weekly schedule at doses ranging between 5 and 15 mg orally or 15 and 75 mg intravenously. Measurements of liver function levels and, possibly, pulmonary function should be performed before initiating MTX therapy to minimize confusion between changes in these parameters caused by the basic disease and the potential hepatic and pulmonary toxicities of the medication. Azathioprine is also useful in many cases.[143] The usual dose of azathioprine is 2 to 3 mg/kg (with the usual maximum of 150 mg) per day in a single oral dose. Results from a randomized crossover study showed that the continuation of weekly oral MTX and daily oral azathioprine may be effective in patients in whom prednisone plus either drug alone has failed.[146] Therefore, this combination should be considered for patients with refractory or treatment-resistant myositis.

Other immunosuppressive agents have been used in steroid-resistant patients.[12,149] Hydroxychloroquine can be used to treat the cutaneous lesions of DM, even in patients with an associated malignancy. However, this drug has no recognized effect on the myositis. Cyclophosphamide given intravenously with concomitant oral prednisone appears to be effective in childhood disease and in some adults, although it has not proved effective in small numbers of patients with longstanding myositis, interstitial pneumonitis, or IBM. Anecdotal reports suggest that 6-mercaptopurine and chlorambucil may be helpful. Low-dose cyclosporine therapy (2.5 to 7.5 mg/kg of body weight daily) has been observed to be very helpful and safe in children and adults who were unresponsive to other treatments.[153] The use of cyclosporine in combination with MTX has also been employed.[154] Plasmapheresis, lymphapheresis, and total body (or total nodal) irradiation have been used but do not appear to have clinical utility.[149]

Intravenous immune globulin is being used increasingly to treat inflammatory myopathies. Based on the theorized mechanisms of therapeutic effect, immune globulin should be most effective in DM. Both the one controlled trial[145] and uncontrolled trials show that this therapy is generally effective in treating DM and may also improve muscular strength in some patients with PM and IBM.[149,155] This therapy is associated with little toxicity but is extremely expensive. Individuals commonly receive 1 to 2 g/kg each month. The long-term utility is not known, and tachyphylaxis has been reported.[156] Controlled trials involving larger numbers of patients are definitely needed to prove a benefit for this and other therapies.

The general approach to the therapy outlined previously can be applied to all the idiopathic inflammatory myopathies. However, special consideration should be given to the subset of patients with IBM. Because this subset has generally been identified as refractory to therapy, some have suggested that treatment is futile. However, steroid therapy has provided mild or transient benefit to some patients with IBM, and a small number have had excellent responses. There is evidence that other immunosuppressive agents may retard the progression of the disease. Therefore, it is worth a therapeutic trial for a limited time for patients with IBM. Initially, prednisone is used as a single agent. If no benefit is found in 6 weeks, a second immunosuppressive drug should be added. If no benefit is witnessed after 6 more weeks, another agent can be substituted. If that trial fails, then treatment with immunosuppressive agents should be abandoned to avoid toxicity. In contrast, patients with an elevated CK level and an associated collagen-vascular disease may have an extremely rapid response to glucocorticoid therapy.[12,116] This, however, is not always the case.

The prognosis for patients with idiopathic inflammatory myopathies has improved with the availability of immunosuppressive therapy. Studies for the adults indicate a 5-year survival of 60 percent in the preglucocorticoid era, 68 percent between 1947 and 1968, and 80 percent in more recent reports. The reasons for the improved survival are not certain but may be related to earlier and more accurate diagnosis, improved treatments for associated problems such as infection, and the earlier use of immunosuppressive agents. In general, children have a better prognosis than adults. Ninety percent of children with juvenile DM who live 10 years after diagnosis lead normal lives. Mortality in children is attributable most often to myocarditis, perforation of a viscus, or infection. Whites have a better prognosis than blacks. Regardless of age or race, the longer the duration of disease and the more severe the weakness at the time when therapy is initiated, the worse the morbidity and mortality. Pharyngeal muscle weakness, aspiration, and interstitial pulmonary fibrosis bode a poor diagnosis. Patients with myositis and malignancy fare the worst. The actual prognosis for patients with IBM is unknown but appears favorable for most[2] because of the recent discovery of the disease and the small number of patients identified. Generally, the course is slow and prolonged. Whereas the weakness becomes fixed in some, in others it continues with a relentless progression leading to severe incapacitation and death. The presence of a circulating MSA helps predict the response to therapy (see Table 80–5). With some exceptions, those with anti–Mi-2 antibodies do well; those with antisynthetase or anti-SRP antibodies respond poorly.[2,6]

REFERENCES

1. Bohan A, Peter JB: Polymyositis and dermatomyositis (first of two parts). N Engl J Med 292:344, 1975.
2. Love LA, Leff RL, Fraser DD, et al: A new approach to the classification of idiopathic inflammatory myopathy: Myositis specific autoantibodies define useful homogeneous patient groups. Medicine 70:360, 1991.
3. Tanimoto K, Nakano K, Kano S, et al: Classification criteria for polymyositis and dermatomyositis. J Rheumatol 22:668, 1995.
4. Targoff IN, Miller FW, Medsger TA Jr, Oddis CV: Classification criteria for the idiopathic inflammatory myopathies. Curr Opin Rheumatol 9:527, 1997.
5. Peng A, Koffman BM, Malley JD, et al: Disease progression in sporadic inclusion body myositis: Observations in 78 patients. Neurol 55:296, 2000.

6. Targoff IN: Autoantibodies. *In* Wortmann RL (ed): Diseases of Skeletal Muscle. Philadelphia, Lippincott, Williams & Wilkins, 2000, pp 267-296.

7. Plotz PH, Rider LG, Targoff IN: Myositis: Immunologic contribution to understanding cause, pathogenesis, and therapy. Ann Intern Med 122:715, 1995.

8. Cronin ME, Plotz PH: Idiopathic inflammatory myopathies. Rheum Dis Clin North Am 16:655, 1990.

9. Phillips BA, Zilko PJ, Mastagalia FL: Prevalence of sporadic inclusion body myositis in western Australia. Muscle Nerve 23:970, 2000.

10. Pachman LM: Inflammatory myopathy in children: Clinical and laboratory indicators of disease activity and chronicity. *In* Wortmann RL (ed): Diseases of Skeletal Muscle. Philadelphia, Lippincott, Williams & Wilkins, 2000, pp 87-110.

11. Bohan A, Peter JB, Bowman BS, Pearson CM: A computer assisted analysis of 153 patients with polymyositis and dermatomyositis. Medicine 56:255, 1977.

12. Oddis C: Idiopathic inflammatory myopathy. *In* Wortmann RL (ed): Diseases of Skeletal Muscle. Philadelphia, Lippincott, Williams & Wilkins, 2000, pp 45-86.

14. Mastaglia FL, Garlepp MJ, Phillips BA, et al: Inflammatory myopathies: Clinical, diagnostic and therapeutic aspects. Muscle Nerve 27:407, 2003.

15. Chauvet E, Sailler M, Carriero M, et al: Symptomatic macroglossia and tongue myositis in polymyositis: Treatment with corticosteroids and intravenous immunoglobulin. Arthritis Rheum 46:2762, 2002.

16. Marie I, Horton P-Y, Hachulla E, et al: Pulmonary involvement in polymyositis and in dermatomyositis. J Rheumatol 25:1336, 1998.

17. Spiera R, Kagan L: Extramuscular manifestations in idiopathic inflammatory myopathies. Curr Opin Rheumatol 10:556, 1998.

18. Ascherman DP: Pulmonary complications of inflammatory myopathy. Curr Rheumatol Rep 4:409, 2002.

19. Anders H-J, Wanders A, Rihl M, et al: Myocardial fibrosis and polymyositis. J Rheum 26:1840, 1999.

20. Yazici Y, Kagen L: Cardiac involvement in myositis. Curr Opin Rheumatol 14:663, 2002.

21. Gran JT, Myklebast G: Adult idiopathic polymyositis without elevation of creatine kinase: Case report and review of the literature. Scand J Rheumatol 22:94, 1993.

22. Tymms KE, Beller EM, Webb J, et al: Correlation between tests of muscle involvement and clinical muscle weakness in polymyositis and dermatomyositis. Clin Rheumatol 9:523, 1990.

23. Mahowald M, David WS: Electrophysiologic evaluation of muscle disease. *In* Wortmann RL (ed): Diseases of Skeletal Muscle. Philadelphia, Lippincott, Williams & Wilkins, 2000, pp 313-332.

24. Mantegazza R, Bernasconi P, Confalonieri P, Cornelio F: Inflammatory myopathies and systemic disorders: A review of immunopathogenetic mechanisms and clinical features. J Neurol 244:277, 1997.

25. Bossen EH: Muscle biopsy. *In* Wortmann RL (ed): Diseases of Skeletal Muscle. Philadelphia, Lippincott, Williams & Wilkins, 2000, pp 338-348.

26. Callen J: Dermatomyositis. Lancet 255:53, 2000.

27. Messner RP: Pathogenesis of idiopathic inflammatory myopathy. *In* Wortmann RL (ed): Diseases of Skeletal Muscle. Philadelphia, Lippincott, Williams & Wilkins, 2000, pp 111-128.

28. Scheja A, Elborgh R, Wildt M: Decreased capillary density in juvenile dermatomyositis and in mixed connective tissue disease. J Rheum 26:1337, 1999.

29. Hansmann G, Herroro C, Cid MC, et al: Immunopathologic study of skin lesions in dermatomyositis. J Am Acad Dermatol 25:225, 1991.

30. Olsen NJ, Park JH, King LE Jr.: Amyotrophic dermatomyositis. Curr Rheumatol Rep 3:346, 2001.

31. Drake LA, Dinehart SM, Farmer ER, et al: Guidelines of care for dermatomyositis. American Academy of Dermatology. J Am Acad Dermatol 34:824, 1996.

32. Ang P, Sugeng MW, Chua SH: Classical and amyopathic dermatomyositis seen at the National Skin Care Centre of Singapore: 3-year retrospective review of their clinical characteristics and association with malignancy. Ann Acad Med Singapore 29:219, 2000.

33. Park JH, Vital TZ, Ryder NM, et al: Magnetic resonance imaging and P31 magnetic resonance spectroscopy provide unique quantitative data useful in the longitudinal management of patients with dermatomyositis. Arthritis Rheum 37:736, 1994.

34. Dourmishev AL, Dourmishev LA: Dermatomyositis and drugs. *In* Mallia A, Uitto J (eds): RheumaDerma. New York, Kluwer Academic/Plenum Publishers, 1999, p 187.

35. Reed AM: Myositis in children. Curr Opin Rheumatol 13:428, 2001.

36. Tse S, Lubelsky S, Gordon M, et al: The arthritis of inflammatory childhood myositis syndromes. J Rheumatol 28:192, 2001.

37. Harel L, Harel G, Korenreich L, et al: Treatment of calcinosis in juvenile dermatomyositis with probenecid: The role of phosphorus metabolism on the development of calcifications. J Rheumatol 28:1129, 2001.

38. Huemer C, Kitson H, Malleson PN, et al: Lipodystrophy in patients with juvenile dermatomyositis: Evaluation of clinical and metabolic abnormalities. J Rheum 28:610, 2001.

39. Plamondon S, Dent PB: Juvenile amyopathic dermatomyositis: Results of a case finding descriptive survey. J Rheumatol 27:2031, 2001.

40. Quartier P, Bonnet D, Fournet J-C, et al: Severe cardiac involvement in children with systematic sclerosis and myositis. J Rheum 29:1767, 2002.

41. Scully RE, Mark EJ, McNeely WF, et al: Case records of the Massachusetts General Hospital. New Engl J Med 345:596, 2001.

42. Zakrzewska-Pniewska B, Jablonska S, Kowalska-Oledzka E, et al: Sympathetic skin response in scleroderma, scleroderma overlap syndromes and inflammatory myopathies. Clin Rheum 18:473, 2000.

43. Greenberg SA, Amato AA: Inflammatory myopathy associated with mixed connective tissue and scleroderma renal crisis. Muscle Nerve 24:1562, 2001.

44. Lindvall B, Bengtsson A, Ernerudh J, et al: Subclinical myopsitis is common in primary Sjörgen's syndrome and is not related to muscle pain. J Rheum 29:717, 2002.

45. Garton MJ, Isenberg DA: Clinical features of lupus myositis versus idiopathic myositis: A review of 30 cases. Br J Rheumatol 36:1067, 1997.

46. Rosenbaum R: Neuromuscular complications of connective tissue diseases. Muscle Nerve 24:154, 2001.

47. Bekkelund SI, Torbergsen T, Husby G, et al: Myopathy and neuropathy in rheumatoid arthritis: A quantitative controlled electromyographic study. J Rheum 26:2348, 1999.

48. Fieschi C, Pitte J-C: Myositis and neoplasia. *In* Schoenfeld Y, Gershwin ME (eds): Cancer and Autoimmunity. Amsterdam, Elsevier, 2000, p 85.

49. Buchcinder R, Hill CL: Malignancy in patients with inflammatory myopathy. Curr Rheum Rep 4:415, 2002.

50. Buchbinder R, Forbes A, Hall S, et al: Incidence of malignant disease in biopsy-proven inflammatory myopathy. Ann Intern Med 134:1087, 2001.

51. Whitmore SE, Rosenshein NB, Provost TT: Ovarian cancer in patients with dermatomyositis. Medicine 73:153, 1994.

52. Askanas V, Engel WN: Sporadic inclusion-body myositis and hereditary inclusion body myopathies: Current concepts of diagnosis and pathogenesis. Curr Opin Rheumatol 10:530, 1998.

53. Oldfors A, Fyhr I-M: Inclusion body myositis: Genetic factors, aberrant protein expression, and autoimmunity. Curr Opin Rheumatol 13:469, 2001.

54. Tawil R, Griggs RC: Inclusion body myositis. Curr Opin Rheumatol 14:653, 2002.

55. Rose MR, McDermott MP, Thornton CA, et al: Prospective natural history of inclusion body myositis: Implications for clinical trials. Neurology 57:548, 2001.

56. Phillips BA, Cala LA, Thickbroom GW, et al: Patterns of muscle involvement in inclusion body myositis: Clinical and magnetic resonance imaging study. Muscle Nerve 24:1526, 2001.

57. Watts RA: Eosinophilia and musculoskeletal disease. Curr Opin Rheumatol 13:57, 2001.

58. Kobayashi Y, Fujimoto T, Shiiki H, et al: Focal eosinophilic myositis. Clin Rheum 20:369, 2001.

59. Costenbader KH, Kieval RI, Anderson RJ: Eosinophilic fasciitis presenting as pitting edema of the extremities. Am J Med 111:318, 2001.

60. Zivkovic SA, Lacomis D, Clemens PR: Chronic eosinophilic perimyositis persistent myalgias. Muscle Nerve 25:461, 2002.

61. Hertzman PA, Clauw DJ, Kaufman LD, et al: The eosinophilia myalgia syndrome: Status of 205 patients and treatment results of treatment 2 years after onset. Ann Intern Med 122:851, 1995.

62. Nuovo MA, Norman A, Chumas J, et al: Myositis ossificans with atypical clinical, radiographic, or pathologic findings: A review of 23 cases. Skeletal Radiol 21:87, 1992.

63. Bridges AJ, Hsu KC, Singh A, et al: Fibrodysplasia (myositis) ossificans progressive. Semin Arthritis Rheum 24:155, 1994.

64. Caunes O, Chevrel G, Miossec P: Focal myositis: A new HLA-DR4 0401 associated disease? J Rheum 26:2502, 1999.

65. Chiba S, Hatanaka Y, Ohkubo Y, et al: Focal Myositis: Magnetic resonance imaging findings and peripheral arterial administration of prednisolone. Clin Rheum 18:495, 2000.

66. Sieb JP, Ries F, Traber, et al: Recurrent focal myositis. Muscle Nerve 20:1205, 1997.

67. Lim KL, Robson K, Powell RJ: Focal myositis: An unusual cause of bilateral upper eyelid swellings. Postgrad Med J 69:876, 1993.

68. Berger C, Sommer C, Meinck H-M: Isolated sarcoid myopathy. Muscle Nerve 26:553, 2002.

69. Herrman DN, Blaivas M, Wald JJ, et al: Granulomatous myositis, primary biliary cirrhosis, pancytopenia, and thymoma. Muscle Nerve 23:1133, 2000.

70. Gherardi RK, Coquet M, Cherin P, et al: Macrophagic myofasciitis: an emerging entity. Lancet 352:347, 1998.

71. Cherin P, Authier RK, Gherardi RK, et al: Gallium-67 scintigraphy in macrophagic myofasciitis. Arthritis Rheum 43:1520, 2000.

72. Gherardi RK: Skeletal muscle involvement in HIV-infected patients. Neuropathol Appl Aeurobiol 20:232, 1994.

73. Ytterberg SR: The relationship of infections agents to inflammatory myositis. Rheum Dis Clin North Am 20:995, 1994.

74. Andersson JA, Englund P, Sunnermark D, et al: CBA/J mice infected with Trypanosoma cruzi: An experiment model for inflammatory myopathies. Muscle Nerve 27:442, 2003.

75. Shamim EA, Rider LG, Janardan PP, et al: Differences in idiopathic inflammatory myopathy phenotyoes and genotypes between Mesoamerican Mestizos and North American Caucasions. Arthritis Rheum 46:1885, 2002.

76. Rider LG, Shamim E, Okada S, et al: Genetic risk and protective factors for idiopathic inflammatory myopathy in Koreans and American whites. Arthritis Rheum 42:1285, 1999.

77. Reed AM, Pachman LM, Hayford JR, et al: Immunogenetic studies in families of children with juvenile dermatomyositis. J Rheumatol 25:1000, 1998.

78. Pachman LM, Liotta-Davis MR, Hong DK, et al: TNF(-308A allele in juvenile dermatomyositis. Arthritis Rheum 43:2368, 2000.

79. Koffman BM, Sivakumar K, Simonis T, et al: HLA allele distribution distinguishes sporadic inclusion body myositis from hereditary inclusion body myopathies. J Neuroimmunol 84:139, 1998.

80. Kok CC, Croager EJ, Witt CS, et al: Mapping a candidate region for susceptibility to inclusion body myositis in the human major histocompatibility complex. Immunogenetics 49:508, 1999.

81. Kok CC, Boyt A, Gaudier S, et al: Mitochondrial DNA variants in inclusion body myositis. Neuromuscul Disord 10:508, 1999.

82. Eisenberg I, Thiel C, Levit, et al: Fine-structure mapping of the hereditary inclusion body myopathy locus. Genomics 55:43, 1999.

83. Askanas V, Engel WK: Sporadic inclusion-body myositis and hereditary inclusion-body myositis: Current concepts of diagnosis and pathogenesis. Curr Opin Rheumatol 10:530, 1998.

84. Martinsson T, Oldforg A. Darin N, et al: Autosomal dominant myopathy: Misuse mutation (Glu-706 to lgs) in the myosin heavy chain IIa gene. Proc Natl Acad Sci U S A 97:14614, 2000.

85. Hohfeld R, Engel AG, Goebels N, et al: Cellular immune mechanisms in inflammatory myopathies. Curr Opin Rheumatol 9:520, 1997.

86. Nagaraju K: Update on immunopathogenesis in inflammatory myopathies. Curr Opin Rheumatol 13:461, 2001.

87. Cid M-C, Grau J-M, Casademont J, et al: Leucocyte/endothelial cell adhesion receptors in muscle biopsies from patients with idiopathic inflammatory myopathies. Clin Exp Immunol 104:467, 1996.

88. Fyher I-M, Moslemi A-R, Mosavia A, et al: Oligoexpression in muscle infiltrating T cells in inclusion body myositis. J Neuroimmunol 79:185, 1997.

89. Amemiya K, Granger RP, Dalakas MC: Clonal Restriction of the T-cell receptor expression by infiltrating lympocytes in inclusion body myositis persists over time: Studies in repeated muscle biopsies. Brain 123:2030, 2000.

90. Fyhr I-M, Oldfors A: Upregulation of tas/fas ligamal in inclusion body myositis. Ann Neurol 43:127, 1998.

91. Inukai A, Kobayashi Y, Ito K, et al: Expression of fas antigen is not associated with apoptosis in human myopathies. Muscle Nerve 20:702, 1997.

92. Askanas V, Engel WK; Newest pathogenic considerations in inclusion-body myositis: Possible role of amyloid-β, cholesterol, relation to aging and to Alzheimer's disease. Curr Rheumatol Rep 4:427, 2002.

93. Askanas V, McFerrin J, Alvarez RB, et al: APP gene transfer into cultured human muscle induces inclusion-body myositis aspects. Neuroreport 8:9, 1997.

94. Banwell BL, Engel AG: αB-crystalin immunolocalization yields new insights into inclusion body myositis. Neurology 54:1033, 2000.

95. Goncalves FGP, Chimelli L, Sallum AME, et al: Immunohistological analysis of CD59 and membrane attack complex of complement in muscle in juvenile dermatomyositis. J Rheum 29:1301, 2002.

96. Lundberg I, Ulfgren A-K, Nyberg P, et al: Cytokine production in muscle tissue of patients with idiopathic inflammatory myopathies. Arthritis Rheum 40:865, 1999.

97. Nyberg P, Wikman A-L, Nennesmo I, et al: Increased expression of interleukin 1α and MHC class I in muscle tissue of patients with chronic, inactive polymyositis and dermatomyositis. J Rheumatol 27:940, 2000.

98. Englund P, Lindroos E, Memmesmo I, et al: Skeletal muscle fibers express major histocompatibility complex class II antigens independently of inflammatory infiltrates in inflammatory myopathies. Am J Pathol 159:1263, 2001.

99. Englund P, Nennesmo I, Klareskog L, et al: Interleukin-1α expression in capillaries and major histocompatibility complex class I expression in type II muscle fibers from polymyositis and dermatomyositis patients. Arthritis Rheum 46:1044, 2002.

100. Lundberg I, Kratz A-K, Alexanderson H, et al: Decreased expression of interleukin-1α, interleukin-1β, and cell adhesion molecules in muscle tissue following corticosteroid treatment in patients with polymyositis and dermatomyositis. Arthritis Rheum 43:336, 2000.

101. Li Y-P, Reid MB: Effect of tumor necrosis factor-α on skeletal muscle metabolism. Curr Opin Rheumatol 13:483, 2001.

102. Hicks JE, Drinkard B, Summers RM, et al: Decreased aerobic capacity in children with juvenile dermatomyositis. Arthritis Rheum 47:118, 2002.

103. Park JH, Niermann KJ, Ryder NM, et al: Muscle abnormalities in juvenile dermatomyositis patients. Arthritis Rheum 43:2359, 2000.

104. Lacomis D: Neuropathic disorders and muscular dystrophy. In Wortmann RL (ed): Diseases of Skeletal Muscle. Philadelphia, Lippincott, Williams & Wilkins, 2000, pp 197-220.

105. Rudnicki SA, Dalmau J: Paraneoplastic syndromes of the spinal cord, nerve, and muscle. Muscle Nerve 23:1800, 2000.

106. Sieb JP, Gillessen T: Iatrogenicand toxic myopathies. Muscle Nerve 27:142, 2003.

107. De Jonghe B, Sharshar T, Lefaucheur J-P, et al: Paresis acquired in the intensive care unit. JAMA 288:2859, 2002.

108. Lacomis D: Critical illness myopathy. Curr Rheum Reports 4:403, 2002.

109. Baker SK, Tarpolsky MA: Statin myopathies: Pathophysiology and clinical perspectives. Clin Invest Med 24:258. 2001.

110. Wortmann RL: Lipid-lowering agents and myopathy. Curr Opin Rheumatol 14:643, 2002.

111. Messner RP: Infections of muscle. In Wortmann RL (ed): Diseases of Skeletal Muscle. Philadelphia, Lippincott, Williams & Wilkins, 2000, pp 129-146.

112. Richardson SJ, Lopez F, Rojas S, et al: Multinodular polymyositis in a patient with human immunodeficiency and hepatitis C virus coinfection. Muscle Nerve 24:433, 2001.

113. Casado E, Olive A, Holgado S, et al: Musculoskeletal manifestations in patients positive for human immunodeficiency virus: Correlation with CD4 count. J Rheum 28:802, 2001.

114. Simpson DM, Slaslor P: Analysis of myopathy in placebo-controlled zidovudine trial. Muscle Nerve 22:382, 1997.

115. Patel SR, Olengenski TP, Perruquet JL, et al: Pyomyositis: Clinical features and predisposing conditions. J Rheum 24:1734, 1667.

116. Rayes AA, Nobre V, Teixeira DM, et al: Tropical pyomyositis and human Toxocariasis: A clinical and experimental study. Am J Med 109:422, 2000.

117. Hoffman JC, Stichtenoth DO, Zeidler H, et al: Lyme disease in a 74-year-old forest owner with symptoms of dermatomyositis. Arthritis Rheum 38:1157, 1995.

118. Bretagne S, Costa R: Lack of Toxoplasma gondii DNA in muscle of patients with inflammatory myopathy and increased anti-Toxoplasma antibodies. Muscle Nerve 17:822, 1994.

119. Miro O, Laguno M, Masanes F, et al: Congenital and metabolic myopathies of childhood or adult onset. Arthritis Rheum 29: 335, 2000.

120. Wortmann RL: Metabolic diseases of muscle. In Wortmann RL (ed): Diseases of Skeletal Muscle. Philadelphia, Lippincott, Williams & Wilkins, 2000, pp 157-188.

121. DiMauro S, Lamperti C: Muscle glycogenoses. Muscle Nerve 24:984, 2001.

122. Wortmann RL, DiMauro S: Differentiating idiopathic inflammatory myopathies from metabolic myopathies. Rheum Dis Clin North Am 28:759, 2002.

123. Vladutiu GD, Bennett MJ, Fisher NM, et al: Phenotypic variability among first-degree relatives with carnitine palmitoyltransferase II deficiency. Muscle Nerve 26:492, 2002.

124. Sabina RL: Myoadenylate dominase deficiency. Neurol Clin 18:185, 2000.

125. Gross M, Rotzer F, Kolle P, et al: A G168-T AMPD1 mutant allele contributes to the high incidence of myoadenylate deaminase deficiency in the Caucasian population. Neuromusc Dis 12:558, 2002.

126. Simon DK, Johns DR: Mitochondrial disorders: Clinical and genetic features. Annu Rev Med 50:111, 1999.

127. Grigoriads E, Fam AG, Starok M, et al: Skeletal muscle infarction in diabetes mellitus. J Rheum 27:1063, 2000.

128. Warren JD, Blumbergs PC, Thompson PD: Rhabdomyolsis: A review. Muscle Nerve 25:332, 2002.

129. Csuka M, McCarty DJ: A simple method for measurement of lower extremity muscle strength. Am J Med 78:77, 1985.

130. Moxley RT: Evaluation of neuromuscular function in inflammatory myopathy. Rheum Dis Clin North Am 20:827, 1995.

131. Wortmann RL, Vladutiu GD: The clinical evaluation off the patient with noninflammatory myopathy. Curr Rheumatol Rep 3:310, 2001.

132. Reijneveld JC, Boekhorst TE, Zonderland ML, et al: Response to exercise of patients with idiopathic hyper-CK-emia. Muscle Nerve 26:832, 2002.

133. Simmons Z, Peterlin BL, Boyer PJ, et al: Muscle biopsy in the evaluation of patients with modestly elevated creatine kinase levels. Muscle Nerve 27:242, 2003.

134. Brouwer R, Hengstman GJD, Vree Egberts W, et al: Autoantibody profiles in the serum of European patients with myositis. Ann Rheum Dis 60:116, 2001.

135. Nardin RA, Rutkove SB, Raynor EM: Diagnostic accuracy of electrodiagnostic testing in the evaluation of weakness. Muscle Nerve 26: 201, 2002.

136. Dorph C, Nennesmo I, Lunberg I: Percutaneous conchotome muscle biopsy: A useful diagnostic and assessment tool. J Rheumatol 28:1591, 2001.

137. Park JH, Olsen NJ: Utility of magnetic resonance imaging in the evaluation of patients with inflammatory myopathies. Curr Rheumatol Reo 3:334, 2001.

138. Dion E, Cherin P, Payan C, et al: Magnetic resonance imaging criteria for distinguishing between inclusion body myositis and polymyositis. J Rheum 29:1897, 2002.

139. Park JH, Olsen NJ: Imaging of skeletal muscle. In Wortmann RL (ed): Diseases of Skeletal Muscle. Philadelphia, Lippincott, Williams & Wilkins, 2000, pp 293-312.

140. Fleckenstein JL, Crues JV, III, Reimers CD (eds): Muscle Imaging in Health and Disease. New York, Springer, 1996.

141. Jacobson JA, van Holsbeeck MT: Musculoskeletal ultrasonography. Orthop Clin North Am 29:135, 1998.

142. Kimball AB, Summers RM, Turner M, et al: Magnetic resonance imaging detection of occult-skin and subcutaneous abnormalities in juvenile dermatomyositis. Arthritis Rheum 43:1866, 2000.

143. Bunch TW, Worthington JW, Combs JJ, et al: Azathioprine with prednisone for polymyositis: A controlled, clinical trial. Ann Intern Med 92:365, 1980.

144. Miller FW, Leitman SF, Cronin ME, et al: A randomized controlled trial of plasma exchange and leukapheresis in polymyositis and dermatomyositis. N Engl J Med 326:1380, 1992.

145. Dalakas MC, Illa I, Dambrosia JM, et al: A controlled trial of high-dose intravenous immune globulin infusions as treatment for dermatomyositis. N Engl J Med 329:1993, 1993.

146. Villalba L, Hicks JE, Adams EM, et al: Treatment of refractory myositis. Arthritis Rheum 41:392, 1998.

147. Miller FW, Rider LG, Chung YL, et al: Proposed preliminary core ser measures for disease outcome assessment in adult and juvenile idiopathic inflammatory myopathies. Rheumatology 40:1262, 2001.

148. Alexanderson HA, Lundberg IE, Stenström CH: Developments of the myositis activities profile: Validity and reliability of a self-administered questionnaire to assess activity limitations in patients with polymyositis/dermatomyositis. J Rheum 29:2386, 2002.

149. Wortmann RL: Idiopathic inflammatory diseases of muscles. In Weisman MH, Weinblatt ME, Louie JS (eds): Treatment of the Rheumatic Diseases. Companion to the Textbook of Rheumatology, 2nd edition. Philadelphia, WB Saunders, 2001, pp 390-403.

150. Wiesinger GF, Quittan M, Aringer M, et al: Improvement in physical fitness and muscle strength in polymyositis/dermatomyositis patients by a training program. Br J Rheumatol 37:1960, 1998.

151. Mahowald ML: The benefits and limitations of a physical training program in patients with inflammatory arthritis. Curr Rheumatol Rep 3:317, 2001.

152. Al-Mayouf S, Al Mazyed A, Bahabri S: Efficacy of treatment of severe juvenile dermatomyositis with intravenous methylprednisolone and methotrexate. Clin Rheumatol 19:138, 2000.

153. Langford CA, Klippel JH, Balow JE, et al: Use of cytotoxic agents and cyclosporine in the treatment of autoimmune disease. I. Rheumatologic and renal diseases. Ann Intern Med 128:1021, 1998.

154. Mitsunaka H, Tokuda M, Hiraishi T, et al: Combined use of cyclosporine A and methotrexate in refractory polymyositis. Scan J Rheumatol 29:192, 2000.

155. Al-Mayouf SM, Laxer RM, Schneider R, et al: Intravenous immunoglobulin therapy for juvenile dermatomyositis: Efficacy and safety. J Rheum 27:2498, 2000.

156. Reimold AM, Weinblatt ME: Tachyphylaxis of intravenous immunoglobulin in refractory inflammatory myopathy. J Rheumatol 21:1144, 1994.

Vasculitis

81 The Classification and Epidemiology of Systemic Vasculitis

JOHN H. STONE

Few disorders within medicine are more challenging in diagnosis and treatment than the systemic vasculitides. These heterogeneous disorders are linked by the common finding of destructive inflammation within the walls of blood vessels. Current classification schemes recognize approximately 20 primary forms of vasculitis, as well as several major categories of secondary vasculitis (e.g., other rheumatologic diseases, malignancy, and infection) (Table 81–1). Over the past half century, numerous comprehensive classification schemes have been attempted.[1] No attempt has been entirely satisfactory, because understanding of these conditions continues to evolve. All vasculitis classification schemes remain works in progress.

Current classification schemes are understood best in light of their nosological predecessors. The first "modern" case of systemic vasculitis was recognized less than 150 years ago by Adolf Kussmaul and Rudolf Maier.[2] That case, which involved medium-sized, muscular arteries, has served as the reference point for classifying many subsequently recognized forms of vasculitis. Because of the importance of that first report in the understanding and classification of vasculitis, the case is described in detail here.

The First Modern Case: "Periarteritis Nodosa"

In 1866, Kussmaul and Maier reported the case of a 27-year-old tailor who died during a month-long hospital confinement.[2,3] Upon presentation, the patient was strong enough to climb two flights of stairs to the clinic, but "afterward felt so weak that he immediately had to go to bed." He complained of numbness on the volar aspect of his thumb and the two neighboring fingers on the right hand. Over the ensuing days, "the general weakness increased so rapidly that he was unable to leave the bed, (and) the feeling of numbness also appeared in the left hand." Muscle paralysis progressed quickly: "Before our eyes, a young man developed a general paralysis of the voluntary muscles...(He) had

to be fed by attendants, and within a few weeks was robbed of the use of most of his muscles."[2,3]

The patient's weakness, caused by vasculitic neuropathy (mononeuritis multiplex), was accompanied by tachycardia, abdominal pains, and the appearance of cutaneous nodules over his trunk. His death was described poignantly: "He was scarcely able to speak, lay with persistent severe abdominal and muscle pains, opisthotonically stretched, whimpering, and begged the doctors not to leave him.... Death occurred ... at 2 o'clock in the morning." At autopsy, grossly visible nodules were present along the patient's medium-sized arteries. Kussmaul and Maier suggested the name "periarteritis nodosa" for this disease, because of the apparent localization of inflammation to the perivascular sheaths and outer layers of the arterial walls, leading to nodular thickening of the vessels. The name was later revised to polyarteritis nodosa (PAN), to reflect both the widespread arterial involvement of this disease and the fact that the inflammation in PAN extends through the entire thickness of the vessel wall.[4,5]

POLYARTERITIS NODOSA AS A REFERENCE POINT

In addition to its status as the first form of vasculitis recognized, several features of PAN make it a logical reference point for the classification of inflammatory vascular disease. Other forms of vasculitis can usually be differentiated from PAN through their contrasts to one or more of the following PAN characteristics:

The general confinement of the disease to "medium-sized" vessels, as opposed to capillaries and postcapillary venules ("small" vessels) and the aorta and its major branches ("large" vessels)
The exclusive involvement of arteries, with sparing of veins
The tendency to form microaneurysms
The absence of lung involvement
The lack of granulomatous inflammation
The absence of associated autoantibodies (e.g., antineutrophil cytoplasmic antibodies [ANCA] or

TABLE 81–1 · CLASSIFICATION SCHEME OF VASCULITIDES ACCORDING TO SIZE OF PREDOMINANT BLOOD VESSELS INVOLVED

Primary Vasculitides

Predominantly large-vessel vasculitides
Takayasu's arteritis
Giant cell arteritis (temporal arteritis)
Cogan's syndrome
Behçet's disease†
Predominantly medium-vessel vasculitides
Polyarteritis nodosa
Cutaneous polyarteritis nodosa
Buerger's disease
Kawasaki's disease
Primary angiitis of the central nervous system
Predominantly small-vessel vasculitides
Immune complex–mediated:
Goodpasture's disease (antiglomerular basement membrane disease)†
Cutaneous leukocytoclastic angiitis (hypersensitivity vasculitis)
Henoch-Schönlein purpura
Hypocomplementemic urticarial vasculitis
Essential cryoglobulinemia‡
Erythema elevatum diutinum
Vasculitis associated with anti-neutrophil cytoplasmic antibodies, (ANCA)
Wegener's granulomatosis‡
Microscopic polyangiitis‡
Churg-Strauss syndrome‡
Renal-limited vasculitis

Secondary Forms of Vasculitis

Miscellaneous small-vessel vasculitides:
Connective tissue disorders‡ (rheumatoid vasculitis, lupus, Sjögren's syndrome, inflammatory myopathies)
Inflammatory bowel disease
Paraneoplastic
Infection
Drug-induced vasculitis: ANCA-associated, other

*May involve small-, medium-, and large-sized blood vessels.
†Immune complexes formed in situ, in contrast to other forms of immune complex–mediated vasculitis
‡Frequent overlap of small- and medium-sized blood vessel involvement
§Not all forms of these disorders are always associated with ANCA.

antiglomerular basement membrane [anti-GBM] antibodies)
The association of some cases with hepatitis B virus (HBV) infection

CLASSIFICATION BY VESSEL SIZE

Because the etiologies of most forms of vasculitis remain unknown, the most valid basis for classifying the vasculitides is the size of the predominant blood vessels involved. Under such classification schemes, the vasculitides are categorized initially by whether the vessels affected are large, medium, or small (see Table 81–1). "Large" generally denotes the aorta and its major branches (as well as the corresponding vessels in the venous circulation in some forms of vasculitis, e.g., Behçet's disease). "Medium" refers to vessels that are smaller than the major aortic branches yet still large enough to contain four elements: 1) an intima; 2) a continuous internal elastic lamina; 3) a muscular media; and 4) an adventitia. In clinical terms, medium-vessel vasculitis (see Table 81–1) is generally macrovascular (i.e., involves vessels large enough to be observed in gross pathologic specimens). Small-vessel vasculitis, which incorporates all vessels below macroscopic disease, includes capillaries, postcapillary venules, and arterioles. Such vessels are all typically less than 500 microns in outer diameter. Because glomeruli may be viewed simply as differentiated capillaries, forms of vasculitis that cause glomerulonephritis are considered to be small-vessel vasculitides. The typical clinical manifestations associated with small-, medium-, and large-vessel vasculitides are shown in Table 81–2.

All discussions of vasculitis classification schemes involving vessel size must acknowledge the frequent occurrence of overlap. For example, although PAN primarily involves medium-sized arteries, palpable purpura—a manifestation of small-vessel disease—clearly is observed in some cases. Despite the possibility of vessel size overlap within individual cases, the categorization of a patient's vasculitis as primarily large-, medium-, or

TABLE 81–2 · TYPICAL CLINICAL MANIFESTATIONS OF LARGE-, MEDIUM-, AND SMALL-VESSEL INVOLVEMENT BY VASCULITIS

Large	Medium	Small
Constitutional symptoms: fever, weight loss, malaise, arthralgias and arthritis (common to vasculitides of all vessel sizes)		
Limb claudication	Cutaneous nodules	Purpura
Asymmetric blood pressures	Ulcers	Vesiculobullous lesions
Absence of pulses	Livedo reticularis	Urticaria
Bruits	Digital gangrene	Glomerulonephritis
Aortic dilation	Mononeuritis multiplex	Alveolar hemorrhage
	Microaneurysms	Cutaneous extravascularnecrotizing granulomas
		Splinter hemorrhages
		Uveitis/episcleritis/scleritis

TABLE 81–3 • CONSIDERATIONS IN THE CLASSIFICATIONS OF SYSTEMIC VASCULITIS

Size of Predominant Blood Vessels Affected
Epidemiologic features
Age
Gender
Ethnic background
Pattern of Organ Involvement
Pathologic Features
Granulomatous inflammation
Immune complex deposition versus "pauci-immune" histopathology
Linear staining along glomerular basement membrane
Presence of ANCA or Anti-GBM Antibodies in Serum
Demonstration of a specific associated infection (hepatitis B or hepatitis C)

small-vessel in nature remains enormously useful in focusing the differential diagnosis, and is the first step in planning the approach to treatment.

ADDITIONAL CONSIDERATIONS IN CLASSIFICATION

Many other considerations are important in the classification of vasculitis (Table 81–3): 1) the patient's demographic profile (see following section on epidemiology); 2) the disease's tropism for particular organs; 3) the presence or absence of granulomatous inflammation; 4) the participation of immune complexes in disease pathophysiology; 5) the finding of characteristic autoantibodies in the patients' serum (e.g., ANCA or anti-GBM antibodies); and, 6) the detection of certain infections known to cause specific forms of vasculitis.

The organ tropisms of these disorders are illustrated by the following examples. Wegener's granulomatosis classically involves the kidneys, upper airways, and lungs. In contrast, Henoch-Schönlein purpura often affects the kidneys but never the nose or sinuses and almost never the lungs. In contrast to both of these forms of vasculitis, Cogan's syndrome is defined by the simultaneous occurrence of ocular inflammation (most often intersititial keratitis) and sensorineural hearing loss (and, in 10% of

TABLE 81–4 • FORMS OF VASCULITIS ASSOCIATED WITH GRANULOMATOUS INFLAMMATION

Giant-cell arteritis
Takayasu's arteritis
Cogan's syndrome
Wegener's granulomatosis
Churg-Strauss syndrome
Primary angiitis of the central nervous system

cases, a large-vessel vasculitis). The histopathologic findings in these three disorders are equally distinctive, ranging from granulomatous inflammation of small-to-medium-sized vessels (Wegener's granulomatosis), to immunoglobulin A (IgA) deposition in small vessels (Henoch-Schönlein purpura), to large-vessel vasculitis centered on the adventitia (Cogan's syndrome).

The granulomatous features of some forms of vasculitis resemble chronic infections (e.g., those caused by fungi or mycobacteria) or the inflammation induced by the presence of a foreign body. Granulomatous inflammation is more likely to be found in some organs—for example, the lung—than in others (e.g., the kidney or skin). Some patients without evidence of granulomatous inflammation at early points in their courses later demonstrate such features as their diseases unfold. Thus, patients initially diagnosed with cutaneous leukocytoclastic angiitis or microscopic polyangiitis may be reclassified as having Wegener's granulomatosis if disease manifestations appear in new organs and granulomatous inflammation is found on biopsy. Forms of vasculitis commonly associated with granulomatous inflammation are shown in Table 81–4.

Immune complexes are essential to the pathophysiology of some small- and medium-vessel vasculitides. Immune complex–mediated tissue injury does not produce a single clinical syndrome, but rather applies to many forms of vasculitis and overlaps with injuries caused by other immune mechanisms. Anti-GBM disease (Goodpasture's disease) is a unique form of immune complex disease in which the immune complexes form in situ rather than in the circulation.[6] Complexes of IgA1 are found in Henoch-Schönlein purpura. Immune complexes comprised of IgG, IgM, complement components, and the hepatitis C virion characterize most cases of mixed cryoglobulinemia. HBV surface antigen/antibody complexes are present in the circulation and involved tissues of patients with HBV-associated PAN.

In contrast, other small- and medium-vessel vasculitides, such as Wegener's granulomatosis, microscopic polyangiitis, and the Churg-Strauss syndrome, are pauci-immune diseases. Pauci-immune refers to the absence of significant Ig or complement deposition within diseased tissues. Many (but not all) patients with pauci-immune forms of vasculitis have ANCA in their serum. Three decades before the description of ANCA, Godman and Churg observed pathologic links between the diseases we now term *pauci-immune vasculitides*,[7] noting that these disorders "group themselves into a compass, (ranging from) necrotizing and granulomatous processes with angiitis, through mixed forms, to vasculitis without granulomata."

ANCA (see Chapter 83) are directed against antigens that reside within the primary granules of neutrophils and monocyte.[8] Two types of ANCA appear to be relevant to vasculitis: 1) ANCA directed against proteinase 3 (PR3), a serine protease found within the primary granules of neutrophils and monocytes; and 2) ANCA directed against myeloperoxidase (MPO), another serine protease found within the same granules. Although rigorous serologic assays for these antibodies are helpful in diagnosis, evidence for a primary etiologic role of these antibodies in human forms of pauci-immune vasculitis remains controversial. In contrast, anti-GBM antibodies have been proven to play a major role in the pathogenesis of Goodpasture's disease.[9]

Finally, although the causes of most forms of vasculitis remain unknown, several infections have been linked definitively with specific forms of these diseases (e.g., HBV with some cases of PAN and hepatitis C with type II mixed cryoglobulinemia).

Historic Attempts at Classification and Nomenclature

For decades after this initial description of vasculitis, most forms of systemic inflammatory vascular disease were termed *periarteritis nodosa*. In the 1900s, two major factors led to the recognition of new forms of vasculitis. First, the use of microscopy in the evaluation of pathologic specimens became routine. Second, horse serum and sulfonamides came to be employed in the treatment of many medical conditions. These new therapies frequently induced small-vessel vasculitides on the basis of serum sickness or "hypersensitivity" phenomena, which were observed readily through the microscope. In some cases, the histopathologic findings of hypersensitivity reactions (e.g., serum sickness) were confused with periarteritis nodosa. The gradual recognition that these syndromes represented departures from PAN spurred interest in the first classification scheme for necrotizing angiitis.

In 1952, Pearl Zeek[10] identified five major categories of necrotizing angiitis. The Zeek classification included: 1) hypersensitivity angiitis; 2) allergic granulomatous angiitis (the Churg-Strauss syndrome); 3) rheumatic arteritis (vasculitis associated with connective tissues disorders); 4) periarteritis nodosa; and, 5) temporal arteritis. This classification scheme omitted several forms of systemic vasculitis that were known but not yet described in the English medical literature (e.g., Wegener's granulomatosis and Takayasu's arteritis).

SOURCES OF CONFUSION IN CLASSIFICATION

Two forms of vasculitis, now termed *microscopic polyangiitis* and *cutaneous leukocytoclastic angiitis*, respectively, have been consistent sources of confusion in vasculitis nosology. In our current understanding of systemic vasculitides, it is clear that these two conditions are separate entities. Microscopic polyangiitis affects capillaries and veins as well as arteries (in contrast to PAN) and is recognized to be a disorder associated with ANCA in approximately 70 percent of cases.[11] In 1923, Friedrich Wohlwill[12] observed unequivocal evidence of small-vessel involvement in cases of vasculitis he still considered part of the spectrum of periarteritis nodosa. Davson and colleagues[13] remarked on two forms of periarteritis nodosa with differential effects on the kidney: one with a predilection for medium-sized, muscular arteries and the other for small vessels, including glomerulonephri-

tis. Davson and colleagues termed this latter form *microscopic periarteritis nodosa*. Unfortunately, swayed by both human and animal models of hypersensitivity that demonstrated small-vessel disease involving the kidneys, lungs, and other organs,[14,15] Zeek chose to group microscopic periarteritis nodosa under the heading of hypersensitivity vasculitis.[10]

Over the next several decades, hypersensitivity vasculitis came to refer to an immune complex–mediated small vasculitis of the skin that spared internal organs and often followed drug exposures.[16] The Chapel Hill Consensus Conference (CHCC)[17] (see following) recommended eliminating the term *hypersensitivity* altogether, because evidence for hypersensitivity is lacking in many cases. Participants in the CHCC preferred the term *cutaneous leukocytoclastic angiitis*, because of the disorder's typical confinement to the skin and the usual predominant cell type: the neutrophil. Although cutaneous leukocytoclastic angiitis can mimic the skin features of microscopic polyangiitis, cutaneous leukocytoclastic angiitis does not involve the kidneys, lungs, peripheral nerves, and other internal organs, and it is not associated with ANCA.

In 1990, the American College of Rheumatology (ACR) performed a study designed to establish criteria for the classification of vasculitis, through the identification of features that distinguish one form of vasculitis from others.[18,19] An important caveat: this study was *not* designed to establish criteria for diagnosis, but rather to facilitate research by permitting the inclusion of similar types of patients in studies. Patients with giant cell arteritis (GCA), Takayasu's arteritis, polyarteritis nodosa, Wegener's granulomatosis, the Churg-Strauss syndrome, Henoch-Schönlein purpura, and hypersensitivity vasculitis were included in this study.[16,20-25] The findings of the ACR study remain useful for the purposes of the study's original intention—the insurance of uniform inclusion criteria for patients in research studies. However, the passage of time and the development of new insights have shown the need for updates. First, because the study was performed before the days of reliable and widely available assays for ANCA, ANCA positivity was not considered as a possible classification criterion. Second, the ACR Classification Criteria study did not include microscopic polyangiitis as a separate disease, but rather lumped such patients under the heading of PAN.[22] Third, the study did not define classification criteria for such rarer forms of vasculitis as Cogan's syndrome and Behçet's disease.

In 1994, the CHCC reviewed the nomenclature of systemic vasculitides. Again, formal diagnostic criteria were not attempted, but definitions were created for 10 forms of vasculitis (in addition to the seven forms of vasculitis included in the ACR study, microscopic polyangiitis, Kawasaki's disease, and essential cryoglobulinemic vasculitis were defined). The CHCC emphasized the important role that ANCA play in the diagnosis of several forms of vasculitis, and they carefully distinguished microscopic polyangiitis from classic PAN. The conference defined classic PAN as necrotizing inflammation of medium-sized or small arteries without glomerulonephritis.[17] Microscopic polyangiitis was defined as a necrotizing vasculitis with few or no immune deposits that: 1) affects small blood vessels (capillaries, venules, or arterioles); 2) often includes glomerulonephritis and pulmonary capillaritis; and, 3) is often associated with either MPO- or PR3-ANCA.

The classification of vasculitis continues to evolve. In the years since the CHCC, it has become clear that hepatitis C plays a major role in 90 percent of cases that formerly were termed *essential* mixed cryoglobulinemia. However, some cases of this syndrome are not associated with hepatitis C infections and probably have some other infectious etiology. Similarly, with the availability of the HBV vaccine, increasingly fewer cases of PAN are associated with this infection. The great majority of PAN cases have no known cause. As emphasized by Churg,[26] cases of PAN currently termed *idiopathic* do not represent a single entity but almost certainly include several different disorders. Some of these, as indicated by low serum complement levels and measurable immune complexes in the blood, are mediated by immune complex deposition. Others may be relatively independent of this mechanism. Finally, although "cutaneous leukocytoclastic angiitis" may be preferable to "hypersensitivity vasculitis" in describing small-vessel vasculitis confined to the skin, the term fails to acknowledge the minority of cases in which lymphocytic infiltrates predominate, even early in the inflammatory lesion.

Epidemiology

Accurate definition of the epidemiology of vasculitis confronts several challenges. These include: 1) the relatively uncommon nature of many forms of vasculitis; 2) the frequent difficulties in making the correct diagnosis of vasculitis (and in distinguishing one form of vasculitis from another); 3) the fact that the etiologies of most types of vasculitis remain unknown; and 4) historic uncertainty with regard to the classification of these conditions. Nevertheless, in recent years, the epidemiology of some forms of vasculitis has been defined with reasonable precision. The major epidemiologic features of several forms of systemic vasculitis are shown in Table 81–5.

GEOGRAPHY

The epidemiologic features of systemic vasculitis vary tremendously by geography. This variation may reflect genetics, differences in environmental exposures dictated by continent and latitude, and the prevalence of other disease risk factors. For example, whereas Behçet's disease[27] is rare in North Americans (affecting only approximately 1 person in 300,000), the condition is perhaps several hundred times more common among inhabitants of countries that border the ancient silk route.[28] Similarly, although Takayasu's arteritis is rare in the United States—on the order of 3 new cases per million people per year—the disease is reportedly the most common cause of renal artery stenosis in India, where the incidence may be as high as 200 to 300 cases per million people per year. Several studies indicate that the prevalence of GCA in Olmsted County, Minnesota is similar to that of Scandinavian countries, with an annual incidence rate of approximately 240 cases for every million individuals over the age of 50.[29] The similar prevalence calculations across these countries probably reflect shared genetic risk factors for this condition, as many of the current inhabitants of Olmsted County are descended from Scandinavia and northern Europe. Based on 2000 U.S. Census data, the prevalence of GCA in the United States as a whole is approximately 160,000 per year.

AGE, GENDER, AND ETHNICITY

Age is an important consideration in the epidemiology of vasculitis. Eighty percent of patients with Kawasaki's disease are younger than age 5.[30] In contrast, GCA virtually never occurs in patients under the age of 50, and the mean age of patients with that disease is 72. Age may also impact disease severity and outcome. In Henoch-Schönlein purpura, the overwhelming majority of cases in children (who comprise 90% of all cases) have self-limited courses, resolving within several weeks. In adults, however, Henoch-Schönlein purpura may have a higher likelihood of chronicity and a greater likelihood of a poor renal outcome.[31]

The distribution of gender varies across many forms of vasculitis. Buerger's disease is the only form of vasculitis

---

TABLE 81–5 · EPIDEMIOLOGY OF SELECTED FORMS OF VASCULITIS

Disease	United States	Elsewhere	Age/Gender/Ethnic Predispositions
Giant cell arteritis	Incidence: 240 per million (Olmsted County, MN)	220-270/million (Scandinavian countries)	Age > 50, mean age 72; females 3:1; Northern European ancestry
Takayasu's arteritis	Incidence: 3 per million	200-300/million (India)	Age < 40; Females 9:1; Asian
Behçet's disease	Prevalence: 3 per million	3,000/million (Turkey)	Silk route countries
Polyarteritis nodosa	Incidence: 7 per million	7/million (Spain)	Slight male predominance
Kawasaki's disease	Incidence: 100 per million*	900/million (Japan)	Children of Asian ancestry
Wegener's granulomatosis	Incidence: 4 per million	8.5/million (United Kingdom)	Caucasians >> blacks
Henoch-Schönlein purpura	Incidence in children: 135-180 per million; In adults: 13 per million		Only 10% of cases occur in adults

From Gonzalez-Gay MA, Garcia-Porrua: Epidemiology of the vasculitides. Rheum Dis Clin North Am 27(4):729-750, 2001.
*Among children less than 5 years of age

with a striking male predominance. The predilection of this disease for males may be explained by the greater prevalence of smoking among males in most societies. In contrast, Takayasu's arteritis has an overwhelming tendency to occur in women (a 9:1 female-male ratio), a fact that presently has no explanation. Pauci-immune forms of vasculitis such as Wegener's granulomatosis occur in males and females with approximately equal frequencies, but there is some evidence for a female predominance in patients with the limited form of the disease and a male predominance among those with severe Wegener's granulomatosis.[32]

For some forms of vasculitis, there are striking variations in tendencies to afflict specific ethnic groups. GCA and Wegener's granulomatosis, for example, occur with an overwhelming predominance in Caucasians.[33-35] Takayasu's arteritis and Kawasaki's disease have higher incidences in patients of Asian ancestry.

GENES AND ENVIRONMENT

Although genetic risk factors are undoubtedly important in the susceptibility to some forms of vasculitis, familial cases are very unusual (with the exception of GCA; see following). The rarity of familial cases in vasculitis indicates that the genetics of these disorders are polygenic and complex. The strongest link between any single gene and vasculitis is the association of HLA-B51 with Behçet's disease. In Behçet's disease, 80 percent of Asian patients have the HLA-B51 gene.[28] The prevalence of HLA-B51 is significantly higher among patients with Behçet's disease in Japan than among nondisease controls (55% versus less than 15%). Among the sporadic cases of Behçet's disease involving Caucasian patients in the United States, however, HLA-B51 occurs in fewer than 15 percent of cases.

In addition to increasing the risk of disease susceptibility in some patients, HLA-B51 also increases disease severity. Patients with this gene are more likely to have posterior uveitis, central nervous system involvement, or other severe manifestations. Reports of familial aggregation in GCA are common. Genetic studies have indicated roles for HLA class II alleles such as HLA-DRB1*0401 and *0101, albeit the specific associations have varied from study to study.[36,37] Other work indicates that certain tumor necrosis factor (TNF) microsatellite polymorphisms may contribute to disease susceptibility.[38] Several environmental and occupational exposures have been linked to the development of vasculitis, but with the exception of Buerger's disease and smoking no true associations between disease and exposure have been confirmed. Associations have been reported but not confirmed between exposure to inhaled silica dust and some types of pauci-immune vasculitis.[39] Precise definitions of the relationships between exposures and vasculitis are complicated by difficulties in obtaining reliable measurements of the levels of such exposures, the likelihood of recall bias among patients who are diagnosed with vasculitis, and the choice of appropriate control groups.

Finally, estimates of disease prevalence in vasculitis may be subject to revision because of changing disease definitions. In the ACR Classification Criteria study, for example, manifestations of both small- and medium-vessel involvement were included in the criteria for PAN.[22] Four years later, the CHCC defined PAN as a form of arterial inflammation limited to medium-sized vessels, sparing capillaries, arterioles, and venules.[17] Under this definition, classic PAN is believed to be a rare condition. Applying the CHCC definition retrospectively, not a single case of classic PAN was reported over a 6-year period in the region of the Norwich Health Authority (United Kingdom), an area that included a population of more than 400,000 people.[40]

The epidemiologic differences among individual types of vasculitis raise compelling questions about the etiologies of these diseases. Ultimately, better insights into the pathogenesis of these conditions should explain these epidemiologic differences and will in turn facilitate the development of more refined classification schemes.

REFERENCES

1. Lie JT: Nomenclature and classification of vasculitis: plus ça change, plus c'est la même chose. Arthritis Rheum 37:181-186, 1994.
2. Kussmaul A, Maier R: Ueber eine bisher nicht beschriebene eigenthümliche Arterienerkrankung (Periarteritis nodosa), die mit Morbus Brightii und rapid fortschreitender allgemeiner Muskellähmung einhergeht. Dtsch Arch Klin Med 1:484-518, 1866.
3. Matteson F: Polyarteritis nodosa: Commemorative translation on the 130-year anniversary of the original article by Adolf Kussmaul and Rudolf Maier. Rochester, Minn., Mayo Foundation, 1996.
4. Ferrari E: Ueber Polyarteritis acuta nodosa (sogenannte Periarteritis nodosa) und ihre Beziehungen zur Polymyositis und Polyneuritis acuta. Beitr Pathol Anat 34:350-386, 1903.
5. Dickson W: Polyarteritis acuta nodosa and periarteritis nodosa. J Pathol Bacterial 12:31-57, 1908.
6. Salama AD, Pusey CD: Immunology of anti-glomerular basement membrane disease. Curr Opin Nephrol Hyperten 11:279-286, 2002.
7. Godman GC, Churg J: Wegener's granulomatosis: Pathology and review of the literature. Arch Pathol 58:533-553, 1954.
8. Hoffman GS, Specks U: Antineutrophil cytoplasmic antibodies. Arthritis Rheum 41(9):1521-1537, 1998.
9. Salama AD, Levy JB, Lightstone L, Pusey CD: Goodpasture's disease. Lancet 358:917-920, 2001.
10. Zeek PM: Periarteritis nodosa: A critical review. Am J Clin Pathol 22:777-790, 1952.
11. Guillevin L, Durand-Gasselin B, Cevallos R, et al: Microscopic polyangiitis: clinical and laboratory findings in 85 patients. Arthritis Rheum 42:421-430, 1999.
12. Wohlwill F: On the only microscopically recognizable form of periarteritis nodosa. Virchow's Archiv für pathologische Anatomie und Physiologie 246:377-411, 1923.
13. Davson J, Ball J, Platt R: The kidney in periarteritis nodosa. Q JM 17:175-192, 1948.
14. Rich AR: The role of hypersensitivity in periarteritis nodosa. Bull JHH LXXI:123-140, 1942.
15. Zeek P, Smith C, Weeter J: Studies on periarteritis nodosa. III. The differentiation between the vascular lesions of periarteritis nodosa and hypersensitivity. Am J Pathol 24:889-917, 1948.
16. Calabrese LH, Michel BA, Bloch DA, et al: The American College of Rheumatology 1990 criteria for the classification of hypersensitivity vasculitis. Arthritis Rheum 33:1094-1100, 1990.
17. Jennette JC, Falk RJ, Andrassy K, et al: Nomenclature of systemic vasculitides: proposal of an international consensus conference. Arthritis Rheum 37(2):187-192, 1994.
18. Hunder GG, Arend WP, Bloch DA, et al: The American College of Rheumatology 1990 criteria for the classification of vasculitis: Introduction. Arthritis Rheum 33:1065-1067, 1990.

19. Bloch DA, Michel BA, Hunder GG, et al: The American College of Rheumatology 1990 criteria for the classification of vasculitis: patients and methods. Arthritis Rheum 33:1068-1073, 1990.

20. Hunder GG, Bloch DA, Michel BA, et al: The American College of Rheumatology 1990 criteria for the classification of giant cell arteritis Arthritis Rheum 33:1122-1128, 1990.

21. Arend WP, Michel BA, Bloch DA, et al: The American College of Rheumatology 1990 criteria for the classification of Takayasu's arteritis. Arthritis Rheum 33:1129-1134, 1990.

22. Lightfoot RW Jr., Michel BA, Bloch DA, et al: The American College of Rheumatology 1990 criteria for the classification of polyarteritis nodosa. Arthritis Rheum 33:1088-1093, 1990.

23. Leavitt RY, Fauci AS, Bloch DA, et al: The American College of Rheumatology 1990 criteria for the classification of Wegener's granulomatosis. Arthritis Rheum 33:1101-1107, 1990.

24. Masi AT, Hunder GG, Lie JT, et al: The American College of Rheumatology 1990 criteria for the classification of Churg-Strauss syndrome (allergic granulomatosis and angiitis). Arthritis Rheum 33:1094-1100, 1990.

25. Mills JA, Michel BA, Bloch DA, et al: The American College of Rheumatology 1990 criteria for the classification of Henoch-Schönlein purpura. Arthritis Rheum 33:1114-1121, 1990.

26. Churg J: Nomenclature of vasculitic syndromes: A historical perspective. Am J Kidney Dis 18(2):148-153, 1991.

27. International Study Group for Behçet's disease: Criteria for diagnosis of Behçet's disease. Lancet 335:1078-1080, 1990.

28. Sakane T, Tekeno M, Suzuki N, et al: Behcet's disease. N Engl J Med 341:1284-1291, 1999.

29. Salvarani C, Gabriel SE, O'Fallon WM, et al: The incidence of giant cell arteritis in Olmsted County, Minnesota: Apparent fluctuations in a cyclic pattern. Ann Intern Med 123:192-194, 1995.

30. Barron KS, Shulman ST, Rowley A, et al: Report of the National Institutes of Health Workshop on Kawasaki's Disease. J Rheumatol 26:170-190, 1999.

31. Blanco R, Martinez-Taboada VM, Rodriguez-Valverde V, et al: Henoch-Schönlein purpura in adulthood and childhood: Two different expressions of the same syndrome. Arthritis Rheum 40:859-864, 1997.

32. The Wegener's Granulomatosis Etanercept Trial Research Group: Limited versus severe Wegener's granulomatosis: Baseline data on patients in the Wegener's Granulomatosis Etanercept Trial. Arthritis Rheum 2003, 48(8): 2299-309.

33. Liu NH, LaBree LD, Feldon SE, Rao NA. The epidemiology of giant cell arteritis a 12-year retrospective study. Ophthalmology 2001, 108(6): 1145-9.

34. Falk RJ, Hogan S, Carey TS, Jennette JC: Clinical course of anti-neutrophil cytoplasmic autoantibody-associated glomerulonephritis and systemic vasculitis. The Glomerular Disease Collaborative Network. Ann Intern Med 113:656-663, 1990.

35. Hoffman GS, Kerr GS, Leavitt RY, et al: Wegener's granulomatosis: an analysis of 158 patients. Ann Intern Med 116:488-498, 1992.

36. Weyand CM, Hunder GG, Hickok KC, et al: HLA-DRB1 alleles in polymyalgia rheumatica, giant cell arteritis, and rheumatoid arthritis. Arthritis Rheum 37:514-520, 1994.

37. Rauzy O, Fort M, Nourhashemi F: Relation between HLA DRB1 alleles and corticosteroid resistance in giant cell arteritis. Ann Rheum Dis 57:380-382, 1998.

38. Mattey DL, Hajeer AH, Dababneh A, et al: Association of giant cell arteritis and polymyalgia rheumatica with different tumor necrosis factor microsatellite polymorphisms. Arthritis Rheum 43:1749-1755, 2000.

39. Hogan SL, Satterly KK, Dooley MA, et al: Silica exposure in anti-neutrophil cytoplasmic autoantibody-associated glomerulonephritis and lupus nephritis. J Am Soc Nephrol 12:134-142, 2001.

40. Watts R, Carruthers D, Scott D: Epidemiology of systemic vasculitis: changing incidence or definition? Semin Arthritis Rheum 25:28-34, 1995.

41. Gonzalez-Gay MA, Garcia-Porrua: Epidemiology of the vasculitides. Rheum Dis Clin North Am 27(4):729-750, 2001.

Giant Cell Arteritis and Polymyalgia Rheumatica

DAVID B. HELLMANN • GENE G. HUNDER

Giant cell arteritis (GCA) and polymyalgia rheumatica (PMR) are discussed together because they are linked conditions that affect similar epidemiologic subsets of patients and often occur together in the same individual.

Definitions

GIANT CELL ARTERITIS

GCA is the most common form of systemic vasculitis in adults.[1] The disease primarily affects the extracranial branches of the carotid artery in patients more than 50 years old. The most feared complication of GCA is the possibility of irreversible visual loss. Because the cause of GCA is unknown, various names—including temporal arteritis, cranial arteritis, and granulomatous arteritis—have been employed to highlight different salient features. All of the designations for this disease have both merits and shortcomings. The designation temporal arteritis or cranial arteritis, for example, conveys how frequently the temporal arteries or other cranial arteries are involved but fails to capture GCA's more widespread nature. Although granulomatous arteritis and GCA pay homage to an important pathologic finding, the names may focus on this more than is deserved because giant cells are absent in about half of the cases and present in other forms of vasculitis. With no perfect name available, this chapter bows to convention in opting to refer to this disease as giant cell arteritis, or GCA.

POLYMYALGIA RHEUMATICA

Polymyalgia rheumatica, a term suggested by Barber,[2] is a syndrome characterized by aching in the proximal portions of the extremities and torso. PMR, a disease without a specific diagnostic test or pathologic finding, is an entity defined by its clinical features. The following features are usually included in most definitions of PMR: 1) aching and morning stiffness lasting half an hour or longer in the shoulder, hip girdle, neck, or some combination of these; 2) duration of these symptoms for 1 month or longer; 3) age greater than 50 years; and 4) laboratory evidence of systemic inflammation (e.g., an elevated erythrocyte sedimentation rate [ESR]).[3] Some definitions have also included a rapid response to small doses of glucocorticoids, such as 10 mg of prednisone daily.[4] The presence of another specific disease other than GCA, such as rheumatoid arthritis (RA), chronic infection, polymyositis, or malignancy, excludes the diagnosis of PMR.

Epidemiology

The incidence of GCA varies widely in different populations, from less than 0.1 per 100,000 to 33 per 100,000 persons aged 50 years and older.[5-15] The greatest risk factor for developing GCA is aging, as the disease almost never occurs before age 50, and its incidence rises steadily thereafter. Nationality, geography, and race are also important, as the highest incidence figures are found in Scandinavians and in Americans of Scandinavian descent. The lowest incidences of GCA are reported in Japanese, Northern Indians, and African Americans. Within Western Europe, GCA is more common in northern latitudes than in southern ones. The incidence of GCA has been increasing over the last 20 to 40 years, possibly because of greater physician awareness.[5] Some studies have reported seasonal variations and clustering of cases with peaks about 7 years apart.[5,14] The prevalence of GCA in Olmsted County, Minnesota, home to many Scandinavian immigrants, is 200 per 100,000 population aged 50 years or older.[13] Autopsy studies suggest that GCA may be more common than is clinically apparent. Östberg[16] found arteritis in 1.6 percent of 889 postmortem cases in which sections of the temporal artery and two transverse sections of the aorta were examined.

Genetic susceptibility to the development of GCA was suggested initially by reports of GCA in families[17-19] and more recently by studies demonstrating an association of GCA with genes in the human leukocyte antigen (HLA) class II region.[20,21] Sixty percent of GCA patients have HLA-DRB1*04 haplotype variants, which have a common sequence motif in the second hypervariable region of the B1 molecule.[21] This motif differs from that found in patients with RA.[21] The low prevalence of these alleles in African Americans may explain why blacks develop GCA relatively infrequently. To date, GCA is the form of systemic vasculitis most closely associated with HLA class II genes.

The role of environmental risk factors in for GCA has been suggested by the geographic clustering of cases noted previously. Smoking appears to increase the risk of developing GCA sixfold in women.[22] Circumstantial evidence links the development of GCA to a variety of infectious agents, including *Mycoplasma* pneumonia, varicella-zoster virus, parvovirus B19, and parainfluenza virus type I.[14,15] The reported association of GCA and *Chlamydia pneumoniae* infection has not withstood close scrutiny.[23]

Gender and health status also influence the development of GCA. Women are affected about twice as often as men.[14] Having diabetes reduces the risk of developing GCA by 50 percent in women.[22] Although patients with GCA have an increased risk of developing thoracic aortic aneurysms, they do not have overall higher mortality rates.[14]

PMR is two to three times more common than GCA.[14,15,24,25] In Olmsted County, Minnesota, 245 cases of PMR were diagnosed during the 22-year period from 1970 through 1991, providing an average annual incidence rate of 52.5 cases per 100,000 persons aged 50 years or older.[25] The prevalence of PMR (active plus remitted cases) was approximately 600 per 100,000 persons aged 50 years and older.[25] PMR is associated with the same HLA-DR4 genes as GCA.[20,21,26]

Etiology, Pathology, and Pathogenesis

ETIOLOGY

The causes of GCA and PMR are unknown. Because pathologic studies have provided important clues to the pathogenesis, however, they are discussed first.

PATHOLOGY

In GCA, inflammation is found most often in medium-sized muscular arteries that originate from the arch of the aorta.[14,16,27] The inflammation tends to affect the arteries in a segmental fashion (possibly leading to "skip lesions" within arteries), but long portions of arteries may be involved.[28] In patients who died during the active phase of GCA, the greatest frequency of severe involvement was noted in the superficial temporal arteries, vertebral arteries, and ophthalmic and posterior ciliary arteries.[29] The internal carotid, external carotid, and central retinal arteries were affected somewhat less frequently.[29] In other postmortem studies, lesions were found commonly in the proximal and distal aorta and internal and external carotid, subclavian, brachial, and abdominal arteries.[16] Because GCA affects vessels with an internal elastic lamina and vaso vasorum, and because intracranial arteries lose these structures after penetrating the dura, it is not surprising that GCA rarely involves intracranial arteries.[29-32] In some patients with GCA, follow-up biopsy or autopsy surveys have shown persistence of mild chronic inflammation even though symptoms had resolved.[33]

Early in the disease, collections of lymphocytes are confined to the region of the internal or external elastic lamina or adventitia. The inflammation may be limited to the vasa vasorum in some cases.[34] Intimal thickening with prominent cellular infiltration is a hallmark of more advanced cases. In heavily involved areas, all layers are affected (Fig. 82–1). Transmural inflammation of portions of the arterial wall (including the elastic laminae) and granulomas containing multinucleated histiocytic and foreign body giant cells, histiocytes, lymphocytes (which are predominantly cell determinant [CD]4+ T cells), and some plasma cells and fibroblasts are found.[35-38] Eosinophils may be seen,

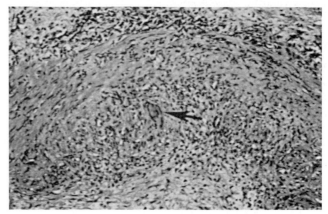

FIGURE 82–1 · Giant-Cell Arteritis (GCA). In transverse section of temporal artery, adventitia is at top and intima is at central portion of bottom. Multinucleated giant cell *(arrow)* is present at junction of media and intima. There is extensive disruption of all layers of vessel wall. (H&E, × 100) (Courtesy of Dr. J.T. Lie.)

but polymorphonuclear leukocytes are rare. Thrombosis may develop at sites of active inflammation; later, these areas may recanalize. The inflammatory process is usually most marked in the inner portion of the media adjacent to the internal elastic lamina. Fragmentation and disintegration of elastic fibers occur, closely associated with an accumulation of giant cells (Fig. 82–2). However, giant cells are seen in only about half of routinely examined specimens and, therefore, are not required for the diagnosis if other features are compatible. In contrast to some other forms of systemic vasculitis (e.g., polyarteritis

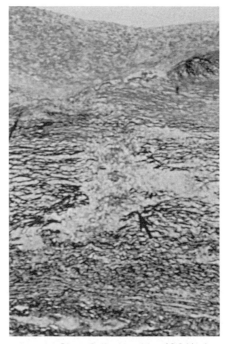

FIGURE 82–2 · Giant-Cell Arteritis (GCA) Involving the Proximal Aorta in a Patient Dying of a Ruptured Ascending Aorta. This section of the ascending aorta is distal to the ruptured portion and shows destruction of elastic fibers *(arrow)*. (Elastic van Gieson stain, × 64) Neighboring sections stained with hematoxylin and eosin showed infiltrations of mononuclear leukocytes in the areas of disrupted fibers.

nodosa, microscopic polyangiitis, and Wegener's granulomatosis), fibrinoid necrosis is rarely if ever observed in GCA.[34]

Immunohistochemical studies have demonstrated inflammatory changes that are specific for each layer of the affected artery.[15,36,43] The adventitia is infiltrated by CD4+ T cells that secrete interferon-γ (IFN-γ) and interleukin-2 (IL-2), and macrophages that secrete IL-1, IL-6, and transforming growth factor-β (TGF-β). This cytokine pattern is characteristic of a T helper type 1 (Th 1) cell–mediated reaction.[40] The advential T cells show evidence of clonal expansion. The media is populated mostly by macrophages that, in contrast to those in other layers, produce matrix metalloproteinases (MMPs) and oxygen free radicals. Closer to the intima, the macrophages secrete nitric oxide and unite to form syncytia—the giant cells—which produce platelet-derived growth factor (PDGF) and substances that stimulate intimal proliferation.[44]

Although microscopic examination of arteries in PMR are usually normal, immunohistochemical studies of apparently uninvolved temporal arteries reveal upregulation of the same macrophage-related inflammatory cytokines found in GCA.[40] The T cell cytokine IFN-γ is abundantly expressed in GCA and is absent in arteries from patients having only PMR.[40] Relatively little else pathologically has been found in PMR. Granulomatous myocarditis and hepatitis have been noted.[45] Muscle biopsy specimens have been normal or have shown nonspecific type II muscle atrophy.[46] However, a number of reports have shown the presence of lymphocytic synovitis in the knees, sternoclavicular joints, and shoulders and evidence of a similar reaction in sacroiliac joints.[47-51] Synovitis (mostly subclinical) has been shown in bone scans demonstrating an increased uptake of technetium pertechnetate in the joints of 24 of 25 patients with PMR.[48] More sensitive studies using magnetic resonance imaging (MRI) and ultrasound have convincingly demonstrated that in PMR, the principal foci of inflammation are the bursa surrounding the shoulder more than the glenohumeral joint itself[52] (Fig. 82–3).

Sera from patients with GCA, PMR, or both demonstrate evidence of systemic inflammation with increased levels of circulating immune complexes during active disease[53,54] and elevated levels of IL-6 and IL-1.[39]

PATHOGENESIS

These observations have been used to propose a model of the immunopathogenesis of GCA[36] (Fig. 82–4). An (unknown) antigen is encountered by T cells in the adventitia, the only arterial layer normally penetrated by the vasa vasorum. Although most speculations have centered on infectious agents, a neoantigen formed during aging is also possible. Following activation, the adventitial CD4+ T cells expand clonally and secrete IFN-γ, which causes macrophages to migrate, differentiate,

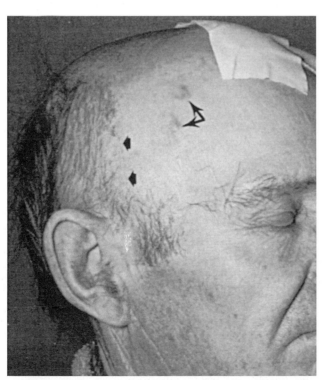

FIGURE 82–3 · Giant-Cell Arteritis (GCA) Involving Temporal Artery. Short segments of curved artery were erythematous and tender *(long arrows)*. Bandage on scalp is over similar artery that was sampled on biopsy and showed GCA. Previous biopsy specimen of a proximal segment of right temporal artery, which was normal on physical examination, was normal histologically. Faint scar of this biopsy can be seen above and anterior to right ear *(short arrows)*.

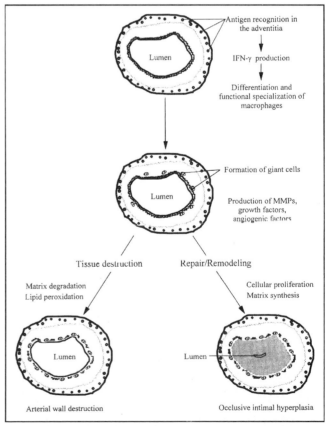

FIGURE 82–4 · Proposed model for the Pathogenesis of Giant cell Arteritis.

and form granuloma. Production of MMPs and lipid peroxidation agents by macrophages in the media results in destruction of elastic laminae. The vessel attempts to counter the tissue destruction by elaborating a variety of growth factors, including PDGF, vascular endothelial growth factor (VEGF), andTGF-β, which prompt smooth muscle cells in the media to revert from a contractile phenotype to a secretory one and to migrate to the intima. Proliferation of the intimal smooth muscle cells results in occlusion of the lumen.[36] PMR appears to result from a similar but less intense innate immune response in blood vessels (as evidenced by the in situ production of many inflammatory cytokines).[40] According to this model, the distinguishing feature of PMR is the absence of T cells producing IFN-γ. Without IFN-γ to stimulate the recruitment and differentiation of macrophages, the level of arterial inflammation in PMR remains subclinical. The constitutional symptoms of PMR and GCA are attributed to the high levels of inflammatory cytokines (e.g., IL-1, IL-6) found in the sera. Whether these serum cytokine elevations result from blood vessel inflammation alone or from some other source of inflammation is not yet clear.

The attractiveness of this model is increased by its ability to explain why subsets of clinical features occur together (see following).

Clinical Features

The mean age at onset of GCA and PMR is approximately 70 years, with a range of about 50 to more than 90 years of age.[14] Younger patients with PMR have been described occasionally. Women are affected about twice as often as men.[1,25] Although the onset of the disease is usually insidious, typically evolving over weeks or months, in one third of cases the disease begins so abruptly that some patients recall the very day they became ill.[14,45]

GIANT CELL ARTERITIS

Classic Manifestations

The most common manifestations of GCA are constitutional symptoms, headache, visual symptoms, jaw claudication, and PMR[14] (Table 82–1). Almost all patients experience one or more constitutional symptoms, including fatigue, weight loss, malaise, and fever.

Beyond constitutional symptoms, headache is the most common symptom in GCA, being present in nearly three quarters of patients.[55] The pain is typically described as boring in quality, of moderate severity, and most commonly appreciated in the temporal area. However, the description of the headache varies enormously. It can be mild to so severe that the patient seeks immediate relief by presenting to the emergency department. The pain may localize to any site of the skull, including the occiput (owing to involvement of the occipital artery).[14,16] The most consistent characteristic is that the patient experiences the headache as something new and unusual. In untreated patients, the

Symptom	Frequency (%)
Headache	76
Weight loss	43
Fever	42
Fatigue	39
Any visual symptom	37
Anorexia	35
Jaw claudication	34
Polymyalgia rheumatica (PMR)	34
Arthralgia	30
Unilateral visual loss	24
Bilateral visual loss	15
Vertigo	11
Diplopia	9

TABLE 82–1 • SYMPTOMS AMONG PATIENTS WITH GIANT CELL ARTERITIS (GCA)*

*Modified from Smetana GW, Shmerling RH: Does this patient have temporal arteritis? JAMA 287:92, 2002. Data from a review of 2475 patients whose data have been reported in the literature. (Reprinted by permission of JAMA)

headache may subside over weeks, even though the disease activity continues. The headache of GCA is often not associated with any particular findings on physical examination. Abnormalities of the temporal artery—including enlargement, nodular swelling, tenderness, or loss of pulse—develop in only about half of patients (Fig. 82–5). Some patients will note tenderness of the scalp, which can be aggravated by brushing or combing the hair.

Visual symptoms are common in GCA, especially visual loss and diplopia. Visual loss can be unilateral or (less commonly) bilateral, transient or permanent, and partial or complete.[56,57] Visual loss lasting more than a

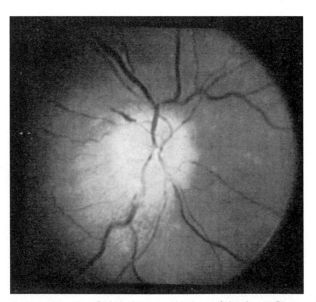

FIGURE 82–5 • Ophthalmoscopic view of the Acute Phase of Ischemic Optic Neuropathy as seen in Patients with Giant cell Arteritis (GCA) and Loss of Vision. The optic disk is pale and swollen, the retinal veins are dilated, and a flame-shaped hemorrhage is visible. (Courtesy of Dr. J. Trautmann.)

few hours usually does not reverse. Loss of vision often reflects an anterior ischemic optic neuropathy (AION) caused by occlusive arteritis of the posterior ciliary artery, the chief blood supply to the optic-nerve head. The posterior ciliary artery is a branch of the ophthalmic artery (which derives, in turn, from the internal carotid artery). Less frequently, visual loss in GCA stems from a retinal artery occlusion. Regardless of the site of the culprit lesion, visual loss in GCA is usually profound, with more than 80 percent of patients unable to see hand waving.[56]

The early funduscopic appearance observed in the setting of blindness caused by AION is that of ischemic optic neuritis—slight pallor and edema of the optic disk, with scattered cotton-wool patches and small hemorrhages[56] (Fig. 82–6). Later, optic atrophy occurs. Blindness may rarely be the initial symptom but tends to follow other symptoms by several weeks or even months. Ophthalmoscopic examination findings in patients without eye involvement are generally normal. In most reports, the incidence of blindness has been 20 percent or less.[4,24,30,54,56,58] In a series of 245 patients from the modern era, 34 (14%) had some permanent visual loss.[58] In 32 of these patients, the visual deficit developed before glucocorticoid therapy was begun. In the other two, the visual loss occurred after therapy was started. Visual loss progressed in 3 of the 32 after therapy was initiated, and in 5 it improved. At 5 years of follow-up, among the patients with visual deficits caused by GCA at the time glucocorticoids were started, the risk of additional visual loss was 13 percent over the follow-up period. If no visual loss had occurred at the beginning of glucocorticoid therapy, there was only a 1-percent risk of new visual loss over the subsequent 5 years.

Another potential ocular complication of GCA is ophthalmoplegia. Diplopia usually results from ocular motor nerve palsies caused by ischemia and usually resolves after therapy is started. Oculomotor nerve involvement in GCA usually spares the pupil.[56] Rarely, arterial lesions cause infarction of the occipital cortex with visual loss.

Intermittent claudication may occur in the muscles of mastication (jaw claudication), the extremities, and occasionally the muscles of the tongue or those involved in swallowing.[14] In the jaw muscles, the discomfort is noted especially when chewing meat and may involve the muscles on one side of the mandible more than those on the other. In some instances, however, facial artery involvement results in spasm of the jaw muscles. More marked vascular narrowing may lead to gangrene of the scalp or the tongue.

Atypical Manifestations of Giant Cell Arteritis

Approximately 40 percent of patients present with disease manifestations that are considered atypical[59-61] (Table 82–2). In these patients, headache, jaw claudication, visual symptoms and PMR do not occur or are less prominent.

Fever occurs in up to 40 percent of patients with GCA, but it is usually low grade and overshadowed by other classic symptoms. However, 15 percent of GCA patients may present with a fever of unknown origin (FUO) in which the temperature spikes are high and dominate the clinical picture.[4,45] Although GCA causes only 2 percent of all cases of FUO, it is responsible for 16 percent of all such fevers in individuals over the age of 65.[45] Approximately two thirds of patients experience shaking chills and drenching sweats, features often attributed to infection or malignancy. The median temperature is 39.1° C, and the maximum 39.8° C. The white blood cell count in GCA-induced FUO is usually normal or nearly so (at least before the initiation of prednisone).

Neurologic problems occur in approximately 30 percent of patients.[31,32] These are diverse, but most common are neuropathies and transient ischemic attacks or strokes. Hemiparesis or brain stem events are due to narrowing or occlusion of the carotid or vertebrobasilar

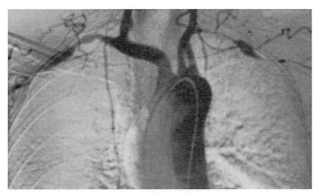

FIGURE 82–6 · Giant Cell Arteritis (GCA) of Large Arteries. Arch aortogram. Both subclavian and axillary arteries are affected. Smooth-walled segmental constrictions alternate with areas of normal caliber or aneurysmal dilation. (From Klein RG, Hunder GG, Stanson AW, Sheps SG: Large artery involvement in giant cell [temporal] arteritis. Ann Intern Med 83:806, 1975. Reprinted by permission of Annals of Internal Medicine.)

TABLE 82–2 · ATYPICAL MANIFESTATIONS OF GIANT CELL ARTERITIS (GCA)

Fever of unknown origin
Respiratory symptoms (especially cough)
Otolaryngeal manifestations
   Glossitis
   Lingual infarction
   Throat pain
   Hearing loss
Large-artery disease
   Aortic aneurysm
   Aortic dissection
   Limb claudication
   Raynaud's phenomenon
Neurologic manifestations
   Peripheral neuropathy
   Transient ischemic attack, (TIA) or stroke
   Dementia
   Delerium
Myocardial infarction
Tumorlike lesions
   Breast mass
   Ovarian and uterine mass
Syndrome of inappropriate antidiuretic hormone secretion (SIADH)
Microangiopathic hemolytic anemia

artery. GCA preferentially involves the posterior circulation; the 3:2 ratio of anterior to posterior strokes and transient ischemic attacks seen in the normal population, reaches nearly 1:1 in patients with GCA.[31] Delirium, reversible dementia, and myelopathy have also been reported.[31] However, the assignment of an exact etiology to ischemic central nervous system events is often challenging, given the older population in which GCA occurs. The neuropathies of GCA include mononeuropathies and peripheral polyneuropathies and may affect the upper or lower extremities. Presumably, they are secondary to involvement of nutrient arteries, but little pathologic documentation is available. Among the vasculitides, GCA has a nearly unique propensity for involving the C5 nerve root, resulting in loss of shoulder abduction.[31] Mononeuropathies affecting the hands and feet, so typical of polyarteritis and other forms of vasculitis, develop less often in GCA.

Prominent respiratory tract symptoms occur in about 10 percent of patients.[63] These include cough with or without sputum, sore throat, and hoarseness. When these symptoms are severe or an initial manifestation of GCA, they may direct the attention of the examining physician away from the underlying arteritis. The vasculitis may induce these symptoms by causing ischemia or hyperirritability of the affected tissues. Otolaryngeal manifestations of GCA include throat pain, dental pain, tongue pain, glossitis, and ulceration or infarction of the tongue.[63,64]

Clinical evidence of large-artery involvement occurs in 10 to 15 percent of cases.[28,50,51,65,66] The findings are upper extremity claudication; bruits over the carotid, subclavian, axillary, and brachial arteries; absent or decreased pulses in the neck or arms; and Raynaud's phenomenon (Fig. 82–7). Angiographic features that suggest GCA are smooth-walled arterial stenoses or occlusions alternating with areas of normal or increased caliber in the absence of irregular plaques and ulcerations, located especially in the carotid, subclavian, axillary, and brachial arteries. Thoracic aortic aneurysms and dissection of the aorta are important late complications in GCA. In one series of 41 patients,

the average time between the diagnosis of GCA and the recognition of this complication was 7 years.[65] Thoracic aortic aneurysms were 17 times more likely to develop in patients with GCA than in persons without this disease. To place this figure in context, this means that thoracic aortic aneurysms are twice as likely to complicate GCA as lung cancer is to result from smoking.[66]

In women, GCA may present as a breast or ovarian mass. The mass lesions in these tissues result from granulomatous inflammation in and around the arteries.[67] Angina pectoris, congestive heart failure, and myocardial infarction secondary to coronary arteritis occur rarely.

Clinical Subsets

Studies suggest that GCA is not just one disease, but rather consists of clinical subsets, which in turn are explained by the differential expression of inflammatory cytokines.[68] Ischemic events, including blindness and large-artery disease, occur more commonly in patients who express high levels of IFN-γ and low levels of IL-6.[68] In contrast, patients who produce high levels of IL-6 are more likely to have strong inflammatory features (such as fever and constitutional symptoms) and are less likely to develop visual loss or other ischemic events.[68-71]

POLYMYALGIA RHEUMATICA

As in GCA, PMR patients are characteristically in good health before their disease begins.[14] Systemic manifestations, such as malaise, low-grade fever, and weight loss, are present in more than half the patients and may be the initial symptoms. High, spiking fevers are uncommon in PMR in the absence of GCA.[45] Arthralgias and myalgias may develop abruptly or evolve insidiously over weeks or months.[3] Malaise, fatigue, and depression, along with aching and stiffness, may be present for months before the diagnosis is made. In most patients, the shoulder girdle is the first to become symptomatic; in the remainder, the hip or neck is involved at the onset.

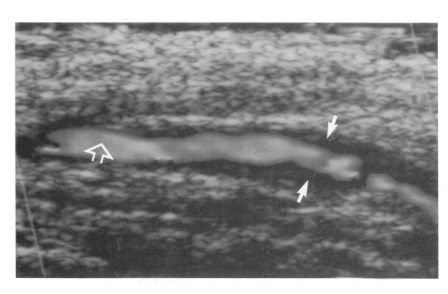

FIGURE 82–7 · Color Duplex Ultrasound Examination of a Swollen, Tender Temporal Artery in a Patient with Giant-cell Arteritis (GCA). The variably thickened artery wall is visible as the clear "halo" (*solid arrows*) around the lumen in the center (*open arrow*).

The discomfort may begin in one shoulder or hip but usually becomes bilateral within weeks. Symptoms center on the proximal limb, axial musculature, and tendinous attachments. Morning stiffness resembling that of RA and "gelling" after inactivity are usually prominent. If the symptoms are severe, aching is more persistent. Although movement of the joints accentuates the pain, it is often felt in the proximal extremities rather than in the joints.[3] Distal joint pain and swelling occur in some cases, including diffuse distal extremity swelling with pitting edema.[72] Pain at night is common, and movement during sleep may awaken the patient. Muscle strength is generally unimpaired, although the pain with movement makes the interpretation of strength-testing maneuvers difficult. Pain with movement also makes it difficult for patients to get out of bed or the bathtub. In the later stages of the syndrome, muscle atrophy may develop, and contracture of the shoulder capsule may result in limitation of passive motion as well as of active motion.

As noted, the presence of bursal inflammation and synovitis in PMR has been described by many authors and is undoubtedly the cause of many of the findings in this condition.[52] A careful examination may reveal transient synovitis of the knees, wrists, and sternoclavicular joints. The shoulders and hips are covered by heavy muscles, and minimal effusions of slight synovitis are not palpable on physical examination. Synovitis has been documented by biopsies, synovial analysis, joint scintiscans, ultrasound, and MRI.[46-51,73]

Relationship Between Polymyalgia Rheumatica and Giant Cell Arteritis

There is abundant evidence that PMR and GCA are related and should be considered different manifestations of a common disease process.[14] The association with age, ethnicity, geographic region, and HLA class II alleles are the same in both disorders. Moreover, both disorders involve overproduction of many of the same inflammatory cytokines. Between 30 and 50 percent of patients with GCA develop PMR. Approximately 10 to 15 percent of patients who appear to have only PMR will have positive temporal-artery biopsies. In the absence of symptoms of GCA (e.g., headache, jaw claudication, visual symptoms, or high fever), PMR by itself does not appear to cause visual loss and responds to low doses of glucocorticoids (see following).[14]

Laboratory Studies

Except for the findings on arterial biopsy, laboratory results in PMR and GCA are similar[24] (Table 82–3). A mild-to-moderate normochromic anemia is usually present in both diseases during their active phases. Leukocyte and differential counts are generally normal. A markedly elevated ESR and C-reactive protein (CRP) level are characteristic of both. ESR above 100 mm in 1 hour (Westergren method) are common, but untreated biopsy-proven cases of GCA may be associated with normal or nearly normal levels. In a study of

TABLE 82–3 · PHYSICAL FINDINGS AND LABORATORY ABNORMALITIES IN GIANT CELL ARTERITIS (GCA)*

Feature	Frequency (%)
Any temporal artery abnormality	65
Prominent or enlarged temporal artery	47
Absent temporal artery pulse	45
Scalp tenderness	31
Any fundoscopic abnormality	31
Abnormal erythrocyte sedimentation rate (ESR)	96
ESR > 50 mm/hr	83
ESR > 100 mm/hr	39
Anemia	44

*Modified from Smetana GW, Shmerling RH: Does this patient have temporal arteritis? JAMA 287:92, 2002. (Reprinted by permission of JAMA)

167 GCA patients, 10.8 percent presented with an ESR of less than 50 mm/hr and 3.6 percent had a rate of less than 30 mm/hr.[74] Rare individuals appear unable to develop an elevated ESR during any inflammatory problem, including active GCA.[74] The ESR is also liable to be relatively low or normal in patients who have been receiving corticosteroids for another condition.[75] Thus, a normal ESR does not exclude GCA, especially in a patient with otherwise classic symptoms and findings. Platelet counts are often increased.

Nonspecific changes in plasma proteins are often present and include a decrease in the concentration of albumin and an increase in α_2-globulins, fibrinogen, and other acute-phase reactant proteins. Slight increases in gamma globulins and complement may be present. Results of tests for antinuclear antibodies (ANAs) and rheumatoid factor (RF) are generally negative.

Results of tests measuring liver function have been found to be mildly abnormal in approximately one third of patients with GCA and in slightly less in PMR.[24,54] An increased alkaline phosphatase level is the most common abnormality, but increases in aspartate aminotransferase and prolonged prothrombin time may also be found.[76] Liver biopsy specimens are generally normal; granulomatous hepatitis has been observed.[45] Renal function and urinalysis are usually normal. Red blood cell casts are found in some instances, but their presence does not correlate with clinical large-artery involvement.[28]

Levels of serum creatine kinase and other enzymes reflecting muscle damage are normal. Electromyograms (EMGs) have usually been reported to be normal, and muscle biopsy shows normal histologic features or only the mild atrophy characteristic of disuse.[46]

Synovial fluid analyses reported in GCA or PMR have shown evidence of mild inflammation, including increased synovial fluid leukocyte counts with a mean of 2900 cells/mm³, but a range from 300 to 20,000 cells/mm³, with 40 to 50 percent being polymorphonuclear leukocytes.[49,73] Synovial fluid complement levels have usually been normal.[77] In some instances, synovial biopsy has shown lymphocytic synovitis.[47-51]

Serum IL-6 levels are elevated in patients with PMR and GCA and appear to closely parallel the inflammatory activity.[78] Factor VIII or von Willebrand's factor levels have been found to be elevated in patients with GCA and PMR.[79,80]

Differential Diagnosis

The diagnosis of GCA should be considered in any patient more than 50 years old who experiences loss of vision, diplopia, new form of headache, jaw claudication, PMR, fever of unknown origin, unexplained constitutional symptoms, anemia, and a high ESR. GCA can cause so many forms of cranial discomfort (e.g., headache, scalp tenderness, jaw claudication, or pain of the throat, gums, and tongue) that the disease should also be considered in any patient older than 50 who develops new, unexplained "above-the-neck" pain. The protean manifestations of GCA means that GCA should also be considered in the differential diagnosis of an older patient presenting with a dry cough, a stroke, arm claudication, or acute C5 radiculopathy accompanied by other classic symptoms or findings of GCA.

Few individual symptoms or findings substantially increase or decrease the likelihood of a patient having this disease[55] (Table 82–4). Only jaw claudication, diplopia, abnormal temporal artery signs, scalp tenderness, or ESR greater than 50 mm/hr increase the likelihood that a patient has GCA.[55] Conversely, the absence of headache or temporal artery abnormalities on physical examination, the presence of synovitis, and a normal ESR reduce the likelihood of GCA.

A large number of disorders can mimic GCA. There are many causes of monocular visual loss besides vasculitis, including arteriosclerosis-induced thromboembolic disease.[56] Patients with nonarteritic visual loss do not have other GCA-related symptoms, signs, or findings. The funduscopic examination may also help by revealing Hollenhorst plaques in cases caused by cholesterol emboli. AION, the most common cause of visual loss in GCA, can also be caused by arteriosclerosis. Nonarteritic AION invariably produces a small optic disk and cup-to-disk ratio, whereas GCA-related AION results in optic disk of variable size.[56] Thus, a normal size or large cup in a patient with AION suggests GCA until proven otherwise.[56]

Constitutional symptoms with anemia and an elevated ESR in an older person—so common in GCA—may also be produced by occult infections (e.g., tuberculosis, bacterial endocarditis, human immunodeficiency virus [HIV]) or malignancy (especially lymphoma and multiple myeloma). These diagnoses highlight the value of selective serologic tests, imaging studies, and immunoelectrophoresis in appropriate patients. Systemic amyloidosis can mimic GCA very closely, being one of the very few disorders besides GCA that cause jaw claudication.[81] The amyloid deposits in the temporal artery may not be detected unless the specimen is stained with Congo red. Polyarthritis in an older patient is much more likely caused by RA than by GCA. In one study of 520 GCA patients, less than 2 percent developed polyarthritis before GCA was diagnosed.[82]

Criteria for the classification of GCA have been formulated and help to differentiate this arteritis from other forms of vasculitis[83] (Table 82–5). Takayasu's arteritis, like GCA, can affect the aorta and the major arterial branches to the head and arms. Takayasu's arteritis, however, is a disease of young women. Wegener's granulomatosis can

TABLE 82–4 • LIKELIHOOD RATIOS FOR SYMPTOMS, SIGNS, AND LABORATORY FINDINGS AMONG PATIENTS WITH GIANT CELL ARTERITIS (GCA)*

		Positive Likelihood Ratio (95% CI)	Negative Likelihood Ratio (95% CI)
Symptoms	Jaw claudication	4.2 (2.8-6.2)	0.72 (0.65-0.81)
	Diplopia	3.4 (1.3-8.6)	0.95 (0.91-0.99)
	Weight loss	1.3 (1.1-1.5)	0.89 (0.79-1.0)
	Any headache	1.2 (1.1-1.4)	0.7 (0.57-0.85)
	Fatigue	NS	NS
	Anorexia	NS	NS
	Arthralgia	NS	NS
	Polymyalgia rheumatica	NS	Ns
	Fever	NS	NS
	Visual Loss	NS	NS
Signs	Beaded temporal artery	4.6 (1.1-18.4)	0.93 (0.88-0.99)
	Tender temporal artery	2.6 (1.9-3.7)	0.82 (0.74-0.92)
	Any temporal artery abnormality	2.0 (1.4-3.0)	0.53 (0.38-0.75)
	Scalp tenderness	1.6 (1.2-2.1)	0.93 (0.86-1.0)
	Synovitis	0.41 (0.23-0.72)	1.1 (1.0-1.2)
	Optic atrophy	NS	NS
Laboratory Findings	ESR abnormal	1.1 (1.0-1.2)	0.2 (0.08-0.51)
	ESR > 50 mm/hr	1.2 (1.0-1.4)	0.35 (0.18-0.67)
	ESR > 100 mm/hr	1.9 (1.1-3.3)	0.8 (0.68-0.95)
	Anemia	NS	NS

Modified from Smetana GW, Shmerling RH: Does this patient have temporal arteritis? JAMA 287:92, 2002. (Reprinted by Permission of JAMA)
*Based on literature review with number of patients for each variable ranging from 68 to 2475.
CI, confidence interval; NS, not significant.

TABLE 82–5 • 1990 CRITERIA FOR THE CLASSIFICATION OF GIANT CELL (TEMPORAL) ARTERITIS (TRADITIONAL FORMAT)*

Criterion	Definition
Age at disease onset ≥50 yr	Development of symptoms or findings beginning at age 50 or older
New headache	New onset of or new type of localized pain in the head
Temporal artery abnormality	Temporal artery tenderness to palpation or decreased pulsation, unrelated to arteriosclerosis of cervical arteries
Elevated erythrocyte sedimentation rate (ESR)	ESR ≥50 mm/h by the Westergren method
Abnormal artery biopsy	Biopsy specimen with artery showing vasculitis characterized by a predominance of mononuclear cell infiltration or granulomatous inflammation, usually with multinucleated giant cells

*For purposes of classification, a patient with vasculitis is said to have giant cell (temporal) arteritis if at least three of these five criteria are present. The presence of any three or more criteria yields a sensitivity of 93.5 percent and a specificity of 91.2 percent.

From Hunder GG, Bloch DA, Michel BA, et al: The American College of Rheumatology 1990 criteria for the classification of giant cell arteritis. Arthritis Rheum 33:1125, 1990. Reprinted by permission of Arthritis and Rheumatism.

TABLE 82–6 • TWO SETS OF DIAGNOSTIC CRITERIA FOR POLYMYALGIA RHEUMATICA (PMR)*

Criteria of Chuang and colleagues[84] (1982)

Age 50 years or older
Bilateral aching and stiffness for 1 month or more and involving two of the following areas: neck or torso, shoulders or proximal regions of the arms, and hips or proximal aspects of the thighs
Erythrocyte sedimentation rate (ESR) greater than 40 mm/hr
Exclusion of all other diagnoses except giant cell arteritis (GCA)

Criteria of Healey[85] (1984)

Pain persisting for at least 1 month and involving two of the following areas: neck, shoulders, and pelvic girdle
Morning stiffness lasting more than 1 hour
Rapid response to prednisone (20 mg/day or less)
Absence of other diseases capable of causing the musculoskeletal symptoms
Age more than 50 years
ESR greater than 40 mm/hr

*For each set of criteria, all the findings must be present for PMR to be diagnosed.

From Salvarani C, Cantini F, Boiardi L, Hunder GG: Polymyalgia rheumatica and giant-cell arteritis. New Engl J Med 347:261, 2002. (Reprinted by permission of New England J Med)

affect the temporal artery and joins systemic amyloidosis as an exception to the rule that jaw claudication is pathognomonic for GCA. Wegener's granulomatosis, however, almost always produces tell-tale involvement of the respiratory tract or kidneys and is associated with antineutrophil cytoplasmic antibodies (ANCA). Polyarteritis nodosa can also affect the temporal artery and should be considered if the biopsy does not contain giant cells and the patient has other features atypical for GCA, such as mesenteric arteritis. Fibrinoid necrosis of the vasa vasorum occurs in polyarteritis but rarely, if ever, in GCA. Primary angiitis of the central nervous system differs from GCA in affecting intracranial arteries.

The diagnosis of PMR is clinical and depends on eliciting the symptoms and findings noted earlier. Two sets of criteria for the diagnosis have been proposed[84,85] (Table 82–6).

Several disorders can mimic PMR. Distinguishing early RA from PMR can be difficult, especially in the 15 percent of patients who are RF negative, and in those few RA patients who have not yet developed prominent synovitis of the small joints of the hands and feet. Patients with polymyositis complain much more of weakness than pain, the exact opposite symptom pattern reported by patients with PMR. In addition, in polymyositis, levels of muscle enzymes are elevated, and EMGs are abnormal. Although patients with neoplasms may have generalized musculoskeletal aching, there is no association between PMR and malignant neoplasia.

Therefore, a search for an underlying tumor is not necessary unless some clinical evidence for a tumor is present or the patient has an atypically poor response to low-dose prednisone.

Some patients with chronic infections, such as bacterial endocarditis, may have findings simulating PMR, and blood cultures should be obtained in patients with fever.[86] Patients with fibromyalgia usually do not have typical morning stiffness and have laboratory test results that are normal or nearly so. Rarely, the stiffness of early Parkinson's disease can be confused with PMR if the bradykinesia and tremor of Parkinson's disease are subtle or absent. Lumbar spinal stenosis sometimes causes patients to complain of hip girdle–area pain and stiffness. The absence of symptoms above the waist helps differentiate it from PMR. Statin drugs for cholesterol lowering can produce myalgia with or without muscle enzyme elevations, but rarely mimic PMR. Hypothyroidism in the elderly can mimic many conditions, including PMR.[86] A peculiar syndrome of remitting, seronegative synovitis with pitting edema (designated RS$_3$PE syndrome) may be difficult to differentiate from PMR.[87] Indeed, they may be related disorders. Patients with the RS$_3$PE syndrome develop acute symmetrical polysynovitis of distal joints with pitting edema of the hands and feet. The RS$_3$PE syndrome and PMR both respond to nonsteroidal anti-inflammatory drugs (NSAIDs) and low-dose prednisone.[14,87]

Diagnostic Evaluation in Giant Cell Arteritis

Temporal artery biopsy is the gold standard for diagnosing GCA.[14,88] Because GCA does not involve the artery in a continuous fashion, temporal artery biopsy should be directed to the symptomatic side, if evident. Removing a small (1- to 2-cm) section of temporal artery is usually adequate in patients who have palpable abnormalities of the vessel. Otherwise, the surgeon should try to excise a 4- to 6-cm sample, and the pathologist should examine multiple sections.[14] In skilled hands, temporal-artery biopsy is virtually free of morbidity or mortality. Scalp necrosis can rarely complicate active GCA but has not developed as a consequence of temporal artery biopsy.[88]

Temporal artery biopsies performed at institutions experienced in treating GCA are sensitive and have a high negative predictive value. At the Mayo Clinic, the sensitivity of temporal artery biopsy is approximately 90 to 95 percent, meaning that only 5 to 10 percent of patients with negative biopsies will subsequently be proven (by additional biopsy, angiography, or autopsy) to have GCA and require corticosteroid therapy.[88,89] The sensitivity figures noted previously include some patients who underwent bilateral temporal-artery biopsy. Estimates of the value of bilateral biopsies vary. Of 234 cases of biopsy-proven GCA, unilateral biopsy was positive in 86 percent and the second biopsy was positive in 14 percent.[88] Other studies indicate that a second temporal-artery biopsy improves the diagnostic yield by only 3 to 5 percent.[90,91]

Management of the patient with a negative unilateral biopsy depends on how strongly the patient's clinical picture suggests GCA (Fig. 82–8). When GCA is still strongly suspected, a second biopsy should be considered. Patients with chiefly occipital headache may be best diagnosed by biopsy of the occipital artery.[92] Patients who have signs of subclavian and axillary disease manifested by arm claudication, unequal arm blood pressures, and supraclavicular or axillary bruits may be diagnosed by angiogram, magnetic resonance angiography, or computed tomography (CT) scan.[68] Typically, patients with extracranial GCA will have smooth, tapered stenosis or occlusion of the subclavian, axillary, and proximal brachial arteries. In one series, temporal artery biopsy was positive in only 58 percent of patients with larger artery involvement.[68] MRI and CT are the best established methods for detecting aortic involvement by GCA.[14]

Other imaging techniques have been proposed to assist in the diagnosis of GCA. Color duplex ultrasonography showed abnormalities of the temporal artery in 28 of 30 patients with GCA (sensitivity 93%).[93] The most characteristic finding was a dark halo around the lumen of the temporal arteries. However, the diagnostic value of ultrasonography remains controversial[94]: One study found that ultrasonography did not improve the diagnostic accuracy of a carefully performed physical examination.[95] Positron emission tomography (PET) is showing promise in detecting occult involvement of the aorta and great vessels by GCA, but remains experimental.[96,97]

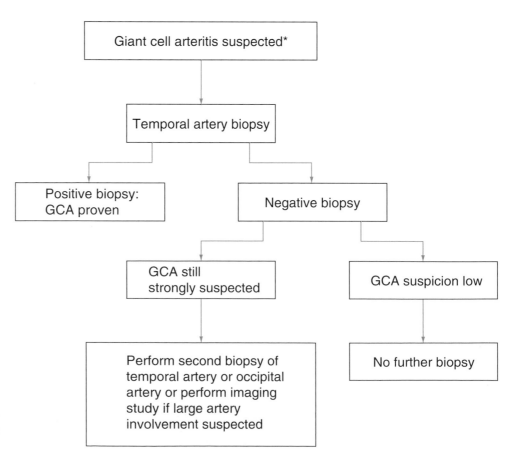

FIGURE 82–8 • Algorithm for the approach to diagnosing giant cell arteritis (GCA).

Treatment and Course

Most authorities recommend starting glucocorticoid therapy as soon as the diagnosis of GCA is strongly suspected. The main goal of treatment is to prevent visual loss. Because visual loss is almost always permanent, it seems prudent to initiate corticosteroid therapy as early as possible, even before the biopsy is performed. Fortunately, the diagnostic yield of temporal-artery biopsy is not altered by corticosteroid therapy for at least 2 weeks and perhaps longer.[98,99]

INITIAL TREATMENT FOR GIANT CELL ARTERITIS

An initial dose of 40 to 60 mg of prednisone daily or equivalent is adequate in nearly all cases.[14] Dividing the dose for the first 1 to 2 weeks may accelerate the rate of improvement. If the patient does not respond promptly, the dose should be increased. High-dose, intravenous-pulse methylprednisolone (e.g., 1000 mg/day) for 3 days can be tried in patients with recent visual loss. Unfortunately, visual loss remains permanent in the vast majority of patients.[100] The occlusive nature of the vasculitides argues against any role of thrombolytic therapy in the treatment of blindness.[38]

Because all patients with GCA will require months of glucocorticoid therapy, measures to prevent osteoporosis should be started early, as outlined in Table 82–7.

SUBSEQUENT TREATMENT FOR GIANT CELL ARTERITIS

The effective initial dose of prednisone should be continued until all reversible symptoms, signs, and laboratory abnormalities have reverted to normal.[14] This usually takes 2 to 4 weeks. After that, the dose can be gradually reduced by a maximum of 10 percent of the total dose each week or every 2 weeks.[14] The decision to reduce prednisone should be based on the composite assessment of the patient's symptoms, signs, and laboratory markers of inflammation. The ESR and serum

concentration of CRP are generally the most convenient and helpful laboratory markers of inflammation. The ESR is reliable only if performed promptly after the blood sample is obtained. Serum level of IL-6 appears to be the most sensitive marker of activity of GCA, but this test is not widely available.[101] At some point in the reduction program, the ESR may rise above normal once again, and further reduction of prednisone may be temporarily interdicted. Subsequent reductions may have to be smaller and made at longer intervals. It is not uncommon to find that it is necessary to continue doses of 10 to 20 mg or more of prednisone daily for several months before further reductions are possible. Gradual reductions allow the identification of the minimal suppressive dose and also help avoid "exacerbation" resulting from tapers of prednisone that are too rapid. Even with gradual reduction of prednisone, more than 50 percent of patients will experience flares of disease activity during the first year.[102,103] These exacerbations can usually be handled by increasing the prednisone 10 mg above the last dose at which the disease was controlled.

GCA tends to run a self-limited course for several months to several years, commonly 1 or 2 years.[14] Glucocorticoids can eventually be reduced and discontinued in some patients. Many patients require low doses of prednisone for several years or more to control musculoskeletal symptoms.

The nearly universal experience of serious side effects associated with daily corticosteroids has prompted the search for steroid-sparing alternative treatments. Unfortunately, to date, none has been convincingly effective. Alternate-day prednisone, for example, is not effective initial therapy for GCA.[104] The combination of low-dose, weekly, oral methotrexate (MTX) and prednisone was steroid sparing in one placebo-controlled, double-blind treatment trial,[103] but not in another.[102] These conflicting results argue against using MTX in combination with prednisone as initial therapy for GCA. MTX may be worth adding to the treatment regimen of a patient who has experienced several exacerbations despite slow tapering of prednisone. Similarly, cytotoxic drugs, dapsone, antimalarials, cyclosporine, and TNF inhibitors have not been clearly shown to be effective, but they may be considered in patients who cannot achieve an acceptably low dose of prednisone.[14]

Whether aspirin should be added to prednisone treatment of GCA is not established. Aspirin is theoretically appealing because in experimental models of GCA it inhibits IFN-γ production more effectively than prednisone.[105] In addition, one retrospective study found that GCA patients taking aspirin had a lower risk of developing an ischemic event, such as visual loss.[106] More research is needed to determine whether aspirin offers a benefit that exceeds its risk of causing gastrointestinal bleeding.

Thoracic aortic aneurysm is greatly increased in patients with GCA.[66] Although it can be present at the outset, aneurysms are usually noted late in the disease course, an average of 7 years after disease onset. Some authorities have recommended annual chest radiographs to detect thoracic aortic aneurysms.[66]

TABLE 82–7 · MEASURES TO PREVENT CORTICOSTEROID-INDUCED OSTEOPOROSIS IN PATIENTS WITH GIANT CELL ARTERITIS (GCA) OR POLYMYALGIA RHEUMATICA (PMR)*

Avoid or stop smoking
Reduce alcohol consumption if excessive
Participate in weight-bearing exercise
Supplement diet with calcium (1000 to 1500 mg/day)
Supplement diet with 800 IU vitamin D per day
Measure bone mineral density (BMD) at lumbar spine and hip
  If BMD is normal, repeat BMD annually
  If BMD is not normal (i.e., T score below −1), then prescribe
    bisphosphonate

*Modified from American College of Rheumatology Ad Hoc Committee on Glucocorticoid-Induced Osteoporosis: Recommendations for the prevention and treatment of glucocorticoid-induced osteoporosis. Arthritis Rheum 44:1496, 2001. (Reprinted by permission of Arthritis Rheum)

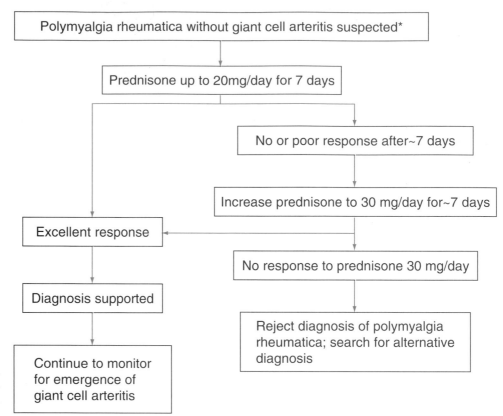

FIGURE 82-9 · Algorithm for the approach to diagnosing polymyalgia rheumatica without giant cell arteritis

TREATMENT FOR POLYMYALGIA RHEUMATICA

Patients with PMR without symptoms or signs or biopsy evidence of GCA are usually initially treated with 5 to 20 mg daily doses of prednisone or equivalent.[107] Salicylates and NSAIDs have been used but are less appealing: Salicylates and NSAIDs adequately control symptoms only in a minority of patients with milder symptoms and add to overall adverse drug reactions when they are used with glucocorticoids.[3,7,108] Prednisone therapy usually results in rapid (often overnight) and dramatic improvement of the musculoskeletal aching and stiffness, and a (more gradual) return of the ESR and CRP level to normal.[109] A minority of patients with isolated PMR fail to respond to prednisone (20 mg/day) after 1 week and may require up to 30 mg of prednisone daily as initial treatment.[110] Studies suggest that the "resistant" cases are more likely to have ESR of greater than 50 mm/hr and very high levels of IL-6.[110] Failure to respond to prednisone (30 mg daily) for 1 week should prompt a search for an alternative diagnosis (Fig. 82–9). Lower doses of prednisone may not suppress an underlying arteritis if it is present. Thus, the patient must be observed carefully even though the aching improves. In patients with PMR, the dose should be reduced gradually as soon as symptoms permit. Pretreatment ESR, CRP, and IL-6 concentrations and initial responses to therapy appear to be helpful in dividing patients into subsets with different treatment requirements.[107,109] If the laboratory test results become normal while the patient is receiving the smaller doses, the likelihood of an underlying active vasculitis would seem to be much less, and the risk of vascular complications is smaller. However, this does not hold in all instances, because active arteritis has been observed even though the ESR was improved.[111]

Once the symptoms, signs, and laboratory abnormalities of PMR have resolved (usually after 2 to 3 weeks of prednisone therapy), the prednisone daily dose can be slowly tapered. Some experts have recommended tapering prednisone by 2.5 mg every week until reaching 10 mg/day when the decrements should be reduced by 1 mg each month.[109] Flares develop commonly and require raising the prednisone dose to achieve remission before attempting a slower taper. The minority of patients with PMR will succeed in tapering off prednisone in less than 1 year.[110] Many require at least 2 years of low-dose prednisone.[112]

REFERENCES

1. Hunder GG, Allen GL: Giant cell arteritis: A review. Bull Rheum 29:980, 1978-1979.
2. Barber HS: Myalgic syndrome with constitutional effects: Polymyalgia rheumatica. Ann Rheum Dis 16:230, 1957.
3. Chaung T-Y, Hunder GG, Ilstrup DM, Kurland LT: Polymyalgia rheumatica: A 10-year epidemiologic and clinical study. Ann Intern Med 97:672, 1982.
4. Healey LA, Wilske KR: The Systemic Manifestations of Temporal Arteritis. New York, Grune & Stratton, 1978.
5. Salvarani C, Gabriel SE, O'Fallon WM, Hunder GG: The incidence of giant cell arteritis on Olmsted County, Minnesota: Apparent fluctuations in cyclic pattern. Ann Intern Med 123:192, 1995.

6. Baldursson O, Steinsson K, Bjornsson J, Lie JT: Giant cell arteritis in Iceland: An epidemiologic and histologic analysis. Arthritis Rheum 37:1007, 1994.

7. Nordborg E, Bengtsson B-A: Epidemiology of biopsy-proven giant cell arteritis (GCA). J Intern Med 227:233, 1990.

8. Jonasson F, Cullen JF, Elton RA: Temporal arteritis: A 14-year epidemiologic, clinical and prognostic study. Scot Med J 24:111, 1979.

9. Boesen P, Sorensen SF: Giant cell arteritis, temporal arteritis and polymyalgia rheumatica in a Danish county: A prospective investigation, 1982-1985. Arthritis Rheum 30:294, 1987.

10. Barrier J, Pion P, Massari R, et al: Epidemiologic approach to Horton's disease in Department of Loire-Atlantique: 110 cases in 10 years (1970–1979). Rev Med Interne 3:13, 1983.

11. Smith CA, Fidler WJ, Pinals RS: The epidemiology of giant cell arteritis: Report of a ten-year study in Shelby County, Tennessee. Arthritis Rheum 26:1214, 1983.

12. Friedman G, Friedman B, Benbassat J: Epidemiology of temporal arteritis in Israel. Isr J Med Sci 18:241, 1986.

13. Machado EBV, Michet CJ, Ballard DJ, et al: Trends in incidence and clinical presentation of temporal arteritis in Olmsted County, Minnesota, 1950-1985. Arthritis Rheum 31:745, 1988.

14. Salvarani C, Cantini F, Boiardi L, Hunder GG: Polymyalgia rheumatica and giant cell arteritis. New Engl J Med 347:261, 2002.

15. Levine SM, Hellmann DB: Giant cell arteritis. Curr Opin Rheumatol 14:3, 2002.

16. Östberg G: On arteritis with special reference to polymyalgia arteritica. Acta Pathol Microbiol Scand (A) Suppl 237:1, 1973.

17. Hunder GG, Lie JT, Goronzy JJ, Weyand CM: Pathogenesis of giant cell arteritis. Arthritis Rheum 36:757, 1993.

18. Liang GC, Simkin PA, Hunder GG, et al: Familial aggregation of polymyalgia rheumatica and giant cell arteritis. Arthritis Rheum 17:19, 1974.

19. Mathewson JA, Hunder GG: Giant cell arteritis in two brothers. J Rheumatol 13:190, 1986.

20. Weyand CM, Hunder NN, Hicok KC, et al: The HLA-DRB1 locus as a genetic component in giant cell arteritis: Mapping of a disease-linked sequence motif to the antigen binding site of the HLA-DR molecule. J Clin Invest 90:2355, 1992.

21. Weyand CM, Hunder NN, Hicok KC, et al: HLA-DRB1 alleles in polymyalgia rheumatica, giant cell arteritis, and rheumatoid arthritis. Arthritis Rheum 37:514, 1994.

22. Duhaut P, Pinede L, Demolombe-Rague S, et al: Giant cell arteritis and cardiovascular risk factors. Arthritis Rheum 41:1960, 1998.

23. Regan MJ, Wood BJ, Hsieh YH, et al: *Chlamydia pneumoniae* and Temporal Arteritis: Failure to detect the organism by PCR in 180 cases and controls. Arthritis Rheum 46:1056, 2002.

24. Calamia KT, Hunder GG: Clinical manifestations of giant cell arteritis. Clin Rheum Dis 6:389, 1980.

25. Salvarani C, Gabriel SE, O'Fallon WM, Hunder GG: Epidemiology of polymyalgia rheumatica in Olmsted County, Minnesota, 1970-1991. Arthritis Rheum 38:369, 1995.

26. Sakkas LI, Loqueman N, Panayi GS, et al: Immunogenetics of polymyalgia rheumatica. Br J Rheumatol 29:331, 1990.

27. Klein RG, Hunder GG, Stanson AW, Sheps SG: Large artery involvement in giant cell (temporal) arteritis. Ann Intern Med 83:806, 1975.

28. Klein RG, Campbell RJ, Hunder GG, Carney JA: Skip lesions in temporal arteritis. Mayo Clin Proc 51:504, 1976.

29. Wilkinson IMS, Russell RWR: Arteries of the head and neck in giant cell arteritis: A pathological study to show the pattern of arterial involvement. Arch Neurol 27:378, 1972.

30. Casselli RJ, Hunder GG, Whisnant JP: Neurologic disease in biopsy-proven giant cell (temporal) arteritis. Neurology 38:352, 1988.

31. Caselli RJ, Hunder GG: Neurologic aspects of giant cell (temporal) arteritis. Rheum Dis Clin North Am 19:941, 1993.

32. Reich KA, Giansiracusa DF, Strongwater SL: Neurologic manifestations of giant cell arteritis. Am J Med 89:67, 1990.

33. Evans JM, Batts KP, Hunder GG: Persistent giant cell arteritis despite corticosteroid treatment. Mayo Clin Prac 69:1060, 1994.

34. Esteban M-J, Front C, Hernández-Rodríguez J, et al: Small-vessel vasculitis surrounding a spared temporal artery. Arthritis Rheum 44:1387, 2001.

35. Cid MC, Campo E, Ercilla G, et al: Immunohistochemical analysis of lymphoid and macrophage cell subsets and the immunological activation markers in temporal arteritis. Arthritis Rheum 32:884, 1989.

36. Weyand CM, Garonzy JJ: Arterial wall injury in giant cell arteritis. Arthritis Rheum 42:844, 1999.

37. Brach A, Gusler A, Martinez-Taboada, et al: Giant cell vasculitis is a T cell-dependent disease. Mol Med 3:530, 1997.

38. Weyand CM, Wagner, AD, Bjornsson J, et al: Correlation of the topographical arrangement and the functional pattern of tissue-infiltrating macrophages in giant cell arteritis. J Clin Invest 98:1642, 1996.

39. Wagner AD, Garonzy JJ, Weyand CM: Functional profile of tissue-infiltrating and circulating CD68+ cells in giant cell arteritis: Evidence for two components of the disease. J Clin Invest 4:1134, 1994.

40. Weyand CM, Hicok KC, Hunder GG, et al: Tissue cytokine patterns in patients with polymyalgia rheumatica and giant cell arteritis. Ann Intern Med 121:484, 1994.

41. Weyand CM, Tetzlaff N, Bjornsson J, et al: Disease patterns and tissue cytokine profiles in giant cell arteritis. Arthritis Rheum 40:19, 1997.

42. Grunewald J, Andersson R, Rydberg L, et al: CD4+ and CD8+ T cell expansions using selected TCR V and J gene segments at the onset of giant cell arteritis. Arthritis Rheum 37(8):1221, 1994.

43. Shiiki H, Shimokama T, Watanabe T: Temporal arteritis: Cell composition and the possible pathogenetic role of cell-mediated immunity. Hum Pathol 20:1057, 1989.

44. Kaiser M, Weyand CM, Bjornsson J, et al: Platelet-derived growth factor, intimal hyperplasia, and ischemic complications in giant cell arteritis. Arthritis Rheum 41:623, 1998.

45. Calamia KT, Hunder GG: Giant cell arteritis (temporal arteritis) presenting as fever of undetermined origin. Arthritis Rheum 24:1414, 1981.

46. Brooke MH, Kaplan H: Muscle pathology in rheumatoid arthritis, polymyalgia rheumatica, and polymyositis: A histochemical study: Arch Pathol 94:101, 1972.

47. Salvarani C, Cantini F, Oliveri I, et al: Proximal bursitis in active polymyalgia rheumatica. Ann Intern Med 127:27, 1997.

48. O'Duffy JD, Hunder GG, Wahner HW: A follow-up study of polymyalgia rheumatica: Evidence of chronic axial synovitis. J Rheumatol 7:685, 1980.

49. Healey LA: Long-term follow-up of polymyalgia rheumatica: Evidence for synovitis. Semin Arthritis Rheum 13:322, 1984.

50. Douglas WA, Martin BA, Morris JH: Polymyalgia rheumatica: An arthroscopic study of the shoulder joint. Ann Rheum Dis 42:311, 1983.

51. Chow CT, Schumacher HR Jr: Clinical and pathologic studies of synovitis in polymyalgia rheumatica. Arthritis Rheum 27:1107, 1984.

52. Cantini F, Salvarani C, Olivieri I, et al: Inflamed shoulder structures in polymyalgia rheumatica with normal erythrocyte sedimentation rate. Arthritis Rheum 44:1155, 2001.

53. Papaioannou CC, Gupta RC, Hunder GG, McDuffie FC: Circulating immune complexes in giant cell arteritis polymyalgia rheumatica. Arthritis Rheum 23:1021, 1980.

54. Smith AJ, Kyle V, Cawston TE, Hazleman BL: Isolation and analysis of immune complexes from sens of patients with polymalgia rheumatica and giant cell arteritis. Ann Rheum Dis 46: 468, 1987.

55. Smetana GW Shmerling RH: Does this patient have temporal arteritis? JAMA 287:92, 2002.

56. Miller NR: Visual manifestations of temporal arteritis. *In* Stone JH, Hellmann DB (eds): Rheumatic Disease Clinics of North America. WB Saunders, 2001, p 781.

57. Mehler MF, Rabinowich L: The clinical neuro-ophthalmologic spectrum of temporal arteritis. Am J Med 85:839, 1988.

58. Aiello PD, Trautmann JC, McPhee TJ, et al: Visual prognosis in giant cell arteritis. Ophthalmology 100:550, 1993.

59. Healy LA, Wilske KR: Presentation of occult giant cell arteritis. Arthritis Rheum 23:641, 1980.

60. Hellmann DB: Occult manifestations of giant cell arteritis. Med Rounds 2:296, 1989.

61. Sonnenblick M, Nesher G, Rosin A: Nonclassical organ involvement in temporal arteritis. Semin Arthritis Rheum 19:183, 1989.

62. Hollenhorst RW, Brown JR, Wagener HP, Shick RM: Neurologic aspects of temporal arteritis. Neurology 10:490, 1960.

63. Larson TS, Hall S, Hepper NGG, Hunder GG: Respiratory tract symptoms as a clue to giant cell arteritis. Ann Intern Med 101:594, 1984.

64. Hamilton CR, Shelley WM, Tumulty PA: Giant cell arteritis: Including temporal arteritis and polymyalgia rheumatica. Medicine 50:1, 1971.

65. Evans JM, Bowles CA, Bjornsson J, et al: Thoracic aortic aneurysm and rupture in giant cell arteritis. Arthritis Rheum 37:1539, 1994.

66. Evans JM, O'Fallon WM, Hunder GG: Increased incidence of aortic aneurysm and dissection in giant cell (temporal) arteritis: A population based study. Ann Intern Med 122:502, 1995.

67. Kariv R, Sidi Y, Gur H: Systemic vasculitis presenting as a tumor-like lesion: Four case reports and an analysis of 79 reported cases. Medicine 79:349, 2000.

68. Brack A, Martinez-Taboada V, Stanson A, et al: Disease pattern in cranial and large-vessel giant cell arteritis. Arthritis Rheum 42:311, 1999.

69. Liozon E, Herrmann F, Ly K, et al: Risk factors for visual loss in giant cell (temporal) arteritis: A prospective study of 174 patients. Am J Med 111:211, 2001.

70. González-Gay MA, Blanco R, Rodríguez-Valverde V, et al: Permanent visual loss and cerebrovascular accidents in giant cell arteritis: Predictors and response to treatment. Arthritis Rheum 41:1497, 1998.

71. Cid MC, Font C, Oristrell J, et al: Association between strong inflammatory response and low risk of developing visual loss and other cranial ischemic complications in giant cell (temporal) arteritis. Arthritis Rheum 41:26, 1998.

72. Salvarani C, Gabriel S, Hunder GG: Distal extremity swelling with pitting edema in polymyalgia rheumatica: Report of nineteen cases. Arthritis Rheum 39:73, 1996.

73. Chou C-T, Schumacher HR Jr: Clinical and pathologic studies of synovitis in polymyalgia rheumatica. Arthritis Rheum 27:1107, 1984.

74. Salvarani C, Hunder GG: Giant cell arteritis with low erythrocyte sedimentation rate: Frequency of occurrence in a population-based study. Arthritis Care Res 45:140, 2001.

75. Wise CM, Agudelo CA, Chmelewski WL, et al: Temporal arteritis with low erythrocyte sedimentation rate: A review of five cases. Arthritis Rheum 34:1571, 1991.

76. Dickson ER, Maldonado JE, Sheps SG, Cain JA Jr: Systemic giant-cell arteritis with polymyalgia rheumatica: Reversible abnormalities of liver function. JAMA 224:1496, 1973.

77. Bunch TW, Hunder GG, McDuffie FC, et al: Synovial fluid complement determination as a diagnostic aid in inflammatory joint disease. Mayo Clin Proc 49:715, 1974.

78. Roche NE, Fulbright JW, Wagner AD, et al: Correlation of inter-leukin-6 production and disease activity in polymyalgia rheumatica and giant cell arteritis. Arthritis Rheum 36:1286, 1993.

79. Persellin ST, Daniels TM, Rings LJ, et al: Factor VIII–von Willebrand factor in giant cell arteritis and polymyalgia rheumatica. Mayo Clin Proc 60:457, 1985.

80. Olsson A, Elling P, Elling H: Serologic and immunohistochemical determination of von Willebrand factor antigen in serum and biopsy specimens from patients with arteritis temporalis and polymyalgia rheumatica. Clin Exp Rheumatol 8:55, 1990.

81. Gertz MA, Kyle RA, Griffing WL, Hunder GG: Jaw claudication in primary systemic amyloidosis. Medicine (Baltimore) 65:173, 1986.

82. Ginsburg WW, Cohen MD, Hall SB, et al: Seronegative polyarthritis in giant cell arteritis. Arthritis Rheum 28:1362, 1985.

83. Hunder GG, Bloch DA, Michel BA, et al: The American College of Rheumatology 1990 criteria for the classification of giant cell arteritis. Arthritis Rheum 33:1122, 1990.

84. Chuang T-Y, Hunder GG, Ilstrup DM, Kurland LT: Polymyalgia rheumatica: a 10-year epidemiologic and clinical study. Ann Intern Med 97:672, 1982.

85. Healey LA: Long-term follow-up of polymyalgia rheumatica: evidence for synovitis. Semin Arthritis Rheum 13:322, 1984.

86. Gonzalez-Gay MA, Garcia-Porrua C, Salvarani C, et al: The spectrum of conditions mimicking polymyalgia rheumatica in Northwestern Spain. J Rheumatol 27:2179, 2000.

87. McCarty DJ, O'Duffy D, Pearson L, Hunter JB: Remitting seronegative symmetrical synovitis with pitting edema. RS$_3$PE Syndrome. JAMA 254:2763, 1985.

88. Hall S, Hunder GG: Is temporal artery biopsy prudent? Mayo Clin Proc 59:793, 1984.

89. Hall S, Lie JT, Kurland LT, et al: The therapeutic impact of temporal artery biopsy. Lancet 2:1217, 1983.

90. Boyev LR, Miller NR, Green WR: Efficacy of unilateral versus bilateral temporal artery biopsies for the diagnosis of giant cell arteritis. Am J Ophthalmol 128:211, 1999.

91. Pless M, Rizzo JF III, Lamkin JC, Lessell S: Concordance of bilateral temporal artery biopsy in giant cell arteritis. J Neuroophthalmol 20:216, 2000.

92. Jundt JW, Mock D: Temporal arteritis with normal erythrocyte sedimentation rates presenting as occipital neuralgia. Arthritis Rheum 34:217, 1991.

93. Schmidt WA, Kraft HE, Vorpahl L, et al: Color duplex ultrasonography in the diagnosis of temporal arteritis. N Engl J Med 337:1336, 1997.

94. Hunder GG, Weyand CM: Sonography in giant cell arteritis. N Engl J Med 337:1385, 1997.

95. Salvarani C, Silingardi M, Ghirarduzzi A, et al: Is duplex ultrasonography useful for the diagnosis of giant-cell arteritis? Ann Intern Med 137:232, 2002.

96. Blockmans D, Stroobants S, Maes A, Mortelmans L: Positron emission tomography in giant cell arteritis and polymyalgia rheumatica: Evidence for inflammation of the aortic arch. Am J Med 108:246, 2000.

97. Turlakow A, Yeung HWD, Pui J, et al: Fludeoxyglucose positron emission tomography in the diagnosis of giant cell arteritis. Arch Intern Med 161:1003, 2001.

98. Ray-Chaudhuri N, Kiné DA, Tijani SO, et al: Effect of prior steroid treatment on temporal artery biopsy findings in giant cell arteritis. Br J Ophthalmol 86:530, 2002.

99. Achkar AA, Lie JT, Hunder GG, et al: How does previous corticosteroid treatment affect the biopsy findings in giant cell (temporal) arteritis? Ann Intern Med 120:987, 1994.

100. Hayreh SS: Steroid therapy for visual loss in patients with giant-cell arteritis. Lancet 355:1572, 2000.

101. Weyand CM, Fulbright JW, Hunder GG, et al: Treatment of giant cell arteritis. Interleukin-6 as a biologic marker of disease activity. Arthritis Rheum 43:1041, 2000.

102. Hoffman GS, Cid MC, Hellmann DB, et al: A multicenter, randomized, double-blind, placebo-controlled trial of adjuvant methotrexate treatment for giant cell arteritis. Arthritis Rheum 46:1309, 2002.

103. Jover JA, Hernández-Garcia C, Morado IC, et al: Combined treatment of giant-cell arteritis with methotrexate and prednisone: A randomized, double-blind, placebo-controlled trial. Ann Intern Med 134:106, 2001.

104. Hunder GG, Sheps SG, Allen GL, Joyce JW: Daily and alternate-day corticosteroid regimens in treatment of giant cell arteritis: comparison in a prospective study. Ann Intern Med 82:613, 1975.

105. Weyand CM, Kaiser M, Yang H, et al: Therapeutic effects of acetylsalicylic acid in giant cell arteritis. Arthritis Rheum 46:457, 2002.

106. Nesher G: Low-dose aspirin and prevention of cranial ischemic complications in giant cell arteritis. Arthritis Rheum, in press.

107. Weyand CM, Fulbright JW, Evans JM, et al: Corticosteroid requirements in polymyalgia rheumatica. Arch Intern Med 159:577, 1999.

108. Gabriel SE, Sunku J, Salvarani C, et al: Adverse outcomes of anti-inflammatory therapy among patients with polymyalgia rheumatica. Arthritis Rheum 40:1873, 1997.

109. Schreiber S, Buyse M: The CRP initial response to treatment as prognostic factor in patients with polymyalgia rheumatica. Clin Rheumatol 14:315, 1995.

110. Weyand CM, Fulbright JW, Evans JM, et al: Corticosteroid requirements in polymyalgia rheumatica. Arch Intern Med 159:577, 1999.

111. Rynes RI, Mika P, Bartholomew LE: Development of giant cell (temporal) arteritis in a patient "adequately" treated for polymyalgia rheumatica. Ann Rheum Dis 36:88, 1977.

112. Narvaez J, Nolla-Sole JM, Clavaguera MT, et al: Longterm therapy in polymyalgia rheumatica: effect of coexistent temporal arteritis. J Rheumatol 26:1945, 1999.

83 Antineutrophil Cytoplasmic Antibody–Associated Vasculitis

LEONARD H. CALABRESE · GEORGE DUNA

In recent years considerable progress has been made in understanding the nature and relationships among the major classes of primary vasculitic syndromes. The discovery of antineutrophil cytoplasmic antibody (ANCA) and its development as a diagnostic tool, as well as its role in nosology of the vasculitides, has been of major clinical and theoretic importance to the field. Three diseases—Wegener's granulomatosis (WG), microscopic polyangiitis (MPA), and Churg Strauss syndrome (CSS)—may now be considered together in view of their sharing a number of pathologic, clinical, and laboratory features.[1] These diseases share histologic features, preferentially involving small vessels (i.e., venules, capillaries, and arterioles). They also share a similar glomerular lesion (i.e., focal necrosis, crescents, and absence or paucity of immunoglobulin [Ig] deposition). All three of these diseases may, at times, also share clinical features, including a propensity to present as pulmonary renal syndromes. Finally, all share a varying prevalence of ANCA positivity. The epidemiology of these disorders reveals a collective incidence approaching two per 100,000 people in the United States and approximately 1 in 10,000 in Sweden.[1] Although each disease, in its characteristic form, may be distinguished from the others on clinical and histologic grounds, quite often the distinctions are blurred and, thus, their consideration as a group is reasonable from the pathologic as well as the clinical perspective.

Antineutrophil Cytoplasmic Antibody

HISTORIC BACKGROUND

ANCAs were first described in 1982 by Davies and colleagues in eight patients with necrotizing pauci-immune glomerulonephritis, suspected of having viral infections.[2] A few years later, Hall and colleagues identified ANCA in four patients with systemic vasculitis.[3] In 1985, Van der Woude and colleagues were the first to suggest an association between ANCA and WG.[4] Since that time, subsequent studies have established a close association between ANCA and three major vasculitis syndromes: WG, MPA, and CSS.[1] ANCAs were originally described based on their immunofluorescence patterns: divided into cytoplasmic (c-ANCA) and perinuclear (p-ANCA) categories. The antigens responsible for these patterns and closely allied with the vasculitic syndromes have also been identified (i.e., proteinase 3 [PR3] for c-ANCA and myleoperoxidase [MPO] for p-ANCA). The last 15 years have yielded more than 1300 reports on ANCA.[5] ANCA testing as a diagnostic tool is now established in the field of systemic vasculitis, and its potential role in pathogenesis of disease and as a target for therapy is still evolving.

METHODOLOGY

As noted previously, ANCAs were originally defined by indirect immunofluorescence (IFA) performed on ethanol-fixed neutrophils as substrate and broadly categorized as c-ANCA or p-ANCA (Fig. 83–1). In patients with vasculitis (i.e., WG, MPA, and CSS), specific immunochemical assays have demonstrated two major antigenic specificities responsible for these immunofluorescent patterns. In the case of c-ANCA reactivity, PR3 is responsible for more than 90 percent of such reactions, although other antigens may occasionally contribute, including bactericidal permeability-inducing protein (BPI) and rarely MPO.[1,5] The p-ANCA pattern is much less closely correlated, being found in less than 10 percent of 620 consecutive p-ANCA–positive sera by immunofluorescence in one laboratory.[6] Other antigens capable of producing p-ANCA reactivity include elastase, azurocidin, cathepsin G lysozyme, lactoferrin, and others.[5] Antinuclear antibodies (ANAs) may also yield a p-ANCA pattern, further compromising IFA as the diagnostic technique of choice.

To circumvent the lack of correlation between immunofluorescent patterns and the antigens of interest (i.e., PR3 and MPO), as well as the inherent interobserver variability of IFA, antigen-specific assays have been developed and are readily available. Clinicians ordering ANCA need to ensure that ANCA by IFA testing is confirmed by antigen-specific testing for both PR3 and MPO. When criteria for a positive ANCA include both positive IFA and an antigen-specific ANCA (PR3-ANCA indicating c-ANCA and confirmatory antigenic testing for PR3 and MPO-ANCA indicating p-ANCA and confirmatory antigenic testing for MPO), the test is highly specific for the vasculitic syndromes currently under discussion, even when tested in patients with connective tissue disease.[7]

ANTINEUTROPHIL CYTOPLASMIC ANTIBODY DISEASE ASSOCIATIONS

Vasculitis

A large number of investigations have attempted to establish the sensitivity of PR3-ANCA and MPO-ANCA in systemic vasculitis, and these have been extensively reviewed.[5] In general PR3-ANCA and MPO-ANCA are

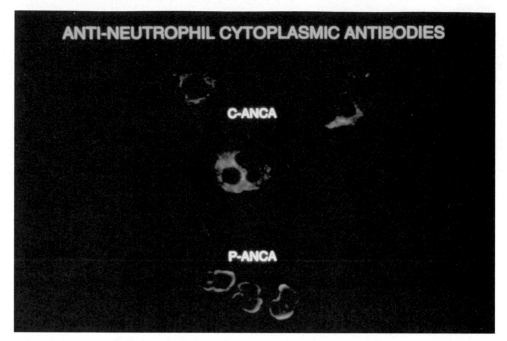

FIGURE 83–1 · Immunoflourescence of diffuse or cytoplasmic antineutrophil cytoplasmic antibody (c-ANCA), which is highly correlated with antibodies to proteinase 3 (PR-3) and the less-specific perinuclear pattern (p-ANCA), which is at times indicative of antibodies to myeloperoxidase (MPO). Although immunoflourescence was historically the standard for ANCA testing, current standards require confirmatory antigen-specific testing for PR3 and MPO. (See color plate 42.)

detected in a limited number of disorders, including the three small vessel vasculitic syndromes, as well as the renal-limited form of vasculitis: idiopathic necrotizing crescentic glomerulonephritis. The sensitivity of ANCA varies in these disorders from 50 to more than 90 percent. A large, multicenter cooperative European trial attempting to standardize ANCA testing has been reported[8] and is summarized in Figure 83–2. The results of this trial emphasize that a significant number of patients with idiopathic small-vessel vasculitis are ANCA negative and, thus, a negative test in no way eliminates the diagnosis in a patient with a high pretest probability of disease. In WG, the disorder most highly associated with PR3-ANCA, the test is most likely to be positive in those patients with triad disease (i.e., upper respiratory, lung, and kidney), which is active and untreated.[5,9,10] Similar correlations of end-organ damage and disease activity with ANCA positivity are less clear in the other vasculitic syndromes.

The specificity of ANCA testing appears dependent on both technical factors and the nature of the control pop-

ulations tested. If IFA results are combined with antigen-specific assays, then the specificity of both PR3-ANCA and MPO-ANCA are exceedingly high. Typical IFA patterns are demonstrated in Figure 83–1. In the European cooperative study of Hagan and colleagues,[8] 184 disease controls were studied, including various forms of glomerulonephritis and granulomatous disease, and specificity for the ANCA-associated small-vessel vasculitides exceeded 99 percent. A study by Merkel and colleagues,[7] utilizing IFA confirmed by antigen-specific assay, examined a large cohort of well-characterized connective tissue disease patients and reported specificity also in excess of 99 percent. An earlier study of ANCA, which also included a large number of disease controls, demonstrated high specificity as well.[11] Salient points from these large, controlled studies include the unreliability of IFA testing, even when performed by highly trained and experienced personnel, and that IFA alone is less specific than IFA combined with antigen-specific testing for PR3 and MPO. Collectively, clinicians using ANCA to diagnose vasculitis must demand

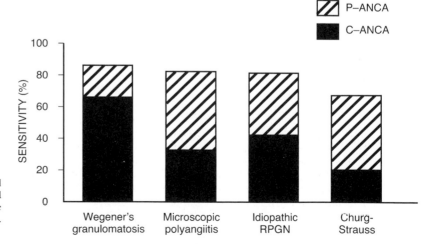

FIGURE 83–2 · Frequency of (antineutrophil cytoplasmic antibody) ANCA reactivity in associated vasculitic conditions divided on the basis of proteinase 3 (PR3) ANCA and myeloperoxidase (MPO) ANCA. RPGN, rapidly progressive glomerutonephritis.

substantial experience from their laboratories and require IFA testing be supplemented by antigen-specific determinations. Even when these technical criteria are met, it must still be appreciated that ANCA, like any laboratory test, provides its optimal diagnostic value only when applied in clinical context.

In general, the specificity of ANCA influences disease phenotype, at least by association. In addition to the predilection of PR3 patients for WG and those with MPO for MPA, a direct comparison of patient populations reveals PR3-positive patients to have more extrarenal manifestations, granuloma formation, and relapses. Even among patients with MPA, those with PR3 specificity are more likely to have a severe outcome or death. Despite substantial overlap, there appear to be distinct clinical and pathologic differences among patients with PR3-ANCA and those with MPO-ANCA, suggesting possible differences in pathogenic mechanisms.[12]

Antineutrophil Cytoplasmic Antibody in Other Diseases

ANCAs have been reported in a wide variety of other conditions.[5] Patients with connective tissue diseases, including rheumatoid arthritis (RA),[7,13,14] systemic lupus erythematosus (SLE),[7] and myositis,[7] may occasionally display ANCA positivity, but these are largely non–MPO-ANCA and non–PR3-ANCA types. Infections such as those found in cystic fibrosis,[15] endocarditis,[16] and human immunodeficiency virus (HIV), among others,[5] are occasionally ANCA positive. These may be of particular clinical importance because infections may mimic systemic vasculitis. As with connective tissue diseases reported to be ANCA positive, most reports of ANCA in infectious diseases are largely non–PR3-ANCA and non–MPO-ANCA, further underscoring the importance of confirmation of IFA by antigen-specific testing.

ANCAs are often encountered in inflammatory bowel disease (IBD) and are more frequent in ulcerative colitis than Crohn's disease.[17,18] The antigenic target is non-PR3 or -MPO and largely unknown, although a multitude of targets have been reported, including cathepsin G, lactoferrin, elastase lysozyme, and BPI.[17-19] Other forms of gastrointestinal (GI) disease reported to be ANCA positive (of the non–PR3-ANCA non–MPO-ANCA variety) include sclerosing cholangitis and autoimmune hepatitis.[20,21]

Drugs may be a particularly important cause of false-positive ANCA reactions, especially because hydrazaline, propylthiouracil, D-penacillamine, and minocycline[22-25] may be associated with high-titer MPO-ANCA reactivity with or without an associated vasculitic syndrome. Minocycline has also been associated with a reversible autoimmune syndrome and MPO-ANCA.[26]

Antineutrophil Cytoplasmic Antibody and Pathophysiology of Small Vessel Vasculitis

Although ANCAs are firmly entrenched in the diagnostic process for vasculitis, their role in the pathophysiology of these conditions is less so. Teleologic objections to a central role include the observation that ANCAs are not detected in a sizable portion of patients with well-documented small vessel vasculitis.[27] Despite such considerable limitations, mounting evidence suggests that ANCA may either induce or augment vascular inflammation. These data have been critically reviewed by several groups.[5,28]

A variety of in vitro observations favor a pathogenic role for ANCA in some forms of vasculitis.

For instance, in neutrophils, both MPO and PR3 are transported from primary granules to the cell membrane during activation and are part of the physiologic response of these cells to inflammatory mediators (i.e., tumor necrosis factor-α [TNF-α] and interleukin-8 [IL-8]).[29-31] Evidence for surface expression of PR3 on circulating neutrophils and MPO release within renal lesions have both been reported in WG.[29,30] The binding of PR3-ANCA, MPO-ANCA, and other ANCAs to their cognate targets on neutrophils augment a variety of activation-related neutrophilic functions, including degranulation, respiratory burst, nitric oxide production, chemotaxis, adhesion molecule expression, and binding to cultured endothelial cells.[29,31-33] Such binding appears to be dependent not only on binding of ANCA via the antigen-binding site but also on engagement of the (Fc-γ) receptor as well.[34] Collectively, these events may contribute to vascular damage. ANCAs also stabilize cell adhesion and promote migration and flow of neutrophils through endothelium.[35]

Whether or not PR3 is synthesized and expressed on endothelial cells is controversial, but PR3 does appear capable of passive binding to the cell surface and, thus, serves as a target for PR3-ANCA. Binding of PR3-ANCA to endothelial cells has been demonstrated to lead to upregulation of adhesion molecule expression and IL-8 production, both of which could well contribute to vessel inflammation and injury.[5,29,34] ANCAs are able to positively or negatively affect the proteolytic activity of PR3 or MPO, depending on epitope restriction.[5,36] Thus, if these enzymes play a homeostatic role in the inflammatory response, ANCAs might have a modulatory effect.

The activity of ANCAs in vivo have been demonstrated in animal models of vascular inflammation,[29,37,38] but these have been often criticized on methodologic grounds, as well on the lack of similarity of the vascular lesions to the human disease. More recently a murine model has strengthened the argument that ANCAs actually cause vasculitis.[39] Anti-MPO antibodies alone have induced glomerulonephritis with crescent formation and systemic vasculitis in mice lacking functional T or B cells, as well as in an immunocompetent wild-type strain C57BL/6J, thus offering strong support for a direct pathogenic role.

Despite the observation that ANCAs are not present in all patients with systemic small vessel vasculitic syndromes, a number of studies have reported correlations between the presence and magnitude of ANCA and a variety of disease manifestations. Among these clinical correlates, supported by many but not all investigations, are those with disease activity and severity,[10,40] risk of relapse,[41] target organ distribution, and response to therapy.[40]

Most of these data stem from studies of PR3-ANCA in patients with WG, whereas supporting data from other diseases such as MPA and CSS are much more limited. Despite such limitations, there is also evidence that MPO-ANCA may play a similar role including the display of MPO on the neutrophil cell membrane and its subsequent engagement leading to degranulation, endothelial-cell adhesion, and injury.[42,43] The pathophysiologic significance of non–PR3- and non–MPO-ANCA are far less clear, but other antigen autoantibody systems, such as lactoferrin, may also lead to inflammatory damage at the neurophil-endothelial interface.[44,45] Collectively, these studies, albeit indirectly, are support-

ive of a direct role of ANCA in the pathogenesis of small vessel vasculitis. Figure 83–3 is a schematic representation of the pathogenic role of ANCA in vascular inflammation.

ANTINEUTROPHIL CYTOPLASMIC ANTIBODY AND DISEASE ACTIVITY

Although the specificity and diagnostic value of ANCA testing is well established, there remains considerable controversy as to the relative worth of such serology in monitoring of disease activity.[5] In a pooled analysis of published data only 48 percent of rises in ANCA titers

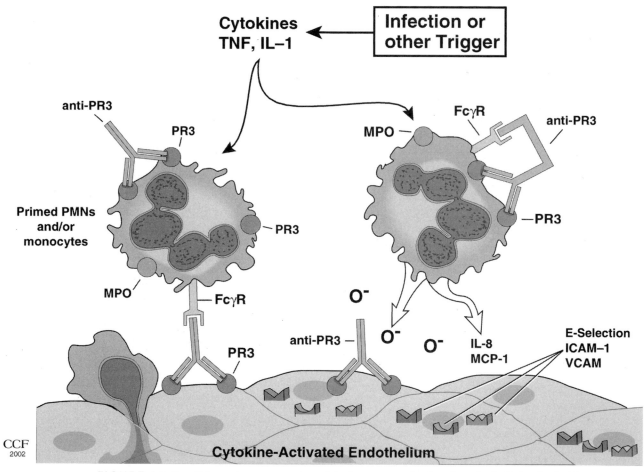

FIGURE 83–3 • Schematic representation of the immune mechanisms hypothetically involved with antineutrophil cytoplasmic antibody (ANCA) enhancement of vascular injury. In this scheme an infectious trigger or other environmental stimuli leads to a burst of cytokines that serve to prime neutrophils or monocytes and may lead to local upregulation of adhesion molecules on endothelium. The priming process within the inflammatory cells leads to enhanced expression of ANCA antigens on the cell surface. Activated neutrophils or monocytes may degranulate and release reactive oxygen species and lysosomal enzymes, leading to endothelial injury and further activation of the endothelial cell surface. The magnitude of this effect is influenced by the specificity of ANCA for proteinase 3 (PR3) or myeloperoxidase (MPO), as well as different epitopes of these respective antigens. The reaction may also be further influenced by immunoglobulin G (IgG) and the (Fcγ) receptor phenotype engaged. Release of products from degranulated inflammatory cells become bound to endothelial cells and further service targets of ANCA. Release of chemotactic chemokines such as interleukin-8 (IL8) and macrophage chemoattractant protein-1 (MCP-1) serve to augment chemotaxis and inflammatory cell transmigration in conjunction with other adhesion molecules. Thus, the scheme provides the prerequisites for endothelial and vascular injury induced by ANCA namely, A) the presence of ANCA, B) the expression of target antigens for ANCA on prime neutrophils and monocytes, C) the interaction between prime neutrophils and endothelium via adhesion molecules and finally D) the activation of endothelial cells and ultimate efflux of inflammatory cells to the extravascular and perivascular tissues. (See color plate 43.)

as measured by IFA were followed by relapse, and only 51 percent of all relapses were preceded by a rise in ANCA.[46] A study of 100 ANCA-positive patients with vasculitis followed serially over a 2-year period found that 92 percent of flares were associated with rises in ANCA. The predicative values were higher for enzyme-linked immunosorbent assay (ELISA) than IFA for both PR3 and MPO. Although a substantial number of patients with rising ANCA did not flare, it was rare to see a flare in the absence of ANCA, which affirms a strong negative predictive value of the test in this setting. As with all tests of high sensitivity, their greatest clinical utility is when they are negative, thus ruling out the disease in question.[47]

▌ Wegener's Granulomatosis

WG is a granulomatous necrotizing vasculitis characteized by its predilection to affect the upper and lower respiratory tracts and, in most cases, the kidneys. The disease was first described in 1931 by Heinz Klinger, a German medical student.[48] In 1936 and 1939, Dr. Friedrich Wegener, a young pathologist, provided detailed information about three patients with a similar illness.[49,50] Both Klinger and Wegener were struck by the unusual distribution of disease in their patients. Involvement of the upper and lower airways was quite unlike the pattern seen in periarteritis nodosa. What later came to be known as WG remained relatively unknown in the American literature until the 1950s, when Godman and Churg published a detailed clinicopathologic description of the disorder.[51] In 1973, Fauci and Wolff, at the National Institutes of Health (NIH), recorded their observations of 18 patients with WG treated with a combination of steroids and cyclophosphamide.[52] Sustained remissions and prolonged survival resulted, marking the beginning of a new era in the treatment of WG.

EPIDEMIOLOGY

Rigorous epidemiologic studies of WG have not been published. The NIH experience suggests that WG affects both sexes equally, occurs in patients of all ages (mean age 41 years; range 9 to 78 years), and is more commonly seen in Caucasian patients (97%).[53] Based on the National Hospital Discharge Survey (NHDS), the 1986 to 1990 period prevalence of WG was estimated to approximate 3.0 per 100,000 persons.[54] Both sexes were equally represented. Only 0.1 percent of patients were less than 19 years of age (vs. 15% in the NIH series). Most patients were Caucasian (80.9%). Seasonal differences in dates of hospitalization were not readily apparent.

It is likely that the prevalence of WG has been underestimated. Only since the early 90's have we come to recognize the existence of mild and more indolent forms of disease and the variability in clinical presentation and course of illness. Future epidemiologic studies need to take such factors into consideration and should extend beyond the hospital setting.

PATHOGENESIS

The etiology of WG is unknown. Sporadic efforts have been made to identify a genetic predisposition to WG. Higher prevalence of human leukocyte antigen (HLA)-DR1[55] and HLA-DQw7[56] were reported among small number of patients with WG. However, larger studies failed to identify any unique genetic markers.[57]

Several attempts to link infectious diseases to the development of WG have been unconvincing. Reports that the onset of disease occurs mostly in winter (a period of presumed increased respiratory illness)[58] have not been confirmed in larger series.[53,54] Analysis of bronchoalveolar lavage fluid and open lung biopsy specimens in patients with recent-onset disease did not reveal bacteria, fungi, mycoplasma, respiratory viruses, or viral-like inclusions.[59]

Although the association of PR3-ANCA antibodies and WG is now well established, the pathogenic role of these antibodies remains unclear. Many of the arguments supporting a pathogenic role were described previously. In addition, several clinical, in vitro, and ex vivo studies provide indirect evidence that these autoantibodies are more than an epiphenomenon. Clinical studies have documented that PR3-ANCA antibodies are highly specific for WG (90 to 97%).[4,9] They are almost always present in active, generalized WG,[53,60] and may be produced by pulmonary lymphoid tissue of patients with active disease, but not those in remission.[61] In vitro and ex vivo studies have shown that activation of polymorphonuclear cells and monocytes leads to translocation of PR3 from the intracellular compartment to the cell surface, where it becomes accessible to circulating antibodies.[62] ANCAs enhance neutrophil activation, degranulation, and respiratory burst, as well as adherence and damage to endothelial cells.[31,32,42] Endothelial cells might also be a direct target for ANCA: PR3 is present in the cytoplasm of untreated human cultured endothelial cells, and stimulation with TNF-leads to a time-dependent translocation of PR3 to the cell surface.[63] These observations suggest, but do not prove, that ANCAs are directly involved in the pathogenesis of WG.

Evidence for T cell involvement in WG is less direct than that supporting the pathogenic effect of ANCA. Biopsies of various tissues reveal the presence of polymorphonuclear and mononuclear infiltrates, the latter consisting of plasma cells, monocytes, and T cells, with a predominance of CD4+ cells.[64,65] Increasing levels of soluble interleukin-2 receptors (sIL-2R), sometimes preceding disease relapse, indicate the presence of activated T cells.[66,67] In addition, autoreactive PR3-specific T cells have been shown to be present in higher percentages in patients with WG compared to controls.[68] The role of PR3-autoreactive T cells in ANCA production, disease activity, and pathogenesis of the granulomatous lesions remains to be established.

Also, as previously mentioned, a recently described animal model of vasculits[39] has provided substantial support implicating a direct pathogenic role for ANCA, by producing lesions in the kidney and lung highly reminiscent of WG, and microscopic polyangiitis, through the action of anti-MPO antibodies alone. In this important model, the production of lesions similar to human disease in the absence of other confounding immuno-logic variables adds an important argument for causa-tion of ANCA.

CLINICAL FEATURES

WG is characterized by its predilection to affect the upper and lower respiratory tracts and, in most cases, the kidneys. Relatively mild forms of WG without renal involvement have been described. The course of illness may be indolent or rapidly progressive. Mild and indo-lent disease may go unrecognized for months to years, leading to delays in diagnosis and institution of appro-priate therapy. Neither clinical nor laboratory markers are able to distinguish which patients will continue to have limited, nonrenal forms of disease and which patients will experience progression in the future.

Unexplained constitutional symptoms are often part of the initial presentation. Fever due to WG is present in about one fourth of patients at disease onset and occurs in up to one half of cases during the course of illness.[53] Weight loss exceeding 10 percent of usual body weight has been reported in 15 percent of patients at onset and 35 percent of patients overall.[53]

The clinical features of WG are presented in the fol-lowing sections, using an organ-oriented approach. For each organ system, we have discussed the following: signs and symptoms of disease, differential diagnoses (when appropriate), clinical and laboratory methods to diagnose and assess disease activity, and aspects of disease-related morbidity.

Upper Airway Manifestations

Upper airway disease is the most common presenting feature of WG, occurring in greater than 70 percent of patients at onset and ultimately developing in more than 90 percent of cases.[53,68-70]

Otologic manifestations may be part of the initial pres-entation in about 25 percent of patients with WG and may occur in up to 60 percent of cases during the course of disease.[53,69-72] Serous otitis media is the most common ear problem encountered (25 to 44%). It may be com-plicated by the presence of a suppurative infection in up to one fourth of cases.[33] Significant degrees of hearing loss (mostly conductive) may result in 14 to 42 percent of patients.[51,69-72] Inner ear manifestations include sen-sorineural hearing loss and, rarely, vertigo.[70,72]

Nasal disease is a prominent presenting feature of WG in about one third of cases, but it eventually develops in 64 to 80 percent of patients.[53,69-71] Symptoms and signs of nasal involvement in WG include mucosal swelling with nasal obstruction, crusted nasal ulcers and septal perfo-rations, serosanguinous discharge, epistaxis (11 to 32%), and external saddle nose deformity (9 to 29%)[53,69-71] (Fig. 83–4).

Sinusitis is present at initial presentation in about one half to two thirds of patients with WG and is seen in 85 percent of cases during the entire course of disease.[53,69] A simple computed tomography (CT) scan of the sinuses (Fig. 83–5) is often anatomically more informative than plain radiographs, especially in the setting of destructive

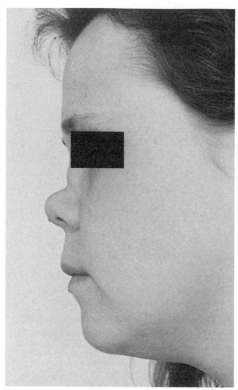

FIGURE 83–4 · Saddle-nose Deformity in a Patient with Wegener's Granulomatosis.

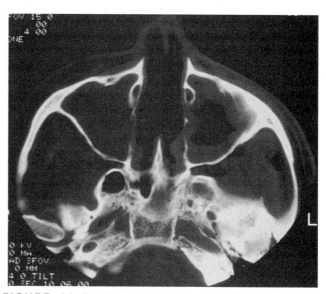

FIGURE 83–5 · Computed Tomography (CT) Scan of the Sinuses Revealing the Presence of Chronic Sinusitis.

or erosive bony changes. Most patients with sinus or nasal disease will eventually develop a secondary infec-tion of these tissues, *Staphylococcus aureus* being the predominant organism identified from cultures.[69]

Although laryngotracheal disease in WG may be asymptomatic, clinical presentations may range from subtle hoarseness to stridor and life-threatening upper airway obstruction.[53,70,73] The most characteristic lesion is that of subglottic stenosis (SGS), which occurs in up to 16 percent of patients.[53,73] It is important to note that in pediatric and adolescent patients with WG the frequency of SGS is dramatically increased, reaching an alarming 48 percent prevalence.[73,74] Direct laryngoscopy may reveal either active erythematous, friable mucosa, or bland scar.[70] Tracheal tomograms, CT and magnetic resonance imaging (MRI) scans may be useful adjuncts in the diagnosis of SGS. Only 20 percent of lesions diminish with immunosuppressive therapy alone, whereas 80 percent are fixed or irreversible due to chronic fibrosis.[73]

Pulmonary Manifestations

Pulmonary involvement is one of the cardinal features of WG. Pulmonary manifestations occur in 45 percent of cases at presentation and in 87 percent during the course of disease.[53] Cough, hemoptysis, and pleuritis are the most common pulmonary symptoms. However, it is important to realize that up to one third of cases with radiographically demonstrable pulmonary lesions may not have lower airway symptoms. The most common radiologic findings include pulmonary infiltrates (67%) and nodules (58%).[53] The pulmonary infiltrates in WG may be quite fleeting, appearing and resolving in some cases even before the institution of therapy.[52] Persistent diffuse interstitial infiltrates are rare (less than 1%) and should suggest other diagnoses. Pulmonary nodules in WG are usually multiple, bilateral, and often cavitate (50%).[52,53,69,71,75-77] CT of the chest (see Fig. 83–6) may

reveal infiltrates and nodules that were undetected by conventional radiographs in 43 to 63 percent of cases.[76-78] Less common pulmonary manifestations of WG include pleural effusions, diffuse pulmonary hemorrhage, and mediastinal or hilar lymph node enlargement or mass.[79,80] Diffuse pulmonary hemorrhage has been reported in up to 8 percent of cases, and it carries a high fatality rate (50%).[52,77,81,82]

In patients presenting with pulmonary symptoms, it is imperative to make every effort to exclude the presence of infection in a timely fashion because pneumonia in an immunocompromised host can yield up to 50 percent mortality. Bronchoscopy is often needed to satisfactorily exclude infection or alternatively establish a microbiologic diagnosis by performing the appropriate stains and cultures. Pneumonia may account for up to 40 percent of serious infections in patients with WG and may be the cause of death in a significant proportion of cases (16%).[53,75]

Pulmonary morbidity in WG is significant. Pulmonary function tests may reveal obstructive defects in up to 55 percent of patients, generally caused by endobronchial lesions and scarring.[83] Restrictive defects with reduced lung volumes and carbon monoxide diffusion capacity are observed in 30 to 40 percent of patients.[83] In more than 17 percent of patients, serial pulmonary function tests may document moderate to severe degrees of progressive pulmonary insufficiency, perhaps as a result of fibrosis following active disease, pneumonia, cyclophosphamide-induced pneumonitis, or some combination of these.[53]

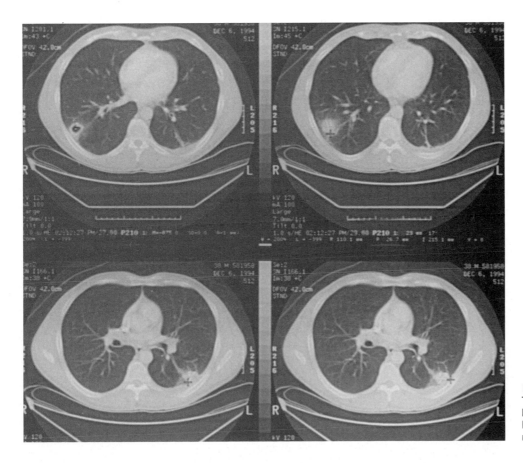

FIGURE 83–6 · Computed Tomography (CT) Scan of the Lungs Revealing the Presence of Nodules. The Rightsided Pulmonary Nodule is Cavitary.

Renal Manifestations

The presence or absence of renal disease defines the subsets of generalized and limited WG, respectively.[84,85] The exact frequency of renal involvement in WG is difficult to ascertain. Limited WG may go undiagnosed in patients with mild disease. By excluding such patients, published series may overestimate the frequency of renal disease in WG. On the other hand, early renal disease may be clinically silent (i.e., kidney biopsies may, on rare occasions, reveal focal inflammatory changes in patients with normal urinary sediment and renal function).[52,84,86] In addition, patients who appear to have limited WG at one time may later develop glomerulonephritis. This observation represents a caution in patients thought to have limited WG and dictates the need for careful and close monitoring of renal status in all patients.

When renal disease is defined by pathologic findings on kidney biopsy or the presence of an active urinary sediment and functional abnormalities, it is then estimated to occur in 11 to 18 percent of patients at presentation and 77 to 85 percent during the entire course of disease.[53,69,80] Extrarenal manifestations often precede renal disease. Once present, renal disease may progress from being asymptomatic and mild to fulminant glomerulonephritis within days or weeks, resulting in end-stage renal failure.[69] If untreated, mean survival time for this subset is about 5 months.[71] Even when appropriate therapy is instituted, initial and recurrent renal damage may lead to chronic renal insufficiency in up to 42 percent of patients, often requiring dialysis (11%) and renal transplantation (5%).[53]

The role of microscopic urinalysis in the evaluation of patients with suspected or proven WG cannot be overemphasized. It remains the most useful tool to assess for the presence of active glomerulonephritis (GN). The freshly collected urinary sediment should be personally and carefully examined by the treating physician. The presence of red blood cell (RBC) casts approaches a 100-percent positive predictive value for GN. In the absence of RBC casts, the presence of hematuria should lead to consideration of lower urinary tract involvement by the vasculitic process, which is uncommon, or presence of cyclophosphamide-induced cystitis.

Ocular Manifestations

Ocular manifestations have been reported to occur in 28 to 58 percent of patients with WG and may be part of the initial presentation in 8 to 16 percent of cases.[80] Any compartment of the eye may be affected. Keratitis, conjunctivitis, scleritis, episcleritis, nasolacrimal duct obstruction, uveitis, retroorbital pseudotumor with proptosis (Fig. 83–7), retinal vessel occlusion, and optic neuritis have all been described.[80] Visual loss has been reported to occur in as many as 8 percent of patients.[53] Although most ocular findings are nonspecific, proptosis is a diagnostically helpful finding,[52,53] as it is a poor prognostic sign for vision. About half of the patients with proptosis in one series lost vision due to optic nerve ischemia.[53] A complete ophthalmologic examination is an important part of the diagnostic evaluation. In

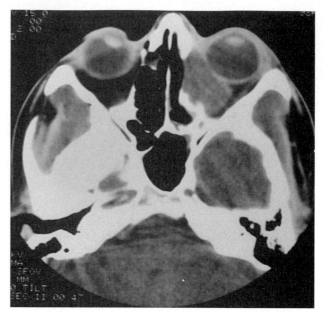

FIGURE 83–7 · Computed Tomography (CT) Scan of the Orbits Revealing the Presence of a Retro-Orbital Mass (Orbital Pseudotumor).

patients with proptosis, CT or MRI of the orbits and sinuses may provide useful anatomic information.[53,87]

Ocular disease may also occur as a complication of therapy. Glucorticoid (GC)-related catatracts occured in 21 percent of patients in one series.[53] GC and cyclophosphamide therapy has been associated with opportunistic ocular infections, including cytomegalovirus (CMV) retinitis, and herpes zoster ophthalmicus.[88]

Cutaneous Manifestations

Cutaneous manifestations have been reported in 40 to 50 percent of patients with WG and may be part of the initial presentation in 13 to 25 percent of cases.[80] The cutaneous manifestations of WG have included ulcers, palpable purpura, subcutaneous nodules, papules, and vesicles. Although cutaneous lesions rarely dominate the clinical picture, they do tend to parallel disease activity in other organs. The presence of active skin lesions is, thus, a reliable clinical marker for active systemic disease and should prompt the clinician to evaluate other organ systems thoroughly.

Musculoskeletal Manifestations

Musculoskeletal symptoms are common in patients with WG, occurring in 32 to 53 percent of cases at presentation and 67 to 76 percent during the course of disease.[80] Although most patients experience only arthalgias and myalgias, arthritis is observed in up to 28 percent of patients.[69,89] When synovitis is present, several patterns can be observed, including monoarticular disease, migratory oligoarthritis, and symmetric or asymmetric polyarthritis of small and large joints.[53,89] Symmetric polyarthritis of small and large joints may be mistaken for RA.[53,89] A positive test for rheumatoid factor (RF) may be observed in as many as 50 to 60 percent of cases, often contributing to an incorrect diagnosis.[53,89] In contrast to RA, the symmetric polyarthritis of WG is generally nonerosive and nondeforming.[53,69,89]

Neurologic Manifestations

Neurologic involvement is rarely a presenting feature of WG, but it may develop during the course of disease in 22 percent to more than 50 percent of cases.[53,69,75,80,90] Multiple neurologic complications may occur in up to 11 percent of patients.[56] Peripheral neuropathy is the most common single neurologic manifestation of WG (10 to 16%).[53,69,75,90] Mononeuritis multiplex is the most frequent clinical pattern (12 to 15%), followed by a distal and symmetric polyneuropathy (2%).[53,90] Electromyography (EMG) and nerve conduction studies may be useful in demonstrating the extent and distribution of involvement and will often identify an overlapping mononeuropathy multiplex that may not be apparent on clinical examination. Biopsy of the involved nerve(s) will reveal the presence of vasculitis, but it is rarely necessary for establishing the diagnosis or making therapeutic decisions.

The overall frequency of central nervous system (CNS) involvement is difficult to estimate because the symptoms, signs, and clinical presentations of CNS disease have been variably defined and accrued in different series. In addition, significant classification overlap exists between the symptoms and signs of CNS, ocular, and sinus disease and treatment complications. Cranial neuropathy occurs in 6 to 9 percent of patients.[53,90] Cerebrovascular events, occuring in up to 4 percent of cases, may include cerebral or brain stem infarction, subdural hematoma, and subarachnoid hemorrhage.[53,75,80,90] Diffuse meningeal and periventricular white matter disease, presumably reflecting CNS vasculitis, has been reported in patients presenting with diffuse and focal CNS symptoms.[91,92]

In patients presenting with symptoms and signs of CNS disease, several diagnostic tests may be considered. CT or MRI of the brain may document the presence of infarcts, hemorrhage, mass lesions, diffuse meningeal enhancement, or periventricular white matter lesions. In some cases, lumbar puncture is necessary to exclude CNS infections and subarachnoid hemorrhage. Cerebral angiography is a test of low diagnostic yield in WG because in most instances, relatively small vessels are involved.[90,92]

Gastrointestinal Manifestations

The frequency of GI involvement in WG is difficult to estimate, perhaps because it is frequently asymptomatic and may, thus, be unrecognized. The literature mainly consists of individual case reports of patients with dramatic or unusual GI presentations. Abdominal pain, diarrhea, and bleeding are the most frequently reported symptoms, and they relate to the presence of ulcerations in the small intestines, large intestines, or both (enterocolitis).[80] Small and large bowel perforations have been described, with dramatic and often fatal presentations.[80] Other unusual presentations have included cholecystitis, unexplained ascites, nonhealing perianal ulcers, recurrent acute pancreatitis, and pancreatic mass with extrahepatic obstruction.[80] Steroid-induced peptic ulcers may occur, but a biopsy would be required to distinguish such lesions from those due to vasculitis. Unexplained elevations of liver enzymes have also been described and may resolve with therapy.[69,93] In autopsy series of patients with WG, the spleen was commonly involved; the majority of cases demonstrated splenic lesions with a combination of necrosis, vasculitis, and granuloma formation.[71] However, clinically apparent splenic disease is rare.

The occurence of GI complaints in a patient with a known or suspected diagnosis of WG (or other systemic vasculitides) represents a medical emergency.[94] In patients with abdominal pain and systemic vasculitis, especially those receiving GCs, the lack of physical signs on abdominal examination should not provide the clinician with a false sense of security. Plain abdominal radiographs may detect the presence of free air, indicative of perforation. Arteriography may not be helpful because WG most often affects small vessels, which are beyond the resolution of this technique.[94] Endoscopic studies (colonoscopy, gastroscopy) may document the presence of ulcerations. Endoscopic biopsies usually demonstrate nonspecific inflammatory changes and may, on rare occasions, reveal granulomatous necrotizing vasculitis, thus establishing a histopathologic diagnosis. Histologic diagnosis is more commonly made on examination of surgical specimens because of the larger amount of tissue available.[95]

Genitourinary Manifestations

Virtually every segment of the genitourinary (GU) tract distal to the kidneys may be involved in WG. The literature mostly consists of individual case reports, suggesting that such manifestations are uncommon. Ureteral obstruction by an extrinsic inflammatory mass has been reported.[96] Hemorrhagic cystitis is more commonly seen in relation to cyclophosphamide therapy, but it may be due to involvement of the bladder wall by necrotizing vasculitis.[62] In an autopsy series, granulomatous or necrotizing prostatitis was found in 7.4 percent of patients with WG.[71] Other GU manifestations have included necrotizing urethritis, orchitis, epididymitis, and penile necrosis.[80]

Microscopic examination of freshly voided urine is the most important diagnostic test. The presence of hematuria in the absence of RBC casts (after adequate review by the clinician) should prompt evaluation of the lower GU tract. Cystoscopy is preferred because it allows direct visualization of abnormal structures and the performance of diagnostic biopsies. This is equally important in the patient receiving long-term cyclophosphamide therapy. Urinary tract infections should always be considered and the appropriate cultures obtained.

Cardiac Manifestations

The frequency of cardiac involvement in WG varies from 6 to 12 percent in clinical series[53,69] and may reach

30 percent in autopsy series.[71] Pericarditis has been the most frequently reported cardiac manifestation in WG.[80] Patients may present with asymptomatic pericardial effusions or complain of chest pain, associated with a pericardial friction rub on physical examination. In the setting of advanced renal disease, the differential diagnosis includes uremic and infectious causes of pericarditis. Pericardial tamponade has rarely been reported and may require pericardiocentesis, pericardiectomy, or both.[53,97,98] Pericarditis is also the most common pathologic finding in the heart, accounting for about 50 percent of histologically documented cardiac disease in WG.[99] Necrotizing vasculitis and granuloma formation may involve the pericardium in a focal or diffuse pattern.[99] Other cardiac manifestations of WG include myocardial ischemia due to coronary vasculitis, myocarditis, endocarditis and valvulitis, arrhythmias, and conduction defects.[80]

LABORATORY DIAGNOSIS

General laboratory abnormalities in untreated patients may include leukocytosis, normocytic normochromic anemia, thrombocytosis, and elevated erythrocyte sedimentation rate (ESR). These are imperfect markers of disease activity and should always be interpreted in relation to organ-specific clinical and laboratory evidence of active disease. The role of ANCA testing in the evaluation of WG and other systemic vasculitides has already been discussed. The sensitivity of PR3-ANCA is about 90 percent in active WG and 40 percent when disease is in remission.[4,60,100] The specificity of PR3-ANCA in the diagnosis of WG exceeds 95 percent.[4,60,100] In general, the presence of high-titer ANCA by IFA combined with confirmatory antigen-specific assay for either PR3 or MPO in the setting of a high index of suspicion for vasculitis (i.e., high pretest probability) is

sufficient for diagnosis, even in the absence of tissue confirmation.

PATHOLOGY

Inflammatory lesions in WG typically include necrosis, granulomatous changes, and vasculitis.[48-50,52,53,69,71] The diagnostic yield of a biopsy varies with the size of the pathologic specimen and how completely it is sectioned and studied.

The small amount of tissue available in head and neck biopsies (mostly from nasal and paranasal sinuses) may make it difficult to identify all of the pathologic features of WG.[101-103] Vasculitis, necrosis, and granulomatous inflammation are each encountered in roughly one third to one half of pathologic specimens.[101-103] Vasculitis and necrosis are seen together in only one fifth of biopsies.[102,103] The frequency of combined vasculitis and granulomatous inflammation is also about one fifth.[102,103] Most importantly, a complete diagnostic triad is only seen in 3 to 16 percent of biopsies.[102,103] Thus, it appears that head and neck biopsies most often reveal findings compatible with, but rarely characteristic of, WG. Awareness of these limitations is required for the correct interpretation of head and neck biopsy results in patients suspected of having WG.

The diagnostic yield of lung biopsies similarly reflects the sample size of pulmonary tissue obtained.[53,65] Transbronchial biopsies are rarely diagnostic (less than 7%), whereas open lung biopsies reveal various combinations of vasculitis, granulomas, and necrosis in about 90 percent of cases[53,65] (Fig. 83–8). Nonetheless, bronchoscopy and transbronchial biopsy remain valuable in the diagnosis or exclusion of bacterial, mycobacterial, or fungal infections that can mimic or complicate WG. Capillaritis, a pathologic finding, has been described in 35 to 45 percent of WG cases in surgical biopsy and

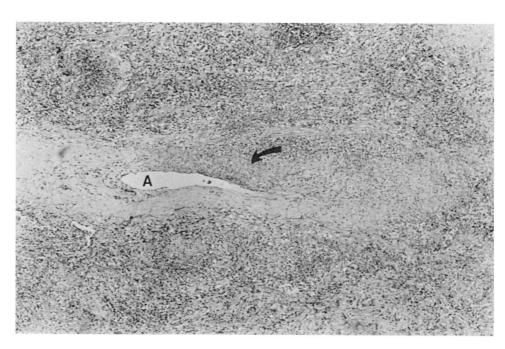

FIGURE 83-8 • Medium-sized artery (A in lumen) with granulomatous vasculitis (arrow) destroying media in a patient with Wegener's granulomatosis. (H & E, ×20)

autopsy series.[104,105] In one study, capillaritis was found in all 11 patients with WG presenting with diffuse pulmonary hemorrhage.[106] However, the finding of capillaritis is not diagnostically specific. Capillaritis has been described in SLE, immune complex–associated vasculitides, dermatomyositis (DM), RA, Henoch-Schöenlein purpura, and even bronchopneumonias.[82]

Pathologically, renal disease in WG is characterized by the presence of focal and segmental GN[52,53,69,71,75,86] (Fig. 83–9). Fibrinoid necrosis and proliferative changes are seen in varying degrees. In patients with irreversible renal impairment, epithelial crescents and sclerotic lesions are commonly encountered.[53,69,71] True vasculitis of medium-sized renal arteries is only occasionally noted (3 to 15%), and granulomatous changes are equally rare (3%).[51-53,69,75] Immune-complex deposition, as demonstrated by immunofluorescence or electron microscopy, is distinctly unusual.[53,86,107] The results of kidney biopsies are, thus, more often compatible with, rather than diagnostic of, WG.

TREATMENT

To manage WG effectively, the clinician must establish the diagnosis without delay, recognize variability in clinical course and severity, critically monitor disease activity, and anticipate disease- and treatment-related morbidity. Therapeutic decision making should be based on a critical assessment of disease activity. Meticulous attention should be paid to complications of therapy, which often lead to permanent morbidity and, sometimes, mortality. In addition, certain complications (infections, drug reactions or toxicity, drug-induced pneumonitis, renal impairment) may be confused with active disease. The significant toxicity of currently available therapeutic agents has been the main driving force for the development of new drugs and innovative approaches to the treatment of WG and other systemic vasculitides.

Glucocorticoids

In WG, GC are most commonly used in combination with cytotoxic agents. Although palliation of limited, indolent disease may be achieved with GC alone, disease progression and relapses usually occur. Patients with generalized WG uniformly fail to achieve remission with GC therapy alone. Treatment is generally initiated with high-dose GC, such as prednisone at 1 mg/kg/day or more. High doses are maintained until all manifestations of active disease have abated (e.g., stabilization of renal function, resolution of pulmonary infiltrates). Tapering GC should follow after WG is well under control, usually about 1 month from initiation of treatment. The literature does not provide a consensus opinion about the subsequent strategy for tapering GC. One approach is to reduce prednisone on an alternate-day basis so that within another 2 to 3 months, in the absence of relapse or exacerbations, a dose of about 1 mg/kg every other day is achieved. During the ensuing 2 to 3 months, tapering of the alternate-day schedule continues until GC therapy is discontinued. Waxing and waning of disease may force alterations in these guidelines. The rationale for this approach is well established.[53,69,108] Another approach during the initiation of therapy is the use of intravenous (IV) "pulse" or "bolus" methylprednisolone (e.g., 1 g daily for 3 days) for immediately life-threatening disease (e.g., diffuse pulmonary hemorrhage, rapidly progressive glomerulonephritis). However, the optimal dose and frequency of administration of IV GC have not been studied in a controlled fashion for systemic vasculitis. In addition, the short-lasting effects of pulse GC do not obviate the need for maintenance therapy.

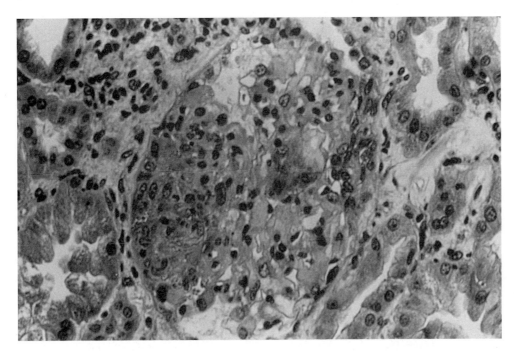

FIGURE 83–9 · Kidney biopsy specimen demonstrating a necrotizing segmental glomerulonephritis with crescent formation. (H & E, × 100)

Prior to the advent of GC, the mean survival time of patients with WG was 5 months. GC alone modestly increased mean survival time to 12 months.[109] Greater than 80 percent 5-year survival rates were not seen until the introduction of aggressive combination therapy with GC and daily cyclophosphamide.

Cyclophosphamide

Combination therapy with oral daily cyclophosphamide (CTX) and GC has been considered the standard therapy for WG.[52,53,69] Oral CTX is generally initiated at doses of 2 mg/kg/day. In life-threatening situations (pulmonary hemorrhage or rapidly progressive glomerulonephritis), CTX doses of 3 to 5 mg/kg/day may be used for about 3 to 4 days, then reduced to the more conventional range. The leukocyte count is used to guide subsequent dosage adjustments (discussed in following section). Tapering and discontinuation of GC generally precede attempts to taper CTX. The latter is continued for at least 1 year after the patient achieves complete remission and is then tapered by 25-mg decrements every 2 to 3 months until discontinuation or until disease recurrence requires an increase in the dose.

Orally administered CTX is well absorbed and completely metabolized within 24 hours by the liver to multiple active and inactive metabolites that are mostly excreted in the urine. One of these metabolites, acrolein, is known to be responsible for hemorrhagic cystitis, bladder fibrosis, and bladder cancer. High oral fluid intake by the patient should be encouraged to dilute this CTX-derived bladder irritant and reduce the incidence of such complications. The time from initial use of CTX to detection of bladder cancer may be as brief as 7 months or as long as 10 to 15 years, even after CTX has been discontinued.[53] Urine cytology is an insensitive diagnostic tool to detect bladder cancer. Cystoscopy is, therefore, necessary in any CTX-treated patient with nonglomerular hematuria. Life-long surveillance for bladder cancer, as well as hematologic malignancies, is indicated in all patients who have been treated with chronic daily CTX therapy.[53] Dose-related bone marrow suppression is a common toxicity caused by CTX, and blood counts should be closely observed in the course of treatment. Leukopenia is the most frequent sign of marrow suppression and should guide dosage adjustments in these patients. The risk of infection is increased even in the absence of leukopenia. Total leukocyte counts of less than $3500/mm^3$ or absolute neutrophil counts of $1500/mm^3$ or less should be avoided. Based on data from recent pharmacokinetic investigations, the dose of CTX should be adjusted downward by 25 to 30 percent in the presence of significant renal impairment.[110] CTX is formally contraindicated during pregnancy, and birth control should be strongly advised in women of childbearing age. When utilized in men considering fatherhood, counsel should be given regarding sperm banking.

In a large series of 158 patients with WG followed at the NIH for up to 24 years (mean follow-up period of 8 years), 84 percent of patients received "standard" therapy with daily CTX and GC.[53] This regimen produced marked improvement in 91 percent of the patients and complete remission in 75 percent of the patients. Disease relapse was seen in 50 percent of patients in this study, with permanent morbidity from disease occurring in 86 percent of them. This included chronic renal insufficiency (42%), hearing loss (35%), cosmetic and functional nasal deformities (28%), tracheal stenosis (13%), and visual loss (8%), with many patients experiencing more than one type of morbidity. Permanent morbidity as a result of treatment with GC and CTX occurred in 42 percent of the patients, including CTX cystitis (43%), bladder cancer (2.8%, which is 33 times the expected rate), lymphoma (1.5%, which is 11 times the expected rate), myelodysplasia (2%), infertility (more than 57% of women), GC-related cataracts (21%), fractures (11%), and aseptic necrosis (3%). Moreover, 46 percent of the patients experienced serious infectious episodes, which required hospitalization and IV antibiotics.

In addition to the significant disease- and treatment-related morbidity, more indolent forms of disease, without significant pulmonary or renal abnormalities, do occur. This reinforces the need to identify effective and less toxic therapeutic interventions that take into consideration the severity and rate of progression of individual cases.

Intermittent High-Dose Intravenous Cyclophosphamide

Studies of intermittent high-dose IV CTX (pulse CTX) were motivated by its demonstrated efficacy in the treatment of lupus nephritis and the anticipation of reduced toxicity. Pulse CTX is only rarely associated with hemorrhagic cystitis and has not been associated with bladder cancer. Several randomized trials of IV pulse CTX (0.7 g/m^2 every 3 weeks) have demonstrated efficacy comparable to oral daily CTX in achieving initial remission in WG[111,112] with fewer associated infections, especially *Pneumocystis carinii* pneumonia (PCP), and lower mortality than oral therapy. Several criticisms of these investigations have been rendered, including an unacceptable overall mortality rate in one trial[111] and a lack of statistical power in the other.[112] To minimize bladder toxicity, some investigators recommend the use of mesna (sodium 2-mercaptoethane sulphate).[113] This may be given intravenously at the time of CTX infusion, but due to a short half-life, it must be administered orally 2 and 4 hours after the infusion to be effective. In addition to having its own toxicities, the technique is cumbersome and, thus, many favor a high oral intake of fluids as an alternative. Until additional studies are performed, pulse CTX is not recommended as standard therapy for WG.[114]

Methotrexate

Low-dose methotrexate (MTX), such as 0.05 to 0.3 mg/kg/week, has been used to treat a variety of autoimmune diseases. MTX-related toxicity is most often mild and can be diminished by either dose reduction or temporary discontinuation of the drug. Folic or folinic acid supplementation may also reduce the incidence of selected MTX side effects without compromising its therapeutic efficacy in RA.[114] Although mild elevations of liver enzymes are common during MTX therapy, cirrhosis rarely occurs with careful monitoring and in the absence of risk factors. MTX appears to be less oncogenic than CTX. Nonetheless, reversible lymphoproliferative disorders have occurred during MTX therapy for RA and DM.[115,116] MTX is teratogenic and causes a high rate of malformation and abortion. Therefore, birth control is mandatory in females and advised in males who are taking the drug.

In an effort to find an effective and safe alternative to CTX for the induction of remission in WG, the NIH initiated an open-label study of weekly low-dose MTX plus GC in 42 patients with biopsy-proven WG.[117] Although none of the patients included in this study had immediately life-threatening disease (serum creatinine above 2.5 mg/dl or acute pulmonary hemorrhage), 50 percent had active glomerulonephritis. Twenty-six patients (62%) had previously received treatment with GC, a cytotoxic agent, or both. These patients were enrolled because of either persistent or relapsing disease, serious toxicity from prior use of cytotoxic drugs, or both. Weekly administration of MTX (0.15 to 0.30 mg/kg/week) and GC produced remission in 71 percent of patients after a median of 4.2 months. Nonetheless, relapses occurred in 36 percent of cases after a median of 29 months. Treatment was not free of serious side effects: Four patients developed PCP, and two of them died. This stresses the need for vigilance in monitoring for opportunistic infections, particularly in patients receiving daily steroids and a cytotoxic agent. PCP prophylaxis should be now be standard in such patients.

Antimicrobial Agents

Since the original report by Wegener,[49] it has been postulated that airway stimulation is necessary for disease expression. Upper or lower airway symptoms are present at disease onset in 90 percent of patients.[53] Neutrophilic alveolitis and increased concentration of IgG c-ANCA in bronchoalveolar lavage fluid is seen in patients with active WG, but not those in remission.[59,61] Most patients with WG develop respiratory tract infections at some point during the course of their disease. Secondary infection of the paranasal sinuses occurs most frequently with *Staphylococcus aureus*.[69] An observational cohort study of 57 patients with biopsy-proven WG has suggested that chronic nasal carriage of *S. aureus* identifies a subgroup of patients who are more prone to relapse.[118] Whether infectious organisms can induce a relapse of disease activity and whether relapses can be prevented by antibiotic prophylaxis remains the subject of speculation. Similarly controversial are several reports advocating the use of trimethoprim/sulfamethoxazole (T/S) as single-drug therapy for WG.[119] In a recent controlled trial, T/S was clearly inferior to MTX for the maintenance of remission in patients with generalized WG.[120] Because T/S seemed to increase the chance of relapse, the authors recommended against using T/S alone or T/S plus prednisone for the maintenance of remission in generalized WG.

Intravenous Immunoglobulin

Treatment with IV immunoglobulins (IVIg) has been used in a wide variety of autoimmune disorders with variable results. In systemic inflammatory diseases, several mechanisms of action have been postulated and reviewed.[121] Of relevance to WG, anti-idiotypic antibodies present in the IVIg preparations may bind to idiotypic determinants on pathogenic autoantibodies, downregulate B cell receptors for antigen, or bind to T cell receptors and influence their activation and regulatory properties.[121,122]

The investigational use of IVIg in the treatment of WG was prompted by the detection of anti-idiotype antibody reactivity with ANCA in IVIg preparations.[122] Several small, open trials and numerous anecdotes have been published utilizing IVIg, but recently Jayne and colleagues have published a small, controlled trial.[123] In this study, 17 patients were randomized to receive IVIg and 17 to receive placebo. Treatment responses were observed in 14 of 17 and 6 of 17 of the IVIg and placebo groups, respectively, as measured by a vasculitis activity scale. This modest treatment effect was only observed for 3 months following a single infusion. Significant decreases in C-reactive protein (CRP) were seen for up to 1 month in the IVIg group but then returned to pretreatment levels. No differences were observed between ANCA levels or cumulative exposure to immunosuppressive drugs. Reversible increases in serum creatinine occurred in four patients from the IVIg group. Thus, IVIg might be an alternative treatment for some forms of systemic vasculitis with persistent disease activity after standard therapy.

Tumor Necrosis Factor Inhibitors

Evidence from animal models and in vitro studies in humans suggest that TNF-α plays a prominent role in the pathogenesis of ANCA-associated vasculitis. Accordingly, there are now a few uncontrolled studies supporting the use of TNF inhibitors in patients with active disease. In an uncontrolled trial of infliximab in six patients with CTX-resistant disease, remission was induced in five individuals and one patient was withdrawn due to infection.[124] In a second study, 10 patients with refractory disease were treated in an open-label fashion, with complete or partial remission observed in all, with minimal toxicity.[125] In the largest of these investigations, Stone and colleagues[126] treated 20 patients with etanercept and found the drug to be safe and well tolerated. Overall, 14 of these 20 patients received only etanercept as an additional therapy to their stable regimens, and disease activity was significantly improved at 6 months. Minor disease flares were did occur in this trial, but importantly, no significant toxicity was ascribed to etanercept. At present there are little data to support initiation of anti-TNF therapy for untreated patients, but this class of drugs will play an increasingly more important role in the setting of treatment-resistant disease.

Apheresis

A small amount of literature on apheresis derived from several small, controlled trials suggests that there might be therapeutic efficacy in a subset of patients with advancing oliguric renal failure.[127] These studies are methodologically diverse and no definitive conclusions can be drawn. At present, apheresis in addition to standard therapy is reasonable in those patients presenting with severe renal involvement with initial creatinine levels over 6 mg/dl who fail to respond to standard therapy.

Remission-Maintenance Strategies

In an effort to take advantage of the potency of CTX as a remission-induction agent and the lower toxicity of antimetabolites, there is currently growing enthusiasm for treatment regimens that combine both, so called "step down" strategies. Two agents have been studied most thoroughly, namely azathioprine and MTX, although other agents have been anecdotally employed, including mycophenolate and leflunomide.[128] In an open-label study of 31 patients at the NIH, the sequential use of CTX followed by MTX was highly effective at maintaining remission. However, 16 percent suffered relapses, some while still on therapy. A limitation of this strategy is the danger of using MTX in settings of changing renal function or when the baseline value is greater than 2 to 2.5 mg/dl. In these situations, azathioprine may be a safer option.[129]

Surgical Interventions

WG is a paradigm for illnesses that require a multidisciplinary approach. For instance, the management of SGS in WG is complex and often requires individualized multimodality interventions to achieve satisfactory results. To plan strategies for treatment, it is extremely important to assess whether stenosis is due to active inflammation, noninflammatory scar tissue, or both. When present, the inflammatory process should always be suppressed concurrent with, or prior to, surgical intervention.[73] Patients with severe SGS may need temporary, and sometimes permanent, tracheostomy. Manual dilation of noninflamed lesions and intralesional steroid injections may be useful, if performed as part of a strategy of progressive tracheal rehabilitation.[73] An open procedure may be necessary if no appreciable progress is made in improving airway function. Laryngotracheoplasty has been used with success in WG patients with SGS.[73] When indicated, microvascular laryngotracheal reconstruction should also be considered.[73]

Patients with WG might also need tympanostomies and drainage tubes for chronic otitis media, irrigation and drainage procedures (maxillary windows, Caldwell-Luc procedure) for impacted sinuses with persistent or recurrent infections, and ocular surgery for orbital pseudotumors or nasolacrimal duct obstruction. Urgent surgical intervention may be needed in patients with severe pulmonary hemorrhage or GI vasculitis. Whether or not surgery is indicated, aggressive medical therapy is required to suppress active inflammatory processes and prevent further damage.

In patients with end-stage renal failure, kidney transplantation is generally successful when recipients have been in sustained remission at the time of surgical engraftment.[52,53,69,130,131] Recurrent GN in the transplanted kidney has been occasionally documented.[53,130]

Microscopic Polyangiitis

MPA was first recognized as a distinct entity by Davson and colleagues in 1948.[132] They described this as subgroup of polyarteritis nodosa, distinguished by the presence of segmental necrotizing glomerulonephritis.

MPA was not included in the American College of Rheumatology (ACR) classification scheme, and it is assumed that most of such patients were labeled as having polyarteritis or, less frequently, WG. The Chapel Hill International Consensus Criteria[1] defined MPA as a necrotizing vasculitis with few or no deposits affecting small vessels (i.e., capillaries, venules, or arterioles). They also noted that MPA frequently is associated with necrotizing glomerulonephritis and pulmonary capillaritis. MPA is also occasionally referred to as "microscopic polyarteritis," but MPA is preferred because it distinguishes the syndrome more clearly.

CLINICAL FEATURES

The general clinical features of MPA, collected from four large clinical series,[133-136] are summarized in Table 83-1 and reflect the propensity for widespread target-organ involvement. The disease tends to affect males more frequently than females, with male-to-female ratios ranging from 1[133] to 1.8.[134] The age of onset is generally in the fourth or fifth decade but can range from early childhood to old age.[137] The onset may be hyperacute with rapidly progressive glomerulonephritis and pulmonary hemorrhage, presenting as the pulmonary renal syndrome, or at times may be extremely insidious with several years if intermittent constitutional symptoms, purpura, mild renal disease, and even periodic bouts of hemoptysis.

Renal Disease

The universal presence of renal disease in most large series[133-136] reflects both the common involvement of the kidney and the ascertainment bias of reporting by nephrology groups. Clearly MPA can be seen in the absence of renal disease, although it is less common. The course of the renal disease is also variable, but a rapidly progressive course has been frequently reported in series reported by nephrology groups. Dialysis has been

TABLE 83–1 • CLINICAL FEATURES OF MICROSCOPIC POLYANGIITIS (PMA)

Clinical Feature	Percentage*
Constitutional symptoms	76-79
Fever	50-72
Renal disease	100
Arthralgias	28-65
Purpura	40-44
Pulmonary disease (hemorrhage, infiltrates, effusion)	50
Neurologic disease (central, peripheral)	28
Ear, nose, throat	30

*Percentage of studied populations totaling 150 patients from four studies[133-136]

required in between 25 and 45 percent of patients in several large series.[134,135] The renal lesion of MPA is that of necrotizing glomerulonephritis. The characteristic features of this lesion are segmental necrosis, crescent formation (extracapillary proliferation), slight or no endocapillary proliferation, slight or no immune deposits by immunohistology, and slight or no electron-dense deposits by electron microscopy.[138] This lesion is clearly distinct from immune complex–mediated glomerulonephritis and antiglomerular basement membrane antibody–mediated disease but is not distinguishable from the glomerular lesion of WG or idiopathic rapidly progressive crescentic glomerulonephritis (see Fig. 83-8).

Pulmonary Disease

Lung involvement is common in MPA and is present in more than half of reported cases in most series. Diffuse alveolar hemorrhage (DAH) is the most serious form of lung involvement and has been reported in 12 to 29 percent of patients in several series.[133-136] The clinical manifestations may range from mild dyspnea and anemia without any hemoptysis to massive hemorrhage and bleeding with profound hypoxia, but the onset is acute in most patients. The radiographic features of DAH are nonspecific, demonstrating alveolar infiltration ranging from patchy to diffuse. The characteristic finding of alveolar infiltrates in the absence of congestive heart failure or infection is helpful, but the clinical differentiation of these disorders in the acutely ill patient may at times be difficult. The absence of frank hemoptysis should never dissuade serious consideration of possible, even massive, DAH, as it may be absent in up to one third of patients.[139] An alternative presentation of lung involvement in MPA is that of interstitial fibrosis based on recurrent episodes DAH. This generally occurs after a prolonged (i.e., many years) history of such events.[139]

The characteristic histopathology of MPA is that of pulmonary capillaritis (Fig. 83-10). In this lesion there is disruption of the alveolar interstitium, leading to loss of integrity of the constituent capillary network and resulting in RBC leakage into the alveolar spaces. The alveolar wall expands and becomes edematous and ultimately undergoes fibrinoid necrosis. Characteristically, there is prominent neutrophilic leukocytosis of the alveolar septum, often accompanied by leucocytoclasia. Immunohistology, similar to the kidney, rarely demonstrates immune deposits. Other findings include capillary thrombosis, type II epithelial cell hyperplasia, and lymphoplasmocytic infiltration.[139] This clinical and histologic picture can be seen in a variety of conditions commonly observed in WG, SLE, and in an isolated form.[139,140] When DAH occurs in an isolated form, it may be in the presence or absence of MPO-ANCA.[139]

Other Disease Manifestations

Other clinical features of MPA are similar to the other major forms of ANCA-associated small vessel vasculitis, as well as classic polyarteritis nodosa. Arthralgia, myalgia, and fever are common (see Table 83–1). Skin involvement is common as well and most frequently manifests as palpable purpura. Peripheral neuropathy is observed in the minority of patients and appears to be less common than the other ANCA-associated syndromes. Involvement of the ears, nose, and throat is infrequent and when present should seriously raise the question of missed WG in which granulomas have either been overlooked or missed by sampling error on biopsy.

DIAGNOSIS

The diagnosis of MPA may at times be problematic. There is a great variability in the presenting manifestations, as well as the intensity of the illness. Clearly MPA

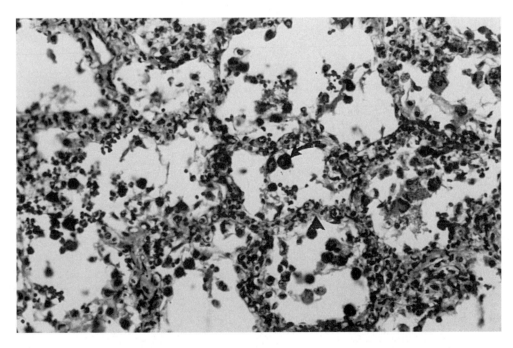

FIGURE 83–10 · Acute inflammatory cells and fibrinoid necrosis diffusely involve the capillaries within the alveolar walls (arrow head) in a patient with acute capilaritis. The presence of numerous hemosiderin-laden macrophages (arrow) confirms a histology of pulmonary hemorrhage. (H & E, × 100)

should be considered in any patient with the general features of a systemic vasculitis, such as prolonged unexplained fever, unexplained multisystem organ involvement (especially renal and pulmonary), and palpable purpura. MPA is prominent in the differential pulmonary renal syndromes along with WG, SLE, and antiglomerular basement membrane disease.

Although the diagnosis of MPA may at times be based on clinical and laboratory findings, it is preferred to secure the diagnosis with histology. The most accessible and rewarding tissues are skin, kidney, and lung. It must be emphasized that in none of the organs is there a specific histopathologic picture of MPA. However, the presence of pulmonary capillaritis, necrotizing pauci-immune glomerulonephritis, or leukocytoclastic vasculitis in skin can secure the diagnosis in the patient with the appropriate degree of pretest probability and the necessary exclusions. As noted, MPO-ANCA is present in 60 to 85 percent of patients, but occasionally, patients may be PR3-ANCA positive. Diagnosis of MPA based solely on a positive MPO-ANCA in a patient with low test probability is fraught with risk, considering the gravity of the therapy.

Differential Diagnosis

Differentiating MPA from classic polyarteritis is often based on the pattern of renal disease, which differs dramatically between the two. In classic polyarteritis, the glomerulus is largely spared and extraglomerular vascular disease (i.e., vascular nephropathy) is common. Pulmonary involvement is uncommon in classic disease, and hemorrhage is virtually never encountered. Hypertension and peripheral neuropathy are much more common in classic polyarteritis as well. From the laboratory perspective, classic polyarteritis is rarely PR3- or MPO-ANCA positive, and MPA is rarely associated with hepatitis B. Angiographically, classic polyarteritis nodosa is far more frequently associated with microaneursyms, which are rare in MPA.[141]

Differentiation from WG may at times be difficult because of the random nature of the granulomas in this condition. Prominent involvement of the upper respiratory tract or the presence of PR3-ANCA should seriously raise the possibility of WG because the occurrence of these findings are unusual, though not unheard of, in MPA.

TREATMENT

The treatment of MPA is based on the same therapeutic principles as those outlined for WG. The majority of information on therapy and prognosis of this disorder is based on retrospective analysis of case series.[134,135,142,143] Most investigators agree that in the presence of serious renal or pulmonary disease, combined therapy with high-dose GC and CTX is indicated. A recent study by the French Vasculitis Study Group,[144] representing the longest follow-up of a cohort including MPA (88.3 months), has reaffirmed that combined GC and CTX is beneficial, especially in severe disease. In this complex study representing a pooled analysis of four prospective trials of different therapeutic agents, there was an overall mortality of 30 percent throughout approximately 7 years of follow-up. Mortality, not surprisingly, was seen in those with a high incidence of renal, GI, cardiovascular, or CNS involvement. Survival rates were superior among the most severely ill patients treated with combination of GC and CTX versus those treated with GC alone. There are limited data supporting a role of apheresis in those with the most advanced renal disease, including those who are dialysis dependent.[145] Lastly there are also uncontrolled reports of successful therapy with IVIg.[146] Whatever therapy is employed, there is a significant risk of relapse in MPA, particularly when therapy is being tapered or after therapy is discontinued.[147] Careful follow-up, including serial monitoring of clinical symptoms and renal function with serial examination of the urinary sediment, is important for long-term management.

◾ Churg-Strauss Syndrome

The syndrome defined by Churg and Strauss in 1951 has undergone several redefinitions but still is ultimately characterized by three histopathologic features: necrotizing vasculitis, infiltration by eosiniphils, and extravascular granulomas.[148] Using only pathologic features to define the disease resulted in making the disorder a diagnostic rarity. In 1984, based on the limitations of defining the disease on strictly pathologic grounds, Lanham and colleagues[149] suggested that the diagnosis be based on clinical and pathologic grounds requiring three criteria: asthma, peak eosinopohil count of greater than 1500 cells/ml, and systemic vasculitis involving two or more organs.[149] In 1994, the International Consensus Conference held in Chapel Hill, North Carolina,[1] defined the disease as an eosinophil-rich and granulomatous inflammation involving the respiratory tract and necrotizing vasculitis involving the medium-sized vessels associated with asthma and eosinophilia. Each component of these definitions (i.e., histopathology, eosinophilia in blood and tissues, asthma) helps to define the disease, but none of these features individually is specific for CSS, and unfortunately, not all are present in every patient. Although most cases can be clearly defined, the concept of partial or incomplete CSS remains necessary.[150]

PATHOGENESIS

The etiology of CSS is unknown, but its association with allergy and atopic disorders is a dominant factor. Nearly 70 percent of patients have a history of allergic rhinitis, often associated with nasal polyposis, and the association with asthma, usually adult onset, is part of most case definitions. Both peripheral blood and tissue eosinophilia are major constituents of the syndrome, and the majority of patients tested have had elevated IgE levels.[149] As will be later discussed, a link between the use of the leukotriene type 1 receptor antagonist zafirulkast and a syndrome resembling CSS has further strengthened this association, but the epidemiologic link between this drug and vasculitis is not proven[151].

The sharing of many of the clinical and pathologic features with the other ANCA-associated small vessel syndromes is also of interest, suggesting a possible etiopathogenic role of ANCA in this syndrome. Unlike MPA and WG, however, the association of CSS with ANCA positivity is much less robust, with sensitivity data based on small numbers of patients tested.

Leukotriene Inhibitors and Churg-Strauss Syndrome

CSS has been reported to occur in asthmatics following use of either lipoxygenase inhibitors or cysteinyl leukotriene receptor type 1 antagonists, thereby raising the concern that leukotriene inhibition might function as an etiologic influence.[152-154] Alternative explanations include an unmasking effect when these drugs are provided to a population with severe airway disease and followed by steroid tapering. To date there are few data to suggest causality, but it is probably prudent to avoid these agents in patients with CSS until more definitive studies become available.

CLINICAL FEATURES

CSS has been viewed by some observers to be characterized by three distinct phases. A prodrome, dominated by allergic features, is common in patients ultimately diagnosed with CSS. Allergic rhinitis and asthma may often precede diagnosis of vasculitis by 3 to 7 years.[149,155] It is interesting and important to note that the asthma can abruptly abate as the patient moves into the vasculitic phase of the illness.

Tissue infiltration by eosinophils, in the form of eosinophilic pneumonia (Loeffler's syndrome) and eosino-philic gastroenteritis, may also occur in the prodrome. Because these patients may have marked constitutional symptoms and high blood eosinophilia, this stage may be difficult to distinguish from the onset of frank vasculitis on other than histologic grounds. The vascultic stage advances, and the clinical picture is dependent on the distribution of target organs. Finally the vasculitic stage abates and allergic disease then dominates the clinical picture. Clearly not all patients express a sequential staging of the illness and may present with only one or two manifestations as described.

Pulmonary Disease

Pulmonary infiltrates may occur in the prodromal phase, vasculitic phase, or both, and their appearance is generally nonspecific. Their radiographic appearance is variable, but lobar, interstitial, and nodular patterns have all been described, with most abnormalities being fleeting in nature. Pleural effusions were reported in 27 percent of patients in one series[149] and typically are rich in eosinophils. Pulmonary hemorrhage is a grave complication and may occur with or without renal involvement.

Nervous System Involvement

Peripheral neurologic involvement often dominates the clinical picture and has been reported in the majority of patients.[141,149,155] It was found in 62 percent of patients in one series.[149] The pattern of involvement may be that of mononeuritis multiplex or symmetric or asymmetric polyneuropathy. Less commonly, cranial neuropathy may be observed.[155] CNS involvement is uncommon and tends to dominate in the latter stages of the illness.[150] Collectively, involvement of the peripheral nervous system is so common that in any patient with asthma who develops neurologic symptoms, CSS should be considered.

Renal Disease

Kidney involvement is less common in CSS than MPA or WG and when present is rarely the cause of death. CSS shares the same renal lesion (i.e., necrotizing crescentic pauci-immune glomerulonephritis) with the other ANCA-associated diseases. A noteworthy feature of CSS is its propensity to involve the lower urinary tract, including the prostate gland.[156] We have seen extremely high levels of prostate-specific antigen in the setting of active CSS normalize during successful treatment. Such lower-tract involvement may at times lead to obstruction.

Other Organs

CSS may involve a wide variety of other target organs, including the skin, heart, skeletal muscle, joints, eye, and GI tract.[142,149] Skin involvement has often led to confusion, for the term *Churg-Strauss granuloma* may be seen in other disorders. Palpable purpura has been observed in nearly 50 percent of CSS patients, and the histopathology may be quite nonspecific. Alternatively, inflammatory nodules with characteristic histopathology (necrotizing vasculitis, eosinophilic infiltration, and extravascular granulomas) are less commonly encountered.[157]

GI involvement may precede the vasculitic phase or coincide with it. Diarrhea, pain, or bleeding are not uncommon. Similar to classic polyarteritis, abdominal complications may at times dominate.[158] Cardiac disease is common in postmortem series[148] and may contribute heavily to morbidity and mortality.[149] The cardiac pathology most frequently demonstrates granulomatous nodules in the epicardium, which may lead to ventricular dysfunction and congestive heart failure.[148] Coronary arteritis may also occur. Lastly, a variety of ocular complications have been described, including conjuctivitis, episcleritis, panuveitis, and marginal corneal ulcerations.[156]

PATHOLOGY

As noted previously, the pathologic features of CSS are necrotizing vasculitis, eosinophilic tissue infiltration, and extravascular granulomas (Fig. 83-11). Unfortunately, depending on the timing and tissue sampling, not all of these features may be present.[11] Necrotizing vasculitis of small vessels accompanied by tissue infiltration with eosinophils is not specific for CSS and also may be seen in WG and polyarteritis nodosa.[150] The extravascular Churg-Strauss granuloma, in its fully developed form, is highly specific for the condition. Its distinctive features include its eosinophilic core, which differenti-

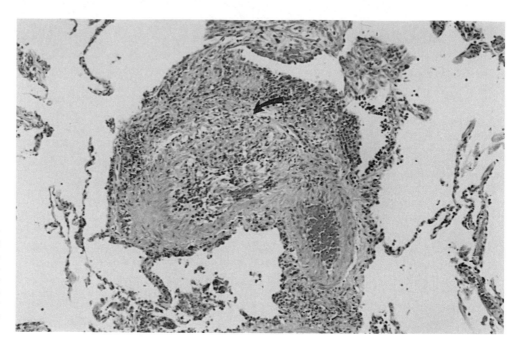

FIGURE 83–11 • Granulomatous inflammation and eosinophils destroying the wall *(arrow)* of a medium-sized muscular artery in a patient with Churg-Strauss syndrome (CSS). Numerous eosinophils are also present within the perivascular acute inflammatory infiltrate. (H & E, × 100)

ates it from the basophilic granuloma (unfortunately also referred to as a Churg-Strauss granuloma), but it is frequently seen in numerous other disorders.[150]

LABORATORY TESTS

Peripheral eosinophilia at levels in excess of 1500 cells/ml^3 often occurs in the prodromal stages of CSS, associated with rhinitis and asthma. Occasionally patients have been described without significant blood eosinophilia but with prominent tissue eosinophilia.[159] There is no definite correlation between eosinophilia and disease activity, for eosinophils often rapidly decrease on initiation of GC therapy.

ANCAs have been reported in as many as 70 percent of patients in some series, although the number of patients tested have been small. The majority of these are MPO-ANCA.[142] A negative ANCA should not dissuade the clinician from the diagnosis of CSS if there is a high pretest probability.

DIAGNOSIS AND DIFFERENTIAL DIAGNOSIS

The diagnosis of CSS should be based on the documentation of necrotizing vasculitis with eosinophils occurring in a patient with adult-onset asthma or allergic rhinitis. The documentation of the presence of extravascular granulomas is of added specificity, although it is not essential. High-yield sites for biopsy include nerve and muscle in patients with clinical evidence of their involvement.

Differentiation of CSS from WG, MPA, and classic polyarteritis nodosa is generally straightforward (Table 83-2). Significant peripheral eosinophilia is uncommon in the latter conditions, although this point is often poorly appreciated. This misconception stems from early reports of such patients derived from series reportedly describing WG but that are contaminated with yet-unrecognized CSS patients. Microaneurysms can be seen in both classic polyarteritis and CSS and, thus, do little to differentiate the conditions. Asthma is uncommon in polyarteritis, as is glomerulonephritis.

TABLE 83–2 • DIFFERENTIAL DIAGNOSTIC FEATURES OF THE ANTINEUTROPHIL CYTOPLASMIC ANTIBODY (ANCA) ASSOCIATED VASCULITIDES

	Wegener's Granulomatosis	Microscopic Polyangiitis	Polyarteritis Nodosa	Churg-Strauss Syndrome	Comments
Pulmonary infiltrates or nodules	+++	++	−	+++	Asthma and eosinophilia in CSS
Alveolar hemorrhage	++	++	−	+	
Glomerulonephritis	+++	+++	−	++	Progressive renal failure uncommon in CSS
Upper airway disease	+++	+	+	++	ENT disease usually favors WG
Skin/purpura	+	+++	−	++	
Peripheral nervous system	++	+	++	+++	Often a prominent feature of CSS
Central nervous system	+	+	+	++	

Abbreviations: CSS, Churg-Strauss syndrome; ENT, ear, nose, and throat; WG, Wegener's granulomatosis.

CSS may at times be difficult to differentiate from eosinophilic infiltrative diseases. Acute (Loeffler's syndrome) and chronic eosinophilic pneumonia are not associated with extrapulmonic disease. Hypereosinophilic syndrome may, however, be associated with eosinophilic infiltration of numerous target organs and may at times be difficult to differentiate from CSS. In this disorder, there is no true vasculitis, and eosinophil counts are often much higher, possibly in excess of 100,000 cells/mm³.

PROGNOSIS AND TREATMENT

The outcome of patients with CSS has been considered by some investigators to be similar to patients with polyarteritis nodosa, but several factors limit these observations. The largest series comparing such patient populations is, by its own admission, contaminated with patients with both the microscopic and classic forms of polyarteritis due the more recent recognition of the former.[160] Other investigators have asserted CSS is a more benign disease.[156,161,162] The work of Guillevin and colleagues has helped to clarify this debate and has demonstrated that, as with polyarteritis, the outcome of patients with CSS is dependent on severity of the disease, which can readily be clinically assessed.[163] Overall the 5-year survival rate for patients with CSS was 78.9 percent, but five factors were associated with poor outcome. These included azotemia (creatinine level greater than 1.58 mg/dl), proteinuria (higher than 1 g/day), GI tract involvement, cardiomyopathy, and CNS involvement. Relative risk of death increased in the presence of these risk factors. Absence of these complications, such as a patient with disease limited to muscle and nerve, carried the best prognosis.

Therapeutic trials have been limited but have demonstrated that both GC alone and GC combined with CTX are efficacious.[164,165] Based on these data and the prognostic studies of Guillevin and colleagues, it would appear reasonable to treat patients with limited disease with GC alone and reserve combined therapy for those with immediately life threatening or major-organ threatening disease. The principles of such therapy are similar to those discussed in the treatment of WG.

REFERENCES

1. Jennette CJ, Falk R: Small vessel vasculitis. New Eng J Med 337:1512, 1997.
2. Davies DJ, et al: Segmental necrotizing glomerulonephritis with antineutrophil antibody: possible arbovirus aetiology. Br Med J 285:606, 1982.
3. Hall JB, et al: Vasculitis and glomerulonephritis: a subgroup with an antineutrophil cytoplasmic antibody. Aust NZ J Med 14:277, 1984.
4. van der Woude FJ, et al: Autoantibodies against neutrophils and monocytes: tool for diagnosis and marker of disease activity in Wegener's granulomatosis. Lancet 1:425, 1985.
5. Hoffman GS, Specks U: Antineutrophil cytoplasmic antibodies [See comments]. Arthritis Rheum 41(9):1521-1537, 1998.
6. Ulmer M, Rautmann A, Gross WL: Immunodiagnostic aspects of autoantibodies against myeloperoxidase. Clin Nephrol 37(4):161, 1992.
7. Merkel A, et al: Prevalence of antineutrophil cytoplasmic antibodies in a large inception cohort of patients with connective tissue disease. Ann Intern Med 126(11):866-873, 1997.
8. Hagen EC, et al: Diagnostic value of standardized assays for antineutrophil cytoplasmic antibodies in idiopathic systemic vasculitis. EC/BCR Project for ANCA Assay Standardization [See comments]. Kidney Int 53(3):743-753, 1998.
9. Nölle B, et al: Anticytoplasmic autoantibodies: their immunodiagnostic value. Ann Intern Med 111:28, 1989.
10. Cohen Tervaert JW, et al: Association between active Wegener's granulomatosis and anticytoplasmic antibodies. Arch Intern Med 149:2461, 1989.
11. Niles JL, et al: Antigen-specific radioimmunoassays for antineutrophil cytoplasmic antibodies in the diagnosis of rapidly progressive glomerulonephritis. J Am Soc Nephrol 2(1):27-36, 1991.
12. Specks U: ANCA subsets: influence on disease specificity. Cleveland Clin J Med 69(Suppl ii):56-59, 2002.
13. Rother E, Schochat T, Peter HH: Antineutrophil cytoplasmic antibodies (ANCA) in rheumatoid arthritis: a prospective study. Rheumatol Int 15(6):231-237, 1996.
14. de Bandt M, et al: Antineutrophil cytoplasmic antibodies in rheumatoid arthritis patients. Br J Rheumatol 35(1):38-43, 1996.
15. Efthimiou J, Spickett G, Lane D: Antineutrophil cytoplasmic antibodies, cystic fibrosis, and infection. Lancet 337:1037, 1994.
16. Soto A, et al: Endocarditis associated with ANCA [See comments]. Clin Exper Rheumatol 12(2):203-204, 1994.
17. Abad E, et al: Relationship between ANCA and clinical activity in inflammatory bowel disease: variation in prevalence of ANCA and evidence of heterogeneity. J Autoimmun 10(2):175-180, 1997.
18. Freeman H, et al: Prospective evaluation of neutrophil autoantibodies in 500 consecutive patients with inflammatory bowel disease. Can J Gastroenterol 11(3):203-207, 1997.
19. Mulder AH, et al: Anti-neutrophil cytoplasmic antibodies (ANCA) in inflammatory bowel disease: characterization and clinical correlates. Clin Exper Immunol 95(3):490-497, 1994.
20. Targan SR, et al: High-titer antineutrophil cytoplasmic antibodies in type-1 autoimmune hepatitis [See comments]. Gastroenterology 108(4):1159-1166, 1995.
21. Gur H, et al: Autoantibody profile of primary sclerosing cholangitis. Pathobiology 63(2):76-82, 1995.
22. Jones BF, Major, G : Crescentic glomerulonephritis in a patient taking penicillamine associated with antineutrophil cytoplasmic antibody. Clin Nephrol 38:393, 1992.
23. Vogt BA, et al: Antineutrophil cytoplasmic autoantibody-positive crescentic glomerulonephritis as a complication of treatment with propylthiouracil in children. J Pediatr 124:986, 1994.
24. Short AK, Lockwood CM: Antigen specificity in hydralazine associated ANCA positive systemic vasculitis. QJM 88(11):775-783, 1995.
25. Choi HK, Merkel A, Niles JL: ANCA-positive vasculitis associated with allopurinol therapy. Clin Exper Rheumatol 16(6):743-744, 1998.
26. Elkayam O, Yaron M, Caspi D: Minocycline induced arthritis associated with fever, livedo reticularis, and pANCA. Ann Rheum Dis 55(10):769-771, 1996.
27. Hoffman GS: Classification of the systemic vasculitides: antineutrophil cytoplasmic antibodies, consensus and controversy. Clin Exper Rheumatol 16(2):111-115, 1998.
28. Hewins P, Tervaer JW, et al: Is Wegener's granulomatosis an autoimmune disease? Curr Opin Rheumatol 12(1):3-10, 2000.
29. Cid MC: New developments in the pathogenesis of systemic vasculitis. Curr Opin Rheumatol 8(1):1-11, 1996.
30. Csemok E, et al: Activated neutrophils express proteinase 3 on their plasma membrane in vitro and in vivo. Clin Exper Immunol 95:244, 1994.
31. Falk RJ, et al: Anti-neutrophil cytoplasmic autoantibodies induce neutrophils to degranulate and produce oxygen radicals in vitro. Proc Nat Acad Sci U S A 87(11):4115-4119, 1990.
32. Keogan MT, et al: Anti-neutrophil cytoplasm antibodies (ANCA) increase neutrophil adhesion to cultured human endothelium. Adv Exper Med Biol 336:115-119, 1993.
33. De Bandt M, et al: Antibodies to proteinase-3 mediate expression of intercellular adhesion molecule-1 (ICAM-1, CD 54). Br J Rheumatol 36(8):839-846, 1997.
34. Ralston DR, et al: Antineutrophil cytoplasmic antibodies induce monocyte IL-8 release: Role of surface proteinase-3, a1-antitrypsin, and Fcg receptors. J Clin Invest 100:1416, 1997.

35. Radford DJ, et al: Antineutrophil cytoplasmic antibodies stabilize adhesion and promote migration of flowing neutrophils on endothelial cells. Arthritis Rheum 44(12):2851-2861, 2001.

36. Griffin SV, et al: The inhibition of myeloperoxidase by ceruloplasmin can be reversed by anti-myeloperoxidase antibodies. Kidney Int 55(3):917-925, 1999.

37. Brouwer E, et al: Antimyeloperoxidase-associated proliferative glomerulonephritis: an animal model. J Exper Med 177:905, 1993.

38. Kobayashi K, Shibata T, Sugisaki T: Aggravation of rat nephrotoxic serum nephritis by anti-myeloperoxidase antibodies. Kidney Int 47(2):454-463, 1995.

39. Xiao H, et al: Antineutrophile cytoplasmic antibodies specific for myeloperoxidase cause glomerulonephritis and vasculitis in mice. J Clin Invest 110(7):955-963, 2002.

40. Jayne DR, et al: ANCA and predicting relapse in systemic vasculitis. QJM 88(2):127-133, 1995.

41. Tervaert JW, Stegeman CA, Kallenberg CG: Serial ANCA testing is useful in monitoring disease activity of patients with ANCA-associated vasculitides. Sarcoid Vascul Diff Lung Dis 13(3):241-245, 1996.

42. Charles LA, et al: Antibodies against granule proteins activate neutrophils in vitro. J Leukocyte Biol 50(6):539-546, 1991.

43. Ewert BH, et al: Antimyeloperoxidase antibodies induce neutrophil adherence to cultured human endothelial cells. Ren Fail 17:125, 1995.

44. Peen E, Sundqvist T, Skogh T: Leucocyte activation by anti-lactoferrin antibodies bound to vascular endothelium. Clin Exper Immunol 103(3):403-407, 1996.

45. Oseas R, et al: Lactoferrin: a promoter of olymorphonuclear leukocyte adhesiveness. Blood 57:939, 1981.

46. Davenport A, Lock RJ, Wallington T: Clinical significance of the serial measurement of autoantibodies to neutrophil cytoplasm using a standard indirect immunofluorescence test. Am J Nephrol 15(3):201-207, 1995.

47. Boomsma MM, et al: Prediction of relapses in Wegener's granulomatosis by measurement of antineutrophil cytoplasmic antibody levels: a prospective study. Arthritis Rheum 43(9):2025-2033, 2000.

48. Klinger H: Grenzformen der periarteritis nodosa. Frankfurt Z Pathol 42:455, 1931.

49. Wegener F: Über eine generalisierte, septische of gefäberkrankungen. Verh Dtsch Pathol Ges 29:202, 1936.

50. Wegener F: Über eine eigenartige rhinogene granulomatose mit besonderer beteilung des arterien systems und der nieren. Beitr Pathol Anat Allg Pathol 36:202-210, 1939.

51. Godman GC, Churg J: Wegener's granulomatosis: Pathology and review of the literature. Arch Pathol Lab Med 6:533, 1954.

52. Fauci AS, Wolff SM: Wegener's granulomatosis: Studies in eighteen patients and a review of the literature. Medicine 52:535, 1973.

53. Hoffman GS, et al: Wegener granulomatosis: An analysis of 158 patients [See comments]. Ann Intern Med 116(6):488-498, 1992.

54. Cotch MF, et al: The epidemiology of Wegener's granulomatosis: Estimates of the five-year period prevalence, annual mortality, and geographic disease distribution from population-based data sources. Arthritis Rheum 39(1):87-92, 1996.

55. Papiha SS, et al: Association of Wegener's granulomatosis with HLA antigens and other genetic markers. Ann Rheum Dis 51:246, 1992.

56. Spencer SJ, et al: HLA class II specificities in vasculitis with antibodies to neutrophil cytoplasmic antigens. Kidney Int 41(4):1059-1063, 1992.

57. Murty GE, et al: HLA antigen frequencies and Wegener's granulomatosis. Clin Otolaryngol 16:448, 1991.

58. Falk RJ, et al: Clinical course of anti-neutrophil cytoplasmic autoantibody-associated glomerulonephritis and systemic vasculitis: The Glomerular Disease Collaborative Network [See comments]. Ann Intern Med 113(9):656-663, 1990.

59. Hoffman GS, et al: Bronchoalveolar lavage analysis in Wegener's granulomatosis: A method to study disease pathogenesis. Am Rev Resp Dis 143(2):401-407, 1991.

60. Specks U, et al: Anticytoplasmic autoantibodies in the diagnosis and follow-up of Wegener granulomatosis. Mayo Clin Proc 64:28, 1989.

61. Baltaro RJ, et al: Immunoglobulin G antineutrophil cytoplasmic antibodies are produced in the respiratory tract of patients with Wegener's granulomatosis. Am Rev Resp Dis 143(2):275-278, 1991.

62. Csernok E, et al: Membrane surface proteinase 3 expression and intracytoplasmic immunoglobulin on neutrophils from patients with ANCA-associated vasculitides. Adv Exper Med Biol 336:45-50, 1993.

63. Mayet WJ, et al: Human endothelial cells express proteinase 3, the target antigen of anticytoplasmic antibodies in Wegener's granulomatosis. Blood 82(4):1221-1229, 1993.

64. Gephardt GN, Ahmad M, Tubbs RR: Pulmonary vasculitis (Wegener's granulomatosis): Immunohistochemical study of T and B cell markers. Am J Med 74:700, 1985.

65. Travis WD, et al: Surgical pathology of the lung in Wegener's granulomatosis: Review of 87 open lung biopsies from 67 patients. Am J Surg Pathol 15(4):315-333, 1991.

66. Schmitt WH, et al: Elevated serum levels of soluble interleukin-2 receptor in patients with Wegener's granulomatosis: Association with disease activity. Arthritis Rheum 35(9):1088-1096, 1992.

67. Stegeman CA, et al: Serum markers of T cell activation in relapses of Wegener's granulomatosis. Clin Exper Immunol 91(3):415-420, 1993.

68. Brouwer E, et al: T cell reactivity to proteinase 3 and myeloperoxidase in patients with Wegener's granulomatosis (WG). Clin Exper Immunol 98(3):448-453, 1994.

69. Fauci AS, et al: Wegener's granulomatosis: Prospective clinical and therapeutic experience with 85 patients for 21 years. Ann Intern Med 98:76, 1983.

70. Murty GE: Wegener's granulomatosis: Otorhinolaryngological manifestations. Clin Otolaryngol 15:385, 1990.

71. Walton EW: Giant-cell granuloma of the respiratory tract (Wegener's granulomatosis). Br Med J 2:265, 1958.

72. McCaffrey TV, et al: Otologic manifestations of Wegener's granulomatosis. Otolaryngol Head Neck Surg 88:586, 1980.

73. Lebovics RS, et al: The management of subglottic stenosis in patients with Wegener's granulomatosis. Laryngoscope 102(12 Pt 1):1341-1345, 1992.

74. Rottem M, et al: Wegener granulomatosis in children and adolescents: clinical presentation and outcome. J Ped 122(1):26-31, 1993.

75. Anderson G, et al: Wegener's granuloma. A series of 265 British cases seen between 1975 and 1985: A report by a sub-committee of the British Thoracic Society Research Committee. QJM 83:427, 1992.

76. Kuhlman JE, Hruban RH, Fishman EK: Wegener granulomatosis: CT features of parenchymal lung disease. J Comp Assist Tomog 15:948, 1991.

77. Cordier JF, et al: Pulmonary Wegener's granulomatosis: A clinical and imaging study of 77 cases. Chest 97:906, 1990.

78. Papiris SA, et al: Imaging of thoracic Wegener's granulomatosis: the computed tomographic appearance. Am J Med 93:529, 1992.

79. George TM, et al: Mediastinal mass and hilar adenopathy: Rare thoracic manifestations of Wegener's granulomatosis. Arthritis Rheum 40(11):1992-1997, 1997.

80. Duna GF, Galperin C, Hoffman GS: Wegener's granulomatosis. Rheum Dis Clin North Am 21(4):949-986, 1995.

81. Leavitt RY, Fauci AS: Pulmonary vasculitis. Am Rev Resp Dis 134:149-166, 1986.

82. Travis WD, Carpenter HA, Lie JT: Diffuse pulmonary hemorrhage: An uncommon manifestation of Wegener's granulomatosis. Am J Surg Pathol 11:702, 1987.

83. Rosenberg DM, et al: Functional correlates of lung involvement in Wegener's granulomatosis: Use of pulmonary function tests in staging and follow-up. Am J Med 69:387, 1980.

84. Carrington CB, Liebow AA: Limited forms of angiitis and granulomatosis of Wegener's type. Am J Med 41:497, 1966.

85. Cassan SM, Coles DT, Harrison EG: The concept of limited forms of Wegener's granulomatosis. Am J Med 49:366, 1970.

86. Horn RG, et al: Renal biopsy pathology in Wegener's granulomatosis. Am J Pathol 74:423, 1974.

87. Duncker G, et al: Orbital involvement in Wegener's granulomatosis. Adv Exper Med Biol 336:315, 1993.

88. Bullen CL, et al: Ocular complications of Wegener's granulomatosis. Ophthalmology 90:279, 1983.

89. Noritake DT, et al: Rheumatic manifestations of Wegener's granulomatosis. J Rheumatol 14:949, 1987.

90. Nishino H, et al: Neurological involvement in Wegener's granulomatosis: An analysis of 324 consecutive patients at the Mayo Clinic. Ann Neurol 33:4, 1993.

91. Stumvoll M, et al: Systemic vasculitis positive for circulating antineutrophil cytoplasmic antibodies and with predominantly neurological presentation. Clin Invest 71(8):613-615, 1993.

92. Weinberger LM, et al: Intracranial Wegener's granulomatosis. Neurology 43:1831, 1993.

93. Hoffman GS: Wegener's granulomatosis. Curr Opin Rheumatol 5(1):11-17, 1993.

94. Hoffman GS, Kerr GS: Gastrointestinal emergencies: vasculitis and the gut. In Tytgat GNJ, Van Blankenstein M (eds): Current Topics in Gastroenterology and Hepatology. Thieme Verlag, 1990, pp 36-54.

95. Lie JT: Vasculitis and the gut: Unwitting partners or strange bedfellows. J Rheumatol 18:647-648, 1991.

96. Hensle TW, et al: Urologic manifestations of Wegener granulomatosis. Urology 12:553, 1978.

97. Meryhew NL, Bache RJ, Messner R: Wegener's granulomatosis with acute pericardial tamponade. Arthritis Rheum 31:300, 1988.

98. Grant SCD, et al: Wegener's granulomatosis and the heart. Br Heart J 71:82, 1994.

99. Forstot JZ, et al: Cardiac complications of Wegener granulomatosis: A case report of complete heart block and review of the literature. Semin Arthritis Rheum 10:148, 1980.

100. Kerr GS, et al: Limited prognostic value of changes in antineutrophil cytoplasmic antibody titer in patients with Wegener's granulomatosis [See comments]. Arthritis Rheum 36(3):365-371, 1993.

101. Colby TV, et al: Nasal biopsy in Wegener's granulomatosis. Hum Pathol 22:101, 1991.

102. Delbuono EA, Flint A: Diagnostic usefulness of nasal biopsy in Wegener's granulomatosis. Hum Pathol 22:107, 1991.

103. Devaney KO, et al: Interpretation of head and neck biopsies in Wegener's granulomatosis: A pathologic study of 126 biopsies in 70 patients. Am J Surg Pathol 14:555, 1990.

104. Myers JI, Katzenstein ALA: Wegener's granulomatosis presenting with massive pulmonary hemorrhage and capillaritis. Am J Surg Pathol 11:895, 1987.

105. Yoshikawa Y, Watanabe T: Pulmonary lesions in Wegener's granulomatosis: A clinicopathologic study of 22 autopsy cases. Hum Pathol 17:401, 1986.

106. Travis WD, et al: A clinicopathologic study of 34 cases of diffuse pulmonary hemorrhage with lung biopsy confirmation. Am J Surg Pathol 14:1112, 1990.

107. Andrassy K, et al: Wegener's granulomatosis with renal involvement: patient survival and correlations between initial renal function, renal histology, therapy and renal outcome. Clin Nephrol 35:139, 1991.

108. Fauci AS: Alternate-day corticosteroid therapy. Am J Med 64:729, 1978.

109. Hollander D, Manning RT: The use of alkylating agents in the treatment of Wegener's granulomatosis. Ann Intern Med 67:393, 1967.

110. Haubitz M, et al: Cyclophosphamide pharmacokinetics and dose requirements in patients with renal insufficiency. Kidney Int 61:1495-1501, 2002.

111. Guillevin L, et al: A prospective, multicenter, randomized trial comparing steroids and pulse cyclophosphamide versus steroids and oral cyclophosphamide in the treatment of generalized Wegener's granulomatosis. Arthritis Rheum 40:2187, 1997.

112. Haubitz M, et al: Intravenous pulse administration of cyclophosphamide versus daily oral treatment in patients with antineutrophil cytoplasmic antibody-associated vasculitis and renal involvement: A prospective, randomized study [See comments]. Arthritis Rheum 41(10):1835-1844, 1998.

113. Richmond R, McMillan TW, Luqmani RA: Optimisation of cyclophosphamide therapy in systemic vasculitis. Clin Pharmacokinet 34(1):79-90, 1998.

114. Hoffman GS: Treatment of Wegener's granulomatosis: time to change the standard of care? [Letter, comment]. Arthritis Rheum 40(12):2099-2104, 1997.

115. Kamel OW, et al: Brief report: reversible lymphomas associated with Epstein-Barr virus occuring during methotrexate therapy for rheumatoid arthritis and dermatomyositis. New Engl J Med 328:1317, 1993.

116. Shiroky JB, et al: Complications of immunosupression associated with weekly low dose methotrexate. J Rheumatol 18:1172, 1991.

117. Sneller MC, et al: An analysis of forty-two Wegener's granulomatosis patients treated with methotrexate and prednisone. Arthritis Rheum 38(5):608-613, 1995.

118. Stegeman CA, et al: Association of chronic nasal carriage of Staphylococcus aureus and higher relapse rates in Wegener granulomatosis [See comments]. Ann Intern Med 120(1):12-17, 1994.

119. DeRemee RA: The treatment of Wegener's granulomatosis with trimethoprim/sulfamethoxazol: Illusion or vision? Arthritis Rheum 31:1068, 1988.

120. de Groot K, et al: Therapy for the maintenance of remission in sixty-five patients with generalized Wegener's granulomatosis: methotrexate versus trimethoprim/sulfamethoxazole. Arthritis Rheum 39:2052, 1996.

121. Ronda N, Hurez V, Kazatckine MD: Intravenous immunoglobulin therapy of autoimmune and systemic inflammatory diseases. Vox Sang 64:65, 1993.

122. Rossi F, et al: Anti-idiotypes against anti-neutrophil cytoplasmic antigen autoantibodies in normal human polyspecific IgG for therapeutic use and in the remission sera of patients with systemic vasculitis. Clin Exper Immunol 83(2):298-303, 1991.

123. Jayne DR, et al: Intravenous immunoglobulin for ANCA-associated systemic vasculitis with persistent disease activity. QJM 93(7):433-439, 2000.

124. Lamprecht Voswinkel J. Lilentaal T. et al: Effectiveness of TNF alpha blockade with infliximab in refractory Wegener's granulomatosis. Rheumatology 41:1303-1307, 2002.

125. Batolucci P., Ramanoelinaj Conen P. et al: Efficacy of anti-TNF antibody infliximab against refractory systemic vasculitides: an open pilot study in 10 patients. Rheumatology 41:1126-1132, 2002.

126. Stone JH, et al: Etanercept combined with conventional treatment in Wegener's granulomatosis: a six-month open-label trial to evaluate safety. Arthritis Rheum 44(5):1149-1154, 2001.

127. Jayne D: Conventional treatment of Wegener's granulomatosis and microscopic polyangiitis. Cleveland Clin J Med 69(suppl II):110-115, 2002.

128. Regan M, Hellmann DB, Stone J: Treatment of Wegener's granulomatosis. Rheum Dis Clin North Am 27:863-886, 2001.

129. Langford CA, et al: A staged approach to the treatment of Wegener's granulomatosis. Arthritis Rheum 42:2666-2673, 1999.

130. Steinman TI, et al: Recurrence of Wegener's granulomatosis after kidney transplantation: Sucessful re-induction of remission with cyclophosphamide. Am J Med 68:458, 1980.

131. Fauci AS, et al: Successful renal transplantation in Wegener's granulomatosis. Am J Med 60:437, 1976.

132. Davson J, Ball J, Platt R: The kidney in periarteritis nodosa. QJM 17:175, 1948.

133. D'Agati V, et al: Idiopathic microscopic polyarteritis nodosa: ultrastructural observations on the renal vascular and glomerular lesions. Am J Kidney Dis 7:95, 1986.

134. Savage COS, et al: Microscopic polyarteritis: Presentation, pathology and prognosis. QJM 56:467, 1985.

135. Adu D, et al: Polyarteritis and the kidney. QJM 62:221, 1987.

136. Serra A, et al: Vasculitis affecting the kidney: presentation, histopathology and long-term outcome. QJM 53:181, 1984.

137. Lhote F, Cohen P, Guillevin L: Polyarteritis nodosa, microscopic polyangiitis and Churg-Strauss syndrome. Lupus 7(4):238-258, 1998.

138. Rosen S, Falk RJ, Jennette JC: Polyarteritis nodosa including microscopic form and renal vasculitis. In Churg A, Churg J (eds): Systemic Vasculitides. New York, Igahu-Shoin, 1991, p 57.

139. Schwarz MI: The nongranulomatous vasculitides of the lung. Semin Resp Crit Care Med 19:47, 1998.

140. Jennings CA, King TE, *** TR Jr: Diffuse alveolar hemorrhage with underlying isolated pauci-immune pulmonary capillaritis. Am J Resp Crit Care Med 155:1101, 1997.

141. Guillevin L, et al: Antineutrophil cytoplasmic antibodies, abnormal angiograms and pathological findings in polyarteritis nodosa and Churg-Strauss syndrome: Indications for the classification of vasculitides of the polyarteritis nodosa grou. Br J Rheumatol 35(10):958-964, 1996.

142. Lhote F, Guillevin L: Treatment of polyarteritis nodosa and microscopic polyangiitis. Annales de Medecine Interne 145(8):550-565, 1994.

143. Rodgers H, et al: Microscopic polyarteritis: clinical features and treatment. Postgrad Med J 65:515, 1989.

144. Gayraud M, et al: Long-term followup of polyarteritis nodosa, microscopic polyangiitis, and Churg-Strauss syndrome: analysis of four prospective trials including 278 patients [See comments]. Arthritis Rheum 44(3):666-675, 2001.

145. Pusey CD, et al: Plasma exchange in focal necrotizing glomerulonephritis without anti-GBM antibodies. Kidney Int 40:757, 1991.

146. Jayne DRW: Intravenous immunoglobulins in the therapy of systemic vasculitis. Transfusion Sci 13:317, 1992.

147. Gordon M, et al: Relapses in patients with a systemic vasculitis. QJM 86:779, 1993.

148. Churg J, Strauss L: Allergic granulomatosis, allergic angiitis and periarteritis nodosa. Am J Pathol 27:277, 1951.

149. Lanham JG, et al: Systemic vasculitis with asthma and eosinophilia: A clinical approach to the Churg Strauss syndrome. Medicine 63:65, 1984.

150. Lanham JG, Churg J: Churg Strauss syndrome. In Churg A, Churg J (eds): Systemic Vasculitides. New York, Ikagu Shoin, 1991, p 101.

151. Wechsler ME, et al: Pulmonary infiltrates, eosinophilia and cardiomyopathy following corticosteroid withdrawal in patient with asthma receiving Zafirlukast. JAMA 279:455, 1998.

152. Gross WL: Churg-Strauss syndrome: update on recent developments. Curr Opin Rheumatol 14(1):11-14, 2002.

153. Bielory L, et al: Asthma and vasculitis: controversial association with leukotriene antagonists. Ann Allergy Asthma Immunol 87(4):274-282, 2001.

154. Jamaleddine G, et al: Leukotriene antagonists and the Churg-Strauss syndrome [See comments]. Semin Arthritis Rheum 31(4):218-227, 2002.

155. Sehgal M, et al: Neurologic manifestations of Churg-Strauss syndrome. Mayo Clin Proc 70:337, 1995.

156. Chumbley LC, Harrison EG, DeRemee RA: Allergic granulomatosis and angiitis (Churg-Strauss syndrome). Mayo Clin Proc 52:477, 1977.

157. Crotty C, DeRemee RA, Winkelmann RK: Cutaneous clinicopathologic correlation of allergic granulomatosis. J Am Acad Dermatol 5:571, 1981.

158. Modigliani R, et al: Allergic granulomatous vasculitis (Churg-Strauss syndrome): Report of a case with widespread digestive involvement. Digest Dis Sci 26:164, 1981.

159. Shields CL, Shields JA, Rozanski TI: Conjunctival involvement in Churg-Strauss syndrome. Am J Ophthalmol 102:601, 1986.

160. Guillevin L, et al: Clinical findings and prognosis of polyarteritis nodosa and Churg-Strauss angiitis: A study in 165 patients. Br J Rheumatol 27:258, 1988.

161. Cohen R, Conn D, Ilstrup D: Clinical features, prognosis and response to treatment in polyarteritis. Mayo Clin Proc 55:146, 1980.

162. Finan MC, Winkelmann RK: The cutaneous extravascular necrotizing granuloma (Churg-Strauss granuloma) and systemic disease: a review of 27 cases. Medicine 62:142, 1983.

163. Guillevin L, et al: Prognostic factors in polyarteritis nodosa and Churg-Strauss syndrome: A prospective study of 342 patients. Medicine 75:17, 1996.

164. Guillevin L, et al: Longterm followup after treatment of polyarteritis nodosa and Churg-Strauss angiitis with comparison of steroids, plasma exchange and cytophosphamide to steroids and plasma exchange: A prospective randomized trial of 71 patients. J Rheumatol 18:567, 1991.

165. Guillevin L, et al: Lack of superiority of steroids plus plasma exchange to steroids alone in the treatment of polyarteritis nodosa and Churg-Strauss syndrome: A prospective, randomized trial in 78 patients. Arthritis Rheum 35:208, 1992.

84

Polyarteritis and Related Disorders

JOHN S. SERGENT

■ Polyarteritis Nodosa

Polyarteritis nodosa (PAN) is a necrotizing vasculitis of medium-sized arteries. Immune deposits are minimal or absent, and test results for antineutrophil cytoplasmic antibodies (ANCAs) are typically negative.

PAN has undergone an impressive change in its definition. For many years, it was used in a generic sense to include most cases of generalized vasculitis, but as our understanding improved, the definitions became tighter. Thus, what was formerly "PAN complicating rheumatoid arthritis" is now called rheumatoid vasculitis, and most cases of "polyarteritis nodosa with lung involvement" are now called Churg-Strauss syndrome (CSS).

However, the most important shift in our thinking came about with the finding that patients with microscopic PAN have ANCAs directed against myeloperoxidase (MPO). This disease is much more common than classic PAN of medium-sized arteries (see Chapter 83), and as a result of the separation of the two, PAN, as currently defined, is a rare disease. In my experience, it accounts for less than 5 percent of all cases of systemic vasculitis and is several-fold less common than Wegener's granulomatosis (WG), although the actual incidence is unknown.

Patients with classic PAN can be any age, including children, but the peak onset is in the fifth or sixth decade. There is approximately a 2:1 male-to-female preponderance in most studies.[1] Although there are reports of polyarteritis that follows infections,[3-7] vaccination,[8,9] serous otitis media,[10] and the use of various drugs, especially amphetamines,[11] no etiology is apparent in most cases. In fact, it is possible that some of the associations mentioned could be random events or that PAN was already present before the exposure.

Onset may be abrupt and catastrophic, but the typical patient has a period of weeks or months of systemic symptoms including fever, abdominal pain, weight loss, and arthralgias. During this period the diagnosis is usually not apparent, and individuals are often treated for presumed diagnoses ranging from infections to systemic juvenile rheumatoid arthritis (RA).[12] In this setting, sudden events may occur, such as intestinal ischemia, digital gangrene, ischemic skin ulcers, infarction of a kidney or other major organ, or sudden loss of multiple nerves (mononeuritis multiplex). Table 84-1 shows the estimated frequency of various findings in PAN. Virtually all are due to ischemia of the area involved.

TABLE 84–1 · SELECTED CLINICAL MANIFESTATIONS OF POLYARTERITIS NODOSA (PAN)

Clinical Feature	Frequency (%)
Muscle pain or weakness	69
Weight loss	67
Mononeuritis multiplex	42
Polyneuropathy	36
Azotemia	40
Hypertension	37
Testicular pain	29
Skin ulcers or infarcts	27
Livedo reticularis	25

From Lightfoot RW, Michel BA, Bloch DA, et al: The American College of Rheumatology 1990 criteria for the classification of polyarteritis nodosa. Arthritis Rheum 33:1088, 1990.

PATHOLOGY

PAN is a patchy disease, with areas of impressive necrosis and inflammation interspersed with unaffected vessels[13,14] (Fig. 84-1). There is a propensity for aneurysm formation, especially in the mesenteric circulation. Other target organs include the kidney, the peripheral nerves, and the heart. There is strong correlation between the amount of fibrinoid necrosis and the number of neutrophils in the vessel wall and surrounding tissues.[15]

Because of this irregular distribution, obtaining a diagnostic biopsy can be difficult. If purpura is present, a skin biopsy may be diagnostic, although a generous sample may be required. Punch biopsy may show only hemorrhage and nonspecific inflammation. In people with few or no localizing findings but in whom PAN is highly suspected, "blind" muscle biopsy is often performed, although about half the patients later shown to have PAN will have a negative biopsy finding.

Mesenteric arteriography showing widespread aneurysms[16] is a most impressive diagnostic finding (Fig. 84-2). It is probably the procedure of choice in patients with significant abdominal pain.

Probably the most popular biopsy site today is the sural nerve.[17] In patients with neuropathy, especially if sural nerve conduction is abnormal, the biopsy finding is positive more than 80 percent of the time. Other areas in which biopsy is occasionally performed include the testicle, especially if it is painful or if a mass is palpable, and the kidney.

Laboratory findings in PAN are nonspecific. Anemia and leukocytosis are typical, and almost all patients

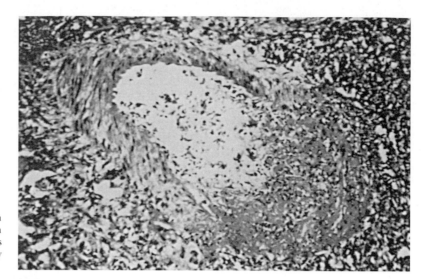

FIGURE 84–1 • Polyarteritis. Right lower portion of arterial wall shows fibrinoid necrosis and formation of "microaneurysm." Intense infiltration of leukocytes is present in and about artery wall. (H&E, × 40) (Courtesy of Dr. J.T. Lie.)

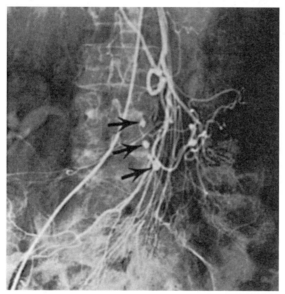

FIGURE 84–2 • Superior Mesenteric Arteriogram in Patient with Polyarteritis. Several small aneurysms *(arrows)* are present in branches of superior mesenteric artery. (Courtesy of Dr. A.W. Stanson.)

have an elevated erythrocyte sedimentation (ESR) rate. Evidence of mild liver dysfunction, such as an elevated alkaline phosphatase, may be seen. There are no specific serologic findings, and ANCAs are absent, almost by definition (see Chapter 83).

SYSTEMS INVOLVED IN POLYARTERITIS NODOSA[18]

Cutaneous manifestations occur in up to one third of patients, usually seen as areas of palpable purpura, sometimes with ulceration (Fig. 84-3). Frequent sites include the fingers, the ankles around the malleoli, and the pretibial areas. In severe cases, there may be widespread digital cyanosis secondary to ischemia. Splinter hemorrhages and livedo reticularis (Fig. 84-4) are also commonly observed.

Hypertension, due to arteritis in the renal circulation, is present in approximately one third of the cases and is occasionally severe. New-onset hypertension in a patient with systemic symptoms such as fever, weight

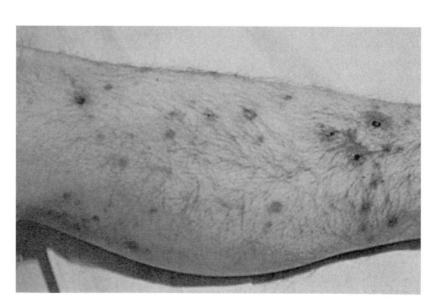

FIGURE 84–3 • Polyarteritis Involving Skin. Sharply circumscribed skin infarcts are 1 to 1.5 cm in diameter and are in various stages of healing.

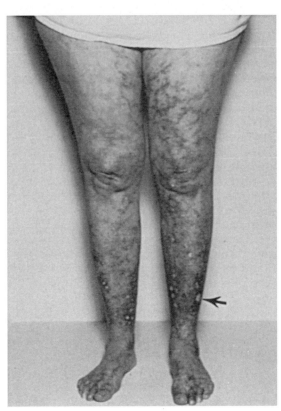

FIGURE 84-4 · Polyarteritis Involving Skin of Legs. Livedo reticularis is most prominent over left anterior region of thigh but is also visible over right thigh, legs below knees, and dorsa of feet. Petechiae and ulcers *(arrow)* are present on anterior and medial portions of lower legs.

loss, and joint pain should be a clue that vasculitis, specifically PAN, may be present.

Mononeuritis multiplex is a term applied to the widespread development of neuropathy involving large, mixed motor and sensory nerves. The loss of each involved nerve may be a sudden event, although many patients describe paresthesias or weakness of the involved area before the total loss of nerve function. Frequently affected nerves include the peroneal, median, ulnar, and sural nerves.[19] The nerve injury is due to ischemia and eventual infarction. The nerve injuries may progress in an asymmetric manner during days to weeks and, thus, are a major cause of long-term morbidity. Less often, a slowly progressive sensory neuropathy in a stocking-glove distribution develops.

Abdominal pain, due to mesenteric vasculitis, is usually dull and constant, but it is often made worse by eating. Some patients exhibit classic findings of mesenteric ischemia, including food avoidance and rapid weight loss. Mesenteric infarction and bowel perforation are infrequent but catastrophic manifestations.

The liver is frequently involved at autopsy, but clinical involvement is uncommon. Occasional patients present with appendiceal or biliary tract involvement, usually cholecystitis,[20] and there are reports of spontaneous splenic rupture as a complication of rupture of vasculitic aneurysms.

The testicle is also a frequent site of involvement in autopsy series, and testicular pain is occasionally seen.

In addition, there are a few patients whose diagnosis was made from prostatic tissue after presentation with symptoms of prostatic hypertrophy or prostatitis.

Kidney involvement is usually manifest only as hypertension, often with mild to moderate azotemia. There is no glomerulitis, and the urinalysis usually shows only moderate proteinuria with modest hematuria, or the sediment may be entirely normal. However, occasional patients have sudden severe flank pain due to renal infarction or spontaneous rupture of intrarenal aneurysms, a life-threatening event.[21]

The musculoskeletal symptoms of PAN are typically nonspecific, with widespread arthralgias and myalgias. Joint pain is occasionally severe and debilitating, although signs of frank arthritis are uncommon.

COURSE

Without treatment, PAN is probably nearly universally fatal, although because of changing definitions, new serologic tests, and the universal treatment of patients in this era, the true natural history is not known. It is highly probable, however, that the majority of patients would die within 1 to 2 years if left untreated.

THERAPY

Whereas occasional patients seem to have limited disease that remains stable with minimal therapy, the risk of major organ involvement necessitates aggressive therapy in nearly all patients once the diagnosis is made. Treatment consists of prednisone, 1 mg/kg/day in divided doses, and, in most cases, an additional agent, usually a cytotoxic drug.

The prednisone dose should be maintained until the patient is clinically stable with no evidence of ongoing active disease. The precise method of steroid reduction is a matter open to individual variation and interpretation, but it is my preference to follow the regimen outlined in Table 84-2.

Although there is no unanimity of opinion, virtually all rheumatologists would add a second drug to corticosteroids if major organs are threatened or if the prednisone dose required to suppress disease activity is regarded as unacceptably high. Guillevin and coworkers[21] have described five prognostic factors that predict a high probability of mortality and, therefore, are considered

---

TABLE 84-2 · PREDNISONE THERAPY IN POLYARTERITIS NODOSA (PAN)

Disease control (4-8 weeks)	Prednisone 1 mg/kg/day in divided doses
Consolidation (1 month)	Gradually change to a single daily dose at 1 mg/kg/day
Rapid tapering (1-2 months)	Decrease by 5-10 mg every 2-4 weeks, observing closely, until dose is 15-20 mg/day
Slow tapering (1-2 months)	Decrease dose in increments of 1-25 mg/day at intervals of 1-2 weeks, continuing close observation

indications for another immunosuppressive drug in addition to prednisone. The factors are proteinuria greater than 1 g/day, azotemia, cardiomyopathy, gastrointestinal (GI) involvement, and central nervous system (CNS) disease. With none of these factors, 5-year mortality is 12 percent. With two or more, 46 percent of patients were dead at 5 years.

Cyclophosphamide has been the drug of choice of Fauci and coworkers[22] at the National Institutes of Health (NIH), and many physicians regard the diagnosis of PAN as an indication for cyclophosphamide therapy. Alternatives to cyclophosphamide are chlorambucil, azathioprine, methotrexate, dapsone, cyclosporine, plasma exchange, and others.[24,25]

Alkylating agents work quickly and are regarded as the agent of choice for seriously ill patients. Cyclophosphamide is used most commonly, although chlorambucil may be equally effective. Both have oncogenic potential; cyclophosphamide has a disproportionate increase in bladder cancer, whereas chlorambucil has a higher incidence of secondary leukemia (see Chapter 60).

If cyclophosphamide is chosen, the usual dose is 2 mg/kg, although doses of up to 4 mg/kg are sometimes used for short periods. Once such an agent is instituted, most rheumatologists maintain their patients with the alkylating agent for 1 to 2 years. An alternative is intermittent intravenous (IV) cyclophosphamide, usually given in doses of 10 to 15 mg/kg monthly, which is less toxic and may be equally effective.[26]

The use of high-dose IV methylprednisolone, in doses up to 1 g/day, is occasionally recommended in cases of fulminant vasculitis.[27] Table 84-3 compares some of the agents that have been used in PAN.

PROGNOSIS

In a rare disease whose definition has undergone considerable changes and whose treatment is not standard, it is difficult to be confident about the prognosis. However, with a combination of prednisone and an alkylating agent, it appears that approximately 80 percent of PAN patients will survive, with the majority of those entering a long-term remission.[28] In classic PAN, the usual approach is to maintain prednisone at

1 mg/kg for 1 to 2 months, then slowly taper over 4 to 6 months. Some favor converting patients to an alternate-day steroid regimen; others maintain daily steroids during the period of dose reduction.

These critical first 6 months of therapy require careful monitoring, both for toxicity of the drugs and for evidence of disease relapse. Most rheumatologists follow blood counts, urinalyses, serum chemistries, and the ESR on at least monthly intervals.

At the end of 6 months or so, the goal is to have the patient in remission (no active disease) and taking little or no steroids. Patients are generally maintained with cyclophosphamide for a full year, and then it is tapered and withdrawn over 3 to 6 months.

■ Cutaneous Polyarteritis Nodosa

Cutaneous (or limited) PAN is a term applied to a small group of patients who have cutaneous manifestations of the disease, with characteristic histopathologic features but no systemic features.[29] Thus, by definition, they have no fever, weight loss, or evidence of disease in any internal organs. Cases have been associated with streptococcal infection,[30] minocycline,[31] and hepatitis C,[32] but the etiology is unknown in most. The disease affects people of all ages, including children, but the peak age at onset seems to be in the thirties.

PATHOLOGY

The lesions, on biopsy, show necrotizing vasculitis with transmural inflammation of small- and medium-sized arteries.[33] As is true of systemic polyarteritis, the definition of cutaneous PAN has also changed during the years, so that many examples in the literature would be classified today as hypersensitivity angiitis, microscopic PAN, or other entities.

CLINICAL FEATURES

The typical patient develops crops of tender subcutaneous nodules over the lower legs, often with scattered lesions elsewhere. Larger nodules may become necrotic,

■ TABLE 84-3 • TREATMENT OF POLYARTERITIS NODOSA (PAN)

Drug	Dose	Comment
Oral prednisone	1 mg/kg/day	Mainstay of therapy
Methylprednisolone	1 g/day for 3-5 days	Used in fulminant disease
Cyclophosphamide	2-4 mg/kg/day PO	Used with major organ involvement or inability to withdraw steroids
Cyclophosphamide	10-15 mg/kg/mo IV	Alternative to oral therapy, less toxic
Chlorambucil	0.1 mg/kg/day	Alternative to cyclophosphamide
Azathioprine	2-4 mg/kg/day	Less toxic and possibly less effective than cyclophosphamide
Methotrexate	15-25 mg PO q wk	Less effective, but often used after 1-2 years of therapy with more potent agents
Plasmapheresis		No proven benefit
Intravenous immune globulin (IVIg)		Proven benefit in vasculitis due to parvovirus B19; may benefit others
Monoclonal antibody		Limited experience
Interferon alfa		Used in vasculitis secondary to hepatitis B
Immunoadsorption[27]		Investigational

and painful ulcers develop about 50 percent of the time.[34] In addition to the lower legs, lesions occur on the arms, buttocks, trunk, and occasionally the head and neck. The lesions usually occur in crops, appearing within a few days of each other. Untreated, they persist 1 to 6 months; occasional lesions persist for years. Livedo reticularis is common, and most patients complain of some joint pain, especially in joints adjacent to the lesions. No synovitis is present, however, and there are no other associated physical findings.

DIAGNOSIS

The results of laboratory studies are typically normal, other than mild elevation of the ESR and occasionally mild leukocytosis. There are a few reports of positive test results for ANCAs, although there are no studies to date to determine whether the presence of these antibodies describes a different set of patients who may, in time, evolve into microscopic PAN.

TREATMENT AND COURSE

The acute lesions usually respond to corticosteroids, although moderate to high doses may be required. For that reason, combined with the tendency of the disease to relapse and remit for many years, a variety of other agents have been used, with variable success. These include anti-inflammatory drugs, sulfapyridine, methotrexate,[35] dapsone,[36] IV immune globulin,[37] tamoxifen,[38] and thalidomide.[39]

The prognosis is generally good, although the painful cutaneous ulcers can be disabling at times. However, most patients have recurrent disease for many years,[40] and frustration with the disease and with the treatment regimen is high. Rarely, patients with cutaneous PAN develop features of systemic PAN, even after many years.[41]

Cogan's Syndrome

This rare disease, consisting of interstitial keratitis, audiovestibular symptoms, and, in most cases, systemic manifestations, has been reported in several hundred patients since Cogan's description of four cases in 1945.[42] Cogan's syndrome is a disease of young people, for the most part, with a median age at onset of 25 years in one large study.[43]

CLINICAL FEATURES

The initial manifestations are usually ocular or audiovestibular, with more than 75 percent of patients developing both eye and ear complications within 4 months of each other. In classic Cogan's syndrome, with interstitial keratitis as the ocular manifestation, systemic vasculitis occurs rarely; other systemic manifestations, especially aortitis with aneurysm formation or aortic insufficiency, occur in about 10 percent of patients.[44]

Atypical Cogan's syndrome, in which the ocular manifestation is something other than interstitial keratitis, has a higher frequency of aortic and other systemic manifestations and a correspondingly worse prognosis.[43] Atypical manifestations of eye disease in Cogan's syndrome include episcleritis, scleritis, iritis, uveitis, and chorioretinitis. Rare cases of optic neuritis are also reported.

The eye symptoms usually begin with photophobia, redness, and local irritation. The audiovestibular symptoms are abrupt in onset with partial or total hearing loss, vertigo, and ataxia. The vestibular symptoms usually improve with time, but the hearing loss rarely returns to normal.

About half the patients have constitutional features, including weight loss, fever, lymphadenopathy, hepatosplenomegaly, and rash. Aortitis, causing both aneurysms and aortic insufficiency, is the most serious manifestation of Cogan's syndrome and accounts for the majority of the deaths. The aortic manifestations may follow the ophthalmic and audiovestibular features by months to several years. Rarely, patients develop widespread vasculitis including purpura and skin necrosis.[45]

PATHOLOGY

The aortic and other vascular lesions are characterized by a mixture of acute and chronic inflammation, often most prominent in the region of the internal elastic lamina. Granulomas containing giant cells have been reported, but many lesions contain a mixture of neutrophils, eosinophils, mononuclear cells, and fibrosis.

DIAGNOSIS

The diagnosis of Cogan's syndrome is entirely clinical because there are no definitive serologic or histologic markers. As would be expected, most patients have leukocytosis, anemia, thrombocytosis, and an elevated ESR during active phases of their disease. Patients with aortitis show aortic root dilatation and aortic insufficiency on aortography. Cases have been reported with anti–endothelial cell antibodies[46] and anti-MPO antibodies.[47] The significance of these, if any, is unknown.

TREATMENT AND COURSE

No prospective studies of treatment regimens have been carried out in this rare disease. The interstitial keratitis usually responds to topical corticosteroids. It is common practice to treat acute audiovestibular symptoms with high doses of corticosteroids. In general, patients respond quickly or not at all, so that after 2 to 4 weeks, the clinician can determine whether chronic therapy is indicated. High-dose corticosteroids along with cytotoxic drugs,[44] methotrexate,[48] and cyclosporine[49] have been used to treat the vasculitis.

The course is variable. Some patients have a single episode and are free of active disease thereafter. The more typical course, however, is one of waxing and waning symptoms for a period of months to years. Virtually all patients sustain some permanent hearing loss, and nearly half are left totally deaf. Aortic valve replacement and surgical repair of aortic aneurysms may be required.

Buerger's Disease

Buerger's disease, also known as thromboangiitis obliterans, is an inflammatory vaso-occlusive disease that primarily affects the lower extremities in young adult male cigarette smokers, although women and older adults are also affected. The average age at onset is 35 years. More recent reports have emphasized a higher percentage of female patients, older age at onset, and perhaps a declining overall incidence.[50]

The role of tobacco, especially cigarette smoking, is clear, but the pathogenesis remains unknown. No consistent human leukocyte antigen (HLA) association has been demonstrated.[51] Antibodies against collagen, elastin, and laminin have been reported in some patients.[52,53] One study demonstrated high levels of anti–endothelial cell antibodies in patients with active disease but not in those in remission.[54] ANCAs directed against MPO, lactoferrin, and elastase have also been associated with severe disease.[55]

PATHOLOGY

In most cases, Buerger's disease is limited to small arteries and veins in the distal extremities. However, there are numerous reports of visceral involvement, including mesenteric, coronary, and pulmonary arteries. Active lesions show a segmental inflammatory response with transmural infiltration of polymorphonuclear leukocytes and lymphocytes and preservation of the internal elastic membrane.[56] Thrombosis is prominent, and microabscesses are seen in the vessel wall and surrounding tissue. The infiltrating cells are enriched in cell determinant (CD) 3T cells, and CD68 macrophages and S-100 dendritic cells have been reported to be increased during disease activity.[57]

CLINICAL FEATURES

Buerger's disease typically begins with bilateral pain and ischemia in both lower extremities, although the upper extremities may be the site of initial symptoms. At onset, the symptoms may be mild, such as paresthesias or pain only with exposure to cold. However, most cases rapidly evolve into a painful condition with digital cyanosis, splinter hemorrhages, vesicles, and severe claudication. Digital ulcers often occur, especially after relatively minor trauma.[58] The disease typically begins distally, with symptoms worse in the tips of the fingers and toes, but it tends to progress to larger, more proximal vessels during a period of several years. Proximal leg claudication is uncommon, however. Superficial phlebitis occurs in about one third of patients and may be the first symptom. Elevated plasma homocysteine levels have been associated with poor prognosis.[59]

DIAGNOSIS

Characteristic angiographic changes include multiple bilateral areas of narrowing or occlusion in the digital, palmar, plantar, ulnar, radial, tibial, and peroneal arteries. Small collateral vessels around the occlusion often take on a corkscrew appearance. More proximal lesions resemble atherosclerotic occlusion. Whereas these findings are typical, they are not pathognomonic; in the absence of pathologic confirmation, the disease must be differentiated from premature atherosclerosis, hyperviscosity syndrome, scleroderma, and other rheumatic diseases; Takayasu's arteritis; embolic disease including cholesterol emboli and atrial myxomas; ergot toxicity; and thoracic outlet syndrome.

TREATMENT AND COURSE

Treatment consists of abstinence from all forms of tobacco. In severely addicted individuals unable to stop smoking, nicotine substitutes may be employed,[60] it is hoped for only a brief period.

Affected limbs must be protected from trauma and cold. Ulcers and cellulitis often require antibiotics and careful debridément. Calcium channel blockers and pentoxifylline have reportedly been beneficial in some patients, as has intra-arterial streptokinase.[61] However, most patients show little or no response to any of these measures. Sympathectomy likewise seems to provide little or no long-term benefit and is not usually recommended. Therapy using the transfer of the gene for vascular endothelial growth factor is under investigation.[62]

In individuals with Buerger's disease who continue to smoke, about half will come to amputation, often multiple times as more proximal vessels are involved. If smoking is stopped, most will stabilize, with amputation required in a minority. However, the ischemic limb may be a source of pain and ulceration for many years. Although most patients are men, the course in affected women is no different from that in men.[63]

Vasculitis due to Viral Infections

The vasculitis due to human immunodeficiency virus (HIV) infection is covered in Chapter 101. Many other viruses have been reported to be associated with vasculitis, but the cases are so infrequent as to render the diagnosis in doubt. However, two viruses, hepatitis B and parvovirus B19, clearly have an association with vasculitis.

HEPATITIS B VASCULITIS

This entity, described simultaneously in 1970 by investigators in the United States and in France,[2,3] is seen in individuals with chronic hepatitis B antigenemia, most of whom have active liver disease. The manifestations vary considerably, from diffuse small-vessel vasculitis predominantly in the skin to larger vessel lesions typical of PAN.[64] Thus, clinical symptoms may include the entire spectrum of vasculitic manifestations from purpura and other rashes to abdominal pain, hypertension, renal disease, and stroke. Patients with cryoglobulinemia almost always have concomitant hepatitis C infection (see Chapter 81).

Treatment of these patients with immunosuppressive drugs has been only moderately successful; many die of either their vasculitis or their liver disease. Trepo and colleagues[65] have reported good results using a combination of plasmapheresis, corticosteroid therapy, and antiviral therapy. Successful treatment with interferon-alpha (IFN-α) has also been reported.

PARVOVIRUS B19 VASCULITIS

Although by far the most common rheumatic manifestation of parvovirus B19 infection is arthritis (see Chapter 102), occasional patients, usually children, have been reported to develop an impressive vasculitis, usually resembling PAN, in the setting of chronic parvovirus B19 infection.[66,67] These children have responded nicely to IV immune globulin (IVIg) therapy, suggesting that they may have a specific immune deficit regarding an inability to mount a normal immune response to parvovirus B19, although there was no other evidence suggesting generalized immunodeficiency.

Isolated Angiitis of the Central Nervous System

Granulomatous angiitis limited to the CNS is a rare disorder. It has been reported in children and in older adults, but the majority of cases are in the fourth and fifth decades. There is a slight male predominance. Although the disorder has been associated with HIV infection[68] and graft-versus-host disease,[69] the majority of cases are idiopathic.

PATHOLOGY

The typical feature is a granulomatous inflammatory response involving arterioles and small veins of the leptomeninges, although lesions may be seen throughout the CNS. Granulomatous findings are not inevitable, and some cases have shown simply necrosis and a lymphocytic or mixed infiltrate.[70] Thrombosis is common and often accounts for many of the symptoms. The cerebrospinal fluid typically shows modest protein elevation and phagocytosis.

CLINICAL FEATURES

The disease may be abrupt in onset or, more commonly, may present with gradual worsening of symptoms over 1 to 3 months. Headache is the most frequent symptom, and it may be severe and associated with nausea and vomiting. Confusion (which may be intermittent), dementia, drowsiness, and coma may develop early in the course of this disease. In addition, focal lesions including cranial neuropathies, stroke-like syndromes, and cerebral hemorrhage may occur. The spinal cord is occasionally involved, and paraplegia may occur in those patients. Seizures have been reported in 10 to 30 percent of patients.[70]

DIAGNOSIS

The only definitive diagnostic procedure is a biopsy of leptomeninges demonstrating granulomatous vasculitis.

Angiographic features are not specific but may be characteristic. Stenosis or occlusion of multiple arteries is the most common abnormality, although dilatation of vessels with discrete aneurysmal change may be seen. However, relying exclusively on angiography to make the diagnosis is somewhat risky, because many other disorders can occasionally have features similar to primary angiitis of the CNS. These include severe hypertension,[71] cerebral amyloid angiopathy,[72] migraine,[73] systemic vasculitis, rheumatic diseases, drug-induced vasculopathy (especially phenylpropanolamine[74]), infection (especially syphilis), malignant neoplasm (including CNS lymphoma), and thrombotic disorders.[75]

TREATMENT AND COURSE

When the diagnosis is confirmed, therapy is similar to that for PAN, using cyclophosphamide and corticosteroids.[76] The course, once therapy is initiated, is variable, but significant morbidity is common.[77,78]

As pointed out by Calabrese and associates,[70] patients with acute focal disease, diagnosis of which is made by angiography alone, often have a benign course. They recommend a short course of corticosteroids plus a calcium channel blocker along with avoidance of vasoconstrictive drugs.

REFERENCES

1. Cohen RD, Conn DL, Ilstrup DM: Clinical features, prognosis, and response to treatment in polyarteritis. Mayo Clin Proc 55:146, 1980.
2. Gocke DJ, Morgan C, Lockshin M, et al: Association between polyarteritis nodosa and Australia antigen. Lancet 2:1149, 1970.
3. Trepo C, Thivolet J: Hepatitis associated antigens and periarteritis nodosa (PAN). Vox Sang 19:410, 1970.
4. Goodman MD, Porter DD: Cytomegalovirus vasculitis with fatal colonic hemorrhage. Arch Pathol 96:281, 1973.
5. Massari M, Salvarani C, Portioli I, et al: Polyarteritis nodosa and HIV infection: No evidence of a direct pathogenic role of HIV. Infection 24:159, 1996.
6. Calabrese LH: Vasculitis and infection with the human immunodeficiency virus. Rheum Dis Clin North Am 17:131, 1991.
7. Wharton CF, Pieroni R: Polyarteritis after influenza vaccination. Br Med J 2:331, 1974.
8. Bani-Sadr F, Gueit I, Humbert G: Vasculitis related to hepatitis A vaccination. Clin Infect Dis 22:596, 1996.
9. Sergent JS, Christian CL: Necrotizing vasculitis after acute serous otitis media. Ann Intern Med 81:195, 1974.
10. Bingham C, Beaman M, Nicholls AJ, et al: Necrotizing renal vasculopathy resulting in chronic renal failure after ingestion of methamphetamine and 3,4 methylenedioxymethamphetamine ("ecstasy"). Nephrol Dial Transplant 13:2654, 1998.
11. Stone JH: Polyarteritis nodosa. JAMA 288:1632, 2002.
12. Moskowitz RW, Baggenstoss AH, Slocumb CH: Histopathologic classification of periarteritis nodosa: A study of 56 cases confirmed at necropsy. Mayo Clin Proc 38:345, 1963.
13. Antonovych TT, Sabnis GG, Tuur SM, et al: Morphologic differences between polyarteritis and Wegener's granulomatosis using light, electron and immunohistochemical techniques. Mod Pathol 24:349, 1989.
14. Cid MC, Grau JM, Casademont J, et al: Immunohistochemical characterization of inflammatory cells and immunologic activation markers in muscle and nerve biopsy specimens from patients with polyarteritis nodosa. Arthritis Rheum 37:1055, 1994.
15. Ewald EA, Griffin D, McCune WJ: Correlation of angiographic abnormalities with disease manifestations and disease severity in polyarteritis nodosa. J Rheumatol 14:952, 1987.

16. Wees SJ, Sunivoo IN, Oh SJ: Sural nerve biopsy in systemic necrotizing vasculitis. Am J Med 71:525, 1981.
17. Lightfoot RW, Michel BA, Bloch DA, et al: The American College of Rheumatology 1990 criteria for the classification of polyarteritis nodosa. Arthritis Rheum 33:1088, 1990.
18. Chang RW, Bell CL, Hallet M: Clinical characteristics and prognosis of vasculitic mononeuropathy multiplex. Arch Neurol 41:618, 1984.
19. Lie JT: Histopathologic specificity of systemic vasculitis. Rheum Dis Clin North Am 21:883, 1995.
20. Smith DL, Wernick R: Spontaneous rupture of a renal artery aneurysm in polyarteritis nodosa: Critical review of the literature and report of a case. Am J Med 87:464, 1989.
21. Guillevin L, Lhote F, Gayraud M, et al: Prognostic factors in polyarteritis nodosa and Churg-Strauss syndrome: A prospective study in 342 patients. Medicine (Baltimore) 75:17, 1996.
22. Fauci AS, Katz P, Haynes BF, et al: Cyclophosphamide therapy of severe systemic necrotizing vasculitis. N Engl J Med 301:235, 1979.
23. Clements PJ, Davis J: Cytotoxic drugs and their clinical application to rheumatic diseases. Semin Arthritis Rheum 15:231, 1986.
24. Guillevin L, Lhote F: Treatment of polyarteritis nodosa and microscopic polyangiitis. Arthritis Rheum 41:2100, 1998.
25. Gayraud M, Guillevin L, Cohen P, et al: Treatment of good-prognosis polyarteritis nodosa and Churg-Strauss syndrome: Comparison of steroids and oral or pulse cyclophosphamide in 25 patients. Br J Rheumatol 36:1290, 1997.
26. Fort JG, Abruzzo JL: Reversal of progressive necrotizing vasculitis with intravenous pulse cyclophosphamide and methylprednisolone. Arthritis Rheum 31:1194, 1998.
27. Leavitt RY, Fauci AS: Therapeutic approach to the vasculitis syndromes. Mt Sinai J Med 53:440, 1986.
28. Moreland LW, Ball GV: Cutaneous polyarteritis nodosa. Am J Med 88:426, 1990.
29. Albornoz MA, Benedetto AV, Korman M, et al: Relapsing cutaneous polyarteritis nodosa associated with streptococcal infections. Int J Dermatol 37:664, 1998.
30. Schaffer JV, Davidson DM, McNiff JM, et al: Perineuclear antineutrophil cytoplasmic antibody-postiive cutaneous polyarteritis nodosa associated with minocycline therapy for acne vulgaris. J Am Acad Dermatol 44:1908, 2001.
31. Soufir N, Descamps V, Crickx B, et al: Hepatitis C virus infection in cutaneous polyarteritis nodosa: a retrospective study of 16 cases. Arch Dermatol 135:1001, 1999.
32. Chen KR: Cutaneous polyarteritis nodosa. Am J Med 88:426, 1990.
33. Diaz-Perez JL, Winkelmann RK: Cutaneous polyarteritis nodosa. Arch Dermatol 110:407, 1974.
34. Jorrizzo JL, White WL, Wise CM, et al: Low-dose weekly methotrexate for unusual neutrophilic vascular reactions: Cutaneous polyarteritis nodosa and Behçet's disease. J Am Acad Dermatol 24:973, 1991.
35. Gibson LE, Su WP: Cutaneous vasculitis. Rheum Dis Clin North Am 16:309, 1990.
36. Uziel Y, Silverman ED: Intravenous immunoglobulin therapy in a child with cutaneous polyarteritis nodosa. Clin Exp Rheumatol 16:187, 1998.
37. Cvancara JL, Meffert JJ, Elston DN: Estrogen-sensitive cutaneous polyarteritis nodosa: Response to tamoxifen. J Am Acad Dermatol 39:643, 1998.
38. Cejudo-Rodriguez C, Hernandez V, Rodriguez R, et al: Thalidomide in mild and severe recurrent cutaneous polyarteritis nodosa. Ann Allergy Astham Immunol 82:128, 1999.
39. Kelleman D, Kempf W, Burg G, et al: Cutaneous polyarteritis nodosa. Vasa 27:54, 1998.
40. Dervar CL, Bellamy N: Necrotizing mesenteric vasculitis after long-standing cutaneous polyarteritis nodosa. J Rheumatol 19:1308, 1992.
41. Cogan DG: Syndrome of nonsyphilitic interstitial keratitis and vestibuloauditory symptoms. Arch Ophthalmol 33:144, 1945.
42. Vollertsen RS, McDonald TJ, Younge BR, et al: Cogan's syndrome: 18 cases and a review of the literature. Mayo Clin Proc 61:344, 1986.
43. Haynes BF, Kaiser-Kupfer MI, Mason P, et al: Cogan syndrome: Studies in thirteen patients, long-term follow-up, and a review of the literature. Medicine (Baltimore) 59:426, 1980.
44. VanDoornum S, McColl G, Walter M, et al: Prolonged prodrome, systemic vasculitis, and deafness in Cogan's syndrome. Ann Rheum Dis 60:69, 2001.
45. Vollertsen RS: Vasculitis and Cogan's syndrome [Review]. Rheum Dis Clin North Am 16:433, 1990.
46. Ottaviani F, Cadoni G, Marinelli L, et al: Anti-endothelial cell autoantibodies in patients with sudden hearing loss. Laryngoscope 109:1084, 1999.
47. Yamanishi Y, Ishioka S, Takeda M, et al: Atypical Cogan's syndrome associated with antineutrophil cytoplasmic antibodies. Br J Rheumatol 35:601, 1996.
48. Richardson B: Methotrexate therapy for hearing loss in Cogan's syndrome. Arthritis Rheum 37:1559, 1994.
49. Hammer M, Witte T, Mugge A, et al: Complicated Cogan's syndrome with aortic insufficiency and coronary stenosis. J Rheumatol 21:552, 1994.
50. Olin JW, Young JR, Graor RA, et al: The changing clinical spectrum of thromboangiitis obliterans (Buerger's disease). Circulation 82(Suppl IV):3, 1990.
51. Olin JW: Thromboangiitis obliterans [Review]. Curr Opin Rheumatol 6:44, 1994.
52. Aclar R, Papa MZ, Halpern Z, et al: Cellular sensitivity to collagen in thromboangiitis obliterans. N Engl J Med 308:1113, 1983.
53. Hada M, Sakihama T, Kamiya K, et al: Cellular and humoral immune responses to vascular components in thromboangiitis obliterans. Angiology 44:533, 1993.
54. Eichhorn J, Sima D, Lindschau C, et al: Antiendothelial cell antibodies in thromboangiitis obliterans. Am J Med Sci 315:17, 1998.
55. Halacheva KS, Manolova IM, Petkov DP, et al: Study of antineutrophil cytoplasmic antibodies in patients with thromboangiitis obliterans (Buerger's disease). Scand J Immunol 48:544, 1998.
56. Lie JT: Diagnostic histopathology of major systemic and pulmonary vasculitic syndromes. Rheum Dis Clin North Am 16:269, 1990.
57. Kobayashi M, Ito M, Nakagawa A, et al: Immunohistochemical analysis of arterial cell wall infiltration in Buerger's disease (endartheritis obliterans). J Vasc Surg 29:451, 1999.
58. Joyce JW: Buerger's disease (thromboangiitis obliterans) (Review). Rheum Dis Clin North Am 16:463, 1990.
59. Olin JW, Childs MB, Bathrolomex JR, et al. Anticardiolipin antibodies and homcysteine levels in patients with thromboangiitis obliterans. Arthritis Rheum 39:547, 1996.
60. Kawallata H, Kanekura T, Gushi A, et al: Successful treatment of digital ulceration in Buerger's disease with nicotine chewing gum (letter). Br J Dermatol 140:187, 1999.
61. Hussein EA, el Douri A: Intra-arterial streptokinase as adjuvant therapy for complicated Buerger's disease: Early trials. Int Surg 78:54, 1993.
62. Isner JM, Baumgartner I, Rauch G, et al: Treatment of thromboangiitis obliterans (Buerger's disease) by intramuscular gene transfer of vascular endothelial growth factor: Preliminary clinical results. J Vasc Surg 28:964, 1998.
63. Sasaki S, Sakuma M, Kunihara T, et al: Current trends in thromboangiitis obliterans (Buerger's disease) in women. Am J Surg 177:316, 1999.
64. Sergent JS, Lockshin MD, Christian CL, et al: Vasculitis with hepatitis B antigenemia. Medicine (Baltimore) 55:1, 1976.
65. Trepo C, Ouzan D, Delmont J, et al: Superiorite d'un nouveau traitement etiopathogenique curateur des periarteritis noueuses induites par le virus de l'hepatite B gra***ce a l'association corticotherapie breve, vidarabine, echanges plasmatiques. Presse Med 17:1527, 1988.
66. Gattorno M, Picco P, Vignola S, et al: Brother and sister with different vasculitides. Lancet 353:728, 1999.
67. Finkel TH, Torok TJ, Ferguson PJ, et al: Chronic parvovirus B19 infection and systemic necrotizing vasculitis: Oppoertunistic infection or aetiological agent? Lancet 343:1255, 1994.
68. Nogueras C, Sala M, Sasal M, et al. Recurrent stroke as a manifestation of primary angiitis of the central neverous system in a patient infected with human immunodeficiency vierus. Arch Neurol 59:468, 2002.
69. Lie JT: Angiitis of the central nervous system. Curr Opin Rheumatol 3:36, 1991.
70. Calabrese LH, Duna GF, Lie JT: Vasculitis in the central nervous system [Review]. Arthritis Rheum 40:1189, 1997.

71. Garner BF, Burns P, Bunning BD, et al: Acute blood pressure elevation can mimic arteriographic appearance of cerebral vasculitis-a postpartum case with relative hypertension. J Rheumatol 17:93, 1990.

72. Gray F, Vinters HV, LeNoan H, et al: Cerebral amyloid angiopathy and granulomatous angiitis: Immunohistochemical study using antibodies to the Alzheimer A4 peptide. Hum Pathol 21:1290, 1990.

73. Solomon S, Lipton RB, Harris PH: Arterial stenosis in migraine: Spasm or arteriopathy? Headache 30:52, 1990.

74. Lake CR, Gallant S, Mason E, et al: Adverse drug effects attributed to phenylpropanolamine: A review of 142 case reports. Am J Med 89:195, 1990.

75. Duna GF, Calabrese LH: Limitations of invasive modalities in the diagnosis of primary angiitis of the central nervous system. J Rheumatol 22:662, 1995.

76. Cupps TR, Moore PM, Fauci AS: Isolated angiitis of the central nervous system. Am J Med 74:97, 1983.

77. Moore PM: Vasculitis of the central nervous system. Semin Neurol 14:313, 1994.

78. Koo EH, Massey EW: Granulomatous angiitis of the central nervous system: Protean manifestations and response to treatment. J Neurol Neurosurg Psychiatry 51:1126, 1988.

85

Cutaneous Small-Vessel Vasculitis

KEITH T. ROTT · EMILIO B. GONZALEZ · DOYT L. CONN

Definitions

CUTANEOUS SMALL-VESSEL VASCULITIS

The primary clinical finding in cutaneous vasculitis is palpable purpura. Pathologically, the disorder is characterized by involvement of small vessels and histopathologically, by leukocytoclastic vasculitis. Cutaneous vasculitis has many causes. It may be a part of a systemic vasculitis, such as Churg-Strauss syndrome (CSS), Wegener's granulomatosis (WG), polyarteritis nodosa (PAN), or microscopic polyangiitis. It may be a manifestation of a systemic rheumatic disease such as rheumatoid arthritis (RA), systemic lupus erythematosus (SLE), Sjögren's syndrome, or dermatomyositis (DM). Cutaneous vasculitis may be associated with a systemic infection, such as subacute bacterial endocarditis or human immunodeficiency virus (HIV), or with a malignancy, usually hematologic. It may also be caused by a drug-associated hypersensitivity reaction, mixed cryoglobulinemia, urticarial vasculitis, or Henoch-Schönlein purpura (HSP). Thus, recognizing the presence of a cutaneous vasculitis is only half of the problem; the clinician must also look for the process underlying the condition. Common causes of cutaneous vasculitis are listed in Table 85-1.

This chapter will deal primarily with cutaneous small-vessel vasculitis that manifests as palpable purpura and is not a part of a systemic vasculitis or rheumatologic disease. Another form of chronic cutaneous vasculitis that can occur in patients with autoimmune diseases, erythema elevatum diutinum, has a distinctive presentation as raised papules and nodules[1] and is discussed further in Chapter 45, which deals with the skin.

Any of the possibilities previously delineated should be kept in mind in the evaluation of the patient with cutaneous vasculitis. The classic skin lesion of a cutaneous vasculitis is palpable purpura, but urticarial lesions, small nodules, or palpable petechiae may also be manifestations of a cutaneous vasculitis. In addition, there may be constitutional signs and symptoms such as arthralgias, myalgias, fever, and malaise. Once the presence of this disorder has been identified, several questions must be addressed to ascertain the underlying cause, as outlined in Table 85-2.

NOMENCLATURE

A Modern, Clinically Useful Approach

There is no uniform classification system to describe small-vessel or cutaneous vasculitis. Existing classification criteria were developed for research studies, not for diagnostic purposes in the individual patient.[2] A more clinically useful approach once a cutaneous vasculitis has been recognized is to determine the underlying cause using the approach in Table 85-2. Aside from any specific classification schemes, the following types of cutaneous vasculitis are discussed in this chapter: hypersensitivity vasculitis, urticarial vasculitis, cutaneous vasculitis associated with infection or malignancy, mixed cryoglobulinemia–associated vasculitis, and HSP.

TABLE 85–1 · TYPES (AND CAUSES) OF CUTANEOUS SMALL-VESSEL VASCULITIS

Associated with a systemic vasculitis	Churg-Strauss syndrome, Wegener's granulomatosis, polyarteritis nodosa, microscopic polyangiitis
Associated with a rheumatic disease	Rheumatoid arthritis, systemic lupus erythematosus, Sjögren's syndrome, dermatomyositis
Hypersensitivity vasculitis	Drugs, vaccinations
Infection	Bacterial, viral
Malignancy	Hematologic or solid tumor
Mixed cryoglobulinemia	Hepatitis C
Urticarial vasculitis	
Henoch-Schönlein purpura	

TABLE 85–2 · QUESTIONS TO BE ADDRESSED IN EVALUATING CUTANEOUS VASCULITIS

1. Is there evidence of a systemic vasculitis (Churg-Strauss syndrome, Wegener's granulomatosis, polyarteritis nodosa, microscopic polyangiitis) as manifested by pulmonary involvement, renal involvement, or peripheral neuropathy?
2. Is there evidence of another rheumatologic disease (rheumatoid arthritis, systemic lupus erythematosus, Sjögren's syndrome, dermatomyositis) as manifested by synovitis, myositis, or other organ involvement?
3. Is there evidence of another systemic condition (bacterial or viral infection, hematologic or solid-tumor malignancy) as the cause of the cutaneous vasculitis?
4. Is there evidence of Henoch-Schönlein purpura as manifested by abdominal pain or renal involvement?
5. Has a new drug been started?
6. Are the lesions urticarial and long lived (e.g., more than 72 hr)?
7. Is there evidence of hepatitis C infection with mixed cryoglobulinemia?

Traditional Nomenclature

The designation *hypersensitivity vasculitis* has been used to describe a number of mainly cutaneous vasculitic syndromes. Specifically, small-vessel vasculitis affecting the skin has been variously termed *allergic angiitis, allergic vasculitis, hypersensitivity angiitis, hypersensitivity vasculitis,* and *small-vessel cutaneous vasculitis*. From a pathogenic standpoint, cutaneous vasculitis associated with serum sickness and drug reactions perhaps best fits the description of hypersensitivity vasculitis, alluding to the possibility of an aberrant immune reaction to an exogenous stimulus.

In 1990, the American College of Rheumatology (ACR) proposed the following criteria for the classification of hypersensitivity vasculitis[3]:

1. Development of symptoms after age 16
2. Tuse of a possible offending drug temporally related to the onset of symptoms
3. Palpable purpura
4. Maculopapular rash
5. Biopsy with evidence of granulocytes around an arteriole or venule

The presence of three or more of these criteria had a sensitivity and specificity of 71 percent and 84 percent, respectively, for the diagnosis of hypersensitivity vasculitis. These criteria cannot distinguish the various forms of cutaneous vasculitis (e.g., serum sickness from HSP).

Several other classification schemes have been proposed. The Chapel Hill Consensus Conference definition takes into account the presence or absence of internal organ involvement[4] and does not include the term *hypersensitivity vasculitis*. For example, patients with isolated skin purpura are said to have cutaneous leukocytoclastic angiitis. On the other hand, those with cutaneous vasculitis as a manifestation of a systemic disease, particularly in the absence of immune deposits in the vessel wall, are considered to have microscopic polyangiitis. The pauci-immune nature of these lesions would distinguish microscopic polyangiitis from HSP and mixed cryoglobulinemia, in which immunoglobulin deposits are seen in the vascular wall.

Several studies have challenged the value of the criteria proposed by the ACR. Watts and coworkers[5] studied an unselected cohort of 84 patients with biopsy-proven cutaneous vasculitis attending a single district hospital in the United Kingdom. Of the 84 patients, 37 fulfilled clinical ACR criteria for HSP, and of these, 27 also satisfied clinical ACR criteria for hypersensitivity vasculitis. Thirty-two patients met the Chapel Hill Consensus Conference definition for cutaneous leukocytoclastic angiitis, and seven met its definition for HSP. The authors concluded by saying that the 1990 ACR criteria for hypersensitivity vasculitis and HSP overlap. In a similar study in the United States, Rao and colleagues[6] testing the ACR classification criteria in a prospective cohort study of 198 consecutive patients having all the major vasculitic syndromes, including hypersensitivity vasculitis, reached a similar conclusion: The ACR classification criteria function poorly in the diagnosis of specific vasculitis.

Epidemiology

Epidemiologic studies of cutaneous vasculitis are difficult to undertake both due to the relatively uncommon occurrence of the disorder and the lack of a clear definition or criteria. A 1998 study of a large, well-defined population in the United Kingdom estimated the annual incidence of cutaneous vasculitis at approximately 40 cases per million, equivalent to the annual incidence of systemic vasculitis in that population.[5] In the mid-1980s in the United States, approximately 9 percent of patients who presented to a rheumatologist with a diagnosis of vasculitis were said to have hypersensitivity vasculitis, and another 9 percent were diagnosed with HSP.[7]

Histopathology

Biopsy of a typical lesion shows inflammation of small cutaneous blood vessels, termed *leukocytoclastic vasculitis* or *leukocytoclastic angiitis*. Usually most prominent in the postcapillary venules, the features are fibrinoid necrosis of the vessel wall, transmural inflammation, polymorphonuclear cell–derived nuclear debris termed *nuclear dust* and neutrophil-rich infiltrates in perivascular areas of the vessel wall (Fig. 85–1). Lymphocytes may predominate in the healing phases of cutaneous vasculitis, although this is not a uniform finding. Leukocytoclastic vasculitis is associated with immunoglobulin A (IgA) immune deposits in HSP and with IgG and IgM immune complexes in the vasculitis associated with mixed cryoglobulinemia.

When a skin biopsy is performed in the evaluation of cutaneous vasculitis, the subcutis should be included. The diagnostic changes present in the dermis or underlying fat may be missed with only a punch biopsy. A skin biopsy cannot distinguish any of the clinical forms of cutaneous vasculitis, with the exception of HSP and its IgA deposition in the vessel wall. The term *leukocytoclastic vasculitis* is a pathologic term, not a clinical diagnosis. Therefore, in every case of biopsy-proven cutaneous leukocytoclastic vasculitis, a complete evaluation of the patient should be undertaken to exclude the possibility of a more serious underlying systemic disease, as discussed previously.

Specific Types of Cutaneous Small-Vessel Vasculitis

HYPERSENSITIVITY VASCULITIS

Clinical Features

Hypersensitivity vasculitis, as classically described by Zeek and coworkers,[8] occurs after an antigenic stimulus induces an Arthus reaction or type III hypersensitivity. The etiology of hypersensitivity vasculitis is often unknown,[9] although drugs seem the most commonly identifiable offenders.[10] Vaccinations have more rarely been associated with hypersensitivity vasculitis.[11] Onset can be abrupt after exposure to the etiologic agent, but it usually ranges from 7 to 21 days after initial expo-

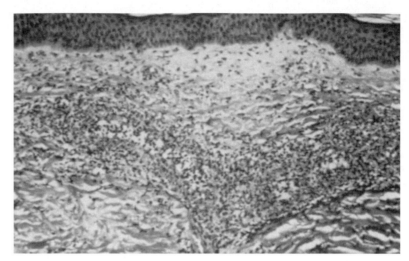

FIGURE 85–1 • Leukocytoclastic Vasculitis. Dermal vessels, probably venules, are sectioned longitudinally. Intense infiltration of inflammatory cells (primarily polymorphonuclear leukocytes) has resulted in narrowing and occlusion of vessel lumen and in necrosis of wall. Fragments of degenerated leukocyte nuclei (nuclear dust) are visible in perivascular areas. (H&E, ×100)

sure.[2] Although almost any medication can be associated with a hypersensitivity vasculitis, certain classes of drugs are more commonly associated with hypersensitivity and are listed in Table 85-3.[2,11,13,52]

Palpable purpura, similar to that seen in Figure 85–2, is the most common clinical finding. The lesions are papular and do not blanche. Early in the disease, the skin lesions may be flat and erythematous, but they progress rapidly to palpable purpura. They are often located in the lower extremities and dependent areas, including the back and gluteal regions. The skin lesions vary from 1 mm to several centimeters in size and may coalesce. It is unusual for palpable purpura of hypersensitivity vasculitis to involve the torso and upper extremities; however, skin trauma (e.g., the area under a waistband) seems to promote or facilitate the eruption. New crops of skin lesions tend to occur episodically; individual lesions last about a week and usually no more than a month. Skin hyperpigmentation can be a sequela. The lesions of palpable purpura are typically not painful, but a prodrome with prurituis or mild pain can occur in the location prior to the appearance of a lesion.

The severity of hypersensitivity vasculitis varies considerably from a few scattered purpuric spots in the lower extremities to an extensive, prolonged, chronic

TABLE 85–3 • SOME DRUGS ASSOCIATED WITH HYPERSENSITIVITY VASCULITIS

Nonsteroidal anti-inflammatory Drugs (NSAIDs)	Including ibuprofen, diclofenac, etodolac, piroxicam, naproxen
Antibiotics	Including β-lactams, macrolides, sulfonamides, quinolones, antivirals
Growth factors	Including G-CSF, GM-CSF
Selective serotonin reuptake inhibitors, (SSRIs)	Including paroxetine, fluoxetine
Antithyroid drugs	Propylthiouracil
Antihypertensive medications	Including thiazides, β-blockers
Anticonvulsants	Including phenytoin
Vaccinations	
Allopurinol	
Aspirin	
Acetaminophen	
Insulin	
Methotrexate	
Anti–tumor necrosis factor agents	Etanercept, infliximab

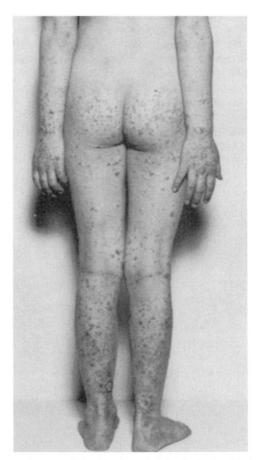

FIGURE 85–2 • Palpable Purpura in Patient with Henoch-Schönlein Purpura (HSP). Palpable purpura is most prominent over extensor surfaces of distal regions of upper and lower extremities and over buttocks. Some small skin infarcts are visible.

purpura. In these chronic cases, the skin lesions may form small nodules, vesicles, and bullae containing bloody fluid, sometimes leading to skin necrosis and ulceration. In the lower extremities, palpable purpura of hypersensitivity vasculitis may be accompanied by edema and ankle swelling. Constitutional symptoms may include fever, malaise, and generalized arthralgias, but true synovitis is uncommon.

The percent of cutaneous vasculitis that is a hypersensitivity vasculitis due to drug exposure is commonly reported as 5 to 10 percent.[2] However, a recent study from Spain, which included patients with milder but biopsy-proven cutaneous vasculitis, showed 24 percent of the cases were due to drug exposure, and most of these cases completely resolved without sequelae.[12] In all studies addressing the incidence of drug-associated hypersensitivity vasculitis, establishing causality is the major issue.[12] Plausible pathologic mechanisms for causing a hypersensitivity vasculitis include conjugation of the drug to serum protein, formation of immune complexes with foreign proteins used for treatment, and induction of autoantibodies such as antineutrophil cytoplasmic antibodies (ANCAs).[2]

It should also be noted that drugs can also induce systemic vasculitis syndromes.[11,13] Thus, the patient with cutaneous vasculitis attributed to a new drug should also be evaluated for evidence of a more serious systemic vasculitis.

Diagnosis

The diagnosis of hypersensitivity vasculitis is made by recognizing the skin lesions of palpable purpura in a dependent distribution in a patient with a history of exposure to a new agent. The offending triggering antigen, usually a drug, is sought by history. The diagnosis of hypersensitivity vasculitis necessitates excluding other causes of cutaneous vasculitis by history and physical examination. It is often not necessary to confirm the pathologic changes of leukocytoclastic vasculitis in characteristic lesions by a skin biopsy, as the histopathology is not unique to this condition.

Treatment

When an exogenous offending agent such as a recently started medication is identified or suspected, that agent should be discontinued. In mild cases in which only a few scattered purpuric lesions are present without systemic organ involvement, no specific treatment other than for symptoms may be needed, particularly when some of the lesions begin to show evidence of healing.

When the skin lesions are extensive or are severe in the form of skin ulceration or bullae, or when there is significant systemic involvement, corticosteroids are indicated. For more severe involvement, a daily dose of 40 to 60 mg of prednisone may be necessary. The dose is gradually tapered to the lowest amount possible to control symptoms and abnormal findings. Antihistamines, pentoxifylline, and dapsone may be helpful in controlling cutaneous vasculitis.[14,15] Colchicine has been tried

successfully by some investigators.[16,17] Combinations of these drugs can also be used. Nonsteroidal anti-inflammatory drugs (NSAIDs) are usually disappointing in the treatment of hypersensitivity vasculitis. Cytotoxic agents such as cyclophosphamide, methotrexate, and azathioprine are usually not indicated for the treatment of hypersensitivity vasculitis limited to the skin.

URTICARIAL VASCULITIS

Urticaria, or hives, may be the predominant skin lesion of a cutaneous vasculitis with or without palpable purpura (Fig. 85–3). Such cases must be differentiated from patients with immune complex–mediated disease and connective tissue disorders, such as SLE, that have urticaria as a manifestation of the underlying disease. Simple hives tend to vanish in less than 48 hours. Hives lasting longer than 3 to 4 days, myalgias, polyarthralgias and polyarthritis, malaise, fever, leukocytosis, and an elevated erythrocyte sedimentation rate (ESR) are features associated with urticarial vasculitis. A biopsy of the urticarial lesions shows necrotizing leukocytoclasia. Immunofluorescent studies typically show deposition of Igs and complement components in and around the vascular wall. In urticarial vasculitis, other organ involvement may be seen, such as glomerulonephritis,[18,19] pseudotumor cerebrii,[19] angioedema, arthritis, and myalgias.

Patients with predominantly urticarial vasculitis have traditionally been classified into two different subgroups: those with serum hypocomplementemia[18] and those whose serum complement level is normal.[20] Davis and colleagues[21] compared features of normocomplementemic

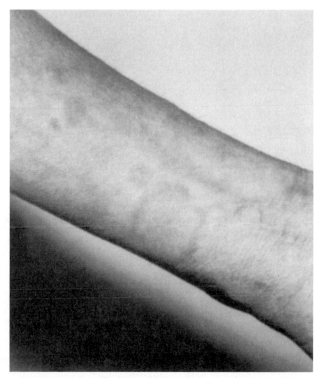

FIGURE 85–3 · Urticarial Vasculitis. Large resolving urticarial lesion on flexor surface of forearm shows central clearing.

patients with those in whom hypocomplementemia was observed. Of the 132 patients, 24 had hypocomplementemia. On direct immunofluorescent testing of lesional skin, 23 of the hypocomplementemic patients (96%) had a continuous, strong granular deposition of immunoreactants along the basement membrane, compatible with the so-called lupus band test of SLE. In fact, systemic lupus was present or occurred in 13 of the hypocomplementemic patients (54%). Only one patient in the normocomplementemic group had direct immunofluorescent staining compatible with the lupus band test. According to these investigators, patients with hypocomplementemic urticarial vasculitis are more likely to be female, have diffuse neutrophilia on biopsy specimens, have findings compatible with the lupus band test, and have a diagnosis of lupus, compared to patients with normocomplementemic urticarial vasculitis.[21] Hypocomplementemic urticarial vasculitis may well be a subset of SLE. Low-molecular-weight IgG precipitins interacting as autoantibodies with C1q and lowering C1q levels seem characteristic of hypocomplementemic urticarial vasculitis.[22]

The therapy for urticarial vasculitis is similar to that outlined previously for hypersensitivity vasculitis. In addition to corticosteroids and dapsone, hydroxychloroquine seems uniquely effective for hypocomplementemic urticarial vasculitis in a dose range of 200 to 400 mg daily.[23]

CUTANEOUS VASCULITIS DUE TO SYSTEMIC INFECTION OR MALIGNANCY

Infection

Numerous bacterial and viral infections have been associated with leukocytoclastic vasculitis. Commonly associated bacterial pathogens include *Neisseria gonorrhoea* and *N. meningitidis*, *Staphylcoccus aureus*, *Streptococcus pneumoniae* and *equisimilus*, and viridans and β–hemolytic *Streptococcus*.[24] Common viral pathogens include cytomegalovirus, hepatitis B virus, hepatitis C virus, HIV, and parvovirus B19.[24] Numerous other bacterial, viral, and even parasitic pathogens have occasionally been reported to be associated with cutaneous vasculitis. Identification of an underlying systemic infection is important for proper treatment (e.g., subacute bacterial endocarditis or HIV infection).

Malignancy

A malignant neoplasm may be the underlying disease in cutaneous vasculitis.[25] The majority of patients with neoplasm-associated vasculitis have hematologic neoplasms such as lymphoma or hairy-cell leukemia, although solid tumors have also been described.[26] Of the solid tumors, the most common have been non–small cell lung cancer and prostate, breast, colon, and renal malignant neoplasms.[25,26] Cutaneous vasculitis and nerve and muscle microvasculitis are the most frequently observed types of vasculitis in malignancies.

MIXED CRYOGLOBULINEMIA

Clinical Features

Cryoglobulins are Igs that precipitate in the cold and dissolve again on rewarming. Three different types of cryoglobulins[27] are known, as outlined in Table 85-4. In type II or mixed essential cryoglobulinemia, 80 to 95 percent of patients have circulating antibodies to the hepatitis C virus, as well as the presence of viral RNA in the plasma. The cryoprecipitate in these cases typically contains polyclonal IgG antibodies against hepatitis C as well as viral RNA.[28-30] Patients with hepatitis C–associated essential cryoglobulinemia need not have evidence of chronic liver disease at the time of presentation.[29] In one prospective study of 226 patients with chronic liver disease, 127 had hepatitis C virus infection, and of these, 69 patients (54%) had serum cryoglobulins.[31] One large study suggested that the triad of necrotizing vasculitis, chronic hepatitis C infection, and cryoglobulinemia occurs late in the course of the viral disease.[32]

The majority of hepatitis C–infected patients with mixed cryoglobulinemia do not have vasculitis (less than 5% in large studies).[33] In general, patients without vasculitis have more type III cryoglobulins at a low titer, whereas patients with vasculitis have type II cryoglobulins at a high titer.[33] Skin is the most commonly involved organ. Rarely, nerves or kidneys may be affected, but hardly ever in the absence of skin involvement.

The clinical features of mixed cryoglobulinemia include leukocytoclastic vasculitis (manifested as palpable purpura), arthralgias and arthritis, lymphadenopathy, hepatosplenomegaly, peripheral neuropathy, and hypocomplementemia, especially decreased C_4 serum levels. Renal disease is present in 20 to 60 percent of the patients and is more likely with type II cryoglobulinemia.[30] Renal biopsies have shown a proliferative glomerulonephritis.[34] Subendothelial deposits, diffuse IgM deposition in the capillary loops on immunofluorescence,

TABLE 85–4 • TYPES OF CRYOGLOBULINEMIAS[28-30]

Type I	Monoclonal Immunoglobulin	Typically seen in myeloproliferative disorders such as multiple myeloma and Waldenström's macroglobulinemia
Type II	Essential mixed cryoglobulin (polyclonal immunoglobulin and a monoclonal rheumatoid factor)	Associated with hepatitis B or C virus infection in most cases
Type III	Mixed polyclonal cryoglobulin (both the immunoglobulin and the rheumatoid factor are polyclonal)	Often seen in autoimmune diseases such as lupus, Sjögren's syndrome, and hematologic malignant neoplasms and with hepatitis C virus or other infections

and intraluminal thrombi composed of precipitated cryoglobulins are typical findings.

Diagnosis

The diagnosis of mixed cryoglobulinemia should be suspected in a patient with cutaneous vasculitis associated with systemic symptoms, particularly in the presence of hypocomplementemia, and especially if liver function test values are elevated.[32] All such patients should undergo testing for hepatitis C virus infection. A positive rheumatoid factor (RF) may indicate the presence of cryoglobulins. For detection of serum cryoglobulins, blood should be obtained in the fasting state to avoid interference by serum lipids. The sample should be transported to the laboratory at once and stored at 37°C. After centrifugation, the sample should be refrigerated at 4°C for 24 to 72 hours. If cryoprecipitate is found, it should rapidly redissolve at 37°C.

Treatment

The decision of how to treat this condition is based on the severity of the vasculitis and the liver disease. Patients can be divided into two groups: mild to moderate and severe to life threatening.[33] In mild-to-moderate cutaneous vasculitis associated with hepatitis C cryoglobulinemia, treatment is directed at the infection with the goal of viral clearance. The treatment of hepatitis C is a rapidly changing clinical area. Current protocols for treatment of hepatitis C virus infection use interferon-α (IFN-α) with or without ribavirin. A recent development is the use of pegylated IFN-α.

Approximately 75 percent of patients with mild-to-moderate hepatitis C–associated cryoglobulinemic vasculitis respond to antiviral therapy initially. Due to the low rate of sustained virologic response, the majority of these patients will have a relapse of their vasculitis after antiviral therapy is stopped. Although low-dose corticosteroids may help with the symptoms, they should be avoided if possible during initial antiviral therapy and are not recommended for long-term use. Response rates for renal or neurologic involvement is much lower. However, the current data do not support the idea that patients with hepatitis C–associated mixed cryoglobulinemia respond less well to antiviral treatment.[33] The specific treatment regimen and the response to treatment are in large part dependent on the virus genotype, with genotypes B and C having a better response rate. Consultation with a hepatologist is recommended.

In severe or life-threatening vasculitis involving large areas of skin or vital organs, treatment is directed at controlling the vasculitis using immunosuppressive agents. Of concern is whether the use of such drugs affects viral replication or liver pathology. Short courses of corticosteroids have been shown to result in increased hepatitis C virus levels, lower ALT values, and no significant change in liver histopathology.[33] The Italian experience treating patients with hepatitis C and glomerulonephritis has resulted in no evidence of acute liver damage in more than 100 patients treated with corticosteroids, cyclophosphamide, and plasmapheresis.[35] In hepatitis C–infected patients with severe cryoglobulinemia-associated vasculitis, oral or intravenous corticosteroids and oral daily cyclophosphamide are recommended for the duration of the acute flare only.[33] Plasmapheresis has also been used in life-threatening cases but often requires concomitant immunosuppressive treatment[33] or antiviral drugs.[36] Rituximab, an anti-CD20 monoclonal antibody that depletes B cells, is also being explored as a therapeutic agent.[37]

There is no benefit of extending immunosuppression beyond the acute flare. After the vasculitis has been controlled, the goal again becomes viral clearance. Relapses in severe or life-threatening disease activity can be retreated with immunosuppressive drugs or plasmapheresis. Only those few patients with frequent flares or chronic severe vasculitis benefit from constant immunosuppression; such patients require close clinical follow-up and frequent monitoring of liver function.

HENOCH-SCHÖNLEIN PURPURA

Clinical Features

HSP is typically a disease of childhood, although adults can be affected as well. Half the affected children are younger than 5 years. The typical clinical findings are a cutaneous rash, arthralgias, abdominal pain, and renal disease.[38] These signs and symptoms can occur in any order during a period of days to weeks. Renal and pulmonary findings with hemoptysis can occur, giving rise to a pulmonary-renal syndrome mimicking WG, microscopic polyangiitis, and Goodpasture's syndrome. The rash can be urticarial or purpuric and is usually in the lower extremities, although facial edema with an associated eruption can be seen in young children.[38] The abdominal pain is probably secondary to an underlying intestinal vasculitis and may be mild to severe, on occasions accompanied by gastrointestinal bleeding. Intussusception may occur, especially in older children. The arthralgias most often affect the lower extremities, sometimes with knee arthritis; on occasion, especially in children, an entire lower extremity becomes edematous. Typically, there are no residual joint deformities in patients with HSP.

HSP is characterized by the tissue deposition of IgA in the skin and kidney and circulating IgA immune complexes.[39] In IgA nephropathy, a similar disease, IgA immune deposits are also present in the kidney. In this regard, both HSP and IgA nephropathy may share a common immunopathogenesis; in fact, both diseases have been observed to occur simultaneously in twins after a viral upper respiratory infection.[40] In older children and adults, the disease tends to be more severe, particularly with regard to renal involvement.[38,41] Although IgA immune deposits are classic for both HSP and IgA nephropathy, the renal lesions may be mediated at least in part by IgG autoantibodies directed against mesangial cell antigens.[42] Of interest, in those patients with HSP but without renal involvement, the IgG autoantibodies appear to be absent.

The renal involvement in HSP is common and tends to relate to the severity of the extrarenal disease. Hematuria and proteinuria occur in 30 to 70 percent of patients.[43] Renal involvement can be seen within a few days to several weeks after the onset of HSP and can recur. Most patients have relatively mild nephritis with mild proteinuria; active urine sediment is accompanied by a normal or slightly elevated serum creatinine concentration. Findings on renal biopsy range from focal mesangial proliferation and varying degrees of cellular proliferation to frank crescent formation. The findings of crescent formation correlate with a worse outcome.[44] Recurrent attacks of skin purpura for weeks to months can be followed by the occurrence of nephritis. Patients with repeated attacks of purpura and persistent hematuria may show findings on biopsy consistent with progressive renal disease.

The renal involvement in HSP differs between children and adults. Overall, the renal prognosis is typically excellent in most children with HSP. In fact, all the manifestations of HSP usually resolve spontaneously in most children. Still, some children who seem to have completely recovered may, after many years, experience clinical deterioration, particularly if they have had persistent urinary abnormalities, such as hematuria.[45]

A study based in Northwest Spain followed all children and adults diagnosed with HSP over a 21-year period.[46] Seventy-three children and 31 adults met criteria for the study. Six of 31 adults (19%) had severe renal manifestations, and an additional four (13%) had renal insufficiency. After an average of 5 years of follow-up, almost 40 percent of the adults had persistent hematuria, with three (10%) having persistent renal insufficiency. Two of these three required hemodialysis. The risk of long-term renal disease is greater in older children and adults with HSP; approximately 10 to 30 percent of these patients progress to chronic renal disease and end-stage renal failure.[44] Adults diagnosed with HSP should be followed for long periods to monitor for renal disease.[47]

Treatment

The treatment of IgA nephropathy, both primary and that associated with HSP, is an area with little clear evidence but much ongoing investigation.[48] Angiotensin-converting enzyme (ACE) inhibitors decrease proteinuria and hypertension, but at present, the long-term efficacy of ACE inhibitors or angiotensin-receptor blockers is unknown. Corticosteroids have been used, with all studies showing reduced proteinuria but only one study showing lack of progression of renal disease. Anecdotal reports exist for numerous other agents in IgA nephropathy, including mycophenylate mofetil, cyclophosphamide, and azathioprine. The utility of steroids with azathioprine is not proven but might be beneficial. Fish oil supplements have yielded mixed results; no specific recommendation can be made at this time.

A renal biopsy is recommended in the presence of pronounced proteinuria, persistently active urine sediment, and prolonged marked hematuria, particularly when accompanied by renal function abnormalities, to determine whether there is crescent formation. These patients carry a worse prognosis, and, therefore, aggressive treatment may be considered. High-dose corticosteroids (e.g., 250 to 1000 mg/day of intravenous methylprednisolone for 3 days followed by oral prednisone, 1 mg/kg/day) were used successfully in one prospective but uncontrolled study of 36 children with HSP and nephrotic syndrome or severe crescentic glomerulonephritis.[49] Azathioprine along with corticosteroids has also been successfully used in an uncontrolled setting.[50] The benefit of plasmapheresis remains uncertain. High-dose IV immune globulin (IVIg) has been used with promising results; however, its potential benefits require further confirmation in controlled studies with greater numbers of patients.[51] Renal transplantation can be done with patient and graft survival comparable to patients without an IgA nephropathy. However, IgA nephropathy recurs in 20 to 60 percent of grafts over time.[48,51]

▮ Summary

The most common cutaneous manifestation of a small-vessel vasculitis is palpable purpura (see Fig. 85–2). A biopsy of such a lesion will reveal leukocytoclastic vasculitis (see Fig. 85–1), which is a pathologic diagnosis, not a specific disease. There are many causes of cutaneous vasculitis (see Table 85-1). Therefore, once a cutaneous vasculitis has been recognized, the clinician must search for the underlying cause (see Table 85-2). Treatment is guided by the underlying cause of the disease and the severity of the vasculitis and is often supportive. As with all of the vasculitidies, the practitioner must balance vigilance for recognizing the presence of a cutaneous small-vessel vasculitis, thoroughness in evaluating the patient for an underlying cause, and judiciousness in matching the treatment to the severity of the disease.

REFERENCES

1. Gibson L, El-Azhary R: Erythema elevatum diutinum. Clin Dermatol 18:295, 2000.
2. Jeanette J, Falk R: Small-vessel vasculitis. N Engl J Med 337:1512, 1997.
3. Calabrese L, Michael B, Bloch D, et al: The American College of Rheumatology 1990 Criteria for the classification of hypersensitivity vasculitis. Arthritis Rheum 33:1108, 1990.
4. Jennette J, Falk R, Andrassy K, et al: Nomenclature of systemic vasculitis: Proposal of an international consensus conference. Arthritis Rheum 37:187, 1994.
5. Watts R, Jolliffe V, Grattan C, et al: Cutaneous vasculitis in a defined population: Clinical and epidemiological associations. J Rheumatol 25:920, 1998.
6. Rao J, Allen N, Pincus T: Limitations of the 1990 American College of Rheumatology criteria in the diagnosis of vasculitis. Ann Intern Med 129:345, 1998.
7. Bloch D, Michel B, Hunder G, et al: The American College of Rheumatology 1990 criteria for the classification of vasculitis. Arthritis Rheum 33:1068, 1990.
8. Zeek P, Smith C, Wector J: Studies on periarteritis nodosa. III. The difference between the vascular lesions of periarteritis nodosa and of hypersensitivity. Am J Pathol 24:889, 1948.
9. Callen J: Cutaneous vasculitis and other neutrophilic dermatoses. Curr Opin Rheumatol 5:33, 1993.

10. Michel B, Hunder G, Bloch D, Calabrese L: Hypersensitivity vasculitis and Henoch-Schönlein purpura: A comparison between the two disorders. J Rheumatol 19:721, 1992.

11. Yung R, Richardson B: Drug-induced rheumatic syndromes. Bull Rheum Dis 51:1, 2002.

12. Garcia-Porrua C, Gonzalez-Gay M, Lopez-Lazaro L: Drug associated cutaneous vasculitis in adults in northwestern Spain. J Rheumatol 26:1942, 1999.

13. Cuellar M: Drug-induced vasculitis. Curr Rheumatol Rep 4:55, 2002.

14. Gibson L, Su W: Cutaneous vasculitis [Review]. Rheum Dis Clin North Am 16:309, 1990.

15. Nurnberg W, Grabbe J, Czarnetzki B: Urticarial vasculitis syndrome effectively treated with dapsone and pentoxifylline. Acta Dermatovenereol 75:54, 1995.

16. Callen J: Colchicine is effective in controlling chronic cutaneous leukocytoclastic vasculitis. J Am Acad Dermatol 13:193, 1985.

17. Sais G, Vidaller A, Jucgla A, et al: Colchicine in the treatment of cutaneous leukocytoclastic vasculitis. Results of a prospective, randomized controlled trial. Arch Dermatol 131:1399, 1995.

18. McDuffie F, Sams W, Maldonado J, et al: Hypocomplementemia with cutaneous vasculitis and arthritis. Mayo Clin Proc 48:340, 1973.

19. Ludivico C, Myers A, Maurer K: Hypocomplementemic urticarial vasculitis with glomerulonephritis and pseudotumor cerebri. Arthritis Rheum 22:1024, 1979.

20. Soter N, Austen K, Gigli I: Urticaria and arthralgias as a manifestation of necrotizing angiitis. J Invest Dermatol 63:489, 1974.

21. Davis M, Daoud M, Kirby B, et al: Clinicopathologic correlation of hypocomplementemic and normocomplementemic urticarial vasculitis. J Am Acad Dermatol 38:899, 1998.

22. Marder R, Rent R, Choi E, et al: C1q deficiency associated with urticaria-like lesions and cutaneous vasculitis. Am J Med 61:560, 1976.

23. Kaplan A: Urticaria and angioedema. In Middleton E Jr, Reed C, Ellis E, et al (eds): Allergy, Principle and Practice, Mosby, 1998, pp 1104-1122.

24. Somer T, Feingold S: Vasculitides associated with infections, immunization, and antimicrobial drugs. Clin Infect Dis 20:1010, 1995.

25. Mertz L, Conn D: Vasculitis associated with malignancy. Curr Opin Rheumatol 4:39, 1992.

26. Kurzrock R, Cohen P, Merkowitz A: Clinical manifestations of vasculitis in patients with solid tumors: A case report and review of the literature. Arch Intern Med 154:334, 1994.

27. Gorevic P, Kassab H, Levo Y, et al: Mixed cryoglobulinemia: Clinical aspects and long-term follow-up of 40 patients. Am J Med 69:287, 1980.

28. Agnello V, Chung R, Kaplan L: A role for hepatitis C virus infection in type II cryoglobulinemia. N Engl J Med 327:1490, 1992.

29. Misiani R, Bellavita P, Fenili D, et al: Hepatitis C virus infection in patients with essential mixed cryoglobulinemia. Ann Intern Med 117:573, 1992.

30. Marti G, Galli M, Invernizzi F, et al: Cryoglobulinemias: A multicentre study of the early clinical and laboratory manifestations of primary and secondary disease. Q J Med 88:115, 1995.

31. Lunel F, Musset L, Cacoub P, et al: Cryoglobulinemia in chronic liver disease: Role of HCV and liver damage. Gastroenterology 106:1291, 1994.

32. Daoud M, el-Azhary R, Gibson L, et al: Chronic hepatitis C, cryoglobulinemia, and cutaneous necrotizing vasculitis: Clinical, pathologic, and immunopathologic study of twelve patients. J Am Acad Dermatol 34:219, 1996.

33. Vassilopoulos D, Calabrese L: Hepatitis C virus infection and vasculitis. Arthritis Rheum 46:585, 2002.

34. D'Amico G, Colasanti G, Ferrario F, Sinico R: Renal involvement in essential mixed cryoglobulinemia. Kidney Int 35:1004, 1989.

35. D'Amico G: Renal involvement in hepatitis C infection: cryoglobulinemic glomerlulonephritis. Kidney Int 54:650, 1998.

36. Guillevin L, Cohen P: Management of virus-induced systemic vasculitides. Curr Rheumatol Rep 4:60, 2002.

37. Zaja F, Russo D, Fuga G, et al: Rituximab for the treatment of type II mixed cryoglobulinemia. Haematologica 84:1157, 1999.

38. Meadow S: Schönlein-Henoch syndrome. In Edelmann C (ed): Pediatric Nephrology. Boston, Little, Brown, 1992, pp 1525-1533.

39. Kauffman R, Herman W, Meyer C, et al: Circulating IgA immune-complexes in Henoch-Schönlein purpura: A longitudinal study of their relationship to disease activity and vascular deposition of IgA. Am J Med 69:859, 1980.

40. Meadow S, Scott D: Berger disease. Henoch-Schönlein purpura without the rash. J Pediatr 106:27, 1985.

41. Blanco R, Martinez-Taboada V, Rodriguez-Valverde V, et al: Henoch-Schönlein purpura in adulthood and childhood: Two different expressions of the same syndrome. Arthritis Rheum 40:859, 1997.

42. O'Donoghue D, Darvill A, Ballardie F: Mesangial cell autoantigens in immunoglobulin A nephropathy and Henoch-Schönlein purpura. J Clin Invest 88:1522, 1991.

43. Cameron J: Henoch-Schönlein purpura: Clinical presentation. Contrib Nephrol 40:246, 1984.

44. Habib R, Niaudet P, Levy M: Schönlein-Henoch purpura nephritis and IgA nephropathy. In Tisher C, Brenner B (eds): Renal Pathology with Clinical and Functional Correlations. Philadelphia, JB Lippincott, 1993, pp 472-523.

45. Goldstein A, White R, Akuse R, Chantler C. Long term follow-up of childhood Henoch-Schönlein nephritis. Lancet 339:280, 1992.

46. Garcia-Porrua C, Calvin M, Lora J, et al: Henoch-Schönlein purpura in children and adults: Clinical differences in a defined population. Sem Arthritis Rheum 32:149, 2002.

47. Ilan Y, Naparstek Y: Henoch Schönlein purpura in children and adults: Is it one entity? Sem Arthritis Rheum 32:139, 2002.

48. Donadio J, Grande J: IgA nephropathy. N Engl J Med 347:738, 2002.

49. Niaudet P, Murcia I, Beaufils H, et al: Primary IgA nephropathies in children: Prognosis and treatment. Adv Nephrol Necker Hosp 22:121, 1993.

50. Bergstein J, Leiser J, Andreoli S: Response of crescentic Henoch-Schönlein purpura nephritis to corticosteroid and azathioprine therapy. Clin Nephrol 49:9, 1998.

51. Rostoker G, Desvaux-Belghiti D, Pilatte Y, et al: High-dose immunoglobulin therapy for severe IgA nephropathy and Henoch-Schönlein purpura. Ann Intern Med 120:476, 1994.

52. McCain M, Quinet R, Davis W: Etanercept and infliximab associated with cutaneous vasculitis. Rheumatology 41:116-117, 2002.

86

Behçet's Disease

RACHEL A. GARTON · JAYASHRI V. GHATE · JOSEPH L. JORIZZO

Behçet's disease is a chronic disease with multisystem involvement characterized clinically by oral and genital aphthae, cutaneous lesions, and ophthalmologic, neurologic, or gastrointestinal manifestations (or some combination of these). The first description of Behçet's disease was probably by Hippocrates in the fifth century BC,[1] and the first modern account was presented in 1937 by the Turkish dermatologist Hulusi Behçet, who reported on a patient with recurrent oral and genital aphthae and uveitis.[2]

Epidemiology

Although Behçet's disease is seen worldwide, the highest prevalence is reported in Japan, the Middle East, and the Mediterranean region (i.e., "the silk route"), and it is relatively uncommon in northern Europe and the United States.[3] The age at which manifestations that fulfill diagnostic criteria occur is typically in the range of the midtwenties to thirties.[4] In the past, Behçet's disease was thought to predominantly affect males, but more current epidemiologic data show a more equal male-to-female ratio.[5] Overall, males are more affected in the Middle East, whereas females predominate in northern Europe and the United States.[5]

Diagnosis and Patient Evaluation

The diagnosis of Behçet's disease is sometimes difficult to confirm, particularly in patients with partial symptomatology. Clinicians and investigators alike must rely on clinical criteria because there are no pathognomonic laboratory findings. Several diagnostic criteria sets have been proposed, including those by O'Duffy and Goldstein,[6] Mason and Barnes,[7] and the Japanese study group.[8] In 1990, the International Study Group established a set of criteria based on the presence of recurrent oral aphthae along with two additional findings from the following list: recurrent genital aphthae, cutaneous lesions, ocular involvement, and a positive result on pathergy testing[9] (Table 86-1). These criteria were found to have a sensitivity of 91 percent and specificity of 96 percent.[9] Although not required by the International Study Group criteria, inflammatory bowel disease (IBD), systemic lupus erythematosus (SLE), Reiter's syndrome, and herpetic infections should first be excluded, because the presenting manifestations of these conditions are often similar to those of Behçet's disease. The O'Duffy-Goldstein criteria also mandate the presence of recurrent oral aphthae plus at least two of the following: genital aphthae, synovitis, posterior uveitis, cutaneous pustular vasculitis, and meningoencephalitis. Patients who have only two of these findings, one being recurrent oral aphthae, are considered to have an incomplete form of Behçet's disease. Another concern over the International Study Group criteria is the inclusion of acneiform lesions, which are a common nonspecific finding in both adolescents and adults. Therefore our group has advocated histologic confirmation of vessel-based histology to exclude acne lesions.[10]

All patients presenting with recurrent oral or genital aphthae should undergo testing for herpes simplex virus (HSV) infection by means of culture or polymerase chain reaction (PCR) assay to rule out this common cause of aphthous lesions. Initial evaluation should also include referral for ophthalmologic consultation to identify insidious ocular involvement. Patients who have arthralgias, gastrointestinal symptoms, or neurologic abnormalities may need

TABLE 86–1 · INTERNATIONAL STUDY GROUP CRITERIA FOR THE DIAGNOSIS OF BEHÇET'S DISEASE*

Recurrent Oral Ulceration
Minor aphthous, major aphthous, or herpetiform ulceration observed by physician or patient that recurred at least three times in one 12-month period *Plus two of the following criteria:*
Recurrent Genital Ulceration
Aphthous ulceration or scarring observed by physician or patient
Eye Lesions
Anterior uveitis, posterior uveitis, or cells in vitreous on slit-lamp examination *or* Retinal vasculitis observed by ophthalmologist
Skin Lesions
Erythema nodosum observed by physician or patient, pseudofolliculitis, or papulopustular lesions *or* Acneiform nodules observed by physician in postadolescent patients not on corticosteroid treatment
Positive Result on Pathergy Testing
Read by physician at 24 to 48 hr

*Findings applicable only in absence of other clinical explanations.

Data from International Study Group for Behçet's Disease: Criteria for the diagnosis of Behçet's disease. Lancet 335:1078-1080, 1990.

further workup such as radiographic studies and evaluation by appropriate specialists. Cutaneous pustular lesions, erythema nodosum–like lesions, and pyoderma gangrenosum–like lesions should be biopsied (both for histologic evaluation and culture) to confirm the diagnosis.

Pathogenesis

The pathogenesis of Behçet's disease remains unknown, but theories include many etiologic factors such as genetics, infections, immune regulation, and inflammatory mediators.

GENETICS

A familial pattern of Behçet's disease has been reported, but there are regional differences throughout the world. Familial occurrence is more common in Korea, Israel, Turkey, and Arab countries, compared to Japan, China, and Europe.[5] Studies have shown a significant association between the human leukocyte antigen (HLA)-B51 and Behçet's disease.[11,12] The relative risk of HLA-B51–positive individuals to develop Behçet's disease varies depending on the geographic region of the world.[5] Moreover, the role of HLA-B51 in the etiology of Behçet's disease is unclear. It may be that HLA-B51 is not directly involved in the etiology of the disease, but instead it may be closely linked to disease-related genes.[13] Candidate genes have been localized to chromosome 6 and include the major histocompatibility complex class I related gene, (MICA), (specifically the MICA6 allele), perth block, (PERB), new organization associated with HLA-B, (NOB), and transporter associated with antigen processing genes, (TAP) genes.[13]

Although Behçet's disease has many features in common with the spondyloarthropathies, especially those associated with IBD, the disorder in IBD patients generally evolves in a pattern resembling Reiter's syndrome, and HLA-B27 is not associated with Behçet's disease.[14] Patients who are HLA-DR1 and HLA-DQw1 positive may have an innate resistance to the development of Behçet's disease.[15]

INFECTIOUS AGENTS

Several studies have suggested a role for various infectious agents in the pathogenesis of Behçet's disease; however, no organisms have been consistently isolated. Antistreptococcal antibodies have been isolated in the serum of patients with Behçet's disease.[16] Higher concentrations of *Streptococcus sanguis* have also been found in the oral flora of patients with Behçet's disease and may play a role in the development of aphthae, which is often the initial manifestation.[17] In addition to streptococcal antigens, other bacteria, such as *Escherichia coli* and *Staphylococcus aureus* may have a role in Behçet's disease through the activation of lymphocytes.[18]

HSV DNA has been isolated from the nuclei of peripheral blood lymphocytes by PCR assay in patients with Behçet's disease.[15] HSV has also been detected by PCR assay in biopsy samples of genital ulcers in these patients.[19] Other studies, however, have shown no difference in the detection of HSV in patients with Behçet's disease with oral aphthae compared to those without aphthae.[20]

IMMUNE MECHANISMS

Immune mechanisms play a major role in Behçet's disease, including heat-shock proteins (HSPs), cytokines, alteration in neutrophil and macrophage activity, and autoimmune mechanisms.[13] HSPs are released in response to stress. HSPs have been found to share a significant sequence homology with microbial HSPs and may be involved in stimulating the immune response.[18] Most of the T lymphocytes thought to be involved in this reaction are of the $\gamma\delta$ type.[21] Cytokines such as interleukin-1 (IL-1), IL-8, and tumor necrosis factor-α (TNF-α) seem to involved in the pathogenesis, and elevated levels may be a marker of disease activity.[13] The production of these proinflammatory cytokines, which are responsible for the chronic inflammation observed, may be the result of activated macrophages.[13,22] In addition to macrophage activation, neutrophil chemotaxis and phagocytosis are increased in lesions of Behçet's disease.[13,23] This overactivity of neutrophils leads to tissue injury in the form of the neutrophilic vascular reaction seen in lesions such as aphthae, pustular lesions, and erythema nodosum–like lesions. Circulating immune complexes also play a role in precipitating the characteristic neutrophilic vascular reaction.[24] Finally, the role of endothelial cell dysfunction in the pathogenesis of Behçet's disease has been suggested by decreased levels of prostacyclin in the serum of Behçet's disease patients. Other abnormalities in the endothelium and with clotting factors have also been found.[25]

Overall, the pathogenesis is not completely understood, but likely an infectious or other environmental agent triggers an inflammatory cascade in a genetically predisposed individual. Please see the recent review by Zouboulis and May for an excellent overview of the pathogenesis of Behçet's disease.[13]

Clinical Features

APHTHAE

Oral aphthae often denote the onset of Behçet's disease and constitute a requisite diagnostic feature (Fig. 86-1), although anecdotally a number of investigators believe that this disease can occur in the absence of oral aphthae. Oral ulcerations may occur in a herpetiform configuration or as individual lesions on the buccal mucosa, gingiva, lips, and tongue. Aphthae tend to be painful and shallow, and they heal without scarring over a period of 1 to 3 weeks.[26] Genital ulcers typically occur on the scrotum and penis in males and on the vulva or vagina in females. These aphthae are similar in appearance to oral lesions, but they have a greater tendency toward scarring and may recur less frequently.[26] Recurrent aphthous stomatitis and complex aphthosis,

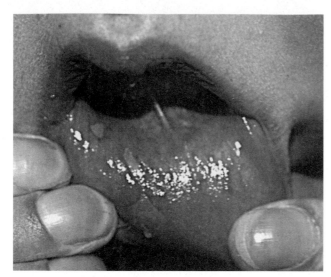

FIGURE 86–1 · Patient with Multiple Aphthae on Oral Mucosa Characteristic of Behçet's Disease.

defined as recurrent oral and genital aphthous ulcers or almost constant, multiple (3 or more) oral aphthae, should be considered in the differential diagnosis of patients presenting with oral or genital aphthae.[27] Also included in the differential diagnosis are HSV infection, Reiter's syndrome, and IBD.

CUTANEOUS LESIONS

Several cutaneous manifestations of Behçet's disease have been described. These include erythema nodosum–like lesions, pyoderma gangrenosum–like lesions (Fig. 86-2), Sweet's syndrome–like lesions, cutaneous small vessel vas-

culitis and pustular lesions including the so-called pathergy lesion.[26] Specimens from all these lesions demonstrate a neutrophilic vascular reaction on histopathologic analysis.[28] Acneiform or pseudofolliculitis lesions should be considered nonspecific, nondiagnostic findings because of their common occurrence in acne and folliculitis.

OPHTHALMOLOGIC FEATURES

A variety of ocular manifestations of Behçet's disease (see Chapter 44) have been reported, including anterior and posterior uveitis, retinal vasculitis, and hypopyon, with secondary glaucoma, cataract formation, decreased acuity and synechiae formation.[29] Ocular involvement occurs in 83 to 95 percent of men and 67 to 73 percent of women with Behçet's disease.[29] Although ocular involvement is not commonly the presenting feature of Behçet's disease, it is a major source of serious morbidity and close ophthalmologic evaluation and follow-up is critical to prevent blindness in these patients.[30]

ARTHRITIS

Patients with Behçet's disease generally present with a nonerosive inflammatory symmetric or asymmetric oligoarthritis, although polyarticular and monarticular forms are also seen. The most commonly involved joints are the knees, wrists, ankles, and elbows.[31] The prevalence of arthritis among different populations ranges from 40 to 60 percent, and destructive joint lesions are not usually observed.[30] Dilsen and colleagues reported that 10 percent of patients with Behçet's disease had a sacroiliitis.[32] However, HLA-B27–positive patients were not excluded from their series. Other studies have shown

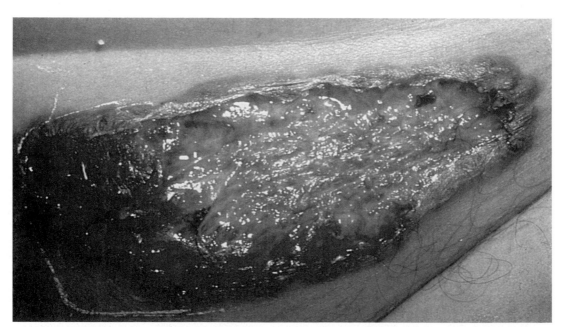

FIGURE 86–2 · Pyoderma Gengrenosum–Like Lesion on the Lower Abdomen of a Patient with Behçet's Disease. (From Manglesdorf HC, White WL, Jorizzo JL: Behçet's disease. Report of twenty-five patients from the United States with prominent mucocutaneous involvement. J Am Acad Dermatol 34:745-750, 1996.)

no significant difference in the occurrence of sacroiliitis between patients with Behçet's disease and the normal population. HLA-B27–positive patients with erosive sacroiliitis should be included in the Reiter's syndrome or enteropathic arthritis disease spectrum due to the erosive axial nature of the arthritis in the HLA-B27 spectrum pattern vs. the non-erosive, non axial nature of the arthritis in Behçet's disease. Both groups may have opthal and ocular lesions. Patients who have had Bilroth II surgery or bowel bypass may present with features similar to those of Behçet's disease, with aphthosis and therefore Goldstein exclusion of patients with IBD is appropriate.

Biopsy specimens of the synovial membrane reveal a neutrophilic reaction with occasional plasma cells and lymphocytes. Immunofluorescence microscopy may show immunoglobulin G (IgG) deposition along the synovial membrane.[30] Reports of synovial fluid analysis in patients with Behçet's disease show leukocyte counts ranging from 300 to 36,200 cells/mm^3, with a predominance of neutrophils and normal glucose levels.[34] Synovitis is included as one of the O'Duffy-Goldstein criteria for the diagnosis of Behçet's disease.[6]

OTHER SYSTEMIC MANIFESTATIONS

Central nervous system (CNS) involvement is most commonly characterized by brain stem or corticospinal tract syndromes (neuro-Behçet syndrome), venous sinus thrombosis, increased intracranial pressure secondary to venous sinus thrombosis or aseptic meningitis, isolated behavioral symptoms, or isolated headache.[35] Rarely, ruptured aneurysms, peripheral neuropathy, optic neuritis, and vestibular involvement can occur.[35] Poor prognosis is associated with a progressive course, parenchymal or brain stem involvement, and cerebrospinal fluid abnormalities.[36]

Patients with Behçet's disease may have gastrointestinal lesions resembling orogenital aphthae, which occur most commonly in the ileocecal region and less often in the ascending or transverse colon or esophagus.[37] Large aphthae may rarely lead to perforation. Presenting symptoms include abdominal pain, diarrhea, and melena. It as important to distinguish IBD from Behçet's disease is discussed above.[37]

Pulmonary abnormalities including pulmonary arterial aneurysms, pulmonary hypertension, embolism, and fibrosis are infrequent manifestations of Behçet's disease. Rupture of a pulmonary artery aneurysm is associated with a high mortality rate.

Renal manifestations of Behçet's disease are uncommon and vary from minimal-change disease to proliferative glomerulonephritis and rapidly progressive crescentic glomerulonephritis.[38] The pathogenesis likely involves immune complex deposition.[38]

Manifestations of cardiac involvement include myocardial infarction, pericarditis, arterial and venous thromboses, and aneurysm formation. Thromboses more commonly involve the venous system, leading to superior and inferior vena cava obstruction.[28] Both cardiac and pulmonary arterial manifestations, either occlusive or aneurysmal, are postulated to occur due to a vasculitis of the vasa vasorum, which induces a thickening of the media and splitting of elastic fibers.[39]

Histopathologic Features

Histopathologic analysis of the lesions of Behçet's disease reveals a neutrophilic vascular reaction or even fully developed leukocytoclastic vasculitis. Microscopic examination of dermal capillary or venule walls shows neutrophilic infiltrates, nuclear dust, and extravasation of erythrocytes with or without fibrinoid necrosis.[40] Immune complex–mediated vasculitis is the likely mechanism in the development of Behçet's disease.[41] A previously reported finding of a lymphocytic vasculitis in patients with Behçet's disease is thought to represent an older lesion.[42]

Prognosis and Clinical Course

Behçet's disease has a variable clinical course in most patients, with a pattern of exacerbations and remissions. A delay in diagnosis after the initial manifestation of Behçet's disease is not uncommon. Most patients present initially with mucocutaneous manifestations, and evidence of ocular and neurologic involvement may appear several years after diagnosis. Patients with the finding of complex aphthosis may represent a forme fruste of Behçet's disease, and the patients should, therefore, be monitored for the development of additional abnormalities fulfilling diagnostic criteria through regular follow-up and referral to appropriate specialists.[27] Mortality is low and usually is related to pulmonary or CNS involvement or bowel perforation.[5] The most common cause of morbidity is ocular involvement, with manifestations such as posterior uveitis, which can cause blindness.

Treatment

Therapeutic options should be based on the degree of involvement[26] (Table 86-2).

MUCOCUTANEOUS DISEASE

Patients with oral and genital aphthae may be treated with intralesional, superpotent, topical or aerosolized (not inhaled) corticosteroids. Topical tacrolimus can also be used, often in combination with superpotent topical corticosteroids. Other palliative therapies include the use of oral tetracycline solutions, topical anesthetics, and rinses containing chlorhexidine gluconate. Oral colchicine, 0.6 mg two to three times daily, can decrease the size and frequency of mucocutaneous lesions.[43,44] Doses may be adjusted according to the degree of gastrointestinal upset experienced by the patient. Dapsone in a dose of 50 to 100 mg/day is often helpful alone[45] or in combination with colchicine.[26] Patients must be monitored for the development of hemolytic anemia and methemoglobinemia; the glucose 6-phosphate dehydro-

TABLE 86-2 • TREATMENT OF BEHÇET'S DISEASE

Mucocutaneous Disease

Topical, intralesional, or aerosolized corticosteroids
Local anesthetics
Topical tacrolimus
Colchicine (0.6 to 1.8 mg/day)
Dapsone (50 to 100 mg/day)
Combinations of these agents

Severe Mucocutaneous Disease

Thalidomide (100 mg/day)
Methotrexate (7.5 to 20 mg/wk)
Prednisone
Interferon alfa (3 to 9 million U/wk)

Systemic Disease

Prednisone (1 mg/kg/day)
Azathioprine
Chlorambucil
Cyclophosphamide
Cyclosporine
Anti–tumor necrosis factor (TNF)-α agents (infliximab [3 mg/kg,
    6 to 8 wk], etanercept [25 mg sq, 2 wk])

genase (G6PD) level should be checked in all patients before beginning therapy with dapsone.

SEVERE MUCOCUTANEOUS DISEASE

Patients who fail to respond to conservative therapy as outlined for mucocutaneous disease may require thalidomide (see Chapter 61), whose mechanism of action is thought to be mediated via modulation of TNF-α and other cytokines. Previous studies have shown that thalidomide is a relatively safe and effective agent for treatment of Behçet's disease.[46,47] Thalidomide is known to cause severe teratogenicity, and all patients and prescribing physicians must adhere to the System for Thalidomide Education and Prescribing Safety (STEPS) protocol, including monthly follow-up visits.[48,49] Patients receiving thalidomide can be monitored for the development of peripheral neuropathy with nerve conduction studies if clinically warranted.

Low-dose weekly oral methotrexate (7.5 to 20 mg/week) and low-dose prednisone are alternatives for patients with severe mucocutaneous involvement.[44,50] Patients receiving methotrexate should be monitored for the development of hepatotoxicity and leukopenia (see Chapter 57). In addition, interferon alpha has been shown to be effective for severe mucocutaneous lesions and some systemic manifestions.[51,52] A review of the safety and efficacy of interferon alfa by Zouboulis and Orfanos recommended a 3-month high-dose regimen of 9 million units 3 times per week, followed by a low, maintenance dose of 3 million units 3 times per week.[51]

SYSTEMIC DISEASE

Patients with systemic disease such as ocular and cardiovascular abnormalities require immunosuppressive ther-

apy, particularly in view of the risk of morbidity and mortality resulting from untreated disease. Systemic corticosteroids may be used alone or in combination with other immunosuppressive agents such as azathioprine, interferon-alpha cyclosporine, cyclophosphamide, and chlorambucil.[44,53] Standard of care for eye disease is prednisone plus azathioprine.[54] If this combination is not successful, one of the aforementioned immunosuppressive agents may be substituted for the azathioprine.[53] Several of these immunosuppressive agents have associated hematologic toxicity, as well as the potential to cause malignancies; therefore, close monitoring is essential. There have also been more recent reports of Behçet's disease treated with the newer anti-TNF agents, infliximab and etanercept.[55] Larger studies looking at the long-term efficacy and safety of these agents are in progress.

REFERENCES

1. Feigenbaum A: Description of Behçet's syndrome in the Hippocratic third book of endemic diseases. Br J Ophthalmol 40:355, 1956.
2. Behçet H: Uber rezidivierende Aphthose durch ein Virus verursachte Geschwure am Mund, am Auge, und an den Genitalien. Dermatol Wochenschr 105:1152-1157, 1937.
3. Dilsen N: History and development of Behçet's disease [Abstract]. Rev Rhum Engl Ed 63:512-519, 1996.
4. Hegab S, Samia A: Immunopathogenesis of Behçet's disease. Clin Immunol 96:174-186, 2000.
5. Zouboulis CC: Epidemiology of Adamantiades-Behçet's disease. In Bang D, Lang E-S, Lee S (eds): Behçet's Disease: Proceedings of the 8th and 9th International Conference on Behçet's disease. Seoul, Design Mecca, 2000, pp 43-47.
6. O'Duffy JD, Goldstein NP: Neurologic involvement in seven patients with Behçet's disease. Am J Med 61:17-18, 1976.
7. Mason RM, Barnes CG: Behçet's syndrome with arthritis. Ann Rheum Dis 28:95-103, 1969.
8. Behçet's Disease Research Committee of Japan: Behçet's disease: A guide to diagnosis of Behçet's disease. Jpn J Ophthalmol 18:291-294, 1974.
9. International Study Group for Behçet's Disease: Criteria for the diagnosis of Behçet's disease. Lancet 335:1078-1080, 1990.
10. Jorizzo JL: Behçet's disease. In Fitzpatrick TB, Eisen AZ, Wolff K, et al (eds): Dermatology in General Medicine, 5th ed. New York, McGraw-Hill, 1999, pp 2161-2165.
11. Yazici H, Chamberlain MA, Schreuder I, et al: HLA antigens in Behçet's disease: A reappraisal by a comparative study of Turkish and British patients. Ann Rheum Dis 39:344-348, 1980.
12. Ohno S, Ohguchi M, Hirose S, et al: Close association of HLA-BW51 with Behçet's disease. Arch Ophthalmol 100:1455-1458, 1982.
13. Zouboulis CC, May T: Pathogenesis of Adamantiades-Behçet's disease. Adv Exp Med Biol 528: 161-71, 2003.
14. O'Duffy JD, Taswell HF, Elveback LR: HLA antigens in Behçet's disease. J Rheumatol 3:1-3, 1976.
15. Jorizzo JL: Behçet's disease: An update based on the 1985 International Conference in London. Arch Dermatol 122: 556-558, 1986.
16. Mizushima Y: Behçet's disease. Curr Opin Rheumatol 3:32-35, 1991.
17. Isogai E, Ohno S, Kotake S, et al: Chemiluminescence of neutrophils from patients with Behçet's disease and its correlation with an increased proportion of uncommon serotypes of *Streptococcus sanguis* in the oral flora. Arch Oral Biol 35:43-48, 1990.
18. Direskeneli H: Behçet's disease: infectious aetiology, new autoantigens, and HLA-B51. Ann Rheum Dis 60:996-1002, 2001.
19. Bang D, Cho YH, Choi H-J, et al: Detection of herpes simplex virus DNA by polymerase chain reaction in genital ulcers of patients with Behçet's disease [Abstract]. Rev Rhum Engl Educ 63:532, 1996.

20. Lee S, Bang D, Cho YH: Polymerase chain reaction reveals herpes simplex virus DNA in saliva of patients with Behçet's disease. Arch Dermatol Res 288:179-183, 1996.

21. Hasan A, Fortune F, Wilson A, et al: Role of gamma delta T cells in the pathogenesis and diagnosis of Behçet's disease. Lancet 347:789-794,1996.

22. Sahin S, Lawrence R, Direskeneli H, et al: Monocyte activity in Behçet's disease. Br J Rheum 35:424-429, 1996.

23. Takeno M, Kariyone A, Yamashita N, et al: Excessive function of peripheral blood neutrophils from patients with Behçet's disease and from HLA-B51 transgenic mice. Arthritis Rheum 38:426-433, 1995.

24. Gupta RC, O'Duffy JD, McDuffie FC, et al: Circulating immune complexes in active Behçet's disease. Clin Exp Immunol 34: 213-218, 1978.

25. Saylan T, Mat C, Fresko I, et al: Behçet's disease in the Middle East. Clin Dermatol 17:209-223, 1999.

26. Ghate JV, Jorizzo JL: Behçet's disease and complex aphthosis. J Am Acad Dermatol 40:1-8, 1999.

27. McCarty MA, Garton RA, Jorizzo JL: Complex aphthosis and Behçet's disease. Dermatol Clin 21:41-48, 2003.

28. Jorizzo JL, Solomon AR, Zanollu MD, et al: Neutrophilic vascular reactions. J Am Acad Dermatol 19:983-1005, 1988.

29. Bhisitkul RB, Foster CS: Diagnosis and ophthalmological features of Behçet's disease. Int Ophthalmol Clin 36:127-134, 1996.

30. Kaklamani VG, Vaiopoulos G, Kaklamanis PG: Behçet's disease. Semin Arthritis Rheum 27:197-215, 1998.

31. Moral F, Hamuryudan V, Yurdakul S, et al: Inefficacy of azapropazone in the acute arthritis of Behçet's syndrome: A randomized, double blind, placebo controlled study. Clin Exp Rheumatol 13:493-495, 1995.

32. Dilsen N, Konice M, Aral O: Why Behçet's disease should be accepted as a seronegative arthritis. *In* Lehner T, Barnes CG (eds): Recent Advances in Behçet's Disease. International Congress and Symposium Series No. 103. London/New York, Royal Society of Medicine Services, 1986, pp 281-284.

33. Jorizzo JL, Apisarnthanarax P, Subrt P, et al. Bowel-bypass syndrome without bowel bypass: Bowel-associated dermatosis-arthritis syndrome. Arch Intern Med 84:572-573, 1976.

34. Yurdakul S, Yazici H, Tuzun Y, et al: The arthritis of Behçet's disease: A prospective study. Ann Rheum Dis 42:505-515, 1983.

35. Siva A, Kantarci OH, Saip S, et al: Behçet's disease: diagnostic and prognostic aspects of neurological involvement. J Neurol 248: 95-103, 2001.

36. Akman-Demir G, Serdaroglu P, Tasçi B, the Neuro-Behçet Study Group: Clinical patterns of neurological involvement in Behçet's disease: evaluation of 200 patients. Brain 122:2171-2181, 1999.

37. Sakane T, Takeno M, Suzuki N, et al: Behçet's Disease. N Engl J Med 341:1284-1291, 1999.

38. El Ramahi KM, Al Dalaan A, Al Shaikh A, et al: Renal involvement in Behçet's disease: review of 9 cases. J Rheumatol 25:2254-2260, 1998.

39. Du LTH, Wechsler B, Piette J, et al: Long-term prognosis of arterial lesions in Behçet's disease. *In* WechslerB, Godeau P (eds): Behçet's disease: Proceedings of the 6th International Conference on Behçet's disease. Paris, France, 30 June -1 July, 1993. Amsterdam, Elsevier Science, 1993, pp 557-562.

40. Ackerman AB: Behçet's disease. *In* Ackerman AB, Chongchitnant N, Sanchez J, et al (eds): Histologic Diagnosis of Inflammatory Skin Diseases. An Algorithmic Method Based on Pattern Analysis, 2nd ed. Baltimore, Williams & Wilkins, 1997, pp 229-232.

41. Jorizzo JL, Soloman AR, Cavaloo T: Behçet's syndrome: Immunopathological and histopathologic assessment of pathergy lesions is useful in diagnosis and follow-up. Arch Pathol Lab Med 109:747, 1985.

42. Lakhanpal S, Tani K, Lie JT, et al: Pathologic features of Behçet's syndrome: A review of Japanese autopsy registry data. Hum Pathol 16:790, 1985.

43. Miyachi Y, Taniguchi S, Ozaki M et al: Colchine in the treatment of cutaneous manifestations of Behçet's disease. Br J Dermatol 104:67-69, 1981.

44. Kaklamani VG, Kaklamanis PG: Treatment of Behçet's disease: An update. Semin Arthritis Rheum 30:299-312, 2001.

45. Sharquie KE, Najim RA, Abu-Raghif AR: Dapsone in Behçet's disease: a double-blind, placebo-controlled, cross-over study. J Dermatol 29:267-279, 2002.

46. Hamuryudan V, Mat C, Saip S, et al: Thalidomide in the treatment of the mucocutaneous lesions of Behçet's syndrome: A randomized double-blinded, placebo controlled trial. Ann Intern Med 128:443-450, 1998.

47. De Wazieres B, Gil H, Vuitton DA, et al: Treatment of recurrent oro-genital ulceration with low doses of thalidomide. Clin Exp Rheumatol 17:393 1999.

48. Housman TS, Jorizzo JL, McCarty AM, et al: Low-dose thalidomide therapy for refractory cutaneous lesions of lupus erythematosus. Arch Dermatol 139:50-54, 2003.

49. Thalidomide STEPS [booklet]. Warren, NJ, Celgene Corporation, 1999.

50. Jorizzo JL, White WL, Wise CM, et al: Low-dose weekly methotrexate for unusual neutrophilic vascular reactions: cutaneous polyarteritis nodosa and Behçet's disease. J Am Acad Dermatol 24:973-978, 1991.

51. Zouboulis CC, Orfanos CE. Treatment of Adamantiades-Behçet disease with systemic interferon alpha. Arch Dermatol 134: 1010-1016, 1998.

52. O'Duffy JD, Calamia K, Cohen S, et al: Alpha interferon treatment of Behçet's disease. J Rheumatol 25:1938-1944, 1998.

53. Green JJ, Jorizzo JL: Behçet disease. *In* Lebwohl M, Heymann WR, Berth-Jones J, Coulson I (eds): Treatment of Skin Disease: Comprehensive Therapeutic Strategies, 1st ed. London, Harcourt Publishers Limited, 2002, pp 86-89.

54. Yazici H, Pazarli H, Barnes CG, et al: A controlled trial of azathioprine in Behçet syndrome. N Engl J Med 322:281-285, 1990.

55. Sfikakis PP: Behçet's disease: a new target for anti-tumour necrosis factor treatment. Ann Rheum Dis 61:ii51-ii53, 2002.

Crystal-induced Inflammation

87

Gout and Hyperuricemia

R O B E R T L . W O R T M A N N · W I L L I A M N . K E L L E Y

Gout has been called the "king of diseases" and the "disease of kings." Today, the term *gout* is used to represent a heterogeneous group of diseases found exclusively in the human species that include:

1. An elevated serum urate concentration (hyperuricemia)
2. Recurrent attacks of acute arthritis in which monosodium urate monohydrate crystals are demonstrable in synovial fluid leukocytes
3. Aggregates of sodium urate monohydrate crystals (tophi) deposited chiefly in and around joints, which sometimes lead to deformity and crippling
4. Renal disease involving glomerular, tubular, and interstitial tissues and blood vessels
5. Uric acid nephrolithiasis

These manifestations can occur in various combinations.[1]

Hyperuricemia is a term representing an elevated level of urate in the blood. This occurs in an absolute (or physiochemical) sense when the serum urate concentration exceeds the limit of solubility of monosodium urate in the serum, which is about 7 mg/dl at 37°C. Thus, a value greater than this represents supersaturation of body fluids. The serum urate concentration is elevated in a relative sense when it exceeds the upper limit of an arbitrary normal range, which is usually defined as the mean serum urate value plus two standard deviations in a sex-and age-matched healthy population. In most epidemiologic studies, the upper limit has been rounded off at 7 mg/dl in men and 6 mg/dl in women. Finally, a serum urate value in excess of 7 mg/dl begins to carry an increased risk of gouty arthritis or renal stones. For these reasons, hyperuricemia is defined as a true serum urate concentration greater than 7 mg/dl.

Epidemiology

Hyperuricemia is fairly common, with a prevalence ranging between 2.3 to 41.4 percent in various populations.[2] A variety of factors appear to be associated with higher serum urate concentrations. In adults, serum urate levels correlate strongly with the serum creatinine and urea nitrogen levels, body weight, height, age, blood pressure, and alcohol intake.[3] In epidemiologic studies, body bulk (as estimated by body weight, surface area, or body mass index) has proved to be one of the most important predictors of hyperuricemia in people of widely differing races and cultures with rare exceptions.[4,5]

Serum urate concentrations vary with the age and sex. Children normally have a concentration in the range of 3 to 4 mg/dl because of high renal uric acid clearance.[6] At puberty, serum urate concentrations increase by 1 to 2 mg/dl in males, with this higher level generally sustained throughout life. In contrast, females exhibit little change in their serum urate concentrations until menopause, when concentrations increase to approach the values seen for adult men.[7] The mechanism of lower serum urate levels in women is a consequence of sex hormones and is related to a higher fractional excretion of urate secondary to lower tubular urate postsecretory reabsorption.[8]

The incidence of gout varies in populations, with an overall prevalence of less than 1 to 15.3 percent[3] and appears to be increasing.[9] The prevalence seems to increase substantially with age and increasing serum urate concentration. The annual incidence rate of gout is 4.9 percent for urate levels greater than 9 mg/dl, 0.5 percent for values between 7 and 8.9 mg/dl, and 0.1 percent for values less than 7 mg/dl.[10] For serum urate values greater than 9 mg/dl, the cumulative incidence of gout reaches 22 percent after 5 years.

Clinical Features

In the complete development of its natural history, gout passes through four stages: 1) asymptomatic hyperuricemia, 2) acute gouty arthritis, 3) intercritical (or interval) gout, and 4) chronic tophaceous gout. The basic pattern of clinical gout begins with acute attacks of intensely painful arthritis. The first attack is usually monarticular and associated with few constitutional symptoms. Later, attacks become polyarticular and associated with fever. Attacks vary in duration but are time limited. The intervals between attacks are termed *inter-critical* (or interval) gout. Over time, attacks recur at shorter intervals, last longer, and eventually resolve incompletely. This leads to the development of chronic arthritis that progresses slowly to a crippling disease on which acute exacerbations are superimposed.

ASYMPTOMATIC HYPERURICEMIA

Asymptomatic hyperuricemia is a situation in which the serum urate level is high, but gout—as manifested by arthritic symptoms, tophi, or uric acid nephrolithiasis—has not yet appeared. Most people with hyperuricemia remain asymptomatic throughout their lifetime. The tendency toward acute gout increases with the serum urate concentration. The risk of nephrolithiasis increases with the serum urate level and with the magnitude of daily urinary uric acid excretion. The phase of asymptomatic hyperuricemia ends with the first attack of gouty arthritis or urolithiasis. In most instances, this occurs after at least 20 years of sustained hyperuricemia. Between 10 and 40 percent of gouty subjects have one or more attacks of renal colic before the first articular event.

ACUTE GOUTY ARTHRITIS

The first attack of acute gouty arthritis usually occurs between ages 40 and 60 years in men and after age 60 years in women.[8] Onset before age 25 should raise the question of an unusual form of gout, perhaps related to a specific enzymatic defect that causes marked purine overproduction, an unusual renal disorder, or the use of cyclosporine.

A single joint is involved in about 85 to 90 percent of first attacks, with the first metatarsophalangeal joint being the most commonly affected site. The percentage of patients in whom the initial attack is polyarticular ranges from 3 to 14 percent. Acute gout is predominantly a disease of the lower extremity, but any joint of any extremity may be involved. Ninety percent of patients experience acute attacks in the great toe at some time during the course of their disease. Next in order of frequency are the insteps, ankles, heels, knees, wrists, fingers, and elbows. Acute attacks rarely affect the shoulders, hips, spine, sacroiliac joints, sternoclavicular joints, acromioclavicular joints, or temporomandibular joints.[11-13] Acute gouty bursitis also occurs and mainly involves the prepatellar or olecranon bursa.[14] Urate deposition and subsequent gout appear to have a predilection for previously damaged joints. Gout occurs in the Heberden nodes of older women.[15]

Some patients report a history of short, trivial episodes of "ankle sprains," sore heels, or twinges of pain in the great toe before the first dramatic gouty attack. In most patients, however, the initial attack occurs with explosive suddenness and commonly begins at night after the individual had gone to sleep feeling well. Within a few hours after onset, the affected joint becomes hot, dusky red, swollen, and extremely tender. Occasionally, lymphangitis may develop. Systemic signs of inflammation may

include leukocytosis, fever, and elevation of the erythrocyte sedimentation rate (ESR). Radiographs usually show only soft tissue swelling during early episodes.

The course of untreated acute gout is highly variable. Mild attacks may subside in several hours or persist for only a day or two and never reach the intensity described for the classic attack. Severe attacks may last days to weeks. The skin over the joint may desquamate as the attack subsides. With resolution, the patient becomes asymptomatic and enters the intercritical period.

Drugs may precipitate acute gout by either increasing or decreasing serum urate levels acutely. The occurrence of gout after the initiation of antihyperuricemic therapy is well established.[16,17] Drug-induced gout secondary to increased serum urate levels occurs on occasion with diuretic therapy, intravenous heparin, and cyclosporine.[18-20] Diuretic therapy in the elderly appears to be a particularly important precipitating factor for gouty arthritis.[18] Other provocative factors include trauma, alcohol ingestion, surgery, dietary excess, hemorrhage, foreign protein therapy, infections, and radiographic contrast exposure.[21,22] The risk of a patient with gout developing an attack during a hospitalization is 20 percent.[23]

The definitive diagnosis of gout is best established by aspiration of the joint and identification of intracellular needle-shaped crystals that have negative birefringence with compensated polarized light microscopy,[23] but criteria have been proposed for the presumptive diagnosis.[24] They include 1) the triad of acute monarticular arthritis, hyperuricemia, and a dramatic response to colchicine therapy; and 2) criteria proposed by the American College of Rheumatology (ACR)[25] (Table 87–1). There are limitations to employing either of these schemes. First, although the diagnosis of acute gouty arthritis can be strongly suggested by the typical picture presentation, not all inflammation of the great toe (podagra) in hyperuremic patients is caused by gout.[26] Second, some patients with gout are normouricemic at

---

TABLE 87–1 • CRITERIA FOR THE CLASSIFICATION FOR ACUTE GOUTY ARTHRITIS

The presence of characteristic urate crystals in the joint fluid, or a tophus proved to contain urate crystals by chemical means or polarized light microscopy, or the presence of 6 of the following 12 clinical, laboratory, and radiographic phenomena:
* More than one attack of acute arthritis
* Maximal inflammation developed within 1 day
* Attack of monarticular arthritis
* Joint redness observed
* First metatarsophalangeal joint painful or swollen
* Unilateral attack involving first metatarsophalangeal joint
* Unilateral attack involving tarsal joint
* Suspected tophus
* Hyperuricemia
* Asymmetric swelling within a joint (radiograph)
* Subcortical cysts without erosions (radiograph)
* Negative culture of joint fluid for microorganisms during attack of joint inflammation

Adapted from Wallace SL, Robinson H, Masi AT, et al: Preliminary criteria for the classification of acute arthritis of primary gout. Arthritis Rheum 20: 895-900, 1977.

the time of an acute attack, a phenomenon related to alcohol use or a consequence of interleukin-6 (IL-6) generation by the acute inflammatory process.[27-29] Next, diseases other than gout that may improve with colchicine therapy include pseudogout, hydroxyapatite calcific tendinitis, sarcoid arthritis, erythema nodosum, serum sickness, rheumatoid arthritis (RA), and familial Mediterranean fever.[30] Finally, the simultaneous presence of both gout and septic arthritis can be confusing clinically, with the former masking the latter.[31]

INTERCRITICAL GOUT

The terms *intercritical gout* and *interval gout* have been applied to the periods between gouty attacks. Some patients never have a second attack. In most patients, a second attack does occur within 6 months to 2 years (but may not develop until after 27 years). In Gutman's[32] series, 62 percent had recurrences within the first year, 16 percent in 1 to 2 years, 11 percent in 2 to 5 years, and 4 percent in 5 to 10 years; 7 percent had experienced no recurrence in 10 or more years. The frequency of gout attacks usually increases with time in untreated patients. Later, attacks have a less-explosive onset, are polyarticular, become more severe, last longer, and abate more gradually. Nevertheless, recovery is complete. Roentgenographic changes may develop during the intercritical period despite no sign of tophi on physical examination. These changes are more likely in those with more severe hyperuricemia and more frequent acute attacks.[23,33]

The diagnosis of gout in a hyperuricemic patient with a history of acute attacks of monarthritis may be difficult or inconclusive during the intercritical phase. Aspiration of an asymptomatic joint, however, can be a useful adjunct in the diagnosis of gout if urate crystals are demonstrated. Joint fluids obtained from gouty patients during the intercritical phase revealed monosodium urate crystals in 12.5 to 90 percent of joints.[34] Such crystals in asymptomatic joints are often associated with mild synovial fluid leukocytosis, which suggests the potential for contribution to joint damage even in the intervals between attacks.

CHRONIC TOPHACEOUS GOUT

Eventually, the patient may enter a phase of chronic polyarticular gout with no pain-free intercritical periods. At this stage, gout may be easily confused with other types of arthritis.[35,36] The time from the initial attack to the beginning of chronic symptoms or visible tophaceous involvement is highly variable in studies of untreated patients. Hench reported intervals ranging from 3 to 42 years, with an average of 11.6 years between the first attack and the development of chronic arthritis.[37] Ten years after the first attack, about half of the individuals were still free of obvious tophi, and most of the remainder had only minimal deposits. Thereafter, the proportion of those with nontophaceous involvement slowly declined, to 28 percent after 20 years. Two percent of the patients had severe crippling disease some 20 years after the initial attack.

The rate of formation of tophaceous deposits correlates with both the degree and the duration of hyperuricemia. The principal determinant is the serum urate level.[23] Gutman found the mean serum urate concentration to be 9.1 mg/dl in 722 patients without tophi, 10 to 12 mg/dl in 456 patients with minimal to moderate tophi, and greater than 11 mg/dl in 11 patients with extensive tophaceous involvement.[38] The rate of tophus formation also increases with the severity of renal disease and the use of diuretics.[18,39]

Tophaceous gout is the consequence of the chronic inability to eliminate urate as rapidly as it is produced. As the urate pool expands, deposits of urate crystals appear in cartilage, synovial membranes, tendons, soft tissues, and elsewhere. Tophi are rarely present at the time of an initial attack[40,41] of primary gout, but have been observed in gout secondary to myeloproliferative diseases, in juvenile gout–complicating glycogen storage diseases (GSDs), in Lesch-Nyhan syndrome, or after allograft transplantation in patients treated with cyclosporine.[30,42]

Tophi can occur in a variety of locations. Tophaceous deposits may produce irregular, asymmetric, moderately discrete tumescence of the fingers (Fig. 87–1), hands, knees, or feet. Tophi also form along the ulnar surfaces of the forearm, as saccular distentions of the olecranon bursa (Fig. 87–2), in the antihelix of the ear (Fig. 87–3), or as fusiform enlargements of the Achilles tendon (Fig. 87–4). The process of tophaceous deposition advances insidiously. Although the tophi themselves are relatively painless, acute inflammation can occur around them at times. Eventually, extensive destruction of the joints and large subcutaneous tophi may lead to grotesque deformities, particularly of the hands and feet, and to progressive crippling. The tense,

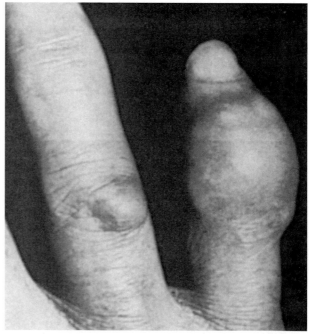

FIGURE 87–1 • Tophus of the Fifth digit, with smaller Tophus over Fourth Proximal Interphalangeal joint.

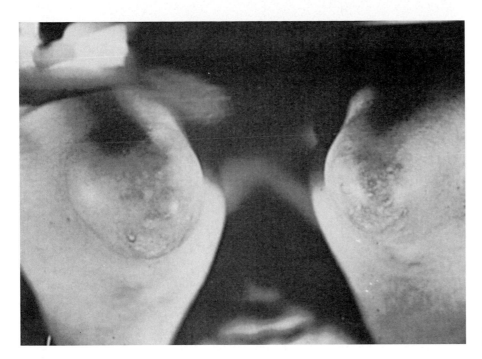

FIGURE 87–2 · Saccular tophaceous enlargements of oclecranon bursae, with small cutaneous deposits of urate.

shiny, thin skin overlying the tophus may ulcerate and extrude white, chalky, or pasty material composed of urate crystals. Secondary infection of tophi is rare.

Typical radiographic changes, particularly erosions with sclerotic margins and overhanging edges, occur with the development of tophi[43,44] (Fig. 87–5). These may be difficult to distinguish from erosions of other causes,[35] but the presence of a thin, overhanging calcified edge is strong evidence of gout. Calcifications can be seen in some tophi, and bony ankylosis may rarely occur. Ultrasonography, magnetic resonance imaging (MRI), and computed tomography (CT) can demonstrate tophi, with the latter providing the more specific images.

Tophi can produce a marked limitation of joint movement by involvement of the joint structure directly or of a tendon serving the joint. Any joint may be involved, although those of the lower extremity are per-

sonally affected. Spinal joints do not escape urate deposition,[45,46] but acute gouty spondylitis is unusual. Symptoms related to nerve or spinal cord compression by tophi have rarely been observed.[12] Tophi may also occur in myocardium, valves,[47] the cardiac conduction system, various parts of the eye, and the larynx. Finally, chronic topahaceous gout can be associated with clinical presentations that can be confused with infectious processes or RA.[35,48]

Genetics of Gout

Since antiquity, gout has been recognized as a familial disorder. The familial incidences reported range from 11 to 80 percent.[30] In two large series, one English and one American, about 40 percent of gouty subjects gave a positive family history of gout. These wide discrepancies may be attributed in part to variations in diligence and pursuit of geneologic data. When all available data are considered, they suggest that serum urate concentrations are controlled by polygenic traits.[2] Several rare forms of hyperuricemia and gout, such as hypoxanthine phosphoribosyltransferase deficiency, increased phosphoribosyl,[1] pyrophosphate synthetase overactivity, and familial hyperuricemia nephropathy, have a genetic basis and will be discussed later.

ASSOCIATED CONDITIONS

The association of gout with obesity and overeating is well recognized. In 6000 subjects, hyperuricemia was found in only 3.4 percent of those with a relative weight at or below the 20th percentile, in 5.7 percent of those between the 21st and 79th percentile, and in 11.4 percent of those at or above the 80th percentile.[49]

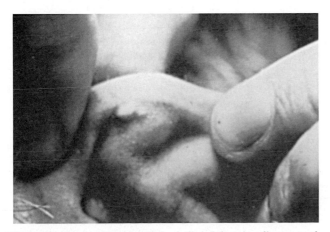

FIGURE 87–3 · Tophus of the helix of the ear adjacent to the auricular tubercle.

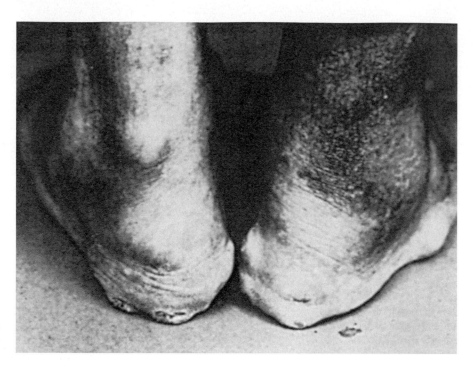

FIGURE 87-4 • Tophi of Achilles tendons and their insertions in a patient with gout.

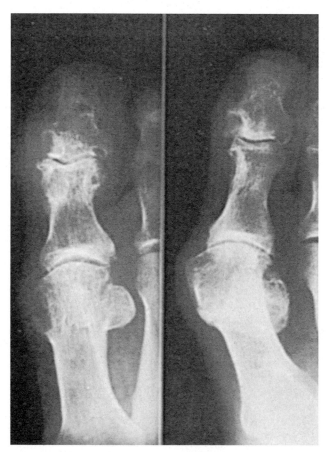

FIGURE 87-5 • These panels show changes typical for bony tophi, including soft tissue distortion, erosions with sclerotic margins, and overwhelming edges. Joint-space narrowing is minimal despite the large erosions. (From Nakayama DA, Barthelemy C, Carrera G, et al: Tophaceous gout: a clinical and radiographic assessment. Arthritis Rheum 27:468, 1984.)

·Hypertriglyceridemia has been reported in 75 to 80 percent of patients with gout,[50] and hyperuricemia is found in more than 80 percent of patients with hypertriglyceridemia.[30] However, studies have been unable to show a correlation between serum urate and cholesterol values or an unique lipid phenotype.[51] It appears that diet and possibly defective clearance of triglyceride may be among the etiologic factors associated with elevated triglyceride and lipoprotein concentrations in gouty individuals. Gouty patients who drink alcohol excessively have mean serum triglyceride levels that are higher than those of their obesity-matched controls and those of non–alcohol drinking gouty patients.[52]

Hyperuricemia has been reported in 2 to 50 percent of patients with diabetes mellitus, and gouty arthritis in less than 0.1 to 9 percent.[53] Abnormal glucose tolerance tests have been noted in 7 to 74 percent of patients with gout,[54] depending, in part, on the criteria used.

Hyperuricemia has been reported in 22 to 38 percent of patients with untreated hypertension. This figure increases to as high as 67 percent when diuretic therapy and renal disease are present.[30] Hyperuricemia may be an indication of potential risk of hypertension for adolescent males.[55-57] Hypertension is present in one fourth to one half of patients with classic gout, but the presence of hypertension is unrelated to duration of gout.[49] Elevated serum urate concentrations are associated with increased tubular reabsorption of sodium.[58] The serum urate concentration also correlates inversely with renal blood flow and urate clearance and directly with both renovascular and total resistance. Therefore, the association between hypertension and hyperuricemia may be related to the reduction of renal blood flow in hypertension. In addition, uric acid causes smooth muscle proliferation in vitro and vascular disease in animal models through a mechanism that involves complex intracellular signaling, mitogen-activated protein (MAP) kinase activation and platelet-derived growth factor (PDGF) expression.[59,60]

The association of hyperuricemia with the manifestations of atherosclerosis has led to speculation that hyperuricemia is a risk factor for coronary artery disease. Some studies show no clear associations between level of blood pressure, blood glucose, or serum cholesterol and serum urate concentration when adjustments were made for effects of age, sex, and relative weight[30,49] and show that the serum urate concentrations of persons with coronary heart disease are not significantly different from the mean levels of the population.[61,62] Other studies, however, maintain that hyperuricemia is an independent risk factor for coronary artery disease.[63,64]

The term *syndrome X* has been applied to a cluster of abnormalities, including resistance to insulin-stimulated glucose uptake, hyperinsulinemia, hypertension, and dyslipoproteinemia, that are characterized by high levels of plasma triglycerides and high-density lipoprotein cholesterol. Hyperuricemia closely correlates with the degree of insulin resistance[65-67] and, therefore, is a likely feature of syndrome X. Syndrome X has been associated with coronary artery disease, and hyperuricemia, as a component of syndrome X, may explain the previously recognized association between coronary artery disease and hyperuricemia.

Hyperuricemia is associated with increased cerebrovascular disease, cardiovascular disease, and cardiovascular mortality.[63,64] It seems likely that in patients with hyperuricemia, clinical correlates such as hypertension, insulin resistance, diabetes mellitus, hyperlipidemia, and obesity contribute meaningfully to the observed association between elevated serum urate concentrations and atherosclerosis. Whether urate levels simply help to identify these patients or play a primary role in the pathogenesis is unclear.

Alcohol consumption has long been associated with hyperuricemia and gout. In susceptible persons, alcohol use can lead to the precipitation of acute gouty arthritis. An epidemiologic study in Saudi Arabia, a country where alcohol consumption is quite rare, revealed a prevalence of hyperuricemia of 8.42 percent of participants but no cases of gout among that group.[68] Both a decrease in the renal excretion of uric acid and an increase in uric acid production seem to be important factors in this association.[69,70] Ethanol increases uric acid production by accelerating the turnover of adenosine triphosphate (ATP). Among alcoholic beverages, beer may have more potent effects on uric acid production because of its high guanosine content.[71]

There appears to be a significant increased prevalence of hypothyroidism among both female patients (25 percent) and male patients with gouty arthritis, in contrast to the rates in control subjects (10 percent and 2 percent, respectively).[72] Hyperuricemia may also be more prevalent in patients with hypothyroidism. Thyroid replacement therapy is associated with a decrease in serum urate concentration caused by an increased uric acid diuresis, a change not explained solely by a change in creatinine clearance.[73] Although the cause of hyperuricemia and gout in patients with hypothyroidism is unknown, it is speculated that urate metabolism is mediated by thyroid-stimulating hormone receptors in extrathyroidal tissues, including the kidney, and that these modulate urate homeostasis.[74]

Studies of acutely ill patients in intensive care units indicate that markedly increased serum urate concentrations, in the range of 20 mg/dl, are associated with hypotensive events and a poor prognosis.[75] This finding may be related to two factors. First, ischemic tissue may foster the degradation of ATP to purine end products, thereby enhancing the production of urate. The finding of increased plasma ATP degradation products associated with hyperuricemia and adult respiratory distress syndrome supports this possibility.[76] Second, the conversion of hypoxanthine to uric acid by xanthine oxidase during ischemia produces oxidant radicals,[77] which are themselves associated with tissue injury. It is possible that inhibition of xanthine oxidase with allopurinol may be a useful therapy in this setting. The substantial antioxidant properties of uric acid have been the subject of speculation[78]; it is possible that these properties may counteract the potent oxidant properties of xanthine oxidase during uric acid synthesis.

Maternal serum urate concentrations normally decrease during pregnancy until the 24th week and then increase until 12 weeks after delivery.[79] An increase in the serum urate level occurs in preeclampsia and toxemia of pregnancy, owing to decrease in the renal clearance of urate.[80] Perinatal mortality is markedly increased when maternal plasma urate levels are raised, usually in association with early-onset preeclampsia. The highest mortality rate is seen with serum urate concentrations higher than 6 mg/dl and diastolic blood pressures greater than 110 mm Hg. Labor itself is associated with an increased serum urate level, with the level remaining elevated for 1 to 2 days after delivery.

Gout is rarely seen in patients with RA, SLE, or ankylosing spondylitis (AS).[81-83] The basis for the decreased concurrence of these disorders is unclear, although the long-term use of nonsteroidal anti-inflammatory drugs (NSAIDs) may mask the clinical features of gout in some of these patients.

Renal Disease

Twenty to 40 percent of patients with gout have albuminuria, which is usually mild and often intermittent. Hyperuricemia alone may be implicated as the cause of renal damage only when the concentration of urate chronically exceeds 13 mg/dl in men or 10 mg/dl in women.[84] Prior to the routine treatment of asymptomatic hypertension, renal failure accounted for 10 percent of the deaths in patients with gout. Today, it appears that moderate hyperuricemia has no direct harmful effect on renal function. Nevertheless, after gouty arthritis, renal problems appear to be the most frequent complication of hyperuricemia. These include urate nephropathy, uric acid nephropathy, and nephrolithiasis.

The term *urate nephropathy* is used to represent the deposition of urate crystals in the interstitium of the medulla

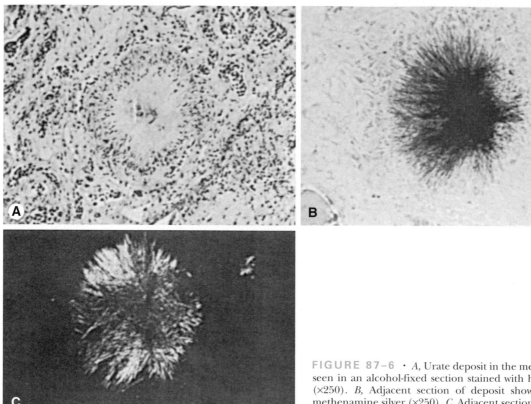

FIGURE 87–6 • *A,* Urate deposit in the medulla of the kidneys as seen in an alcohol-fixed section stained with hemotoxylin and eosin (×250). *B,* Adjacent section of deposit shown in *A,* stained with methenamine silver (×250). *C,* Adjacent section of deposit shown in *A* as seen with polarized light (×250).

and pyramids with a surrounding giant cell reaction, a distinctive histologic finding characteristic of the gouty kidney (Fig. 87–6). Factors such as coexistent hypertension, chronic lead exposure ischemic heart disease, and primary preexistent renal insufficiency, probably play important roles in the pathogenesis of this pathology. Although urate nephropathy appears to exist as a distinct entity, it is not believed to be an important contributor to defining renal function in most gouty patients.[30,85]

In contrast, *uric acid nephropathy* is the term used to represent acute renal failure resulting from the precipitation of large quantities of uric acid crystals in the collecting ducts and ureters. This complication most commonly occurs in patients with leukemia and lymphomas as a result of rapid malignant cell turnover, often during chemotherapy.[86,87] This syndrome (also termed *acute tumor lysis syndrome*) has been more clearly defined as hyperuricemia, lactic acidosis, hyperkalemia, hyperphosphatemia, and hypocalcemia and is most commonly observed in patients with aggressive, rapidly proliferating tumors, including lymphoproliferative disorders and metastatic medulloblastoma.

Uric acid nephropathy is less commonly found with other neoplasms, after epileptic seizures, after vigorous exercise with heat stress, and after angiography and coronary artery bypass surgery.[88]

The large amount of nucleic acid in nucleotides liberated with massive cytolysis is converted rapidly to uric acid. Typically, there is marked hyperuricemia, with a mean serum urate level of 20 mg/dl (range is 12 to 80 mg/dl). The pathogenesis of acute renal failure in uric acid nephropathy is related to the precipitation of uric acid in the distal tubules and collecting ducts, the sites of maximal acidification and concentration of the urine. Oliguria, or even anuria, as well as azotemia may occur. There may be "gravel" or "sand" noted in the urine. The ratio of urinary uric acid to creatinine in these patients typically exceeds 1; in patients with most other causes of acute renal failure, the ratio is 0.4 ± 0.3.[87]

Nephrolithiasis occurs in 10 to 25 percent of patients with primary gout, a prevalence greater than that in the general population. The likelihood of stones in a given patient with gout increases with the serum urate concentration and with amounts of urinary uric acid excretion.[89] It exceeds 50 percent with a serum urate value above 13 mg/dl or with urinary uric acid excretion rates in excess of 1100 mg every 24 hours.

Uric acid calculi, which account for approximately 10 percent of all stones in patients in the United States, range from as low as 5 percent in some countries to 40 percent in Israel and Australia.[30] Uric acid stones do occur in patients with no history of gouty arthritis, and only 20 percent of this group are hyperuricemic. Other renal stone disease is associated with hyperuricemia and gout. Gouty subjects also have an increased incidence of stones that contain calcium. In addition, about 30 percent of patients with recurrent calcium stone disease have either an increased urinary uric acid excretion rate or hyperuricemia. An etiologic link between uric acid and recurrent calcium oxalate stones is provided by the reports of reduced stone frequency in such patients treated with allopurinol.

Finally, the report of uric acid as the major constituent of a stone obtained from a patient with no apparent abnormalities of uric acid metabolism should suggest the possibility that the constituent is actually 2,8-dihydroxyadenine and that the patient has adenine phosphoribosyltransferase deficiency.[90] This is because radiographic diffraction is required to distinguish uric acid from 2,8-dihydroxyadenine.

The characteristics of familial juvenile hyperuricemic nephropathy include a high incidence of hyperuricemia with gout beginning at a young age, hypertension, and renal disease leading to death before 40 years of age.[91-93] These urilital familial urate nephropathies are the result of a defect in a gene that resides in chromosome 1b, passed on by an autosomal dominant mode of inheritance and affecting both women and men.[94] Although no evidence for a metabolic abnormality that increases uric acid production has been discovered, there is evidence showing impaired renal excretion due to severely reduced fractional excretion of uric acid.[93] Identification of this disease early is important because presymptomatic treatment with allopurinol retards disease progression and morbidity due to renal failure.

Hyperuricemia has been associated with other familial nephropathies, such as medullary cystic disease,[95] focal tubulointerstitial disease,[96] and polycystic kidney disease. In fact, gout develops in 24 to 36 percent of individuals with polycystic kidney disease.[97,98] The hyperuricemia and gouty arthritis appear to precede the development of renal failure. Although the basis of this association remains unclear, altered renal handling of uric acid may be an early manifestation of the underlying renal lesion.

Lead Intoxication

Hyperuricemia and gout are well-recognized complications of chronic lead intoxication, with the prevalence of gout in patients with plumbism ranging between 6 and 50 percent.[99] Although a renal defect appears to be present, it has not been well defined.[100,101] Some patients with primary gout have increased blood lead levels, compared to age-and sex-matched controls, despite the absence of a history of overt lead exposure.[102] This suggests that occult chronic lead intoxication may play an etiologic role in some cases of primary gout (up to 36 percent of some gout populations[99]). In addition, patients with gout who have renal impairment, compared to gouty patients with normal renal function, seem to have an increased quantity of mobilized lead. These observations suggest an important role for lead in the pathogenesis of gouty nephropathy.[102,103] On the other hand, in a study of patients with a history of moonshine ingestion, no correlation was found between the extent of depression in clearance of uric acid or creatinine and the amount of lead excretion after ethylenediaminetetraacetic acid (EDTA) infusion.[104]

Cyclosporine-Induced Hyperuricemia and Gout

Cyclosporine interferes with urinary uric acid excretion. Hyperuricemia and gout occur with increased frequency among transplant recipients treated with cyclosporine,[42,105] and even more often when diuretics are employed concomitantly. However, the serum urate levels do not correlate directly with cyclosporine levels or with degrees of hypertension or renal insufficiency. The onset of gout may occur soon after transplantation, with a mean of about 17 months. Gouty attacks may be typical and monarticular but also may affect unusual sites, such as the shoulder, hip, or sacroiliac joints. Polyarticular attacks and an accelerated course with early development of tophi may also be observed. Nephrolithiasis develops in about 3 percent of renal transplantations. All calculi from azathioprine-treated patients are composed of calcium compounds, whereas 60 percent of the calculi from those treated with cyclosporine contain uric acid.[106]

Purine Metabolism

Uric acid is a purine base composed of a six-membered pyrimidine ring fused to a five-membered imidazole ring (Fig. 87-7). Purine nucleosides are composed of a purine base plus a pentose joined to the base by an N-glycosyl bond between carbon atom 1 of the pentose and nitrogen atom 9 of the purine base. There are two series of nucleosides: the ribonucleosides, which con-

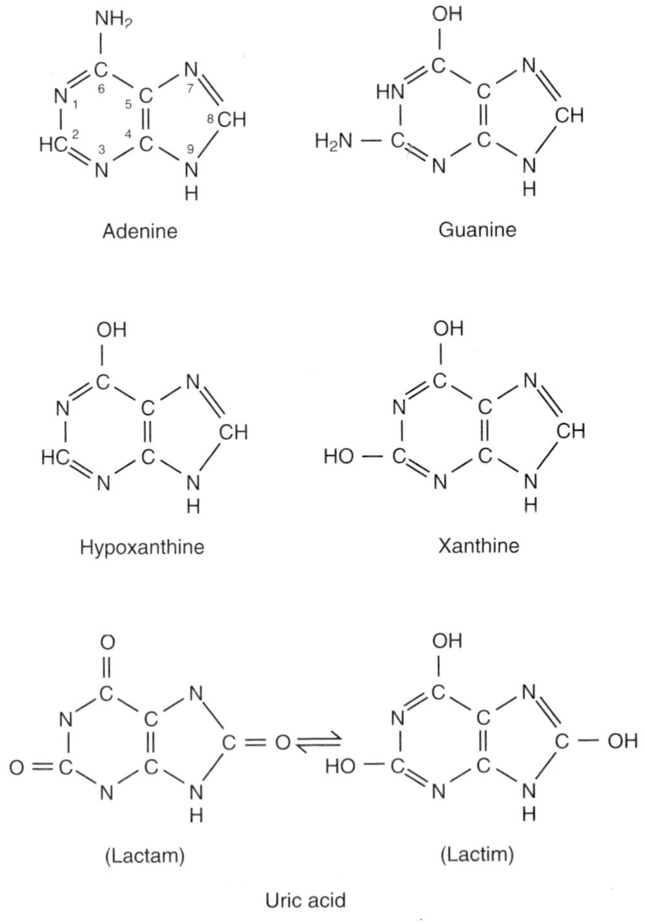

FIGURE 87-7 · Structure of Uric Acid. All purine bases may exist in the lactam form in a reversible manner, as shown for uric acid.

tain D-ribose as the sugar component, and the deoxyribonucleosides, which contain 2'-deoxy-D-ribose (Fig. 87–8). Purine nucleotides and deoxynucleotides consist of a nucleoside of deoxynucleoside with a phosphate group and ester linkage with carbon 5 of the pentose (Fig. 87–9). The nucleosides and deoxynucleosides exist as 5'-monophosphates, 5'-diphosphates, and 5'-triphosphates (Fig. 87–10). These compounds serve as building blocks for RNA and DNA; as precursors of the cyclic nucleotides adenosine-3', 5'-cyclic-phosphate, and guanosine-3', 5'-cyclic-phosphate; as a source of chemical energy; and as precursors of various purine cofactors and coenzymes, such as nicotinamide adenine dinucleotide.

Xanthine oxidase is a flavoprotein containing both iron and molybdenum that oxidizes a wide variety of

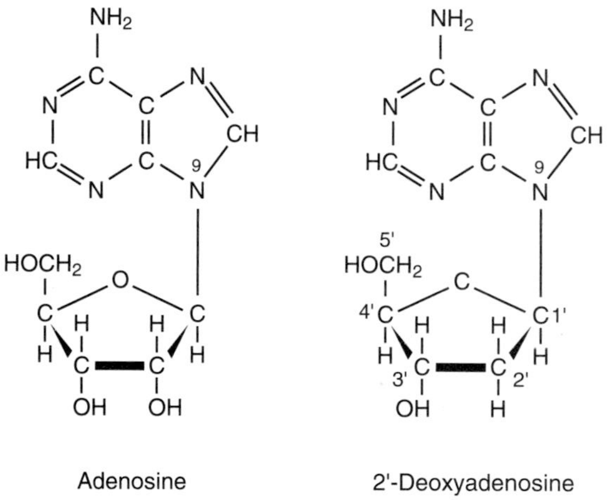

FIGURE 87–8 · Structures of adenosine and 2'-deoxydenosine as examples of nucleosides and 2'-deoxynucleosides, respectively.

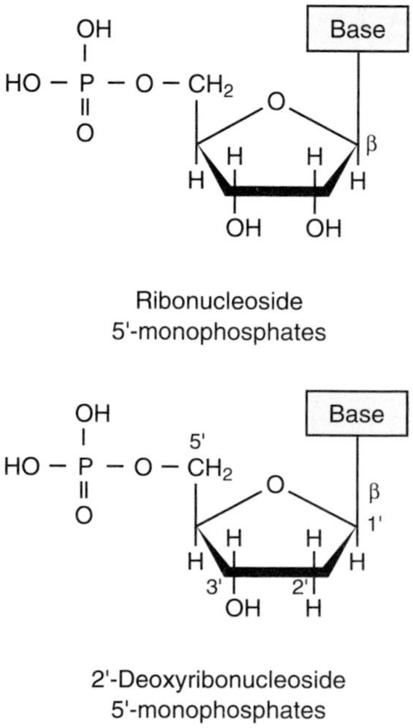

FIGURE 87–9 · General structures of nucleosides and deoxynucleoside 5'-monophosphates.

$$Hypoxanthine + H_2O + 2O_2 \longrightarrow$$
$$Xanthine + 2O^{2-} + 2H^+$$

$$Hypoxanthine + H_2O + O_2 \longrightarrow Xanthine + H_2O_2$$

$$Xanthine + H_2O + 2O_2 \longrightarrow Uric\ Acid +$$
$$2O^{2-} + 2H^+$$

or

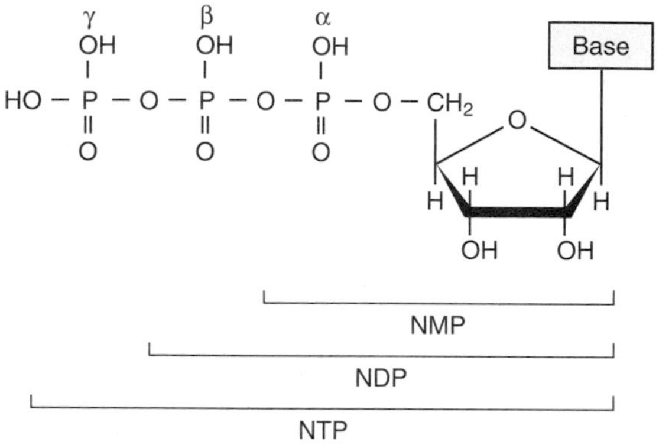

FIGURE 87–10 · Comparison of the structures of nucleoside, monophosphates, diphosphates, and triphosphates.

purines and pteridines. A soluble form of the enzyme that has dehydrogenase activity (xanthine dehydrogenase or D-form) is found in high activity in liver and small intestine and is responsible for the formation of uric acid as the final metabolic product in human purine metabolism. This enzyme converts hypoxanthine to xanthine and xanthine to uric acid (Fig. 87–11).

Purines can be synthesized de novo in cells.[30] The initial and rate-limiting step of this biosynthestic process is the conversion of phosphoribosylpyrophosphate (PRPP) to 5'-phosphoribosylamine. This step is catalyzed by the enzyme amidophosphoribosyltransferase, and it is regulated by the concentrations of nucleoside monophosphates and PRPP. Adenylic acid (AMP) and guanylic acid (GMP) are feedback inhibitors of the enzyme. Under normal conditions, depletion of PRPP decreases the rate of purine biosynthesis de novo. Elevation of PRPP is associated with an increased rate of purine biosynthesis de novo.

The first branch point in the pathway leading to the synthesis de novo of AMP and GMP (see Fig. 87–11) occurs with the synthesis of inosinic acid (IMP). IMP is used to form AMP and GMP, and these steps may be governed by the intracellular concentration of guanylic acid triphosphate (GTP). GTP is a substrate of adenylosuccinate synthetase and an inhibitor of IMP dehydrogenase. As IMP is formed, it is used for the synthesis of xanthylic acid, guanylic acid, guanylic acid diphosphate, and GTP. As GTP reaches a critical concentration in the cell, it may then increase the activity of adenylosuccinate synthetase, allowing IMP to be effectively used in the synthesis of AMP. When accelerated purine biosynthesis de novo results in production of surplus IMP, there is a rapid conversion of the excess ribonucleotide to uric acid rather than a continued expansion of the pools of adenyl and guanyl nucleotides.

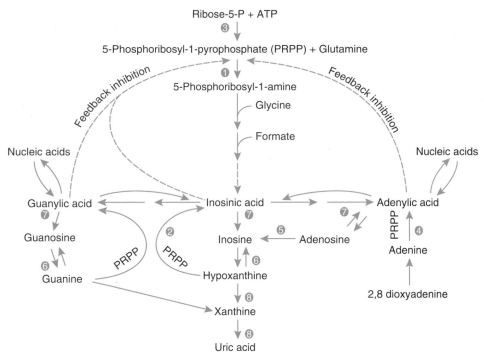

FIGURE 87–11 · Outline of Purine Metabolism: 1) amidophosphoribosyltransferase; 2) hypoxanthine-guanine phosphoribosyltransferase; 3) phosphoribosylpyrophosphate (PRPP) synthetase; 4) adenine phosphoribosyltransferase; 5) adenosine deaminase; 6) purine nucleoside phosphorylase; 7) 5′ nucleotidase; 8) xanthine oxidase. (From Seegmiller JE, Rosenbloom RM, Kelley WN: Enzyme defect associated with sex-linked human neurological disorder and excessive purine synthesis. Science 155:1682, 1967.) Model of interconversion of small (active) and large (inactive) forms of amidophosphoribosyltransferase. (From Kelley WN, Holmes EW, Van der Weyden MB: Current concepts on the regulation of purine biosynthesis de novo in man. Arthritis Rheum 18:673, 1975.) Abbreviated scheme of purine nucleoside monophosphate metabolism. 1, AMP deaminase. 2, 5′ Nucleotidase. 3, Nonspecific acid and alkaline phosphatases. 4, AMP (adenylate) kinase. 5, Adenylosuccinic acid synthetase. 6, IMP dehydrogenase. AMP, Adenylic acid; GDP, guanylic acid diphosphate; GMP, guanylic acid; GTP, guanylic acid triphosphate; IMP, inosinic acid; XMP, xanthylic acid.

Nucleotide breakdown is regulated in a complex manner. Regulation of nucleotide degradation is critically controlled by AMP deaminase and 5′-nucleotidase activities. Release of inhibition of AMP deaminase results in accelerated production of uric acid. Regulation of dephosphorylation is complex, involving three soluble 5′-nucleotidase activities. The nucleosides formed by nucleotidase reactions are converted to the bases adenine, guanine, or hypoxanthine. These bases can be "salvaged" by reconversion to nucleosides catalyzed by purine nucleoside phosphorylase activity (hypoxanthine and guanine) or conjugated with PRPP to form ribonucleotides by phosphoribosyltransferase activities (all three). If not salvaged, they are degraded to uric acid.

Exogenous purines also significantly contribute to the total body urate pool. The magnitude of this contribution depends on the amount and type of purine in the diet, but it is often considerable. When healthy young men were given an isocaloric, purine-free formula diet, serum urate values declined in 10 days from about 4.9 to 3.1 ± 0.4 mg/dl, and urinary excretion of uric acid declined from between 500 and 600 to 336 ± 39 mg/day.[107] Urinary uric acid excretion declines to constant low values after 5 to 7 days of dietary purine elimi-

nation or severe restriction. Mean values then range from 336 ± 39 to 426 ± 81 mg every 24 hours. These values reflect the continued synthesis and turnover of endogenous purines. The urinary uric acid excretion, however, accounts for only a part of the daily disposition of uric acid. The true rate of endogenous purine turnover cannot accurately be determined by measurement of urinary uric acid excretion but requires the use of isotope-dilution techniques in subjects in whom the exogenous contribution has been reduced to a minimum by severe dietary purine restriction.

Uric Acid Elimination and Excretion

Because less than two percent of the turnover of the total body urate pool can be attributed to tissue uricolysis, most uric acid is eliminated from the body by renal and extrarenal routes. Extrarenal routes include saliva, gastric juice, pancreatic secretions, and bowel. These routes account for about one third of the uric acid normally turned over each day. The percentage of extrarenal excretion increases, however, when serum urate concentrations rise above 12 to 14 mg/dl.

Most investigations support a four-component model for renal handling of uric acid.[30,108] This consists of glomerular filtration, early proximal tubular reabsorption, tubular secretion, and finally postsecretory tubular reabsorption. Glomerular ultrafiltration of uric acid in humans is believed to be complete, with urate concentrations in the glomerular fluid being the same as those in plasma. Although some urate may be bound to plasma protein, this fraction is thought to be small, perhaps less than 5 percent. At least 90 to 93 percent of filtered urate is reabsorbed in the proximal tubule. Distal tubular fluid, however, contains a greater fraction of filtered urate than does final urine. This finding may signify reabsorption of a small fraction of filtered or secreted urate in collecting ducts. Therefore, although net urate reabsorption occurs largely in the proximal tubule, the possibility exists of reabsorption in more distal segments.

Urate reabsorption occurs by a mechanism of active transport, although there may also be a passive mechanism. This active transport mechanism has been shown to have saturable kinetics, indicating that the urate reabsorption in the proximal tubule is probably carrier mediated. In humans, the concentration of uric acid in urine may approach one tenth the concentration in plasma during diuresis and inhibition of urate secretion with pyrazinoate. Therefore, urate reabsorption may occur against a concentration gradient.

There is a close link between reabsorption of sodium and reabsorption of a number of other components of the glomerular filtrate, such as glucose, phosphate, calcium, bicarbonate, and uric acid. In conditions associated with an increase in proximal reabsorption of sodium, the clearance of uric acid is reduced (Table 87–2); in conditions leading to decreased proximal reabsorption of sodium, the uric acid clearance is increased (Table 87–3). In addition, sodium reabsorption per nephron is decreased and uric acid excretion per nephron is increased in chronic renal failure.

Net tubular secretion of urate occurs in humans under certain conditions. The biphasic effect of salicylate on uric acid excretion has been interpreted as representing inhibition of urate secretion with urate retention at low salicylate doses plus inhibition of urate reabsorption with urate diuresis at higher salicylate doses. The apparent paradoxical effect of salicylate on uric acid excretion has been attributed to inhibition of reabsorption by salicylate itself, with inhibition of secretion resulting from action of a metabolite, salicylurate. A number of organic acids inhibit uric acid excretion in animals and humans. These include lactate, β-hydroxybutyrate, acetoacetate, and branched-chain ketoacids. These effects have been interpreted as representing inhibition of tubular secretion of urate.

TABLE 87–2 • CONDITIONS ASSOCIATED WITH HYPERURICEMIA OR REDUCED RENAL URIC ACID CLEARANCE

Condition	Δ Serum Urate	Δ Uric Acid Clearance	Δ Extracellular Fluid Volume	Δ Filtration Fraction	Predicted Δ Proximal Tubular Sodium Reabsorption*
Salt restriction	↑	↓	↓	–	↑
Diuretic therapy without salt replacement	↑	↓	↓	–	↑
Diabetes insipidus	↑	↓	↓	↑	↑
Hypertension	↑	↓	–	↑	↑
Angiotension infusion (without increased lactate or ketones)	–	↓	–	↑	↑
Norepinephrine (without increased lactate or ketones)		↓	–	↑	↑

Proximal tubular sodium reabsorption was not evaluated directly in the reported studies; the changes listed represent a prediction from the observed changes in extracellular fluid volume and filtration fraction.

From Holmes EW, et al: The kidney and uric acid excretion in man. Kidney Int 2:115, 1972.

TABLE 87–3 • CONDITIONS ASSOCIATED WITH REDUCTION IN SERUM URATE LEVELS

Condition	Δ Serum Urate	Δ Uric Acid Clearance	Δ Extracellular Fluid Volume	Δ Filtration Fraction	Predicted Δ Proximal Tubular Sodium Reabsorption*
Salt	↓	↑	↑	–	↓
Diuretic therapy with salt replacement	↓	↑	↑	–	↓
Inappropriate secretion of ADH	↓	↑	↑	–	↓
Pregnancy (early)	↓	↑	↑	–	↓

From Holmes EW, et al: The kidney and uric acid excretion in man. Kidney Int 2:115, 1972.

Pyrazinamide has significant effects on uric acid excretion. In patients with Wilson's or Hodgkin's disease and hypouricemia associated with raised renal urate clearance values, pyrazinamide suppresses the hyperuricosuria. The uricosuric response to probenecid is virtually abolished by pretreatment with pyrazinamide or pyrazinoate. Finally, the uricosuric response to intravenous chlorothiazide or volume expansion with hypertonic sodium chloride is substantially diminished by pretreatment with pyrazinamide. A model that accounts for these observations postulates extensive postsecretory reabsorption of urate. In this model, the effects of pyrazinamide are explained in terms of reduced secretory delivery to the late reabsorptive sites.

A variety of factors influence the renal clearence of uric acid, including urine flow, estrogens, surgery, and the autonomic nervous system. Uric acid excretion increases by more than 25 percent as urine flow doubles in response to oral and intravenous fluid loading in humans. Changes in clearance are at least partially responsible for lower concentrations of serum urate in children and women before menopause.[6,7] An increase in the excretion of uric acid in urine occurs in patients undergoing abdominal surgery, with little or no change taking place in the serum urate concentration. Factors such as anesthesia, increased endogenous steroids, intravenous fluids, intestinal manipulation, and vagotomy are suggested as possibly affecting urate clearance. Several anticholinergic agents increase renal clearance of uric acid, indicating that the parasympathetic nervous system plays a role in controlling the renal excretion of uric acid.

Physical Properties of Uric Acid

The weakly acidic nature of uric acid results from ionization of hydrogen ions at position 9 ($pKa_1 = 5.75$) and position 3 ($pKa_2 = 10.3$). The ionized forms of uric acid readily form salts, which are monosodium and disodium or potassium urates. In extracellular fluids in which sodium is the principal cation, approximately 98 percent of uric acid is in the form of the monosodium salt at pH 7.4. When the solubility limits of the body fluids are exceeded, the crystals that occur in the synovial fluid or the tophi of gouty patients are composed of monosodium urate monohydrate. Actual determinations of solubility of monosodium urate in human plasma (or serum) indicate that saturation occurs at concentrations of about 7 mg/dl. Considerably higher concentrations of monosodium urate in plasma can be achieved in supersaturated solutions. Stable supersaturated solutions of monosodium urate ranging up to 40 to 90 mg/dl have been observed in patients with leukemia or lymphoma after aggressive therapy with cytotoxic drugs in the absence of allopurinol therapy.[87] The factors responsible for enhanced urate solubility in such patients are not clear and may include both the natural tendency for urate to form stable supersaturated solutions and an increase in plasma of substances capable of solubilizing urate. Studies of urate binding disclose that no more than 4 to 5 percent of urate is bound to plasma protein, indicating that the binding of uric acid to plasma proteins at 37°C is small and probably of little physiologic significance.

As the urine is acidified along the renal tubule, a portion of urinary urate is converted to uric acid. The solubility of uric acid in aqueous solutions is substantially less than that of urate. At pH 5, urine is saturated with uric acid at 15 mg/dl; at pH 7, urine accommodates 158 to 200 mg/dl in solution. The limited solubility of uric acid in urine of pH 5 is of particular significance in patients with gout, many of whom display a tendency toward excretion of unusually acidic urine.

Monosodium urate occurs as a monohydrate and forms crystals in tissue and joint fluids that are needle shaped or rod shaped. Urate crystals are insoluble in ethanol, sparingly soluble in water, and markedly soluble in formalin. Free uric acid crystallizes from pure solutions in an orthorhombic system, forming rhombic plates. Crystals formed in urine incorporate pigments and exist in a variety of crystalline forms. Tissue deposits are composed of monosodium urate monohydrate, whereas urinary stones are largely uric acid. Both urate and uric acid crystals are birefringent, with strong negative elongation when viewed under compensated polarized light. These features should permit ready identification of urate crystals in synovial fluid, leukocytes, or tissue deposits and, therefore, constitute an important diagnostic aid.[109]

Classification and Pathogenesis of Hyperuricemia and Gout

The concentration of uric acid in body fluids is determined by the balance between rates of urate production and its elimination. The development of hyperuricemia may be caused by an excessive rate of urate production, a decrease in the renal excretion of uric acid, or a combination of both events.

Hyperuricemia and gout may be classified as follows (Table 87–4):

Primary: These are cases that appear to be innate, neither secondary to another acquired disorder nor the result of a subordinate manifestation of an inborn error that leads initially to a major disease unlike gout; although some cases of primary gout have a genetic basis, others do not.
Secondary: These are cases that develop in the course of another disease or as a consequence of drug use.
Idiopathic: These are cases in which a more precise classification cannot be assigned.

Further subdivisions within each major category are based on the identification of overproduction, underexcretion, or both, as responsible for the hyperuricemia. Evidence of overproduction of urate is provided by determination of the 24-hour urinary uric acid excretion.[110] For adults ingesting a purine-free diet, a total excretion of up to 600 mg/day is considered within the normal range.[111] With patients on regular diets, a value in excess of 1000 mg/day is clearly abnormal and an indication of overproduction, and values between 800 to 1000 mg/day are considered border-

TABLE 87–4 • CLASSIFICATION OF HYPERURICEMIA AND GOUT

Type	Metabolic Disturbance	Inheritance
Primary		
Molecular defects undefined		
Underexcretion (90% of primary gout)	Not established	Polygenic
Overproduction (10% of primary gout)	Not established	Polygenic
Associated with specific enzyme defects	Overproduction of PRPP and of uric acid	X-linked
PRPP synthetase variants; increased activity		
HPRT deficiency, partial	Overproduction of uric acid; increased purine biosynthesis de novo driven by surplus PP-ribose-P; Kelley-Seegmiller syndrome	
Secondary		
Associated with increased purine biosynthesis de novo		
HPRT deficiency, "virtually complete"	Overproduction of uric acid; increased purine biosynthesis de novo driven by surplus PRPP; Lesch-Nyhan syndrome	X-linked
Glucose-6-phosphatase deficiency or absence	Overproduction plus underexcretion of uric acid; glycogen storage disease, type I (von Gierke's disease)	Autosomal recessive
Fructose-1-phosphate aldolase deficiency	Overproduction plus underexcretion of uric acid	Autosomal recessive
Associated with increased ATP degradation		
Associated with increased nucleic acid turnover	Overproduction of uric acid	Most not familial
Associated with decreased renal excretion of uric acid	Decreased filtration of uric acid; inhibited tubular secretion of uric acid; or enhanced tubular reabsorption of uric acid	Some autosomal dominant; some not familial; most unknown
Idiopathic		Unknown

Abbreviations: ATP, adenosine triphosphate; HPRT, hypoxanthine-guanine phosphoribosyltransferase; PRPP, phosphoribosylpyrophosphate.

line. It has been suggested that overproduction of uric acid can be assessed simply by determining the ratio of uric acid to creatinine in the urine or the $C_{urate}/C_{creatinine}$ ratio. However, comparison of these two ratios with the 24-hour urinary uric acid excretion reveals a poor correlation in most patients.[110,112] Exceptions include patients with specific enzymatic deficiencies or with rapid cell lysis during chemotherapy for leukemia or lymphoma.

Primary Gout

Renal mechanisms are responsible for the hyperuricemia in most cases of gout. Genetic factors exert an important control in the renal clearance of uric acid.[113] A careful comparison of uric acid clearances and excretion rates over a wide but comparable range of filtered loads of urate indicates that most gouty subjects have a lower ratio of urate to inulin clearance (C_{urate}/C_{inulin} ratio) than do nongouty subjects.[111,113-117] The excretion rates and the capacity of the excretory mechanism for uric acid are the same for gouty subjects and nongouty individuals (Fig. 87–12). The excretion curve, however, is shifted: Gouty subjects require serum urate values 2 or 3 mg/dl higher than those of controls to achieve equivalent uric acid

excretion rates. Theoretically, the shift in the excretion curve in gouty subjects may result from reduced filtration of uric acid, enhanced reabsorption, or decreased secretion. Attempts to localize the site of the defect of uric acid transport in the nephron have been unsuccessful. No unequivocal data exist to establish any one of these three mechanisms. Patients classified as exhibiting an overproduction of uric acid represent less than 10 percent of the gouty population.

Secondary Gout

Numerous secondary causes of hyperuricemia and gout can be attributed to a decrease in the renal excretion of uric acid. A reduction in the glomerular filtration rate leads to decrease in the filtered load of uric acid and consequently to hyperuricemia. Patients with renal disease are hyperuricemic on this basis. Other factors, such as decreased secretion of uric acid, have been postulated in patients with some types of renal disease (e.g., polycystic kidney disease, lead nephropathy). Gout is a rare complication of the secondary hyperuricemia that results from renal insufficiency. When it occurs in this setting, there is likely to be a positive family history.

Diuretic therapy currently represents one of the most important causes of secondary hyperuricemia in humans.

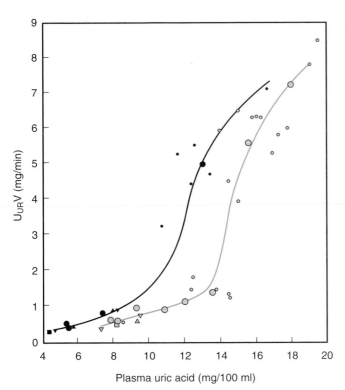

FIGURE 87-12 · Rate of uric acid excretion at various plasma urate levels in nongouty *(solid symbols)* and gouty *(open symbols)* subjects. Large symbols represent mean values; small symbols represent individual data of a few mean values selected to illustrate the degree of scatter within groups. Studies were conducted under basal conditions, after RNA feeding, and after infusions of lithium urate. (Data from Nugent and Tyler,[114] Seegmiller et al,[111] Yu et al,[115] and Latham and Rodnan.[116]) (From Wyngaarden JB: Gout. Adv Metabol Dis 2:2, 1965. Reproduced by permission of Academic Press.)

Diuretic-induced volume depletion leads to enhanced tubular reabsorption of uric acid, as well as decreased filtered load of uric acid. Decreased secretion of uric acid has also been postulated as a possible mechanism in diuretic-induced hyperuricemia. A number of other drugs lead to hyperuricemia by a renal mechanism, although the nature of the abnormality remains less clear. These agents include lower-dose aspirin, pyrazinamide, nicotinic acid, losartan, ethambutol, ethanol, and cyclosporine.

Decreased renal excretion of uric acid is thought to be an important mechanism for the hyperuricemia associated with several disease states. Volume depletion may be an important factor in patients with hyperuricemia associated with adrenal insufficiency or nephrogenic diabetes insipidus. An accumulation of organic acids on any basis is thought to competitively inhibit uric acid secretion and thereby lead to hyperuricemia. This is the case in starvation, alcoholic ketosis, diabetic ketoacidosis, maple syrup urine disease, and lactic acidosis of any cause (e.g., hypoxemia, respiratory insufficiency, chronic beryllium disease, acute alcohol intoxication). The renal basis of the hyperuricemia in conditions such as chronic lead intoxication, hyperparathyroidism, hypoparathyroidism, pseudohypoparath-yroidism, and hypothyroidism remains unclear.

Secondary gout can also result from urate overproduction. Four specific defects cause urate overproduction as a consequence of accelerated de novo purine biosynthesis. These include hypoxauthine phosphorbosal transferase (HPRT) deficiency, PRPP synthetase overactivity, glucose-6-phosphatase deficiency, and fructose-1-phosphate aldolase deficiency.

A complete deficiency of the enzyme HPRT, the Lesch-Nyhan syndrome, is characterized by choreoathetosis, striking growth, mental retardation, spasticity, self mutilation, and marked hyperuricemia with excessive uric acid production and uric acid crystalluria[119-121] (Figs. 87-13 and 87-14). Adolescent and adult patients with a "partial" rather than a "complete" deficiency of HPRT, the Kelley-Seegmiller syndrome, present with uric acid calculi or gouty arthritis but do not have the devastating neurologic and behavioral features characteristic of the children with a complete enzyme deficiency.[122] Both the complete and partial deficiencies are inherited in an X chromosome–linked manner.

The level of HPRT activity in patients with each syndrome is the same within a family but often differs between families, with values ranging from 0.01 to almost 70 percent of normal. More than 50 different mutations have been defined.[30,123] Among these, major and minor deletions and rearrangements, as well as base substitutions, are represented. The excessive production of urate that is characteristic of partial HPRT deficiency results from an accelerated rate of purine biosynthesis de novo. This is caused by a decreased consumption of PRPP and the decreased reutilization of hypoxanthine through at least three mechanisms. First, the deficiency leads to enhanced purine synthesis by virtue of decreased concentrations of either IMP or GMP, because these nucleotides are normally important inhibitors of de novo purine synthesis. Second, the loss of hypoxanthine reutilization leads to decreased consumption of PRPP and increased intracellular concentrations of this compound. The resulting increased concentrations of PRPP increase de novo purine biosynthesis by providing more substrate for amido-phosphoribosyltransferase, the enzyme that catalyzes the presumed limiting step of this pathway. Third, in the absence of HPRT activity, hypoxanthine cannot be salvaged and is therefore oxidized to urate.

Increased PRPP synthetase activity causes accelerated PRPP formation. (Fig. 87-15) This, in turn, results increased de novo purine biosynthesis and excessive overproduction of urate.[124,125] Transmitted by X-linked inheritance, male subjects have clinical gout with typical onset between ages 21 and 39 years and can have renal calculi with onset as early as 18 years of age.[126]

Patients with glucose-6-phosphatase deficiency (von Gierke's disease, GSD type I) uniformly exhibit an increased production of uric acid as well as an accelerated rate of purine biosynthesis de novo. A major cause of increased uric acid synthesis is accelerated breakdown of ATP.[127]

In patients with hereditary fructose intolerance caused by fructose-1-phosphate aldolase deficiency, hyperuricemia develops in part because of accelerated purine nucleotide catabolism. In homozygotes, vomiting

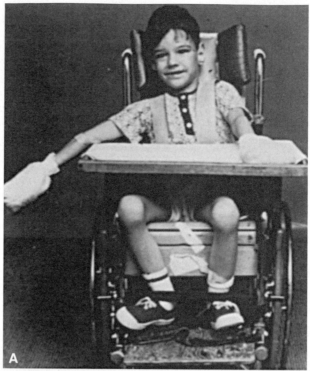

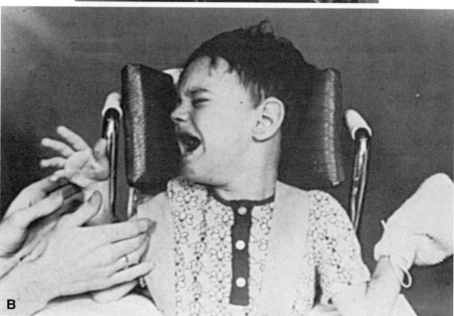

FIGURE 87-13 • A, Patient with HPRT deficiency. B, Example of self-multilative behavior Note agitated appearance and the attempt by the patient to bite his fingers after the wrapping is removed from his hands.

and hypoglycemia after fructose ingestion can proceed to hepatic failure and proximal tubular dysfunction. Ingestion of fructose causes an accumulation of fructose-1-phosphate, the substrate for the enzyme, which, in turn, results in ATP depletion. Both lactic acidosis and renal tubular acidosis also contribute to urate retention. Heterozygous carriers develop hyperuricemia, and perhaps one third develop gout.[128]

In most patients with secondary hyperuricemia caused by an overproduction of uric acid, the predominant abnormality appears to be an increased turnover of nucleic acids. A number of diseases, including the myeloproliferative and lymphoproliferative dis-

orders, multiple myeloma, secondary polycythemia, pernicious anemia, certain hemoglobinopathies, thalassemia, other hemolytic anemias, infectious mononucleosis, and some carcinomas, may be associated with increased marrow activity or increased turnover and associated increased turnover of nucleic acids. The increased turnover in nucleic acid, in turn, leads to hyperuricemia, hyperuricaciduria, and a compensatory increase in the rate of purine biosynthesis de novo.

An important cause of overproduction of uric acid in secondary hyperuricemia appears to be related to the acceleration of ATP degradation to uric acid. This can occur with excessive alcohol consumption, myocardial

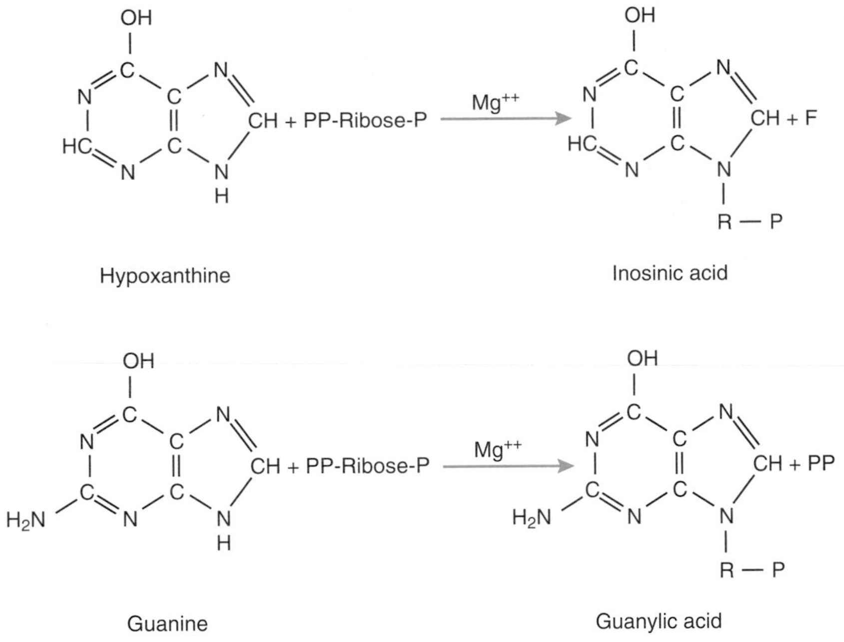

FIGURE 87-14 · Reactions Catalyzed by Hypoxanthineguanine Phosphoribosyltransferase.

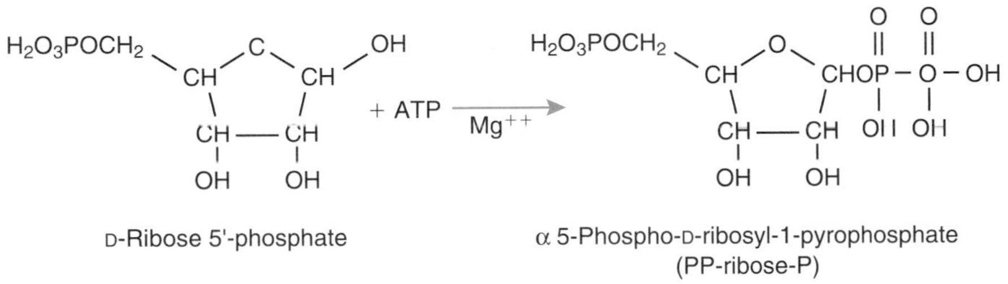

FIGURE 87-15 · Reaction Catalyzed by Phosphoribosylpyrophosphate Synthetase.

infarction, acute smoke inhalation, respiratory failure, status epilepticus, and strenuous exercise.[71,128] This can lead to increased serum urate levels, which can be substantial with extreme exercise, as seen in status epilepticus. Myogenic hyperuricemia has been reported in patients with muscle involvement either in the basal state or after exercise in three GSDs[129]: debranching enzyme deficiency (GSD type III), myophosphorylase deficiency (GSD type V), and muscle phosphofructokinase deficiency (GSD type VII) (Fig. 87–16). Excessive formation of ATP degradation products also can occur in carnitine palmitoyltransferase deficiency, myoadenylate deaminase deficiency[130,131] and medium-chain acyl–coenzyme A dehydrogenase deficiency.[132]

▪ Acute Gouty Arthritis

Urate crystals are almost always present in acute gouty arthritis. At the height of the response, the majority of crystals in the synovial fluid are intracellular.[133] The extracellular proportion increases as inflammation subsides. Urate crystals may also rarely occur in synovial fluid in a sphere-like form. Urate crystals and microtophi are present in the synovial membranes 2 days after the onset of a first attack of acute gout.[134] This

finding and others suggest that acute gout may be superimposed on a joint in which urate deposition and low-grade chronic inflammation may have developed silently at an earlier time. The crystals of the synovium are often in a superficial location near the joint space. Therefore, crystals may "flake off" the synovial membrane into the synovialfluid, triggering an inflammatory attack when phagocytized by polymorphonuclear or synovial cells.

The factors leading to precipitation of monosodium urate crystals in tissues and the mechanisms whereby those crystals induce inflammation are complex and incompletely understood. A relationship between the process by which the acute attack is triggered and that by which visible urate deposits form is not yet established. Supersaturation of serum or synovial fluid with monosodium urate is a necessary, but not sufficient, precondition for the development of acute gouty arthritis. In addition, acute gouty arthritis may develop at a time when the serum urate concentration is well below saturation.[27-29] In subjects with gouty synovitis, the concentration of urate in the synovial fluid is usually similar to that in serum. Urate has less of a tendency to precipitate in plasma than in synovial fluid, because plasma is a significantly better solvent for monosodium urate. Therefore, an important question

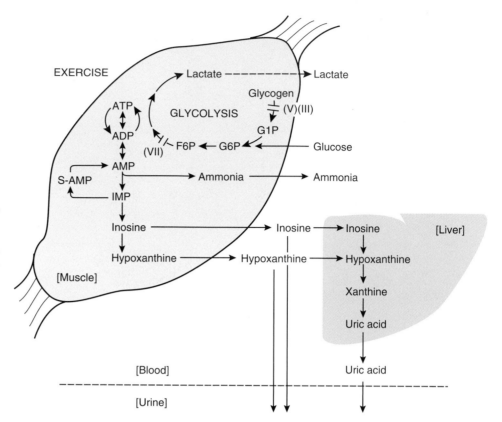

FIGURE 87–16 · Mechanism of Myogenic Hyperuricemia in Glycogen Storage Diseases (GSDs). In the three GSDs associated with metabolic myopathy, there is impairment of the metabolic pathways providing the substrate necessary for adenosine triphosphate (ATP) synthesis. Thus, when ATP is consumed by muscle contraction, accelerated degradation of ATP may occur. (Adapted from information appearing in Mineo I, Kono N, Hara N, et al: Myogenic hyperuricemia: A common pathophysiologic feature of glycogenosis types III, V, and VII. N Engl J Med 317:75. 1987. Used by permission.)

is what makes monosodium urate crystals form in some subjects, but not in others, despite similar serum urate concentrations.

Factors that may regulate the deposition of urate in human tissues include lower intra-articular temperature, gamma globulins, type I collagen, proteoglycans, changes in pH, reduced binding of urate to plasma protein, trauma, aging, connective tissue turnover, and dysequilibrium, which can result from extracellular fluid reabsorption from the joint space at a faster rate than urate.[30,135] It has been suggested that urate crystals can act as antigens mediating the production of antibodies that can behave as a nucleation matrix for new urate crystallization.[136]

Although urate crystals are a virtual constant in acute gouty arthritis, the factors that initiate the inflammatory response are not well understood. Monosodium urate crystals can be found in synovial fluid from asymptomatic patients, and these fluids may also contain increased numbers of neutrophils.[34,137] During the asymptomatic period, 99.5 percent of intracellular crystals are found within mononuclear cells in synovial fluid and synovium.[138,139] Therefore, despite the absence of clinical symptoms, there appears to exist a basal level of low-grade inflammation in some patients with gout. The lack of symptoms is at least partially due to the ability of macrophages to phagocytose urate crystals without releasing inflammatory mediators; instead they release anti-inflammatory cytokines such as transforming growth factor-β (TGF-β).[140,141]

The phlogistic properties of the crystals seem to vary with surface characteristics and are related to their capacity to induce the production of serum proteins and release of chemotactic factors and inflammatory mediators from cells, including neutrophils, macrophages, synovial lining cells, chondrocytes, and endothelial cells.[142] Surface characteristics, which include the physical properties of surface-bound proteins, play a significant role. Urate spherulytes, which may represent newly crystallizing monosodium urate, are less phlogistic than most needle-shaped forms of urate crystals.[143] Monosodium urate crystals from tophi are more active in stimulating neutrophils than uncoated synthetic urate crystals.[144] Crystals heavily coated with IgG appear to be the most inflammatory.[146] Conversely, if serum is added to the crystals taken from tophi, if crystals from tophi are treated with protease, or if crystals are coated with apolipoprotein A, they are less inflammatory.[144,146,147] Crystals collected from tophi have significant concentrations of ionizable iron.[148] The addition of the iron chelator deferoxamine decreases their inflammatory potential.

The symptomatic inflammatory response to urate crystals involves a host of cellular and chemical mediators. But mononuclear cells are involved as well. Monocytes can secrete proinflammatory cytokines such as TNF-α, IL-1, IL-6, and IL-8.[139,149,150] TNF-α and IL-1 released by peripheral blood monocytes can activate vascular endothelial cell expression of E-selectin, intercellular adhesion molecule-1 (ICAM-1), and vascular cell adhesion molecule-1 (VCAM-1) and thereby stimulate both recruitment of neutrophils to the site of crystal deposition and amplification of the inflammatory response.[150] Neutrophils are also attracted to the synovial fluid by crystal-induced chemotactic factor, the activated fifth component of complement (C5a), leukotriene B$_4$ (LTB$_4$), and

IL-8.[151] Crystal-induced activation of neutrophils can occur through both tyrosine kinase activity and phosphatidylcholine-specific phospholipase D activity.[152-154]

There appears to be no correlation between crystal size, shape, or number and the intensity of the inflammation. Protein-coated crystals of sodium urate are taken up within the phagosomes of polymorphs and merged with lysosomes. The interaction between the crystals and the lysosomal membranes involves binding and then membranolysis with accompanying generation of free radicals and protease release. A variety of serum factors appear to mediate the inflammatory response. The complement system appears to play an important role. More than 30 polypeptides associated with crystal-induced inflammation have been identified, including C1q, C1r, C1s, fibronectin, fibrinogen, IgG, lysosomal enzymes, apolipoproteins, and TGF-β.[155]

Other mediators released from polymorphonuclear leukocytes appear to have important roles in urate-induced inflammation. These include LTB_4, kinins, latent collagenase, kallikrein, prostaglandin E_2 (PGE_2), and 6-keto-PGF_1-α, and IL-1.[156,157] The further metabolism and deactivation of LTB_4, an important local mediator of inflammation, is partially inhibited by monosodium urate crystals, potentiating its activity.[158]

Additional cell types also contribute to the inflammatory response.[151,159-162] Synovial cells exposed to crystals can synthesize and release LTB_4, TNF-α, IL-1, latent collagenase, and PGE_2.[163] Phagocytosis of crystals by endothelial cells results in superoxide oxygen free radical generation.[164] TNF-α and IL-1 can induce chondrocytes to release IL-8 and monocyte chemoattractant protein-1.[165]

The acute gout attack continues as long as neutrophils are present and is terminated with their disappearance through apoptosis. In most acute inflammatory responses, TNF-α has a proapoptotic effect on neutrophils.[166] It appears that opsonized urate crystals override the TNF-α–induced signal transduction, thereby extending the duration of the attack.[167] Proteins exuding into the joint space (e.g., apolipoprotein B) or materials released by the lysis of leukocytes may displace IgG from the surface of the crystals and thereby decrease their phlogistic properties.[147]

Other factors also appear to contribute to the termination of the acute attack. The increased heat of inflammation may increase urate solubility, decreasing the tendency toward new crystal formation and favoring dissolution of existing crystals. Increased blood flow may help transport urate away from the joint and lessen the tendency toward formation of local regions of supersaturation. Some of the ingested crystals may be destroyed by leukocyte myeloperoxidase, diminishing the load of crystals released by ruptured cells that are capable of perpetuating the inflammatory response. Adrenocorticotropic hormone (ACTH), secreted as part of the alarm reaction of the acute attack, may suppress the inflammatory process. Superoxide anion generated by crystal-leukocyte interaction during the acute attack may alter crystal properties and the proteins bound to the crystals.

Finally, the differentiation of monocytes to mature macrophages may also be significant. Mature macrophages are capable of ingesting urate crystals and apoptotic neutrophils without generating proinflammatory factors. In addition, they can release TGF-β, an anti-inflammatory cytokine.[141,168] Therefore, the state of maturation of the monocytic cells proximate to the urate crystals in synovial fluid or synovium may modulate the level of inflammatory response.

Treatment of Gout

The therapeutic aims in gout are as follows:

1. To terminate the acute attack as promptly and gently as possible
2. To prevent recurrences of acute gouty arthritis
3. To prevent or reverse complications of the disease resulting from deposition of sodium urate or uric acid crystals in joints, kidneys, or other sites
4. To prevent or reverse associated features of the illness that are deleterious, such as obesity, hypertriglyceridemia, and hypertension

ASYMPTOMATIC HYPERURICEMIA

The presence of hyperuricemia is rarely an indication for specific antihyperuricemic drug therapy. Rather, the finding of hyperuricemia should cause the following questions to be addressed:

1. What is the cause of the hyperuricemia?
2. Are associated findings present?
3. Has damage to tissues or organs occurred as a result?
4. What, if anything, should be done?

Hyperuricemia may be the initial clue to the presence of a previously unsuspected disorder. In 70 percent of hyperuricemic patients, an underlying cause of the hyperuricemia can be readily defined by history and physical examination. The nature of the underlying cause may be useful in predicting the potential consequence, if any, of the elevated serum urate concentration. Therefore, the possibility of an underlying cause should be explored in every patient with hyperuricemia. A schema for investigating the cause of hyperuricemia, including the secondary causes, is summarized in Figure 87–17.

The decision whether to treat hyperuricemia uncomplicated by articular gout, urolithiasis, or nephropathy is an exercise in clinical judgment about which there is less than universal agreement. When considering whether to treat asymptomatic hyperuricemia with urate-lowering agents, the following data are pertinent:

1. Renal function is not adversely affected by elevated serum urate concentrations.
2. The renal disease that accompanies hyperuricemia most often is related to inadequately controlled hypertension.
3. Correction of hyperuricemia has no apparent effect on renal function or the development of heart disease.

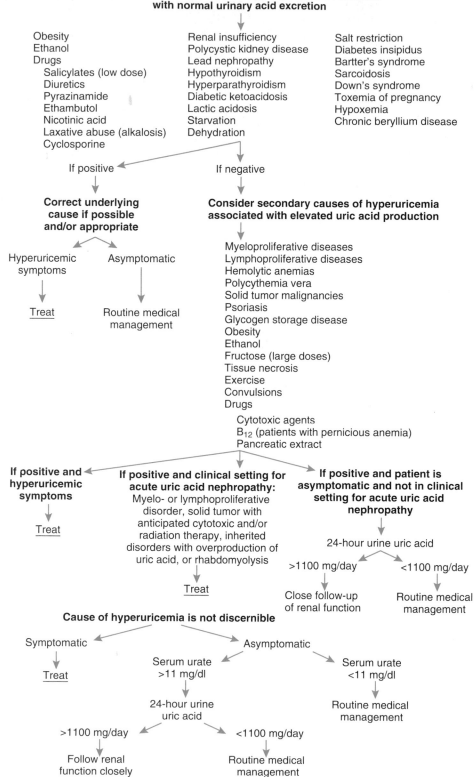

FIGURE 87–17 · Evaluation of Patients with Hyperuricemia.

Thus, it seems prudent to not treat asymptomatic hyperuricemia with specific antihyperuricemic agents until symptoms attributable to the hyperuricemia develop. Rare exceptions include individuals with a known hereditary cause of uric acid overproduction or patients at risk for acute uric acid nephropathy. It is, however, strongly recommended that the cause of hyperuricemia be determined and any associated factors related to the process, such as obesity, hyperlipidemia, alcoholism, and, especially, hypertension, be addressed.

ACUTE GOUTY ARTHRITIS

The acute gouty attack may be successfully terminated by any of several drugs. For practical purposes, the choice in most situations is among colchicine, an NSAID, or a corticosteroid preparation. The time of initiation of therapy is more important then the choice of drug.[169] With any of these agents, the sooner the drug is started, the more rapidly a complete response will be attained. Generally, colchicine is preferred for patients in whom the diagnosis of gout is not confirmed, whereas NSAIDs are preferred when the diagnosis is secure. If a patient cannot take medications by mouth or has active peptic ulcer disease, the choice is among intravenous colchicine, intra-articular glucocorticoid, or parenteral glucocorticoids. Local application of ice packs may help control the pain of an acute attack.[170] In some cases, analgesics, including narcotics, may be added as well. Drugs that affect serum urate concentrations, including antihyperuricemic agents, should not be changed (either started or stopped) during an acute attack. Just as sudden fluctuations in serum urate levels may tend to precipitate an acute attack, an inflammatory reaction already in progress may be made substantially worse by a major change in the serum urate concentration.

COLCHICINE

Colchicine can be administered by oral or intravenous routes.[171] Orally, a dose of 0.5 or 0.6 mg is taken hourly until one of three things occurs: 1) joint symptoms ease; 2) nausea, vomiting, or diarrhea develops; or 3) the patient has taken a maximum of 10 doses. If 10 doses are taken without benefit, the clinician should question the accuracy of the diagnosis. Peak plasma concentrations occur within 2 hours of oral administration. Although its plasma half-life is 4 hours, levels can be detected in neutrophils 10 days after ingestion. Colchicine has a low therapeutic index with steady-state plasma concentrations after acute treatment ranging between 0.5 and 3.0 ng/ml and with toxic effects occurring at approximately 3 ng/ml.[172] Therefore, in most patients, the side effects precede or coincide with improvement in joint symptoms. These side effects develop in 50 to 80 percent of patients and include increased peristalsis, cramping abdominal pain, diarrhea, nausea, or vomiting. The drug must be stopped promptly at the first sign of gastrointestinal side effects.[173]

Colchicine derives its effectiveness from its ability to interfere with acute inflammatory reactions in a variety of ways many of which are mediated by effects on neutrophil microtubules. Colchicine inhibits E-selectin–mediated adhesiveness for neutrophils[173] and diminishes neutrophil L-selectin expression, random motility, chemotaxis, PLA_2 activation, and IL-1 expression, as well as the stimulated elaboration of PLAF (platelet-activating factor) and the chemotactic factors CCF and LTB4. Colchicine also inhibits endothelial cell ICAM-1 expression, mast cell histamine release, and downregulates TNF-α receptors on macrophages and endothelial cells.

Colchicine can also be given intravenously. When used properly, the drug abolishes the acute attack with a low incidence of gastrointestinal side effects (provided that the patient is not also taking colchicine by mouth). An initial dose of 1 or 2 mg can be followed by one or two additional 1-mg doses administered at 6-hour intervals, if needed. The total dose of intravenous colchicine should not exceed 4 mg.[173] The colchicine should be diluted with 20 ml of normal saline before administration and given slowly into an established venous access to minimize sclerosis of the vein. In addition, oral colchicine should be discontinued and no additional colchicine should be given for at least 7 days because of the slow excretion of this drug.

The use of intravenous colchicine is associated with some risk. The most common complication is local extravasation during or immediately after injection. This can lead to inflammation and necrosis and may be extremely painful. The drug should not be given to patients who are neutropenic or to those with significant liver or renal disease. Although this form of therapy is effective, the reports of severe toxicity and death caused by inappropriate use of the medication are too plentiful.[174,175]

NONSTEROIDAL ANTI-INFLAMMATORY DRUGS

In the patient with an established diagnosis of uncomplicated gout, the preferred agent of choice is an NSAID. Indomethacin has been the traditional choice of agents in this class. Although this drug may be effective in doses as low as 25 mg given four times a day, an initial dose of 50 to 75 mg, followed by 50 mg every 6 to 8 hours with a maximum dose of 200 mg in the first 24 hours, has generally been recommended. To prevent relapse, it is reasonable to continue this dose for an additional 24 hours, then taper to 50 mg every 4 to 8 hours for the next 2 days. Clinical trials have also shown that oral naproxen, fenoprofen, ibuprofen, sulindac, piroxicam, and ketoprofen, as well as intramuscular ketorolac, are also effective.[169] In fact, all members of this family of drugs can be highly effective in the treatment of acute gouty arthritis, including the cyclooxygenase-2 (COX-2) selective agents.[176]

GLUCOCORTICOIDS

Intra-articular glucocorticoids are useful in the treatment of acute gout limited to a single joint or bursa.[177,178] Oral glucocorticoid usage along with a single intramuscular or intravenous injection of a parenteral glucocorticoid can also provide relief. None of these approaches has been systematically studied. Anecdotally, rebound attacks have been reported as steroids were withdrawn. ACTH has been used effectively, especially in attacks in patients following surgery.

PROPHYLAXIS

The practice of giving small daily doses of colchicine as prophylaxis to prevent acute attacks is up to 85 percent effective.[179] The use of colchicine at 0.6 mg once to three times a day is generally well tolerated, although the drug may produce a reversible axonal neuromyopathy.[180] Rhabdomyolysis may also occur in these settings.[181] This complication causes proximal muscle weakness with or without painful paresthesia and elevated serum levels of creatine phosphokinase. This is most often seen in patients also using diuretics with hypertension, renal dysfunction, or liver disease. Rhabdomyolysis may also occur in these settings.[181] In patients who are unable to tolerate even one colchicine tablet per day, indomethacin or another NSAID has been used prophylactically at low doses (e.g., 25 mg indomethacin two times per day) with some success. A program of maintenance colchicine or an NSAID may make the difference between frequent incapacitation and uninterrupted daily activities. Prophylaxis usually is continued until the serum urate value has been maintained well within the normal range and there have been no acute attacks for a period of 3 to 6 months. It is important to warn patients that colchicine discontinuation may be followed by an exacerbation of acute gouty arthritis and advise them what to do should an attack occur. Finally, prophylactic treatment is not recommended unless the clinician also uses urate-lowering agents. Prophylactic colchicine may block the acute inflammatory response but does not alter the deposition of crystals in tissues. With continued deposition without the warning signs of recurrent bouts of acute arthritis, tophi and destruction to cartilage and bone can occur without notice.

CONTROL OF HYPERURICEMIA

Elimination of hyperuricemia with antihyperuricemic agents can prevent as well as reverse urate deposition. Today, a spectrum of opinions exists as to when in the course of gout the clinician should start antihyperuricemic therapy. Some physicians regard the first gouty attack as a late event in a disorder marked by years of antecedent silent deposition of urate crystals in cartilage and other connective tissue. There is some morphologic evidence for this position.[134] Others believe that because tophi and symptomatic chronic gouty arthritis develop only in a minority of cases and ordinarily develop very slowly after many years of recurrent acute attacks, unnecessary or premature medication can be avoided without demonstrable penalty. Indeed, some patients never have a second attack, even in the absence of therapy. The probability of such a "benign" course is greatest in patients who have only minimally elevated serum urate concentrations and normal 24-hour urinary uric acid values. Arguably, a case can be made for initiating antihyperuricemia therapy after the second attack in most patients.[182]

Antihyperuricemic drugs provide a definitive method for controlling hyperuricemia. Although it is important to treat and prevent acute attacks of gouty arthritis with anti-inflammatory agents, it is the long-term control of hyperuricemia that ultimately modifies the manifestations of the gouty diathesis. In general, the aim of antihyperuricemic therapy is to reduce the serum urate concentration to 6.0 mg/dl or less, well below the concentration at which monosodium urate saturates extracellular fluid. When this is achieved, urate deposits resolve.

In general, the lower the serum urate level achieved during antihyperuricemic therapy, the faster the reduction in tophaceous deposits.[183] Reduction to target levels may be achieved pharmacologically by the use of xanthine oxidase inhibitors or uricosuric agents. Xanthine oxidase, the enzyme that catalyzes the oxidation of hypoxanthine to xanthine and xanthine to uric acid, is inhibited by allopurinal and oxypurinal. Probenecid, sulfinpyrazone, and benzbromarone are uricosuric agents that reduce serum urate concentrations by enhancing the renal excretion of uric acid. These antihyperuricemic drugs do not have anti-inflammatory properties.

Once initiated, the use of antihyperuricemic agents is ordinarily carried on indefinitely. For those patients with gout who excrete less than 800 mg of uric acid per day and have normal renal function, reduction of serum urate concentration can be achieved equally well with a xanthine oxidase inhibitor or a uricosuric drug. These agents are equally effective in preventing deterioration of renal function in patients with primary gout.[184] In most cases, allopurinol is probably the drug of choice because it can be used with fewer restrictions compared to uricosuric agents.

In general, the candidate for uricosuric agents is the gouty patient who is younger than 60 years of age and has normal renal function (creatinine clearance greater than 80 ml/min), uric acid excretion of less than 800 mg/24 hours on a general diet, and no history of renal calculi. Patients prescribed uricosuric agents should be counseled to avoid salicylate use at doses greater than 81 mg per day.[118]

In certain situations, an inhibitor of xanthine oxidase is clearly the drug of choice in the gouty patient (Table 87–5). Gouty individuals who excrete larger quantities of uric acid in their urine or who have a history of renal calculi of any type should be treated with allopurinol. The incidence of renal calculi is about 35 percent in patients with primary gout who excrete more than 700 mg/day of uric acid.[89] There is also greater risk for uric acid stones on initiation of uricosuric therapy. In addition, patients with tophi generally should receive this agent to decrease the load of uric acid that must be handled by the kidney. Patients with gout and mild renal insufficiency may be given either type of agent, but

---

TABLE 87–5 • INDICATIONS FOR ALLOPURINOL

Hyperuricemia associated with increased uric acid production
Urinary uric acid excretion of 1000 mg or more in 24 hours
Hyperuricemia associated with HPRT deficiency or PRPP synthetase overactivity
Uric acid nephropathy
Nephrolithiasis
Prophylaxis before cytolytic therapy
Intolerance or reduced efficacy of space uricosuric agents
Gout with renal insufficiency (GFR <60 ml/min)
Allergy to uricosurics

Abbreviations: GFR, glomerular filtration rate; HPRT, hypoxanthine-guanine phosphoribosyltransferase; PRPP, phosphoribosylpyrophosphate.

probenecid and sulfinpyrazone would not be expected to work when the glomerular filtration rate is less than 30 ml/min. Allopurinol is effective in the presence of renal insufficiency, but doses may have to be decreased in that situation. A final indication for a xanthine oxidase inhibitor is the failure of uricosuric agents to produce a serum urate concentration lower than 6 mg/dl or patient intolerant to the uricosuric agent. Allopurinol and a uricosuric drug may be used in combination for the patient with tophaceous gout in whom it is not possible to reduce the serum urate below 6 mg/dl with a single agent. In most settings, if allopurinol does not cause the serum urate to drop below 6 mg/dl, it is the result of insufficient dosing or poor patient compliance.

▌Xanthine Oxidase Inhibitors

Allopurinol is presently the only xanthine oxidase inhibitor approved for use, but others are under development. Allopurinol is also a substrate for xanthine oxidase and is converted to oxipurinol by that enzyme activity. Oxipurinol is also an inhibitor of xanthine oxidase. Allopurinol is metabolized in the liver and has a half-life of 1 to 3 hours, but oxipurinol, which is excreted in the urine, has a half-life of 12 to 17 hours. Because of these pharmacokinetic properties, allopurinol is dosed on a daily basis, and the dosage required to reduce serum urate levels is lower in patients with decreased glomerular filtration rates.[185]

Allopurinol should be used at the lowest does that lowers the serum urate level below 6 mg/dl. This most often achieved with doses of 300 mg per day, but a maximum of 800 mg can be used (Figure 87–18). The sudden lowering of serum urate concentrations that accompanies initiation of allopurinol therapy may trigger acute gout attacks. This risk can be minimized by beginning prophylactic colchicine or NSAID (see previous discussion) 2 weeks before the first dose of allopurinol. As an alternative, the clinician can start the allopurinol at a dose of 100 mg per day and increase by 100-mg increments on a weekly basis.

About 20 percent of patients who take allopurinol report side effects, with 5 percent of patients discontinuing the medication. More common side effects include gastrointestinal intolerance and skin rashes. The occurrence of a rash does not necessarily mean the drug should be discontinued. If the rash is not severe, the allopurinol can be withheld temporarily and resumed after the rash has cleared. Oxipurinol has been tried in patients sensitive to allopurinol, but its use is limited by poor gastrointestinal absorption and a high prevalence of cross-reactivity with allopurinol. Oral and intravenous protocols for desensitization to allopurinol have been proven successful for some patients following cutaneous reactions.[186,187]

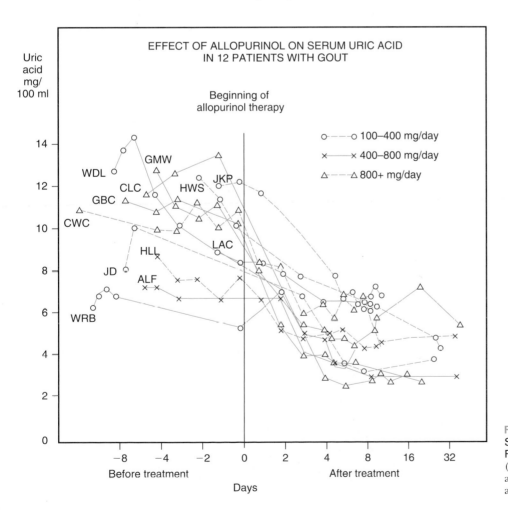

FIGURE 87–18 · Reductions in Serum Urate Concentrations in Patients Receiving Allopurinol. (From Wyngaarden JB, Kelley WN: Gout and Hyperuricemia. New York, Grune and Stratton, 1976, p. 478.)

Other adverse reactions include fever, toxic epidermal necrolysis, alopecia, bone marrow suppression with leukopenia or thrombocytopenia, agranulocytosis, aplastic anemia, granulomatous hepatitis, jaundice, sarcoidlike reaction, and vasculitis. The most serve reaction is the allopurinol hypersensitivity syndrome that consists of a constellation of findings and may include fever, skin rash, eosinophilia, hepatitis, progressive renal insufficiency, and death.[188,189] Autopsies reveal diffuse vasculitis involving multiple organs. This is most likely to develop in individuals with preexisting renal dysfunction and those taking diuretics.

Allopurinol is involved in relatively few drug-drug interactions. Its use will potentiate the actions of other agents that are inactivated by xanthine oxidase. The most important of these are azathioprine and 6-mercaptopurine. In addition, allopurinol can reduce the activity of hepatic microsomal drug-metabolizing enzymes and prolong the half-lives of warfarin and theophylline. Rash may be more common in patients using allopurinol and ampicillin, and bone marrow suppression may be increase in those also taking cyclophosphamide.

Uricosuric Agents

A uricosuric agent increases the rate of renal uric acid excretion.[190] In the kidney, there are separate transport systems for the secretion and reabsorption of organic ions, including uric acid. Because urate is reabsorbed by a renal tubular brush border anion transporter, the reabsorption of urate can be inhibited when uricosuric agents are present in the lumen and compete with urate for the transporter. This inhibition of reabsoptive anion transporter requires higher dose of uricosuric agents. Because the secretory transport system is quantitatively much smaller than that for reabsorption and is located in the basolateral membrane of the tubule, when uricosuric agents are taken in very low doses, they actually decrease the renal excretion of uric acid and raise serum urate levels by inhibiting the secretory transport system.

Probenecid and sulfinpyrazone are the most widely used uricosuric agents available in the United States; benzbromarone is used for this purpose in other countries as well. However, many other agents can reduce serum urate levels by enhancing the renal excretion of uric acid (Table 87–6).

Probenecid is readily absorbed from the gastrointestinal tract. Its half-life in plasma is dose dependent, varying from 6 to 12 hours. This can be prolonged by the concomitant use of allopurinol. Probenecid is metabolized in vivo, with less than 5 percent of the administered dose recovered in the urine. The maintenance dosage of probenecid ranges from 500 mg to 3 g per day and is administered on a twice or three-times-a-day schedule. Acute gouty attacks may accompany the initiation of this medication, as with all other antihyperuricemic agents, and, as with all uricosuric agents, patients using probenecid are at increased risk for developing renal calculi. With long-term use, up to 18 percent of individuals develop gastrointestinal complaints, and 5 percent develop hypersensitivity and rash. Although serious toxicity is rare, approximately one third of individuals eventually become intolerant of probenecid and discontinue its use. Probenecid alters the metabolism of several other agents by several mechanisms (Table 87–7). Concomitant use of probenecid can increase the potency of some agents by decreasing their renal excretion, delaying their metabolism, or impairing their hepatic uptake. In others it may decrease their effectiveness by reducing their volume of distribution.

Sulfinpyrazone is completely absorbed from the gastrointestinal tract and has a half-life of 1 to 3 hours. Most of the drug is excreted in the urine as the parahydroxyl metabolite, which is also uricosuric. Sulfinpyrazone is

TABLE 87–6 • DRUGS SHOWN TO BE URICOSURIC IN HUMANS

Acetoheximide	Glycerol guaiacolate
Amflutizole	Glycine
Ascorbic acid	Glycopyrrolate
Azapropazone	Iodopyracet
Azauridine	Iopanic acid
Benzbromarone	Losartan
Calcitonin	Meclofenamic acid
Calcium ipodate	Orotic acid
Citrate	Outdated tetracyclines
Dicumarol	Phenolsulfonphthalein
Diflunisal	Probenecid
Estrogens	Salicylates
Fenofibrate	Sulfinpyrazone

TABLE 87–7 • EFFECTS OF PROBENECID ON METABOLISM OF OTHER DRUGS

Decreased Renal Excretion

p-Aminohippuric acid
Phenolsulfophthalein
Salicylic acid and its acyl and phenolic glucuronides
Phlorizin and its glucuronide
Acetazolamide
Dapsone and its metabolites
Sulfinpyrazone and its parahydroxyl metabolite
Indomethacin
Ampicillin
Penicillin
Cephradine

Reduced Volume of Distribution

Ampicillin
Ancillin
Nafcillin
Cephaloridine

Impairment of Hepatic Uptake

Bromsulfophthlein
Indocyanin green
Rifampicin

Delayed Metabolism

Heparin

usually maintained at a daily dosage of 300 to 400 mg per day given in three to four divided doses. The rates of tolerability and types of adverse reactions are similar to those with probenecid.

Benzbromarone is a potent uricosuric.[184] It is more potent than probenecid and sulfinpyrazone. It is well tolerated and effective in cyclosporine-treated renal-transplant patients. It can be used with moderate renal dysfunction (creatinine clearance is approximately 25 ml./min).

COMPLIANCE AND TREATMENT OF GOUT

Because the disease processes involved in gout are so well understood, the diagnosis can be definitively established, and available therapies are so effective that gout should be a readily treated and easily managed disease. However, too many patients, including those who are accurately diagnosed, do not do well. Failure of antihyperuricemic therapy to attain the target urate level is due to improper prescribing or poor compliance.[185] Compliance is often a problem when treating chronic asymptomatic conditions, and associated alcoholism can be a factor. Perhaps more important is the fact that patients may need to take up to three different medications on three different schedules to appropriately control their symptoms and treat the disease.

It is believed that if patients understand why they are taking medications they are more likely to be compliant. To this end, an analogy has been developed that helps some patients become more compliant.[191] In this analogy, urate crystals are compared to matches. The patient is told that "when the match strikes," it causes a gout attack. "To put out the fire" the patient takes an NSAID or colchicine, but although this resolves the attack "the matches are still there." To eliminate future attacks the patient is given prophylactic colchicine, "which makes the matches damp and harder to strike," and allopurinol (or a uricosuric agent), "which actually removes the matches from the body."

MANAGEMENT OF GOUT AFTER ORGAN TRANSPLANTATION

The management of patients with gout after organ transplantation requires careful consideration. The use of glucocorticoids, azathioprine, or cyclosporine and the precarious status of renal function in many patients pose complex problems. Colchicine and NSAIDs may be inappropriate for management of acute gouty arthritis in this setting because of their potential toxicities. Intrarticular glucocorticoid injections may be most helpful, and one may be forced to rely more heavily on the use of pain medications in this setting. Prophylactic colchicine can be used in patients with normal renal function, but treatment must be monitored closely. The combination of colchicine and cycloporine has induced rhabdomyolysis.[181]

When considering chronic therapy, it should be helpful to lower the doses of cyclosporine and eliminate the use of diuretics if possible. Uricosuric agents can be used safely, but their usefulness declines if renal func-

tion is poor. Allopurinol can be used in patients with abnormal renal function, but the dose may need to be reduced. Allopurinol, however, has potential severe interaction with azathioprine. Azathioprine is metabolized by xanthine oxidase. Because allopurinol inhibits that enzyme, the breakdown of azathioprine is slowed, increasing the effective dose. If care is not taken, significant bone marrow toxicity can result. If azathioprine and allopurinol are used together, they can be started at 25 and 50 mg/day, respectively.[192] Complete blood counts and serum urate level concentrations are then monitored weekly, and the allopurinol dose is adjusted to bring the serum urate concentration to less than 6 mg/dl. Mycophenolate mofetil, as an alternative to azathioprine, has been used effectively with allopurinol in some transplant patients.[193]

Urate oxidase has been used to drastically lower serum urate levels and shrink tophi in a small number of patients with gout after cardiac transplantation.[194] This treatment has been associated with significant allergic reactions, including anaphylaxis, bronchospasm, and hemolytic anemia, but newer preparations of uricase formulated with polycthylene glycol may avoid those complications and prove more effective.[195]

ANCILLARY FACTORS

In addition to anti-inflammatory agents, colchicine prophylaxis, and antihyperuricemic therapy, other factors may be decisive in determining whether recurrent attacks, chronic gouty arthritis, kidney stones, or nephropathy develops. Today, dietary purine restriction solely to control serum urate levels is rarely necessary. A diet totally restricted in purine content can reduce the urinary excretion of uric acid by only 200 to 400 mg/day and lower the mean serum urate value by about 1 mg/dl.[196] In addition, the antihyperuricemic agents available today are so effective that the clinician rarely needs to resort to this kind of dietary manipulation. Nevertheless, beneficial results have been reported with a diet of moderate calorie and carbohydrate restriction and increased proportional intake of protein and unsaturated fat.[196] Some subjects with gout are susceptible to acute attacks after the use of alcoholic beverages or consumption of rich foods. Others describe idiosyncratic responses, such as acute gout after eating a particular food, but such relationships are rare and questionable. A diet designed to avoid indiscretions known to be associated with the precipitation of an acute gouty attack in a particular individual is recommended.

In addition, diet is very important with regard to other medical problems.[197] Many gouty patients are overweight, and restoration of ideal body weight through regulated caloric restriction is recommended. In addition, at least 75 percent of patients with primary gout have hypertriglyceridemia. The initial step in management of hypertriglyceridemia is reduction to ideal body weight and elimination of alcohol ingestion.

Many patients with gout consume liberal amounts of alcohol. Acute excesses may lead to exacerbations of hyperuricemia secondary to the temporary hyperlactacidemia, and chronic ingestion of alcohol may stimulate increased purine production.[69] The added purine load resulting from regular ingestion of beer may also be a contributing factor. The patient should be instructed in the deleterious effects of excessive alcohol intake. Compliance with medication is also much worse among patients who consume alcohol.

About one third of gouty subjects are hypertensive. The complications of hypertension are potentially more serious than those of hyperuricemia, and the clinician should not hesitate to use whatever drugs are necessary to control the hypertension. Many hypertensive gouty patients require a thiazide diuretic. If this medication is needed to control hypertension, it should be used, with the recognition that the dosage of concomitant antihyperuricemic therapy may need to be adjusted to maintain appropriate control of serum urate levels.

REFERENCES

1. Wyngaarden JD, Kelley WN: Gout and Hyperuricemia. New York, Grune & Stratton, 1976.
2. Ghei M, Mihailescu M, Levinson J, et al.: Pathogenisis of hyperuricemia: recent advances. Curr Rheumatol Rep 4:270, 2002.
3. Chang H-Y, Pan W-H, Yeh W-T, et al: Hyperuricemia and gout in Taiwan: results of the nutritional and health survey in Taiwan. J Rheum 28:1640, 2001.
4. Wortmann RL: zGout and hyperuricemia. Curr Opin Rheumatol 14:281, 2002.
5. Darmawan J, Valkenburg HA, Muirden KD, Wigley RD: The epidemiology of gout and hyperuricemia in a rural population in Java. J Rheumatol 19:1595, 1992.
6. Cameron JS, Moro F, Simmonds HA: Gout, uric acid, and purine metabolism in pediatric nephrology. Pediatr Nephrol 7:105, 1993.
7. Park YB, Park YS, Lee WK, et al: Clinical manifestations of Korean female gouty patients. Clin Rheumatol 19:142, 2000.
8. Marinello E, Giuseppe RS, Marcolongo R: Plasma follicle-stimulating hormone, luteinizing hormone, and sex hormones in patients with gout. Arthritis Rheum 28:127, 1985.
9. Arromlee E, Michet CJ, Crowson CS, et al: Epidemiology of gout: is the incidence rising? J Rheumatol 29:2403, 2002.
10. Campion EW, Glynn RJ, deLabry LO: Asymptomatic hyperuricemia: the risks and consequences. Am J Med 82:421, 1987.
11. Parhami N, Feng H: Gout in the hip joint. Arthritis Rheum 36:1026, 1993.
12. Yasuhara K, Tomita Y, Takayama A, et al: Thoracic myelopathy due to compression by the epidural tophas: a case report. J Spinal Disord 7:82, 1994.
13. Musgrave DS, Ziran BH: Monoarticular acromiclavicular joint gout. Am J Orthoped 29:544, 2000.
14. Recht MP, Saragini F, Kramer J, et al: Isolated or dominant lesions of the patella in gout: a report of seven patients. Skeletal Radiol 23:113, 1994.
15. Lally EV, Zimmerman B, Ho G, Kaplan SR: Urate-mediated inflammation in nodal osteoarthritis: clinical and roentgenographic correlations. Arthritis Rheum 32:86, 1989.
16. Kuzell WC, Glover RP, Gibbs JD, et al: Effect of sulfinpyrazone on serum acid and gout. Geriatrics 19: 894, 1964.
17. Rundles RW, Metz EN, Silberman HR: Allopurinol in the treatment of gout. Ann Intern Med 64:229, 1966.
18. Gurwitz JH, Kalish SC, Bohn RL, et al: Thiazide diuretics and the initiation of anti-gout therapy. J Clin Epidemiol 50:953, 1977.
19. Khalifa P, Sereni D, Boissonnas A, et al: Attacks of gout and thromboembolic disease: role of heparin therapy. Ann Intern Med 136:582, 1985.
20. Tiller DJ, Hall BM, Horvath JS, et al: Gout and hyperuricemia in patients on cyclosporin and diuretics [Letter]. Lancet 1:453, 1985.
21. Kalia KK, Moossy JJ: Carpal tunnel release complicated by acute gout. Neurosurgery 33:1102, 1993.
22. Williamson SC, Roger DJ, Petrera P, Glockner F: Acute gouty arthropathy after total knee arthroplasty: a case report. J Bone Joint Surg Am 76:126, 1994.
23. Nakayama DA, Barthelemy C, Carrera G, et al: Tophaceous gout: a clinical and radiographic assessment. Arthritis Rheum 27:468, 1984.
24. Wallace SL, Bernstein D, Diamond H: Diagnostic value of the colchicine therapeutic trial. JAMA 199:525, 1967.
25. Wallace SL, Robinson H, Masi AT, et al: Preliminary criteria for the classification of acute arthritis of primary gout. Arthritis Rheum 20:897, 1977.
26. Bonal J, Schumacher HR: Podagra is more than gout. Bull Rheum Dis 34:1, 1984.
27. Vandenberg MK, Moxley G, Breitbach SA, et al: Gout attacks in chronic alcoholics occur at lower serum urate levels than in nonalcoholics. J Rheumatol 21:700, 1994.
28. Tsutani H, Yoshio N, Takanori U: Interleukin 6 reduces serum urate concentrations. J Rheumatol 27:554 2000.
29. Urano W, Yamanaka H, Tsutani H, et al: The inflammatory process in the mechanism of decreased serum uric acid concentration during acute gouty arthritis. J Rheumatol 29:1950, 2002.
30. Wortmann RL, Kelley WN: Gout and Hyperuricemia. In Ruddy S, Harris ED Jr., Sledge CB (eds): Kelley's Textbook of Rheumatology, 6th ed. Philadelphia, WB Saunders, 2001, p 1339.
31. Rogachefsky RA, Cameiro R, Altman RD, et al: Gout presenting as infectious arthritis. J Bone Surg Am 76:269, 1994.
32. Gutman AB: Gout. In Beeson PB, McDermott W (eds): Textbook of Medicine, 12th ed. Philadelphia, WB Saunders, 1958, p 595.
33. McCarthy GM, Barthelemy CR, Verum JA, et al: Influence of antihyperuricemia therapy and radiographic progression of gout. Arthritis Rheum 34:1489, 1991.
34. Pascual E, Batlle-Gualda E, Martinez A, et al: Synovial fluid analysis for diagnosis of intercritical gout. Ann Intern Med 131:756, 1999.
35. Cobb, KL, Mendez EA, Espinoza LR: Gouty arthritis mimicking rheumatoid arthritis. J Clin Rheumatol 4:225, 1998.
36. Kini S, Mittal G, Balakrishna C, et al: An unusual systemic presentation of gout. JAPI 48:354, 2000.
37. Hench PS: The diagnosis of gout and gouty arthritis. J Lab Clin Med 220:48, 1936.
38. Gutman AB: The past four decades of progress in the knowledge of gout, with an assessment of the present status. Arthritis Rheum 16:431, 1973.
39. Scott JT, Higgens CS: Diuretic induced gout: a multifactoral condition. Ann Rheum Dis 51:259, 1992.
40. Wernick R, Winkler C, Campbell S: Tophias, the initial manifestation of gout: report of six cases and review of the literature. Arch Intern Med 152:873, 1992.
41. Lopez Redondo MJ, Requena L, Macia M, et al: Fingertip tophi without gouty arthritis. Dermatology 187:140, 1993.
42. Beathge BA, Work J, Landreneau MD, et al: Tophaceous gout in patients with renal transplants treated with cyclosporine A. J Rheumatol 20:718, 1993.
43. Barthelemy CR, Nakayama DA, Carrera GF, et al: Gouty arthritis: a prospective radiographic evaluation of sixty patients. Skeletal Radiol 11:1, 1984.
44. Gerster JC, Landry M, Dufresne L, et al: Imaging of tophaceous gout: computed tomography provider specific images compared to magnetic resonance imaging and ultrasonography. Ann Rheum Dis 61:52, 2002.
45. Vaccaro AR, An HS, Cotler JM, et al: Recurrent cervical sublaxationsin a patient with gout and endstage renal disease. Orthopedics 16:1273, 1993.
46. Hausch R, Wilkerson M, Singh E, et al: Tophaceous gout of the thoracic spine presenting as back pain and fever. J Clin Rheumatol 5:335, 1999.
47. Gawoski JM, Balogh K, Landis WJ: Aortic valvular tophus: identification by x-ray diffraction of urate and calcium phosphates. J Clin Pathol 38:873, 1985.
48. Schapira D, Stahl S, Izhak OB, et al: Chronic tophaceous gouty arthritis mimicking rheumatoid arthritis. Semin Arthritis Rheum 29:56, 1999.

49. Myers A, Epstein FH, Dodge HJ, et al: The relationship of serum uric acid to risk factors in coronary heart disease. Am J Med 45:520, 1968.

50. Takahashi S, Yamamoto T, Moriwaki Y, et al: Impaired lipoprotein metabolism in patients with primary gout: influence of alcohol intake and body weight. Br J Rheumatol 33:731, 1994.

51. Collantes E, Tinahones FJ, Cisnal A, et al: Variability of lipid phenotypes in hyperuricemic-hyperlipidemic patients. Clin Rheumatol 13:244, 1994.

52. Tsutsumi S, Yamamoto T, Moriwaki Y, et al: Decreased activities of lipoprotein lipase and hepatic trglyceride lipase in patients with gout. Metabolism 50:952, 2001.

53. Mikkelsen WM: The possible association of hyperuricemia and/or gout with diabetes mellitus. Arthritis Rheum 8:853, 1965.

54. Denis G, Launay MP: Carbohydrate intolerance in gout. Metabolism 18:770, 1969.

55. Selby JV, Friedman GD, Quesenberry CP: Precursors of essential hypertension: pulmonary function, heart rate, uric acid, serum cholesterol, and other serum chemistries. Am J Epidemiol 131:1017, 1990.

56. Goldstein HS, Manowitz P: Relation between serum uric acid and blood pressure in adolescents. Ann Hum Biol 20:423, 1993.

57. Jossa F, Farinaro E, Panico S, et al: Serum uric acid and hypertension: The Olivetti Heart Study. J Hum Hypertens 8:677, 1994.

58. Cappuccio FP, Stazzullo P, Farinaro E, Trevisan M: Uric acid metabolism and tubular sodium handling: results from a population based study. JAMA 270:354, 1993.

59. Kang DH, Nakagawa T, Feng L, et al: A role for uric acid in the progression of renal disease. J Am Soc Nephrol 13:1288, 2002.

60. Mazzali M, Kanellis J, Han L, et al: Hyperuricemia induces primary renal arteriolopathy in rats by a blood pressure–independent mechanism. Am J Physical Renal Physiol 282:F991, 2002.

61. Grundy SM, Balady GJ, Criqui MH, et al: Primary prevention of coronary heart disease: guidance from Framingham. a statement of healthcare professionals from the AHA task force on risk reduction. Circulation 97.1876, 1998.

62. Culleton BF, Larson MG, Kannal WB, et al: Serum uric acid and risk of cardiovascular disease and mortality: The Framingham Heart Study. Ann Int Med 131:7, 1999.

63. Fang J, Alderman MH: Serum uric acid and cardiovascular mortality: The NHANES I Epidemiologic Follow-up Study, 1971-1992. JAMA 283:2404, 2000.

64. Verdecchia P, Schillaci G, Reboldi GP, et al: Relation between serum uric acid and risk of cardiovascular disease in hypertension: The PIUMA Study. Hypertension 36:1072, 2000.

65. Vuorinen-Markkola H, YkiJarvinen H: Hyperuricemia and insulin resistance. J Clin Endocrinol Metab 78:25, 1994.

66. Chou P, Lin K-C, Lin Y-H, et al: Gender differences in the relationship of serum uric acid with fasting serum insulin and plasma glucose in patients without diabetes. J Rheumatol 28:571, 2001.

67. Takahashi S, Moriwaki Y, Tsutsuni Z, et al: Increase visceral fat accumulation further aggravates the risks of insulin resistance in gout. Metabolism 50:393, 2001.

68. Al-Arfaj AS: Hyperuricemia in Saudi Arabia. Rheumatol Int 20:61, 2001.

69. Faller J, Fox IH: Ethanol-induced hyperuricemia: evidence for increased urate production by activation of adenine nucleotide turnover. N Engl J Med 307:1598, 1982.

70. Puig JG, Fox IH: Ethanol-induced activation of adenine nucleotide turnover: evidence for a role of acetate. J Clin Invest 74:936, 1984.

71. Gibson T, Rodgers AV, Simmonds HA, Toseland P: Beer drinking and its effect on uric acid. Br J Rheumatol 23:203, 1984.

72. Erickson AR, Enzenauer RJ, Nordstrom DM, Merenich JA: The prevalence of hypothyroidism in gout. Am J Med 97:231, 1994.

73. Nordstrom DM, Merenich JA: The relationship of gout to hyperthyroidism [Abstract]. Arthritis Rheum 32:S68, 1989.

74. Staub JJ, Althaus BU, Engler H, et al: Spectrum of subclinical and overt hypothyroidism: effects of thyrotropin, prolactin, and thyroid reserve, and metabolic impact on peripheral target tissues. Am J Med 92:631, 1992.

75. Woolliscroft JO, Fox IH: Increased body fluid purines during hypotensive events: evidence for ATP degradation. Am J Med 81:472, 1986.

76. Grum CM, Simon RH, Dantzker DR, Fox IH: Biochemical indicators of cellular hypoxia in critically ill patients: evidence for ATP degradation. Chest 88:763, 1985.

77. McCord J: Oxygen-derived free radicals in postischemic tissue injury. N Engl J Med 312:159, 1985.

78. Meadows J, Smith RC, Reeves J: Uric acid protects membranes and linolenic acid from ozone-induced oxidation. Biochem Biophys Res Commun 137:536, 1986.

79. Lind T, Godfrey KA, Otun H: Changes in serum uric acid concentrations during normal pregnancy. Br J Obstet Gynaecol 91:128, 1984.

80. Liedholm H, Montan S, Aberg A: Risk grouping of 113 patients with hypertensive disorders during pregnancy, with respect to serum urate, proteinuria and time of onset of hypertension. Acta Obstet Gynecol Scand 118(Suppl):43, 1984.

81. Wooten MD, Lipsmeyer E: Gout accompanying rheumatoid arthritis: a comparison of affected women and men. J Clin Rheumatol 4:220, 1998.

82. Wall BA, Agudelo CA, Weinblatt ME, et al: Acute gout and systemic lupus erythematosus: report of 2 cases and literature review. J Rheumatol 9:305, 1982.

83. Wong DMT, Chambers IM: Coexistent acute gouty arthritis and ankylosing spondylitis: a rare occurrence. J Rheumatol 21:773, 1994.

84. Fessel WJ: Renal outcomes of gout and hyperuricemia. Am J Med 67:74, 1979.

85. Yu TF, Berger L: Renal function in gout: Its association with hypertensive vascular disease and intrinsic renal disease. Am J Med 72:95, 1982.

86. Cohen LF, Balow JE, Poplack DG, et al: Acute tumor lysis syndrome: a review of 37 patients with Burkitt's lymphoma. Am J Med 68:486, 1980.

87. Kelton J, Kelley WN, Holmes EW: A rapid method for the diagnosis of acute uric acid nephropathy. Arch Intern Med 138:612, 1978.

88. Gutman AB, Yu TF: Uric acid nephrolithiasis. Am J Med 45.756, 1968.

89. Yu TF, Gutman AB: Uric acid nephrolithiasis in gout: predisposing factors. Ann Intern Med 67:1133, 1967.

90. Simmonds HA, Sahota AS, Van Acker KJ: Adenine phosphoribosyltransferase deficiency and 2,8-dihydroxyadenine lithiasis. In Scriver CR, Beaudet AC, Sly WS, Valle D (eds): The Metabolic and Molecular Bases of Inherited Disease, 7th ed. New York, McGraw-Hill, 1995, pp 1655-1670.

91. Calabrese G, Simmonds HA, Cameron JS, Davies PM: Precocious familial gout with reduced fractional urate clearance and normal purine enzymes. Q J Med 75:441, 1990.

92. Puig JG, Miranda ME, Matcos FA, et al: Hereditary nephropathy associated with hyperuricemia and gout. Arch Intern Med 153:357, 1993.

93. McBride MB, Rigden S, Haycock GB, et al: Presymptomatic detection of familial juvenile hyperuricemia nephropathy in children. Pediatr Nephrol 12:357, 1998.

94. Kamatani N, Maritani M, Yamanaka H, et al: Localization of the gene for familial juvenile hyperuricemia nephropathy causing underexcretion-type gout to 16p2 by genome-wide linkage analysis of a large family. Arthritis Rheum 43:925, 2000.

95. Stavrou C, Pierides A, Zouvani I, et al: Medullary cystic kidney disease with hyperuricemia and gout in a large Cypriot family: no allelism with nephronophthisis type I. Am J Med Genet 77:149, 1998

96. Leumann EP, Wegmann W: Familial nephropathy with hyperuricemia and gout. Nephron 34:51, 1983.

97. Hosoya T, Ichida K, Tabe A, Sakai O: A study of uric acid metabolism and gouty arthritis in patients with polycystic kidney. Nippon Jinzo Gakkai Shi 35:43, 1993.

98. Gabow PA: Autosomal dominant polycystic kidney disease. N Engl J Med 329:332, 1993.

99. Halla JT, Ball GV: Saturnine gout: a review of 42 patients. Semin Arthritis Rheum 11:307, 1982.

100. Lin J-L, Tan D-T, Ho H-H, et al: Environmental lead exposure and urate excretion in the general population. Am J Med 113:563, 2002.

101. Marsden PA: Increased body lead burden-cause or consequence of chronic renal insufficiency? N Eng J Med 348:345, 2002.

102. Batuman V: Lead nephropathy, lead, and hypertension. Am J Med Sci 305:241, 1993.
103. Lin JL, Huang PT: Body lead stores and urate excretion in men with chronic renal disease. J Rheumatol 21:705, 1994.
104. Reynolds PP, Knapp MJ, Baraf HSB, Holmes EW: Moonshine and lead: relationship to the pathogenesis of hyperuricemia in gout. Arthritis Rheum 26:1057, 1983.
105. Burack DA, Griffith BP, Thompson ME, Kahl LE: Hyperuricemia and gout among heart transplant recipients receiving cyclosporine. Am J Med 92:141, 1992.
106. Cantarell MC, Capdevila L, Morlans M, Piera L: Uric acid calculus in renal transplant patients treated with cyclosporine. Clin Nephrol 35:288, 1992.
107. Griebsch A, Zollner N: Effect of ribonucleotides given orally on uric acid production in man. In Sperling O, de Vries A, Wyngaarden JB (eds): Purine Metabolism in Man. Vol 41B. New York, Plenum Press, 1974, p 443.
108. Maesaka JK, Fishbane S: Regulation of renal urate excretion: a critical review. Am J Kidney Dis 32:917, 1998.
109. Segal JB, Albert D: Diagnosis of crystal-induced arthritis by synovial fluid examination: lessons from and imperfect test. Arthritis Car Res 12:376, 1999.
110. Wortmann RL, Fox IH: Limited value of uric acid to creatinine ratios in estimating uric acid excretion. Ann Intern Med 93:822, 1980.
111. Seegmiller JE, Grayzel AI, Howell RR, et al: The renal excretion of uric acid in gout. J Clin Invest 41:1094,1962.
112. Moriwaki Y, Yamamoto T, Takahashi S, et al: Spot urine uric acid to creatinine ratio used in the estimation of uric acid excretion in primary gout. J Rheumatol 28:1306, 2001.
113. Emmerson BT, Nagel SL, Duffy DL, Martin NG: Genetic control of the renal clearance of urate: a study of twins. Ann Rheum Dis 51:375, 1992.
114. Nugent CA, Tyler FH: The renal excretion of uric acid in patients with gout and in nongouty subjects. J Clin Invest 38:1890, 1959.
115. Yu TF, Berger L, Gutman AB: Renal function in gout. II. Effect of uric acid loading on renal excretion of uric acid. Am J Med 33:829, 1962.
116. Latham W, Rodnan GP: Impairment of uric acid excretion in gout. J Clin Invest 41:1955, 1962.
117. Vecchio PC, Emmerson BT: Gout due to renal disease. Br J Rheumatol 31:63, 1992
118. Caspi D, Lubert E, Graft E, et al: The effect of mini-dose aspirin on renal function and uric acid handling in elderly patients. Arthritis Rheum 43:103, 2000.
119. Lesch M, Nyhan WL: A familial disorder of uric acid metabolism and central nervous system function. Am J Med 36:561, 1964.
120. Seegmiller JE, Rosenbloom RM, Kelley WN: An enzyme defect associated with a sex-linked human neurological disorder and excessive purine synthesis. Science 155:1682, 1967.
121. Kelley WN: Hypoxanthine guanine phosphoribosyltransferase deficiency in the Lesch-Nyhan syndrome and gout. Fed Proc 27:1060, 1968.
122. Kelley WN, Rosenbloom EM, Henderson JF, et al: A specific enzyme defect in gout associated with overproduction of uric acid. Proc Natl Acad Sci U S A 57:1735, 1967.
123. Chang SJ, Chang JG, Chen CJ, et al: Identification of a new single nucleotide substitution on the hypoxanthine-guanine phosphoribosyltransferase gene (HPRT[Tsou]) from a Taiwanese aboriginal family with severe gout. J Rheumatol 26:1802, 1999.
124. Sperling O, Eilam G, Persky-Brosh S, et al: Accelerated erythrocyte 5'-phosphoribosylpyrophosphate synthesis: a familial abnormality associated with excessive uric acid production and gout. Biochem Med 6:310, 1972.
125. Becker MA, Losman MJ, Itkin P, et al: Gout with superactive phosphoribosylpyrophosphate synthetase due to increased enzyme catalytic rate. J Lab Clin Med 99:495, 1982.
126. Takeuchi F, Hanaoka F, Yano E, et al: The mode of genetic transmission of a gouty family with increased phosphoribosylpyrophosphate synthetase activity. Hum Genet 58:322, 1981.
127. Cohen JL, Vinik A, Faller J, Fox IH: Hyperuricemia in glycogen storage disease type I: contributions by hypoglycemia and hyperglucagonemia to increased urate production. J Clin Invest 75:251, 1985.
128. Seegmiller JE, Dixon RM, Kemp GJ, et al: Fructose-induced aberration of metabolism in familial gout identified by ^{31}P magnetic resonance spectroscopy. Proc Natl Acad Sci USA 87:8326, 1990.
129. Mineo I, Kono N, Hara N, et al: Myogenic hyperuricemia: A common pathophysiologic feature of glycogenosis types III, V, and VII. N Engl J Med 317:75, 1987.
130. Bertorini TE, Shively V, Taylor B, et al: ATP degradation products after ischemic exercise: Hereditary lack of phosphorylase or carnitine palmitoyltransferase. Neurology 35:1355, 1985.
131. Sabina RL, Swain JL, Olanow CW, et al: Myoadenylate deaminase deficiency: functional and metabolic abnormalities associated with disruption of the purine nucleotide cycle. J Clin Invest 73:720, 1984.
132. Davidson-Mundt A, Luder AS, Greene CL: Hyperuricemia in medium-chain acylcoenzyme A dehydrogenase deficiency. J Pediatr 120:444, 1992.
133. McCarty DJ Jr: Phagocytosis of urate crystals in gouty synovial fluid. Am J Med Sci 243:288, 1962.
134. Agudelo CA, Schumacher HR: The synovitis of acute gouty arthritis: a light and electron microscopic study. Hum Pathol 4:265, 1973.
135. McGill NW, Dieppe PA: The role of serum and synovial fluid components in the promotion of urate crystal formation. J Rheumatol 18:1042, 1991.
136. Kam M, PerlTreves D, Caspi D, Addadi L: Antibodies against crystals. FASEB J 6:2608, 1992.
137. Pascual E, Castellano JA: Treatment with colchicine decreases the white blood cell counts in the synovial fluid of asymptomatic knees which contain monosodium urate crystals. J Rheumatol 19:600, 1992.
138. Pascual E, Jovani V: A quantitative study of phagocytosis of urate crystals in the synovial fluid of asymptomatic joints of patients with gout. Br J Rheumatol 34:724, 1995.
139. Schweyor S, Hemmerlein H, Radzun HJ, et al: Continuous recruitment, co-expression of tumor necrosis-α; and matrix metalloproteinases, and apoptosis of macrophages on gout tophi. Vinchows Arch 437:534, 2000.
140. Liote F, Prudhommeaux F, Schiltz C, et al: Inhibition and prevention of monosodium urate monohydrate crystal-induced acute inflammation in vivo by transforming growth factor β1, Arthritis Rheum 39:1192, 1996.
141. Yagnik DR, Hillyer P, Marshall D, et al: Noninflammatory phagocytosis of monosodium urate monohydrate crystals by mouse macrophages: implication for the control of joint inflammation in gout. Arthritis Rheum 43:1779, 2000.
142. Weinberger A: Gout, uric acid metabolism, and crystal-induced inflammation. Curr Opin Rheumatol 7:359, 1995.
143. Fam AG, Schumacher HR Jr., Clayburne G, et al: A comparison of five preparations of synthetic monosodium urate monohydrate crystals. J Rheumatol 19:780, 1992.
144. Stankovic A, Front P, Barbara A, Mitrovic DR: Tophus-derived monosodium urate monohydrate crystals are biologically much more active than synthetic counterpart. Rheumatol Int 10:221, 1991.
145. Burt HM, Jackson JK: Cytosolic Ca^{2+} concentration determinations in neutrophils stimulated by monosodium urate and calcium pyrophosphate crystals: effect of protein adsorption. J Rheumatol 21:138, 1994.
146. Ortiz-Bravo E, Schumacher HR: Components generated locally as well as serum after the phlogistic effect of monosodium urate crystals in vivo. J Rheumatol 20:1162, 1993.
147. Ortiz-Bravo E, Sieck MS, Schumacher HR: Changes in the proteins coating monosodium urate crystals during active and subsidiary inflammation: Immuno-gold studies of synovial fluid from patients with gout and of fluid obtained using the rat subcutaneous air pouch model. Arthritis Rheum 36:1274, 1993.
148. Ghio AJ, Kennedy TP, Rao G, et al: Complexation of iron cation by sodium urate crystals and gouty inflammation. Arch Biochem Biophys 313:215, 1994.
149. Hachicha M, Naccache PH, McColl SR: Inflammatory microcrystals differentially regulate the secretion of macrophage inflammatory protein 1 and interleukin 8 by human neutrophils: a possible mechanism of acutrophil recruitment to sites of inflammation in synovitis. J Exp Med 182:2019, 1995.

150. Chapman PT, Yarwood H, Harrison, et al: Endothelial activation ion monosodium monohydrate crystal-induced inflammation: in vitro and in vivo studies on the roles of tumor necrosis factor ∝ and interleukin 1. Arthritis Rheum 40:955, 1977.

151. Verburgh CA, Hart MHL, Aarden LA, Swaak AJG: Interleukin-8 (IL-8) in synovial fluid of rheumatoid and nonrheumatoid joint effusions. Clin Rheumatol 12:494, 1993.

152. Smallwood JL, Malawista SE: Colchicine, crystals, and neutrophil tyrosine phosphorylation. J Clin Invest 92:1602, 1993.

153. Naccache PH, Bourgoin S, Plante E, et al: Crystal induced neutrophil activation. II. Evidence for the activation of a phosphatidylcholine-specific phospholipase D. Arthritis Rheum 36:117, 1993.

154. Burt HM, Jackson JK, Salari H: Inhibition of crystal-induced neutrophil activation by a protein tyrosine kinase inhibitor. J Leukoc Biol 55:112, 1994.

155. Terkeltaub R, Smeltzer D, Curtiss LK, Ginsberg MH: Low density lipoprotein inhibits the physical interaction of phlogistic crystals and inflammatory cells. Arthritis Rheum 29:363, 1986.

156. Roberge CJ, Brassi J, de Medicis R, et al: Crystal-neutrophil interactions lead to interleukin-synthesis. Agents Actions 34:38, 1994

157. Roberge CJ, de Medicis R, Dayer JM: Crystal-induced neutrophil activation. V. Differential production of biologically active IL-1 and IL-1 receptor antagonist. J Immunol 152:5485, 1994.

158. Hering FG, Lam EWN, Burt HM: A spin label study of the membranolytic effects of crystalline monosodium urate monohydrate. J Rheumatol 13:623, 1986.

159. Terkeltaub R, Zachariae C, Santoro D, et al: Monocyte-derived neutrophil chemotactic factor/IL-8 is a potential mediator of crystal-induced inflammation. Arthritis Rheum 34:894, 1991.

160. Digiovine FS, Malawista SF, Thornton E, et al: Urate crystals stimulate production of tumor necrosis factor-alpha from human blood monocytes and synovial cells: Cytokine messenger RNA and protein kinetics and cellular distribution. J Clin Invest 87:1375, 1991.

161. Hachicha M, Naccache PH, McColl SR: Inflammatory microcrystals differentially regulate secretion of MIP-1 and IL-8 by human neutrophils. J Exp Med 182:2019, 1995.

162. Terkeltabu R, Baird S, Sears P, et al: The murine homolog of the interleukin-8 receptor CXCR-2 is essential for the occurrence of neutrophilic inflammation in the air pouch model of acute crystal-induced gouty synovitis. Arthritis Rheum 41:900, 1998.

163. Wigley FM, Fine IT, Newcombe DS: The role of the human synovial fibroblast in monosodium urate crystal-induced synovitis. J Rheumatol 10:602, 1983.

164. Falasca GF, Ramachandrula A, Kelley KA, et al: Superoxide anion production and phagocytosis of crystals by cultured endothelial cells. Arthritis Rheum 36:105, 1993.

165. Villiger PM, Terkeltaub R, Lotz M: Monocyte chemoattractant protein-1 (MCP-1) expression in human cartilage: induction by leukemia inhibitory factor (LIF) and differential regulation by dexamethasone and retinoic acid. J Clin Invest 90:488, 1992.

166. Gon S, Gatanaga T, Sendo F: Involvment of two types of TNF receptor in TNF-α induced neutropohil apoptosis. Microbiol Immunol 40:463, 1996.

167. Tudan C, Fong D, Duronio V, et al: The inhibition of spontaneous and tumor necrosis factor-α induced neutrophil apoptosis by crystals of calcium pyrophosphate dihydrate and monosodium urate monohydrate. J Rheumatol 27:2463, 2000.

168. Landis RC, Yagnik DR, Florey O, et al: Safe disposal of inflammatory monosodium urate monohydrate crystals by differentiated macrophages. Arthritis Rheum 46:3026, 2002.

169. Schlesinger N, Baker DG, Schumacher HR Jr.: How well have diagnostic tests and therapies for gout been evaluated? Curr Opin Rheumatol 11:441, 1999.

170. Schlesinger N, Detry MA, Holland BK, et al: Local ice therapy during bouts of acute gouty arthritis. J Rheumatol 29:331, 2002.

171. Lange U, Schumann C, Schmidt KL: Current aspects of colchicine therapy: classical indications and new therapeutic uses. Eur J Med Res 6:150, 2001.

172. Molad Y: Update on colchicines and its mechanism of action. Curr Rheum Reports 4:252, 2002.

173. Iacobuzio-Donahue CA, Lee EL, Abraham SC, et al: Colchicine toxicity. distinct morphologic findings in gastrointestinal biopsies. Am J Surg Path 25:1067, 2001.

174. Wallace SL, Singer JZ: Review: Systemic toxicity associated with the intravenous administration of colchicines: guidelines for use. J Rheumatol 15:495, 1988.

175. Evans TI, Wheeler MT Small RE, et al: A comprehensive investigation of inpatient colchicines use shows more education is needed. J Rheumatol 23:143, 1996.

176. Schumacher HR, Boice HA, Daikh, et al: Randomized double blind trial of etoricoxib and indomethacin in treatment of acute gouty arthritis. BMJ 324:1488, 2002.

177. Schumacher HR: Crystal induced arthritis: an overview. Am J Med 100:46S, 1996.

178. Fernandez C, Moguera R, Gonzalez JA, et al: Treatment of acute attacks of gout with a small dose of intraarticular triameenalone acetonide. J Rheumatol 26:2285, 1999.

179. Yu TF, Gutman AB: Efficacy of colchicine prophylaxis: prevention of recurrent gouty arthritis over a mean period of five years in 208 gouty subjects. Ann Intern Med 55:179, 1961.

180. Kunck RW, Duncan G, Watson D, et al: Colchicine myopathy and neuropathy. N Engl J Med 316:1562, 1987.

181. Chattopadhyay I, Shetty HMG, Routledge PA et al: Cochincine induced rhabdomyolysis. Postgrad Med J 77:191, 2001.

182. Ferraz MB, O'Brien B: A cost effectiveness analysis of urate lowering drugs in nontophaceous recurrent gouty arthritis. J Rheumatol 22:908, 1995.

183. Perez-Ruiz F, Calabozo M, Pijoan JI, et al: Effect of urate-lowering therapy on the velocity of size reduction of tophi in chronic gout. Arthritis Rheum (Arthritis Care Res) 47:356, 2002.

184. Perez-Ruiz F, Calabozo C, Herrero-Betes A, et al: Improvement in renal function in patients with chronic gout after proper control of hyperuricemia and gouty bouts. Nephron 86:287, 2000.

185. Stamp L, Sharples K, Gow P, et al: The optional use of allopurinol: an audit of allopurinol use in South Auckland. Aust NZJ Med 30:567, 2000.

186. Fam AG, Dunne SM, Iazzetta J, et al: Efficacy and safety of desensitization to allopurinol following cutaneous reactions. Arthritis Rheum 44:231, 2001.

187. Fam AG: Difficulty gout and new approaches for control of Hyperuricemia to allopurinal-allergic patients. Curr Rheum Reports 3:29, 2001.

188. Hande KR, Noone RM, Stone WJ: Severe allopurinol toxicity: description and guidelines for presentation in patients with renal insufficiency. Am J Med 76:47, 1984.

189. Singer JZ, Wallace SL: The allopurinol hypersensitivity syndrome: unnecessary morbidity and mortality. Arthritis Rheum 29:82, 1986.

190. Weiner IM, Mudge GH: Inhibitors of tubular transport of organic compounds. In Gillman AG, Rall TW, Nies AW, Taylor P (eds): The Pharmacologic Basis of Therapeutics, 8th ed. New York, Pergamon Press, 1990, p 920.

191. Wortmann RL: The treatment of gout: The use of an analogy. Am J Med 105:513, 1998.

192. Perez-Ruiz F, Alonso-Ruiz A, Calabozo M, Duruelo J: Treatment of gout after transplantation. Br J Rheumatol 37:580, 1998.

193. Jacobs F, Mamzer-Bruneel MF, Skhir H, et al: Safety of the mycophenolate mofetil-allopurinol combination in kidney transplant recipients with gout. Transplantation 64:1087, 1997.

194. Rozenberg S, Koeger AC, Bourgeois P: Urate-oxydase for gouty arthritis in cardiac transplant recipients. J Rheumatol 20:2171, 1993.

195. Bomalaski JS, Holtsberg FW, Ensor CM, et al: Uricase formulated with polyethyleneglycol (uricase-PEG 20): biochemical rationale and preclinical studies. J Rheumatol 29:1942, 2002.

196. Dessein PH, Shipton EA, Stanwix AE, et al: Beneficial effects of weight loss associated with moderate calorie/carbohydrate restriction, and increased proportional intake of protein and unsaturated fat on serum urate and lipoprotein levels in gout. a pilot study. Ann Rheum Dis 59:539, 2000.

197. Fam AG: Gout, diet and the insulin resistance syndrome. J Rheumatol 29:1350, 2002.

Diseases Associated with Articular Deposition of Calcium Pyrophosphate Dihydrate and Basic Calcium Phosphate Crystals

88

R. TERKELTAUB

Definition and Criteria

The loose, avascular connective tissue matrices of articular hyaline cartilage, fibrocartilaginous menisci, and of certain ligaments and tendons are particularly susceptible to calcification. Calcium-containing crystals deposited in the pericellular matrix of cartilage are often in the form of calcium pyrophosphate dihydrate (CPPD). The chemical formula is $Ca_2P_2O_7{\cdot}H_2O$, and the substance has a calcium-to-phosphate ratio of 1.0. The related disorder is commonly termed *chondrocalcinosis* or *pyrophosphate arthropathy*, and, when associated with acute arthritis, it may be called *pseudogout*. Crystals of basic calcium phosphate (BCP), including partially carbonate-substituted hydroxyapatite (HA), also may be deposited pathologically in articular cartilage, particularly in osteoarthritis (OA). The chemical formula for HA is $Ca_5(PO_4)3OH{\cdot}2H_2O$, and it has a calcium-to-phosphate ratio of 1.67. Importantly, physiologic (and noninflammatory) deposition of HA is essential, as HA is the principal mineral laid down in growth cartilage and in bone.

Inflammatory conditions also may result from deposition of HA and the closely related BCP crystals octacalcium phosphate (chemical formula $Ca_8H_2[PO_4]_6{\cdot}5H_2O$; calcium:phosphate ratio 1.33) and tricalcium phosphate or "whitlockite" (chemical formula $Ca_3[PO_4]_2$; calcium:phosphate ratio 1.5) in periarticular structures, such as the rotator cuff (calcific tendinitis) and subacromial bursa of the shoulder. CPPD and BCP crystal deposition, which are reviewed in this chapter, are by far the most prevalent arthropathies associated with calcium-containing crystals. Articular calcium oxalate crystal deposition, which is less common, is reviewed in Chapter 109.

Proposed diagnostic criteria for CPPD deposition disease are summarized in Table 88–1. The diagnosis is based on detection of CPPD crystals by one or more methods. These include not only standard, clinically applied radiography that detects calcifications characteristic of CPPD, but also detection of typical CPPD crystals via compensated polarized light microscopic analysis of synovial fluids or tissue sections. On occasion, specialized crystal analytic approaches including radiographic energy spectroscopy and powder diffraction analysis[1,2] or atomic force microscopy[3] may be helpful in establishing or confirming CPPD crystal deposition. In assessing the form of deposited crystals in calcifications, determination of the calcium-to-phosphate ratios and the spacing of radiographic powder diffraction lines provide the most specific information.

Consensus clinical diagnostic criteria for articular BCP crystal deposition disorders are not in place. Importantly, BCP crystals are not birefringent. Hence, diagnosis is predicated on detection of: 1) radiographic detection of calcifications characteristic of BCP crystals, 2) synovial fluid crystals that stain strongly for the calcium-binding dye Alizarin Red S (which only weakly stains CPPD crystals), and 3) BCP crystals confirmed by transmission electron microscopy or specialized crystal analytic approaches (including those mentioned previous for CPPD and discussed in following sections).

Epidemiology

Studies of the prevalence of both CPPD crystal deposition disease and various forms of articular BCP crystal deposition disease have been predominantly based on characteristic plain radiographic features of the disease in limited numbers of joints. This is an incompletely sensitive and specific approach. Other studies have been

 TABLE 88–1 • PROPOSED DIAGNOSTIC CRITERIA FOR CALCIUM PYROPHOSPHATE DIHYDRATE (CPPD) CRYSTAL DEPOSITION DISEASE

Criteria:

I. Demonstration of CPPD crystals, obtained by biopsy or aspirated synovial fluid, by definitive means (such as characteristic radiographic diffraction powder pattern)

II. A. Identification of monoclinic or triclinic crystals showing a weak positive birefringence (or no birefringence) by compensated polarized light microscopy
   B. Presence of typical calcifications on radiographs (as discussed in text): heavy punctate and linear calcifications in fibrocartilages, articular (hyaline) cartilages, and joint capsules, especially if bilaterally symmetric

III. A. Acute arthritis, especially of knees or other large joints
   B. Chronic arthritis, especially of knee, hip, wrist, carpus, elbow, shoulder, and metacarpophalangeal joints, particularly if accompanied by acute exacerbations

Diagnostic Categories:

A. Definite: Criteria 1 or 11(A) must be fulfilled
B. Probable: Criteria IIA or IIB must be fulfilled
C. Possible: Criteria IIIA or IIIB suggests possible underlying CPPD deposition disease

Adapted from McCarty DJ: Crystals and arthritis. Dis Month 6:255, 1994.

based on results of synovial fluid analyses and pathologic findings on examination of articular cartilages. As such, the true prevalence of both CPPD crystal deposition disease and pathologic articular BCP crystal deposition are not known. There is no obvious race predilection. Women may be somewhat more commonly affected than men.[4] Chondrocalcinosis, including asymptomatic disease, increases progressively in prevalence with aging.[5,6] Idiopathic or sporadic chondrocalcinosis is quite uncommon before age 50, particularly in the absence of a history of joint trauma or knee meniscectomy.

In a classic study, knee meniscal calcification was detected in 16 percent of 55 women aged 80 to 89 and in 30 percent of 53 women older than 89,[7] figures comparable to those obtained in other studies.[8,9] For example, in a radiographic survey study of hands, wrists, pelvises, and knees of patients admitted to a geriatrics ward, there was a 44-percent prevalence of chondrocalcinosis in patients older than 84, a 36-percent prevalence in the 75 to 84 year olds, and a prevalence of 15 percent in 65 to 74 year olds.[10] Most elderly patients with chondrocalcinosis of the knee also have detectable chondrocalcinosis in other joints.[7]

▌ Etiology

Supersaturation of certain solutes in body fluids may culminate in the deposition of distinct crystals and calculi, exemplified by pathologic crystallization within extracellular fluids such as the biliary and urinary tracts. In addition, pathologic crystallization can occur in the extracellular matrix of certain connective tissues such as the artery wall, in subjects with atherosclerosis or chronic renal failure,[11] and in the synovium and articular cartilage in gout (see Chapter 87). Significantly, articular cartilage, unlike growth plate cartilage, is specialized to avoid the process of matrix calcification.[12] But the matrix of articular hyaline cartilage, like that of fibrocartilaginous menisci, lends itself well to pathologic calcification,[13] particularly in association with certain changes in matrix composition in aging and OA.[14]

Articular cartilage matrix calcification can reflect deficiencies of certain physiologic calcification inhibitors or upregulation of mediators that actively drive stereotypical patterns of tissue injury, culminating in calcification within degenerating cartilage.[12,15,16] Alteration of the concentrations of calcium, inorganic phosphate (P_i), inorganic pyrophosphate(PP_i), and the solubility products of these ions clearly are at work in promoting CPPD and BCP crystal formation.[13-16] The levels of ambient magnesium and the composition of the chondrocyte pericellular matrix influence the dynamics of CPPD crystal formation and help to determine whether monoclinic or triclinic CPPD crystals are predominantly formed in the cartilage matrix.[14,15] Enhanced formation of monoclinic CPPD crystals could be significant, as such CPPD crystals may be more inflammatory than triclinic CPPD crystals.[17]

Besides physical effects of calcium, P_i, and PP_i on crystal nucleation and propagation, these solutes exert a variety of mineralization-regulating effects on gene expression, differentiation, and viability in chondrocytes, mediated partly by calcium-sensing receptors and sodium-dependent phosphate cotransporters in chondrocytes.[12,18-23] Noxious effects of excess PP_i on chondrocytes, including induction of matrix metalloproteinase-13 (MMP-13) expression[24] and promotion of apoptosis[25] support the long-standing use of the term *pyrophosphate arthropathy* to describe the chronic cartilage degenerative manifestations of CPPD crystal deposition disease.

DYSREGULATED PP$_i$ METABOLISM IN PATHOLOGIC ARTICULAR CARTILAGE CALCIFICATION AND THE ROLE OF PC-1/NPP1

PP_i is a potent inhibitor of the nucleation and propagation of BCP crystals.[12,15] Concordantly, maintenance of physiologic extracellular PP_i levels by chondrocytes and certain other cells serves to suppress calcification with HA, as illustrated in certain mouse models of deficient PP_i generation and transport,[19,26,27] as well as a variant of human infantile arterial calcification associated with periarticular calcification.[28] But the relatively unique capacity of chondrocytes to produce copious amounts of extracellular PP_i is double edged (Fig. 88–1), as it is a major factor in promoting CPPD crystal deposition.[12,29-31] Furthermore, excess PP_i generation can promote HA crystal deposition by providing a source for increased P_i generation via PP_i hydrolysis by inorganic pyrophosphatase and alkaline phosphatase activities[29,31] (see Fig. 88–1). Depending on cartilage adenosine triphosphate (ATP) and PP_i concentrations, and the level of activity of P_i-generating ATPases and pyrophosphatases, CPPD and HA crystal formation may be jointly promoted in cartilage, an event that commonly occurs clinically in OA, as will be discussed later. In addition, alterations in PP_i transport by the multiple-pass plasma membrane protein ANK[16,24,26] are implicated in the pathogenesis of chondrocalcinosis, as discussed in detail in the upcoming section on familial chondrocalcinosis. Increased ANK expression in OA cartilage clearly factors into promotion of secondary chondrocalcinosis[24] (see Fig. 88–1).

There is a strong linkage of sporadic, aging-associated CPPD crystal deposition disease with excess chondrocyte PP_i-generating nucleoside triphosphate pyrophosphohydrolase (NTPPPH) activity and augmented PP_i generation by chondrocytes that promotes cartilage supersaturation with PP_i.[12,29-34] In this context, NTPPPH generates PP_i by hydrolysis of nucleoside triphosphates including ATP.[16,29,30] A substantial portion of ATP used by chondrocytes to generate extracellular PP_i is provided by the mitochondria.[16] Free synovial fluid ATP levels have been reported to be elevated in subjects with idiopathic chondrocalcinosis.[35] Furthermore, cartilage NTPPPH activity and PP_i levels may average approximately double those of normal subjects in idiopathic chondrocalcinosis.[36]

The NTPPPH plasma cell membrane glycoprotein-1 (PC-1) (see Fig. 88–1) plays a central role in sustaining and augmenting extracellular PP_i in chondrocytes and certain other cells.[11,16,28-30] PC-1 (also known as nucleotide pyrophoshatae pyrophosphohydrolase 1 [NPP1]) is one of three highly homologous NPP family isoenzymes

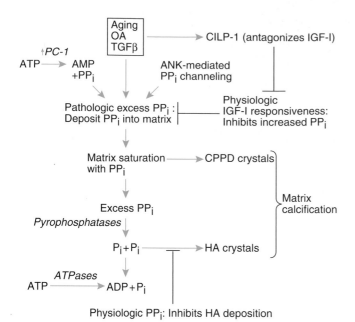

FIGURE 88-1 · Proposed PP$_i$-dependent mechanisms stimulating calcium pyrophosphate dihydrate (CPPD) and hydroxyapatite (HA) crystal deposition in aging and osteoarthritis (OA). Roles of adenosine triphosphate (ATP) and PP$_i$ metabolism and inorganic phosphate (P$_i$) generation in pathologic cartilage calcification. This model accounts for the association of extracellular PP$_i$ excess with both CPPD and basic calcium phosphate (BCP) (HA) crystal deposition in OA and chondrocalcinosis, as well as the paradoxical association of extracellular PP$_i$ deficiency (from defective ANK or PC-1/NPP1 expression) with pathologic calcification of articular cartilage with HA crystals in vivo. Excess PP$_i$ generation in aging cartilages in idiopathic CPPD deposition disease of aging, and in osteoarthritic cartilages, is mediated in part by marked increases in nucleoside triphosphate pyrophosphohydrolase (NTPPPH) activity and in part by the NTPPPH isozyme PC-1/NPP1. In idiopathic chondrocalcinosis of aging, mean cartilage PP$_i$ and NTPPPH levels are twice normal. As discussed in the text, PC-1 is markedly upregulated at sites of meniscal cartilage calcification in vivo, and PC-1/NPP1 not only directly induces elevated PP$_i$ but also matrix calcification by chondrocytes in vitro. Depending on extracellular availability of substrate PP$_i$ and the activity of pyrophosphatases, the availability of substrate ATP and the activity of ATPases, and other factors such as substantial local Mg^{++} concentrations, HA crystal deposition, as opposed to CPPD deposition, may be stimulated. In this model, excess extracellular PP$_i$ also may result from heightened "leakiness" of intracellular PP$_i$ via increased ANK expression in OA and abnormal ANK function in familial chondrocalcinosis, as well as from deficient activity of pyrophosphatases (such as tissue-nonspecific alkaline phosphatase [TNAP] and possibly inorganic pyrophosphatase) in certain primary metabolic disorders. Also illustrated is the role in cartilage calcification in OA and aging of increased expression of cartilage intermediate layer protein-1 (CILP-1), which inhibits the capacity of insulin-like growth factor I (IGF-I) to suppress elevation of extracellular PP$_i$, as discussed in the text.

that share NTPPPH catalytic activity and type II transmembrane ectoenzyme structures.[16,37,38] However, PC-1/NPP1 plays a far greater role than autotaxin/NPP2 and B10/NPP3 in augmenting extracellular PP$_i$ in chondrocytes.[29,30] Significantly, cultured PC-1/NPP1 knockout cells have up to 50 percent less extracellular PP$_i$.[18]

Upregulated PC-1/NPP1 expression is associated with both calcification and apoptosis in degenerative human cartilages.[29] Direct upregulation of PC-1/NPP1 in chondrocytic cells stimulates calcification, as well as apoptosis.[25] These effects are not shared by B10/NPP3, which likely has other intracellular "housekeeping" functions in chondrocytes.[25,29] Autotaxin/NPP2, which is also expressed in normal cartilages, functions more actively as a P$_i$-generating T-type ATPase and as a lysophospholipase D and only modestly stimulates chondrocytes to calcify.[29,40]

PC-1/NPP1 expression is stimulated by the chondrocyte growth factor transforming grown factor-β (TGF-β), which markedly elevates chondrocyte extracellular PP$_i$.[41] PC-1/NPP1 expression and subcellular movement toward the plasma membrane play a major role in the capacity of TGF-β to elevate chondrocyte extracellular PP$_i$.[30,41] Conversely, interleukin-1 (IL-1) suppresses both PC-1/NPP1 expression and extracellular PP$_i$ in chondrocytes and blocks the effects of TGF-β on PP$_i$.[30,41] The capacity of TGF-β to raise chondrocyte PP$_i$ rises with aging,[33] as does TGF-β–stimulated NTPPPH activity.[42] At the same, the beneficial growth-promoting effects of TGF-β decrease with aging in articular chondrocytes.[33] These effects likely reflect altered signal transduction with chondrocyte aging. It is noteworthy, in this context, that protein kinase C and protein kinase A signaling differentially affect extracellular PP$_i$ levels of chondrocytes.[34]

Cartilage intermediate layer protein (CILP) (see Fig. 88–1), a secreted matrix molecule unrelated to the NPP family NTPPPH isoenzymes was initially reported to be an NTPPPH, based on apparent artefacts of chromatographic purification.[44,45] This claim was refuted in detailed studies using recombinant CILP isoforms CILP-1 and CILP-2, which are both cartilage expressed.[46] Interestingly, CILP expression rises in aging and OA, is induced by TGF-β, and is most abundant in the middle zone of articular cartilage where CPPD crystal deposition is most prevalent.[47,48] The chondrocyte anabolic growth factor insulin-like growth factor I (IGF-I), which induces CILP expression,[49] normally suppresses basal extracellular PP$_i$ in chondrocytes and also interferes with the ability of TGF-β to increase extracellular PP$_i$ in chondrocytes[46,50] (see Fig. 88–1). Significantly, CILP-1, but not the CILP-2 isoform, indirectly promotes increased extracellular PP$_i$ in chondrocytes by acting as an antagonist of IGF-I at the receptor level.[46] Moreover, the common finding of chondrocyte IGF-I resistance in OA and aging cartilages[46] suggests a role for CILP-1 in pathogenesis of both OA and chondrocalcinosis (see Fig. 88–1).

DYSREGULATED PP$_i$ METABOLISM IN CALCIUM PYROPHOSPHATE DIHYDRATE DEPOSITION DISEASE SECONDARY TO PRIMARY METABOLIC DISORDERS

Hypophosphatasia, hypomagnesemic conditions (including the Gitelman's variant of Bartter's syndrome), hemochromatosis, and hyperparathyroidism are the best-characterized primary metabolic disorders linked to secondary CPPD crystal deposition disease.[51] Increased joint fluid PP$_i$ levels in each of these conditions suggests at least one common thread in the pathogenesis of chondrocalcinosis via cartilage PP$_i$ excess.[52] In this context, magnesium is a cofactor for pyrophosphatase activity, and iron excess can suppress pyrophosphatase activity. Hypercalcemia may promote CPPD crystal deposition in hyperparathyroidism by effects beyond cartilage matrix supersaturation with ionized calcium, such as calcium function as a cofactor in PC-1/NPP1 NTPPPH activity, as well as chondrocyte-activating effects mediated by the calcium-sensing receptor.[20,21] In addition, normal articular chondrocytes express parathyroid hormone (PTH) and parathyroid hormone–related protein (PTHrP) receptors, and functional responses of chondrocytes to PTH can promote proliferation, altered matrix synthesis, and mineralization.[53,54]

Hypophosphatasia is due to deficient activity of the ectoenzyme tissue-nonspecific alkaline phosphatase (TNAP), whose activities include hydrolysis of PP_i to generate P_i.[19] TNAP is a major physiologic antagonist of PC-1/NPP1–mediated elevation of extracellular PP_i.[19,55] Conversely, physiologic PC-1/NPP1–induced PP_i generation antagonizes the essential promineralizing effects of TNAP mediated by P_i generation.[19,55] Significantly, articular cartilage PP_i excess and chondrocalcinosis are associated with hypophosphatasia, Conversely, PC-1/NPP1 knockout mice and mice homozygous for the PC-1 truncation mutant *ttw* demonstrate marked articular cartilage calcification with HA and OA, as well as ankylosing spinal ligament hyperostosis and synovial joint ossific fusion.[19,27] Furthermore, PP_i levels and mineralization disturbances in tissues of PC-1/NPP1 knockout and TNAP knockout mice are mutually corrected by crossbreeding to generate double knockout mice.[19] Disordered growth plate chondrocyte organization in TNAP knockout mice also are corrected, in large part, by breeding onto the PC-1 null background.[19] These findings have reinforced the paradigm for critical regulation of calcification by PP_i (see Fig. 88–1) and illuminated interactive effects on chondrocyte differentiation of PC-1, TNAP, and PP_i metabolism.

FAMILIAL CALCIUM PYROPHOSPHATE DIHYDRATE CRYSTAL DEPOSITION DISEASE AND THE ROLE OF ANK MUTATIONS IN PATHOLOGIC ARTICULAR CARTILAGE CALCIFICATION

Familial chondrocalcinosis is clinically heterogeneous.[56] For example, prominent CPPD and HA crystal deposits and cartilage and periarticular calcifications in association with OA were described in a kindred not yet linked to a specific chromosomal locus.[57] A syndrome of spondyloepiphyseal dysplasia tarda, brachydactyly, precocious OA, and intra-articular calcifications with CPPD crystals, HA crystals, or both, as well as periarticular calcifications, was linked to mutation of the procollagen type II gene in indigenous natives of the Chiloe Island region of Chile.[58] This population has a high prevalence of familial CPPD deposition disease.[56,58]

Two major chromosomal linkages, 8q and 5p, have been identified in studies of familial CPPD deposition disease.[56] Linkage with chromosome 8q of both early-onset OA and chondrocalcinosis in a New England fam-

ily was given the designation CCAL1.[59] Chromosome 5p-linked chondrocalcinosis (CCAL2) is broadly distributed and has been studied in greater detail than 8q chondrocalcinosis.[60-65] Linkage of familial CPPD crystal deposition disease to the ANKH gene on chromosome 5p has been established in these studies.[60-65] A search for ANKH gene mutation in 95 subjects with sporadic chondrocalcinosis uncovered a unique mutation in only one subject.[64]

The ANKH gene product ANK is a multiple-pass transmembrane protein that functions in PP_i channeling[26,66] (Fig. 88–2). Transport of PP_i generated intracellularly by PC-1/NPP1[24] is one of the means used by chondrocytes to regulate extracellular PP_i levels.[16] Modeling of the PP_i channeling function of human ANK has posited 10 or 12 membrane-spanning domains in ANK with an alternating inside/out orientation and with a central channel to accommodate the passage of PP_i[26,66] (see Fig. 88–2). Mutations at different locations in ANK can affect function and the skeleton in a manner including autosomal dominant chondrocalcinosis[64,65] and certain other phenotypes[26,66,67] (see Fig. 88–2). Clinical heterogeneity, even for chondrocalcinosis associated with human ANK mutations,[64,65] suggests differing functional effects of ANK mediated by specific regions of the molecule.

In 5p familial chondrocalcinosis, subtle "gain of function" of intrinsic ANK PP_i-channeling activity may lead to chronic, low-grade chondrocyte "PP_i leakiness", thereby causing matrix supersaturation with PP_i, CPPD crystal deposition, and cartilage degeneration.[64,65] However, marked intracellular PP_i elevation in cell lines from the French chromosome 5p familial chondrocalcinosis kindred may be discordant with this hypothesis.[68,69] With respect to chondrocalcinosis in OA and aging, it is clear that expression of wild-type ANK is highly regulated, comparable to regulation of PC-1/NPP1, and that ANK expression is upregulated in OA and chondrocalcinotic cartilage.[24,45] Thus, secondary alterations in chondrocyte expression of both wild-type ANK and PC-1/NPP1 likely drive PP_i supersaturation in cartilage in idiopathic or sporadic and OA-associated CPPD crystal deposition disease (see Fig. 88–1).

ALTERED CHONDROCYTE DIFFERENTIATION, INFLAMMATION, AND TISSUE TRANSGLUTAMINASE IN CALCIFICATION

Dysregulated PP_i metabolism synergizes with substantial joint pathology (Fig. 88–3) in driving pathologic cartilage calcification.[12] Regulated changes in chondrocyte differentiation and viability appear to be mechanistically unified processes that promote both OA and pathologic articular cartilage CPPD and HA crystal deposition.[12] Such changes include development of chondrocyte hypertrophy associated with expression of stereotypic bone matrix proteins (see Chapter 91) and the presence of hypertrophy and apoptosis of chondrocytes adjacent to cartilage calcifications[70,71] (see Fig. 88–3D). Chondrocyte hypertrophy is associated with dysregulated matrix synthetic reparative responses (see Chapter 91), heightened PP_i generation,[72] and increased production of calcifying cell fragments known as matrix vesicles.[73] Altered TGF-β

FIGURE 88-2 • Model for multiple-pass membrane protein structure of ANK (ANKH gene product) and for ANK mutations associated with distinct skeletal phenotypes. The putative multiple-pass transmembrane protein structure of ANK/ANKH appears to function in PP_i channeling from the cytosol to the extracellular space. Distinct mutations in ANK promote distinct phenotypes. As illustrated, impairment of ANK function via homozygosity for a C-terminal cytosolic domain *ank* truncation mutation in murine progressive ankylosis *ank/ank* mice leads to a decrease in extracellular PP_i, resulting in deposition of hydroxyapatite (HA) crystals in articular cartilage, osteoarthritis (OA), and peripheral synovial and intervertebral bony ankyloses. PC-1/NPP1 deficient mice (*ttw/ttw* mice and PC-1 knockout mice) have a remarkably similar phenotype to that of *ank/ank* mice, linked by decreased extracellular PP_i. Sites of known ANKH gene mutations associated with autosomal dominant familial chondrocalcinosis (CPPD crystal deposition disease) and with sporadic chondrocalcinosis, in one subject, are also shown. It has been proposed that some of the described ANK mutations linked to human chondrocalcinosis promote chronic, low-grade extracellular PP_i excess resulting in CPPD crystal formation. The sites of autosomal dominant ANKH gene mutations implicated in craniometaphyseal dysplasia (CMD) also are depicted. CMD is a pediatric disorder characterized by progressive thickening and increased mineral density of craniofacial bones and hyperostotic flaring at metaphyses in long bones, as well as the classic "mask" facies. The effects of the ANK CMD mutations on PP_i transport (or other potential functions of ANK) are not currently understood but may involve dysregulated intramembranous bone formation.

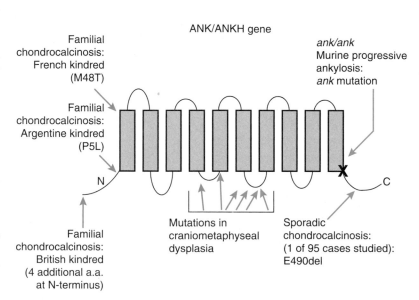

signal transduction in aging and OA may be involved, as expression of a truncated, kinase-defective TGF-β receptor type II promotes hypertrophy and terminal chondrocyte differentiation, along with cartilage degeneration in vivo.[74] Moreover, aging human knee chondrocytes demonstrate decreased growth responses to TGF-β.[33]

Upregulation of local PTHrP expression also may be one of the shared features driving sequential chondrocyte proliferation and altered differentiation in growth plate chondrocytes and articular chondrocytes.[53,54] In addition, P_i and calcium can modulate chondrocyte hypertrophic differentiation and apoptosis.[16,22,75] Chondrocyte apoptosis also promotes calcification partly through the calcifying potential of matrix vesicle–like apoptotic bodies released from dying chondrocytes.[25,76-78] Mitochondrial dysfunction, a central factor in tissue aging, also can stimulate cartilage matrix degeneration and calcification, as mitochondria are remarkably specialized to regulate calcification, and apoptosis is critically regulated by mitochondrial function.[78]

Inflammatory mediators that promote degradation of the articular cartilage matrix may also stimulate calcification in OA. In this context, nitric oxide (NO), a mediator of OA pathogenesis (see Chapter 91), stimulates apoptosis in chondrocytes and NO donor treatment of chondrocytes stimulates calcification.[76-78] IL-1 is upregulated in OA cartilage and stimulates articular chondrocytes to calcify their matrix.[42,79] IL-1 stimulates inducible nitric oxide synthase (iNOS), expression and increased NO generation, as well as expression of other cytokines and of MMPs that can alter matrix composition to potentially favor calcification (see Chapter 91).

IL-1 also stimulates chondrocytes to express the protein cross-linking enzymes factor XIIIA, transglutaminase (TGase), and tissue TGase (tTGase or TG2).[42,79] IL-1 (as well as tumor necrosis factor-α [TNF-α], donors of NO, and the potent oxidant peroxynitrite) also induce increased chondrocyte TGase cross-linking activity.[42]

TG2 and FXIIIA are markers of growth plate chondrocyte hypertrophy.[42,79] Significantly, there is marked upregulation of TG2 and Factor XIIIA expression in hypertrophic cells in the superficial and deep zones of knee OA articular cartilage and the central (chondrocytic) zone of OA menisci.[42] Moreover, increased factor XIIIA and TG2 activities both directly stimulate calcification by chondrocytes.[42] Because TGase activity promotes activation of latent TGF-β,[80] it is noteworthy that TGase activity and extracellular PP_i levels are concurrently elevated in association with articular cartilage aging.[42] In addition, OA severity–related, donor age-dependent, and marked age-dependent IL-1–induced increases in TGase activity occur in chondrocytes from human knee menisci.[42] The TG2 TGase isoenzyme is essential for IL-1 to stimulate articular chondrocytes to calcify their matrix in vitro.[79] In addition, the closely related inflammatory chemokines IL-8 and GROα, which are both upregulated in OA cartilage, stimulate increased TGase activity attributed specifically to TG2.[81] Furthermore, IL-8 and GROα stimulate chondrocyte hypertrophic differentiation and calcification in a manner that requires TG2 expression.[81] Therefore, inflammation-induced TGase activity promotes pathologic cartilage calcification in OA.

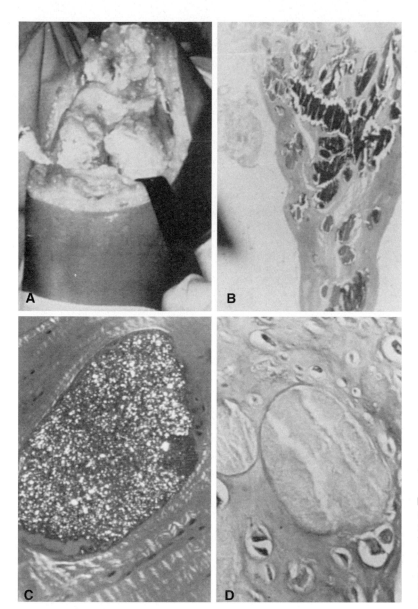

FIGURE 88–3 · *A,* Chalky calcium pyrophosphate dihydrate (CPPD) crystal deposits oberved on synovium, menisci, and hyaline cartilage of a 35-year-old patient with familial calcium pyrophosphate deposition disease. *B,* Menisci showing black-stained crystalline deposits under von Kossa's stain. *C,* Crystalline pyrophosphate deposits in articular cartilage. (Compensated polarized light, × 300.) *D,* Hypertrophic chondrocytes surrounding CPPD deposits. (H&E × 400)

SPECIAL PATHOGENIC ASPECTS OF ARTICULAR AND PERIARTICULAR BASIC CALCIUM PHOSPHATE CRYSTAL DEPOSITION

CPPD and BCP crystal deposition can develop in different zones of articular cartilage and probably in distinct phases of cartilage degenerative disease, such as ongoing loss of viability in hypertrophic chondrocytes. In addition, abundant cartilage NO production may promote mitochondrial dysfunction, chondrocyte extracellular ATP depletion, and lowering of extracellular PP_i, consequently favoring HA over CPPD crystal deposition.[82] The observation that OA and HA crystal deposition in articular cartilage (and arteries)[11,28] are promoted by extracellular PP_i deficiency states strikingly illustrates the deleterious effects of deprivation of physiologic extracellular PP_i levels.[16] However, it is noted that joint fluid PP_i and NTPPPH levels are elevated in HA-associated shoulder arthropathy ("Milwaukee shoulder syndrome"),[83] consistent with the model in Figure 88–1.

Pathologic BCP crystal deposition may occur in periarticular sites, as well as numerous organs and soft tissues.[11] Significantly, the shoulder is the most common articular region affected by symptomatic BCP crystal deposition, in part reflecting unique shoulder-structure function. Degenerative changes promoted by biomechanic stress promote calcific tendinitis in the body of the rotator cuff.[84] Such tendon calcifications can remain asymptomatic and also can eventually resorb, but the degenerative changes can predispose to tendon rupture (see Chapter 38). Osteopontin, a factor that normally restrains BCP crystal deposition (and is regulated by PP_i and P_i),[18] can be detected in fibroblast-like cells and multinucleated macrophages surrounding areas of calcification in calcific tendinitis.[85] In this regard, osteopontin promotes MMP activation, as well as macrophage recruitment and osteoclast activation.[18] The presence of multinucleated cells with cathepsin K expression and osteoclast-like functions at sites of tendon calcification[86] suggests a mechanism for both resorption of BCP crystal deposits and tendon degeneration.

CALCIUM PYROPHOSPHATE DIHYDRATE AND HYDROXYAPATITE CRYSTAL–INDUCED INFLAMMATION

Some of the crystals deposited in cartilage can subclinically traffic to joint fluid and synovium, and the crystals can directly stimulate chondrocytes, synovial lining cells, and intra-articular leukocytes.[87-89] Inflammation triggered by CPPD and HA crystals thereby contributes to cartilage degradation and can potentiate worsening of OA.[87-89] Many proinflammatory mechanisms active in gout likely mediate synovitis and cartilage degeneration associated with CPPD and HA crystal deposition.[87-89] In this regard, CPPD and HA crystals activate cells partly via nonspecific activation of signal transduction pathways (e.g., mitogen-activated protein kinase [MAPK] activation) and induce cellular release of cyclooxygenase (COX)- and lipoxygenase-derived metabolites of arachidonic acid and cytokines including TNF-α, IL-1, and IL-8.[87-89] The ingress of neutrophils into the joint is central in triggering acute pseudogout.[86] Effects on neutrophil-endothelial interaction likely represent a major locus for the prophylactic and therapeutic effects of colchicine.[90] IL-8 and related chemokines that bind the IL-8 receptor CXCR2 (including GROα) appear to be critical in initiating and perpetuating neutrophil ingress in acute crystal-induced inflammation.[91] Despite the fact that BCP and CPPD crystals share the capacity to activate certain cell-signaling pathways and to induce several MMPs,[92] BCP crystals generally trigger much less neutrophil influx into the joint than do CPPD crystals. Concordantly, free intra-articular BCP crystals likely induce less proinflammatory cytokine expression than do CPPD and monosodium urate crystals.[93-95]

Clinical Features

CLINICAL PRESENTATIONS OF CALCIUM PYROPHOSPHATE DIHYDRATE DEPOSITION DISEASE

Most elderly individuals with CPPD deposition disease in the United States have a primary (idiopathic or sporadic) disorder (Table 88–2). Idiopathic chondrocalcinosis generally appears only after the fifth decade of life. However, patients with a history of repetitive joint trauma of knee meniscectomy may present with nonsystemic (monoarticular) chondrocalcinosis prior to age 50. Familial forms of CPPD crystal deposition disease also have been widely documented, as will be discussed. The clinical presentation of familial chondrocalcinosis is often manifest in the third and fourth decades of life, but familial disease can sometimes be detected before age 20, or it may first present clinically at advanced age. CPPD crystal deposition disease also is a common manifestation of a variety of hereditary and metabolic conditions (including hyperparathyroidism, dialysis-dependent renal failure, and

TABLE 88–2 • COMMON ETIOLOGIES OF CALCIUM PYROPHOSPHATE DIHYDRATE (CPPD) CRYSTAL DEPOSITION DISEASE

High Prevalence
Idiopathic in association with aging (most frequent)
Complication of primary osteoarthritis
Long-term consequence of mechanic joint trauma or knee meniscectomy

Moderate Prevalence
Familial
Associated with systemic metabolic disease (hyperparathyroidism, dialysis-dependent renal failure, hemochromatosis, hypomagnesemia)

Low Prevalence (Largely Based on Case Reports)
X-linked hypophosphatemic rickets
Familial hypocalciuric hypercalcemia
Ochronosis
Gout
Articular amyloidosis
Myxedematous hypothyroidism
Osteochondrodysplasias and spondyloepiphyseal dysplasias
Neuropathic joints
Wilson's disease

hemochromatosis)[51] in which the CPPD-related arthropathy can present prior to age 50. For unclear reasons, hemochromatosis can present predominantly with CPPD crystal deposition disease or as OA, as is discussed in Chapter 109. The weight of evidence from controlled studies suggests that hypothyroidism (with the probable exception of myxedematous hypothyroidism) is not associated with a significantly increased prevalence of CPPD crystal deposition disease, although both disorders are clearly prevalent in aging.[51,96,97] It has been suggested that initiation of thyroxine supplementation therapy may trigger pseudogout.[98]

The clinical manifestations of CPPD deposition disease vary widely[99] (Table 88–3, Fig. 88–4). Quite commonly, the disease can be asymptomatic. Alternatively, it can mimic OA ("pseudo-osteoarthritis"), gout ("pseudogout"), acute-onset or insidious rheumatoid arthritis (RA) ("pseudorheumatoid arthritis"), or it may present as "pseudoneuropathic" arthropathy. Patients with CPPD crystal deposition disease also commonly present with episodes of hemarthrosis, often post-traumatic and in the knee.[100] The contributions of the forms of CPPD deposited (e.g., monoclinic versus triclinic crystals[17]) and of host factors to these wide differences in clinical manifestations are not clear. Overall, only a small fraction of patients with CPPD deposition disease have prolonged, recurring polyarticular inflammation. Progressive degenerative arthropathy is more common. Though CPPD deposition disease appears to be a common and significant public health problem in the elderly, the "disease impact" and the long-term course of CPPD-associated degenerative arthropathy in an unselected population have not been adequately evaluated.

TABLE 88-3 • COMMON CLINICAL PRESENTATIONS OF CALCIUM PYROPHOSPHATE DIHYDRATE (CPPD) CRYSTAL DEPOSITION DISEASE

Asymptomatic or incidental finding (e.g., asymptomatic knee fibrocartilage chondrocalcinosis in the elderly)

Recurrent acute inflammatory monoarticular arthritis ("pseudogout") (e.g., wrist or knee arthritis, sometimes provokes by trauma, concurrent medical or surgical illness, or intra-articular hyaluronan) "pseudoseptic arthritis"

Recurrent acute hemarthrosis

Chronic degenerative arthritis ("pseudo-osteoarthritis" or "pseudoneuropathic arthritis")

Chronic symmetric inflammatory polyarthritis ("pseudorheumatoidarthritis")

Systemic illness ("pseudopolymyalgia rheumatica", fever of unknown origin)

Destructive arthritis in dialysis-dependent renal failure

Carpal tunnel syndrome

Tumoral and pseudotophaceous CPPD crystal deposits

Central nervous system disease complicating ligamentum flavum or transverse ligament of atlas involvement (cervical canal stenosis, cervical myelopathy, meningismus, foramen magnum syndrome, odontoid fracture)

ACUTE SYNOVITIS

Pseudogout is a major cause of acute monoarticular or oligoarticular arthritis in the elderly. The attacks typically involve a large joint, most often the knee, and less often the wrist or ankle, and, unlike gout, rarely the first metatarsophalangeal joint. Acute attacks of inflammatory pseudogout in patients with CPPD deposition disease typically have a sudden onset and can be excruciatingly painful, with pronounced periarticular erythema, warmth, and swelling comparable to gout (see Fig. 88-4). In addition, arthritis in some attacks of pseudogout can be migratory or can be additive, polyarticular, and bilateral. Polyarticular pseudogout is particularly common in association with familial chondrocalcinosis and hyperparathyroidism.

Pseudogout can be provoked by minor trauma or intercurrent medical or surgical conditions, including pneumonia, myocardial infarction, cerebrovascular accident, and pregnancy. Parathyroid surgery for hyperparathyroidism frequently triggers pseudogout attacks. In addition, pseudogout of the knee can be precipitated by arthroscopy or by intra-articular administration of hyaluronan[101-103] that could reflect proinflammatory mechanisms triggered through the hyaluronan receptor CD44.[104,105] Parenteral administration of granulocyte colony-stimulating factor (G-CSF)[106] and of bisphosphonates[107,108] also can trigger pseudogout, the former

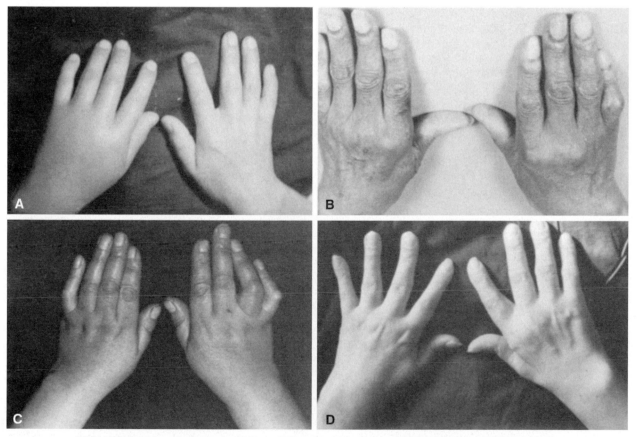

FIGURE 88-4 • *A*, Acute pseudogout. *B*, Pseudo-osteoarthritis. *C*, Pseudo-rheumatoid arthritis with boutonnière deformity. *D*, Pseudo-rheumatoid arthritis showing ulnar deviation, interosseous muscle atrophy, and metacarpophalangeal and wrist joint involvement. The patients in *A*, *C*, and *D* are siblings.

likely by ignition of smoldering intra-articular inflammation, the latter theoretically via pyrophosphatase inhibition.

Acute and subacute pseudogout can be associated with fever, chills, elevated erythrocyte sedimentation rate (ESR), and systemic leukocytosis, particularly with polyarticular involvement and in the elderly.[109] Leukocyte counts in the synovial fluid are substantially elevated and intraleukocytic CPPD crystals are most often (but not universally) detectable by compensated polarized light microscopy in pseudogout. The attacks typically last for 7 to 10 days, but they also can be clustered and may last for weeks to months. Occasionally the leukocyte count in pseudogout can exceed 50,000 per mm³ (a condition known as "pseudoseptic arthritis").

CHRONIC DEGENERATIVE AND INFLAMMATORY ARTHROPATHIES

Acute pseudogout attacks may be interspersed with chronic arthropathy in CPPD crystal deposition disease. Chronic degenerative arthropathy in CPPD deposition disease commonly affects certain joints that are typically spared in primary OA (e.g., metacarpophalangeal joints, wrists, elbows, glenohumeral joints). The development of cartilage degenerative changes in CPPD deposition disease in both typical and atypical joints for primary OA suggests one or more systemic abnormalities.

Degenerative cartilage disease associated with sporadic CPPD crystal deposition disease may present as destructive arthropathy of the knees, hips, shoulders, or some combination of these, particularly in elderly females (Fig. 88–5A,B). The CPPD crystal arthropathy-associated degenerative disease can be less or more destructive than that observed in primary OA. For example, patients with primary OA and CPPD crystals have been reported to require knee replacement surgery more often than those with primary OA without crystals.[110] In another study, 60 percent of patients undergoing joint replacement had pathologic calcium crystals, CPPD or BCP crystals, in their knee synovial fluids, and higher mean radiographic scores correlated with the presence of calcium-containing crystals.[111] However, prospective analysis of CPPD deposition disease that principally involved the knee has suggested that radiographic worsening of degenerative changes may be slow.[112] The disease also may not appear to be clinically progressive in the involved knee after substantial periods of follow-up in a subset of patients, although clinical involvement may spread to other joints in the same time frame.[112] Most patients develop changes in radiographic extent of chon-

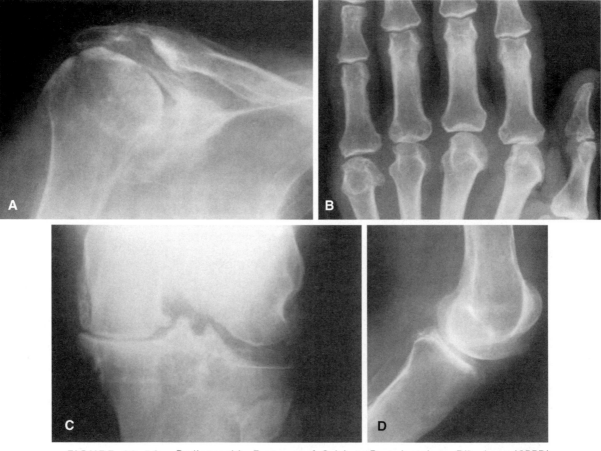

FIGURE 88–5A • Radiographic Features of Calcium Pyrophosphate Dihydrate (CPPD) Arthropathy. *A,* Destructive shoulder arthropathy. *B,* Metacarpophalangeal joint arthropathy. *C,* Knee degenerative joint disease with large subchondral bone cyst. *D,* Wraparound patella of the same patient shown in *A.*

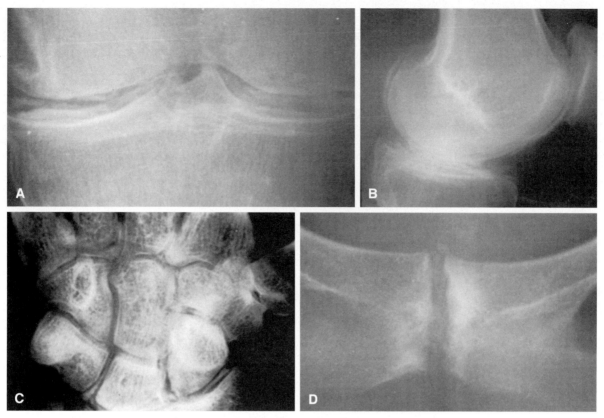

FIGURE 88-5B · Chondrocalcinosis of the Most Commonly Attected Joints in Calcium Pyrophosphate Dihydrate (CPPD) Deposition Disease. *A*, Lineal calcifications observed in knee menisci and fibrocartilage. *B*, Lateral view showing calcification of the articular cartilage as a line parallel to femoral condyles. *C*, Calcification of intercarpal joints and triangular ligament. *D*, Calcification of the symphysis pubis fibrocartilage associated with subchondral bone erosions and subchondral increased bone density.

drocalcinosis over time.[112] However, there is no clear correlation between the extent of calcification and progression of CPPD deposition arthropathy. There may be a relatively good prognosis for initial presentation of CPPD deposition disease in the knee as acute pseudo-gout attacks alone.[112]

Pseudorheumatoid involvement in a small subset of patients with CPPD deposition disease presents as a chronic, bilateral, symmetric deforming inflammatory polyarthropathy (see Fig. 88-4 C and D). Many of these patients have bilateral wrist and metacarpophalangeal joint involvement. Wrist tenosynovitis and carpal tunnel syndrome, cubital tunnel syndrome, and tendon rupture may develop. Ingestion of CPPD crystals by synovial lining cells, and lysosomal catabolism of such ingested crystals, stimulates synovial proliferation, in part via solubilization of the crystalline calcium. Such effects may contribute to regional synovial and periarticular tenosynovial proliferation promoted by CPPD crystal deposition.[88]

OTHER CLINICAL FORMS OF CALCIUM PYROPHOSPHATE DIHYDRATE CRYSTAL DEPOSITION

Concentrated (tumoral or pseudotophaceous) CPPD crystal deposition can occur in periarticular structures including tendons, ligaments, bursae, and occasionally

in bone.[99,113] CPPD deposits in tendons (e.g., the Achilles, triceps, and obturator tendons) are usually fine and linear on radiographs. Pseudotophaceous deposits of CPPD crystals have been detected in the temporal bone, around the knee and hip, and in the acromio-clavicular, temporomandibular, elbow, and small hand joints.[113] Peripheral tumoral CPPD crystal deposits may sometimes present with acute arthritic attacks. Rarely, tumoral CPPD deposits around the knee can mimic osteonecrosis.[114]

Axial skeletal CPPD crystal deposition occasionally involves the intervertebral disks, sacroiliac joints, and lumbar facet joints, and radiographic findings such as linear calcification and spinal ankylosis may appear.[115] Meningismus and clinical manifestations resembling herniated intervertebral disk, ankylosing spondylitis, and acute pseudogout of lumbar facet joints have been observed.[115,116] In addition, CPPD deposits within the ligamentum flavum or the transverse ligament of atlas can be sizeable and can progress to cause cervical canal stenosis, cervical myelopathy, and foramen magnum syndrome.[117-120] Odontoid fracture due to the calcification of the atlantoaxial joint may occur in CPPD deposition disease.[117-120] Thus, CPPD deposition disease can be a factor in the differential diagnosis of patients with neurologic disturbances and painful cervical mass, especially in the elderly.

FAMILIAL CHONDROCALCINOSIS

Familial CPPD deposition disease has been described in numerous countries and ethnic groups, including kindreds from Spain, Czechoslovakia, Holland, France, England, Germany, Sweden, Israel, the United States, Canada, Chile, and Japan.[56] In one English kindred with CPPD disease linked to ANKH gene mutation on chromosome 5p, recurrent childhood seizures were strongly associated with later development of CPPD deposition disease.[121] Familial chondrocalcinosis may be most prevalent in Spain and Chile. It is possible that certain mutations originating in Spain may have been spread across Europe and into South America along military and trade routes highly traveled in the seventeenth century.[56]

The pattern of inheritance and clinical presentation of familial CPPD deposition disease is variable, even for linkages to chromosome 5p.[65,66] Some families manifest early-onset polyarthritis, which can include ankylosing intervertebral and sacroiliac joint disease. In others, a late-onset chondrocalcinosis occurs, and the disease can be oligoarticular, mild in intensity and destructiveness, and nearly indistinguishable from idiopathic CPPD deposition disease.[121] Kindreds from Argentina and the Alsace region of France linked to 5p did share similar phenotypic features of chondrocalcinosis, including early age at onset (third decade of life), common but not universal premature OA, some cases of pseudorheumatoid arthritic peripheral joint disease, and radiographic evidence of fibrocartilage and hyaline cartilage calcifications typical of CPPD deposition.[61,62] The most commonly affected joints in these kindreds were the knees and wrists, with involvement of the pubic symphysis and intervertebral disks also described.[61,62]

CLINICAL FEATURES OF PATHOLOGIC BASIC CALCIUM PHOSPHATE CRYSTAL DEPOSITION AT THE JOINT

Unlike the case for urate and CPPD crystal deposition, acute synovitis due to HA crystal deposition is unusual.[122] However, acute inflammatory syndromes, including subacromial bursitis (see Chapter 38) and a form of pseudopodagra described in young women,[123] may occur in association with periarticular HA crystal deposition in bursae, tendons, ligaments, and soft tissues. Patients with advanced chronic renal failure, particularly those on dialysis, may develop symptomatic articular and periarticular BCP crystal deposition, which may be destructive and involve the axial skeleton.[124-126] In some cases of dialysis-dependent renal failure, destructive arthropathy associated with BCP crystal deposition may resemble or be associated with CPPD deposition disease,[126] and monosodium urate crystal deposits in the joint also may occur in the setting. Hyperparathyroidism can promote BCP-associated arthropathy.[127] Clinically significant periarticular HA crystal deposition also may occur in certain post-traumatic conditions and the systemic autoimmune diseases scleroderma and dermatomyositis[128] (Fig. 88–6).

BCP crystal deposition has a particular predilection for the shoulder, where it may manifest as calcific tendinitis of the rotator cuff (see Chapter 38) or as a destructive process associated with rotator cuff tear, which is most prevalent in the elderly and more common in females.[129] Abundant intra-articular BCP crystalline material is typically present in the distinctive noninflammatory syndrome of rotator cuff tear and marked cartilage degeneration, an entity termed *Milwaukee shoulder syndrome* (MSS), *cuff tear arthropathy*, or *apatite-associated destructive arthritis*[57,83,129,130] (see Fig. 88–6 C). The process may be bilateral but is generally worse on the side of the dominant hand. Substantial glenohumeral joint effusions are typically seen, and synovial fluid is often blood-stained but contains, at most, relatively low numbers of mononuclear leukocytes. Joints other than the shoulder, such as the knee and hip, can be affected by a condition similar to MSS, sometimes in the same individual with shoulder involvement.[57,129,131] In contrast to primary OA, lateral tibiofemoral compartment involvement is common in BCP-associated destructive knee arthropathy. Concurrent CPPD deposition, biomechanic abnormalities, chronic renal failure, and neuropathic factors appear to be predisposing factors. A kindred with familial OA and apparent Milwaukee shoulder-knee syndrome (MSKS) had an unusual type of degenerative joint disease with both intra-articular and periarticular calcifications[57] (see Fig. 88–6 C and D).

Studies of synovial fluids and cartilage specimens from OA have indicated that intra-articular BCP crystalline material, including HA in the pericellular matrix of chondrocytes, is frequently detectable in the disease.[70,111] Synovial fluid HA crystals are frequently present in conjunction with CPPD crystals in OA, particularly in advanced disease of the knee at the time of total joint replacement.[111,132] Subchondral bone shards in OA cartilage that are comprised of BCP crystalline material could contribute to a fraction of such crystal-positive specimens. In addition, the traffic of crystals from articular cartilage to synovium[88,89] can promote calcific synovial crystal deposits at or just beneath the synovial surface, and synovium-derived rice bodies can give rise to BCP crystal deposits released into the joint space.[133,134] Therefore, it is difficult to quantify the precise prevalence of HA crystal deposits in articular cartilage in OA. Both HA and CPPD crystal–induced synovial proliferation, cytotoxic effects on chondrocytes, and synovial and chondrocyte MMP expression can promote OA progression.[88,89]

▊ Differential Diagnosis

CPPD deposition disease can imitate a number of other conditions and vice versa (see Table 88–3), which mandates attention to fulfillment of diagnostic criteria for CPPD deposition disease (see Table 88–1). Conversely, it is important to note that presence of radiographic evidence for chondrocalcinosis is a common finding in the aged and does not necessarily indicate that the patient's symptomatic articular problem is due to CPPD deposition disease, which often is asymptomatic.

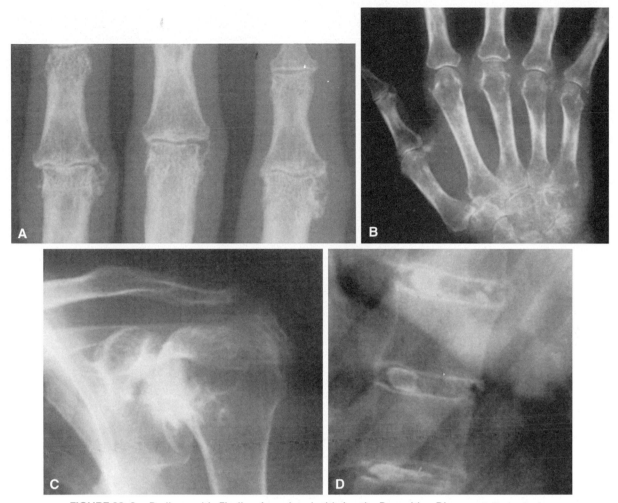

FIGURE 88-6 · Radiographic Finding Associated with Apatite Deposition Disease. *A*, Periarticular apatite deposit in proximal interphalangeal joints. (From Reginato AJ, Schumacher HR: Crystal associated arthritis. Clin Geriatric Med 4:295-322, 1988.) *B*, Periarticular finger joint calcified deposits in a patient with systemic sclerosis. *C*, Destructive shoulder arthropathy associated secondary to rotator cuff tear in a member of an Italo-Argentinean family. (Courtesy of B. PonsEstel.) *D*, Intervertebral disk calcification in a sibling of the family in *C* with erosive osteoarthritis, mild spondyloepiphyseal dysplasia, and apatite deposition. (Courtesy of J.C. Marcos.)

The demonstrable presence of CPPD crystals in synovial fluid or in tissues using compensated polarized light microscopy (as discussed previously for gout versus pseudogout) is definite evidence for CPPD deposition disease. Although weakly birefringent relative to urate crystals and often rhomboid in shape, CPPD crystals can be rod-shaped and intracellular, and thereby resemble urate crystals. Thus, the use of compensated polarized light microscopy is essential to confirm the presence of positively birefringent CPPD crystals, although it should be noted that some CPPD crystals are nonbirefringent.[135] The appearance and number of CPPD crystals can change with storage. Therefore, clinicians should examine relatively fresh specimens collected in vials free of calcium-chelating anticoagulants such as EDTA.

The ability of pseudogout to mimic septic arthritis ("pseudoseptic arthritis") and vice versa underscores the diagnostic importance of arthrocentesis with appropriate synovial fluid crystal analysis and, in many instances, concomitant exclusion of joint infection. This measure is important as crystal deposits can be "enzymatically strip-mined" by inflammation associated with joint sepsis. Hence, CPPD (as well as other crystals) may be observed free in the joint fluid and within synovial-fluid leukocytes in an infected joint.

Chronic arthritis in CPPD deposition disease has several clinical and plain radiographic features helpful in differentiating it from OA. These include involvement at sites uncommon for primary OA, such as the wrist, metacarpophalangeal joints, elbow, or shoulder, as well as radiographic heavy punctate and linear calcifications in fibrocartilages, articular (hyaline) cartilages, and joint capsules, especially if bilaterally symmetric (Fig. 88-7). It should be noted that faint or atypical calcifications may be due to BCP-related vascular calcifications. Deposition of nonpathologic dicalcium phosphate dihydrate (DCPD), which has a chemical formula of $CaHPO_4 \cdot 2H_2O$, a calcium-to-phosphate ratio of 1.0, and is also known as "brushite" crystals, has been thought to cause some atypical calcifications, but it should be noted that brushite crystals can arise as an artifact of preparation of calcified tissue for pathologic analyses.[136]

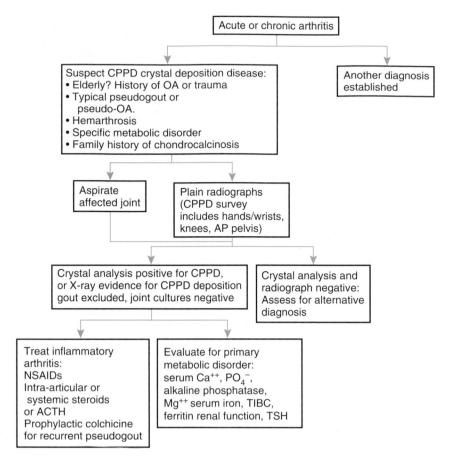

FIGURE 88–7 · Algorithm for Evaluation and Treatment of Calcium Pyrophosphate Dihydrate Deposition Disease.

Patients with arthritis in whom CPPD deposition disease is part of the differential diagnosis can be adequately screened radiologically by obtaining an anteroposterior (AP) view of each knee, an AP view of the pelvis (to detect symphysis pubis involvement, which is quite common), and posteroanterior (PA) views of both hands that include visualization of both wrists (see Figs. 88–5B and 88–7). Calcific deposits may or may not be detectable by radiographic screening of these areas in CPPD deposition disease. In this circumstance, radiographic evidence other than chondrocalcinosis may point to the correct diagnosis.[137] For example, radiographic findings suggestive of CPPD deposition disease, as opposed to primary OA, include radiocarpal or marked patellofemoral joint-space narrowing, especially if isolated (such as the patella "wrapped around" the femur), as well as scaphoid-lunate widening and femoral cortical erosion superior to the patella. Severe progressive degeneration in the knee, with subchondral bony collapse (microfractures), and fragmentation, with formation of intra-articular radiodense bodies is a feature of CPPD presenting as a "pseudoneuropathic" joint. CPPD deposition disease involving the metacarpophalangeal joints can be distinguished radiographically from RA by metacarpal squaring associated with "beak-like" osteophytes and subchondral cyst formation. Tendon calcifications (e.g., Achilles, triceps, and obturator tendons) are a valuable differential diagnostic feature of CPPD deposition. Osteophyte formation is more variable with CPPD deposition disease than with OA.

Diagnosis of CPPD deposition disease prior to age 50, particularly if CPPD deposition is widespread, should prompt differential diagnostic consideration of a primary metabolic or familial disorder (see Table 88–2). In the elderly, presentation of CPPD deposition as diffuse pain and fever of unknown origin[109] can mimic infection, polymyalgia rheumatica, and RA. A false positive rheumatoid factor (RF) test is common in the elderly (30% or greater positivity). Thus, patients with pseudorheumatoid CPPD deposition disease are often RF seropositive.

BCP crystals may be detected as nonbirefringent globular clumps within leukocytes in some synovial fluids, and BCP crystal clumps stain with the calcium binding dye Alizarin red S under light microscopy.[122,132] CPPD crystals also can be detected using Alizarin red S, but they stain more weakly than BCP crystals. Relative paucity of osteophytes (so-called "atrophic degenerative arthritis") and the sizeable glenohumeral joint effusions with abundant synovial-fluid BCP crystalline material associated with MSS help distinguish MSS from primary OA of the glenohumeral joint. However, destructive, neuropathic shoulder arthropathy due to syringomyelia or alcoholism[138] sometimes merits consideration in the differential diagnosis of MSS. Oxalate crystal deposition arthropathy can be a major differential diagnostic consideration with BCP-associated arthritis and periarticular calcifications in dialysis-dependent renal failure.[139] Differential diagnosis of calcific tendinitis of the shoulder is discussed in Chapter 38.

Evaluation

A thorough laboratory evaluation of the newly diagnosed CPPD-disease patient routinely includes serum levels of calcium, phosphorus, magnesium, alkaline phosphatase, ferritin, iron and total iron binding capacity, and TSH (see Fig. 88–7). Conventional radiography is usually the first method used to evaluate patients with suspected chondrocalcinosis, but radiographic findings may not correlate with pathologic and clinical manifestations. For example, the correlation between radiographic and pathologic findings was only 39.2 percent in a study of patients via knee arthroscopy.[140] Radiographic diagnostic approaches to CPPD deposition disease other than conventional radiographs with the potential to improve sensitivity include computed tomography (CT), magnetic resonance imaging (MRI), and ultrasonography (US), which can detect CPPD (as well as BCP) crystals, particularly in the knee.[137,141,142] Specialized techniques beyond Alizarin red S staining, such as radiographic diffraction or transmission electron microscopy showing electron-dense clumps of needle-like crystals, may be needed to confirm BCP crystal deposition.[2]

Under conditions in which synovial fluid specimens are not fresh (or stored at 4°C for analysis after significant delay[143]), Gram stain and Diff Quick staining methods for crystal analysis in synovial fluids have been suggested to provide information beyond that from compensated polarized light microscopy.[144,145] Demonstration of CPPD crystals in articular tissues (see Fig. 88–3) can be difficult in specimens stained with hematoxylin and eosin (H&E), as the acidity of hematoxylin solutions promotes decalcification. But the decalcifying effect of hematoxylin can be diminished by limiting the staining period with Mayer's hematoxylin to 3 minutes.[146]

Treatment

CALCIUM PYROPHOSPHATE DIHYDRATE DEPOSITION DISEASE

As in gout, therapeutic approaches to patients with CPPD deposition disease involve treatment and prophylaxis of acute arthritic attacks, as well as therapy to lessen chronic and anatomically progressive sequelae of crystal deposition (Table 88–4). Reduced meniscal calcification was reported over a 10-year period in association with administration of oral magnesium to a patient with secondary CPPD deposition disease due to hypomagnesemia.[147] However, there is no specific treatment for idiopathic CPPD deposition disease. In addition, the potential benefits for prevention of chondrocalcinotic cartilage degeneration in the appropriate treatment of hemochromatosis and hyperparathyroidism are unclear, because the ability to detect chondrocalcinosis radiologically is usually indicative of advanced crystal deposition disease.

Episodes of pseudogout generally respond to nonsteroidal anti-inflammatory drugs (NSAIDS) including COX-2 inhibitors, intraarticular steroids, or both, although sometimes more slowly than in gout. ACTH[148] and systemic glucocorticosteroids,[149] generally given as

TABLE 88–4 · THERAPEUTICS FOR CALCIUM PYROPHOSPHATE DIHYDRATE (CPPD) CRYSTAL DEPOSITION DISEASE

Proven Benefits
Nonsteroidal anti-inflammatory drugs (NSAIDS) or cyclooxygenase-2 (COX-2) inhibitors
Intra-articular corticosteroids
Systemic corticosteroids
Adrenocortiotrophic hormone (ACTH)
Prophylactic low-dose colchicine

Possible Benefits Already Observed Clinically
Hydroxychloroquine
Oral magnesium (for patients with hypomagnesemia)

Theoretical Benefits
ANK anion channel blockade (probenicid)
PC-1 inhibition
TG2 transglutaminase inhibition
Phosphocitrate
Polyphosphates
Promotion of crystal dissolution by alkaline phosphatase or polyamines

described for acute gout (see Chapter 87), are effective in most cases of acute pseudogout. The response to colchicine bolus is less consistent than that usually seen in acute gout and intravenous (IV) colchicine is not recommended as treatment for pseudogout; it can be quite dangerous in elderly patients. Pseudogout episodes can be diminished in frequency by low-dose daily colchicine prophylaxis, as for gouty arthritis. The self-limited nature of most acute pseudogout attacks in the knee can sometimes be accelerated by simple arthrocentesis and thorough drainage of the joint effusion, but there are currently no data for measures such as tidal irrigation.

In a short trial, hydroxychloroquine was suggested to be of some benefit to patients with chronic polyarticular CPPD deposition disease.[150] In addition, pseudorheumatoid CPPD crystal deposition disease is potentially responsive to methotrexate. However, effective cartilage-preserving therapy is still lacking in idiopathic chronic progressive CPPD deposition disease. Some reports have suggested that OA patients with cartilage calcification respond distinctly to arthroscopic irrigation and daily low-dose colchicine,[151-153] but further substantiation is needed. There is currently no evidence to support arthroscopic debridement as a treatment modality for CPPD deposition disease. There is insufficient evidence for beneficial effects of intra-articular hyaluronate therapy in CPPD deposition disease of the knee, and the risks of precipitating pseudogout appear to be significant with this treatment modality, as discussed previously.

BASIC CALCIUM PHOSPHATE CRYSTAL ARTHROPATHIES

NSAIDS and local glucocorticoid injection (Table 88–5) are effective treatment options for BCP crystal–associated calcific tendinitis and subacromial bursitis (see

TABLE 88–5 • THERAPEUTICS FOR ARTICULAR AND PERIARTICULAR BASIC CALCIUM PHOSPHATE CRYSTAL DEPOSITION

Proven Benefits
Nonsteroidal anti-inflammatory drugs (NSAIDS) or cyclooxygenase-2 (COX-2) inhibitors
Local corticosteroid injection
Local irrigation
Ultrasonography (US)

Theoretical Benefits
Phosphocitrate
Modulators of ANK (e.g., probenecid), PC-1/NPPI1, or TG2 transglutaminase

Chapter 38). BCP crystal–associated inflammation of the rotator cuff and subacromial bursa of the shoulder can be successfully treated using needle aspiration, irrigation, and steroid injections. Ultrasound-guided techniques, which promote resorption of rotator cuff and bursal calcifications, can enhance the success of such approaches.[154,155]

FOUNDATION FOR NOVEL THERAPIES

The potential to develop therapies for both CPPD and BCP crystal–associated arthropathies based on new molecular targets has been elevated by the identification of ANK, PC-1, and TG2 TGase as specific molecular mediators of cartilage calcification, as discussed previously. Intriguingly, the anion transport inhibitor probenecid suppresses ANK-induced and TGF-β–induced increases in extracellular PP_i in vitro.[26,65,156] Prevention of CPPD deposition by polyphosphates or promotion of CPPD dissolution by depot alkaline phosphatase and by pyrophosphatase activation–promoting polyamines could provide alternative therapeutic approaches.[157,158] The PP_i analogue phosphocitrate, a natural compound in mammalian mitochondria and in the urinary tract, is a potent inhibitor of HA crystal formation.[159] Phosphocitrate inhibits NO-induced calcification of cartilage[77] and also inhibits both HA and CPPD crystal–associated cell stimulation, including induction of MMP-3 in fibroblasts.[160] Systemic phosphocitrate treatment suppresses ankylosing ossification in murine progressive ankylosis of *ank/ank* mice.[161] Further clinical development of phosphocitrate has been slowed in part by low bioavailability unless given parenterally.[159] The use of bisphosphonates as PP_i analogues can be beneficial in some cases of idiopathic infantile arterial and periarticular calcification, including disease associated with PC-1/NPP1 deficiency.[11,28]

Summary and Conclusion

CPPD and BCP crystal deposition are common disorders and frequently require rheumatologic evaluation. This chapter has reviewed newly identified central basic mechanisms governing cartilage calcification and their relationship to aging and OA. These include the identification of mutations in the ANKH gene associated with disordered PP_i transport in some kindreds with familial chondrocalcinosis linked to chromosome 5p, the role of the PP_i-generating NTPPPH ectoenzyme PC-1/NPP1 in chondrocalcinosis, and the linkage of low-grade inflammation to expression and activation of TG2 TGase with chondrocyte hypertrophic differentiation and stimulation of calcification. Diagnostic and therapeutic advances pertaining to CPPD and HA crystal deposition in the joint have arisen in step with new imaging approaches and detailed clinical assessment of subjects with degenerative joint disease. Novel molecular-based therapeutics could see future application for CPPD and BCP crystal deposition arthropathies.

REFERENCES

1. Pritzker KP, Cheng PT, Grynpas MD, et al: Crystal associated diseases: role of scanning electron microscopy in diagnosis. Scanning Microsc 2:1471-1478, 1988.
2. Pritzker KP, Cheng PT, Renlund RC: Calcium pyrophosphate crystal deposition in hyaline cartilage: Ultrastructural analysis and implications for pathogenesis. J Rheumatol 15:828-835, 1988.
3. Luisiri P, Blair J, Ellman MH: Calcium pyrophosphate dihydrate deposition disease presenting as tumoral calcinosis (periarticular pseudogout). J Rheumatol 23:1647-1650, 1996.
4. Felson DT, Anderson JJ, Naimark A, et al: The prevalence of chondrocalcinosis in the elderly and its association with knee osteoarthritis: The Framingham Study. J Rheumatol 16:1241-1245, 1989.
5. Zitnan D, Sitaj S: Chondrocalcinosis articularis Section I. Clinical and radiological study. Ann Rheum Dis 22:142-169, 1963.
6. Ellman MH, Brown NL, Levin B: Prevalence of knee chondrocalcinosis in hospital and clinic patients aged 50 or older. J Am Geriatr Soc 29:189-192, 1981.
7. Ellman MH, Levin B: Chondrocalcinosis in elderly persons. Arthritis Rheum 18:43-47, 1975.
8. Mitrovic DR, Stankovic A, Iriarte-Borda O, et al: The prevalence of chondrocalcinosis in the human knee joint: An autopsy survey. J Rheumatol 15:633-641, 1988.
9. Mccarty DJ Jr., Hogan JM, Gatter RA, et al: Studies on pathological calcifications in human cartilage. I. Prevalence and types of crystal deposits in the menisci of two hundred fifteen cadavera. J Bone Joint Surg Am 48:309-325, 1966.
10. Wilkins E, Dieppe P, Maddison P, et al: Osteoarthritis and articular chondrocalcinosis in the elderly. Ann Rheum Dis 42:280-284, 1983.
11. Rutsch F, Terkeltaub R: Parallels between arterial and cartilage calcification: What understanding artery calcification can teach us about chondrocalcinosis. Curr Op Rheum, 15:302-310, 2003.
12. Terkeltaub R: What does cartilage calcification tell us about osteoarthritis? J Rheumatol 29:411-415, 2002.
13. Mandel N, Mandel G: Calcium pyrophosphate crystal deposition in model systems. Rheum Dis Clin North Am 14:321-340, 1988.
14. Hunter GK, Grynpas MD, Cheng PT, et al: Effect of glycosaminoglycans on calcium pyrophosphate crystal formation in collagen gels. Calcif Tissue Int 41:164-170, 1987.
15. Cheng PT, Pritzker KP: Pyrophosphate, phosphate ion interaction: Effects on calcium pyrophosphate and calcium hydroxyapatite crystal formation in aqueous solutions. J Rheumatol 10:769-777, 1983.
16. Terkeltaub R: Inorganic pyrophosphate (PP_i) generation and disposition in pathophysiology. Am J Physiol: Cell Physiol 281:C1-C11, 2001.
17. Swan A, Heywood B, Chapman B, et al: Evidence for a causal relationship between the structure, size, and load of calcium pyrophosphate dihydrate crystals, and attacks of pseudogout. Ann Rheum Dis 54:825-830, 1995.
18. Johnson K, Goding J, van Etten D, et al: Linked deficiencies in extracellular inorganic pyrophosphate and osteopontin

expression mediate pathologic calcification in PC-1 null mice. Am J Bone Min Res, 18:994-1004.

19. Hessle L, Johnson KA, Anderson HC, et al: Tissue-nonspecific alkaline phosphatase and plasma cell membrane glycoprotein-1 are central antagonistic regulators of bone mineralization. Proc Natl Acad Sci U S A 99:9445-9449, 2002.

20. Chang W, Tu C, Chen TH, et al: Expression and signal transduction of calcium-sensing receptors in cartilage and bone. Endocrinology 140:5883-5893, 1999.

21. Chang W, Tu C, Pratt S, et al: Extracellular Ca(2+)-sensing receptors modulate matrix production and mineralization in chondrogenic RCJ3.1C5.18 cells. Endocrinology 143:1467-1474, 2002.

22. Adams CS, Mansfield K, Perlot RL, et al: Matrix regulation of skeletal cell apoptosis: Role of calcium and phosphate ions. J Biol Chem 276:20316-20322, 2001.

23. Wang D, Canaff L, Davidson D, et al: Alterations in the sensing and transport of phosphate and calcium by differentiating chondrocytes. J Biol Chem 276:33995-34005, 2001.

24. Johnson K, Van Etten D, Terkeltaub R: ANK and PC-1 regulate cartilage matrix calcification by synergistically controlling extracellular PPi. Arthritis Rheum 44:S162, 2001.

25. Johnson K, Pritzker K, Goding J, et al: The nucleoside triphosphate pyrophosphohydrolase (NTPPPH) isozyme PC-1 directly promotes cartilage calcification through chondrocyte apoptosis and increased calcium precipitation by mineralizing vesicles. J Rheumatol 28: 2681-2691, 2001.

26. Ho A, Johnson M, Kingsley DM: Role of the mouse ank gene in tissue calcification and arthritis. Science 289:265-270, 2000.

27. Okawa A, Nakamura I, Goto S, et al: Mutation in Npps in a mouse model of ossification of the posterior longitudinal ligament of the spine. Nat Genet 19:271-273, 1998.

28. Rutsch F, Vaingankar S, Johnson K, et al: PC-1 nucleoside triphosphate pyrophosphohydrolase deficiency in idiopathic infantile arterial calcification. Am J Pathol 158:543-554, 2001.

29. Johnson K, Hashimoto S, Lotz M et al: Up-regulated expression of the phosphodiesterase nucleotide pyrophosphatase family member PC-1 is a marker and pathogenic factor for knee meniscal cartilage matrix calcification. Arthritis Rheum 44:1071-1081, 2001.

30. Johnson K, Vaingankar S, Chen Y et al: Differential mechanisms of inorganic pyrophosphate production by plasma cell membrane glycoprotein-1 and B10 in chondrocytes. Arthritis Rheum 42:1986-1997, 1999.

31. Terkeltaub R: Inorganic pyrophosphate generation and disposition in pathophysiology. Am J Physiol:Cell Physiol 281:C1-C11, 2001.

32. Rosenthal AK, Cheung HS, Ryan LM: Transforming growth factor beta 1 stimulates inorganic pyrophosphate elaboration by porcine cartilage. Arthritis Rheum 34:904-911, 1991.

33. Rosen F, McCabe G, Quach J, et al: Differential effects of aging on human chondrocyte responses to transforming growth factor beta: increased pyrophosphate production and decreased cell proliferation. Arthritis Rheum 40:1275-1281, 1997.

34. Ryan LM, Kurup IV, Cheung HS: Transduction mechanisms of porcine chondrocyte inorganic pyrophosphate elaboration. Arthritis Rheum 42:555-560, 1999.

35. Ryan LM, Rachow JW, McCarty DJ: Synovial fluid ATP: a potential substrate for the production of inorganic pyrophosphate. J Rheumatol 18:716-720, 1991.

36. Pattrick M, Hamilton E, Hornby J, et al: Synovial fluid pyrophosphate and nucleoside triphosphate pyrophosphatase: comparison between normal and diseased and between inflamed and non-inflamed joints. Ann Rheum Dis 50:214-218, 1991.

37. Bollen M, Gijsbers R, Ceulemans H, et al: Nucleotide pyrophosphatases/phosphodiesterases on the move. Crit Rev Biochem Mol Biol 35:393-432, 2000.

38. Goding JW: Ecto-enzymes: physiology meets pathology. J Leukoc Biol 67:285-311, 2000.

39. Johnson K, Goding J, van Etten D, et al: Linked deficiencies in extracellular inorganic pyrophosphate and osteopontin expression mediate pathologic calcification in PC-1 null mice. Am J Bone Min Res, in press.

40. Tokumura A, Majima E, Kariya Y, et al: Identification of human plasma lysophospholipase D, a lysophosphatidic acid-producing enzyme, as autotaxin, a multifunctional phosphodiesterase. J Biol Chem 277:39436-39442, 2002.

41. Lotz M, Rosen F, McCabe G, et al: Interleukin 1 beta suppresses transforming growth factor-induced inorganic pyrophosphate [PPi] production and expression of the PPi-generating enzyme PC-1 in human chondrocytes. Proc Natl Acad Sci USA 92:10364-10368, 1995.

42. Johnson K, Hashimoto S, Lotz M, et al: IL-1 induces pro-mineralizing activity of cartilage tissue transglutaminase and factor XIIIa. Am J Pathol 159:149-163, 2001.

43. Ryan LM, Kurup IV, Cheung HS: Transduction mechanisms of porcine chondrocyte inorganic pyrophosphate elaboration. Arthritis Rheum 42:555-560, 1999.

44. Masuda I, Hamada J, Haas AL, et al: A unique ectonucleotide pyrophosphohydrolase associated with porcine chondrocyte-derived vesicles. J Clin Invest 95:699-704, 1995.

45. Hirose J, Ryan LM, Masuda I: Up-regulated expression of cartilage intermediate-layer protein and ANK in articular hyaline cartilage from patients with calcium pyrophosphate dihydrate crystal deposition disease. Arthritis Rheum 46:3218-3229, 2002.

46. Johnson K, Farley D, Hu S-I, Terkeltaub R: One of two chondrocyte-expressed isoforms of Cartilage Intermediate Layer Protein functions as an IGF-I antagonist. Arthritis Rheum, 48:1302-14, 2003.

47. Masuda I, Iyama KI, Halligan BD, et al: Variations in site and levels of expression of chondrocyte nucleotide pyrophosphohydrolase with aging. J Bone Miner Res 16:868-875, 2001.

48. Lorenzo P, Bayliss MT, Heinegard D: A novel cartilage protein (CILP) present in the mid-zone of human articular cartilage increases with age. J Biol Chem 273:23463-23468, 1998.

49. Hirose J, Masuda I, Ryan LM: Expression of cartilage intermediate layer protein/nucleotide pyrophosphohydrolase parallels the production of extracellular inorganic pyrophosphate in response to growth factors and with aging. Arthritis Rheum 43:2703-2711, 2000.

50. Olmez U, Ryan LM, Kurup IV, et al: Insulin-like growth factor-1 suppresses pyrophosphate elaboration by transforming growth factor beta1-stimulated chondrocytes and cartilage. Osteoarthritis Cartilage 2:149-154, 1994.

51. Jones AC, Chuck AJ, Arie EA, et al: Diseases associated with calcium pyrophosphate deposition disease. Semin Arthritis Rheum 22:188-202, 1992.

52. Doherty M, Belcher C, Regan M, et al: Association between synovial fluid levels of inorganic pyrophosphate and short term radiographic outcome of knee osteoarthritis. Ann Rheum Dis 55:432-436, 1996.

53. Terkeltaub R, Lotz M, Johnson K, et al: Parathyroid hormone related protein (PTHrP) expression is abundant in osteoarthritic cartilage, and the PTHrP 1-173 isoform is selectively induced by TGFβ in articular chondrocytes, and suppresses extracellular inorganic pyrophosphate generation. Arthritis Rheum 41:2152-2164, 1998.

54. Goomer R, Johnson K, Burton D, et al: A tetrabasic C-terminal motif determines intracrine regulatory effects of PTHrP 1-173 on PPi metabolism and collagen synthesis in chondrocytes. Endocrinology 141:4613-4622, 2000.

55. Johnson KA, Hessle L, Vaingankar S, et al: Osteoblast tissue-nonspecific alkaline phosphatase antagonizes and regulates PC-1. Am J Physiol Regul Integr Comp Physiol 279:R1365-R1377, 2000.

56. Maldonado I, Reginato AM, Reginato AJ: Familial calcium crystal disease: What have we learned? Curr Opin Rheum 13:225-233, 2001.

57. Pons-Estel BA, Gimenez C, Sacnun M, et al: Familial osteoarthritis and Milwaukee shoulder associated with calcium pyrophosphate and apatite crystal deposition. J Rheumatol 27:471-480, 2000.

58. Reginato AJ, Passano GM, Neumann G, et al: Familial spondyloepiphyseal dysplasia tarda, brachydactyly, and precocious osteoarthritis associated with an arginine 75—>cysteine mutation in the procollagen type II gene in a kindred of Chiloe Islanders. I. Clinical, radiographic, and pathologic findings. Arthritis Rheum 37:1078-1086, 1994.

59. Baldwin CT, Farrer LA, Adair R, et al: Linkage of early-onset osteoarthritis and chondrocalcinosis to human chromosome 8q. Am J Hum Genet 56:692-697, 1995.

60. Hughes AE, McGibbon D, Woodwar E, et al: Localization of a gene for chondrocalcinosis to chromosome 5p. Hum Mol Genet 4:1225-1228, 1995.

61. Andrew LJ, Brancolini V, Serrano de la Pena L, et al: Refinement of the chromosome 5p locus for familial calcium pyrophosphate dihydrate deposition disease. Am J Hum Genet 64:136-145, 1999.

62. Rojas K, Serrano de la Pena L, Gallardo T, et al: Physical map and characterization of transcripts in the candidate interval for familial chondrocalcinosis at chromosome 5p15.1 Genomics 62:177-183, 1999.

63. Reginato AJ, McCarty DJ, Serrano de la Pena L, et al: Linkage of a North American kindred with primary calcium pyrophosphate deposition disease [CPPDD] linked to chromosome 5p. Arthritis Rheum 42:S159, 1999.

64. Pendleton A, Johnson MD, Hughes A, et al: Mutations in ANKH cause chondrocalcinosis. Am J Hum Genet 71:933-940, 2002.

65. Williams JC, Zhang Y, Timms A, et al: Autosomal dominant familial calcium pyrophosphate dihydrate deposition disease is caused by mutation in the transmembrane protein ANKH. Am J Hum Genet 71:985-991, 2002.

66. Nurnberg P, Thiele H, Chandler D, et al: Heterozygous mutations in ANKH, the human ortholog of the mouse progressive ankylosis gene, result in craniometaphyseal dysplasia. Nat Genet 28:37-41, 2001.

67. Reichenberger E, Tiziani V, Watanabe S, et al: Autosomal dominant craniometaphyseal dysplasia is caused by mutations in the transmembrane protein ANK. Am J Hum Genet 68:1321-1326, 2001.

68. Lust G, Faure G, Netter P, et al: Evidence of a generalized metabolic defect in patients with hereditary chondrocalcinosis: Increased inorganic pyrophosphate in cultured fibroblasts and lymphoblasts. Arthritis Rheum 24:1517-1521, 1981.

69. Lust G, Faure G, Netter P, et al: Increased pyrophosphate in fibroblasts and lymphoblasts from patients with hereditary diffuse articular chondrocalcinosis. Science 214:809-810, 1981.

70. Kirsch T, Swoboda B, Nah H: Activation of annexin II and V expression, terminal differentiation, mineralization and apoptosis in human osteoarthritic cartilage. Osteoarthritis Cartilage 8:294-302, 2000.

71. Masuda I, Ishikawa K, Usuku G: A histologic and immunohistochemical study of calcium pyrophosphate dihydrate crystal deposition disease. Clin Orthop 263:272-287, 1991.

72. Rosenthal AK, Henry LA: Thyroid hormones induce features of the hypertrophic phenotype and stimulate correlates of CPPD crystal formation in articular chondrocytes. J Rheumatol 26:395-401, 1999.

73. Kirsch T, Nah HD, Shapiro IM, et al: Regulated production of mineralization competent matrix vesicles in hypertrophic chondrocytes. J Cell Biol 137:1149-1160, 1997.

74. Serra R, Johnson M, Filvaroff EH, et al: Expression of a truncated, kinase-defective TGF-beta type II receptor in mouse skeletal tissue promotes terminal chondrocyte differentiation and osteoarthritis. J Cell Biol 139:541-552, 1997.

75. Adams CS, Shapiro IM: The fate of the terminally differentiated chondrocyte: evidence for microenvironmental regulation of chondrocyte apoptosis. Crit Rev Oral Biol Med 13:465-473, 2002.

76. Hashimoto S, Ochs RL, Rosen F, et al: Chondrocyte-derived apoptotic bodies and calcification of articular cartilage. Proc Natl Acad Sci U S A 95:3094-3099, 1998.

77. Cheung HS, Ryan LM: Phosphocitrate blocks nitric oxide-induced calcification of cartilage and chondrocyte-derived apoptotic bodies. Osteoarthritis Cartilage 7:409-412, 1999.

78. Terkeltaub R, Johnson K, Murphy A, et al: The mitochondrion in osteoarthritis. Mitochondrion 1:301-319, 2002.

79. Johnson K, Van Etten D, Nanda N, et al: Distinct Trans-glutaminase II/TG2-independent and TG2-dependent pathways mediate articular chondrocyte hypertrophy. J Biol Chem 278:18824-321, 2003.

80. Rosenthal AK, Gohr CM, Henry LA, et al: Participation of transglutaminase in the activation of latent transforming growth factor beta1 in aging articular cartilage. Arthritis Rheum 43:1729-1733, 2000.

81. Merz D, Liu R, Johnson K, Terkeltaub R, IL-8/CXCL8 and growth-related oncogene alpha/CXCL1 induce chondrocyte hypertrophic differentiation. J Immunol 171:4406-15, 2003.

82. Johnson K, Jung AS, Andreyev A, et al: Mitochondrial Oxidative Phosphorylation is a downstream regulator of nitric oxide effects on chondrocyte matrix synthesis and mineralization. Arthritis Rheum 43:1560-1570, 2000.

83. Rachow JW, Ryan LM, McCarty DJ, et al: Synovial fluid inorganic pyrophosphate concentration and nucleotide pyrophosphohydrolase activity in basic calcium phosphate deposition arthropathy and Milwaukee shoulder syndrome. Arthritis Rheum 31:408-413, 1988.

84. Sano H, Ishii H, Trudel G, et al: Histologic evidence of degeneration at the insertion of 3 rotator cuff tendons: a comparative study with human cadaveric shoulders. J Shoulder Elbow Surg 8:574-579, 1999.

85. Takeuchi E, Sugamoto K, Nakase T, et al: Localization and expression of osteopontin in the rotator cuff tendons in patients with calcifying tendinitis. Virchows Arch 438:612-617, 2001.

86. Nakase T, Takeuchi E, Sugamoto K, et al: Involvement of multinucleated giant cells synthesizing cathepsin K in calcified tendinitis of the rotator cuff tendons. Rheumatology (Oxford) 39:1074-1077, 2000.

87. Liu R, O'Connell M, Johnson K, et al: Extracellular signal-regulated kinase 1/extracellular signal-regulated kinase 2 mitogen-activated protein kinase signaling and activation of activator protein 1 and nuclear factor kappaB transcription factors play central roles in interleukin-8 expression stimulated by monosodium urate monohydrate and calcium pyrophosphate crystals in monocytic cells. Arthritis Rheum 43:1145-1155, 2000.

88. Morgan MP, McCarthy GM: Signaling mechanisms involved in crystal-induced tissue damage. Curr Opin Rheumatol 14:292-297, 2002.

89. Sun Y, Wenger L, Brinckerhoff CE, et al: Basic calcium phosphate crystals induce matrix metalloproteinase-1 through the Ras/mitogen-activated protein kinase/c-Fos/AP-1/metalloproteinase 1 pathway. Involvement of transcription factor binding sites AP-1 and PEA-3. J Biol Chem 277:1544-1552, 2002.

90. Cronstein BN, Molad Y, Reibman J, et al: Colchicine alters the quantitative and qualitative display of selectins on endothelial cells and neutrophils J Clin Invest 96:994-1002, 1995.

91. Terkeltaub R, Baird S, Sears P, et al: The murine homolog of the interleukin-8 receptor CXCR-2 is essential for the occurrence of neutrophilic inflammation in the air pouch model of acute urate crystal-induced gouty synovitis. Arthritis Rheum 41:900-909, 1998.

92. Halverson PB, Carrera GF, McCarty DJ: Milwaukee shoulder syndrome: Fifteen additional cases and a description of contributing factors. Arch Intern Med 150:3, 677-682, 1990.

93. Carroll GJ, Stuart RA, Armstrong JA, et al: Hydroxyapatite crystals are a frequent finding in osteoarthritic synovial fluid, but are not related to increased concentrations of keratan sulfate or interleukin 1 beta. J Rheumatol 18:861-866, 1991.

94. Alwan WH, Dieppe PA, Elson CJ, et al: Hydroxyapatite and urate crystal induced cytokine release by macrophages. Ann Rheum Dis 48:476-482, 1989.

95. Di Giovine FS, Malawista SE, Nuki G, et al: Interleukin 1 (IL 1) as a mediator of crystal arthritis: Stimulation of T cell and synovial fibroblast mitogenesis by urate crystal-induced IL 1. J Immunol 138:3213-3218, 1987.

96. Chaisson CE, McAlindon TE, Felson DT, et al: Lack of association between thyroid status and chondrocalcinosis or osteoarthritis: The Framingham Osteoarthritis Study. J Rheumatol 23:4, 711-715, 1996.

97. Job-Deslandre C, Menkes CJ, Guinot M, et al: Does hypothyroidism increase the prevalence of chondrocalcinosis? Br J Rheumatol 32:3, 197-198, 1993.

98. Benito-Lopez P, Ramos-Rolon G, Ysamat-Marfa R, et al: Pseudogout caused by thyroid hormone replacement therapy. Rev Clin Esp 163:349-350, 1981.

99. Canhao H, Fonseca JE, Leandro MJ, et al: Cross-sectional study of 50 patients with calcium pyrophosphate dihydrate crystal arthropathy. Clin Rheumatol 20:119-122, 2001.

100. Stevens LW, Spiera H: Hemarthrosis in chondrocalcinosis (pseudogout). Arthritis Rheum 15:651-653, 1972.

101. Disla E, Infante R, Fahmy A, et al.: Recurrent acute calcium pyrophosphate dihydrate arthritis following intraarticular hyaluronate injection. Arthritis Rheum 42:1302-1303, 1999.

102. Bernardeau C, Bucki B, Liote F: Acute arthritis after intra-articular hyaluronate injection: Onset of effusions without crystals. Ann Rheum Dis 60:518-520, 2000.

103. Kroesen S, Schmid W, Theiler R: Induction of an acute attack of calcium pyrophosphate dihydrate arthritis by intra-articular injection of hylan G-F 20. Clin Rheumatol 19:147-149, 2000.

104. Fujii K, Tanaka Y, Hubscher S, et al: Crosslinking of CD44 on rheumatoid synovial cells augment interleukin 6 production. Lab Invest 79:1439-1446, 1999.

105. Mikecz K, Dennis K, Shi M, et al: Modulation of hyaluronan receptor (CD44) function in vivo in a murine model of rheumatoid arthritis. Arthritis Rheum 42:659-668, 1999.

106. Sandor V, Hassan R, Kohn E: Exacerbation of pseudogout by granulocyte colony-stimulating factor. Ann Intern Med 125:781, 1996.

107. Malnick SD, Ariel-Ronen S, Evron E, et al: Acute pseudogout as a complication of pamidronate. Ann Pharmacother 31:499-500, 1997.

108. Gallacher SJ, Boyle IT, Capell HA: Pseudogout associated with the use of cyclical etidronate therapy. Scott Med J 36:49, 1991.

109. Mavrikakis ME, Antoniades LG, Kontoyannis SA, et al: CPPD crystal deposition disease as a cause of unrecognised pyrexia. Clin Exp Rheumatol 12:419-221, 1994.

110. Reuge L, Lindhoudt DV, Geerster J: Local deposition of calcium pyrophosphate crystals in evolution of knee osteoarthritis. Clin Rheumatol 20:428-431, 2001.

111. Derfus BA, Kurian JB, Butler JJ, et al: The high prevalence of pathologic calcium crystals in pre-operative knees. J Rheumatol 29:570-574, 2002.

112. Doherty M, Dieppe P, Watt I: Pyrophosphate arthropathy: a prospective study. Br J Rheumatol 32:189-196, 1993.

113. Yamakawa K, Iwasaki H, Ohjimi Y, et al: Tumoral calcium pyrophosphate dihydrate crystal deposition disease. Pathology 197:499-506, 2001.

114. Kwak SM, Resnick D, Haghighi P: Calcium pyrophosphate dihydrate crystal deposition disease of the knee simulating spontaneous osteonecrosis. Clin Rheumatol 18:390-393, 1999.

115. el Maghraoui A, Lecoules S, Lechavalier D, et al: Acute sacroiliitis as a manifestation of calcium pyrophosphate dihydrate crystal deposition disease. Clin Exp Rheumatol 17:477-478, 1999.

116. Fujishiro T, Nabeshima Y, Yasui S, et al: Pseudogout attack of the lumbar facet joint: A case report. Spine 27:396-398, 2002.

117. Pascal-Moussellard H, Cabre P, Smadja D, et al: Myelopathy due to calcification of the cervical ligamenta flava: A report of two cases in the West Indian patients. Euro Spine J 8:238-240, 1999.

118. Cabre P, Pascal-Moussellard H, Kaidomar S, et al: Six cases of ligamentum cervical flavum calcification in blacks in the French West Indies. Joint Bone Spine 68:158-165, 2001.

119. Assaker R, Louis E, Boutry N, et al: Foramen magnum syndrome secondary to calcium pyrophosphate crystal deposition in the transverse ligament of atlas. Spine, 26:1396-1400, 2001.

120. Kakitsubata Y, Boutin RD, Theodorou DJ, et al: Calcium pyrophosphate dihydrate crystal deposition in and around the atlantoaxial joints: Association with type 2 odontoid fractures in nine patients. Radiology 216:213-219, 2000.

121. Doherty M, Hamilton E, Henderson J, et al: Familial chondrocalcinosis due to calcium pyrophosphate dihydrate crystal deposition in English families. Br J Rheumatol 30:10-15, 1991.

122. Schumacher HR, Smolyo AP, Tse RL, et al: Arthritis associated with apatite crystals. Ann Intern Med 87:411-416, 1977.

123. Fam AG, Rubenstein J: Hydroxyapatite pseudopodagra: A syndrome of young women. Arthritis Rheum 32:741-747, 1989.

124. Grinlinton FM, Vuletic JC, Gow PJ: Rapidly progressive calcific periarthritis occurring in a patient with lupus nephritis receiving chronic ambulatory peritoneal dialysis. J Rheumatol 17:8, 1100-1103, 1990.

125. Ferrari AJ, Rothfuss S, Schumacher HR Jr.: Dialysis arthropathy: Identification and evaluation of a subset of patients with unexplained inflammatory effusions. J Rheumatol 24:1780-1786, 1997.

126. Braunstein EM, Menerey K, Martel W, et al: Radiologic features of a pyrophosphate-like arthropathy associated with long-term dialysis. Skeletal Radiol 16(6):437-441, 1987.

127. ter Borg EJ, Eggelmijer F, Jaspers PJ, et al: Milwaukee shoulder associated with primary hyperparathyroidism. J Rheumatol 22:561-562, 1995.

128. Fam AG, Pritzker KP: Acute calcific periarthritis in scleroderma. J Rheumatol 19:1580-1585, 1992.

129. Halverson PB, Carrera GF, McCarty DJ: Milwaukee shoulder syndrome: Fifteen additional cases and a description of contributing factors. Arch Intern Med 150:677-682, 1990.

130. Antoniou J, Tsai A, Baker D, et al: Milwaukee shoulder: correlating possible etiologic variables. Clin Orthop:79-85, 2003.

131. Doherty M, Holt M, MacMillan P: A reappraisal of 'analgesic hip'. Ann Rheum Dis 45:272-276, 1986.

132. Paul H, Reginato AJ, Schumacher HR: Alizarin red S staining as a screening test to detect calcium compounds in synovial fluid. Arthritis Rheum 26:191-200, 1983.

133. van Linthoudt D, Beutler A, Clayburne G, et al: Morphometric studies on synovium in advanced osteoarthritis: is there an association between apatite-like material and collagen deposits? Clin Exp Rheumatol 15:493-497, 1997.

134. Li-Yu J, Clayburne GM, Sieck MS, et al: Calcium apatite crystals in synovial fluid rice bodies. Ann Rheum Dis 61:387-390, 2002.

135. Ivorra J, Rosas J, Pascual E: Most calcium pyrophosphate crystals appear as non-birefringent. Ann Rheum Dis 58:582-584, 1999.

136. Keen CE, Crocker PR, Brady K, et al: Intraosseous secondary calcium salt crystal deposition: an artefact of acid decalcification. Histopathology 27:181-185, 1995.

137. Steinbach LS, Resnick D: Calcium pyrophosphate dihydrate crystal deposition disease: imaging perspective. Curr Prob Diag Radiol 29:209-229, 2000.

138. Hatzis N, Kaar TK, Wirth MA, et al: Neuropathic arthropathy of the shoulder. J Bone Joint Surg Am 80:1314-1319, 1998.

139. Maldonado I, Prasad V, Reginato AJ: Oxalate crystal deposition disease. Curr Rheumatol Rep 4:257-264, 2002.

140. Fisseler-Eckhoff A, Muller KM: Arthroscopy and chondrocalcinosis. Arthroscopy 8:98-104, 1992.

141. Sofka CM, Adler RS, Cordasko FA: Ultrasound diagnosis of chondrocalcinosis in the knee. Skeletal Radiol 31:43-45, 2002.

142. Foldes K: Knee chondrocalcinosis an ultrasonographic study of the hyaline cartilage. J Clin Imaging 26:194-196, 2002.

143. Galvez J, Saiz E, Linares LF, et al: Delayed examination of synovial fluid by ordinary and polarized light microscopy to detect and identify crystals. Ann Rheum Dis 61:444-447, 2002.

144. Petrocelli A, Wong AL, Sweezy RL: Identification of pathologic synovial fluid crystals on Gram stains. J Clin Rheumatol 4:103-105, 1998.

145. Selvi E, Manganelli S, Catenaccio M, et al: Diff Quik staining method for detection and identification of monosodium urate and calcium pyrophosphate crystals in synovial fluids. Ann Rheum Dis 60:194-198, 2001.

146. Ohira T, Ishikawa K: Preservation of calcium pyrophosphate dihydrate crystals: effect of Mayer's haematoxylin staining period. Ann Rheum Dis 60:80-82, 2001.

147. Smilde TJ, Haverman JF, Schipper P, et al: Familial hypokalemia/hypomagnesemia and chondrocalcinosis. J Rheumatol 21:1515-1519, 1994.

148. Ritter J, Kerr LD, Valeriano-Marcet J, et al: ACTH revisited: effective treatment for acute crystal induced synovitis in patients with multiple medical problems. J Rheumatol 21:696-699, 1994.

149. Roane DW, Harris MD, Carpenter MT, et al: Prospective use of intramuscular triamcinolone acetonide in pseudogout. J Rheumatol 24:1168-1170, 1997.

150. Rothschild B, Yakubov LE: Prospective 6-month, double-blind trial of hydroxychloroquine treatment of CPPD. Compr Ther 23:327-331, 1997.

151. Kalunian KC, Ike RW, Seeger LL, et al: Visually-guided irrigation in patients with early knee osteoarthritis: A multicenter randomized, controlled trial. Osteoarthritis Cartilage 8:412-418, 2000.

152. Das SK, Mishra K, Ramakrishnan S, et al: A randomized controlled trial to evaluate the slow-acting symptom modifying effects of a regimen containing colchicine in a subset of patients with osteoarthritis of the knee. Osteoarthritis Cartilage 10:247-252, 2002.

153. Das SK, Ramakrishnan S, Mishra K, et al: A randomized controlled trial to evaluate the slow-acting symptom modifying effects of colchicine in osteoarthritis of the knee: A preliminary report. Arthritis Care Res 47:280-284, 2002.

154. Farin PU, Rasenen H, Jaroma H, et al: Rotator cuff calcifications: Treatment with ultrasound-guided percutaneous needle aspiration and lavage. Skeletal Radiol 25:551-554, 1996.

155. Ebenbicher G, Erdogmus C, Resch K, et al: Ultrasound therapy for calcific tendonitis of the shoulder. N Engl J Med 340: 1533-1538,1999.

156. Rosenthal AK, Ryan LM: Probenecid inhibits transforming growth factor-beta 1 induced pyrophosphate elaboration by chondrocytes. J Rheumatol 21:896-900, 1994.

157. Cini R, Chindamo D, Catenaccio M, et al: Dissolution of calcium pyrophosphate crystals by polyphosphates: An in vitro and ex vivo study. Ann Rheum Dis 60:962-967, 2001.

158. Shinozaki T, Pritzker KP: Polyamines enhance calcium pyrophosphate dihydrate crystal dissolution. J Rheumatol 22:1907-1912, 1995.

159. Cheung HS: Phosphocitrate as a potential therapeutic strategy for crystal deposition disease. Curr Rheumatology Reports 3: 24-28, 2001.

160. Nair D, Misra RP, Sallis JD, et al: Phosphocitrate inhibits a basic calcium phosphate and calcium pyrophosphate dihydrate crystal-induced mitogen-activated protein kinase cascade signal transduction pathway. J Biol Chem 272:18920-18925, 1997.

161. Krug HE, Mahowald ML, Halverson PB, et al: Phosphocitrate prevents disease progression in murine progressive ankylosis. Arthritis Rheum 36:1603-1611, 1993.

Bone, Cartilage, and Heritable Connective Tissue Disorders

89 Biology, Physiology, and Morphology of Bone

CLINTON T. RUBIN • JANET E. RUBIN

Bone is an extremely complex tissue that regulates its mass and architecture to meet two critical and competing responsibilities, one structural and the other metabolic. In the first case, the skeleton provides a sophisticated framework for the body: It protects vital organs and facilitates locomotion. Second, it serves as a mineral reservoir containing 99 percent of the body's total calcium and 85 percent of its phosphorus. It is this dual responsibility that creates conflicting goals and competing stimuli in the catabolic and anabolic regulation of skeletal tissues. Metabolic aberrations, such as hypocalcemia, hyperparathyroidism, renal failure, and aging, can cause impairment in the structural integrity of the skeleton while regulatory controls struggle to maintain calcium homeostasis. On the other hand, the skeleton perceives another set of regulatory controls over its structural morphology and adapts to meet altered functional demand. This structural adaptation can proceed apace, ignoring potential consequences of rapid fluctuations in serum calcium levels (e.g., renal lithiasis, hypercalcemia). However, despite what appear to be independent sets of regulatory controls for metabolic and structural needs of the organism, skeletal integrity and the viability of the organism are critically dependent on maintaining an intricate balance between them.

The balance between structural and metabolic responsibilities is achieved via the complex and tightly regulated cellular processes of formation and resorption of bone tissue. Beginning at the level of the cell, this chapter covers local and systemic factors that influence bone turnover and growth of the skeleton, the composition and mineralization of the matrix, the architecture and material properties of the tissue, and the adaptive capacity of the skeleton. This multilevel, multidisciplinary overview is intended to provide the reader with an appreciation of not only the complexity of bone but also its success in meeting its wide-ranging responsibilities.

Cellular Basis of Bone Remodeling

The constant modeling and remodeling of skeletal tissue is necessary during growth as well as for the repair of skeletal defects caused by fracture and inflammation. Remodeling is also essential for the rapid mobilization of mineral required for metabolic homeostasis and for the fine adjustment of skeletal mass and morphology needed to achieve an effective and efficient supporting structure. The skeleton's capacity to adapt to changes in both its functional and metabolic milieu is achieved through its sophisticated network of osteoregulatory cells. These cells—osteoblasts, osteocytes, and osteoclasts—mediate the remodeling balance of the skeleton as well as provide the cellular machinery necessary for the maintenance of calcium homeostasis in the extracellular fluid.

OSTEOBLASTS

Function

The primary function of the plump, cuboidal osteoblast is to synthesize and mineralize the extracellular matrix. Osteoblasts are connected to one another via extended cell processes that are interconnected via gap junctions,[1] establishing a single, continuous blanket of cells on the bone surface (Fig. 89-1). The cytoplastic elements of the osteoblast include abundant endoplasmic reticulum with cisternae, a well-developed Golgi body, and numerous free ribosomes that are responsible for the basophilia seen in sections stained with hematoxylin and eosin (H&E). These features help to distinguish osteoblasts from the thin, flat mesenchymal precursors (preosteoblasts) that are also found on bone surfaces. Together, these two cell types are known as *bone-lining* cells. Morphologically, the tight canopy of the lining cells enables the selective isolation of the mineralized surface from the extracellular milieu, which is critical for the site-specific control of mineralization or resorption.[2]

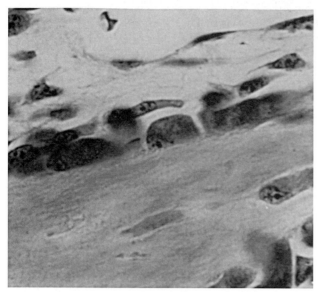

FIGURE 89–1 · Polyhedral Osteoblasts lying on the Surface of Newly formed Bone Mmatrix. (Courtesy of Dr. B. Boothroyd.)

TABLE 89–1 · COMPOSITION OF BONE OSTEOID

Collagen
Type I, some types III, V, XI, XIII
Proteoglycans
Biglycan, decorin, hyaluronan
Glycoproteins
Osteonectin, bone sialoprotein, osteopontin, thrombospondin, fibronectin, γ-carboxyglutamic acid–containing proteins (osteocalcin, matrix *gla* protein)
Enzymes
Alkaline phosphatase, collagenase, cysteine proteinases, plasminogen activator, tissue inhibitor of metalloproteinases
Growth factors
Fibroblast growth factor (FGF), insulin-like growth factor (IGF), transforming growth factor (TGF), bone morphogenetic protein (BMP), α_2–human serum glycoprotein
Proteolipids

In forming bone, the osteoblast first secretes an extracellular matrix termed *osteoid* (see section on composition of bone matrix), which is subsequently mineralized. Although it is unclear whether mineralization itself necessitates the presence of the osteoblast (see Chapter 1), this cell's secretion of a panel of secretory proteins, including type I collagen, several noncollagenous proteins, and proteoglycans, is critical to the appropriate orchestration of the remodeling response (Table 89-1). Many of these proteins, whether secreted or displayed by osteoblasts have signaling roles in bone remodeling, such as the role of osteocalcin to recruit osteoclasts[3]; the initiation of collagen breakdown by plasminogen activator[4]; and the signal for osteoclast recruitment by expression of receptor activator of nuclear factor kappa B (NFκB) ligand (RANKL).[5] Other proteins, such as osteopontin and bone sialoprotein, are critical components of osteoid, strongly binding ionic calcium and serving as cell attachment factors.[6]

The functional life of the osteoblast varies in different species from 3 days in young rabbits[7] to up to 8 weeks in human osteoblasts.[8] A typical active osteoblast in humans produces a seam of osteoid about 15-μm thick, at a rate of 0.5 to 1.5 μm/day,[9] suggesting the average osteoblast life in humans to be 15 days. Although osteoid seams can exceed 70 mm,[10] such a seam width can also indicate a disruption or flaw in the mineralization process (e.g., rickets or osteomalacia). Several reports suggest that a contraction of the life span of the osteoblast might underlie pathophysiologic conditions. For instance, in the presence of glucocorticoids, an increased rate of programmed cell death, or apoptosis, is seen, which may account for the decrease in bone quality recognized in patients with glucocorticoid excess.[11]

Differentiation

Studies of the molecular mechanisms involved in osteoblast maturation have revealed a complex set of interacting factors. A specific helix-loop-helix nuclear factor termed *RUNX2/cbfa1* directs entry of the pluripotent mesenchymal stem cell into the osteoblast lineage both in vitro[12] and in vivo where heterozygous loss of RUNX2 in several human kindreds causes cleidocranial dysplasia. Osteoblast expression of both osteopontin and type I collagen is delayed, with resultant late ossification of the clavicle.[13] This condition, defined by short stature and hypoplasia of the clavicles,[14] predicted a similar phenotype generated by targeted disruption of the RUNX2 gene in mice.[15] In the transgenic RUNX2 knockout mouse, however, the cartilaginous skeleton never ossifies, emphasizing how necessary RUNX2 is to the normal skeleton. Since the description of the RUNX2-null transgenic mouse, other genes have been shown to be important to osteoblast differentiation and function, with proof-of-concept in transgenic animals.

Transgenic Models Inform Osteoblast Pathophysiology

Although this chapter cannot document all the genes necessary for osteoblast function, a few, besides RUNX2, deserve mention. A second transcription factor, osterix, was discovered while scientists attempted to learn more about the role bone morphogenetic proteins (BMPs) play in osteoblast function. Although osterix appears to function distal to RUNX2, its absence precludes osteoblasts and bone tissue in osterix-null transgenic animals.[16] Interestingly, the cartilaginous skeleton in the absence of osterix is normal.

Scientists seeking to understand human kindreds with very high bone mineral densities uncovered the involvement of the Wnt pathway in osteoblast function and perhaps differentiation. These kindreds turned out to have mutations of the Lrp5 protein, which inhibits signaling by the developmental protein Wnt.[17,18] Knockout of Lrp5 in mice caused a decrease in osteoblast proliferation and osteopenia.[19] Because soluble mediators can interact with the Wnt signaling pathway, manipulation of this pathway will surely offer itself as a means of controlling osteoblast function in the future.

Other genes have been linked to abnormalities in mesenchymal condensation and differentiation, including phenotypes with extra digits. One of these is synpolydactyly, which involves an abnormal HOXD-13 gene.[20] As with other members of the Hox gene family, HOXD-13 is involved in skeletal patterning. Fibrodysplasia ossificans progressiva is a disabling disorder characterized by a gradual and continuous heterotopic ossification of soft tissues. This autosomal-dominant disorder appears to be associated with misexpression of the growth factor BMP-4, which is also secreted by osteoblasts.[21]

OSTEOCYTES

As mineralization proceeds, the osteoblast may become engulfed in its own calcifying osteoid matrix, thereby becoming the osteocyte.[22] Osteocytes are connected to each other via cytoplasmic extensions that pass through a network of catacombs radiating outward from the central vascular canal (Fig. 89-2). The volume of bone occupied by this syncytium is approximately 5 percent for the canalicular network and 2 percent for the lacunar spaces.[23] These interconnecting canaliculi are ideal pathways for chemical, electric, and stress-generated fluid communication through the dense bone matrix.[24] Importantly, the processes themselves are interconnected by gap junctions composed of the protein connexin 43, which facilitates the integration of many of these regulatory messages.[25] The surface area of the lacunar and canalicular system is at least 250 m²/liter of calcified bone matrix and communicates with a submicroscopic, interfibrillar space, representing 35,000 µm²/mm³. Thus, exchange of mineral, nutrients, and chemical and physical stimuli through this enormous network is certainly facilitated, which is critical considering the need for rapid mobilization of mineral in the homeostatic control of the skeleton. As well, this cell syncytium deteriorates markedly with increasing age and may contribute to the age-related insensitivity of bone tissue to chemical and physical signals.

Although osteoblasts and osteoclasts are largely responsible for executing the appropriate modeling-remodeling responses, given the time required to recruit these cells in the adult skeleton, it is likely that the extensive network of resident cells, the osteocytes and bone-lining cells, actually orchestrate the adaptive response. Past work has provided strong evidence that the osteocyte is capable of rapidly responding to changes in the bone's chemical and mechanic environment. For example, mechanic strain increases osteocyte levels of glucose-6-phosphate dehydrogenase activity[26] as well c-fos mRNA levels within 60 minutes of loading, evidence that osteocytes are intimately—and rapidly—involved in the osteogenic response to mechanic signals.[27] Physiologic levels of mechanic strain, furthermore, reduce the rate of osteocyte apoptosis, suggesting that matrix deformation affects cell survival.[28] When bone is subject to disuse, osteocytes are capable of expressing collagenase,[29] emphasizing that this cell has the ability to regulate the recruitment of bone-forming and -resorbing cells, as well as to modulate its own immediate microenvironment.

OSTEOCLASTS

Function

The osteoclast, functioning as the bone's specific macrophage, is found wherever existing bone tissue is being removed. This large, multinucleated cell migrates on the bone surface, creating irregular, scalloped cavities termed *Howship's lacunae* (Fig. 89-3). Activated osteo-

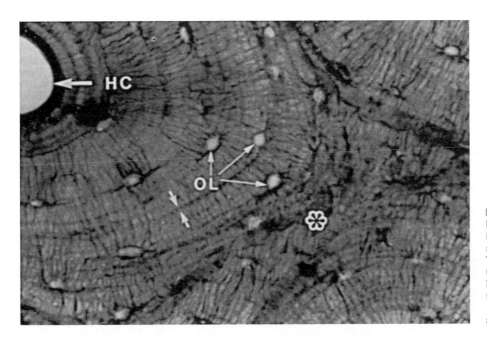

FIGURE 89-2 · Ground section of bone photographed in normal light showing empty osteocyte lacunae (OL) connected by fine, darkly stained canaliculi. The central haversian canal (HC) is seen in the upper left hand corner; the reversal line (*) marking the junction between two adjacent osteons and the cement line (→ ←) separating adjacent lamellae can also be seen.

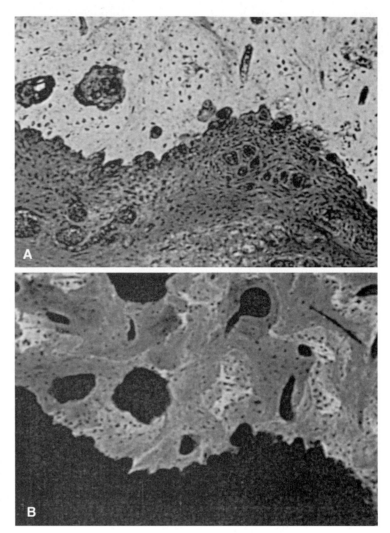

FIGURE 89–3 · *A*, Paragon-stained mineralized section with large, multinucleate osteoclasts lying along the pale-staining bone surface. *B*, Microradiograph of the same area showing Howship's lacunae in the areas of osteoclastic resorption. (From Jowsey J, Gordan G. *In* Bourne GH [ed]: The Biochemistry and Physiology of Bone, 2nd ed. Vol III. New York, Academic Press, 1972, pp 201-238.)

clasts can travel up to 100 μm/day, resorbing a cavity 300 μm in diameter and excavating 200,000 μm^3 of bone. The reclamation of this volume of bone requires 7 to 10 generations of working osteoblasts to fill the resorption space.[30] An absence of osteoclasts or a population of dysfunctional osteoclasts leads to osteopetrosis, or marble bone disease, which can be fatal in childhood secondary to pancytopenias due to decreased marrow space.[31]

Through the interactions of systemic and local factors, a cellular symbiosis exists in which an integrated "activation, resorption, reversal, and formation" (ARRF) occurs, reflecting an intricate control of both osteoblasts and osteoclasts.[32] To initiate this sequence, osteoclasts are activated by chemical or physical signals that recruit them to specific remodeling areas. Once activated and attached to the matrix, they begin the resorption cycle and create the Howship's lacunae. When resorption is completed, new bone formation begins within the cavity, a process that leaves a boundary, which is visible in histologic sections as a reversal line.[33] This "pocket" of new bone is known as a bone structural unit.[34] A similar line, called a cement line, is seen between adjacent lamellae of bone (see Fig. 89-2).

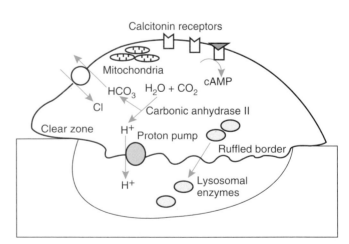

FIGURE 89–4 · The osteoclast is a polarized cell that adheres to bone, generating a subosteoclastic space where bone resorption occurs. Into this space the osteoclast pumps hydrogen ions and lysosomal enzymes. The protons that create the acid pH in the resorption space derive from the action of carbonic anhydrase II on bicarbonate, which has entered the cell via a chloride bicarbonate exchanger on the marrow side of the cell. Calcitonin receptors distinguish this cell, as does the characteristic ruffled border seen on electron micrographs.

Mature osteoclasts possess several unique ultrastructural characteristics that allow their very active functional phenotype (Fig. 89-4). These include abundant pleomorphic mitochondria, vacuoles, and lysosomes, which store the multiple secretory products necessary for the digestion of bone substance.[35] The apical membrane of the osteoclast is tightly sealed to the calcified matrix, creating a clear zone that has no cellular organelles but is rich in contractile proteins. Toward the center of the cell, the membrane becomes deeply folded, creating the characteristic ruffled border.[36] Under the ruffled border is the resorption pit, where the osteoclast secretes lysosomal enzymes and generates an acid environment by secreting protons through a vacuolar proton pump.[37] Protons are generated for the pump through the actions of carbonic anhydrase II, an enzyme subtype also associated with vacuolar proton pumps in the renal cortex and the gastric parietal cell. Deficiencies in carbonic anhydrase II lead to a mild form of osteopetrosis.[38] The bicarbonate resulting from this activity is transported via a chloride bicarbonate exchanger on the marrow-facing side of the osteoclast. The osteoclast's highly polarized nature allows unidirectional secretion of protons into the resorption bay at its basal membrane, and transport of resorbed products out its apical region.[39] Protons accumulate within the confined subosteoclastic space, lowering the pH to a level sufficient to dissolve the mineral phase of the matrix (pH of 2 to 4) and activate osteoclastic hydrolytic enzymes. Osteoclast acid secretion can be inhibited through regulation of calmodulin kinase; tamoxifen, an antiestrogen that prevents postmenopausal bone loss, can directly inhibit this kinase and prevent osteoclast acidification.[40] The remaining organic matrix is subsequently dissolved by lysosomal enzymes (e.g., cathepsin B), leaving the osteoclast's signature scalloped resorption cavity.[41] As the excavation proceeds, the ionized calcium levels just beyond the clear zone rise from a base level of 1 to 2 mM to as high as 20 mM.[42] Other clinically useful modulators of osteoclast development and function include the bisphosphonates. Several congeners are now widely used to prevent osteoporotic fractures.[43] Bisphosphonates are incorporated into bone mineral in place of phosphate and prevent osteoclast recruitment and activity, increasing bone mineral density by slowing resorption.[44]

Differentiation

Osteoclast precursors arise from hematopoietic stem cells in the bone marrow.[45] The processes controlling osteoclast differentiation can be reduced, at least in tissue culture, to three basic elements. These include the osteoclast precursor cell, which arises out of the macrophage lineage of hematopoietic stem cells; macrophage colony-stimulating factor (M-CSF), which is necessary for the differentiation, proliferation, and survival of cells of macrophage lineage; and RANKL.[46,47] Loss of M-CSF action engenders deficiencies of both osteoclasts and macrophages: the osteopetrotic op/op mouse secretes a prematurely terminated and dysfunctional M-CSF protein molecule.[48] Interestingly, after "rescue" with M-CSF infusions early in life, the op/op mouse no longer requires

M-CSF for normal bone remodeling.[49] It has been reported that the op/op mouse can also be rescued by vascular endothelial growth factor (VEGF), suggesting that this growth factor and perhaps others may be able to substitute for M-CSF under certain conditions.[50] In any case, M-CSF alone is unable to generate osteoclasts from progenitor cells; further progression into the osteoclast lineage (appearance of functional osteoclast characteristics such as calcitonin receptor and carbonic anhydrase II expression) requires other local stimuli including, importantly, the physical presence of bone stromal or osteoblast cells.[51-53] The requirement for physical contact between stromal cells and osteoclast precursors is for monocytic precursors expressing RANK-receptors to bind RANKL, which is displayed on the stromal or osteoblast membrane.[46,47] In the absence of RANKL, normal osteoclastogenesis does not progress, as shown by the RANKL-null transgenic animal.[54] The importance of RANKL is underscored by the presence of a soluble factor termed *osteoprotegerin* (OPG), which serves as a "decoy receptor", essentially inhibiting RANKL action. Overexpression of osteoprotegerin leads to an inhibition of osteoclastogenesis and decreased bone turnover.[55]

The list of factors that influence the progression of osteoclast differentiation is growing. For instance, systemic factors 1,25-dihydroxyvitamin D, parathyroid hormone (PTH), and tumor necrosis factor (TNF) are able to enhance the development of osteoclasts from hematopoietic progenitor cells in the presence of stromal elements from bone.[52] In fact, each of these three factors induce the expression of RANKL by bone cells. Cytokines such as interleukin-6 (IL-6) and IL-11 also influence osteoclast development and may have particular significance in pathogenic states such as postmenopausal osteoporosis[56] and Paget's disease.[57]

Transgenic Models Inform Osteoclast Pathophysiology

Many other cofactors participating during osteoclast lineage selection have been discovered due to gene dysfunction or knockout experiments. For example, knockout of the murine tyrosine kinase c-fos gene inhibits the divergence of cells from macrophage lineage into that of osteoclasts, despite normal levels of both M-CSF and RANKL.[58] Knockout of the transcription factor PU.1 inhibits early osteoclast precursor development by disallowing entry into the macrophage lineage,[59] and the abnormal function of the helix-loop-helix factor MITF inhibits late differentiation of osteoclasts.[60] Knockout of signaling cascades necessary for RANKL action (i.e., NFκB) also result in deficient osteoclast differentiation.[61] On the other hand, upregulation of signal cascades that enhance osteoclastic differentiation and function should increase bone turnover, as is evidenced by knockout of the src homology 2-containing inositol-5'-phosphatase (SHIP). The SHIP-null transgenic mouse has increased numbers of osteoclast precursors and overactive osteoclasts, resulting in an osteoporotic skeleton.[62] The unexpected finding of osteopetrosis after homologous knockout of the ubiquitous src protein kinase in the mouse[63] has precipitated study of the roles of osteoclast attachment and movement. The src-deficient mouse has osteoclasts, but these cells are unable to resorb bone. The src tyrosine kinase is important in the downstream signaling required for osteoclast function at the bone surface.[64] Scientists have also begun to examine the motility of the osteoclast, as well as its ability to transcytose resorbed materials liberated from the mineralized matrix.[39] The motility of the osteoclast is under the control of many factors, including those recognized by its polarized basal surface connected to the mineral and matrix by an integrin such as vitronectin.[65] As might be predicted, knockout of the beta-3 integrin subunit leads to dysfunction of osteoclasts and osteosclerosis in transgenic mice.[66]

▌ Development of the Skeleton

GROWTH

Most of the bones of the skeleton appear first in the embryo as cartilaginous models, which are later resorbed and replaced by bone tissue. The cartilage template, or anlage, is formed by the condensation of mesenchymal cells in the developing limb bud. Although the shape of the anlage resembles that of the adult bone and appears to be genetically determined, the bone that replaces the cartilage template is greatly influenced by physical factors (e.g., weight-bearing, muscle pull) and is constantly modeled and remodeled as these forces change according to the dictums of Wolff's Law.[67]

The cartilage anlage, or template, expands and elongates by interstitial growth, in which chondrocytes divide, enlarge, and surround themselves with the new matrix. At about the same time, cells in the connective tissues surrounding the anlage (perichondrium) begin to lay down bone tissue and form a collar of bone around the center of the cartilage model. At the time it is formed, the anlage is pierced by a capillary that begins the process of matrix excavation and allows entry of osteoblast precursors that replace cartilage with bone. This process of vascular invasion of the cartilage model, followed by bone deposition, is referred to as enchondral ossification. The process continues until the entire shaft of the anlage is replaced by marrow and bone, confining the growth process of chondrocyte multiplication to the epiphyseal ends of the bone, away from the primary center of ossification. As the epiphysis swells, the central chondrocytes find themselves too remote from the blood supply to survive solely by means of diffusion. Cartilage canals facilitate the diffusion of nutrients and provide conduits for subsequent capillary ingrowth. The hypertrophic chondrocytes survive and elaborate angiotrophic substances.

Parathyroid-related peptide (PTHrp) has emerged as one of the most important factors controlling the complex process of embryologic bone growth and maturation. PTHrp, which has long been known to be the most common causative factor in neoplastic hypercalcemia, binds to the PTH receptor.[68] During fetal development of the cartilaginous anlage, the product of the Indian hedgehog gene (Ihh) is released by hypertrophic chondrocytes in the growth plate. The Ihh protein induces PTHrp release by the perichondrium at the end of the long bones.[69] PTHrp then binds to receptors in the proliferating chondrocytes, causing a delay of their maturation and, thus, allowing further elongation of the anlage before entry of osteoblasts and ossification. In the absence of PTHrp, the developing bone ossifies prematurely and ends up foreshortened. The interplay of Ihh and PTHrp, which has such profound effects during embryologic development, may have a subtler role in the adult skeleton involved in the modulation of osteoblast response to the continual need for bone maintenance.

Although growth in length occurs at the growth plate, growth in diameter occurs by the centrifugal proliferation of cartilage cells along the groove of Ranvier,[70] an anatomic structure bordered outwardly by a continuation of the fibrous periosteum and inwardly by the physeal cartilage. When swelling of the cartilaginous anlage first begins, a condensed layer of mesenchyme develops around it as a membrane of cells and collagen, called perichondrium. As the cartilage is replaced by bone, this membrane is renamed periosteum. In the growing skeleton, this periosteum is clearly divided into an inner cellular layer and an outer fibrous layer, which merges gradually into the surrounding muscle. Muscles take origin from the periosteum; collagen bundles can be traced flowing from tendon and ligament through the periosteum to anchor directly into the bone via Sharpey's fibers.[71]

Along with the genetic regulation discussed previously, there are epigenetic regulatory mechanisms including control by mechanic stresses as proposed by Roux.[72] General considerations of how mechanic stress might control skeletal growth abound, including the proposal of Carter and coworkers.[73] They proposed that intermittently applied shear stresses promote enchondral ossification and that intermittent hydrostatic compression inhibits cartilage degeneration and ossification. The contribution of mechanic stresses to bone growth is not yet understood.

Rosenberg and coworkers[74] characterized the changes that occur during ossification of the anlage, including the deposition of a 35,000-MW protein (probably osteocalcin) and the modification of existing proteoglycans. Mineral deposition begins in the matrix vesicles located in the columns between the last hypertrophic chondrocytes on the extreme metaphyseal end of the physis.[75] Invasion by osteoblasts and osteoclasts results in the resorption of this woven bone and its replacement by mature lamellar bone.[76] The hydroxyapatite formed during primary ossification is a rather rough crystal whose imperfections may render it more vulnerable to resorption,[77] which also implies the facility with which woven bone is removed.

Important in the regulation of both growth and the cascade of processes leading to adequate mineralization of bone by osteoblasts are a number of cell-secreted factors. Urist's identification of a factor in demineralized bone powder that initiated bone formation has led to the cloning and sequencing of at least seven bone morphogenetic proteins (BMPs) belonging to the transforming

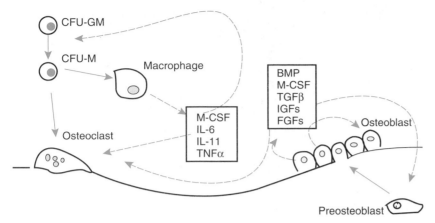

FIGURE 89-5 · Osteoclasts and Osteoblasts Interact Through Cytokines Released into the Bone Micromilieu. Macrophages secrete macrophage colony-stimulating factor (M-CSF), various interleukins (IL), and tumor necrosis factor (TNF), all of which promote osteoclast differentiation from hematopoietic stem cells, from the colony-forming unit for granulocyte-macrophages (CFU-GM) and the CFU for macrophage (CFU-M) to terminal osteoclast phenotype. Osteoblasts interact by secreting factors that affect osteoclasts, including M-CSF and transforming growth factor-β (TGF-β) as well as factors affecting bone mineralization and progression of their own phenotype, such as insulin-like growth factors (IGFs) and basic fibroblast growth factors (FGFs).

growth factor-β (TGF-β) family of growth potentiators.[78] These polypeptide factors appear to be important regulators of bone growth and repair through their ability to activate migration of mesenchymal cells and induce osteoblastic differentiation followed by proliferation.[79] TGF-β itself is abundant in bone matrix. In vitro cell work has shown that TGF-β has both positive and negative effects on osteoblast proliferation, differentiation, and matrix synthesis.[80-82] TGF-β is released during the process of osteoclastic bone resorption[83] and may initiate the formative part of the bone-remodeling unit, the "coupling" of formation to resorption.[84] The differential effects of the various BMPs to induce cartilage and bone formation in vivo are being examined to determine their potential to accelerate the healing of complex fractures and to improve the rate of allograft and autograft successes.[85] BMP-4, for instance, initiates the sequential gene expression of osteopontin and osteocalcin in chondrocytes and osteoblasts.[86] BMP-6 may be involved in the earliest part of the differentiation of osteoblast cells.[87]

Osteoblasts also produce a number of growth factors and cytokines that are critical to the process of bone formation, remodeling, and repair (Fig. 89-5). Many of these soluble products are also released by circulating macrophages and lymphocytes. For example, insulin-like growth factor-I (IGF-I), or somatomedin C, directly stimulates osteoblast replication and function[88] and also may increase remodeling by inducing RANKL.[89] Many of these regulatory compounds are discussed later, in the section on bone remodeling.

GENETIC ABNORMALITIES

Many genetic diseases have predominant skeletal phenotypes, including at least 150 osteochondrodysplasias. The fact that dysfunction of many single genes is likely to cause skeletal manifestations arises from the great number of genes involved in the complex processes of skeletal development, growth, and remodeling. Interestingly, a number of genes not previously suspected to be associated with skeletal physiology generate abnormal skeletal phenotypes when deleted from transgenic mice. Examples are the ubiquitous c-src tyrosine kinase[63] and the intranuclear factor c-fos[58]; deletion of either gene leads to osteopetrosis. The association of genes with processes critical to normal skeletal physiology is a growing area of research; only a few striking examples are offered here.

A receptor for fibroblast growth factor (FGF) has been implicated in achondroplasia, the most common form of chondroplasia in humans. This disease is characterized by short-limbed dwarfism combined with a large head. Gene abnormalities in multiple subjects consist of point mutations in the FGF receptor-3.[20] Most of these mutations involve single base changes resulting in a constitutively active receptor,[90] indicating that FGF limits the expansion of the growth plate. Another gene regulating elongation of the growth plate is PTHrp; interruption of PTHrp action causes a shortening of long bone.[91] In comparison, increasing PTHrp action, as seen in the constitutively activated PTHrp receptor associated with Jansen's metaphyseal chondrodysplasia, causes metaphyseal abnormalities.[92]

Alterations in either the organic (e.g., collagen) or inorganic (e.g., hydroxyapatite) matrix components will bring about changes in the bone structure, some of which are indirect and some of which can be catastrophic. An entire spectrum of bone diseases, including osteogenesis imperfecta, is discussed in Chapter 90.

With even this briefest of presentations, the reader should be aware of the virtual explosion of our knowledge base with regard to the genes controlling skeletal growth and homeostasis. Targeted disruption of genes in animals, genetic studies of human kindreds with abnormal skeletal phenotypes, and the sequencing of the human genome will rapidly lead to a fuller understanding of the many heritable diseases affecting the skeleton.

■ Systemic Regulation of Bone Remodeling

CALCIUM METABOLISM

Calcium is critical to many processes in the body, including most signaling cascades and synaptic signaling, creating a requirement for tight control of systemic calcium concentrations. As stated in the introduction, the skeleton is the reservoir for calcium, and bone remodeling is one of the processes critical to calcium regulation. Thus, hormones involved in calcium homeostasis have profound effects on the skeleton.

Parathyroid Hormone

The primary function of PTH is to maintain serum ionized calcium levels within a narrow physiologic range. PTH secretion rises as calcium levels drop below 8 mg/dl, controlled by decreased binding of the calcium ion to the calcium receptor on the parathyroid cell.[93] Thus, when a serum calcium value above 10 mg/dl accompanies a high level of serum PTH, a diagnosis of hyperparathyroidism can be made.[94] Other circulating factors such as vitamin D, TNF-α, and prostaglandins are also involved in regulating calcium balance.

By stimulating osteoclast activity and, in turn, bone resorption, PTH provides calcium and phosphate for mineral homeostasis. Membrane receptors for PTH on osteoblasts stimulate substantial morphologic and metabolic changes in these cells and subsequently in osteoclasts.[95] The distal effects of PTH occur by increases in levels of intracellular cyclic adenosine monophosphate (cAMP) and mobilization of cytosolic calcium ion.[96] Although PTH receptors probably do not exist on osteoclasts,[97] these cells are activated within minutes of osteoblast exposure to PTH. PTH also targets renal 1α-hydroxylase, which is the final step in the activation of vitamin D. Thus, PTH contributes to maintaining serum calcium levels by both direct and indirect interactions with the skeleton.

Vitamin D

Vitamin D has effects on both bone remodeling and calcium homeostasis. A 10-minute exposure of the skin to ultraviolet light from the sun causes endogenous production of sufficient quantities of vitamin D_3 from 7-dehydrocholesterol to allow normal calcium balance. Vitamin D_3 is first hydroxylated to 25-hydroxyvitamin D in the liver, followed by 25-hydroxyvitamin D hydroxylation in the kidney. Often referred to as calcitriol, the active metabolite, 1,25-dihydroxyvitamin D, stimulates intestinal absorption of calcium, thus providing the mineral necessary to build bone. An absence of vitamin D action, such as in either vitamin D–resistant rickets due to mutations in the vitamin D receptor[98] or in pseudovitamin D rickets due to an abnormality of the 1α-hydroxylase,[99] leads to hypocalcemia and severe ricketic bone disease. Even though adequate levels of 1, 25-dihydroxyvitamin D are necessary to provide calcium for bone formation, supraphysiologic levels induce bone resorption by stimulating the differentiation of osteoclast precursors.[100] This occurs through 1,25-dihydroxyvitamin D's effect of increasing bone stromal cell production of both M-CSF[101] and RANKL expression.[102]

Besides vitamin D's role in ensuring calcium acquisition from the intestine, vitamin D has subtle effects on the formation and resorption of bone.[103] An Australian cohort of white women found to have certain allelic variants of the vitamin D receptor (VDR) appeared to have lower bone densities as measured by absorptiometry.[104] This area has generated great controversy, beginning with another group's failure to confirm this relationship.[105] Another study of VDR polymorphisms in 189 dizygotic American twins showed no association with bone density.[106] In a 1997 paper by Sainz and associates,[107] three allelic variants of VDR were examined in normal prepubescent girls of Mexican descent. In this study, VDR gene alleles predicted the density of femoral and vertebral volumetric bone density. Full understanding of vitamin D's role in skeletal development will require continued epidemiologic and basic studies.

Calcitonin and Other Calcium-Regulating Factors

Calcitonin is a calcium regulatory hormone that works independently of PTH and vitamin D and possesses a potent capacity to modulate serum calcium and phosphate levels.[108] Like the control of PTH secretion from parathyroid cells, serum calcium levels regulate the secretion of calcitonin from parafollicular or C cells of the thyroid. In contrast to the secretion of PTH, which is secreted in inverse proportion to serum calcium levels, calcium ion directly stimulates the secretion of calcitonin[109] by its binding to the calcium receptor on the parafollicular C cells.[110] The binding of calcitonin to receptors on osteoclasts[111] causes a marked decrease in osteoclast metabolic activity along with cell retraction.[112,113] For these reasons, calcitonin has been used successfully in the acute treatment of the humoral hypercalcemia of malignancy and in Paget's disease; the use of calcitonin in the treatment of hyperresorptive osteoporosis is also salutary.[114] The response to calcitonin is transitory, however, as it downregulates its cognate receptor within hours.[115]

Osteoblasts also secrete prostaglandin E_2 (PGE$_2$) in response to hormonal or mechanic stimuli. PGE$_2$ can stimulate both bone formation and resorption, as well as serve as a chemotactic factor for osteoclasts.[116] Although PGE$_2$ and PTH stimulate the same second messengers in osteoblasts, PGE$_2$ directly affects osteoclasts through its ubiquitous receptor. PGE$_2$ stimulates several second-messenger responses in bone cells, including an increase in cytosolic calcium, elevated cAMP production, and activation of the phosphatidyl inositol pathway.[117] In the anabolic response to loading, prostaglandins may be particularly important, as prostaglandin levels increase during loading and can reproduce some specific responses of load when given in vitro.[118]

MATURATION: SEX STEROIDS

The rapid decline of skeletal mass after menopause underscores the critical regulatory role of sex steroids in bone cell metabolism. The expression of estrogen receptors,[119,120] as well as androgen receptors,[121] within osteoblasts designates bone cells as targets of these sex steroids. Elevated estrogen levels both increase osteoblast proliferation[122] and attenuate the osteoblast response to PTH.[123] In addition, estrogens increase both osteoblastic collagen gene expression[122] and IGF-II production[124] and may even directly regulate the production of osteoclastic lysosomal enzymes.[125] It has also been recognized that IL-6 can stimulate osteoclastic bone resorption only in the estrogen-deficient state.[56] Recently, estrogen has been shown to have effects on the RANKL-osteoprotegerin equilibrium. Estrogen deficiency, although not changing RANK expression on osteoclast precursors, blunts the intracellular signaling stimulated by RANKL binding, essentially decreasing osteoclastogenesis.[126] As well, estrogen has been shown to increase osteoprotegerin in the circulation, thereby diminishing RANKL effect by preventing its access to potential osteoclasts.[127]

Further appreciation of estrogen action has emerged with evidence of effects on the male skeleton. A unique male patient shown to be unresponsive to estrogen because of an abnormal estrogen receptor never fused his epiphyses, despite an intact androgen axis.[128] A second patient, still growing taller at the age of 30 years, was found to lack estrogen action in bone, in this case through the complete absence of the cytochrome P-450 aromatase necessary to convert androgen to estradiol.[129] Interestingly, this patient was noted to have extremely low bone mineral density. Treatment with low doses of estradiol not only caused epiphyseal fusion but increased bone mineral density by nearly 10 percent over the first year of treatment, with a continued rise during the subsequent 3 years.[130] These concepts have led workers in osteology to promote a "unifying model" suggesting that bone mineral density in men as well as women is dependent on sufficient estrogen levels and that androgen may have completely separate, and unknown, effects on skeletal growth and mass.[131]

REGULATION OF BONE MINERAL DENSITY

Humans attain a mature skeleton by the age of 30 years, when bone mineral density peaks. The peak bone mineral density is largely controlled by hereditary factors, which are not well understood.[132,133] After this peak, our long-lived peers are subject to a continual decline in mineral status, increasing skeletal susceptibility to fracture. With much attention to osteoporosis in the last several decades, clinicians have recognized that some pathologic conditions can prevent the achievement of peak bone mass and others can promote the normal decline in bone mineral density after maturity. Although a significant discussion of this complex and thoroughly studied process is beyond the scope of this chapter, several points can be made. First, as suggested previously, normal sex steroids are required to attain peak bone mass, as shown by the failure of young hypogonadal adults to reach normal peak bone mineral density.[134] Deficiency of either estrogen or testosterone after attaining adult bone mass increases the rate of mineral loss, largely through increased resorption.[135] IGF-I, a critical factor for bone development and mineralization, appears to enhance normal mineralization,[136] but may also promote bone remodeling by decreasing osteoprotegerin and increasing RANKL.[89] Certain medical conditions are associated with both increased resorption and decreased bone formation, such as excess glucocorticoids, either iatrogenic or in Cushing's disease.[137] Increased loss of bone mineral density is also associated with any coexisting illness,[138] undoubtedly due to multifactorial causes, including the inevitable decline in exercise that parallels aging, which in turn stimulates bone loss due to decreased function.[139,140]

One of the most exciting discoveries regarding the genetics of bone mineral density (discussed previously) is the involvement of the Wnt pathway in osteoblast function and bone mineral content. Two kindreds with increased bone mineral density with abnormalities in Lrp5 protein, which leads to enhanced Wnt signaling, have so far been described.[17,18]

BIOPHYSICAL STIMULI

Working systemically or locally, chemical factors such as sex steroids, vitamin D, M-CSF, or TGF-β, for instance, play vital roles in the regulation of skeletal modeling and remodeling. There is increasing evidence that the ultimate role these "mediators of change" play may be orchestrated by local factors that are *not* chemical in origin. One of the most potent influences of the development and maintenance of the skeleton is by-products of function (during use), referred to as biophysical factors (i.e., mechanic-electric; discussed in detail at the end of this chapter). Whether it is an increase in bone mass due to exercise or work habits, or a decrease in bone mass due to bed rest, cast immobilization, or space flight, physical factors are key to determining the ultimate structural success of the skeleton. Indeed, it is essential to keep the role of chemical mediators in perspective and acknowledge physical factors as a critical control mechanism in the regulation of tissue differentiation, growth, repair, and remodeling.[141] Although the molecular mechanisms are not well understood, studies proving an effect of biophysical stimuli on bone microstructure and mineral density are increasing in number.[142,143] Physical stimuli as potent determinants of skeletal morphology have even been postulated as primary regulators of chondro-osseous morphogenesis,[144] yet the specific mechanic parameters that control the process have yet to be determined. Nevertheless, recent studies have documented the potential efficacy of biophysical stimuli in improving bone quantity and quality; departing from the premise that larger signals are necessarily better, extremely small mechanical strains, below 10 microstrain, were shown to be strongly anabolic to trabecular bone, indicating the potential for a nonpharmacologic intervention for osteoporosis.[145]

Composition of Bone Matrix

Bone is composed of inorganic mineral (70 percent of weight), organic matrix and cells (25 percent), and water (5 percent). Before its calcification, newly synthesized bone matrix is essentially completely organic and is called *osteoid*. Collagen is the predominant organic component in bone, accounting for approximately 94 percent of the unmineralized matrix (see Table 89–1). Other noncollagenous proteins unique to bone are found in osteoid, accounting for approximately 4 percent of its weight. These include glycoproteins and phosphoproteins such as osteonectin,[146] sialoproteins, which are predominantly osteopontin,[147] osteocalcin,[148] and BMP.[149] Extracts of bone also include enzymes, hormones, growth factors, and other metabolites essential for bone metabolism.[150] Bone cells, for all their responsibility to mineral and structural homeostasis, constitute only 2 percent of the organic tissue.[151]

COLLAGEN AND PROTEOGLYCANS

The major protein secretory product of the osteoblast is collagen, whose complex primary, secondary, and tertiary structure lends strength to bone and allows the seeding of hydroxyapatite (HA) crystals from a supersaturated extracellular fluid. Collagen is a critical element of the skeleton, and abnormalities in its structure and regulation lead to severe skeletal phenotypes. Because of its importance, collagen metabolism occupies a chapter of its own in this text (see Chapter 2) and is not discussed in detail here.

Osteoblast formation of collagen is typified by crosslinking of lysine and proline residues to form procollagen trimers. The processed collagen is organized into parallel fiber sheets of tropocollagen.[152] Within each

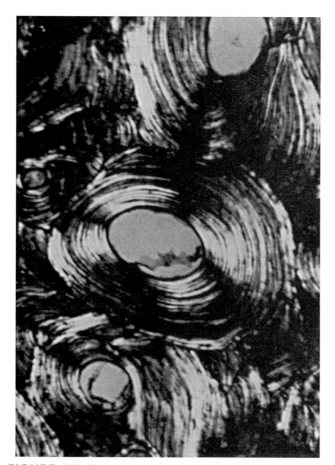

FIGURE 89–6 · Ground section of bone photographed with polarized light showing the concentric lamellar structure of the basic unit of mature bone, the osteon. The central vascular canal (empty in this preparation) is surrounded by multiple lamellae of bone. The adjacent lamellae are composed of collagen bundles with differing orientations, giving rise to alternating light and dark bands in polarized light.

sheet, or lamella, the fibers lie parallel to each other,[153] whereas the fibril orientation on adjacent lamellae runs in directions distinct from this axis (Fig. 89-6), contributing to the strength of bone, as in the structure of plywood. This structure also facilitates the seeding of HA crystals from a supersaturated extracellular fluid.

Bone collagen is primarily type I and resembles other type I collagens found in skin and tendon. The basic unit of bone collagen, the tropocollagen molecule, is a triple helix of three polypeptide α-chains, each with approximately 1000 amino acids.[154] By stabilization of these soluble molecules with cross-links of hydroxylysine and lysine, the bone collagen fibrils become insoluble.[155] Type I collagen differs from the type II collagen of cartilage in several salient aspects. Each of the three α-chains of type II collagen is identical to the others, yet their amino acid composition is different from that of any of the three (one pair, one unique) α-chains of the type I tropocollagen of bone.[156] Compared to the chains of type I collagen, the chains of type II collagen contain much more glycosylated hydroxylysine, making cartilage all the more resistant to degradation by collagenase.

The triple helix of type I collagen forms a linear molecule approximately 300-nm long.[157] Each molecule is aligned parallel to the next, producing a collagen fibril. Within the collagen fibril, gaps called *hole zones* exist between the end of one molecule and the beginning of the next. It is thought that noncollagenous proteins reside in these spaces, which chemotactically attract and initiate the mineralization process.[151] The fibrils are further grouped in bundles to form the collagen fiber.

Proteoglycans constitute the principal noncollagenous protein in the mineralized matrix and, again, because of their importance for rheumatology, occupy a full chapter early in this text (see Chapter 3). Bone proteoglycan is similar in structure to that found in cartilage, consisting of a thin protein core with multiple covalently bound glycosaminoglycan chains.[158] Although the role of these proteins in bone has not been determined, it has been proposed that they may actually store load information after functional activity, serving as a form of strain memory.[159] These molecules deform rapidly in response to load, yet reestablish their original relative orientation after unloading. Although somewhat speculative, this matrix cell interaction may well serve as a signal transduction mechanism to transfer mechanic information from the matrix to the entombed osteocytes.

OSTEOCALCIN

Also present in the matrix are substantial quantities of osteocalcin, a protein found almost exclusively in bone, which comprises 1 to 2 percent of the total bone protein. Osteocalcin synthesis takes place in the osteoblasts during the carboxylation of glutamate, a vitamin K–dependent reaction.[160] 1,25-dihydroxyvitamin D enhances the synthesis of this noncollagenous protein.[161] The function of this protein remains unclear, but it has been postulated to play a role in both osteoclast recruitment and bone formation.[88] The osteocalcin knockout mouse, which required that three gene isoforms be deleted to achieve the unique phenotype, is characterized by a late-onset increase in bone mineral density, suggesting that an absence of the osteocalcin signal for activation of osteoclasts results in a thicker, less remodeled, bone.[12] Osteocalcin also appears to have a role in regulating mineral properties.[162]

HYDROXYAPATITE

Bone mineral is generically referred to as HA ($Ca_{10}[PO_4]_6[OH]_2$), a plate-like crystal 20- to 80-nm long and 2- to 5-nm thick. Bone HA is quite different from naturally occurring apatite, as it contains a number of impurities, including sodium, fluorine, strontium, lead, and radium. It is smaller in size than natural apatites (10 versus 40 nm) and more reactive and soluble because of its less-perfect atomic arrangement.[163] The nucleation sites of bone mineral may not be the plates of HA but the more energetically favorable crystal spicules such as amorphous calcium phosphate and octacalcium phosphate.[164] It is believed these unstable precursors are formed first and gradually transformed to the more crystalline HA.[165] Mineral exchange is facilitated by the enormous surface area of amorphous calcium phosphate, including its hydration shell. This is reflected in the greater avidity of new bone for "bone-seeking" isotopes (e.g., technetium, fluorine, strontium). The bone mineral continues to mature throughout an individual's lifetime,[166] becoming more and more "perfect" and, thus, exposing less surface area for a given volume of mineral. Indeed, the process of crystal maturity may contribute to the etiology of osteopenia;[167] not only would greater levels of systemic factors be needed to liberate calcium from the more stable crystal, but stress-generated electrical charge in the form of zeta potentials would attenuate as a function of the diminished surface area of the mineral constituents. The magnitude of these stress-generated potentials, produced by the ionic constituents of the fluid flowing by the charged phase of the mineral, drops proportionally as less mineral is exposed at the microboundary layer. In elderly persons, therefore, the same degree of functional strain would generate a weaker regulatory signal.

BONE MARKERS AND MEASUREMENT OF BONE MINERAL

Alkaline phosphatase has long been used as a crude marker of bone turnover, as it is released during osteoblast function. In an effort to refine markers of bone remodeling, measurement of other products of bone formation and breakdown found in the blood and urine has been attempted. One of the first was osteocalcin, which can be used to reflect bone formation activity.[168] Separation of bone alkaline phosphatase from total serum alkaline phosphatase has also been achieved, enhancing sensitivity for marking increased osteoblast activity. Measurements of bone breakdown have also been pursued to give the clinician a better marker than bone density to follow the progress of patients. These include serum and urine markers for collagen breakdown products such as N telopeptides,[169] and pyridinolines[170] (see Chapter 50).

Despite their usefulness in large pharmaceutical trials to reflect generalized changes in bone remodeling, none of these markers has demonstrated much utility as an indicator of bone turnover for a specific patient because of the heterogeneity of response. However, there is some indication that during treatment of high bone-turnover states, decreases in markers of bone breakdown such as N-telopeptide might be a reasonable sign that remodeling has been restrained.[171]

The "gold standard" of measurement of bone mineral density remains dual-energy x-ray absorptiometry (DEXA). The density units are given in grams per centimeter squared, as opposed to cubed, and they are indicative more of an apparent—rather than real—density as the two-dimensional rendering does not fully account for the bone size.[172] In contrast, quantitative computed tomography (QCT) measurement is a true volumetric measure of bone mineral density, but it is used infrequently because of the necessity of technical expertise, radiation exposure, and cost. Although promising, there are not yet any large-scale longitudinal studies using QCT to monitor bone changes in an adult or elderly population. Ultimately, to determine bone's true physical properties, assays such as transcutaneous ultrasound may provide more specific information as to both the quantity and quality of the bone.[173]

◼ Mineralization of Bone Tissue

The mineralization of bone begins 10 to 15 days after the organic osteoid matrix has been laid down.[174] At this point, mineral increases almost immediately to 70 percent of the ultimate content, whereas deposition of the final 30 percent takes several months.[175] The process of mineralization is extremely complex and temporally dynamic.[176] There is emerging evidence that HA deposition and seeding of mineralization are strongly interdependent on both cartilage- and bone-derived macromolecules, such as osteonectin, phosphoproteins, and proteolipids. Surprisingly, the initial sites of calcium phosphate nucleation in growing bone, fracture callus, and calcifying cartilage appear to be not at the bone surface but on the processes of matrix vesicles.[177] Matrix vesicles are small, round, extracellular lipid–bilaminar bound organelles that bud from hypertrophic chondrocytes or osteoblasts undergoing the process of apoptosis,[178] as well as from cell processes originating from the plasma membrane.[179] There is a definite polarity to the vesicles, with mineralization occurring in a predictable and organized way adjacent to the requisite phosphatases on the inner leaflet of the membrane.[180] The matrix vesicles contain alkaline phosphatase, adenosine triphosphatase (ATPase), inorganic pyrophosphatase, 5′-nucleotidase, and adenosine triphosphate (ATP)-pyrophosphohydrolase[181] in addition to phospholipids (especially phosphatidyl serine), which have a strong affinity for calcium ions.[182] It is believed that these ions accumulate in the matrix vesicle because of their affinity for the phospholipids and because of a membrane-bound calcium pump. At a point of supersaturation, nucleation of the mineral begins.[183]

In retrospect, the question of whether mineralization is an active or passive process remains to be answered. In a fascinating process, Stupp and colleagues have created nanofibers that assemble in structures reminiscent of the osteoid matrix. These assembled nanofibers are actually able to direct mineralization of HA in the absence of cells.[184] Thus, the osteoblast may enable passive mineralization entirely through production of the extracellular matrix.

NUCLEATION

Alkaline phosphatase, a biosynthetic product of osteoblasts, is present in very high concentrations during development and osteoid production.[185] The regulatory role of this disulfide-linked dimer is not known, but its presence may increase local concentrations of phosphate and thereby facilitate HA deposition.[186] Increasing the concentration of phosphate in the micromilieu exceeds the local solubility product and catalyzes deposition along the inner leaflet of the vesicle.

After this accretion, the destruction of the membrane has been attributed to an increasing concentration of lysophospholipids within the matrix vesicles, which suggests that they are programed to self destruct.[187] After dissolution of the matrix vesicle membrane, the HA crystals are exposed to the extravesicular environment, where additional mineral accretes to the newly formed crystal.[188] The crystal is then believed to chemotactically move toward and preferentially bind at the hole zones between collagen fibrils, precipitated by the nesting osteonectin[189] and fibronectin.[190] Mineralization proceeds and extends over the collagen matrix, with the long axis of the HA crystal parallel to the collagen fiber. The arrangement of the collagen matrix that is synthesized during osteoblast activity ultimately determines the orientation of the bone mineral crystal.[153]

In the extravesicular milieu, glycosaminoglycans inhibit the calcification process by modulating the advancing mineral front.[191] Indeed, it may be just these proteoglycan macromolecules, found in high concentrations in noncalcifying collagenous structures such as ligament, tendon, and skin, that may prevent mineral deposition.[192] Other theories for the lack of calcification of dense connective tissues include the tighter packing of their collagen fibrils, limited access of phosphate ions to the interfibrillar nucleation sites, and the existence of crystallization inhibitors, such as pyrophosphate, present in synovial fluid, plasma, and urine at concentrations sufficient to prevent deposition of calcium carbonates.[193] Once the concentration of these inhibitors reaches a threshold, mineralization is halted, leaving a thin layer of osteoid between the lining cells and the mineralization front. This establishes the syncytium, or cellular canopy, which must be retracted to expose the mineral and reinitiate the remodeling cycle.

TURNOVER

In undecalcified ground sections, microradiography demonstrates subtle differences in the calcium content of the bone tissue, thus allowing separation into "old"

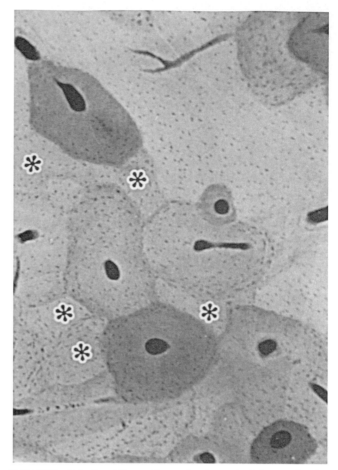

FIGURE 89-7 • Microradiograph of cortical bone showing osteons in varying degrees of mineralization with numerous interstitial fragments (*).

and "new" bone on the basis of contrast intensity (Fig. 89-7). For example, young osteons, in the process of formation, have large central vascular canals that narrow with infilling, showing progressively less mineralization toward the center. This contrasts sharply with the active tunneling process of resorption, in which case the inside rim of the osteon appears equally mineralized as with the outer rings. Static remodeling parameters, such as the osteoid seam width, the number of resorptive events, and the number of formative events, can, thus, be inferred from these morphologic characteristics. By using double-fluorescent labels (e.g., tetracyclines) administered at known intervals, the clinician can determine dynamic parameters of bone remodeling (i.e., rates of turnover, infilling, and formation). Static and dynamic histomorphometric studies, quantified by means of biopsy specimens harvested from such areas as the iliac crest, are extremely powerful means of evaluating the systemic state of the skeleton.[194]

The complex, composite nature of bone achieved through the secretion of the collagen matrix and its subsequent mineralization is a product of the synergistic interrelationships of the cell types, the systemic regulators of calcium metabolism, and the matrix-bound proteins that locally control bone remodeling. The product of this sophisticated and interdependent process is an extremely successful tissue that serves both as a structural organ and as a mineral reservoir. Importantly, many substitutes for bone, derived from calcium phosphate and HA mixtures (e.g., coral), have been used successfully in the clinic as bone substitutes in allografts or as an osteoconductive surface on implants.

Architecture of Bone

MACROSCOPIC ORGANIZATION

Bones are remarkably well suited for their structural role. At the gross level, as hollow tubes they derive maximal strength from minimal weight.[195] At the next-lower structural level, cortical and cancellous morphology is strategically arranged to evenly distribute functional stresses.[196] Lower still, the arrangement of the collagen within the cancellous or cortical bone, combined with the two-phase composite matrix of the collagen and mineral, provides both tensile and compressive strength.[197] The ultimate tensile strength of bone approaches that of cast iron, and its capacity to absorb and release energy is twice that of oak, yet the weight of bone is only one third that of steel. And while proving a resilient and resistant material, this tissue's capacity to remodel, adapt, and repair itself—without leaving a scar—is what identifies bone as the ultimate biomaterial. An excellent review of the architecture of bone can be found in the monograph by Martin and colleagues.[198] The structural success of skeletal morphology can be examined at a series of levels:

1. Gross anatomy and functional responsibility
2. Ultrastructural morphology (cortical or cancellous)
3. Microscopic organization (lamellar or woven)
4. Mineralization process (enchondral or intramembranous)

At the gross structural level, each bone has diverse and distinct morphologic features. Regardless of function, each bone is composed of dense cortical tissue (e.g., diaphyseal shaft) and cancellous tissue, such as the trabecular cascades found in the neck of the femur or the metaphysis of the proximal tibia (Fig. 89-8). At the microscopic level, two types of bone are identified: the disorganized, hypercellular woven bone and the highly organized, relatively hypocellular lamellar bone. Essentially, all bone tissue can be described by one of these two morphologic patterns, whether mature, growing, pathologic, or healing.

Woven bone is a product of rapid bone formation. Architecturally, it has an irregular, disorganized pattern of collagen orientation and osteocyte distribution (Fig. 89-9). Although woven bone is characteristic of embryonic and fetal development, it is also found in the healthy adult skeleton at ligament and tendon insertions as well as in specific disease states, such as Paget's disease, osteogenic sarcoma, and metastases. Under less severe pathologic conditions (fracture callus, inflammatory responses, stress fractures), woven bone is usually reabsorbed and replaced by lamellar bone within a few weeks of its deposition.[199] Mechanical stimulation, if potent enough, can even cause a rapid production of woven bone, which ultimately remodels into dense lamellar bone.[200] Many consider woven bone an aberrant response. That it is laid down so quickly and is so readily remodeled, however, distinguishes this type of bone as a wise strategy in accommodating new, intense structural challenges.

Lamellar, or mature, bone can be packed tightly to form the dense cortex of a bone, or it can be organized as the trabecular struts in cancellous bone. In contrast to the random and disorganized structure of woven bone, the lamellar appearance of this mature bone is the product of highly organized mineralized plates. In cancellous bone, the lamellae run parallel to the trabeculae. In cortical bone, several patterns occur. The predominant one is that found in osteons, which are composed of small, concentric lamellar cylinders sur-

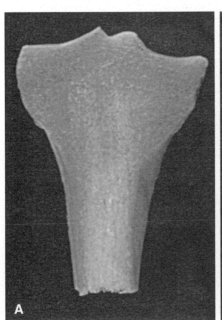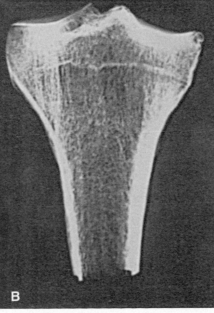

FIGURE 89-8 · *A*, Macerated preparation of the human knee showing the trabecular structure that supports the flared articular surface. *B*, Radiograph of the specimen shown in *A*.

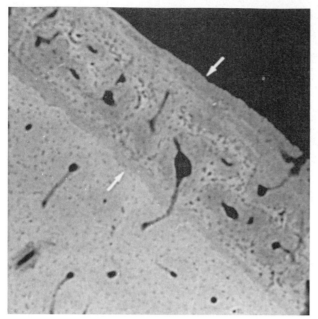

FIGURE 89-9 • Outer cortex of bone showing the results of rapid periosteal bone formation producing woven bone *(arrows)*, followed by the slower formation of primary osteons surrounding blood vessels.

rounding a central vascular channel, not unlike the rings in a tree trunk (Fig. 89-10). Osteons are typically 200 to 300 μm in diameter, consisting of up to six or seven concentric osteocyte rings, which are composed of up to 20 lamellar plates.[201] Canaliculi in lamellar bone are consistent in diameter and orientation and, in total, contain fewer osteocytes per unit volume than woven bone (20,000 cells/μm³ vs. 80,000 cells/μm³).

During growth in diameter, new bone must be added appositionally. After the formation of the periosteal cuff about the primary center of ossification, bone increases its diameter by one of two methods. During rapid growth, spicules of new woven bone are formed perpendicular to the surface, which allows maximal radial expansion with minimal material. The gaps between the spicules are subsequently filled in and consolidated by the formation of lamellar bone. In this process, individual periosteal blood vessels that lie in the valley of the spicules are surrounded by the encroaching new lamellar formation, creating primary osteons parallel to the long axis of the bone. An osteon that has formed de novo, as in the woven bone consolidation process just described, is known as a primary osteon. If this occurs intracortically by a resorptive process to replace preexisting bone tissue, it is referred to as a secondary osteon, or haversian system, and constitutes the bulk of adult human bone.[202]

When slow diametric growth occurs, seams of new bone are laid appositionally on the existing surface. As discussed previously, the birefringent pattern of both circumferential lamellae and single osteons is believed to arise through directional changes between collagen bundles in layers, therefore maximizing strength in a number of different planes. Although the collagen bundles within each of these lamellar plates are highly oriented, individual fibers often traverse interlamellar spaces. Such a composite integration increases both the individual osteon's resistance to external loads and the effective strength of the bone structure.[203]

An alternative theory for the polarized light birefringence of an osteon is based on fiber-rich, fiber-poor lamellar rings, in which the thinner (1- to 2-μm) plates contain

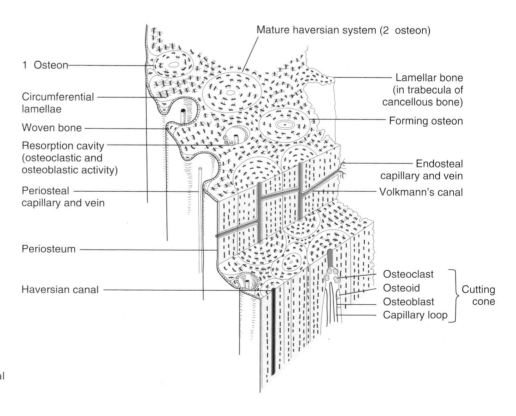

FIGURE 89-10 • Architectural Organization of Cortical Bone.

a greater degree of glycosaminoglycans (ground substance) than the adjacent 5- to 7-μm collagen-rich layers.[204] These glycosaminoglycans are thought to be continuous from the "thin" lamellar plate, through the cement line, to interdigitate with the ground substance of the "thick" plate. This architecture, with a true continuity between plates, would produce an increase in the stiffness of each osteon or each circumferential plate. Perhaps the morphology of lamellar bone will prove to be some combination of these two postulations, thus maximizing both the stiffness of the material (continuity of ground substance) and its toughness (integration of collagen layers).

CORTICAL DRIFTS: FLEXURAL NEUTRALIZATION

If periosteal surface modeling were to occur in the absence of endosteal resorption, the overall thickness of the cortex would increase with increasing age, leaving too much bone and too little marrow space. This is avoided by coordinating the increasing periosteal diameter with a concomitant increase in the diameter of the endosteal envelope, which is achieved through resorption at this inner surface.[205] Although these rapid surface drifts diminish in the mature skeleton, they rise again in elderly persons. In the aged skeleton, the rate of surface erosion of the endosteal surface exceeds the formation rate of the periosteum, resulting in a net decrease in total bone mass. However, this age-related expansion of the cortex establishes a biomechanical compensatory mechanism by the concurrent increase in the cross-sectional moments of inertia, which results in an increased capacity of the bone to resist bending loads.[206]

METAPHYSEAL RESHAPING

During growth in length, the changes in periosteal and endosteal compartments are altered toward, instead, periosteal resorption accompanied by endosteal extension. As the metaphysis and diaphysis elongate, resorption at the periosteal surface must be closely coordinated with deposition at the endosteum, a process known as metaphyseal reshaping.[207] Under these circumstances, some of the cortical bone within the epiphyseal shell is spared and subsequently becomes a component of the cancellous structure within the metaphysis. Where fragments of osteons as well as new lamellae and abundant cement lines are seen, the ultrastructural organization of trabeculae reflects their cortical origin.

HAVERSIAN REMODELING

Bone remodeling is a process of "real-time" tissue replacement. In places, trabeculae are covered with osteoblasts making new bone; in others, osteoclasts are eroding the surface. This process of resorption and formation can rapidly alter the orientation of the trabeculae to accommodate changes in the manner of loading or shifts in alignment secondary to disease or fracture.[208] To remodel cortical bone so that intracortical damage or dead tissue can be replaced, the cortex must first be resorbed from within, thus creating a surface for apposi-

tion. When haversian systems replace or remodel existing bone, this is not necessarily achieved through the identical pathway of the original osteon. Indeed, these secondary osteons can persist directly through an existing arrangement of osteons and circumferential lamellae, leaving only remnants of these preexisting structures. These fragments of lamellar or woven bone are called interstitial lamellae. Because the structural integrity of the bone must be preserved during this remodeling, the replacement process requires close integration between resorption and formation. Thus, the cutting cone of the osteoclast must be followed rapidly by capillary invasion and the simultaneous intrusion of a population of osteoblasts infilling the lamellar rings of the secondary osteon. As discussed previously, matrix-bound proteins, such as TGF-β, which are released by the resorption process, may be critical to the retention of the close integration of this coupling process.

Although levels of intracortical remodeling may be elevated by changes in the organism's nutritional status (e.g., calcium deficiency[209]), endocrine imbalance (hyperparathyroidism, menopause[210]), or even aging (osteopenia[167]), one of the most potent stimuli for remodeling is a change in the level of physical activity.[211] If physical demands are altered (e.g., an increased or decreased level of activity), or if the manner in which the bone is loaded is changed (e.g., distribution of strain or loading rate), the bone remodels internally to adapt to the new demands.[212] Evidence of this osteonal turnover has been demonstrated in rabbits, in which a 150-percent increase in the number of labeled secondary osteons arose in the subchondral plate of the proximal tibia subjected to repetitive impulsive loads.[213]

Not only does loading activate modeling and remodeling, but by-products of loading are also believed to influence morphology. For example, one of the strongest correlates to elevated intracortical turnover is an increased strain rate.[214] Another alternative to strain magnitude, strain frequency, is a potent determinant of bone morphology.[215] This sensitivity to discrete components of the biophysical milieu opens several distinct avenues for the treatment of musculoskeletal disorders, including induced electric fields,[216] low-intensity ultrasound,[217] and low-magnitude, high-frequency mechanic stimulation.[218]

BLOOD SUPPLY OF BONE

Bone is extremely vascular and requires approximately 10 percent of the cardiac output.[219] Blood supply to the cortical diaphysis is derived from the nutrient artery and the periosteal vessels. In the metaphyseal ends of the bone, where metabolism is most active, the periosteal vessels are large and abundant and are also referred to as metaphyseal arteries, although they are entirely analogous to the periosteal capillaries. The third set of vessels, the epiphyseal arteries, supplies the subarticular ends of the bones and assumes special importance because of the growth process in this area and the vulnerability of these vessels to injury.

During infancy and adolescence, the epiphyseal plate serves as a barrier separating the epiphysis from

A   **B**

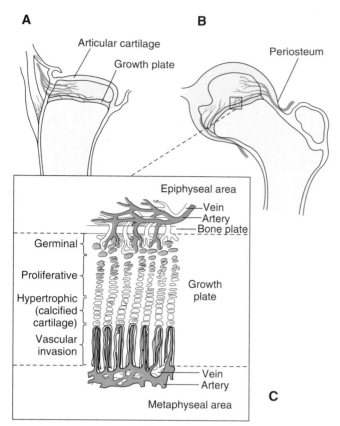

FIGURE 89–11 · Epiphyseal Blood Supply of Growing Bone. *A,* The blood supply of most secondary centers of ossification is abundant by virtue of the numerous soft tissue attachments. *B,* Certain secondary centers, such as the proximal femur, are devoid of soft tissue attachments, and the blood supply, therefore, follows a tenuous route through the joint, where it is liable to injury. *C,* The blood supply to the growth plate showing the contribution of the epiphyseal artery to the germinal portion of the growth plate. (From Sledge CB: Biology and development of the growth plate. *In* Cave EF [ed]: Trauma Management. Chicago, Year Book Medical Publishers, 1974.)

the metaphysis. Although a few vessels crossing the plate have been described, it is widely accepted that there is no effective circulation across the plate. Essentially, therefore, the epiphyses have an isolated blood supply via the epiphyseal arteries, but those few vessels do present a potential route for the spread of infection or tumor from the metaphysis into the epiphysis. In most joints, there are abundant soft tissue attachments to the epiphyses (muscles, ligaments, capsule), so that numerous vessels supply the bone through these attachments (Fig. 89-11). In a few locations, such as the proximal femur, the entire epiphysis may be intra-articular and, therefore, may be covered by articular cartilage. Because neither the articular nor the growth cartilage is penetrated by vessels, the few epiphyseal arteries must pass alongside the growth plate, covered by a thin layer of periosteum, to perforate the epiphysis.[220] This route of blood supply is extremely vulnerable to trauma (fractures through the growth plate), increased intra-articular pressure (joint infections or bleeding into the joint), or idiopathic interruption (Legg-Perthes disease in children, avascular necrosis in adults).

Epiphyseal vessels arborize within the bony nucleus to supply the marrow, cancellous bone, and the dividing chondrocytes in the microepiphyseal plates in the depths of the articular cartilage, as well as the growth plate itself. Because of this, interruption of the vessels leads to cessation of longitudinal growth and diametric growth of the epiphysis and joint surface.

Within the cortex of bone, capillaries travel primarily in the longitudinal direction within haversian canals. Occasional branching is seen, and lateral communication with the periosteal vessels through Volkmann's canals provide collateral circulation. The usual haversian system is 100 mm or less in diameter; thus, individual osteocytes are not more than 50 mm from their blood supply. The rich system of canaliculi radiating out from the central canal enhances microcirculation to the most distant osteocytes.

Mechanical Properties of Bone

Even considering the elaborate cell kinetics, mineralization process, and morphology of bone, its success as a structure is ultimately a product of bone's mechanic properties: how stiff it is, how resilient it is to fatigue, and how effectively it withstands the extremes of physical activity. The skeleton's structural success can be jeopardized by genetic disorders such as osteogenesis imperfecta, metabolic diseases such as Paget's disease, or even the bone loss that parallels the aging process (i.e., osteopenia). To appreciate the structural risks that accompany metabolic bone diseases, several interdependent concepts of bone's biomechanic properties must be considered.[221]

The mechanic strength of fully mature osteonal bone is greater than that of immature bone, which is composed of circumferential lamellae and a few osteons that may only be partially mineralized.[222] Values for the mechanic properties of individual osteons range from a tensile elastic modulus of 12 gigapascals (GPa) and 114 megapascals (MPa) ultimate tensile strength for a fully mature, mineralized osteon, to less than half that modulus and only 75 percent of the ultimate tensile strength for a younger, less mineralized osteon. For normal tensile or compressive loading, the stiffness of the material, or elastic modulus, shows human haversian bone to be about 17 GPa in the longitudinal direction, 11.5 GPa in the transverse direction, and 3.3 GPa in shear.[223] The degree of mineralization (young bone) or porosity (old bone) compromises the stiffness of the bone and thereby lowers the elastic modulus. However, the "effective" modulus of the bone can compensate for decreased stiffness by changes in morphology (e.g., periosteal expansion).

STRENGTH

A major contributor to the strength of bone is derived through its composite nature of haversian, circumferential, and interstitial lamellae that works synergistically to avoid yield, or ultimate strain. Strain, a dimensionless unit of change in length divided by its original length, is used in bone physiology as 10^{-6} strain, or microstrain. The yield strain of bone, or that degree of deformation reached at which the bone does not elastically recover, is approximately 7000 microstrain; that is, a 0.7-percent change in length causes irreversible damage to the tissue. Ultimate strain in bone, or that degree of deformation at which the material actually fractures, is 15,000 microstrain.[224]

An analogy of a bundle of straws versus a solid stick illustrates how a composite structure, such as bone, can prove more successful in resisting loads by avoiding yield and the ultimate strain of the material. The solid stick breaks with relatively little bending, because relatively high strains are generated within the periphery of the material. In contrast, the bundle of straws composed of the same mass and subjected to the same bending conditions continues to deform (strain) rather than break, as each independent element slips relative to adjacent bundles. By dissipating the strains generated by identical forces, the chance of exceeding yield strains or ultimate failure is greatly diminished.

This analogy is often put into practice with the use of multistranded wire rather than single-stranded wire. During flexion, each individual strand slips relative to its neighbor rather than straining, thus minimizing the generation of potentially damaging levels of strain. In the same manner, individual lamellae "slip" relative to adjacent lamellae, dissipating energy and minimizing strain levels within the material, thus allowing the entire system to react in a more elastic manner, rather than sustain brittle failure or ultimate fracture.

TOUGHNESS

As an organ, bone needs to be both stiff (to resist deformation) and tough (to prevent crack propagation). However, there is a compromise between these two objectives, as they are attained through a balance of the composite between the resiliency to crack propagation provided by collagen and the resiliency to deformation provided by mineral. Comparatively small changes in the mineral content of bone tissue can have substantial effects on its properties as a material, as demonstrated by Curry[225] in his determination of the mechanic properties of diverse types of bone. By comparing the bovine femur, the deer antler, and the whale tympanic bulla, he illustrated that as the morphologic responsibility of the skeletal element changed, so did its mineral content. In the extreme, the mineral content ranged from 86 percent in the bulla, which requires high acoustic impedance, to 59 percent in the antler, which must be resilient to high-impact loads. The consequence of this high mineral content is revealed by comparing the relative work-to-fracture ratio of these bones; the work-to-fracture ratio of the bulla is only 3 percent that of the antler.

The material properties of the appendicular skeleton, however, remain remarkably consistent through a wide range of animals.[226] Over an animal mass range of 0.09 to 700 kg, the bending strength of those bones relegated to traditional load-bearing responsibilities remains approximately 200 to 250 MPa, with an elastic modulus consistently approaching 20 GPa. To adapt to changes in the physical demands placed on it, it appears that the appendicular skeleton responds not by changing its material properties but by altering its shape and morphology.[227] This is achieved by functionally regulated alterations in bone mass and architecture.

STRUCTURAL ADAPTATION IN BONE

Bone tissue has the capacity to adapt to its functional environment such that its morphology is "optimized" for its mechanic demand. Indeed, the concept proposed in 1892—that the course and balance of bone remodeling can be affected by mechanic function—is one of the oldest in modern medicine and is widely referred to as Wolff's law.[67] But what component of the functional environment is osteoregulating, and what is the structural objective of bone morphology? Strains measured during functional activity should indicate what the architecture of the skeleton is trying to amplify or suppress. Loads can be sustained with the smallest strains if they are applied axially. However, the axial component of functional activity is responsible for only a small percentage of the total strain measured at the bone surface; the femur, humerus, radius, ulna, and tibia all show that well over 80 percent of the measured strain is caused by bending moments.[228] As the neutral axis of strain typically passes across the marrow cavity, a significant portion of the tissue is in fact subjected to tension.[229] Although bending moments cannot be extinguished, their effect would be minimized if the bone's longitudinal curvature were oriented such that the moment created by curvature counteracted those externally imposed by activity. Surprisingly, long bone curvature does not appear directed toward the neutralization of bending, and in some cases this curvature is oriented such that bending is increased.[230] Perhaps bone curvature, a morphologic modification attributable to functional loading,[231] acts to accentuate bone strain rather than cancel it.

Similarity of Peak Strain Magnitudes in Functionally Loaded Bone

Contrary to our normal interpretation of Wolff's law, it appears that minimizing strain is not the ultimate goal of adaptation; instead, skeletal morphology strives to generate a certain type of strain. But what kind of strain is morphology trying to achieve? Although vertebrate design and function are diverse, at the level of small volumes of tissue all loads and bending moments resolve into strain. Peak strain magnitudes measured in adult species, including horse, human, lizard, sheep, goat, goose, pig, macaque, turkey, sunfish, and dog, are remarkably similar, ranging from 2000 to 3500 microstrain. This relationship has been called dynamic strain similarity and suggests that skeletal morphology and locomotion character combine to elicit a very specific and perhaps beneficial level of strain.[232]

This limited range of strain has implications beyond the maintenance of a twofold safety factor within the bone material. Although the structural benefit of a safety factor cannot be denied, it is difficult to imagine a cellular process that could monitor how close to deleterious strain levels the skeleton came during activity and then adjust the tissue's mass simply to avoid them. It seems reasonable that the cell population responsible for adjusting skeletal mass can respond only to the strains to which it is subjected, not the potential strain it might see should an aberrant loading incident occur. Instead, perhaps the safety factors within bone are simply a valuable by-product of a tissue that strives for some cytologic benefit generated by this common strain milieu. The interspecies similarity in strain magnitudes is strong evidence for the existence of a common strain-sensitive cellular population within the skeletal tissues of each of these animals. Further, it suggests the existence of a generic cellular mechanism that strives toward a common, strain-determined structural goal that is desired by and beneficial to the bone cell population.

Strain-Regulated Adaptation

Although the nature of this structure-function relationship is only poorly understood, it has been proposed that bone remodeling is continually influenced by the level and distribution of the functional strains within the bone.[233] One striking example of the skeleton's capacity to adapt to its functional environment has been demonstrated in professional tennis players. By comparing the humeral mass of the racquet arm to the side that simply throws the ball into the air, Jones and colleagues[234] observed a 35-percent increase in men and a 28-percent increase in women in the cortical thickness of the more active humerus.

The converse can also be demonstrated, as immobilization and bed rest can cause negatively balanced bone remodeling either locally or within the entire skeleton. Healthy men restricted to complete bed rest for up to 36 weeks showed a total body calcium loss averaging 4.2 percent. However, bone mineral content measurements of the calcaneus showed a mean decrease of 34 percent; in one case, 45 percent bone mineral was lost,[235] demonstrating that at specific weight-bearing sites the negatively balanced bone remodeling stimulated by diminished demand can be severe.

Attempts to identify those aspects of the skeleton's functional milieu that are responsible for generating and controlling this adaptive response have demonstrated that alterations in bone mass, turnover, and internal replacement are sensitive to changes in the magnitude,[236] distribution,[237] and rate of strain[214] generated within the bone tissue. A loading regimen must be dynamic; static loads do not influence bone morphology,[238] yet its full osteogenic potential is achieved after only an extremely short exposure to this stimulus.[239] The potency of the stimulus is proportional to the magnitude of the strain.[236] As strain levels that are acceptable in one location induce adaptive remodeling in others, each region of each bone may be genetically programmed to accept a particular amount and pattern of intermittent strain as normal. Deviation from this optimal strain environment stimulates changes in the bone's remodeling balance, resulting in adaptive increases or decreases in its mass.

It is not clear whether a discrepancy in strain is picked up at the level of each individual osteocyte, whether the cell has the ability to manipulate the structural milieu of its adjacent space, or whether the osteocyte network somehow spatially integrates the load information across the cortex.[29,240] However, bone mass is substantially influenced by strain situations engendered by short periods of particularly osteogenic activity (e.g., vigorous and diverse exercise) rather than by the strain situation experienced during a predominant activity (e.g., walking) or by the fatigue damage that this might produce.

Isolating specific components of the physical milieu that regulate skeletal morphology has been difficult; no single parameter of the mechanic environment has been shown to reliably predict bone remodeling in all naturally observed or experimentally created conditions.[212] Perhaps our limited success in identifying these elusive stimuli has in part been due to our presumption that structural efficiency (minimal strain with minimal mass) is an essential goal of skeletal morphology. That the skeleton has "optimized" its structure is supported by the similarity in peak strains generated in the cortex regardless of animal or activity (2000 to 3000 microstrain), indicating a common, peak strain–determined goal. Contrasting with this perspective, however, is the nonuniform, but consistent distribution of normal and shear strains that exist throughout the stance phase, leaving large areas of the diaphyseal shaft subjected only to extremely low levels of strain-energy density.[241] Further, rather than a signal to repair accumulated damage, a new strain milieu needs to be applied for only a very short time to maximize the tissue response.[236] Perhaps the engineering perspective that strain is harmful to bone and that remodeling is a repair-driven process needs to be reconsidered. Instead, there may be some by-product of strain, such as stress-generated potentials, piezoelectric currents, or increased perfusion, that enhances the viability of the bone cell population.[242]

Perhaps a principal objective of tissue adaptation is to promote and regulate some specific aspect of the functional milieu such that the matrix or cells within the tissue enjoy some direct or indirect benefit of strain.[241] Indeed, it may not even be the predominant components of the physical milieu that regulate these processes. Very low intensity electric fields (less than 10 μV/cm [243]) as well as low-magnitude strains (less than 10 microstrain [244]), when induced within a specific, hyperphysiologic (10- to 50-Hz) frequency band, influence bone mass as effectively as stimuli of greater intensity induced at more "physiologic" frequencies. Importantly, strains at this frequency and magnitude are induced as by-products of muscle contractions, which resonate between 20 and 50 Hz, and they imply that skeletal diseases such as osteopenia may result not only from dysfunction of the bone cell population, but from the decline of the musculature, as is the case with sarcopenia.[245] Perhaps we should be more hesitant to presume skeletal morphology to be a product of dominant strain parameters with the structural goal of minimizing strain and instead consider the matrix and cellular advantages of a tissue exposed to a dynamic functional milieu.

BIOELECTRIC STIMULI

Although these data demonstrate some relationship of function to form, they do not suggest the means by which the physical signal is transduced by the cell and extracellular matrix into the adaptive process. One potential mechanism for the coupling of mechanic deformation and control of cellular metabolic activity may be the stress-generated electric potential. A change in the bone's level or type of activity in turn alters the magnitude of this potential charge at the bone-fluid interface. Vascular channels within haversian systems, combined with the lacunae and canaliculi occupied by cells and the microporosity of the matrix, may consume as much as 10 percent of the bone tissue's volume, are filled with fluids or cellular components, or both. The deformation of the skeleton caused by functional activity initiates this fluid to flow, similar to the way in which water flows through a sponge that is stretched or compressed. Although at one level this fluid behavior may contribute to increased perfusion and nutrient delivery, the ionic constituents of the fluid interact with the charged nature of the mineral to generate electrokinetic potentials.[246] In 1962, Bassett and Becker[247] hypothesized that a primary step in translating functional load-bearing to an adaptive cellular response was linked to the electric potential generated by the mechanic deformation of the bone tissue. This postulation has been supported by many subsequent investigators, showing the relationship between electric potential and the regulation of bone cell activity. Several excellent reviews are available.[216,248]

Because fluid pressure gradients and the resultant streaming potentials affect primarily those cells confined within the cortices of the extracellular matrix (osteocytes), and changes in the "normal" electrokinetic signal would be generated by alterations in the type or amplitude of function, or both, this "intracortical syncytium" might be a key regulator of bone cell activity. This electric potential in turn may act to effect proliferation of osteoprogenitor cells[249] or catalyze the production[250] or mineralization[251] of the extracellular matrix. Indeed, electric fields of extremely low magnitude can affect both differentiation of osteoblasts[252] and recruitment of osteoclasts.[253]

Whatever the signal transduction pathway of transforming physical information to something the cell population can perceive and respond to, it is clear that the capacity of bone tissue to adapt to its functional demands is critical to the skeleton's structural success. Indeed, as we attempt to evaluate the cellular mechanisms responsible for the positive control of bone mass, the osteogenic potential of physical stimuli cannot be ignored.

▮ Summary

This chapter has provided an overview of the cells responsible for the regulation of bone mass as well as the local and systemic factors that influence their activity. Clearly, the cells and matrix that make up the tissue of bone reflect a sophisticated interaction of organic and inorganic constituents that contribute to the skeleton's admirable capacity to serve as both a mineral reservoir and a structural entity. The process of cell proliferation and differentiation, matrix synthesis and mineralization, growth and adaptation all contribute to this elaborate balance of modeling and remodeling. It is hoped that this chapter has diminished the skeleton's reputation as a static entity and has demonstrated its critical role in the dynamic process of mineral homeostasis and its unparalleled capacity to facilitate locomotion. It is neither solely a reservoir of minerals nor uniquely a structure. The skeleton represents an extremely complex and successful combination of these responsibilities.

REFERENCES

1. Doty S: Morphological evidence of gap junctions between bone cells. Calcif Tiss Int 33:509-512, 1981.
2. Rodan GA, Martin TJ: Role of osteoblasts in hormonal control of bone resorption: A hypothesis. Calcif Tissue Int 33:349-351, 1981.
3. Owen TA, Aronow M, Shalhoub V, et al: Progressive development of the rat osteoblast phenotype in vitro: Reciprocal relationships in expression of genes associated with osteoblast proliferation and differentiation during formation of the bone extracellular matrix. J Cell Physiol 143:420-430, 1990.
4. Martin TJ, Allan EH, Fukumoto S: The plasminogen activator and inhibitor system in bone remodeling. Growth Regul 3:209-214, 1993.
5. Yasuda H, Shima N, Nakagawa N, et al: Osteoclast differentiation factor is a ligand for osteoprotegerin/osteoclastogenesis-inhibitory factor and is identical to TRANCE/RANKL. Proc Natl Acad Sci USA 95:3597-3602, 1998.
6. Reinholt FP, Hultenby K, Oldberg A, Heinegard D: Osteopontin: A possible anchor of osteoclasts to bone. Proc Natl Acad Sci USA 87:4473-4475, 1990.
7. Owen M: Cellular dynamics of bone. In Bourne GH (ed): The Biochemistry and Physiology of Bone, 2nd ed. Vol III. New York, Academic Press, 1972, p 271.
8. Jaworski ZFG: Lamellar bone turnover system and its effector organ. Calcif Tissue Int 36S:46, 1984.
9. Jowsey J: Metabolic Diseases of Bone. Philadelphia, WB Saunders, 1977, p 61.
10. Parfitt AM: Osteomalacia and related disorders. In Avioli LV, Krane SM (eds): Metabolic Bone Disease and Clinically Related Disorders. Philadelphia, WB Saunders, 1990, p 329.
11. Weinstein RS, Jilka RL, Parfitt AM, Manolagas SC: Inhibition of osteoblastogenesis and promotion of apoptosis of osteoblasts and osteocytes by glucocorticoids: Potential mechanisms of their deleterious effects on bone. J Clin Invest 102:274-282, 1998.
12. Ducy P, Desbois C, Boyce B, et al: Increased bone formation in osteocalcin-deficient mice. Nature 382:448-452, 1996.
13. Huang LF, Fukai N, Selby PB, et al: Mouse clavicular development: Analysis of wild-type and cleidocranial dysplasia mutant mice. Dev Dyn 210(1):33-40, 1997.
14. Mundlos S, Otto F, Mundlos C, et al: Mutations involving the transcription factor CBFA1 cause cleidocranial dysplasia. Cell 89:773-779, 1997.
15. Otto F, Thornell AP, Crompton AD, et al: CBFA1, a candidate gene for cleidocranial dysplasia syndrome, is essential for osteoblast differentiation and bone development. Cell 89:765-771, 1997.
16. Nakashima K, Zhou X, Kunkel G, et al: The novel zinc finger-containing transcription factor osterix is required for osteoblast differentiation and bone formation Cell 108:17-29, 2002.
17. Little RD, Carulli JP, Del Mastro RG, et al: A mutation in the LDL receptor-related protein 5 gene results in the autosomal dominant high-bone-mass trait. Am J Hum Genet 70:11-19, 2002.
18. Boyden L, Mao M, Belsky J, et al: High bone density due to a mutation in LDL-receptor-related protein 5. New Engl J Med 346:1513-1521, 2002.
19. Kato M, Patel M, Levasseur S, et al: Cbfa1-independent decrease in osteoblast proliferation, osteopenia, and persistent embryonic eye vascularization in mice deficient in Lrp5, a Wnt coreceptor. J Cell Biol 157:303-314, 2002.

20. Mundlos S, Olsen BR: Heritable diseases of the skeleton. FASB J 11:227-233, 1997.

21. Shafritz AB, Shore EM, Gannon FH, et al: Overexpression of an osteogenic morphogen in fibrodysplasia ossificans progressiva. N Engl J Med 335:555-561, 1996.

22. Menton DN, Simmons DJ, Chang SL, Orr BY: From bone lining cell to osteocyte: An SEM study. Anat Rec 209:29-39, 1984.

23. Rubin JE, Rubin CT: The osteoblast, osteoclast and osteocyte. Curr Opin Orthop 8:34-42, 1997.

24. Curtis TA, Ashrafi SH, Weber DF: Canalicular communication in the cortices of human long bones. Anat Rec 212:336-344, 1985.

25. VanderMolen M, Rubin C, Donahue H: Decreased hormonal responsiveness in gap junction deficient osteoblasts. Trans 41st Orthop Res Soc 20:295, 1995.

26. Skerry T, Bitensky L, Chayen J, Lanyon L: Early strain-related changes in enzyme activity in osteocytes following bone loading in vivo. J Bone Miner Res 4:783-788, 1989.

27. Inaoka T, Lean JM, Bessho T, et al: Sequential analysis of gene expression after an osteogenic stimulus: C-FOS expression is induced in osteocytes. Biochem Biophys Res Com 217:264-270, 1995

28. Noble B, Stevens H, Mosley J, et al: Bone loading changes the number and distribution of apoptotic osteocytes in cortical bone. J Bone Miner Res 12s:36, 1997.

29. Rubin C, Sun Y-Q, Hadjiargyrou M, McLeod K: Increased expression of MMP-1 in osteocytes precedes bone resorption as stimulated by disease: Evidence for autoregulation of the cell's mechanical environment? J Orthop Res 17:354-361, 1999.

30. Albright JA, Skinner C: Bone: Structural organization and remodeling dynamics. In Albright JA, Brand RA (eds): The Scientific Basis of Orthopaedics, 2nd ed. East Norwalk, Conn, Appleton & Lange, 1987, pp 161-198.

31. Felix R, Hofstetter W, Cecchini MG: Recent developments in the understanding of the pathophysiology of osteopetrosis. Eur J Endocrinol 134:143-156, 1996.

32. Parfitt AM: The coupling of bone resorption to bone formation: A critical analysis of the concept and of its relevance to the pathogenesis of osteoporosis. Metab Bone Dis Relat Res 4:1-6, 1982.

33. Bain SD, Impeduglia TM, Rubin CT: Cement line staining in undecalcified thin sections of cortical bone. Stain Tech 65:159-163, 1990.

34. Parfitt AM: The cellular basis of bone remodeling: The quantum concept re-examined in light of recent advances in cell biology of bone. Calcif Tissue Int 36(Suppl):S37-S45, 1984.

35. Walker DG: Enzymatic and electron microscopic analysis of isolated osteoclasts. Calcif Tissue Res 9:296, 1972.

36. Baron R: Polarity and membrane transport in osteoclasts. Connect Tissue Res 20:109-120, 1989.

37. Blair HC, Teitelbaum SL, Chiselli R, Gluck S: Osteoclastic bone resorption by a polarized vacuolar proton pump. Science 245:855-857, 1989.

38. Biskobing D, Nanes M, Rubin J: 1,25(OH)$_2$D is required for protein kinase C upregulation of carbonic anhydrase II in a monomyelocytic cell line. Endocrinology 139:1493-1498, 1994.

39. Nesbitt SA, Horton MA: Trafficking of matrix collagens through bone-resorbing osteoclasts. Science 276:266-269, 1997.

40. Williams JP, Blair H, Jordan S, McDonald JM: Tamoxifen inhibits osteoclastic bone resorption and H$^+$-ATPase activity by an estrogen receptor independent mechanism. J Bone Miner Res 9:62, 1994.

41. Jones SJ, Boyde A, Ali NN, Maconnachie E: A review of bone cell substratum interactions. Scanning 7:5-24, 1985.

42. Silver A, Murrills RJ, Etherington DJ: Microelectrode studies on the acid microenvironment beneath adherent macrophages and osteoclasts. Exp Cell Res 175:266-276, 1988.

43. Rodan GA: Bone mass homeostasis and bisphosphonate action. Bone 20:1-4, 1997.

44. David P, Nguyen H, Barbier A, Baron R: The bisphosphonate tiludronate is a potent inhibitor of the osteoclast vacuolar H(+)-ATPase. J Bone Miner Res 11:1498-1507, 1996.

45. Kahn AJ, Simmons DJ: Investigation of cell lineage in bone using a chimaera of chick and quail embryonic tissue. Nature 258:325, 1975.

46. Yasuda, H, Shima N, Nakagawa N, et al: Osteoclast differentiation factor is a ligand for osteoprotegerin/osteoclastogenesis-inhibitory factor and is identical to TRANCE/RANKL. Proc Natl Acad Sci USA 95:3597-3602, 1998.

47. Lacey DL, Timms E, Tan HL, et al: Osteoprotegerin ligand is a cytokine that regulates osteoclast differentiation and activation. Cell 93:165-176, 1998.

48. Felix R, Cecchini M, Fleisch H: MCSF restores in vivo bone resorption in the op/op osteopetrotic mouse. Endocrinology 127:2592, 1990.

49. Hume DA, Favot P: Is the osteopetrotic mouse completely deficient in expression of MCSF? J Interferon Cytokine Res 15:279-284, 1995.

50. Niida S, Kaku M, Tanne K, et al: Vascular endothelial growth factor can substitute for M-CSF in the support of osteoclast bone resorption. J Exp Med 190:293-298, 1999.

51. Fan X, Biskobing DM, Fan D, et al: Macrophage colony stimulating factor downregulates MCSF-receptor expression and entry of progenitors into the osteoclast lineage. J Bone Miner Res 12:1387-1395, 1997.

52. Suda T, Takahashi N, Martin TJ: Modulation of osteoclast differentiation. Endocr Rev 13:66-80, 1992.

53. Biskobing DM, Fan D, Fan X, Rubin J: Induction of carbonic anhydrase II expression in osteoclast progenitors requires physical contact with stromal cells. Endocrinology 138:4852-4857, 1997.

54. Kong YY, Yoshida H, Sarosi I, et al: OPGL is a key regulator of osteoclastogenesis, lymphocyte development and lymph-node organogenesis. Nature 397:315-323, 1999.

55. Simonet WS, Lacey DL, Dunstan CR, et al: Osteoprotegerin: a novel secreted protein involved in the regulation of bone density. Cell 89:309-319, 1997.

56. Jilka RL, Hangoc G, Girasole G, et al: Increased osteoclast development after estrogen loss: Mediation by interleukin-6. Science 257:88-91, 1992.

57. Roodman G, Kurihara N, Ohsaki Y, et al: Interleukin 6: A potential autocrine/paracrine factor in Paget's disease of bone. J Clin Invest 98:46-52, 1992.

58. Grigoradis AE, Wang A, Cecchini MG, et al: c-Fos: A key regulator of osteoclast-macrophage lineage determination and bone remodeling. Science 266:443-448, 1994.

59. Tondravi MM, McKercher SR, Anderson K, et al: Osteopetrosis in mice lacking haematopoietic transcription factor PU.1. Nature 386:81-84, 1997.

60. Steingrimsson E, Nii A, Fisher DE, et al: The semidominant Mi(b) mutation identifies a role for the HLH domain in DNA binding in addition to its role in protein dimerization. EMBO J 15:6280-6289, 1996.

61. Iotsova V, Caamano J, Loy J, et al: Osteopetrosis in mice lacking NF-kappaB1 and NF-kappaB2. Nat Med 3:1285-1289, 1997.

62. Takeshita S, Namba N, Zhao JJ, et al: SHIP-deficient mice are severely osteoporotic due to increased numbers of hyper-resorptive osteoclasts. Nat Med 8(9):943-949, 2002.

63. Soriano P, Montgomery C, Geske R, Bradley A: Targeted disruption of the c-src protooncogene leads to osteopetrosis in mice. Cell 64:693, 1991.

64. Tanaka S, Amling M, Neff L, et al: c-Cbl is downstream of c-Src in a signalling pathway necessary for bone resorption. Nature 383:528-531, 1996.

65. Miyauchi A, Alvarez J, Greenfield EM, et al: Recognition of osteopontin and related peptides by an $\alpha_v\beta_3$ integrin stimulates immediate cell signals in osteoclasts. J Biol Chem 266:20,369-20,374, 1991.

66. McHugh KP, Hodivala-Dilke K, Zheng MH, et al: Mice lacking beta3 integrins are osteosclerotic because of dysfunctional osteoclasts. J Clin Invest 105(4):433-440, 2000.

67. Wolff J: The Law of Remodeling. Maquet P, Furlong R (trans). Berlin, Springer Verlag, 1986 (original manuscript 1892).

68. Dunbar E, Wysolmerski J, Broadus E: Parathyroid hormone-related protein: From hypercalcemia of malignancy to developmental regulatory molecule. Am J Med Sci 312: 287-294, 1996.

69. Vortkamp A, Lee K, Lanske B, et al: Regulation of rate of cartilage differentiation by Indian Hedgehog and PTH-related protein. Science 27:613-663, 1996.

70. Shapiro F, Holtrop ME, Glimcher MJ: Organization and cellular biology of the perichondrial ossification groove of Ranvier. J Bone Joint Surg Am 59:703, 1977.

71. Cooper RR, Misol S: Tendon and ligament insertion: A light and electron microscopic study. J Bone Joint Surg Am 52:1, 1970.

72. Roux W: Gesammelte Abhandlungen_uber Entwicklungsmechanik der Organismen. Vol I and II. Leipzig, Wilhelm Engelmann, 1895.

73. Carter DR, Orr TE, Fyhrie DP, Schurman DJ: Influences of mechanical stress on prenatal and postnatal skeletal development. Clin Orthop 219:237, 1987.

74. Rosenberg LC, Choi HU, Poole AR: Biological processes involved in endochondral ossification. In Rubin RT, Weiss GB, Putney JB (eds): Calcium in Biological Systems. New York, Plenum, 1985, pp 617-624.

75. Eggli PS, Herrmann W, Hunziker EB, Schenk RK: Matrix compartments in the growth plate of the proximal tibia of rats. Anat Rec 211:246, 1985.

76. Floyd WE, Zaleske DJ, Schiller AL, et al: Vascular events associated with the appearance of the secondary center of ossification in the murine distal femoral epiphysis. J Bone Joint Surg Am 69:185, 1987.

77. Trelstad RL, Silver FH: Matrix assembly. In Hay ED (ed): Cell Biology of Extracellular Matrix. New York, Plenum, 1981, pp 179-215.

78. Urist MF, Mikulski A, Lietze A: Solubilized and insolubilized bone morphogenetic protein. Proc Natl Acad Sci USA 76:1828-1832, 1979.

79. Wozney JM: Bone morphogenetic protein family and osteogenesis. Mol Reprod Dev 32:160-167, 1992.

80. Elima K: Osteoinductive proteins. Ann Med 24:395-402, 1993.

81. Noda M, Camilliere JJ: In vivo stimulation of bone formation by transforming growth factor-beta. Endocrinology 124:2991-2994, 1989.

82. Chenu C, Pfeilschifter J, Mundy GR, Roodman GD: Transforming growth factor-β inhibits formation of osteoclast-like cells in long-term human marrow cultures. Proc Natl Acad Sci USA 85:5683-5687, 1988.

83. Pfeilschifter JP, Seyedin S, Mundy GR: Transforming growth factor-β inhibits bone resorption in fetal rat long bone cultures. J Clin Invest 82:680-685, 1988.

84. Takaishi T, Matsui T, Tsukamoto T, et al: TGF-β induced macrophage colony-stimulating factor gene expression in various mesenchymal cell lines. Am J Physiol 267:C25-C31, 1994.

85. Stevenson S, Cunningham N, Toth J, et al: The effect of osteogenin (a bone morphogenetic protein) on the formation of bone in orthotopic segmental defects in rats. J Bone Joint Surg Am 76:1676-1687, 1994.

86. Hirota S, Takaoka K, Hashimoto J, et al: Expression of mRNA of murine bone-related proteins in ectopic bone induced by murine bone morphogenetic protein 4. Cell Tissue Res 277:27-32, 1994.

87. Boden SD, Hair G, Titus L, et al: Glucocorticoid-induced differentiation of fetal rat calvarial osteoblasts is mediated by bone morphogenetic protein-6. Endocrinology 138:2820-2828, 1997.

88. Canalis E, McCarthy T, Centrella M: Growth factors and the regulation of bone remodeling. J Clin Invest 81:277-281, 1988.

89. Rubin J, Ackert-Bicknell C, Zhu L, et al: Insulin like growth factor-I (IGF-I) regulates osteoprotegerin (OPG) and RANK Ligand (RANKL) in vitro and osteoprotegerin in vivo. J Clin Endo Met 87:4273-4279, 2002.

90. Rousseau F, Bonaventure J, Legeai-Mallet L, et al: Mutations in the gene encoding FGFR3 in achondroplasia. Nature 371:252-254, 1994.

91. Karaplis AS, Luz A, Glowacki J, et al: Letal skeletal dysplasia from targeted disruption of PTHrp gene. Genes Dev 8:277-289, 1994.

92. Schipani E, Kruse K, Juppner H: A constitutively active mutant PTH-PTHrp receptor in Jansen-type metaphyseal chondrodysplasia. Science 268:90-100, 1995.

93. Brown, EM, Gamba G, Riccardi D, et al: Cloning and characterization of an extracellular Ca²⁺-sensing receptor from bovine parathyroid. Nature 366:575-580, 1993.

94. Diagnosis and management of asymptomatic primary hyperparathyroidism: Consensus Development Conference Statement. Ann Intern Med 1145:593-597, 1991.

95. McSheehy PMJ, Chambers TJ: Osteoblast-like cells in the presence of parathyroid hormone release soluble factor that stimulates osteoclastic bone resorption. Endocrinology 119:1654-1659, 1986.

96. Donahue HJ, Fryer MJ, Eriksen EF, Heath H III: Differential effects of parathyroid hormone and its analogues on cytosolic calcium ion and cAMP levels in cultured rat osteoblast-like cells. J Biol Chem 263:13,522-13,527, 1988.

97. Rouleau MF, Warshawsky H, Goltzman D: Parathyroid hormone binding in vivo to renal, hepatic, and skeletal tissues of the rat using a radioautographic approach. Endocrinology 118:919-931, 1986.

98. Hughes MR, Malloy TJ, Kieback DG, et al: Point mutations in the human vitamin D receptor gene associated with hypocalcemic rockets. Science 242:1702-1705, 1988.

99. Kitanaka S, Takeyama K, Murayama A, et al: Inactivating mutations in the 25-hydroxyvitamin D3 1-hydroxylase gene in patients with pseudovitamin D–deficiency rickets. N Engl J Med 338:653-661, 1998.

100. Pharoah MJ, Heersche JNM: 1,25-Dihydroxyvitamin D₃ causes an increase in the number of osteoclast-like cells in cat bone marrow cultures. Calcif Tissue Int 37:276-281, 1985.

101. Rubin J, Fan X, Thornton D, et al: Regulation of murine osteoblast macrophage colony-stimulating factor secretion by 1,25(OH)₂D₃. Calcif Tissue Int 59:291-296, 1996.

102. Horwood NJ, Elliott J, Martin TJ, Gillespie MT: Osteotropic agents regulate the expression of osteoclast differentiation factor and osteoprotegerin in osteoblastic stromal cells. Endocrinology 139:4743-4750, 1998.

103. Stern PH: Vitamin D and bone. Kidney Int 38:S17-S21, 1990.

104. Morrison NA, Qi JI, Tokita A, et al: Prediction of bone density from vitamin D receptor alleles. Nature 367:284-287, 1994.

105. Hustmyer FG, Peacock M, Hui S, et al: Bone mineral density in relation to polymorphism at the VDR gene locus. J Clin Invest 94:2130-2134, 1994.

106. Arden NK, Keen RW, Lanchbury JS, Spector TD: Polymorphisms of the VDR gene do not predict quantitative ultrasound of the calcaneus of hip axis length. Osteoporosis Int 6:334-337, 1996.

107. Sainz J, Tornout J, Loro L, et al: Vitamin D-receptor gene polymorphisms and bone density in prepubertal American girls of Mexican descent. N Engl J Med 337:77-82, 1997.

108. Austin LA, Heath H III: Calcitonin: Physiology and pathophysiology. N Engl J Med 304:269-278, 1981.

109. Arnaud CD, Kolb FO: The calciotropic hormones and metabolic bone disease. In Greenspan FS, Forsham PH (eds): Basic and Clinical Endocrinology. Los Altos, Calif, Lange Medical, 1983, pp 187-250.

110. Garret JE, Tamir H, Kifor O, et al: Calcitonin-secreting cells of the thyroid gland express and extracellular calcium-sensing receptor gene. Endocrinology 136:5202-5211, 1995.

111. Nicholson GC, Moseley JM, Sexton PM, et al: Abundant calcitonin receptors in isolated rat osteoclasts: Biochemical and autoradiographic characterization. J Clin Invest 78:355-360, 1986.

112. Chambers TJ, Athanasou NA, Fuller K: Effect of parathyroid hormone and calcitonin on the cytoplasmic spreading of isolated osteoclasts. J Endocrinol 102:281, 1984.

113. Murrills RJ, Dempster DW: The effects of stimulators of intracellular cyclic AMP on rat and chick osteoclasts in vitro: Validation of a simplified light microscope assay of bone resorption. Bone 11:333-344, 1990.

114. Raisz LG: Local and systemic factors in the pathogenesis of osteoporosis. N Engl J Med 318:818-828, 1988.

115. Takahashi S, Goldring S, Katz M, et al: Downregulation of calcitonin receptor mRNA expression by calcitonin during human osteoclast-like cell differentiation. J Clin Invest 95:167-171, 1995.

116. Raisz LG, Niemann I: Effect of phosphate, calcium and magnesium on bone resorption and hormonal responses in tissue culture. Endocrinology 85:446-452, 1969.

117. Yamaguchi DT, Hahn TJ, Beeker TG, et al: Relationship of cAMP and calcium messenger systems in prostaglandin-stimulated UMR-106 cells. J Biol Chem 263:10,745-10,753, 1988.

118. Cheng MZ, Zaman G, Rawlinson SC, et al: Mechanical loading and sex hormone interactions in organ cultures of rat ulna. J Bone Miner Res 11:502-511, 1996.

119. Eriksen EF, Colvard DS, Berg NJ, et al: Evidence of estrogen receptors in normal human osteoblast-like cells. Science 241:84-86, 1988.

120. Komm B, Terpening C, Benz D, et al: Estrogen binding, receptor mRNA, and biologic response in osteoblast-like osteosarcoma cells. Science 241:81-84, 1988.

121. Colvard DS, Eriksen EF, Keeting PE, et al: Identification of androgen receptors in normal human osteoblast-like cells. Proc Natl Acad Sci USA 86:854-857, 1989.

122. Ernst M, Schmid CH, Froesch ER: Enhanced osteoblast proliferation and collagen gene expression by estradiol. Proc Natl Acad Sci USA 85:2307-2310, 1988.

123. Rouleau MF, Warshawsky H, Goltzman D: Parathyroid hormone binding in vivo to renal, hepatic, and skeletal tissues of the rat using a radioautographic approach. Endocrinology 118:919-931, 1986.

124. Gray TK, Mohan S, Linkhart TA, Baylink DJ: Estradiol stimulates in vitro the secretion of insulin-like growth factors by the clonal osteoblastic cell line, UMR 106. Biochem Biophys Res Commun 158:407-412, 1989.

125. Oursler MJ, Pederson L, Pyfferoen J, et al: Estrogen modulation of avian osteoclast lysosomal gene expression. Endocrinology 132:1373-1380, 1993.

126. Shevde NK, Bendixen AC, Dienger KM, Pike JW: Estrogens suppress RANK ligand-induced osteoclast differentiation via a stromal cell independent mechanism involving c-Jun repression. Proc Natl Acad Sci USA 97(14):7829-7834, 2000.

127. Khosla S, Atkinson EJ, Dunstan CR, O'Fallon WM: Effect of estrogen versus testosterone on circulating osteoprotegerin and other cytokine levels in normal elderly men. J Clin Endocrinol Metab 87(4):1550-1554, 2002.

128. Smith EP, Boyd J, Frank GR, et al: Estrogen resistance caused by a mutation in the estrogen-receptor gene in a man. N Engl J Med 16:1056-1061, 1994.

129. Carani C, Qin K, Simoni M, et al: Effect of testosterone and estradiol in a man with aromatase deficiency. N Engl J Med 337:91-95, 1997.

130. Bilzekian JP, Morishima A, Bell J, Grumbach MM: Increased bone mass as a result of estrogen therapy in a man with aromatase deficiency. N Engl J Med 339:599-603, 1998.

131. Riggs BL, Khosla S, Melton LJ: A unitary model for involutional osteoporosis. J Bone Miner Res 13:763-773, 1998.

132. Christian JC, Yu P, Slemenda CW, Johnston CC: Heritability of bone mass. Am J Hum Genet 44:429-433, 1989.

133. Pocock NA, Eisman JA, Hopper JL, et al: Genetic determinants of bone mass in adults. J Clin Invest 80:706-710, 1987.

134. Finkelstein JS, Klibanski A, Neer RM: A longitudinal evaluation of bone mineral density in adult men with histories of delayed puberty. J Clin Endocrinol Metab 81:1152-1155, 1996.

135. Han ZH, Palnitkar S, Sudhaker Rao D, et al: Effects of ethnicity and age or menopause on the remodeling and turnover of iliac bone: Implications for mechanisms of bone loss. J Bone Miner Res 12:498-508, 1997.

136. Zhao G, Monier-Faugere MC, Langub MC, et al: Targeted overexpression of insulin-like growth factor I to osteoblasts of transgenic mice: increased trabecular bone volume without increased osteoblast proliferation. Endocrinology 141(7):2674-2682, 2000.

137. Adachi JD: Corticosteroid-induced osteoporosis. Am J Med Sci 313:41-49, 1997.

138. Mussolino ME, Looker AC, Madans JH, et al: Risk factors for hip fracture in white men: The NHANES I epidemiologic follow-up study. J Bone Miner Res 13:918-924.

139. Nguyen TV, Sambrook PN, Eisman JA: Bone loss, physical activity and weight change in elderly women: The Dubbo osteoporosis epidemiology study. J Bone Miner Res 13:1458-1467, 1998.

140. Zerwekh JE, Ruml LA, Gottschalk F, Pak CYC: The effects of 12 weeks of bed rest on bone histology, biochemical markers of bone turnover, and calcium homeostasis in 11 normal subjects. J Bone Miner Res 13:1594-1601, 1998.

141. Rubin CT, Hausman MR: The cellular basis of Wolff's law: Transduction of physical stimuli to skeletal adaptation. Rheum Dis Clin North Am 14:503-517, 1988.

142. Marcus R: Exercise: Moving in the right direction. J Bone Miner Res 13:1793-1796, 1998.

143. Bradney M, Pearce G, Naghton G, et al: Moderate exercise during growth in prepubertal boys: Changes in bone mass, size volumetric density and bone strength—A controlled prospective study. J Bone Miner Res 13:1814-1821, 1998.

144. Carter D, Wong A: Mechanical stresses and endochondral ossification in chondroepiphysis. J Orthop Res 6:148, 1988.

145. Rubin C, Turner AS, Bain S, et al: Anabolism. Low mechanical signals strengthen long bones. Nature 412:603-604, 2001.

146. Fisher LW, Gehron RP, Tuross N, et al: The Mr 24,000 phosphoprotein from developing bone is the NH_2-terminal propeptide of the α chain of type I collagen. J Biol Chem 262: 13,457-13,463, 1987.

147. Noda M, Yoon, Prince CW, et al: Transcriptional regulation of osteopontin production in rat osteosarcoma cells by type β transforming growth factor. J Biol Chem 263:13,916, 1988.

148. Price PA, Otsuka AS, Poser JW, et al: Characterization of gamma-carboxyglutamic acid containing protein from bone. Proc Natl Acad Sci USA 73:1447, 1976.

149. Urist MR, Juo YK, Brownell AG, et al: Purification of bovine bone morphogenetic protein by hydroxyapatite chromatography. Proc Natl Acad Sci USA 81:371, 1984.

150. Termine JD, Belcourt AB, Conn KM, et al: Mineral and collagen-binding proteins of fetal calf bone. J Biol Chem 256:10,403, 1981.

151. Robey PG, Bosky A: The biochemistry of bone. In Marcus R, Feldman D, Kelsey J: Osteoporosis. San Diego, Calif, Academic Press, 1996, pp 95-183.

152. Pritchard JJ: General histology of bone. In Bourne GH (ed): The Biochemistry and Physiology of Bone, 2nd ed. Vol I. New York, Academic Press, 1972, p 15.

153. Ascenzi A, Bonucci E: Relationship between ultrastructure and "pin test" in osteons. Clin Orthop 121:275, 1976.

154. Eyre DR: Collagen: Molecular diversity in the body's protein scaffold. Science 207:1315, 1980.

155. Boskey AL, Posner AS: Bone structure, composition and mineralization. Orthop Clin North Am 15:597, 1984.

156. Veis A, Sharkey M, Dickson I: Non-collagenous proteins of bone and dentin extracellular matrix and their role in organized mineral deposition. In Wasserman RH (ed): Calcium Binding Proteins and Calcium Function. New York, Elsevier, 1977, pp 409-418.

157. Glimcher MJ: Studies of the structure, organization and reactivity of bone collagen. In Gibson T (ed): Proceedings of the International Symposium on Wound Healing. Nice, France, Montreaux Foundation of International Cooperative Medical Science, 1975, p 253.

158. Herring GM: The chemical structure of tendon cartilage, dentin and bone matrix. Clin Orthop 60:261, 1968.

159. Skerry TM, Suswillo R, ElHaj AJ, et al: Load-induced proteoglycan orientation in bone tissue in vivo and in vitro. Calcif Tissue Int 46:318-326, 1990.

160. Hauschka PV, Lian JB, Cole DEC, Gundberg CM: Osteocalcin and matrix Gla protein: Vitamin K-dependent protein in bone. Physiol Rev 69:990-1047, 1988.

161. Lian JB, Coutts M, Canalis E: Studies of hormonal regulation of osteocalcin synthesis in cultured fetal rat calvariae. J Biol Chem 260:8706-8710, 1985.

162. Boskey AL, Gadaleta S, Gundberg C, et al: Fourier transform infrared microspectroscopic analysis of bones of osteocalcin-deficient mice provides insight into the function of osteocalcin. Bone 23:187-196, 1998.

163. Weiner S, Traub W: Bone structure: From angstroms to microns. FASEB J 6:879-885, 1992.

164. Posner AS: Crystal chemistry of bone mineral. Physiol Rev 49:760, 1969.

165. Moradian-Oldak J, Weiner S, Addadi L, et al: Electron imaging and diffraction study of individual crystals of bone, mineralized tendon and synthetic carbonate apatite. Connect Tissue Res 25:219-228, 1991.

166. Bonar LC, Roufosse AH, Sabine WK, et al: X-ray diffraction studies of the crystallinity of bone mineral in newly synthesized and density fractionated bone. Calcif Tissue Int 35:202-209, 1983.

167. Rubin CT, Bain S, McLeod KJ: Suppression of the osteogenic response in the aging skeleton. Calcif Tissue Int 50:306-313, 1992.

168. Lian JB, Gundberg CM: Osteocalcin: Biochemical considerations and clinical applications. Clin Orthop 262:267-291, 1988.

169. Rosen CJ, Chesnut CH III, Mallinak NJ: The predictive value of biochemical markers of bone turnover for bone mineral density in early postmenopausal women treated with hormone replacement or calcium supplementation. J Clin Endocrinol Metab 82:1904-1910, 1997.

170. Ross PD, Knowlton W: Rapid bone loss is associated with increased levels of biochemical markers. J Bone Miner Res 13:297-302, 1998.

171. Greenspan SL, Parker RA, Ferguson L, et al: Early changes in biochemical markers of bone turnover predict the long-term response to alendronate therapy in representative elderly women: A randomized clinical trial. J Bone Miner Res 13:1431-1438, 1998.

172. Seemon E: From density to structure: Growing up and growing old on the surfaces of bone. J Bone Miner Res 12:509-521, 1997.

173. Howard GM, Nguyen TV, Harris M, et al: Genetic and environmental contributions to the association between quantitative ultrasound and bone mineral density measurements: a twin study. J Bone Miner Res 13:1318-1327, 1998.

174. Christoffersen J, Landis WJ: A contribution with review to the description of bone and other calcified tissues in vivo. Anat Rec 230:435-450, 1991.

175. Jowsey J: Microradiography: A morphologic approach to quantitating bone turnover. Excerpta Medica International Congress Series No. 270. Amsterdam, Excerpta Medica Foundation, 1972, p 114.

176. Glimcher MJ, Lian JB (eds): The Chemistry and Biology of Mineralized Tissues. Proceedings of the Third International Conference on the Chemistry and Biology of Mineralized Tissues. New York, Gordon and Breach Science, 1988.

177. Wuthier RE, Jajeska RJ, Collins GM: Biosynthesis of matrix vesicles in epiphyseal cartilage. I. In vivo incorporation of ^{32}P-orthophosphate into phospholipid of chondrocyte, membrane and matrix vesicle fractions. Calcif Tissue Res 23:135-139, 1977.

178. Kerr JFR, Wyllie AH, Currie AR: Apoptosis: A basic biological phenomenon with wide ranging implications in tissue kinetics. Br J Cancer 26:239, 1972.

179. Russell RGG, Caswell AM, Hearn PR, Sharrard RM: Calcium in mineralized tissues and pathological calcification. Br Med Bull 42:435, 1986.

180. Anderson HC: Electron microscopic studies of induced cartilage development and calcification. J Cell Biol 35:81, 1967.

181. Anderson HC: Matrix vesicle calcification: Review and update. In Peck WA (ed): Bone and Mineral Research. Vol 3. New York, Elsevier, 1985, p 109-150.

182. Wuthier RE: Lipid composition of isolated cartilage cells, membranes and matrix vesicles. Biochim Biophys Acta 409:128, 1975.

183. Endo A, Glimcher MJ: The potential role of phosphoproteins in the in vitro calcification of bone collagen. In Goldberg VM (ed): Transactions of the 32nd Meeting of Orthopaedic Research Society. Chicago, Adept Printing, 1986, p 221.

184. Hartgerink JD, Beniash E, Stupp SI: Self-assembly and mineralization of peptide-amphiphile nanofibers. Science 294(5547): 1684-1688, 2001.

185. Puzas JE: Phosphotyrosine phosphatase activity in bone cells: An old enzyme with a new function. Adv Protein Phosphatases 3:237-256, 1986.

186. Anderson HC: Biology of disease: Mechanism of mineral formation in bone. Lab Invest 60:320, 1989.

187. Wuthier RE: The role of phospholipids in biological calcification: Distribution of phospholipase activity in calcifying epiphyseal cartilage. Clin Orthop 90:191, 1973.

188. Peress NS, Anderson HC, Sajdcra SW: The lipids of matrix vesicles from bovine fetal epiphyseal cartilage. Calcif Tissue Res 14:275, 1974.

189. Termine JD, Belcourt AB, Conn KM, et al: Mineral and collagen-binding proteins of fetal calf bone. J Biol Chem 256:10,403, 1981.

190. Hynes RO: The molecular biology of fibronectin. Annu Rev Cell Biol 1:67, 1985.

191. Glimcher MJ, Krane SM: The organization and structure of bone and the mechanism of calcification. In Ramachandran GN, Gould BS (eds): Treatise on Collagen. Vol 11B. Biology of Collagen. New York, Academic Press, 1968, p 221.

192. Baylink D, Wengedal J, Thompson E: Loss of protein polysaccharides at sites where bone mineralization is initiated. J Histochem Cytochem 20:279, 1972.

193. Glimcher MJ: Composition, structure and organization of bone and other mineralized tissues and the mechanism of calcification. In Handbook of Physiology: Endocrinology. Vol VII. Baltimore, Williams & Wilkins, 1976, p 25.

194. Parfitt AL: Bone histomorphometry: Proposed system for standardization of nomenclature, symbols and units. Calcif Tissue Int 42:284-286, 1988.

195. Hayes WC, Gerhart TN: Biomechanics of bone: Applications for assessment of bone strength. In Peck WA (ed): Bone and Mineral Research, 3rd ed. New York, Elsevier, 1985, p 259.

196. Lanyon LE: Analysis of surface bone strain in the calcaneus of sheep during normal locomotion: Strain analysis of the calcaneus. J Biomech 6:41-49, 1973.

197. Ascenzi A: The micromechanics versus the macromechanics of cortical bone: A comprehensive presentation. J Biomech Eng 110:357-363, 1988.

198. Martin RB, Burr DB, Sharkey N: Skeletal Tissue Mechanics. New York, Springer-Verlag, 1998.

199. Jones BH, Harris J McA, Vinh TN, Rubin CT: Exercise-induced stress fractures and stress reactions of bone: Epidemiology, etiology, and classification. Exerc Sport Sci Rev 17:379-422, 1989.

200. Rubin CT, Gross T, McLeod K, Bain SD: Morphologic stages in lamellar bone formation stimulated by a potent mechanical stimulus. J Bone Miner Res 10:488-495, 1995.

201. Albright JA, Skinner HCW: Bone: Structural organization and remodeling dynamics. In Albright JA, Brand RA (eds): The Scientific Basis of Orthopaedics, 2nd ed. East Norwalk, Conn, Appleton & Lange, 1987, pp 161-198.

202. Frost HM: Secondary osteon population densities: An algorithm for estimating the missing osteons. Yearbook Phys Anthropol 30:221-238, 1987.

203. Ascenzi A, Benvenuti A: Orientation of collagen fibers at the boundary between two successive osteonic lamellae and its mechanical interpretation. J Biomech 19:455-463, 1986.

204. Schaffler MB, Burr DB, Fredrickson RG: Morphology of the osteonal cement line in human bone. Anat Rec 217:223-228, 1987.

205. Garn SM: The course of bone gain and the phases of bone loss. Orthop Clin North Am 3:503, 1972.

206. Ruff CV, Hayes WC: Subperiosteal expansion and cortical remodeling of the human femur and tibia with aging. Science 217:945, 1982.

207. Enlow DH: Principles of Bone Remodeling. Springfield, Ill, Charles C Thomas, 1963.

208. Koch JC: The laws of bone architecture. Am J Anat 21:177, 1917.

209. Lanyon LE, Rubin CT, Baust G: Modulation of bone loss during calcium insufficiency by controlled dynamic loading. Calcif Tissue Int 38:209-216, 1986.

210. Bain SD, Rubin CT: Metabolic modulation of disuse osteopenia: Endocrine-dependent site specificity of bone remodeling. J Bone Miner Res 5:1069-1075, 1990.

211. Rubin CT: The benefits and consequences of structural adaptation in bone. In Fitzgerald R (ed): Non-Cemented Total Hip Arthroplasty. New York, Raven Press, 1988, pp 41-48.

212. Brown TD, Pedersen DR, Gray ML, et al: Toward an identification of mechanical parameters initiating periosteal remodeling: A combined experimental and analytic approach. J Biomech 23:893-905, 1990.

213. Radin EL, Martin RB, Burr DB, et al: Effects of mechanical loading on the tissues of the rabbit knee. J Orthop Res 2: 221-234, 1984.

214. O'Connor JA, Lanyon LE, MacFie H: The influence of strain rate on adaptive bone remodeling. J Biomech 15:767-781, 1982.

215. Rubin C, Gross T, Donahue H, et al: Physical and environmental influences on bone formation. In Brighton CT, Friedlaender GE, Lane JM (eds): Bone Formation and Repair. Rosemont, Ill, American Academy of Orthopaedic Surgeons, 1994, pp 61-78.

216. Bassett CA: Fundamental and practical aspects of therapeutic uses of pulsed electromagnetic fields (PEMFs). Crit Rev Biomed Eng 17:451-529, 1989.

217. Heckman J, Ryaby J, McCabe J, et al: Acceleration of tibial fracture healing by noninvasive low intensity ultrasound. J Bone Joint Surg Am 76:165-174, 1994.

218. Rubin C, Turner AS, Muller R, et al: Quantity and quality of trabecular bone in the femur are enhanced by a strongly anabolic, noninvasive mechanical intervention. J Bone Miner Res 17:349-357, 2002.

219. Shim SS: Physiology of blood circulation of bone. J Bone Joint Surg Am 50:812, 1968.

220. Sledge CB: Epiphyseal injuries. In Cave EF, Burke JF, Boyd RJ (eds): Trauma Management. Chicago, Year Book Medical, 1974, pp 152-161.

221. Cowin SC: Bone Mechanics. Boca Raton, Fla, CRC Press, 2001.

222. Ascenzi A, Bell GH: Bone as a mechanical engineering problem. *In* Bourne GH (ed): The Biochemistry and Physiology of Bone. Vol 1: Structure. New York, Academic Press, 1972, p 311.

223. Reilly DT, Burstein AH: The elastic and ultimate properties of compact bone tissue. J Biomech 8:393-405, 1975.

224. Carter DR, Harris WH, Caler WE: The mechanical and biological response of cortical bone to in vivo strain histories. *In* Cowin SC (ed): Mechanical Properties of Bone. Vol 45. New York, American Society of Mechanical Engineers, 1981, pp 81-92.

225. Curry JD: Mechanical properties of bone with greatly differing functions. J Biomech 12:313, 1979.

226. Lanyon LE, Rubin CT: Functional adaptation in skeletal structures. *In* Hildebrand M, Bramble DM, Leim KF, Wake DB (eds): Functional Vertebrate Morphology. Cambridge, Harvard University Press, 1985, pp 1-25.

227. Woo SLY: The relationships of changes in stress levels on long bone remodeling. *In* Cowen S (ed): Mechanical Properties of Bone, AMD. Vol 45. New York, American Society of Mechanical Engineers, 1981, p 107.

228. Rubin CT, Lanyon LE: Limb mechanics as a function of speed and gait: A study of functional strains in the radius and tibia of horse and dog. J Exp Biol 101:187-211, 1982.

229. Gross T, McLeod K, Rubin C: Characterizing bone strain distributions in vivo using three triple rosette strain gages. J Biomech 25:1081-1087, 1992.

230. Rubin CT: Skeletal strain and the functional strain significance of bone architecture. Calcif Tissue Int 36:S11-S18, 1984.

231. Lanyon LE: The influence of function on the development of bone curvature: An experimental study on the rat tibia. J Zool Lond 192:457-466, 1980.

232. Rubin CT, Lanyon LE: Dynamic strain similarity in vertebrates: An alternative to allometric limb bone scaling. J Theor Biol 107:321-327, 1984.

233. Rubin CT, Lanyon LE: Osteoregulatory nature of mechanical stimuli: Function as a determinant for adaptive remodeling in bone. J Orthop Res 5:300-310, 1987.

234. Jones HH, Pries JD, Hayes WC, et al: Humeral hypertrophy in response to exercise. J Bone Joint Surg Am 59:204-208, 1977.

235. Donaldson CL, Hulley SB, Vogel JM, et al: Effect of prolonged bed rest on bone mineral. Metabolism 19:1071, 1970.

236. Rubin CT, Lanyon LE: Regulation of bone mass by mechanical loading. Calcif Tissue Int 37:411, 1985.

237. Lanyon LE, Goodship AE, Pye C, MacFie H: Mechanically adaptive bone remodeling: A quantitative study on function adaptation in the radius following ulna osteotomy in sheep. J Biomech 15:141-154, 1982.

238. Lanyon LE, Rubin CT: Static versus dynamic loads as an influence on bone remodeling. J Biomech 17:897, 1984.

239. Rubin CT, Lanyon LE: Regulation of bone formation by applied dynamic loads. J Bone Joint Surg Am 66:397-402, 1984.

240. Sun Y, McLeod K, Rubin C: Upregulation of collagen type 1 mRNA following mechanical loading as measured by in situ RT PCR. Trans 41st Orthop Res Soc 20:290, 1995.

241. Rubin CT, McLeod KJ: Biologic modulation of mechanical influence in bone remodeling. *In* Mow VC, Ratcliffe A, Woo SLY (eds): Biomechanics of Diarthrodial Joints. Vol II. New York, Springer-Verlag, 1990, pp 97-118.

242. You L, Cowin SC, Schaffler MB, Weinbaum S: A model for strain amplification in the actin cytoskeleton of osteocytes due to fluid drag on pericellular matrix. J Biomech 34:1375-1386, 2001.

243. McLeod KJ, Rubin CT: The effect of low frequency electric fields on osteogenesis. J Bone Joint Surg Am 74:920-929, 1992.

244. Rubin CT, Sommerfeldt DW, Judex S, Qin Y: Inhibition of osteopenia by low magnitude, high-frequency mechanical stimuli. Drug Discov Today 6:848-858, 2001.

245. Fritton SP, McLeod KJ, Rubin CT: Quantifying the strain history of bone: Spatial uniformity and self-similarity of low-magnitude strains. J Biomech 33:317-325, 2000.

246. Berretta D, Pollack SR: Ion concentration effects on the zeta potential of bone. J Orthop Res 4:337-345, 1986.

247. Bassett CA: Biophysical principles affecting bone structure. *In* Bourne GH (ed): The Biochemistry and Physiology of Bone. Vol 3. New York, Academic Press, 1971, pp 1-76.

248. Brighton CT, McCluskey WP: Cellular response and mechanism of action of electrically induced osteogenesis. *In* Peck WA (ed): Bone and Mineral Research, 4th ed. New York, Elsevier, 1986, p 213-254.

249. Ashihara T, Kagawa K, Kamich M, et al: ³H-Thymidine autoradiographic studies of the cell proliferation and differentiation in electrically stimulated osteogenesis. *In* Brighton CT, Black J, Pollack SR (eds): Electrical Properties of Bone and Cartilage. New York, Grune & Stratton, 1979, pp 401-426.

250. McLeod KJ, Lee RD, Ehrlich HP: Frequency dependence of electric field modulation of fibroblast protein synthesis. Science 236:1465-1469, 1987.

251. Otter M, McLeod K, Rubin C: Electromagnetic fields in experimental fracture healing. Clin Orthop 355:90-104, 1998.

252. McLeod K, Fontaine MA, Donahue HJ, Rubin CT: Electric fields modulate bone cell function in a density dependent manner. J Bone Miner Res 8:977-983, 1993.

253. Rubin J, McLeod K, Titus L, et al: Formation of osteoclast-like cells is suppressed by low frequency, low intensity electric fields. J Orthop Res 14:7-15, 1996.

90

Metabolic Bone Disease

NANCY LANE · MERYL S. LEBOFF

Osteoporosis is characterized by low bone density and a deterioration of bone microarchitecture that reduces bone strength and increases the risk of fracture. The hallmark of osteoporosis is the loss of both of bone mineral and bone matrix with the maintenance of a normal mineral-to-matrix ratio. Bone consists of organic matrix (collagen and noncollagenous proteins) and an inorganic mineral component (calcium and phosphate in hydroxyapatite [HA] crystals). Normally, bone turnover is tightly coupled with osteoclast-mediated bone resorption followed by osteoblast-stimulated bone formation; this delicate balance in bone remodeling results in no net change in skeletal mass. Osteoblasts synthesize osteoid, bone that subsequently undergoes mineralization and becomes mature bone matrix. The skeleton contains approximately 80 percent cortical bone, which is concentrated in the appendicular skeleton and femoral neck, and 20 percent more metabolically active trabecular bone, which is located in the spine, epiphyses, and pelvis. Osteoporosis is characterized by reduced bone mass; osteomalacia encompasses disorders in which there is decreased mineralization of bony matrix. Paget's disease is a skeletal disorder characterized by increased rates of bone turnover with the development of disorganized woven bone.

Osteoporosis

EPIDEMIOLOGY AND CLINICAL SIGNS

Osteoporosis, the most common metabolic bone disease, affects 200 million individuals worldwide. Approximately 28 million Americans have osteoporosis or are at risk for osteoporosis. Osteoporosis, or porous bone, is a "disease characterized by low bone mass and structural deterioration of bone tissue, leading to bone fragility and an increased susceptibility to fractures, especially of the hip, spine and wrist."[1] Although usually asymptomatic, osteoporosis can produce the clinical signs and symptoms of loss of height, pain, a dowager's hump, and an increased risk of fracture. After 50 years of age, there is an exponential rise in fractures such that 40 percent of women and 13 percent of men develop one or more osteoporotic fractures in their lifetime. In the United States alone, there are more than 1.5 million osteoporotic fractures annually, including 250,000 hip, 250,000 wrist, and 500,000 vertebral fractures. Hip fractures are associated with a 12- to 24-percent mortality rate in women and a 30-percent mortality rate in men within the first year of fracture, and 50 percent of patients are unable to ambulate independently and require long-term nursing home care.[2] These numbers should continue to grow exponentially as the elderly population of industrialized nations increases over the next 10 years. Bone accretion occurs during adolescence, when there is a large increment in bone mass. Peak bone density is normally achieved after puberty and into the third decade of life. However, by age 22, most individuals have achieved their peak bone mass. At menopause, an acceleration of bone loss usually occurs over approximately 5 to 8 years, with an annual 2- to 3-percent loss of trabecular and 1- to 2-percent loss of cortical bone. Both men and women lose bone with age. Over a lifetime, women lose approximately 50 percent of trabecular and 30 percent of cortical bone, whereas men generally lose two thirds of these amounts.[3] Osteoporosis was previously thought to be a silent disease that was part of the normal aging process; however, the advent of bone densitometry has made it possible to identify patients at risk for osteoporosis accurately and reproducibly so that prevention and treatment strategies can be instituted to reduce this sharp rise in fractures with age. With a health care expenditure of $13.8 billion annually for osteoporosis-related fractures and a projected threefold rise in these costs over the next 40 years in the United States, the institution of effective prevention and treatment strategies to reduce fractures is of great importance.[1,4]

PATHOPHYSIOLOGY OF MENOPAUSAL AND AGE-RELATED BONE LOSS AND OSTEOPOROSIS

Bone is constantly undergoing remodeling, with areas of resorption produced by osteoclastic action being replaced by bone laid down by osteoblasts. Osteoporosis results from an imbalance between bone resorption and formation. The initiation of bone remodeling is still being debated. However, the osteocytes, or terminally differentiated osteoblasts, located within the bone matrix and connected to each other and the bone surface may release chemical mediators that attract osteoclasts to the bone surface (Figs. 90–1A, 90–1B). Osteoclasts originate from the colony-forming unit granulocyte-monocytes (CFU-GMs), are attracted to the bone surface, attach to bone matrix, and resorb the bone tissue. Generally, bone resorption is rapid and a resorption pit is made within 10 to 14 days. After resorption is complete, osteoblasts, derived from the bone marrow stromal cells, attach to the resorbed bone surface and produce osteoid, which is then mineralized. Bone formation can take up to 3 or 4 months. Therefore, a normal bone remodeling cycle in

BONE REMODELING

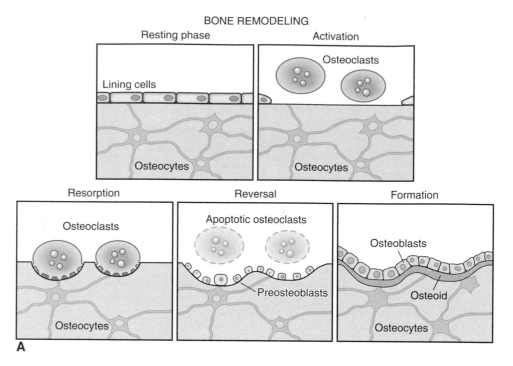

FIGURE 90-1A · The Bone Remodeling Cycle. Osteocytes most likely release chemicals to the bone surface that attract osteoclasts. Osteoclasts attach to the bone matrix, create a tight ring, and release acid that lowers the pH and dissolves the mineral from the bone matrix. After the mineral is released, the demineralized matrix is broken down. The osteoclast leaves the bone surface and an osteoblast is attracted to the area of the bone that was resorbed. The resorption phase is about 10 to 14 days. Osteoblasts produce new bone, or osteoid, that fills in the resorption pit. Also, some of the osteoblasts are left within the bone matrix as osteocytes. The osteoid mineralizes over time, about 3 months, and the bone remodeling cycle is complete.

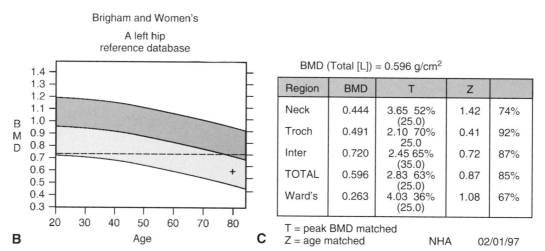

FIGURE 90-1B · *A,* Dual x-ray absorptiometry (DXA) bone mineral density (BMD) measurement in the proximal femur of a postmenopausal woman. *B* and *C,* The patient's bone density is compared with both the mean young, normal bone density and age-matched and gender-matched controls. The T-score and Z-score represent the number of standard deviations below young, normal and age-matched controls, respectively. Because the bone density provides a gradient of risk of fracture, therapies may be instituted to prevent the development of osteoporosis or to treat patients at increased risk for a fracture.

adults can last 4 to 6 months (Fig. 90–1A). A number of metabolic changes such as estrogen deficiency, immobilization, metabolic acidosis, hyperparathyroidism, and systemic and local inflammatory diseases can increase osteoclast number and activity, uncoupling bone turnover. This results in greater bone resorption than bone formation and a net loss of bone tissue. Recently, there are new data that show that a number of local factors in bone affect the regulation of bone formation and resorption and the coupling of these processes; these include prostaglandins, insulin-like growth factors (IGFs), interleukins (IL-1, IL-6, and IL-11), tumor necrosis factor

(TNF), and transforming growth factor (TGF).[5] Animal studies have shown that IL-1, IL-6, and TNF knockout mice do not lose bone with estrogen deficiency.[6] In addition, inflammatory arthritis animal models find that TNF, IL-1, and IL-6 are all strong stimulators of osteoclastic bone resorption. This link between the immune system and the maintenance of bone mass is very intriguing but requires additional work.

A number of mechanisms underlie primary osteoporosis, including a low peak bone mass as a young adult and rapid bone loss during menopause. Factors contributing to age-related bone loss, in turn, include impaired calcium absorption with age, a compensatory rise in parathyroid hormone (PTH) levels, and greater resorption than formation of bone. Estrogen deficiency is associated with the release of cytokines IL-1, IL-6, TNF, and receptor activator of NFκB ligand (RANKL), which leads to the recruitment and stimulation of osteoclasts in the marrow and increased production of bone-resorptive cytokines that may contribute to menopause-related bone loss.[5] Estrogen therapy, however, inhibits IL-1 release, and in oophorectomized rats an inhibitor of IL-1 (the IL-1 receptor antagonist) suppresses bone loss.[6] IL-6 levels also increase with age in human marrow cultures[7] and in peripheral monocytes. IL-1 and TNF induce the production of IL-6 from osteoblasts and stromal cells. Further evidence supporting a role of IL-6 in bone turnover includes data showing that oophorectomized IL-6 knockout transgenic mice do not lose bone. Recently, two other proteins have been identified that influence osteoclast activity: osteoprotegerin (OPG) and RANKL, which are produced by osteoblasts.[8] Estrogen deficiency increases osteoblast production of RANKL, which stimulates maturation and activity of osteoclasts by attaching to RANK on the surface of immature and mature osteoclasts. Simultaneously, estrogen deficiency decreases osteoblast production of OPG, the decoy receptor that reduces RANKL production and activity. Adenoviral delivery of OPG ameliorates bone resorption in a mouse ovariectomy model of osteoporosis.[8]

In addition, a number of genetic, nutritional, and lifestyle risk factors predispose to the development of osteoporosis. Caucasians and Asians are at risk for low bone mass and osteoporosis, whereas African Americans have a higher bone density and one-third to one-half the number of fractures.[1,8,9] Some studies show that African Americans have lower vitamin D and urinary calcium levels, higher PTH levels, and skeletal resistance to the effects of PTH on bone.[9,10,11] Studies in twins and families show that up to 80 percent of the variance in bone mass is accounted for by genetic factors.[12] A maternal history of a hip fracture, for example, is associated with a twofold increased risk of a hip fracture.[13] Data from Uitterlinden and colleagues show that the gene encoding collagen type IA1 is associated with low bone density with increasing age and an increased risk of fracture.[14] In the ss allele group, bone density was 12 percent lower at the femoral neck and 20 percent lower at the lumbar spine than that in the SS group, indicating an increased gene-dose effect with increasing age. However, *COLIA1* is associated with a lower baseline bone density and not an increased rate of bone loss. Furthermore, genetically determined architectural features of bone such as a long hip axis length may contribute to increased fracture risk; conversely, a short hip axis length confers some protective effect on the risk of hip fracture.[15] Recently, a family has been described that have very high bone mass and are otherwise phenotypically normal. This family has a mutation (an amino acid change) in the low-density lipoprotein receptor–related protein 5 (LRP5). Using in situ hybridization to a rat tibia, expression of the LRP5 was detected in areas of bone involved in remodeling. Additional studies have reported that this LRP5 mutation increases Wnt signaling, which may alter bone mass through a primary defect on bone formation. Individuals affected with this mutation demonstrated normal levels of bone resorption but specific markers of bone formation were strikingly elevated. The observation that LRP5 is expressed at high levels in osteoblasts is consistent with its having a role in this area. Further work is now required to determine if other mutations in the chromosome containing the LRP5 segment are associated with variation in bone density in the general population.[16,17]

Other risk factors for osteoporosis, as outlined in Table 90–1, include low body weight and reduced gonadal steroid levels.[12] Lifestyle factors that may contribute to the development of osteoporosis include cigarette smoking, excessive alcohol intake, reduced physical activity, and inadequate calcium intake, according to some reports. Cigarette smokers have poorer health than nonsmokers, have impaired calcium absorption, exercise less, and have lower estrogen levels, earlier menopause, and more fractures; smoking cessation reverses this risk of osteoporosis.

In a large, prospective study of 9516 women older than 65 years, the following lifestyle factors significantly increased the risk of a hip fracture: no walking for exercise, intake of more than two cups of coffee daily, current use of long-acting benzodiazepines and anticonvulsant drugs, current weight less than weight at age 25 years, height greater than 5 feet 7 inches, age older than 80 years, fracture since age 50 years, inability to stand from a chair without using arms, poor depth perception, and self evaluation of health as fair to poor.[13] Low bone density in conjunction with a fall or trauma predisposes the individual to a fracture. Poor health and compromise of neuromuscular function increase the risk of osteoporosis and falls, which, in turn, increases the risk of hip fracture.[13] Importantly, elderly Caucasian women with both a low bone mass and more than two risk factors show nearly a 20-fold increased risk for a fracture. Secondary causes of bone loss that can affect women and men of all ages and races are listed in Table 90–2. Glucocorticoid therapy is the most common secondary cause of bone loss; osteoporotic fractures develop in an estimated 30 to 50 percent of glucocorticoid-treated patients.[18] Glucocorticoid therapy causes bone loss through a number of different mechanisms, including producing negative calcium balance through impaired intestinal calcium absorption, increasing urinary calcium excretion, decreasing bone

---

TABLE 90–1 · RISK FACTORS FOR OSTEOPOROSIS

Primary
  Previous fracture at <50 yr, parent or sibling with previous fractures, cigarette smoking, weight <127 lb or height >5 ft, 7 in
Secondary
  Nonmodifiable
    White race, advanced age, frailty or poor health, dementia
  Modifiable
    Low calcium intake, eating disorder, low testosterone levels (men), premenopausal estrogen deficiency (amenorrhea >1 yr or menopause at age <45 yr), excessive alcohol intake, physical inactivity, impaired vision, neurologic disorders, lack of sunlight exposure

TABLE 90–2 • MEDICAL DISORDERS OR MEDICATIONS ASSOCIATED WITH BONE LOSS AND OSTEOPOROSIS

Primary osteoporosis	Juvenile osteoporosis, postmenopausal osteoporosis (type I), involutional osteoporosis (type II)
Endocrine abnormalities	Glucocorticoid excess, thyroid hormone excess (supraphysiologic), hypogonadism including prolactinomas or anorexia nervosa, hyperparathyroidism, hypercalciuria
Processes affecting the marrow	Multiple myeloma, leukemia, Gaucher's disease
Immobilization	Space flight
Gastrointestinal diseases	Gastrectomy, primary biliary cirrhosis, celiac disease
Connective tissue disorders	Osteogenesis imperfecta, homocystinuria, Ehlers-Danlos syndrome
Rheumatologic disorders	Ankylosing spondylitis, rheumatoid arthritis
Other medications	Anticonvulsants, heparin, methotrexate, Cytoxan (cyclophosphamide) and GnRH agonists (hypogonadism), lithium, cyclosporine, aluminum, excessive alcohol, premenopausal tamoxifen

Abbreviation: GnRH, Gonadotropin-releasing hormone.

Modified from LeBoff MS: Calcium and metabolic bone disease. *In* Medical Knowledge Self Assessment Program (MKSAP X). Philadelphia, American College of Physicians, 1995.

formation, increasing bone resorption by stimulating osteoclast activity by macrophage colony-stimulating factor (M-CSF), and suppression of endogenous gonadal steroid production.[18] Therapy with glucocorticoids leads to an early and, in some instances, dramatic loss of trabecular bone, with less effect on cortical bone. In hyperthyroidism (e.g., Graves' disease or toxic nodule) or supraphysiologic therapy with thyroid hormone, the ensuing accelerated bone turnover may produce a reduction in bone mass when the thyroid-stimulating hormone level is suppressed, even when thyroid hormone levels are within the normal range.[19] Athletic amenorrhea, anorexia nervosa, and other hypogonadal states, including the use of gonadotropin-releasing hormone agonists,[20,21] may result in bone loss. In addition to estrogen deficiency, women with anorexia nervosa have low levels of IGF-I and reduced levels of adrenal androgen dehydroepiandrosterenedione that may contribute to the development of osteoporosis.[22]

Patients with rheumatoid arthritis (RA) experience periarticular and generalized bone loss, with an increased incidence of fractures compared to the general population.[23] Both T lymphocytes and tissue macrophages, and probably fibroblasts, release both inflammatory cytokines (IL-1, TNF, IL-6,) and RANKL that stimulate preosteoclasts in the bone marrow and synovium to mature actively resorb bone.[24,25] In an animal model of inflammatory arthritis induced with collagen, animals pretreated with OPG did not have bone loss within the periarticular bone or the presence of erosions.[26] Additional factors that may contribute to osteoporosis in RA include decreased mobility and glucocorticoid therapy.[27] Some data, however, show that low-dose glucocorticoid therapy in women with RA does not have adverse skeletal effects, possibly because of a decrease in disease activity in association with suppression of inflammatory cytokines and improved physical activity and function.[28,29] Ankylosing spondylitis (AS) is also associated with fractures and reduced bone density in the spine and proximal femur, even early in the disease.[30] Infiltrative processes in the marrow, such as multiple myeloma, mastocytosis, and Gaucher's disease, may produce osteoporosis. Patients with Gaucher's disease show an accumulation of glucocerebrosides in macrophages in the spleen, liver, and bone marrow, which causes hepatosplenomegaly, anemia, thrombocytopenia, bone infarcts and infections, fractures, and aseptic necrosis.[31] The immunosuppressant drug Cytoxan (cyclophosphamide) induces amenorrhea and hypogonadism, which may increase the risk of bone loss. In rodent models, the immunosuppressive drug cyclosporine produces a time- and dose-dependent bone loss[32]; in contrast, azathioprine (Imuran) and rapamycin (Sirolimus) do not appear to affect skeletal homeostasis adversely.[33] Therapy with both cyclosporine and prednisone in transplant recipients is associated with early accelerated bone loss after the initiation of treatment with these immunosuppressant agents and the development of osteoporosis and fractures with continued exposure.[34]

Vitamin D deficiency may also manifest as osteopenia and fractures, but this condition is both preventable and treatable.[35] Unlike the situation in osteoporosis, very low vitamin D levels are often characterized by a mineralization defect and osteomalacia. Vitamin D deficiency may be present in up to 50 percent of women with hip fractures.[35]

DIAGNOSTIC MEASUREMENTS TO ASSESS BONE DENSITY AND OSTEOPOROTIC RISK

Osteoporosis may first be diagnosed on a radiograph with signs of demineralization or evidence of compression fractures of vertebral bodies on a spinal film. Because an estimated 25 to 50 percent of bone mass must be lost to show osteopenia on radiographs, conventional radiography is an insensitive technique for diagnosing bone loss. Radiographs may demonstrate signs of secondary causes of osteoporosis, such as the presence of subperiosteal resorption in hyperparathyroidism, characteristic lytic changes or bone infarcts in Gaucher's disease, local sites of lytic destruction in malignancy, and pseudofractures in osteomalacia. Bone densitometry makes it possible to measure the amount of bone in the relevant fracture sites of the spine, forearm, and proximal femur as well as the total body.

Techniques for evaluating bone mass have included the use of dual-energy x-ray absorptiometry (DEXA) and quantitative computed tomography (CT) scanning of the spine.[1,2] Bone density evaluations using DEXA incorporate the attenuation of soft tissue and bone by x-rays to calculate the bone mineral density (BMD). DEXA is both precise and safe, with a very low radiation exposure. With reproducibility errors of approximately 0.6 to 1.5 percent, this technique is able to detect small changes over time.[2,36,37] Furthermore, newer DEXA techniques measure bone density rapidly in 0.5 to 2.5 minutes. It is possible to determine the BMD of the central trabecular portion of the spine using DEXA, excluding osteophytes or extraskeletal calcifications that may falsely raise the bone density in the standard anteroposterior projection. Quantitative CT scanning has made it possible to measure directly the loss of trabecular bone in the central region of the spine, but the procedure entails a comparatively high radiation exposure and time, with precision errors that are usually higher than those of DEXA.

Figure 90–2 shows BMD in a patient compared to that of young healthy controls to determine whether there is reduction in BMD compared with peak bone mass (percentage of young healthy controls expressed as a T-score) and with age-matched controls to assess whether BMD is diminished relative to an age-matched cohort (percentage of age-matched controls expressed as a Z-score). There is an inverse relationship between bone density and the gradient of risk for fracture.[38] Prospective studies show that bone densitometry identifies patients with an increased gradient of risk for fracture. In 8134 women, a 1–standard deviation (SD) decrement in the bone density of the spine and the femoral neck compared with age-adjusted controls was associated with a 1.6- and 2.6-fold increased risk of hip fracture, respectively.[39] Measurement of bone density in the hip is more predictive of a hip fracture than is measurement at another site. Studies show that in women older than 65 years, hip bone density is predictive of a spine and hip fracture and that conventional spine density does not add to the diagnostic utility of a single hip bone–density test in assessing the risk of fracture.

Although bone densitometry provides a quantitative measure of bone mass, in vitro studies using ultrasonography indicate that this technique also provides information about the mechanic properties of bone, including both density and elasticity—qualities that are strong predictors of bone strength. Ultrasound techniques include speed-of-sound and broad-band ultrasound attenuation methods; the speed-of-sound technique reflects bone density and elasticity, and broad-band ultrasound attenuation is an indicator of bone density, bone structure, and composition. Approved for clinical use by the U.S. Food and Drug Administration (FDA), both ultrasound techniques have been shown to discriminate between normal and osteoporotic patients at increased fracture risk.[40] T-score parameters in use by some ultrasound machines do not correspond to the T-score levels by DEXA. Although ultrasonography is a radiation-free technique that may provide information regarding the risk of fracture and bone quality, the reproducibility of this technique and the measurement sites of mainly cortical bone or low-weight-bearing locations may make it unsuitable for the monitoring of small changes in bone over time. Therefore, ultrasound measurements cannot reliably be utilized to monitor response to osteoporosis therapies. Further data are necessary to validate the clinical utility of ultrasonography.

On the basis of the guidelines of the Scientific Advisory Board of the National Osteoporosis Foundation, bone densitometry is useful in determining which patients might benefit from therapy to protect the skeleton, including patients who have a deficiency of gonadal hormones (postmenopausal women younger than 65 years with one or more risk factors or older than 65 years regardless of risk factors), postmenopausal fracture, evidence of osteopenia or a vertebral abnormality on a radiograph, hyperparathyroidism, or exposure to supraphysiologic doses of glucocorticoids (Table 90–3). Bone densitometry is also used to facilitate the decision for some women to commence therapy for osteoporosis and to assess the clinical response to a therapeutic intervention.[35] Screening normal premenopausal women is not cost effective.

The World Health Organization (WHO) has published criteria for osteoporosis based on bone density[1,41]:

1. Osteopenia (low bone mass) is defined by a bone density measurement between 1 and 2.5 SD below the young-adult mean (T-score between −1 and −2.5).

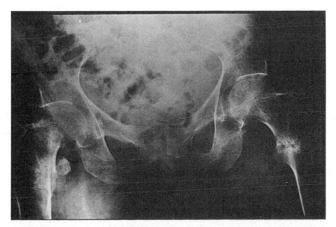

FIGURE 90–2 · Osteomalacia and Fractures in a 65-year-old Woman with Malabsorption. Shown are a pseudofracture of the left lesser trochanter *(arrow)* and an avulsion of the right lesser trochanter *(arrow head)*. This patient also had previous bilateral pubic rami fractures.

TABLE 90–3 · INDICATIONS FOR BONE DENSITOMETRY

- All postmenopausal women <65 yr who have one or more additional risk factors for osteoporosis, besides menopause
- All women >65 yr regardless of additional risk factors
- Documenting reduced bone density in a patient with a vertebral abnormality or osteopenia on a radiograph
- Estrogen-deficient women at risk for low bone density, considering use of estrogen or an alternative therapy, if bone density would facilitate the decision
- Women who have been on estrogen replacement therapy for prolonged periods or to monitor the efficacy of a therapeutic intervention or interventions for osteoporosis
- Diagnosing low bone mass in glucocorticoid-treated individuals
- Documenting low bone density in patients with asymptomatic primary or secondary hyperparathyroidism

2. Osteoporosis is defined as a bone density measurement less than 2.5 SD below young, healthy controls (T-score less than 2.5).
3. Established osteoporosis is defined as a T-score of less than 2.5 and the presence of a fracture.

Therapy to prevent bone loss is recommended if the T-score is −1.5 or less in a patient with risk factors or previous fracture, or if the T-score is −2 or less with no risk factors. Treatment of osteoporosis is recommended for those in groups 2 and 3 as defined by the previous list. T-score cutoffs for diagnosis and treatment do not apply to secondary osteoporosis.[41]

Markers of Bone Turnover

The development of sensitive biochemical markers of bone turnover makes it possible to analyze changes in bone formation and resorption at a given time point. Osteocalcin, a noncollagenous matrix protein in bone, is produced exclusively by osteoblasts. It is a marker of bone formation that correlates with histomorphometric bone measurements. In most conditions, bone resorption and formation are tightly coupled, and osteocalcin levels reflect bone turnover. Other markers of bone formation include levels of bone-specific alkaline phosphatase and procollagen I carboxyl- and amino-terminal peptides.

Sensitive indicators of bone resorption derived from the degradation of mature collagen include the older urinary hydroxyproline and hydroxylysine amino acids, which are no longer used clinically, and the newer urinary (and recently serum) pyridinoline and deoxypyridinoline collagen cross-links and cross-linked N telopeptides or C telopeptides for type I collagen. Urinary pyridinoline cross-link levels correlate with histomorphometric determinations of bone resorption; these biomarkers increase with menopause and are high in patients with a variety of disorders characterized by accelerated bone turnover, including Paget's disease and osteoporosis.[42,43] Urinary excretion of N telopeptides is inversely related to the total hip and spinal bone density and, according to some studies, may be a more specific index of bone resorption than urinary pyridinoline levels.[44] However, the within-subject variability for this marker of bone resorption is high, requiring large changes in a disease process or therapeutic intervention to detect significant changes. The Epidimiologie de l'Ostioporose Study, (EPIDOS), study in elderly women showed that elevated C telopeptide and deoxypyridinoline levels are associated with an increased risk of hip fracture independent of BMD (odds ratio of 2), and when it is coupled with a T score less than −2.5, there is an increased risk of fracture, with an odds ratio of 4.8.[45] Rosen and associates found that N telopeptides and osteocalcin were the most sensitive predictors of change in spine BMD after 1 year of estrogen replacement therapy or calcium supplementation.[46] In clinical studies, antiresorptive agents such as estrogen and bisphosphonates induce a significant decrease in markers of resorption (ranging from 30 to 70%) and formation within 3 to 6 months, earlier for resorption than for formation markers. Resorption markers decrease before formation markers and correlate with either a maintenance or increase in BMD. A significant change in bone markers can be observed within months of antiresorptive therapy, before there are changes in BMD.[46] Further long-term, prospective studies of large numbers of women are necessary to determine whether selective biochemical markers of bone turnover can predict changes in BMD or fracture risk and whether these tests should be used in the standard clinical care of patients.

The majority of bone turnover marker data is derived from large studies of antiresorptive agents. However, recently a bone-building anabolic agent, PTH, has been approved for the treatment of osteoporosis. PTH's action is to stimulate osteoblast activity; therefore, osteocalcin and other markers of bone formation increase rapidly, within a few weeks of initiation of treatment. However, activation of the osteoblast over time results in RANKL production, which stimulates osteoclast activity. With continued treatment with PTH, markers of osteoclast activity also increase to levels equal to the formation markers. Because the overall result is an increase in bone mass, the bone turnover markers during PTH therapy reflect significant bone remodeling, both on the trabecular and cortical bone surfaces. A few small studies have found that increases in both bone formation and resorption markers predict an increase in bone mass with PTH treatment.[47,48]

Evaluation for Secondary Bone Loss

The workup for osteoporosis is directed toward excluding secondary causes of bone loss and includes determination of serum calcium, phosphate, supersensitive thyroid-stimulating hormone, 25-hydroxyvitamin D (25-OHD), and urine calcium and creatinine levels. Also, a complete blood cell (CBC) count and alkaline phosphatase and liver function tests, and in some cases an intact PTH level, erythrocyte sedimentation rate (ESR), and serum and urine protein electrophoresis, may be necessary (Table 90–4).

■ **TABLE 90–4 • WORKUP FOR OSTEOPOROSIS**

For all patients
Laboratory tests including SMA, complete blood cell count, supersensitive TSH, ±PTH, alkaline phosphatase, 25-hydroxyvitamin D levels, and 24-hour urinary calcium measurement; +/– serum and urine protein electrophoresis and ESR

For selected patients (children, premenopausal women, men younger than 60 yr, African Americans, patients with rapidly progressive disease)
Definitive tests for endocrine, neoplastic, and gastrointestinal disorders
Bone biopsy under calcified sections with double tetracycline label
In selected patients, markers of bone turnover to identify patients at risk for increased bone loss

Abbreviations: ESR, Erythrocyte sedimentation rate; PTH, parathyroid hormone; SMA, sequential multiple analysis; TSH, thyroid-stimulating hormone.

Further tests to rule out neoplastic or endocrinologic disorders and a bone biopsy (decalcified bone specimen is obtained after a double tetracycline label with two different fluorescent labels) should be considered in certain patients with progressive bone loss and in those in whom osteoporosis is unlikely. Identification and appropriate therapy for underlying secondary causes of osteoporosis are important. For example, treatment of vitamin D deficiency is best accomplished with vitamin D supplements. Parathyroidectomy in patients with hyperparathyroidism characterized by hypercalcemia, hypercalciuria, nephrolithiasis, an age less than 50 years, or low cortical BMD (Z-score 2 or less) was associated with a large (4 to 12.8%) increase in bone density over 4 years.[49] Bone density was, however, stable for up to 6 years in patients with mild hyperparathyroidism.[50] In addition, treatment of hyperthyroidism, hypercortisolism, and a variety of other disorders that may cause osteoporosis can produce increments in bone mass.

TREATMENT

Calcium

The goals of therapy for osteoporosis are to reduce bone resorption and to enhance bone formation, if possible. Bone loss occurs when the calcium intake and absorption are insufficient to balance the daily calcium losses. Prospective data show that calcium stabilizes bone.[51]

Table 90–5 shows the current recommendations for optimal calcium intake for women and men from the 1997 Report of the Institute of Medicine to the National Academy of Sciences.[52] In the absence of kidney stones or an underlying disorder of calcium metabolism, these calcium intakes are safe. To prevent negative calcium balance, premenopausal women require 1000 mg and postmenopausal women 1200 mg of total elemental calcium daily.[53] Children have increasing calcium requirements during adolescence, and data show increased

TABLE 90–5 • OPTIMAL CALCIUM REQUIREMENTS RECOMMENDED BY THE NATIONAL ACADEMY OF SCIENCES 1997

Age Group	Optimal Daily Intake of Calcium (mg)
Infants	
Birth-6 mo	400
6 mo-1 yr	600
Children	
1-8 yr	500-800
Adolescents, 9-18 yr	
Pregnant and nursing females	1300
Men and women	
19-50 yr	1000
Older than 50 yr (men and women)	
+/– hormone replacement therapy	1200

Modified from Atkinson SA, Abrams SA, Dawson-Hughes B, et al: Calcium. In Young V (ed): Dietary Reference Intake for Calcium, Phosphorus, Magnesium, Vitamin D and Fluoride. Washington, DC, National Academy Press, 1997, pp 91-143.

bone accretion with increased calcium intake in prepubesent and pubertal children. Calcium carbonate contains 40 percent elemental calcium and should be taken with meals because of poor absorption in achlorhydric patients in the absence of food. Calcium citrate is a more bioavailable and readily absorbed calcium preparation that contains 24 percent elemental calcium[54]. It is also absorbed well on an empty stomach in patients with achlorhydria.

Estrogen

Hormone replacement therapy (HRT) was the mainstay of treatment in osteoporosis because estrogen inhibits bone resorption, produces a small rise in bone density, and reduces the risk of fracture by approximately 50 percent in retrospective observational studies. Cardiovascular disease is the leading cause of death in postmenopausal women. Previous data suggest that estrogen replacement has a beneficial effect on reducing primary and secondary cardiac events in postmenopausal women. However, in 1998, data were published from the 4-year Heart and Estrogen/Progestin Replacement Study of secondary prevention of coronary heart disease in postmenopausal women.[55] In this study, 2763 postmenopausal women with a previous history of heart disease were randomized to receive estrogen (0.625 mg) plus progestin (2.5 mg) or placebo alone. Results show that the treatment group had no reduction in the overall rate of coronary heart disease, CHD events, and in fact, an early increase in risk of CHD events was noted, possibly related to increased coagulability.[56] In addition, data from a large, multicenter, longitudinal study by the Women's Health Initiative (WHI)—in which 162,000 women aged 50 to 79 years were randomized into a placebo group, an HRT group if a woman's uterus was intact, or an estrogen-only group if a woman did not have a uterus—was terminated early due to an increased risk of breast and cardiovascular events. The research questions for the WHI were to determine the effects of HRT, diet modification, and calcium and vitamin D supplements on heart disease, osteoporosis, colorectal cancer risk. After a mean follow-up of 5.3 years in a 8.5-year study, the HRT group had a increased risk of seven more CHD events per 10,000 women taking the drug for a year, eight more invasive breast cancers, eight more strokes, and eight more pulmonary emboli, but six fewer colorectal cancers, and five fewer hip fractures.[57] At this time, the general recommendations for HRT are that it is only to be used for vasomotor symptoms that occur at the time of menopause. When these symptoms abate, it is recommended that estrogen replacement with HRT (combined estrogen and progestin for women with a uterus intact) be stopped because the perceived cardiovascular benefits have not been substantiated and the cardiovascular disease and breast cancer risk make the benefit to risk ratio unacceptable for most women. It is important to acknowledge that, at this time, the estrogen-only arm of the WHI study is continuing. Therefore, it will be a few years before all the results of estrogen use alone in women without a uterus is known.

If a woman and her physician decide she is going to take HRT or estrogen alone for vasomotor symptoms, in those with an increased risk of coagulability, transdermal estrogen replacement should be considered. Estrogen has also been shown to potentially reduce the risk or progression of Alzheimer's disease and the development and progression of diabetes mellitus, although data from large, prospective studies are necessary to confirm these findings.

Selective Estrogen Receptor Modulators

The ideal estrogen replacement therapy would confer the beneficial effects of estrogen on bone and cardiovascular disease without an increased risk of breast or uterine cancer. Selective estrogen receptor modulators (SERMs) are a nonsteroidal class of drugs that bind to the estrogen receptor and differ from each other in their actions on estrogen-responsive tissues, acting selectively as agonists or antagonists. Tamoxifen, the first available SERM, is an estrogen antagonist that binds to the estrogen receptor and also has estrogen-agonist effects on bone, lipids, clotting factors, and endometrium. Tamoxifen therapy in women with breast cancer produced a small increase in bone density of the spine over 2 years, with no effect on radial bone density in association with reductions in both low-density lipoprotein (LDL) and total cholesterol.[58] The Breast Cancer Prevention Trial studied 13,388 women at increased risk for breast cancer, comparing treatment with tamoxifen (20 mg daily) to placebo for 5 years.[59] Tamoxifen reduced the risk of invasive and noninvasive breast cancer by 50 percent, and a decreased risk of fracture was observed—45 percent reduction at the hip and 29 percent at the spine. An increased incidence of low-grade endometrial cancer was noted, but there was no change in the risk of ischemic heart disease.[59]

Raloxifene,[60] now FDA-approved for the prevention and treatment of osteoporosis, is a SERM that acts as an estrogen agonist on bone, with antagonist effects on the breast and uterus, compared to placebo.[61] Raloxifene (60 mg per day over a 2-year study period) increased BMD in the lumbar spine by 2.4 percent, in the total hip by 2.4 percent, and in the total body by 2 percent, with a reduction in fracture risk at 2 years similar to treatment with estrogen or alendronate (5 mg). Over a 2-year study period, raloxifene produced a significant reduction in vertebral fractures; fractures were present in 1.6 percent of raloxifene-treated women compared to 2.9 percent of those in the placebo group; fractures recurred in 7.6 percent of treated women with a previous fracture compared to 14.3 percent of those in the placebo group.[62] Endometrial thickness is not increased by raloxifene, but menopausal symptoms may be made worse. Raloxifene has been shown to decrease LDL cholesterol by 12 percent with a nonsignificant increase in HDL_2 cholesterol; cardiovascular protection has not yet been determined.[63] However, raloxifene, unlike estrogen, does not change C-reactive protein (CRP) levels, and elevated levels of this protein are associated with an elevated risk of a cardiovascular event.[64,65] Raloxifene also decreased the incidence of breast cancer by 76 percent in patients with osteoporosis who were enrolled in a clinical study of osteoporosis, with breast cancer incidence studied as a secondary end point.[60] Studies are now underway to assess the effect of raloxifene on cardiovascular disease raloxifene use in the heart, (RUTH), breast cancer compared to tamoxifen Study of Tamoxifen and raloxifene, (STAR), and raloxifene to prevent the development of breast cancer raloxifene to prevent breast cancer study, (CORE), Depending on the results of these studies, this class of drug will have a significant impact on the diseases of elderly women. At this time, there is no information on the use of raloxifene in men. Therefore, we do not recommend it at this time for men.

Testosterone

Men with osteoporosis with hypogonadism and symptoms of low libido may potentially benefit from testosterone replacement therapy. This may be administered as testosterone cypionate or enanthate (50 to 400 mg intramuscularly every 2 to 4 weeks) or as a transdermal testosterone replacement patch, which is now administered transscrotally (Testoderm, 4 to 6 mg daily) or transcutaneously (Androderm, 2.5 or 5 mg daily).[66] Most studies find that bone-mass increases observed with testosterone replacement are observed when levels of testosterone are very low at the initiation of the therapy.

Calcitonin

Calcitonin, a 32–amino acid peptide synthesized by the C cells of the thyroid gland, is a potent inhibitor of osteoclast-mediated bone resorption. Although human and salmon calcitonin are commercially available, salmon calcitonin is most commonly used because it is of greater potency. On the basis of data showing an increase in total body calcium, parenteral calcitonin was approved by the FDA for the treatment of osteoporosis in 1984, and calcitonin in a nasal spray was approved for the treatment of postmenopausal osteoporosis in 1995. Parenteral calcitonin (100 IU subcutaneously or intramuscularly three times a week or daily) can maintain bone density or produce a small increase in bone mass in the spine, and in some instances the forearm, particularly in patients with a high bone turnover.[67] Nasal spray calcitonin is absorbed through the nasal mucosa and is approximately 40 percent as potent as the parenterally administered drug (e.g., 50 to 100 IU of injectable calcitonin is comparable to 200 IU of nasal spray calcitonin).[68] In osteoporotic women more than 5 years past menopause, nasal calcitonin (200 IU daily) increases spinal bone density 2 to 3 percent compared to placebo without an effect on proximal femur bone mass; higher doses are necessary in the early menopausal period.[68,69] Nasal spray–calcitonin therapy in patients with osteoporosis is associated with a 36-percent reduction in vertebral fractures over 5 years.[69]

Although the adverse effects of parenteral calcitonin include nausea, flushing, and local irritation at the injection site, calcitonin given intranasally is well tolerated, with rhinitis and nasal symptoms such as dryness and crusts as potential side effects. Patients treated with parenteral and nasally administered calcitonin may also show a beneficial analgesic response in the presence of osteoporotic fractures.

Bisphosphonates

Bisphosphonates are analogues of pyrophosphate, with a P-C-P rather than a P-O-P core, that are absorbed by the HA of bone and suppress bone resorption. Modification of the side chains can result in the development of a variety of compounds with differing abilities to inhibit bone resorption (Table 90–6). Some bisphosphonates have been administered intermittently because of a long skeletal half-life and prolonged retention in bone. These compounds must be taken on an empty stomach because gastrointestinal absorption is less than 10 percent.

Bisphosphonates have been used for the treatment of patients with Paget's disease of bone, hypercalcemia of malignancy, osteoporosis, and for the prevention and treatment of glucocorticoid-induced osteoporosis. Etidronate (Didronel) administered intermittently (400 mg daily for 2 weeks in 3-month cycles) produced an approximately 5-percent increase in bone density of the spine and a 50-percent reduction in vertebral fractures at 2 years. Longer follow-up did not reveal a significant reduction in fractures compared to baseline, except in a post hoc analysis of patients with three or more fractures and low bone density.[70] Etidronate is not approved by the FDA for the treatment of osteoporosis.

Alendronate (Fosamax) is FDA-approved for the prevention and treatment of osteoporosis. Data in postmenopausal women with bone density 2.5 SD below peak bone mass or less show that alendronate (10 mg daily) compared to placebo produces an 8.8- and 7.8-percent increase in bone density in the spine and femoral trochanter, respectively, and a 5.9 percent increase in the femoral neck after 3 years of therapy[71]; there are smaller rises (2.3 to 4.4 percent) in bone density in the spine and proximal femur in women within 0.5 to 3 years of menopause. Fosamax treatment in women with osteoporosis (T-score less than 2.5) yields a

significant reduction in spine and hip fractures compared to the placebo-treated patients.[72] Prevention of bone loss with alendronate (5 mg per day) over 2 years increases BMD in the lumbar spine by 2.9 percent and hip by 1.3 percent, compared to estrogen-progestin therapy, which increases BMD in these locations by 4 percent and 1.8 percent, respectively.[73] Alendronate did not reduce the incidence of clinical fractures in women who had low bone mass but without osteoporosis, although longer studies may be necessary.[74] Alendronate treatment is also effective in increasing bone mass in the spine, hip, and total body and helps prevent vertebral fractures and height loss in men with osteoporosis.[75] Adverse effects of bisphosphonates include gastrointestinal symptoms such as stomach pain and esophagitis (caution is advised regarding their use in patients with active symptoms or a history of ulcer disease). Recently, a once-a-week alendronate preparation of alendronate (70 mg) has been approved for the treatment of osteoporosis. This preparation increased spinal and hip bone mass similarly to alendronate (10 mg/day over a 2-year study period). However, the once-a-week preparation is well tolerated by patients, and administering the medication once a week has become quite acceptable.[76]

Risedronate, another oral bisphophonate, is approved for the prevention and treatment of osteoporosis. Risedronate, administered at 5 mg/day, increased bone mass and reduced the risk of new vertebral fractures 50 percent more than placebo.[77-79] In addition, a separate study performed to assess the effect of risedronate on hip fractures found that women with osteoporosis defined by a femoral neck T-score of −4.0 or less had a significant reduction in the risk of a hip fracture.[80] Recently, risedronate (35 mg once a week) has been approved for the prevention and treatment of osteoporosis.[81] Risedronate is FDA approved for the treatment of Paget's disease at 30 mg daily for 2 months, with retreatment if relapse occurs after 2 months.[82] Studies show that risedronate may be well tolerated even in patients with mild gastrointestinal symptoms. Bisphosphonates may also reduce bone pain.

Studies of other new bisphosphonates in the prevention and treatment of osteoporosis are under way. Zoledronic acid (Zometa), a potent bisphosphonate, is approved for the treatment of hypercalcemia of malignancy. Recently a phase II, dose-ranging study of zoledronic acid for the treatment of postmenopausal osteoporosis was completed. A dose of 4 mg given at the beginning of the study increased lumbar spine bone mass by nearly 5 percent, and biochemical markers of bone resorption remained suppressed nearly 70 percent below baseline levels at the 12-month point. This one dose, given only at baseline, has similar efficacy to less or equal doses given every 3 or 6 months. Although there was no apparent dose response, and no information about reduction in fracture risk in this phase II trial, it did suggest that some bisphosphonates may be able to be administered much less frequently than is our current practice. Two large, phase III studies are now underway to determine the safety and efficacy of once-yearly zolendronate on both vertebral and hip fracture risk.[83]

■ **TABLE 90–6** • RELATIVE POTENCY OF VARIOUS BISPHOSPHONATES TO INHIBIT METAPHYSEAL BONE RESORPTION IN VIVO

Chemical Modifications	Examples	Antiresorptive Potency
First-generation: short alkyl or halide side chain	Etidronate	1
	Clodronate	10
Second-generation: NH$_2$-terminal group	Tiludronate*	10
	Pamidronate	100
	Alendronate	100-1000
Third-generation: cyclic side chain	Risedronate	1000-10,000
	Ibandronate	1000-10,000
	Zoledronate	10,000+

*Tiludronate has a cyclic side chain, not an NH$_2$-terminal group, but is generally classified as a second-generation compound based on its time of development and potency.

Adapted from Watts NB: Treatment of osteoporosis with bisphosphonates [Review]. Endocrinol Metab Clin North Am 27:419-439, 1998.

Fluoride

Fluoride stimulates osteoblast proliferation and the formation of bone. Although studies show that high doses of sodium fluoride (75 mg/day) produced large increases in BMD of the spine and proximal femur, vertebral fractures did not significantly decrease and nonvertebral fractures increased—indications that bone strength was not improved. Furthermore, adverse effects of sodium fluoride were common at high doses, including lower-extremity pain, gastrointestinal irritation, and impaired mineralization of bone (osteomalacia). In contrast, a low-dose, slow-release fluoride preparation (25 mg twice daily) with calcium supplements for 1 year has been shown to increase bone mass and reduce the individual vertebral fracture rate in postmenopausal women with osteoporosis.[84] Bone mass of the spine and femoral neck rose 4 percent and 2.38 percent each cycle, respectively, for 4 years; forearm bone density did not change. The reduction in the vertebral fracture rate was greater in patients with bone density of the lumbar spine that was 65 percent or more of that of young, healthy controls. Although not FDA-approved, slow-release fluorides, unlike sodium fluoride, that do not produce toxic levels of circulating fluoride may prove beneficial in patients with mild to moderate bone loss.

Parathyroid Hormone

Small randomized studies have been performed to assess the anabolic effects of Parathyroid hormone, (PTH), on changes in bone mass. PTH 1-34 (400 to 500 IU subcutaneously daily) with 1,25-dihydroxyvitamin D (1,25-[OH]$_2$D) (0.25 mg daily) produced large increases in spinal bone density, although there was a small loss of cortical bone. The use of parenteral PTH (40 µg daily) alone in women who had endometriosis treated with gonadotropin-releasing hormone agonists for 12 months produced a 7.5-percent rise in lateral spinal bone density and prevented bone loss from the femoral neck, trochanter, and total body, despite severe estrogen deficiency over this time interval.[85] Lindsay and coworkers have shown that PTH 1-34 (25 µg daily) increases bone density and decreases vertebral fractures in postmenopausal women taking estrogen replacement therapy.[86] Over a 3-year period, bone density increased 13 percent in the vertebrae, 2.7 percent in the hip, and 8 percent in the total body. Markers of bone formation increased by 55 percent, and markers of bone resorption increased 20 percent, demonstrating uncoupling of bone turnover with an overall increase in formation.

A recombinant human (rhPTH) composed of the 34 amino acids from the amino terminal end of the hormone (known as Forteo) has now been approved for the treatment of postmenopausal osteoporosis. A large, muticenter international study of osteoporotic women with the presence of a fracture were randomized to either rhPTH 1-34 at 20 µg/day or 40 µg/day or placebo for an average time of 21 months. Lumbar spine bone mass increased between 9 and 13 percent in the rhPTH 1-34–treated subjects compared to the placebo-treated ones. Hip bone mass also increased a few percent. Most importantly, the risk of new vertebral fractures was reduced nearly 70 percent in both sets of rhPTH 1-34–treated subjects and nonvertebral low-trauma fractures were reduced nearly 50 percent compared to the placebo-treated patients.[87] This study was initially planned to be a 3-year study. However, it was stopped at approximately 21 months because of preclinical evidence of malignant bone tumors in animal models. Additional studies of osteoporosis in men have performed with rhPTH 1-34 and significant gains in bone mass were reported.[88]

RhPTH 1-34, or Forteo, has recently been approved by the FDA for the treatment of postmenopausal osteoporosis. This is a special label that states that this medication should not be used in individuals other than those specifically stated on the label. Also, the medication needs to be given for at least 18 months before there are any fracture-reduction benefits. RhPTH 1-34 is given as a daily injection. Individuals using this medication may experience headache, nausea, and flushing with the initiation of the injections. These side effects generally become less severe after a few weeks.

A number of studies are currently underway comparing the effects of rhPTH 1-34 or PTH 1-84 alone and in combination with bisphosphonates.[89] The results of these studies, when available, provide valuable information on how best to use this new anabolic bone-building agent to increase bone mass and maintain it in osteoporotic patients.

Vitamin D

Physiologic doses of vitamin D are important to ensure normal bone mineralization. In individuals between 50 and 70 years of age and those older than 70 years, the recommended 400 and 600 IU, respectively, of vitamin D daily should be taken as a multivitamin or combined with a calcium supplement. Hypovitaminosis D is common in the elderly population, with one study demonstrating that 57 percent of patients in a general medical ward were vitamin D deficient.[90] Low vitamin D levels increase the risk of bone loss and fracture. LeBoff and associates found that 50 percent of patients admitted with acute femur fractures had vitamin D deficiency (25-OHD level less than 12 ng/ml), and 36.7 percent had secondary hyperparathyroidism.[35] Data show seasonal variations in vitamin D levels, with low 25-OHD levels during the winter and spring that are associated with decreases in bone density.

Although 200 IU of vitamin D prevented bone loss in the spine, data show that a higher daily vitamin D intake (800 IU) was necessary to diminish bone loss in the hip during the winter and spring seasons. Treatment with 700 IU of cholecalciferol and 500 mg of calcium carbonate per day reduced the rate of bone loss significantly in femoral neck, spine, and total body and decreased the incidence of nonvertebral fractures by 50 percent.[91] Therefore, patients require a vitamin D intake greater than 200 IU daily (400 IU to perhaps 800 IU daily in some instances) to maintain skeletal health.

Although this dramatic effect on fractures in the elderly population may represent a correction of vitamin

D insufficiency, this study underscores how adequate vitamin D replacement can effectively diminish fractures in older individuals. Use of the active vitamin D metabolite 1,25-(OH)$_2$D (known as Rocaltrol) may stimulate the absorption of calcium and, at pharmacologic doses, bone formation. Whereas some studies show that high doses of 1,25-(OH)$_2$D produce a rise in bone mineral density, other studies indicate that 1,25-(OH)$_2$D is ineffective in the treatment of osteoporosis. Because 1,25-(OH)$_2$D is not under feedback regulation, it has a narrow therapeutic window, and patients must be carefully monitored for the potential risks of hypercalcemia and hypercalciuria. Insufficient calcium and low 25-OHD levels are common in ambulatory patients and should be identified and treated before antiresorptive or other therapy for osteoporosis is initiated.

Dehydroepiandrosterone Sulfate

Anorexia nervosa is associated with a decrease in bone density, and in chronic disease there is an increased incidence of fractures and osteoporosis. In anorexia nervosa, excessive exercise and weight loss lead to amenorrhea with estrogen deficiency and subnormal adrenal steroid levels of dehydroepiandrosterone (DHEA) sulfate. In a study by Gordon and coworkers, 15 patients with anorexia nervosa were randomized in a double-blind study to receive 50, 100, or 200 mg of micronized DHEA daily for 3 months.[22] At 3 months, urine N telopeptide levels had decreased and osteocalcin levels had increased significantly without any adverse effects. More than 50 percent of the patients resumed menses. These results suggest that DHEA sulfate may normalize bone turnover in patients with anorexia nervosa at risk of bone loss. Previously, Luo and colleagues showed that rats treated for 280 days with a pure antiestrogen had a significant increase in bone density of the hip, spine, and total body when treated concurrently with DHEA (10 mg daily).[92] However, we await future studies to determine the long-term effects of DHEA on bone density and its therapeutic role.

PREVENTIVE MEASURES

Because bone loss is not completely reversible with existing therapies, prevention is essential for optimizing skeletal health. Strategies directed at increasing peak bone mass, reducing risk factors for bone loss (e.g., hypogonadism, decreased body fat, cigarette smoking, inactivity, or excessive alcohol intake), and reversing the secondary causes of osteoporosis may prevent bone loss. Patients should be advised, therefore, to consume adequate vitamin D and calcium and to participate in a regular weight-bearing exercise program. Weight-bearing exercise increases muscle strength and may stabilize or modestly increase bone density. On the basis of emerging data showing that increased calcium intake and exercise can add to bone accretion during adolescence and that interventions such as vitamin D and calcium and other therapeutic interventions can reduce fractures in older patients, it is never too early or too late to institute preventive strategies or therapies to diminish fractures that rise exponentially with age.

GLUCOCORTICOID-INDUCED OSTEOPOROSIS

Bone loss is a common sequela of therapy with glucocorticoids.[15] Rheumatic diseases are associated with an increased risk of bone loss and fracture, which is determined by a high cumulative glucocorticoid dose, an age greater than 50 years, a menopausal status, or a combination of these factors.[18] The severity of the bone loss in glucocorticoid-treated patients may vary from an approximately 3 to 20 percent decrease in bone density over 1 to 2 years. Glucocorticoid therapy is associated with increased fractures of the ribs and vertebrae, sites that contain predominantly trabecular bone, and it triples the risk of hip fracture in one third of patients after 5 to 10 years of treatment.[93] In adults, alternate-day glucocorticoid therapy does not prevent bone loss. In patients with rheumatic diseases, concerns over the development of glucocorticoid-induced osteoporosis limit treatment decisions regarding the dose and duration of glucocorticoid therapy.

The lowest possible glucocorticoid dose should be used, along with general preventive strategies such as a regular weight-bearing exercise program, adequate calcium and vitamin D intake, and reduction of other risk factors that might contribute to the development of osteoporosis. However, data show that even patients on 5 mg of prednisone daily have accelerated bone loss compared to controls. General prophylactic

TABLE 90–7 · RECOMMENDATIONS FOR THE PREVENTION AND TREATMENT OF GLUCOCORTICOID-INDUCED OSTEOPOROSIS (GIOP)

Prevention

Patients initiating glucocorticoid (GC) therapy at a dose equivalent to 5 mg or more of prednisone/day for 3 months or more should:

Modify risk factors for osteoporosis (stop smoking, decrease excessive alcohol consumption)
Start regular weight-bearing physical exercise
Initiate intake of calcium (total 1500 mg/day) and vitamin D (400-800 IU/day)
Consider bone mineral density (BMD) testing to predict risk of fracture and bone loss
Initiate bisphosphonate therapy (alendronate [5 mg/day or 35 mg/week] or risedronate [5 mg/day or 35 mg/week])

Treatment

Patients on long term GC therapy should be tested for osteoporosis using BMD measurement. If T-score less than –1, and consider:

Risk-factor modification including reducing risk of falls
Regular weight-bearing physical exercises
Calcium and vitamin D supplementation
Replacing gonadal steroids, if deficient
Bisphosphonate therapy (alendronate [10 mg/day or 70 mg/week] or risedronate [5 mg/day or 35 mg/week]); if bisphosphonates are contraindicated or not tolerated, consider calcitonin as second-line agent, intravenous bisphosphonate (pamidronate or zolendronate), or PTH 1-34
Repeat BMD measurement annually or biannually

Adapted from Recommendations for the prevention and treatment of glucocorticoid-induced osteoporosis 2001 update. Arthritis Rheum 44:1496-1503, 2001.

measures to prevent glucocorticoid-induced osteoporosis are shown in Table 90–7. To offset the impaired intestinal calcium absorption in glucocorticoid-treated patients, early studies showed that vitamin D (50,000 IU two to three times weekly) or 25-OHD produced an increase in bone density of the forearm. Because administration of supraphysiologic doses of vitamin D requires careful monitoring of the serum and urinary calcium concentrations in patients at a high risk for bone loss (with a normal urinary calcium level and no history of nephrolithiasis), an alternative approach in patients at risk for osteoporosis receiving long-term glucocorticoid therapy is to raise the 25-OHD level into the upper normal range to ensure adequate intestinal calcium absorption. This can usually be accomplished by administering vitamin D at 800 IU per day.

Because of the enhanced bone resorption in patients treated with glucocorticoids, investigators have examined the effects of inhibitors of bone resorption. Several short-term studies show that calcitonin maintains or produces a small increase in bone density in glucocorticoid-treated subjects compared to placebo-treated controls.[95] In a multicenter, placebo-controlled study, preliminary analysis shows that parenteral calcitonin increased spinal bone density 3.7 percent, with continued bone loss in the control group. In another study, calcium (1 g daily) and 1,25-$(OH)_2D$, (0.6 mcg daily) with or without 400 IU of nasal calcitonin prevented vertebral bone loss in glucocorticoid-treated patients, with bone loss occurring in the calcium only–treated group. The calcitonin-treated group had a sustained effect in the second year after treatment and was discontinued.[96]

The use of bisphosphonates in patients receiving chronic glucocorticoid therapy has also been shown to be quite beneficial. The use of alendronate (5 and 10 mg daily for 1 year) in patients receiving glucocorticoid therapy[97] increased lumbar spine BMD by 2.1 and 2.9 percent, respectively, and increased femoral neck BMD by 1.2 and 1 percent, respectively (p <0.001). After 1 year of treatment there was a insignificant reduction in new vertebral fractures, but after 2 years of treatment, there was nearly a 40-percent reduction in new vertebral fracture risk.[98] Risedronate, at a dose of 5 mg per day, was also found to be effective in the prevention and treatment of glucocorticoid-induced bone loss.[99,100] Both alendronate and risedronate are approved by the FDA to reduce bone loss in glucocorticoid-treated patients.

In a prospective pilot study in glucocorticoid-treated patients, intravenous (IV) infusions of pamidronate (30 mg every 3 months) increased spinal bone density 3.4 percent in 1 year.[101] Studies of new, more potent bisphosphonates for the prevention and treatment of glucocorticoid-induced bone loss are in progress.

Traditionally, postmenopausal women on glucocorticoids have been treated with HRT, and there is some data to support prevention of bone loss in these women.[102] However, because the WHI results have shown unacceptable cardiovascular and cancer risks associated with HRT therapy, it is no longer the standard of care for the treatment of glucocorticoid-induced bone loss. However, recent data from SLE subjects treated with DHEA find an increase in lumbar spine and hip bone mass compared to placebo-treated patients.[103,104] DHEA may soon be approved for the treatment of SLE, and bone mass may increase in the presence of glucocorticoids when the patient is on this medication. The mechanism for the effect of DHEA on bone mass is not yet known. Investigators have suggested the bone mass preservation results from DHEA metabolism to estrogen, or by direct effects on IGF-I bone-promoting factors. Additional studies are now in progress to determine whether this agent is effective for the prevention of bone loss in glucocorticoid-treated SLE patients.

In addition, men on glucocorticoids can have a lowering of their testosterone levels.[105] Generally they are asymptomatic, but if men on glucocorticoids have evidence of low serum testosterone levels and symptoms of low libido, they can be safely treated with testosterone. Bone-mass increases have been observed in men who had low testosterone levels on glucocorticoids and were treated with testosterone.[106] However, because there are risks associated with testosterone treatment, unless there are symptoms of low libido present, it is more prudent to treat these patients with a bisphosphonate medication.

Although glucocorticoids alter bone metabolism via a number of different mechanisms, inhibition of osteoblast life span and activity is the most significant. Whereas calcium and vitamin D supplementation and antiresorptive therapies can prevent bone loss and reduce fracture risk, they do not significantly alter osteoblast activity in the presence of glucocorticoids. Because a bone anabolic agent, hPTH 1-34 can increase osteoblast activity and increase bone mass in postmenopausal osteoporosis, Lane and colleagues tested the hypothesis that hPTH 1-34 could override the suppressive effects of glucocorticoids on osteoblast activity and reverse the bone loss. Data from a 12-month randomized trial of human PTH 1-34 in postmenopausal women with osteoporosis currently taking glucocorticoids and estrogen replacement therapy showed an 11 percent increase in lumbar BMD compared to 0 percent in the estrogen-only group.[107] After 1 year of treatment and 1 year of follow-up, total and femoral neck BMD increased nearly 5 percent when the there was not much change in the estrogen-only group. In this study, QCT of the lumbar spine, a measure of only trabecular bone, found nearly a 35-percent increase in PTH-treated patients compared to the estrogen-only group after 12 months of therapy.[108] This information demonstrated that the major effect of PTH is to increase bone mass is by thickening the existing trabeculae. In addition, 1 year of hPTH 1-34 treatment increased the vertebral cross-sectional area, most likely by thickening the periosteal envelope.[109] Studies are now underway comparing rhPTH 1-34 to alendronate for the treatment of osteoporosis. Currently, there is no fracture information for PTH and glucocorticoid-induced bone loss.

In addition to a stimulatory effect on bone resorption, glucocorticoid therapy is associated with a suppression of bone formation; thus, investigators have examined the use of fluoride therapy for the treatment of glucocorticoid-induced bone loss. In a short study over 24 weeks, Rickers and colleagues found no effect of fluoride, calcium, and vitamin D in attenuating glucocorticoid-induced bone loss of the forearm.[110] In a prospective study in patients receiving long-term, moderate doses of glucocorticoids, sodium monofluorophosphate (26 mg of elemental fluoride daily) and calcium therapy over 18 months produced a significant rise in spinal bone density with no effect on femoral neck or femoral shaft bone density when compared to controls.[111] Long-term prospective studies are necessary to establish that fluoride therapy reduces fractures in glucocorticoid-treated patients.

To prevent bone loss in patients with pulmonary diseases requiring glucocorticoid therapy, treatment with inhaled glucocorticoids has been studied. Treatment with inhaled glucocorticoids appears to uncouple bone turnover and increase bone loss; however, this is dose dependent. Less than 800 mcg/day of inhaled budesonide dipropionate does not increase the risk of osteoporosis, but more than 800 μg/day does. A group of 36 patients were randomized to receive prednisone or deflazacort (a prednisolone derivative) in equipotent anti-inflammatory doses.[112] Both glucocorticoids induced a significant decrease in trabecular bone by biopsy, although deflazacort caused significantly less. In a study of kidney transplantation patients, lumbar spine BMD decreased more in prednisone-than in deflazacort-treated patients (9.1% vs. 3%). The total body bone density was preserved by deflazacort, but hip density decreased equally in both groups.[112] Studies of deflazcort as a bone-sparing glucocorticoid have been discontinued, because when the anti-inflammatory potency of deflazacort and prednisone were made equivalent, deflazacort has no bone-sparing effects

Because patients receiving glucocorticoids may lose a dramatic amount of bone, it is important to monitor the efficacy of a treatment intervention, assess the need for further diagnostic evaluation for other secondary causes of bone loss, and consider alternative treatment strategies if a given therapy is ineffective in preventing bone loss or fractures. In patients at increased risk of fracture, therapy with a potent bisphosphonate is highly recommended to slow bone loss and the rate of new fractures. Alendronate or risedronate are available for use, and future studies of more potent bisphosphonates and PTH are awaited.

Osteomalacia

Osteomalacia is characterized by impaired mineralization of bony matrix. Calcium, phosphate, and vitamin D are necessary for the normal mineralization of bone. Normally, there is a steep inverse relationship between the serum calcium and PTH concentrations. A small decrease in the serum calcium concentration leads to a rise in PTH release that promotes distal renal calcium reabsorption, proximal tubulorenal phosphorus excretion, and the resorption of calcium from bone. Vitamin D is produced in the skin in the presence of ultraviolet light or absorbed in the intestine from dietary or supplemental sources. Activation of vitamin D to 25-OHD occurs in the liver and to 1,25-(OH)$_2$D in the proximal tubules of the kidney; PTH, hypocalcemia, and hypophosphatemia

stimulate the renal 1-hydroxylase enzyme that converts 25-OHD to 1,25-(OH)$_2$D, which in turn indirectly enhances intestinal calcium absorption.

Osteomalacia results from reduced availability of calcium or phosphate for incorporation into the HA of bone or from deficient absorption or activation of vitamin D.[112,113] The term *rickets* applies to the defective mineralization of bone and the cartilaginous growth plate in growing children. As shown in Table 90–8, osteomalacia or rickets may result from decreased availability of vitamin D as a consequence of insufficient ultraviolet light exposure, insufficient vitamin intake, or malabsorption in patients with gastrointestinal or biliary disorders. Reduced levels of 25-OHD are caused by severe liver disease, increased renal excretion of vitamin D metabolites due to nephrotic syndrome, or accelerated metabolism of 25-OHD caused by anticonvulsant drugs. Decreased activation of 1,25-(OH)$_2$D is seen in patients with renal insufficiency due to increased phosphate levels, and the resultant lower ionized calcium levels lead to secondary or tertiary hyperparathyroidism.

A careful history is important in the diagnosis of osteomalacia or vitamin D insufficiency. For example, a history of a malabsorptive process such as a gastrectomy, intestinal resection, sprue, primary biliary cirrhosis, or pancreatic deficiency may lead to the identification of vitamin D deficiency and osteomalacia.[113] Patients with osteomalacia may present with generalized pain involving the pelvis, spine, ribs, or lower extremities or with

TABLE 90–8 · CAUSES OF OSTEOMALACIA AND RICKETS

Vitamin D deficiency or dysfunction
Reduced availability
  Nutritional deficit
  Reduced exposure to ultraviolet light
  Malabsorption (gastrointestinal or biliary disease, surgical resection)
Alteration in metabolism of vitamin D
  Reduced 25-hydroxyvitamin D—liver or gastrointestinal disease, nephrotic syndrome, anticonvulsant drugs
  Reduced 1,25-dihydroxyvitamin D—renal disease, vitamin D–dependent rickets type I
Alteration in action of vitamin D on target tissues—
  Vitamin D–dependent rickets type II
Phosphate deficiency
Decreased availability—dietary deficiency, phosphate-binding antacids
Decreased renotubular phosphate reabsorption
  Familial: X-linked hypophosphatemic rickets, adult-onset vitamin D–resistant osteomalacia
  Acquired: Hypophosphatemic osteomalacia (phosphate diabetes), oncogenic osteomalacia
  Generalized renotubular disorders
Acidosis
  Renotubular acidosis, ureterosigmoidostomy, carbonic anhydrase inhibitors (acetazolamide)
Miscellaneous mineralization defects
  Inhibitors of mineralization—fluoride, bisphosphonates (e.g., etidronate), chronic renal failure (aluminum)
  Hypophosphatasia

Modified from LeBoff MS, Brown EM: Metabolic bone disease. *In* Hare JW (ed): Signs and Symptoms in Endocrine and Metabolic Disorders. Philadelphia, JB Lippincott, 1986, pp 239-260.

skeletal deformities such as bowing of the long bones, kyphoscoliosis, or pelvic abnormalities. Another clinical sign of osteomalacia in the adult includes proximal muscle weakness that may result in an antalgic or waddling gait and difficulty ambulating.

Pain may be elicited by deep palpation of the tibia, ribs, or pubic ramus.[113] One of the radiologic signs of osteomalacia is the presence of pseudofractures, or Looser's zones, which are transverse lines of rarefaction through the cortices, with incomplete healing in the ribs, scapulae, long bones (see Fig. 90–2), or pubic rami. Pseudofractures, however, may be indistinguishable from those associated with osteogenesis imperfecta or Paget's disease. Other radiologic findings in osteomalacia are vertebral fractures or protrusio acetabuli. Vitamin D deficiency may result in irreversible cortical bone loss.[113] In subtle cases of osteomalacia, a bone biopsy with a double tetracycline label may be necessary; characteristic histomorphometric findings in this disorder include increased osteoid and delayed mineralization of bone.

Rickets causes abnormalities of the epiphyseal growth plate, and the clinical signs include an inability to ambulate, growth disturbances, bowing of the long bones, and short stature. Bony deformities of the skull and ribs may develop with widened cranial sutures (craniotabes), thickened costochondral junctions (rachitic rosary), or indentation of the margins of the ribs (Harrison's grooves).

The biochemical parameters in patients with osteomalacia reflect the underlying pathophysiologic process and the compensatory biologic responses. In vitamin D–deficiency states, the serum calcium levels are usually normal or slightly decreased because PTH levels rise rapidly as a compensatory response to impaired calcium absorption.[114] In renal insufficiency phosphate retention, impaired renal production of $1,25-(OH)_2D$, hypocalcemia and skeletal resistance to PTH are thought to lead to the development of hyperparathyroidism and the resultant renal osteodystrophy, mixed osteomalacia, and osteitis fibrosa cystica[115]; aluminum intoxication may present with pure osteomalacia or adynamic bone disease.[114,116] Chronic vitamin D deficiency may increase the secretory demands of the parathyroid glands, thereby producing secondary, or in some instances tertiary, hyperparathyroidism. In patients with osteomalacia without hepatobiliary disease, alkaline phosphatase levels are often elevated.[113]

Osteomalacia may be associated with a deficiency of phosphate, principally in patients with decreased renotubular reabsorption of phosphate. Familial hypophosphatemic vitamin D–resistant rickets in children or osteomalacia in adults usually presents with a renal phosphate leak, hypophosphatemia, rachitic or osteomalacial changes, and an inappropriately normal or low-normal $1,25-(OH)_2D$ level for the degree of hypophosphatemia. This X-linked dominant disorder may present in young children with the inability to walk followed by progressive bowing and skeletal deformities, without signs of proximal myopathy. Data map the genetic locus for X-linked hypophosphatemic rickets to Xp22.1, and the gene is named *PHEX* (phosphate regulating gene with homology to endopeptidases on the X chromosome).[117]

Oncogenic osteomalacia or rickets is a vitamin D–resistant process associated with certain neoplasias, principally with small, benign mesenchymal or endodermal tumors and, infrequently, with certain malignant tumors (e.g., multiple myeloma and prostatic, oat cell, and breast carcinomas).[118,119] Such patients typically present with decreased renotubular phosphate reabsorption, hypophosphatemia, muscle weakness, diminished 1,25-$(OH)_2D$ levels, and normocalcemia. The benign tumors tend to be small and difficult to identify on physical examination or radiographic-imaging studies. Surgical removal of these tumors results in a rise in the phosphate and $1,25-(OH)_2D$ levels and resolution of the skeletal process. Osteomalacia may also be associated with generalized renotubular disorders and the use of certain drugs that contain inhibitors of mineralization (e.g., fluoride, etidronate, and aluminum). The evaluation of a patient in whom osteomalacia is suspected is shown in Table 90–9.

Osteomalacia is often a treatable disease, but the diagnosis may be overlooked. Vitamin D deficiency may be treated with physiologic doses of vitamin D, but higher doses (1000 to 2000 IU/day) may hasten the healing of bone. In the presence of intestinal malabsorption, and until the underlying malabsorptive process is corrected, very large doses of vitamin D (ranging from 50,000 IU once weekly to three or more times weekly) are often required. Careful monitoring of the serum and urinary calcium levels and 25-OHD concentrations is necessary to prevent vitamin D intoxication. Use of the active metabolite of 25-OHD (Calderol) may occasionally be necessary in resistant patients or in those with severe liver disease who cannot achieve activation of this metabolite. The potential advantages of using 25-OHD are a more stable bioavailability, shorter half-life, and greater potency than the parent compound,[113] although the cost is greater.

In patients with hypophosphatemia and disorders of renotubular phosphate reabsorption, mineralization of bone occurs with phosphate therapy and moderately high doses of $1,25-(OH)_2D$, the latter being necessary to prevent the secondary hyperparathyroidism associated with phosphate therapy. In patients with renal insufficiency or failure, a phosphate binder (calcium acetate or calcium carbonate) should be used after meals to decrease intestinal phosphate absorption. Calcium citrate therapy should not be used, as it augments aluminum absorption. In those with renal fail-

---

TABLE 90–9 • WORKUP FOR OSTEOMALACIA

Calcium, phosphorus, alkaline phosphatase, urinary calcium levels, 25-Hydroxyvitamin D and intact parathyroid hormone levels
In selected patients
  1,25-Dihydroxyvitamin D levels (e.g., renal insufficiency or vitamin D–resistant osteomalacia or rickets)
  Vitamin D absorption test: obtain 25-hydroxyvitamin D levels at 0, 4, and 8 hr (for some instances of malabsorption)
  Tubular reabsorption of phosphate (e.g., vitamin D–resistant osteomalacia or rickets)
Bone biopsy with double tetracycline labels

ure, 1,25-$(OH)_2$D therapy administered orally[114,120] (or intravenously in some dialysis patients) suppresses parathyroid cell secretion and proliferation; a threefold elevation of the PTH level is advocated by some investigators to prevent adynamic bone disease.[115] Analogues of 1,25-$(OH)_2$D that do not produce hypercalcemia but decrease levels of PTH are now available and may be useful in patients with renal insufficiency.

Paget's Disease of Bone

Paget's disease affects approximately 2 to 3 percent of the population older than 50 years and is uncommon in individuals younger than 40 years.[121] Paget's disease of bone is characterized by enhanced resorption of bone by giant, multinucleated osteoclasts followed by the formation of disorganized woven bone by osteoblasts. The resultant bone is expanded, weak, and vascular, so that affected bones may become enlarged and deformed, and the overlying skin may confer increased warmth to the touch.[122]

ETIOLOGY

The cause of Paget's disease is uncertain, although available data showing the presence of viral inclusion particles in giant pagetic osteoclasts support a viral cause, possibly associated with measles, respiratory syncytial, or canine distemper viruses. Paget's disease tends to aggregate in families in an autosomal dominant pattern, and 40 percent of patients have at least one other family member affected.[90] Recently, in a family with juvenile Paget's disease, the disease was found to be associated with a polymorphism in the OPG allele.[123] Study of additional families with this mutation may lead to the etiology of Paget's disease.

CLINICAL FEATURES

Although many patients with Paget's disease are asymptomatic and the disease is detected by the incidental finding of an elevated alkaline phosphatase level or characteristic radiographic abnormality, other patients present with a range of symptoms that include bone pain, skeletal deformities (bowing of long bones, enlarged skull, or pelvic alterations), pathologic fractures, increased cardiac output (with extensive disease), and nerve compression. Paget's disease typically includes a lytic phase, the common combined lytic and blastic mixed phase of the disease, and the sclerotic, or "burned out," phase found late in the disease process.

Radiologic signs of the three stages of Paget's disease may be present at different sites in the same patient.[121] The skeletal sites commonly involved with Paget's disease include the skull (Fig. 90–3), vertebrae, pelvis, sacrum, and lower extremities. Degenerative joint disease may develop adjacent to the bones and cause pain that may obscure the symptoms associated with Paget's disease.[121] Ten to 30 percent of patients with Paget's disease may experience fractures that present initially as asymptomatic or painful short fissure fractures travers-

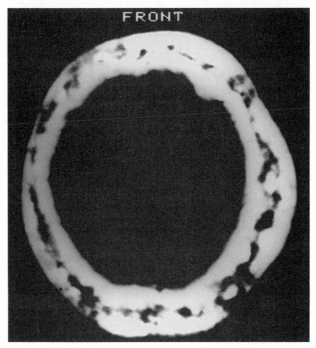

FIGURE 90–3 · Paget's Disease of the Skull in a Woman with Signs of Increasing Head Size and Progressive Hearing Loss. The alkaline phosphatase level was 2100 units/liter. Shown on this computerized axial tomogram is marked thickening of the inner and outer skull tables with osteoblastic pagetoid changes. Audiologic evaluation revealed bilateral hearing loss.

ing the bony cortex (Fig. 90–4). Complete fractures of the bones, such as the "chalk stick" fracture, also occur; fractures of the long bones may be a serious complication because the increased vascularity of pagetic bone may lead to excessive blood loss. Healing of fractures in pagetic bone usually occurs normally, although there have been reports of nonunion. A rare complication of Paget's disease of bone is sarcomatous degeneration in less than 1 percent of patients (with osteogenic sarcomas or, less commonly, fibrosarcomas or chondrosarcomas), who generally have a poor prognosis. The development of a sarcoma may be heralded by the presence of a soft tissue mass, localized pain, and a rise in the alkaline phosphatase level.

Neurologic symptoms generally result from compression of the nerves by pagetic bone. Hearing loss is common and is caused by sensory loss and conduction abnormalities due to pagetic involvement of the bones of the inner ear. Paget's disease of the skull may also produce ocular and other cranial nerve palsies. Compression of the base of the skull may lead to basilar invagination, cerebellar dysfunction, or obstructive hydrocephalus, with symptoms of nausea, ataxia, incontinence, gait disturbances, and dementia. Neurologic compromise of the thoracic or lumbar spine may lead to spinal cord compression or, in the latter instance, a cauda equina syndrome.

LABORATORY FINDINGS

Biochemical indices in patients with Paget's disease usually show normal serum calcium and phosphate

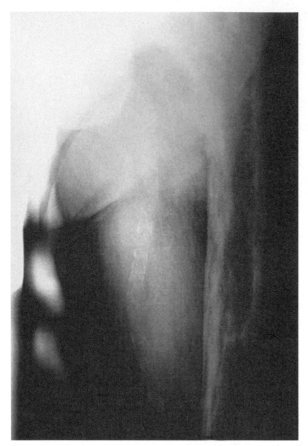

FIGURE 90–4 • Paget's Disease of the Proximal Femur. Note the coarse trabeculae, thickened cortices, lateral fissure fracture *(arrow heads)*, and expanding lytic region characteristic of the "blade-of-grass" lesion.

levels, although hypercalcemia may develop with immobilization when there is an uncoupling of bone resorption and formation. Patients with Paget's disease may also be hypercalcemic if they coincidentally acquire primary hyperparathyroidism, which can further increase bone remodeling and worsen the disease process. Secondary hyperparathyroidism may develop in approximately 10 to 15 percent of patients with Paget's disease, presumably because of inadequate calcium intake to meet the skeletal demands of the heightened bone remodeling.[121]

Alkaline phosphatase levels of bone origin are commonly elevated in patients with significant Paget's disease because of the increased osteoblastic activity combined with bone breakdown. In the absence of liver disease, the alkaline phosphatase level typically correlates with the extent of the pagetic involvement of bone, although it may be more elevated in Paget's disease of the skull (see Fig. 90–3).

Unexpectedly, circulating osteocalcin levels do not reflect disease activity in patients with Paget's disease as well as alkaline phosphatase levels do. Markers of bone resorption, such as urinary collagen cross-links and N telopeptides, are also elevated in active Paget's disease. These, newer, more sensitive markers of bone resorption may prove useful in monitoring the response to therapy in patients with Paget's disease.

Other laboratory abnormalities in patients with Paget's disease include hypercalciuria, hyperuricuria, and hyperuricemia, possibly related to the increased turnover of osteoclasts. Serum uric acid levels should be measured periodically because of the association of Paget's disease with gouty arthritis.

DIAGNOSIS

Bone scans are valuable tools for assessing the extent of Paget's disease and are, therefore, useful as part of the initial evaluation.[122] As diagnostic tests, however, bone scans in general are sensitive but not specific for a number of skeletal processes. Radiographs show characteristic radiologic findings such as transverse lucent areas, osteoporosis circumscripta, enlargement of the bones, expanding lytic changes, the "blade-of-grass" lesion shown in Figure 90–4, thickened cortices, a coarse trabecular pattern, or sclerotic changes.

In patients with involvement of the skull and changes in mental status, a skull radiograph, magnetic resonance imaging (MRI), or QCT may be useful to diagnose platybasia and flattening of the base of the skull, basilar invagination, or the infrequent complication of hydrocephalus. Audiologic evaluation may reveal hearing loss in patients with pagetic involvement of the skull.

TREATMENT

The indications for treatment of Paget's disease (Table 90–10) include pain, hypercalcemia, fractures, high-output failure (rare), and neurologic compromise. Therapy can also be used to prevent the progression of deformity or risk of nerve compression when there is pagetic involvement of the skull, a vertebral body, or a weight-bearing bone (femur) or disease adjacent to a major articular joint.

Treatment of symptomatic Paget's disease is usually directed at suppression of the enhanced bone resorption and skeletal turnover with calcitonin or bisphosphonates.[121,124] Response to therapy is monitored by the reduction of symptoms and maintenance of the alkaline phosphatase levels in a mid-normal range with retreatment once values rise 25 percent above normal.

Calcitonin

Salmon calcitonin and human calcitonin inhibit the function of the osteoclasts, which are active in the

TABLE 90–10 • INDICATIONS FOR TREATMENT OF PAGET'S DISEASE OF BONE

Pain
Hypercalcemia
Fractures
High-output failure (rare)
Skull involvement
Neurologic compromise
Periarticular disease
Prevention of progression of Paget's disease

pagetic process; both calcitonin preparations are FDA-approved therapies for patients with Paget's disease in an injectable form.[125] Salmon calcitonin therapy is usually initiated at a low dose to ensure patient tolerance and increased to a daily dose of 100 Medical Research Council units (intramuscularly or subcutaneously). After 6 months of therapy, the patient may be maintained on 50 to 100 Medical Research Council units daily.[121] Approximately two thirds of patients show a decrease in alkaline phosphatase levels of 50 percent or more in 2 to 6 months. Some patients experience resistance to the effects of calcitonin, which may be reversed in some instances by switching the therapy from salmon calcitonin to human calcitonin. Calcitonin is a safe drug.

Calcitonin is useful in patients with expanding lytic lesions, particularly of a weight-bearing bone, or for preoperative therapy before elective orthopedic procedures. The use of calcitonin nasal spray has few systemic side effects but is not FDA approved for the treatment of Paget's disease.

Bisphosphonates

Several bisphosphonates are currently approved by the FDA for the treatment of Paget's disease; they include 1) etidronate (Didronel), 2) pamidronate (Aredia), 3) alendronate (Fosamax), 4) tiludronate, and 5) risedronate (Actonel).

Etidronate is an orally administered form of therapy that produces a clinical and biochemical response similar to that of calcitonin. Therapy for Paget's disease is provided at a dose of 5 mg/kg/day (400 mg/day or a minimum of 200 mg/day for smaller patients) for 6 months and is then stopped; etidronate therapy is reinstituted after 6 months of no treatment for 6-month cycles of therapy.[126] As mentioned previously, higher doses of etidronate are associated with defective mineralization of bone and osteomalacia with symptoms of pain and fractures. Measurement of alkaline phosphatase levels at 3- to 6-month intervals is useful to ensure suppression of bone turnover; an estimated 25 percent of patients may become resistant to etidronate.[121] However, newer, more potent bisphosphonates are very effective for the treatment of Paget's disease.

Pamidronate as a parenteral therapy is also approved for the treatment of symptomatic Paget's disease of bone in patients with a threefold or greater elevation of alkaline phosphatase concentrations. This more potent bisphosphonate is useful in patients who acquire resistance to etidronate or in patients with more severe disease; an advantage of this therapy is that the alkaline phosphatase levels may be reduced into the normal range, with a sustained response for a prolonged period (e.g., up to a year or more).[121,127]

The FDA-recommended dose of pamidronate for patients with Paget's disease is 30 mg/day as a 4-hour infusion on 3 sequential days (total dose 90 mg), with retreatment possible if necessary. Other regimens for the treatment of Paget's disease include 60 mg of pamidronate daily (infused over 3 hours) once a week for 1 or 2 weeks in patients with alkaline phosphatase levels between 300 and 400 U/liter. For more extensive disease, three or four infusions of pamidronate every 1 to 2 weeks may be necessary; to assess the efficacy of these regimens for Paget's disease, clinical symptoms should be reviewed and alkaline phosphatase levels measured 2 to 3 months later.[89]

Some patients treated with pamidronate may experience a transient fever, musculoskeletal and flulike symptoms, and hypocalcemia; calcium supplementation (500 mg twice daily in vitamin D–replete patients) can offset the hypocalcemia that results from the suppression of bone resorption. Pamidronate is available only as a parenteral drug, which restricts the use of this therapy.

Alendronate has been approved for the oral treatment of Paget's disease at a dose of 40 mg daily for 6 months. Therapy with alendronate is recommended for patients with at least a two-fold elevation in alkaline phosphatase levels or for those in whom there are specific indications for therapy (e.g., those shown in Table 90–9). The use of alendronate produces a normalization, or a 60 percent or greater reduction, in the alkaline phosphatase level in approximately 85 percent of patients, and studies indicate that this therapy is more effective than etidronate. (All bisphosphonates must be taken correctly to minimize gastrointestinal side effects.)

Risedronate is another potent bisphosphonate (see Table 90–5) that is FDA approved for the treatment of Paget's disease. Siris and colleagues treated 162 patients with moderate to severe Paget's disease with oral risedronate (30 mg daily for 84 days followed by 112 days without treatment).[90] This cycle was repeated if the serum alkaline phosphatase level did not normalize or increased more than 25 percent from its nadir value. After the first and second cycles, the serum alkaline phosphatase level decreased 65 percent and 69 percent, respectively, and urine markers decreased 50 percent and 66.9 percent, respectively. The serum alkaline phosphatase level normalized in 53.8 percent of patients, and a significant decrease in bone pain was noted. Risedronate is well tolerated and has few adverse effects, including a flulike syndrome, gastrointestinal symptoms, and rarely iritis. Other groups have shown a decrease in serum alkaline phosphatase levels of 79 percent and 86 percent, with an 85 percent and 100 percent decrease in urine markers.[128] There is no evidence of osteomalacia in bone biopsies from patients treated with 30 mg of risedronate. Patients who have become resistant to etidronate appear to respond to risedronate. Patients must be instructed to have an adequate intake of calcium and vitamin D while taking risedronate.

Thus, the newer, more potent bisphosphonates are very effective in Paget's disease, and some of the newer agents may potentially produce a remission of the disease. Therapy with plicamycin (formerly mithramycin), a treatment reserved for severe, refractory Paget's disease, is rarely necessary. In addition to antiresorptive therapies, nonsteroidal anti-inflammatory drugs (NSAIDs) and aspirin are useful therapeutic modalities to alleviate associated joint pain and symptoms that result from degenerative joint disease. Lastly, surgical intervention is sometimes warranted in patients with Paget's disease and bony deformities, pathologic fractures, nerve compression, or degenerative arthritis. Orthopedic procedures, such as total joint replacement and osteotomies, are associated with a reduced risk of intraoperative bleeding or other complications if patients are treated medically (e.g., calcitonin or other bisphosphonates) to reduce the disease activity and vascularity for at least 6 weeks before the procedure.

REFERENCES

1. National Osteoporosis Foundation: Osteoporos Int 4(Suppl): S7-S80, 1998.
2. Riggs BL, Melton LJI: The prevention and treatment of osteoporosis. N Engl J Med 327:620-627, 1992.
3. Riggs BL, Wahner HW, Dunn WL, et al: Differential changes in bone mineral density of the appendicular and axial skeleton with aging: Relationship to spinal osteoporosis. J Clin Invest 67:328, 1981.
4. National Osteoporosis Foundation: Physician's Guide to Prevention and Treatment of Osteoporosis. Belle Mead, NJ, Excerpta Medica, 1998.
5. Manolagas SC, Jilka RL: Bone marrow, cytokines, and bone remodeling. N Engl J Med 332:305-311, 1995.
6. Kimble RB, Kitazawa R, Vannice JL, et al: Persistent bone-sparing effect of interleukin-1 receptor antagonist: A hypothesis on the role of IL-1 in ovariectomy-induced bone loss. Calcif Tissue Int 55:260-265, 1996.
7. Cheleuitte D, Mizuno S, Glowacki J: In vitro secretion of cytokines by human bone marrow: Effects of age and estrogen status. J Clin Endocrinol Metab 83:2043-2051, 1998.
8. Boyce BF, Hughes RD, Wright KR: Recent advances in bone biology provide insights in the pathogenesis of bone disease. Lab Invest 79:83-94, 1999.
9. Nevitt MC: Epidemiology of osteoporosis. Osteoporosis 20:535-554, 1994.
10. El-Hajj Fuleihan G, Gundberg CM, Gleason R, et al: Racial differences in parathyroid hormone dynamics. J Clin Endocrinol Metab 79:1642-1647, 1994.
11. Bell NH, Shary J, Stevens J: Demonstration that bone mass is greater in black than in white children. J Bone Miner Res 6:719-723, 1991.
12. Sambrook PN, Kelly PJ, Morrison NA, et al: Scientific review. Genetics of osteoporosis. Br J Rheumatol 33:1007-1011, 1994.
13. Cummings SR, Nevitt MC, Browner WS, et al: Risk factors for hip fracture in white women. N Engl J Med 332:767-773, 1995.
14. Uitterlinden AG, Burger H, Huang Q, et al: Relation of alleles of the collagen type 1α1 gene to bone density and the risk of osteoporotic fractures in postmenopausal women. N Engl J Med 338:1016-1021, 1998.
15. Faulkner KG, Cummings SR, Black D, et al: Simple measurement of femoral geometry predicts hip fracture: the study of osteoporotic fractures. J Bone Miner Res 8:1211-1217, 1993.
16. Little RD, Carulli JP, Del Mastro RG, et al: A mutation in the LDL receptor-related protein 5 gene results in the autosomal dominant high-bone mass trait. Am J Hum Genet 70(1):11-19, 2002.
17. Boyden LM, Mao J, Belsky J, et al: High bone density due to a mutation in LDL-receptor protein 5. New Engl J Med 346(20):1513-1521, 2002.
18. Lane NE, Lukert BP: The science and therapy of glucocorticoid-induced osteoporosis. Endocrinol Metab Clin North Am 27:465-483, 1998.
19. Ross DS, Neer RM, Ridgway EC: Subclinical hyperthyroidism and reduced bone density as a possible result of prolonged suppression of the pituitary-thyroid axis with L-thyroxine. Am J Med 82:1167-1170, 1987.
20. Biller BMK, Saxe V, Herzog DB, et al: Mechanisms of osteoporosis in adult and adolescent women with anorexia nervosa. J Clin Endocrinol Metab 68:548-551, 1989.
21. Friedman AJ, Daly M, Juneau-Norcross M, et al: A prospective, randomized trial of gonadotropin-releasing hormone agonist plus estrogen-progestin add-back regimens for women with leiomyomata uteri. J Clin Endocrinol Metab 76:1439-1445, 1993.
22. Gordon CM, Grace E, Emans SJ, et al: Changes in bone turnover markers and menstrual function after short-term oral DHEA in young women with anorexia nervosa. J Bone Miner Res 14:136-145, 1999.
23. Sambrook PN, Ansell BM, Foster S, et al: Bone turnover in early rheumatoid arthritis. II. Longitudinal bone density studies. Ann Rheum Dis 44:580-584, 1985.
24. Rehman Q, Lane NE: Therapeutic approaches for preventing bone loss in inflammatory arthritis. Arthritis Res 3(4):221-227, 2001.
25. Gravallese EM, Goldring SR: Cellular mechanisms and the role of cytokines in bone erosions in rheumatoid arthritis. Arthritis Rheum 43(10):2143-2151, 2000.
26. Kong YY, Yoshida H, Sarosi I, et al: OPGL is a key regulator of osteoclastogenesis, lymphocyte development and lymph-node organogenesis. Nature 397: 316-323, 1999.
27. American College of Rheumatologists Task Force on Osteoporosis Guidelines: Recommendations for the prevention and treatment of glucocorticoid-induced osteoporosis 2001 update. Arthritis Rheum 44:1496-1503, 2001.
28. Hansen M, Florescu A, Stoltenberg M, et al: Bone loss in rheumatoid arthritis: Influence of disease activity, duration of the disease, functional capacity, and corticosteroid treatment. Scand J Rheumatol 25(6):367-376, 1996.
29. LeBoff MS, Wade JP, Mackowiak S, et al: Low dose prednisone does not affect calcium homeostasis or bone density in postmenopausal women with rheumatoid arthritis. J Rheumatol 18:339-344, 1991.
30. Hunter T, Dubo HI: Spinal fractures complicating ankylosing spondylitis: A longterm follow-up study. Arthritis Rheum 26:751-759, 1983.
31. Stowens DW, Teitelbaum SL, Kahn AJ, et al: Skeletal complications of Gaucher disease. Medicine 64:310-322, 1985.
32. Movsowitz C, Epstein S, Fallon M, et al: Cyclosporin-A in vivo produces severe osteopenia in the rat: Effect of dose and duration of administration. Endocrinology 123:2571-2577, 1988.
33. Bryer HP, Isserow JA, Armstrong EC, et al: Azathioprine alone is bone sparing and does not alter cyclosporin A-induced osteopenia in the rat. J Bone Miner Res 10:132-138, 1995.
34. Rich GM, Mudge GH, Laffel GL, et al: Cyclosporine A and prednisone-associated osteoporosis in heart transplant recipients. J Heart Lung Transplant 11:950-958, 1992.
35. LeBoff MS, Kohlmeier L, Hurwitz S, et al: Occult vitamin D deficiency in postmenopausal U.S. women with acute hip fracture. JAMA 281:1505-1511, 1999.
36. Johnston CC Jr., Slemenda CW, Melton LJ III: Clinical use of bone densitometry. N Engl J Med 324:1105-1109, 1991.
37. El-Hajj Fuleihan G, Testa MA, Angell JE, et al: Reproducibility of DXA absorptiometry: A model for bone loss estimates. J Bone Miner Res 10:1004-1014, 1995.
38. Melton LJ, Atkinson EJ, O'Fallon WM, et al: Long-term fracture prediction by bone mineral assessed at different skeletal sites. J Bone Miner Res 8:1227-1233, 1993.
39. Cummings SR, Black DM, Nevitt MC, et al: Bone density at various sites for prediction of hip fractures: The Study of Osteoporotic Fractures Research Group. Lancet 341:72-75, 1993.
40. Stewart A, Reid DM, Porter RW: Broadband ultrasound attenuation and dual energy x-ray absorptiometry in patients with hip fractures: Which technique discriminates fracture risk? Calcif Tissue Int 54:466, 1994.
41. Kanis JA, Melton LJ III, Christiansen C, et al: Perspective: The diagnosis of osteoporosis. J Bone Miner Res 9:1137-1141, 1994.
42. Uebelhart D, Schlemmer A, Johansen JS, et al: Effect of menopause and hormone replacement therapy on the urinary excretion of pyridinium cross-links. J Clin Endocrinol Metab 72:367-373, 1991.
43. Delmas PD, Schlemmer A, Gineyts E, et al: Rapid publication: Urinary excretion of pyridinoline crosslinks correlates with bone turnover measured on iliac crest biopsy in patients with vertebral osteoporosis. J Bone Miner Res 6:639-644, 1991.
44. Rosen HN, Dresner-Pollak R, Moses AC, et al: Specificity of urinary excretion of cross-linked N-telopeptides of type I collagen as a marker of bone turnover. Calcif Tissue Int 54:26-29, 1994.

45. Garnero P, Hausherr E, Chapuy MC, et al: Markers of bone resorption predict hip fracture risk in elderly women: The EPIDOS Prospective Study. J Bone Miner Res 11:1531-1538, 1996.

46. Rosen CJ, Chestnut CH III, Mallinak NJ: The predictive value of biochemical markers of bone turnover for bone mineral density in early postmenopausal women treated with hormone replacement or calcium supplementation. J Clin Endocrinol Metab 82:1904-1910, 1997.

47. Lane NE, Sanchez S, Genant HK, et al: Short-term increases in bone turnover markers predict parathyroid hormone-induced spinal bone mineral density gains in postmenopausal women with glucocorticoid-induced osteoporosis. Osteoporos Int 11:434-442, 2000.

48. Cosman F, Nieves J, Woeflert I: Alendronate does not block the anabolic effect of PTH in posmenopausal osteoporotic women. J Bone Miner Res 13:1051-1055, 1998.

49. Silverberg SJ, Gartenberg F, Jacobs TP, et al: Increased bone mineral density after parathyroidectomy in primary hyperparathyroidism. J Clin Endocrinol Metab 80:729-734, 1995.

50. Silverberg SJ, Gartenberg F, Jacobs TP, et al: Longitudinal measurements of bone density and biochemical indices in untreated primary hyperparathyroidism. J Clin Endocrinol Metab 80:723-728, 1995.

51. Dawson-Hughes B, Dallal GE, Krall EA, et al: A controlled trial of the effect of calcium supplementation on bone density in postmenopausal women. N Engl J Med 323:878-883, 1990.

52. Atkinson SA, Abrams SA, Dawson-Hughes B, et al: Calcium. In Young V (ed): Dietary Reference Intake for Calcium, Phosphorus, Magnesium, Vitamin D and Fluoride. Washington, DC, National Academy Press, 1997, pp 91-143.

53. Optimal calcium intake: NIH Consensus Conference. JAMA 272:1942-1947, 1994.

54. Nicar MJ, Pak CYC: Calcium bioavailability from calcium carbonate and calcium citrate. J Clin Endocrinol Metab 61:391-393, 1985.

55. Hulley S, Grady D, Bush T, et al: Randomized trial of estrogen plus progestin for secondary prevention of coronary heart disease in postmenopausal women. JAMA 280:605-613, 1998.

56. Grady D, Herrington D, Bittner V, et al: Cardiovascular disease outcomes during a 6.8 years of hormone therapy: Heart and Estrogen/Progestin Replacement Study follow-up (HERS II). JAMA 288(1):58-66, 2002.

57. Writing Group for the Women's Health Initative Investigators: Risk and benefits of estrogen plus progestin in healthy postmenopausal women: Principal results from the Women's Health Initiative randomized controlled trial. JAMA 288:321-333, 2002.

58. Love RR, Mazess RB, Barden HS, et al: Effects of tamoxifen on bone mineral density in postmenopausal women with breast cancer. N Engl J Med 326:852-856, 1992.

59. Fisher B, Costantino JP, Wicherham DL, et al: Tamoxifen for prevention of breast cancer: Report of the National Surgical Adjuvant Breast and Bowel Project P-1 Study. J Natl Cancer Inst 90:1371-1388, 1998.

60. Cummings SR, Eckert S, Krueger KA, et al: The effect of raloxifene on risk of breast cancer in postmenopausal women: Results from the MORE randomized trial. Multiple Outcomes of Raloxifene Evaluation. JAMA 281:2189-2197, 1999.

61. Delmas P, Bjarnason NH, Mitlak B, et al: Effects of raloxifene on bone mineral density, serum cholesterol concentrations, and uterine endometrium in postmenopausal women. N Engl J Med 337:1641-1647, 1997.

62. Ettinger B, Black D, Mitlak B, et al: Reduction of vertebral fracture risk in postmenopausal women with osteoporosis treated with raloxifene: Results from 3 year randomized clinical trial (MORE). JAMA 282:637-645, 1999.

63. Walsh BW, Kuller LH, Wild RA, et al: Effects of raloxifene on serum lipids and coagulation factors in healthy postmenopausal women. JAMA 279:1445-1451, 1998.

64. Walsh BW, Paul S, Wild RA, et al: The effects of hormone replacement therapy and raloxifene on C-reactive protein and homocystein in healthy postmenopausal women: A randomized controlled trial. J Clin Endocrinol Metab 85(1):214-218, 2000.

65. Ridker PM, Buring JE, Shin J, et al: Prospective study of C-reactive protein and the risk of furture cardiovascular events among apparently healthy women. Circulation 98(8):731-733, 1998.

66. Tenover JL: Male hormone replacement therapy including "Andropause." Endocrinol Metab Clin North Am 27:969-988, 1998.

67. Gennari C, Chierichetti SM, Bigazzi S, et al: Comparative effects on bone mineral content of calcium and calcium plus salmon calcitonin given in two different regimens in postmenopausal osteoporosis. Curr Ther Res 38:455-464, 1985.

68. Overgaard K, Riis BJ, Christiansen C, et al: Nasal calcitonin for treatment of established ostcoporosis. Clin Endocrinol 30:435-442, 1989.

69. Chesnut C, Silverman S, Andriono K, et al: A randomized trial of nasal spray salmon calcitonin in postmenopausal women with established osteoporosis: the prevent recurrence of osteoporotic fractures study. PROOF Study group. Amer J Med 109:267-276, 2000.

70. Harris ST, Watts NB, Jackson RD, et al: Four-year study of intermittent cyclic etidronate treatment of postmenopausal osteoporosis: Three years of blinded therapy followed by one year of open therapy. Am J Med 95:557-567, 1993.

71. Liberman UA, Weiss SR, Broll J, et al: Effect of oral alendronate on bone mineral density and the incidence of fractures in postmenopausal osteoporosis. N Engl J Med 333:1437-1443, 1995.

72. Black DM, Cummings SR, Karpt DB, et al: Randomized trial of effect of alendronate on risk of fracture in women with existing vertebral fractures. Lancet 348:1535-1541, 1996

73. Hosking D, Chilvers CE, Christiansen C, et al: Prevention of bone loss with alendronate in postmenopausal women under 60 years of age. N Engl J Med 338:485-492, 1998.

74. Cummings SR, Black DM, Thompson DE, et al: Effect of alendronate on risk of fracture in women with low bone density but without vertebral fractures. JAMA 280:2077-2082, 1998.

75. Orwoll E, Ettinger M, Weiss S, et al: Alendronate for the treatment of osteoporosis in men. New Engl J Med 343(9):604-610, 2000.

76. Schnitzer T, Bone HG, Crepaldi G, et al: Therapeutic equivalence of alendronate 70mg once-weekly and alendronate 10mg daily in the treatment of osteoporosis. Aging 12(1):1-12, 2000.

77. Harris ST, Watts NB, Genant HK, et al: Effects of risedronate treatment on vertebral and nonverterbal fractures in women with postmenopausal osteoporosis: A randomized controlled trial. Vertebral Efficacy With Risedronate Therapy (VERT) Study Group. JAMA 282:1344, 1999.

78. Heaney RP, Zizic TM, Fogelman I, et al: Risedronate reduces the risk of first vertebral fracture in osteoporotic women. Osteoporos Int 13:501-505, 2002.

79. Reginster J-Y, Minne HW, Sorensen O, et al: Randomized trial of the effects of risedronate on vertebral fractures in women with postmenopausal osteoporosis. Osteoporos Int 11:83-91, 2000.

80. McClung MR, Geusens P, Miller PD, et al: Effect of risedronate on the risk of hip fracture in elderly women. New Engl J Med 344:333-340, 2001.

81. Risedronate Delaney M, Harwitz S, Shaw J, LeBoff Ms. Bone density changes with once weekly risedronate in postmenopausal women J. Clin. Densitrom, 2003; 6(1). 45-50.

82. Miller PD, Brown JP, Siris ES: A randomized double-blind trial of risedronate and etirdonate in the treatment of Paget's disease of bone. Am J Med 106:513-520, 1999.

83. Reid IR, Brown JP, Burckhardt P, et al: Intravenous zoledronic acid in postmenopausal women with low bone density. New Engl J Med 346(9):653-661, 2002.

84. Pak CYC, Sakhaee K, Adams-Huet B, et al: Treatment of postmenopausal osteoporosis with slow-release sodium fluoride. Ann Intern Med 123:401-408, 1995.

85. Finkelstein JS, Klibanski A, Arnold A, et al: Prevention of estrogen deficiency-related bone loss with human parathyroid hormone-(1-34). JAMA 280:1067-1073, 1998.

86 Lindsay R, Nieves J, Formica C, et al: Randomized controlled study of effect of parathyroid hormone on vertebral-bone mass and fracture incidence among postmenopausal women on oestrogen with osteoporosis. Lancet 350:550-555, 1997.

87. Neer RM, Arnaud CD, Zanchetta JR, et al: Effect of parathyroid hormone (1-34) on fractures and bone mineral density in postmenopausal women with osteoporosis. New Engl J Med 344:1434-1441, 2001.

88. Kurland ES, Cosman F, McMahon DJ, et al. Parathyroid hormone as a therapy for idiopathic osteoporosis in men: effects on bone

mineral density and bone markers. J Clin Endocrinol Metab 85:2129-2134, 2000.

89. Rittmaster RS, Bolognese M, Ettinger MP: Enhancement of bone mass in osteoporotic women with parathyroid hormone followed by alendronate. J Clin Endocrinol Metab 85:2129-2134, 2000.

90. Thomas MK, Lloyd-Jones DM, Thadhani RI, et al: Hypovitaminosis D in medical inpatients. N Engl J Med 338:777-783, 1998.

91. Dawson-Hughes B, Harris SS, Krall EA, et al: Effect of calcium and vitamin D supplementation on bone density in men and women 65 years of age or older. N Engl J Med 337:670-676, 1997.

92. Luo S, Labrie C, Belanger A, Labrie F: Effect of DHEA and the pure antiestrogen EM-800 on bone mass, serum lipids, and the development of dimethylbenz(a)-anthracene (DMBA)-induced mammary carcinoma in the rat [Abstract P1-527]. The Endocrine Society, 1997.

93. Adinoff AD, Hollister JR: Steroid-induced fractures and bone loss in patients with asthma. N Engl J Med 309:265-268, 1983.

94. American College of Rheumatology Ad Hoc Committee on published journal Glucocorticoid-Induced Osteoporosis: Recommendations for the prevention and treatment of glucocorticoid-induced osteoporosis: 2001 Update. Arthritis Rheum 44:1496-1503, 2001.

95. Montemurro L, Schiraldi G, Fraioli P, et al: Prevention of corticosteroid-induced osteoporosis with salmon calcitonin in sarcoid patients. Calcif Tissue Int 49:71-76, 1991.

96. Sambrook P, Birmingham J, Kelly P, et al: Prevention of corticosteroid osteoporosis: A comparison of calcium, calcitriol, and calcitonin. N Engl J Med 328:1747-1752, 1993.

97. Saag HG, Emkey R, Schnitzer TJ, et al: Aledronate for the prevention and treatment of glucocorticoid-induced osteoporosis. N Engl J Med 339:292-299, 1998.

98. Adachi JD, Saag KG, Delmas PD, et al: Two-year effects of alendronate on bone mineral density and vertebral fracture in patients receiving glucocorticoids: A randomized, double-blind, placebo-controlled extension trial. Arthritis Rheum 44(1):202-211, 2001.

99. Cohen S, Levy RM, Keller M, et al: Risedronate therapy prevents corticosteroid-induced bone loss. Arthritis Rheum 42(11):2309-2318, 1999.

100. Reid DM, Hughes RA, Laan R, et al: Efficacy and safety of daily risedronate in the treatment of corticosteroid-induced osteoporosis in men and women: A randomized trial. J Bone Miner Res 15:1006-1013, 2000.

101. Boutsen Y, Jamart J, Esselinckx W, Devogelaer JP: Primary prevention of glucocorticoid-induced osteoporosis with intravenous pamidronate and calcium: A prospective controlled 1-year study comparing a single infusion, an infusion given once every 3 months, and calcium alone. J Bone Miner Res 16:104-112, 2001.

102. Lukert BP, Johnson BE, Robinson RG: Estrogen and progesterone replacement therapy reduces glucocorticoid-induced bone loss. J Bone Miner Res 7:1063-1069, 1992.

103. Petri MA, Lahita RG, Van Vollenhoven RF, et al: Effects of prasterone on corticosteroid requirements of women with systemic lupus erythematosus: A double blind, randomized, placebo-controlled trial. Arthritis Rheum 46(7):1820-1829, 2002.

104. Meese PJ, Ginzler EM, Gluck OS, et al: Improvement in bone mineral density in steroid-treated SLE patients during treatment with prasterone (DHEA). Arthritis Rheum 43(Suppl I):S206, 2000.

105. Reid IR, Ibbertson HK, France JT, et al: Plasma testosterone concentrations in asthmatic men treated with glucocorticoids. BMJ 291:574, 1985.

106. Reid IR, Wattie DJ, Evans MC, et al: Testosterone therapy in glucocorticoid-treated men. Arch Intern Med 156:1173-1178, 1996.

107. Lane NE, Sanchez S, Modin GW, et al: Parathyroid hormone treatment can reverse corticosteroid-induced osteoporosis. J Clin Invest 102:1627-1633, 1998.

108. Lane NE, Sanchez S, Genant HK, et al: Bone mass continues to increase at the hip after parathyroid hormone treatment is discontinued in postmenopausal women with glucocorticoid-induced osteoporosis. J Bone Miner Res 15(5): 994-951.

109. Rehman Q, Lang T, Lane NE: Daily treatment with parathyroid hormone is associated with an increase in vertebral cross-sectional area in postmenopausal women with glucocorticoid-induced osteoporosis. Osteoporos Int, 41(5):374-382, 2003.

110. Rickers H, Deding A, Christiansen C, et al: Corticosteroid-induced osteopenia and vitamin D metabolism: Effect of vitamin D2, calcium phosphate and sodium fluoride administration. Clin Endocrinol (Oxford) 16:409, 1982.

111. Reginster JY, Meurmans L, Zegeks B, et al: The effect of sodium monofluorophosphate plus calcium on vertebral fracture rate in postmenopausal women with moderate osteoporosis. Ann Intern Med 129:1-8, 1998.

112. Lippuner K, Casez JP, Horber FF, et al: Effects of deflazacort versus prednisone on bone mass, body composition, and lipid profile: A randomized, double blind study in kidney transplant patients. J Clin Endocrinol Metab 83:3795-3802, 1998.

113. Frame B, Parfitt AM: Osteomalacia: Current concepts. Ann Intern Med 89:966-982, 1978.

114. Streeten EA, Levine MA: Hyperparathyroidism and hypoparathyroidism. In Rakel RE (ed): Conn's Current Therapy. Philadelphia, WB Saunders, 2000, pp 627-634.

115. Hruska KA, Teitelbaum SL: Renal osteodystrophy. N Engl J Med 333:166-174, 1995.

116. Felsenfeld AJ, Llach F: Parathyroid gland function in chronic renal failure. Kidney Int 43:771-789, 1993.

117. Econs MJ, Rowe PS, Francis F, et al: Fine structure mapping of the human X-linked hypophosphatemic rickets gene locus. J Clin Endocrinol Metab 79:1351-1354, 1994.

118. Ryan EA, Reiss E: Oncogenous osteomalacia: Review of the world literature of 42 cases and report of two new cases. Am J Med 77:501-512, 1984.

119. Drezner MK, Lyles KW, Haussler MR, et al: Evaluation of a role for 1,25-dihydroxyvitamin D_3 in the pathogenesis and treatment of X-linked hypophosphatemic rickets and osteomalacia. J Clin Invest 66:1020-1032, 1980.

120. Quarles LD, Davidai GA, Schwab SJ, et al: Oral calcitriol and calcium: Efficient therapy for uremic hyperparathyroidism. Kidney Int 34:840-844, 1988.

121. Siris ES: Extensive personal experience: Paget's disease of bone. J Clin Endocrinol Metab 80:335-338, 1995.

122. Siris ES, Chines AA, Altman RD, et al: Risedronate in the treatment of Paget's disease of bone: An open label, multicenter study. J Bone Miner Res 13:1032-1038, 1998.

123. Whyte MP, Obrecht SE, Finnegan PM, et al: Osteoprotegrin deficiency and juvenile Paget's disease. New Engl J Med 347(3):175-184, 2002.

124. LeBoff MS, El-Hajj Fuleihan G, Brown EM: Osteoporosis and Paget's disease of bone. In Branch WT (ed): Office Practice of Medicine, 3rd ed. Philadelphia, WB Saunders, 1994, pp 700-714.

125. DeRose J, Singer FR, Avramides A, et al: Response of Paget's disease to porcine and salmon calcitonins: Effects of long-term treatment. Am J Med 56:858-866, 1974.

126. Krane SM: Etidronate disodium in the treatment of Paget's disease of bone. Ann Intern Med 96:619-625, 1982.

127. Gallacher SJ, Boyce BF, Patel U, et al: Clinical experience with pamidronate in the treatment of Paget's disease of bone. Ann Rheum Dis 50:930-933, 1991.

128. Hosking DJ, Eusabio RA, Chines AA: Paget's disease of bone: Reduction of disease activity with oral risedronate. Bone 22:51-55, 1998.

91

Pathogenesis of Osteoarthritis

PAUL E. DI CESARE · STEVEN B. ABRAMSON

Osteoarthritis (OA) is a degenerative joint disease, occurring primarily in older persons, characterized by erosion of the articular cartilage, hypertrophy of bone at the margins (i.e., osteophytes), subchondral sclerosis, and a range of biochemical and morphologic alterations of the synovial membrane and joint capsule. Pathologic changes in the late stages of OA include softening, ulceration, and focal disintegration of the articular cartilage; synovial inflammation also can occur. Typical clinical symptoms are pain and stiffness, particularly after prolonged activity.

In industrialized societies OA is the leading cause of physical disability, increase in health care utilization, and impaired quality of life. The impact of arthritic conditions is expected to grow as the population both increases and ages in the coming decades.[1] Despite its prevalence, the precise etiology, pathogenesis, and progression of OA remain beyond our understanding, primarily due to confounding factors in human epidemiologic studies, including individual variations in physical activity, diet, and medical history; the poor correlation between symptoms of OA and radiographic lesions; and our inability to detect early disease. Furthermore, because arthritic human tissue for study is typically obtained at surgery from patients with severe OA, it may not manifest those pathologic or biochemical changes that occur early in the disease process. Without a clear-cut picture of how OA arises at the cellular or molecular level, many still consider it a result of "wear and tear," an inevitable consequence of aging.

Although the etiology of OA is incompletely understood, the accompanying biochemical, structural, and metabolic changes in joint cartilage have been well documented. It is now known, for example, that cytokines, mechanic trauma, and altered genetics are involved in its pathogenesis and that these factors can initiate a degradative cascade that results in many of the characteristic alterations of articular cartilage in OA. More recently it has become apparent that OA is a disease process that affects the entire joint structure, including cartilage, synovial membrane, subchondral bone, ligaments, and periarticular muscles. OA is, thus, better thought of as a group of overlapping disorders with varied etiologies and arising from a combination of systemic (e.g., genetic) and local factors (e.g., biomechanically or biochemically mediated events) that gradually converge to produce a condition with definable morphologic and clinical outcomes and end-stage commonalities.

OA may be classified as primary or secondary according to its cause or major predisposing factor; what all OA has in common is altered cartilage physiology. Primary OA is the most common type and has no identifiable etiology or predisposing cause. Secondary OA, although it has an identifiable underlying cause, is pathologically indistinguishable from primary OA. The most common causes of secondary OA are metabolic conditions (e.g., calcium crystal deposition, hemochromatosis, acromegaly), anatomic factors (e.g., leg length inequality, congenital hip dislocation), traumatic events (e.g., major joint trauma, chronic joint injury, joint surgery), or the sequelae of inflammatory disorders (e. g., ankylosing spondylitis, septic arthritis). In the case of secondary OA arising from inflammatory joint disease, cartilage degeneration most likely results initially from degradative enzymes released from the synovium or leukocytes within the joint space and later from the mechanic disruption of a biomechanically altered extracellular matrix. Distinguishing between primary and secondary OA may be difficult because the clinical presentation and symptoms are often so similar.

Etiologic Factors in Osteoarthritis

Major factors affecting degree of risk for developing OA include age, joint location, obesity, genetic predisposition, joint malalignment, trauma, and gender.

AGE

Age is the single risk factor most strongly correlated with OA.[2,3] OA is, in fact, the most common chronic disease in later life; more than 80 percent of persons over age 75 years are affected, and OA increases progressively with age at all joint sites. Radiologic changes in OA increase as individuals age,[4] although these changes do not always correlate with clinical symptoms or disability.[5,6] Although clearly an age-related disease, OA is not an inevitable consequence of aging.

Age-related morphologic and structural changes in articular cartilage include fraying, softening, and thinning of the articular surface, decreased size and aggregation of matrix proteoglycans, and loss of matrix tensile strength and stiffness. These age-related tissue changes are most likely due to a decrease in the ability of chondrocytes to maintain and repair the tissue, as chondrocytes themselves undergo age-related decreases in mitotic and synthetic activity, exhibit decreased responsiveness to anabolic growth factors, and synthesize smaller and less uniform large aggregating proteoglycans and fewer functional link proteins. Cultured chondrocytes have been shown to exhibit an age-related decline in response to insulin-like growth factor-I (IGF-I), a growth factor that stimulates the production of proteoglycans, collagen, and integrin cell receptors. Progressive chondrocyte senescence (as reflected in expression of the senescence-associated enzyme β-galactosidase), erosion of chondrocyte telomere length, and mitochondrial degeneration due to oxidative damage also contribute to the age-related reduction in chondrocyte function.[3]

JOINT LOCATION

Although OA occurs most commonly in weight-bearing joints,[7] age affects joints differently.[8] A study comparing tensile fracture stress of cartilage in the femoral head and in the talus showed that it decreased progressively with age in the former but not in the latter.[9] Joint-specific, age-related changes in articular cartilage may explain why OA is more common in hip and knee joints with increasing age but occurs rarely in the ankle.

Alterations in chondrocyte responsiveness to cytokines also appear to vary depending on the joint. For example, studies show that knee chondrocytes exhibit more interleukin-1 (IL-1) receptors than ankle chondrocytes and that knee chondrocytes express mRNA for matrix metalloproteinase-8 (MMP-8), whereas chondrocytes from the ankle do not.[10-12]

OBESITY

Obesity is another important risk factor for OA.[13-15] Greater body mass index in both women and men has been associated with an increased risk of knee (but not hip) OA.[6,16,17] In a study that examined 715 paired radiographs (index and 4-year follow-up), Hart and colleagues reported that obesity significantly increased the risk of knee symptoms and radiographic osteophytes.[18]

An increase in mechanical forces across weight-bearing joints is probably the primary factor leading to joint degeneration. Obesity not only increases the forces at weight-bearing joints, but may also change posture, gait, and physical activity level, any or all of which may further contribute to altered joint biomechanics.[19] The majority of obese patients exhibit varus knee deformities, which result in increased joint reactive forces within the medial compartment of the knee that accelerate the degenerative process.[20]

Particularly in elderly obese individuals, heavy physical activity is an additional risk factor for the development of knee OA, whereas light to moderate activity does not appear to increase risk for knee OA and may, in fact, alleviate symptomatic knee OA by reducing body mass index.[6,16,17] Similarly, weight loss can reduce both radiographic knee OA progression and clinical symptoms.

GENETIC PREDISPOSITION

Because of the prevalence of OA in the general population and its extensive clinical heterogeneity, the genetic contribution to its pathogenesis has been difficult to analyze.[21,22] In the 1960s, Kellgren reported that generalized nodal OA, characterized by multiple joint involvement, including the presence of Heberden's nodes and knee OA, was twice as likely to occur in first-degree relatives than in controls.[23] Population studies of patients with radiographic evidence of OA followed in two major cohorts (the Framingham Study and the Baltimore Longitudinal Study on Aging) clearly support a significant genetic contribution to OA, with evidence for a major recessive gene and a multifactorial component, representing either polygenic or environmental factors.[24,25] Twin-pair and family-risk studies have indicated that the hereditable component of OA may be on the order of 50 to 65 percent.[22,26,27] Moreover, family, twin, and population studies have indicated differences among genetic influences that determine the site of OA (hip, spine, knee, hand).[25,28,29] Further evidence supporting a genetic predisposition to OA is the demonstration of a significantly higher concordance for OA between monozygotic twins than between dizygotic twins. Genetic studies have identified multiple gene variations associated with an increased risk of OA.[30]

Structural genes are clearly important for the maintenance and repair of articular cartilage, as well as regulation of chondrocyte proliferation and gene expression; in some cases (e.g., chondrodysplasias), structural genes are the identifiable causes of OA. Several candidate genes encoding for structural proteins of the extracellular matrix of the articular cartilage have been associated with early-onset OA.[31,32] Although likely of limited importance in most cases of OA, the discovery of a point mutation (Arg519 → Cys in exon 31) in the cDNA coding for type II collagen found in articular cartilage in several generations of a family with spondyloepiphyseal dysplasia and polyarticular OA[31,32] has focused attention on this area.

In addition to the point mutation in type II collagen, which was identified in the family noted previously,[32] inherited forms of OA may be caused by mutations in several other genes that are expressed in cartilage, including those encoding types IV, V, and VI collagen, as well as cartilage oligomeric matrix protein (COMP).[33] Moreover, candidate genes in OA have been identified that are not structural proteins. The haplotype of a vitamin D receptor (VDR) that plays a vital role in controlling bone mineral density (BMD) appears to be associated with a twofold risk of knee OA[34]—although the VDR locus is very close to the COL2A1 locus on chromosome 12q, so that the association may be due to linkage disequilibrium with the latter.[21] In addition, the locus of the *IGF-I* gene has been associated with radiographic OA, as has an aggrecan polymorphic allele with hand OA.[21] Evidence from patients as well as from animal models indicates that disorders characterized by calcium crystal deposition may predispose to OA. The defect in the progressive ankylosis (ank) mouse is in a gene that encodes a transmembrane protein that controls levels of inorganic phosphate, an inhibitor of matrix calcification.[35] Joints in the ank mouse contain hydroxyapatite (HA) crystals in articular cartilage, with accompanying joint-space narrowing, cartilage erosion, and osteophyte formation, all hallmarks of OA.

In recent population studies, genome-wide linkage scans have highlighted up to seven chromosomal regions that may harbor OA-susceptibility genes.[36] Chromosome 2q was positive in several scans, suggesting that this chromosome is likely to harbor one or more susceptibility genes. In a study of affected sibling pairs, a region of linkage stretching from 2q12 to 2q21 was reported for OA of the distal interphalangeal joint, and a previous study of affected sibling pairs in the United Kingdom demonstrated a broader region of linkage, stretching from 2q12 to 2q31.[36,37] Two IL-1 genes (*IL-1A* and *IL-1B*) and the gene encoding IL-1Ra (*IL1RN*) are located on chromosome 2q13 within a 430-kb genomic fragment. Given the importance of IL-1 in the perpetuation of cartilage damage in OA, it is possible that a proportion of the genetic susceptibility to OA may be encoded for by variation in the activity of cytokines, and that for chromosome 2q this susceptibility could reside within the IL-1 gene clusters. Loughlin and colleagues, however, have provided evidence that the IL-1 gene cluster harbors susceptibility for knee OA, but not for hip OA.[36] These and other epidemiologic studies have highlighted potential differences in the degree of OA heritability among different joint groups and between the two sexes.[38]

Genomic and postgenomic technology, in addition to defining susceptibility genotypes, will also lead to the discovery of genes and gene products that are overexpressed in OA tissues and that contribute to disease pathogenesis and progression.[39,40] Studies of differential gene expression in diseased tissue, in addition to elucidating pathogenic processes that lead to novel therapies, could also have two additional benefits: 1) identification of unique biomarkers that can be used for OA diagnosis or management; and 2) identification of candidate susceptibility genotypes, such as polymorphic variations of cytokines or growth factors, that may predispose to disease progression.[41]

JOINT MALALIGNMENT AND TRAUMA

Joint malalignment or trauma may lead to rapid development of OA, or it may initiate a slow process that results in symptomatic OA years later. Probably as a result of progressive reduction in periarticular blood flow and the resultant decrease in rate of remodeling at the osteochondral junction, joints become increasingly congruent with age.[42,43] Altered joint geometry may interfere with nutrition of the cartilage, or it may alter load distribution, either of which may result in altered biochemical composition of the cartilage, irrespective of age.[44,45] Local factors, such as stresses related to joint use and joint deformity, also influence the development of OA. A previously injured joint is very susceptible to development of OA.

Joint incongruence (e.g., malreduced intra-articular fractures, developmental dysplasia of the hip, recurrent dislocation of the patella) can lead to early-onset OA.[46] Repetitive, high-impact sports are strongly associated with joint injury and increase the risk for lower limb OA.[47] Repetitive trauma at a subfracture level has been shown to accelerate remodeling in the zone of calcified cartilage, with reduplication of the tidemark and thinning of the noncalcified zone resulting in stiffening of the subchondral bone, increased wear of the overlying

cartilage, and ultimately development of OA.[48-50] Regular exercise is important in maintaining articular cartilage structure and metabolic function. Recreational running and low-impact activities have not been shown to increase the risk of OA.

Articular cartilage is remarkably resistant to damage by shear forces; it is, however, highly vulnerable to repetitive impact loading.[51] When joints are subjected to in vitro cyclic loads that are easily borne by subchondral bone, cartilage degeneration still results.[52] This vulnerability could account for the high frequency of OA in shoulders and elbows of pneumatic drill operators and baseball pitchers, ankles of ballet dancers, metacarpophalangeal joints of boxers, and knees of basketball players. The major forces on articular cartilage, in addition to weight-bearing, are due to the contraction of the muscles that stabilize or move the joint.[53] For example, in normal walking, four to five times the body weight, and in squatting up to 10 times the body weight, is transmitted through the knee.[54] Articular cartilage is believed to be too thin to be an effective shock absorber under these high loads. What protects the joint under physiologic conditions of impact loading is joint motion, with the associated lengthening of muscles under tension and deformation of the subchondral bone.[55,56] Cancellous subchondral bone functions as a major shock absorber due to its material properties.[50] Two thirds of subchondral bone stiffness derives from bony trabeculae and about one third from intraosseous fluid.[57] In the normal, unloaded joint, the opposing surfaces are not congruous; under loading, both the cartilage and the bone deform so that a larger proportion of the opposing surfaces comes into contact, increasing joint congruity and resulting in force distribution over the largest possible area.[58] Excessive loads may cause microfractures of subchondral trabeculae that heal via callus formation and remodeling, resulting in stiffer-than-normal bone that is less effective as a shock absorber and predisposing articular cartilage to excessive impact loading and, eventually, degeneration.

Whether subchondral sclerosis precedes the onset of OA or is a change secondary to cartilage degeneration is not known. Indirect evidence supports the theory that biomechanical changes in subchondral bone may be important in OA.[57,59,60] Foss, for example, reported cases of unilateral femoral osteoporosis (which is associated with softening and greater compliance of the subchondral bone) that may have protected the hip from OA.[61] Conversely, in vitro studies have shown that stiffening of the cancellous bone with methacrylate, which reduces its deformability, leads to cartilage degeneration with repetitive impact loading.[62]

GENDER

Women are about twice as likely as men to develop OA. Although women have a lower prevalence of OA than men before age 50 years, there is a marked increase in prevalence among women after 50, particularly in the knee.[63] Women have a greater number of joints involved and are more likely to exhibit clinical symptoms of morning stiffness, joint swelling, and nocturnal pain. The gender differences in OA incidence after age 50 may be the result of postmenopausal estrogen deficiency. Articular chondrocytes possess functional estrogen receptors, suggesting that these cells can be regulated by estrogen. Nuclear estrogen receptors (ERs) have been detected in articular chondrocytes of humans,[64,65] rats,[65,66] monkeys,[65,67] and pigs[68] and in human growth-plate chondrocytes.[69] Chondrocytes express two isoforms of ER—ER-α and ER-β—that may have different organ-specific roles; ER-α is expressed more predominantly in cortical bone and ER-β in cartilage[65] and cancellous bone.[70] One direct effect of estrogen on cultured chondrocytes is upregulation of ER,[67] and an increase in ER has been associated with increased proteoglycan synthesis in rats.[66]

Recent epidemiologic studies have linked estrogen replacement therapy (ERT) with a lower-than-expected risk of knee and hip OA in postmenopausal women. Clinical investigations of the association between OA and hormonal level in women have involved measurement of circulating estrogen levels in postmenopausal women, general radiographic evaluation of postmenopausal women, and examination of the effect of ERT on such variables as knee OA and cartilage volume.[71-74] In a study of more than 4000 women aged 65 years or older that assessed pelvis radiographs for hip OA, Nevitt and colleagues[71] showed that women using oral estrogen faced a significantly reduced risk of hip OA. Estrogen users for 10 years or longer had a greater reduction in risk of developing hip OA than users for less than 10 years. Using weight-bearing radiographs in female participants in the Framingham Osteoarthritis Study ($n = 831$, mean age 73 years, age range 63 to 93) to study the prevalence of knee OA, a modest but insignificant protective effect for radiographically detected OA was demonstrated for women who were on ERT.[75] Zhang and colleagues[73] performed a prospective cohort study using anteroposterior weight-bearing knee radiographs of women (mean age 71 years, age range 63 to 91 years) from the Framingham Study; they categorized their sample into three groups according to estrogen use at biennial examination: never users ($n = 349$), past users ($n = 162$), and current users ($n = 40$). When both incident and progressive radiographic knee OA cases were combined, current ERT users were found to have 60-percent less risk for knee OA than never users. In a cross-sectional study of postmenopausal women from the Chingford Study ($n = 606$) using standard anteroposterior radiographs of hands and knees, ERT was shown to have a significant protective effect against knee OA and a similar but not significant effect for hand OA.[76] Interestingly women who had discontinued ERT for more than 1 year had no overall protective effect of the ERT for OA. In studies of the longer-term use of ERT and its association with knee cartilage volume in postmenopausal women (measured by magnetic resonance imaging [MRI]), it was reported that after adjusting for confounders, women using long-term ERT had more knee cartilage than controls.[74] Beneficial effects of ERT on the severity of knee OA in ovariectomized monkeys has also been demonstrated.[77]

Further clinical evidence of the role of estrogen in OA came from a case control study to determine whether an association existed between ER gene polymorphisms and generalized OA.[78] The investigators analyzed 65 women with generalized OA and compared them to 318 healthy female controls for the Pvu II and Xba I restriction fragment length polymorphisms of *ER* gene. The result showed that the ER genotype PpXx, with the combination of the Pvu II and Xba I RFLP, was a significant risk factor for generalized OA and was most prevalent in younger patients with severe radiographic changes.

Overall, these human and animal studies show that women taking ERT may have a lower incidence of OA, although prospective randomized trials to confirm these observations have not been performed.

Changes in Osteoarthritis

MORPHOLOGIC CHANGES

In early OA, the articular cartilage surface becomes irregular, and superficial clefts within the tissue become apparent; proteoglycan distribution is altered, as revealed by histochemical staining. As the condition worsens, the clefts deepen, surface irregularities increase, and the articular cartilage eventually ulcerates, exposing the underlying bone. Attempts at local self-repair can be seen as an initial increase in the number of chondrocytes in the form of clusters or clones, with as many as 50 or more cells in a cluster[54] (Fig. 91–1). Marginal osteophytes form, representing production of new bone, capped by newly formed, irregularly shaped hyaline and fibrocartilage.

BIOCHEMICAL CHANGES

The biochemical changes that occur in the articular cartilage vary from early to later stages in the disease process. In early OA the water content of the articular cartilage significantly increases, causing the tissue to swell and altering its biomechanic properties. This phenomenon suggests that there has been weakening of the collagen network; the type II collagen fibers in early OA have a smaller diameter than those in normal cartilage, and the normally tight weave in the midzone is slackened and distorted.[79-84] In later stages of OA, type I collagen concentration within the extracellular matrix increases and the proteoglycan concentration falls to 50 percent or less of normal, with less aggregation and shorter glycosaminoglycan side chains.[81,84,85] Keratan sulfate concentration decreases, and the ratio of chondroitin-4-sulfate to chondroitin-6-sulfate increases, reflecting synthesis by chondrocytes of a proteoglycan profile more characteristic of immature cartilage.[86] Proteoglycan concentration in the cartilage diminishes progressively until the end stages, when histologic staining detects little or none.[87]

Calcium crystals (e.g., calcium pyrophosphate dihydrate, basic calcium phosphate crystals) are commonly found in the cartilage of the elderly, and often crystal arthropathy coexists with OA.[88] It is unclear, however, whether these crystals are directly involved in the patho-

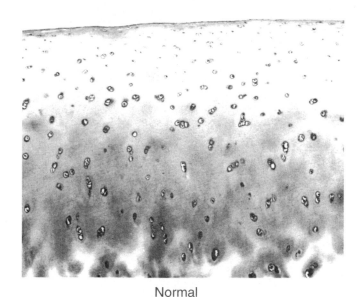

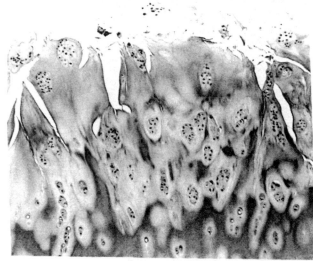

Normal   Osteoarthritis

FIGURE 91–1 · Histologic sections of normal (left) and osteoarthritic (OA) (right) articular cartilage obtained from the femoral head. The OA cartilage demonstrates surface irregularities, with clefts to the radial zone and cloning of chondrocytes.

genesis of OA or are merely a byproduct or marker of the disease. That calcium crystals play a role in causing or worsening OA is supported by clinical and laboratory studies, but the relationship is complex.[89] Pyrophosphate (PP) is produced from adenosine triphosphate (ATP) by the exoenzyme nucleoside pyrophosphohydrolase.[90] In normal cartilage basal zones, strong staining for alkaline phosphatase and matrix vesicles is indicative of cartilage calcification.[91] Human OA cartilage cultured in vitro also produces large quantities of alkaline phosphatase and PP.[91] Synovial fluid from OA patients shows high levels of PP similar to those in calcium pyrophosphate dihydrate (CPPD) crystal deposition disease—levels that correlate directly with severity of joint damage.[92,93] Young or proliferating chondrocytes are a major source of PP, whereas resting chondrocytes from normal adult cartilage secrete little.[90] It has thus been theorized that the increased PP secretion in OA cartilage may be an indication of increased chondrocyte metabolic activity toward matrix repair.[94] The presence of CPPD may alter the biomechanical properties of the cartilage extracellular matrix and lead to cartilage breakdown. Hemochromatosis (hemosiderin), Wilson's disease (copper), ochronotic arthropathy (homogentisic acid polymers), gouty arthritis (crystals of monosodium urate), and CPPD crystal deposition disease are further examples of conditions in which the abnormal entity may alter the net intermolecular charges in cartilage extracellular matrix, leading to either direct or indirect chondrocyte injury by increasing the stiffness of the tissue and thereby precipitating the development of OA.

METABOLIC CHANGES

As the severity of OA progresses, the synthesis and secretion of matrix-degrading enzymes by chondrocytes markedly increase[87,95] (Fig. 91–2). Early cartilage degeneration in OA is most likely the result of the action of enzymes from the MMP family of proteinases that degrade both proteoglycans (aggrecanases) and collagen (collagenases).[96-98] Collagenases typically make the first cleavage in triple-helical collagen, allowing its further degradation by other proteases. Aggrecanases in conjunction with other MMPs degrade aggrecan. Serine- and cysteine-dependent proteases (e.g., plasminogen activator/plasmin system and cathepsin B, respectively), as well as membrane-type MMPs act primarily as MMP activators.[99-101] The control of these enzymes is complex, with regulation occurring at three different levels: synthesis and secretion, activation of latent enzyme, and inactivation by proteinase inhibitors.[101a] In OA, the expression and production of proteinases is increased. Native collagen has been shown to be cleaved by MMP-1, -8 and -13; the resultant fragments may then be susceptible to cleavage by such other enzymes as MMP-2 (gelatinase A), MMP-9 (gelatinase B), MMP-3 (stromelysin 1), and cathepsin B. Of the three major MMPs that degrade native collagen, MMP-13 may be the most important in OA, because it preferentially degrades type II collagen.[102] It has also been shown that expression of MMP-13 greatly increases in OA[103]; overall collagenase activity also markedly increases in human OA cartilage cultures, suggesting that it is a major factor in OA progression and cartilage matrix degradation.[104,105] MMPs can degrade other cartilage extracellular matrix molecules in addition to collagen; if combined with plasmin (from plasminogen), MMPs can rapidly destroy cartilage altogether. In OA, collagenase, stromelysin, and gelatinase are secreted as proenzymes by the chondrocyte and are upregulated by IL-1 or tumor necrosis factor (TNF).[106,107] These proenzymes, each exhibiting a zinc-binding catalytic sequence, contain three histidine residues and a glutamine residue, all of which must be activated by proteolytic cleavage of their amino terminal sequence (see Chapter 4).

The aggrecanases belong to a family of extracellular proteases known as a disintegrin and metalloprotease with

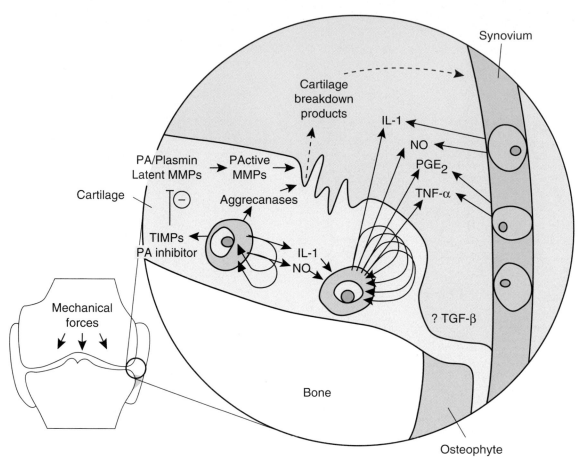

FIGURE 91–2 • Schematic of Pathogenic Mechanisms of Osteoarthritis (OA). Mechanical stress initiates altered metabolism characterized by the release of metalloproteinases (MMPs), proinflammatory cytokines, and mediators such as nitric oxide (NO) and prostaglandins (PGs). Cartilage breakdown products play a role by stimulating the release of cytokines from synovial lining cells, and by inducing MMP production by chondrocytes. Perpetuation of cartilage damage is amplified by the autocrine and paracrine actions of interleukin-1β (IL-1β) and tumor necrosis factor-α (TNF-α) produced by chondrocytes.

thrombospondin motifs (ADAMTS).[108] Two aggrecanases, ADAMTS-4 and ADAMTS-5, appear to be major enzymes in cartilage degradation in arthritis.[109] Recombinant ADAMTS-4 and ADAMTS-5 cleave aggrecan at five distinct sites along the core protein, and all resultant fragments have been identified in cartilage explants undergoing matrix degradation. Aggrecanase proteolytic activity can be modulated by altered expression, by activation by proteolytic cleavage at a furin-sensitive site, by binding to the aggrecan substrate through the C-terminal thrombospondin motif, by activation through post-translational processing of a portion of the C terminus, and by inhibition of activity by the endogenous inhibitor tissue inhibitor of metalloproteinases-3 (TIMP-3). ADAMTS-4 and ADAMTS-5 activity has also been detected in joint capsule and synovium and may be upregulated in arthritic synovium at either the message level or through post-translational processing. In addition to aggrecan, aggrecanases have been shown to degrade the nonaggrecated chondroitin-sulfate proteoglycans known as brevican and versican. The G1 region of aggrecan is highly resistant to proteases; however, a glutamate-alanine bond within the extended region between G1 and G2 is remarkably susceptible to proteolytic degradation.[110] Low concentrations of stromelysin readily cleave the region between G1 and G2 domains, resulting in disruption of the proteoglycan, (PG), aggregate structure and increased loss of PGs from the extracellular matrix. A specific hyaluronidase has not been found in articular cartilage, but one or several lysosomal enzymes that can cleave both hyaluronic acid and chondroitin-6-sulfate have been implicated.[99] The decrease in chondroitin sulfate chain length in OA cartilage may be due to digestion by synovial fluid hyaluronidase, which may diffuse into the matrix as its permeability increases.[86] Evidence to support this theory is the finding that the hyaluronic acid concentration in OA cartilage is low, even though its rate of synthesis is considerably greater than normal.[87,95] These degradative enzymes serve to disrupt the proteoglycan aggregate. The early result of the MMP-induced tissue degradation is thinning of the collagen fibers, loosening of the tight collagen network, and the consequent cartilage matrix swelling seen in OA.

Many investigators consider IL-1β a prime mediator in cartilage matrix degradation (see Fig. 91–2). IL-1 is synthesized by mononuclear cells (including synovial lining cells) in the inflamed joint and by chondrocytes as an autocrine activity.[111-113] IL-1 stimulates the synthesis and secretion of many degradative enzymes in cartilage, including latent collagenase, latent stromelysin, latent gelatinase, and tissue plasminogen activator.[114-117] With regard to aggrecanases, it appears that ADAMTS-5 is constitutively expressed, whereas IL-1 and TNF can induce ADAMTS-4.[118] Plasminogen, synthesized by the chondrocyte or entering the matrix by diffusion from the synovial fluid, is the substrate for tissue-type plasminogen activator (tPA).

The balance of active and latent enzymes is controlled to some extent by at least two enzyme inhibitors: TIMP and plasminogen activator inhibitor-1 (PAI-1).[97,119,120] TIMP and PAI-1 are synthesized in increased amounts under the regulation of transforming growth factor-β (TGF-β).[121-123] If insufficient concentrations of (or degraded) TIMP or PAI-1 are present in the matrix along with active enzymes, increased matrix degradation occurs.

Early OA is characterized by increases in the synthesis of proteoglycans, collagen, noncollagenous proteins, hyaluronate, and DNA (indicating cell replication and accounting for the observed chondrocyte clones or clusters).[87,95] Anabolic and catabolic processes increase as cells attempt to repair or maintain tissue integrity.[81] This explains why OA typically is slowly progressive and at times static by morphologic criteria. Eventually OA progresses; when the cell number declines, proteoglycan synthesis declines sharply, and the chondrocytic anabolic repair processes cannot keep pace with catabolic processes, resulting in the further degeneration of cartilage extracellular matrix.[81,87]

The imbalance between proteoglycan synthesis and degradation is important in the pathogenesis of cartilage breakdown.[124] OA cartilage is relatively deficient in TIMP content. Increased proteoglycan synthesis in early OA is further compromised by the fact that OA chondrocytes synthesize proteoglycans in a manner different from that of normal chondrocytes with respect to the composition and distribution of their glycosaminoglycans, the size of the proteoglycan subunit, and their ability to aggregate with hyaluronic acid.[81,83,86,100,125]

MATRIX CHANGES

Much of what is known about changes in the extracellular matrix in early OA comes from animal models (e.g., the rabbit partial meniscectomy model, the canine anterim cruciate ligament, (ACL), deficient model).[126,127] These animal models represent secondary OA, produced by internal derangement of the joint, and, therefore, may not precisely simulate the state of affairs in primary OA.

In the dog model, the first alteration seen within days after joint destabilization is an increase in cartilage water content.[128] Initially, water content increases locally, in the tibial plateau and femoral condyle cartilage, but it soon spreads to the entire joint cartilage. Proteoglycans are more readily extractable from the matrix of experimental animals than from that of controls. These matrix changes are also seen in spontaneously occurring dog and steer OA and in experimentally induced rabbit OA.[128-130] The increase in water content in OA cartilage is due to loss of the collagen network's elastic restraint, enabling the hydrophilic polyanionic proteoglycans to swell more than normal.[131] In early-stage OA, proteogly-

can concentration may increase, and the cartilage may consequently become thicker than normal and exhibit increased staining for proteoglycans.[132-134] Very shortly after the increase in cartilage water, newly synthesized proteoglycans are characterized by a higher proportion of chondroitin sulfate and a lower proportion of keratan sulfate, and proteoglycan aggregation is impaired.[127,128] These abnormal changes in extracellular matrix occur before fibrillation or any other gross morphologic changes are evident and result in a generalized decrease in stiffness that occurs in grossly normal cartilage adjacent to fibrillated areas.[135] As OA progresses, focal cartilage ulcerations develop. Proteoglycan loss is accompanied by a decrease in its ability to aggregate, persistence in abnormal glycosaminoglycan composition, and a decrease in chondroitin sulfate chain length. Once proteoglycan loss reaches a critical threshold, water content, which initially increased, falls below normal.[136]

BIOMECHANICAL CHANGES

Two long-standing biomechanis theories of the pathogenesis of OA hold that mechanical stresses injure chondrocytes, causing them to release degradative enzymes, and that mechanical stresses initially damage the collagen network (as opposed to the cells per se)[137,138]—in either case, resulting in a breakdown of the matrix. Extracellular matrix breakdown in OA cartilage leads to 1) loss of compressive stiffness and elasticity, resulting in greater mechanical stress on chondrocytes; and 2) an increase in hydraulic permeability, resulting in loss of interstitial fluid during compression and increased diffusion of solutes through the matrix, as well as the movement of degradative enzymes and their inhibitors. One important consequence of this is disruption of normal fluid film joint lubrication and loading dynamics due to alterations in inflammatory synovial fluid.[139-142] Joint friction, wear, lubrication, and contact mechanics are further negatively affected by the loss of cartilage proteoglycans.[143-146]

OSTEOPHYTE FORMATION

Osteophytes—bony proliferations at the joint margins and in the floor of cartilage lesions—are in part responsible for the pain and restriction of joint movement in OA. Human OA joint osteophytes synthesize cartilage with significant amounts of type I collagen and nonaggregating proteoglycans.[147] In experimentally induced OA, osteophytes may develop even though the articular cartilage appears grossly normal.[148] Because osteophytes may increase the joint surface available for load bearing, they may contribute to some cases of regression of the early OA cartilage changes.[149] It has been theorized that osteophytes occur as a result of penetration of blood vessels into the basal layers of degenerating cartilage or as a result of abnormal healing of stress fractures in the subchondral trabeculae near the joint margins.[150,151] In the OA dog model, periarticular osteophyte formation begins in the marginal zone, where synovium merges with periosteum and articular cartilage, as early as 3 days after induction of knee instability.[152] TGF-β is a known anabolic growth factor that increases the expression of several types of collagen and proteoglycans.[153] When introduced into the joint in experimental animals, however, TGF-β induces osteophyte formation,[154] and TGF-β expression is observed in osteophytes in patients with OA.[155]

Bony proliferation may result from venous congestion; in human hip OA, phlebography has demonstrated the formation of medullary varices, presumably due to changes in the medullary sinusoids, which may be compressed by subchondral cysts and thickened subchondral trabeculae.[156,157] Subchondral cysts in OA may be created by entry of synovial fluid under pressure through defects in the cartilage or may develop in necrotic areas of subchondral bone.[158] The increased venous pressure caused by the cysts and remodeled trabeculae may account for some of the pain in OA. Immobilization and glucocorticoids (but not bisphosphonates) have been shown to decrease the size and prevalence of osteophytes in experimental models of OA.[159-162]

Biomechanics and Disease Mechanisms of Osteoarthritis

RESPONSE OF CARTILAGE TO MECHANICAL INJURY

The response of normal articular cartilage to injury typically results in suboptimal repair; these injuries can often result in secondary OA.[163,164] Unlike tissues that have the ability to regenerate injured regions with new cells and extracellular matrices that closely resemble the original tissue, articular cartilage produces a repair tissue with neither the original structure nor properties of normal cartilage.[165-168] Chondrocytes in areas surrounding an injured zone are unable to migrate, proliferate, repopulate, or regenerate repair tissue that has the structure, function, and biomechanical properties of normal hyaline cartilage.[136,165,169]

That articular cartilage lacks regenerative power has a long history of documentation.[170] Redfern, in 1851, reported that articular cartilage wounds healed with fibrous tissue, which he believed arose from chondrocyte intercellular substance.[171] Fisher and Ito in the 1920s proposed that cartilage repair is effected by fibrous tissue resulting from proliferation of cells from bone marrow, synovial membrane, and occasionally surrounding articular cartilage.[172,173] It was later observed that the fibrous-tissue regenerate subsequently transforms into fibrocartilage, with occasional foci of imperfect hyaline cartilage.[174-178] The common findings of these investigators were that articular cartilage lacks regenerative potential and that the regenerative fibrous tissue and fibrocartilage tissue must have originated from undifferentiated mesenchymal tissue arising from bone marrow, synovium, or the superficial layer of articular cartilage.[170]

One reason the reparative process of cartilage significantly differs from those of other tissues is that it is avascular. The healing response in vascularized tissues consists of three main phases: necrosis, inflammation, and repair.[163,168] Cartilage undergoes the initial phase of necrosis in response to injury, although typically less cell death occurs than in vascularized tissues because of chondrocytes' relative insensitivity to hypoxia.[163,168] The inflammatory phase, primarily mediated (in other tissues) by the vascular system, is largely absent in partial-thickness injuries (i.e., lesions that do not cross the tidemark), and the repair phase is severely limited given the lack of vascularity and a preceding inflammatory response. Thus, no local hyperemia results, no fibrin network is produced, no subsequent clot develops to act as a scaffold for the ingrowth of repair tissue, no mediators nor cytokines are released that can stimulate cellular migration and proliferation, and no inflammatory cells—which have mitotic and reparative potential—are recruited.[136,168] In lesions that do not cross the tidemark, the burden of repair falls on the chondrocytes[168] in a process that has been termed *intrinsic repair*.[179] Although fetal cartilage is capable of mitotic activity and replication, adult chondrocytes have little potential for replication and intrinsic repair.[176-178] Articular cartilage lesions that cross the tidemark may undergo extrinsic repair via differentiation and proliferation of mesenchymal stem cells from para-articular connective tissues; typically, however, fibrocartilage with inadequate biomechanical properties compared to true hyaline cartilage is the result.[179]

There are three categories of articular cartilage injury: 1) microdamage or repetitive trauma to the matrix and cells; 2) partial-thickness or superficial injuries or chondral fractures—articular surface injuries that do not penetrate the subchondral plate; and 3) osteochondral (full-thickness or deep, penetrating) injuries, which extend through the tidemark and into the underlying subchondral bone.[163,165,168] The host response to each type of injury differs in both timing and quality of repair.

Microdamage to the chondrocytes or extracellular matrix without gross disruption of the articular surface can be caused by a single severe impact or by repetitive blunt trauma.[163,165,168] Repetitive loading of rabbit cartilage produces a surface loss of proteoglycans and an increase in chondrocyte metabolic activity.[180] Proteoglycans become more easily extractable from the articular cartilage, with a greater percentage of nonaggregated forms.[136] Several investigators have observed that cellular, metabolic, and biochemical changes after repetitive blunt trauma resemble those in the early stages of OA: increased hydration, cellular degeneration or death, disruption of the collagen ultrastructure resulting in marked variation in the size and arrangements of fibers, fissuring and ulceration of the articular surface, thickening of the subchondral bone, and softening of the cartilage with loss of its compressive and tensile stiffness.[136,165,181-183] Trauma induces the release of degradative enzymes and proinflammatory factors (e.g., nitric oxide [NO], TNF, IL-1) that frequently cause degradation of the surrounding matrix.[180,184,185] Eventually the material properties of the cartilage are altered—cartilage matrix thins and subchondral bone stiffens—which, in turn, often accelerate the degenerative process.[136] The point at which accumulated microdamage becomes irreversible is unknown, although it has been demonstrated that lost proteoglycans and matrix components may be restored if damage to chondrocytes and the collagen network is limited and the repetitive trauma is halted.[165]

Necrosis of neighboring chondrocytes follows chondral fractures and superficial lacerations, injuries that do not cross the tidemark.[163,168,186] Within 48 to 72 hours, surviving chondrocytes bordering the defect exhibit increased synthesis rates of extracellular matrix molecules and type II collagen, sometimes accompanied by cell proliferation and formation of clusters or clones in the periphery of the injured zone.[136,168,186,187] The increased metabolism and mitotic activity is transient, however, and is followed by a fall in metabolic rate back to normal levels, typically resulting in a suboptimal repair.[136,168] Chondrocytes proliferating on the border of the injured zone do not migrate into the defect that remains unfilled by the newly synthesized matrix.[136,165,169] In some cases, superficial lacerations in otherwise normal joints may not progress to full-thickness loss of cartilage or OA.[136]

Lesions that cross the articular cartilage tidemark and disrupt the underlying subchondral plate elicit the three-phase repair response normally encountered in vascularized tissues: A hematoma forms in the defect, and it becomes organized into a fibrin clot, activating an inflammatory response. Transformation of the fibrin clot into vascular fibroblastic repair tissue[168,187] is accompanied by release of cytokines important in stimulating a repair response (e.g., TGF-β, platelet-derived growth factor [PDGF], IGF, bone morphogenic proteins [BMPs]).[166] These cytokines help set in motion the recruitment, proliferation, and differentiation of undifferentiated cells into a fibrin network that serves as a scaffold for fibrocartilaginous repair tissue.[166,188,189] The origin of these mesenchymal stem cells has been determined to be the underlying bone marrow rather than the adjacent residual articular surface.[187,189,190] These cells progressively differentiate into chondroblasts, chondrocytes, and osteoblasts and synthesize cartilage and bone matrices. At 6 to 8 weeks postinjury, the repair tissue contains a high proportion of chondrocyte-like cells surrounded by a matrix consisting of proteoglycans and type II collagen, with a lesser amount of type I collagen.[190-192] Cells in the deeper layers of the defect differentiate into osteoblasts and subsequently undergo endochondral ossification to heal the subchondral bone defect.[136]

This regenerative tissue eventually undergoes a transformation to a more fibrocartilaginous repair accompanied by a shift in the synthesis of collagen from type II to type I.[169,186,188,189,192] Typically, within 1 year of injury, the repair tissue resembles a mixture of fibrocartilage and hyaline cartilage, with a substantial component (20 to 40 percent) of type I collagen.[191] The size of the osteochondral defect is an important factor in the quality of repair; as a general rule, the smaller the defect the better the repair.[193] Depending on the joint, there exists a critical size for defects, and if larger than this they will not repair. Fibrocartilaginous repair is susceptible to early degenerative changes, as it lacks the biomechanical properties to withstand normal physiologic joint loads.[189,191]

MECHANOTRANSDUCTION AND GENE EXPRESSION

Chondrocytes can sense and respond to mechanical and physicochemical stimuli via several regulatory pathways (e.g., upstream signaling, transcription, translation, post-translational modification, vesicular transport).[194] Physical forces may also influence the synthesis, assembly, and degradation of the extracellular cartilage matrix. Normal stimuli help chondrocytes maintain the extracellular matrix; abnormal stimuli can disrupt this balance.

Mechanotransduction influences the cell-mediated feedback between physical stimuli, the molecular structure of newly synthesized matrix molecules, and the resulting biomechanic tissue properties.[195] Cell-matrix interactions are believed to be one of the important mediators in mechanotransduction in chondrocytes. In a study on the expression of cartilage oligomeric matrix protein (COMP) as it relates to long-term cyclic compression, it was found that with uniaxial unconfined dynamic compression, COMP expression was significantly upregulated; incubation with anti–β1-integrin blocking antibodies abolished the mechanosensitivity of COMP expression.[196] Studies of cyclic and static unconfined compression of bovine articular cartilage explants showed that cyclic loading increased protein synthesis by as much as 50 percent above free-swelling controls, but it had an inhibitory influence on proteoglycan synthesis; static compression was associated with a dose-dependent decrease in biosynthetic activity.[197] Fibronectin and COMP were the most affected noncollagenous extracellular proteins; static compression caused a significant increase in fibronectin synthesis versus free-swelling control levels, and cyclic compression caused a significant increase in synthesis of COMP and fibronectin. These results support the theory that chondrocytes can remodel extracellular matrix in response to alterations in functional demand.

Human articular chondrocytes use the $\alpha_5\beta_1$ integrin as a mechanoreceptor: Mechanic stimulation initiates a signal cascade involving stretch-activated ion channels, the actin cytoskeleton, and tyrosine phosphorylation of the focal adhesion complex molecules pp125, focal adhesion kinase and paxillin, and β-catenin.[198] Autocrine secretion of IL-4 ensues. After binding to its type II receptors, IL-4 induces membrane hyperpolarization of chondrocytes from normal human knee joint articular cartilage. The result is an anabolic response, manifested by increased levels of aggrecan mRNA following mechanic stimulation and decreased levels of MMP-3. Mechanically induced release of the chondroprotective cytokine IL-4 from chondrocytes acts in both an autocrine and paracrine manner and represents an important regulator of articular cartilage structure and function; dysfunction of this pathway may be implicated in OA. Although the mechanoreceptor in OA chondrocytes is also the $\alpha_5\beta_1$ integrin, downstream signaling pathways in OA chondrocytes differ and may contribute to changes in chondrocyte behavior, leading to increased cartilage breakdown.[199] Integrins and integrin-associated signaling pathways are at least partly regulated by mechanic stimulation by activation of plasma membrane apamin-sensitive Ca^{2+}-activated K^+ channels; the result is membrane hyperpolarization after cyclic mechanic stimulation.[200] Chondrocytes from normal articular cartilage exhibit membrane hyperpolarization in response to cyclical pressure-induced strain, whereas chondrocytes from OA cartilage respond by membrane depolarization and exhibit no changes in aggrecan or MMP-3 mRNA following mechanical stimulation.[201,202] These findings suggest that chondrocytes derived from OA cartilage have a different signaling pathway via the $\alpha_5\beta_1$ integrin in response to mechanical stimulation; these may play a role in the chondroyte phenotypic changes seen in diseased cartilage.

Another study used cDNA array analysis to compare the expression profiles of mRNA from hydrostatic pressurized and nonpressurized human chondrosarcoma cells.[203] Several immediate-early and regulating cell cycle and growth genes were upregulated in response to high pressure, whereas a decrease was observed in osteonectin, fibronectin, and collagen types VI and XVI mRNAs.

Fluid flow during dynamic compression of cartilage explants can stimulate proteoglycan and protein synthesis independent of changes in cell shape. A study using a tissue shear-loading model to uncouple fluid flow from cell and matrix deformation demonstrated that deformation of cells and pericellular matrix alone stimulated protein synthesis by approximately 50 percent and proteoglycan synthesis by approximately 25 percent; thus, even in the absence of macroscopic tissue-level fluid flow, chondrocytes can respond to a change in shape.[204]

Indian hedgehog (Ihh) protein is a key signaling molecule that controls chondrocyte proliferation and differentiation and may also be an essential mediator of mechanotransduction in cartilage: Cyclic mechanical stress has been shown to induce Ihh expression by chondrocytes.[205]

▌ Role of Inflammatory Mediators in Disease Progression

Although OA is not considered an inflammatory disease, mediators classically associated with inflammation (cytokines, prostaglandins (PGs), NO, proteases) perpetuate cartilage damage that ensues from repeated mechanical injury (see Fig. 91–2). These products of synovial cells and chondrocytes represent potential targets for the development of disease-modifying agents in OA.

ALTERATIONS IN SYNOVIAL TISSUE

One reason OA is classified as a noninflammatory arthritis is that the synovial fluid leukocyte count in OA is typically fewer than 2000 cells/mm³. To the extent that synovial fluid leukocytic inflammation does occur in OA, it may be the result of crystal-induced synovitis (either calcium apatite or CPPD). Low-grade inflammatory processes nevertheless occur in OA synovial tissues that contribute to disease pathogenesis. Even in early OA, some degree of synovitis has been observed.[206] Many of the clinical symptoms and signs seen in OA joints clearly

reflect synovial inflammation (e.g., joint swelling and effusion, stiffness, occasionally redness). Synovial histologic changes include synovial hypertrophy and hyperplasia with an increased number of lining cells, often accompanied by infiltration of the sublining tissue with scattered foci of lymphocytes.

Cartilage breakdown products, derived from the articular surface as a result of mechanical or enzymatic destruction of the cartilage, can provoke the release of collagenase and other hydrolytic enzymes from synovial cells and macrophages[207,208] (see Fig. 91–2). Cartilage breakdown products are also believed to result in mononuclear cell infiltration and vascular hyperplasia in the synovial membrane in OA.[209-211] A consequence of these low-grade inflammatory processes is the induction of synovial IL-1β and TNF-α, which are likely contributors to the degradative cascade.[212] Although less prominent than in rheumatoid arthritis (RA), deposits of immunoglobulin (Ig) and complement can be found in the collagenous network of the superficial zone of the articular cartilage, suggesting that deposition of immune complexes, perhaps containing breakdown products of the cartilage as antigens, may play a role in the chronicity of the inflammatory reaction in the joint.[213] There are also reports of increased numbers of immune cells in synovial tissue, including activated B cells and T lymphocytes, as well as evidence that OA patients express cellular immunity to the cartilage proteoglycan link protein and C1 domain.[214,215]

Inflammatory processes may contribute to the progression of cartilage damage.[76,216-218] Areas of increased radionuclide uptake ("hot spots") on bone scintigraphy have also been reported to identify joints more likely to progress by radiographic criteria—or to require surgical intervention—over a 5-year period.[216] Recently, reports by Dougados and coworkers suggest that arthroscopic evidence of synovitis in OA is a risk factor for progressive cartilage degeneration[218,219] (Fig. 91–3). Several biologic markers (e.g., COMP, C-reactive protein [CRP], hyaluronic acid) may be associated with OA synovial inflammation,[212] and there appears to be a correlation of high disease activity with more rapid OA progression.

COMP, a member of the thrombospondin gene family,[220] is an abundant noncollagenous extracellular matrix protein in cartilage[221-223] and is present in relatively high concentrations in articular cartilage (–0.1% wet weight). Several recent studies[224-227] suggest that monitoring of COMP levels (in both joint fluid and serum) can assess the potential for, presence of, and progression of arthritis.[225,226,228-232] Synovial-fluid COMP levels were found to be higher in individuals with knee pain or injury,[229] anterior cruciate ligament or meniscal injury,[225,229] and OA[226,229] than in comparably healthy individuals. The degradation and tissue distribution of COMP in normal and OA human knee articular cartilage exhibits marked differences in tissue distribution from COMP in normal cartilage. COMP in normal cartilage is predominantly localized to the interterritorial matrix throughout all zones of the matrix, with increased staining in the deeper cartilaginous zones. COMP in OA cartilage is predominantly localized to the superficial zones of fibrillated

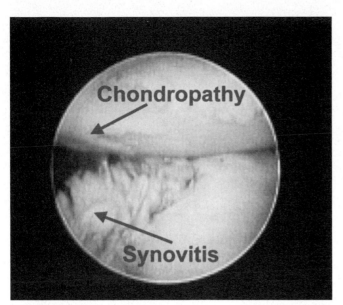

FIGURE 91–3 · Arthroscopic view of osteoarthritic (OA) lesion of the femoral condyle, designated "Chondropathy." Note that proliferative synovitis is localized to the area of the OA lesion. (Courtesy of Maxime Dougados.)

cartilage, with little to no immunostaining in the midzones and relatively poor staining in the deeper cartilaginous zones. In areas of fibrocartilaginous repair in OA, the repair matrix stained poorly for proteoglycans but strongly for COMP. Some fibrocartilaginous cells stained positively for COMP, suggesting that these cells were actively synthesizing COMP.[233] Once believed to be a cartilage-specific molecule, COMP has also been localized in tendon, bone (osteoblasts only), and human synovium. Because activated synovial cells synthesize COMP, it has been theorized that the elevated COMP levels in OA may also be due to active synovitis. Recently, it was shown that synovitis exerts a significant effect on serum COMP levels as measured by a monoclonal antibody (mAb 17-C10) in OA patients.[234]

Elevated levels of CRP, a marker of inflammation, appear to be predictive of radiographic progression of long-term knee OA.[235] It appears that continued low-grade inflammation is part of the etiology and progression of early OA of the knee. An elevation in CRP in women was found to be predictive of progression of mild to moderately severe knee OA.[76] In a study of 1025 women, higher serum CRP levels were associated with a statistically significant increase in both prevalent and incident knee OA and greater knee-OA severity; women with bilateral knee OA had higher CRP levels than those with unilateral knee OA. Compared to women who did not develop knee OA, those that did had a higher baseline CRP at their index test 2.5 years earlier.[235] In a study of women (aged 44 to 67 years), CRP levels were statistically greater in 105 women with knee OA than in 740 women without OA. These and other studies report that CRP levels are modestly but significantly increased in women with early knee OA and that higher levels are predictive of OA that will progress over time.[76]

The glycosaminoglycan hyaluronic acid has been investigated as a marker of cartilage degradation that can be detected in body fluids.[236] The level of hyaluronate present in synovial fluid and serum may be reflective of cartilage metabolism, although the majority of circulating hyaluronate actually originates from extracartilaginous sources. It has become clear that hyaluronic acid levels reflect synovial activity, whereas proteoglycan levels reflect cartilage turnover. Elevated levels of hyaluronate have been detected in both OA and RA, with significantly higher levels in RA.[236,237] In addition, higher serum hyaluronic acid levels correlated with the number of joints involved and degree of clinical disability. These findings support the theory that serum hyaluronic acid levels reflect synovial hyperactivity. An animal model in which the anterior cruciate ligament was transected to induce OA also demonstrated a rise in serum hyaluronate level within 7 days after joint injury, a rise sustained at 13 weeks; the rise in the synovial fluid hyaluronic acid levels correlated with serum levels.[238] Serum hyaluronic acid levels may also serve as a predictor of OA disease progression.[239] Serum hyaluronic acid levels in OA patients were found to correlate with radiographic evidence of disease progression during a 5-year time interval. Patients whose disease progressed had higher levels at the outset.[240]

Verbruggen and Veys[241] demonstrated that patients with distal or proximal interphalangeal OA are generally asymptomatic when the disease is nonerosive and become symptomatic during inflammatory episodes (associated with erosive OA changes). OA patients have been shown to express cellular immunity to the cartilage proteoglycan link protein, and C1 domain and immune complexes containing antibodies to type II collagen have been detected in the superficial layer of OA cartilage.[242] Histologic changes in OA synovium usually demonstrate mild or moderate synovitis characterized by an increase in the number of inflammatory mononuclear cells in the sublining tissue, including activated B cells and T lymphocytes.[243-248]

Inflammation in OA may be the result of crystal-induced synovitis (either calcium apatite or CPPD). "Milwaukee shoulder syndrome" represents a rapidly destructive form of OA with evidence of inflammation in the synovial membrane but minimal synovial fluid leukocytosis. It is typically associated with rotator-cuff degeneration, severe shoulder OA, and HA crystal deposition in the synovial membrane.[249] The synovial fluid typically contains few cells and high levels of active collagenase. It is theorized that crystals released from the degenerating tendons trigger the release of collagenase from synovial mononuclear cells, which leads to cartilage breakdown; cartilage-breakdown products then further activate release of enzymes from the synovium. Joint inflammation is typically associated with increases in synovial IL-1 and TNF that further proteinate the degradative cascade.[250]

ALTERATIONS IN CARTILAGE

Chondrocytes obtained from patients with OA actively produce inflammatory mediators, including NO, PGs, IL-1β, TNF-α, IL-6, and IL-8.[39,212] Because articular cartilage is avascular and aneural, the production of such mediators by chondrocytes is not associated with the classic signs of inflammation. There is evidence, however, that these mediators act within cartilage in an autocrine or paracrine fashion to promote a catabolic state that leads to progressive cartilage damage in OA[39,212] (see Fig. 91–2).

Proinflammatory Cytokines

The proinflammatory cytokines IL-1β and TNF-α are produced by OA chondrocytes and appear to be of major importance in cartilage destruction[251] (Fig. 91–4). Both cytokines exert comparable catabolic effects on chondrocyte metabolism, decreasing proteoglycan collagen synthesis and increasing aggrecan release via the induction of degradative proteases.[39,98,212,252-255] IL-1β and TNF-α also induce chondrocytes and synovial cells to produce other inflammatory mediators, such as IL-8, IL-6, NO, and prostaglandin E_2 (PGE_2). Catabolic activities are further amplified because IL-1β and TNF-α act in an autocrine or paracrine fashion to stimulate their own production.

The actions of IL-1 are regulated by the engagement of two specific cell-surface receptors (IL-1R), designated type I and type II.[256] The type I receptor, which spans the plasma membrane, is responsible for signal transduction, whereas the type II receptor is a "decoy" receptor, expressed at the cell membrane but unable to signal. IL-1 receptor antagonist (IL-1Ra) is a competitive inhibitor of the IL-1/IL-1R complex. A relative deficit of the ratio of IL-1Ra to IL-1 has been described in OA synovial tissue, which may permit increased IL-1 activity.[256,257] Addition of IL-1Ra, or soluble type I and II

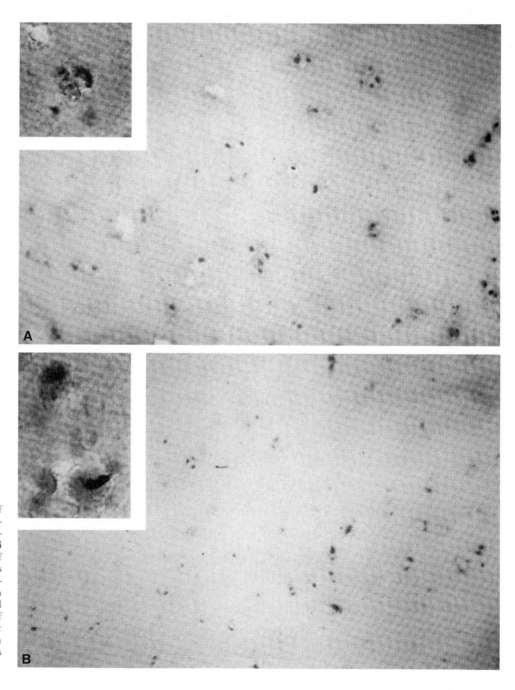

FIGURE 91–4 · Immunostaining of osteoarthritic (OA) cartilage specimen for inducible nitric oxide synthase (iNOS) (A) and interleukin-1β (IL-1β) (B). Note intense staining of chondrocytes in the superficial zones for both inflammatory proteins. (Reproduced with permission from Melchiorri C, et al: Enhanced and coordinated in vivo expression of inflammatory cytokines and nitric oxide synthase by chondrocytes from patients with osteoarthritis. Arthritis Rheum 41(12):2165-2174, 1998.)

IL-1 receptors, to OA explant cultures blocks PGE_2 synthesis, collagenase production, and NO production.[39,255] Such observations confirm that IL-1β, spontaneously produced by OA chondrocytes, acts within cartilage to induce the production of other catabolic mediators. IL-1β is, therefore, considered central to the perpetuation of OA and is a potential target for future treatment strategies designed to inhibit cartilage degradation. Encouraging results have been reported in vivo, where the intra-articular administration of IL-1Rα, either by repeated injection or gene therapy, has been shown to retard the progression of experimental OA.[258]

IL-1β is synthesized as a precursor and released extracellularly in an active form. A protease designated IL-1β–converting enzyme (ICE), or caspase-1, and located in the plasma membrane, is responsible for generating the mature form of this cytokine.[259] The expression of this enzyme has been shown to be upregulated in both OA synovium and cartilage. Similarly, the proteolytic cleavage of the proform of TNF-α takes place at the cell surface via a TNF-α–converting enzyme (TACE), which belongs to a subfamily of proteases named adamalysin.[260] Like the expression ICE, that of TACE is upregulated in OA cartilage.[261,262] Inhibitors of both ICE and TACE are of interest as future therapeutic small-molecule antagonists of IL-1β and TNF-α, respectively.

Also upregulated in OA cartilage is the production of both CXC and CC chemokines, including IL-8, monocyte chemoattractant protein-1 (MCP-1), regulated on activation, normal T cell–expressed and secreted (RANTES) chemokine, and the receptors CCR-2 and CCR-5.[212,219,263] The expression of chemokines is low or undetectable in normal chondrocytes unless stimulated with such cytokines as IL-1 or IL-17.[264] Chemokines are detected by immunohistochemistry in the superficial and mid zones of the tissue, as has been demonstrated for such other inflammatory mediators as inducible nitric oxide synthase (iNOS), IL-1β, and TNF-α.[219] RANTES induces expression of its own receptor, CCR-5, suggesting an autocrine or paracrine pathway of the chemokine within the cartilage. MCP-1 and RANTES promote chondrocyte catabolic activities, including induction of iNOS, increased MMP-3 expression, inhibition of proteoglycan synthesis, and enhancement of proteoglycan release.[219,263] Consistent with these effects, treatment of normal articular cartilage with RANTES increases the release of glycosaminoglycans and profoundly reduces the intensity of Safranin O staining.[219]

The expression and degradation of noncollagenous proteins and nonaggregating proteoglycans are also altered in OA cartilage and may have a direct or indirect effect on modulating the catabolic state of the chondrocyte.[265] These groups of molecules, which have only been sparsely characterized, are likely to have important structural functions, biologic functions, or both.[266,267] Via their interactions with other extracellular matrix constituents they can influence the supramolecular assembly of the cartilage matrix and, as a result, affect the physical properties of the tissue; by interacting directly with the chondrocytes, neighboring cells, or both, they can provide biologic signals on matrix properties and thereby influence cellular function.[268] For example, there is increased expression of fibronectin, osteonectin, and osteopontin in OA cartilage compared to normal.[269] Homandberg and others have demonstrated that fragments of fibronectin (but not the intact fibronectin molecule) induce the production of MMPs and other catabolic factors in cartilage, in a process that in part depends on IL-1 induction.[270-272] Recent studies indicate that fibronectin fragments stimulate type II collagen cleavage via enhanced MMP-13 and MMP-3 production.[273] The chondrolytic effects of the fragments were blocked by the addition of either a preferential MMP-13 inhibitor or IL1-Rα.

Nitric Oxide

NO, produced by the inducible isoform of iNOS, is a major catabolic factor produced by chondrocytes in response to proinflammatory cytokines such as IL-1-β and TNFα.[212] Considerable evidence indicates that the overproduction of NO by chondrocytes plays a major role in the perpetuation of cartilage destruction in OA[274-277] (see Fig. 91–2). Increased concentrations of nitrites have been demonstrated in the synovial fluids of patients with OA, and iNOS has been demonstrated in OA synoviocytes and chondrocytes by in situ hybridization and immunohistochemistry.[76,278,279] OA cartilage explants spontaneously produce large amounts of NO, whereas normal cartilage does not express iNOS nor produce NO without stimulation by cytokines such as IL-1.[274]

NO exerts multiple effects on chondrocytes that promote the degradation of articular cartilage.[280] These include the following:

1. Inhibition of collagen and proteoglycan synthesis[281]
2. Activation of MMPs[282]
3. Increased susceptibility to injury by other oxidants (e.g., hydrogen peroxide [H_2O_2],[283]
4. Apoptosis[284]

Chondrocyte apoptosis is a particular feature of progressive OA, and several studies have implicated nitric oxide, (NO), as an important mediator in this process.[283,285] Immuno-histochemistry of joint tissue obtained from patients with OA reveals colocalization of iNOS protein and apoptosis in articular cartilage cells.[286] There is evidence that apoptosis results from the formation of peroxynitrite, a toxic free radical produced by the reaction of NO and superoxide anion. Peroxynitrite reacts with tyrosine residues on proteins, which can be detected by antibodies to nitrotyrosine. Immunostaining of OA cartilage reveals that chondrocytes that are highly positive for IL-1β also stain for nitrotyrosine, consistent with overproduction of peroxynitrate and oxidative damage.[279] The importance of NO has been corroborated in animal models of OA. In the Pond-Nuki canine model, the inhibition of NO reduced the progression of cartilage lesions.[287] The protective effect of NO inhibition was also reflected in decreased levels in articular cartilage of MMPs, caspace-2, and IL-1β, and decreased chondrocyte apoptosis. Van den Berg et al.[288] has demonstrated that iNOS-deficient mice are protected against experimental OA. OA pathology, including cartilage lesions and osteophyte formation, were both reduced in the mutant mice.

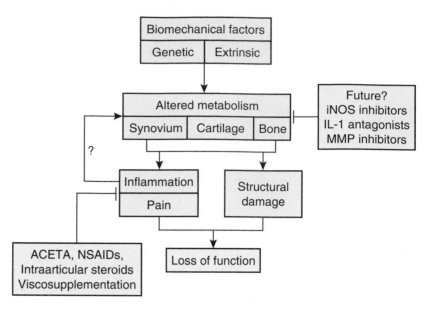

FIGURE 91–5 · Multiple Factors That Predispose to, Initiate, and Perpetuate Osteoarthritis (OA). In the future, structure-modifying treatments will be targeted to the biochemical processes that promote disease progression. ACETA, acetaminophen; NSAIDs, nonsteroidal anti-inflammatory drugs; viscosupplementation, hyaluronans.

NO also plays an important role in bone-cell function, which could have implications for OA insofar as it contributes to alterations in subchondral bone. The endothelial isoform endothelial cell nitric oxide synthase (ecNOS) is constitutively expressed in bone, where it seems to play a key role in regulating osteoblast activity and bone formation. ecNOS also mediates the effects of mechanic loading on the skeleton, where it acts along with prostaglandins to promote bone formation and suppress bone resorption.[289] In contrast, such proinflammatory cytokines as IL-1 and TNF induce iNOS in bone cells, and NO derived from this pathway potentiates bone loss.[212]

Prostaglandins

The expression of the inducible cyclooxygenase-2 (COX-2) is increased in OA chondrocytes, which spontaneously produce PGE_2 ex vivo.[261] The effects of prostaglandins on chondrocyte metabolism are complex and include enhanced type II collagen synthesis, activation of MMPs, and promotion of apoptosis.[290] In cartilage explants, IL-1β induces COX-2 expression and PGE_2 production coordinate with proteoglycan degradation. COX-2 inhibition prevents IL-1β–induced proteoglycan degradation, which can be reversed by the addition of PGE_2 to cultures.[291] In contrast, in vitro evidence has accumulated that selected nonsteroidal anti-inflammatory drugs (NSAIDs) may interfere with proteoglycan synthesis.[292] No convincing randomized studies in patients have been conducted to determine whether chronic COX-2 inhibition affects disease progression in OA. Because of the widespread chronic use of COX-2 inhibitors in clinical practice, however, this is an area that merits further investigation, including the assessment of structural outcome studies in patients with OA.[293]

■ Summary

OA, although classically conceived of as a degenerative consequence of aging, is a disease with an increasingly well-characterized molecular pathophysiology. Biomechanical factors, particularly in the context of genetic predisposition, obesity, and malalignment, result in chemical alterations within the joint that promote cartilage degradation (see Fig. 91–2). Early anabolic changes, characterized by proliferation of chondrocytes and increased matrix production, are followed by a predominantly catabolic state, characterized by decreased matrix synthesis, increased proteolytic degradation of matrix, and chondrocyte apoptosis. Many of the features of the catabolic chondrocyte are related to the production of inflammatory mediators by synovium and chondrocytes that act locally to perpetuate cartilage degradation. Although current treatments improve the signs and symptoms of disease, further characterization of the altered metabolism in synovium, cartilage, and bone that promote disease progression should lead to future treatments that can prevent structural damage in OA (Fig. 91–5).

REFERENCES

1. Herndon JH, Davidson SM, Apazidis A: Recent socioeconomic trends in orthopaedic practice. J Bone Joint Surg Am 83-A(7): 1097-1105, 2001.
2. Peyron JG: The epidemiology of osteoarthritis. In Moskowitz RW, Howell DS, Goldberg YM, et al (eds): Osteoarthritis: Diagnosis and Management Philadelphia, WB Saunders, 9-27, 1984.
3. Martin JA, Buckwalter JA: Aging, articular cartilage chondrocyte senescence and osteoarthritis. Biogerontology 3(5):257-264, 2002.
4. Lawrence JS: Rheumatism in Populations. London, Heinemann Medical, 1977.

5. Forman MD, Kaplan DA, Muller GF, et al: The epidemiology of osteoarthritis of the knee, in Epidemiology of Osteoarthritis, ed. JG Peyron. Ciba-Geigy, Paris. 243, 1980.

6. Brandt KD, Flusser D: Osteoarthritis, in Prognosis in the Rheumatic Diseases, ed. N. Bellamy. Kluwer Academic Publishers: Lancaster, UK 11, 1991.

7. Cole AA, Kuettner KE: Molecular basis for differences between human joints. Cell Mol Life Sci 59(1): 19-26, 2002.

8. Kerin A, Patwari P, Kuettner K, et al: Molecular basis of osteoarthritis: biomechanical aspects. Cell Mol Life Sci 59(1): 27-35, 2002.

9. Kempson GE: Age-related changes in the tensile properties of human articular cartilage: A comparative study between the femoral head of the hip joint and the talus of the ankle joint. Biochim Biophys Acta 1075(3): 223-30, 1991.

10. Huch K, Kuettner KE, Dieppe P: Osteoarthritis in ankle and knee joints. Semin Arthritis Rheum 26(4): 667-74, 1997.

11. Hauselmann HJ, Mok SS, Fleechtenmacher J, et al: Chondrocytes from human knee and ankle joints show differences in response to IL-1 and IL-1 receptor inhibitor. Orthop Trans 17: 710, 1993.

12. Chubinskaya S, Huch K, Mikecz K, et al: Chondrocyte matrix metalloproteinase-8: Up-regulation of neutrophil collagenase by interleukin-1 beta in human cartilage from knee and ankle joints. Lab Invest 74(1): 232-40, 1996.

13. Anderson JJ, Felson DT: Factors associated with osteoarthritis of the knee in the first national Health and Nutrition Examination Survey (HANES I). Evidence for an association with overweight, race, and physical demands of work. Am J Epidemiol 128(1): 179-89, 1988.

14. Felson DT, Zhang Y, Hannan MT, et al: The incidence and natural history of knee osteoarthritis in the elderly. The Framingham Osteoarthritis Study. Arthritis Rheum 38(10): 1500-5, 1995.

15. Hunter DJ, March L, Sambrook PN: Knee osteoarthritis: the influence of environmental factors. Clin Exp Rheumatol 20(1): 93-100, 2002.

16. Kellgren JH, Lawrence JS, Bier F: Genetic factors in generalized osteoarthritis. Ann Rheum Dis 22: 237-55, 1963.

17. Saville PD, Dickson J: Age and weight in osteoarthritis of the hip. Arthritis Rheum 11(5): 635-44, 1968.

18. Hart DJ, Doyle DV, Spector TD: Incidence and risk factors for radiographic knee osteoarthritis in middle-aged women: The Chingford Study. Arthritis Rheum 42(1): 17-24, 1999.

19. Jadelis K, Miller ME, Ettinger WH Jr, et al: Strength, balance, and the modifying effects of obesity and knee pain: Results from the Observational Arthritis Study in Seniors (oasis). J Am Geriatr Soc 49(7): 884-91, 2001.

20. Leach RE, Baumgard S, Broom J: Obesity: Its relationship to osteoarthritis of the knee. Clin Orthop 93: 271-3, 1973.

21. Newman B, Wallis GA: Is osteoarthritis a genetic disease? Clin Invest Med 25(4): 139-49, 2002.

22. Loughlin J: Genetic epidemiology of primary osteoarthritis. Curr Opin Rheumatol 13(2): 111-6, 2001.

23. Kellegren J, Lawrence J, Bier F: Genetic factors in generalized osteoarthrosis. Ann Rheum Dis 22: 237-255, 1963.

24. Felson DT, Couropmitree NN, Chaisson CE, et al: Evidence for a Mendelian gene in a segregation analysis of generalized radiographic osteoarthritis: The Framingham Study. Arthritis Rheum 41(6): 1064-71, 1998.

25. Hirsch R, Lethbridge-Cejku M, Hanson R, et al: Familial aggregation of osteoarthritis: Data from the Baltimore Longitudinal Study on Aging. Arthritis Rheum 41(7): 1227-32, 1998.

26. MacGregor AJ, Antoniades L, Matson M, et al: The genetic contribution to radiographic hip osteoarthritis in women: Results of a classic twin study. Arthritis Rheum 43(11): 2410-6, 2000.

27. Cicuttini FM, Spector TD: What is the evidence that osteoarthritis is genetically determined? Baillieres Clin Rheumatol 11(4): 657-69, 1997.

28. Spector TD, Cicuttini F, Baker J, et al: Genetic influences on osteoarthritis in women: A twin study. Bmj 312(7036): 940-3, 1996.

29. Bijkerk C, Houwing-Duistermaat JJ, Valkenburg HA, et al: Heritabilities of radiologic osteoarthritis in peripheral joints and of disc degeneration of the spine. Arthritis Rheum 42(8): 1729-35, 1999.

30. Reginato AM, Olsen BR: The role of structural genes in the pathogenesis of osteoarthritic disorders. Arthritis Res 4(6): 337-45, 2002.

31. Knowlton RG, Katzenstein PL, Moskowitz RW, et al: Genetic linkage of a polymorphism in the type II procollagen gene (COL2A1) to primary osteoarthritis associated with mild chondrodysplasia. N Engl J Med 322(8): 526-30, 1990.

32. Ala-Kokko L, Baldwin CT, Moskowitz RW et al: Single base mutation in the type II procollagen gene (COL2A1) as a cause of primary osteoarthritis associated with a mild chondrodysplasia. Proc Natl Acad Sci U S A 87(17): 6565-8, 1990.

33. Jimenez SA, Williams CJ, Karasick, D: Hereditary osteoarthritis, in Osteoarthritis, ed. KD Brandt, M Doherty, LS Lohmander. Oxford University Press, Oxford 31-49, 1998.

34. Uitterlinden AG, Burger H, van Duijn CM, et al: Adjacent genes, for COL2A1 and the vitamin D receptor, are associated with separate features of radiographic osteoarthritis of the knee. Arthritis Rheum 43(7): 1456-64, 2000.

35. Ho AM, Johnson MD, Kingsley DM: Role of the mouse ank gene in control of tissue calcification and arthritis. Science 289(5477): 265-70, 2000.

36. Loughlin J, Dowling B, Mustafa Z et al: Association of the interleukin-1 gene cluster on chromosome 2q13 with knee osteoarthritis. Arthritis Rheum 46(6): 1519-27, 2002.

37. Leppavuori J, Kujala U, Kinnunen J, et al: Genome scan for predisposing loci for distal interphalangeal joint osteoarthritis: evidence for a locus on 2q. Am J Hum Genet 65(4): 1060-7, 1999.

38. Loughlin J: Genome studies and linkage in primary osteoarthritis. Rheum Dis Clin North Am 28(1): 95-109, 2002.

39. Attur MG, Patel IR, Patel RN, et al: Autocrine production of IL-1 beta by human osteoarthritis-affected cartilage and differential regulation of endogenous nitric oxide, IL-6, prostaglandin E2, and IL-8. Proc Assoc Am Physicians 110(1): 65-72, 1998.

40. Attur MG, Dave MN, Clancy RM, et al: Functional genomic analysis in arthritis-affected cartilage: yin-yang regulation of inflammatory mediators by alpha 5 beta 1 and alpha V beta 3 integrins. J Immunol 164(5): 2684-91, 2000.

41. Moos V, Rudwaleit M, Herzog V, et al: Association of genotypes affecting the expression of interleukin-1beta or interleukin-1 receptor antagonist with osteoarthritis. Arthritis Rheum 43(11): 2417-22, 2000.

42. Bullough PG: The geometry of diarthrodial joints, its physiologic maintenance, and the possible significance of age-related changes in geometry-to-load distribution and the development of osteoarthritis. Clin Orthop (156): 61-6, 1981.

43. Lane LB, Villacin A, Bullough PG: The vascularity and remodelling of subchondrial bone and calcified cartilage in adult human femoral and humeral heads. An age- and stress-related phenomenon. J Bone Joint Surg Br 59(3): 272-8, 1977.

44. Day WH, Swanson SA, Freeman MA: Contact pressures in the loaded human cadaver hip. J Bone Joint Surg Br 57(3): 302-13, 1975.

45. Slowman SD, Brandt KD: Composition and glycosaminoglycan metabolism of articular cartilage from habitually loaded and habitually unloaded sites. Arthritis Rheum 29(1): 88-94, 1986.

46. Schumacher HR: Secondary osteoarthritis, in Osteoarthritis: Diagnosis and Management, ed. RW Moskowitz, DS Howell, VM Goldberg et al. WB Saunders: Philadelphia. 235, 1984.

47. Conaghan PG: Update on osteoarthritis part 1: current concepts and the relation to exercise. Br J Sports Med 36(5): 330-3, 2002.

48. Donahue JM, Oegema TR Jr, Thompson RG. Jr: The zone of calcified cartilage: the focal point of changes following blunt trauma to articular cartilage. Trans Orthop Res Soc 11: 233, 1986.

49. Oegema TR, Thompson RC Jr: Cartilage-bone interface (tidemark), in Cartilage Changes in Osteoarthritis, ed. KD Brandt. Indiana University School of Medicine: Indianapolis. 43, 1990.

50. Radin EL: Mechanical factors in the etiology of osteoarthrosis, in Epidemiology of Osteoarthrosis, ed. JG Peyron. Ciba-Geigy, Paris. 136, 1981.

51. Linn FC, Radin EL: Lubrication of animal joints. III. The effect of certain chemical alterations of the cartilage and lubricant. Arthritis Rheum 11(5): 674-82, 1968.

52. Radin EL, Paul IL: Response of joints to impact loading. I. In vitro wear. Arthritis Rheum 14(3): 356-62, 1971.

53. Reilly DT, Martens M: Experimental analysis of the quadriceps muscle force and patello-femoral joint reaction force for various activities. Acta Orthop Scand 43(2): 126-37, 1972.

54. Sokoloff L: The Biology of Degenerative Joint Disease. Chicago: University of Chicago Press, 1969.

55. Radin EL, Paul IL: Does cartilage compliance reduce skeletal impact loads? The relative force-attenuating properties of articular cartilage, synovial fluid, periarticular soft tissues and bone. Arthritis Rheum 13(2): 139-44, 1970.

56. Hill AV: Production and absorption of work by muscle. Science 131: 897-903, 1960.

57. Ochoa JA, Heck DA, Brandt KD et al: The effect of intertrabecular fluid on femoral head mechanics. J Rheumatol 18(4): 580-4, 1991.

58. Bullough P, Goodfellow J, O'Conner J: The relationship between degenerative changes and load-bearing in the human hip. J Bone Joint Surg Br 55(4): 746-58, 1973.

59. Todd RC, Freeman MA, Pirie, CJ: Isolated trabecular fatigue fractures in the femoral head. J Bone Joint Surg Br 54(4): 723-8, 1972.

60. Fazzalari NL, Vernon-Roberts B, Darracott J: Osteoarthritis of the hip. Possible protective and causative roles of trabecular microfractures in the head of the femur. Clin Orthop (216): 224-33, 1987.

61. Foss MV, Byers PD: Bone density, osteoarthrosis of the hip, and fracture of the upper end of the femur. Ann Rheum Dis 31(4): 259-64, 1972.

62. Radin EL: Mechanical aspects of osteoarthrosis. Bull Rheum Dis 26(7): 862-5, 1976.

63. Wluka AE, Cicuttini FM, Spector TD: Menopause, oestrogens and arthritis. Maturitas 35(3): 183-99, 2000.

64. Ushiyama T, Ueyama H, Inoue K, et al: Expression of genes for estrogen receptors alpha and beta in human articular chondrocytes. Osteoarthritis Cartilage 7(6): 560-6, 1999.

65. Pelletier G, El-Alfy M: Immunocytochemical localization of estrogen receptors alpha and beta in the human reproductive organs. J Clin Endocrinol Metab 85(12): 4835-40, 2000.

66. Ng MC, Harper RP, Le CT, et al: Effects of estrogen on the condylar cartilage of the rat mandible in organ culture. J Oral Maxillofac Surg 57(7): 818-23, 1999.

67. Richmond RS, Carlson CS, Register TC, et al: Functional estrogen receptors in adult articular cartilage: Estrogen replacement therapy increases chondrocyte synthesis of proteoglycans and insulin-like growth factor binding protein 2. Arthritis Rheum 43(9): 2081-90, 2000.

68. Claassen H, Hassenpflug J, Schunke M, et al: Immunohistochemical detection of estrogen receptor alpha in articular chondrocytes from cows, pigs and humans: In situ and in vitro results. Ann Anat 183(3): 223-7, 2001.

69. Nilsson LO, Boman A, Savendahl L, et al: Demonstration of estrogen receptor-beta immunoreactivity in human growth plate cartilage. J Clin Endocrinol Metab 84(1): 370-3, 1999.

70. Bord S, Vedi S, Beavan SR, et al: Megakaryocyte population in human bone marrow increases with estrogen treatment: a role in bone remodeling? Bone 27(3): 397-401, 2000.

71. Nevitt MC, Cummings SR, Lane NE, et al: Association of estrogen replacement therapy with the risk of osteoarthritis of the hip in elderly white women. Study of Osteoporotic Fractures Research Group. Arch Intern Med 156(18): 2073-80, 1996.

72. Sowers M, Crutchfield M, Bandekar R, et al: Bone mineral density and its change in pre- and perimenopausal white women: The Michigan Bone Health Study. J Bone Miner Res 13(7): 1134-40, 1998.

73. Zhang Y, McAlindon TE, Hannan MT, et al: Estrogen replacement therapy and worsening of radiographic knee osteoarthritis: The Framingham Study. Arthritis Rheum 41(10): 1867-73, 1998.

74. Wluka AE, Davis SR, Bailey M, et al: Users of oestrogen replacement therapy have more knee cartilage than non-users. Ann Rheum Dis 60(4): 332-6, 2001.

75. Hannan MT, Felson DT, Anderson JJ, et al: Estrogen use and radiographic osteoarthritis of the knee in women. The Framingham Osteoarthritis Study. Arthritis Rheum 33(4): 525-32, 1990.

76. Spector TD, Hart DJ, Nandra D, et al: Low-level increases in serum C-reactive protein are present in early osteoarthritis of the knee and predict progressive disease. Arthritis Rheum 40(4): 723-7, 1997.

77. Ham KD, Loeser RF, Lindgren BR, et al: Effects of long-term estrogen replacement therapy on osteoarthritis severity in cynomolgus monkeys. Arthritis Rheum 46(7): 1956-64, 2002.

78. Ushiyama T, Ueyama H, Inoue K, et al: Estrogen receptor gene polymorphism and generalized osteoarthritis. J Rheumatol 25(1): 134-7, 1998.

79. Maroudas AI: Balance between swelling pressure and collagen tension in normal and degenerate cartilage. Nature 260(5554): 808-9, 1976.

80. Maroudas A: Transport through articular cartilage and some physiological implications, in Normal and Osteoarthrotic Articular Cartilage, ed. SY Ali, MW Elves, DH Leaback. Institute of Orthopaedics, London 33, 1974.

81. Mankin HJ, Brandt KD: Biochemistry and metabolism of articular cartilage in osteoarthritis, in Osteoarthritis: Diagnosis and Medical/Surgical Management, ed. RW Moskowitz, DS Howell, VM Goldberg, et al. WB Saunders, Philadelphia 109-54, 1992.

82. Herbage D, Huc A, Chabrand D et al: Physicochemical study of articular cartilage from healthy and osteo-arthritic human hips. Orientation and thermal stability of collagen fibres. Biochim Biophys Acta 271(2): 339-46, 1972.

83. Muir H: Current and future trends in articular cartilage research and osteoarthritis, in Articular Cartilage and Biochemistry, ed. KE Kuettner, R Schleyerbach, VC Hascall. Raven Press, New York. 423-40, 1986.

84. Mankin HJ, Lippiello L: Biochemical and metabolic abnormalities in articular cartilage from osteo-arthritic human hips. J Bone Joint Surg Am 52(3): 424-34, 1970.

85. Inerot S, Heinegard D, Audell L et al: Articular-cartilage proteoglycans in aging and osteoarthritis. Biochem J 169(1): 143-56, 1978.

86. Bollet AJ, Nance JL: Biochemical findings in normal and osteoarthritic articular cartilage. II. Chondroitin sulfate concentration and chain length, water, and ash contents. J Clin Invest 44: 1170-1177, 1966.

87. Mankin HJ, Dorfman H, Lippiello L et al: A: Biochemical and metabolic abnormalities in articular cartilage from osteoarthritic human hips. II. Correlation of morphology with biochemical and metabolic data. J Bone Joint Surg Am 53(3): 523-37, 1971.

88. Jaovisidha K, Rosenthal AK: Calcium crystals in osteoarthritis. Curr Opin Rheumatol 14(3): 298-302, 2002.

89. Ryan LM, Cheung HS: The role of crystals in osteoarthritis. Rheum Dis Clin North Am 25(2): 257-67, 1999.

90. Howell DS, Muniz OE, Morales S: 5′ Nucleotidase and pyrophosphate (Ppi)-generating activities in articular cartilage extracts in calcium pyrophosphate deposition disease (CPPD) and in primary osteoarthritis (OA), in Epidemiology of Osteoarthritis, ed. JG Peyron. Ciba-Geigy, Paris. 99, 1980.

91. Howell DS, Muniz O, Pita JC, et al: Extrusion of pyrophosphate into extracellular media by osteoarthritic cartilage incubates. J Clin Invest 56(6): 1473-8, 1975.

92. Altman RD, Muniz OE, Pita JC et al: Articular chondrocalcinosis: Microanalysis of pyrophosphate (PPi) in synovial fluid and plasma. Arthritis Rheum 16(2): 171-8, 1973.

93. Silcox DC, McCarty DJ Jr: Elevated inorganic pyrophosphate concentrations in synovial fluids in osteoarthritis and pseudogout. J Lab Clin Med 83(4): 518-31, 1974.

94. Tenenbaum J, Muniz O, Schumacher HR, et al: Comparison of phosphohydrolase activities from articular cartilage in calcium pyrophosphate deposition disease and primary osteoarthritis. Arthritis Rheum 24(3): 492-500, 1981.

95. Ryu J, Treadwell BV, Mankin HJ: Biochemical and metabolic abnormalities in normal and osteoarthritic human articular cartilage. Arthritis Rheum 27(1): 49-57, 1984.

96. Mort JS, Billington CJ: Articular cartilage and changes in arthritis: matrix degradation. Arthritis Res 3(6): 337-41, 2001.

97. Murphy G, Docherty AJP: Molecular studies on the connective tissue metalloproteinases and their inhibitor TIMP, in The

Control of Tissue Damage, ed. AM Galuert. Elsevier, Oxford 223, 1988.

98. Mankin HJ, Thrasher AZ: Water content and binding in normal and osteoarthritic human cartilage. J Bone Joint Surg Am, 57(1): 76-80, 1975.

99. Sandy JD, Lark MW: Proteolytic degradation of normal and osteoarthritic cartilage matrix, in Osteoarthritis, ed. KD Brandt, M Doherty, LS Lohmander. Oxford University Press, Oxford 84, 1998.

100. Morales TI, Kuettner, KE: The properties of the neutral proteinase released by primary chondrocyte cultures and its action on proteoglycan aggregate. Biochim Biophys Acta 705(1): 92-101, 1982.

101. Sapolsky AI, Howell DS: Further characterization of a neutral metalloprotease isolated from human articular cartilage Arthritis Rheum 25(8): 981-8, 1982.

102. Knauper V, Lopez-Otin C, Smith B, et al: Biochemical characterization of human collagenase-3. J Biol Chem 271 (3): 1544-50, 1996.

103. Tetlow LC, Adlam DJ, Woolley DE: Matrix metalloproteinase and proinflammatory cytokine production by chondrocytes of human osteoarthritic cartilage: Associations with degenerative changes. Arthritis Rheum 2001, 44(3): 585-94.

104. Ehrlich MG, Mankin HJ, Jones H, et al: Collagenase and collagenase inhibitors in osteoarthritic and normal cartilage. J Clin Invest 59(2): 226-33, 1977.

105. Ehrlich MG, Houle PA, Vigliani G et al: Correlation between articular cartilage collagenase activity and osteoarthritis. Arthritis Rheum 21(7): 761-6, 1978.

106. Xie DL, Hui F, Meyers R et al: Cartilage chondrolysis by fibronectin fragments is associated with release of several proteinases: Stromelysin plays a major role in chondrolysis. Arch Biochem Biophys 311 (2): 205-12, 1994.

107. Campbell IK, Piccoli DS, Butler DM, et al: Recombinant human interleukin-1 stimulates human articular cartilage to undergo resorption and human chondrocytes to produce both tissue- and urokinase-type plasminogen activator Biochim Biophys Acta 967(2): 183-94, 1988.

108. Tang BL: ADAMTS: a novel family of extracellular matrix proteases. Int J Biochem Cell Biol 33(1): 33-44, 2001.

109. Arner, EC: Aggrecanase-mediated cartilage degradation. Curr Opin Pharmacol 2(3): 322-9, 2002.

110. Hardingham T, Bayliss M: Proteoglycans of articular cartilage: changes in aging and in joint disease. Semin Arthritis Rheum 20(3 Suppl 1): 12-33, 1990.

111. Campbell IK, Wojta J, Novak U et al: Cytokine modulation of plasminogen activator inhibitor-1 (PAI-1) production by human articular cartilage and chondrocytes. Down-regulation by tumor necrosis factor alpha and up-regulation by transforming growth factor-B basic fibroblast growth factor. Biochim Biophys Acta 1226(3): 277-85, 1994.

112. Ollivierre F, Gubler U, Towle CA, et al: Expression of IL-1 genes in human and bovine chondrocytes: A mechanism for autocrine control of cartilage matrix degradation. Biochem Biophys Res Commun 141(3): 904-11, 1986.

113. Rath NC, Oronsky AL, Kerwar SS: Synthesis of interleukin-1-like activity by normal chondrocytes in culture. Clin Imm Immunopathol 47(1): 39-46, 1988.

114. Kandel RA, Dinarello CA, Biswas, C: The stimulation of collagenase production in rabbit articular chondrocytes by interleukin-1 is increased by collagens. Biochem In 15(5): 1021-31, 1987.

115. Pujol JP, Loyau G: Interleukin-1 and osteoarthritis. Life Sci 41(10): 1187-98, 1987.

116. Dodge GR, Poole AR: Immunohistochemical detection and immunochemical analysis of type II collagen degradation in human normal, rheumatoid, and osteoarthritic articular cartilages and in explants of bovine articular cartilage cultured with interleukin 1. J Clin Invest 83(2): 647-61, 1989.

117. Ratcliffe A, Tyler JA, Hardingham TE: Articular cartilage cultured with interleukin 1: Increased release of link protein, hyaluronate-binding region and other proteoglycan fragments. Biochem J 238(2): 571-80, 1986.

118. Tortorella MD, Malfait AM, Deccico C et al: The role of ADAM-TS4 (aggrecanase-1) and ADAM-TS5 (aggrecanase-2) in a model of cartilage degradation. Osteoarthritis Cartilage 9(6): 539-52, 2001.

119. Dean DD, Woessner JF, Jr: Extracts of human articular cartilage contain an inhibitor of tissue metalloproteinases. Biochem J 218(1): 277-80, 1984.

120. Yamada H, Stephens RW, Nakagawa T et al: Human articular cartilage contains an inhibitor of plasminogen activator. J Rheumatol 15(7): 1138-43, 1988.

121. Malemud CJ: The role of growth factors in cartilage metabolism. Rheumatic Diseases Clinics of North America 19(3): 569-80, 1993.

122. Hardingham TE, Bayliss MT, Rayan V et al: Effects of growth factors and cytokines on proteoglycan turnover in articular cartilage. Br J Rheumatol 31(Suppl 1): 1-6, 1992.

123. Morales TI: Transforming growth factor-beta and insulin-like growth factor-1 restore proteoglycan metabolism of bovine articular cartilage after depletion by retinoic acid. Arch Biochem Biophys 315(1): 190-8, 1994.

124. Dean DD, Azzo W, Martel-Pelletier J, et al: Levels of metalloproteases and tissue inhibitor of metalloproteases in human osteoarthritic cartilage. J Rheumatol 14 Spec No: 43-4, 1987.

125. Teshima R, Treadwell BV, Trahan CA et al: Comparative rates of proteoglycan synthesis and size of proteoglycans in normal and osteoarthritic chondrocytes. Arthritis Rheum 26(10): 1225-30, 1983.

126. Moskowitz RW, Davis W, Sammarco J, et al: Experimentally induced degenerative joint lesions following partial meniscectomy in the rabbit. Arthritis Rheum 16(3): 397-405, 1973.

127. Muir H: Heberden Oration, 1976. Molecular approach to the understanding of osteoarthrosis. Ann Rheum Dis 36(3): 199-208, 1977.

128. McDevitt CA, Muir H: Biochemical changes in the cartilage of the knee in experimental and natural osteoarthritis in the dog. J Bone Joint Surg Br 58(1): 94-101, 1976.

129. Brandt KD: Enhanced extractability of articular cartilage proteoglycans in osteoarthrosis. Biochem J 143(2): 475-8, 1974.

130. Moskowitz RW, Howell DS, Goldberg VM, et al: Cartilage proteoglycan alterations in an experimentally induced model of rabbit osteoarthritis. Arthritis Rheum 22(2): 155-63, 1979.

131. Maroudas A, Katz EP, Wachtel EJ, et al: Physiochemical properties and functional behavior of normal and osteoarthritic human cartilage, in Articular Cartilage Biochemistry, ed. R Schleyerbach, KE Kuettner, VC Hascall. Raven Press, New York 311-30, 1986.

132. Adams ME, Brandt KD: Hypertrophic repair of canine articular cartilage in osteoarthritis after anterior cruciate ligament transection. J Rheumatol 18(3): 428-35, 1991.

133. Bywaters EGL: Metabolism of joint tissue. J Pathol Bacteriol 44: 247, 1937.

134. Johnson LD: Kinetics of osteoarthritis. Lab Invest 8: 1223, 1959.

135. Kempson GE, Spivey CJ, Swanson SA et al: Patterns of cartilage stiffness on normal and degenerate human femoral heads. J Biomech 4(6): 597-609, 1971.

136. Mankin HJ, Mow VC, Buckwalter JA, et al: Form and function of articular cartilage, in Orthopaedic Basic Science, ed. S Simon. American Academy of Orthopaedic Surgeons, Chicago 1-44, 1994.

137. Bollet AJ: Connective tissue polysaccharide metabolism and the pathogenesis of osteoarthritis. Adv Intern Med 13: 33-60, 1967.

138. Freeman MAR: Discussion on pathogenesis of osteoarthrosis, in Normal and Osteoarthrotic Articular Cartilage, ed. SY Ali MW Elves, DH Leaback. Institute of Orthopaedics, London 301, 1974.

139. Hlavacek M: The role of synovial fluid filtration by cartilage in lubrication of synovial joints. I. Mixture model of synovial fluid. J Biomech 26(10): 1145-50, 1993.

140. Hlavacek M: The role of synovial fluid filtration by cartilage in lubrication of synovial joints. II. Squeeze-film lubrication: Homogeneous filtration. J Biomech 26(10): 1151-60, 1993.

141. Mow VC, Ateshian GA, Spilker RL: Biomechanics of diarthrodial joints: A review of twenty years of progress. J Biomech Eng 115(4B): 460-7, 1993.

142. Unsworth A: Tribology of human and artificial joints. Proc Inst Mech Eng [H] 205(3): 163-72, 1991.

143. Hlavacek M: The role of synovial fluid filtration by cartilage in lubrication of synovial joints. IV. Squeeze-film lubrication: The central film thickness for normal and inflammatory synovial fluids for axial symmetry under high loading conditions. J Biomech 28(10): 1199-205, 1995.

144. Hlavacek M, Novak J: The role of synovial fluid filtration by cartilage in lubrication of synovial joints—III. Squeeze-film lubrication: Axial symmetry under low loading conditions. J Biomech 28(10): 1193-8, 1995.

145. Hlavacek M: Squeeze-film lubrication of the human ankle joint with synovial fluid filtrated by articular cartilage with the superficial zone worn out. J Biomech 33(11): 1415-22, 2000.

146. Hlavacek M: The influence of the acetabular labrum seal, intact articular superficial zone and synovial fluid thixotropy on squeeze-film lubrication of a spherical synovial joint. J Biomech 35(10): 1325-35, 2002.

147. Malemud CJ, Goldberg VM, Moskowitz RW, et al: Biosynthesis of proteoglycan in vitro by cartilage from human osteochondrophytic spurs. Biochem J 206(2): 329-41, 1982.

148. Marshall JL, Olsson SE: Instability of the knee: A long-term experimental study in dogs. J Bone Joint Surg Am 53(8): 1561-70, 1971.

149. Danielsson LG: Incidence and prognosis of coxarthrosis. 1964: Clin Orthop (287): 13-8, 1993.

150. Trueta J: Studies of the Development and Decay of the Human Frame. Philadelphia, WB Saunders 1968.

151. Swanson SAV, Freeman MAR: The mechanics of synovial joints, in Modern Trends in Biomechanics, ed. DC Simpson. Butterworths, London 239, 1970.

152. Gilbertson EM: Development of periarticular osteophytes in experimentally induced osteoarthritis in the dog: a study using microradiographic, microangiographic, and fluorescent bone-labelling techniques. Ann Rheum Dis 34(1): 12-25, 1975.

153. Shuler FD, Georgescu HI, Niyibizi C, et al: Increased matrix synthesis following adenoviral transfer of a transforming growth factor beta1 gene into articular chondrocytes. J Orthop Res 18(4): 585-92, 2000.

154. Bakker AC, van de Loo FA, van Beuningen HM, et al: Overexpression of active TGF-beta-1 in the murine knee joint: evidence for synovial-layer-dependent chondro-osteophyte formation. Osteoarthritis Cartilage 9(2): 128-36, 2001.

155. Uchino M, Izumi T, Tominaga T, et al: Growth factor expression in the osteophytes of the human femoral head in osteoarthritis. Clin Orthop (377): 119-25, 2000.

156. Bernstein MA: Experimental production of arthritis by artificially produced passive congestion. J Bone Joint Surg 15: 661, 1933.

157. Phillips RS: Phlebography in osteoarthritis of the hip. J Bone Joint Surg Br 48(2): 280-8, 1966.

158. Landells JW: The bone cysts of osteoarthritis. J Bone Joint Surg 35: 643, 1953.

159. Palmoski MJ, Brand KD: Immobilization of the knee prevents osteoarthritis after anterior cruciate ligament transection. Arthritis Rheum 25(10): 1201-8, 1982.

160. Butler M, Colombo C, Hickman L, et al: A new model of osteoarthritis in rabbits. III. Evaluation of anti-osteoarthritic effects of selected drugs administered intraarticularly. Arthritis Rheum 26(11): 1380-6, 1983.

161. Pelletier JP, Martel-Pelletier J: Protective effects of corticosteroids on cartilage lesions and osteophyte formation in the Pond-Nuki dog model of osteoarthritis. Arthritis Rheum 32(2): 181-93, 1989.

162. Myers SL, Brand KD, Burr DB, et al: Effects of a bisphosphonate on bone histomorphometry and dynamics in the canine cruciate deficiency model of osteoarthritis. J Rheumatol 26(12): 2645-53, 1999.

163. Chen FS, Frenkel SR, Di Cesare PE: Repair of articular cartilage defects. part I. Basic Science of cartilage healing. Am J Orthop 28(1): 31-3, 1999.

164. Frenkel SR, Di Cesare PE: Degradation and repair of articular cartilage. Front Biosci 4: D671-85, 1999.

165. Buckwalter JA, Mow VC, Ratcliffe A: Restoration of Injured or Degenerated Articular Cartilage. J Am Acad Orthop Surg 2(4): 192-201, 1994.

166. Buckwalter JA, Lohmander S: Operative treatment of osteoarthrosis: Current practice and future development. J Bone Joint Surg Am 76(9): 1405-18, 1994.

167. Coletti JM Jr, Akeson WH, Woo SL: A comparison of the physical behavior of normal articular cartilage and the arthroplasty surface. J Bone Joint Surg Am 54(1): 147-60, 1972.

168. Mankin HJ: The response of articular cartilage to mechanical injury. J Bone Joint Surg Am 64(3): 460-6, 1982.

169. Hamerman D: Prospects for medical intervention in cartilage repair, in Joint Cartilage Degradation: Basic and Clinical Aspects, ed. JF Woessner, D Howell. Marcel Dekker, Inc, New York 529-546, 1993.

170. Campbell CJ: The healing of cartilage defects. Clin Orthop 64: 45-63, 1969.

171. Redfern P: On the healing of wounds in articular cartilage. Clin Orthop Rel Res 64: 4-6, 1969.

172. Fisher T: Some researches into the physiological principles underlying the treatment of injuries and diseases of the articulations. Lancet 2: 541-548, 1923.

173. Ito LK: The nutrition of articular cartilage and its method of repair. Brit J Surg 12: 31-42, 1924.

174. Carlson H: Reactions of rabbit patellary cartilage following operative defects. Acta Orthop Scand Suppl 28: 1-118, 1957.

175. Gilmer WS, Jr, Calandruccio R: Proliferation, regeneration, and repair of articular cartilage of immature animals. J Bone Joint Surg AM 44: 431-455, 1962.

176. Mankin HJ: Localization of tritiated thymidine in articular cartilage of rabbits. I.: Growth in immature cartilage. J Bone Joint Surg AM 44 (682-688): 1962.

177. Mankin HJ: Localization of tritiated thymidine in articular cartilage of rabbits. II.: Repair in immature cartilage. J Bone Joint Surg AM 44: 688-698, 1962.

178. Mankin HJ: Localization of tritiated thymidine in articular cartilage of rabbits. III.: Mature articular cartilage. J Bone Joint Surg AM 45: 529-540, 1963.

179. Grande DA, Singh IJ, Pugh J: Healing of experimentally produced lesions in articular cartilage following chondrocyte transplantation. Anat Rec 218(2): 142-8, 1987.

180. Radin EL, Ehrlich MG, Chernack R, et al: Effect of repetitive impulsive loading on the knee joints of rabbits. Clin Orthop (131): 288-93, 1978.

181. Berm GM, Fu FH: Classification and treatment of DJD of the knee. Orthop Spec Educ 2(1): 31-35, 1996.

182. Dekel S, Weissman SL: Joint changes after overuse and peak overloading of rabbit knees in vivo. Acta Orthop Scand 49(6): 519-28, 1978.

183. Lee SH, Abramson SA: Stepped-care guide to osteoarthritis therapy. Orthop Spec Educ 2(2): 7-10, 1996.

184. Farrell AJ, Blake DR, Palmer RM et al: Increased concentrations of nitrite in synovial fluid and serum samples suggest increased nitric oxide synthesis in rheumatic diseases. Ann Rheum Dis 51(11): 1219-22, 1992.

185. Yoshimi T, Kikuchi T, Obara T, et al: Effects of high-molecular-weight sodium hyaluronate on experimental osteoarthrosis induced by the resection of rabbit anterior cruciate ligament. Clin Orthop (298): 296-304, 1994.

186. Cheung HS, Cottrell WH, Stephenson K et al: In vitro collagen biosynthesis in healing and normal rabbit articular cartilage. J Bone Joint Surg Am 60(8): 1076-81, 1978.

187. DePalma AF, McKeever CD, Subin DK: Process of repair of articular cartilage demonstrated by histology and autoradiography with tritiated thymidine. Clin Orthop 48: 229-42, 1966.

188. Mitchell N, Shepard N: The resurfacing of adult rabbit articular cartilage by multiple perforations through the subchondral bone. J Bone Joint Surg Am 58(2): 230-3, 1976.

189. Shapiro F, Koide S, Glimcher MJ: Cell origin and differentiation in the repair of full-thickness defects of articular cartilage. J Bone Joint Surg Am 75(4): 532-53, 1993.

190. Cheung HS, Lynch KL, Johnson RP et al: In vitro synthesis of tissue-specific type II collagen by healing cartilage. I. Short-term repair of cartilage by mature rabbits. Arthritis Rheum 23(2): 211-9, 1980.

191. Furukawa T, Eyre DR, Koide S et al: Biochemical studies on repair cartilage resurfacing experimental defects in the rabbit knee. J Bone Joint Surg Am 62(1): 79-89, 1980.

192. Hjertquist SO, Lemperg R: Histological, autoradiographic and microchemical studies of spontaneously healing osteochondral articular defects in adult rabbits. Calcif Tissue Res 8(1): 54-72, 1971.

193. Convery FR, Akeson WH, Keown, GH: The repair of large osteochondral defects. An experimental study in horses. Clin Orthop 82: 253-62, 1972.

194. Mobasheri A, Carter SD, Martin-Vasallo P et al: Integrins and stretch activated ion channels; putative components of functional cell surface mechanoreceptors in articular chondrocytes. Cell Biol Int 26(1): 1-18, 2002.

195. Grodzinsky AJ, Levenston ME, Jin M et al: Cartilage tissue remodeling in response to mechanical forces. Annu Rev Biomed Eng 2: 691-713, 2000.

196. Giannoni P, Siegrist M, Hunziker EB et al: The mechanosensitivity of cartilage oligomeric matrix protein (COMP). Biorheology 40(1,2,3): 101-109, 2003.

197. Wong M, Siegrist M, Cao X: Cyclic compression of articular cartilage explants is associated with progressive consolidation and altered expression pattern of extracellular matrix proteins. Matrix Biol 18(4): 391-9, 1999.

198. Lee HS, Millward-Sadler SJ, Wright MO, et al: Integrin and mechanosensitive ion channel-dependent tyrosine phosphorylation of focal adhesion proteins and beta-catenin in human articular chondrocytes after mechanical stimulation. J Bone Miner Res 15(8): 1501-9, 2000.

199. Salter DM, Millward-Sadler SJ, Nuki G et al: Differential responses of chondrocytes from normal and osteoarthritic human articular cartilage to mechanical stimulation. Biorheology 39(1-2): 97-108, 2002.

200. Millward-Sadler SJ, Wright MO, Lee H, et al: Integrin-regulated secretion of interleukin 4: A novel pathway of mechanotransduction in human articular chondrocytes. J Cell Biol 145(1): 183-9, 1999.

201. Millward-Sadler SJ, Wright MO, Davies LW, et al: Mechanotransduction via integrins and interleukin-4 results in altered aggrecan and matrix metalloproteinase 3 gene expression in normal, but not osteoarthritic, human articular chondrocytes. Arthritis Rheum 43(9): 2091-9, 2000.

202. Millward-Sadler SJ, Wright MO, Lee H, et al: Altered electrophysiological responses to mechanical stimulation and abnormal signalling through alpha5beta1 integrin in chondrocytes from osteoarthritic cartilage. Osteoarthritis Cartilage 8(4): 272-8, 2000.

203. Sironen RK, Karjalainen HM, Torronen K, et al: High pressure effects on cellular expression profile and mRNA stability. A cDNA array analysis. Biorheology 39(1-2): 111-7, 2002.

204. Jin M, Frank EH, Quinn TM, et al: Tissue shear deformation stimulates proteoglycan and protein biosynthesis in bovine cartilage explants. Arch Biochem Biophys 395(1): 41-8, 2001.

205. Wu Q, Zhang Y, Chen Q: Indian hedgehog is an essential component of mechanotransduction complex to stimulate chondrocyte proliferation. J Biol Chem 276(38): 35290-6, 2001.

206. Rizkalla G, Reiner A, Bogoch E et al: Studies of the articular cartilage proteoglycan aggrecan in health and osteoarthritis. Evidence for molecular heterogeneity and extensive molecular changes in disease. J Clin Invest 90(6): 2268-77, 1992.

207. Evans CH: Cellular mechanisms of hydrolytic enzyme release in proteoglycan. Semin Arthritis Rheum 11: 93, 1981.

208. Evans CH, Mears DC, McKnight JL: A preliminary ferrographic survey of the wear particles in human synovial fluid. Arthritis Rheum 24(7): 912-8, 1981.

209. Haraoui B, Pelletier JP, Cloutier JM, et al: Synovial membrane histology and immunopathology in rheumatoid arthritis and osteoarthritis. In vivo effects of antirheumatic drugs. Arthritis Rheum 34(2): 153-63, 1991.

210. Farahat MN, Yanni G, Poston R et al: Cytokine expression in synovial membranes of patients with rheumatoid arthritis and osteoarthritis. Ann Rheum Dis 52(12): 870-5, 1993.

211. Smith MD, Triantafillou S, Parker A, et al: Synovial membrane inflammation and cytokine production in patients with early osteoarthritis. J Rheumatol 24(2): 365-71, 1997.

212. Pelletier JP, Martel-Pelletier J, Abramson SB: Osteoarthritis, an inflammatory disease: potential implication for the selection of new therapeutic targets. Arthritis Rheum, 44(6): 1237-47, 2001.

213. Cooke TD: Significance of immune complex deposits in osteoarthritic cartilage. J Rheumatol 14 Spec No: 77-9, 1987.

214. Krenn V, Hensel F, Kim HJ, et al: Molecular IgV(H) analysis demonstrates highly somatic mutated B cells in synovialitis of osteoarthritis: A degenerative disease is associated with a specific, not locally generated immune response. Lab Invest 79(11): 1377-84, 1999.

215. Nakamura H, Yoshino S, Kato T, et al: T-cell mediated inflammatory pathway in osteoarthritis. Osteoarthritis Cartilage 7(4): 401-2, 1999.

216. Dieppe P, Cushnaghan J, Young P et al: Prediction of the progression of joint space narrowing in osteoarthritis of the knee by bone scintigraphy. Ann Rheum Dis 52(8): 557-63, 1993.

217. Ayral X, Dougados M, Listrat V, et al: Arthroscopic evaluation of chondropathy in osteoarthritis of the knee. J Rheumatol 23(4): 698-706, 1996.

218. Ayral X, Pickering EH, Woodworth TJ, et al: Synovitis predicts the arthroscopic progression of medial tibiofemoral knee osteoarthritis (OA). Ann Rheum Dis 60: 57, 2001.

219. Alaaeddine N, Olee T, Hashimoto S, et al: Production of the chemokine RANTES by articular chondrocytes and role in cartilage degradation. Arthritis Rheum 44(7): 1633-43, 2001.

220. Oldberg A, Antonsson P, Lindblom K et al: COMP (cartilage oligomeric matrix protein) is structurally related to the thrombospondins. J Biol Chem 267(31): 22346-50, 1992.

221. DiCesare PE, Morgelin M, Mann K et al: Cartilage oligomeric matrix protein and thrombospondin 1. Purification from articular cartilage, electron microscopic structure, and chondrocyte binding. Eur J Biochem 223(3): 927-37, 1994.

222. Hedbom E, Antonsson P, Hjerpe A, et al: Cartilage matrix proteins. An acidic oligomeric protein (COMP) detected only in cartilage. J Biol Chem 267(9): 6132-6, 1992.

223. Morgelin M, Heinegard D, Engel J et al: Electron microscopy of native cartilage oligomeric matrix protein purified from the Swarm rat chondrosarcoma reveals a five-armed structure. J Biol Chem 267(9): 6137-41, 1992.

224. Clark AG, Jordan JM, Vilim V, et al: Serum cartilage oligomeric matrix protein reflects osteoarthritis presence and severity: The Johnston County Osteoarthritis Project. Arthritis Rheum 42(11): 2356-64, 1999.

225. Lohmander LS, Ionescu M, Jugessur H et al: Changes in joint cartilage aggrecan after knee injury and in osteoarthritis. Arthritis Rheum 42(3): 534-44, 1999.

226. Neidhart M, Hauser N, Paulsson M, et al: Small fragments of cartilage oligomeric matrix protein in synovial fluid and serum as markers for cartilage degradation. Br J Rheumatol 36(11): 1151-60, 1997.

227. Saxne T, Heinegard D: Cartilage oligomeric matrix protein: a novel marker of cartilage turnover detectable in synovial fluid and blood. Br J Rheumatol 31(9): 583-91, 1992.

228. Dahlberg L, Roos H, Saxne T, et al: Cartilage metabolism in the injured and uninjured knee of the same patient. Ann Rheum Dis 53(12): 823-7, 1994.

229. Lohmander LS, Saxne T, Heinegard, DK: Release of cartilage oligomeric matrix protein (COMP) into joint fluid after knee injury and in osteoarthritis. Ann Rheum Dis 53(1): 8-13, 1994.

230. Mansson B, Carey D, Alini M, et al: Cartilage and bone metabolism in rheumatoid arthritis. Differences between rapid and slow progression of disease identified by serum markers of cartilage metabolism. J Clin Invest 95(3): 1071-7, 1995.

231. Petersson IF, Boegard T, Svensson B, et al: Changes in cartilage and bone metabolism identified by serum markers in early osteoarthritis of the knee joint. Br J Rheumatol 37(1): 46-50, 1998.

232. Sharif M, Saxne T, Shepstone L, et al: Relationship between serum cartilage oligomeric matrix protein levels and disease progression in osteoarthritis of the knee joint. Br J Rheumatol 34(4): 306-10, 1995.

233. DiCesare P, Hauser N, Lehman D, et al: Cartilage oligomeric matrix protein (COMP) is an abundant component of tendon. FEBS Lett 354(2): 237-40, 1994.

234. Vilim V, Vytasek R, Olejarova M, et al: Serum cartilage oligomeric matrix protein reflects the presence of clinically diagnosed synovitis in patients with knee osteoarthritis. Osteoarthritis Cartilage 9(7): 612-8, 2001.

235. Sowers M, Jannausch M, Stein E, et al: C-reactive protein as a biomarker of emergent osteoarthritis. Osteoarthritis Cartilage 10(8): 595-601, 2002.

236. Hedin PJ, Weitoft T, Hedin H, et al: Serum concentrations of hyaluronan and proteoglycan in joint disease: Lack of association. J Rheumatol 18(10): 1601-5, 1991.

237. Goldberg RL, Huff JP, Lenz ME, et al: Elevated plasma levels of hyaluronate in patients with osteoarthritis and rheumatoid arthritis. Arthritis Rheum 34(7): 799-807, 1991.

238. Manicourt DH, Cornu O, Lenz ME, et al: Rapid and sustained rise in the serum level of hyaluronan after anterior cruciate ligament transection in the dog knee joint. J Rheumatol 22(2): 262-9, 1995.

239. Sinigaglia L, Varenna M, Binelli L, et al: Urinary and synovial pyridinium crosslink concentrations in patients with rheumatoid arthritis and osteoarthritis. Ann Rheum Dis 54(2): 144-7, 1995.

240. Sharif M, George E, Dieppe PA: Correlation between synovial fluid markers of cartilage and bone turnover and scintigraphic scan abnormalities in osteoarthritis of the knee. Arthritis Rheum 38(1): 78-81, 1995.

241. Verbruggen G, Veys EM: Numerical scoring systems for the anatomic evolution of osteoarthritis of the finger joints. Arthritis Rheum 39(2): 308-20, 1996.

242. Mort JS, Caterson B, Poole AR et al: The origin of human cartilage proteoglycan link-protein heterogeneity and fragmentation during aging. Biochem J 232(3): 805-12, 1985.

243. Roughley PJ, Lee ER: Cartilage proteoglycans: structure and potential functions. Microsc Res Tech 28(5): 385-97, 1994.

244. Neame PJ, Sandy JD: Cartilage aggrecan: biosynthesis, degradation and osteoarthritis. J Fla Med Assoc 81(3): 191-3, 1994.

245. Perkins SJ, Nealis AS, Dudhia J et al: Immunoglobulin fold and tandem repeat structures in proteoglycan N-terminal domains and link protein. J Mol Biol 206(4): 737-53, 1989.

246. Williams AF, Barclay AN: The immunoglobulin superfamily: Domains for cell surface recognition. Annu Rev Immunol 6: 381-405, 1988.

247. Rosenberg LC: Structure and function of dermatan sulfate proteoglycans in articular cartilage, in Articular Cartilage and Osteoarthritis, ed. KE Kuettner, R Schleyerbach, JG Peyron, et al. Raven Press, New York. 45-62, 1992.

248. Noyori K, Jasin HE: Inhibition of human fibroblast adhesion by cartilage surface proteoglycans. Arthritis Rheum 37(11): 1656-63, 1994.

249. McCarty DJ, Halverson PB, Carrera GF, et al: "Milwaukee shoulder": Association of microspheroids containing hydroxyapatite crystals, active collagenase, and neutral protease with rotator cuff defects. I. Clinical aspects. Arthritis Rheum 24(3): 464-73, 1981.

250. Shlopov BV, Smith GN Jr, Cole AA et al: Differential patterns of response to doxycycline and transforming growth factor beta1 in the down-regulation of collagenases in osteoarthritic and normal human chondrocytes. Arthritis Rheum 42(4): 719-27, 1999.

251. Melchiorri C, Melicon R, Frizziero L, et al: Enhanced and coordinated in vivo expression of inflammatory cytokines and nitric oxide synthase by chondrocytes from patients with osteoarthritis. Arthritis Rheum 41(12): 2165-74, 1998.

252. Martel-Pelletier J, di Battista JA, Lajeunesse D: Biochemical factors in joint articular tissue degradation in osteoarthritis, in Osteoarthritis: Clinical and experimental aspects, ed. JY Reginster, JP Pelletier, J Martel-Pelletier, Y Henrotin. Springer-Verlag, Berlin 156-187, 1999.

253. Caron JP, Fernandes JC, Martel-Pelletier J, et al: Chondroprotective effect of intraarticular injections of interleukin-1 receptor antagonist in experimental osteoarthritis: suppression of collagenase-1 expression. Arthritis Rheum 39(9): 1535-44, 1996.

254. van de Loo, FA, Joosten LA, van Lent PL, et al: Role of interleukin-1, tumor necrosis factor alpha, and interleukin-6 in cartilage proteoglycan metabolism and destruction: Effect of in situ blocking in murine antigen- and zymosan-induced arthritis. Arthritis Rheum 38(2): 164-72, 1995.

255. Attur MG, Dave M, Cipolletta C, et al: Reversal of autocrine and paracrine effects of interleukin 1 (IL-1) in human arthritis by type II IL-1 decoy receptor: Potential for pharmacological intervention. J Biol Chem 275(51): 40307-15, 2000.

256. Slack J, McMahan CJ, Waugh S, et al: Independent binding of interleukin-1 alpha and interleukin-1 beta to type I and type II interleukin-1 receptors. J Biol Chem 268(4): 2513-24, 1993.

257. Martel-Pelletier J, Alaaeddine N, Pelletier JP: Cytokines and their role in the pathophysiology of osteoarthritis. Front Biosci 4: D694-703, 1999.

258. Pelletier JP, Caron JP, Evans C, et al: In vivo suppression of early experimental osteoarthritis by interleukin-1 receptor antagonist using gene therapy. Arthritis Rheum 40(6): 1012-9, 1997.

259. Kronheim SR, Mumma A, Greenstreet T, et al: Purification of interleukin-1 beta converting enzyme, the protease that cleaves the interleukin-1 beta precursor. Arch Biochem Biophys 296(2): 698-703, 1992.

260. Black RA, Rauch CT, Kozlosky CJ, et al: A metalloproteinase disintegrin that releases tumor-necrosis factor-alpha from cells. Nature 385: 729-733, 1997.

261. Amin AR, Attur M, Patel RN, et al: Superinduction of cyclooxygenase-2 activity in human osteoarthritis-affected cartilage: Influence of nitric oxide. J Clin Invest 99(6): 1231-7, 1997.

262. Amin AR: Regulation of tumor necrosis factor-alpha and tumor necrosis factor converting enzyme in human osteoarthritis. Osteoarthritis Cartilage 7(4): 392-4, 1999.

263. Yuan GH, Masuko-Hongo K, Sakata M, et al: The role of C-C chemokines and their receptors in osteoarthritis. Arthritis Rheum 44(5): 1056-70, 2001.

264. Honorati MC, Bovara M, Cattini L, et al: Contribution of interleukin 17 to human cartilage degradation and synovial inflammation in osteoarthritis. Osteoarthritis Cartilage 10(10): 799-807, 2002.

265. Aigner T, McKenna L: Molecular pathology and pathobiology of osteoarthritic cartilage. Cell Mol Life Sci 59(1): 5-18, 2002.

266. Scher DM, Stolerman ES, Di Cesare, PE: Biologic markers of arthritis. Am J Orthop 25(4): 263-72, 1996.

267. Heinegard D, Oldberg A: Structure and biology of cartilage and bone matrix noncollagenous macromolecules. Faseb J 3(9): 2042-51, 1989.

268. Roughley PJ: Articular cartilage and changes in arthritis: noncollagenous proteins and proteoglycans in the extracellular matrix of cartilage. Arthritis Res 3(6): 342-7, 2001.

269. Attur MG, Dave MN, Stuchin S, et al: Osteopontin: an intrinsic inhibitor of inflammation in cartilage. Arthritis Rheum 44(3): 578-84, 2001.

270. Arner EC, Tortorella MD: Signal transduction through chondrocyte integrin receptors induces matrix metalloproteinase synthesis and synergizes with interleukin-1. Arthritis Rheum 38(9): 1304-14, 1995.

271. Homandberg GA, Hui F, Wen C, et al: Fibronectin-fragment-induced cartilage chondrolysis is associated with release of catabolic cytokines. Biochem J 321(Pt 3) 751-7, 1997.

272. Homandberg GA, Meyers R, Williams JM: Intraarticular injection of fibronectin fragments causes severe depletion of cartilage proteoglycans in vivo. J Rheumatol 20(8): 1378-82, 1993.

273. Yasuda T, Poole AR: A fibronectin fragment induces type II collagen degradation by collagenase through an interleukin-1-mediated pathway. Arthritis Rheum 46(1): 138-48, 2002.

274. Amin AR, Di Cesare PE, Vyas P, et al: The expression and regulation of nitric oxide synthase in human osteoarthritis-affected chondrocytes: Evidence for up-regulated neuronal nitric oxide synthase. J Exp Med 182(6): 2097-102, 1995.

275. Pelletier JP, Mineau F, Ranger P, et al: The increased synthesis of inducible nitric oxide inhibits IL-1ra synthesis by human articular chondrocytes: possible role in osteoarthritic cartilage degradation. Osteoarthritis Cartilage 4(1): 77-84, 1996.

276. McInnes IB, Leung BP, Field M, et al: Production of nitric oxide in the synovial membrane of rheumatoid and osteoarthritis patients. J Exp Med 184(4): 1519-24, 1996.

277. Grabowski PS, Wright PK, Van `t Hof RJ, et al: Immunolocalization of inducible nitric oxide synthase in synovium and cartilage in rheumatoid arthritis and osteoarthritis. Br J Rheumatol 36(6): 651-5, 1997.

278. Hayashi T, Abe E, Yamate T, et al: Nitric oxide production by superficial and deep articular chondrocytes. Arthritis Rheum 40(2): 261-9, 1997.

279. Loeser RF, Carlson CS, Del Carlo M et al: Detection of nitrotyrosine in aging and osteoarthritic cartilage: Correlation of oxidative damage with the presence of interleukin-1beta and

with chondrocyte resistance to insulin-like growth factor 1. Arthritis Rheum 46(9): 2349-57, 2002.

280. Abramson SB, Attur M, Amin AR et al: Nitric oxide and inflammatory mediators in the perpetuation of osteoarthritis. Curr Rheumatol Rep 3(6): 535-41, 2001.

281. Taskiran D, Stefanovic-Racic M, Georgescu H Nitric oxide mediates suppression of cartilage proteoglycan synthesis by interleukin-1. Biochem Biophys Res Commun 200(1): 142-8, 1994.

282. Hirai Y, Migita K, Honda S, et al: Effects of nitric oxide on matrix metalloproteinase-2 production by rheumatoid synovial cells. Life Sci 68(8): 913-20, 2001.

283. Clancy RM, Abramson SB, Kohne C et al: Nitric oxide attenuates cellular hexose monophosphate shunt response to oxidants in articular chondrocytes and acts to promote oxidant injury. J Cell Physiol 172(2): 183-91, 1997.

284. Alaaeddine N, DiBattista JA, Pelletier JP, et al: Osteoarthritic synovial fibroblasts possess an increased level of tumor necrosis factor-receptor 55 (TNF-R55) that mediates biological activation by TNF-alpha. J Rheumatol 24(10): 1985-94, 1997.

285. Lotz M: The role of nitric oxide in articular cartilage damage. Rheum Dis Clin North Am 25(2): 269-82, 1999.

286. van't Hof RJ, Hocking L, Wright PK et al: Nitric oxide is a mediator of apoptosis in the rheumatoid joint. Rheumatology (Oxford) 39(9): 1004-8, 2000.

287. Pelletier JP, Jovanovic D, Fernandes JC, et al: Reduced progression of experimental osteoarthritis in vivo by selective inhibition of inducible nitric oxide synthase. Arthritis Rheum 41(7): 1275-86, 1998.

288. van den Berg WB, van de Loo F, Joosten LA, et al: Animal models of arthritis in NOS2-deficient mice. Osteoarthritis Cartilage, 7(4): 413-5, 1999.

289. van't Hof RJ, Ralston SH: Nitric oxide and bone. Immunology 103(3): 255-61, 2001.

290. Amin AR, Abramson SB: The role of nitric oxide in articular cartilage breakdown in osteoarthritis. Curr Opin Rheumatol 10(3): 263-8, 1998.

291. Hardy MM, Seibert K, Manning PT, et al: Cyclooxygenase 2-dependent prostaglandin E2 modulates cartilage proteoglycan degradation in human osteoarthritis explants. Arthritis Rheum 46(7): 1789-803, 2002.

292. Dingle JT: The effect of nonsteroidal antiinflammatory drugs on human articular cartilage glycosaminoglycan synthesis. Osteoarthritis Cartilage 7(3): 313-4, 1999.

293. Abramson SB: The role of COX-2 produced by cartilage in arthritis. Osteoarthritis Cartilage 7(4): 380-1, 1999.

92

Clinical Features of Osteoarthritis

MAXIME DOUGADOS

Osteoarthritis (OA) is a heterogeneous condition with a variety of patterns of expression. The objective of this chapter is to describe the clinical features of OA to assist the physician in the management of this disease in daily practice. For some aspects of clinical features, this chapter will refer to the data obtained at a group level for research purposes (e.g., classification criteria, outcome measures, epidemiologic findings).

■ Is the Patient Suffering from Osteoarthritis?

CLINICAL RESEARCH

In clinical research studies, patients fulfill a set of criteria that differentiate them from a normal population. These criteria are usually applied to patients with advanced disease. However, they are very specific (patients that fulfill these criteria are likely to suffer from the disease) and not very sensitive (patients who do not fulfill these criteria may actually suffer from the disease). These criteria are based on clinical descriptions,, radiographic descriptions, or both. Radiographic definitions are most widely used for epidemiologic studies. The major radiologic signs of OA are summarized in Figure 92–1. Narrowing of joint-space width is usually the main radiologic feature to evaluate the severity of the disease. The presence of osteophytes seems to be the most important feature to consider in identifying OA in the general population.[1]

Identification of OA based on clinical symptoms alone is sometimes used for epidemiologic or therapeutic studies, especially for the knee and hand joints. Figure 92–2 summarizes the main clinical symptoms found in OA. Research studies, and in particular therapeutic trials, typically refer to a set of criteria combining both clinical and radiologic definitions. Table 92–1 summarizes the characteristics of the set of criteria proposed by the American College of Rheumatology (ACR) concerning the two main localizations of OA (e.g., hip and knee).[2-4]

DAILY PRACTICE

- Which subjective symptoms suggest OA?[5]
  - Pain is undoubtedly the most important symptom of OA.[6] The time of occurrence of pain is the main feature to take into account, well before severity or localization. In contrast to inflammatory rheumatic disorders, in which the pain is most severe at night or in the morning, use-related pain is the most frequently described symptom in OA. Pain related to

activity usually begins within a few minutes of start of joint use and may persist for hours after the activity has ceased. Young patients in particular complain of maximum pain levels several hours after physical activities. On the other hand, pain occurring at night can be accounted for in various situations:
- Patients with mild OA who have used joints for several hours (e.g., those who play sports)
- Patients with advanced OA with severe destructive changes in bone and cartilage breakdown
- During an inflammatory episode of the disease (see later)
  - Joint stiffness is rarely the sole reason for a visit, but is frequently associated with pain.
  - Tenderness occurs on waking in the morning and resolves within a few minutes (usually less than 10), contrasting with the long-standing tenderness (usually more than 30 minutes) seen in inflammatory

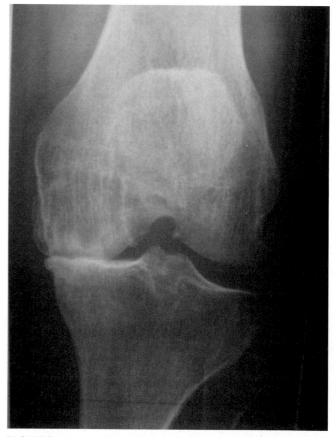

FIGURE 92–1 · Main Radiologic Signs in Osteoarthritis (OA).

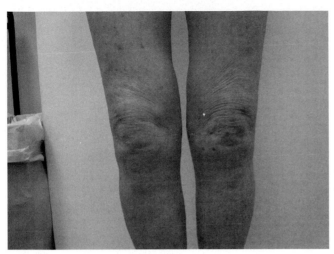

FIGURE   92-2 · Main Clinical Signs and Symptoms Observed in Osteoarthritis (OA) of the Knee.

TABLE 92–1 · AMERICAN COLLEGE OF RHEUMATOLOGY (ACR) RADIOLOGIC AND CLINICAL CRITERIA FOR KNEE AND HIP OSTEOARTHRITIS (OA)*

Knee Osteoarthritis [2]
⇒ Set of criteria:
    Knee pain
    AND
    One of the following features
        Age >50 years
        Morning stiffness <30 minutes
        Crepitus
        AND
        Radiologic osteophytes
⇒ Performance
    Sensitivity = 91%
    Specificity = 86% [4]
Hip Osteoarthritis
⇒ Set of criteria:
    Hip pain
    AND
    At least two of the following features:
        Erythrocyte sedimentation rate (ESR) <20 mm 1st hour
        Radiologic osteophytes
        Radiologic joint-space narrowing
⇒ Performance
    Sensitivity = 91%
    Specificity = 89%

*Reference 2.

rheumatic disorders. Tenderness may also occur after periods of inactivity.
○ Loss of movement is also rarely a reason for consultation. The complaint is expressed as a difficulty in moving the joint throughout its range—for example, the inability to kneel (knee OA) or to cut one's toenails (hip OA).
○ Instability is a frequent complaint of OA patients. This symptom seems to originate from abnormal strength and functioning of the muscles rather than from mechanic defects of the joints.
• Which clinical findings at physical examination are suggestive of OA?

○ A normal physical examination does not rule out the diagnosis of OA. Physical examination can remain normal throughout the first years of the disease.
○ A decrease in joint mobility is the first physical abnormality to occur in the course of the disease. Examples include a decrease in the internal rotation of the hip, a decrease in the external rotation of the shoulder, and a decrease in the flexion of the knee.
○ Bony swelling and crepitus stand out as the best signs for clinical differentiation at an advanced stage of the disease. [2]
○ Joint deformities reflect advanced joint destruction that may involve the surrounding bone and soft tissues, such as the capsule and ligaments. Such destruction is responsible for malalignment (e.g., varus angulation of the knee due to damage of the medial compartment), joint instability (e.g., at the distal interphalangeal joints), and leg shortening.
○ Joint effusion is thought to be caused by inflammation of the synovial membrane. The aspirated fluid has a high viscosity, a low cell count, and no crystals. [7] Effusion can be seen in patients complaining of chronic mechanical pain, but is seen more often during an acute painful episode of the disease together with symptoms suggestive of inflammation.
• Which investigations are necessary to confirm the diagnosis of OA?

Before answering this question, the clinician should whether there any need to confirm this diagnosis.

The diagnosis of OA is often obvious after the interview and physical examination of the patient. In some cases, the diagnosis is sufficiently obvious that no particular investigation is necessary (e.g., hand OA and forefoot OA). Investigations appear necessary for some localizations (such as the hip) because of the possibility of other diseases that could benefit from a specific treatment (e.g., Paget's disease of the pelvis). However, the clinician should bear in mind that certain investigations provide a measurement of structural parameters that can help predict the evolution of the disease, indicate specific treatments, and provide a baseline value for subsequent evaluations of the structural damage of OA.

This is an important aspect that must guide the choice of the investigation to be performed.

○ Radiographic investigations are the most common investigation performed. When prescribing such investigation, the clinician should keep in mind the recommendations concerning the view and film to be performed. For example, how many angles are needed and should the joint be weight-bearing or not?
○ Other investigations are rarely prescribed to confirm a diagnosis of OA (positive approach). But investigations performed to rule out other diagnoses (negative approach) can also help visualize some or all of the structural abnormalities of OA. Such investigations include the following:
    ■ Arthroscopy, which can show cartilage and synovial membrane abnormalities and also detect osteophytes [8]

- Magnetic resonance imaging (MRI), which can show cartilage breakdown and bone abnormalities[9]; more importantly, MRI can detect signs of inflammation of the bone or the synovial membrane[10]
- Computed tomography (CT) scan and arthro-CT scan, which both can show bone abnormalities; arthro-CT scan is the gold standard to detect and describe cartilage abnormalities[11]
- Ultrasonography, which can easily detect effusion and synovitis but is considered less accurate for detecting and quantifying cartilage abnormalities[12]

In daily practice, such investigations are not useful for a patient in whom the diagnosis of OA is obvious.[13] Conversely, patients who present with articular pain should have their previous investigations carefully scanned. In particular, the reports of these investigations (e.g., arthroscopy, MRI) should ideally include a section related to the presence or lack of cartilage breakdown, specifying its exact localization (e.g., femoral condyle versus tibial plateau) and trying to quantify the cartilage breakdown.

Who Is Suffering (or Will Suffer) from Osteoarthritis?

PREVALENCE

Figures regarding the prevalence of OA vary widely according to localization and diagnosis methodology. Data concerning both radiologic and symptomatic diagnosis of OA are available for knee, hip, and hand OA (Fig. 92–3).

PREDISPOSING FACTORS

Clinicians can differentiate between the predisposing factors of occurrence of OA that are useful at a population level and those that are more useful at an individual level. Clinicians should also distinguish "nonmodifiable" factors, which are valuable from a pathophysiologic point of view and at a group level, and "modifiable" factors, which are more valuable from a therapeutic point of view and at an individual level. Table 92–2 summarizes the main predisposing factors that have been recognized

in epidemiologic studies. Data are mostly available for hip and knee localizations and for risk factors of occurrence as opposed to risk factors of progression.

A question remains as to whether the treatment of a predisposing factor will have any effect on the progression of the disease. No randomized, controlled trial has yet addressed this question. To our knowledge, there is only one epidemiologic study concerning obesity in knee OA that suggests that a reduction of weight in obese patients will result in a decrease in the risk of occurrence of OA.[38] What remains to be proven is whether a reduction of weight in obese OA patients will result in a decrease in the rate of radiologic joint-space narrowing.

This lack of accurate information has important implications in daily practice:

- Is it advisable to treat a malalignment in a non-OA patient or in an OA patient at an early stage of the disease?
- Should hormone replacement therapy be recommended in postmenopausal women because of a risk of OA?
- Should serum vitamin D be assessed for every patient over 50 years of age?
- Who can benefit from vitamin D supplementation? The whole population? People with low serum vitamin D levels? Patients in an early stage of OA?

Three "nonmodifiable" factors are also important to consider: age, gender, and genetic makeup.

- *Age.* This is undoubtedly the strongest predictor for both occurrence and progression of OA. Of particular interest in daily practice is the recognition at an early stage of the very rapidly destructive OA that usually occurs in the very elderly.
- *Gender.* Generalized OA is more common in women, and the rate of progression of OA in women seems to be more rapid. The underlying mechanisms (sex hormones? genetics?) are unknown.
- *Genetic factors.* The role of genetic factors in the development of OA has been known for more than 50 years and has received considerable attention during the last decade, sustained by the rapidly expanding knowledge of molecular biology.[39] Based on the concordance rates for OA between monozygotic and dizygotic twin pairs, the heritable component was between 39 and 65 percent, depending on which joint was considered. Gene-association studies in genetically complex polygenic conditions such as OA entail many difficulties, including case definition, late age of phenotype expression, and adjustment for other constitutional and environmental risk factors. Nevertheless, associations and suggested linkages have been demonstrated. Ongoing studies are likely to give important insights into the pathogenesis of OA.

How Do We Describe an Osteoarthritis Patient?

Standardizing the description of an OA patient can greatly enhance communication between physicians.

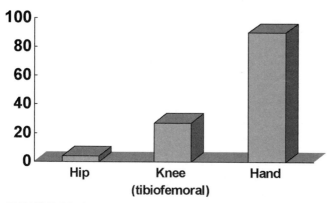

FIGURE 92–3 · Radiographic prevalence of osteoarthritis (OA) in elderly patients (65 years old or older).

TABLE 92–2 • RISK FACTORS OF INCIDENT AND PROGRESSION OF OSTEOARTHRITIS (OA) IN KNEES, HIPS, AND HANDS

Disease Progression	Localization		
	Knee	*Hip*	*Hand*
Occurrence of OA	Age[14]	Age[14]	Age[14]
	Female[14]	Physical activity[32,33]	Grip strength[27]
	Physical activity[15-17]	BMI[32,34]	BMI[36]
	BMI[16,19]	Previous injury	Occupation[37]
	Bone density[20]	Intensive sport activities[28]	Intensive sport activities[37]
	Previous injury[16-21]		
	HRT[19,22,23]		
	Vitamin D[24]		
	Smocking (protective)[25]		
	Alignment[26]		
	Quadriceps strength (protective)[27]		
	Intense sport activities[28]		
Progression of OA	Age[29]	Age	?
	Vitamin D[24]	Symptomatic activity[35]	
	HRT[30]	Gender[35]	
	Alignment[26]	Intensive sport activities[28]	
	Hydarthrodial OA[29]		
	Intensive sport activities[28]		
	Subchondral bone edema (MRI findings)[31]		

Abbreviations: BMI, Body Mass Index; HRT, Hormone Replacement Therapy; MRI, magnetic resonance imaging.

At least five characteristics are of interest: 1) localization, 2) etiology, 3) radiologic aspect, 4) existence of an inflammatory episode, and 5) level of symptomatic and structural severity.

LOCALIZATION

Specific Joint Localization

Localization of OA to a specific joint is rarely mentioned, even in specialized literature. It is nonetheless of high importance both in clinical research and daily practice. For example, in knee OA, the risk of handicap is much greater in case of medial femorotibial OA than in lateral tibiofemoral or patellofemoral involvement. In the hip, OA with a superolateral migration of the femoral head is at higher risk of structural progression and of need for surgery than that with a mediolateral migration. In the hand, involvement of the proximal interphalangeal (PIP) or the metacarpophalangeal (MCP) joint more frequently results in disability than involvement of the distal interphalangeal (DIP) joint.

Generalized Osteoarthritis

Whatever the localization, the handicap will be greater if OA involves other joints. In knee OA, generalized OA has been suggested as a predisposing factor for structural progression of the disease. There is, unfortunately, to date no simple tool to classify a patient as suffering from generalized OA. There are no strictly validated criteria for generalized OA. Polyarticular OA (including the presence of Heberden's nodules) as a marker of gener-

alized OA has been studied in different populations.[40] This localization (hand OA) indicating generalized OA has been confirmed in a prospective, trans-sectional epidemiologic study of more than 1000 patients who consulted their rheumatologist for hand, back, hip, or knee OA.[41] The results of the multivariate analysis of this study are summarized in Figure 92–4. This study also emphasized the importance of spinal OA and of toe involvement. Hallux valgus was present in 17 percent of the 516 patients with localized OA and in 41 percent of the 416 patients with generalized OA; hammer toes were present in 9 percent of the 516 patients with localized OA and in 24 percent of the patients with generalized OA.

ETIOLOGY AND PREDISPOSING FACTORS

Secondary Osteoarthritis

It is not easy to distinguish between etiologic and predisposing factors. A concomitant disease in the target joint is generally considered an etiologic factor, and the OA is thereafter tagged "secondary" OA. The list of concomitant diseases proposed by a group of European experts who created recommendations for conducting clinical trials in OA[42] Respect of Ethics and Excellence in Scince, (GREES), is summarized in Table 92–3. In daily practice, consider these practical points: A history of septic arthritis raises the question of whether or not to treat the patient with intra-articular injections (with either corticosteroids or hyaluronic acid). In which patients must treatable metabolic diseases, such as gout, acromegaly, haemochromatosis, or Wilson's disease, be investigated? Using a pragmatic approach, the following advice can be given:

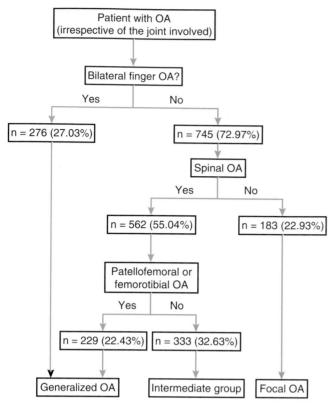

FIGURE 92–4 · Criteria to classify a patient suffering from generalized osteoarthritis (OA). (From Dougados M, Nakache JP, Gueguen A: Criteria for generalized and focal osteoarthritis. Rev Rhum 63:569-575, 1996.)

- Paget's disease, which requires a specific treatment, should systematically be searched for by a radiologic evaluation of the pelvis and knees.
- There is sufficient evidence to propose a blood evaluation of iron and copper in case of polyarticular involvement including MCP and PIP in young OA patients (<50 years old).
- Questions remain as to the necessity of recognizing a potential primary osteochondromatosis at an early stage of OA, which would require specific investigations such as arthrography or arthro-CT scan. The answer seems to be yes in case of knee OA and probably no in case of hip OA and depends mostly on the specific treatment of the underlying disease (in this case, synovectomy followed by intra-articular injection of radioisotopes).[43] This treatment is obviously of interest in case of knee OA seen at an early stage. In case of hip OA, arthrotomy might interfere with the prognosis of potential subsequent hip arthroplasty.

Primary Osteoarthritis

If the concomitant diseases listed in Table 92–3 are absent, the disease is usually called "primary OA." Predisposing factors may coexist, such as obesity in knee OA or dysplasia in hip OA. Identifying predisposing factors in progression of OA is important and further treatment may be required to address them. The decision to add treatment is easy in the case of nonaggressive treatments such as weight reduction, but it is more difficult in

TABLE 92–3 · ARTICULAR DISEASES THAT ARE ETIOLOGIC FACTORS FOR OSTEOARTHRITIS (OA)

Septic arthritis
Inflammatory joint disease
Gout
Recurrent episodes of pseudogout
Paget's disease
Ochronosis
Acromegaly
Hemochromatosis
Wilson's disease
Primary osteochondromatosis

Adapted from Dougados M, Nakache JP, Gueguen A: Criteria for generalized and focal osteoarthritis. Rev Rhum 63:569-575, 1996.

cases of aggressive therapy such as osteotomy to treat malalignment.

RADIOGRAPHIC APPEARANCE

At least for the hip, OA can be separated into two main types: the hypertrophic type characterized by extensive osteophytosis and subchondral bone sclerosis, and the atrophic type in which bone response is absent.[44]

The hypertrophic type is commonly observed in patients with diffuse idiopathic skeletal hyperostosis.[45] A rapidly progressive form of hip OA has been described in elderly patients with a reduction of at least 50 percent of the radiologic joint-space width within 2 years.[46-48] In these patients, bone sclerosis and osteophytes are rare. Question remains as to whether this particular feature should be considered a distinct disease (a rapidly destructive arthropathy) or an extremely severe aspect of OA.

INFLAMMATORY FLARES

Despite the fact that OA is considered as primarily due to a degenerative process or biomechanic disorders, an increasing amount of data strongly support the idea that articular inflammation may interfere with the natural history of the disease, especially with cartilage breakdown. Inflammation can occur within the cartilage itself, but it is more easily and frequently seen in the synovial membrane or the subchondral bone.

For clinicians, post-traumatic chondromalacia (swelling of the cartilage after trauma) can be considered an inflammatory process. Chondromalacia occurring without trauma is sometimes considered to be the first stage of OA.[49] Moreover, chondrocytes (via their cytokines and enzymes) have the ability to create inflammation (chondritis). Inflammation of the synovial membrane is responsible for a thickening of the synovial membrane and for hydarthrodial effusion.

In the subchondral bone, MRI signal abnormalities or "hot" bone at scintigraphy may be suggestive of an inflammatory process. In longitudinal epidemiologic studies, the presence of inflammation (defined either by bone scintigraphy,[31,50] MRI signal abnormalities, presence of hydarthrodial effusion, or macroscopical synovitis) has been correlated with a subsequent rapid structural progression of the disease. These abnormalities (hot bone scintigraphy and MRI abnormalities) can also be explained by a process other than inflammation, such as a microfracture.[51]

In OA, synovitis has a patchy distribution that contrasts with the diffuse distribution seen in the synovitis of inflammatory rheumatic disorders such as rheumatoid arthritis (RA). Within the joint cavity, synovitis seems to be closely related to chondropathy in OA, as is illustrated in Figure 92–5.

It is important to identify inflammatory flares and treat them, because data from epidemiologic studies clearly show a correlation between inflammation and subsequent chondrolysis.[52] Treating inflammatory bouts may slow down subsequent cartilage breakdown.

Several clinical symptoms are usually considered suggestive of inflammation:

- Sudden increase in pain
- Night pain
- Morning stiffness of at least 30 minutes' duration

In the hip, physical examination often detects no sign of inflammation. In the knee, effusion has been found to correlate with synovitis.[53] In finger joints, the typical signs of inflammation are usually present: rubor (redness), calor (heat), dolor (pain), and tumor (swelling). Questions remain as to whether specific investigations are necessary in daily practice to assess inflammatory flares in the hip or knee. MRI and bone scintigraphy are costly and are difficult to access in certain countries. Ultrasonography might be an accurate and inexpensive alternative.

▌ Is the Disease Severe?

WHY EVALUATE THE SEVERITY OF THE DISEASE?

The severity of the disease can be considered either at the symptomatic or structural level.

The level of symptomatic severity is related both to the structural damage and the inflammatory process. It is, thus, important to take into account symptoms evaluating symptomatic severity (pain after physical activities, functional impairment), symptoms evaluating the inflammatory process (night pain, duration of morning stiffness, effusion) and structural severity (mainly by performing plain radiographs).

Another reason to separately evaluate symptoms and structure is the weak correlation that exists between them. This is important in practice because some indications of therapy, such as surgery, are based on both types of information.

Evaluation of Symptomatic Severity

Domains To Be Evaluated

Two main domains are important to consider in this evaluation, both in daily practice and in clinical research.[54]

Pain occurring after physical activities is usually evaluated in clinical trials either with a single, general question (e.g., What is the level of pain you have after physical activities in your daily life?) or by specific questions, such as four of the five (1, 2, 4, and 5) included in the Western Ontario and McMaster Universities (WOMAC) questionnaire pain subscale[55] (Table 92–4).

Functional impairment is usually evaluated in clinical trials using the WOMAC function subscale, which is a questionnaire including 17 items related to daily activities. Another possibility is to use Lequesne's algo-functional index (Table 92–5), which is a composite index including questions related to inflammation (night pain, morning stiffness), pain (while walking, sitting down), performance (walking distance), and functional impairment (four questions).[56]

TABLE 92–4 · WOMAC

1. **Pain subscale (5 questions)**
   How much pain do you have...
   Walking on a flat surface?
   Going up or down stairs?
   At night while in bed?
   Sitting or lying?
   Standing upright?
2. **Stiffness subscale (2 questions)**
   How severe is your stiffness after first waking in the morning?
   How severe is your stiffness after sitting, lying, or resting later in the day?
3. **Function subscale (17 questions)**
   What degree of difficulty do you have with...
   Descending stairs?
   Ascending stairs?
   Rising from sitting?
   Standing?
   Bending to floor?
   Walking on flat surface?
   Getting in and out of car?
   Going shopping?
   Putting on socks or stockings?
   Rising from bed?
   Taking off socks/stockings?
   Lying in bed?
   Getting in and out of bath?
   Sitting?
   Getting on and off of toilet?
   Heavy domestic duties?
   Light domestic duties?

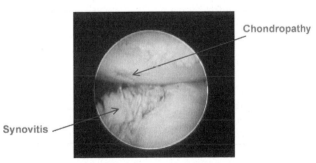

FIGURE 92–5 · Close Relationship Between Synovitis and Chondropathy in Osteoarthritis (OA).

TABLE 92–5 • LEQUESNE

Pain or Discomfort	Points
During nocturnal bedrest	
None or insignificant	0
Only on movement or in certain positions	1
With no movement	2
Morning stiffness or regressive pain after rising	
1 minute or less	0
More than 1 but less than 15 minutes	1
After standing for 30 minutes	0 or 1
While ambulating	
None	0
Only after ambulating some distance	1
After initial ambulation and increasingly with	
continued ambulation	2
With prolonged sitting (2 hours)	0 or 1
Maximum distance walked (may walk with pain)	
Unlimited	0
More than 1 km, but limited	1
About 1 km (0.6 mi) in about 15 min	2
From 500 to 600 m (1640 to 2952 ft or 0.31	
to 0.56 mi) in about 8 to 15 min	3
From 300 to 500 m (987 to 1640 ft)	4
From 100 to 300 m (328 to 984 ft)	5
Less than 100 m (328 ft)	6
With one walking stick or crutch	1
With two walking sticks or crutches	2
Activities of daily living*	
Put on socks by bending forward	0 or 2
Pick up an object from the floor	0 or 2
Climb up and down a standard flight of stairs	0 or 2
Can get into and out of a car	0 or 2

*Code: without difficulty, 0; with difficulty, 1 (or 0.5 or 1.5); unable, 2.

Other domains can also be considered to evaluate symptomatic severity (e.g., patient's overall assessment, range of motion, and performance).

Implementation in Clinical Research Studies

Outcome Measures for Rheumatic Arthritis Clinical Trials (OMERACT) is a scientific society that proposes outcome measures for rheumatic disorders trials. Meetings have taken place every 2 years since 1992. At the OMERACT III meeting (1996, Cairns, Australia), a session focused on the domains identified as core variables to be included in clinical trials involving OA: pain, function, and patient's global assessment.[26] One of the first problems was how to identify patients suffering from severe OA, thereby specifying inclusion criteria for studies. There is no strong consensus in this field. A pain level greater than 30 in a 0 to 100 scale (in which 0 is absence of pain and 100 is maximum level of pain) is generally accepted as the threshold to initiate a study drug.

Application in Daily Practice

Simply by interviewing the patient, the physician evaluates symptomatic severity at each visit. It is not clear whether the use of tools, such as visual analog scale (VAS) for pain, Lequesne's index, or WOMAC for function, are of interest. However, these tools clearly con-

tribute to better communication between physicians and between the patient and his physician.

A recent cluster randomization trial suggested that although the use of these tools improves the satisfaction of the patient regarding health care, it does not improve symptomatic severity.

If these tools prove useful, question remains as to how to implement them in daily practice. To evaluate pain, a VAS is generally considered relevant. To evaluate function, the question of the number of items to collect is important. It appears that the 17 questions of the WOMAC function subscale are more sensitive than Lequesne's index in clinical research studies.[57] In daily practice, a total of 10 questions is usually the maximum accepted by physicians. To this end, attempts are being made to reduce the number of items in the WOMAC function subscale.

Evaluation of Structural Severity

Definition of Structure

Defining structure is more complicated than it appears. It is agreed that cartilage breakdown is the most important structural severity index, but the tools to evaluate cartilage breakdown are still a matter of debate. Other structural conditions can also be considered, including synovitis (arthroscopy, MRI, ultrasound), osteophytes (plain radiographs, MRI, arthroscopy), subchondral bone cysts (plain radiographs, MRI), subchondral bone sclerosis (plain radiographs, MRI), subchondral bone edema (MRI, bone scintigraphy), and laboratory markers. Some of the tools that can be used to evaluate cartilage breakdown are plain radiographs to measure joint-space width at the narrowest point, digitized radiographs to measure joint-space surface, arthroscopy to evaluate the cartilage surface, MRI to evaluate the cartilage surface, cartilage volume, and contents of the cartilage (water, glucosamine glycans, etc.).

Application in Clinical Research Studies

Structural severity is usually evaluated with the Kellgren and Lawrence classification score, a composite index of the presence and severity of joint-space narrowing and the degree of joint-space narrowing (commonly the radiologic interbone distance at the narrowest point).[58]

Application in Daily Practice

Most physicians use a "personal," semiquantitative, typically three-scale variable: minimal, moderate, and severe. This is probably sufficient for single-visit therapeutic decisions, but it is inaccurate for long-term monitoring of structural damage.

How Will the Disease Progress?

The natural history of OA can vary widely for various joint sites and patients. However, a three-grade classification system has been proposed and is summarized in Figure 92–6. In most cases, the condition takes years to develop.

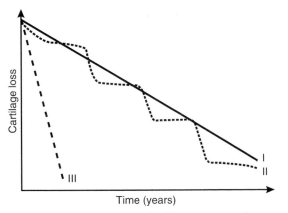

FIGURE 92–6 · Three-grade classification system for progression of osteoarthritis (OA).

Symptoms are sometimes continuous (type I). Most of the time, the evolution is punctuated by inflammatory "flares" that can last days or months, in which pain and functional disability are particularly severe and signs of inflammation might be observed (type II). These "flares" are thought to be responsible for chondrolysis. Rapid-progression OA (defined by a 50% joint-space narrowing within 24 months) occurs in a minority of patients (type III).

How Is Disease Progression Monitored?

Monitoring is well specified for clinical trials, but no consensus is available for the management of patients in daily practice.

CLINICAL RESEARCH STUDIES

Symptomatic Outcome Variables

OMERACT III and other scientific societies such as the GREES and the OsteoArthritis Research Society International (OARSI)[59] have provided recommendations for determining symptomatic outcome. These recommendations involve 1) the domains to be evaluated; 2) the tool used to evaluate each domain; 3) for each tool, a cutoff above which a treatment has to be considered and that defines active disease; 4) for each tool, a cutoff below which the disease is considered acceptable by the patient and that defines inactive disease; 5) for each tool, the definition of a clinically relevant change (improvement or deterioration).

It is not clear whether the two cutoffs mentioned (items 3 and 4) are superimposable. Preliminary studies evaluating pain using a 0 to 100 mm VAS suggest that the cut-off defining active disease is higher (approximately 40 to 50) than that defining acceptable disease (approximately 30). For the definition of a clinically relevant change (item 5), a change of at least 30 percent was chosen for comparing different treatment modalities when establishing the European League Against Rheumatism (EULAR) recommendations for the treatment of knee OA.[60] For most variables, this type of detailed information is still missing.

The OMERACT and OARSI societies recommend considering at least the three following domains: pain, function, and patient's global assessment.

Whereas defining a core set of domains to be measured represents an advance in defining and standardizing the conduct of OA clinical trials, the analysis and reporting of results continues to be based on average improvement for the study population on each of the outcome measures. Another possibility is to present the results in terms of percentage of patients with a clinically relevant change in each of the outcome measures or, at the end of therapy, the percentage of patients with a value in each outcome measure below the cutoff defining an active disease. A multivariate response set of criteria including information from the three main domains has recently been proposed by the OMERACT-OARSI society and is summarized in Figure 92–7. With this set of criteria, trial results can be presented as a dichotomous variable (responder states yes or no).

Structural Outcome Variables

Plain Radiographs

The measure of radiologic interbone distance at the narrowest point is considered the gold standard in this field. However, as in the case of symptomatic variables, the clinical relevance of this measure is unknown. The first step in the evaluation of the clinical relevance of a change in a structural variable is to transform a continuous variable (e.g., change in joint-space width in millimeters) into a dichotomous variable (e.g., presence or absence of radiologic progression). Some preliminary data in this field suggest that a change in the radiologic joint-space width of at least 0.5 mm could be clinically relevant. The clinical relevance of a treatment effect remains poorly evaluated. For example, a 56 percent progression rate in a placebo group compared to 47 percent in an active treatment group (9% treatment effect) is difficult to interpret in terms of clinical relevance.[61]

Other Tools

Many tools, including laboratory markers, ultrasonography, MRI, and arthroscopy are potentially interesting but require further investigation.

DAILY PRACTICE

Several domains should be considered in daily practice, not only to evaluate the effect of a treatment, but also to indicate particular treatments.

Monitoring should include:

- The amount of symptomatic treatment taken by the patient
- The presence of inflammation
- The degree of symptomatic severity
- The degree of structural severity
- The presence of muscle atrophy or vicious attitude at physical examination

We have previously discussed inflammation and symptomatic severity.

OMERACT-OARSI SET OF RESPONDER CRITERIA

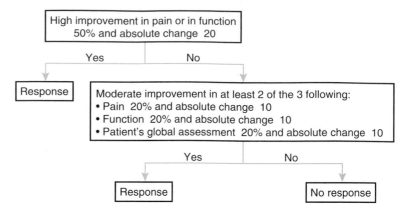

FIGURE 92-7 • OMERACT-OARSI criteria.

The amount of symptomatic treatment (analgesics, NSAIDs, and local therapy) required by the patient's condition can be collected with simple tools such as the number of days per week drug intake is required.[62]

The degree of structural severity has also been discussed. This information is obviously of interest to indicate a treatment such as articular replacement, but its interest in daily practice to monitor a treatment is still a matter of debate. The new chondromodulating drugs will probably modify this situation because continuing these drugs might be tied to the absence of radiographic progression after a period of treatment intake (24 to 48 weeks).

All these variables are similar to those used in clinical research studies. Other variables are important to consider in daily practice to indicate specific treatment modalities:

- Periarticular muscle atrophy indicates a need to reinforce physiotherapy.
- Flexion contracture or malalignment may require specific treatments such as joint lavage, physiotherapy in a rehabilitation center, osteotomy, and insoles.
- Patient's desire and presence of concomitant diseases are important to evaluate when surgery is required because of symptomatic and structural severity.

Questions Related to Specific Localization

OA can affect any joint, but it primarily affects four localizations: the hip, the knee, the hand, and the spine.

HIP OSTEOARTHRITIS

Radiologic Investigation

In daily practice, an anteroposterior view of the pelvis with the patient in a standing position and an internal rotation of the feet (15 to 20 degrees) is the most accurate. However, clinicians should keep in mind that involvement in the posterior pole cannot be captured by this view and necessitates an oblique view. For clinical research studies,

there is still a debate as to whether the pelvic film is as useful as a film focused on the target hip.[63]

Localization

Several distribution patterns of hip OA have been described (Fig. 92–8). Involvement of the superior pole is common (50%) and often results in superolateral migration of the femoral head.

Involvement of the medial pole (20%) is more frequently seen in women and is usually well tolerated as it has a slower progression rate.

Etiology and Risk Factors

Dysplasia, avascular osteonecrosis, and trauma are the most frequent causes.[64] Overuse, particularly intensive sports activities, is also a predisposing factor.

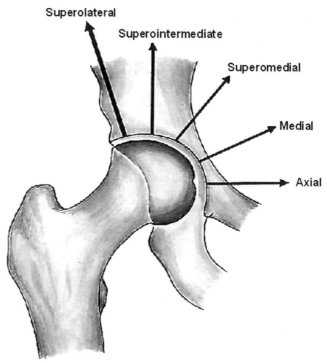

FIGURE 92–8 • Patterns of Osteoarthritis (OA) of the Hip.

Radiologic Appearance

The "hypertrophic" aspect of OA is often seen in males suffering from concomitant Forestier's disease or who have a long history of sports participation. The "atrophic" aspect is commonly observed in rapidly progressive OA.

Inflammation

Inflammation of the hip is difficult to describe from a clinical point of view because effusion and other cardinal signs of inflammation cannot be directly observed at physical examination. In case of sudden increase in pain or morning stiffness, the clinician should consider further investigations such as ultrasonography, bone scintigraphy, or MRI.

Severity

Of particular concern in a case of hip OA are possible quadriceps atrophy and fixed external rotation and loss of extension. These conditions may require intensive physiotherapy.

KNEE OSTEOARTHRITIS

Radiologic Investigation

In daily practice, the most important requirement is a comparative analysis of the two knees. There is a consensus concerning the requirement of the patient in a standing position when evaluating the tibiofemoral compartment. The patellofemoral compartment is accurately evaluated by performing a sky view. Because the OA process usually begins at the posterior part of the tibiofemoral compartment and because the standard standing anteroposterior radiograph of the extended knee does not capture this part of the joint (Fig. 92–9), a view performed while the knees are flexed has been recommended. The different techniques used to perform such flexed view are summarized in Figure 92–10. It is our experience that the "schuss" view (see Fig. 92–10E) is the most accurate.[65]

Localization

The medial tibiofemoral joint has been extensively studied. This localization is usually the one selected for clinical trials because this pattern is more homogeneous than the two others (i.e., lateral tibiofemoral and patellofemoral). Moreover, the level of disability due to advanced disease in this area is more important than that observed when the disease is affecting the other compartments.

The radiologic evaluation of the lateral tibiofemoral area is less reliable than that of the medial tibiofemoral area. This localization occurs preferentially in women.

The patellofemoral localization is probably the most frequent and is usually well tolerated; however, it can be responsible for disability resulting in the requirement of total knee replacement.

Etiology and Risk Factors

Obesity, malalignment, and trauma are the most frequent etiologies.

Radiologic Appearance

The "hypertrophic" appearance (obvious osteophytes) contrasting with a normal joint-space width on an anteroposterior film view can result from Forestier's disease, but it also can be the expression of concomitant advanced patellofemoral OA.

Inflammation

Inflammation at the knee level is easily recognized when an effusion is observed.

Severity

At an advanced stage of the disease, an increase in malalignment, flexion contracture, and quadriceps muscle atrophy can be observed.

HAND OSTEOARTHRITIS

Radiologic Investigation

A posteroanterior view of the two hands including the wrists is the conventional film. This view permits the evaluation of the DIP, PIP, MCP, and trapezometacarpal joints.[66,67]

Localization

Thumb OA is sometimes considered a specific pattern of hand OA. Such localization is frequent and is responsible for pain and functional disability, especially in case of fixed adduction. DIP involvement is the most frequent, but it is rarely responsible for functional impairment.[68,69]

PIP and MCP involvement are less frequent but can result from a specific etiology and can be responsible for substantial disability.

Etiology and Risk Factors

The genetic factors are probably the most important to consider (familial aggregation). In case of PIP involvement, MCP involvement, or both, a metabolic disorder should be considered.

Radiologic Appearance

An "erosive" aspect has been proposed as a distinct entity, in contrast to the "hypertrophic" aspect usually observed. In fact, the longitudinal studies have clearly shown that an erosive aspect is not a specific pattern of

Standing position
(standing-extended view)

Flexion
(Schuss view)

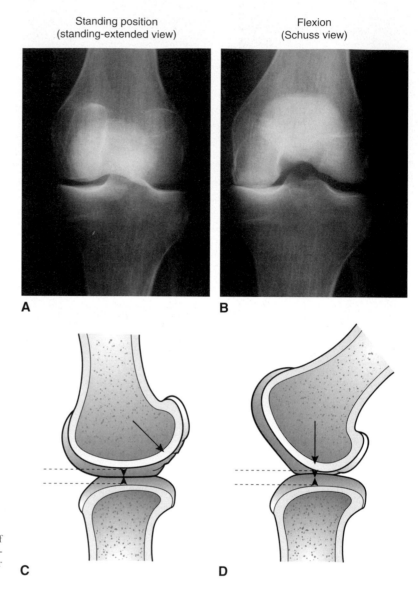

A

B

C

D

FIGURE 92–9 • Fixed and anterioposterior views of the knee with patient in a standing position do not capture the osteoarthritis (OA) process at the posterior level.

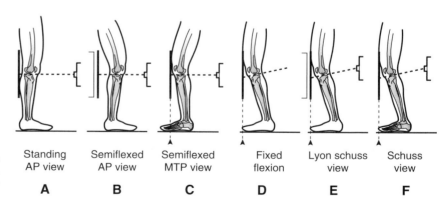

FIGURE 92–10 • Radiographic techniques to evaluate the tibiofemoral compartment and adequately capture the posterior part of the compartment.

Standing AP view	Semiflexed AP view	Semiflexed MTP view	Fixed flexion	Lyon schuss view	Schuss view
A	B	C	D	E	F

hand OA but a transient phenomenon in the long-term natural history of the disease.[70-72]

Inflammation

Inflammation at the hand level is easily recognized because the cardinal signs (rubor, calor, tumor, dolor) can be observed.

Severity

At an advanced stage of the disease, the patient may complain of esthetic impairment due to the deformities (especially in case of DIP involvement) or esthetic and functional impairment (especially in case of concomitant PIP and MCP involvement).

SHOULDER OSTEOARTHRITIS[73]

Radiologic Investigation

Both an anteroposterior (AP) and oblique view of both shoulders are required to accurately evaluate the disease.

Localization, Etiology, Risk Factors, and Radiologic Appearance

OA of the glenohumeral joint occurs less commonly than that of the weight-bearing joints. Apart from OA occurring in the natural course of muscular osteonecrosis of the humeral head, two main categories of the disease are commonly described (Fig. 92–11):

- Central or eccentric OA, sometimes called "primary OA"
- Noneccentric OA, usually considered a complication of degenerative lesions of the rotator cuff; such lesions

result in an ascension of the humoral head and subsequently lead to a "secondary" OA of the shoulder

These classifications are of high clinical relevance because the long-term outcome of shoulder prosthesis is better in cases of eccentric disease.[74]

Inflammation

Inflammation at the shoulder level is difficult to recognize and usually requires specific investigations.

Severity

At an advanced stage of the disease, the functional disability and level of pain can be so advanced that a total articular replacement can be considered.

SPINAL OSTEOARTHRITIS

The different clinical features of back disorders are described in detail in Chapter 39. However, we would like to emphasize here the similarities existing between spinal arthrosis and arthrosis occurring in a peripheral joint.[75]

Diarthrodial joints (in which cartilage and synovial tissue are clearly identified) are present at the spinal level in the apophyseal joints. There is growing evidence that the degenerative process occurring at the intervertebral disk level is very similar to that occurring in the diarthrodial joints. Therefore, the different aspects discussed in this chapter, and especially the presence of flare due to an inflammatory process, have to be investigated because rapidly destructive diskopathies have been observed concurrently with features (MRI abnormalities) suggestive of subchondral bone inflammation.

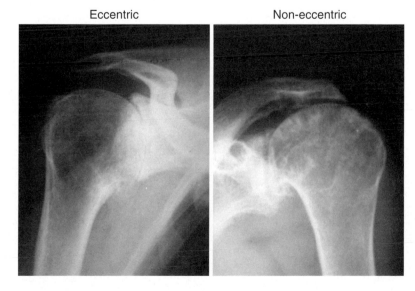

Eccentric   Non-eccentric

FIGURE 92–11 • Eccentric (primary) and noneccentric (secondary) shoulder osteoarthritis (OA).

REFERENCES

1. Spector TD, Cooper C: Radiological assessment of osteoarthritis in population studies: whither Kellgren & Lawrence? Osteoart Cartilage 1:203-206, 1994.
2. Altman R, Asch E, Bloch D, et al: Development of criteria for the classification of osteoarthritis of the knee. Arthritis Rheum 29:1039-1049, 1986.
3. Lequesne M: La coxarthrose: critères de diagnostic; étiologie sur 200 cas; rôle de la dysplasie congénitale. In Peyron JG (ed): Epidémiologie de l'arthrose, Paris, CIBA-GEIGY, 1980, pp 198-210.
4. Altman R, Alarcon G, Appelrouth D, et al: The American College of Rheumatology criteria for the classification and reporting of osteoarthritis of the hip. Arthritis Rheum 34:505-514, 1991.
5. Peat G, Croft P, Hay E: Clinical assessment of the osteoarthritis patient: Best practice and Research. Clin Rheumatol 15:527-544, 2001.
6. Altman RD, Dean D (eds): Pain in osteoarthritis. Semin Arthritis Rheum 18(Suppl 2)1-104, 1989.
7. Dougados M: Synovial fluid cell analysis. Baillière's Clin Rheumatol 10:519-534, 1996.
8. Ike RW: Diagnostic arthroscopy. Baillière's Clin Rheumatol 10:495-519, 1996.
9. Peterfy CG: Scratching the surface: articular cartilage disorders in the knee. Magn Reson Imaging Clin N Am 2:409-430, 2000.
10. Peterfy CG: Magnetic resonance imaging in rheumatoid arthritis: current status and future directions. J Rheumatol 5:1134-1142, 2001.
11. Drape JL, Chevrot A, Godefroy D, et al: CT scans and arthro-CT scans. Baillière's Clin Rheumatol 10:615-634, 1996.
12. Grassi W, Lamanna G, Farina A, Cervini C: Sonographic imaging of normal and osteoarthritic cartilage. Sem Arthritis Rheum 6:398-403, 1999.
13. RCR Working Party: Making the Best Use of a Department of Clinical Radiology. Guidelines for Doctors, 4th ed. London, The Royal College of Radiologists, 1998.
14. van Saase JL, van Romunde LK, Cats A, et al: Epidemiology of osteoarthritis: Zoetermeer survey. Comparison of radiological osteoarthritis in a Dutch population with that in 10 other populations. Ann Rheum Dis 48:271-280, 1989.
15. McAlindon TE, Wilson PW, Aliabadi P, et al: Level of physical activity and the risk of radiographic and symptomatic knee osteoarthritis in the elderly: The Framingham study. Am J Med 106:151-157, 1999.
16. Cooper, Snow S, McAlindon TE, et al: Risk factors for the incidence and progression of radiographical knee osteoarthritis. Arthritis Rheum 43:995-1000, 2000.
17. Felson D, McAlindon CT, Anderson JJ, et al: Defining radiographical osteoarthritis for the whole knee. Osteoart Cartilage 5:241-220, 1997.
18. Zhang Y, Hannan MT, Chaisson CE, et al: Bone mineral density and risk of incident and progressive radiographical knee osteoarthritis in women: The Framingham study. J Rheumatol 27:1032-1037, 2000.
19. Hart DJ, Doyle DV, Spector TD: Incidence and risk factors for radiographic knee osteoarthritis in middle-aged women: the Chingford study. Arthritis Rheum 42:17-24, 1999.
20. Felson DR, Lawrence RC, Dieppe PA, et al: Level of physical activity and the risk of radiographic and symptomatic knee osteoarthritis in the elderly: The Framingham study. Am J Med 106:151-157, 1999.
21. Rohrbough JT, Mudge MK, Schilling RC, Jansen C: Radiographic oseoarthritis in the hands of rock climbers. Am J Orthop 27:734-738, 1998.
22. Nevitt MC, Cummings SR, Lane NE, et al: Association of estrogen replacement therapy with the risk of osteoarthritis of the hip in elderly white women: Study of Osteoporotic Fractures Research Group. Arch Int Med 156:2073-2080, 1996.
23. Zhang Y, McAlindon TE, Hannan MT, et al: Estrogen replacement therapy and worsening of radiographic knee osteoarthritis: The Framingham study. Arthritis Rheum 41:1867-1873, 1998.
24. McAlindon TE, Felson DT, Zhang Y, et al: Relation of dietary intake and serum levels of vitamin D to progression of osteoarthritis of the knee among participants in The Framingham study. Ann Int Med 125:353-359, 1996.
25. Felson DR, Zhang Y, Hannan MT, et al: Risk factors for incident radiographic knee osteoarthritis in the elderly: The Framingham study. Arthritis Rheum 40:728-733, 1997.
26. Sharma L, Song J, Felson DT, et al: The role of knee alignment in disease progression and functional decline in knee osteoarthritis. JAMA 286:188-195, 2001.
27. Chaisson CE, Zhang Y, Sharma L, et al: Grip strength and the risk of developing radiographical hand osteoarthritis: results from The Framingham study. Arthritis Rheum 42:33-38, 1999.
28. Lequesne MG, Dang N, Lane NE: Sport practice and osteoarthritis of the limbs. Osteoart Cartilage 2:75-86, 1997.
29. Dougados M, Gueguen A, Nguyen M, et al: Longitudinal radiologic evaluation of osteoarthritis of the knee. J Rheumatol 19:378-384, 1992.
30. Nevitt MC, Felson DT: Sex hormones and the risk of osteoarthritis in women: epidemiological evidence. Ann Rheum Dis 55:673-676, 1996.
31. Felson DT, Chaisson CE, Hill CL, et al: The association of bone marrow lesions with pain in osteoarthritis. Ann Med Int 7:541-549, 2001.
32. FlugsrudGB, Nordsletten L, Espehaug B, et al: Risk factors for total hip replacement due to primary osteoarthritis: a cohort study in 50,034 persons. Arthritis Rheum 46:675-682, 2002.
33. Coggon D, Kellingray S, Inskip H, et al: Osteoarthritis of the hip and occupational lifting. Am J Epidemiol 147:523-528, 1998.
34. Croft P: The occurrence of osteoarthritis outside Europe. Ann Rheum Dis 55:661-664, 1996.
35. Dougados M, Gueguen A, Nguyen M, et al: Radiological progression of hip osteoarthritis: definition, risk factors and correlations with clinical status. Ann Rheum Dis 55:356-362, 1996.
36. Carman WJ, Sowers M, Hawthorne VM, Weissfeld LA: Obesity as a risk factor for osteoarthritis of the hand and wrist: a prospective study. Am J Epidemiol 139-29, 1994.
37. Lawrence J: Rheumatism in Populations. London, Heineman, 1977.
38. Felson DT, Zhang Y, Anthony JM, et al: Weight loss reduces the risk for symptomatic knee osteoarthritis in women: The Framingham Study. Ann Intern Med 116:535-539, 1992.
39. Spector TD, Cicuttini F, Baker J, et al: Genetic influences on osteoarthritis in women: a twin study. Br Med J 312:940-943, 1996.
40. Kellgren JH, Moore R: Generalized osteoarthritis and Heberden's nods. British Medical Journal:181-187, 1952.
41. Dougados M, Nakache JP, Gueguen A: Criteria for generalized and focal osteoarthritis. Rev Rhum 63:569-575, 1996.
42. Group for the Respect of Ethics and Excellence in Science (GREES): Osteoarthritis section: Recommendations for the registrations of drugs used in the treatment of osteoarthritis. Ann Rheum Dis 55:552-557, 1996.
43. Langguth DM, Kleston A, Denaro C: Synovial osteochondromatosis. Intern Med J 32:419-420, 2002.
44. Dougados M, Gueguen A, Nguyen M, et al: Radiographic features predictive of radiographic progression of hip osteoarthritis. Rev Rheum 64:795-803, 1997.
45. Arlet J, Jacqueline F, Depeyre M, et al: La hanche dans l'hyperostose vertébrale. Rev Rhum Mal Osteoart 45:17-26, 1978.
46. Lequesne M: Les coxopathies destructrices. Rev Rhum Mal Osteoart 37:711-719, 1970.
47. Edelman J, Own EJ: Acute progressive osteoarthropathy of large joints. J Rheumatol 8:482-485, 1981.
48. Rosenberg ZS, Shankman S, Steiner G, et al: Rapid destructive osteoarthritis: clinical, radiographic and pathologic features. Radiology 182:213-216, 1992.
49. Bentley G, Dowd G: Current concepts of etiology and treatment of chondromalacia patellae. Clin Orthop Rel Res 189:209-228, 1984.
50. Dieppe P, Cushnagan J, Young P, Kirwan J: Prediction of the progression of joint space narrowing of the knee by bone scintigraphy. Ann Rheum Dis 52:557-563, 1993.
51. Schneider R, Bullough P, Mintz D, Di Carlo E: Subchondral insufficiency and impaction fractures of the femoral head as a cause of rapidly destructive osteoarthritis of the hip. Arthritis Rheum 46(Suppl 9):1553, 2002.
52. Ayral X, Ravaud P, Bonvarlet JP, et al: Arthroscopic evaluation of post-traumatic patellofemoral chondropathy. J Rheumatol 26:1140-1147, 1999.

53. Ayral X, Pickering EH, Woodworth TG, et al: Synovitis predicts the arthroscopic progression of medial tibiofemoral knee osteoarthritis. Arthritis Rheum 44(Suppl 9):S101, 2001.

54. Bellamy N, Kirwan J, Altman R, et al: Recommendations for a core set of outcome measures for future phase III clinical trials in knee, hip and hand osteoarthritis: Results of consensus development at OMERACT III. J Rheumatol 24:799-804, 1997.

55. Bellamy N, Buchanan WW, Goldsmith CH, et al: Validation of WOMAC: a health status instrument for measuring clinically important patients relevant outcomes to antirheumatic drug therapy in patients with osteoarthritis of the hip or knee. J Rheumatol 15:1833-1840, 1995.

56. Lequesne M, Mery C, Samson M, Gerard P: Indexes of severity for osteoarthritis of the hip and knee. Scand J Rheuamtol 65:85-89, 1987.

57. Gentelle S, Le Claire P, Mezieres M et al: Comparison of the responsiveness of symptomatic outome measures in knee osteoarthritis. Arthritis Care Res 13:280-285, 2000.

58. Ravaud P, Dougados M: Radiographic assessment in osteoarthritis. J Rheumatol 4:786-791, 1997.

59. Altman R, Brandt K, Hochberg M, et al: Design and conduct of clinical trials of patients with osteoarthritis: Recommendations from a task force of the Osteoarthritis Research Society—results of a workshop. Osteoart Cartilage 4:217-243, 1996.

60. Pendleton A, Arden N, Dougados M, et al: EULAR recommendations for the management of knee osteoarthritis: report of a task force of the Standing Committee for International Studies including therapeutic trials. Ann Rheum Dis 59:936-944, 2000.

61. Dougados M, Nguyen M, Berdah L, et al: Evaluation of the structure-modifying effects of diacerein in hip osteoarthritis: ECHODIAH, a three year placebo controlled trial. Arthritis Rheum 11:2539-2547, 2001.

62. Constant F, Guillemin F, Herbeth B, et al: Measurement methods of drug consumption as a secondary judgment criterion for clinical trials in chronic rheumatic diseases. Am J Epidemiol 145:826-833, 1997.

63. Auleley GR, Duche A, Drape JL, et al: Measurement of joint space width in hip osteoarthritis: influence of joint positioning and radiographic procedure. Rheumatology 40:414-419, 2001.

64. Harris W: Etiology of osteoarthritis of the hip. Clin Orthop 213:20-33, 1986.

65. Vignon E, Piperno M, Hellio MP, et al: Measurement of radiographic joint space width in the tibiofemoral compartment of the osteoarthritis knee: Comparison of standing anteroposterior and Lyon Schuss views. Arthritis Rheum 48:378-384, 2003.

66. Kellgren JH, Lawrence JS: Radiological assessment of osteoarthrosis. Ann Rheum Dis 16:494-502, 1957.

67. Verbruggen G, Veys E: Numerical scoring systems for the anatomic evolution of osteoarthritis of the finger joints. Arthritis Rheum 39:308-320, 1996.

68. Swanson AB, de Groot-Swanson G: Osteoarthritis in the hand. Clin Rheum Dis 11:393-420, 1985.

69. Docken WP: Clinical features and medical management of osteoarthritis at the hand and wrist. Hand Clin 3:337-349, 1987.

70. Pattrick M, Aldridge S, Hamilton E, et al: A controlled study of hand function in nodal and erosive osteoarthritis. Ann Rheum Dis 48:978-982, 1989.

71. Cobby M, Cushnaghan J, Creamer P, et al: Erosive osteoarthritis: is it a separate disease entity? Clin Radiol 42:258-263, 1990.

72. Smith D, Braunstein EM, Brandt KD, Katz PB: A radiographic comparison of erosive osteoarthritis and idiopathic nodal osteoarthritis. J Rheumatol 19:896-904, 1992.

73. Chard M, Hazleman B: Shoulder disorders in the elderly. Ann Rheum Dis 46:684-689, 1987.

74. Fardet L, Messow M, Maillefert JF, Dougados M: Primary glenohumeral degenerative joint disease: Factors predisposing to arthroplasty. Clin Exp Rheumatol 21:13-18, 2003.

75. Revel M, Poiraudeau S, Lefevre-Colau MM, Mayoux-Benhamou MA: La discopathie destructrice rapide. Rev Rhum (Educ Fr) 67(Suppl 4):266-269, 2000.

93

Management of Osteoarthritis

CARLOS J. LOZADA

Osteoarthritis (OA) is the most common form of arthritis. It's often referred to by other names such as "arthrosis", "osteoarthrosis", or simply "arthritis." Because its incidence increases with age, OA will become an increasing health issue with the "graying" of the world's population.

OA can be defined radiologically or clinically. The most useful definition, however, requires symptoms from OA as well as radiographic changes. If a pure radiologic definition is used, it can be demonstrated that almost all individuals past age 75 have OA.[1] Although the epidemiology of OA is well covered in Chapter 92, Clinical Features of OA, it has been estimated that between 10 and 30 percent of those affected with OA are significantly disabled, making OA the leading cause of chronic disability in the United States.[2] This leads to heavy direct and indirect costs.

Traditional treatment paradigms for OA have conceded the inexorable progression of the disease and concentrated on pain management.[3] The importance of training physicians in the management of OA has been underscored by the development of guidelines. These have focused on the symptomatic management of OA. With the relatively rapid recent evolution in the field of rheumatology, some of the guidelines have already required revision. A simplistic but potentially useful guideline is provided in Figure 93–1. As the population ages, there will be increasing societal pressures on physicians, particularly rheumatologists, to improve on available treatment alternatives for OA.[4-6] Researchers have now turned to the investigation of agents that might delay the progression of OA. Potential future interventions include the use of collagenase inhibitors, polysaccharides, and growth factor and cytokine manipulation.[7]

Assessment of the Patient with Osteoarthritis

Appropriate management of OA begins with an accurate diagnosis. As with most rheumatic illnesses, obtaining a good history is of paramount importance. Symptoms should be carefully described, particularly pain. Duration, location, and any alleviating or exacerbating factors should be ascertained. Distinct features of presentation such as stiffness or gelling and description of events such as "locking" or "giving way" of a joint can help the physician in directing the physical examination.

The physical examination then seeks to confirm the diagnostic suspicion and establish the causes of symptomatology. Laboratory evaluations are not helpful in establishing the diagnosis of OA but can help in excluding alternative diagnoses. They are useful in deciding which therapeutic approaches are appropriate to employ in a particular patient, as conditions such as renal insufficiency or anemia can be identified.

Radiographs are not necessary for diagnosis in a majority of patients but can identify co-occurring conditions such as chondrocalcinosis that may lead to further workup or to modification of the therapeutic plan.

Sources of Pain in Osteoarthritis

The main symptom in OA is pain. It has many potential sources in and around the joint. These include focal synovitis, synovial effusions, subchondral bone pain receptors, and periarticular tendons and bursae. Factors complicating the determination of the source of pain may include varus or valgus deformity, weight issues, and the emotional impact of chronic pain. Once the source(s) of the pain is (are) accurately identified, a treatment plan can be formulated.

Management of Osteoarthritis

The management of OA can be divided into nonpharmacologic interventions (Table 93–1), pharmacologic interventions and surgical options. Pharmacologic interventions can be further subdivided into symptomatic therapy and potential structure- or disease-modifying therapy.

NONPHARMACOLOGIC INTERVENTIONS

Psychosocial Interventions

As in other types of arthritis, patient education is an important first step in OA therapy. The patient should be an integral part of the decision making team. To do this effectively, the patient should understand the nature of OA, including its natural history and treatment options. It is often reassuring for the patient to realize that OA is a very common, slowly progressive ailment and is not typically as disabling or deforming as the inflammatory arthritides. A significant number of patients have already tried nonprescription medication or nutriceutical remedies for their symptoms prior to seeing the physician and will want to discuss these. Emphasis should be given to the fact that treatment includes nonpharmacologic as well as pharmacologic interventions. Organizations such

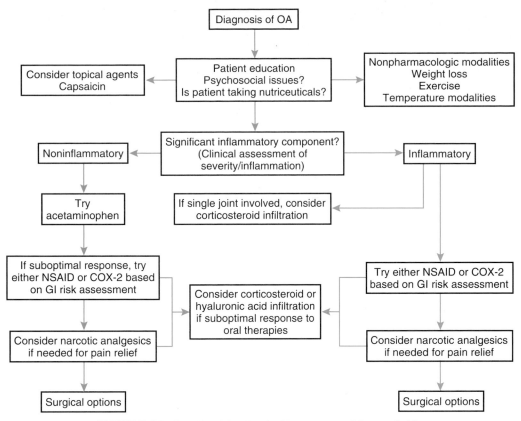

FIGURE 93-1 · Algorithm for the Management of Osteoarthritis

as the Arthritis Foundation can be valuable sources of information geared to patients, such as reading materials.

Some patients may develop significant emotional disturbances related to the pain and change in normal daily activities that can stem from OA. These may include mood disorders, such as depression, or sleep disorders. A suspicion of either of these should lead to the evaluation by a psychiatrist or a primary physician that regularly manages these types of disorders.

Weight Loss

Obesity in an important risk factor in the development of OA of the knee.[8,9] Furthermore, higher body mass index (BMI) has been associated to an increased risk of progression of OA of the knee.[10] This can be compounded by malalignment, namely varus and valgus deformities, that modulate the effect of weight on knee OA.[11] In one study, BMI was associated with OA severity in those with varus deformity but not those with valgus.

Regimens of weight loss and exercise have been associated with improvement in pain and disability in OA of the knee.[12] Weight loss alone has been associated with a decrease in the odds of developing symptomatic knee OA.[13] One study has suggested that a reduction in percent body fat, rather than weight, may be significant in reducing pain from OA of the knee.[14]

Temperature Modalities

Topical applications of heat or cold can be a helpful adjunct to the therapeutic plan for the OA patient. These are more effectively used in superficial joints, such as the knees, than in deep ones, such as the hip. An acute injury, such as a sprained ankle, calls for cold

---

■ **TABLE 93-1 · NONPHARMACOLGIC MANAGEMENT OF OSTEOARTHRITIS (OA)**

Conventional Options in the Management of OA
Patient education
Arthritis self-help courses
Weight loss
Temperature modalities
Exercise
Orthotics
Modified activities of daily living

Unconventional Options for OA
Transcutaneous electrical nerve stimulation (TENS)
Pulsed electromagnetic fields
Static magnets
Acupuncture
Spa therapy
Yoga

applications in the initial 2 to 3 days.[15] In a setting of chronic pain, most patients prefer warm applications, although if superior pain relief is obtained from cold applications, these can be continued.

Warm applications can be in the form of warm soaks or heating pads. Individual sessions should not exceed a temperature of 45° C or a length of approximately 30 minutes.[16] They should be avoided over certain areas, such as close to the testicles, or in patients that have poor vascular supply, neuropathies, or cancer. Benefits of warm applications include decreased pain and stiffness along with relief of muscle spasm and prevention of contractures.

Exercise

Periarticular structures, particularly muscles, influence the expression of OA. This is likely due to their role in providing stability to the joints and in dampening some of the forces acting across joints. Quadriceps-muscle weakness has been postulated as a risk factor for OA of the knee.[17] Quadriceps strengthening exercises, on the other hand, have been advanced as fundamental to the management of conditions such as chondromalacia patella.[18]

Both the dynamic and isometric exercise arms of a 16-week study of patients with knee OA had equivalent improvement of symptoms and physical functioning.[19] Walking can be beneficial. Supervised fitness-walking regimens have been shown to improve function in OA of the knee.[20] Home-based exercise interventions have also been shown to significantly improve symptoms in those with knee OA.[21] Finally, community-based aquatic exercise programs, such as aquatic aerobics programs, have merit and can also be implemented.[22]

Orthotics and Bracing

Orthotics can be effective in symptomatic relief of OA and are probably underused by most physicians. They range from insoles to braces. Studies have demonstrated that lateral wedged insoles provide substantial relief to those with medial compartment knee OA, particularly those with varus deformity.[23] In some studies, those with milder symptoms have obtained the greater benefit.[24] Knee braces have been evaluated as well. Valgus bracing of patients with medial compartment OA has been found to reduce pain and increase levels of activity.[25] In one study, medial taping of the patella relieved the pain of those with patellofemoral compartment OA by 25 percent.[26]

Heel lifts have been tried in those with hip OA. In one uncontrolled study, most patients reported diminished symptoms. Time to improvement lengthened with the radiologic stage of OA.[27] For those with calcaneal spurs, or foot joint OA in general, appropriate athletic-type footwear should be recommended. A good athletic shoe should provide medial arch support and calcaneal cushioning, as well as good mediolateral stability.

Those with carpometacarpal, (CMC), joint arthritis should initially be offered conservative management including the use of splints. In one trial, 70 percent of patients treated with a 7-month intervention including the use of splints were able to improve their symptoms considerably and avoided surgical intervention.[28]

The Cane

The appropriate use of a cane can be an important adjunct, particularly in OA of the hip. It has been estimated that a cane can provide up to 40-percent reduction in hip contact forces during ambulation.[29] The cane should be used in the hand contralateral to the affected hip and should be advanced with the affected limb while walking. The appropriate cane size is that which results in about a 20-degree flexion of the elbow during use.[30] A useful approximation is a cane that is equal to the length from the floor to the patient's greater trochanter.

Modification in Activities of Daily Living

Physician advice and occupational therapy may provide useful insights to the patient that can be put to use in modifying daily activities and, thus, reduce symptomatology from OA. These interventions can be varied and range from using an elevated toilet seat or shower bench in someone with lower extremity OA to using appliances designed to help with the opening of jars in a patient with hand OA. Assistance in these modifications from occupational therapists can be valuable.

Other Interventions

Other modalities have been tried in OA. These are unconventional and include magnetic-field application, acupuncture, and yoga-based regimens. These are not accepted as standard therapy for OA, but some are deserving of further study. A significant number of these are being used by patients on their own and should be formally studied not only for evidence of any benefit but to ensure that there are no potential harmful effects.

Studies of transcutaneous electrical nerve stimulation (TENS) have generally been small. A recent review of TENS studies in OA of the knee concluded that a trend toward symptom-improvement existed, warranting larger, well-controlled studies.[31] In one randomized, controlled study, patients had an initial symptom reduction over placebo, but at 1 year follow-up only two patients continued to use the device.[32]

Pulsed electromagnetic fields have been tested in double-blind, placebo-controlled trials. These fields are applied through the daily use of a brace-type device. In one study, a primary end point of pain reduction was not achieved.[33]

The use of static magnets in chronic knee pain has become quite popular with some patients. In one double-blind, randomized, placebo-controlled trial of 43 patients, the Western Ontario McMaster Osteoarthritis Index (WOMAC) pain and physical function subscales, along with a 50-foot walk, demonstrated a statistically significant benefit of static magnets at 2 weeks.[34] The potential mechanism for any such effect remains unclear and larger, longer-term studies are needed before any clinical effect can be postulated.

Acupuncture is being formally tested in a National Institutes of Health (NIH)-sponsored, multicenter clinical trial. In testing acupuncture's clinical efficacy, development of appropriate controls has been difficult. Most recent studies have tried to employ "sham" methods in the control arm. One such method has been the employment of blunted, telescopic needles.[35] Early clinical trials[36,37] and one literature review[38] have concluded that there is promise in treating pain from OA of the knee.

Spa therapy also has advocates. It has been touted for low back pain and for lower extremity osteoarthritis.[39] However, randomized, controlled studies are lacking.[40] Yoga has also shown some symptomatic benefit for OA of the hands in limited testing.[41]

PHARMACOLOGIC INTERVENTIONS IN OSTEOARTHRITIS

Topical Agents

Topical agents for the management of OA are available without a prescription in the United States (Table 93–2). The two most widely used types are preparations containing capsaicin and those containing topical nonsteroidal anti-inflammatory drugs (NSAIDs).

Capsaicin is a pungent ingredient found in red peppers (such as hot chili peppers). The mechanism of action is thought to be through selective stimulation of unmyelinated type C afferent neurons, causing the release of substance P. Such a release reversibly depletes the stores of substance P, a neurotransmitter of peripheral pain sensations.[42] Capsaicin preparations are available in concentrations of .025 or .075 percent in either ointment or, more recently, "roll on" form, and they can be applied up to four times daily. They have been tested in controlled, double-blind studies in OA of the hands and knees.[43,44] Patient response is quite variable, with some obtaining significant pain relief and others not being able to tolerate the burning or stinging sensations produced by its application. Usually the counterirritant sensation decreases gradually with repeated use, but pain relief remains. Although very safe overall, capsaicin products can be quite irritating if in contact with mucosal surfaces, particularly the eyes. Patients using them should wear disposable gloves, if possible, while applying them. There can also be some reddening of the skin in the area where the compound is applied.

Topical NSAID preparations are popular as treatments for OA in many countries around the world.[45,46] Safety concerns with the traditional oral NSAIDs[47] have been the driving force in the use of these topical treatments, although questions remain as to absorption and degree of relief obtained. Results of placebo-controlled trials in OA of the knee have been conflicting. Some have shown benefit of gels containing NSAIDs, such as diclofenac,[48] whereas others have shown only trends favoring the NSAID, or no difference at all.

One double-blind, placebo-controlled study enrolled 237 European patients with knee OA.[49] Patients were randomized to receive eltenac or placebo gel over 4 weeks. Eltenac is a nonselective NSAID that has structural similarities to diclofenac. The primary end point was global pain on a visual analogue scale (VAS). At 4 weeks, there was a trend, but no statistical difference, favoring the eltenac gel. Two patients in the active treatment group and two in the placebo group had local itching, reddening, or both in the application area.

There are menthol- and salicylate-based over-the-counter topical preparations, but there are no published trials supporting their use in OA.

Systemic Agents

Non-Narcotic Analgesics

Acetaminophen (paracetamol) has often been touted as the initial systemic intervention for the management of OA. This is mainly due to its favorable side-effect profile but also to a perception of equivalent efficacy to NSAIDs. This perception derives from studies of OA in which patients have not been stratified as to degree of symptomatology. In one study, acetaminophen at 4 g/day was equivalent to ibuprofen at 1200 or 2400 mg/day, with the notable exception of pain at rest.[50] More recently, it has been noted that NSAIDs may have superior efficacy in patients with more symptomatic or inflammatory presentations, as acetaminophen has no anti-inflammatory effects at approved doses.[51] Particular concerns in those taking acetaminophen include the concomitant use of alcohol or of over-the-counter products containing acet-

TABLE 93–2 • SYMPTOM-RELIEVING PHARMACOLOGIC THERAPIES FOR OSTEOARTHRITIS (OA)

Topical
Capsaicin
Topical nonsteroidal anti-inflammatory drug (NSAID) preparations

Systemic
Acetaminophen
Nonselective NSAIDs
Cyclooxygenase-2 (COX-2)–specific inhibitors
Tramadol
Narcotic analgesics

Intra-articular
Corticosteroids
Hyaluronic-acid derivatives

TABLE 93–3 • NUTRICEUTICALS FOR OSTEOARTHRITIS (OA)

Glucosamine
Chondroitin sulfate
Ginger extracts
Avocado and soy unsaponifiables
Cat's claw
Shark cartilage
s-Adenosyl-L-methionine (SAMe)

aminophen. Either of these situations can lead to enhanced possibility of hepatic toxicity through toxic metabolites.

Nonsteroidal Anti-Inflammatory Drugs

NSAIDs are the most commonly prescribed medications for the treatment of OA. Nonselective NSAIDs work through nonspecific inhibition of cyclooxygenase isoforms 1 and 2 (COX-1 and COX-2). COX-1 is constitutively expressed in renal and gastrointestinal tissues, among others. COX-2 is inducible in inflammatory responses. The major side effects of NSAIDs are gastrointestinal (GI) toxicities (gastritis, peptic ulcer disease) and renal (interstitial nephritis, prostaglandin inhibition–related renal insufficiency) toxicities. As GI tissues have a higher expression of COX-1, a selective COX-2 inhibitor would potentially spare patients the GI side effects. Unfortunately, COX-2 is expressed in renal tissue and COX-2–specific drugs, such as traditional NSAIDs, have potential adverse renal effects. This is especially so in those with baseline renal insufficiency. Alternative mechanisms of action of NSAIDs, such as interference with receptors in the cell membrane phospholipid bilayers, have been proposed.[52] Further discussion of NSAIDs can be found in Chapter 56, Nonsteroidal Anti-inflammatory Drugs.

Nonselective NSAIDs are used widely for the management of OA. They include ibuprofen, naproxen, diclofenac, and others. NSAIDs are usually analgesic at lower doses but have both analgesic and anti-inflammatory effects at their higher, recommended doses. They are prescribed either in fixed doses or "as needed" and are quite effective as symptom modifiers; however, they have no structure-or disease-modifying effects. NSAIDs should be used in the smallest dose that will provide satisfactory symptom relief, as GI toxicity has been linked to dosage. GI adverse events have also been linked to age of patient, previous history of peptic ulcers or bleeding, and the presence of comorbid conditions such as heart disease.

To reduce the potential for GI events, misoprostol can be added to the therapeutic regimen. It is a prostaglandin E2 (PGE_2) analogue that has been shown to reduce GI adverse events from NSAIDs when used at 200 mcg q.i.d.[53] Diarrhea is a potential side effect. The use of a concomitant proton pump inhibitor has also been shown to reduce upper GI endoscopic ulceration rates from NSAIDs, although no study has attempted to show a decrease in events such as symptomatic ulcers or bleeds.[54] Over-the-counter doses of histamine receptor 2, (H-2), blockers and antacids have not been shown to reduce either endoscopic or serious clinical GI events. The use of COX-2–specific inhibitors is the latest attempt at reducing the GI adverse event profile of OA therapy.

COX-2–specific inhibitors are highly selective for COX-2 in vitro. Currently, three such agents are available: celecoxib, rofecoxib, and valdecoxib. Others are in various stages of investigation. All of the available agents have reported reduction of more than 50 percent in the rates of endoscopic ulceration when compared to nonselective NSAIDs. Rofecoxib and celecoxib have also reported significant reduction in the rates of symptomatic ulcers, bleeds, perforations, and obstructions in patients not concurrently on aspirin.[55,56] It remains unclear how substantial the benefits of these compounds are to those on aspirin. As COX-2–specific agents can inhibit endothelial prostacyclin but do not affect platelet thromboxane, cardiovascular safety remains an area of investigation.[57,58]

Combination COX/lipoxygenase inhibitors are in development. It remains to be seen how these will compare with traditional NSAIDs and with COX-2 inhibitors in terms of both safety and efficacy.[59] Animal studies have hinted at the possibility of a structure- and disease-modifying effect.[60]

Narcotic Analgesics

Although several options exist for management of pain in OA, for some these provide suboptimal pain relief. If a patient has failed to respond to other nonpharmacologic and pharmacologic modalities and has no additional identifiable causes of pain (such as fibromyalgia), a narcotic analgesic should be considered.

The pain of OA is generally responsive to narcotic analgesics. Because of concerns such as potential addiction, appropriate patient selection is important. Narcotic analgesics, such as codeine and propoxyphene, have been used effectively in patients with OA, especially in combination with non-narcotic analgesics (e.g., acetaminophen). Potential side effects include nausea, constipation, and somnolence.

Tramadol is an oral medication with mild suppressive effects on the μ opioid receptor. It also inhibits the uptake of norepinephrine and serotonin[61] and is not thought to have significant addictive tendencies.[62] It is available alone or in combination with acetaminophen and is not a controlled-schedule medication in the United States.[63] Tramadol has been used for the symptomatic relief of OA.[64] Seizures and allergic reactions are potential side effects.[65] The incidence of nausea can be reduced by slowly escalating the dose until the desired pain relief is achieved.

One study compared tramadol and acetaminophen to the combination of codeine and acetaminophen.[66] Patients with OA or chronic low back pain were randomized to receive tramadol and acetaminophen (37.5 mg and 325 mg, respectively) or codeine and acetaminophen (30 mg and 300 mg, respectively) for 4 weeks. Pain relief and changes in pain intensity were equivalent in both groups. Those on codeine and acetaminophen had a significantly higher incidence of somnolence (24 vs. 17 percent) and constipation (21 vs. 11 percent).

Intra-articular Agents

Corticosteroids

Although there is no role for systemic corticosteroids in OA, local intra-articular corticoid preparations have a long history in the management of OA. Corticosteroids have been shown to downregulate expression of adhesion molecules. This, in turn, could reduce cellular infiltration into the joint and subsequent inflammation. Corticosteroid injections have been shown to slow macrophage-like cell infiltration of the synovium in OA.[67] The dose of steroid injected is determined by the volume of the joint being injected, with larger joints such as the knees receiving higher doses. The risk of joint infection is very low if proper technique is employed. Postinjection flares due to corticosteroid crystal synovitis can occur.

There is a relative dearth of clinical trial–based information on intra-articular corticosteroid injections. However, in one trial, symptomatic benefit from corticosteroid injection in OA of the knee was demonstrated in a double-blind trial at 1 and 4 weeks postinjection.[68] The specific corticosteroid compound used, frequency of injections, and other particulars related to the use of corticosteroid injections in OA vary widely and are heavily influenced by the training program the rheumatologist attended and where he or she practices.[69] In general, corticosteroid injections are believed to be most effective in patients with evidence of inflammation, effusions, or both. Because of concerns over possible deleterious effects, usually no more than four corticosteroid injections per year are given in a particular joint. Further discussion of arthrocentesis can be found in Chapter 47, Arthrocentesis and Injections of Joints and Soft Tissues.

Hyaluronic-Acid Derivatives

Synthetic and naturally occurring hyaluronic-acid derivatives are administered intra-articularly. Two of these agents—Hyalgan and Synvis—are approved in the United States for use in OA of the knees. They require multiple-injection courses, with the injections spaced 1 week apart. One medication requires three injections per course of treatment (Synvisc), the other five (Hyalgan). Although often mentioned as potential "structure-modifying" agents, these products are presently considered symptom-modifying drugs. Their molecular weights vary (from less than 100,000 to more than 1 million Svedberg units) depending on the preparation. They have been reported to reduce pain for prolonged periods of time and, potentially, to improve mobility.[70] Improvement in overall physical functioning has also been reported.[71] The mechanism(s) of action are not known. However, there is evidence for an anti-inflammatory effect (particularly at high molecular weight), a short-term lubricant effect, an analgesic effect by directly buffering of synovial nerve endings, and a stimulating effect on synovial lining cells leading to production of normal hyaluronic acid.[72]

In one study, three weekly hyaluronic acid intra-articular injections provided comparable pain relief to a single depocorticosteroid intra-articular injection at 1 week follow-up; at 45 days follow-up, hyaluronic acid was superior to the depocorticosteroid.[73] In a Canadian study, 102 patients with OA of the knee were randomized to three weekly intra-articular injections of Hylan G-F (Synvisc), Hylan G-F plus an NSAID, or to the NSAID alone. At 26 weeks, both groups receiving hylan G-F were significantly better than the group receiving NSAIDs alone.[74]

Substantial clinical responses to the saline injections used as placebo in hyaluronic acid trials have sometimes made interpretation of the data in those studies challenging. In a double-blind, placebo-controlled trial, 495 patients with knee OA were randomized to receive five intra-articular injections of hyaluronic acid (Hyalgan) given 1 week apart, placebo, or naproxen (500 mg p.o. b.i.d.) and followed for 26 weeks.[75] Patients on the group receiving hyaluronic acid improved significantly more with respect to pain on the 50-foot walk compared to placebo and more of them had a 20-mm or greater reduction in pain as judged with a VAS. At trial conclusion, more hyaluronic acid–treated patients (47.6%) had slight pain or were pain free in contrast to placebo-treated (33.1%) or naproxen-treated (36.9%) patients. As expected, GI adverse events were significantly more common in the naproxen group than the hyaluronic acid or placebo groups.

One multicenter, randomized, double-blind study, reported as an abstract, revisited the issue of disease modification with hyaluronic acid. Patients received three courses of three intra-articular knee injections of either hyaluronan or saline over the course of 1 year. Joint-space width (JSW) was assessed using standing, weight-bearing radiographs; 273 patients completed the trial and had complete data collection. In those with greater JSW at entry, hyaluronan use led to slightly less joint-space narrowing than saline.[76] These results have not been confirmed in other trials.

Hyaluronic acid products are also being actively investigated in shoulder joint OA, periarthritis,[77] and adhesive capsulitis.[78]

Nutriceuticals

A pair of nutritional supplements, namely glucosamine and chondroitin sulfate, have received significant attention (Table 93–3). Health food stores and the lay press have been touting them as "cures for arthritis." The mechanism of action of glucosamine sulfate is uncertain. Some in vitro experiments have shown stimulation of the synthesis of cartilage glycosaminoglycans and proteoglycans.[79,80] Others have shown that glucosamine and N-Acetylglucosamine inhibit interleukin-1β (IL-1β)– and tumor necrosis factor-α (TNF-α)–induced nitric oxide (NO) production in normal human articular chondrocytes.[81] N-Acetylglucosamine also suppressed production of IL-1β and stimulated IL-6 and COX-2.

Urinary excretion of glucosamine (and other glycosaminoglycans) has been investigated and found to be elevated in both OA and rheumatoid arthritis (RA).[82] Supplementation with glucosamine sulfate, an intermediate in mucopolysaccharide synthesis, has been tried both orally and intramuscularly as therapy for OA. Glucosamine sulfate (400 mg twice weekly intramuscularly for 6 weeks) reduced the severity of disease as judged by the Lequesne index when compared to placebo.[83] A randomized, double-blind, parallel-group study in knee OA compared 500 mg p.o. t.i.d. of glucosamine sulfate to 400 mg p.o. t.i.d. of ibuprofen for 4 weeks. The response to ibuprofen was more rapid, but at 4 weeks, there was no statistically significant difference in the response rate (reduction of at least 2 points in the Lequesne index).[84] No group in the study received higher, anti-inflammatory doses of ibuprofen.

An NIH-sponsored trial is currently underway in the United States to more thoroughly study the symptom-relieving and possible structural-modification properties of glucosamine. Meanwhile, some already advocate the use of glucosamine as part of the first line of therapy for symptomatic OA.[85]

Two European trials have tried to address the subject of disease modification with glucosamine. In one study, 212 patients with OA of the knee were randomized to receive placebo or glucosamine sulfate (1500 mg/day) and were followed prospectively for 3 years.[86] Fluoroscopically positioned, standing anteroposterior (AP) radiographs of the knees were taken at enrollment, 1 year, and 3 years. At 3 years, the treatment group had a joint-space reduction of .06 mm, whereas the placebo group had a reduction of .31 mm. Whether this is a clinically meaningful difference in joint space is unclear. Those taking glucosamine also showed symptomatic benefit on the order of 20 to 25 percent, whereas those taking placebo had a slight worsening of symptoms, as judged by the WOMAC. There were no significant adverse events attributed to the use of the glucosamine sulfate.

A second group of researchers randomized 202 patients to receive placebo or glucosamine sulfate (1500 mg/day for 3 years).[87] The width of the narrowest medial joint space of the tibiofemoral joint was measured serially, using visual assessments with a 0.1-mm graduated magnifying glass on standardized, full extension, weight-bearing AP radiographs of each knee. At 3 years, there was a significant difference in JSW, with a decrease of .19 mm in the JSW of the placebo group and an increase of .04 mm in JSW in the glucosamine sulfate group. Also seen were significantly greater improvements in the WOMAC score and the Lequesne index in the glucosamine group.

The favorable results of these studies have been brought into question because of the radiographic technique employed to assess joint space. At issue is whether the joint space seen on standing films of the knee could be significantly affected by the symptomatology of OA (i.e., pain) and whether a semiflexed film would be a preferred method for use in these studies. In one study, investigators obtained baseline radiographs (after analgesic or NSAID washout) using both standing-extended and semiflexed, fluoroscopically positioned techniques in 19 patients with knee OA.[88] Radiographs were then repeated 2 to 8 weeks later after reinstitution of analgesic or NSAID therapy. JSW increased upon effective pain relief in highly symptomatic patients, if measured through standing-extended view radiographs. Using the semiflexed technique, there were no changes in JSW related to degree of severity or responsiveness to pain therapy. This suggests that data obtained using the standing-extended radiographic technique may need to be revisited, as the results may represent a therapeutic intervention's effect on symptoms (pain), rather than a disease-modifying effect. More recent, ongoing trials have changed to the semiflexed, fluoroscopically positioned knee radiograph in assessing potential disease modification.

Oral chondroitin sulfate, a glycosaminoglycan composed of units of glucosamine with attached sugar molecules (molecular mass of around 14,000), has also been used as therapy for hip and knee OA. Its mechanism of action is unknown. A double-blind, placebo-controlled study included a 3-month treatment phase followed by a 2-month treatment-free phase. The major outcome parameter was NSAID consumption. Those receiving chondroitin sulfate used fewer NSAIDs than the controls at both the completion of the treatment and in the treatment-free phase.[89] Another study compared chondroitin sulfate to diclofenac sodium. One group received chondroitin sulfate (400 mg t.i.d.) and the other diclofenac sodium (50 mg t.i.d.). Each group also received placebo in place of the other medication. The chondroitin group received the active drug for 3 months, whereas the diclofenac group received it only for 1 month and was then switched to placebo. Both groups took placebo only from month 4 through month 6. The diclofenac group had quicker response to therapy, whereas the chondroitin group had a more prolonged improvement as measured by the Lequesne index, VAS for pain, four-point scale for pain, and paracetamol use (rescue medication).[90] This study raises questions because of the different lengths of treatment with active drug in each group. Further studies are needed.

Combination products containing both glucosamine and chondroitin have become quite popular in the United States despite a dearth of clinical trial data. One small, placebo-controlled trial randomized patients with knee OA to a receive regimen of glucosamine hydrochloride (1000 mg), chondroitin sulfate (800 mg), and manganese ascorbate (152 mg) twice a day or placebo.[91] Patients were evaluated at baseline and then every 2 months for 6 months using the Lequesne index of OA severity. At 4 and 6 months, those with mild to moderate radiographic OA of the knee showed significant improvement by Lequesne index when compared to those on placebo. In those with severe radiographic OA of the knee, no significant symptomatic benefit could be demonstrated. The study did not evaluate patients for structure or disease modification.

Ginger extracts have been popular in the list of "natural" remedies for OA for some time.[92] Most of the world's production of ginger comes from China. Its "medicinal" use dates back more than 2000 years. Ginger actually contains very small amounts of salicylate.[93] In some animal models, ginger has been shown to have inhibitory effects on COX and lipooxygenase.[94] One study with 247 evaluable patients revealed a small but statistically significant reduction in knee pain on standing (63 vs. 50%; $p = 0.048$) after taking ginger.[95] Reduction in knee pain after a 50-foot walk was also significant. Use of acetaminophen was reduced in the ginger-extract group but the difference was not statistically significant. The extract was well tolerated, except for GI events such as dyspepsia, nausea, and eructation, which were increased over placebo. The question remains as to whether benefits observed represent a clinically relevant effect.

Some of the more unusual agents proposed as structure or disease modifiers in OA are oral preparations of avocado and soy unsaponifiables (ASU). These compounds are derived from unsaponifiable residues of avocado and soya oils mixed in a 1:2 ratio. In vitro studies on cultured chondrocytes have shown partial reversal of IL-1β effects. IL-1β roles in OA are thought to include inhibition of prostaglandin synthesis by chondrocytes and stimulation of matrix metalloproteinases (MMPs) and NO production. MMPs and NO can degrade cartilage matrix and cause chondrocyte apoptosis. Use of ASU also reportedly results in inhibited production of IL-6, IL-8, MMPs and stimulation of collagen synthesis. The mechanism through which these effects occur is unknown, as is the active ingredient in ASU.[96] Symptomatic benefit in double-blind human trials in OA of the hip and knee has also been reported.[97] Some abstract presentations have suggested structure or disease modification in human hip OA.[98]

Other "nutritional supplements" entrenched in regional and international popular cultures, such as cat's claw and shark cartilage, are used, often with limited or no data to support their use. A small, placebo-controlled trial showed improvement of OA pain on activity in those taking cat's claw extracts.[99] Shark cartilage also contains a small amount of chondroitin sulfate.[100]

S-Adenosyl methionine (SAMe), a methyl group donor and oxygen radical scavenger, is also often touted as a remedy for OA, although little evidence of an effect has been published.[101,102] In one double-blind, placebo-controlled study, the two centers reported differing results. One center reported reductions in overall pain and rest pain, whereas the other showed no significant difference between the test group and placebo.[103] There is insufficient evidence to recommend the use of these products in the treatment of OA.

POTENTIALLY STRUCTURE- OR DISEASE-MODIFYING THERAPIES FOR OSTEOARTHRITIS

The term *chondroprotective* has been used to describe structure- or disease-modifying agents. This is a misnomer, however, because the goal is to protect the entire joint (not only the cartilage) from the arthritic process. A workshop of the Osteoarthritis Research Society (OARS)[104] recommended that the term *structure-modifying drugs* be used to describe medications that would previously have been classified as chondroprotective. These drugs are intended to prevent, retard, stabilize, or even reverse the development of OA. Any

---

TABLE 93–4 • POTENTIALLY STRUCTURE- AND DISEASE-MODIFYING DRUGS IN OSTEOARTHRITIS (OA)

Tetracyclines
Metalloproteinase or collagenase inhibitors
Glucosamine
Diacerein
Growth factor and cytokine manipulation (interleukin-1 receptor antagonist [IL-1Ra], transforming growth factor-β [TGF-β])
Gene therapy (IL-1Ra, IL-1RII)
Chondrocyte and stem cell transplants

---

benefits from them, it appears, are evident after prolonged observation, given the typically slow progression of OA (Table 93-4). Therefore, clinical trials in this area have been challenging, with most having been designed for at least 3 years of follow-up. Progress in the methodology used to assess for structure and disease modification may shorten the length of these trials.

Measures used to identify structure and disease modification include radiographic assessments of joint space, such as fluoroscopically positioned AP radiographs of the knee or magnetic resonance imaging (MRI).[105] Unfortunately, to date, no drug has been conclusively proven to be structure or disease modifying. As already noted, two European trials have hinted at glucosamine sulfate being such an agent, although methodologic issues with those studies remain.

Although the chapter focuses on medication-based therapies, other approaches, such as osteochondral grafts of chondrocytes, stem cells, or both, with eventual differentiation into bone and cartilage, are in various stages of development.[106]

Potentially structure or disease modifying interventions under investigation include collagenase inhibitors, polysaccharides, and growth factor and cytokine manipulations.

Tetracyclines, apart from any antimicrobial effect, are inhibitors of tissue metalloproteinases. This could be due to their ability to chelate calcium and zinc ions. There has also been investigation into the potential role of nitric oxide in the mechanism of action of the tetracyclines.[107] Minocycline, a tetracycline-family antibiotic, has been used in the management of RA.[108] Doxycycline, another tetracycline derivative, has been shown to inhibit articular cartilage collagenase activity.[109,110]

Doxycycline has also reduced the severity of OA in canine models. In one study, there was preservation of medial femoral condyle cartilage in treated dogs compared to the untreated group. Other lesions, such as medial trochlear ridge cartilage damage, superficial fibrillation of the medial tibial plateau, and osteophytosis, were unaffected by treatment. Collagenolytic and gelatinolytic activity, however, were reduced to one-fifth and one-fourth their previous levels, respectively, when compared to the untreated dogs. In an in vitro model, not only did doxycycline reduce collagenase and gelatinase activity in cartilage, it also prevented proteoglycan loss, cell death, and deposition of type X collagen matrix.[111]

A multicenter, double-blind, placebo-controlled trial using doxycycline for structure or disease modification in obese female subjects with OA of the knee is ongoing. Other compounds with collagenase-inhibiting properties are being developed and investigated as structure- or disease-modifying agents not only in OA, but also in RA.[112]

Glycosaminoglycan polysulfuric acid (GAGPS), known as Arteparon or Adequan, is purported to work through reducing the activity of collagenase. It is a highly sulfated glycosaminoglycan, ranging from 2,000 to 16,000 in molecular weight,[113] which is derived from bovine tracheal cartilage. In a canine model of OA, GAGPS was administered intra-articularly twice weekly for 4 weeks.[114]

Four weeks after completion of the GAGPS, medial femoral condylar lesions had developed to a lesser degree in the treated group than in saline-treated dogs. Furthermore, swelling, an indicator of collagen network integrity, remained near control levels in the treatment group. In humans, OA of the knee was studied in a 5-year trial. There was improvement in multiple measured parameters, including less time lost from work.[115] Another double-blind, placebo-controlled trial evaluated GAGPS in 80 patients with OA of the knee; patients received two series of five intra-articular injections of 25 mg (0.5 ml) GAGPS at 1-week intervals. At 14 weeks, 31 percent of the GAGPS group had improvement as judged by the Lequesne index, compared to 15 percent in the placebo group.[116] Potential allergy and heparin-like effects were observed. GAGPS is available in the United States for equine, but not human, use.

Another extract, a glycosaminoglycan-peptide complex (GP-C), known as Rumalon, is an intramuscularly administered, highly sulfated polysaccharide derived from bovine tracheal cartilage and bone marrow.[117] It has been shown to increase the levels of tissue inhibitor of metalloproteinases (TIMP).[118] A randomized, placebo-controlled trial selected patients with hip or knee OA to receive 10 courses of injections of placebo or GP-C (2 ml) over 5 years (two courses/yr). Each course consisted of 15 injections given twice weekly. GP-C failed to demonstrate a structure- or disease-modifying effect.[119] In addition, there were no statistical differences favoring the active treatment group when measured by Lequesne index, pain on passive motion, or consumption of NSAIDs. GP-C is available in parts of Europe and South America.

Pentosan polysulfate (Cartrofen) is a purified extract of beech hemicellulose administered intramuscularly, or orally as a calcium salt. It can inhibit granulocyte elastase. Experimental studies in animal models have suggested that it helps preserve cartilage proteoglycan content and retards cartilage degradation.[120,121] However, a recent blinded, placebo-controlled study using an oral preparation in a dog model failed to demonstrate either a symptomatic benefit or a structure- or disease-modifying effect.[122]

Diacerein[123] and its active metabolite rhein are anthraquinones related to senna compounds. They inhibit the synthesis of IL-1β in human OA synovium in vitro, as well as the expression of IL-1 receptors on chondrocytes.[124] No effects have been reported on TNF or its receptors. Collagenase production and articular damage have been reduced in animal models.[125-127] Early human clinical trials have shown improved pain scores as compared to placebo and comparable efficacy to NSAIDs but slower onset of action. Diarrhea is the main potential side effect. On the strength of these prior trials, diacerein has been proposed as a slow-acting symptom-modifying and perhaps structure- or disease-modifying drug for OA.

A double-blind, randomized, placebo-controlled trial looking at the efficacy and safety of diacerein in OA of the knee enrolled 484 patients with symptomatic knee OA.[128] They were randomized to receive placebo, diacerein (25 mg twice a day), diacerein (50 mg twice a day), or diacerein (75 mg twice a day). Using intent-to-treat analysis, diacerein (100 mg/day) was significantly superior to placebo (p < 0.05) by the primary end point, patients' assessment of pain on movement at week 24 (−18.3 ± 19.3 mm vs. −10.9 ± 19.3 mm). It was also superior by WOMAC and disability scores. However, no statistical difference was detected in the primary end point between placebo and 50 mg/day diacerein (−15 ± 21.0 mm) or 150 mg/day diacerein (−14.3 ± 23.7 mm).

There have also been investigations into the potential structure- or disease-modifying attributes of diacerein in OA.[129] Patients (n = 507) with OA of the hip (according to American College of Rheumatology [ACR] criteria) were randomized to receive either diacerein (50 mg p.o. b.i.d.) or placebo for 3 years. Patients were followed with yearly pelvic radiographs to assess for hip joint space. Using completer analysis, the diacerein patients showed a significantly lower rate of radiographic progression (.18 mm/yr vs. .23 mm/year). Using intent-to-treat analysis, a smaller proportion of those taking diacerein had significant joint space loss (defined as loss of 0.5 mm of joint space or more) during the study (50.7 vs. 60.4 percent).

Unfortunately, almost 50 percent of the patients failed to complete the 3-year study. In the placebo group, the principal reason for discontinuation was lack of efficacy, whereas in the diacerein group, it was adverse effects such as diarrhea. Curiously, the symptom-relieving effect of diacerein observed in prior studies could not be confirmed in this one.

Additional areas for future intervention in OA include growth factor and cytokine manipulation.[130] Cytokines, such as IL-1 and TNF-α, are produced by the synovium and contribute to the inflammation within the OA joint.[131] Moreover, there might be deficient expression of naturally occurring anti-inflammatory compounds such as IL-1 receptor antagonist (IL-1Ra) by the chondrocytes of patients with OA.[132] In some, increased NO production by OA articular chondrocytes may inhibit IL-1Ra synthesis.[133]

In a dog model of OA, IL-1Ra therapy has been shown to reduce expression of collagenase-1 in cartilage.[134] The severity of cartilage lesions is also diminished.[135] In a rabbit model of OA, transfer of the IL-1Ra gene to joints has prevented OA progression.[136] The effect of IL-1 blockade in humans with OA through the use of IL-1Ra is currently being investigated.

Induction of repair in partial-thickness articular cartilage lesions by timed release of transforming growth factor-β (TGF-β) using liposomes has been attempted in an animal model. There was an increase in the cellularity of the defects. These were populated by cells of mesenchymal origin from the synovial membrane. The appearance of the repaired cartilage resembled hyaline cartilage, and its integrity persisted up to 1 year after surgery.[137] Combination therapy is another alternative. In a study of canine induced OA, sodium pentosan polysulfate, when combined with insulin-like growth factor I (IGF-I), reduced stromelysin activity and increased TIMP.[138]

Attempts at gene therapy have proceeded as well. The control of genes such as TIMP and MMPs would, in theory, provide the opportunity to modulate the patient's disease. As previously noted, gene expression of IL-1Ra has already been tried in rabbits and dogs, as well as in an equine model of OA using an adenovirus vector.[139] Use of gene transfer–mediated overexpression of IL-1β decoy receptor (IL-1RII) has also been contemplated.[140]

Chondrocyte and stem cell transplants into articular cartilage defects have been tried as well. Chondrocytes transplanted (expressing previously transfected beta-galactosidase gene) into human cartilage explants survived up to 45 days in vitro in one trial.[141] Transfection of chondrocytes with the galactosidase gene has been successful both before and after the transplantation.

SURGICAL INTERVENTION IN OSTEOARTHRITIS

Surgical interventions in OA usually are in the form of osteotomies or joint replacements. Osteotomies can be effective pain-relieving interventions and can delay the need for joint-replacement surgery in selected patients. These tend to be younger subjects with OA.

Joint-replacement surgery (joint arthroplasty) is effective in providing pain relief and restoring function in many patients with OA. Hip and knee joint replacements are most common. Indications for surgery include symptomatology (i.e., pain) that is refractory to the previoulsy discussed interventions and significant impairment of the patient's daily life secondary to the OA and its symptoms. Therefore, patients should be the key decision makers as they are the ones that can relate the severity of symptoms and impairment.

If deciding to undergo replacement surgery, the patient should be deemed able to undertake the rehabilitation necessary to regain reasonable use of the joint involved. Infections are rare but do occur. Joint replacements have a typical life span of between 10 and 15 years. Revision surgery may be necessary, particularly in a relatively young patient who outlives the useful life span of the prosthesis.

Other potential rationales for surgical intervention in OA include removal of loose bodies, stabilization of joints, redistribution of joint forces (e.g., osteotomy), and relief of neural impingement (e.g., spinal stenosis, herniated disk). The value of arthroscopic debridément or lavage in OA has been questioned. A recent randomized, blinded trial failed to demonstrate significant symptomatic benefit in OA of the knee.

▌ Conclusion

In summary, the treatment of OA includes a variety of possible nonpharmacologic and pharmacologic interventions. Treatment should be tailored to the individual and will consist of a combination of available modalities. These provide symptom relief but have no proven effect on the progression of disease.

Structure and disease modification has yet to be achieved in OA. Trials underway, could provide an answer as to whether this is a realistic goal. Claims of

structure or disease modification in OA should not be made for any drugs until well-designed, double-blind, placebo-controlled trials demonstrate this.

Some of the drugs being tested for structure and disease modification, however, could provide symptom relief and could add to our armamentarium in that capacity, even if not successful as structure- or disease-modifying agents.

REFERENCES

1. Lawrence JS, Bremmer JM, Bier F: Osteo-arthrosis: prevalence in the population and relationship between symptoms and x-ray changes. Ann Rheum Dis 25:1-24, 1966.
2. Peyron JG, Altman RD: The epidemiology of osteoarthritis. In Moskowitz RW, Howell DS, Goldberg M, Mankin HI (eds): Osteoarthritis: Diagnosis and Medical/Surgical Management. 2nd ed. Philadelphia, WB Saunders, 1992, pp 15-37.
3. Lozada CJ, Altman RD: Osteoarthritis: A comprehensive approach to management. J Musculoskeletal Med 14:26-38, 1997.
4. Hochberg MC, Altman RD, Brandt RD, et al: Guidelines for the medical management of osteoarthritis. I. Osteoarthritis of the hip. Arthritis Rheum 38:1535-1540, 1995.
5. Hochberg MC, Altman RD, Brandt KD, et al: Guidelines for the medical management of osteoarthritis. II: Osteoarthritis of the knee. Arthritis Rheum 38:1541-1546, 1995.
6. American College of Rheumatology Subcommittee on osteoarthritis guidelines: Recommendations for the medical management of osteoarthritis of the hip and knee: 2000 update. Arthritis Rheum 43:1905-1915, 2000.
7. Lozada CJ, Altman RD: Management of osteoarthritis. In Koopman WJ (ed): Arthritis and Allied Conditions. 13th ed. Baltimore, Williams & Wilkins, 1997, pp 2013-2025.
8. Coggon D, Reading I, Croft P, et al: Knee osteoarthritis and obesity Int J Obes Relat Metab Disord 25:622-627, 2001.
9. Sturmer T, Gunther KP, Brenner H: Obesity, overweight and patterns of osteoarthritis: The Ulm Osteoarthritis Study. J Clin Epidemiol 53:307-313, 2000.
10. Cooper C, Snow S, McAlindon TE, et al: Risk factors for the incidence and progression of radiographic knee osteoarthritis. Arthritis Rheum 43:995-1000, 2000.
11. Sharma L, Lou C, Cahue S, Dunlop DD: The mechanism of the effect of obesity in knee osteoarthritis: The mediating role of malalignment. Arthritis Rheum 43:568-575, 2000.
12. Messier SP, Loeser RF, Mitchell MN, et al: Exercise and weight loss in obese older adults with knee osteoarthritis: A preliminary study. J Am Geriatr Soc 48:1062-1072, 2000.
13. Felson DT, Zhang Y, Anthony JM, et al: Weight loss reduces the risk for symptomatic knee osteoarthritis in women. Ann Intern Med 116:535-539, 1992.
14. Toda Y, Toda T, Takemura S, et al: Change in body fat, but not body weight or metabolic correlates of obesity, is related to symptomatic relief of obese patients with knee osteoarthritis after a weight control program. J Rheumatol 25:2181-2186, 1998.
15. Swezey RL: Essentials of physical management and rehabilitation in arthritis. Semin Arthritis Rheum 3:349-368, 1974.
16. Lehman JF, DeLateur BJ: Diathermy and superficial heat, laser, and cold therapy. In Kottke FJ, Lehman JF (eds): Krusen's Handbook of Physical Medicine and Rehabilitation, 4th ed. Philadelphia, WB Saunders, 1990, pp 283-367.
17. Slemenda C, Heilman DK, Brandt KD, et al: Reduced quadriceps strength relative to body weight: A risk factor for knee osteoarthritis in women? Arthritis Rheum 41:1951-1959, 1998.
18. Bentley G, Dowd G: Current concepts of etiology and treatment of chondromalacia patellae. Clin Orthop 189:209-228, 1984.
19. Topp R, Woolley S, Hornyak J III, et al: The effect of dynamic versus isometric resistance training on pain and functioning among adults with osteoarthritis of the knee. Arch Phys Med Rehabil 83(9):1187-1195, 2002.

20. Kovar PA, Allegrante JP, MacKenzie R, et al: Supervised fitness walking in patients with osteoarthritis of the knee. Ann Int Med 116:529-534, 1992.

21. Thomas KS, Muir KR, Doherty M, et al: Home based exercise programme for knee pain and knee osteoarthritis: Randomised controlled trial. BMJ 325:752, 2002.

22. Belza B, Topolski T, Kinne S, et al: Does adherence make a difference? Results from a community-based aquatic exercise program. Nurs Res 51:285-291, 2002.

23. Kerrigan DC, Lelas JL, Goggins J, et al: Effectiveness of a lateral-wedge insole on knee varus torque in patients with knee osteoarthritis. Arch Phys Med Rehabil 83:889-893, 2002.

24. Keating EM, Faris PM, Ritter MA, Kane J: Use of lateral heel and sole wedges in the treatment of medial osteoarthritis of the knee. Orthop Rev 22:921-924, 1993.

25. Pollo FE, Otis JC, Backus SI, et al: Reduction of medial compartment loads with valgus bracing of the osteoarthritic knee. Am J Sports Med 30:414-421, 2002.

26. Cushnaghan J, McCarthy C, Dieppe P: Taping the patella medially: A new treatment for osteoarthritis of the knee joint? BMJ 308:753-755, 1994.

27. Ohsawa S, Ueno R: Heel lifting as a conservative therapy for osteoarthritis of the hip: Based on the rationale of Pauwels' intertrochanteric osteotomy. Prosthet Orthot Int 21:153-158, 1997.

28. Berggren M, Joost-Davidsson A, Lindstrand J, et al: Reduction in the need for operation after conservative treatment of osteoarthritis of the first carpometacarpal joint: A seven year prospective study. Scand J Plast Reconstr Surg Hand Surg 35:415-417, 2001.

29. Brand RA, Crowninshield RD: The effect of cane use on hip contact force. Clin Orthop 147:181-184, 1980.

30. Blount WP: Don't throw away the cane. J Bone Joint Surg Am 38:695-708, 1956.

31. Osiri M, Welch V, Brosseau L, et al: Transcutaneous electrical nerve stimulation for knee osteoarthritis. Cochrane Database Syst Rev 4:CD002823, 2000.

32. Taylor P, Hallett M, Flaherty L: Treatment of osteoarthritis of the knee with transcutaneous electrical nerve stimulation. Pain 11:233-240, 1981.

33. Pipitone N, Scott DL: Magnetic pulse treatment for knee osteoarthritis: a randomised, double-blind, placebo-controlled study. Curr Med Res Opin 17:190-196, 2001.

34. Hinman MR, Ford J, Heyl H: Effects of static magnets on chronic knee pain and physical function: a double-blind study. Altern Ther Health Med 8:50-55, 2002.

35. White AR, Filshie J, Cummings TM: International Acupuncture Research Forum: Clinical trials of acupuncture: consensus recommendations for optimal treatment, sham controls and blinding. Complement Ther Med 9:237-245, 2001.

36. Tillu A, Tillu S, Vowler S: Effect of acupuncture on knee function in advanced osteoarthritis of the knee: A prospective, non-randomised controlled study. Acupunct Med 20:19-21, 2002.

37. Berman BM, Singh BB, Lao L, et al: A randomized trial of acupuncture as an adjunctive therapy in osteoarthritis of the knee. Rheumatology (Oxford) 38:346-354, 1999.

38. Ezzo J, Hadhazy V, Birch S, et al: Acupuncture for osteoarthritis of the knee: a systematic review. Arthritis Rheum 44:819-825, 2001.

39. Guillemin F, Virion JM, Escudier P, et al: Effect on osteoarthritis of spa therapy at Bourbonne-les-Bains. Joint Bone Spine 68:499-503, 2001.

40. Ernst E, Pittler MH: [How effective is spa treatment? A systematic review of randomized studies] Dtsch Med Wochenschr 123:273-277, 1998.

41. Garfinkel M, Schumacher HR Jr: Yoga. Rheum Dis Clin North Am 26:125-132, 2000.

42. Rains C, Bryson HM: Topical capsaicin: A review of its pharmacological properties and therapeutic potential in post-herpetic neuralgia, diabetic neuropathy and osteoarthritis. Drugs Aging 7:317-328, 1995.

43. McCarthy GM, McCarty DJ: Effect of topical capsaicin in the therapy of painful osteoarthritis of the hands. J Rheumatol 19:604-607, 1992.

44. Deal CL, Schnitzer TJ, Lipstein E, et al: Treatment of arthritis with topical capsaicin: A double-blind trial. Clin Ther 13(3):383-395, 1991.

45. Dreiser RL, Tisne-Camus M: DHEP plasters as a topical treatment of knee osteoarthritis: A double-blind placebo-controlled study. Drugs Exper Clin Res 19:117-123, 1993.

46. Rolf C, Engstrom B, Beauchard C, et al: Intra-articular absorption and distribution of ketoprofen after topical plaster application and oral intake in 100 patients undergoing knee arthroscopy. Rheumatology 38:564-567, 1999.

47. Goodman LS, Gilman A: The Pharmacological Basis of Therapeutics. New York, Pergamon Press, 1990.

48. Grace D, Rogers J, Skeith K, Anderson K: Topical diclofenac versus placebo: a double blind, randomized clinical trial in patients with osteoarthritis of the knee. J Rheumatol 26:2659-2663, 1999.

49. Sandelin J, Harilainen A, Crone H, et al: Local NSAID gel (eltenac) in the treatment of osteoarthritis of the knee: A double blind study comparing eltenac with oral diclofenac and placebo gel. Scand J Rheumatol 26:287-292, 1997.

50. Bradley JD, Brandt KD, Katz BP, et al: Comparison of an antiinflammatory dose of ibuprofen, an analgesic dose of ibuprofen, and acetaminophen in the treatment of patients with osteoarthritis of the knee. N Eng J Med 325:87-91, 1991.

51. Pincus T, Koch GG, Sokka T, et al: A randomized, double-blind crossover clinical trial of diclofenac plus misoprostol versus acetaminophen in patients with osteoarthritis of the hip or knee. Arthritis Rheum 44:1587-1598, 2001.

52. Abramson SB, Weissmann G: The mechanism of action of nonsteroidal antiinflammatory drugs. Arthritis Rheum 32:1, 1989.

53. Graham DY, Agrawal NM, Roth SH: Prevention of NSAID-induced gastric ulcer with misoprostol: multicenter, double-blind, placebo-controlled trial. Lancet 2:1277-1280, 1988.

54. Hawkey CJ, Karrasch JA, Szczepanski L, et al: Omeprazole compared with misoprostol for ulcers associated with nonsteroidal antiinflammatory drugs: Omeprazole versus Misoprostol for NSAID-induced Ulcer Management (OMINUM) Study Group. N Engl J Med 338:727-734, 1998.

55. Bombardier C, Laine L, Reicin A, et al: Comparison of upper gastrointestinal toxicity of rofecoxib and naproxen in patients with rheumatoid arthritis: VIGOR Study Group. N Engl J Med 343:1520-1528, 2000.

56. Silverstein FE, Faich G, Goldstein JL, et al: Gastrointestinal toxicity with celecoxib vs nonsteroidal anti-inflammatory drugs for osteoarthritis and rheumatoid arthritis: The CLASS study—randomized controlled trial: Celecoxib Long-term Arthritis Safety Study. JAMA 284:1247-1255, 2000.

57. Cheng Y, Austin SC, Rocca B, et al: Role of prostacyclin in the cardiovascular response to thromboxane A2. Science 296:539-541, 2002.

58. Mukherjee D, Nissen SE, Topol EJ: Risk of cardiovascular events associated with selective COX-2 inhibitors. JAMA 286:954-959, 2001.

59. Jovanovic DV, Fernandes JC, Martel-Pelletier J, et al: In vivo dual inhibition of cyclooxygenase and lipoxygenase by ML-3000 reduces the progression of experimental osteoarthritis: Suppression of collagenase 1 and interleukin-1beta synthesis. Arthritis Rheum 44:2320-2330, 2001.

60. Boileau C, Martel-Pelletier J, Jouzeau JY, et al: Licofelone (ML-3000), a dual inhibitor of 5-lipoxygenase and cyclooxygenase, reduces the level of cartilage chondrocyte death in vivo in experimental dog osteoarthritis: Inhibition of pro-apoptotic factors. J Rheumatol 29:1446-1453, 2002.

61. Raffa RB, Friederichs E, Reimann W, et al: Opioid and non-opioid components independently contribute to the mechanism of action of tramadol, an "atypical" opioid analgesic. Jour Pharmacol Exp Thera 260:275-285, 1992.

62. Katz WA: Pharmacology and clinical experience with tramadol in osteoarthritis. Drugs 52(Suppl 3):39-47, 1996.

63. Silverfield JC, Kamin M, Wu SC, et al: Tramadol/acetaminophen combination tablets for the treatment of osteoarthritis flare pain: a multicenter, outpatient, randomized, double-blind, placebo-controlled, parallel-group, add-on study. Clin Ther 24:282-297, 2002.

64. Roth SH: Efficacy and safety of tramadol HCl in breakthrough musculoskeletal pain attributed to osteoarthritis. J Rheumatol 25:1358-1363, 1998.

65. Goeringer KE, Logan BK, Christian GD: Identification of tramadol and its metabolites in blood from drug-related deaths and drug-impaired drivers. J Anal Toxicol 21:529-537, 1997.

66. Mullican WS, Lacy JR, and TRAMAP-ANAG-006 Study Group: Tramadol/acetaminophen combination tablets and codeine/acetaminophen combination capsules for the management of chronic pain: a comparative trial. Clin Ther 23:1429-1445, 2001.

67. Young L, Katrib A, Cuello C, et al: Effects of intraarticular glucocorticoids on macrophage infiltration and mediators of joint damage in osteoarthritis synovial membranes: Findings in a double-blind, placebo-controlled study. Arthritis Rheum 44:343-350, 2001.

68. Ravaud P, Moulinier L, Giraudeau B, et al: Effects of joint lavage and steroid injection in patients with osteoarthritis of the knee: results of a multicenter, randomized, controlled trial: Arthritis Rheum 42:475-482, 1999.

69. Centeno LM, Moore ME: Preferred intraarticular corticosteroids and associated practice: A survey of members of the American College of Rheumatology. Arthritis Care Res 7:151-155, 1994.

70. Peyron JG: Intraarticular hyaluronan injections in the treatment of osteoarthritis: state-of-the art review. J Rheumatol 20(Suppl 39):10-15, 1993.

71. Petrella RJ, DiSilvestro MD, Hildebrand C: Effects of hyaluronate sodium on pain and physical functioning in osteoarthritis of the knee: a randomized, double-blind, placebo-controlled clinical trial: Arch Intern Med 162:292-298, 2002.

72. Kuiper-Geertsma DG, Bijlsma JW: Intra-articular injection of hyaluronic acid as an alternative option to corticosteroid injections for arthrosis. Ned Tijdschr Geneeskd 144:2188-2192, 2000.

73. Leardini G, Mattara L, Franceschini M, Perbellini A: Intra-articular treatment of knee osteoarthritis: A comparative study between hyaluronic acid and 6-methyl prednisolone acetate. Clin Exp Rheumatology 9:375-381, 1991.

74. Adams ME, Atkinson MH, Lussier AJ, et al: The role of viscosupplementation with hylan G-F 20 (Synvisc) in the treatment of osteoarthritis of the knee: A Canadian multicenter trial comparing hylan G-F 20 alone, hylan G-F 20 with non-steroidal antiinflammatory drugs (NSAIDs) and NSAIDs alone. Osteoarthritis Cartilage 3:213-225, 1995.

75. Altman RD, Moskowitz R: Intraarticular sodium hyaluronate (Hyalgan) in the treatment of patients with osteoarthritis of the knee: a randomized clinical trial—Hyalgan Study Group. J Rheumatol 25:2203-2212, 1998.

76. Jubb RJ, Piva S, Beinat I, et al: Structure modifying study of hyaluronan (500-730kDA Hyalgan) on osteoarthritis of the knee [Abstract #617]. Arthritis Rheum 44(9):S155, 2001.

77. Itokazu M, Matsunaga T: Clinical evaluation of high-molecular-weight sodium hyaluronate for the treatment of patients with periarthritis of the shoulder. Clin Ther 17:946-955, 1995.

78. Rovetta G, Monteforte P: Intraarticular injection of sodium hyaluronate plus steroid versus steroid in adhesive capsulitis of the shoulder. Int J Tissue React 20:125-130, 1998.

79. Karzel K, Domenjoz R: Effects of hexosamine derivatives and uronic acid derivatives on glycosaminoglycan metabolism of fibroblast cultures. Pharmacology 5:337-345, 1971.

80. Bassleer C, Reginster JY, Franchimont P: Effects of glucosamine on differentiated human chondrocytes cultivated in clusters [Abstract]. Rev Esp Reumatol 20(Suppl 1):96, 1993.

81. Shikhman AR, Kuhn K, Alaaeddine N, Lotz M: N-Acetylglucosamine prevents IL-1 beta-mediated activation of human chondrocytes. J Immunol 166(8):5155-5160, 2001.

82. Krajickova J, Macek J: Urinary proteoglycan degradation product excretion in patients with rheumatoid arthritis and osteoarthritis. Ann Rheum Dis 47(6):468-471, 1988.

83. Reichelt A, Forster KK, Fischer M, et al: Efficacy and safety of intramuscular glucosamine sulfate in osteoarthritis of the knee: A randomiscd, placebo-controlled, double-blind study. Arzneimittel Forschung-Drug Research 44:75-80, 1994.

84. Muller-Fabender H, Bach GL, Haase W, et al: Glucosamine sulfate compared to ibuprofen in osteoarthritis of the knee. Osteoarthritis Cartilage 2:61-69, 1994.

85. Hochberg MC: What a difference a year makes: reflections on the ACR recommendations for the medical management of osteoarthritis. Curr Rheumatol Rep 3:473-478, 2001.

86. Reginster JY, Deroisy R, Rovati LC, et al: Long-term effects of glucosamine sulphate on osteoarthritis progression: a randomised, placebo-controlled clinical trial. Lancet 357:251-256, 2001.

87. Pavelka K, Gatterova J, Olejarova M, et al: Glucosamine sulfate use and delay of progression of knee osteoarthritis: a 3-year, randomized, placebo-controlled, double-blind study. Arch Intern Med 162:2113-2123, 2002.

88. Mazzuca SA, Brandt KD, Surber J: Reduction of severe joint pain increases joint space width (JSW) in standing extended-view X-rays of patients with knee osteoarthritis (OA) [Abstract #614]. Arthritis Rheum 44(9):S155, 2001.

89. Mazieres B, Loyau G, Menkes CJ, et al: Chondroitin sulfate in the treatment of gonarthrosis and coxarthrosis: 5-month results of a multicenter double-blind controlled prospective study using placebo. Revue du Rhumatisme 59:466-472, 1992.

90. Morreale P, Manopulo R, Galati M, et al: Comparison of the antiinflammatory efficacy of chondroitin sulfate and diclofenac sodium in patients with knee osteoarthritis. J Rheumatol 23(8):1385-1391, 1996.

91. Das A Jr., Hammad TA: Efficacy of a combination of FCHG49 glucosamine hydrochloride, TRH122 low molecular weight sodium chondroitin sulfate and manganese ascorbate in the management of knee osteoarthritis. Osteoarthritis Cartilage 8:343-350, 2000.

92. Srivasta KC, Mustafa T: Ginger (Zingiber officinale) in rheumatism and musculoskeletal disorders. Med Hypotheses 39(4):342-348, 1992.

93. Swain AR, Duton SP, Truswell AS: Salicylates in foods. J Am Diet Assoc 85:950-960, 1985.

94. Mustafa T, Srivastava KC, Jensen KB: Drug development: Report 9. Pharmacology of ginger, Zingiber officinale. J Drug Dev 6:25-89, 1993.

95. Altman RD, Marcussen KC: Effects of a ginger extract on knee pain in patients with osteoarthritis. Arthritis Rheum 44:2531-2538, 2001.

96. Henroitin YE, Labasse AH, Jaspar JM, et al: Effects of three avocado/soybean unsaponifiable mixtures on metalloproteinases, cytokines and prostaglandin E2 production by human articular chondrocytes. Clin Rheumatol 17:31-39, 1998.

97. Maheu E, Mazieres B, Valat JP, et al: Symptomatic efficacy of avocado/soybean unsaponifiables in the treatment of osteoarthritis of the knee and hip: A prospective, randomized, double-blind, placebo-controlled, multicenter clinical trial with six-month treatment period and two-month follow-up demonstrating a persistent effect. Arthritis Rheum 41:81-91, 1998.

98. Lequesne M, Maheu E, Cadet C, et al: Effect of avocado/soya unsaponifiables (ASU) on joint space loss in hip osteoarthritis (HOA) over 2 years: A placebo controlled trial: Arthritis Rheum 39(Suppl 9):S227, 1996.

99. Piscoya J, Rodriguez Z, Bustamante SA, et al: Efficacy and safety of freeze-dried cat's claw in osteoarthritis of the knee: Mechanisms of action of the species Uncaria guianensis. Inflamm Res 50:442-448, 2001.

100. Nadanaka S, Clement A, Masayama K, et al: Characteristic hexasaccharide sequences in octasaccharides derived from shark cartilage chondroitin sulfate D with a neurite outgrowth promoting activity. J Biol Chem 273:3296-3307, 1998.

101. Barcelo HA, Wiemeyer JC, Sagasta CL, et al: Experimental osteoarthritis and its course when treated with S-adenosyl-L-methionine. Rev Clin Esp 187:74-78, 1990.

102. Montrone F, Fumagalli M, Sarzi Puttini P, et al: Double-blind study of S-adenosyl-methionine versus placebo in hip and knee arthrosis. Clin Rheumatol 4:484-485, 1985.

103. Bradley JD, Flusser D, Katz BP, et al: A randomized, double blind, placebo controlled trial of intravenous loading with S-adenosylmethionine (SAM) followed by oral SAM therapy in patients with knee osteoarthritis. J Rheumatol 21:905-911, 1994.

104. Altman R, Brandt K, Hochberg M, et al: Design and conduct of clinical trials in patients with osteoarthritis: recommendations from a task force of the Osteoarthritis Research Society. Osteoarthritis Cartilage 4:217-243, 1996.

105. Lozada CJ, Altman RD: Chondroprotection in osteoarthritis. Bull Rheum Dis 46:5-7, 1997.

106. Brittberg M, Lindahl A, Nilsson A, et al: Treatment of deep cartilage defect in the knee with autologous chondrocyte transplantation. New Engl J Med 331:889-895, 1994.

107. Amin AR, Attur MG, Thakker GD, et al: A novel mechanism of action of tetracyclines: effects on nitric oxide synthases. Proc Natl Acad Sci USA 93:14014-14019, 1996.

108. Tilley BC, Alarcon GS, Heyse SP, et al: Minocycline in rheumatoid arthritis: A 48-week, double-blind, placebo-controlled trial. Ann Int Med 122:81-89, 1995.

109. Cole AD, Chubinskaya S, Luchene LJ, et al: Doxycycline disrupts chondrocyte differentiation and inhibits cartilage matrix degradation. Arthritis Rheum 32:1727-1734, 1994.

110. Yu LP Jr, Smith GN Jr, Hasty KA, Brandt KD: Doxycycline inhibits type XI collagenolytic activity of extracts from human osteoarthritic cartilage and of gelatinase. J Rheumatol 18(10): 1450-1452, 1991.

111. Brandt KD, Yu LP, Amith G, et al: Therapeutic effect of doxycycline (doxy) in canine osteoarthritis (OA). Osteoarthritis Cartilage 1:14, 1993.

112. Lewis EJ, Bishop J, Bottomley D, et al: Ro32-3555, an orally active collagenase inhibitor, prevents cartilage breakdown in vitro and in vivo. Br J Pharmacol 121:540-546, 1997.

113. Burkhardt D, Ghosh P: Laboratory evaluation of antiarthritic drugs as potential chondroprotective agents. Semin Arthritis Rheum 17(Suppl1):3-34, 1987.

114. Altman RD, Dean DD, Muniz OE, Howell DS: Prophylactic treatment of canine osteoarthritis with glycosaminoglycan polysulfuric acid ester. Arthritis Rheum 32:759-766, 1989.

115. Rejholec V: Long-term studies of antiosteoarthritic drugs: An assessment. Semin Arthritis Rheum 17(Suppl 1):35-53, 1987.

116. Pavelka K Jr., Sedlackova M, Gatterova J, et al: Glycosaminoglycan polysulfuric acid (GAGPS) in osteoarthritis of the knee. Osteoarthritis Cartilage 3(1):15-23, 1995.

117. Moskowitz RW, Reese JH, Young RG, et al: The effects of Rumalon, a glycosaminoglycan peptide complex, in a partial meniscectomy model of osteoarthritis in rabbits. J Rheumatol 18:205-209, 1991.

118. Howell DS, Altman RD: Cartilage repair and conservation in osteoarthritis. Rheum Dis Clin North Am 19:713-724, 1993.

119. Pavelka K, Gatterova J, Gollerova V, et al: A 5-year randomized controlled, double-blind study of glycosaminoglycan polysulphuric acid complex (Rumalon) as a structure modifying therapy in osteoarthritis of the hip and knee. Osteoarthritis Cartilage 8:335-342 , 2000.

120. Golding JC, Ghosh P: Drugs for osteoarthrosis. I. The effects of pentosan polysulphate (SP54) on the degradation and loss of proteoglycans from articular cartilage in a model of osteoarthrosis induced in the rabbit knee joint by immobilization. Curr Ther Res 32:173-184, 1983.

121. Smith MM, Ghosh P, Numata Y, et al: The effects of orally administered calcium pentosan polysulfide on inflammation and cartilage degradation produced in rabbit joints by intra-articular injection of a hyaluronate-polylysine complex. Arthritis Rheum 37:125-136, 1994.

122. Innes JF, Barr AR, Sharif M: Efficacy of oral calcium pentosan polysulphate for the treatment of osteoarthritis of the canine stifle joint secondary to cranial cruciate ligament deficiency. Vet Rec 146:433-437, 2000.

123. Spencer CM, Wilde MI: Diacerein. Drugs 53:98-108, 1997.

124. Martel-Pelletier J, Mineau F, Jolicoeur FC, et al: In vitro effects of diacerhein and rhein on interleukin 1 and tumor necrosis factor-alpha systems in human osteoarthritic synovium and chondrocytes. J Rheumatol 25:753-762, 1998.

125. Carney SL, Hicks CA, Tree B, Broadmore RJ: An in vivo investigation of the effect of anthraquinones on the turnover of aggrecans in spontaneous osteoarthritis in the guinea pig. Inflamm Res 44:182-186, 1995.

126. Brun PH: Effect of diacetylrhein on the development of experimental osteoarthritis: A biochemical investigation [Letter]. Osteoarthritis Cartilage 5:289-291, 1997.

127. Brandt K, Smith G, Kang SY, et al: Effects of diacerein in an accelerated canine model of osteoarthritis. Osteoarthritis Cartilage 5:438-449, 1997.

128. Pelletier JP, Yaron M, Haraoui B, et al: Efficacy and safety of diacerein in osteoarthritis of the knee. Arthritis Rheum 43:2339-2348, 2000.

129. Dougados M, Nguyen M, Berdah L, et al: Evaluation of the structure-modifying effects of diacerein in hip osteoarthritis: ECHODIAH, a three-year, placebo-controlled trial: Evaluation of the Chondromodulating Effect of Diacerein in OA of the Hip. Arthritis Rheum 44:2539-2547, 2001.

130. Pelletier JP, Roughley PJ, DiBattista JA, et al: Are cytokines involved in osteoarthritic pathophysiology? Semin Arthritis Rheum 20(Suppl 2):12-25, 1991.

131. Smith MD, Triantafillou S, Parker A, et al: Synovial membrane inflammation and cytokine production in patients with early osteoarthritis. J Rheumatol 24:365-371, 1997.

132. Attur MG, Dave M, Cipolletta C, et al: Reversal of autocrine and paracrine effects of interleukin 1 (IL-1) in human arthritis by type II IL-1 decoy receptor: Potential for pharmacological intervention. J Biol Chem 275:40307-40315, 2000.

133. Pelletier JP, Mineau F, Ranger P, et al: The increased synthesis of inducible nitric oxide inhibits IL-1ra synthesis by human articular chondrocytes: possible role in osteoarthritic cartilage degradation. Osteoarthritis Cartilage 4:77-84, 1996.

134. Caron JP, Fernandes JC, Martel-Pelletier J, et al: Chondroprotective effect of intraarticular injections of interleukin-1 receptor antagonist in experimental osteoarthritis: Suppression of collagenase-1 expression. Arthritis Rheum 39:1535-1544, 1996.

135. Pelletier JP, Caron JP, Evans C, et al: In vivo suppression of early experimental osteoarthritis by interleukin-1 receptor antagonist using gene therapy. Arthritis Rheum 40:1012-1019, 1997.

136. Fernandes J, Tardif G, Martel-Pelletier J, et al: In vivo transfer of interleukin-1 receptor antagonist gene in osteoarthritic rabbit knee joints: prevention of osteoarthritis progression. Am J Pathol 154:1159-1169, 1999.

137. Hunziker EB, Rosenberg L: Induction of repair in partial thickness articular cartilage lesions by timed release of TGF-beta. Transactions of the 40th Annual Meeting of the Orthopaedic Research Society. Vol.19. Sec.1.236, 1994.

138. Rogachefsky RA, Dean DD, Howell DS, Altman RD: Treatment of canine osteoarthritis with insulin-like growth factor-1 (IGF-1) and sodium pentosan polysulfate. Osteoarthritis Cartilage 1: Orthopaedic Research Society, Rosemont, IL 105-114, 1993.

139. Frisbie DD, Ghivizzani SC, Robbins PD, et al: Treatment of experimental equine osteoarthritis by in vivo delivery of the equine interleukin-1 receptor antagonist gene. Gene Ther 9: 12-20, 2002.

140. Attur MG, Dave MN, Leung MY, et al: Functional genomic analysis of type II IL-1beta decoy receptor: potential for gene therapy in human arthritis and inflammation. J Immunol 168: 2001-2010, 2002.

141. Doherty PJ, Zhang H, Tremblay L, et al: Resurfacing of articular cartilage explants with genetically-modified human chondrocytes in vitro. Osteoarthritis Cartilage 6:153-159, 1998.

142. Moseley JB, O'Malley K, Petersen NJ, et al: A controlled trial of arthroscopic surgery for osteoarthritis of the knee. N Engl J Med 347:81-88, 2002.

94

Relapsing Polychondritis

JEAN-CHARLES PIETTE · PHILIPPE VINCENEUX

Definition and Criteria

Relapsing polychondritis is a rare, long-lasting, and potentially life-threatening disorder characterized by recurrent inflammatory episodes affecting the cartilaginous structures of the external ears, nose, larynx, and tracheobronchial tree, sometimes leading to their destruction.[1-5] Systemic manifestations involving auricles, eyes, skin, inner ears, and vessels are frequently associated. Among several sets of clinical diagnostic criteria,[1-3] the most commonly used are listed in Table 94-1. Biopsy confirmation is not required for diagnosis, except for atypical cases.

Epidemiology

Since its first description by Jaksch-Wartenhorst in 1923, less than 800 cases of polychondritis have been published, including two series of 100 or more.[3,6] Epidemiologic data are scarce. Most of reported patients are Caucasians, but the disease has been found in all ethnic groups. Though polychondritis may develop at any age,[5,7] it usually occurs in mid-adulthood, with a mean age of onset of 43 years, slightly higher in men. Sex distribution is usually said to be equal, but a female predominance has been reported in recent series,[4,6] leading to a female-to-male ratio of 1.2:1 established on 600 patients. Familial cases are extremely rare.[8] The maternofetal transmission of polychondritis, reported only once,[9] has never occurred in our experience[10]

Pathophysiology

The etiology of polychondritis remains unknown. A history of mechanic insult to cartilage is infrequent. Cartilage destruction by degradative enzymes is supported by peculiar animal models[8] and by electron microscopic studies.[11] Their release is thought to result from autoimmune reactions. The pathogenetic role of the immune system is suggested by the presence of a lymphocytic infiltrate and of immune deposits in tissue lesions,[1,8,12] humoral[13-17] and cell-mediated[18,19] responses to cartilage components, frequent overlaps with various autoimmune disorders, and principally by recent advances on animal models. Polychondritis has been induced in rats and mice by immunization with type II collagen[20,21] or with matrilin-1, a noncollagenous cartilage matrix protein.[22] The importance of the genetic background is attested by a double-transgenic mouse model[21] and by the association of human polychondritis with human leukocyte antigen (HLA)-DR4.[23] Finally, a two-step process has been suggested, the starter of which remains to be determined among matrilin-1, type II collagen, or other proteins.[20,24]

Clinical Features

The onset of polychondritis is usually abrupt, with highly variable presenting manifestations including isolated general symptoms.[1,18] The occurrence of chondritis may be delayed from months to years.[4] Table 94-2 indicates the main cumulative clinical features.

TABLE 94–1 · EMPIRICAL DIAGNOSTIC CRITERIA FOR RELAPSING POLYCHONDRITIS*

Major Criteria

Proven inflammatory episodes involving auricular cartilage
Proven inflammatory episodes involving nasal cartilage
Proven inflammatory episodes involving laryngotracheal cartilage

Minor Criteria

Ocular inflammation (conjunctivitis, keratitis, episcleritis, uveitis)
Hearing loss
Vestibular dysfunction
Seronegative inflammatory arthritis

*Diagnosis is made by two major criteria or one major and two minor. Histologic examination of affected cartilage is not required.

From Michet CJ Jr., McKenna CH, Luthra HS, O'Fallon WM: Relapsing polychondritis. Survival and predictive role of early disease manifestations. Ann Intern Med 104:74-78, 1986.

TABLE 94–2 · MAIN CUMULATIVE CLINICAL FEATURES OF RELAPSING POLYCHONDRITIS*

Feature	Frequency (%)
Auricular chondritis	85
Nasal chondritis	65
Laryngotracheobronchial chondritis	48
Costal chondritis	38
Arthropathy	78
Ocular inflammation	60
Fever 38° C or higher	38
Hearing loss	33
Dermatologic manifestations	33
Cardiovascular manifestations	30
Vestibular dysfunction	22
Renal involvement	13

*Compiled from published series and our personal experience, totaling more than 500 patients. Data should be regarded as approximations.

CHONDRITIS

Auricular chondritis is a key manifestation and is rarely absent in the course of the disease. Acute episodes manifest with pain, tenderness, swelling, warmth, and marked redness affecting the helix, antihelix, or sometimes tragus on one or both sides, but sparing the soft lobule, which lacks cartilage. Attacks resolve spontaneously or with treatment within days, but relapses invariably occur sooner or later, their features being attenuated by steroids. Recurrent inflammation may lead to permanent sequelae: either a drooping, "cauliflower" ear or more frequently an induration of the pinna (Fig. 94-1). A prior history of inflammatory episodes is necessary to confirm the diagnosis of chondritis in patients with a "flat" auricle, devoid of its normal relief.

Nasal chondritis is far less obvious than auricular chondritis during acute episodes. Symptoms are restricted to nose pain, tenderness, mild swelling, and infrequent redness, sometimes accompanied by fullness, crusting, rhinorrhea, and rare epistaxis. On the contrary, a suggestive saddle-nose deformity resulting from cartilage collapse (Fig. 94-2) may progressively develop in the absence of patent prior acute attacks, especially in women.[3,25]

Laryngeal, tracheal, or bronchial chondritis, which may extend to the subsegmental level, are frequently associated together and worsen the patient's prognosis.[1,5,25-28] Laryngeal chondritis is responsible for hoarseness or aphonia, tenderness over the thyroid cartilage, and inspiratory dyspnea with stridor. Subglottic stenosis mainly occurs in women[3] and may require emergency tracheostomy. Tracheobronchial manifestations (i.e., cough,

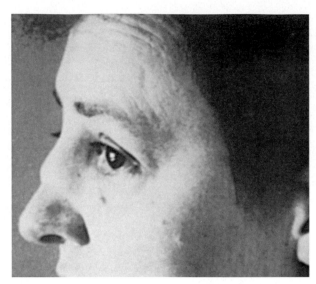

FIGURE 94-2 · Destruction of the nasal cartilage in a patient with relapsing polychondritis, creating the characteristic "saddle-nose" deformity. (From McKay DAR, Watson PG, Lyne AJ, et al: Relapsing polychondritis and eye disease. Br J Ophthalmol 58:600, 1974.)

chest pain, expiratory dyspnea, wheezing, and frequent infections due to inability to clear secretions) are nonspecific. When polychondritis presents with isolated lower respiratory tract involvement, the diagnosis may be delayed by months.[29] Severe respiratory failure resulting from permanent stenoses, expiratory collapse, or both due to tracheobronchomalacia may lead to death.

Costal chondritis provokes localized parietal pain and costochondral tumefactions, but it rarely results in depression of the anterior chest wall.[30]

OTHER MANIFESTATIONS

Aside from chondritis, diverse symptoms may occur as presenting features or later in the disease course.

Joint manifestations vary from arthralgias to an oligo- or polyarthritis, either acute and episodic and migratory or, less frequently, chronic, nonerosive, nondeforming, and not accompanied by nodules.[31-33] Peripheral arthropathy is usually asymmetric and mainly affects the wrists, metacarpophalangeal and proximal interphalangeal joints, elbows, knees, ankles, and parasternal joints. Synovial fluid may be paucicellular. Tenosynovitis and other para-articular manifestations are common, as are cervical or lumbar inflammatory pain.[31] The presence of radiographic abnormalities on peripheral joints or spine is infrequent and suggestive of an overlap, mainly with spondylarthropathies[34] or rheumatoid arthritis (RA).[23,35]

Eye involvement results from polychondritis itself or from associated Sjögren's syndrome (SS).[36,37] Recurrent episcleritis and scleritis or conjunctivitis are more frequent than keratitis or uveitis. Vision is rarely threatened by retinal vasculitis, optic neuropathy, or necrotizing scleritis. Frank proptosis obligates the clinician to rule out Wegener's granulomatosis (WG) and lymphoma.[38]

Audiovestibular manifestations are frequent.[2] Hearing impairment may result from stenosis of the external

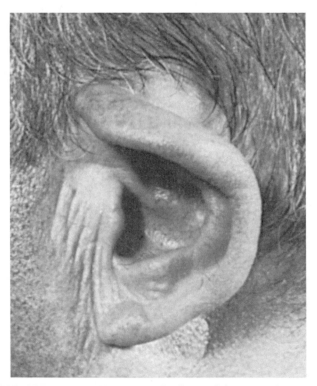

FIGURE 94-1 · Distortion and collapse of the external ear in a patient with relapsing polychondritis.

auditory meatus, otitis media caused by eustachian tube chondritis, or more specifically from neurosensory lesions due to vasculitis of the internal auditory artery. In the latter, deafness is abrupt, uni- or bilateral, of variable magnitude, accompanied by buzzing, and inconstantly reverses under prompt high-dose steroids. Transient vertigo may be associated or may occur independently.

Vascular involvement is uncommon but extremely diverse and frequently multifocal. It carries a negative prognosis. Acquired inflammatory aneurysms usually affecting the ascending thoracic aorta may progressively develop late in the course of polychondritis.[39-43] Large arteries at various sites may also be affected by aneurysms, stenosis, or both.[44] A microvasculitic process sometimes involves the skin; organs such as kidney, brain, sclera, inner ear, or testes; or both.[3,39,45] Its implication in most cases of polychondritis remains disputed. Thrombophlebitis is occasionally related to antiphospholipid antibodies.[46]

Cardiac lesions include aortic failure due to dilated aortic annulus associated with ascending aortic aneurysms, mitral valve failure (sometimes resulting from active inflammation), steroid-sensitive conduction disturbances, myocarditis, pericarditis, and coronary aneurysms.[1,3,41,43,47-49]

Dermatologic manifestations consist of oral or complex aphthosis, nodules, purpura, papules, sterile pustules, superficial phlebitis, livedo, ulcerations, and distal necrosis.[6] Histologic findings include leukocytoclastic vasculitis, neutrophil infiltrates, or thrombosis. These lesions frequently occur in association with myelodysplasia,[6] and sometimes resemble those of Behçet's syndrome. The acronym "MAGIC Syndrome" (mouth and genital ulcers with inflamed cartilage) has been proposed for this overlap.[50,51]

Kidney involvement, attested by microscopic hematuria, proteinuria, and sometimes severe loss of renal function, is usually attributed by biopsy to a crescenting pauci-immune glomerulonephritis within an accompanying micropolyangiitis.[45] Less frequently, immune complex nephritis is related to overlapping systemic lupus or cryoglobulinemia.

Neurologic manifestations consist of peripheral or cranial neuropathies, hemiplegia, seizures, rhombencephalitis, and lymphocytic or aseptic neutrophilic meningitis.[52,53]

Flares are accompanied by fever, asthenia, weight loss, and sometimes liver or lymph node enlargement.[1]

The clinical picture may be modified by various associated conditions such as thyroiditis or ulcerative colitis.[4]

▌ Laboratory Findings

To date, the contribution of laboratory findings to diagnosis remains limited. A major elevation of acute-phase reactants and erythrocyte sedimentation rate (ESR) is observed during flares, with few exceptions, associated with mild to moderate anemia of chronic disease, leukocytosis, and thrombocytosis.[1,5] Polyclonal elevation of serum immunoglobulin A (IgA), IgG, or IgM is not rare. Tests for rheumatoid factors (RFs) or antinu-

clear antibodies (ANAs) may be positive, but high titers suggest an overlap with RA, SS, or systemic lupus erythematosus (SLE).[4,23,54,55] Antineutrophil cytoplasmic antibodies (ANCAs) devoid of proteinase 3–specificity are present in some patients.[56] Antibodies to cartilage detected by indirect fluorescence staining are not routinely determined.[13] Though initially claimed sensitive and specific,[14] tests for antibodies to type II collagen have limited clinical significance.[20] Preliminary data on antibodies to matrilin-1 appear promising, but require confirmation.[16,17]

Histologic examination of an affected cartilage, mainly auricular, is considered suggestive when it shows the association of degenerative changes with the presence of an inflammatory infiltrate (Fig. 94-3). The infiltrate containing cell determinant (CD)4+ lymphocytes, macrophages, polymorphonuclear cells, and capillaries penetrate the cartilage from its outer surface to its depth.[1,8,12] Loss of basophilic staining of the matrix reflects proteoglycan depletion. Chondrocytes become vacuolated and die. The destroyed cartilage is replaced by fibrous tissue in which calcification or even ossification may occur. Degenerative changes are commonly found in normal subjects aged 40 or older, and the biopsy must be performed during an acute flare to objectivate the infiltrate.

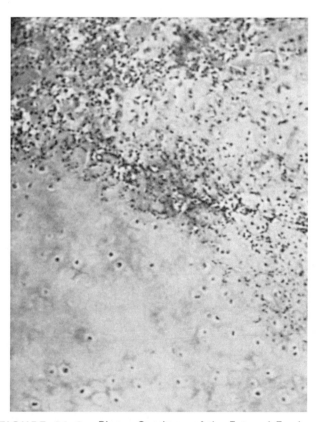

FIGURE 94–3 · Biopsy Specimen of the External Ear in a Patient with Relapsing Polychondritis. Specimen demonstrates necrotizing chondritis with inflammatory cell infiltrate, depletion of matrix proteoglycans, chondrocyte degeneration, and fibrosis. (Original magnification, ×400.) (From Herman JH, Dennis MV: Immunopathologic studies in relapsing polychondritis. J Clin Invest 52:549, 1973; by copyright permission of the American Society for Clinical Investigation.)

Acquired myelodysplasia frequently occurs in males with late-onset polychondritis.[6,57,58] Chronic macrocytic nonregenerative anemia requiring regular tranfusions is sometimes accompanied by leukopenia and thrombocytopenia. Myeloproliferative disorders and other forms of hematologic malignancies have also been reported.[3,38]

Differential Diagnosis

Auricular chondritis is frequently misdiagnosed as infectious perichondritis, although infection does not spare the lobule and occurs in peculiar circumstances.[2,8] Confusing aspects of the auricle may be observed in leprosy, leishmaniasis, and after repeated traumas in rugby players.

A saddle-nose deformity may result from congenital syphilis, direct trauma, nasal septal perforation, and mainly WG. Rare differential diagnoses of nasal chondritis include the recessive genetic defect affecting expression of the transporter associated with antigen-presentation genes[59] and two pediatric disorders: the chronic infantile neurologic cutaneous and articular syndrome (CINCA)[60] and an autosomal, dominant degenerative chondropathy.[61]

Lower respiratory tract involvement may be confused with asthma or chronic bronchitis. Stenoses occur in amyloidosis, sarcoidosis, inflammatory bowel disorders (IBDs), tracheobronchopathia osteochondroplastica, rhinoscleroma in endemic areas, and mainly WG.[62,63]

Arterial involvement shares similarities with those of closely related Takayasu's arteritis, Behçet's disease, and Cogan's syndrome.[40,50] Involvement of the aortic root also occurs in Marfan or Ehlers-Danlos syndrome, syphilis, medial cystic necrosis, or spondylarthropathies.[49]

Taken altogether, WG remains the main differential diagnosis of polychondritis. Both disorders share acquired saddle-nose deformity, subglottic stenosis, scleritis, and sometimes audiovestibular involvement or pauci-immune glomerulopathy. Furthermore, auricular chondritis has been described in WG,[45] and proptosis or nasal septum perforation in polychondritis.[44] Key features suggestive of WG are pansinusitis, parenchymal lung involvement, mononeuritis multiplex, granulomatous vasculitis, and ANCAs directed to proteinase 3. Conversely, diffuse tracheomalacia is a distinctive feature of polychondritis. Although these disorders are distinct entities, their frontiers remain imprecise, and overlaps probably exist.[39,64,65]

Evaluation, Course, and Prognosis

Evaluation of airway disease is of major importance. Pulmonary function tests using forced inspiratory and expiratory flow volume-loop studies quantify the deficit and localize the structures involved.[26,28] Tracheobronchoscopy may worsen hypoxia and even lead to death.[26,28] In most cases, it should be replaced by computed tomography (CT) or magnetic resonance imaging (MRI).[26,27,66,67] Reconstruction techniques, including virtual endoscopy, and dynamic studies easily visualize the respiratory tree without the hazards of real endoscopy.

Routine echocardiograms check the valves and ascending aorta. Repeated vascular imaging is needed in patients with large artery involvement, given that lesions are frequently multiple and tend to recur.[40,43] The use of nontraumatic methods, such as MRI angiograms, prevents the development of false aneurysms induced by arterial puncture.[50]

The course of polychondritis is highly variable. Disease remains smoldering in a minority of patients, whereas most experience flares affecting cartilage, joints,[33] or vessels independently,[40] and very few undergo a progressive downhill course refractory to therapy. Although durable remissions may occur, polychondritis rarely evolves to extinction. Pregnancy has no influence on disease activity.[10] The discrimination between tracheobronchial flare and superimposed infection may be difficult, given that both may coexist. Functional impairment, either disease or treatment related, frequently develops with time.

The severity of prognosis reflects the frequent requirement of high-dose steroids and the extreme duration of polychondritis. The 5- and 10-year probabilities of survival after diagnosis were 74 and 55 percent, respectively, in a Mayo Clinic series.[3] Recent data[4] and our experience are much more encouraging. The leading causes of death are airway obstruction, pneumonia, or both in women and specific cardiovascular involvement in men.[3,5] In patients less than 51 years old, saddle-nose deformity and systemic vasculitis were the worst prognostic factors.[3] For older patients, only anemia predicted outcome. Indeed, survival is limited when repeated transfusions are required for myelodysplasia.[57]

Treatment

Systemic treatment is empirical and should be adapted to disease activity and severity.[4] Minor cases may respond to nonsteroidal anti-inflammatory drugs (NSAIDs), colchicine, or dapsone.[4,5,68] Prednisone remains the cornerstone for a majority of patients. Initial doses vary from 0.5 to 1 mg/kg/day. Methylprednisolone "pulses" (1 g/day for 3 days) are used in frank respiratory flares, recent neurosensorial hearing loss, or systemic microvasculitis.[69] Progressive tapering is frequently limited by the requirement for substantial maintenance doses. Combined immunosuppression is indicated either initially, in severe respiratory or vasculitic involvement, or secondarily to improve disease control and allow steroid tapering. Methotrexate (0.3 mg/kg/week) is frequently effective[4,70] and carries no risk of secondary myelodysplasia. Cyclophosphamide, azathioprine, chlorambucil, and mycophenolate mofetil have also been used, as has cyclosporine in cases of preexisting cytopenias.[1,4,5,44,45,71] In our experience, cyclophosphamide is more potent. Infliximab has been recently reported to be effective in two cases,[72] but our results in six patients with refractory polychondritis have been disappointing. Such patients, who do not respond to plasmapheresis or high-dose Igs, might be candidates for experimental regimens such as toleragens[7] or autologous stem cell transplantation.[73]

Focal steroid treatment includes eye drops, intra-articular injections, and inhaled steroids sometimes associated with ephedrine.[74] Propanolol is used empirically to limit aortic dilatation. Airway obstruction may require tracheostomy, mechanic ventilation, tracheal surgery, or stenting.[26,29,75,76] Sustained disease control allows successful nasal reconstruction. The initial fair results of heart or arterial surgery are frequently jeopardized in the long term by valve desinsertion or relapsing aneurysms that occur despite immunosuppression.[39-41,49,50] A careful preoperative anesthesia evaluation is mandatory.[77]

■ Summary and Conclusion

Although early recognition and conventional management have improved the prognosis of relapsing polychondritis in the last decade, a better comprehension of its pathophysiology is needed to elaborate targeted intervention.

REFERENCES

1. McAdam LP, O'Hanlan MA, Bluestone R, Pearson CM: Relapsing polychondritis. Prospective study of 23 patients and a review of the literature. Medicine (Baltimore) 55:193-215, 1976.
2. Damiani JM, Levine HL: Relapsing polychondritis. Report of ten cases. Laryngoscope (St. Louis) 89:929-946, 1979.
3. Michet CJ Jr., McKenna CH, Luthra HS, O'Fallon WM: Relapsing polychondritis. Survival and predictive role of early disease manifestations. Ann Intern Med 104:74-78, 1986.
4. Trentham DE, Le CH: Relapsing polychondritis. Ann Intern Med 129:114-122, 1998.
5. Vinceneux P, Pouchot J, Piette JC: Polychondrite atrophiante. In Kahn MF, Peltier AP, Meyer O, Piette JC (eds): Maladies et Syndromes Systémiques. Paris, Flammarion Médecine-Sciences, 2000, pp 623-649.
6. Francès C, el Rassi R, Laporte JL, et al: Dermatologic manifestations of relapsing polychondritis. A study of 200 cases at a single center. Medicine (Baltimore) 80:173-179, 2001.
7. Navarro MJ, Higgins GC, Lohr KM, Myers LK: Amelioration of relapsing polychondritis in a child treated with oral collagen. Am J Med Sci 324:101-103, 2002.
8. Arkin CR, Masi AF: Relapsing polychondritis: review of current status and case report. Semin Arthritis Rheum 5:41-61, 1975.
9. Arundell FW, Haserick JR: Familial chronic atrophic polychondritis. Arch Dermatol 82:439-440, 1960.
10. Papo T, Wechsler B, Bletry O, et al: Pregnancy in relapsing polychondritis: twenty-five pregnancies in eleven patients. Arthritis Rheum 40:1245-1249, 1997.
11. Giroux L, Paquin F, Guerard-Desjardins MJ, Lefaivre A: Relapsing polychondritis: an autoimmune disease. Semin Arthritis Rheum 13:182-187, 1983.
12. Riccieri V, Spadaro A, Taccari E, Zoppini A: A case of relapsing polychondritis: pathogenetic considerations. Clin Exp Rheumatol 6:95-96, 1988.
13. Ebringer R, Rook G, Swana GT, et al: Autoantibodies to cartilage and type II collagen in relapsing polychondritis and other rheumatic diseases. Ann Rheum Dis 40:473-479, 1981.
14. Foidart JM, Abe S, Martin GR, et al: Antibodies to type II collagen in relapsing polychondritis. N Engl J Med 299:1203-1207, 1978.
15. Yang CL, Brinckmann J, Rui HF, et al: Autoantibodies to cartilage collagens in relapsing polychondritis. Arch Dermatol Res 285:245-249, 1993.
16. Buckner JH, Wu JJ, Reife RA, et al: Autoreactivity against matrilin-1 in a patient with relapsing polychondritis. Arthritis Rheum 43:939-943, 2000.
17. Hansson AS, Heinegard D, Piette JC, et al: The occurrence of autoantibodies to matrilin 1 reflects a tissue-specific response to

18. Alsalameh S, Mollenhauer J, Scheuplein F, et al: Preferential cellular and humoral immune reactivities to native and denaturated collagen types IX and XI in a patient with fatal relapsing polychondritis. J Rheumatol 20:1419-1424, 1993.
19. Buckner JH, Van Landeghen M, Kwok WW, Tsarknaridis L: Identification of type II collagen peptide 261-273-specific T cell clones in a patient with relapsing polychondritis. Arthritis Rheum 46:238-244, 2002.
20. Cremer MA, Rosloniec EF, Kang AH: The cartilage collagens: a review of their structure, organization, and role in the pathogenesis of experimental arthritis in animals and in human rheumatic disease. J Mol Med 76:275-288, 1998.
21. Bradley DS, Das P, Griffiths MM, et al: HLA-DQ6/8 double transgenic mice develop auricular chondritis following type II collagen immunization: a model for human relapsing polychondritis. J Immunol 161:5046-5053, 1998.
22. Hansson AS, Heinegard D, Holmdahl R: A new animal model for relapsing polychondritis, induced by cartilage matrix protein (matrilin-1). J Clin Invest 104:589-598, 1999.
23. Zeuner M, Straub RH, Rauh G, et al: Relapsing polychondritis;clinical and immunogenetic analysis of 62 patients. J Rheumatol 24:96-101, 1997.
24. Hansson AS, Holmdahl R: Cartilage-specific autoimmunity in animal models and clinical aspects in patients-focus on relapsing polychondritis. Arthritis Res 4:296-301, 2002.
25. McCaffrey TV, McDonald TJ, McCaffrey LA: Head and neck manifestations of relapsing polychondritis: review of 29 cases. Otolaryngology 86:473-478, 1978.
26. Eng J, Sabanathan S: Airway complications in relapsing polychondritis. Ann Thorac Surg 51:686-692, 1991.
27. Davis SD, Berkmen YM, King T: Peripheral bronchial involvement in relapsing polychondritis: demonstration by thin-section CT. AJR 153:953-954, 1989.
28. Tillie-Leblond I, Wallaert B, Leblond D, et al: Respiratory involvement in relapsing polychondritis. Clinical, functional, endoscopic, and radiographic evaluations. Medicine (Baltimore) 77:168-176, 1998.
29. Sarodia BD, Dasgupta A, Mehta AC: Management of airway manifestations of relapsing polychondritis: case reports and review of literature. Chest 116:1669-1675, 1999.
30. Lim MC, Chan HL: Relapsing polychondritis–a report on two Chinese patients with severe costal chondritis. Ann Acad Med Singapore 19:396-403, 1990.
31. O'Hanlan M, McAdam LP, Blueston R, et al: The arthropathy of relapsing polychondritis. Arthritis Rheum 19:191-194, 1976.
32. Balsa A, Espinosa A, Cuesta M, et al: Joint symptoms in relapsing polychondritis. Clin Exp Rheumatol 13:425-430, 1995.
33. Gunaydin I, Daikeler T, Jacki S, et al: Articular involvement in patients with relapsing polychondritis. Rheumatol Int 18:93-96, 1998.
34. Pazirandeh M, Ziran BH, Khandelwal BK, et al: Relapsing polychondritis and spondylarthropathies. J Rheumatol 15:630-632, 1988.
35. Rajace A, Voossoghi AA: Classical rheumatoid arthritis associated with relapsing polychondritis. J Rheumatol 16: 1263-1265, 1989.
36. Isaak BL, Liesegang TJ, Michet CJ Jr.: Ocular and systemic findings in relapsing polychondritis. Ophthalmology 93:681-689, 1986.
37. Letko E, Zafirakis P, Baltatzis S, et al: Relapsing polychondritis: a clinical review. Semin Arthritis Rheum 31:384-395, 2002.
38. Lichauco JJ, Lauer S, Shigemitsu HH, et al: Orbital mucosa-associated lymphoid tissue (MALT)-type lymphoma in a patient with relapsing polychondritis. Arthritis Rheum 44:1713-1715, 2001.
39. Michet CJ Jr.: Vasculitis and relapsing polychondritis. Rheum Dis Clin North Am 16:441-444, 1990.
40. Piette JC, Vinceneux P, Francès C: Vascular manifestations in relapsing polychondritis. In Asherson RA, Cervera R, Abramson S, et al (eds): Vascular Manifestations of Systemic Autoimmune Diseases. Boca Raton, Fla., CRC Press, 2001, pp 351-359.
41. DelRosso A, Petix NR, Pratesi M, Bini A: Cardiovascular involvement in relapsing polychondritis. Semin Arthritis Rheum 26: 840-844, 1997.
42. Selim AG, Fulford LG, Mohiaddin RH, Sheppard MN: Active aortitis in relapsing polychondritis. J Clin Pathol 54:890-892, 2001.

43. Barretto SN, Oliveira GH, Michet CJ Jr., et al: Multiple cardiovascular complications in a patient with relapsing polychondritis. Mayo Clin Proc 77:971-974, 2002.

44. Esdaile J, Hawkins D, Gold P, et al: Vascular involvement in relapsing polychondritis. Canad Med Assoc J 116:1019-1022, 1977.

45. Chang-Miller A, Okamura M, Torres VE, et al: Renal involvement in relapsing polychondritis. Medicine (Baltimore) 66:202-217, 1987.

46. Empson M, Adelstein S, Garsia R, Britton W: Relapsing polychondritis presenting with recurrent venous thrombosis in association with anticardiolipin antibody. Lupus 7:132-134, 1998.

47. Bowness P, Hawley IC, Dearden A, Walport MJ: Complete heart block and severe aortic incompetence in relapsing polychondritis;clinicopathologic findings. Arthritis Rheum 34:97-100, 1991.

48. Buckley LM, Ades PA: Progressive aortic valve inflammation occurring despite apparent remission of relapsing polychondritis. Arthritis Rheum 35:812-814, 1992.

49. Lang-Lazdunski L, Hvass U, Paillole C, et al: Cardiac valve replacement in relapsing polychondritis: a review. J Heart Valve Dis 4:227-235, 1995.

50. Le Thi Huong D, Wechsler B, Piette JC, et al: Aortic insufficiency and recurrent valve prosthesis dehiscence in MAGIC syndrome. J Rheumatol 20:397-398, 1993.

51. Imai H, Motegi M, Mizuki N, et al: Mouth and Genital Ulcers with Inflamed Cartilage (MAGIC Syndrome): A case report and literature review. Am J Med Sci 314:330-332, 1997.

52. Hanslik T, Wechsler B, Piette JC , et al: Central nervous system involvement in relapsing polychondritis. Clin Exp Rheumatol 12:539-541, 1994.

53. Kothare SV, Chu CC, VanLandingham K, et al: Migratory leptomeningeal inflammation with relapsing polychondritis. Neurology 51:614-617, 1998.

54. Kitridou RC, Wittmann AL, Quismorio FP: Chondritis in systemic lupus erythematosus: clinical and immuno-pathologic studies. Clin Exp Rheumatol 5:349-353, 1987.

55. Piette JC, El-Rassi R, Amoura Z: Antinuclear antibodies in relapsing polychondritis. Ann Rheum Dis 58:656-657, 1999.

56. Papo T, Piette JC, Le Thi Huong D, et al: Antineutrophil cytoplasmic antibodies in polychondritis. Ann Rheum Dis 52:384-385, 1993.

57. Piette JC, Papo T, Chavanon P, et al: Myelodysplasia and relapsing polychondritis. J Rheumatol 22:1208-1209, 1995.

58. Diebold J, Rauh G, Jäger K, Löhrs U: Bone marrow pathology in relapsing polychondritis: high frequency of myelodysplastic syndromes. Br J Haematol 89:820-830, 1995.

59. Moins-Teisserenc HT, Gadola SD, Cella M, et al: Association of a syndrome resembling Wegener's granulomatosis with low surface expression of HLA class-I molecules [erratum in Lancet 356:170, 2000]. Lancet 354:1598-1603, 1999.

60. Prieur AM, Griscelli C, Lampert F, et al: A chronic, infantile, neurological, cutaneous and articular (CINCA) syndrome. A specific entity analysed in 30 patients. Scand J Rheumatol 66(Suppl): 57-68, 1987.

61. Kurien M, Seshadri MS, Zacharia A: Inherited degenerative chondropathy-an autosomal dominant new clinical entity: report on two cases and follow-up of four cases. J Laryngol Otol 109: 433-436, 1995.

62. Loehrl TA, Smith TL: Inflammatory and granulomatous lesions of the larynx and pharynx. Am J Med 111(Suppl 8A):113S-117S, 2001.

63. Prince JS, Duhamel DR, Levin DL, et al: Nonneoplastic lesions of the tracheobronchial wall: radiologic findings with bronchoscopic correlation [erratum in Radiographics 23:191, 2003]. Radiographics 22(Spec No):S215-S230, 2002.

64. Case records of the Massachusetts General Hospital (Case 26-1985). N Engl J Med 312:1695-1703, 1985.

65. Cauhape P, Aumaitre O, Papo T, et al: A diagnostic dilemna: Wegener's granulomatosis, relapsing polychondritis or both? Eur J Med 2:497-498, 1993.

66. Behar JV, Choi YW, Hartman TA, et al: Relapsing polychondritis affecting the lower respiratory tract. Am J Roentgenol 178: 173-177, 2002.

67. Heman-Ackah YD, Remley KB, Goding GS Jr.: A new role for magnetic resonance imaging in the diagnosis of laryngeal relapsing polychondritis. Head Neck 21:484-489, 1999.

68. Barranco VP, Minor DB, Solomon M: Treatment of relapsing polychondritis with dapsone. Arch Dermatol 112:1286-1288, 1976.

69. Lipnick RN, Fink CW: Acute airway obstruction in relapsing polychondritis: treatment with pulse methylprednisolone. J Rheumatol 18:98-99, 1991.

70. Park J, Gowin KM, Schumacher HR Jr.: Steroid sparing effect of methotrexate in relapsing polychondritis. J Rheumatol 23: 937-938, 1996.

71. Svenson KLG, Holmdahl R, Klareskog L, et al: Cyclosporin A treatment in a case of relapsing polychondritis. Scand J Rheumatol 13:329-333, 1984.

72. Saadoun D, Deslandre CJ, Allanore Y, et al: Sustained response to infliximab in 2 patients with refractory relapsing polychondritis. J Rheumatol 30:1394-1395, 2003.

73. Rosen O, Thiel A, Massenkeil G, et al: Autologous stem-cell transplantation in refractory autoimmune diseases after in vivo immunoablation and ex vivo depletion of mononuclear cells. Arthritis Res 2:327-336, 2000.

74. Gaffney RJ, Harrison M, Blayney AW: Nebulized racemic ephedrine in the treatment of acute exacerbations of laryngeal relapsing polychondritis. J Laryngol Otol 106:63-64, 1992.

75. Adliff M, Ngato D, Keshavjee S, et al: Treatment of diffuse tracheomalacia secondary to relapsing polychondritis with continuous positive airway pressure. Chest 112:1701-1704, 1997.

76. Dunne JA, Sabanathan S: Use of metallic stents in relapsing polychondritis. Chest 105:864-867, 1994.

77. Biro P, Rohling R, Schmid S, et al: Anesthesia in a patient with acute respiratory insufficiency due to relapsing polychondritis. J Clin Anesth 6:59-62, 1994.

Heritable Disorders of Structural Proteins

JAY R. SHAPIRO · DAVID ROWE · PAUL SPONSELLER

The heritable disorders of connective tissue are the result of genetic defects that alter the quantity or structure of extracellular matrix proteins. These diseases, originally defined by McKusick,[1] primarily affect the musculoskeletal systems, including bone, tendon and ligaments, and the connective tissue matrix in several organs such as the eye, heart valve, blood vessels, and the lung. Mutations involving several extracellular matrix proteins have been associated with these disorders. These include specific collagens (osteogenesis imperfecta [OI], Ehlers-Danlos syndrome [EDS]), fibrillins (Marfan syndrome [MFS]), elastin (pseudoxanthoma elazticum), and other noncollagenous extracellular matrix proteins and proteoglycans. The inborn metabolic disorder homocystinuria is the result of alterations in the synthesis of sulfoproteins and is grouped with heritable disorders of connective tissue because of the shared phenotype due to involvement of bone and ligament matrix.

The enhanced understanding of these disorders has been the direct result of advances in molecular biology and protein chemistry that have identified these components of the extracellular matrix and defined mutations in their genes. The application of new techniques involving transgenic animal models is providing unparalleled insight into the basic function of matrix gene products, including transcription factors, growth and differentiating factors, and cytokines that independently and interactively modulate connective tissue development and organization. The challenge in the future will be to relate the mutation of a specific gene to a clinical phenotype, with the hope that understanding the pathophysiologic impact of the mutation will lead to rational therapeutic strategies. Although we currently lack that insight, therapies have been developed to ameliorate many of the clinical problems expressed in individuals with these disorders.

The goal of this chapter is to relate principles of connective tissue biology to the heritable disorders that occur when a mutation disrupts function of an essential component of the extracellular matrix. The basic elements of extracellular matrix biochemistry and gene structure are presented in Chapters 2 and 3.

Biochemical, Molecular, and Cellular Aspects of Heritable Disorders of Connective Tissue

RELATION OF COLLAGEN AND OTHER MATRIX MOLECULES TO HERITABLE DISORDERS

Collagens contribute to the structural integrity and function of several organs, including the eye, heart muscle and valves, blood vessels (including the great vessels), skeletal muscle, ligaments, tendons, intervertebral disk, the interstitium of the kidneys, and the cartilage lining of joints. Defects in these organs are expressed in the clinical phenotype as a consequence of defective extracellular matrix synthesis. The family of collagen proteins is large and diverse, with 20 distinct collagen types recognized, representing 38 separate genes dispersed among 12 chromosomes.[2-4] The collagen proteins are divided into two major classes, fibrillar collagens and nonfibrillar collagens.[5] The fibrillar group includes types I, II, III, V, and XI collagens. The proteins provide structural support to bone, ligaments, tendons, muscle bundles, skin, blood vessels, and heart valve and nerves. The fibrous capsules of many organs are composed of fibrillar collagens. Nonfibrillar collagens include fibril-associated collagens (types IX, XII, and XIV), basement membrane collagens (types IV and VII), and short-chain collagens (types VIII and X). Type XIII collagen has been identified at the genomic level, but its function is unknown. Type VI collagen has three α-chains that are largely noncollagenous with a short triple-helical domain.[5]

This bewildering array of proteins is further diversified through mechanisms of alternative splicing of segments of the transcribed gene or through the use of alternative promoters that transcribe a separate ribonucleic acid (RNA). Functional adaptation is further achieved as major collagen types are modified by the association with minor collagens and noncollagenous proteins in the extracellular matrix. This concept, that the primary protein is modified by specialized or minor collagens, portrays the connective tissue as an alloy of a number of components assembled to meet

TABLE 95–1 • COLLAGEN TYPES GROUPED INTO FAMILIES OF PROTEINS WITH COMMON STRUCTURAL PROPERTIES

Functional Component	Type I Family (Tensile CT)	Type II Family (Compressive CT)	Type IV Family (Barrier CT)
Primary collagen	I(2^3)*	II(1,as^4)	IV(5$^{5-7}$)
Integral with primary protein	V(3)	XI(3)	
Surrounding the primary protein	XII(1^8)	IX(2,ap^9)	
Anchoring	VI(3, as^{10,11})	VI(as)	VII(1)
Specialized tissue distribution	III(1)—in viscera and blood vessels Elastin (as^{12})—microfibrilin	X(1^{13})—in hypertrophic chondrocytes	VIII(1^{14})—in blood vessels, neural tissue
Uncertain	XII(as^{15})		Short chain^{16}

*The number within the parentheses is the number of genetically distinct chains that comprise the collagen molecule; (as) indicates that the messenger RNA is alternatively spliced; and (ap) indicates an alternative promoter.

Abbreviation: CT, Connective tissue.

the functional demands of a specific connective tissue. These requirements include tensile strength, resistance to compressive forces, and a barrier-filtration function typified by collagen types IV in the glomerular basement membrane (Table 95–1).

Connective tissues providing the tensile strength of skin, tendons, and ligaments are represented by the type I collagen family. Within the fibers of type I collagen are small amounts of type V collagen,[6] and type XII collagen is distributed on the surface of the fiber bundles.[7] Collagen type VI is distributed throughout this matrix and is thought to help anchor interstitial collagen to surrounding structures. The diversity of structural properties within this family of collagens is achieved by interaction with noncollagenous proteins. For example, the matrix proteoglycan decorin is bound to collagen[8] and may function by binding transforming growth factor-β (TGF-β) molecules to the surface of the fiber.[9] In bone, the presence of noncollagen matrix proteins, such as phosphoprotein and osteocalcin, permits the accumulation of highly ordered plates of hydroxyapatite (HA) crystals that give bone the properties of reinforced concrete. Type III collagen in visceral tissues and blood vessels is associated with connective tissue of smooth muscle cells. The second structural demand of connective tissue is resistance to compressive forces, such as those that occur in intervertebral disks and joints. The intervertebral disk contains predominately types I and II collagens, but types V, VI, IX, XI XII, and XIV also contribute to disk matrix.[10] Type II collagen has been identified in the nucleolus pulposus of intervertebral disks. Type II collagen is the major constituent of articular cartilage, and its fibers are modified by association with types XI and type IX collagens.[11] It is also a major component of the nose, auricle of the ear, and the vitreous of the eye.

Similar to members of the type I collagen family, type VI collagen is distributed throughout cartilage, allowing anchoring of this tissue to surrounding structures. Type X collagen, a short-chain collagen, is primarily expressed by hypertrophic chondrocytes at the epiphyseal growth plate of long bones. It is considered to play a role in the late stages of endochondral ossification.

The third function of connective tissue is to provide a barrier between cell types, yet still allow the passage of molecules. This filtration function is met by the basement membrane, which is composed primarily of type IV collagen with types XV and XVIII collagens also present.[12] Type IV collagen forms a complex scaffold that serves as a framework for basement membrane. This collagen interacts with a variety of noncollagenous components, including laminin and heparin sulfate proteoglycan. A short-chain collagen has been identified in basement membrane, and it may be analogous to the minor collagens that interact with the fibrillar collagen types I and II. Type VII collagen has the important function of anchoring basement membrane to adjacent tissues. Type VIII collagen may represent a specialized component that is present primarily in blood vessels and neural tissue. The functions of these collagens underscore the alloy nature of connective tissues within the basement membrane,[13] occurring in tissues as diverse as the cornea of the eye, the endothelium of a blood vessel, and the glomerulus of the kidney, where they are involved in filtration.

Beyond the structural properties of each collagen family, the extracellular matrix responds to the environment of tissue and the cells it supports. The important aspects of this interaction are detailed in Chapter 3 and include the noncollagenous components such as fibronectin, tenascin, and proteoglycans in the interstitial space and the family of heterodimeric cell surface receptors, the integrins.[14] A new class of collagen molecule (types XV and XVII) was discovered in which a portion is buried within the surface of the cell and the helical domain extends out from the cell. Type XV and type XVIII collagens are classified as part of multiplexin collagen superfamily and their C-terminal parts, endostatin and restin, respectively, have been shown to be antiangiogenic in vivo and in vitro. Nonvascular basement membranes are mainly one of two types: type XVIII in subepithelial basement membranes and type XV in skeletal and cardiac muscles. Basement membranes surrounding smooth muscle cells in vascular tissues contain one or both of these collagens, depending on their location.[15]

In an undefined manner, the extracellular matrix changes to meet growth and repair of tissue by relaying signals back to the cells through transmembrane integrin receptors. Biologic function is encoded within the primary sequence of the structural proteins. The complexity of function represented in the connective tissue proteins includes short protein sequences within an extracellular matrix protein interacting with cell-surface integrin receptors to alter the state of differentiation of the cells, growth factor–like signals to specific cells,[14] and components of the blood-clotting cascade. It can be anticipated that mutations within genes that encode such diversity of structural and biologic functions will present as highly pleomorphic clinical phenotypes.

RELATION OF MOLECULAR CONTROL OF COLLAGEN BIOSYNTHESIS TO CLINICAL DISEASE

The synthesis of type I collagen and the diseases that result from defects in this pathway have become the paradigm for studying mutations affecting all the fibrillar collagens and will be useful in approaching mutations of those collagens with more complex and interrupted structures. Mutations in collagen genes or deficiencies in specific enzymes catalyzing post-translational or extr cellular modifications of collagen protein have been described in several disorders, including OI, several chondrodysplasias, subtypes of EDS, the X-linked Alport syndrome, and forms of epidermolysis bullosa.[16] Collagen mutations have been reported in a limited number of patients with apparent juvenile osteoporosis and in patients who have familial aortic aneurysm.[17,18] Families with early-onset osteoarthritis (OA) as a manifestation of underlying chondrodysplasia express COL2A1 gene mutations.[19] However, several studies have failed to reveal type I collagen mutations in individuals with idiopathic (familial) osteoporosis.[20]

COLLAGEN SYNTHESIS

The type I collagen genes that code for the 1 and 2 procollagen chains are present as one allele per haploid set of chromosomes. Compared to other mammalian genes, both type I collagen genes are large, complex, and distributed throughout 50 or 51 exons. The level of activity of the collagen gene is determined by its promoter, which contains DNA elements responsive to a wide variety of transcriptional factors (Fig. 95–1, step 1). These elements are located at the distal end of the coding region of the gene (5′ upstream region) and within the body of the gene (intron sequence).[21] Analysis of the regulatory domains of the collagen promoter in transgenic mice has revealed that different type I collagen–producing cells use different regions of the collagen promoter. An element required for expression primarily in bone can be distinguished from one that is active in tendon, skin, and vascular smooth muscle. This may explain how a single collagen gene is expressed in such divergent ways in different cell types.

The initial collagen messenger RNA (mRNA) transcribed is an exact copy of the gene containing both introns and exons (see Fig. 95–1, step 2). In keeping

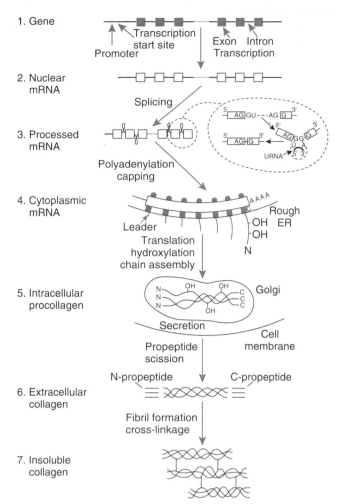

FIGURE 95–1 · Steps of Collagen Biosynthesis Relevant to the Heritable Diseases of Collagen. The structure of the gene *(step 1)* is represented by darkened squares for the exons and by a line for the introns. The RNAs *(steps 2 to 4)* are represented by open squares. See text for the narrative description. mRNA, messenger ribonucleic acid.

with the composition of the type I heterodimer, $[\alpha1(I)]$, $\alpha2(I)$, twice as much 1(I) as 2(I) mRNA is transcribed from each gene.[22] The intervening sequences are removed through a splicing mechanism similar to those in other eukaryotic mRNAs.[23] The recognition sequences at the boundaries of the intron exon junction are complementary to a small nuclear RNAs (U 1–6 RNAs) that identify each exon and act to bring the ends of the introns into alignment for removal and subsequent joining of the adjacent exons (see Fig. 95–1, step 3). The entire intron sequence must be removed, because its presence would alter the reading frame of the RNA or substitute inappropriate amino acids into the encoded protein. In those cases in which the reading frame is altered, a stop codon prior to the terminal exon (premature stop codon) is encountered. Premature stop codons also can be introduced as a point mutation within an exon. In either case, this type of mutation leads to rapid destruction of the RNA by a recently described cellular process called nonsense-mediated RNA decay.[24,25] This process appears to be an important mechanism for preventing a truncated

TABLE 95–2 • CLASSIFICATION OF MUTATIONS OF TYPE I COLLAGEN BASED ON FUNCTIONAL CONSEQUENCE OF THE PRODUCTION OF COLLAGEN PROTEIN

Null Mutations*	Helix-Disrupting Mutations
Inactivation of transcription control sequences	Gene deletion removing complete exons and producing a truncated chain
Gene deletion or duplication of partial exons producing a frame shift	Gene duplication adding complete exons
Splicing that results in an RNA that is out of frame or that contains premature stop codons	Exon skipping secondary to abnormal splicing
Increased rate of collagen mRNA degradation	Activation of cryptic splice sites that produce a retained in-frame intron sequence
Mutations that prevent incorporation of α_1(I)-chain into the molecule	Point mutation of first position of Gly-codons of the Gly-X-Y triplet

*Null mutations produce a reduced quantity of a structurally normal product, whereas mutations within the coding domains of the gene can result in a protein with abnormal structure or function.

protein from expression, thus saving the cell from proteins with unintended function. The net result is a reduction of normal mRNA productively synthesized from the affected allele. Such a defect is considered a "regulatory" mutant because it results in a nonfunctional, or null, allele (Table 95–2). Small amounts of collagen are synthesized, but the collagen produced from the remaining normal allele is structurally normal.[26] Other examples of regulatory mutations include those altering sequences in the promoter and large gene deletions.

Upon reaching the rough endoplasmic reticulum, mRNA is translated into a polypeptide α-chain (see Fig. 95–1, step 4). Abnormalities in the primary sequence of the mRNA include a base change that codes for a premature stop codon in the terminal exon. All the amino acids beyond the frame-shift mutations required for the collagen chain to assemble into the collagen triple helix are altered, rendering the mutant allele null.

POST-TRANSLATIONAL MODIFICATION AND CHAIN ASSEMBLY

As the collagen mRNA is translated, certain prolyl residues become hydroxylated, and specific lysines are hydroxylated and then glycosylated (see Fig. 95–1, steps 4 and 5). The hydroxyproline residues appear to enhance the stability of the collagen triple helix at physiologic temperatures. Prolyl hydroxylase has been cloned, and its activity parallels the rate of collagen synthesis. Lysyl hydroxylase acts on lysine residues important for the formation of stable interchain cross-links in bone and cartilage. The function of the glycosylated hydroxylysine, or the heterosaccharide unit of the C-terminal propeptide, is uncertain. Polyl and lysyl hydroxylases act on nascent procollagen chains and are unable to hydroxylate after the procollagen chain assumes the helical conformation. Excessive lysyl hydroxylation is associated with mutations that impair the rate of helix formation.

Within the Golgi apparatus, the individual procollagen chains initiate self assembly from the C-terminal propeptide toward the N-terminal end[27] (see Fig. 95–1, step 5). There is a highly conserved region within the C-terminal propeptide in all the collagen α-chains that is essential for initial chain alignment and subsequent assembly. A mutation in this region of the molecule inhibits incorporation of the abnormal chain into the triple helix and reduces total collagen synthesis (i.e., null mutation).[28]

The most common mutation of the collagen gene associated with a clinical disease is a single base substitution, particularly affecting the first position glycine residues of the Gly-X-Y triplet. Glycine residues permit the polypeptide chain to maintain the tight helical conformation. The replacement of this glycine molecule as a result of a point mutation in the glycine codon interferes with the formation of the triple helix[29] or induces a kink within the helical domain.[30] Molecules that contain such a defect are slow to assemble, are poorly secreted, and have an increased susceptibility to tissue proteases. Mutations of this type can lead to enhanced intracellular or interstitial degradation of collagen α-chains and a lower net rate of collagen production. The presence of an α-chain with impaired incorporation into the collagen helix appears to induce synthesis of intracellular chaperone proteins that may determine whether the mutant molecules are secreted or degraded intracellularly. The presence of the mutant α-chain compromises the function of the normal chains that associate with it. All molecules that interact with molecules containing the defective chain are compromised, which greatly amplifies the destructive effect of the mutant chain. Other examples of mutations that have similar adverse effects on helix stability and subsequently lead to protein suicide are deletion of a small region of the helical domain due to a small gene deletion or exon skipping and insertion of an extraneous helical[31] or nonhelical sequence due to a partial gene duplication or a mutation of splicing that retains a small sequence of intron[32] (see Table 95–2).

FIBER FORMATION AND CROSS-LINKING

The assembled procollagen molecule is secreted, followed by removal of the N- and C-terminal propeptides (see Fig. 95–1, step 6). Commercially available radio immunoassays for these propeptides have provided a valuable clinical tool for assessing rates of collagen synthesis in specific disorders, such as growth defects, or for assessing the response of collagen synthesis to hormonal intervention. Genetic defects involving the N-terminal propeptide region have been defined in humans and animals. In this situation, type VII EDS or dermatosparaxis in

TABLE 95–3 • SITES OF MUTATIONS THAT AFFECT THE QUANTITY AND QUALITY OF THE EXTRACELLULAR MATRIX

Mutation Site	Functional Consequence of the Mutation	Clinical Example (Recognized or Suspected)	Anticipated Inheritance
Primary gene defects	Abnormal structure	Small deletions or point mutations that disrupt the collagen fiber (OI and EDS IV)	Dominant or sporadic
	Decreased production	Reduced synthesis, but the product has normal structure (OI)	Dominant or sporadic heritability may not be recognized
Modifiers of gene activity	Excessive activity	?Keloids, gingival hyperplasia	Dominant or sporadic, may not be recognized
	Diminished activity	?Familial osteoporosis	?Probably only recognized in a recessive manner
Modifiers of collagen chains	Intracellular modifiers	Prolyl and lysyl hydroxlase hydroxlase (EDS VI)	Recessive
	Extracellular modifiers	Procollagen peptidases (EDS VII), lysyl oxidase (cutic laxa)	Recessive
Proteins that interact with collagen fibers	Collagen-like	Minor collagens	?Dominant
	Noncollagenous	Proteoglycans, fibronectin, elastin	?
	Cell-associated	Integrins	?

Abbreviations: EDS, Ehlers-Danlos syndrome; OI, osteogenesis imperfecta.

animals, a failure to cleave the N-terminal propeptide, interferes with the organization of the collagen fiber[33] (Table 95–3). Genetic defects involving removal of the C-terminal propeptide have not been reported.

The final step in the formation of a mature collagen fiber is the assembly of the individual molecules into the collagen polymer and its subsequent stabilization by intermolecular and intramolecular cross-links (see Fig. 95–1, step 7). The assembly process appears to be directed by information within exposed areas of the triple-helical molecule, because fiber formation can occur in vitro. The proper alignment of microfibrils is essential for the enzyme lysyl oxidase (LO) to initiate cross-link formation between adjacent molecules by converting the ε-amino group of exposed lysine residues to a chemically reactive aldehyde group. Mutations that disrupt helix alignment further weaken the connective tissue because of a deficiency in collagen cross-linking.[34] Agents that block cross-link formation (e.g., penicillamine, aminopropionitrile) result in enhanced tissue friability, bowing of the bones, and aortic aneurysms (i.e., lathyrism).

The gene for LO was cloned and localized to chromosome 5.[35] Previously, a number of X-linked disorders that resulted in impaired cross-link formation were thought to arise from a mutation within this enzyme. However, no genetic abnormality of cross-link formation has been demonstrated. Cross-links are initially bifunctional but become trifunctional with age, leading to a highly cross-linked structure. Commercial assays for these trifunctional cross-links, pyridinium and hydroxypyridinium, are widely used in clinical disorders to assess the turnover of a mature connective tissue. Assays are also available to measure a section of the N-telopeptide region adjacent to the pyridinoline cross-link as a indicator of tissue collagen turnover.[36] Nonenzymatic ligation with subsequent oxidation of ε-amino groups with glucose can further increase the

cross-linkage and insolubility of the collagen, which may account for the fibrosis and endothelial changes associated with aging and diabetes mellitus.[37] In the initial phase of this reaction, referred to as glycation, glucose reacts with the free amino group of proteins, resulting in Schiff base formation followed by rearrangement to an Amadori product. In human studies, glycation of collagen has been found to increase modestly with age and to be associated with decreased collagen solubility in several tissues.

Controlled removal of the extracellular matrix is essential to tissue remodeling during growth and wound repair. The earliest step in the removal of collagen is its scission at a specific site within the helical region by mammalian collagenase. Once cut, the helix unwinds and then becomes a substrate for other gelatinases and proteolytic enzymes. Failure to remove matrix can occur on a genetic basis, as in osteoporosis due to a defect in the maturation or activity of the osteoclast or when glycosylated collagen cross-links accumulate in patients with diabetes. An interesting theoretical mechanism was demonstrated experimentally in mice. A mutation was placed in the collagen helix at the site where mammalian collagenase acts. The mice developed a condition resembling systemic sclerosis.[38]

Genetic Aspects of Connective Tissue Diseases

PATTERN OF INHERITANCE

Dominant traits are recognized as a result of one allele's being affected, whereas recessive traits require that both alleles are affected. This separation becomes less distinct as individual traits are examined more closely, and heterozygous carriers of recessive traits have minor consequences. In general, for the connective tissue proteins, mutations that affect the structure or the amount of the extracellular matrix protein are inherited as dominant traits. In many cases, a strong dominant pedigree can be discerned within a family; when present, it is an asset to diagnosis. Similar mutations can arise spontaneously, however, and in this case, they can manifest in a sporadic manner without a prior dominant pedigree. Subsequent offspring, if biologically possible, would reveal the dominant character of the mutation. There is increasing realization that one normal parent can produce two or more severely affected individuals, suggesting a recessive inheritance pattern. However, molecular analysis has shown that such a pedigree usually results from germinal mosaicism in one parent rather than a recessively expressed codominant trait.[39]

IDENTIFYING NEW GENETIC LOCI

The remarkable progress in identifying new genes or unsuspected known genes that cause specific heritable disorders of connective tissue is based on studies using DNA linkage. In this procedure, a small segment of DNA that is unique to the entire genome is identified, and its presence or absence is scored within a pedigree or a population of individuals. If this segment is always present in individuals with a disorder and absent from those lacking the disorder, the DNA in proximity to the fragment is likely to harbor the locus causing the disorder. Because recombination between alleles can occur during meioses, a small number of individuals do not show linkage. The closer the unique fragment is to the disease locus, the more likely cosegregation will occur. A mathematic analysis is performed that yields a logarithm of the odds (lod) score that indicates the statistic probability that there is cosegregation of this DNA fragment to a disease or genetic trait. The higher the lod score, the closer the DNA fragment is to the disease locus.

The Human Genome Initiative has developed thousands of unique fragments and has mapped them to segments of every chromosome at an approximate interval of 1 million bases (1 centimorgan). Some of the unique fragments are restriction sites within known genes, but most are variable dinucleotide repeats. Fragments of unique DNA surrounding a dinucleotide repeat can be identified and amplified from the entire chromosome using the polymerase chain reaction (PCR) based on sequence-specific oligonucleotide primers. Because the number of repeats is genetically inherited and highly polymorphic within a family, these PCR fragments are almost always useful for linkage. Prior methods using enzyme restriction sites for localization (i.e., restriction-fragment linkage polymorphism) often failed to be informative for purposes of linkage.

Once linkage to a segment of a specific chromosome is determined, the next problem is identifying the disease locus. Candidate genes may be suggested by the proximity of a known (candidate) gene to the locus. When this fails, strategies to further subdivide and determine DNA sequence for genes in the region eventually identify the locus, although this is an extremely labor-intensive approach. With completion of the human genome sequence, candidate genes frequently are suggested from the presence of a linkage analysis. This was the approach used in the identification of the genetic loci for fibrillin associated with cases of MFS and fibroblast growth factor (FGF) receptor loci related to achondroplasia.

The heritable disorders of connective tissue discussed in this chapter all arise from a single gene defect. However, attention is now turning to complex genetic traits in which more than one gene contributes to the phenotype. The best example is postmenopausal osteoporosis, in which several candidate genes have been associated with low bone mineral density (BMD) in several populations. The identification of these genes is defined based on the presence of specific allelic fragments (i.e., polymorphisms) within the region of the specific gene and demonstration of its linkage to individuals and families with osteoporosis. Examples of polymorphisms of current interest include vitamin D receptor alleles, polymorphisms associated with the Sp1 transcription factor site in the $\alpha 1(I)$ collagen first intron, and estrogen receptor polymorphisms.[40] This type of analysis requires large cohorts of individuals and pedigrees, and it requires statistical analysis to show that the DNA fragment associated with this allele is contributing to a complex phenotype.

IDENTIFYING MUTATIONS IN KNOWN GENES

Proof that a genetic locus is encoding a disease phenotype is the demonstration that the gene harbors a mutation that would alter the function of the gene product. Several techniques are capable of identifying a single base change within DNA. The method that has received widespread application is sequence-specific conformational polymorphism.[41] Several variations on this basic method have been reported.[42] Demonstration that the DNA fragment harbors the mutation requires that the fragment be molecularly cloned and that the normal and mutated genes be identified by DNA sequencing.

After the mutation within a specific pedigree has been identified, the recurrence of the same mutation in other family members can be rapidly identified by DNA sequencing of the fragment surrounding the mutation or by the use of small oligonucleotide fragments (i.e., allele-specific oligonucleotides) specific for the normal and the mutant allele. Laboratories that offer molecular diagnostic tests for many of the heritable disorders can be found in the United States and in Europe.

■ Heritable Disorders of the Type I Collagen Family

OSTEOGENESIS IMPERFECTA

OI refers to a generalized disorder of connective tissue that predominantly affects the skeletal system.[43,44] It is estimated to affect between 20 and 50 million persons in the United States. The gene prevalence of OI is calculated as 4 to 5 per 100,000 persons. These estimates may fall short of OI's true prevalence because of the number of very mild cases that are undiagnosed or diagnosed late in life. In the discussion that follows, the clinical classification of Sillence[45] has been supplemented with recent reports of skeletal disorders that share phenotypic features with the sillence OI types I through IV. As will be described, type I collagen mutations have been reported in types I through IV phenotypes but not in recently reported types V, VI, and VII phenotypes (vide infra). This nosologic debate will require future deliberation to clarify (Table 95–4). A useful Web site, which compiles most of the known mutations resulting in OI, can be found at *http://www.le.ac.uk/genetics/collagen/*. This Web site presents information about the locus of the molecular defects recognized in each major clinical OI variant.

Mild Osteogenesis Imperfecta (Sillence Types I A and B)

Affected individuals with type I disease (Sillence types 1A and 1B) have OI of mild to moderate severity in terms of their clinical course, the extent of skeletal deformity, and the radiologic appearance of the skeleton (Fig. 95–2A). The type designations A and B refer to individuals with normal dentition (A) or those expressing dentinogenesis imperfecta (DI) (B). These subjects are usually short for their age, although normal stature occurs in a few individuals. They may have little or no skeletal deformity in spite of having experienced multiple fractures of their extremities.

The disorder is transmitted as an autosomal dominant trait, but it may first appear as a new mutation (i.e., sporadic). Parental gonadal or somatic mosaicism, in which the parents appear clinically unaffected, may confuse interpretation of the pattern of inheritance.[46] Type I disease accounts for approximately 60 percent of OI patients. A diagnostic problem is the differentiation of these individuals from those with juvenile osteoporosis or adult idiopathic osteoporosis.[47]

Type I subjects have a characteristic triangular facial shape caused by mild prominence of the frontal bones and narrowing of the mandible anteriorly. The skin of patients with mild OI has normal elasticity but is occasionally thin and somewhat smooth in texture. The sclerae are blue, with the tint varying from a deep, blue-gray hue to pale blue. Patients have reported that the color of their sclerae varies over time; in general, deeper hues are seen in children. Arcus senilis not related to lipid abnormalities occur in many patients during their middle years. Other reported ocular defects include scleromalalcia, keratoconus, and retinal detachment.[48] The pseudoglioma osteoporosis syndrome, which is related to mutations in the lipoprotein receptor–related protein 5 (LRP5) gene, is a separate entity from OI. Different mutations in LRP5 have been associated with both decreased and increased bone mass. (Osteoporosis-Pseudoglioma Syndrome Collaborative Group, *Cell*, 107: 513, 2001) Although the occurrence of DI (OI type IB disease) has not been observed in this group, a subgroup of patients with OI was reported on by Levin.[49] During the second and third decades of life, a characteristic high-frequency sensorineural or mixed hearing loss can

be detected.[47,50] Several neurologic complications have been reported in OI, including—in severe disease—the presence of basilar invagination[47,50-52] (see following). These include both obstructive and communicating hydrocephalus in infants and cervical spinal cord compression syndromes with paresthesias, peripheral weakness, and loss of bladder control in adults.[53] Basilar impression with compression of the posterior fossa occurs in 10 percent of type I subjects, usually in the absence of neurologic signs that may occur in more severe OI phenotypes.[53] However, pain syndromes including complex central pain syndromes (reflex sympathetic dystrophy syndrome) may occur in OI patients following multiple episodes of trauma.

Connective tissue laxity extends to cardiac structures. The incidence of mitral valve prolapse is not increased in these patients compared to the population at large, but individual kindreds with increased diameter of the aortic root or subjects with aortic regurgitation have been reported.[54] Corrective aortic surgery has been performed in several OI patients.[55] Many patients have hyperextensible joints as children, but this tends to be less marked in adults. Joint dislocation is infrequent in OI compared to the EDS subgroups.

Patients with OI complain of hypermetabolism with diaphoresis. The frequency and cause of this is unexplained. Although many patients complain of easy bruising, detailed studies of clotting function in OI patients have not revealed a consistent abnormality. Hypercalciuria has been reported in 36 percent of a pediatric OI population.[56] We have not observed this in an adult population, although renal calculus formation has been observed in several adult patients. Although hypercalciuria appears to be related to the severity of disease, evaluation of renal function disclosed no impairment of renal function or evidence of nephrocalcinosis on renal ultrasound in this cohort of hypercalciuric patients. However, renal calculi have been described in many OI patients, including both infants and adults in the our clinic and other international clinics.

Mildly affected patients may not have fractures at birth, although there is occasionally a fracture of a clavicle or extremity during delivery. Prenatal diagnosis by ultrasound is not helpful in the mild form of OI because intrauterine fractures and deformity are not recognized. The first fracture may occur in the newborn nursery with daily handling or as the infant starts to crawl. The frequency of fracture thereafter depends on the child's activity, the need for immobilization after lower extremity fractures, and the attitude of the family toward independent activity. In general, these patients may experience 5 to 15 major fractures before puberty, as well as several minor traumatic fractures of the digits or the small bones of the feet. Poor alignment or repeated immobilization, as in a spica cast, leads to recurrent fractures, which may lead to bowing, with shortening of a limb and subsequent gait disturbance.

Characteristically, the fracture rate falls dramatically after puberty, only to increase during later life (Patterson). Mild scoliosis approximating 20 degrees is common. Osteopenia is observed in vertebral bodies and the peripheral skeleton and progresses with age. It is remark-

TABLE 95–4 • CHARACTERISTICS OF OSTEOGENESIS IMPERFECTA (OI)

Sillence Type	Clinical Features	Frequency (%)	Inheritance	No. of Fractures	Scleral Color	Presence of Dentinogenesis Imperfecta (DI)	Anticipated Inheritance
I	No major skeletal deformities	50	Dominant, occasionally sporadic	5 to 15	Blue	Infrequent	Null mutation of α1(I) gene
II	Lethal; severely deformed	5	Dominant new mutation or germinal mosaicism	Multiple in utero and at birth	Blue or gray	Occurs, but prevalence is uncertain	Mutations of α2(I) that disrupt the integrity of the helical domain of collagen
III	Major skeletal deformities; very osteopenic; usually not ambulatory	20	Dominant new mutation or germinal mosaicism; possible genetic compound	30 to 60	Usually white, occasionally blue	25%	Mutations of α1(I) or α2(I) that disrupt the integrity of the helical domain of collagen
IV	Moderate osteopenia and bony deformity; usually ambulatory with mechanic support	25	Dominant, occasionally sporadic	10 to 25	White or gray	25%	Mutations of α2(I) that affect the stability of the helical domain of collagen

able that despite multiple fractures, in persons with type I OI, the long bones usually heal with no significant deformity. When compared to more severe phenotypes, children with type I OI only infrequently require the insertion of intramedullary rods and almost never experience nonunion at a fracture site. Similar to other variants, the frequency of fractures diminishes markedly after puberty, an observation that is not explained by the level of activity or the child's ability to protect against trauma.

Although osteopenia with rarefaction of the medullary space and cortical thinning are observed in radiographs, many type I cases are so mild as to be missed on routine radiographic examination. The diagnosis may be first suspected when a parent with unrecognized disease is found to have a child suffering repeated fractures. Unfortunately, this situation has led to the accusation of child abuse (vide infra).[57]

Measurement of BMD by dual-energy x-ray absorptiometry (DEXA) at any age discloses a significant decrease in bone mass.[58] This is the case for mild disease, in which BMD is reported to be 76 percent of that of an age-matched control in the spine and 71 percent of control in the femoral neck.[59] T scores (i.e., standard deviation from the young-adult mean BMD) are frequently in the range of −2.5 to −4.0 at the lumbar spine or proximal femur, consistent with the diagnosis of osteoporosis as defined by the World Health Organization (WHO). Low BMD in children with recurrent fractures may assist in identifying those with OI.

An examination of iliac crest bone biopsy specimens is occasionally warranted to define the extent of histologic abnormality or to exclude alternate diagnoses in patients suspected of having type I OI.[60] To permit analysis of bone biopsy specimens for static and dynamic histomorphometric parameters, tetracyclines are administered to label osteon or trabecular mineralization fronts. Usually, a 12-day hiatus is allowed between the 2-day oral administration of tetracycline and demethylchlortetracycline, agents that bind to the mineralization front but fluoresce as different colors, permitting calculation of rates of mineralization. Light microscopy in a patient with type I OI shows lamellar bone with an absence of the woven bone present in more severe OI types.[61] Osteocyte number is increased. In mild OI, bone turnover is low, as is evident by reduced eroded surfaces and reduced osteoid surfaces.[62] Although no mineralization defect is apparent, mineralization apposition rate and bone formation rates as determined by histomorphometry are shortened.[63]

Molecular Pathology

As in other phenotypes, type I OI is the result of mutations affecting the α1(I) and α2(I) polypeptide chains of type I collagen. Cultured fibroblasts from individuals with mild OI synthesize low amounts (approximately one half) of the expected amounts of type I collagen. The underproduction of a normal type I collagen molecule is a consequence of failure to process and secrete the product of a mutant allele (i.e., null allele). Type III

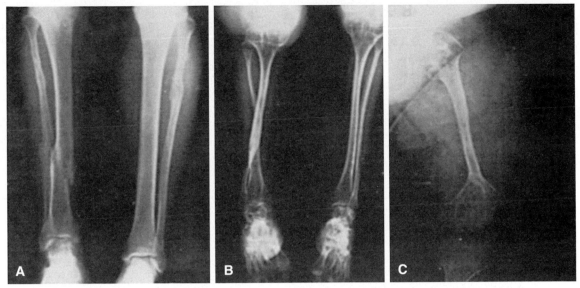

FIGURE 95–2 · These Radiographs Illustrate Skeletal Differences Among Variants of Osteogenesis Imperfecta (OI). *A*, Dominant: mild, with minimal deformity. *B*, Moderate OI: mild epiphyseal dysplasia. *C*, Severe OI: marked diaphyseal narrowing and widening of the metaphysis with severe epiphyseal dysplasia. Lethal OI is not illustrated.

collagen production is normal. The ratio of type III to type I collagen, therefore, is elevated in cultured dermal fibroblast cells[64] and in collagens extracted from skin biopsy specimens.

The molecular basis for the low production of type I collagen appears to be diminished activity of one of the $\alpha1(I)$ or $\alpha2(I)$ collagen alleles. Because collagen molecules composed of more than one $\alpha2$-chain are unstable, the rate of $\alpha1$-chain synthesis determines the rate of type I collagen production. The unincorporated $\alpha2$-chains are degraded.[65] The level of $\alpha1(I)$ collagen mRNA is one half of that expected, suggesting a nonfunctional $\alpha1(I)$ collagen gene or instability of its mRNA. Examination of 1(I) mRNA in the nuclear compartment of cultured fibroblasts has demonstrated excessive accumulation of an $\alpha1(I)$ mRNA containing an unspliced intron, and in another patient, a Gly-to-Arg expressed point mutation was found in the nuclear and cytoplasmic compartments.[66] Another mechanism for a null $\alpha1(I)$ gene is the nonsense and frame-shift mutations that lead to premature stop mutations in the mutant RNA transcript.[67] In certain strains, these mutations influence RNA splicing and induce skipping of the exon that contains the nonsense codon. Two OI type IB patients have been reported to show large multiexon deletions in the *COL1A2* gene for the $\alpha2(I)$ chain.[68]

Consistent with the phenotype of a null mutation of the $\alpha1(I)$ gene is the demonstration that the heterozygous (and phenotypically normal) MOV13 mouse has osteopenia, reduced bone strength, and a hearing deficit similar to patients with type I OI.[69] Mutations near or within the helical domain can also result in OI that is mild and nondeforming. These represent the mildest spectrum of mutations that can alter normal

triple-helical interactions, perhaps forming the bridge between OI and familial osteoporosis syndromes.[47]

Lethal Osteogenesis Imperfecta

Approximately 10 percent of OI patients have the severe neonatal form of the disease—lethal osteogenesis imperfecta (Sillence type II)—which is usually incompatible with survival. Approximately 1 in 20,000 to 60,000 neonates is affected. Most cases result from new somatic mutations, although cases suggesting a recessive inheritance pattern have been observed and probably represent germinal or somatic cell mosaicism in one of the parents.[39] In these cases, the involved parent appears unaffected or only mildly affected.[70]

Birth weight and length are usually decreased. These infants are born with severe bone fragility and present with multiple intrauterine fractures at various stages of healing. Hydrops fetalis has been reported in type II OI neonates. Because of the severity of the underlying collagen defect, dismemberment of the head or a limb may occur during delivery. The sclerae are deep blue. The calvarium is markedly undermineralized, which increases the risk of intracerebral bleeding. The skull appears large compared to the shortened trunk and deformed extremities.[71] Wormian changes involving the occipital, parietal, and temporal bones can be seen on radiographs. The extremities may be bowed and foreshortened due to intrauterine fractures and the effects of muscle tension on soft bones.

Radiographs of these children reveal a characteristic beading of the ribs, representing callus over multiple fractures (Table 95–5). Based on these findings, the phenotypes have been subdivided into groups A, B or C.

TABLE 95–5 • RADIOGRAPHIC CLASSIFICATION OF TYPE II OSTEOGENESIS IMPERFECTA (OI) OR PERINATAL LETHAL SILLENCE TYPE II, 1988

Group A	Broad, "crumpled" long bones and beaded ribs; generally associated with perinatal death
Group B	Broad, crumpled long bones; ribs show minimal or no beading; survival is reported for this category
Group C	Thin, cylindrical, dysplastic bones; thin, beaded ribs

(Sillence 1984) Group A has short, crumpled, broad long bones and continuously beaded ribs. Group B has similar long bones but thin normal ribs, whereas group C has narrow or thin long bones with thin, beaded ribs.

The Apgar score in these patients reflects pulmonary insufficiency. Respiratory reserve is limited by the small thorax and probably underdeveloped thoracic musculature. Death usually ensues within a day for 60 percent of these infants and by the end of the first month for 80 percent,[72] although there are reported instances of survival of an infant with this severe phenotype among the group B patients.

Histologic examination of the affected neonate reveals the presence of woven bone. Type II OI has recently been associated with neuropathologic changes, including abundant perivenous microcalcification and defective neuroblastic cell migration indicated by focal aggregates of germ cells within white matter, suggesting that collagen mutations may alter the development of neural and neurovascular tissues.[73,74] Prenatal diagnosis by ultrasound is possible starting at about week 16 of pregnancy and should be used in families with a previously affected infant. The diagnosis of type II OI has been established using fetal magnetic resonance imaging (MRI).[75] Chorionic villus biopsy can be used to provide DNA for collagen sequence analysis.

Molecular Pathology

Most cases occur sporadically, although germinal or somatic mosaicism has been reported.[68] The recurrence rate varies from less than 1 percent in group A patients to 7.7 percent in group B patients.[76]

Type I procollagen assembles in a direction from the C- to the N-terminal regions of the triple-helical molecule. C-terminal mutations, therefore, should be more disruptive on polypeptide chain assembly and more disruptive of collagen secretion and extracellular matrix development.

The biochemical abnormality common to the lethal form of OI is a severely impaired ability to synthesize and secrete type I collagen.[77] As a result, the amount of type I collagen in bone is low, whereas the quantity of the minor collagen types III and V is relatively high. Bone collagen fibers are distinctly smaller than the fibers in age-matched normal infants, and retained collagen is observed within dilated endoplasmic reticulum.

The biochemical basis of the lack of collagen secretion appears to reside within the primary structures of the $\alpha 1$(I)- or the $\alpha 2$(I)-chains. In the best studied case, which resulted from a partial gene deletion encoding three exons, the shortened $\alpha 1$(I)-chains compromised helix formation of all molecules containing the shortened α-chain.[71,78] In this manner, a defective α-chain can lead to impaired secretion, decreased helical stability, abnormal fiber formation, impaired interactions with other matrix molecules, and defective cross-link formation. This cascade of events resulting from the incorporation of one mutant chain into an interactive supramolecular structure has been aptly called "protein suicide."[79]

Small helical deletions resulting from mutations that impair splicing of the collagen mRNA and lead to exon skipping have a similar outcome. A single glycine substitution with the Gly-X-Y triplet is equally severe.

There appears to be a correlation between the length of the destabilized helix and the severity of the phenotype when the proα1-chain is involved, although inconsistencies with this rule are seen with the proα2-chain.[80]

Severely Deforming Osteogenesis Imperfecta

The deforming variant of osteogenesis imperfecta (Sillence type III) is the classic form of OI and accounts for about 20 percent of cases. The disease usually appears sporadically, although several families have been reported with more than one affected child, normal parents, and an absence of consanguinity.

This variant is characterized by severe deformity of the limbs and marked kyphoscoliosis, with foreshortened deformity of the thorax and growth retardation. Although this was called "progressive deforming OI" by Sillence, the deformities are fully established by the age of 5 years and remain relatively unchanged until the middle years, when kyphoscoliosis may worsen. Pulmonary function is diminished because of distortion of the spine and chest cage, and this may worsen in adulthood.

The extent of growth retardation is remarkable in that many patients' height may not surpass 3 feet (90 to 100 cm). Cranial molding occurs in utero and during infancy, producing frontal bossing and a characteristic occipital "overhang" called the *helmet deformity*. Patients who are immobilized with poor head control may have flattening of the cranium in the anterior-to-posterior dimension. Wormian bones and delayed closure of fontanelles may be observed well into the first decade. Triangular faces occurs in type III OI, as does widening of the orbital fissures, which leads to the eyes appearing in a "sunset" position. Platybasia due to soft bone at the base of the skull may cause the external ear canals to slant upward as the base of the skull sinks on the cervical vertebrae. This may lead to communicating or obstructive hydrocephalus, cranial nerve palsies, and upper and lower motor neuron lesions. Headache, diplopia, nystagmus, cranial nerve neuralgia, decline in motor function, urinary dysfunction, and respiratory compromise are complications of basilar invagination.[52]

Most patients have white sclerae as adults, although bluish discoloration is apparent in childhood, and this may persist in some patients. Approximately 25 percent of patients with type III OI have DI, necessitating constant dental care throughout childhood. Severe hearing impairment occurs in 10 percent of patients, although milder degrees of hearing loss are more common. An unusual and characteristic feature is a high-pitched voice.

The skeleton in these patients is significantly osteoporotic, which leads to multiple fractures in the upper and lower extremities and vertebral bodies, particularly prior to puberty. Unlike type I OI in which fractures tend to heal without deformity, fractures in type III OI frequently lead to increased limb, pelvis, and spinal deformity. Because of their small trunk size and the presence of scoliosis, these patients' chest volume is diminished, and cardiopulmonary insufficiency may become an increasing problem during adulthood. Pulmonary function testing may indicate a restrictive pattern. Sleep apnea may further complicate pulmonary function. These children tend to be hypotonic and have hyperextensible joints so that head control and motor development are delayed. Because of defective bone remodeling associated with marked osteoporosis and excessively thin femur shafts, or the broad bone variant, patients are usually wheelchair bound. Fractures of the clavicle or long bones and vertebral bodies are frequently present at birth. Spontaneous fractures occur with little stress, and infants may experience 20 or more fractures during the first 1 to 3 years of life. The necessity for half-body casting, as may occur after proximal femur fractures, leads to additional loss of bone.

Radiographs of the skeleton reveal marked osteopenia, thinning of cortical bone, narrowing of the diaphysis, and widening of the metaphysis, which merges into a dysplastic epiphyseal zone filled with whorls of partially calcified cartilage (i.e., popcorn deformity)[81] (see Fig. 95–2C). Osteoporosis leads to collapse of vertebral end plates, and scoliosis is marked. Pectus excavatum or pectus carinatum adds to thoracic deformity. Lack of weight-bearing increases the severity of osteoporosis and increases the risk of fracture. Nevertheless, spontaneous fractures do not occur as frequently after puberty. Trauma, however, such as an automobile accident or falling from a wheelchair, can be disastrous. Despite these complications, patients do survive and may have gainful employment into their sixties.

Pulmonary Function in Severe Osteogenesis Imperfecta

Pulmonary insufficiency is a leading cause of death in subjects with severe OI. Chest wall deformity and scoliosis are constant features in these subjects. Basilar invagination with brain stem deformity can also impair pulmonary function. It is the degree of scoliosis, and not the extent of chest wall deformity or kyphosis, that relates to decreased pulmonary function in these patients.[112] Scoliosis predicts the development of restrictive pulmonary disease. Vital capacity is significantly decreased in subjects with scoliotic curves of 60 degrees or greater. Spirometry and lung volume studies are essential for evaluation of pulmonary function. Sleep studies (polysomnography) may disclose problems of gas exchange and sleep apnea that are not apparent with conventional pulmonary function studies. Individuals with hypoxemia but without hypercapnea may require supplemental oxygen. Positive pressure ventilation in the form of biphasic positive airway pressure may be helpful for patients with advanced pulmonary insufficiency. Bracing or spinal fusion has been found to arrest progressive pulmonary dysfunction in certain patients.

Molecular Pathology

Prenatal diagnosis in the first trimester has been achieved using ultrasound or identification of type I collagen mutations using chorionic villus biopsies or aspirated amniotic cells.[71] The best studied case of severe deforming OI showed a complete deficiency of α2(I)-chain synthesis, producing a homotrimeric collagen molecule of three α1(I)-chains.[82] The absence of α2(I)-chains in the collagen molecule results from a four-base deletion in the α2(I)-gene that "frame shifts" the C-terminal propeptide, such that synthesized chains fail to get incorporated into a triple-helical structure. Other cases are the result of helix destabilization by mutations in the molecule similar to those of lethal OI.[83,84] It is not clear whether all defects in this group are collagen related or if there are mutations in other bone-related proteins.

Osteogenesis Imperfecta of Moderate Severity

Clinically, the phenotype of patients with moderately severe OI (Silence type IV) overlap with those with the more severe forms of type I disease. Furthermore, Glorieux and colleagues have separated one variant of type IV disease, which is termed *type V* (see following). The condition is inherited as a dominant trait, with sporadic cases representing new mutations or unrecognized mosaicism; mosaicism contributes to this group as with other OI types. Fractures may be present at birth, but the frequency may be variable; some patients may not have the initial fracture until later in the first decade. However, the extent of skeletal deformity involving the spine, thorax, and extremities is usually intermediate between that of types I and III OI. These patients have short stature. Their sclerae tend to be white, although families have been observed in which sclerae were blue at birth but lightened to white with age; some patients retain blue sclerae as adults. In our limited series, these patients appeared to have more molding of the skull, and an occipital overhang may be palpable. Hearing loss occurs less frequently than in persons with type I disease. Significant kyphoscoliosis is common and may progress during adolescence. Perhaps related to ligamentous laxity, type IV patients have hyperextensible joints and pes planus.

Most fractures occur during childhood, and these may recur during the postmenopausal period in women or in men older than age 50 years. Long bone deformity tends to develop after fractures, which leads to a difficulty in ambulation not typically encountered in the mildly affected (OI type I) subjects. Type IV patients may require the use of a cane, crutches, or a wheelchair at times.

Radiographs of the long bones and vertebral bodies demonstrate marked osteopenia with vertebral collapse involving the thoracic and lumbar vertebrae. Although there is marked cortical thinning, bowing, and coarsening of trabeculae, the overall architecture of the bone remains intact (see Fig. 95–2B). Irregular dysplastic areas, possibly a consequence of fracture healing, may be seen in appendicular bones. Scoliosis, ranging from mild to severe, appears in radiographs of most type IV subjects.

Molecular Pathology

The first structural abnormality of the $\alpha2(I)$-chain to be demonstrated in this form of OI was a 15–amino acid deletion in the N-terminal helical region of the $\alpha2(I)$-chain, which resulted from a splicing abnormality that skipped exon 12.[83] An alteration in molecular stability, analogous to that observed in lethal OI from mutations in the $\alpha2(I)$- or the $\alpha1(I)$-chain, results from glycine point mutations within the helical domain.[75] Additional mutations associated with type IV disease have involved a 9-bp pair deletion of nucleotides 3418 to 3427.

DI has been used as one of the criteria for separating individual patient phenotypes within categories I, III and IV.[85,86] DI is inherited as a dominant trait. The genetic relation between OI and DI has not been precisely defined. The deciduous and permanent teeth have an opalescent and translucent appearance, which tends to darken with age. Primary teeth are more severely affected. The enamel is normal, but the dentin is dysplastic; chipping of enamel occurs, and the teeth are subjected to erosion and breakage. On radiographs, there is an exaggerated constriction at the coronal junction and obliteration of pulpal spaces. Early consideration should be given to capping affected teeth to minimize wear and breakage.

The moderately severe form of OI represents a heterogeneous grouping clinically and biochemically. Restriction fragment length polymorphism (RFLP) analysis has demonstrated linkage of OI type I to the $\alpha1(I)$ and $\alpha2(I)$ genes. This method has been used in prenatal diagnosis of OI type IV.[87]

Type V Osteogenesis Imperfecta

This phenotype was reported by Glorieux and colleagues[88] in 2000 as a variant within the heterogeneous group under type IV OI. In the initial report of seven OI patients, the phenotype was distinguished by the following criteria:

- The patients had a moderate to severe fracture history due to increased bone fragility involving their extremities and vertebral bodies.
- Four of seven children had hyperplastic callus.
- The patients had limitation of forearm pronation and supination due to calcification of the forearm interosseous membrane.
- The disorder was transmitted as an autosomal dominant trait.
- None of the patients had blue sclerae or DI.
- Bone biopsy specimens showed a meshlike appearance of irregularly spaced lamellae.
- Unlike other phenotypes, no type I collagen mutation was identified.

Two issues are important relative to the description of this phenotype: 1) In terms of frequency, this may be more prevalent in the Canadian population of brittle bone subjects; as this group of signs has not been common in the author's clinical experience, and 2) the etiology of the disorder is not defined at this time.

Type VI Osteogenesis Imperfecta[88]

This brittle bone phenotype was also reported among the heterogeneous type IV group of OI patients. Characteristic of the initial group of eight subjects was the occurrence of first fracture at an early age (4 to 18 months of age). Bone appeared severely brittle. Sclerae were white or faintly blue. All patients had vertebral compression fractures. No radiologic evidence of classic rickets was present, but serum alkaline phosphatase levels were elevated. No type I collagen mutation was identified. Of importance was the observation of increased lamellar osteoid and a prolonged mineralization lag time in the absence of clinical signs of a mineralization defect. The etiology of this brittle bone disorder and its relationship to the typical OI phenotype remains unclear.

Type VII Osteogenesis Imperfecta

As noted previously, Glorieux and coworkers[88] have reported additional brittle bone syndromes under the OI classification. Type VII, also named by this group, was found in a small First Nations community in northern Quebec, Canada.[89] This is an autosomal recessive disorder identified in four children and four adults. The phenotype, which includes fractures at birth, blue sclerae, and osteopenia, is described as moderate to severe. It includes rhizomelia, deformity of the lower extremities, and coxa vara. The disorder has been localized to chromosome 3p22-24.[90] A type I collagen mutation was not identified in these individuals. The basis of the disorder remains to be determined.

Mortality Statistics in Osteogenesis Imperfecta

The mortality of 743 patients from England and Wales with OI types I, III, and IV was investigated by Singer and colleagues.[91] The mortality of type II OI is 100 percent, although certain cases are reported to have survived with exceptional supportive care. More than 50 percent of the patients had type I OI, 16 percent had type III OI, and 22 percent had type IVA or IVB. In this series, mean attained age was 24 years for males and 26.8 years for females. Excess mortality was not increased for type IA patients. With groups 1B, IVA, and IVB combined, excess mortality expressed as mortality ratio (MR) was significantly higher for males (MR 295%) but not for females (MR 133%). Almost all the deaths in subjects under age 35 were in the type III group. Extremely high MR was found for children under 15 years, with a MR of 26,000 for children aged 0 to 4 years.

Histopathology of Bone in Osteogenesis Imperfecta

HA crystals in cortical OI bone are smaller than normal, particularly in children and adolescents with type II disease.[92] Bone crystal size was reported to increase with increasing age in OI patients and children. Studies of crystal size and alignment in cortical bone of the animal model oim/oim mouse have similarly shown smaller crystals with variable crystal alignment.[93]

The range of histologic appearances of bone in the different OI phenotypes is as variable as the clinical phenotypes and is illustrated by examination of bone samples using scanning electron microscopy or transmission electron microscopy. Undermineralization and overmineralization of bone have been recognized within the same specimen. Variability in structural composition is evident in that regions of loose, unconnected, and undermineralized type I collagen fibers are seen with overmineralized fibers that probably contain small, unorganized HA crystals.[94] Bone morphology may appear relatively normal in mild OI types, but osteopenia due to thin lamellar plates and diminished cortical width is evident. Immature woven bone and lamellar disarray are characteristic of more severe OI phenotypes.[94]

Some reports indicate that bone turnover measured by histomorphometry is elevated in children younger than 15 years with severe OI types (III, IV). Decreased trabecular number and increased cortical porosity was characteristic of these specimens. In contrast, histologic and histomorphometric analysis of bone from patients 34 to 64 years of age with type IA OI revealed low bone turnover, as illustrated by low eroded surface and reduced osteoid surfaces. Histologic examination showed low bone volume with decreased cortical width, but trabecular connectedness was generally intact.[95] Osteocyte numbers appear increased compared to normal; the mechanisms involved in this consistent finding are unknown.

Examination of iliac crest bone biopsies in children and adults between the ages of 1. 9 and 22. 9 years revealed abundant osteocytes.[96] Compared with controls, bone from children with types III and IV OI showed markedly sparse and very cellular cortical and lamellar bone. Consistent with the findings of other studies, packets of bone tissue showed higher than normal mineralization, which was considered to contribute to the brittleness characteristic of OI bone.

Tetracycline labeled iliac crest bone biopsies from 70 children aged 1.5 to 13 years with OI types I, III and IV, have been reported by Rauch and colleagues.[97] Bone mass was decreased in each group as reflected in decreased core width, cortical width, and cancellous bone volume. Decrease in trabecular number and lower trabecular thickness were both observed. Compared to age-related controls, there was a lesser annual increase in trabecular thickness (5.8 microns versus 3.6 microns in OI), and no increase in thickness was found for types III and IV OI.

Serum and Urinary Biomarkers in Osteogenesis Imperfecta

Considerable uncertainty exists about rates of bone turnover in OI patients of different ages and having different phenotypes. The measurement of blood and urine proteins reflecting bone matrix collagen turnover or osteoblastic activity has been applied to patients with OI. In general, such measurements are useful diagnostic modalities, although it is recognized that these determinations in specific bone disorders may not always reflect the actual rate of bone turnover. Included are parameters of osteoblastic bone formation: serum total alkaline phosphatase or bone-specific alkaline phosphatase, serum osteocalcin, serum C-terminal propeptide of procollagen I (PICP), and the serum procollagen N-terminal propeptide (PINP). The excretion of specific and poorly metabolized urine collagen cross-link products, the N-telopeptide or pyridinoline and deoxypyridinoline cross-links, has replaced the excretion of hydroxyproline as the measure of collagen breakdown.

Increased excretion of urinary collagen cross-link products along with elevated values for serum osteocalcin has suggested the presence of increased bone turnover in approximately 20 percent of patients. Bone turnover is elevated in children with OI, which may in part reflect expected high rates of bone remodeling in children. Diminished bone biomarkers indicating low bone turnover have also been identified in children with OI. Reduced serum levels of PICP were reported in a large family with type IA OI.[98] Pyridinoline and deoxypyridinoline excretion tend to be normal or low in mild cases but may be elevated in those with more severe disease. However, most studies, including those based on histomorphic measurements of tetracycline-labeled bone biopsies, suggest that bone turnover is low rather than high in most adults.[95]

THERAPY

Medical Treatment of Osteogenesis Imperfecta

Over the years, there have been multiple attempts to treat OI with a variety of vitamins, hormones, and drugs, none of which has been successful. The list includes administration of mineral supplements, fluoride, androgenic steroids, ascorbic acid, and vitamin D. Calcitonin has been reported helpful in certain studies, but it has not been administered to numbers of patients adequate to prove its significance.

During the past 5 years, and in a departure from earlier results, treatment with bisphosphonates, administered parenterally or orally to children and adults, has demonstrated favorable results. The intravenously administered bisphosphonate pamidronate increased bone mass, decreased skeletal pain, and decreased fracture incidence in children with severe OI ages 3 to 15 years studied by Glorieux and colleagues.[99] This regimen was also successful in children under the age of 3 years.[100] Similar results involving cyclic administration of pamidronate have been reported by other investigators.[101,102] Dosage regimens in different series for children and adults have varied from 1 mg/kg to 3 mg/kg, administered intravenously at 2- to 4-month intervals, and lower-dosage regimens also have been reported.[103] We have used a dose of 1.5 mg/kg administered at 3-month intervals in children over 3 years of age and a maximum dose of 60 mg administered to adults at 3-month intervals. In general, reports indicate a significant increase in bone mass in children that may approximate or exceed 50 to 100 percent during the first 2 years of treatment, as well as a 50-percent decrease in fracture rate. The effect is most marked in the spine, where vertebral remodeling may improve vertebral height. Metabolic studies by Rauch and coworkers[60] have demonstrated a decrease in serum ionized calcium and increase in serum parathyroid hormone (PTH) of 30 percent. Urinary excretion of N-telopeptide as an index of bone resorption decreased 61 to 73 percent. Of importance is the study by Zacharin and colleagues[104] in which pamidronate was administered at a dose of 1 mg/kg for 3 days every 4 months. Although a decreased fracture rate and a decrease in musculoskeletal pain were observed, there was no correlation between the phenotypic severity, age at start of treatment, and treatment response. Although fracture incidence is more difficult to quantify in adults than in children, treatment with pamidronate in a series of adult OI patients has increased bone mass as measured in iliac crest bone biopsies.[63] In our experience, the oral administration of alendronate has increased bone mass in adult OI patients. It appears, however, that treatment results are more impressive in children than in adults, perhaps because of higher rates of bone turnover in the younger patients. The major side effects of intravenous (IV) bisphosphonate treatment involve the acute-phase response (24 hours after infusion) and the occurrence of otitis and vestibular imbalance in a small number of patients. The currently recommended treatment regimen includes the use of a bisphosphonate, with adequate calcium and vitamin D supplementation to avoid the occurrence of hypercalciuria and to maintain serum vitamin D levels within normal limits.

The use of surgery to correct deformities and to facilitate weight-bearing has been the subject of several reviews.[105,106] Multiple osteotomies and realignment of a deformed bone over intramedullary rods is an option for many children with severe bowing.[107] Indications include frequent fractures at the apex of the bow, impaired standing, or limb-length inequality due to bowing.[108] The ideal age for this intervention is some time after the age 2 to 3 years, when the growth rate slows and the child's physical potential can be better assessed.[107] In some cases, the physician can take advantage of the "down time" of a fracture to perform correction. Contraindications include absence of identifiable cortex or lack of standing potential. Expanding (telescoping) rods are best for growing children, for they require fewer revisions. There are several variations in design, but all incorporate the concept of total intramedullary splinting from proximal epiphysis to distal epiphysis. This eliminates stress concentration at the end of the metal device, such as is seen in plates or rods that do not span the entire bone. Persons with OI are at increased risk of premature OA for reasons that are not completely clear. Total joint arthroplasty is usually successful in these patients, so referral to a specialist is appropriate when symptoms become severe enough to impair quality of life.[109] The procedure should be done by experts experienced in genetic disorders. Acetabular protrusion, small implant size, and risk of stress risers make the surgeon's job more complex.

Spinal deformities are common and usually progressive.[110-112] They include basilar invagination, as well as scoliosis and kyphosis of the thoracolumbar spine. Brace treatment has no significant role in any of these problems, except in children ages 6 to 10 years with scoliosis and mild type I OI.[110] Early basilar invagination may be halted with prophylactic posterior fusion of the occipital-cervical junction with plate fixation.[114] Patients with severe brain stem compression may require anterior transoral decompression, as well as posterior instrumented fusion. Severe scoliosis may impair pulmonary function and cause pain. Surgical stabilization is most advisable in the teen years or early adulthood when patients are best able to tolerate these complex reconstructions (see figures). Some patients with extreme osteoporosis are not candidates for spine surgery. Intramedullary rods have been placed in the lower or upper extremities in many children with cosmetic and functional salutary effects. However, single and expanding rods have been associated with significant complications (e.g., migration from the bone, breakage) after extended use and have required replacement in a large proportion of cases.[113] Every child with OI benefits from appropriate rehabilitative therapy.[115] Bracing with lightweight plastics as the child begins to walk can minimize microfracture and bowing of the upper femurs. Muscle-strengthening exercises are essential as primary care and after immobilization for fracture. Perhaps the most beneficial programs have been developed around swimming, preferably in heated pools, and as part of a planned program of continuous rehabilitative medical care.

EHLERS-DANLOS SYNDROME

The heterogenous group of disorders grouped as EDS illustrates the genetic and clinical variability that is so characteristic of the heritable disorders of connective tissue. The hallmark of these disorders is the presence joint hypermobility, associated with an increase in skin elasticity and skin fragility. Ten EDS types had previously been defined based solely on clinical signs. However, recent advances in discovery of molecular lesions have raised uncertainty about the inclusion of certain phenotypes in the EDS syndrome. This will undoubtedly be resolved as studies progress. In 1997, a simplified classification was proposed dividing EDS into six major clinical types, including genetic defects where known.[116] This classification grouped EDS types I and II into the classic type; former type III EDS into the hypermobility type; EDS type IV into the vascular type; kyphoscoliosis type includes EDS VI; and former types VII A and VII B are now grouped into the arthrochalasia type. Several poorly differentiated EDS types are grouped into "other forms" pending biochemical confirmation of their identity. These include human dermatosparaxis (EDS VIIC), X-linked EDS type V, EDS VIII associated with periodontitis, and EDS type X or fibronectin-deficient EDS associated with prominent bruising. Type IX EDS (occipital horn syndrome), an X-linked recessive disorder, shares biochemical features with the Menkes disease and has been categorized as a disorder of copper metabolism.

Classic Types of Ehlers-Danlos Syndrome

These autosomal dominant forms of EDS account for about 80 percent of the reported cases.[117] Clinically, they are the most difficult to separate because of considerable overlap in phenotype. Up to 50 percent of individuals with clinical signs of EDS do not fit into any current classification.

The prototypic forms of EDS (Fig. 95–3) are characterized by varying degrees of hyperextensibility of large and small joints and present the classic findings of EDS. They are distinguished from each other in that the joint laxity and skin fragility are less severe in type II EDS.

Beighton has presented a clinically useful classification of joint laxity[116] (Fig. 95–4):

1. Passive dorsiflexion of the fifth digit beyond 90 degrees = one point for each hand
2. Passive apposition of the thumbs to the flexor surface of the radius = one point for each hand
3. Hyperextension of the elbows beyond 10 degrees = one point for each side
4. Hyperextension of the knees beyond 10 degrees = one point for each knee
5. Flexion of the trunk forward so that the palms are placed flat on the ground = one point

A score of five or more points is defined as joint hypermobility.

Large-joint hyperextensibility is marked in EDS type I and is mild and limited to the hands and feet in EDS type II. At times, it is difficult to decide whether limited hyperextensibility is present in an older sibling or parent, because joint laxity decreases with increasing age. Recurrent joint dislocations, periodic joint effusion

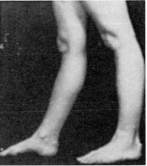
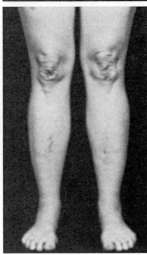

FIGURE 95–3 · Ehlers-Danlos Syndrome (EDS I). Tissue elasticity, joint hypermobility, and tissue fragility are demonstrated by the patient's ability to extend her tongue to the tip of the nose (Gorlin's sign), by hyperextensibility at the knee (genu recurvatum), and by characteristic "cigarette paper" or papyraceous scars of the knees and tibial skin. (Courtesy of V. McKusick, M.D.)

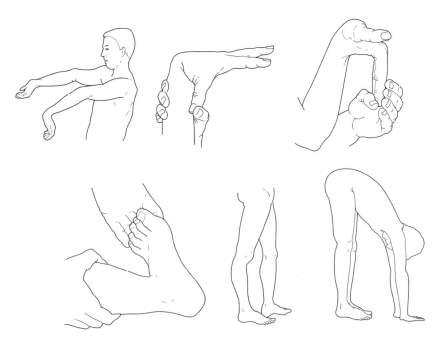

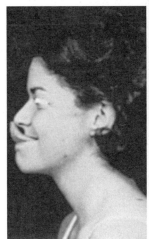

FIGURE 95–4 · Maneuvers that may be used to establish the presence of clinically significant joint laxity found in the Ehlers-Danlos syndrome (EDS). It is not unusual to find extreme laxity of the small joints and less laxity in large joints. Laxity decreases with age, so the dominant nature of most of these syndromes may not be appreciated when examining older family members. (Redrawn and modified from Wynne-Davies R: Acetabular dysplasia and familial joint laxity: two etiological factors in congenital dislocation of the hip—a review of 589 patients and their families. J Bone Joint Surg Br 52:704, 1970.)

related to trauma, and the eventual appearance of OA pose significant management problems. Bilateral synovial thickening has been observed in EDS, along with the accumulation of small masses of crystalline material in synovial villi. Osborn and coworkers[118] observed that EDS types II and III constituted 5 percent of cases in a pediatric arthritis clinic population. Infants may be born prematurely to affected mothers because of early rupture of membranes and are found to be hypotonic and floppy, with articular hyperextensibility. Prematurity is less common in EDS type II. Peripheral neuropathy secondary to stress on the brachial or lumbosacral plexus is another consequence of joint laxity. As these children grow, their muscle strength tends to improve, although strength is decreased in many adults.

Patients with EDS have characteristic parrot-like faces, with a broad nasal root and epicanthal folds. They may be floppy-eared, and traction on the ears or elbows reveals skin hyperextensibility. A gaping, "fish-mouth" wound may appear when skin is traumatized. In EDS the skin has a characteristic soft or "velvety" feel that can be appreciated by stroking the forearms. Thin, atrophic corrugated and hyperpigmented scars are found on the forehead, under the chin, and on the lower extremities (known as cigarette paper or papyraceous scars). Typically, skin lesions heal slowly after injury or surgery. The ability to touch the tip of the tongue to the nose (Gorlin's sign) is also evidence of tissue hyperextensibility. Molluscoid pseudotumors (violaceous subcutaneous tumors ranging in size from 0.5 to 3 cm) may be palpated in tissue over the forearms and lower extremities and may be seen on radiographs. Pseudotumors are calcified fat-containing cysts that occur over pressure points such as the elbows.

Although many patients claim to bruise easily, ecchymoses distributed on the extremities are found only in patients with the more severe forms of the disorder. Severe bilateral varicose veins are a common problem but are less frequent in type II disease.

Associated pulmonary complications of EDS are spontaneous pneumothorax, pneumomediastinum, and subpleural blebs.[119] Mitral valve prolapse and tricuspid valve insufficiency may complicate EDS type I.[120] Aortic root dilatation has been reported in subjects with types I, II, and III EDS.[121] The spectrum of skeletal findings in EDS I and II has been summarized by Coventry.[122] These may include thoracolumbar kyphoscoliosis; a long, giraffe-like neck; downward sloping of the ribs of the upper part of the thorax; and a tendency toward reversal of the normal cervical, thoracic, and lumbar curves. Anterior wedging of thoracic vertebral bodies occasionally is seen. Osteopenia has been recognized in several EDS phenotypes, but little data is available in regard to the mechanisms of bone loss involved in these syndromes.

Hypermobility Syndrome

The hypermobile type of EDS is a dominantly inherited disorder that presents as marked joint and spine hypermobility, recurrent joint dislocations, and the typical soft skin that is neither hyperextensible nor velvety: EDS III individuals may have virtually normal skin.[123] Because of the extent of joint laxity affecting both large and small joints, these patients experience multiple dislocations and may require surgical repair. The shoulders, patellae, and temporomandibular joints are frequently sites of dislocation. Musculoskeletal pain may mimic that of the fibromyalgia syndrome. Pregnancy in the type III EDS syndrome represents a high-risk problem.[124]

Benign Hypermobility Syndrome

In 1967, Kirk and colleagues[125] applied the term *hypermobility syndrome* to patients with generalized joint laxity associated with musculoskeletal complaints. Also apparent was a strong familial tendency, with dominant inheritance and variable expression. Although most persons with this syndrome have no symptoms, many have rheumatologic complaints that pose problems in diagnosis and therapy. There is also added anxiety about the relationship of physical activity to joint trauma, a factor that may adversely limit a patient's lifestyle.[126] There had been a familial joint hypermobility syndrome that was termed *EDS XI*, but it was subsequently removed from EDS classification.

It may be diagnostically important, when evaluating the heritable disorders of connective tissue, to carefully differentiate small-joint extensibility from combined large- and small-joint extensibility. Using a goniometer, Boone and Zane[127] measured the arcs of active joint motion in males between the ages of 18 months and 54 years and found that joint laxity diminishes with age in the normal population. By definition, patients with hypermobility syndrome lack the excessive skin laxity and the other stigmata of EDS or Marfan syndrome. Although hypermobility is usually apparent in early childhood, symptoms generally develop, and patients seek medical advice, during their twenties and thirties. Finsterbush and Pogrund[128] documented musculoskeletal complaints in 100 patients with generalized joint hypermobility, of whom 51 were female and 49 were male. Fifty-six patients had localized complaints, and 44 had more generalized musculoskeletal complaints, including episodic acute knee pain, patellar dislocation, and patellofemoral arthritis with effusion. Bilateral ankle instability, progressive scoliosis with back pain, and pain due to hyperextension at the elbow were also seen. Recurrent dislocation at several joints—sternoclavicular, shoulder, and hip—was particularly frequent in infants. Hypermobile joints were found in 65 percent of first-degree relatives. In the severely affected kindred described by Horton and colleagues[129] as exhibiting "familial joint instability," chronic sequelae included hypoplasia of the femoral heads and acetabulae with the formation of pseudoacetabulae. An association between hypermobility and OA has been suggested.[130]

Structural and Molecular Pathology of Classic and Hypermobile Type of Ehlers-Danlos Syndrome

Abnormally large, small, or frayed dermal collagen fibrils and disordered elastic fibers have been observed in these EDS patients by electronmicroscopy.[131] The ultrastructural findings appear similar in types I, II, and III EDS.

The role that the minor collagens might play in EDS has been strongly implicated based on an experiment in mice. A mutation within the endogenous 2(V) gene was introduced into embryonic stem cells by homologous recombination, and a breeding line expressing this mutation was established. The mice had fragile skin containing grossly deformed collagen fibrils. They developed severe kyphoscoliosis, presumably as a result of ligamentous laxity.

Recent evidence indicates that type V collagen is causally linked to EDS I and II. Type V collagen, a member of the group of fibrillar collagens, is composed of three α polypeptide–chains [1(V)2-2(V)], which are products of the COL5A1, COL5A2, and COL5A3 genes located on chromosomes 9p and 2q31-32, respectively. Type V collagen may stabilize type I collagen by coassembling with that protein. Evidence to date indicates that EDS types I and II, which show phenotypic overlap, may sometimes be allelic.[132] The initial mutation described in EDS I and II was an 1(V) mutation involving substitution of the most 5′ C-propeptide cysteine residue by serine.[133] Splicing defects in EDS I and II were also reported. Mutations affecting the 2(V) chain were reported in two unrelated patients with EDS I; the first was a 7-bp deletion that caused skipping of exon 27, whereas the second, a single nucleotide substitution, caused a skip of exon 28.[134] An arginine for glycine substitution (G934R) in the triple-helical domain was demonstrated in three affected members of an EDS type II family.[135] A unique point mutation at a lariat branch site in intron 32 (IVS32T-25G), which plays a major role in the splicing mechanism and induces exon 32 skip, has also been identified in EDS II.[132]

Mutations in other type I collagen interacting proteins can also produce an EDS I or II phenotype. Tenascin-X has been recently associated with a recessive form of EDS,[136] which is mimicked by a mouse tenascin-X knockout model.[137] Knockout of other noncollagenous proteins expressed in skin results in an EDS model,[138,139] suggesting that similar mutation will be found in humans.

Vascular Type

The clinical characteristic in EDS IV, the most severe form of EDS, is repeated arterial rupture, commonly involving iliac, splenic, or renal arteries or the aorta and resulting in either massive hematomas or death.[140,141] Arterial rupture may lead to stroke or intracompartmental bleeding in a limb. These patients have thin, soft, transparent skin, through which a prominent venous pattern is seen. They are also susceptible to rupture of internal viscera and may experience repeated rupture of diverticula on the antimesenteric border of the large bowel. Problems with pregnancy vary from preterm delivery to uterine rupture, although delivery is uneventful in many instances.[142] However, pregnancy may be complicated by vascular rupture, uterine rupture, and tearing of perineal tissues.[143] Typical causes of death in

EDS families have included gastrointestinal rupture, peripartum uterine rupture, and rupture of the hepatic artery.

In contrast to the other forms of EDS, EDS IV is not associated with hyperextensiblity of large joints, although small joints may be minimally hypermobile. Although the skin is thin, it is not hyperelastic. Excessive bruisability may occur. EDS IV includes, as a subgroup, patients who have been described as acrogyric.[144] These individuals have characteristic thin faces, prominent eyes, and extremities that lack subcutaneous fat, giving the appearance of premature aging. Peripheral joint contractures and acro-osteolysis have been described. Spontaneous hemopneumothorax associated with hemoptysis and mitral valve prolapse occurs frequently. Periodontitis with tooth loss can suggest overlap with EDS VIII.[145]

Surgical repair of ruptured vessels or internal viscera is extremely difficult because of friable tissues. Anesthetic and surgical difficulties related to intubation, spontaneous arterial bleeding during surgery, and the ligation of vessels that tear under pressure complicate surgical maneuvers. Similarly, arteriography may be dangerous in these subjects.

Molecular Pathology

Although EDS IV was clinically recognized as a disorder distinct from the other forms of EDS, the finding by Pope and colleagues[140] that tissues from these individuals were deficient in type III collagen clearly distinguished this as a separate form of EDS. Type III collagen is a homotrimer [1(III)₃] found in skin, blood vessels, and the uterus. Mutations in COL3A1 affect both the synthesis and secretion of type III collagen. Subsequent studies have shown both clinical and biochemical heterogeneity[146,147]; however, there is no correlation between the type of collagen III mutation and the clinical phenotype.[141]

These mutations include point substitutions, exon skipping mutations, and exon deletions. Thus, the mechanisms underlying faulty type III collagen are similar to those affecting type I collagen synthesis in OI. The first defect is decreased or absent production of an electrophoretically normal type I procollagen molecule, suggestive of a null allele due to abnormal RNA splicing. This defect is associated with a milder phenotype. The second category of defects includes mutations that interrupt the helical domain of a1 (III) molecules and result in severe disease. Fibroblastic cells derived from these individuals contain dilated rough endoplasmic reticulum with retained type III procollagen that is inefficiently secreted and is more susceptible to proteolytic digestion.

The majority of mutations involve point substitutions of arginine, serine, valine, aspartic acid, or glutamic acid for glycine in the triple-helical domain.[140,148-150] In addition, a number of mutations leading to exon skipping have been reported to involve exons 7, 8, 14, 16, 18, 20, 24, 25, 27, 34, 37, 41, 42, and 45.[140,150,151] Small genomic deletions and multiple exon deletions have also been reported.[152,153]

Most of the patients studied have a dominant pedigree consistent with a primary defect in one of the type III collagen alleles. However, both new mutations and germinal mosaicism give rise to patients with no family histories of the disease.[154] The recessive forms, representing only a small portion of EDS, tend to be more severe than forms that are dominantly inherited. Polymorphic restriction site analysis can be used to identify individuals at risk for the disease because of the dominant mode of transmission.[140] Biochemical analysis of the amount of type III collagen produced by dermal fibroblasts has proven a useful diagnostic test for EDS IV.[155]

Therapy

Obviously, there is no specific therapy directed at the molecular defect in the dominantly inherited forms of EDS. Supportive therapy, however, is essential for preservation of normal joint function and alleviation of joint pain.[156] Planned exercise programs and muscle-strengthening exercises are useful and do much to maintain a positive outlook in these individuals, who may have a poor prognosis if joint stability and articular surfaces are compromised by excessive activity or chronic trauma.[157] The presence of multiple ecchymoses raises concern about a bleeding diathesis, particularly at the time of elective surgery. Although no consistent basis for the hemorrhagic tendency in EDS I has been identified, caution is advised in patients with strong histories of easy bruisability. The recent discovery of von Willebrand–like protein sequences within certain matrix proteins lends credence to the clinical impression of a mild defect in hemostasis.[158]

Arthrochalasia Type

Type VII EDS is the result of different mutations involving faulty processing of the amino terminal end of type I collagen involving either the proα1(I)-chains (type VIIA) or proα2(I)-chains (type VIIB). The dermatosparactic form is caused by a deficiency of the procollagen 1 N-terminal peptidase, in contrast to the arthrochalastic form, which involves the enzyme cleavage site. The arthrochalstic form is inherited as an autosomal dominant disorder; the dermatsoparatctic form is inherited as an autosomal recessive disorder.

EDS VII is marked by pronounced and generalized joint hypermobility, moderate cutaneous elasticity, moderate bruising, a characteristic round facies with midface hypoplasia, and short stature. Kyphoscoliosis and muscle hypotonia are frequently present. These patients experience multiple dislocations, particularly involving large joints, such as the hips. This may manifest as congenital bilateral hip dislocations. Their tissues are highly friable, a factor that complicates orthopedic procedures. Their skin has a doughy feel and is fragile and hyperelastic. In EDS VIIC the skin is fragile, soft, and doughy with easy bruising. The phenotype includes blue sclerae, marked joint hypermobility, micrognathia, large umbilical hernia, and mild hirsuitism.[159] Premature rupture of fetal membranes may occur.

Molecular Pathology

This group of disorders classified as EDS type VIIA and EDS VIIB are the result of mutations involving the N-terminal α-chain propeptide cleavage site.[160] EDS VII C, the homologue of dermatospraxasis in sheep and cattle, is a result of defects in the converting enzyme procollagen N-peptidase.[161,162]

EDS VII has provided insight into the process of normal fiber formation. The initial observation was of an accumulation of unprocessed procollagen within the dermis of affected children. With subsequent recognition that procollagen had both N- and C-terminal extension propeptides and that separate enzymes were responsible for their removal, the syndrome became more sharply defined as an accumulation of procollagen with the N-terminal peptides still attached (pN collagen). Interference of the extension propeptide with normal extracellular fiber formation probably accounts for the clinical disorder.[163]

Of the two distinctly different genetic abnormalities resulting in procollagen accumulation, the more frequent form is the mutational resistance of a procollagen cleavage site to the action of the N-terminal procollagen peptidase. The resistance probably results from an amino acid substitution or deletion in the pro1α- or pro2α-chain (type VIIA and VIIB, respectively), leading to half of the pro x-chains containing an abnormal N-terminal extension.[164] In EDS VIIA this involves a complete or partial exon 6 skipping mutation that deletes the N-proteinase cleavage site in COL1A1, whereas in EDS VIIB, the exon 6 mutation involves the COL1A2 gene. Thus, one dose of the abnormal gene deranges collagen structure sufficiently to be recognized as a dominant trait. Byers and colleagues[160] have pointed out that the COL1A1 mutations appear to produce the more severe phenotype. Overlapping syndromes of EDS VII and mild OI may be explained by mutations within the helical domain of the collagen chain, placing the N-terminal cleavage site out of register for enzymatic cleavage of the propeptide.

Kyphoscoliosis Type

The first description of a biochemical defect related to collagen biosynthesis in EDS was presented by Pinnell in 1972.[159] This report described hydroxylysine-deficient collagen in two sisters with severe kyphoscoliosis, recurrent joint dislocations, and hyperextensible skin and joints. This is now recognized as due to a deficiency of lysyl hydroxylase. Premature rupture of fetal membranes had occurred at the birth of one of the children. Both were "floppy" at birth due to muscular hypotonia, with poor respiratory movements and subsequent bouts of pneumonia. Spinal deformity was apparent, as was easy bribability. Early growth and motor development were delayed, and muscle mass was diminished. Their skin was described as pale, translucent, and velvety, and it showed typical gaping, fish-mouth wounds after trauma.

The range of clinical manifestations of EDS VI is broadly representative of that of EDS. One exception is involvement of the ocular tissues, with microcornea, retinal detachment, and glaucoma that may lead to blindness. The eye is particularly susceptible to trauma because of scleral fragility that may lead to enucleation. However, trauma to the eye may not be as great a risk as initially assumed because a survey of patients with this disorder did not find abnormalities of the eye other than myopia.[241] Mild arachnodactyly; chest wall deformity associated with narrow shoulders; molluscoid pseudotumors; thin, atrophic scars; and easy bruisability also occur. Hyperextensibility of joints is marked. Severe kyphoscoliosis may lead to cardiorespiratory failure. Gastrointestinal hemorrhage may also occur.

Molecular Pathology

Kyphoscoliotic EDS is transmitted in an autosomal recessive mode. In the original description of EDS VI, it was found that the hydroxylysine content of collagen in skin and tendons was less than 1 residue per 1000 total amino acids in contrast to 4 residues per 1000 in control tissue.[165] The hydroxylysine content was somewhat less than normal in bone and was normal in cartilage. Subsequently, a number of investigators demonstrated low lysyl hydroxylase or even normal activity in fibroblasts obtained from certain individuals with this form of EDS.[166]

The mechanism of the low activity was shown to result from an altered affinity (Km) for ascorbic acid, the cofactor of the enzyme. Although these studies suggested that at higher levels of ascorbic acid the enzyme activity would increase, no systematic study has demonstrated the effectiveness of ascorbic acid in this disease. A variety of mutations within the lysyl hydroxylase gene have been defined and include premature stop codons, amino acid substitutions, internal deletions, and compound heterozygotes. Heikkinen and coworkers[167] have reported that a homozygous duplication of 8.9 kb in the lysyl hydroxylase gene caused by homologous recombination of Alu sequences in introns 9 and 16 occurred with a frequency of 19.1 percent in 35 type VI families. This wide array of mutations may explain the variability in disease severity observed in this disorder.

Defective lysyl hydroxylase impairs the conversion of lysyl residues to hydroxylysine on procollagen peptides. The consequence of deficient hydroxylysine content of collagen is related to the role of this amino acid in cross-link formation. Hydroxylysine-containing cross-links are able to undergo a stabilizing change (Amadori rearrangement), which is particularly common to the types of cross-links found in bone. Although individuals with EDS VI do form reducible cross-links, many appear to lack the hydroxylysine residue[168] that enters into the formation of the hydroxypyridinium cross-links. A practical clinical test for the presence of EDS VI is based on the lack of urinary excretion of hydroxypyridinium cross-links.

Enzyme levels in amniotic fluid fibroblasts may be useful in prenatal diagnostic studies. Exclusion of the diagnosis has been accomplished by screening fetal DNA for mutations in the lysyl hydroxylase gene.[169]

Other Ehlers-Danlos Syndrome Types

X-Linked Ehlers-Danlos Syndrome (Type V)

A phenotype similar to type II EDS with the added feature of intramuscular hemorrhage has been identified in two families.[170] X-linked recessive inheritance was invoked to explain transmission of the disorder. However, there is question as to whether this is a separate entity. A deficiency of LO was suggested based on studies with cultured dermal fibroblasts; however, this has not been supported by all investigators.[156]

Ehlers-Danlos Syndrome VIII

As reported by Stewart[171] and others,[172] the characteristics of EDS VIII, a dominantly inherited syndrome, include 1) a severe resorptive periodontitis that leads to early loss of teeth and 2) marked fragility of the skin in the absence of hyperelasticity that leads to dystrophic scarring. Joint hypermobility is mild. Even the limited number of reported cases suggests that clinical variability, as occurs in the other EDS types, will also be seen in EDS VIII. The dental findings, however, have been rather uniform.

The previously categorized EDS IX is a rare X-linked condition characterized by skeletal dysplasia, characteristic occipital "horns" that appear during adolescence, diarrhea due to increased bowel motility, and obstructive uropathy due to bladder diverticulae that appear during the first decade.[117] Arterial aneurysms may occur in these patients.[173] This condition is allelic with Menkes disease and, along with Wilson's disease, is one of the three hereditary disorders of copper metabolism.[174] Cells from patients with these disorders have elevated levels of intracellular copper due to defective copper transport. A defective copper-transporting adenosine triphosphatase (ATPase) gene demonstrated in Menkes syndrome may underlie the mechanism of this disease.[175] This is associated with severe reduction in the activity of copper-dependent LO as a consequence of decreased synthesis of the enzyme.[176] X-linked cutis laxa has been reclassified as a variant of the occipital horn syndrome.[146]

Ehlers-Danlos Syndrome X

In the original case report of EDS X, or fibronectin-deficient EDS, the proband had hypermobile joints, easy bruising, fish-mouth scars on her extremities, and mitral valve prolapse.[177] Although this presentation clinically resembled EDS II or III, the characteristic velvety feel of the skin was absent, as were striae. Platelets obtained from this patient revealed resistance to aggregation in response to collagen and adenosine diphosphate (ADP), whereas the responses to serotonin, thrombin, and epinephrine were diminished. Because normal plasma or cryoprecipitate was found to correct the clotting defect, it was suggested that a qualitative deficiency of fibronectin caused the abnormality. Molecular confirmation of this suggestion is lacking.

Progeroid Ehlers-Danlos Syndrome

This rare syndrome, a defect in chondroitin and dermatan sulfate proteoglycan synthesis, is characterized by progeroid facies, mild mental retardation, multiple nevi, skin hyperextensibility, increased bruising, and joint laxity mainly affecting the digits.[178,179] The progeroid phenotype is caused by mutations leading to a deficiency in galactotransferase I, which catalyzes the glycosyl transfer in the assembly of dermatan sulfate.[180,181]

MARFAN SYNDROME

One of the most common inherited disorders of connective tissue, MFS is an autosomal dominant disorder with a reported incidence of 1 in 10,000 to 20,000 individuals.[182] There is a wide range of clinical severity associated with MSF. Although many clinicians view the disorder in terms of classic ocular, cardiovascular, and musculoskeletal abnormalities, these patients also demonstrate significant involvement of pulmonary tissues, skin, and the central nervous system (CNS). A severe and rapidly progressive form of MFS may present at birth.

MFS has attracted increasing interest for two major reasons: 1) the discovery that many cases of the Marfan phenotype involve mutations of the fibrillin-1 (FBN-1) gene and 2) the emergence of an aggressive medical and surgical approach to therapy.

MFS shares the stage with other heritable disorders of connective tissue in which different mutations involving a specific connective-tissue protein have been demonstrated.[183] Patients with the typical Marfan phenotype harbor different mutations involving the FBN-1 gene.[184] However, it is well recognized that FBN-1 mutations occur across a wide range of milder phenotypes that overlap the classic Marfan phenotype.[185]

Clinical Features

Because of a recognized tendency to overdiagnose MFS in index cases or family members, stringent criteria for this diagnosis were proposed in 1996.[186] The 1996 criteria rely on the recognition of both "major" and "minor" clinical manifestations involving the skeletal, cardiovascular, dura, and ocular systems Major criteria include four of eight typical skeletal manifestations, ectopia lentis, aortic root dilatation involving the sinuses of Valsalva or aortic dissection, and lumbosacral dural ectasia by computed tomography (CT) or magnetic resonance imaging (MRI). Major criteria for establishing the diagnosis in a family member include having a parent, child, or sibling who meets major criteria independently, the presence of an FBN-1 mutation known to cause the syndrome, or a haplotype around FBN-1 inherited by descent and identified in a familial Marfan patient. To unequivocally establish the diagnosis in the absence of a family history requires a major manifestation from two systems and involvement of a third system. If a mutation known to cause MFS is identified, the diagnosis requires one major criterion and involvement of a second organ system. To establish the diagnosis in a relative of an index case requires the presence of a major criterion in the family history and one major criterion in a organ system with involvement of a second organ system. Illustrative of this problem in definition is the recent report of Montgomery and colleagues[187] who examined the FBN-1 genotypes and clinical phenotypes in three families and segregated MFS with marked intrafamilial clinical variability or with mild overlapping phenotypes in which the manifestations failed to meet stringent criteria for diagnosis of MSF. In one family, clinically similar but genetically distinct syndromes segregated independently with MSF. In another, somatic mosaicism was associated with a mild subdiagnostic phenotype, whereas in a third family, mild mitral valve prolapse syndrome cosegregated with an FBN-1 mutation different from those associated with the classic MSF phenotype.

Aortic disease leading to the formation of aneurysmal dilatation and dissection is the main cause of morbidity and mortality in the MFS.[188] Dilatation of the aorta is found in 50 percent of children, and this progresses with time. Echocardiography demonstrates that 60 to 80 percent of adult patients have dilatation of the aortic root that may involve other segments of the thoracic aorta, the abdominal aorta, or even the carotid and intracranial arteries. Studies indicate that the aorta tends to be stiffer and less distensible in MFS than in controls, but there is only variable correlation between these parameters and aortic distension. Dissection usually begins above the coronary ostia and extends the entire length of the aorta. Sixty to 70 percent of MFS patients have mitral valve prolapse with regurgitation. Heart failure and myocardial infarction may complicate the course of MSF patients. Pregnant women are at particular risk for aortic dissection, particularly those who already have aortic root dilatation.[189]

Arachnodactyly occurs in 90 percent of patients but this is not diagnostic, because elongation of hands and feet may occur in otherwise normal individuals. Confirmation of arachnodactyly may be sought using the following techniques:

1. *The thumb.* The Steinberg test is positive when the thumb, enclosed in the clenched fist, extends beyond the hypothenar border.
2. *The wrist.* The Walker-Murdoch sign is positive when there is overlap of the thumb and fifth digit as they encircle the opposite wrist.
3. *The metacarpal.* The metacarpal index is the mean value of the lengths divided by the midpoint widths of the second, third, and fourth metacarpals. In normal subjects, the metacarpal index ranges from 5.4 to 7.9, whereas this range is 8.4 to 10.4 in patients with MFS.

Thoracic kyphosis may be associated with reduced lung capacity and residual volume that may lead to pulmonary insufficiency. Dural ectasia, which may occur in as many as 40 percent of patients, results from enlargement of the spinal canal owing to progressive ectasia of dura and neural foramina and erosion of vertebral bone. This usually involves the lower spine.[190,191] Diminished bone mineral density (BMD) has recently been reported in several patients with MFS.[192,193]

Ectopia lentis occurs in 50 to 80 percent of patients with MFS. Subluxation of the lens is usually bilateral and appears by the age of 5 years. Although the lens is typically displaced upward, displacement into any quadrant may occur. Visual acuity is diminished in many patients because of lens subluxation or secondary acute glaucoma. Secondary myopia, retinal detachment, and iritis with loss of vision contribute to most of the ocular-related morbidity.[194]

MFS patients have been found to develop large epidural venous plexuses in the lumbar and cervical regions, a major diagnostic criterion for the syndrome. These probably form secondarily to as-yet-undefined structural abnormalities in venous wall.[195] These engorged venous plexuses, which are visualized by MRI myelography, have, in turn, been associated with the syndrome of spontaneous intracranial hypotension, which is also associated with dural tears. Clinical signs of this are severe headache, back and leg pain, radiculopathies, and incontinence secondary to cerebral displacement.[196]

Spinal abnormalities in MFS include increased inter-pedicle distance of nonrotated vertebrae, vertebral inversion (flattening of the normal kyphosis at the dorsal level and kyphosis or disappearance of the physiologic lordosis at the lumbar level), and vertebral dysplasia (dolichospondylia, elongated vertebral bodies with increased concavity). Scoliosis constitutes one of the major management problems in MFS. In one series, the average age of onset was 10.5 years (range of 3 to 15 years), with rapid progression during adolescence.[197] If mechanic bracing or physical therapy fails to halt progression, spinal fusion should be considered, particularly when the curvature exceeds 45 to 50 degrees.

Differential Diagnosis

Homocystinuria

Homocystinuria, which shares several skeletal and ocular features with MFS, is the prime diagnostic consideration. This is an autosomal recessive disease. The characteristic features of this metabolic disorder of sulfur metabolism are marfanoid phenotype with joint laxity, scoliosis, lens dislocation, early-onset osteoporosis, vascular thrombosis affecting arteries and veins due to increased clotting activity and the cytotoxic effect of homocysteine on vascular endothelial cells, and mild mental retardation.[198]

Cystathionine beta synthase (CBS) deficiency is the most common cause of homocystinuria. Rarely, patients develop homocystinuria due to methylene tetrahydrofolate reductase deficiency. The diagnosis of homozygous homocystinuria can be made by measurement of plasma sulfur amino acid concentrations, especially total homocysteine, which is elevated to the range of 100 to 300 μM. Methionine levels are also elevated, whereas cystathionine and cysteine levels in blood are decreased.[199] The CBS gene has been mapped to chromosome 21q.22.3. More than 90 CBS mutations have been reported. The two most common are 833T→C, which results in a mild phenotype, and 919G→A, which results in a more severe phenotype.[200] In Australian patients, two mutations, I278I→T and 307G→S, were most common.[201] Approximately 50 percent of patients respond to the administration of pyridoxine, a low-methionone diet, and betaine.

The mitral valve prolapse-aorta, or mild aortic root dilatation-skeleton-skin (MASS), syndrome may not be linked to the fibrillin genes.[202,203] Also to be differentiated are other genetic disorders of the elastic fiber system with marfanoid features, including ectopia lentis syndrome, isolated skeletal features of MFS, the Shprintzen-Goldberg syndrome, and congenital contractual arachnodactyly, which is caused by mutations in the FBN-2 gene.

Molecular Biology Marfan Syndrome

Fibrillin-1 protein is an important component of both elastic and nonelastic connective tissues throughout the body.[204,205] It is the main protein of a group of connective tissue microfibrils that are essential for normal elastic fibrillogenesis. In nonelastic tissues, the fibrillin-1–containing microfibril functions as an anchoring fiber. FBN-1 is a large gene (65 exons, 250 kb, Human Genome Sequencing Project NT 034890 sequence) located at chromosome 15q-21.1.[206,207] The gene is characterized by the presence of many cysteine-rich sequences homologous to epidermal growth factor (EGF)-like module or the transforming growth factor-β1 (TGF-β1)–binding protein-like module, and a third module called "hybrid modules," which have features of both the EGF- and TGF-β1–binding protein-like modules.[204] EGF-like modules contain multiple important calcium-binding sequences (cbEGF-like modules). Since the first report of an FBN-1 mutation in MFS in 1991, more than 500 different FBN-1 mutations have been described in MFS and related disorders.[208] FBN-1 mutations occur across a wide range of milder phenotypes that overlap the classic Marfan phenotype, including dominantly inherited ectopia lentis, the Shprintzen-Goldberg syndrome, and familial or isolated forms of aortic aneurysms.[204,209] The majority of these occur as nonrecurring mutations, with the exception of the clustering of mutations between exons 24 and 26 and exon 32 in cases of severe neonatal MFS. More than 25 pecent of cases represent a probable new mutation.[208,210,211] Four basic mechanisms result in these mutations: 1) missense mutations, 2) premature terminations caused by nonsense mutation or frame shifts, 3) splice-site deletions and insertions, and 4) intron splice-site changes leading to alternate splicing and in-frame exon skipping or deletion.[211] Several genetic polymorphisms have also been described. To date, although no correlation between the specific type of FBN-1 mutation and clinical phenotype has been recognized, patients with exon skipping tend to have more severe disease, whereas those showing premature termination causing reduced levels of a shortened mutant transcript tend to have milder disease.[212]

Mutations involving a second fibrillin protein, fibrillin-2, a product of the FBN-2 gene located on chromosome 5, have been described in patients with congenital contractual arachnodactly. This disorder is characterized by multiple contractures, arachnodactly, and external ear malformations.[210] The syndrome of annuloaortic ectasia and the dominantly inherited ectopia lentis syndrome have also been linked to the FBN-1 locus on chromosome 15.[213]

Treatment

The life span of untreated patients with classic MFS was about 32 years in 1972. However, careful monitoring, including echocardiographic monitoring every 6 months when the aortic root diameter exceeds 45 mm, and early surgical intervention has resulted in the life expectancy increasing to 41 years in 1993 and 61 years in 1996. Interestingly, survival is lower in men than in women. Treatment with β-adrenergic blockage has been proposed for several years: Reports of its effectiveness have only been available since 1994.[214] In that randomized study, treatment with propanolol (average dose 212 mg/day) resulted in a significantly slower rate of increase in mean aortic root diameter (0.023 vs. 0.084 cm/year). Treatment with a β-blocker at a dose that keeps heart rate less than 110 beats/min after submaximal exercise should be considered in all patients, including children. Women with MFS contemplating pregnancy should have a screening transthoracic echocardiogram (ECG) for assessment of aortic root dimensions. Elective repair is recommended before conception for an aneurysm greater than 50 mm.[215]

ECG monitoring is performed yearly until the aortic root diameter exceeds 45 mm, at which time monitoring is performed every 6 months. Elective repair of aortic root disease before enlargement to 6 cm has occurred is preferable to emergency repair required for marked dilatation or dissection. Surgical intervention is considered when the aortic root diameter approaches twice the upper limit of normal for body surface area or the absolute measurement exceeds 50 to 55 mm.[216] Total aortic root replacement with a composite valve graft (Bentall procedure) and coronary artery implantation have become the surgical procedures of choice and are associated with an 81-percent 10-year survival rate and a 75-percent 20-year survival rate.[217,218] Mitral valve replacement and coronary artery implantation may be accomplished during the same procedure.

Correction of scoliosis may be attempted with bracing; however, surgical repair should be considered when the curve exceeds 40 degrees. Progressive scoliosis in MFS may require fixation with rods, and complications of joint laxity may require orthopedic correction. Arthropathy associated with excessive joint mobility may require orthopedic intervention. Dislocated lenses should not be removed surgically unless more conventional means of correcting vision are ineffective.

Congenital Contractural Arachnodactyly

Congenital contractural arachnodactyly (CCA) is an autosomal dominant condition that includes tall stature, arachnodactyly, dolichostenomelia, and multiple contractures involving large joints.[219] There is a characteristic "crumpled ear" deformity due to a flattened helix with partial obliteration of the concha. Osteopenia occurs frequently. Marked deformity of the chest cage also occurs, and scoliosis may be progressive and severe. For unknown reasons, the contractures tend to become less severe with age. The ocular and typical cardiac lesions of classic MFS are absent. The observation that dolichostenomelia and arachnodactyly can occur in relatives lacking the marfanoid habitus suggests variable expression of the *CCA* gene.

Molecular Pathology

In 1990, two lines of research converged to demonstrate that mutations arising within the FBN gene were responsible for classic MFS. At the time when immunofluorescent studies showed abnormalities in elastin-associated microfibrillin protein in individuals with MFS, a consortium of geneticists localized the disease locus to a region of chromosome 15, which harbors the FBN gene. At the time the initial discovery of the FBN gene was made on chromosome 15, a second highly homologous gene *(FBN-2)* was found on chromosome 5. *CCA* has been linked to this gene.[220] It encodes a similar protein that is expressed earlier in development and may play a greater role in defining the pattern of elastin deposition than as a structural component of mature elastin elastic tissue. *FBN-2* mutations have been observed to cluster in a limited region of the gene and to occur in *FBN-2* locations corresponding to *FBN-1* mutations that have been reported in cases of severe, neonatal MFS.[220]

Cutis Laxa

The term *cutis laxa* refers to a group of generalized connective tissue disorders in which the common clinical feature is lax, redundant, inelastic skin.[221] The skin of these patients is wrinkled and sags in loose folds, imparting a prematurely aged appearance. Acquired cutis laxa may follow penicillamine ingestion, inflammatory skin disease, or a nonspecific febrile illness.

The autosomal dominant form of cutis laxa is mild and largely limited to the dermis and, thus, is compatible with a normal life span. Dermal changes may be present in infancy but usually are not marked until the second or third decade, when tissues loosen and become redundant on the face and extremities. Unlike the case with EDS, the skin in cutis laxa does not recoil when stretched. Several patients have been found to harbor bronchiectasis or mild pulmonary emphysema. Aside from pulmonary infections in childhood and the occurrence of inguinal hernias, these patients remain in good health. The joints are not hyperextensible in this disease. The recessive variety is more severe, as evidenced by diagnosis at birth or shortly thereafter and the early development of severe cardiopulmonary complications. The X-linked variety of cutis laxa appears to be intermediate in severity between the autosomal recessive and the autosomal dominant forms and is included as another X-linked form of EDS IX.[222]

Recently a mouse knockout of the *fibulin-5* gene demonstrated the importance of this elastin-binding protein to the elastic properties of skin, blood vessels, and the lung.[223,224] This serves as confirmation that mutations of this locus can result in a severe autosomal recessive form of the disease.[225]

Molecular Pathology

Microscopic examination of the dermis in cutis laxa reveals alterations in both elastic fibers and collagen. Fine elastic fibers that normally rise into the dermal papillae may be absent. Individual elastic fibers that vary greatly in diameter are short, globular in outline, and less compact; the elastica may be more abundant at deeper levels of the dermis. Globular, fragmented, and clumped elastic fibers have also been observed in the lung and aorta. Fibroblasts derived from these patients appear to have normal levels of lysyl oxidase and possibly increased expression of an elastolytic activity. The level of elastin mRNA appears to be reduced but responds to stimulation with TGF-β.[226] Zhang and coworkers[227] have reported frame-shift mutations in elastin gene exon 30, leading to missense C-termini. *Fibulin-5*, a recently discovered ligand for cell surface integrins, is essential for normal elastin-fiber organization. A homozygous *fibulin-5* missense mutation has been reported in a severe recessive form of cutis laxa.[225]

Therapy

Treatment is limited to plastic surgery, which can significantly improve the patient's appearance. Unlike in EDS, surgery in cutis laxa is not complicated by excessive bleeding or tissue fragility.

Pseudoxanthoma Elasticum

A rare disorder, pseudoxanthoma elasticum (PXE) is characterized by degeneration and calcification of elastic fibers in the skin, retina, and blood vessels.[228] PXE is inherited primarily as an autosomal recessive trait and less frequently as an autosomal dominant.[229] Sporadic occurrence of the disease is recognized. In its classic form, PXE is recognized by the presence of asymptomatic, symmetric, yellowish-white xanthomatoid papules in flexural skin folds, which appear during the second or third decade of life. These occur earlier in recessive forms. Lesions initially involve the skin of the neck and axilla and progress to other areas, where they coalesce to give the skin a redundant, thickened appearance. Mucocutaneous lesions may also occur on the buccal mucosa of the lower lip. Ocular disease develops in almost every patient. Angioid streaks of the retina, radially oriented and resembling vessels, are the result of a break in Bruch's membrane.[230] Druzen, mottling of the retinal pigment epithelium, and a "peau d'orange" lesion may occur. Retinal lesions may be demonstrated with fluorescence angiography. Visual loss in PXE, which varies from mild loss to legal blindness, is the result of maculopathy and retinal hemorrhage. In the lung, lesions are associated with dyspnea and include vascular calcification and intimal fibrosis due to damage of the elastic laminae in arteries, arterioles, and venules. Calcific deposits occur in alveolar lumina and may be seen on radiographs. Involvement of the heart may cause angina, dyspnea, and arrhythmias, suggestive of a cardiomyopathy.[231] Both angina and accelerated atherosclerosis may occur at an early age. Endomyocardial biopsy and postmortem specimens have revealed fragmented and mineralized elastic fibers similar to those seen in the skin. Intimal fibrosis may compromise the coronary circulation. Mitral valve prolapse is a common occurrence. Genitourinary and uterine bleeding may complicate the clinical course of PXE. Bleeding into joints may occur. Arteries of the gastrointestinal tract are particularly susceptible to rupture, which occurred in 14 percent of patients in one series.[232]

Wound healing is generally normal in PXE until late in the course of the disease, when dermal calcification may be extensive. Hyperextensibility may lead to dislocations of both large and small joints.

Histologic evidence of calcification and fragmentation of elastin fibers is essential for the diagnosis of PXE. Acquired forms of PXE have been recognized. These include the use of D-penicillamine and saltpeter-induced skin lesions (Table 95–6).

Molecular Pathology

In cases of PXE, dermal elastic fibers are frayed, swollen, and clumped and appear to be increased in number. The centers of elastin fibers are replaced by an electron-dense material, which appears to disrupt the fiber, leading to calcification. Analysis of this material indicates the presence of several matrix proteins; vitronectin, alkaline phosphatase, and bone sialoprotein were localized in polymorphous material inside the elastic fibers.[234,235] This material is immunologically positive for most of the expected components of skin but negative for elastin. Nonaffected skin in PXE has also been shown to contain increased quantities of this dense material.

Families segregating either autosomal dominant or autosomal recessive PXE have been mapped to chromosome 16p13.1.[236,237] Recent reports have demonstrated that PXE results from mutations in a gene of the ABC transporter family, coding for a membrane-embedded ABC transporter protein, ABCC6 (MRP6).[238] As demonstrated with human mutants, loss-of-function mutations in ABCC6 impair transport of several organic anions, including glutathione conjugates.[239] However, the relation of these defects to the PXE lesion is undefined.

TABLE 95–6 • CRITERIA FOR THE DIAGNOSIS OF PSEUDOXANTHOMA ELASTICUM (PXE)[233]

Major Criteria:
1. Characteristic skin involvement (yellow cobblestone lesions in flexural locations)
2. Characteristic histopathologic features of lesional skin (elastic tissue and calcium or von Kossa stains)
3. Characteristic ocular disease (angoid streaks, peau d'orange or maculopathy) in adults older than 20 years of age

Minor Criteria:
1. Characteristic histopathologic features of nonlesional skin (elastic tissue and calcium or von Kossa stains)
2. Family history of PXE in first-degree relatives

Supervalvular Aortic Stenosis and Williams Syndrome

Although these two conditions have not classically been included in chapters of heritable diseases of connective tissue, they now need to be mentioned because they have recently been shown to contain mutations or deletions within the elastin gene. Williams syndrome is usually obvious in the newborn period because of the characteristic elfin-like faces and transient hypercalcemia.[240] About one third have supervalvular aortic stenosis, which often occurs as an isolated cardiac finding with a dominant mode of inheritance. In both forms, the stenosis can become hemodynamically significant as a result of valvular stenosis or can compromise the aortic valve aorta, leading to aortic insufficiency or aortic dissection. Surgical correction is usually possible.

Molecular Pathology

Williams syndrome represents a continuous gene deletion disorder involving the human chromosome 7q11.23 segment. At least 17 gene deletions have been reported, including a 1.5 million – bp inversion polymorphism in families with this syndrome.[241] Screening of the elastin gene for mutations in supravalvular aortic stenosis has revealed a C to G transversion with the acceptor splice site of exon 16.[242] Both skipping of exon 16 and an intronic 44 bp insertion in exon 16 have been described.[242] In another large kindred, a point mutation in exon 18 and a stop codon in exon 22 of the elastin gene were described.[243] Examples of two recently reported deletions include the deletion of the *BCL7B* member of the *BCL7* gene family and deletion of a known transcription factor, *GTF21*.[244,245]

■ Heritable Diseases of the Type II Collagen Family

Remarkable progress has been made in the past few years in defining the molecular basis of the heritable diseases of cartilage (chondrodystrophies). The epiphyseal and diaphyseal cartilage are the best examples of the ordered maturation of a connective tissue cell. At the base of the epiphysis, the resting undifferentiated prechondrocyte enters a phase of proliferation and differentiation to a chondrocyte, which continues to progress into highly ordered columns of hypertrophic chondrocytes. Because the skeleton is initially modeled in chondrogenic tissue, it is chondrocytes that first respond to the patterning genes that determine the mature skeleton. There is an increasing number of homeobox genes that are implicated in this complex regulatory pathway in somatic pattern formation. As the chondrocytes start to proliferate and mature, they synthesize type II, IX, and XI collagen. Subsequently, they form columns of hypertrophic chondrocytes. Type X collagen production is one of the hallmarks of the hypertrophic chondrocyte. The transition zone between hypertrophic chondrocytes and osteoblasts develops in the region where blood vessels invade and provide the environment for osteogene-

sis to begin. Mutated genes expressed at a particular stage in the maturation of the epiphysis or metaphysis induce a distinctly different phenotype.

The following is not meant to be an exhaustive clinical description of the complex chondrodystrophies but a summary of how approaching these disorders from a genetic perspective of the extracellular matrix can provide a clearer understanding of the clinical presentation.

ACHONDROPLASIA FAMILY OF DISORDERS

Achondroplasia

Achondroplasia is the most common of the chondrodysplasias in man.[246] It is characterized by short-limbed dwarfism, a normal-sized trunk, waddling gait, thoracolumbar gibbus, and a large head with fontal bossing. It is inherited as an autosomal dominant trait, although most cases are sporadic, new mutations. Hypochondroplasia has many of the same features as achondroplasia, although it is much milder and usually is not apparent until late childhood. Achondroplasia occurs with an estimated frequency of 1 in 15,000 to 40,000 live births.

The gene for achondroplasia has been mapped using linkage techniques. Francomano[247] localized the gene to 4p16.3 using 18 multigenerational families with achondroplasia and 10 short, tandem-repeat polymorphic markers from this region. The fFGF receptor 3 gene *(FGFR3)* was also known to be situated in this area. Subsequently, mutations affecting the *FGFR3* gene in achondroplasia were reported in 1994.[248,249] *FGFR3* is a negative regulator of bone growth. Unlike the diverse representation of mutations in other heritable disorders (e.g., OI), in 97 percent of cases, achondroplasia was found associated with one of two mutations—a G to A transition at nucleotide 1138 or a G to C mutation at nucleotide 1138—affecting the transmembrane domain of the *FGFR3* gene by substituting arginine for glycine at position 380 of the protein. These apparently occur on the paternally derived chromosome in sporadic cases of achondroplasia.[250] Although a G to C mutation was observed in another case,[248] Rosseau[249] and colleagues also found that 23 mutations in achondroplasia cases resulted from the same G to A transition at nucleotide 1138. A single case bore a novel G to T transition at codon 375.[251] Ikegawa[252] and coworkers also reported a G to T transition at condon 375, which resulted in the substitution of a cysteine for a glycine. These mutations frequently occur in a cytosine phosphate (Cp) next to guanine, a CpG dinucleotide that is known to be a mutational "hot spot."

Although the biologic consequences of the mutations in the *FGFR3* gene are not yet understood, FGF does play an important role in regulating the lineage pathway of the chondrocyte. It appears to prevent full chondrocyte differentiation during the phase of early chondrocyte proliferation. The dominant inheritance pattern of achondroplasia suggests the mutation is a gain of function. It is the presence of the mutation that may inhibit the differentiation process of the chondrocytes. The histologic examination of the epiphyseal cartilage in achondroplasia shows a poorly organized hypercellular matrix. The chondrocytes are enlarged, with dilated endoplasmic reticulum reminiscent of the dilated, rough endoplasmic reticulum seen in OI osteoblasts expressing a mutant type I collagen chain. The same mechanism proved to be the case for the epiphyseal dysplasias (SED).

Spinal Chondrodysplasia Associated with Early-Onset Osteoarthritis

Recently, COL2A1 mutations have been reported in patients with mild forms of spinal chondrodysplasia associated with the precocious onset of generalized OA. Ala-Kokkoand colleagues reported the isolation of a cosmid clone for an allele of the type II procollagen gene in a family with premature OA.[253] A single base mutation that converted the codon for arginine 519 of the α1(II)-chain to a codon for cysteine was found in affected members of a large family. Subsequent studies have verified the presence of this arg519-to-cys mutation in several other families with the same clinical picture.[254] A type II procollagen mutation consisting of an exon 11 substitution (arginine 75 to cysteine) was also reported in a family demonstrating mild sponsyloepiphyseal dysplasia and precocious OA.[255] Mild deafness was present in the proband and his 21-year-old daughter. This mutation has been recognized in other families; the pattern of mutations suggest the possibility of mutation "hot spots" on COL2A1 related to hypermutability of the cytosine-guanine doublet.[256]

Spondyloepiphyseal dysplasia (SED) congenita is the most widely recognized form of this heterogenous group of disorders. It is characterized by a small trunk, short neck, barrel chest, and long extremities out of proportion to the trunk. The epiphyses are irregular, and the vertebral bodies are deformed. The most severe members of this family are achondrogenesis and hypochondrogenesis. Infants with these conditions have large heads, soft crania, barrel-shaped chests, and little radiographic evidence of ossification. A milder form is recognized as Kneist's dysplasia. All forms are inherited as an autosomal dominant trait. Recently, an aggressive form of degenerative arthritis has been described that also fits into the family because it results from mutations within the same gene. Ikewaga has reported a mutation in COL11A1 in SED consisting of Gly595Glu.[257]

Multiple epiphyseal dysplasia and the Stickler's syndrome are other clinical variants of the epiphyseal dysplasia family of cartilage disease.[258] Both are associated with degenerative arthritis and short stature, but the extremities are not inappropriately long. Stickler's syndrome has the unusual additional features of severe myopia and choroidoretinal and vitreous degeneration.

The molecular basis for these two conditions was initially suggested from transgenic mouse studies. Transgenic mice expressing either a mutant COL9A1 collagen or fully inactivated endogenous COL9A1 gene develop a mild degenerative arthritis.[259]

Recently, one human pedigree with multiple epiphyseal dysplasia was genetically linked to the COL9A2 locus.[260] The cho mouse strain arose from a naturally occurring mutation and was maintained as a homozygous recessive and lethal trait. Linkage studies in mice pointed to the COL11A1 gene. The mutation produces a null allele, which probably accounts for the fact that it is not seen as a dominant trait.

Stickler's syndrome is an autosomal dominant disorder with ophthalmologic and orofacial features, deafness, and OA that develops in the third or fourth decade.[261] There is joint hypermobility that declines with age. Mild SED is often present. The majority of patients have mutations in the COL2A1 gene. A mutation of the COL11A2 gene has now been described in two individuals with Stickler's syndrome.[262] In one case, the inheritance was dominant, and in the other it was recessive. These cases point to the importance of type IX and Xl collagens in the formation of normal type II collagen fibrils. Further molecular characterization should clarify some of the clinical heterogeneity seen in these conditions.[263]

METAPHYSEAL CHONDRODYSPLASIA FAMILY

Three different forms of metaphyseal dysplasia are recognized. They all have the common feature that osteogenesis does not progress normally at its junction with the hypertrophic chondrocyte.[264]

Jansen's type is most severe and is recognizable at birth by short limbs, enlarged joints, and shortened long bones with marked flaring of the metaphyses. Occasionally, these infants have hypercalcemia. The junction between the forming bone and hypertrophic chondrocyte is uneven, with a suggestion that there is a failure of new bone invasion. The molecular basis of this form of metaphyseal dysplasia was initially suggested by a gene knockout of the parathyroid hormone (PTH) and parathyroid hormone–related peptide (PTHRP) receptor. Subsequently, two activating mutations (H223R and I458R) were found in a patients with Jansen's metaphyseal dysplasia.[265]

Schmid's type of metaphyseal dysplasia, which affects long-bone metaphyses, presents in young children at the time of walking, when they are found to have bowing and a waddling gait. Although they have the features of rickets, they do not have the associated metabolic findings. Histology is similar to that of Jansen's type, but it is less severe and bone mineralization appears to be better. Experimental mice that express a mutated form of type X collagen (COLXA1) have an abnormal hypertrophic chondrocyte-osteogenic interface characteristic of a metaphyseal dysplasia. Several mutations of the type X gene, particularly of the C-terminal globular domain, have been seen in Schmid's type metaphyseal chondrodysplasia.[266,267]

The third type of metaphyseal dysplasia is known as McKusick's type, or cartilage-hair hypoplasia. This is a recessively inherited disorder due to mutations in the untranslated RMRP gene on chromosome 9p13-12. (70A—G) that encodes the RNA component of Rnase MRP endoribonuclease.[268,269] These children have short extremities, enlarged joints, and metaphyseal flaring. Unlike the other chondrodystrophies, their hair tends to be finely textured and blond. They have anemia, and due to an immune defect, they are particularly prone to viral and bacterial infections. In vitro colony formation in the myeloid lineage is abnormal in these patients. Osteogenesis at the site of epiphyseal hypertrophic chondrocytes is also impaired. These cases suggest a complex interaction between the hypertrophic chondrocyte and the invading osteoblast. Perhaps the hypertrophic chondrocyte prepares the matrix for the subsequent steps in bone formation, which is lost when mutant type X collagen accumulates or when the degree of cellular differentiation is altered in PTH and PTHRP receptor knockout mice. Clearly, much is yet to be learned about the interaction as more naturally occurring and induced mutations are investigated.

INHERITED DISORDERS WITHIN THE TYPE IV COLLAGEN FAMILY

Although diseases of basement membrane of the kidney or the skin are not of primary interest to the rheumatologist, brief mention of the progress in this area is useful to demonstrate the broad spectrum of heritable diseases of extracellular matrix proteins. The basement membrane complex varies widely among different tissues based on specific structural and functional needs.

Alport's Syndrome

Type IV collagen is a main constituent of basement membrane. Six genes are identified as belonging to the type IV collagen gene family. Sado and colleagues have divided these into three sets: COL4A1/COL4A2, COL4A3/COL4A4, and COL4A5/COL4A6.[270] These are localized on chromosomes 13, 2, and X, respectively. Alpha-chains 3, 4, and alpha 5/alpha and 6 chains are part of basement membrane. Alport's syndrome is an X-linked heritable disease of the kidney basement membrane that is characterized by hematuria leading to progressive renal failure. It is associated with sensorineural hearing loss, ocular defects (lenticonus), and (recently described) leiomyomatosis involving smooth muscle cells of the esophagus and tracheobronchial tree. Approximately 85 percent of patients with Alport's syndrome have mutations in the X-chromosome COL4A5 gene. The remaining cases are autosomal with mutations in COL4A3 or COL4A4 genes.[271,272] Although a mutation within a basement membrane collagen was suspected for some time, it was only when the minor basement membrane collagens (α5[IV]- and α6[148]-chains) were located on the X chromosome that the Alport's locus was identified. Subsequently, a wide variety of expressed and null mutations have been shown to cause this disease. Studies in 50 randomly chosen patients led to identification of the COL4A5 mutation in 41.[272] A variety of mutations have been found: missense, nonsense, splicing, small and large deletions and insertions.[273] The less common autosomal recessive form, accounting for about 15 percent of that population, has been shown to be caused by mutations within the α3(IV)- and (α4(IV)-chains.[274,275] Linkage analysis using highly polymorphic markers is

the best method for defining the disease in autosomal recessive disease, as well as in X-linked disease.[274] No mutations of the major α1(IV) and α2(IV) genes of type IV collagen have yet been described, presumably because they are incompatible with embryogenesis.

The disorder benign familial hematuria is associated with mutations in the COL4A3 and A4 genes.[276]

TYPE 7 COLLAGEN: EPIDERMOLYSIS BULLOSA

Remarkable progress has been made in understanding the molecular basis of the various clinical subtypes of epidermolysis bullosa, which is a devastating skin disease.[277] From the basic knowledge of the protein structure of the dermal basement membrane, mutations in specific proteins that compose the various layers of the epidermal-dermal junction have been correlated with the clinical subtype. At least 10 diverse dermal proteins have been reported to be mutated, including hemidesmosomes, anchoring filaments and fibrils, laminin 5 genes, integrin genes, and the keratin 14 gene in epidermolysis bullosa simplex.[278,279] The dystrophic form of epidermolysis bullosa causes bullae and blistering within the dermis of the skin. This has been shown to result from different mutations of COL7A1 that encodes for type VII collagen—the collagen that forms anchoring fibrils that tether the dermis to the epidermal basement membrane.[280,281] Approximately 100 mutations have been revealed in the type VII collagen gene in these patients. In analogy to other heritable connective tissue disorders, these include mutations leading to stop codons, substitutions, and deletions. The type VII mutations appear exceptional in that the severity of expressed mutations is wide ranging and includes those that may be associated with minimal phenotype or no phenotype at all.[277] Dystrophic epidermolysis bullosa is inherited either as a dominant or recessive trait, based on the severity of the mutation within the COL7A1 gene.[282]

REFERENCES

1. McKusick V: Mendelian Inheritance in Man. XI: Baltimore, Johns Hopkins University Press, 1994.
2. Vuorio E, deCrombrugghe B: The family of collagen genes. Annu Rev Biochem 59:837, 1990.
3. Myllyharju J, Kivirikko K: Collagens and collagen-related diseases. Ann Med 33:7, 2001.
4. Rossert J, deCrombrugghe B: Type I collagen: Structure, synthesis and regulation. In Bilezikian J, Raisz L, Rodan G (eds): Principles of Bone Biology. San Diego, Academic Press, 1996, p 127.
5. Patino M, Neiders M, Andreana S, et al: Collagen: an Overview. Implant Dentistry 11:28084, 2002.
6. Birk D, Fitch J, Babiarz J, et al: Collagen type I and type V are present in the same fibril in the avian corneal stroma. J Cell Biol 106:999, 1988.
7. Gordon M, Gerecke D, Dublet B, et al: Type XII collagen: A large multidomain molecule with partial homology to type IX collagen. J Biol Chem 264:1989.
8. Rousslahti E, Yamaguchi Y: Proteoglycans as modulators of growth factor activities. Cell 64:867, 1991.
9. Takeuchi Y, Kodama Y, and Matsumoto T: Bone matrix decorin bonds transforming growth factor-beta and enhances its bioactivity. J Biol Chem 251:7683, 1994.
10. Eyre D, Matsui Y, and Wu J: Collagen polymorphisms of the intervertebral disc. Biochem Soc Trans 30:844, 2001.

11. Mendler M, Eich-Bender S, Vaughan L, et al: Cartilage contains mixed fibrils of collagen types II, IX, and XI. J Cell Biol 108:191, 1989.

12. Ortega N, Werb Z: New functional roles for non-collagenous domains of basement membrane collagens. J Cell Sci 115:4201, 2002.

13. Kittelberger R, Davis P, Greenhill N: Immunolocalization of type VIII collagen in vascular tissue. Biochem Biophys Res Commun 159:414, 1989.

14. Cox D, Aoki T, Seki J, et al: The pharmacology of integrins. Med Res Rev 14:195, 1994.

15. Tomono Y, Naito I, Ando K, et al: Epitope-defined monoclonal antibodies against multiplexin collagens demonstrate that type XV and XVIII collagens are expressed in specialized basement membranes. Cell Struct Funct 27:9-20, 2002.

16. Kivirikko K: Collagens and their abnormalities in a wide spectrum of diseases. Ann Med 25:113, 1993.

17. Dawson P, Kelly T, Marini J: Extension of phenotype associated with structural mutations in type I collagen: siblings with juvenile osteoporosis have an alpha 2(I)Gly436→Arg substitution. J Bone Min Res 14:449, 1999.

18. van Keulen C, van de Akker E, Pals G, et al: Role of type III collagen in the development of familial abdominal aortic aneurysms. Eur J Vasc Endovasc Surg 18:65, 1999.

19. Ritvaniemi P, Korko J, Bonaventure J, et al: Identification of COL2A1 mutations in patients with chondrodysplasia and familial osteoarthritis. Arthritis Rheum 38:999, 1995.

20. Spotila LS, Colige A, Sereda L, et al: Mutation analysis pf coding sequences for type I procollagen in individuals with low bone density. J Bone Min Res 9:923, 1994.

21. Ramirez F, Did Liberto M: Complex and diversified regulatory programs control the expression of vertebrate collagen genes. FASEB J 4:1616, 1990.

22. Sandmeyer S, Gallis B, Bornstein P: Coordinate transcriptional regulation of type I procollagen genes by Rous Sarcoma virus. J Biol Chem 256:5022, 1981.

23. Aebi M, Weissman C: Precision and orderliness in splicing. Trends Genet 3:102, 1987.

24. Maquat L: Nonsense-mediated mrna decay. Curr Biol 12:R196, 2002.

25. Frischmeyer P, van Hoof A, O'Donnell K, et al: An mrna surveillance mechanism that eliminates transcripts lacking termination codons. Science 295:2258, 2002.

26. Rowe D, Shapiro J, Poirier M, et al: Diminished type I collagen synthesis and reduced al(l) collagen mRNA in cultured fibroblasts from patients with dominantly inherited (type I) osteogenesis imperfecta. J Clin Invest 71:689, 1985.

27. Rosenbloom J, Endo R, Harsch M: Termination of procollagen chain synthesis by puromycin: Evidence that assembly and secretion require a COOH-terminal extension. J Biol Chem 241:2070, 1976.

28. Bateman J, Lamande S, Dahl H, et al: A frameshift mutation results in a truncated non-functional carboxylterminal proalpha 1(1) propeptide of type I collagen in osteogenesis imperfecta. J Biol Chem 264:10960, 1989.

29. Baker A, Ramshaw J, Chan D, et al: Changes in collagen stability and folding in lethal perinatal osteogenesis imperfecta: The effect of al(I)-chain glycine-to-arginine substitutions. Biochem J 261:253, 1989.

30. Vogel BE, Doeiz R, Kadler KE, et al: A substitution of cysteine for glycine 748 of the al chain produces a kink at this site in the procollagen I molecule and an altered pN-proteinase cleavage site over 225 nm away. J Biol Chem 263:1924, 1988.

31. Wenstrup R, Cohn D, Cohen T, et al: Arginine for glycine substitution in the triple-helical domain of the products of one a2(1) collagen allele (COLIA2) produces the osteogenesis imperfecta type IV phenotype. J Biol Chem 263:7734, 1988.

32. Kuivaniemi H, Kontusaa S, Tromp G, et al: Identical G + I to A mutations in three different introns of the type III procollagen gene (COLD 1) produce different patterns of RNA splicing in three variants of Ehlers-Danlos syndrome IV: An explanation for exon skipping with some mutations and not others. J Biol Chem 265:2067, 1990.

33. Weil D, D'Alessio M, Ramirez F, et al: Structural and functional characterization of a splicing mutation in the pro-alpha2(1) collagen gene of an Ehlers-Danlos type VII patient. J Biol Chem 265:16007, 1990.

34. Hollister D: Clinical features of Ehlers-Danlos syndrome types VIII and IX. In Akeson W, Bornstein P, Glimcher V (eds): AAOS Symposium on Heritable Disorders of Connective Tissue. St. Louis, Mosby, 1982, p 102.

35. McAlinden T, Smith D, Smith S, et al: Isolation and characterization of a 1 Mb region of 5q23.3-q31.2 surrounding the human lysyl oxidase gene. J Mol Cell Cardiol 27:2409, 1995.

36. Parviainen M, Jaaskelainen K, Kroger H, et al: Urinary bone resorption markers in monitoring treatment of symptomatic osteoporosis. Clin Chim Acta 279:145, 1999.

37. Buckingham B, Reiser KM: Relationship between the content of lysyl oxidase dependent cross-links in skin collagen, nonenzymatic glycosylation, and long-term complications in type I diabetes mellitus. J Clin Invest 86:1046, 1990.

38. Liu X, Wu H, Byrne M, et al: A targeted mutation at the known collagenase cleavage site in mouse type I collagen impairs tissue remodeling. J Cell Biol 130:227, 1995.

39. Cohn D, Starman B, Blumberg B, et al: Recurrence of lethal osteogenesis imperfecta due to parental mosaicism for a dominant mutation in a human type I collagen gene (COLIAI). Am J Hum Genet 46:591, 1990.

40. Rogers J, Mahaney M, Beamer W, et al: Beyond one gene-one disease: alternative strategies for deciphering genetic determinants of osteoporosis. Calcif Tissue Int 60:225, 1997.

41. MacKay K, Byers P, Dalgleish R: An RT-PCR-SSCP screening strategy for detection of mutations in the gene encoding the al chain of type I collagen: Application to four patients with osteogenesis imperfecta. Hum Mol Genet 2:1155, 1993.

42. Korkko J, Annunen S, Pihlajama T, et al: Conformation sensitive gel electrophoresis for simple and accurate detection of mutations: comparison with denaturing gradient gel electrophoresis and nucleotide sequencing. Proc Nat Acad Sci USA 95:1681, 1998.

43. Rowe D, Shapiro J: Osteogenesis imperfecta. In Avioli L, Krane S (eds): Metabolic Bone Disease. Philadelphia, WB Saunders, 1990, p 659.

44. Rowe D: Osteogenesis imperfecta. In Heersche IN (ed): Bone and Mineral Research, K.J.a.1~ Amsterdam, Elsevier Science, 1991, p 209.

45. Sillence D: Osteogenesis imperfecta: an expanding panorama of variants. Clin Orthop Ret Res 159:11, 1981.

46. Edwards M, Wenstrup R, Byers P, et al: Recurrence of lethal osteogenesis imperfecta due to parental mosaicism for a mutation in the COL1A2 gene of type I collagen: the mosaic parent exhibits phenotypic features of a mild form of the disease. Hum Mutat 1:47, 1992.

47. Shapiro J: Osteogenesis imperfecta and other defects of bone development as occasional causes of adult osteoporosis. In Marcus R, Feldman D, Kelsey J (eds): Osteoporosis. San Diego, Academic Press, 1996, p 899.

48. Madigan W, Wertz D, Cockerham G, et al: Retinal detachment in osteogenesis imperfecta. J Pediatr Ophthal Strab 31:268, 1994.

49. Levin L: The dentition in the osteogenesis imperfecta syndromes. Clin Orthop 159:64, 1981.

50. Pedersen U: Osteogenesis imperfecta clinical features, hearing loss, and stapedectomy: Biochemical osteodensitometric, comcometric and histological aspects in comparison with otosclerosis. Acta Otolaryngol 415:1, 1985.

51. Charnas L, Hopkin E, Koby M, et al: Basilar invagination: frequency, detection, progression and treatment in children with OI. Am J Hum Genet 1996.

52. Charnas L, Marini J: Communicating hydrocephalus, basilar invagination and other neurologic features in osteogenesis imperfecta. Neurology 43:2603, 1993.

53. Sillence D: Craniocervical abnormalities in osteogenesis imperfecta: genetic and molecular considerations. Pediatr Radiol 24:4278, 1994.

54. Hortop J, Tsipouras P, Hanley J, et al: Cardiovascular involvement in osteogenesis imperfecta. Circulation 73:54, 1986.

55. Zegdi R, D'Attellis N, Fornes P, et al: Aortic valve surgery in osteogenesis imperfecta: report of two cases and review of the literature. J Heart Valve Dis 7:510, 1998.

56. Chines A, Boniface A, McAlister W, et al: Hypercalciuria in osteogenesis imperfecta: a follow-up study to assess renal effects. Bone 16:333, 1995.

57. Gahagan S, Rimsza M: Child abuse or osteogenesis imperfecta: How can we tell? Pediatrics 8:987, 1991.

58. Davie M, Haddaway M: Bone mineral content and density in healthy subjects and in osteogenesis imperfecta. Arch Dis Child 70:331, 1994.

59. Zionts L, Nash J, Rude R, et al: Bone mineral density in children with mild osteogenesis imperfecta. J Bone Joint Surg Br 77:143-147, 1995.

60. Rauch F, Plotkin H, Travers R, et al: Osteogenesis imperfecta types I, III and IV: effect of pamidronate therapy on bone and mineral metabolism. J Clin Endocrinol Metab 88:986, 2003.

61. Cassella J, Stamp T, Ali S: A morphological and ultrastructural study of bone in osteogenesis imperfecta. Calcif Tissue Int 58:155, 1996.

62. Shapiro JR, McCarthy EF, Earnest K, et al: Bone turnover is low in type I osteogenesis imperfecta. J Bone Min Res 10:S301, 1995.

63. Shapiro J, McCarthy E, Rossiter K, et al: The effect of intravenous pamidronate on bone mineral density, bone histomorphometry and parameters of bone turnover in adults with type IA osteogenesis imperfecta. Calcif Tissue Int 72:103, 2003.

64. Brenner R, Vetter U, Nerlich A, et al: Altered collagen metabolism in osteogenesis imperfecta fibroblasts: A study on 33 patients with diverse forms. Eur J Clin Invest 20:c3, 1990.

65. Wenstrup R, Willing M, Starman B, et al: Distinct biochemical phenotypes predict clinical severity in nonlethal variants of osteogenesis imperfecta. Am J Hum Genet 46:975, 1990.

66. Redford-Badwal D, Stover M, Valli M, et al: Nuclear retention of COL1A1 messenger RNA identifies null alleles causing mild osteogenesis imperfecta. J Clin Invest 97:1035, 1996.

67. Willing M, Cohn D, Byers P: Frameshift mutation near the 3′ end of the COLIAI gene of type I collagen predicts an elongated proalpha(1) chain and results in osteogenesis imperfecta type I. J Clin Invest 85:282, 1990.

68. Mundlos S, Chan D, Weng Y, et al: Multiexon deletions in the type I collagen COL1A2 gene in osteogenesis imperfecta type IB. J Biol Chem 271:21068, 1996.

69. Bonadio J, Saunders T, Tsai E, et al: Transgenic mouse model of the mild dominant form of osteogenesis imperfecta. Proc Natl Acad Sci USA 87:7145, 1990.

70. Constantinou-Deltas C, Ladda R, Prockop D: Somatic cell mosaicism: another source of phenotypic heterogeneity in nuclear families with osteogenesis imperfecta. Am J Med Genet 45:246, 1993.

71. Bonadio J, Holbrook K, Gelinas R, et al: Altered triple helical structure of type I procollagen in lethal perinatal osteogenesis imperfecta. J Biol Chem 260:1734, 1985.

72. Byers P, Tsipouras P, Bonadio J, et al: Perinatal lethal osteogenesis imperfecta (OI type II): A biochemically heterogenous disorder usually due to new mutations in the genes for type I collagen. Am J Hum Genet 42:237-248, 1988.

73. Emery S, Karpinski N, Hansen L, et al: Abnormalities in central nervous system development in osteogenesis imperfecta type II. Pediatr Dev Pathol 2:124, 1999.

74. Verkh Z, Russell M, Miller C: Osteogenesis imperfecta type II: micro vascular changes in the CNS. Clin Neuropathol 14:154, 1999.

75. Teng S, Guo W, Sheu M, et al: Initial experience using magnetic resonance imaging in prenatal diagnosis of osteogenesis imperfecta type II. Clin Imaging 27:55, 2003.

76. Thompson FM, Young ID, Hall CM, et al: Recurrence risks and prognosis in severe sporadic osteogenesis imperfecta. J Med Genet 24:390-405, 1986.

77. Byers P: Brittle bones–fragile molecules: Disorders of collagen gene structure and expression. Trends Genet 6:293, 1990.

78. Chu M, Williams C, Pepe G, et al: Internal deletion in a collagen gene in perinatal lethal form of osteogenesis imperfecta. Nature 304:78, 1984.

79. Prockop D: Osteogenesis imperfecta: Phenotypic heterogeneity, protein suicide, short and long collagen. Am J Hum Genet 36:499, 1984.

80. Wenstrup R, Shrago-Howe A, Lever L, et al: The effects of different cysteine for glycine substitutions within alpha2(1) chains:

Evidence of distinct structural domains within the type I collagen triple helix. J Biol Chem 266:2590, 1991.

81. Bullough P, Davidson D, Lorenzo J: The morbid anatomy of the skeleton in osteogenesis imperfecta. Clin Orthop 159:42, 1981.

82. Nicholls A, Pope F: Biochemical heterogeneity of osteogenesis imperfecta: A new variant. Lancet 1:1193, 1979.

83. Cohen-Solal L, Bonaventure J, Maroteaux P: Dominant mutations in familial lethal and severe osteogenesis imperfecta. Hum Genet 87:297, 1991.

84. Cole W, Dalgleish R: Perinatal lethal osteogenesis imperfecta. J Med Genet 32:284, 1995.

85. Lindau B, Dietz W, Hoyer I, et al: Morphology of dental enamel and dentine-enamel junction in osteogenesis imperfecta. Int J Pediatric Den 9:13, 1999.

86. O'Connell A, Marini J: Evaluation of oral problems in an osteogenesis imperfecta population. Oral Surg Oral Med Oral Pathol Oral Radiol Endod 87:189, 1999.

87. Tsipouras P, Swartz R, Goldberg J, et al: Prenatal prediction of osteogenesis imperfecta (OI type IV): Exclusion of inheritance using a collagen gene probe. J Med Genet 24:406, 1987.

88. Glorieux F, Rauch F, Plotkin H, et al: Type V osteogenesis imperfecta: a new form of brittle bone disease. J Bone Mineral Res 15:1650, 2000.

89. Ward L, Rauch F, Travcers R: Osteogenesis imperfecta type VII: an autosomal recessive form of brittle bone disease. Bone 31:12, 2002.

90. Labuda M, Morissette J, Ward L, et al: Osteogenesis imperfecta type VII maps to the short arm of chromosome 13. Bone 31:9, 2002.

91. Singer R, Ogston S, Paterson C: Mortality in various types of osteogenesis imperfecta. J Insurance Med 33:216, 2001.

92. Vetter U, Eanes ED, Kopp JB, et al: Changes in apatite crystal size in bones of patients with osteogenesis imperfecta. Calcif Tissue Int 49:248, 1992.

93. Fratzl P, Paris O, Klaushofer K, et al: Bone mineralization in an osteogenesis imperfecta mouse model studied by small-angle x-ray scattering. J Clin Invest 97:396, 1996.

94. Traub W, Arad T, Vetter U, et al: Ultrastructural studies of bones from patients with osteogenesis imperfecta. Matrix Biol 14:337, 1994.

95. McCarthy E, Earnest K, Rossiter K, et al: Bone histomorphometry in adults with type IA osteogenesis imperfecta. Clin Orthop 336:254, 1997.

96. Jones S, Glorieux F, Travers R, et al: The microscopic structure of bone in normal children and patients with osteogenesis imperfecta: a survey using backscattered electron imaging. Calcif Tissue Int 64:8, 1999.

97. Rauch F, Travers R, Parfitt A, et al: Static and dynamic bone histomorphometry in children with osteogenesis imperfecta. Bone 26:581, 2000.

98. Minisola S, Picconi A, Russo R, et al: Reduced levels of carboxy-terminal propeptide of human type I procollagen in a family with type 1A osteogenesis imperfecta. Metabolism 43:1261, 1994.

99. Glorieux F, Bishop N, Plotkin H, et al: Cyclic administration of pamidronate in children with severe osteogenesis imperfecta. N Engl J Med 339:947, 1998.

100. Plotkin H, Rauch F, Bishop N, et al: Pamidronate treatment of severe osteogenesis imperfecta in children under 3 years of age. J Clin Endocrinol Metab 85:1846, 2000.

101. Devogelaer J: New uses of bisphosphonates: osteogenesis imperfecta. Curr Opin Pharmacol 2:748, 2002.

102. Bembi B, Parma A, Bottega M, et al: Intravenous pamidronate treatment in osteogenesis imperfecta. J Pediatr 131:622, 1997.

103. Gonzalez E, Pavia C, Ros J, et al: Efficacy of low dose schedule pamidronate infusion in children with osteogenesis imperfecta. J Pediatr Endocrinol Metab 14:529, 2001.

104. Zacharin M, Bateman J: Pamidronate treatment of osteogenesis imperfecta-lack of correlation between clinical severity, age at onset of treatment, predicted collagen mutation and treatment response. J Pediatr Endocrinol Metab 15:163, 2002.

105. Wilkinson J, Scott B, Clarke A, et al: Surgical stabilization of the lower limb in osteogenesis imperfecta using the Sheffield Telescopic Intramedullary Rod System. J Bone Joint Surg Br 80:999, 1998.

106. Janus G, Vanpaemel L, Engelbert R, et al: Complications of the Bailey-Dubow elongating nail in osteogenesis imperfecta: 34 children with 110 nails. J Pediatr Orthop B 8:203, 1999.

107. Zeitlin L, Fassier F, Glorieux F: Modern approach to children with osteogenesis imperfecta. Pediatr Orthop B 12:77, 2003.

108. Naudie D, Hamdy R, Lutter F, et al: Complications of limb-lengthening in children who have an underlying bone disorder. J Bone Joint Surg Am 80:18, 1998.

109. Papagelopoulos P, Morrey B: Hip and knee replacement in osteogenesis imperfecta. J Bone Joint Surg Am 75:572, 1993.

110. Hanscom D, Winter R, Lutter L, et al: Osteogenesis imperfecta: Radiographic classification, natural history and treatment of spinal deformities. J Bone Joint Surg Am 80:598, 1992.

111. Widman R, Laplaza F, Bitan F, et al: Quality of life in osteogenesis imperfecta. Int Orthop 26:3, 2002.

112. Widmann R, Bitran F, Laplaza F, et al: Spinal deformity, pulmonary compromise and quality of life in osteogenesis imperfecta. Spine 24:1673, 1999.

113. Zionts L, Ebramzadeh E, Stott N: Complications in the use of the Bailey-Dubow extensible nail. Clin Orthop 348:186, 1998.

114. Sawin P, Menezes A: Basilar invagination in osteogenesis imperfecta and related osteochondrodysplasias: medical and surgical management. J Neurosurg 86:950, 1997.

115. Binder H, Conway A, Gerber L: Rehabilitation approaches to children with osteogenesis imperfecta: a ten-year experience. Arch Phys Med Rehabil 74:386, 1993.

116. Beighton P, DePape A, Steinmann B, et al: Ehlers-Danlos syndrome: revised nosology, Villefranche, 1997. Ehlers-Danlos National Foundation (USA) and Ehlers-Danlos Support Group (UK). Am J Med Genet 77:31, 1998.

117. Hollister D: Heritable disorders of connective tissue: Ehlers-Danlos syndrome. Pediatr Clin North Am 25:575, 1978.

118. Osborn T, Lichenstein J, Moore T, et al: Ehlers Danlos syndrome presenting as rheumatic manifestations in the child. J Rheumatol 8:79, 1981.

119. Ayres J, Pope P, Reidy J, et al: Abnormalities of the lungs and thoracic cage in Ehlers-Danlos syndrome. Thorax 40:300, 1985.

120. Leier CV, Call TD, Tulkerson PK, et al: The spectrum of cardiac defects in the Ehlers-Danlos syndrome types I and III. Ann Intern Med 92:171, 1980.

121. Tiller GE, Cassidy SB, Wensel C, et al: Aortic root dilatation in Ehlers-Danlos syndrome types I, II, and III: A report of five cases. Clin Genet 53:460-465, 1998.

122. Coventry M: Some skeletal changes in the Ehlers-Danlos syndrome. J Bone Joint Surg Am 13:855, 1961.

123. Goffin H, Pierard-Franchimont C, Pienard GE: Mechanical properties of skin in Ehlers-Danlos syndrome, types I, II and III. Pediatr Dermatol 13:464, 1996.

124. Morales-Rosello J, Hernandez-Yago J, Pope M: Type III Ehlers-Danlos syndrome and pregnancy. Arch Gynecol Obstet 261:39, 1997.

125. Kirk J, Ansell B, Bywaters K: The hypermobility syndrome. Ann Rheum Dis 26:419, 1967.

126. Beighton S, De Paepe A, Danks D, et al: International nosology of heritable disorders of connective tissue. Am J Med Genet 29:581, 1988.

127. Boone D, Zane S: Normal range of motion of joints in male subjects. J Bone Joint Surg Am 61:756, 1979.

128. Finsterbush A, Pogrund H: The hypermobility syndrome. Clin Orthop 168:124, 1982.

129. Horton W, Collins D, De Smet A, et al: Familial joint instability syndrome. Am J Med Genet 6:2221, 1980.

130. Lewkonia R: Does generalized articular hypermobility predispose to generalized osteoarthritis? Clin Exp Rheumatol 4:115, 1986.

131. Holbrook K, Byers P: Skin is a window on heritable disorders of connective tissue. J Med Genet 34:105, 1989.

132. Burrows N, Nicholls A, Richards A, et al: A point mutation in an intronic branch site results in aberrant splicing of COL5A1 and in Ehlers-Danlos syndrome type II in two British families. Am J Hum Genet 63:390-398, 1998.

133. de Paepe A, Nuytinck L, Hausser I, et al: Mutations in the COL5A1 gene are causal in the Ehlers-Danlos syndromes I and II. Am J Hum Genet 60:547, 1997.

134. Michalickova K, Susic M, Willig M, et al: Mutations of the alpha 2(V) chain of type V collagen impair matrix assembly and produce Ehlers Danlos syndrome type I. Hum Mol Genet 7:249, 1998.

135. Richards A, Martin S, Nicholls A, et al: A single base mutation in COL5A2 causes Ehlers-Danlos syndrome type II. J Med Genet 35:846, 1998.

136. Schalkwijk J, Zweers M, Steijlen P, et al: A recessive form of the Ehlers-Danlos syndrome caused by tenascin-x deficiency. N Engl J Med 345:1167, 2001.

137. Mao J, Taylor G, Dean W: Tenascin-x deficiency mimics Ehlers-Danlos syndrome in mice through alteration of collagen deposition. Nat Genet 30:421, 2002.

138. Jepson K, Wu F, J. H. Peragallo J: A syndrome of joint laxity and impaired tendon integrity in lumican- and fibromodulin-deficient mice. J Biol Chem 277:35532, 2002.

139. Corsi A, Xu X, Chen A, et al: Phenotypic effects of biglycan deficiency are linked to collagen fibril abnormalities, are synergized by decorin deficiency, and mimic Ehlers-Danlos-like changes in bone and other connective tissues. J Bone Miner Res 17:1180, 2002.

140. Byers P: Disorders of collagen biosynthesis and structure. In Scriver C, et al (eds): The Metabolic and Molecular Basis of Inherited Disease. New York, McGraw-Hill, 1995, pp 4051-4061.

141. Hamel B, Pals G, Engels C, et al: Ehlers-Danlos syndrome and type III collagen abnormalities: a variable clinical spectrum. Clin Genet 53:440, 1998.

142. Gilchrist D, Schwarze U, Shields K, et al: Large kindred with Ehlers-Danlos syndrome type IV due to a point mutation (G571S) in the COL3A1 gene of type III procollagen: low risk of pregnancy complications and unexpected longevity in some affected relatives. Am J Med Genet 82:305, 1999.

143. Rudd N, Nimrod C, Holbrook K, et al: Pregnancy complications in type IV Ehlers-Danlos syndrome. Lancet 1:50, 1983.

144. Pope F, Narcisi P, Nicholls A, et al: Clinical presentations of Ehlers-Danlos syndrome type IV. Arch Dis Child 63:1016, 1988.

145. Dowton S, Pincott S, Demmer L: Respiratory complications of Ehlers-Danlos syndrome type IV. Clin Genet 50:510, 1996.

146. Byers P: Ehlers-Danlos Syndrome: recent advances and current understanding of the clinical and genetic heterogeneity. J Invest Dermatol 103:47S-52S, 1994.

147. Super-Furga A, Steinmann B, Ramirez F, et al: Molecular defects of type III procollagen in Ehlers-Danlos syndrome type IV. Hum Genet 82:104, 1989.

148. Anderson D, Thakker-Varia S, Tromp G, et al: A glycine (415) to serine substitution results in impaired secretion and decreased thermal stability of type III procollagen in a patient with Ehlers-Danlos syndrome type IV. Hum Mut 9:62-63, 1997.

149. McCrory J, Weksberg R, Thorner P, et al: Abnormal extracellular matrix in Ehlers-Danlos syndrome type IV due to the substitution of glycine 934 by glutamic acid in the triple helical domain of type III collagen. Clin Genet 50:442, 1996.

150. Smith LT, Schwarze U, Goldstein J, et al: Mutations in the COL3A1 gene result in the Ehlers-Danlos syndrome type IV and alterations in the size and distribution of the major collagen fibrils of the dermis. J Invest Dermatol 108:241, 1997.

151. Schwarze U, Goldstein J, Byers P: Splicing defect in the COL3A1 gene: marked preference for 5' (donor) splice-site mutations in patients with exon skipping mutations and Ehlers Danlos syndrome type IV. Am J Hum Genet 61:1276, 1997.

152. Richards A, Lloyd J, Narcisi P, et al: A 27-bp deletion from one allele of the type III collagen gene (COL3A1) in a large family with Ehlers-Danlos syndrome type IV. Hum Genet 83:325, 1992.

153. Vissing H, D'Alessio M, Lee B, et al: Multiexon deletion in the procollagen III gene is associated with mild Ehlers-Danlos syndrome type IV. Am J Hum Genet 48:5244, 1991.

154. Milewicz D, Witz A, Smith A, et al: Parental somatic and germline mosaiism for a multiexon deletion with unusual endpoints in a type III collagen (COL3A1) allele produces Ehlers-Danlos syndrome type IV in the heterozygous offspring. Am J Hum Genet 53:62, 1993.

155. Milewicz D: Molecular genetics of Marfan syndrome and Ehlers-Danlos type IV. Curr Opin Cardiol 13:198, 1998.

156. Steinmann B, Royce PM, A S-F: The Ehlers-Danlos syndrome. In Royce P, Steinmann B (eds): Connective Tissue and Its

Heritable Disorders: Molecular, Genetic and Medical Aspects. New York, Wiley-Liss, 1993, p 351.

157. Bilkey W, Baxter T, Kottke F, et al: Muscle function in Ehlers-Danlos syndrome. Arch Phys Med Rehabil 62:444, 1981.

158. Takagi J, Kasahara K, Sehya F, et al: A collagen-binding glycoprotein from bovine platelets is identical to propolypeptide of von Willebrand factor. J Biol Chem 264:10425, 1989.

159. Wertelecki W, Smith L, Byers P: Initial observations of human dermatospraxis: Ehlers-Danlos syndrome type VIIIC. J Pediatr 121:558, 1992.

160. Byers P, Duvic M, Atkinson M, et al: Ehlers-Danlos syndrome type VIIA and VIIB result from splice junction mutations or genomic deletions that involve exon 6 in the COL1A1 and COL1A2 genes of type I collagen. Am J Med Genet 72:94-105, 1997.

161. Colige A, Sieron A, Li S, et al: Human Ehlers-Danlos syndrome type VII C and bovine dermatosparaxis are caused by mutations in the procollagenase I N-proteinase gene. Am J Hum Genet 65:1999.

162. Nusgens B, Verellen-Dumoulin C, Hermanns-Le T, et al: Evidence for a relationship between Ehlers-Danlos type VIIIC in humans and bovine dermatospraxis. Nature 1:214, 1992.

163. Wirtz M, Keene D, Hori H, et al: In vivo and in vitro nonconvalent association of excised alpha 1(1) amino terminal propeptides with mutant pN alpha 2(1) collagen chains in native mutant collagen in a case of Ehlers-Danlos syndrome, type VII. J Biol Chem 265:6312, 1990.

164. D'Alessio M, Ramirez F, Blumberg B, et al: Characterization of a COL1A1 splicing defect in a case of Ehlers-Danlos syndrome type VII: Further evidence of molecular homogeneity. Am J Hum Genet 49:400, 1991.

165. Pinnell S, Krane S, Kenzora J, et al: A heritable disorder of connective tissue: Hydroxylysine-deficient collagen disease. N Engl J Med 286:1013, 1972.

166. Krane S, Pinnell S, Erbe R: Lysyl-protocollagen hydroxylase deficiency in fibroblasts from siblings with hydroxylysine-deficient collagen. Proc Natl Acad Sci USA 69:2899, 1972.

167. Heikkinen J, Toppinen T, Yeowell H, et al: Duplication of seven exons in the lysyl hydroxylase gene is associated with longer forms of a repetitive sequence within the gene and is a common cause for the type VI variant of Ehlers-Danlos syndrome. Hum Genet 60:48, 1997.

168. Eyre D, Glimcher M: Reducible cross-link in hydroxylysine-deficient collagens of a heritable disorder of connective tissue. Proc Natl Acad Sci U S A 69:2594, 1972.

169. Yeowell HN, Walker L: Prenatal exclusion of Ehlers-Danlos syndrome type VI by mutational analysis. Proc Assoc Am Physicians 111:57-62, 1999.

170. Beighton P, Curtis D: X-linked Ehlers-Danlos syndrome. Clin Genet 27:476, 1985.

171. Stewart R, Hollister P, Rimoin D: A new variant of Ehlers-Danlos syndrome: An autosomal dominant disorder of fragile skin, abnormal scarring and generalized peridontitis. Birth Defects 13:85, 1977.

172. Hartsfield JJ, Kousseff B: Phenohypic overlap of Ehlers-Danlos syndrome types IV and VIII. Am J Med Genet 37:465, 1990.

173. Mentzel H, Siedel J, Vogt S, et al: Vascular complications (splenic and hepatic artery aneurysms) in the occipital horn syndrome: report of a patient and review of the literature. Peadiar Radiol 29:19, 1999.

174. Camakaris J, Danks D, Ackland L, et al: Altered copper metabolism in cultured cells from human Menkes' syndrome and mottled mouse mutants. Biochem Genet 18:117, 1980.

175. Tumer Z: Menkes disease: recent advances and new insights into copper metabolism. Ann Med 28:121, 1996.

176. Kuivaniemi H, Peltonen L, Kivirikko K: Type IX Ehlers-Danlos syndrome and Menkes syndrome: the decrease in lysyl oxidase activity is associated with a corresponding deficiency in the enzyme protein. Am J Hum Genet 37:798, 1985.

177. Arneson M, Hammerschmidt E, Furcht T, et al: A new form of Ehlers-Danlos syndrome. JAMA 244:144, 1980.

178. Hernandez A, Aguirre-Negrete M, Gonzalez-Flores S, et al: Ehlers-Danlos features with progeroid faces and mild mental retardation: further delineation of the syndrome. Clin Genet 30:456, 1986.

179. Quentin E, Gladen A, Roden L, et al: A genetic defect in the biosynthesis of dermatan sulfate proteoglycan: galactosyltransferase I deficiency in fibroblasts from a patient with progeroid syndrome. Proc Nat Acad Sci U S A 87:1342, 1990.

180. Furukawa K, Okajima T, al e: Galactosyltransferase is a gene responsible for progeroid variant of Ehlers-Danlos syndrome: Molecular cloning and identification of mutations. Biochim Biophys Acta 1573:377, 2002.

181. Okajima T, Fukumoto S, Furukawa K, et al: Molecular basis for the frogeroid variant of Ehlers-Danlos syndrome: Identification and characterization of two mutations in galactosyltransferase gene. J Biol Chem 274:28841, 1999.

182. Ramirez F, Godfrey M, Lee B: Marfan syndrome and relate disorders. In: Scriver C, Beaudet A, Sly W (eds): The Metabolic and Molecular Basis of Inherited Disease. New York, McGraw Hill, 1995, p 4079.

183. Sakai L, Keene D, Glanville R, et al: Purification and partial characterization of fibrillin, a cysteine-rich structural component of connective tissue microfibrils. J Biol Chem 266:14763, 1991.

184. Dietz H, Cutting G, Pyritz R, et al: Marfan syndrome caused by a recurrent de novo missense mutation in the fibrillin gene. Nature 352:337, 1991.

185. Dietz H, Ramirez F, Sakai L: Marfan's syndrome and other microfibrillar diseases. In: Harris H, Hirschhorn K (eds): Advanced Human Genetics. New York, Plenum Press, 1994, p 153.

186. de Paepe A, Devereux R, Deitz H, et al: Revised diagnostic criteria for the Marfan syndrome. J Med Genet 62:417, 1996.

187. Montgomery R, Geraghty M, Bull E, et al: Multiple molecular mechanisms underlying subdiagnostic variants of Marfan syndrome. Am J Hum Genet 63:1703, 1998.

188. Adams J, Trent R: Aortic complications of Marfan's syndrome. Lancet 352:1722, 1999.

189. Elkayam U, Ostrzega E, Shotan A, et al: Cardiovascular problems in pregnant women in the Marfan syndrome. Ann Int Med 123:117, 1995.

190. Pyritz R, McKusick V: The Marfan syndrome: diagnosis and management. N Engl J Med 300:772, 1978.

191. Pyritz R, Fishman E, Bernhardt B, et al: Dural extasia is a common feature of the Marfan syndrome. Am J Hum Genet 43:726, 1988.

192. Kohlmeier L, Gasner C, Bachrach L, et al: The bone mineral status of patients with the Marfan syndrome. J Bone Min Res 10:1550, 1995.

193. Gray J, Bridges A, Mole P, et al: Osteoporosis and the Marfan syndrome. Postgrad Med J 69:373, 1993.

194. Maumenee I: The eye in the Marfan syndrome. Trans Am Ophthalmol Soc 79:684, 1981.

195. Ho N, Hadley D, Jain P, et al: Case 47: Dural ectasia associated with Marfan syndrome. Radiology 223e:767, 2002.

196. Nallamshetty L, Ahn N, Ahn U, et al: Dural ectasia and back pain: review of the literature and case report. J Spinal Discord Tech 15:326, 2002.

197. Savini R, Cervellati S, Beroaldo E: Spinal deformities in Marfan's syndrome. Ital J Orthop Traumatol 1:19, 1980.

198. Mudd S, Levy H, Kraus J: Disorders of transsulfation. In Scriver C, et al (eds): The Metabolic and Molecular Bases of Inherited Disease. New York, McGraw Hill, 2001, pp 2007-2056.

199. Fowler B, Jacobs C: Post- and pre-natal diagnostic methods for the homocystinurias. Eur J Pediatr 157(Suppl 2):S88, 1998.

200. Kraus J, Janosik M, Kozich V, et al: Cystathionine α-synthase mutations in homocystinuria. Hum Mut 13:362, 1999.

201. Gaustadnes M, Wilcken B, Oliveriusova J, et al: The molecular basis of cystathionine β-synthase deficiency in Australian patients: genotype-phenotype correlation and response to treatment. Hum Mut 20:117, 2002.

202. Glesby M, Pyritz R: Association of mitral valve prolapse and systemic abnormalities of connective tissue: a phenotypic continuum. JAMA 262:523, 1989.

203. Boileau G, Babron MC, et al: Autosomal dominant Marfan-like connective tissue disorder and skeletal anomalies not linked to the fibrillin genes. Am J Hum Genet 53:46, 1993.

204. Collod-Beroud G, Bioleau C: Marfan syndrome in the third millennium. Eur J Hum Genet 10:673, 2002.

205. Sakai LY, Keene DR: Fibrillin: monomers and microfibrils. Methods Enzymol 245:29, 1994.

206. Corson G, Chalberg S, Dietz H, et al: Fibrillin binds calcium and is coded by cDNAs that reveal a multidomain structure and alternatively spliced exons at the 5′ end. Genomics 17:476, 1993.
207. Magenis R, Maslen C, Smith L, et al: Localization of the fibrillin (FBN) gene to chromosome 15, band q21.1. Genomics 11:346, 1991.
208. Hayward C, Porteous M, Brock D: Mutation screening of all 65 exons of the fibrillin-1 gene in 60 patients with Marfan syndrome: Report of 12 novel mutations. Hum Mutat 10:280, 1997.
209. Stoll C: Shprintzen-Goldberg marfanoid syndrome: a case followed up for 24 years. Clin Dysmorphol 11:1, 2002.
210. Putnam E, Cho M, Zinn A, et al: Delineation of the Marfan phenotype associated with mutations in exons 23-32 of the FBN-1 gene. Am J Med Genet 6:233, 1996.
211. Hayward C, Brock D: Fibrillin-1 mutations in Marfan syndrome and other type-1 fibrillinopathies. Hum Mutat 10:415, 1997.
212. Ramirez F, Gayraud B, Pereira L: Marfan syndrome: new clues to genotype-phenotype correlations. Ann Med 31:202, 1999.
213. Tsipouras P, Del Mastro R, Sarfarazi M, et al: Genetic linkage of the Marfan syndrome, ectopia lentis and congenital contractural arachnodactyly on the fibrillin genes on chromosomes 15 and 5: The International Marfan Syndrome Collaborative Study. New Eng J Med 326:905, 1992.
214. Shores J, Berger K, Murphy E, et al: Progression of aortic dilatation and the benefit of long-term beta-adrenergic blockade in Marfan's syndrome. N Eng J Med 330:1335, 1994.
215. Bonow R, Carabello B, de Leon A: Guidelines for the management of patients with valvular heart disease: A report of the American College of Cardiology/AHA Task Force on Practice Guidelines. J Am Coll Cardiol 32:1486, 1998.
216. Gott V, Pyritz R, McGovern G, et al: Surgical treatment of aneurysms of the ascending aorta in the Marfan syndrome. N Eng J Med 314:1070, 1986.
217. Finkbohner R, Johnston D, Crawford S, et al: Marfan syndrome: long term survival and complications after aortic aneurysm repair. Circulation 91:728, 1995.
218. Treasure T: Elective replacement of the aortic root in Marfan's syndrome. Br Heart J 69:101, 1993.
219. Ramos-Arrovo M, Weaver D, Beak R: Congenital contractural arachnodactyly. Clin Genet 27:570, 1985.
220. Park E, Putnam E, Chitayat D, et al: Clustering of FBN2 mutations in patients with congenital contractural arachnodactyly indicates an important role of the domains encoded by exons 24 through 34 during human development. Am J Med Genet 78:350, 1998.
221. Meinecke P: Marfan-like features and congenital contractural arachnodactyly. J Pediatr 100:1006, 1982.
222. Byers P, Siegel R, Holbrook K, et al: X-linked cutis laxa; defective cross-link formation due to decreased lysyl oxidase activity. N Engl J Med 202:61, 1980.
223. Yanagisawa H, Davis EC, Starcher BC, et al: Fibulin-5 is an elastin-binding protein essential for elastic fiber development in vivo. Nature 415:168, 2002.
224. Nakamura T, Lozano P, Ikeda Y, et al: Fibulin-5/dance is essential for elastogenesis in vivo. Nature 415:171, 2002.
225. Loeys B, Van Maldergem G, Mortier P, et al: Homozygosity for a missense mutation in fibulin-5 (fbln5) results in a severe form of cutis laxa. Hum Mol Genet 11:2113, 2002.
226. Uitto J, Ryhanen L, Abraham P, et al: Elastin in diseases. J Invest Dermatol 79:1605, 1982.
227. Zhang M, He L, Giro M, et al: Cutis laxa arising from frameshift mutations in exon 30 of the elastin gene (ELN). J Biol Chem 274:981, 1999.
228. McKusick V: Pseudoxanthoma elasticum. In Akeson WH, Bomstein P, Glimcher G (eds): Heritable Disorders of Connective Tissue. St. Louis, Mosby, 1972, p 475.
229. Pope F: Historical evidence for the genetic heterogeneity of pseudoxanthoma elasticum. Br J Dermatol 92:493, 1985.
230. Gurwood A, Mastrangelo D: Understanding angoid streaks. J Am Optom Assoc 68:309, 1997.
231. Przybojewski I, Miritz F, Tiedt F, et al: Pseudoxanthoma elasticum with cardiac involvement. South Afr Med J 59:268, 1981.
232. Cunningham J, Lippman S, Reine W, et al: Pseudoxanthoma elasticum: Treatment of gastrointestinal hemorrhage by arterial embolization and observations on autosomal dominant inheritance. Johns Hopkins Med J 147:168, 1980.
233. Lebwohl M, Nelkdner K, Pope M, et al: Classification of pseudoxanthoma elasticum. J Am Acad Dermatol 30:103, 1994.
234. Truter S, Rosenbaum-Fiedler J, Sapadin A, et al: Calcification of elastic fibers in pseudoxanthoma elasticum. M Sinai M Med 63:210-215, 1996.
235. Contri M, Boraldi F, Taparelli F, et al: Matrix proteins with high affinity for calcium ions are associated with mineralization within the elastic fibers of pseudoxanthoma elasticum dermis. Am J Pathol 148:569, 1996.
236. van Soest S, Swart J, Tijmes N, et al: A locus for autosomal recessive pseudoxsanthoma elasticum with penetrance of vascular symptoms in carriers, maps to chromosome 16p13.1. Genome Res 7:830, 1997.
237. Bale S: Recent advances in gene mapping of skin diseases. Pseudoxanthoma elasticum: a satisfying sibling study. J Cutan Med Surg 3:154, 1999.
238. LeSaux O, Urbvan Z, Tschuch C, et al: Mutations in a gene encoding an ABC transporter cause pseudoxanthoma elasticum. Nat Genet 25:223, 2000.
239. Ilias A, Urban Z, Seidl T: Loss of ATP-dependent transport activity in pseudoxanthoma elasticum-associated mutants of human abcc6 (mrp6). J Biol Chem 277:16860, 2002.
240. Metcalfe K: Williams syndrome: an update on clinical and molecular aspects. Arch Dis Child 81:198, 1999.
241. Osborne L, Pober B, Chitayat D, et al: A 1.5 million-base inversion polymorphism in families with Williams-Beuren syndrome. Nat Genet 29:321, 2001.
242. Urban Z, Michels V, Thibodeau S, et al: Supravalvular aortic stenosis: a splice site mutation within the elastin gene results in reduced expression of two aberrantly spliced transcripts. Hum Genet 104:135-142, 1999.
243. Boeckel T, Dierks A, Vergopoulos A, et al: A new mutation in the elastin gene causing supravalular aortic stenosis. Am J Cardiol 83:1141, 1999.
244. Osborne L, Campbell T, Daradich A, et al: Identification of a putative transcription factor gene (WBSCR11) that is commonly deleted in Williams-Beuren syndrome. Genomics 57:279, 1999.
245. Jadayel D, Osborne L, Coignet L, et al: The BCL7 gene family: deletion of BCL7B, in Williams syndrome. Gene 22:35, 1998.
246. Tanaka H: Achondroplasia: Recent advances in diagnosis and treatment. Acta Pediatr Jpn 39:514, 1997.
247. Francomono C, DeLuna O, Hefferon T, et al: Localization of the achondroplasia gene to the distal 2.5 Mb of human chromosome 4p. Human Mol Genet 3:787, 1994.
248. Shiang R, Thompson L, Zhu Y, et al: Mutations in the transmembrane domain of FGFR3 cause the most common genetic form of dwarfism, achondroplasia. Cell 78:335, 1994.
249. Rousseau F, Bonaventure J, Legeai-Mallet L, et al: Mutations in the Gene encoding fibroblast growth factor receptor-3 in achondroplasia. Nature 3721:252, 1994.
250. Wilkin D, Szabo J, Cameron R, et al: Mutations in fibroblast growth-factor receptor 3 in sporadic cases of achondroplasia occur exclusively on the paternally derived chromosome. Am J Hum Genet 63:711, 1998.
251. Ikegawa S, Fukusima Y, Isomura M, et al: Mutations of the fibroblast growth factor receptor-3 gene in one familial and six sporadic cases of achondroplasia in Japanese patients. Hum Genet 96:309, 1995.
252. Francomono C: The genetic basis of dwarfism. N Eng J Med 332:58, 1995.
253. Ala-Kokko L, Baldwin C, Moskowitz R, et al: Single base mutation in the type II procollagen gene (COL2A1) as a cause of primary osteoarthritis associated with a mild chondrodysplasia. Proc Nat Acad Sci USA 87:6565, 1990.
254. Pun Y, Moskowitz R, Lie S, et al: Clinical correlations of osteoarthritis associated with a single-base mutation (arginine 519 to cysteine) in type II procollagen gene: A newly defined pathogenesis. Arthritis Rheum 37:264, 1994.
255. Bleasel J, Bisagni-Faure A, Holderbaum D, et al: Type II procollagen gene (COL2A1) mutation in exon 11 associated with spondyloephpysdeal dysplasia, tall stature and precocious osteoarthritis. J Rheumatol 22:255, 1995.
256. Bleasel J, Holderbaum D, Mallock V, et al: Hereditary osteoarthritis with mild sponsyloepiphyseal dysplasia: are there "hot spots" on COL2A1? J Rheumatol 23:1594, 1996.

257. Ikegawa S, Nishimura G, Nagai T, et al: Mutation of the type X collagen gene (COL10A1) causes spondylometaphyseal dysplasia. Am J Hum Genet 63:1998.

258. Deere M, Blanton S, Scott C, et al: Genetic heterogeneity in multiple epiphyseal dysplasia. Am J Hum Genet 56:698, 1995.

259. Hagg R, Hedbom E, Mollers U, et al: Absence of the alpha1(IX) chain leads to a functional knock-out of the entire collagen IX protein in mice. J Biol Chem 27:20650, 1997.

260. Holden P, Canty E, Mortier G, et al: Identification of novel pro-alpha2(IX) collagen gene mutations in two families with distinctive oligo-epiphyseal forms of multiple epiphyseal dysplasia. Am J Hum Genet 65:31, 1998.

261. Snead M, Yates J: Clinical and molecular genetics of Stickler syndrome. J Med Genet 36:353, 1999.

262. Martin S, Richards A, Yates J, et al: Stickler syndrome: further mutations in COL11A1 and evidence for additional locus heterogeneity. Eur J Hum Gene 7:807, 1999.

263. Wordsworth P, Ogilvie D, Priestley L, et al: Structural and segregation analysis of the type II collagen gene (COL2A1) in some heritable chondrodysplasias. J Med Genet 25:521, 1988.

264. Olsen B: Mutations in collagen genes resulting in metaphyseal and epiphyseal dysplasias. Bone 17(2 Suppl):45S, 1995.

265. Schipani E, Langman C, Hunzelman J, et al: A novel parathyroid hormone (PTH/PTH-related peptide) receptor mutation in Jansen's metaphyseal chondrodysplasia. J Clin Endocrinol Metab 84:3052, 1999.

266. McLaughlin S, Conn S, Bulleid N, et al: Folding and assembly of type X collagen mutants cause metaphyseal chondrodysplasia type Schmid: Evidence for co assembly of the mutant and wild-type chains and binding to molecular chaparones. J Biol Chem 12:7570, 1999.

267. Chan D, Jacenko O: Phenotypic and biochemical consequences of collagen X mutations in mice and humans. Matrix Biol 17:169, 1998.

268. Ridanpaa M, Sostonen P, Rockas S: Worldwide mutation spectrum in cartilage-hair hypoplasia: Ancient founder origin of the major 70àG mutation of the untranslated RMR. Eur J Hum Genet 10:439, 2002.

269. Sulisalo T, Francomano CA, Sistonen P, et al: High-resolution genetic mapping of the cartilage-hair hypoplasia (CHH) gene in Amish and Finnish families. Genomics 20:347, 1994.

270. Sado Y, Kagawa M, Nalto I, et al: Organization and expression of basement membrane collagen IV genes and their roles in human disorders. J Biochem (Tokyo) 123:767-776, 1998.

271. Gross O, Netzer K, Lambfracht R, et al: Meta-analysis of genotype-phenotype correlation in X-linked Alport syndrome: impact on clinical counseling. Nephrol Dial Transplant 17:1218, 2002.

272. Martin P, Heiskari N, Zhou J, et al: High mutation detection rate in the COL4A5 collagen gene in suspected Alport syndrome using PCR and direct DNA sequencing. J Am Soc Nephrol 12:2291, 1998.

273. Plant K, Green P, Vetrie D, et al: Detection of mutations in COL4A5 in patients with Alport syndrome. Hum Mutat 13:124, 1999.

274. Nomura S, Naitro I, Fukushima T, et al: Molecular genetic and immunohistochemical study of autosomal recessive Alport's syndrome. Am J Kidney Dis 31:E4, 1998.

275. Torra R, Badenas C, Cofan F, et al: Autosomal recessive Alport syndrome: linkage analysis and clinical features in two families. Nephrol Dial Transplant 14:627-630, 1999.

276. Badenas C, Praga M, Tazon B, et al: Mutations in the COL4A4 and COL4A3 genes cause familial benign hematuria. J Am Soc Nephrol 13:1248, 2002.

277. Bruckner-Tuderman L: Hereditary skin diseases of anchoring fibrils. J Dermatol Sci 20:122, 1999.

278. Lanschuetzer C, Klausegger A, Pohla-Gubo G, et al: A novel homozygous nonsense deletion insertion mutation in the keratin 14 gene (Y248XC:delC/insAG) causes recessive epidermolysis bullosa simplex type Kobner. Clin Exp Dermatol 28:77, 2003.

279. Pulkkinen L, Uitto J: Mutation analysis and molecular genetics of eipdermolysis bullosa. Matrix Biol 18:29, 1999.

280. Uitto J, Pulkkinen L, Ringpfeil F, et al: Progress in molecular genetics of heritable skin diseases: the paradigm of epidermolysis bullosa and pseudoxanthoma elasticum. J Invest Dermatol Symp Proc 7:6, 2002.

281. Bruckner-Tuderman L, Hofpner B, Hammami-Hauasli N: Biology of anchoring fibrils: lessons from dystrophic eipdermolysis bullosa. Matrix Biol 18:43-54, 1999.

282. Gardella R, Castiglia D, Posteraro P, et al: Genotype-phenotype correlation in Italian patients with dystrophic epidermolysis bullosa. J Invest Derm 119:1456, 2002.

Rheumatic Diseases of Childhood

96   Juvenile Rheumatoid Arthritis

JAMES T. CASSIDY

Definition and Classification

Juvenile rheumatoid arthritis (JRA) is the most frequent chronic arthritis of children[1] (Table 96–1). It is one of the more common chronic illnesses of childhood and is a major cause of functional disability and eye disease leading to blindness. Early diagnosis is facilitated by recognition of three major types of presentation: oligoarthritis (60 percent), polyarthritis (30 percent), and systemic-onset disease (10 percent). In JRA, in contrast to adult rheumatoid arthritis (RA), large joints such as the knees, wrists, and ankles are more prominently involved than small joints, and there are less frequent complaints of joint pain. Subcutaneous nodules and rheumatoid factor (RF) seropositivity are unusual, but antinuclear antibody (ANA) seropositivity is a hallmark of the disease. Inflammation and ankylosis of the posterior apophyseal joints of the upper cervical spine are particularly characteristic, as is atlantoaxial subluxation, although neurologic sequelae are rare. Management of the disease in the child is affected to a large extent by recognition of the importance of fostering normal growth patterns, both physical and psychologic. The type of onset is associated to some extent with the future unfolding of the clinical disease.[2,3] Soon after onset, the course of JRA is especially unpredictable; the course tends to be more predictable after the pattern of the disease is established. In general, 70 to 90 percent of children enter adulthood without serious disability.[4-7] A small percentage of children will have a recurrence of arthritis as adults.

There is no worldwide agreement on the use of diagnostic terms for this type of arthritis in children or on criteria for classification.[8] There are two principal sets of classification criteria for children with chronic arthritis of the peripheral joints of unknown etiology; criteria for "juvenile rheumatoid arthritis" developed by the American College of Rheumatology (ACR) have been extensively validated,[2,9] and a number of iterations of criteria have been proposed for "juvenile idiopathic arthritis" by the International League of Associations for Rheumatology[10] (Table 96–2).

Epidemiology

By arbitrary definition, JRA begins at or before the age of 16 years. Even though onset before 6 months of age is unusual, the age at onset is characteristically young (1 to

TABLE 96–1 · FREQUENCY OF THE MAJOR PEDIATRIC CONNECTIVE TISSUE DISEASES IN CHILDREN

Disease	Number	Percent
Juvenile rheumatoid arthritis (JRA)	7368	65.2
Systemic lupus erythematosus (SLE)	1214	10.7
Juvenile dermatomyositis	658	5.8
Systemic scleroderma	90	0.8
Localized scleroderma	340	3.0
Polyarteritis nodosa	42	0.4
Kawasaki's disease	259	2.3
Henoch-Schönlein purpura	838	7.4
Other vasculitides	491	4.3

Data on 57,729 diagnoses from 48,934 consecutive patients entered into the Pediatric Rheumatic Disease Registry of the Pediatric Rheumatology Database Research Group, 1992-2002. Courtesy of Suzanne Bowyer, M.D.

TABLE 96–2 · COMPARISON OF CLASSIFICATION CRITERIA FOR CHRONIC ARTHRITIS IN CHILDREN

Characteristic	ACR (JRA)	ILAR (JIA)
Onset types	3	6
Course subtypes	9	1
Age at onset of arthritis	<16 yr	<16 yr
Duration of arthritis	≥6 wk	≥6 wk
Includes JAS	No	Yes
Includes JPsA	No	Yes
Includes IBD	No	Yes
Includes reactive arthritis	No	No
Exclusion of other diseases	Yes	Yes

Abbreviations: ACR, American College of Rheumatology; ILAR, International League of Associations for Rheumatology; IBD, inflammatory bowel disease; JAS, juvenile ankylosing spondylitis; JRA, juvenile rheumatoid arthritis; JIA, juvenile idiopathic arthritis; JPsA, juvenile psoriatic arthritis.

3 years). A substantial number of cases begin throughout childhood[11] (Fig. 96–1). Systemic onset is an exception, with no increased frequency at any particular age. Girls account for the majority of patients in the early peak of the distribution curve and are affected overall at least twice as often as boys, except, again, for systemic onset, in which the female-to-male ratio is 1:1.

A number of studies suggest that a working estimate of the incidence of JRA is 10 to 20 cases per 100,000 children.[11-14] The minimal incidence of the disease was 9.2 per 100,000 children at risk in a report from Michigan[11]; in Finland, 18.2 per 100,000 (confidence limits 10.8 to 28.7)[12]; in Sweden, 11 per 100,000[13]; and in Minnesota, 13.9 per 100,000 (confidence limits 9.9 to 18.8).[14] The prevalence of JRA was 65 per 100,000 children in Michigan[11]; 86 per 100,000 in the Swedish study[13]; and 84 per 100,000 in Minnesota.[14] The highest estimates of incidence (22.6 per 100,000) and prevalence (148 per 100,000) were reported from Norway and Australia (400 per 100,000).[15] A more recent study from Minnesota suggested that the incidence of JRA has been decreasing during the past several decades, from 15 per 100,000 for 1960 through 1969 to 7.8 per 100,000 for 1980 through 1993.[16] Seasonal variation was also observed in this investigation, as it was in one from Manitoba.[17] This trend was not confirmed in a larger study from Canada.[18]

Etiology

The etiology and pathogenesis of JRA are unclear in spite of numerous investigations.[19-21] JRA may represent not a single disease but a syndrome of diverse causes. Both abnormal immunoregulation and cytokine production may play a role.[22,23] Antibodies and cellular immune reactivity to type II collagen have been demon-

strated. An arthritis is associated with the clinical course of many viral diseases such as rubella and parvovirus B19.[24] Persistent rubella virus infection has been implicated as a potential cause of this disease. An increased frequency of JRA was documented after an epidemic of influenza A.[25] A role for immunodeficiency in the pathogenesis of arthritis in children is underlined by the frequent occurrence of chronic arthritis in children with immunoglobulin (Ig) and complement component deficiencies.[1] In children with oligoarthritis, T lymphocyte proliferative responses to heat-shock protein (HSP) 60 are associated with remission of the inflammatory disease.[26] A recent study of 144 families has established the association of several tumor necrosis factor-α (TNF-α) single-nucleotide polymorphisms (SNPs) with juvenile oligoarthritis.[27]

Although JRA seldom occurs in siblings, data on human leukocyte antigen (HLA) segregation underscore a hereditary basis for the immunopathogenesis of the disease.[28,29] There is a striking increase in the frequency of HLA-A2 and specific HLA-DR, -DQ, and -DP genotypes associated with the type of onset and course subtype: The HLA antigens DR5 (DRB1*1104), DRw6, DRw8, DQwl (DQA1*0501), and DQw2 (DPB1*0201) are associated with development of persistent oligoarthritis at an early age in young girls with ANA seropositivity,[30-34] and DR4 (DRB1*0401 and 0404) is increased in frequency in older children who have polyarthritis and are RF seropositive.[35,36] Impressive risk and protective effects of these immunogenetic profiles appear to be age related.[37] T cell receptor (TCR) polymorphisms or antigen-processing genes may also be associated with patterns of disease.[38] A 44-percent concordance has been reported in identical twins and a 4-percent rate in dizygotic twins.[28] Similar patterns of onset of JRA and course of the disease have been found in families and sibling pairs.[39,40]

A number of studies of SNPs implicate genes separate from those associated with the major histocompatibility complex (MHC) in the pathogenesis of specific features of JRA. In systemic-onset disease, interleukin (IL)-6-174G is overrepresented in transcriptional regulation of the IL-6 gene and is associated with resistance to glucocorticoid therapy.[41,42] Also in systemic-onset disease, high levels of macrophage inhibitory factor (MIF) in serum and synovial fluid are associated with a G to C SNP at position 173 of the MIF gene that leads to glucocorticoid resistance, persistence of arthritis, and a relatively poor outcome.[43] Children with chronic arthritis have elevated levels of osteoprotegerin, a decoy receptor, which inhibits differentiation and activation of osteoclasts. This abnormality is related to a TC >> CC genotype that correlates with low bone mass and bone erosions.[44]

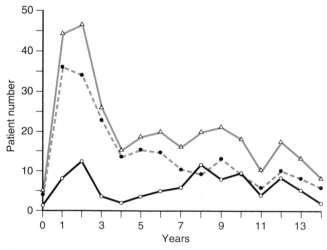

FIGURE 96–1 • Age at onset (0 to 14 years) for a group of 300 children with juvenile rheumatoid arthritis (JRA) (Δ), and for girls (l) and boys (o) separately. For the total group, a single large peak at 1 to 2 years is present. Age at onset for boys, however, has a bimodal distribution, with the first peak at 2 years and the second at 8 years. Age at onset for girls does not clearly show a second peak. No definite accentuation in frequency of onset was seen at 10 to 14 years of age.

Clinical Features

PATHOLOGY

JRA is characterized by many of the same histologic abnormalities that have been identified in RA, and characteristics of the synovitis do not differ among subtypes. There is villous hypertrophy of the synovium and hyperplasia of the synovial lining layer. The subsynovial tissues are edematous and hyperemic, and often there is prominent vascular endothelial hyperplasia and infiltration of lymphocytes and plasma cells. Pannus formation may result and the articular cartilage and later contiguous bone become progressively eroded and destroyed.

The rash of JRA is one of the most characteristic features of the disease. Histologically, there is an infiltration of lymphocytes surrounding capillaries and venules in the subdermal tissues. A neutrophilic perivasculitis may accompany the more flagrant lesions. Rheumatoid nodules in children do not differ in pathologic characteristics from the nodules of RA. The serosal lining surfaces of the major cavities (pleura, pericardium, and peritoneum) may develop a nonspecific fibrous serositis that is characterized clinically by pain, exudation, and effusions. Nonspecific follicular hyperplasia results in enlargement of lymph nodes and spleen. A nonspecific periportal collection of inflammatory cells and hyperplasia of Kupffer cells occurs in the liver.

LABORATORY EXAMINATION

Many children with polyarthritis or systemic disease have a normocytic, hypochromic anemia during periods of active disease. This anemia of chronic disease may be moderately severe, with hemoglobin values in the range of 7 to 10 g/dl. Leukocytosis is common with active disease, especially in children with systemic onset. White blood cell (WBC) counts of 30,000 to 50,000/mm^3 are not uncommon; polymorphonuclear neutrophils (PMNs) predominate. Thrombocytosis parallels the activity of disease and often occurs as a prelude to an exacerbation.

The erythrocyte sedimentation rate (ESR) is a useful measure of the acute-phase reaction and is occasionally helpful in monitoring therapeutic efficacy along with determination of C-reactive protein (CRP) levels. Increases in serum concentrations of Igs are also correlated with inflammatory activity. Serum complement components, especially C3, are usually elevated. Serum amyloid A (AA) protein is increased in concentration as a nonspecific indicator of inflammation.

Tests for ANAs are positive in approximately 40 percent of children. The pattern of fluorescent staining on HEp-2 cells is usually homogeneous or speckled, and the standardized serum-dilution titer is generally low to moderate (less than or equal to 1:256). The frequency of ANA seropositivity is increased in girls with a younger age at onset and decreased in older boys and in children with systemic disease; seropositivity reaches its highest prevalence (65 to 85 percent) in young girls who have an oligoarticular onset and develop uveitis.

The latex fixation test or sensitized sheep-cell agglutination assay for RFs is positive less frequently than in RA. Less than 4 percent of children with JRA are seropositive at the onset of disease. RF seropositivity is more likely in the child in whom disease occurs at a later age; in an older child, in the presence of subcutaneous rheumatoid nodules or articular erosions; or in the child in a poorer functional class. Children who are strongly seropositive for RFs may constitute a subset of patients with JRA.[9] Soluble immune complexes can be detected in the sera of certain children, particularly in those with systemic-onset disease.

Synovial fluid examination is usually typical of inflammatory fluid. As in RA, levels of synovial fluid glucose are low. Complement levels are not as characteristically or uniformly depressed as in adult disease. Findings on urinalysis are usually normal in children with JRA, except for proteinuria associated with fever. Persistent proteinuria is often the first indication of amyloidosis in reports from Europe.[15] Intermittent hematuria may occur, especially at onset, and represent a mild glomerulitis associated with JRA, drug toxicity (interstitial nephritis or renal papillary necrosis), or the development of another disease such as systemic lupus erythematosus (SLE). Hematuria can also result from hypercalciuria, which is not common.

RADIOLOGIC EXAMINATION

Early radiographic changes consist of soft tissue swelling, juxta-articular osteoporosis, and periosteal new-bone formation.[46] Premature epiphyseal closure may lead to stunting of bone growth, especially in the phalanges. Conversely, there may be accelerated epiphyseal development stimulated by local inflammatory changes (Fig. 96–2). Marked bony overgrowth due to enlargement of

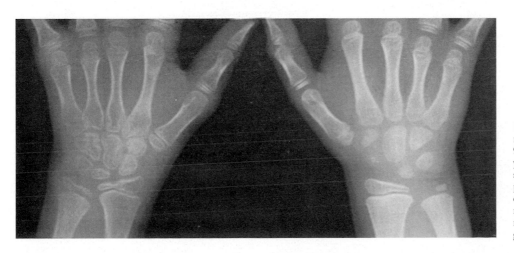

FIGURE 96–2 · Accelerated maturation of the left carpus in a 9-year-old girl with arthritis of 7 years' duration. Marked osteoporosis and atrophy of soft tissues are present. Although the individual carpal bones on the left appear more mature than those on the right, they are smaller, and eventual growth is already stunted.

the epiphyses occurs at the interphalangeal joints. Widening of the phalanges from periosteal new-bone apposition is another characteristic feature of the disease. Marginal erosions and narrowing of the cartilaginous space occur in arthritis of long duration. Magnetic resonance imaging (MRI) is a much more sensitive technique for detecting bone destruction than is standard radiography.[47]

Fusion of the upper cervical apophyseal joints is the most characteristic change in the cervical spine (Fig. 96–3). Atlantoaxial subluxation is a potential complication. The upper limit of the atlantoaxial space in young children is 4 mm, measured at the base of the atlas on a lateral film with the neck in flexion. The odontoid is often eroded and can impinge posteriorly on the upper cervical cord or migrate superiorly (Fig. 96–4). Vertebral bodies at areas of fusion fail to grow normally and are smaller than contiguous vertebrae or have an altered height-to-width ratio. The intervertebral spaces at these levels are also narrowed. Apophyseal joint dis-

ease also occurs in the thoracic and lumbar spine but is less often recognized clinically or radiologically. Sacroiliac arthritis is not characterized by the degree of reactive sclerosis that occurs in juvenile ankylosing spondylitis (AS). Recurrent vertebral compression fractures are also a potential complication. Fractures related to generalized osteopenia are all too frequent in young children, particularly if they have had severe disease, periods of relative immobilization, or glucocorticoid therapy.

TYPES OF ONSET

The diagnosis of JRA has been immeasurably aided by recognition of three major types of disease onset[2,3] (Table 96–3). These are defined by a constellation of clinical signs and symptoms during the first 6 months of illness.[2] Morning stiffness, "gelling" following inactivity, and night pain are probably encountered frequently in JRA; however, children may not directly communicate these symptoms, and their presence may be suspected only by careful observation of the child or questioning of the parent.[48,49] Fatigue and low-grade fever are common at onset of disease. Anorexia, weight loss, failure to grow, and psychologic regression to a more infantile pattern of behavior are present in many children with more severe disease.

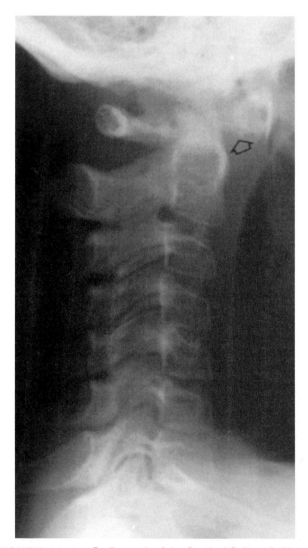

FIGURE 96–3 · Radiograph of the Cervical Spine of a Young Girl with Polyarthritis. There is an atlantoaxial subluxation *(arrow)* and fusion of the C2C3 apophyseal joint. Three years later, subluxation developed at the C3-C4 vertebral interspace.

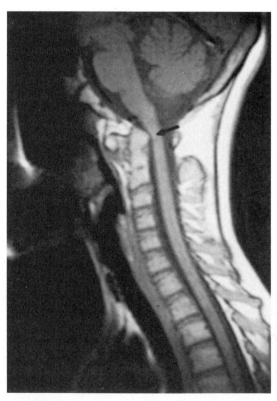

FIGURE 96–4 · Magnetic resonance image (MRI) of the cervical spine in a 10-year-old girl with severe polyarticular juvenile rheumatoid arthritis (JRA) and an atlantoaxial subluxation of 11 mm. The *arrow* points to the odontoid, which has encroached on the upper cervical cord.

TABLE 96–3 • COMPARISON OF ONSET TYPES IN JUVENILE RHEUMATOID ARTHRITIS (JRA)

Feature	Polyarthritis	Oligoarthritis	Systemic-Onset Disease
Relative frequency	30%	60%	10%
Number of joints involved	≥ 5	≤ 4	Variable
Female:male ratio	3:1	5:1	1:1
Extra-articular involvement	Moderate	Not present	Prominent
Chronic uveitis	5%	5 to 15%	Rare
Seropositivity			
Rheumatoid factors	10% (increases with age)	Rare	Rare
Antinuclear antibodies	40 to 50%	75 to 85%*	10%
Clinical course	Systemic disease generally mild; possible unremitting articular involvement	Systemic disease absent; major cause of morbidity is uveitis	Systemic disease often self-limited; arthritis chronic and destructive in half
Prognosis	Guarded to moderately good	Excellent except for eyesight	Moderate

*In girls with uveitis.

Oligoarthritis

The onset of JRA in more than half the children involves four or fewer joints, in particular the knees and ankles. In one third to one half of these children, arthritis begins in a single joint only. Any joint may be affected, but the knee is involved in 75 percent of patients (Figs. 96–5 and 96–6). A limp may be the only sign of disease. Hip involvement is almost never present at onset. Extra-articular disease, except for chronic uveitis, is unusual.

The course of the disease in children with oligoarthritis remains or becomes monarticular or is confined to the joints of initial involvement in one-third of affected children. Another third develop involvement of one or two additional joints. In some children, the disease progresses after 6 months to an articular pattern similar to that described for polyarthritis (Table 96–4). Because of the limited nature of the joint involvement in the majority of children with this pattern of disease, serious functional disability is uncommon, and these children have a generally excellent prognostic outlook if uveitis does not develop. However, in a series from Cincinnati, 41 percent of patients with oligoarticular onset still had active arthritis at 10 years or more after onset.[50]

Polyarthritis

JRA begins in five or more joints in one third of affected children and usually involves at least 10 to 20. The onset

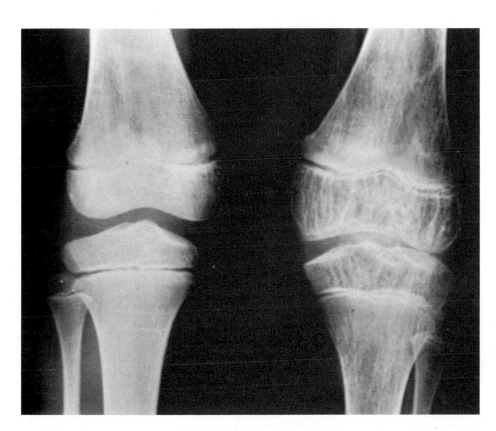

FIGURE 96–5 • Radiographs of the Knees of a Boy with Monarthritis of the Left Knee. There is marked osteoporosis on the left with coarsening of the trabeculae and enlargement of the epiphyses. The joint space is narrowed laterally, and there is lengthening of the left leg with a moderate valgus deformity. Erosions are not present.

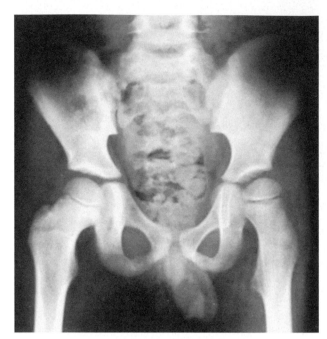

FIGURE 96-6 • Pelvis of the Same Child as in Figure 96–5. Coxa valga is present on the left, and moderate stunting of growth of the ischium is secondary to arthritis of the left knee. The hip was not involved in the inflammatory process; however, its deformity accounts in part for the ipsilateral leg-length discrepancy.

side of the body may be affected. The joints are swollen and warm but are not usually erythematous. Often, the child does not complain of pain[48,49]; however, the joints may be tender or painful on motion. Presentation may be one of increased irritability, assumption of a posture of guarding the joints, or refusal to walk. Systemic manifestations in polyarthritis are usually not as acute or persistent as in children with systemic-onset JRA. Low-grade fever, moderate hepatosplenomegaly, and lymphadenopathy may be present. Clinically evident pericarditis is infrequent, and chronic uveitis occurs in 5 percent of patients or less.

The pattern of small joint involvement of the hands is not remarkably different from that observed in RA; however, terminal interphalangeal joints are affected in 10 to 45 percent of children. Radial deviation at the metacarpophalangeal joints is more frequent than ulnar drift. The wrist is the most commonly involved joint of the upper extremity, with ulnar rotation and subluxation of the carpus (Fig. 96–7). Palpable synovial cysts around large joints are an unusual complication of JRA. Ultrasonography may aid in their identification. These cysts are not confined to polyarticular disease but are also seen in systemic-onset disease and occasionally in oligoarthritis. Tenosynovitis and myositis are also manifestations of active disease. Inflammation of the tendon sheaths develops principally over the dorsa of the wrists and around the ankles. Loss of extension of the fingers results from a stenosing synovitis of the flexor tendon sheaths, sometimes accompanied by nodule formation. Atrophy of muscles around involved joints is characteristic of established disease.

may be acute but is often insidious. The arthritis generally involves large joints—knees, wrists, elbows, and ankles—but may include small joints of the hands or feet either early or late in the course. The pattern of joint involvement is most often symmetric, but only one

TABLE 96–4 • CLINICAL OUTCOME IN JUVENILE RHEUMATOID ARTHRITIS (JRA) BY ONSET TYPE AND COURSE SUBTYPES

Onset Type (N)	Course Subtype (N)	Profile	Outcome
Polyarthritis (78)	RF seropositive (16)	Female Older age Hand-wrist involvement Erosions Nodules Unremitting	Poor
	ANA seropositive (38)	Female Young age	Good
	Seronegative (24)	Variable	Good
Oligoarthritis (121)	ANA seropositive (66)	Female Young age Chronic uveitis	Excellent (except eyes)
	RF seropositive (8)	Polyarthritis Erosions Unremitting	Poor
	HLA-B27 positive (12)	Male Older age	Good
	Seronegative (35)	Variable	Excellent
Systemic disease (51)	Oligoarthritis (30)	Variable	Good
	Polyarthritis (21)	Erosions	Poor

Abbreviations: ANA, antinuclear antibodies; HLA, human leukocyte antigen; RF, rheumatoid factor.
From Cassidy JT, Levinson JE, Bass JC, et al: A study of classification criteria for a diagnosis of juvenile rheumatoid arthritis. Arthritis Rheum 29:274, 1986.

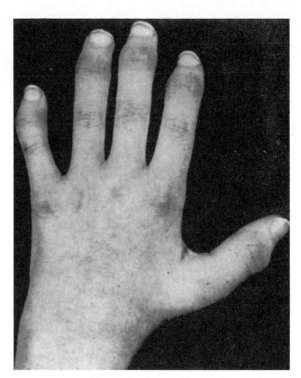

FIGURE 96–7 · Hand of a 7-year-old girl with marked inflammatory involvement of the interphalangeal joint of the thumb and the terminal interphalangeal joints of the fingers. Arthritis began as systemic disease at 5.5 years of age, with fever, maculopapular rash, hepatosplenomegaly, and arthritis of the hands, feet, and left knee.

Arthritis of the apophyseal joints of the spine is common and occurs in half the children with polyarthritis. The neck is usually painful and stiff; an alarmingly rapid loss of extension and rotation may follow. Occasionally, torticollis is encountered. Children with atlantoaxial subluxation or fusion of apophyseal joints of the cervical spine present special challenges in general anesthesia and should not be intubated without careful review of the risks involved. Forced extension of the neck (from intubation or an automobile accident) has resulted in respiratory arrest and death. Temporomandibular joint involvement, which may be asymmetric, is relatively common in children with polyarthritis and leads to limitation of bite and micrognathia. Ankylosis is uncommon.

Although involvement of the vocal cords by rheumatoid nodules can occur, cricoarytenoid arthritis is rare. Subcutaneous rheumatoid nodules are not as common as in RA (occurring in 5 to 10 percent of the cases versus 35 percent). These lesions are associated with RF seropositivity and are typically seen in children with polyarthritis. Benign rheumatoid nodules occur in a rare child without arthritis. At least some of these nodules, however, represent subcutaneous granuloma annulare. Rheumatoid polyarteritis has been described in a few instances, usually in the older child with RF seropositivity, and is a very serious complication of the disease.

The child most at risk to enter adulthood with significant functional disability is the one with polyarthritis that has onset at a later age in childhood, early involvement of the small joints of the hands or feet, rapid appearance of erosions, unremitting inflammatory activity unresponsive to therapy, prominent systemic manifestations, RF seropositivity, and subcutaneous nodules (Table 96–4). Although the small joints may be involved in any of the various types of onset, widespread symmetric involvement of the metacarpophalangeal and proximal interphalangeal joints of the hands—the so-called adult pattern of RA—is characteristically associated with a poorer prognostic outlook. Hip disease is a major cause of disability in JRA and is justifiably interpreted as a relatively poor prognostic sign (Fig. 96–8). The Cincinnati data indicated that 45 percent of patients with polyarticular disease still had active disease at 10 years or more after onset.[50]

Systemic-Onset Disease

A hallmark of systemic onset is the high, spiking fever, which, in combination with the rheumatoid rash, is virtually diagnostic of the disease. Daily (quotidian) or twice daily temperatures of up to 39° C or higher with a rapid return to baseline are characteristic (Fig. 96–9). The fever may occur at any time of the day but is characteristically seen in the late afternoon, evening, or early morning hours. The children are often strikingly ill while febrile but surprisingly well the rest of the day. A few children have severe constitutional and systemic involvement at onset that may precede development of overt arthritis by a variable period of time. Arthritis may appear concurrent with the systemic signs or many weeks to months, and occasionally years, later. The systemic pattern of disease generally establishes this subtype at onset and does not appear later during the course of the other two types of JRA.

The rheumatoid rash consists of discrete, 2- to 5-mm erythematous morbilliform macules and is most commonly seen on the trunk and proximal extremities and over pressure areas (Fig. 96–10). It may occur on the face, palms and soles, and in the axillae. A signal characteristic is its evanescent nature. Lesions are of short duration in any specific location, and the rash tends to be migratory. Each macule is often surrounded by a zone of pallor, and larger lesions demonstrate central clearing. The rash may resemble urticaria but is seldom pruritic. Individual lesions are often induced by rubbing or scratching the skin (i.e., Koebner phenomenon or isomorphic response). A hot bath or psychologic stress may also precipitate the rash.

Systemic-onset disease is also accompanied by prominent manifestations of visceral involvement, such as hepatosplenomegaly, lymphadenopathy, and pericarditis or other evidence of serositis. A true hepatitis not related to nonsteroidal drug therapy may occur; however, even impressive hepatomegaly is usually associated with only mild derangement of laboratory measures of liver function. Enlargement of the spleen, which occurs in a quarter of affected children, is generally most prominent in the first year of disease. The degree of splenomegaly may be extreme but is not usually associated with the hematologic abnormalities of Felty's syndrome, which is rare. Lymphadenopathy, particularly in

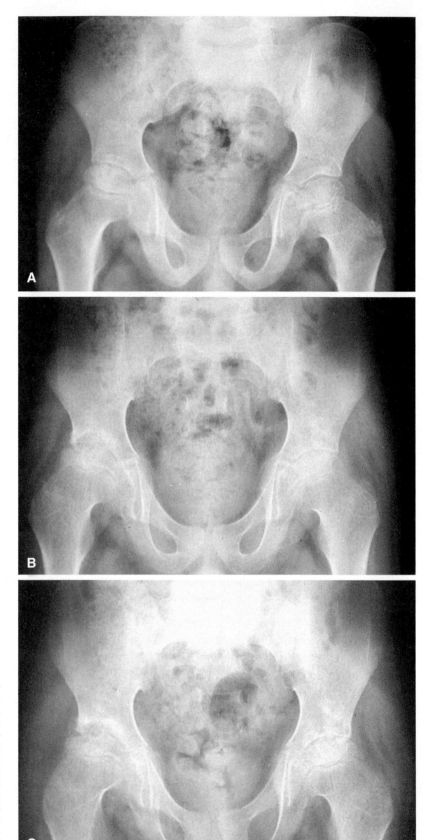

FIGURE 96–8 • *A*, Pelvis at age 5 years in a boy with severe, systemic disease and polyarthritis. Bilateral hip disease, narrowing of the joint spaces, and remodeling of the femoral head are present. *B*, Two years later, destructive hip disease has progressed, and there is more marked involvement of the acetabular bone with sclerosis and multiple cystic lucencies, also seen now along the margins of the femoral heads. *C*, After another year, generalized osteopenia is marked, coxa valga on the right is more extreme, and subluxation of the right femoral head is beginning. Clinically, this child had severe pain in the hips on weight-bearing and virtually no rotation. Flexion contractures with limitation of motion to approximately 35 degrees were present bilaterally.

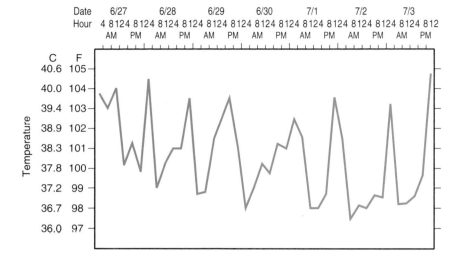

FIGURE 96-9 · Intermittent Fever in a 3-Year-Old Girl with Systemic Onset of Juvenile Rheumatoid Arthritis (JRA). Most of the febrile spikes occurred in the late evening to early morning hours and were accompanied by a rheumatoid rash.

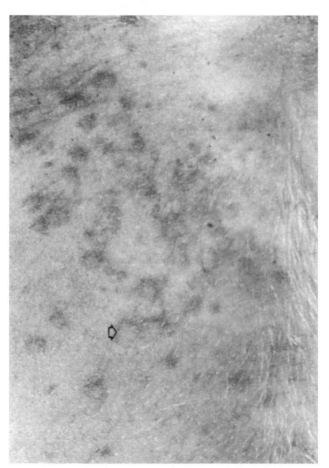

FIGURE 96-10 · Rheumatoid Rash in the Same Patient as in Figure 96-9. This was a faintly erythematous (salmon-colored), macular rash that was most prominent over the back but involved the extremities and face as well. The individual lesions were transient, appeared in crops, and generally conformed to a linear distribution. Some of the lesions were characterized by central clearing (*arrow*).

the cervical, axillary, and epitrochlear areas, may be marked and is usually symmetric.

Pericarditis, often subclinical and detected only by echocardiography, is especially common in systemic-onset disease.[51] It is unusual for pericarditis to precede the development of arthritis, but it may occur at any time during the course of JRA and is usually accompanied by a systemic exacerbation. Each episode generally persists for a week to a few months; pericarditis may be recurrent in the child with poorly controlled disease. Pericardial effusion does not usually progress to tamponade and rarely results in chronic constrictive pericarditis. Myocarditis is much less common but may lead to cardiac enlargement and congestive failure. Valvular lesions, although rare, have been reported. Rheumatoid nodules have been described on valve leaflets and visceral pericardium

Other rare extra-articular manifestations include diffuse interstitial pulmonary fibrosis and central nervous system (CNS) disease. Although CNS involvement has been described in children with JRA, this complication is more likely to be related to drug toxicity, viral infection, fever, embolism, or another systemic disease.

The acute manifestations of systemic-onset JRA are of variable duration, lasting from weeks to months or even years, and tend to recur during the initial years of the disease, usually in association with exacerbations of the arthritis. About half the children with systemic onset will eventually recover completely, especially if only a limited number of joints are involved (see Table 96-5). The other half develop progressive arthritis and moderate-to-severe disability. Systemic symptoms alone are not often a cause of permanent disability and seldom persist longer than 5 years.[2,9] The articular disease may be much more persistent, and in the Cincinnati series 48 percent of the patients still had active disease at 10 years or longer after onset.[50]

Differential Diagnosis

JRA is often a diagnosis of exclusion.[2,52] Because many of the other types of juvenile arthritis may be confused with JRA, serious consideration must initially be given to the possibility of other rheumatic and connective tissue diseases, especially rheumatic fever, SLE, and spondyloarthropathy. Particular attention must also be accorded the possibility of infectious arthritis, serum sickness, Henoch-Schönlein purpura, inflammatory enteropathies, and hematologic diseases, especially leukemia, sickle cell anemia, and hemophilia.

OLIGOARTHRITIS

The child with oligoarthritis will have involvement of one to four joints, generally including the knees. The joint is swollen with effusion but generally not very painful, tender, or red. If a child with limited joint disease has an acutely painful and erythematous monarthritis or systemic signs of illness, a septic process should be suspected, such as one due to *Staphylococcus aureus* or gonococci. Synovial fluid aspiration is almost always indicated in these children to exclude pyogenic synovitis. A nonreactive tuberculin skin test virtually eliminates tuberculosis as a consideration. Needle biopsy of the synovial membrane is occasionally useful in monarthritis to exclude other possible diagnoses. Internal derangements of the knee are not common in children, nor is persistent effusion due to trauma. However, episodic effusions, especially of the knee, are frequent in hypermobile children. Tumors that present as monarticular disease, such as pigmented villonodular synovitis, are rare. The finding of chronic nongranulomatous uveitis in a child with oligoarthritis almost always confirms the diagnosis of JRA. Other causes of uveitis must be considered, however, such as psoriatic arthritis or sarcoidosis.[53]

Lyme disease presents diagnostic difficulties in endemic geographic areas such as the northeastern and upper midwestern United States and Europe.[1,54] It most often has its onset in the summer, and the characteristic rash (erythema migrans) occurs coincident with the tick bite in half the children. Arthritis is often delayed until 1 to 2 months later and is usually a monarthritis or oligoarthritis. It is recurrent and episodic in two thirds of children. Occasionally polyarthritis occurs; 10 percent of children develop a chronic arthritis with erosions. Both chronic and acute anterior uveitis are associated complications.

Onset of hip disease in the very young child may represent a septic process or congenital dislocation of the hip. In the somewhat older child, aseptic necrosis of the femoral head (Legg-Calvé-Perthes disease) is a consideration. In the adolescent, particularly a boy who is obese, a slipped capital femoral epiphysis may initially mimic JRA. Transient synovitis of the hip is a self-limited condition of uncertain origin; results of laboratory and radiologic studies are normal. Osgood-Schlatter disease of the tibial tubercle can be easily distinguished clinically from involvement of the knee in JRA.

The child with juvenile AS will usually develop arthritis in the lower extremities initially, accompanied by enthesitis within the first 6 months after onset, rather than lumbar pain or stiffness.[55] Pain in the groin or buttock may be an early sign. Remittent oligoarthritis is most frequent, and involvement of the wrists or joints of the hands is rare. Two thirds of patients with juvenile AS are boys. Other helpful diagnostic points include onset after the age of 7 to 9 years, infrequent cervical spine involvement, seronegativity for RFs or ANAs, and a family history of similar disease. Approximately 92 percent of these children in North America will be positive for HLA-B27. A firm diagnosis depends on demonstration of characteristic radiologic abnormalities in the sacroiliac joints. Arthritis involving either the peripheral joints or the spine is seen in 5 to 15 percent of children with inflammatory bowel disease (IBD).

POLYARTHRITIS

The child with SLE can present with an arthritis that resembles JRA, and the correct diagnosis may not be evident until one of the more characteristic clinical findings of SLE occurs. The arthropathy of SLE is usually nondeforming and nonerosive. Serologic tests to confirm the presence of SLE should always be performed when a diagnostic question arises. Children with immunologic deficiencies, particularly selective IgA deficiency, common variable immunodeficiency, X-linked agammaglobulinemia, and C2 complement component deficiency may develop an arthritis that mimics JRA.[1] Therefore, it is mandatory in any child with chronic arthritis who has other features of unexpected autoimmunity or infection (e.g., sinopulmonary disease) to obtain studies for immunologic deficiency.

SYSTEMIC-ONSET DISEASE

Although the child with systemic-onset disease has many of the manifestations of an acute infectious process, the presence of the characteristic intermittent fever, rheumatoid rash, or typical and sometimes subtle arthritis, will suggest a diagnosis of JRA. Rare causes of fever and arthritis in infancy, such as neonatal-onset multisystem inflammatory disease (chronic infantile neurologic cutaneous and articular syndrome), should be considered.[1] The periodic fever syndromes should be suggested by the presence of their associated systemic features, ethnicity, and family history.[56] A sustained remittent fever that is readily responsive to salicylate therapy is more characteristic of acute rheumatic fever. A pericardial effusion in conjunction with evidence of endocarditis such as a diastolic murmur would point away from JRA and toward rheumatic fever or infectious endocarditis. The onset of acute rheumatic fever in developed countries usually occurs between the ages of 5 and 15 years. The arthritis is characteristically acute, painful, asymmetric, polyarticular, and migratory or additive, and involves the peripheral joints without permanent sequelae.[57] The total duration of a single attack is usually less than 6 weeks and seldom as long as 3 months. An elevated level of the antistreptolysin O titer should not be taken as an indication of recent streptococcal infection without a documented rise or fall in the titer and confirmation by other antibodies, such as the anti-DNAse B titer.

Certain malignancies, such as neuroblastoma, leukemia, and Langerhans cell histiocytosis, enter into the differential diagnosis. Bone pain on weight-bearing may be a clue to the presence of acute leukemia. The articular pain of leukemia is often out of proportion to the observed swelling. Sickle cell anemia can result in a periarthritis or dactylitis that mimics a true arthritis (the hand-foot syndrome).

▌ Evaluation and Management

GROWTH RETARDATION

Disturbances of growth are characteristic and predictable features of JRA. Linear growth is usually retarded during periods of active disease. There is often delayed puberty and development of secondary sexual characteristics. Growth retardation may also occur in specific areas such as the jaw (Fig. 96–11). Secondary growth deformities are frequent in children with limited joint disease, especially involving the knee, and result in unequal leg lengths, with the involved leg growing longer. Early during active disease, development of the ossification centers or epiphyses is accelerated, and later stunting, dwarfing, and premature fusion of the involved bones results. Brachydactyly of the digits develops from premature closure of the epiphyseal growth plates.

OSTEOPENIA

Osteopenia has emerged as a major determinant of functional outcome in children with JRA. Children with chronic arthritis develop a diminished bone mass and are, therefore, at increased risk of fracture in adulthood and an earlier onset of more severe osteoporosis.[58] An important determinant of future fracture risk is peak bone mass, defined as that present at the end of skeletal maturation, which is nearly complete by the late years of adolescence. A failure to undergo the normal increase in bone mass during puberty is common in children with JRA. A review of the acquisition of skeletal mass for children with JRA has been summarized in a number of publications.[59,60] The appendicular skeleton is predominantly affected, although bone mineral density (BMD) may be decreased at all sites. Osteopenia is characterized by inadequate bone formation for age, low bone turnover, and depressed formation instead of increased resorption.

CHRONIC UVEITIS

One of the most devastating complications of JRA is a chronic nongranulomatous uveitis.[61] Uveitis is especially likely to occur in girls who are ANA seropositive with oligoarthritis developing at a young age. Because onset of chronic uveitis is usually insidious and asymptomatic, ophthalmologic examination must be performed at the time of initial diagnosis and should be repeated at frequent intervals during the first years of the disease. Approximately two thirds of children with uveitis have bilateral disease. If initial involvement is unilateral, the second eye will often be affected within a year.

The earliest manifestations of inflammation are a proteinaceous flare on slit-lamp examination, an increased number of cells in the anterior chamber, and a punctate keratic precipitate on the posterior surface of the cornea (Fig. 96–12). Inflammation that is inadequately controlled results in the formation of posterior synechiae, which produce an irregular or poorly reactive pupil. Band keratopathy occurs as a late, degenerative lesion. Cataracts, secondary glaucoma, and phthisis bulbi are still encountered in a few children with chronic uveitis in spite of vigorous long-term treatment.

▌ Treatment

BASIC PROGRAM

Conservative management of children with JRA attempts to control the clinical manifestations of the

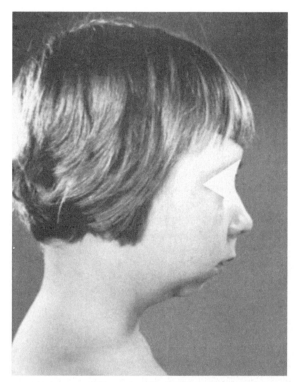

FIGURE 96–11 · **Micrognathia in an 11-Year-Old Girl Whose Polyarthritis Began at 18 Months of Age.** There was no restriction of motion of the temporomandibular joints. Extension, rotation, and lateral binding of the cervical spine were absent, and flexion was limited to 10 degrees.

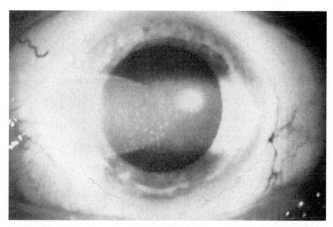

FIGURE 96–12 · A slit-lamp examination demonstrating a "flare" in the fluid of the anterior chamber (caused by increased protein content) and keratic precipitates on the posterior surface of the cornea, representing small collections of inflammatory cells. (Courtesy of Dr. HJ Kaplan.)

disease and to prevent deformity. It ideally involves a coordinated, multidisciplinary team supervising a program that is family-centered, community-based, and coordinated. Treatment in most children is prolonged over many years. This long duration of therapy must be accepted ultimately by the family and the child and judged reasonably safe by the physician.

It is vitally important that the parents and child, if cognitively possible, understand the disease and share in its management.[62,63] A considerable amount of time and effort must be expended in explaining the nature of JRA, reasonable expectations during initial therapy, and the course of the disease. These educational efforts must be an ongoing process; it is useful to ask a parent to write down problems and questions and bring the list to the next appointment. A priority in the management of the child with JRA is to foster normal psychologic and social development. Attendance at school is strongly encouraged; only rarely is home instruction indicated.

The philosophy of management is to begin with the simplest, safest, and most conservative measures. If this approach proves inadequate, the physician should choose other therapeutic modalities in an orderly fashion[1] (Fig. 96–13). Therapy is generally continued for 1 to 2 years after all manifestations of disease activity have been suppressed to avoid the error of stopping anti-inflammatory therapy during short, self-limited remissions. In children, potentially toxic regimens such as prolonged steroid use and immunosuppressive drugs should be employed only for life-threatening disease. Nutrition is an important aspect of long-term management. Dietary supplementation is often wise, especially with vitamin D and calcium.

Nonsteroidal Anti-inflammatory Drugs

Although seldom used in North America, aspirin, on a worldwide basis, is the single most useful and inexpensive nonsteroidal anti-inflammatory drug (NSAID). Treatment is started at 75 to 90 mg/kg/day (depending on the child's age and weight), given in divided doses four times a day with meals and at bedtime with milk to minimize gastrointestinal irritation. Salicylate blood levels are occasionally useful as a guide to correct dosage or when signs of toxicity such as tinnitus or inattention develop. Epidemiologic studies have demonstrated a potential association between the administration of aspirin and the development of Reye's syndrome.[64] As a general rule, any NSAID should be discontinued in a sick child who is vomiting or who potentially has influenza or varicella. Some children develop a transaminasemia related to NSAID therapy, although clinical manifestations of liver disease are uncommon. Transient elevation of these enzymes in a child who is not otherwise showing signs of toxicity is not an indication for stopping the drug.

Among NSAIDs approved for use in North America, naproxen (15 to 20 mg/kg/day twice daily), ibuprofen (35 mg/kg/day four times daily), and tolmetin (25 mg/kg/day four times daily), have been extensively used. The first two medications are also available

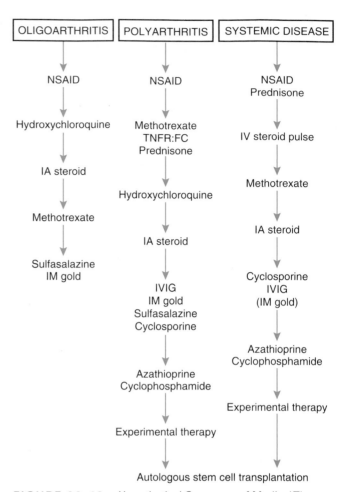

FIGURE 96–13 · Hypothetical Sequence of Medical Therapy in Children with Juvenile Rheumatoid Arthritis (JRA). Addition of medications and alteration of the therapeutic plan are based on the type of onset and course of the disease, its activity and severity, and the clinical response to each sequential therapeutic maneuver.

as suspensions for younger children who have difficulty swallowing tablets (the dose for ibuprofen suspension is 45 mg/kg/day). An unusual toxic result of naproxen therapy and, less commonly of the other NSAIDs, has been the occurrence of pseudoporphyria as an exaggerated photosensitivity reaction. A few children with JRA may develop signs of analgesic nephropathy. These are often children who are severely disabled, confined to wheelchairs, or dependent on adults for their needs and undoubtedly are chronically dehydrated.

The response to NSAIDs varies among children with JRA, but satisfactory treatment of the arthritis will be achieved in about 50 percent. A child may respond to one drug better than another. Introduction of the cyclooxygenase-2 (COX-2) inhibitors may herald an era of more specific and effective therapy when they are approved for use in children.

Methotrexate

When children do not respond adequately to an initial trial of NSAIDs, a number of other medications should be considered as additions to the antirheumatic program.[65] Methotrexate (MTX) is currently the most frequently prescribed drug in children who have failed to respond to NSAIDs, based on the results of an international double-blind trial and subsequent experience.[66,67] The advantages of this medication are its efficacy at relatively low oral doses and its apparent lack of oncogenicity or production of sterility.[68] Potential systemic manifestations of toxicity include bone marrow suppression, gastrointestinal ulceration and diarrhea, headache, acute interstitial pneumonitis, alopecia, dermatitis, and hepatic fibrosis or cirrhosis. Cirrhosis of the liver is not an expected sign of toxicity in children on weekly therapy.[69] MTX should be avoided, however, in children with risk factors such as malnutrition, viral hepatitis, diabetes mellitus, obesity, smoking, or alcohol consumption. As some NSAIDs may interfere with the protein binding and excretion of MTX, their dosage should be kept constant during treatment. Folic acid (1 mg/day) is given during treatment in addition to a multivitamin.

Baseline studies performed before therapy include a complete blood count (CBC), urinalysis, determination of renal and hepatic functions and serum albumin levels, and a chest roentgenogram, if clinically indicated. MTX is given as a single weekly dose on an empty stomach with clear liquids 60 minutes before breakfast. The injectable preparation (25 mg/ml) can be used orally in children to prescribe the correct amount. The minimum starting dose is 10 mg/m^2 weekly (0.35 to 0.45 mg/kg). Monitoring during the course of treatment includes a CBC and assays of liver function every 4 to 8 weeks. The guidelines recommended by the ACR should be observed.[70] The drug should be administered subcutaneously when used in higher dosage (0.65 to 1.0 mg/kg) with a maximum dose of approximately 30 mg per week.[71] MTX therapy should be continued for approximately 1 year after a sustained remission of the disease is achieved. Tapering of the dose may include an every-two-week schedule. Early withdrawal has resulted in an exacerbation of the arthritis, and reinstitution of the drug does not always result in a satisfactory clinical response.[72]

Glucocorticoids

Systemic glucocorticoids are sometimes required in the treatment of JRA that is resistant to more conservative forms of therapy. They are usually combined with an NSAID and often with other antirheumatic drugs. Initial control of inflammatory disease is sometimes aided by the addition of low-dose prednisone in the mornings for a short period of time ("bridge therapy"). For uncontrolled systemic disease with marked disability, prednisone is given as a single morning dose of 0.1 to 1 mg/kg/day (less than or equal to 40 mg total) or in divided doses for more severe disease. After satisfactory control is reached, or it is obvious that adequate control is not going to be achieved, the drug should be gradually decreased and eventually discontinued. "Steroid pseudorheumatism" may make even slow withdrawal of the drug difficult.

Growth retardation is the most significant untoward effect of steroid toxicity. A dose of 5 mg/day is usually inhibitory; as little as 3 mg in a child weighing less than 25 kg may be suppressive. Over time, a child may regain some loss in height, be it the result of either disease or therapy, but this does not happen readily if a significant growth deficit has occurred.

To minimize the daily steroid requirement or avoid it altogether, intravenous (IV) steroid pulse therapy has been introduced for treatment of the more severe manifestations of JRA. Methylprednisolone is the drug of choice, given in a dose of 10 to 30 mg/kg per pulse, administered in a variety of protocols that have consisted of a single IV pulse to three pulses on alternate days. IV steroid pulse therapy should be administered and monitored with caution because it can result in serious and fatal complications involving electrolyte and fluid imbalance and cardiac arrhythmia.

Triamcinolone hexacetonide (5 to 40 mg depending on the size of the joint) is the long-acting intra-articular preparation preferred therapeutically for use in one or two joints that do not respond satisfactorily to a conservative program or as a short-term aid to physical therapy.[73,74] Intra-articular injections should not be given more than a limited number of times if satisfactory results are not achieved—for example, three times in a single joint during a 6-month period.

Etanercept

Etanercept consists of two TNF-α receptor monomer chains fused to the fragment crystallizable (Fc) domain of human IgG$_1$. It binds TNF-α in the vascular and extracellular compartments and inhibits its activity. The controlled trial of etanercept in children with polyarticular JRA who had failed therapy with MTX indicated that 74 percent demonstrated improvement at 3 months on a subcutaneous dose of 0.4 mg/kg twice a week.[75] After randomization, children who began placebo injections had significant differences in clinical exacerbations compared to the group that continued on the active drug (81 vs. 28 percent) and in time to flare (28 vs. 116 days). Observed toxicity included injection site reactions and an increased frequency of upper respiratory tract infections. A 2-year follow-up indicated that the overall response rate of improvement was 79 percent, and remissions occurred in 37 percent.

The long-term safety of TNF-α blockade is unknown. It is associated with a potentially increased frequency of systemic infection and should not be used in children with recurrent or chronic infections. Tuberculosis should always be excluded before beginning therapy. Current monitoring of clinical status and laboratory studies (CBC with differential and platelet counts, biochemistry panel, ESR, and CRP level) should be performed every 1 to 2 months while on therapy.

Infliximab is a monoclonal antibody that has the capacity to bind TNF-α in both the extracellular and vascular compartments but also on the cell surface. A pediatric trial is currently in progress to evaluate the safety and efficacy of this drug in JRA. Another biologic response modifier is anakinra (r-metHuIL-1ra), which interferes with the actions of IL-1 in the inflammatory response.

OTHER ADVANCED THERAPY

Hydroxychloroquine

A large, multicenter study studied the use of hydroxychloroquine and D-penicillamine in the treatment of JRA during a 12-month trial.[76] In the presence of NSAIDs, neither drug was shown to be superior to placebo. However, hydroxychloroquine is often considered a useful adjunctive therapeutic agent in the older child. The initial dose is 5 mg/kg/day (400 mg total). An ophthalmologic examination with evaluation of color vision must be performed before institution of therapy and periodically thereafter. Although it would be unusual and rare for retinal toxicity to occur with currently recommended doses, the drug should be discontinued when any suspicion of retinopathy is present because its effects are cumulative.

Gold Compounds

Intramuscular administration of gold compounds (aurothioglucose, aurothiomalate) is an effective treatment but one that is used much less frequently since the introduction of MTX (with which it may be combined). It is given in conjunction with an NSAID and often with hydroxychloroquine.

A CBC and urinalysis must be obtained before each administration, and clinical assessment for evidence of toxicity, especially stomatitis, dermatitis, bone marrow suppression, hematuria, or proteinuria, should be performed. Renal and hepatic panels are ordered approximately every 6 weeks. Children with systemic-onset disease may be at greater risk for reactions from any of the medications used to treat JRA, especially gold compounds, with neutropenia and diffuse intravascular coagulation as the predominant manifestations of toxicity (the macrophage activation syndrome).[77] In a pediatric trial, auranofin (triethylphosphine gold) was well tolerated but not necessarily more effective than an NSAID.[78]

D-Penicillamine

Indications for the use of D-penicillamine are the same as those for gold compounds; these two agents should not be combined therapeutically.[76] The maintenance dose is 10 mg/kg/day (approximately 750 mg/day). Important side effects are drug-induced lupus, dermatitis, thrombocytopenia, and proteinuria.

Intravenous Immunoglobulin

Intravenous immunoglobulin (IVIg) has been proposed as adjunctive therapy for polyarticular-onset and systemic-onset JRA.[79-81] Double-blind multiclinic trials have not confirmed its complete efficacy, especially in systemic-onset disease, although patient numbers were small.[80]

Sulfasalazine

Although there are few published studies on the use of sulfasalazine in JRA, this agent appears to be effective and relatively safe, with a clinical response evaluable at approximately 6 to 8 weeks.[82] Sulfasalazine should not be used in children with known hypersensitivity to sulfa or salicylate, impaired renal or hepatic function, or specific contraindications such as porphyria or glucose-6-phosphate dehydrogenase deficiency.

Immunosuppressive and Cytotoxic Therapy

Immunosuppressive and cytotoxic agents should be used only in approved protocols for life-threatening illness or unremitting progression of arthritis and disability.[83] The drugs most commonly employed are azathioprine, cyclophosphamide, and chlorambucil. Bone marrow suppression may result from any of these agents. Development of malignancy and mutagenic effects are the most important long-term considerations. Sterility and amenorrhea have been associated with most of the immunosuppressive agents, particularly those of the alkylating variety. A unique indication for the use of immunosuppressive therapy in children with JRA may be the development of amyloidosis.

Other experimental approaches have included cyclosporine, which may have unique therapeutic value in the macrophage activation syndrome.[77,84] Autologous stem cell transplantation is being evaluated in a small number of children with severe disease.[85]

SPECIFIC TREATMENT CONSIDERATIONS

Growth Retardation

Adequate nutrition, exercise, and control of the inflammatory disease are prerequisites for restoring a semblance of normal growth in the moderately to severely affected child. Recombinant growth hormone therapy may not result in "catch-up" growth and may not be cost effective for some of these patients.[86] Leg-length discrepancy should be compensated by adjustments of the shoe height of the shorter leg.

Osteopenia

Onset of accelerated skeletal maturation with puberty is a critical period of potential medical intervention for osteopenia. Conversely, therapeutic maneuvers later during adolescence offer less promise of reversal of inadequate bone mineralization. Increasing attention needs to focus on the development of osteopenia during periods of active disease and on approaches to its prevention and management. Increased intake of calcium and vitamin D corrected metabolic abnormalities but did not affect measures of bone mineralization in a short-term study.[87] Alendronate, a bisdiphosphonate, in one pediatric trial produced impressive benefits in children with rheumatic diseases,[88] but it is not yet approved for use in the United States in this age-group.

Chronic Uveitis

The treatment of chronic uveitis should be supervised by an experienced ophthalmologist. Initial therapy consists of glucocorticoid eye drops and mydriasis. It is sometimes advisable to use supplemental oral prednisone in low dosage (2 to 4 mg once a day). Although evidence of inflammation on slit-lamp examination may abate soon after treatment is initiated, it is inadvisable to stop steroids at that time because of the frequent reappearance of signs of uveitis. The management of complicated disease and glaucoma remains unsatisfactory, but results with lensectomy or vitrectomy for complicated cataract are improving. Administration of MTX is a potentially effective mode of therapy in children with severe uveitis that has failed on other forms of treatment.[89]

Macrophage Activation Syndrome

Treatment of this acute emergency characterized by a marked increase in systemic toxicity and evidence of hemophagocytosis demands precise attention to measures of intensive care and vascular support. IV steroid pulse therapy combined with cyclosporine is usually the recommended approach.[77,84]

PHYSICAL AND OCCUPATIONAL THERAPY

Maintenance of function and prevention of deformity by exercises and splinting cannot be overemphasized and are vitally important in management. Atrophy of the extensor muscles and later of the flexors begins early, and a program to strengthen these muscle groups should be instituted as soon as possible. Passive and then active motion of selected joints must be begun early, because weight-bearing is sometimes difficult because of pain, weakness, or contractures. Heat, and occasionally the use of ice packs, aid in relief of joint pain and stiffness and prepares a child for the exercise program.

A balanced program of increased rest at night or after school is advisable in many children. Children will usually best determine their own level of activity. Normal play should be encouraged, and the only activities that are potentially undesirable are those that place unacceptable levels of stress on weight-bearing joints that are inflamed. Tricycle riding and swimming are almost always helpful and avoid undue load and impact on involved joints.

Cockup splints for the wrists and night splints for the elbows or knees are used to prevent malpositioning or as aids in the long-term correction of deformity. The effects on gait of leg-length discrepancy should be minimized by a heel or sole lift for the shorter extremity. If the hips are involved, use of a prone-lying board will help prevent flexion contractures. For severe contractures of a knee, elbow, or wrist, serial casting after intra-articular steroid injection with active exercises every 2 to 4 days each time the cast is removed may be tried; forced extension should be avoided. Malpositioning of the cervical spine may be minimized by the use of a soft collar and a desk with a tilt top on which the child can do homework. If atlantoaxial subluxation is present, a firm collar should be worn while riding in an automobile.

ORTHOPEDIC SURGERY

Synovectomy does not affect the long-term course of JRA but may be useful in selected children for relief of mechanic impairment of joint motion related to synovial hypertrophy, joint pain, or decreased range of motion. Open arthrotomy should be avoided if at all possible, as remobilization of a postsurgical joint in a child is often difficult. Arthroscopic surgery offers an attractive alternative. Tenosynovectomy may be indicated to decrease the risk of tendon rupture over the dorsum of the wrist or for adhesive tenosynovitis and a trigger finger. A well-thought-out plan of reconstructive surgery can be of crucial importance in patients who enter the late teenage years or adulthood with marked disability. Total joint replacement, particularly of the hip or knee, is usually undertaken only after bone growth has ceased (e.g., 18 years of age or older). Children with micrognathia may benefit from orthodontic management.

▌ Summary and Conclusions

A child's potential for growth is an important factor working in favor of the pediatric rheumatologist and the therapeutic program. To a large extent, it is this endowment for future physical and psychologic development that enables so much to be accomplished in the majority of children with JRA. Analyses from the 1991 Cincinnati study confirmed that active disease was still present in 45 percent of patients at 15 to 20 years, and 17 percent were in functional capacities III and IV.[50] Recent publications have reviewed currently expected outcomes in children with JRA according to type of onset and course,[90-92] which can be compared to those summarized in the ACR classification of 1986.[2] Death has occurred historically in 2 to 7 percent of children with JRA, especially in children with systemic-onset disease, but this is currently the outcome in less than 1 percent of children in North America. Errors of steroid management during periods of stress and infections are particular risks.

Kanski's data on children with uveitis from 1990 indicated that visual prognosis was good in 25 percent and only fair in 50 percent of patients.[93] The remaining 25 percent of patients developed visual impairment from cataract or glaucoma. The prognosis for sight in children with chronic uveitis is, however, probably improving because of earlier detection and better management. The frequency and severity of uveitis may also be decreasing.[94,95]

Sequential measurements of health status on standardized instruments of assessment are useful in judging a child's functional adaptations.[96] A number of studies have indicated that young adults with a past history of JRA function less well than matched controls and have more residual pain syndromes, even though their arthritis is no longer active.[97,98]

REFERENCES

1. Cassidy JT, Petty RE: Textbook of Pediatric Rheumatology, 4th ed. Philadelphia, WB Saunders, 2000.
2. Cassidy JT, Levinson JE, Bass JC, et al: A study of classification criteria for a diagnosis of juvenile rheumatoid arthritis. Arthritis Rheum 29:274-281, 1986.
3. Prieur AM, Ansell BM, Bardfeld R, et al: Is onset type evaluated during the first 3 months of disease satisfactory for defining the sub-groups of juvenile chronic arthritis? A EULAR Cooperative Study (1983-1986). Clin Exp Rheumatol 8:321-325, 1990.
4. Ansell BM, Wood PHN: Prognosis in juvenile chronic polyarthritis. Clin Rheum Dis 2:397, 1976.
5. Ruperto N, Levinson JE, Ravelli A, et al: Long-term health outcomes and quality of life in American and Italian inception cohorts of patients with juvenile rheumatoid arthritis. I. Outcome status. J Rheumatol 24:945-951, 1997.
6. Ruperto N, Ravelli A, Levinson JE, et al: Long-term health outcomes and quality of life in American and Italian inception cohorts of patients with juvenile rheumatoid arthritis. II. Early predictors of outcome. J Rheumatol 24:952-958, 1997.
7. Flato B, Aasland A, Vinje O, et al: Outcome and predictive factors in juvenile rheumatoid arthritis and juvenile spondyloarthropathy. J Rheumatol 25:366-375, 1998.
8. Cassidy JT: What's in a name? Nomenclature of juvenile arthritis: A North American view. J Rheumatol 20(Suppl 40):4-8, 1993.
9. Cassidy JT, Levinson JE, Brewer EJ Jr: The development of classification criteria for children with juvenile rheumatoid arthritis. Bull Rheum Dis 38:1-7, 1989.
10. Petty RE, Southwood TR, Baum J, et al: Revision of the proposed classification criteria for juvenile idiopathic arthritis: Durban, 1997. J Rheumatol 25:1991-1994, 1998.
11. Sullivan DB, Cassidy JT, Petty RE: Pathogenic implications of age of onset in juvenile rheumatoid arthritis. Arthritis Rheum 18:251-255, 1975.
12. Kunnamo I, Kallio P, Pelkonen P: Incidence of arthritis in urban Finnish children: A prospective study. Arthritis Rheum 29:1232-1238, 1986.
13. Gare BA: Juvenile Chronic Arthritis: A Population Based Study on Epidemiology, Natural History and Outcome. Goteborg, Sweden, University of Goteborg, 1994.
14. Towner SR, Michet CJ Jr, O'Fallon WM, et al: The epidemiology of juvenile arthritis in Rochester, Minnesota 1960-1979. Arthritis Rheum 26:1208-1213, 1983.
15. Moe N, Rygg M: Epidemiology of juvenile chronic arthritis in northern Norway: A ten-year retrospective study. Clin Exp Rheumatol 16:99-101, 1998.
15a. Manners PJ, Diepeveen DA: Prevalence of Juvenile chronic arthritis in a population of 12-year-old children in urban Australia. Pediatrics 98:84-90, 1996.
16. Peterson LS, Mason T, Nelson AM, et al: Juvenile rheumatoid arthritis in Rochester, Minnesota 1960-1993: Is the epidemiology changing? Arthritis Rheum 39:1385-1390, 1996.
17. Oen K, Fast M, Postl B: Epidemiology of juvenile rheumatoid arthritis in Manitoba, Canada, 1975-92: Cycles in incidence. J Rheumatol 22:745-750, 1995.
18. Feldman BM, Birdi N, Boone JE, et al: Seasonal onset of systemic-onset juvenile rheumatoid arthritis. J Pediatr 129:513-518, 1996.
19. Lang BA, Shore A: A review of current concepts on the pathogenesis of juvenile rheumatoid arthritis. J Rheumatol 17(Suppl 21):1-15, 1990.
20. Jarvis JN: Pathogenesis and mechanisms of inflammation in the childhood rheumatic diseases. Curr Opin Rheumatol 10:459-467, 1998.
21. Grom AA, Giannini EH, Glass DN: Juvenile rheumatoid arthritis and the trimolecular complex (HLA, T cell receptor, and antigen): Differences from rheumatoid arthritis. Arthritis Rheum 37:601-607, 1994.
22. De Benedetti F, Ravelli A, Martini A: Cytokines in juvenile rheumatoid arthritis. Curr Opin Rheumatol 9:428-433, 1997.
23. Grom AA, Murray KJ, Luyrink L, et al: Patterns of expression of tumor necrosis factor alpha, tumor necrosis factor beta, and their receptors in synovia of patients with juvenile rheumatoid arthritis and juvenile spondylarthropathy. Arthritis Rheum 39:1703-1710, 1996.
24. Petty RE, Tingle AJ: Arthritis and viral infection. J Pediatr 113:948-949, 1988.
25. Pritchard MH, Matthews N, Munro J: Antibodies to influenza A in a cluster of children with juvenile chronic arthritis. Br J Rheumatol 27:176-180, 1988.
26. Prakken ABJ, van Eden W, Rijkers GT, et al: Autoreactivity to human heat-shock protein 60 predicts disease remission in oligoarticular juvenile rheumatoid arthritis. Arthritis Rheum 39:1826-1832, 1996.
27. Zeggini E, Thomson W, Kwiatkowski D, et al: Linkage and association studies of single-nucleotide polymorphism—tagged tumor necrosis factor haplotypes in juvenile oligoarthritis. Arthritis Rheum 46:3304-3311, 2002.
28. Nepom B: The immunogenetics of juvenile rheumatoid arthritis. Rheum Dis Clin North Am 17:825-842, 1991.
29. De Inocencio J, Giannini EH, Glass DN: Can genetic markers contribute to the classification of juvenile rheumatoid arthritis? J Rheumatol [20] (Suppl 40):12-18, 1993.
30. Melin-Aldana H, Giannini EH, Taylor J, et al: Human leukocyte antigen-DRB1*1104 in the chronic iridocyclitis of pauciarticular juvenile rheumatoid arthritis. J Pediatr 121:56-60, 1992.
31. Malagon C, Van Kerckhove C, Giannini EH, et al: The iridocyclitis of early onset pauciarticular juvenile rheumatoid arthritis: Outcome in immunogenetically characterized patients. J Rheumatol 19:160-163, 1992.
32. Haas JP, Truckenbrodt H, Paul C, et al: Subtypes of HLA-DRB1*03, *08, *11, *12, *13 and *14 in early onset pauciarticular juvenile chronic arthritis (EOPA) with and without iridocyclitis. Clin Exp Rheumatol 12(Suppl 10):S7-S14, 1994.
33. Van Kerckhove C, Luyrink L, Taylor J, et al: HLA-DQA1*0101 haplotypes and disease outcome in early onset pauciarticular juvenile rheumatoid arthritis. J Rheumatol 18:874-879, 1991.
34. Haas JP, Kimura A, Andreas A, et al: Polymorphism in the upstream regulatory regions of DQA1 genes and DRB1, QAP, and DQB1 haplotypes in the German population. Hum Immunol 39:31-40, 1994.
35. Vehe RK, Begovich AB, Nepom BS: HLA susceptibility genes in rheumatoid factor positive juvenile rheumatoid arthritis. J Rheumatol 17(Suppl 26):11-15, 1990.
36. Fernandez-Vina MA, Fink CW, Stastny P: HLA antigens in juvenile arthritis: Pauciarticular and polyarticular juvenile arthritis are immunogenetically distinct. Arthritis Rheum 33:1787-1794, 1990.
37. Murray KJ, Moroldo MB, Donnelly P, et al: Age-specific effects of juvenile rheumatoid arthritis associated HLA alleles. Arthritis Rheum 42:1843-1853, 1999.
38. Nepom BS, Malhotra U, Schwarz DA, et al: HLA and T cell receptor polymorphisms in pauciarticular-onset juvenile rheumatoid arthritis. Arthritis Rheum 34:1260-1267, 1991.
39. Rosenberg AM, Petty RE: Similar patterns of juvenile rheumatoid arthritis within families. Arthritis Rheum 23:951-953, 1980.
40. Moroldo MB, Tague BL, Shear ES, et al: Juvenile rheumatoid arthritis in affected sibpairs. Arthritis Rheum 40:1962-1966, 1997.
41. Oglivie EM, Fife MS, Thompson SD, et al: TDT association study confirms the IL6-174 SNP confers susceptibility to systemic JIA. Arthritis Rheum 46(Suppl):S578, 2002.
42. Jefferey R, Luong L, Ogilvie E, et al: The-174 single nucleotide polymorphism (SNP) of the interleukin-6 gene associated with systemic arthritis is functionally significant in the control of common haplotypes, alters transcription factor binding and repression by glucocorticoids. Arthritis Rheum 46(Suppl):S578, 2002.
43. De Benedetti F, Meazza C, Vivarelli M, et al: Functional and prognostic significance of the-173 polymorphism of the macrophage migration inhibitory factor (MIF) gene in systemic JIA. Arthritis Rheum 46(Suppl):S580, 2002.
44. Falcini F, Simonini G, Cimaz R, et al: Osteoprotegerin serum levels and osteoprotegerin polymorphism in juvenile idiopathic arthritis: Correlations with articular erosions and low bone mass. Arthritis Rheum 46(Suppl):S579, 2002.
45. David J: Amyloidosis in juvenile chronic arthritis. Clin Exp Rheumatol 9:73-78, 1991.

46. Reed MH, Wilmot DM: The radiology of juvenile rheumatoid arthritis: A review of the English language literature. J Rheumatol 18(Suppl 31):2-22, 1991.

47. Verbruggen LA, Shahabpour M, Van Roy P, et al: Magnetic resonance imaging of articular destruction in juvenile rheumatoid arthritis. Arthritis Rheum 33:1426-1430, 1990.

48. Ilowite NT, Walco GA, Pochaczevsky R: Assessment of pain in patients with juvenile rheumatoid arthritis: Relation between pain intensity and degree of joint inflammation. Ann Rheum Dis 51:343-346, 1992.

49. Hagglund KJ, Schopp LM, Alberts KR, et al: Predicting pain among children with juvenile rheumatoid arthritis. Arthritis Care Res 8:36-42, 1995.

50. Wallace CA, Levinson JE: Juvenile rheumatoid arthritis: Outcome and treatment for the 1990s. Rheum Dis Clin North Am 17:891-905, 1991.

51. Goldenberg J, Ferraz MB, Pessoa AP, et al: Symptomatic cardiac involvement in juvenile rheumatoid arthritis. Int J Cardiol 34:57-62, 1992.

52. Cassidy JT: Miscellaneous conditions associated with arthritis in children. Pediatr Clin North Am 33:1033-1052, 1986.

53. Petty RE: Juvenile psoriatic arthritis, or juvenile arthritis with psoriasis? Clin Exp Rheumatol 12(Suppl 10):S55-S58, 1994.

54. Athreya BH, Rose CD: Lyme disease. Curr Probl Pediatr 26:189-207, 1996.

55. Burgos-Vargas R, Pacheco-Tena C, Vazquez-Mellado J: Juvenile-onset spondyloarthropathies. Rheum Dis Clin North Am 23:569-598, 1997.

56. Dode C, Andre M, Bienvenu T, et al: The enlarging clinical, genetic, and population spectrum of tumor necrosis factor receptor-associated periodic syndrome. Arthritis Rheum 46:2181-2188, 2002.

57. Ayoub EM, Ahmed S: Update on complications of group A streptococcal infections. Curr Probl Pediatr 27:90-101, 1997.

58. Zak M, Hassager C, Lovell DJ, et al: Assessment of bone mineral density in adults with a history of juvenile chronic arthritis: a cross-sectional long-term followup study. Arthritis Rheum 42:790 798, 1999.

59. Cassidy JT, Hillman LS: Abnormalities in skeletal growth in children with juvenile rheumatoid arthritis. Rheum Dis Clin North Am 23:499-522, 1997.

60. Cassidy JT: Osteopenia and osteoporosis in children. Clin Exp Rheumatol 17:245-250, 1999.

61. Edelsten C, Lee V, Bentley CR, et al: An evaluation of baseline risk factors predicting severity in juvenile idiopathic arthritis associated uveitis and other chronic anterior uveitis in early childhood. Br J Ophthalmol 86:51-56, 2002.

62. Hobbs N, Perrin JM, Ireys HT: Chronically Ill Children and Their Families. Problems, Prospects, and Proposals From the Vanderbilt Study. San Francisco, Jossey-Bass, 1985.

63. Brewer EJ Jr, Angel KC: Parenting a Child with Arthritis. Los Angeles, Lowell House, 1992.

64. Hurwitz ES, Barrett MJ, Bregman D, et al: Public Health Service study of Reye's syndrome and medications: Report of the main study. JAMA 257:1905-1911, 1987.

65. Giannini EH, Cassidy JT, Brewer EJ, et al: Comparative efficacy and safety of advanced drug therapy in children with juvenile rheumatoid arthritis. Semin Arthritis Rheum 23:34 46, 1993.

66. Giannini EH, Brewer EJ, Kuzmina N, et al: Methotrexate in resistant juvenile rheumatoid arthritis: Results of the U.S.A.-U.S.S.R. double-blind, placebo-controlled trial—The Pediatric Rheumatology Collaborative Study Group and The Cooperative Children's Study Group. N Engl J Med 326:1043-1049, 1992.

67. Lovell DJ: Ten years of experience with methotrexate. Past, present and future. Rev Rhum Engl Ed 64:186S-188S, 1997.

68. Giannini EH, Cassidy JT: Methotrexate in juvenile rheumatoid arthritis: Do the benefits outweigh the risks? Drug Saf 9:325-339, 1993.

69. Hashkes PJ, Balistreri WF, Bove KE, et al: The long-term effect of methotrexate therapy on the liver in patients with juvenile rheumatoid arthritis. Arthritis Rheum 40:2226-2234, 1997.

70. Kremer JM, Alarcon GS, Lightfoot RW Jr, et al: Methotrexate for rheumatoid arthritis: Suggested guidelines for monitoring liver toxicity—American College of Rheumatology. Arthritis Rheum 37:316-328, 1994.

71. Wallace CA, Sherry DD: Preliminary report of higher dose methotrexate treatment in juvenile rheumatoid arthritis. J Rheumatol 19:1604-1607, 1992.

72. Gottlieb BS, Keenan GF, Lu T, et al: Discontinuation of methotrexate treatment in juvenile rheumatoid arthritis. Pediatrics 100:994-997, 1997.

73. Sparling M, Malleson P, Wood B, et al: Radiographic followup of joints injected with triamcinolone hexacetonide for the management of childhood arthritis. Arthritis Rheum 33:821-826, 1990.

74. Dent PB, Walker N: Intra-articular corticosteroids in the treatment of juvenile rheumatoid arthritis. Curr Opin Rheumatol 10:475-480, 1998.

75. Lovell DJ, Giannini EH, Reiff A, et al: Etanercept in children with polyarticular juvenile rheumatoid arthritis. N Engl J Med 342:763-769, 2000.

76. Brewer EJ, Giannini EH, Kuzmina N, et al: Penicillamine and hydroxychloroquine in the treatment of severe juvenile rheumatoid arthritis. Results of the U.S.A.-U.S.S.R. double-blind placebo-controlled trial. N Engl J Med 314:1269-1276, 1986.

77. Prieur AM, Stephan JL: Macrophage activation syndrome in rheumatic diseases in children. Rev Rhum Engl Ed 61:385, 1994.

78. Giannini EH, Barron KS, Spencer CH, et al: Auranofin therapy for juvenile rheumatoid arthritis: Results of the five-year open label extension trial. J Rheumatol 18:1240-1242, 1991.

79. Silverman ED, Cawkwell GD, Lovell DJ, et al: Intravenous immunoglobulin in the treatment of systemic juvenile rheumatoid arthritis: A randomized placebo controlled trial—Pediatric Rheumatology Collaborative Study Group. J Rheumatol 21:2353-2358, 1994.

80. Uziel Y, Laxer RM, Schneider R, et al: Intravenous immunoglobulin therapy in systemic onset juvenile rheumatoid arthritis: A follow-Up study. J Rheumatol 23:910-918, 1996.

81. Giannini EH, Lovell DJ, Silverman ED, et al: Intravenous immunoglobulin in the treatment of polyarticular juvenile rheumatoid arthritis: A phase I/II study—Pediatric Rheumatology Collaborative Study Group. J Rheumatol 23:919-924, 1996.

82. van Rossum MA, Fiselier TJ, Franssen MJ, et al: Sulfasalazine in the treatment of juvenile chronic arthritis: A randomized, double-blind, placebo-controlled, multicenter study. Dutch Juvenile Chronic Arthritis Study Group. Arthritis Rheum 41:808-816, 1998.

83. Lehman TJ: Aggressive therapy for childhood rheumatic diseases: When are immunosuppressives appropriate? Arthritis Rheum 36:71-74, 1993.

84. Ostensen M, Hoyeraal HM, Kass E: Tolerance of cyclosporine A in children with refractory juvenile rheumatoid arthritis. J Rheumatol 15:1536-1538, 1988.

85. Wulffraat NM, Kuis W: Autologous stem cell transplantation: A possible treatment for refractory juvenile chronic arthritis? Rheumatology (Oxford) 38:764-766, 1999.

86. Davies UM, Rooney M, Preece MA, et al: Treatment of growth retardation in juvenile chronic arthritis with recombinant human growth hormone. J Rheumatol 21:153-158, 1994.

87. Cassidy JT, Popescu M, Chanetsa F, et al: Effect of treatment with calcium and vitamin D in children with juvenile rheumatoid arthritis (JRA): Program of the Fifth International Symposium: Clinical Advances in Osteoporosis. March 6-9:39, 2002.

88. Bianchi ML, Cimaz R, Bardare M, et al: Efficacy and safety of alendronate for the treatment of osteoporosis in diffuse connective tissue diseases in children: a prospective multicenter study. Arthritis Rheum 43:1960-1966, 2000.

89. Weiss AH, Wallace CA, Sherry DD: Methotrexate for resistant chronic uveitis in children with juvenile rheumatoid arthritis. J Pediatr 133:266-268, 1998.

90. Ansell BM: Prognosis in juvenile arthritis. Adv Exp Med Biol 455:27-33, 1999.

91. Guillaume S, Prieur AM, Coste J, et al: Long-term outcome and prognosis in oligoarticular-onset juvenile idiopathic arthritis. Arthritis Rheum 43:1858-1865, 2000.

92. Lomater C, Gerloni V, Gattinara M, et al: Systemic onset juvenile idiopathic arthritis: a retrospective study of 80 consecutive patients followed for 10 years. J Rheumatol 27:491-496, 2000.

93. Kanski JJ: Juvenile arthritis and uveitis. Surv Ophthalmol 34:253-267, 1990.

94. Sherry DD, Mellins ED, Wedgwood RJ: Decreasing severity of chronic uveitis in children with pauciarticular arthritis. Am J Dis Child 145:1026-1028, 1991.

95. Cabral DA, Petty RE. Malleson PN, et al: Visual prognosis in children with chronic anterior uveitis and arthritis. J Rheumatol 21:2370-2375, 1994.

96. Duffy CM, Duffy KN: Health assessment in the rheumatic diseases of childhood. Curr Opin Rheumatol 9:440-447, 1997.

97. Peterson LS, Mason T, Nelson AM, et al: Psychosocial outcomes and health status of adults who have had juvenile rheumatoid arthritis: A controlled, population-based study. Arthritis Rheum 40:2235-2240, 1997.

98. Aasland A, Flato B, Vandvik IH: Psychosocial outcome in juvenile chronic arthritis: a nine-year follow-up. Clin Exp Rheumatol 15:561-568, 1997.

97

Systemic Lupus Erythematosus, Juvenile Dermatomyositis, Scleroderma, and Vasculitis

JAMES T. CASSIDY

This chapter covers four of the major connective tissue diseases of children—systemic lupus erythematosus (SLE), juvenile dermatomyositis (JDM), scleroderma, and vasculitis—as well as their variants. Discussion is limited to aspects of these diseases important or unique to children,[1] avoiding repetition of data presented elsewhere in this text. Studies on the incidence and prevalence of these diseases are not as complete as are those for juvenile rheumatoid arthritis (JRA). However, data are available from a number of referral clinics in North America that provide reasonable estimates of the relative frequency of these disorders (Table 97–1).

Systemic Lupus Erythematosus

DEFINITION AND CLASSIFICATION

SLE is an episodic multisystem disorder characterized by persistent antinuclear antibody (ANA) seropositivity, widespread inflammation, and immune-complex deposition in key target organs. It is a prototype of autoimmune diseases in humans that results from altered immunologic reactivity and a genetic predisposition.

The 11 criteria developed by the American College of Rheumatology (ACR) for the classification of SLE are applicable to children.[2] The presence of four criteria has a sensitivity of 90 percent and a specificity of 98 percent. A skin biopsy is occasionally helpful diagnostically in difficult cases. Soluble immune complexes containing immunoglobulin G (IgG) and C3 are deposited in the vascular endothelium and along the dermoepidermal junction in both involved and uninvolved skin (determined by lupus band test).

EPIDEMIOLOGY

The incidence of SLE in children has been estimated at 0.6 per 100,000.[3] The disease is probably more frequent in Asians, Polynesians, Native Americans, and blacks in the United States than in whites. It is generally regarded as more serious in children than in adults.[4] Onset of SLE is unusual in a child younger than 4 years of age and becomes increasingly more common from age 9 through the teenage years. The female-to-male ratio in this age-group is approximately 4.3:1; in the younger age-group relatively more boys are affected. SLE accounts for 8 percent of patients referred to pediatric rheumatology clinics.

ETIOLOGY

The basic pathogenesis of SLE is complex, with abnormal immunologic homeostatic control of reactivity to nuclear and cytoplasmic antigens that may be antigen driven.[5] Defective antigen presentation, immune-complex clearance, and Fas-mediated apoptotic cell death may also be involved. An environmental trigger such as sun exposure, drug reaction, or a slow virus infection may precipitate onset of the disease in a genetically susceptible host. Female hormones (estrogen, prolactin) are associated with development of SLE in humans and the F_1 hybrid NZB/NZW mouse.

Genetics

Another connective tissue disease occurs in approximately 1 of 10 families in which a person is afflicted with SLE, an observation that emphasizes the heritability of this disorder, but susceptibility is polygenic. Lupus has been described in identical twins with a concordance rate of 24 percent, compared to 2 percent in dizygotic twins.[6] It is also associated with selective

TABLE 97–1 · CLINICAL MANIFESTATIONS OF SYSTEMIC LUPUS ERYTHEMATOSUS (SLE) IN CHILDHOOD

Manifestation	Occurrence (%)
Skin	15 to 80
Malar erythema	55
Photosensitivity	40
Raynaud's phenomenon	25
Alopecia	20
Kidneys	85 to 100
Hypertension	30
Renal failure	10
Musculoskeletal system	20 to 95
Arthritis	75
Myositis	20
Cardiopulmonary system	30 to 50
Pericarditis	45
Pleuritis	35
Pulmonary hemorrhage	5
Gastrointestinal tract	5 to 20
Oral or nasopharyngeal ulcerations	15
Mesenteric thrombosis	10
Sterile peritonitis	5
Hepatosplenomegaly	45
Nervous system	30 to 40
Central	30
Peripheral	5

immunoglobulin A (IgA) deficiency and inherited deficiencies of complement components such as C2, C1q, C1r, and C1 esterase inhibitor. The C4A null allele is strongly associated with SLE; human leukocyte antigen (HLA)-DR3 is increased in frequency in whites, and HLA-DR2 is increased in blacks.

Drug-Induced Lupus

Acute SLE is precipitated by a drug reaction in some children. Often-implicated medications include anticonvulsant drugs, hydralazine, D-penicillamine, isoniazid, penicillin, minocycline, and the sulfonamides. Most of these disorders are self-limited and abate on withdrawal of the offending agent. The most frequent clinical manifestations are fever, dermatitis, and pleuropericardial disease. Antibodies to double-stranded DNA (ds-DNA) are usually not present; however, ANA reactivity specific for histones is characteristic (but is also found in children with idiopathic SLE). The serum complement concentration typically remains normal, and central nervous system (CNS) disease and nephritis are rare.

Pathology

The basic inflammatory lesion of SLE is an immune-complex vasculitis with fibrinoid necrosis, inflammatory cell infiltrates, and sclerosis of collagen. Vascular deposition of immune complexes affects both arterioles and venules and is widespread throughout the parenchymal organs and in supporting tissues underlying the dermis and mucosal and serosal surfaces. In the kidney, immune complexes are deposited initially in the mesangium and then in subendothelial spaces beneath the glomerular basement membrane. Diffuse proliferative glomerulonephritis represents a more severe form of focal proliferative nephritis, and progression from one to the other has been identified in sequential biopsies. In membranous glomerulonephritis, which is uncommon in children, immune complexes form along the subepithelial surface of the glomerular basement membrane and obliterate the foot processes.

CLINICAL FEATURES

SLE is an extremely variable disease clinically and may develop in any degree of severity, ranging from an acute, rapidly fatal illness to insidious, chronic disability with repeated exacerbations (see Table 97–1). Constitutional symptoms such as fever, malaise, and weight loss are common. Mucocutaneous involvement and a malar erythematous rash in a butterfly pattern are characteristic of acute disease. Hepatomegaly and splenomegaly are common. Lupus hepatitis is an infrequent complication.

Arthritis affects most children with SLE and involves both large and small joints. Characteristics of this arthritis are its transient character and the fact that it may be migratory. Pain is often more severe than seems warranted by objective signs of inflammation. However, the arthritis of SLE does not often result in permanent deformity. SLE may evolve, however, from JRA. Raynaud's phenomenon with digital vasculitic ulcerations is a common finding and often present at onset. Ischemic necrosis of bone, particularly of the femoral heads and tibial plateaus, is frequent in long-standing disease, especially after treatment with glucocorticoids. Pericarditis is the most common manifestation of cardiac involvement, although asymptomatic abnormalities of myocardial perfusion may be more common than has generally been suspected.[7] Valvular insufficiency may occur; Libman-Sacks verrucous endocarditis is particularly characteristic and, by echocardiographic studies, is more common than was previously thought before that diagnostic modality became available. Abnormalities of pulmonary function and pleuritis along with a basilar pneumonitis are frequent. Pulmonary hemorrhage, mesenteric thrombosis, and acute pancreatitis are often life-threatening events.

The two systems whose involvement correlates most closely with survivorship are the central nervous system, (CNS), and the kidneys. Disease of the CNS and the peripheral nervous system is a common cause of morbidity in children. Severe recurrent headaches, seizures, chorea closely resembling that of acute rheumatic fever, and psychiatric manifestations ranging from disordered personality to frank psychosis occur. A labile, inappropriate affect is particularly characteristic in older children and adolescents. Intracranial hemorrhage and cerebral vein thrombosis may result from hypertension, thrombocytopenia, or the presence of antiphospholipid antibodies. Pseudotumor cerebri may be a complication of SLE or of glucocorticoid therapy. Magnetic resonance imaging (MRI) and single photon emission computed tomography (CT) aid in differentiating functional and potentially reversible lesions from organic defects. Systemic polyneuropathy, Guillain-Barré syndrome, transverse myelopathy, and involvement of the cranial nerves all have been reported. The so-called cytoid body of retinal vasculitis is often associated with CNS vasculitis or lupus crisis.

Lupus nephritis is present to some degree in virtually all children with SLE. Even severe nephritis may not be reflected initially in changes in the creatinine clearance, proteinuria, or an abnormal urinary sediment. Evidence of immune-complex disease, however, such as increased levels of anti–ds-DNA antibodies or hypocomplementemia, correlates with active nephritis in most children. It is generally agreed that prognostically important renal lesions are more common in young patients than in adults, and the prognosis of children with renal disease is more guarded. Clinically evident nephritis, if it is going to develop, usually declares itself during the first 2 years after onset.

Persistent leukopenia is particularly characteristic of SLE in general. Most children are leukopenic at onset with a predominance of neutrophils in the peripheral count. Often, leukocytosis does not develop to an appropriate degree even with septicemia. SLE may present as thrombocytopenic purpura with or without hemolytic anemia. Coombs' antibodies are often present in these children. Other causes of anemia besides systemic disease include posthemorrhagic conditions, septicemia, and gastrointestinal bleeding.

Antibodies found in children with SLE include those that are tissue specific (such as antiplatelet antibodies) that result in specific manifestations of the disease, such as thrombocytopenia, and with other antibodies acute hemolytic anemia and leukopenia. Antigen-antibody complex deposition leads to widespread vasculopathy and lupus nephritis. ANAs are a hallmark of the immunologic abnormalities of SLE and are present in nearly all children with the disease.[8] They generally occur in high titer in a homogeneous or peripheral immunofluorescence pattern on the indirect immunofluorescent test. The peripheral nuclear pattern is characteristic of the presence of anti–ds-DNA antibodies, which are associated with active disease, and especially with nephritis.

The lupus anticoagulant, a specificity of antiphospholipid antibodies, is directed against cardiolipin used in the serologic reaction for syphilis. A young person with a false-positive result on these tests for syphilis is at risk for development of SLE. An elevated partial thromboplastin time may signal the presence of this reactivity. Antiphospholipid antibodies also lead to recurrent thromboses (10% or less) and are associated with the development of neuropsychiatric lupus and chorea[9] (see Chapter 77). Antiribosomal P antibodies are also found in children with CNS disease and psychosis.[10,11] Rheumatoid factors (RFs) are often present in high titer. Cold agglutinins and cryoglobulins may also be present, resulting in peripheral anoxic phenomena and gangrene.

Both the classic and alternative complement pathways are activated in the immune-complex vasculitis of SLE.[12] A depressed whole hemolytic complement determination (CH50 assay) reflects the status of the total complement cascade; a low concentration of C3 or C4 is usually a reliable indicator of active disease. Dyslipoproteinemia is characteristic of active disease and also is a consequence of glucocorticoid therapy.[13]

DIFFERENTIAL DIAGNOSIS

A number of other diseases should be considered in the differential diagnosis of a child with suspected SLE. Among these are polyarticular or systemic-onset JRA, acute poststreptococcal glomerulonephritis, idiopathic hemolytic anemia, immune thrombocytopenic purpura, leukemia, allergic or contact dermatitis, an idiopathic seizure disorder, mononucleosis, acute rheumatic fever, septicemia, and infectious endocarditis. Sjögren's syndrome is a multisystem disorder that may be misdiagnosed as SLE, in particular because of the presence of high titers of multiple autoimmune antibodies (Ro/La). It is often insidious in onset and slowly progressive. Primary Sjögren's syndrome is very rare in children and may present as recurrent parotid and lacrimal swelling, dry mouth, and persistent keratoconjunctivitis.

EVALUATION AND MANAGEMENT

Because SLE is an extremely serious disease, most children with this disorder benefit from management by the same multidisciplinary medical team over the course of their illness. Long-term supportive care should include adequate nutrition, prompt treatment of infections, and control of hypertension if present. Unnecessary restraints on a child's general level of activity and psychosocial peer group interactions are undesirable. The prophylactic measures of avoiding unnecessary drug exposure, transfusion, and excessive sunlight should be emphasized. Appropriate clothing and sunscreens are prescribed to minimize exposures to ultraviolet radiation.

Nonsteroidal anti-inflammatory drugs (NSAIDs) are helpful in treating minor manifestations of SLE, such as arthralgia and myalgia. Hydroxychloroquine is used as an adjunctive medication to control dermatitis or to moderate glucocorticoid dosage[14] (see Chapter 96). Glucocorticoids are the mainstay of treatment. Prednisone is the preferred analog for oral administration. As low a dose as possible should be used to achieve the objectives of the treatment program. Initial therapy usually requires a split-dosage regimen. Low-dose therapy, defined as 0.5 mg/kg/day, is used to treat persistent fever, dermatitis, arthritis, or serositis. These manifestations are often suppressed promptly. A period of weeks is usually required for control of anemia and achievement of a serologic remission with suppression of anti–ds-DNA antibodies and return of serum complement levels toward normal. A low-dose program is often sufficient to control clinical disease in children with mesangial or focal glomerulonephritis. Treatment of children with active SLE is monitored by clinical course and by periodic assessment of anti–ds-DNA antibodies and serum complement levels. Exacerbation of the disease during steroid tapering may be signaled by a deterioration of the serologic indices and clinical measures of disease activity.

High-dose prednisone therapy, defined as 1 to 2 mg/kg/day in divided doses, is used for lupus crisis, CNS disease, acute hemolytic anemia, and the more severe forms of nephritis. Intravenous (IV) pulse therapy with methylprednisolone is advocated for acute exacerbations in a variety of protocols at a dose of 10 to 30 mg/kg. Although the approach to diagnosis and therapy of nephritis is a controversial area, the precise glucocorticoid regimen and the decision to add immunosuppressive drugs may need to be based on the degree and type of involvement of the kidneys. Renal biopsy is warranted in most children with significant SLE nephritis to establish the classification of type, activity, and chronicity of the disease.

In addition to glucocorticoids, immunosuppressive agents are necessary in some children.[15] Although azathioprine has been employed extensively and methotrexate (MTX) more recently,[16] data suggest that IV cyclophosphamide pulse therapy is preferable (500 to 750 mg/m[2] every 4 weeks for 6 months followed by maintenance therapy) in patients with severe nephritis.[17,18] Dialysis and kidney transplantation have been successfully used in end-stage renal disease.[19]

SUMMARY AND CONCLUSIONS

SLE is characterized by repeated exacerbations and remissions; active disease is often prolonged over many years. Prognosis for a specific child is unpredictable and generalizations about outcome are especially unreliable during the first 1 to 2 years. Later, a more realistic estimate can be discussed with the family, depending on the degree of systemic activity and the response of the disease to therapy.

Outcome is poorest in children with diffuse proliferative nephritis or with development of an organic brain syndrome; it is best in children with minimal or controlled systemic disease or mesangial nephritis or in those who have a prompt response, to steroid therapy. Morbidity is often underestimated.[20] Although the course of the disease and its severity are highly variable, prognosis has improved dramatically during the past 24 years.[21] Life table analysis in a study from Minnesota, 1982, indicated that survivorship (death, dialysis, or transplantation) in 21 children with diffuse proliferative glomerulonephritis was only 70 percent at 10 years.[22] In a more recent study, 2002, survival can be expected in 94 percent of children for at least 11 years.[23] Although nephritis and CNS disease have been leading causes of death, infection has replaced them in some series as the most common preterminal event. Functional asplenia may contribute by predisposing the child to an increased risk of septicemia. Accelerated atherosclerosis of the coronary arteries is a late complication and cause of death.

Neonatal Lupus Syndromes

Children of mothers who have active SLE, or are at risk to develop it, may present with lupus-like syndromes in the neonatal period related to transplacental passage of maternal IgG ANAs.[24] Neonatal lupus is classified into two types: 1) a transient syndrome and 2) complete congenital heart block.[25]

The transient neonatal lupus syndrome results from transplacental transport of maternal anti-Ro/La antibodies. In some infants, malar erythema develops in conjunction with discoid or annular lesions either immediately after birth or within the first few months of life (Fig. 97–1). In most babies, there is no associated systemic disease, and serologic abnormalities abate in the first few months of life with metabolic decay of maternal Ig. Thrombocytopenia may be present along with mild hemolytic anemia or leukopenia. Usually, this form of the syndrome requires no specific treatment. Occasionally, glucocorticoids are indicated for severe dermatologic disease or gastrointestinal bleeding. A rheumatic disease may develop in young adults who have had neonatal lupus.[26]

Complete congenital heart block, alone or associated with other cardiac defects, such as myocarditis, septal and endocardial cushion defects, and endomyocardial fibroelastosis, has been described as a distinct and permanent neonatal lupus syndrome.[25] Complete congenital heart block can be diagnosed in utero by fetal echocardiography. Extreme bradycardia results in fetal hydrops. The correct obstetric approach to the disorder is unclear but includes treating the mother with glucocorticoids (dexamethasone) and potentially plasma-

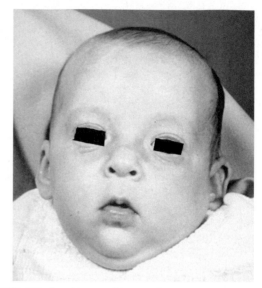

FIGURE 97–1 • Neonatal Lupus. Four-month-old girl with the erythematous rash of neonatal lupus across the bridge of the nose, lower eyelids, and superior forehead. This baby was born at 33 weeks of gestation with complete congenital heart block. Her mother had high titers of anti-Ro antibody.

pheresis. Neonatal death is approximately 15 percent and survivorship at 3 years is only 20 percent. Most of the remaining children will require a pacemaker.

Approximately one third of affected babies are born to mothers who have or are at risk for development of SLE or an associated autoimmune disease.[27,28] More than 90 percent of these mothers are HLA-DR3 positive. Anti-Ro (SSA) antibodies directed against a small cytoplasmic RNA protein complex,[25] and in most cases antibodies to the La (SSB) ribonucleoprotein complex, have been found in virtually every child and mother with this syndrome who have been studied.[29] The predominant anti-Ro specificity is for the 52-kD peptide. These antibodies result in absence or degeneration of the atrioventricular node, resulting in heart block during maturation of the fetal heart at approximately 16 to 18 weeks of age.

Juvenile Dermatomyositis

DEFINITION AND CRITERIA

JDM is a multisystem disease characterized by nonsuppurative inflammation of striated muscle, skin, and gastrointestinal tract.[30,31] It is characterized early in its course by an immune-complex vasculitis of varying severity and later by the development of calcinosis.

An acute onset of proximal muscle weakness accompanied by the characteristic dermatitis is pathognomonic for JDM. The 25 percent of children who do not have the classic rash almost invariably have an atypical rash that still suggests this diagnosis. Polymyositis—that is, inflammatory myositis without dermatitis—is a rare presentation in children. Serum "muscle" enzymes, especially creatine kinase and aldolase, are elevated in 98 percent of the children, and sequential determinations of these are important for diagnosis and in monitoring the effectiveness of the therapeutic program. Electromyography (EMG) is often not done in children because of difficulty obtaining cooperation during an otherwise painful procedure. Notable electromyographic changes are those of myopathy and denervation. Atrophy, fatty infiltration, or signal abnormalities indicative of active disease can also be demonstrated by MRI. A muscle biopsy is sometimes indicated in initial evaluation of a child for assessment of prognosis and to provide support for instituting long-term glucocorticoid therapy or immunosuppressive drugs. The muscle to undergo biopsy should be clinically involved but not atrophied. The best site is generally the deltoid or quadriceps.

Diagnostic histopathologic changes involve the striated muscles, skin, and gastrointestinal tract. The initial lesion is an acute patchy inflammatory lymphocytic infiltration (Fig. 97–2). Concomitant degeneration and regeneration of striated muscle fibers follow, resulting in a moderate variation in fiber size. Areas of focal necrosis are replaced during the healing phase by an interstitial proliferation of connective tissue and fat. An immune-complex necrotizing vasculitis occurs in arterioles, capillaries, and venules and is especially characteristic of this disorder in children. Diffuse linear and occasionally granular deposits of IgM, C3d, and fibrin are present in the areas of noninflammatory vasculopathy.

EPIDEMIOLOGY

JDM is a relatively uncommon rheumatic disease, accounting for approximately 6 percent of children with a major connective tissue disease in pediatric rheumatology clinics (see Table 96–1). Incidence in a study from the United Kingdom and Ireland was 0.19 per 100,000 (95% confidence limits 0.14 to 0.26).[32] The disease is more frequent in girls than in boys. Onset is especially common from the fourth to the tenth year of childhood.

ETIOLOGY

Although the etiology of JDM remains unknown, immune-complex vasculitis may be an important initiating or perpetuating event.[33] Igs and complement are deposited in the walls of small blood vessels in skeletal muscle. HLA-DQA1*0501 is increased in frequency in JDM in white children.[34] This specificity is also associated with an increase in the tumor necrosis factor-α (TNF-α)-308A allele.[35] JDM has occurred after infections, vaccinations, hypersensitivity reactions to drugs, and sunburn. Acute transient inflammatory myositis has been reported after viral and parasitic infections (e.g., coxsackievirus B, influenza, toxoplasmosis) in otherwise normal children. A fatal myositis has been described in children with agammaglobulinemia in association with echovirus infection. JDM has been reported in patients with selective IgA deficiency and C2 complement component deficiency.

CLINICAL FEATURES

Children with JDM present with proximal muscle weakness, dermatitis, fever, and constitutional symptoms such as fatigue, malaise, weight loss, and anorexia[30] (Table 97–2). The proximal limb girdle muscles of the lower extremities are affected initially, followed by the shoulder girdle and proximal arm muscles. Affected muscles are occasionally edematous and indurated. A child may also complain of muscle pain, tenderness, or stiffness, or

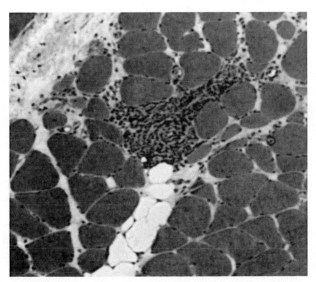

FIGURE 97–2 · Muscle Biopsy Specimen (H&E, ×100). In the center is a perivascular mononuclear cell inflammatory infiltrate with arterial thickening and prominent endothelial cells.

TABLE 97–2 · CLINICAL MANIFESTATIONS OF JUVENILE DERMATOMYOSITIS (JDM)

Manifestation	Occurrence (%)
Musculoskeletal system	100
Muscle weakness in:	
Proximal pelvic girdle	95
Proximal shoulder girdle	75
Neck flexors	60
Pharyngeal muscles	45
Distal muscles of the extremities	30
Facial and extraocular muscles	5
Arthritis	25
Skin	85 to 100
Periungual and articular rash (Gottron's papules)	80
Heliotrope rash of eyelids and periorbital edema	15
Malar rash	40
Photosensitivity	40
Ulcerations	25
Raynaud's phenomenon	15
Calcinosis	40
Gastrointestinal tract	10 to 60
Pharyngitis	40
Dysphagia	10
Hemorrhage	5
Lungs	15 to 80
Restrictive disease	80
Fibrosis	less than 1

stop walking or be unable to climb stairs or dress. An inability to get up off the floor without the classic Gower's maneuver or to get out of bed is common.

It has been proposed that the course of JDM in most children can be divided into four clinical phases[36]:

1. A prodromal period of weeks to months with non-specific symptoms
2. Progressive muscle weakness and dermatitis that lasts days to weeks
3. Persistent myositis and dermatitis of 1 to 2 years' duration
4. Recovery with residual muscle atrophy and contractures with or without calcinosis

Although muscle weakness may be impressive, deep-tendon reflexes are preserved. Weakness of the anterior neck flexors and back leads to an inability to hold the head upright or maintain a sitting posture. Facial and extraocular muscles are uncommonly involved. Ten percent of children develop pharyngeal, hypopharyngeal, or palatal muscle weakness. Dysphonia results along with dysphagia, which may also be related to esophageal hypomotility. These children are at risk for sudden aspiration, which can be fatal. Palatal speech and nasal regurgitation of liquids are early warning signs of potential respiratory compromise. Profound involvement of the thoracic and respiratory muscles is seen in a few children. Later in the disease, or in children with an especially acute onset, the distal muscles of the extremities may be affected. Rarely, there is generalized acute inflammation of the entire striated musculature, a type of onset that may be more characteristic of infantile onset.

Most children have the classic rash of JDM over the malar area, the upper eyelids with periorbital edema, and the dorsal surfaces of the knuckles (Fig. 97–3), elbows, and knees. The basic cutaneous lesion is an angiitis. At onset, indurative edema of the skin and subcutaneous tissues is often present. Later there is epidermal thinning and atrophy of the accessory structures with loss of hair and telangiectases. Vasculitic ulcers at the corners of the eyes, around the axillae, and in "stretch marks" may become a serious problem. Although a few patients have calcinosis at onset of the disease, development of calcification is more characteristic of the healing phase of the disease. Nail-fold capillary loop abnormalities are identifiable through the +40 lens of an ophthalmoscope in half of the children and have prognostic importance. The nail folds show simultaneous dilation of isolated loops, dropout of surrounding vessels, and an arborized cluster of capillary loops—distinctive features of JDM (Fig. 97–4).

Serum concentrations of the muscle enzymes—creatine kinase, aldolase, aspartate aminotransferase, and alanine aminotransferase—are elevated in active disease. The extent of the increase is variable, but levels can range from 20 to 40 times normal for creatine kinase or aspartate. Detection of MB bands on the creatine kinase isozyme pattern is usually evidence of regeneration of striated muscle and not of cardiac damage. Nonspecific tests of inflammation tend to correlate

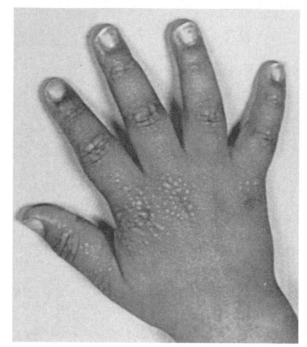

FIGURE 97–3 • Gottron's papules, present since the age of 18 months, in a 4-year-old girl with juvenile dermatomyositis (JDM). There is a remarkable development of raised hypopigmented papules on an erythematous base over the dorsum of the hand, with accentuation over the metacarpophalangeal, proximal interphalangeal, and distal phalangeal joints.

with the degree of clinical activity. Leukocytosis and anemia are uncommon at onset, except in children with associated gastrointestinal bleeding. The occurrence of RFs and ANAs is variable. Myositis-specific and myositis-associated antibodies have been described in

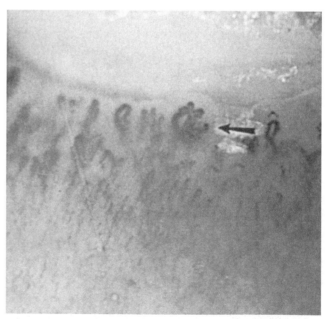

FIGURE 97–4 • Abnormal Nail-Fold Capillary Pattern (×100). The vessels are thickened and tortuous and show a peripheral pattern of arborization (*arrow*). There are clear areas of capillary dropout. (Courtesy of Dr. Jay Kenik.)

only a minority of children.[31,37] Half of the affected children have circulating immune complexes. The serum concentration of von Willebrand factor VIII antigen is elevated in active disease as evidence of vasculitis,[38] as is the serum neopterin concentration.

DIFFERENTIAL DIAGNOSIS

Considerations in the differential diagnosis include the other connective tissue diseases that present as multisystem illnesses. JDM presenting predominantly with arthritis may be confused with either JRA of acute systemic onset or SLE. Scleroderma poses unique diagnostic problems in that approximately 25 percent of children with this disorder have a primary myositis. Although early cutaneous abnormalities of scleroderma and JDM are quite different, the skin changes tend to merge in character later in the course of the two diseases.

In children with muscular dystrophy, there is a selective pattern of muscle weakness, insidious onset of progressive or remitting illness, and a positive family history. Dermatitis is absent. The serum creatine kinase concentration is elevated in first-degree relatives, especially in the mothers of children with X-linked disease. Congenital myopathies, myotonias, hypotonic syndromes, and the metabolic and endocrine myopathies, especially hypothyroidism, must also be considered. Paroxysmal myoglobulinuria and thyrotoxic myopathy may occasionally be encountered. Myasthenia gravis is rare in children.

Rhabdomyolysis may be a complication of an acute infection, trauma, or extreme muscular exertion. Onset is abrupt and is characterized by profound weakness, myoglobinuria, and occasionally oliguria and renal failure. Trichinosis and toxoplasmosis cause myositis of varying severity, and severe pustular acne may occasionally be associated with inflammatory disease of muscle. Influenza B, coxsackievirus B infection, poliomyelitis, and the Guillain-Barré syndrome are other diagnostic considerations.

EVALUATION AND MANAGEMENT

Clinical severity of the vasculitis is an important prognostic factor in the survival of children with JDM. The presence of a noninflammatory vasculopathy is associated with a poorer outcome.[39] Zonal loss of the capillary bed, areas of focal infarction of muscle, lymphocytic non-necrotizing vasculopathy, and a noninflammatory endarteropathy have been associated with progressive infarction of muscle and gastrointestinal tract and cutaneous ulcerations. Except for isolated vasculitis, smooth muscle is not affected. The heart is generally not involved in the primary pathologic process. A few children with cardiac disease have been described with focal myocardial fibrosis and contraction-band necrosis.

Introduction of glucocorticoids into the management of JDM has dramatically improved the prognostic outlook. General supportive care and a coordinated team approach are important and should include individualized rest and positioning. Muscle strengthening should be added to the exercise program only when clinical evidence of acute inflammation has subsided. During the convalescent phase, the physical therapy program is focused on normalizing function as much as possible and minimizing development of contractures secondary to muscle weakness or atrophy.

For initial treatment of acute disease, it is generally necessary to use 2 mg/kg/day of prednisone in four divided doses for at least the first month; then, if indicated by clinical response and a decrease in the serum muscle enzyme concentrations, a lower dose in the range of 1 mg/kg/day can be prescribed. Thereafter, the daily steroid dose is slowly tapered in amount and frequency of administration as determined by improvement in the clinical status of the child, degree of muscle weakness by repeated testing on a 0 to 5 scale, and level of the serum muscle enzymes. Satisfactory control is not achieved until enzyme levels have returned to normal or nearly normal levels and remain there during tapering of the steroid dose and an increase in the child's level of physical activity. Intravenous (IV) pulse steroid therapy is used for acute exacerbations and should be considered as initial treatment to minimize the daily steroid dose. Alternate-day steroid therapy may be useful late in the recovery phase. Addition of hydroxychloroquine aids in controlling the dermatitis and appears to be steroid sparing.

Acute complications such as cutaneous ulcerations and failure of the disease to respond to steroid management may be indications for the use of immunosuppressive agents. Regimens that include MTX, IV cyclophosphamide, cyclosporine, IV immunoglobulin (IVIg), plasmapheresis, and extracorporeal photochemotherapy have been used in resistant disease.[39-42] Many approaches to the therapy of calcinosis have been advocated, including surgery and the administration of colchicine, probenecid, aluminum salts, warfarin, and the bisdiphosphonates. None of these has met with uniform success in studies with adequate numbers of patients. Surgical excision of calcific tumors in areas of ulceration or pressure remains an option. Chronicity of the disease process and pathologic calcifications have been associated with presence of the TNF-α-308A allele.[35] Hypercalcemia has been described during resolution of the calcinosis.[43]

SUMMARY AND CONCLUSIONS

The basic inflammatory nature of JDM, its initial response to treatment, and the presence or absence of vasculitis or progressive involvement of other organ systems, such as the gastrointestinal tract and pulmonary system, are major factors that influence outcome. Durations of active myositis as short as 8 months have been reported: In up to 60 percent of children, the disease course lasts about 2 years and consists of only one or two exacerbations. The remaining 40 percent continue to have acute exacerbations and remissions; a disease that is more typical of systemic vasculitis eventually develops in a few. In a small number of children late in the course, sclerodactyly and cutaneous atrophy may appear, or areas of lipoatrophy and insulin resistance may develop. Acanthosis nigricans or a recurrence of arthritis may occur. Even years after onset, some children have persistent elevations of the serum muscle enzymes, especially creatine kinase, and characteristic histopathologic features of the disease may be noted on rebiopsy.

The course of the dermatitis often does not follow that of the myositis. Many clinicians are convinced that children who have a generalized rash and cutaneous ulcerations have the worst prognoses.[39] The characteristic nail-fold loop abnormalities of thickening and arborization along with a noninflammatory vasculopathy correlate prognostically with more severe disease. During the healing phase of the myositis, calcium salts (hydroxyapatite [HA] or fluorapatite) are deposited in skin and subcutaneous tissues, around the joints, and within interfascial planes of the muscles in up to half of the children. Later, calcification may be slowly resorbed spontaneously (Figs. 97–5 and 97–6). It has been proposed that early use of IV pulse steroid therapy may minimize later development of calcinosis.[31]

Despite these findings, the average child progressively improves to achieve functional recovery[44] (Table 97–3). Most children should be able to function independently as adults, although some have residual atrophy of skin or muscle groups. Difficulties during pregnancy have been described in women who have had JDM. In the preglucocorticoid era, JDM was associated with a mortality rate that approached 50 percent. Surviving children often had devastating residual problems, including contractures, muscle atrophy, and widespread calcinosis. At present, the long-term survival rate approaches 90 percent,

and functional outcome has been greatly improved. The greatest risk of death is within the first 2 years after onset. Outcome is best in children who are seen early after onset and receive vigorous treatment. An acute gastrointestinal complication or respiratory insufficiency leading to hypoxia with or without aspiration is a serious, often preterminal event.

Scleroderma

The sclerodermas are systemic or localized connective tissue diseases of unknown etiology. Often, their development goes unrecognized initially because these disorders are so rare. A classification is presented in Table 97–4. Systemic disease is divided into diffuse cutaneous scleroderma and limited cutaneous scleroderma. The localized forms of the disease, such as morphea or linear scleroderma,[45] often are regarded

TABLE 97–3 • OUTCOME FOR CHILDREN WITH JUVENILE DERMATOMYOSITIS (JDM)

Outcome	Occurrence (%)
Complete functional recovery	65
Minimal disease (atrophy or contracture)	25
Calcinosis	20 to 40
Significant disability or dependence	5
Death	7

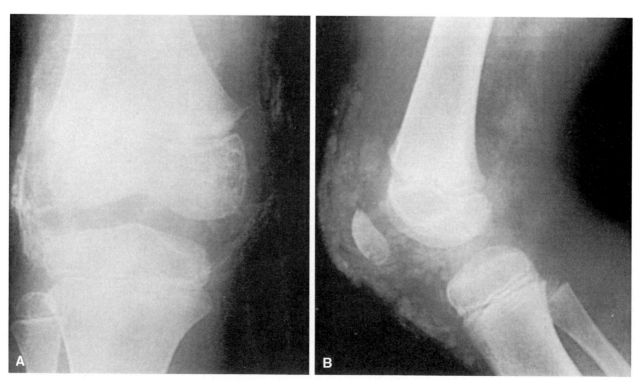

FIGURE 97–5 • Massive Deposits of Calcium Salts in the Subcutaneous Tissue and Fascia About the Right Knee in an 11-Year-Old Boy. Calcinosis followed the acute phase of juvenile dermatomyositis (JDM) by 3 years. A, Anteroposterior view. B, lateral view.

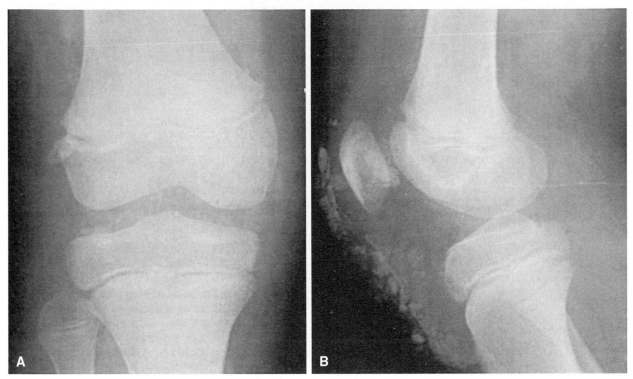

FIGURE 97-6 · Same Patient as in Figure 97-5. Two years later, much of the calcification has been resorbed spontaneously. *A*, Anteroposterior view. *B*, lateral view.

TABLE 97-4 · CLASSIFICATION OF SCLERODERMA

Systemic disease
  Scleroderma
    Diffuse
    Limited
  Overlap syndromes
    Sclerodermatomyositis or other connective tissue diseases
    Mixed connective tissue disease
Localized disease
  Morphea
  Generalized morphea
  Linear scleroderma
  Eosinophilic fasciitis

as more dermatologic than rheumatic in nature. Some rheumatologists also include disorders such as mixed connective tissue disease and eosinophilic fasciitis in this category.

DIFFUSE CUTANEOUS SYSTEMIC SCLERODERMA

The early clinical presentation of diffuse cutaneous systemic scleroderma (DCSS) is often subtle. Although not validated in children, the ACR classification criteria seem applicable to these age-groups.[46,47]

Epidemiology

DCSS is very rare and accounts for 1 percent or less of major connective tissue disorders in pediatric rheumatology clinics[48] (see Table 96–1). Girls are affected more frequently than boys by a ratio of 3:1, except in the youngest age-group.[1] There is no peak age at onset during childhood and no racial predilection.

Etiology

Pathogenesis of DCSS is unknown. There is an increased number of high collagen-producing fibroblasts in the skin. Endothelial perturbation is present with accelerated endothelial cell apoptosis and anti–endothelial cell antibodies. The similarities of scleroderma to graft-versus-host disease in bone marrow transplant recipients has led to investigation of the hypothesis that prolonged persistence of fetal progenitor cells and microchimerism may be involved in pathogenesis.[49,50]

Scleroderma-like disease is seen in children with insulin-dependent (type 1) diabetes mellitus, phenylketonuria, and progeria and has developed following exposure to vinyl chloride, bleomycin, and pentazocine. It occurred in an epidemic in Spain related to a toxin in rapeseed oil.

An angiitis is regarded as the basic initial lesion in DCSS. The skin and gastrointestinal tract are involved early, along with the lungs, heart, and kidneys. Perivascular infiltrates of mononuclear cells are often present and have been identified in some studies to consist predominantly of T lymphocytes. Arterioles eventually undergo hyalinization and fibrosis (Fig. 97–7). In the skin, there is thinning of the epidermis, loss of the rete pegs, and atrophy of the dermal appendages. In the deeper layers, homogenization of the collagen fibers with loss of structural detail, an increased density and thickness of collagen deposition, and a predominance of embryonal fibers are characteristic.

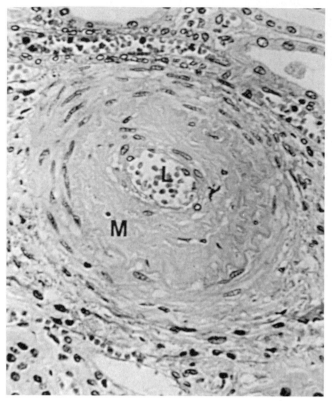

FIGURE 97–7 · Renal Arteriole from a Patient Who Died of Scleroderma and Hypertensive Crisis. There is virtual obliteration of the vessel lumen (L) by intimal proliferation and medial mucoid hyperplasia (M).

Clinical Features

Clinical manifestations of DCSS are summarized in Table 97–5. The onset is often marked by the appearance of Raynaud's phenomenon; tightening, thinning,

and atrophy of the skin of the hands and face; or the appearance of cutaneous telangiectases about the face, upper trunk, and hands. There is often a diagnostic delay of years because of the subtle, insidious nature of the presentation in this disease.

Raynaud's phenomenon occurs in most children with DCSS and may antedate the onset of cutaneous abnormalities. It is characterized by obstructive digital arterial disease and sympathetic hyperactivity. Vascular spasm within viscera such as the esophagus may accompany the peripheral vasoconstriction. Digital gangrene may supervene with the development of small, atrophic pits on the fingertips.

Characteristic abnormalities of the nail-fold capillaries have been identified in children with DCSS.[51] There is a reduction in the number of vessels and a marked tortuosity and "puddling" of the remaining capillaries. Scattered white fibrotic areas are prominent. Skin tightening is virtually universal and tends to become more generalized with time. Hypopigmentation and hyperpigmentation are characteristic, as are subcutaneous calcification and deposition of calcium salts around joints (Fig. 97–8). Erythema and ulcerations may develop over the elbows, knees, and malleoli.

Many children have contractures about joints and a few have objective evidence of arthritis. A crepitant tenosynovitis develops in others. Muscle pain and tenderness are present in approximately 25 percent of patients. Elevation of the serum muscle enzymes tends to be mild to moderate and not as striking as in JDM. Dyspnea on exertion may be related to skin tightness, muscle weakness, or interstitial pulmonary fibrosis. Myocarditis and cardiomyopathy also lead to dyspnea,

TABLE 97–5 • CLINICAL MANIFESTATIONS OF SYSTEMIC SCLERODERMA IN CHILDHOOD

Manifestation	Occurrence (%)
Skin	100
Raynaud's phenomenon	75
Digital ulcerations	60
Telangiectases	30
Subcutaneous calcification	25
Pigmentary changes	20
Gastrointestinal tract	75 to 100
Abnormal esophageal motility	75
Dysphagia	20
Colonic sacculations	20
Duodenal dilatation	5
Lungs	75 to 100
Dyspnea	20
Abnormal diffusion	75
Decreased vital capacity	70
Musculoskeletal system	25 to 75
Joint contractures	75
Resorption of digital tufts	75
Muscle weakness and pain	40
Heart	15 to 30
Electrocardiographic abnormalities and arrhythmias	30
Cardiomegaly	15
Congestive failure	15

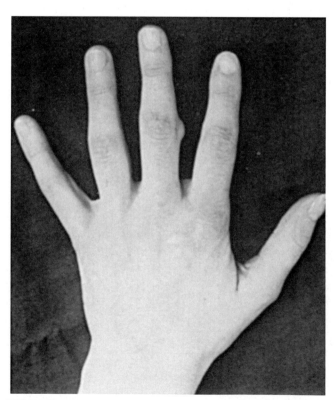

FIGURE 97–8 · Subcutaneous nodule of periarticular calcification in a teenage girl with acrosclerosis.

arrhythmia, and signs of heart failure. Although widespread gastrointestinal involvement occurs in most children, symptomatic disease is often confined to the esophagus with complaints of dysphagia or reflux esophagitis. Esophageal ulceration and constriction may develop. Malabsorption may become severe, leading to a fatal outcome.

High-titer ANAs with speckled patterns are found in most children. Distinct antigenic specificity may be present with anticentromere in limited disease, anti–Scl 70 (topoisomerase 1) in diffuse disease, or ANAs. Pulmonary diffusion testing and spirometry are sensitive measures of involvement of the respiratory tract and document a decrease in the timed vital capacity and forced expiratory flow, an early decrease in diffusion, and an increase in functional residual volume. High-resolution CT may confirm the presence of pulmonary disease even with a normal chest radiograph.

Even in early asymptomatic disease, upper gastrointestinal films often document disordered peristalsis of the distal esophagus. Esophageal motility studies by manometry, however, are more sensitive indicators of functional abnormalities, and a 24-hour pH probe study for potential reflux is helpful. Dilation of the second portion of the duodenum and pseudodiverticula of the colon may also be present. Acro-osteolysis of the digits accompanied by focal areas of soft tissue calcification may be present on radiographs of the hands (Fig. 97–9).

Plethysmography confirms abnormal vascular responses in affected digits in children with Raynaud's phenomenon and documents both the obstructive vascular disease and overactivity of the sympathetic nervous system.

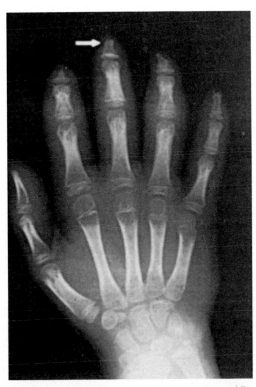

FIGURE 97–9 · Hand of a Girl with Complaints of Raynaud's Phenomenon for 2 Years. Arrow points to early resorption of the tuft of a distal phalanx (acro-osteolysis).

Differential Diagnosis

Considerations in differential diagnosis include JDM, SLE, and less frequently JRA. Patients with limited disease may have the features of the previously designated CREST syndrome (*c*alcinosis, *R*aynaud's phenomenon, *e*sophageal dysmotility, *s*clerodactyly, and *t*elangiectases), which is now referred to as limited cutaneous systemic scleroderma. Other overlap syndromes, mixed connective tissue disease, and eosinophilic fasciitis should also be considered.

Evaluation and Management

No uniformly effective therapy is available for DCSS.[1] NSAIDs may relieve some of the musculoskeletal symptoms. Vigorous physical therapy is important in most patients to prevent or minimize joint contractures. D-Penicillamine or colchicine may be useful in management of the cutaneous manifestations if prescribed early. MTX has been used for arthralgias.[52] Angiotensin-converting enzyme (ACE) inhibitors are effective in treatment of the hypertension and may have some beneficial effect on abnormalities of the skin and subcutaneous tissues.[53] Glucocorticoid drugs are considered to be contraindicated in most children, because these agents may exacerbate small blood vessel disease and renal involvement with hypertension. Malignant hypertension demands urgent lowering of the blood pressure to normal and merits expert intensive care.

Raynaud's phenomenon is best managed with calcium channel blockers such as nifedipine or blocking agents such as phenoxybenzamine or prazosin. Prostacyclin analogues are being evaluated for the treatment of severe vaso-occlusive disease. Biofeedback training has been advocated for the management of less threatening vasospasm. Children with Raynaud's phenomenon must also dress appropriately for the season and avoid cold liquids and objects that exacerbate peripheral arteriolar constriction.

Summary and Conclusions

The prognosis for pediatric patients with DCSS is poor, especially for those with diffuse disease. Death is often related to cardiopulmonary failure or gastrointestinal complications, including severe inanition. Cardiac arrhythmias may develop during the course of the disease secondary to myocardial fibrosis, and congestive heart failure is often a terminal event. Pulmonary interstitial disease and vascular lesions are probably universal. Renal failure or acute hypertensive encephalopathy supervenes as a potentially fatal outcome in a few children; at least in the adult literature, these processes seem more likely to occur early in the course of the disease. A child may live decades after onset of systemic scleroderma, however; therefore, an optimistic but realistic attitude should prevail in discussions with parents. Patients with limited disease (CREST syndrome), were originally thought to have a more favorable prognosis, but evidence for this judgment is not present in studies of children because of the rarity of this diagnosis.

LOCALIZED SCLERODERMAS

The localized sclerodermas are three times as common as systemic disease in children and adolescents (accounting for 3% or less of referrals), and linear scleroderma is approximately twice as frequent as morphea, which has been estimated to have an incidence of 2.7 per 100,000 children.[45,54] Linear scleroderma develops primarily in the first two decades of life. Laboratory abnormalities are few, with the exception of ANAs in about half of the children.[55] Antibodies to centromere or Scl 70 are generally not present in the localized syndromes. In these disorders, fibrosis of the connective tissues is limited to the dermis, subdermis, and superficial striated muscle. Morphea can be subdivided into five types: 1) single or multiple plaques, 2) smaller lesions in a more generalized distribution (guttate morphea), 3) bullous, 4) linear, and 5) deep.[56] All of these subtypes demonstrate homogenization of collagen bundles. In early disease, acute inflammatory erythema and edema are present in one or more circumscribed lesions, followed later by hypopigmentation and induration surrounded by areas of hyperpigmentation (Fig. 97–10). Lesions may be located anywhere on the trunk or extremities. The patches may coalesce or enlarge centrifugally to involve larger areas of the body. Paresthesia or pain may be present over these lesions.

Linear scleroderma is characterized by the presence of one or more areas of linear involvement of the skin of the head, trunk, or extremities. Underlying bone is often affected with resultant growth abnormalities or joint contractures. Because linear lesions of the face or scalp may have the appearance of dueling scars, the term *en coup de sabre* has been used. Linear scleroderma often affects only one side of the body, producing hemiatrophy of involved areas. Indeed, it is this lack of normal development, such as in hemifacial atrophy and failure of an extremity to grow in proportion to its opposite member, that causes the most severe disabili-

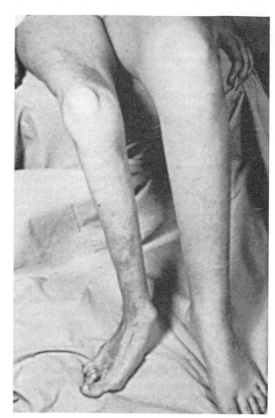

FIGURE 97–11 • Linear scleroderma, affecting the right leg of a 14-year-old girl, began at the age of 6 years and resulted in severe atrophy and shortening of the extremity.

ties (Fig. 97–11). Linear scleroderma is also associated with syndromes of progressive facial hemiatrophy (Parry-Romberg syndrome) or uveitis.[57,58]

D-Penicillamine may be effective if used early in the more generalized form of morphea. Hydroxychloroquine has been recommended by some experts. Local emollients and steroid ointments may result in cutaneous improvement. Localized scleroderma may regress spontaneously without treatment, or fibrosis of the involved skin and subcutaneous tissues may progress to produce "hide binding" and marked contractures of an extremity. Active disease is often characterized by exacerbations and remissions occurring over many months to a few years. Prognosis is generally excellent in the absence of systemic involvement. Occasionally, visceral disease or a seizure disorder develops late in the course of linear scleroderma. In a few children, the disease may evolve into an overlap syndrome with another connective tissue disease, such as SLE.

EOSINOPHILIC FASCIITIS

Controversy continues over whether eosinophilic fasciitis is a distinct clinicopathologic entity or an unusual variant of scleroderma.[59] Eosinophilic fasciitis is also associated with morphea in some children.[60] The primary disorder has been exceptionally rare in the pediatric population. Affected children present with marked induration of cutaneous and subcutaneous tissues of the upper or lower extremities and occasionally the trunk or face. Onset of the disease may be preceded

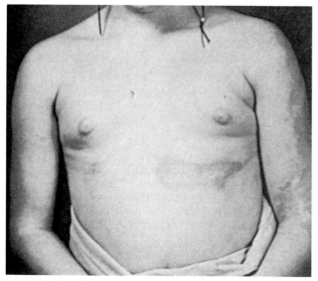

FIGURE 97–10 • Lesions of morphea with central hypopigmentation and active borders on the thorax of a young girl. Another extensive lesion is present on the outer left arm.

by unusual physical exertion. Raynaud's phenomenon, nail-fold capillary abnormalities, and visceral disease are absent. Diagnosis is confirmed by a full-thickness biopsy of skin, fascia, and muscle. Inflammation is present in all layers, but the most characteristic features are 1) thickened fascia with infiltration of histiocytes and often eosinophils and 2) a prominent perivascular infiltrate of lymphocytes and plasma cells. IgG, IgM, and C3 may be deposited in areas of inflammation. Associated laboratory findings include hypergammaglobulinemia and a remarkable peripheral eosinophilia of 40 to 60 percent. Eosinophilic fasciitis should be differentiated from the eosinophilia-myalgia syndrome.

As originally reported, eosinophilic fasciitis was self limited with spontaneous resolution after months to years. There was often marked relief with the administration of low-dose glucocorticoids. Occasionally, a more severe form of the disease with hematologic abnormalities evolved. These complications may be more common with childhood-onset disease.

MIXED CONNECTIVE TISSUE DISEASE

Mixed (undifferentiated) connective tissue disease (MCTD) was initially reported as a disorder associated with a favorable prognosis and an excellent initial response to relatively low-dose glucocorticoid therapy. It had a frequency of 0.3 percent in the U.S. Pediatric Rheumatology Data Base. Children present with arthritis, myositis, and cutaneous disease characteristic of scleroderma, SLE, or JDM. Progression to a more scleroderma-like disease has occurred, with sclerodactyly and gastrointestinal involvement, or an SLE-like disease may evolve.[61-63] Nephritis may be more frequent and more severe in children than in adults. Children often have less pulmonary disease (hypertension) and more hematologic complications (thrombocytopenia) than adults. ANAs are present in very high titers, often in a speckled pattern, to an extractable nuclear antigen (ENA) and ribonucleoprotein (RNP). Epitope specificity is to U_1RNP and the associated 70-kD A and C polypeptides, and in some instances to U_1RNA.[64] The predominant HLA associations in these patients are with DR2 and DR4. Other ANAs delineate a subset of children with an overlap syndrome who have the immune-complex characteristics of SLE. Antibodies to ds-DNA and to the Sm nuclear antigen are present in this latter group.

▪ Vasculitis

Inflammatory vasculitis is a prominent component of virtually all of the systemic connective tissue diseases.[65,66] Classification of idiopathic vasculitis is somewhat unsatisfactory but can be based on the size of the vessels that are predominantly involved, the type of visceral involvement, and whether the predominant histopathologic feature is vessel wall necrosis or a granulomatous response. All forms of vasculitis, except for Henoch-Schönlein purpura and Kawasaki's disease, are rare in children (see Table 97-1). A major study of classification criteria for the vasculitic diseases (predominantly in adults) has been published by a committee of the ACR[67] with modification by a consensus conference.[68]

NECROTIZING VASCULITIS OF MEDIUM AND SMALL ARTERIES

Definition

Medium-sized muscular arteries are involved in necrotizing vasculitis, and the predominant histopathologic change is fibrinoid necrosis of the entire thickness of the vessel wall.[66,69] Lesions tend to be segmental with a predilection for bifurcations of the vessels. Biopsy specimens usually show vasculitis in all stages of development from acute to chronic.

Polyarteritis Nodosa

The classic form of polyarteritis nodosa (PAN) was initially described more than a century ago,[70] and reports of small numbers of cases have periodically appeared in the pediatric literature. The classic disease remains rare and accounts for only 0.5 percent of referrals to pediatric rheumatology clinics. The course and progression of this disease are highly variable, and multisystem involvement leads to confusion with numerous other disorders. Early diagnosis and correct classification are often difficult. Age-specific criteria based on a study of 31 Turkish children have been proposed.[71]

Clinical Features

The onset of PAN is frequently insidious, and constitutional symptoms of fever and weight loss are often the presenting complaints. Disease of the renal, gastrointestinal, and cardiac systems is prominent, along with involvement of both the central and peripheral nervous systems (Table 97–6). The initial clinical diagnosis may be renovascular hypertension or a surgical abdomen. Severe sensorimotor peripheral neuropathy—so-called mononeuritis multiplex—may be observed. Cutaneous lesions are frequent and include purpura, peripheral gangrene, and nodular vasculitis (Fig. 97–12).

The degree and extent of multisystem involvement are often reflected in anemia, leukocytosis, marked elevation of the erythrocyte sedimentation rate (ESR), urinary sediment changes, and abnormalities in serum Ig

TABLE 97–6 · CLINICAL MANIFESTATIONS OF POLYARTERITIS NODOSA (PAN) IN CHILDHOOD

Manifestation	Occurrence (%)
Hypertension	80
Gastrointestinal tract	70
Musculoskeletal system	75
Skin	70
Nervous system	45
Central nervous system	40
Peripheral neuropathy	10
Heart	20
Kidneys	25
Lungs	10

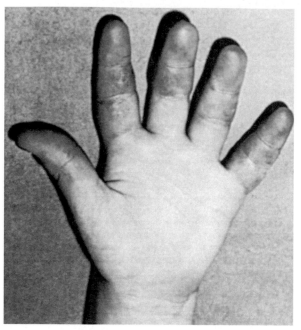

FIGURE 97–12 · Marked Digital Cyanosis and Swelling Were Present in a Young Boy with Polyarteritis Nodosa (PAN). The digital anoxia was accompanied by chronic pain that was exacerbated during acute vasospastic episodes.

concentrations. RF and ANA seropositivity are unusual. Levels of von Willebrand factor VIII antigen and β-thromboglobulin are associated with activity of the vascular disease. Immune complexes may be present. A few children (less than 5 percent) demonstrate seropositivity for hepatitis B– or C–associated antigens. A firm diagnosis depends on confirmation by biopsy of an involved, accessible site (skin, muscle, nerve) or an angio-gram that demonstrates aneurysms in the celiac or renal vasculature.[69]

Management

Glucocorticoid therapy is the mainstay of treatment. Suppressive amounts of prednisone are indicated in the range of 1 to 2 mg/kg/day in divided doses. The aggressiveness of the therapeutic program must be monitored according to the extent of cardiac and renal involvement and the presence of hypertension. A child may not respond adequately to the use of oral prednisone alone or to IV steroid pulse therapy. Extensive systemic involvement, particularly of the abdominal vasculature with aneurysms and thrombosis, is generally accepted as an indication for the use of intermittent IV pulse therapy with cyclophosphamide in conjunction with glucocorticoids.

Summary

PAN is characterized by a chronic relapsing course of many years' duration with eventual remission possible in some children.[72] Mortality has varied widely from study to study. Death is most commonly secondary to renal failure, myocardial infarction, or hypertensive encephalopathy.

Kawasaki's Disease

Definition and Criteria

An acute febrile illness associated with systemic vasculitis that primarily affects infants and young children was initially reported in 1967 by Kawasaki in Japan.[73] The first descriptions in the English literature appeared in 1974 under the designation "mucocutaneous lymph node syndrome." Previously, a number of very young infants with a febrile illness that lasted for a few weeks to months were described with a syndrome referred to as "infantile polyarteritis nodosa," which probably represented undiagnosed Kawasaki's disease. Clinical criteria were established by Japanese investigators in 1974 to aid in the diagnosis of Kawasaki's disease. The revised criteria are listed in Table 97–7.

Epidemiology

Kawasaki's disease has occurred sporadically and in mini epidemics in the United States.[74] An incidence of 6 to 7.6 per 100,000 children younger than 5 years of age has been reported for this country.[75,76] The disease accounts for approximately 3 percent of referrals to U.S. pediatric rheumatology clinics. In Japan, an incidence of 90 per 100,000 children has been recorded.[77] The disease is distinctly more common among Japanese people. In the United States, the risk of development of Kawasaki's disease for children of Japanese ancestry is 17 times that for white children. Within North America, a seasonal variation is often present, with most cases occurring in the spring. The mean age at onset is around 1.5 years, and the male-to-female ratio is 1.5:1. Not only is Kawasaki's disease more common in very young boys, the single most important complication, coronary aneurysms, is most frequent in these children. Furthermore, this disease rarely occurs after the age of 11 years. The occurrence of Kawasaki's disease in

TABLE 97–7 · CRITERIA FOR A DIAGNOSIS OF KAWASAKI'S DISEASE

Criterion*	Occurrence (%)
1. Fever lasting 5 days or more	100
2. Changes of lips and oral cavity	90
a. Dry, red, vertically fissured lips	
b. Strawberry tongue	
c. Diffuse erythema of mucous membranes	
3. Bilateral, nonsuppurative, bulbar conjunctivitis	85
4. Polymorphous rash (primarily on trunk)	80
5. Changes of peripheral extremities	70
a. Erythema of palms and soles	
b. Indurative edema of hands and feet	
c. Desquamation from digital tips	
6. Acute nonpurulent enlargement of cervical Clymph node to more than 1.5 cm in diameter	70

*Five criteria are required for diagnosis or four criteria plus coronary aneurysms on echocardiography. For criteria 2 and 5, any one of the three findings will suffice.

Modified from Sakaguchi M, Taka A, Endo M, et al: On the mucocutaneous lymph node syndrome or Kawasaki disease. *In* Yu PN, Goodwin JF (eds): Progress in Cardiology 13. Philadelphia, Lea & Febiger, 1985, p 97.

adults has been problematic: Patients who have been reported may represent this disease or another similar disorder, such as toxic shock syndrome or severe scarlet fever.

Etiology

The epidemiology of Kawasaki's disease suggests an infectious vector that is currently unidentified; however, secondary cases in a home are unusual. Many etiologic factors have been suggested but none proved. A relationship to heat-shock proteins (HSPs), mycobacterial antigens, staphylococcal toxins, or EB virus has been postulated. A recent study demonstrated IgA-secreting plasma cells in the vasculature of children who died with Kawasaki's disease.[78] Numerous immunologic abnormalities have been reported.[79-81] Kawasaki's disease probably represents a generalized stimulation of the inflammatory response, with increased production of cytokines resulting in cytokine-mediated endothelial damage. The extreme thrombocytosis that is observed (550,000 to 1,000,000/mm³) may contribute to thrombus formation on a damaged vascular endothelium. Factor VIII–related antigen concentrations are elevated in children with active vasculitis. There is no simple relation to antigens of the major histocompatibility complex (MHC) in North American white children. A similar disease can be induced in mice by intraperitoneal injection of *Lactobacillus casei*.[82]

Clinical Features

The usual monocyclic course of Kawasaki's disease has been divided into three phases that aid in diagnosis and approach to treatment.[74] The acute febrile onset of the disease has already been described. The subacute period begins with return of the temperature to normal and elevation of the platelet count. The convalescent phase follows with a return of the platelet count to normal. Recurrences are unusual.[21,83] In rare instances, systemic involvement continues in a pattern indistinguishable from that of PAN.

Fever is universal at onset and is usually sustained and remittent. Temperatures of 40° C are common and may be higher. The febrile phase lasts 5 to 25 days with a mean of about 10 days. Young children may present with a febrile seizure, although other causes for CNS involvement must be carefully excluded. Cerebrospinal fluid (CSF) protein may be elevated and pleocytosis is common. Extreme irritability is also common.

Mucocutaneous changes are prominent at onset. Nonsuppurative conjunctival injection may persist for several weeks. Erythema of the lips, with cracking, peeling, and bleeding, is present in most children. Pharyngeal erythema and a strawberry tongue often accompany these changes. A polymorphous rash develops in most children and represents a small blood vessel vasculitis and perivasculitis of the dermis and subcutaneous tissues. This rash accompanies the fever throughout the acute phase of the disease and then gradually fades. Pruritus is frequently present; vesiculation and purpura do not occur. Painful ery-thema and edema of the hands, fingers, feet, and toes occur within a few days after onset, and the child may refuse to walk. During recovery, desquamation of the hands and feet occurs, with peeling of the skin beginning underneath the tips of the nails. This feature is most commonly seen during the third week after onset and persists for 1 to 2 weeks. Desquamation and indurative edema can also occur elsewhere, including the perineal area early in the course (a valuable diagnostic clue). Beau's lines of the nails develop 1 to 2 months after onset of Kawasaki's disease.

Although lymphadenopathy occurs in about half the children, it is often not prominent and resolves rapidly toward the end of the febrile period. Involvement of the cervical nodes is common and may be unilateral; a sentinel cervical node 1 to 2 cm in diameter is the most characteristic physical finding. Involvement of almost any system can occur in Kawasaki's disease. Relatively common at presentation and during the initial course are pneumonitis, otitis, meningitis, photophobia with uveitis, diarrhea, meatitis and sterile pyuria, and arthritis or arthralgia. Relatively uncommon clinical findings are pleural effusions, abdominal colic, hydrops of the gallbladder, jaundice, and tonsillar exudate. The kidneys are not involved in Kawasaki's disease.

The most serious manifestations are myocarditis and coronary vasculitis. It is assumed that a panmyocarditis is universal during the acute febrile phase of the disease. In a variable number of children, the disease progresses to development of coronary vasculitis with vessel wall necrosis, aneurysm formation, or thrombosis. Coronary artery aneurysms are often present at onset of the disease or appear as early as the second week of the illness. These aneurysms reach their peak development during the subacute period, are usually multiple, and are found in approximately 20 percent of children with Kawasaki's disease in the United States. In children with the risk factors for coronary artery aneurysms (i.e., male age at onset 18 months or younger, Japanese ancestry, and an acute toxic febrile course with early clinical myocarditis), the frequency increases to more than 50 percent. Aneurysms also occur in arteries other than the coronary arteries, such as the brachial, subclavian, and axillary vessels.

The acute-phase indices are elevated early in the course of Kawasaki's disease. Abnormalities of the transaminase enzymes and sterile pyuria may be present. Two-dimensional echocardiography is the most sensitive technique for delineating proximal coronary vasculitis and aneurysms (Fig. 97–13). This study should be performed immediately in a febrile child in whom Kawasaki's disease is suspected. Echocardiography should be repeated during the course of Kawasaki's disease—for example, at 1 week, 6 weeks, and 3 months—with the timing and frequency dependent on characteristics of the course and whether aneurysms were initially detected. A committee of the American Heart Association has issued general recommendations based upon severity of the disease.[84] Angiography in selected children may demonstrate multiple lesions of the proximal or peripheral cardiac vessels. Abnormal lipoprotein patterns have been described.[85]

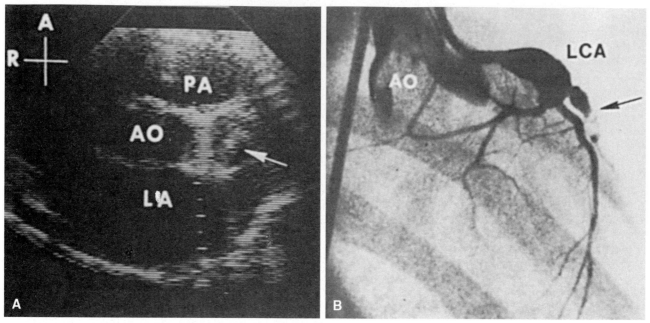

FIGURE 97–13 · *A*, Echocardiographic demonstration of an aneurysm of the left coronary artery *(arrow)* in a young boy with Kawasaki's disease. *B*, Angiogram of this giant aneurysm *(arrow)*. AO, aorta; LA, left atrium, LCA, left coronary artery; PA, pulmonary artery.

Evaluation and Management

The current approach to treatment is divided into two parts: 1) initial administration of aspirin in antiinflammatory doses, and then as an antiplatelet agent, and 2) the use of IVIg.[86] In the presence of developing, progressive, or unstable cardiac disease, close observation of the child in the hospital with cardiac monitoring is extremely important. Only by detecting the initial signs of cardiac decompensation or arrhythmia can appropriate emergency measures be taken to save the life of a severely affected child. High-dose aspirin therapy (e.g., 100 mg/kg/day in divided doses) is traditionally instituted during the acute phase of the illness, although recently this practice has been questioned.[87] With onset of the subacute period (resolution of the fever and development of thrombocytosis), antiplatelet dosages are employed (e.g., 5 mg/kg/day in a single dose). This dosage is continued for months or even years in children with or at risk for coronary artery involvement.

High-dose IVIg (2000 mg/kg) has been used in controlled studies and has been shown to be efficacious in children with Kawasaki's disease.[86,88] In general, this therapy is probably most effective if given within the initial 10 days of the illness. Children often have a dramatic response to IVIg in terms of fever, constitutional symptoms, and general well-being. In addition, IVIg therapy reduces the frequency, size, and severity of coronary aneurysms and improves the outcome compared to that in control groups. Glucocorticoids are generally contraindicated because of early studies in Japan that reported an increase in the frequency of coronary aneurysms in children who received steroids compared to children receiving no therapy or aspirin alone. Use of these agents may be considered in recurrent disease or in severe active myocarditis.[89] Thrombolytic therapy with tissue plasminogen activator or urokinase should be considered in acute coronary thrombosis.

Summary and Conclusions

Almost all of the early deaths and most cases of long-term disability are related to cardiac involvement.[75,90-92] Myocardial infarction was described in approximately 2.5 percent of reported cases; this event occurred most commonly in the subacute phase of the disease. Death may be due to infarction, coronary thrombosis, or rupture of an aneurysm. Giant aneurysms (larger than 8 mm) represent an especially serious development.[93] Late death has occurred as a result of rupture of an aneurysm several years after onset of the disease or from myocardial small blood vessel occlusion and premature atherosclerosis.[94] Extensive scarring, arterial calcification, multiple areas of stenosis, or recanalization may develop in children who have survived an initial severe coronary insult.[90,95] Progressive myocardial dysfunction results from these changes. A child who has had an infarction may be a candidate for coronary bypass surgery.

A careful history to evaluate the occurrence of previous Kawasaki's disease is indicated in all older children and young adolescents who present for physical examinations before participating in a sport, as there may be long-term persistence of vascular abnormalities.[90] If the history includes a febrile illness accompanied by features suggestive of Kawasaki's disease, the examination must include specific measures of cardiac function (e.g., stress testing and echocardiography).

NECROTIZING VASCULITIS OF SMALL VESSELS

Necrotizing vasculitis that affects smaller vessels, including postcapillary venules, is referred to as "leukocytoclastic vasculitis."[69] In these disorders, the vessel wall is infiltrated with polymorphonuclear leukocytes, and nuclear debris is scattered around the lesions. Fibrinoid necrosis is present and deposition of Ig and complement can often be demonstrated by fluorescent microscopy. This form of vasculitis may be encountered as a sequela to drug hypersensitivity, infectious endocarditis, or hematologic malignancy. Cryoglobulinemia, either essential or secondary to another disease, causes an immune-complex vasculitis that mimics various forms of vasculopathy.

Henoch-Schönlein Purpura

Definition and Criteria

Henoch-Schönlein purpura occurs commonly in children and adolescents[69,96] as a putative IgA-mediated immune vasculitis. Diagnosis is based on the clinical tetrad of arthritis, abdominal pain, hematuria, and nonthrombocytopenic purpura.[97] The classic purpuric skin rash (palpable purpura) is generally regarded as essential for diagnosis (Fig. 97–14).

Epidemiology

An incidence of Henoch-Schönlein purpura in 13.5 per 100,000 children was reported from Belfast, Northern Ireland.[98] Henoch-Schönlein purpura accounts for 8 percent of less of new patient referrals (see Table 97–1). It commonly occurs after an upper respiratory tract infection or other illness, often in the spring. Streptococcal disease has been implicated in some cases, and other

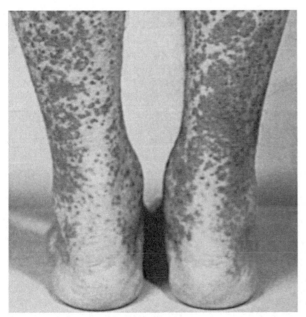

FIGURE 97-14 · Petechial and papular rash over the lower extremities of a teenage boy with Henoch-Schönlein purpura.

reports have been related to vaccination, varicella, hepatitis B infection, insect bites, dietary allergens, malignancy, or mycoplasmal disease. Occasionally, a familial occurrence is reported, but no definite HLA association has been demonstrated. Henoch-Schönlein purpura also occurs in children with C2 complement component deficiency.[99]

Clinical Features

Onset of the disease is often acute, with sequential manifestations appearing over a few days to weeks. A leukocytoclastic vasculitis with deposition of IgA, IgG, fibrin, C3, and properdin occurs in all affected organs,[69] although the skin, gastrointestinal tract, joints, and kidneys are the primary organs and structures affected. The CNS may be involved, and an isolated cerebral vasculitis has been described. Pulmonary disease with hemorrhage can occur.

Purpura is the first sign in more than half of the children. The buttocks and lower extremities are most often affected; the trunk is usually spared. The lesions often appear in crops; some may have central hemorrhage or ulceration, and others mimic urticaria. Individual purpuric lesions often coalesce to form larger areas of involvement interspersed with petechiae. Subcutaneous edema is observed in 25 percent of the children with Henoch-Schönlein purpura. It commonly involves the dorsa of the hands and feet and less commonly the scalp, forehead, periorbital areas, perineum, and scrotum. Extensive edema is most common in children under the age of 2 years. Acute hemorrhagic edema of infancy may be a variant of Henoch-Schönlein purpura.

More than 85 percent of affected children have gastrointestinal signs and symptoms. These include colicky abdominal pain, melena, ileus, vomiting, and hematemesis. Extensive submucosal and mucosal edema, hemorrhage, perforation, and intussusception occur in fewer than 5 percent of children and are more common in children older than 4 years of age. Clinical evidence of glomerulitis is found in up to 50 percent of cases.[98,100] The degree of renal involvement varies from mild endocapillary glomerulitis to extensive crescentic disease. Mesangial involvement is prominent at onset and is similar to that seen in adults in Berger's nephropathy.[101]

Arthritis that is symmetric or asymmetric and predominantly involves the larger joints is a prominent finding in about 75 percent of children with Henoch-Schönlein purpura. Although often painful at onset with limitation of motion, it may be less dramatic and is usually not migratory. The knees and ankles are most commonly affected, but wrists, elbows, and fingers may also be involved, with prominent periarticular swelling and tenderness, usually without erythema or warmth. Joint effusions per se are unusual. The arthritis is transient, often resolves within a few days, and leaves no residual damage.

A moderate leukocytosis occurs, along with a normocytic, normochromic anemia that may be related in part to gastrointestinal blood loss. The platelet count is normal. Activated C3d is present in the circulation, and the concentrations of properdin and factor B are decreased in half of the children during the acute illness. Serum IgA and IgM concentrations are elevated in half of the patients. Fibrin split products are increased in the circulation and urine as evidence of involvement of the fibrinolytic system.

Differential Diagnosis

Henoch-Schönlein purpura must be differentiated from a wide variety of other illnesses of childhood, including poststreptococcal glomerulonephritis, rheumatic fever, SLE, septicemia, and disseminated intravascular coagulation. Other causes of an acute surgical abdomen or gastrointestinal bleeding must be considered along with intussusception or pancreatitis. CT may delineate the cause of abdominal pain in Henoch-Schönlein purpura by demonstrating multifocal areas of bowel wall thickening, mesenteric edema, vascular engorgement, or intussusception. Although traditionally the presence of purpura is held to be necessary for a diagnosis of Henoch-Schönlein purpura, there are undoubtedly children who either do not develop purpura or do not have it at disease onset. Biopsy of a cutaneous lesion may be diagnostic in difficult cases if it demonstrates a leukocytoclastic vasculitis characterized by deposition of IgA and C3.

Evaluation and Management

General measures of support are critically important in seriously ill children with Henoch-Schönlein purpura. In general, glucocorticoids have potential therapeutic value only for management of gastrointestinal vasculitis and hemorrhage or in severe symptomatic disease. The response to their use in these cases may be dramatic. Prednisone (1 to 2 mg/kg/day in divided doses) is used for at least a week and is then gradually tapered based on clinical improvement and extent of bleeding. There is no concrete evidence that prednisone otherwise modifies clinical expression of the disease, shortens its course, or has any direct effect on the frequency or severity of renal involvement. Clinical studies have not thoroughly evaluated the efficacy of steroids administered early to children with nephritis; however, in children with progressive renal disease, consideration should be given to the use of these agents, as well as cytotoxic agents and antiplatelet drugs. A kidney biopsy is generally not indicated except to clarify the extent and nature of renal disease in children who are severely affected. IVIg has also been recommended for severe nephritis. Renal transplantation has been successfully performed in children with renal failure related to Henoch-Schönlein purpura. Nephritis does not generally recur in the allografts.[102]

Summary and Conclusions

Henoch-Schönlein purpura is usually self-limited and often consists of a single episode of clinical involvement. In most children, the course of disease is 4 to 6 weeks in duration. Although about 30 percent of young children have a second or third exacerbation, an increasing percentage of older children have recurrences. The younger the child and the shorter the course, the fewer the recurrences expected. Exacerbations usually occur within the initial 6-week period. An unusual child may develop recurrences for as long as 2 years after onset. Prognosis is generally excellent and depends on the extent of systemic involvement and the age of the child, being better in younger children. Morbidity and mortality are predominantly related to involvement of the gastrointestinal tract or kidneys.[98,100,103] Mortality was less than 1 percent in the Belfast study, and the morbidity rate was 1.1 percent.[98]

Other Forms of Leukocytoclastic Vasculitis

The smaller blood vessels, including arterioles, capillaries, and venules, are typically involved in hypersensitivity angiitis.[69,96] A form of this disease, serum sickness, was previously more common than at present; it occurred secondary to the therapeutic use of heterologous antisera and introduction of the sulfa drugs and penicillin. In addition to these medications, many other medications have been implicated in the pathogenesis of this disorder. Cutaneous disease is common and consists of painful, palpable purpura or hemorrhagic infarcts. The inflammatory lesions are at similar stages of evolution in all involved vessels, and the cellular infiltrate often contains many eosinophils. Immune complexes can be demonstrated in the circulation of many affected children. Arthritis is usually a prominent component of the clinical presentation. Hypersensitivity angiitis is characterized by a variable course whose outcome is often determined by the presence and severity of cardiac, pulmonary, or renal abnormalities. Prednisone is usually effective in suppressing this disorder and in preventing severe complications or death. The disease generally runs its course over approximately 6 weeks.

An isolated cutaneous vasculitis is occasionally seen in a child who presents with palpable purpura, painful nodules, or ridges that develop along the course of involved vessels without systemic or constitutional symptoms.[104] The clinical course is variable and is characterized by remissions and recurrences, often over many years. A few patients have systemic involvement. Although each exacerbation may respond to glucocorticoids, or occasionally even to aspirin, this disease is frequently of such long duration that it is difficult to treat a growing child with prednisone during the entire course. Alternate-day dosage may offer a more acceptable approach to therapy. Hypocomplementemic urticarial vasculitis, although seen primarily in young women, has also been described in children.[105] The eruption affects principally the face, upper extremities, and trunk but also occurs on the palms and soles. The urticarial lesions last for 1 to 3 days with each exacerbation and then fade without scarring. Systemic features of variable severity accompany the cutaneous disease (arthritis, myositis, uveitis, serositis, and involvement of the lungs or kidneys). The degree of hypocomplementemia parallels the severity of the illness. In some patients the condition warrants treatment with glucocorticoid drugs.

Microscopic polyarteritis is a very rare form of vasculitis and glomerulonephritis in children. It is often associated with perinuclear antineutrophil cytoplasmic antibodies (ANCAs).[106] Many of the children progress to end-stage renal disease.[107] Therapy generally includes administration of glucocorticoids and cyclophosphamide.

GIANT CELL ARTERITIS

Characteristic features of giant cell arteritis (GCA) are involvement of the aorta and its major branches with a disruption of the internal elastic lamina, intimal proliferation, and infiltration of vessel walls with mononuclear cells and giant cells. Systemic GCA is rare and involves major branches or segments of the aorta at single or multiple locations. The child may present with constitutional symptoms, fever of unknown origin, or hypertension. A diagnosis is established by angiography combined with biopsy of a vessel if accessible (Fig. 97–15). Vascular occlusion leads to peripheral anoxia, cyanosis, and gangrene. Recanalization may occur spontaneously or during treatment with glucocorticoid drugs.

Cranial or temporal arteritis is generally a disease of older adults, but it has been described in children and is characterized by a persistent, severe headache and localized pain and tenderness over a cranial or temporal vessel. The ESR is dramatically elevated. The threat

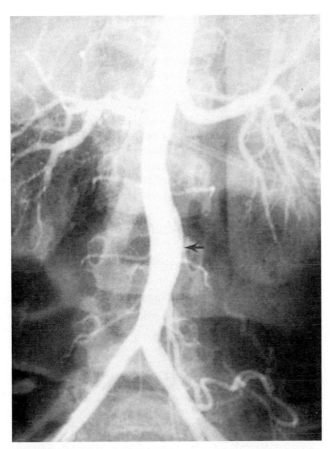

FIGURE 97-15 · Angiogram demonstrating tortuosity and dilation of the lower aorta (*arrow*) in a 6-year-old girl with giant cell arteritis (GCA) of the abdominal vessels. Note involvement of the right renal artery.

of blindness from involvement of the ophthalmic and central retinal arteries is an important consideration and an indication for prompt initiation of glucocorticoid therapy. Diagnosis is established by biopsy of an affected vessel with care taken to secure a generous specimen.

Takayasu's arteritis is a GCA seen predominantly in children and young women, especially teenage girls (female-to-male ratio is 8:1). It involves the aorta and its major branches and the pulmonary arteries.[108,109] Features of the disease include stenosis, occlusion, dilation, and aneurysms. Takayasu's arteritis has been referred to as "pulseless disease" because of the characteristic obliteration of the radial pulses or "reverse coarctation." These signs of peripheral vascular insufficiency often direct attention to the correct diagnosis, which is confirmed by angiography, ultrasonography, MRI, or magnetic resonance angiography. Criteria for diagnosis have been developed by the ACR.[110]

This disorder is more common in Asians, Hispanics, Sephardic Jews, and blacks. It occasionally occurs in families of children with other connective tissue diseases and in conjunction with other rheumatic disorders, and it has been reported in monozygotic twin sisters. Hypertension is frequent during the course of the disease and is in part related to stenosis of the renal arteries. Calcification is sometimes identified in affected vessels on plain films.

The course of the disease may be short, about 3 to 6 months, or as long as many years.[111] It is generally believed that glucocorticoids are effective if used early, before stenosis and thrombosis have developed (after verification of a negative result on cutaneous PPD testing because of a possible association with tuberculosis in some areas of the world), but sufficient clinical studies have not been reported to confirm the efficacy of either this therapeutic approach or the use of cyclophosphamide or MTX. NSAIDs are useful to relieve symptoms during the early phases of the illness. Anticoagulants and antiplatelet agents may be indicated if there is widespread chronic occlusion of vessels. Vessel grafts have been successful late in the course of the disease.

Granulomatous Arteritis

Wegener's granulomatosis (WG) is a rare example of granulomatous arteritis in children.[69,112,113] Onset of the disease has been described as early as 3 months of age. Constitutional symptoms are prominent. Unexplained pain, rhinorrhea, mucosal ulceration, or bleeding from the upper respiratory tract is characteristic. Destruction of nasal cartilage may result in a saddle nose. Hemoptysis and pleuritic pain are frequent. Chest radiographs demonstrate multiform pulmonary infiltrates; pulmonary disease may progress to hemorrhage, obstruction, atelectasis, or repeated episodes of infection. More than 80 percent of the children have renal disease, which may become rapidly progressive, although hypertension is less common than in other types of nephritis. Necrotizing granulomata also occur in skin, heart, CNS, gastrointestinal tract, and synovia. Limited forms of WG have been described, possibly including midline granuloma, which is exceedingly rare in children.

The differential diagnosis includes berylliosis, Loeffler's syndrome, tuberculosis, syphilis, and lymphoma. Goodpasture's syndrome, lymphomatoid granulomatosis, relapsing polychondritis, and other forms of vasculitis are sometimes confused with WG. Sarcoidosis can occur in children with systemic necrotizing vasculitis, cutaneous vasculitis, or granulomatous arteritis.

Biopsy of an affected site, generally nasal mucosa or lung, is essential to early diagnosis. Necrotizing granulomas with leukocytic, lymphocytic, and giant cell infiltration are seen.[69] Overt vasculitis may not be evident. ANCAs in a cytoplasmic pattern are characteristic of WG.[114,115] The perinuclear pattern of staining is less specific and has been described in other forms of vasculitis and connective tissue diseases.

In untreated children, death from renal or pulmonary complications usually occurs in a matter of months, but long-term survival in the absence of specific therapy has been reported. Glucocorticoid drugs and trimethoprim-sulfamethoxazole may be effective early in the disease, but studies confirm that cyclophosphamide is essential for effective treatment.[113] The use of MTX as an alternative immunosuppressive agent has been proposed to avoid the long-term morbidity associated with the use of cyclophosphamide.[116]

Allergic granulomatosis (Churg-Strauss syndrome [CSS]) is a systemic vasculitis that occurs predominantly in males with a background of chronic asthma and peripheral eosinophilia.[69] Other manifestations of this syndrome are similar to those seen in PAN, especially in the gastrointestinal tract, CNS, and musculoskeletal system. Renal disease is, however, less frequent. Pulmonary involvement is often the single most important manifestation. The histopathologic pattern in biopsy specimens is that of a necrotizing vasculitis with an eosinophilic infiltrate and extravascular necrotizing granulomas. Administration of glucocorticoid drugs is the main approach to treatment, occasionally in combination with cyclophosphamide. Prognosis is variable; death often involves cardiopulmonary failure.

REFERENCES

1. Cassidy JT, Petty RE: Textbook of Pediatric Rheumatology, 4th ed. Philadelphia, WB Saunders, 2000.
2. Tan EM, Cohen AS, Fries JF, et al: The 1982 revised criteria for the classification of systemic lupus erythematosus. Arthritis Rheum 25:1271-1277, 1982.
3. Fessel WJ: Epidemiology of systemic lupus erythematosus. Rheum Dis Clin North Am 14:15-23, 1988.
4. Tucker LB, Menon S, Schaller JG, et al: Adult-and childhood-onset systemic lupus erythematosus: A comparison of onset, clinical features, serology, and outcome. Br J Rheumatol 34:866-872, 1995.
5. Kimberly RP: Prospects for autoimmune disease: Research advances in systemic lupus erythematosus. JAMA 285:650-652, 2001.
6. Deapen D, Escalante A, Weinrib L, et al: A revised estimate of twin concordance in systemic lupus erythematosus. Arthritis Rheum 35:311-318, 1992.
7. Gazarian M, Feldman BM, Benson LN, et al: Assessment of myocardial perfusion and function in childhood systemic lupus erythematosus. J Pediatr 132:109-116, 1998.
8. Massa M, De Benedetti F, Pignatti P, et al: Anti-double stranded DNA, anti-histone, and anti-nucleosome IgG reactivities in children with systemic lupus erythematosus. Clin Exp Rheumatol 12:219-225, 1994.
9. Ravelli A, Martini A: Antiphospholipid antibody syndrome in pediatric patients. Rheum Dis Clin North Am 23:657-676, 1997.
10. Press J, Palayew K, Laxer RM, et al: Antiribosomal P antibodies in pediatric patients with systemic lupus erythematosus and psychosis. Arthritis Rheum 39:671-676, 1996.
11. West SG, Emlen W, Wener MH, et al: Neuropsychiatric lupus erythematosus: A 10-year prospective study on the value of diagnostic tests. Am J Med 99:153-163, 1995.
12. Ting CK, Hsieh KH: A long-term immunological study of childhood onset systemic lupus erythematosus. Ann Rheum Dis 51:45-51, 1992.
13. Ilowite NT: Hyperlipidemia and the rheumatic diseases. Curr Opin Rheumatol 8:455-458, 1996.
14. The Canadian Hydroxychloroquine Study Group: A randomized study of the effect of withdrawing hydroxychloroquine sulfate in systemic lupus erythematosus. N Engl J Med 324:150-154, 1991.
15. Lehman TJ: Aggressive therapy for childhood rheumatic diseases: When are immunosuppressives appropriate? Arthritis Rheum 36:71-74, 1993.
16. Ravelli A, Ballardini G, Viola S, et al: Methotrexate therapy in refractory pediatric onset systemic lupus erythematosus. J Rheumatol 25:572-575, 1998.
17. Steinberg AD, Steinberg SC: Long-term preservation of renal function in patients with lupus nephritis receiving treatment that includes cyclophosphamide versus those treated with prednisone only. Arthritis Rheum 34:945-950, 1991.
18. Lehman TJ: A practical guide to systemic lupus erythematosus. Pediatr Clin North Am 42:1223-1238, 1995.
19. Nossent HC, Swaak TJ, Berden JH: Systemic lupus erythematosus after renal transplantation: Patient and graft survival and disease activity—The Dutch Working Party on Systemic Lupus Erythematosus. Ann Intern Med 114:183-188, 1991.
20. Lacks S, White P: Morbidity associated with childhood systemic lupus erythematosus. J Rheumatol 17:941-945, 1990.
21. Urowitz MB, Gladman DD, Abu-Shakra M, et al: Mortality studies in systemic lupus erythematosus: Results from a single center. III. Improved survival over 24 years. J Rheumatol 24:1061-1065, 1997.
22. Platt JL, Burke BA, Fish AJ, et al: Systemic lupus erythematosus in the first two decades of life. Am J Kidney Dis 2:212-222, 1982.
23. Hagelberg S, Lee Y, Bargman J, et al: Longterm followup of childhood lupus nephritis. J Rheumatol 29:2635-2642, 2002.
24. Silverman ED, Laxer RM: Neonatal lupus erythematosus. Rheum Dis Clin North Am 23:599-618, 1997.
25. Buyon JP: Neonatal lupus. Curr Opin Rheumatol 8:485-490, 1996.
26. Neiman AR, Lee LA, Weston WL, et al: Cutaneous manifestations of neonatal lupus without heart block: characteristics of mothers and children enrolled in a national registry. J Pediatr 137: 674-680, 2000.
27. Press J, Uziel Y, Laxer RM, et al: Long-term outcome of mothers of children with complete congenital heart block. Am J Med 100:328-332, 1996.
28. Waltuck J, Buyon JP: Autoantibody-associated congenital heart block: outcome in mothers and children. Ann Intern Med 120:544-551, 1994.
29. Silverman ED, Buyon J, Laxer RM, et al: Autoantibody response to the Ro/La particle may predict outcome in neonatal lupus erythematosus. Clin Exp Immunol 100:499-505, 1995.
30. Pachman LM: Juvenile dermatomyositis. Pathophysiology and disease expression. Pediatr Clin North Am 42:1071-1098, 1995.
31. Rider LG, Miller FW: Classification and treatment of the juvenile idiopathic inflammatory myopathies. Rheum Dis Clin North Am 23:619-655, 1997.
32. Symmons DP, Sills JA, Davis SM: The incidence of juvenile dermatomyositis: Results from a nation-wide study. Br J Rheumatol 34:732-736, 1995.
33. Pachman LM: Juvenile dermatomyositis: Immunogenetics, pathophysiology, and disease expression. Rheum Dis Clin North Am 28:579-602, 2002.
34. Reed AM, Pachman LM, Hayford J, et al: Immunogenetic studies in families of children with juvenile dermatomyositis. J Rheumatol 25:1000-1002, 1998.

35. Pachman LM, Fedczyna TO, Lechman TS, et al: Juvenile dermatomyositis: the association of the TNF alpha-308A allele and disease chronicity. Curr Rheumatol Rep 3:379-386, 2001.

36. Spencer CH, Hanson V, Singsen BH, et al: Course of treated juvenile dermatomyositis. J Pediatr 105:399-408, 1984.

37. Feldman BM, Reichlin M, Laxer RM, et al: Clinical significance of specific autoantibodies in juvenile dermatomyositis. J Rheumatol 23:1794-1797, 1996.

38. Guzman J, Petty RE, Malleson PN: Monitoring disease activity in juvenile dermatomyositis: The role of von Willebrand factor and muscle enzymes. J Rheumatol 21:739-743, 1994.

39. Crowe WE, Bove KE, Levinson JE, et al: Clinical and pathogenetic implications of histopathology in childhood polydermatomyositis. Arthritis Rheum 25:126-139, 1982.

40. Pistoia V, Buoncompagni A, Scribanis R, et al: Cyclosporin A in the treatment of juvenile chronic arthritis and childhood polymyositis-dermatomyositis: Results of a preliminary study. Clin Exp Rheumatol 11:203-208, 1993.

41. Lang BA, Laxer RM, Murphy G, et al: Treatment of dermatomyositis with intravenous gammaglobulin. Am J Med 91:169-172, 1991.

42. Sansome A, Dubowitz V: Intravenous immunoglobulin in juvenile dermatomyositis: four year review of nine cases. Arch Dis Child 72:25-28, 1995.

43. Ostrov BE, Goldsmith DP, Eichenfield AH, et al: Hypercalcemia during the resolution of calcinosis universalis in juvenile dermatomyositis. J Rheumatol 18:1730-1734, 1991.

44. Miller LC, Michael AF, Kim Y: Childhood dermatomyositis: Clinical course and long-term follow-up. Clin Pediatr (Phila) 26:561-566, 1987.

45. Nelson AM: Localized scleroderma including morphea, linear scleroderma, and eosinophilic fasciitis. Curr Probl Pediatr 26:318-324, 1996.

46. Subcommittee for Scleroderma Criteria of the American Rheumatism Association Diagnostic and Therapeutic Criteria Committee: Preliminary criteria for the classification of systemic sclerosis (scleroderma). Arthritis Rheum 23:581, 1980.

47. LeRoy EC, Medsger TA Jr: Criteria for the classification of early systemic sclerosis. J Rheumatol 28:1573-1576, 2001.

48. Uziel Y, Miller ML, Laxer RM: Scleroderma in children. Pediatr Clin North Am 42:1171-1203, 1995.

49. Nelson JL, Furst DE, Maloney S, et al: Microchimerism and HLA-compatible relationships of pregnancy in scleroderma. Lancet 351:559-562, 1998.

50. Johnson KL, Nelson JL, Furst DE, et al: Fetal cell microchimerism in tissue from multiple sites in women with systemic sclerosis. Arthritis Rheum 44:1848-1854, 2001.

51. Spencer-Green G, Schlesinger M, Bove KE, et al: Nailfold capillary abnormalities in childhood rheumatic diseases. J Pediatr 102:341-346, 1983.

52. Bode BY, Yocum DE, Gall EP, et al: Methotrexate in scleroderma: Experience in ten patients. Arthritis Rheum 33:S66, 1990.

53. Steen VD, Costantino JP, Shapiro AP, et al: Outcome of renal crisis in systemic sclerosis: Relation to availability of angiotensin converting enzyme (ACE) inhibitors. Ann Intern Med 113:352-357, 1990.

54. Peterson LS, Nelson AM, Su WP, et al: The epidemiology of morphea (localized scleroderma) in Olmsted County 1960-1993. J Rheumatol 24:73-80, 1997.

55. Rosenberg AM, Uziel Y, Krafchik BR, et al: Antinuclear antibodies in children with localized scleroderma. J Rheumatol 22:2337-2343, 1995.

56. Peterson LS, Nelson AM, Su WP: Classification of morphea (localized scleroderma). Mayo Clin Proc 70:1068-1076, 1995.

57. Lehman TJ: The Parry Romberg syndrome of progressive facial hemiatrophy and linear scleroderma en coup de sabre: Mistaken diagnosis or overlapping conditions? J Rheumatol 19:844-845, 1992.

58. Goldenstein-Schainberg C, Pereira RM, Gusukuma MC, et al: Childhood linear scleroderma "en coup de sabre" with uveitis. J Pediatr 117:581-584, 1990.

59. Grisanti MW, Moore TL, Osborn TG, et al: Eosinophilic fasciitis in children. Semin Arthritis Rheum 19:151-157, 1989.

60. Miller JJ III: The fasciitis-morphea complex in children. Am J Dis Child 146:733-736, 1992.

61. Michels H: Course of mixed connective tissue disease in children. Ann Med 29:359-364, 1997.

62. Yokota S, Imagawa T, Katakura S, et al: Mixed connective tissue disease in childhood: A nationwide retrospective study in Japan. Acta Paediatr Jpn 39:273-276, 1997.

63. Mier R, Ansell B, Hall MA, et al: Long term follow-up of children with mixed connective tissue disease. Lupus 5:221-226, 1996.

64. Hoffman RW, Cassidy JT, Takeda Y, et al: U1-70-kd autoantibody-positive mixed connective tissue disease in children: A longitudinal clinical and serologic analysis. Arthritis Rheum 36:1599-1602, 1993.

65. Athreya BH: Vasculitis in children. Pediatr Clin North Am 42:1239-1261, 1995.

66. Dillon MJ: Childhood vasculitis. Lupus 7:259-265, 1998.

67. Hunder GG, Arend WP, Bloch DA, et al: The American College of Rheumatology 1990 criteria for the classification of vasculitis. Introduction. Arthritis Rheum 33:1065-1067, 1990.

68. Jennette JC, Falk RJ, Andrassy K, et al: Nomenclature of systemic vasculitides: Proposal of an international consensus conference. Arthritis Rheum 37:187-192, 1994.

69. Lie JT, American College of Rheumatology Subcommittee on Classification of Vasculitis: Illustrated histopathologic classification criteria for selected vasculitis syndromes. Arthritis Rheum 33:1074-1087, 1990.

70. Kussmaul A, Maier R: Ueber eine bisher nicht beshriebene eigenthümliche Arterienerkrankung (Periarteritis nodosa), die mit Morbus Brightii und rapid fortschreitender allgemeiner Muskellähmung einhergeht. Deutsches Arch Klin Med 1:484, 1866. (Translated into English by Matteson E: On a previously undescribed peculiar arterial disease (Periarteritis nodosa), accompanied by Bright's disease and rapidly progressive general muscle weakness. Mayo Foundation, Rochester, MN 1996.)

71. Ozen S, Besbas N, Saatci U, et al: Diagnostic criteria for polyarteritis nodosa in childhood. J Pediatr 120:206-209, 1992.

72. Maeda M, Kobayashi M, Okamoto S, et al: Clinical observation of 14 cases of childhood polyarteritis nodosa in Japan. Acta Paediatr Jpn 39:277-279, 1997.

73. Kawasaki T: Acute febrile mucocutaneous syndrome with lymphoid involvement with specific desquamation of the fingers and toes in children. Jpn J Allergy 16:178-222, 1967.

74. Wortmann DW, Nelson AM: Kawasaki syndrome. Rheum Dis Clin North Am 16:363-375, 1990.

75. Taubert KA, Rowley AH, Shulman ST: Nationwide survey of Kawasaki disease and acute rheumatic fever. J Pediatr 119:279-282, 1991.

76. Rowley AH, Shulman ST: Kawasaki syndrome. Clin Microbiol Rev 11:405-414, 1998.

77. Yanagawa H, Nakamura Y, Yashiro M, et al: Update of the epidemiology of Kawasaki disease in Japan: From the results of 1993-94 nationwide survey. J Epidemiol 6:148-157, 1996.

78. Rowley AH, Eckerley CA, Jack HM, et al: IgA plasma cells in vascular tissue of patients with Kawasaki syndrome. J Immunol 159:5946-5955, 1997.

79. Falcini F, Trapani S, Turchini S, et al: Immunological findings in Kawasaki disease: An evaluation in a cohort of Italian children. Clin Exp Rheumatol 15:685-689, 1997.

80. Leung DY, Schlievert PM, Meissner HC: The immunopathogenesis and management of Kawasaki syndrome. Arthritis Rheum 41:1538-1547, 1998.

81. Cuttica RJ: Vasculitis, Kawasaki disease, and pseudovasculitis. Curr Opin Rheumatol 9:448-457, 1997.

82. Lehman TJ, Walker SM, Mahnovski V, et al: Coronary arteritis in mice following the systemic injection of group B Lactobacillus casei cell walls in aqueous suspension. Arthritis Rheum 28:652-659, 1985.

83. Nakamura Y, Yanagawa H, Ojima T, et al: Cardiac sequelae of Kawasaki disease among recurrent cases. Arch Dis Child 78:163-165, 1998.

84. Dajani AS, Taubert KA, Takahashi M, et al: Guidelines for long-term management of patients with Kawasaki disease: Report from the Committee on Rheumatic Fever, Endocarditis, and Kawasaki Disease, Council on Cardiovascular Disease in the Young, American Heart Association. Circulation 89:916-922, 1994.

85. Weng KP, Hsieh KS, Huang SH, et al: Serum HDL level at acute stage of Kawasaki disease. Chung Hua Min Kuo Hsiao Erh Ko I Hsueh Hui Tsa Chih 39:28-32, 1998.

86. Newburger JW, Takahashi M, Beiser AS, et al: A single intravenous infusion of gamma globulin as compared with four

infusions in the treatment of acute Kawasaki syndrome. N Engl J Med 324:1633-1639, 1991.

87. Durongpisitkul K, Gururaj VJ, Park JM, et al: The prevention of coronary artery aneurysm in Kawasaki disease: A meta-analysis on the efficacy of aspirin and immunoglobulin treatment. Pediatrics 96:1057-1061, 1995.

88. Yanagawa H, Nakamura Y, Sakata K, et al: Use of intravenous gamma-globulin for Kawasaki disease: Effects on cardiac sequelae. Pediatr Cardiol 18:19-23, 1997.

89. Wright DA, Newburger JW, Baker A, et al: Treatment of immune globulin-resistant Kawasaki disease with pulsed doses of corticosteroids. J Pediatr 128:146-149, 1996.

90. Kato H, Sugimura T, Akagi T, et al: Long-term consequences of Kawasaki disease: A 10-to 21-year follow-up study of 594 patients. Circulation 94:1379-1385, 1996.

91. Nakano H, Saito A, Ueda K, et al: Clinical characteristics of myocardial infarction following Kawasaki disease: Report of 11 cases. J Pediatr 108:198-203, 1986.

92. Nakamura Y, Yanagawa H, Kato H, et al: Mortality rates for patients with a history of Kawasaki disease in Japan: Kawasaki Disease Follow-up Group. J Pediatr 128:75-81, 1996.

93. Inoue O, Alkagi T, Kato H: Fate of giant coronary aneurysms in Kawasaki disease: Long-term follow-up study. Circulation 80(Suppl II):262, 1989.

94. Fukushige J, Takahashi N, Ueda K, et al: Long-term outcome of coronary abnormalities in patients after Kawasaki disease. Pediatr Cardiol 17:71-76, 1996.

95. Burns JC, Shike H, Gordon JB, et al: Sequelae f Kawasaki disease in adolescents and young adults. J Am Coll Cardiol 28:253-257, 1996.

96. Michel BA, Hunder GG, Bloch DA, et al: Hypersensitivity vasculitis and Henoch-Schönlein purpura: A comparison between the 2 disorders. J Rheumatol 19:721-728, 1992.

97. Mills JA, Michel BA, Bloch DA, et al: The American College of Rheumatology 1990 criteria for the classification of Henoch-Schönlein purpura. Arthritis Rheum 33:1114-1121, 1990.

98. Stewart M, Savage JM, Bell B, et al: Long term renal prognosis of Henoch-Schönlein purpura in an unselected childhood population. Eur J Pediatr 147:113-115, 1988.

99. Atkinson JP: Complement deficiency: Predisposing factor to autoimmune syndromes. Am J Med 85:45-47, 1988.

100. Goldstein AR, White RH, Akuse R, et al: Long-term follow-up of childhood Henoch-Schönlein nephritis. Lancet 339:280-282, 1992.

101. Blanco R, Martinez-Taboada VM, Rodriguez-Valverde V, et al: Henoch-Schönlein purpura in adulthood and childhood: Two different expressions of the same syndrome. Arthritis Rheum 40:859-864, 1997.

102. Hasegawa A, Kawamura T, Ito H, et al: Fate of renal grafts with recurrent Henoch-Schönlein purpura nephritis in children. Transplant Proc 21:2130-2133, 1989.

103. Bunchman TE, Mauer SM, Sibley RK, et al: Anaphylactoid purpura: characteristics of 16 patients who progressed to renal failure. Pediatr Nephrol 2:393-397, 1988.

104. Sheth AP, Olson JC, Esterly NB: Cutaneous polyarteritis nodosa of childhood. J Am Acad Dermatol 31:561-566, 1994.

105. Martini A, Ravelli A, Albani S, et al: Hypocomplementemic urticarial vasculitis syndrome with severe systemic manifestations. J Pediatr 124:742-744, 1994.

106. Nash MC, Dillon MJ: Antineutrophil cytoplasm antibodies and vasculitis. Arch Dis Child 77:261-264, 1997.

107. Valentini RP, Smoyer WE, Sedman AB, et al: Outcome of antineutrophil cytoplasmic autoantibodies-positive glomerulonephritis and vasculitis in children: A single-center experience. J Pediatr 132:325-328, 1998.

108. Morales E, Pineda C, Martinez-Lavin M: Takayasu's arteritis in children. J Rheumatol 18:1081-1084, 1991.

109. Hall S, Barr W, Lie JT, et al: Takayasu arteritis: A study of 32 North American patients. Medicine (Baltimore) 64:89-99, 1985.

110. Arend WP, Michel BA, Bloch DA, et al: The American College of Rheumatology 1990 criteria for the classification of Takayasu arteritis. Arthritis Rheum 33:1129-1134, 1990.

111. Subramanyan R, Joy J, Balakrishnan KG: Natural history of aortoarteritis (Takayasu's disease). Circulation 80:429-437, 1989.

112. Leavitt RY, Fauci AS, Bloch DA, et al: The American College of Rheumatology 1990 criteria for the classification of Wegener's granulomatosis. Arthritis Rheum 33:1101-1107, 1990.

113. Rottem M, Fauci AS, Hallahan CW, et al: Wegener granulomatosis in children and adolescents: Clinical presentation and outcome. J Pediatr 122:26-31, 1993.

114. Ellis EN, Wood EG, Berry P: Spectrum of disease associated with anti-neutrophil cytoplasmic autoantibodies in pediatric patients. J Pediatr 126:40-43, 1995.

115. Hoffman GS: Classification of the systemic vasculitides: Antineutrophil cytoplasmic antibodies, consensus and controversy. Clin Exp Rheumatol 16:111-115, 1998.

116. Gottlieb BS, Miller LC, Ilowite NT: Methotrexate treatment of Wegener granulomatosis in children. J Pediatr 129:604-607, 1996.

Arthritis Caused by Bacteria or Their Components

GEORGE HO, JR. · SUE JOAN JUE · PAUL PENISTON COOK

The normal diarthrodial joint is very resistant to bacterial infection because of local and systemic host defenses. However, bacteria can reach the synovial-lined joint via the hematogenous route and result in septic arthritis. The large joints are affected more commonly than the small joints, and monoarticular infection is the rule with polyarticular infection, more than one joint involved, in less than 20 percent of cases. A prospective series from a community-based population in the Netherlands reflected a representative distribution of joint involvement: knee 55 percent, ankle 10 percent, wrist 9 percent, shoulder 7 percent, hip 5 percent, elbow 5 percent, sternoclavicular, (SC) joint 5 percent, sacroiliac (SI) joint 2 percent, and foot joint 2 percent.[1]

Bacterial infections of the joint are curable with treatment, but the morbidity and mortality are still significant in patients with underlying rheumatoid arthritis (RA), patients with prosthetic joints, the elderly, and those who have severe and multiple comorbidities. Goldenberg wrote in 1994, "Treatment and outcome (of septic arthritis) have not improved substantially over the past 20 years."[2] This statement is probably still true today. However, incremental knowledge of the pathogenesis of septic arthritis caused by two common organisms, *Neiserria gonorrhoeae* and *Staphylococcus aureus,* and understanding the pathobiology of prosthetic devises may lead to innovations in the management and prevention of bacterial joint infections.

Epidemiology and Pathogenesis

The incidence of septic arthritis varies between 2 and 5 per 100,000 per year in the general population, 5.5 and 12 per 100,000 per year in children, 28 and 38 per 100,000 per year in patients with RA, and 40 and 68 per 100,000 per year in patients with joint prosthesis.[3,4] The organisms causing bacterial arthritis depend on the epidemiologic circumstances. For instance, monoarthritis of a prosthetic joint in an elderly man is likely due to *Staphylococcus* species, whereas a migratory arthritis in a

sexually active woman with skin lesions is likely due to disseminated gonococcal infection.

Most cases of septic arthritis result from hematogenous seeding of the synovial membrane. The abundant vascular supply of the synovium, as well as the lack of a limiting basement membrane, allows organisms to target joints during bacteremia. Less common causes of septic arthritis include direct inoculation following joint aspiration or corticosteroid injection of a joint[5]; animal or human bites; nail puncture wounds or plant thorn injury[6]; joint surgery, especially hip and knee arthroplasties; and spread by contiguous osteomyelitis, cellulitis, or septic bursitis. Arthrocentesis is a very common procedure frequently used in conjunction with corticosteroid administration in patients with various forms of joint diseases. Septic arthritis following joint aspiration and injection is extremely rare, occurring in 0.0002 percent of patients.[7] Arthroscopic surgery is also a common procedure that is complicated by a very low incidence of septic arthritis (less than 0.5% of procedures).[8,9] Staphylococcal species, coagulase positive and negative, account for more than 87 percent of these infections. Recently, the Centers for Disease Control (CDC) reported septic arthritis of the knee related to anterior cruciate ligament repair.[10] Cultures yielded gram-negative organisms, such as *Pseudomonas aeruginosa, Citrobacter* species, *Klebsiella oxytoca,* and mixed infection with *S. aureus, Enterococcus faecalis,* and *P. aeruginosa.* In these rare cases, the tissue allografts were identified as the source of the infection.

Acute bacterial arthritis is usually designated gonococcal or nongonococcal. In the case of gonococcal arthritis, *N. gonorrhoeae* possesses a variety of virulence factors on the cell surface. *N. gonorrhoeae* is able to attach to cell surfaces via filamentous outer-membrane appendages, or pili. Another outer membrane protein, Protein I, has forms IA and IB. Protein IA binds the host factor H and inactivates complement component, C3b, thereby circumventing the host's complement system.[11] Protein IA also prevents phagolysosomal fusion in neutrophils, thus enabling survival of the organism within the phagocytes.

Lipooligosaccharide (LOS) is a gonococcal molecule similar to the lipopoly-saccharide (LPS) of other gram-negative bacteria and possesses endotoxin activity, which contributes to the joint damage seen in gonococcal arthritis.[12]

S. aureus is the most common organism causing nongonococcal arthritis. The virulence of *S. aureus* is associated with its ability to attach to host tissue within the joint, evade host defenses, and cause damage to the joint. Some of these virulence factors and their mechanisms of action are listed in Table 98–1. The attachment of *S. aureus* to the joint tissues is facilitated by microbial surface components recognizing adhesive matrix molecules (MSCRAMMs). MSCRAMMs are embedded in the cell wall peptidoglycan of *S. aureus*[13,14] (Fig. 98–1). They bind to host matrix proteins, including collagen, fibrinogen, elastin, vitronectin, laminin, and fibronectin. Knockout gene experiments in animal models showed that the gene coding for the protein that binds collagen is an important virulence factor for *S. aureus* joint infections.[15] Most *S. aureus* isolates also express the fibronectin-binding proteins, FnbpA and FnbpB. Disruption of the respective genes, *fnbpA* and *fnbpB*, by knockout gene experiments completely obliterates adherence of *S. aureus* to fibronectin-coated surfaces (e.g., prosthetic joints).[16]

The genes of several *S. aureus* cell surface proteins (e.g., protein A, fibronectin-binding proteins, coagulase) and exotoxins (e.g., TSST-1, enterotoxin B, proteases, and hemolysins) are regulated by the accessory gene regulator *agr*.[17,18] At low cell numbers, such as at the time of infection, production of cell surface proteins for attachment to host tissues is facilitated by the *agr* gene. Once the cells have attached to tissue or an orthopedic device and have passed from exponential to stationary phase of growth, *agr* then represses the expression of genes coding for cell surface proteins and activates genes coding for exotoxins and tissue-destroying exoenzymes. Because of this complex effect on the different stages of infection, inhibitors of *agr* may reduce tissue destruction but actually enhance tissue colonization. This effect could have implications for chronic infections such as occur with prosthetic joints.

Adherence receptors may allow for the intracellular movement of *S. aureus* into host cells (e.g., osteoblasts,

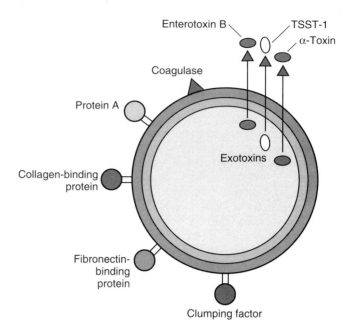

FIGURE 98–1 · Schematic Diagram of *Staphlococcus Aureus*. Many of the cell-surface proteins are regulated by the *agr* locus (see text). At low cell concentrations, *agr* facilitates the production of the cell-surface proteins, which facilitate attachment to tissue. At higher cell concentrations, as occurs with establishment of infection, *agr* downregulates production of the cell-surface proteins and activates genes coding for exotoxins.

endothelial cells, and neutrophils).[19] Once internalized, the organism is protected from the host's immune system and from antimicrobial agents. Following adherence to the joint tissue, the bacteria activate the host immune response. Opsonization and phagocytosis are key defenses to eradicate the organism. *S. aureus* possesses two virulence factors, protein A and capsular polysaccharide, which interfere with these defenses. Protein A interferes with binding of complement by binding to the fragment crystallizable (Fc) portion of immunoglobulin G (IgG). The gene coding for protein A had been experimentally disrupted, and joint infection due to the altered strain in a mouse model resulted in less joint destruction than infection caused by the wild-type strain.[20] Capsular polysaccharide interferes with both opsonization and phagocytosis. Of the 11 reported capsule serotypes of *S. aureus*, types 5 and 8 account for up to 85 percent of clinical infections.[21] The capsule of these two serotypes is thinner, which facilitates the attachment to host fibronectin and fibrin.[22] Once attached to these host proteins, capsule production is upregulated to form a thicker capsule, which makes the bacteria more resistant to opsonization and phagocytosis. The thicker capsule is also able to conceal the highly immunogenic adherence proteins (MSCRAMMs).[23] A mutant of the type 5 capsule in a murine model had a lower rate of infection and resulted in less-severe arthritis compared to mice infected with the wild-type strain.[24] A vaccine consisting of type 5 and 8 polysaccharide reduced *S. aureus* bacteremia by more than half in 1804 hemodialysis patients.[25] The duration of protection was approximately 40 weeks following a single vaccination.

TABLE 98–1 · VIRULENCE FACTORS OF *STAPHYLOCOCCUS AUREUS* AND THEIR MECHANISMS OF ACTION

Virulence Factor	Mechanism of Action
Collagen-binding protein	Binds collagen
Clumping factor A and B	Binds fibrinogen
Fibronectin-binding protein A and B	Binds fibronectin
Capsular polysaccharide	Antiphagocytic
Protein A	Binds fragment crytallizable (Fc) portion of immunoglobulin G (IgG)
Toxic Shock Syndrome Toxin-1, (TSST-1)	Superantigen
Enterotoxins	Superantigens

S. aureus exotoxins (e.g., TSST-1 and enterotoxins) act as superantigens that bind to host major histocompatibility complex (MHC) class II molecules and T cell receptors (TCR), resulting in clonal expansion and activation of some T cells. This activation triggers the release of numerous cytokines, including interleukin-2 (IL-2), interferon-γ (IFN-γ), and tumor necrosis factor-α (TNF-α).[26] Upregulation of these cytokines results in systemic toxicity and joint damage. The stimulated T cells initially proliferate, but later disappear, likely due to apoptosis, and result in immunosuppression.[27] Internalized organisms that had been protected from this inflammatory response may then cause fulminant or persistent infection. Mice injected with strains of *S. aureus* lacking both TSST-1 and enterotoxins rarely develop arthritis; moreover, when arthritis is induced, it is much milder compared to animals injected with the wild-type strain.[26] Furthermore, vaccination of mice with a mutated, recombinant form of enterotoxin A devoid of superantigenicity was associated with a significant reduction in mortality.[28]

In response to bacterial infection of the joint space, the host releases a variety of cytokines and inflammatory mediators. Initially, IL-1β and IL-6 are released into the joint space, leading to an influx of inflammatory cells. These neutrophils and macrophages engulf invading bacteria and release additional cytokines, including TNF-α, IL-1, IL-6, and IL-8. Blocking TNF-α with a monoclonal antibody and IL-1 with an IL-1 receptor antagonist (IL-1Ra) inhibited leukocyte infiltration into the joint by 80 percent in a rabbit model of *S. aureus*–induced arthritis when the cytokine inhibitors were given simultaneously with *S. aureus*.[29] However, when the same inhibitors were given 24 hours following infection, there was no effect on leukocyte infiltration, suggesting the crucial roles of TNF-α and IL-1 in the early stages of *S. aureus*–induced arthritis. Release of IFN-γ is associated with the influx of T cells, which occurs a few days following infection. In a mouse model of *S. aureus* septic arthritis, IFN-γ has been associated with a worsening of the severity of arthritis, while, on the other hand, protecting the animals from septicemia.[30] Thus, the host's early cytokine response may aid the clearance of organisms and limit infection in the host. On the other hand, a late cytokine response may amplify the destructiveness of an established infection.

Clinical Presentation and Differential Diagnosis

Acute bacterial arthritis is most commonly monoarticular. Polyarticular infection occurs in 5 to 8 percent of pediatric cases and in 10 to 19 percent of adult nongonococcal cases.[31,32] The differential diagnosis of acute monoarthritis overlaps with many causes of polyarthritis because virtually any arthritic disorder can initially present as a single swollen joint. The three main etiologies to consider when a patient presents with acute monoarticular arthritis are trauma, infection, and crystal-induced synovitis such as gout or pseudogout. Less commonly, systemic inflammatory disorders such as the spondyloarthropathies can

present as acute monoarthritis. RA, systemic lupus erythematosus (SLE), and other connective tissue diseases are even less-common causes of monoarthritis.

Disseminated gonococcal infection (DGI) occurs in 1 to 3 percent of patients infected with *N. gonorrhoeae*. Gonococcal arthritis is the most common cause of acute monoarthritis in sexually active young adults. In the preantibiotic era, gonococcal arthritis was a well-recognized illness in neonates. DGI is three times more common in women than men. Patients with gonococcal joint disease typically present as one of two forms. The first is characterized by fever, shaking chills, vesiculopustular skin lesions, tenosynovitis, and polyarthralgias. Blood cultures are frequently positive, whereas synovial fluid cultures are rarely positive. *N. gonorrhoeae* can be cultured from genital, rectal, and pharyngeal sites. Tenosynovitis of multiple tendons of the wrist, fingers, ankle, and toes is a unique feature of this form of DGI and distinguishes it from other forms of infectious arthritis. In the other form of gonococcal infection, patients have purulent arthritis, most commonly of the knee, wrist, or ankle, and more than one joint can be infected simultaneously. *N. gonorrhoeae* can frequently be cultured from the synovial fluid.[33]

The classic presentation of nongonococcal septic arthritis is the acute onset of pain and swelling in a single joint. Large joints are affected most commonly. In adults, the knee is involved in more than 50 percent of cases, and hip, ankle, and shoulder infections are less common.[34] In infants and small children, hips are more often involved.[35] Patients with septic arthritis often have underlying illnesses and predispositions to infections. Many are immunocompromised, are intravenous (IV) drug abusers, have prosthetic joints, and have diseases such as neoplasia, renal failure, and RA. Table 98–2 lists the risk factors that predispose to septic arthritis.[3,5,36-38]

Most patients with bacterial arthritis are febrile, although chills are unusual. Fever may be absent in the

---

TABLE 98–2 • RISK FACTORS FOR THE DEVELOPMENT OF SEPTIC ARTHRITIS

Age older than 80 years[3]
Diabetes mellitus[3]
Presence of a prosthetic joint in the knee or the hip[3]
Recent joint surgery[3]
Skin infection[3]
Previous septic arthritis[36]
Recent intra-articular injection[5]
Human immunodeficiency virus (HIV) or acquired immune deficiency syndrome (AIDS)
Intravenous (IV) drug abuse
End-stage renal disease on hemodialysis
Advanced hepatic disease
Hemophilia with or without AIDS
Sickle cell disease
Underlying malignancy
Hypogammaglobulinemia (susceptible to mycoplasma infections)[38]
Late complement-component deficiency (susceptible to neisserial infections)[37]
Low social economic status confounded by high rate of comorbidities[36]

elderly. In children, septic arthritis is usually accompanied by fever, malaise, poor appetite, and irritability, as well as progressive reluctance to use the affected limb. Physical examination typically reveals warmth and tenderness of the affected joint, joint effusion, and limited active and passive range of motion. Septic arthritis among patients with RA has been a special challenge to clinicians because of the high incidence of infection and the poor outcome. Newer series of rheumatoid patients with septic arthritis are reported,[39] but they do not add new insights to the literature of a decade or more ago.[40-43] It is well recognized that septic arthritis in patients with RA is associated with poor joint outcome and mortality as high as 56 percent in those with polyarticular infection.[31] Does more aggressive drainage of an infected joint already damaged by rheumatoid disease result in a better outcome? How can the risk of infection in a host with RA be reduced and how can infection in a prosthetic joint of a rheumatoid patient be prevented? How can rheumatoid flare be differentiated from septic arthritis complicating rheumatoid disease? Whenever bacterial arthritis is suspected, the most important diagnostic procedure is arthrocentesis and examination of the synovial fluid. For those joints that are deep and more difficult to aspirate, ultrasound- or fluoroscopy-guided needle aspiration should be performed.

Synovial Fluid Analysis

Normal joints contain a small amount of synovial fluid that is clear, is highly viscous, and has very few white blood cells (WBCs). The protein concentration is approximately one-third that of plasma, and the glucose concentration is similar to that of plasma. Infected fluid is usually purulent, with an elevated leukocyte count, usually greater than 50,000 WBC/mm^3 and often exceeding 100,000 WBC/mm^3, composed of mainly neutrophils. Synovial fluid levels of glucose, lactate dehydrogenase, and total protein are of limited value in the diagnosis of septic arthritis. Although a low synovial fluid glucose (less than 40 mg/dl or less than half the serum glucose concentration) and an elevated lactate dehydrogenase are suggestive of bacterial infection, they are not sufficiently sensitive or specific for the diagnosis of septic arthritis.[44] Figure 98–2 shows the algorithm for synovial fluid analysis and Table 98–3 is the differential diagnosis of septic arthritis and lists the known causes of pseudoseptic arthritis.[5,45,46]

A definite diagnosis of bacterial arthritis can only be made by visualizing bacteria on a Gram-stained smear or by culturing bacteria from the synovial fluid. In patients not previously treated with antibiotics, synovial fluid cultures are positive in 70 to 90 percent of cases of nongonococcal bacterial arthritis.[47,48] Blood cultures are positive in 40 to 50 percent of cases of septic arthritis and are the only method of identifying the pathogen in about 10 percent of cases. An extra-articular site of infection offers a clue to the etiologic organism infecting the joint. Examples include septic arthritis in association with pneumococcal pneumonia, Escherichia coli urinary tract infection, or cellulitis due to staphylococci

or streptococci. Gram-positive cocci are identified in 50 to 75 percent of synovial fluid Gram-stained smears, but gram-negative bacilli are identified less than 50 percent of the time in culture-proven cases.[48]

Culture for N. gonorrhoeae is almost always negative in skin lesions and is positive in less than 50 percent of synovial fluids and in less than one third of blood cultures. This may be the result of the fastidious growth requirements of N. gonorrhoeae, but the organism can be easily recovered from other sites (i.e., the genitourinary tract). Alternatively, immune response to the organism or its components may be responsible for some of the clinical manifestations of DGI. Thus, the tenosynovitis and dermatitis associated with DGI may not yield viable organisms. Polymerase chain reaction (PCR) techniques have detected gonococcal DNA in the synovial fluid of some culture-negative cases of suspected gonococcal arthritis.[49,50]

When culturing the synovial fluid, it should be brought directly to the laboratory and placed on conventional broth and solid media or into aerobic and anaerobic blood culture bottles. Inoculating blood culture bottles with 5 to 10 ml of joint fluid or smaller volumes into isolator tubes may increase the yield of positive cultures beyond that of standard techniques.[51,52] Synovial fluid culture using the BACTEC Peds Plus/F bottle and the BACTEC 9240 instrument Becton Dickonson Diagnostic Instrument Systems, Sparks, Md.detected significantly more pathogens and fewer contaminants than culture by the agar-plate method.[53]

Microbiology

Table 98–4 breaks down the organisms that cause joint infections according to the age of the patient and whether the joint is native or prosthetic.[54] Overall, S. aureus is the most common etiologic agent among children of all age-groups, followed by group A streptococci and S. pneumoniae. Neonates and infants less than 2 months old are more susceptible to group B streptococcus and gram-negative enteric bacilli than older children. Rarely, Pseudomonas species, N. gonorrhoeae, and Candida albicans may be responsible in the very young. Since the introduction of the Haemophilus influenzae type b, (Hib), vaccine, the incidence of septic arthritis due to Haemophilus influenzae has declined dramatically.[55,56] In sexually active adolescents, N. gonorrhoeae must be considered.[57] P. aeruginosa and Candida species are potential pathogens in adolescent IV drug abusers. Patients with sickle cell anemia are prone to develop Salmonella arthritis, and immunocompromised children are at higher risk for infection with gram-negative bacilli. Other unusual joint pathogens in children include Neisseria meningitidis, anaerobes, Brucella Species, and Kingella kingae.

The organisms causing nongonococcal septic arthritis in adults are 75 to 80 percent gram-positive cocci and 15 to 20 percent gram-negative bacilli.[58] S. aureus is the most common organism in both native and prosthetic joint infections. Staphylococcus epidermidis is common in prosthetic joint infections but is a rare cause of native joint infections. The streptococci, including

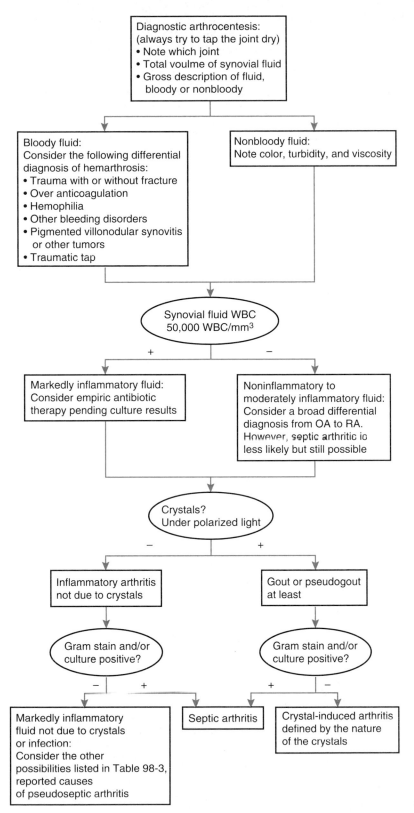

FIGURE 98–2 · Algorithm for Synovial Fluid Analysis in Septic Arthritis.

S. pneumoniae, are the next most common group of gram-positive aerobes. *Streptococcus pyogenes* is followed by groups B, G, C, and F in frequency. Patients with non–group A streptococcal disease often have comorbidities such as immunosuppression, diabetes mellitus, malignancy, and severe genitourinary or gastrointestinal infections.[59] Group B streptococcal arthritis in adults is uncommon, but it can be a serious infection in adult diabetics and patients with late prosthetic hip infections.[60] Aggressive polyarthritis due to group B streptococci resulted in serious functional damage and permanent morbidity.[61,62] Patients predisposed to gram-negative bacillary infections include those with a history of IV drug abuse, who are at extremes of age, or

TABLE 98–3 • DIFFERENTIAL DIAGNOSIS OF SEPTIC ARTHRITIS OR REPORTED CAUSES OF PSEUDOSEPTIC ARTHRITIS[*,5,45,46]

Partially treated septic arthritis
Rheumatoid arthritis (RA)
Juvenile rheumatoid arthritis (JRA)
Gout
Pseudogout
Apatite-related arthropathy
Reiter's syndrome
Psoriatic arthritis (PsA)
Systemic lupus erythematosus (SLE)
Sickle cell disease
Dialysis-related amyloidosis
Transient synovitis of the hip
Plant thorn synovitis
Metastatic carcinoma
Pigmented villonodular synovitis
Hemarthrosis
Neuropathic arthropathy
Synovitis following injection of hylan

[*]Extremely inflammatory synovitis with negative culture is referred to as pseudoseptic arthritis. Typically, synovial fluid analysis shows 50,000 white blood cells (WBC)/mm³ or greater. Often the WBC count exceeds 100,000 WBC/mm³.

who are immunocompromised.[63] The most common gram-negative organisms are *E. coli* and *P. aeruginosa*.

Anaerobes account for 5 to 7 percent of septic arthritis.[1,3,47] Common anaerobes include *Bacteroides* species, *Proprionibacterium acnes*, and various anaerobic gram-positive cocci. Predisposing factors include wound infections, joint arthroplasty, and immunocompromised hosts. Foul-smelling synovial fluid or air in the joint space should raise the suspicion of anaerobic infection, and appropriate cultures should be obtained and held for at least 2 weeks. Anaerobes and coagulase-negative staphylococci are more common in prosthetic joint infections.

Polyarticular septic arthritis is much less common than monoarticular infection.[31,64] Many of the patients have one or more comorbidity, and some have been IV drug abusers. Its occurrence is high in patients with RA and averages 25 percent (ranging from 18 to 35 percent).[65] Although *S. aureus* is the most common pathogen, group G streptococci, *H. influenzae*, *S. pneumoniae*, or mixed aerobic and anaerobic bacteria have been responsible for polyarticular infections. Involvement of more than one joint can also occur in certain patient populations, such as neonates and patients with sickle cell anemia, or with certain organisms such as *N. gonorrhoeae*, *N. meningitidis*, and *Salmonella* species.[66]

Polymicrobial (two or more bacterial species) polyarticular (two or more joints) septic arthritis is a rare clinical entity. Large joints are usually affected. Among five reported cases, the knee was affected in four cases (bilaterally in two); elbow and wrist in three; and the shoulder in two. The mean number of joints infected was three. Bacteremia was present in all but one case (80 percent) and always involved the same organisms that were in the synovial fluids. Most bacterial species isolated were the usual organisms seen in septic arthritis. Combinations of gram-positive aerobic and anaerobic organisms were

TABLE 98–4 • ETIOLOGIC ORGANISMS CAUSING JOINT INFECTION IN VARIOUS HOSTS[54]

Adults	Children = 5 yr old	Children > 5 yr old	Neonates	Prosthetic
Common	*Common*		*Common*	*Common*
Staphylococcus aureus Streptococcus pneumoniae	S. aureus, Haemophilus influenzae[*]	S. aureus Group A streptococcus	S. aureus Group B streptococcus	Coagulase-negative staphylococci Staphylococcus aureus
β-Hemolytic streptococci (mainly Lancefield groups A, G, and B)	Group A streptococcus Streptococcus pneumoniae		Enterobacteriaceae	
Neisseria gonorrhoeae				
Enterobacteriaceae (age older than 60 or predisposing condition)				
Salmonella spp				
	Adolescent (sexually active) Neisseria gonorrhoeae			
Rare	*Rare*		*Rare*	*Less common*
Pseudomonas spp	Salmonella spp		Pseudomonas spp	Corynebacteria spp
Mycobacterium tuberculosis	H. influenzae		H. influenzae	Enterococci and streptococci
Haemophilus influenzae	N. meningitidis		N. gonorrhoeae	Pseudomonas aeruginosa
Neisseria meningitidis	N. gonorrhoeae			Enterobacteriaceae
Pasteurella spp	Kingella kingae			Propronibacterium spp
Anaerobes	M. tuberculosis			Other anaerobes
Mycoplasma/Ureaplasma	B. burgdorferi			Candida spp.
Fungi (Sporothrix, dimorphic fungi, Cryptococcus)				M. tuberculosis
Borrelia burgdorferi				

[*]Rare in children immunized with Hib vaccine.

Adapted with permission from Atkins BL, Bowler IC: The diagnosis of large joint sepsis. J Hosp Infect 40:263-274, 1998.

common. A characteristic of most cases (80 percent) was the extension of locally destructive processes due to the contiguous spread of infection from the affected joints, such as osteomyelitis, fasciitis with compartment syndrome, and abscess or sinus tract formation. Systemic complications, including septic shock, multi-organ failure and toxic-shock syndrome were noted in 60 percent of cases. The mortality rate of polymicrobial polyarticular septic arthritis in this small series was 60 percent.[67]

Unusual organisms are continuously being reported as causes of septic arthritis, and a few noteworthy examples are listed here. *Achromobacter xylosoxidans*, an opportunistic, gram-negative, flagellated bacillus, was cultured from the blood and knee fluid of a 41-year-old woman with SLE.[68] *Moraxella catarrhalis* was isolated from the blood of a 41-year-old man with presumed DGI and septic arthritis.[69] Another gram-negative diplococcus, *N. meningitidis*, was the cause of a septic knee in a 32-year-old human immunodeficiency virus (HIV)-negative homosexual man.[70] *Corynebacterium xerosis* was isolated from the left knee of a 74-year-old man several weeks following vascular surgery for popliteal artery aneurysm in the same limb.[71] Group G-2 coryneform microorganism was responsible for endocarditis and septic arthritis of a wrist joint in a 52-year-old woman with cutaneous SLE complicated by extensive desquamation and palmoplantar erythema with bullae formation.[72] A case of spondylodiscitis caused by *Streptococcus equisimilis* was reported in a healthy 37-year-old man with no history of exposure to animals.[73] Finally, a fatal case of *Vibrio vulnificus* presented as septic arthritis in a man with underlying liver disease.[74]

Imaging

Plain radiographs in septic arthritis are usually normal early in the course of the infection, but baseline films should be obtained to look for evidence of other disease and contiguous osteomyelitis. Radiographs often demonstrate nonspecific changes of inflammatory arthritis, including periarticular osteopenia, joint effusion, soft tissue swelling, and joint-space loss. In more advanced infection, periosteal reaction, marginal or central erosions, and destruction of subchondral bone may be seen. Bony ankylosis is a late sequela of septic arthritis. Dislocation or subluxation of the femoral head is unique to hip infection of neonates.[35]

Ultrasound of the hip is the modality of choice to detect fluid collections in this deep joint and can serve as a guide in its aspiration. Ultrasound can be similarly used in other joints such as the popliteal cyst of the knee, shoulder, acromioclavicular (AC), or sternoclavicular Sternoclavicular, (SC), joints. Triple-phase bone scan using technetium-99 is often done in children to identify an associated metaphyseal osteomyelitis or avascular necrosis of the femoral head. Whole-body bone scan is preferred in young children because, despite focal symptoms, septic arthritis and ostemyelitis may be multifocal in this age-group.[75] In septic arthritis of all age-groups, the periarticular distribution of increased uptake is seen both on the early "blood-pool" phase and the delayed images of the joint. Bone scans, however, only provide nonspecific information and cannot differentiate septic from noninfectious causes of joint inflammation. Therefore, a suggestive bone scan must be interpreted in the proper clinical context and supported by microbiologic data for a definitive diagnosis of joint or bone infection.

In joints that are difficult to evaluate otherwise or that have complex anatomic structures, computed tomography (CT) and magnetic resonance imaging (MRI) can provide useful images to delineate the extent of the infection.[76] MRI is highly sensitive in early detection of joint fluid and is superior to CT in the delineation of soft tissue structures. These images can demonstrate early bone erosion, reveal soft tissue extension, and facilitate arthrocentesis of joints such as shoulders, hips, AC,[77] SC, and SI, as well as facet joints of the spine.

Treatment

Treatment of septic arthritis must begin immediately once the clinical evaluation is complete and all appropriate cultures taken. A serious clinical suspicion of a joint infection warrants the initiation of antibiotic therapy before culture confirmation is available. Delays in treatment allow the infection to become more established in the joint and damage permanently the articular cartilage. Untreated, there is the opportunity for the joint infection to spread to other body sites via the hematogenous route and become more widespread and more difficult to cure.

The principles of treatment of an infected joint, either natural or prosthetic, follow those of treatment of an infected body cavity in which antibiotics must be used in conjunction with adequate drainage of the infected closed space. In the case of an infected prosthesis, the foreign material will often need to be removed before complete eradication of the infection can be achieved. The clinical circumstances and the preliminary laboratory data aid the selection of antibiotic agents. Host factors, any extra-articular sites of infection and the Gram-stained smear of the synovial fluid are the best early guides for the antibiotic agents with which to start. Table 98–5 lists antibiotic agents for adults[78-82] and Table 98–6 lists agents for children.[66] Narrow antibiotic coverage is indicated if gram-positive cocci are found in the synovial fluid and the clinician suspects a primary source of staphylococcal infection from the skin. Appropriate monotherapy in this case may be a penicillinase-resistant penicillin or vancomycin if methicillin resistance is likely. If gram-negative bacilli are noted in the synovial fluid and the patient has a kidney infection, specific agents (e.g., ampicillin or a cephalosporin) against *E. coli* and other common urinary tract pathogens may be used. In an otherwise healthy sexually active person, tenosynovitis of a wrist follows 2 days of migratory joint pain, and the Gram-stained smear of the wrist fluid reveals no visible bacteria. Initiating monotherapy in this patient with penicillin or ceftriaxone against gonococcal infection is appropriate after culturing all portals of possible infec-

TABLE 98–5 • ANTIBIOTIC AGENTS USED IN ADULTS[78-82]

Synovial Fluid Gram Stain	Organism	Antibiotic	Dose
Gram-positive cocci (clusters)	*Staphylococcus aureus* (methicillin-sensitive)	Nafcillin/oxacillin or	2 g IV q4hr
		cefazolin	1-2 g IV q8hr
	Staphylococcus aureus (methicillin-resistant)	Vancomycin or	1 g IV q12
		clindamycin or	900 mg IV q8hr
		linezolid	600 mg IV q12hr
Gram-positive cocci (chains)	*Streptococcus* species	Nafcillin or	2 g IV q4hr
		penicillin or	2 million units IV q4hr
		cefazolin	1-2 g IV q8hr
Gram-negative diplococci	*Neisseria gonorrhoeae*	Ceftriaxone or	2 g IV q24hr
		cefotaxime or	1 g IV q8hr
		ciprofloxacin	400 mg IV q12hr
Gram-negative bacilli	Enterobacteriaceae (*E. coli*, Proteus, Serratia)	Ceftriaxone or	2 g IV q24hr
		cefotaxime	2 g IV q8hr
	Pseudomonas species	Cefepime or	2 g IV q12hr
		piperacillin or	3 gIV q6hr
		imipenem plus	500 mg IV q6hr
		gentamicin	7 mg/kg IV q24hr
Polymicrobial infection	*S. aureus, Streptococcu,* gram-negative bacilli	Nafcillin/Oxacillin plus	2 g IV q4hr
		ceftriaxone or	2 g IV q24hr
		cefotaxime or	2 g IV q8hr
		ciprofloxacin	400 mg IV q12hr
		If penicillin allergic, Vancomycin plus 3rd-generation cephalosporin or ciprofloxacin	

tion. However, in an elderly, debilitated patient with an acute monoarthritis, if the Gram-stained smear of the synovial fluid is nonrevealing, and no clue is found after searching for an extra-articular source of infection, broad antibiotic coverage against a wide variety of organisms should be given initially. A typical regimen includes an antistaphylococcal agent, an aminoglycoside against gram-negative bacilli and an antipseudomonal penicillin or a third-generation cephalosporin.

Once the identity and the sensitivities of the organism are known, antibiotic therapy should continue with the most efficacious agent that has the best safety profile and the lowest cost. The parenteral route of antibiotic administration is the preferred initial treatment. Continued antibiotic therapy may be switched to oral agents if adequate blood levels can be achieved and maintained by this route. There is no evidence that the direct intra-articular instillation of drugs is necessary or preferable in septic arthritis because there is no barrier

against the free diffusion of antibiotic agents from the blood to the synovial fluid. In cases where uncertainty exists, serum and synovial fluid levels of antibiotic drugs can be measured to ensure that therapeutic levels are reached.

Drainage of the infected joint space must be adequate to relieve pain, eradicate the infection, and hasten recovery of lost function. During the initial few days, immobilization of the affected joint and effective analgesic medication will ensure patient comfort. Physical therapy, starting with passive then graduating to active motion, should be instituted as soon as the patient can tolerate mobilization of the inflamed joint. Repeated needle aspirations may prove adequate in those patients in whom sterilization of the joint space can be achieved rapidly. In most instances, a trial with needle aspirations is warranted, unless there is an urgency to decompress the infected joint because of compromised blood flow to the adjacent bone (e.g., the hip).[83] However, if needle aspira-

TABLE 98–6 · ANTIBIOTIC AGENTS USED IN CHILDREN[66]

Age	Likely Pathogen	Antibiotic	Dosage mg/kg/day	doses/day
Neonate	Staphylococcus aureus Group B streptococcus gram-negative bacilli	Nafcillin plus cefotaxime or gentamicin	100 150 5-7.5	4 3 3
Child < 5 yr old	Staphylococcus aureus Haemophilus influenzae[*] Group A streptococcus Streptococcus pneumoniae	Nafcillin[†] plus cefotaxime or ceftriaxone or cefuroxime	150 100-150 50 150-200	4 3-4 1-2 3-4
Child > 5 yr old	Staphylococcus aureus Group A streptococcus	Nafcillin[b] or cefazolin	150 50	4 3-4
Adolescent (sexually active)	Previous organisms Neisseria gonorrhoeae	ceftriaxone	50	1-2

[*]Decreased incidence in children fully immunized with Hib vaccine.
[†]If patient is penicillin allergic, alternatives include vancomycin (40 mg/kg/day divided into four doses) or clindamycin (20 to 40 mg/kg/day divided into four doses).

Adapted with permission from Gutierrez KM: Infectious and inflammatory arthritis. *In* Long SL, Pickering LK, Prober CG (eds): Principles and Practice of Pediatric Infectious Diseases. New York, Churchill Livingstone, 1997, pp 537-545.

tion is technically difficult or does not provide thorough drainage of the joint, if sterilization of the joint fluid is delayed, if the infected joint is already damaged by pre-existing rheumatoid disease, or if infected synovial tissue or bone needs débridement, surgical drainage should be considered sooner rather than later. Tidal lavage to wash out the joint and arthroscopic procedures are intermediate steps that may benefit some patients and help avoid the morbidity of arthrotomy. Involving the orthopedic surgeon and the physical therapist early on in the course of treatment will facilitate the best choice of drainage procedure and result in the best functional outcome.

The optimal duration of antibiotic treatment has not been prospectively studied. For native joint infections, antibiotic administration can be as brief as 2 weeks for uncomplicated infection by susceptible microorganisms. However, the treatment duration is typically more prolonged, between 4 and 6 weeks, for more serious infection in the compromised host. For prosthetic joint infections, the antibiotic course is usually quite protracted. In most cases of late prosthetic joint infection, the prosthesis is removed and antibiotic treatment is continued until the site is sterile before reimplantation is considered.

Prognosis

In the 21st century, patients with septic arthritis as a group are becoming older, with more risk factors for infection and more comorbidities. The number of patients with prosthetic joints is increasing as the population of older patients grows and people live longer. Therefore, it is not surprising to see more cases of infection in total joint replacements. However, the

organisms have not changed significantly. Staphylococci (44 to 66 percent) are still the dominant organism followed by streptococci (18 to 28 percent) and gram-negative bacilli (9 to 19 percent).[84] The emerging challenges in the treatment of septic arthritis are how to improve outcome, how to deal with resistant organisms, and how to overcome host factors that portend a poor prognosis.

The outcome of the treatment of septic arthritis can be measured as mortality, as the functional outcome of the infected joint, or as short-term and long-term outcomes. Certainly death from the infection is a poor outcome. Among the survivors, loss of articular cartilage, loss of motion, or increase in pain in the affected joint would be considered poor functional outcomes. Loss of the limb to infection or need for surgery to fuse the joint or restore function are also poor outcomes. Most studies report the outcome at the time of hospital discharge, and long-term data on adults with septic arthritis are not available. For example, the rate of development of degenerative joint disease, the rate of relapse or recurrence of infection, and the rate of progression of functional impairment in the affected joint over time have not been well studied.

Many retrospective studies have characterized features that may increase the chance of a poor outcome at the time of hospital discharge[36,42,64,85-87] (Table 98–7). One prospective community-based study of adults and children found poor joint outcome in 33 percent of survivors among 154 patients with bacterial arthritis and noted older age, preexisting joint disease, and an infected joint containing synthetic material as negative prognostic factors by univariate analysis.[87] These investigators noted no association between poor outcome

TABLE 98–7 • FACTORS THAT MAY PORTEND A POOR OUTCOME IN SEPTIC ARTHRITIS[36,42,64,85-87]

Older age
Preexisting arthritis, especially rheumatoid arthritis (RA) but also osteoarthritis (OA) and tophaceous gout
Presence of synthetic material (i.e., total joint replacement)
Delay in diagnosis or long duration of symptoms before seeking medical attention
Polyarticular infection, especially if more than three joints (four to nine) and small hand joints are affected
Presence of bacteremia
Infection caused by virulent or difficult to treat organisms (e.g., Staphylococcus aureus, Pseudomonas aeruginosa or some gram-negative bacilli)
Patients receiving immunosuppressive therapy
Serious underlying comorbidities (e.g., liver, kidney, or heart diseases)
Peripheral leukocytosis at presentation
Worsening renal function

and young age, comorbidity, immunosuppressive medication, functional class, multiple infected joints, type of organism, or treatment delay.

Some Unique Aspects of Specific Joints

The shoulder joint is not as commonly infected (3 to 12 percent) as the large, lower extremity joints (61 to 79 percent). Most septic hip joints are surgically drained, and many infected knees are drained by repeated needle aspirations without need for surgery. However, the optimal means of draining the shoulder joint is more controversial. Good results have been achieved with repeated needle aspirations if the diagnosis of septic arthritis is not delayed. However, if there has been a long duration of infection before treatment is initiated or if there is underlying arthritis before the infection, immediate surgical drainage may provide a better outcome.[88-90] Therefore, arthroscopic drainage or arthrotomy should be considered when treating a patient with a septic shoulder who has underlying arthritis in that joint, who has experienced long delay in diagnosis, or if needle aspirations fail to adequately drain the shoulder.

The facet joints throughout the spine may become infected, causing pain in the neck to the low back.[6,91] Infection of the symphysis pubis can cause pelvic or lower abdominal pain. The SI joint is a deep joint that is partially lined by synovial membrane. Patients with bacterial arthritis of the SI joint usually present with symptoms of back and buttock pain that mimic a herniated disk or muscular strain.[91-93] Focal tenderness over the buttock and SI area, limited straight-leg raising, and pain with pelvic compression are often present. Fever is present in 40 to 60 percent of cases, and blood cultures are positive in 60 percent. Because symptoms are poorly localized, delays in diagnosis are common. Scintigraphy, MRI, or CT scans are useful in detecting and localizing the site of infection. Whereas percutaneous joint aspira-

tion may be attempted, open biopsy is often necessary to obtain joint fluid and isolate the pathogen.

Infection of the manubriosternal joint is an uncommon cause of pathology at this site.[94] The AC[77] and SC[91] joints are unusual sites of bacterial infection. Septic arthritis of these sites is most often seen in IV drug abusers, dialysis patients, diabetics, and patients with RA. Infection of the AC joint should be suspected in a patient who presents with shoulder pain, and ultrasound of the glenohumeral joint is normal. A common complaint of SC joint infection is anterior chest discomfort. On physical examination there may be obvious swelling over the joint with restricted range of motion of the shoulder. CT is the most sensitive technique to visualize early changes in the joint and document the extent of infection. Approximately 20 percent of patients with SC joint septic arthritis develop an abscess of the chest wall or intrathoracic extrapleural space, which should be drained.[91]

The temporomandibular joint (TMJ) is another uncommon location for septic arthritis and is very rare in children. There have been five cases of TMJ septic arthritis in children and 20 cases in adults. S. aureus is the most common organism in both age-groups. In adults, N. gonorrhoeae is also an important pathogen. The organisms in 22 reported cases of TMJ infection were S. aureus (9 patients), two each for N. gonorrhoeae and Proteus mirabilis, one each for S. pyogenes, Staphylococcus albus, Enterococcus species, Peptostreptococcus species and five patients with unknown pathogens.[95] Common symptoms are pain on moving the jaw, limitation of jaw opening, facial swelling, malocclusion, and contralateral mandibular deviation. In some cases needle aspiration is sufficient to drain the TMJ. However, surgical irrigation and débridement are often necessary.[95,96] Complications include spread of infection, postinfectious changes, and fibrous or bony ankylosis of the TMJ.

Animal Bites and Zoogenesis

In the United States, more than 5 million people are bitten by animals each year. Dogs (85 percent) and cats (10 percent) cause the majority of these bites.[97] Bites that extend into the tendons and joint spaces or bones may be complicated by tenosynovitis and septic arthritis or osteomyelitis, respectively. Organisms most likely to cause infection in dog or cat bites include Pasturella multocida, S. aureus, streptococci, and anaerobes. P. multocida is more prevalent in a cat's oral flora (70 to 90 percent) and is the major pathogen isolated from cat bites. Dog bites have the lowest infection rate of all mammalian bites, and with good local care infection only occurs in 2 to 5 percent of bite cases. However, due to the sharp, slender teeth of cats, higher carriage rate of P. multocida, and more frequent involvement of tendons and joints, the infection rate from a cat bite is higher (30 to 50 percent).[98,99] P. multocida infection is characterized by the rapid development of localized cellulitis and purulent discharge within 24 hours of the injury in 70 percent of cases and within 48 hours in 90 percent of patients who develop an infection. Wounds in proximity to bones or joints may be associated with septic arthritis, osteomyelitis, or tenosynovitis.

Other mammalian pets that inflict bites include mice, rats, hamsters, gerbils, guinea pigs, and rabbits. Most pets carry *Salmonella* species and *Campylobacter* species. Rabbits also carry *P. multocida*. Rats carry *Spirillium minus* and *Streptobacillus moniliformis*. Rat bite fever due to *S. moniliformis* may be due to a rat bite or to exposure to contaminated milk or water. It is characterized by fever, maculopapular or petechial rash, and arthritis of the large joints. Cases of knee and hip infections have responded to penicillin or cephalosporin plus drainage.[100]

Brucellosis caused by infection with *Brucella* species is a contagious disease of animals (zoonosis) that is transmittable to humans.[101] In the United States, there are less than 100 cases reported each year. Four of the six species are human pathogens (*B. abortus, B, melitensis, B. suis,* and *B. canis*). Humans contract the disease by direct contact with infected animals, their secretions, or their carcasses. Individuals at risk include farmers, veterinarians, abattoir workers, meat inspectors, and laboratory personnel. Another way to contract the disease is by ingesting unpasteurized infected milk or milk products (e.g., goat cheese). Brucellosis presents with nonspecific symptoms of fever, malaise, night sweats, anorexia, weight loss, arthralgia, myalgia, abdominal pain, and headache. These symptoms begin 2 to 4 weeks after exposure and are accompanied by lympadenopathy and hepatosplenomegaly. Arthritis, spondylitis, osteomyelitis, tenosynovitis, and bursitis are osteoarticular complications of brucellosis and have been reported in 20 to 60 percent of cases.[102] Arthritis is the predominant manifestation in children and affects the large peripheral joints, such as knees, hips, and ankles.[103] In contrast, sacroiliitis predominates in adults with brucellosis.[104] Synovial fluids show a predominance of mononuclear cells and the organism is recovered in about half of the cases. Isolation of *Brucella* species from blood, bone marrow, or other tissue establishes a definitive diagnosis.[105] A presumptive diagnosis can be made by serologic testing.

▌ Prosthetic-Joint Infections

Total joint replacement for advanced arthritis is one of the major advances in medicine in the 20th century. Infection of prosthetic joints is an uncommon but devastating complication of joint replacement surgery. Approximately 600,000 joint replacements are done each year in the United States, with an infection rate between 1 and 3 percent.[106] The infection rate is much higher in patients undergoing reimplantation because of infection of the initial prosthesis.

Prosthetic joint infections are divided into early onset (< three 3 months after placement) and late onset (> 3 months after placement). Early infections are usually related to surgical contamination at the time of the implantation, whereas late infections usually result from hematogenous seeding of the joint. In the former case, *S. epidermidis* is the predominant pathogen, whereas

S. aureus accounts for most late infections. The risk of infection is related to a number of factors. In a retrospective study of 462 infected orthopedic implants, the most important risks for infection included 1) a surgical-site infection at a site other than the prosthesis (odds ratio 35.9); 2) a score of 2 on the National Nosocomial Infections Surveillance System surgical patient risk index (odds ratio 3.9); 3) the presence of a malignancy (odds ratio 3.1); and 4) a history of joint arthroplasty (odds ratio 2.0).[107] Certain patient populations are at increased risk of infection because of comorbid conditions (e.g., diabetes mellitus and RA).

Orthopedic implants adversely affect host defenses. Prosthetic devices impair opsonic activity and diminish neutrophils' ability to kill bacteria.[108] Second, polymorphonuclear leukocytes release lysosomal enzymes and superoxide into the area surrounding the prosthesis, resulting in tissue damage and local devascularization.[109] Third, phagocytes may be focused on removal of the foreign body such that fewer cells are available to fight infection.[110] Finally, polymethylmethacrylate bone cement can inhibit both neutrophil and complement functions, and the heat produced by the polymerization of polymethylmethacrylate can damage adjacent cortical bone and result in a devascularized necrotic area, which is ideal for bacterial growth. Following implantation, prosthetic joints are immediately coated by host proteins, including albumin, fibrinogen, and fibronectin. It is not surprising, therefore, that *S. aureus*, which possesses a number of host-protein binding receptors (MSCRAMMs) is the most common pathogen in late-onset infection of prosthetic joints.

Another phenomenon critical to development of infection is the ability of organisms to form biofilms on the surface of the prosthetic device. A biofilm is defined as "an assemblage of microbial cells that is irreversibly associated with a surface and enclosed in a matrix of primarily polysaccharide material."[111] Biofilm formation is a natural process. Organisms grow on indwelling medical devices, potable water system pipes, and living tissues. *S. epidermidis* is particularly adept at attaching to and forming biofilms on foreign bodies such as prosthetic joints. Small numbers of these organisms from the patient's skin or mucous membranes, or from the hands of the surgeons or clinical staff, contaminate and colonize the orthopedic device at the time of implantation. Staphylococcal surface proteins, SSP-1 and SSP-2, are fimbria-like polymers that facilitate adherence of *S. epidermidis* to polystyrene.[112] *S. epidermidis* produces a polysaccharide/adhesin (PS/A) substance critical to the formation of this extracellular matrix known as slime. PS/A mutants have been shown to be less virulent than the wild-type strain in a rabbit model of endocarditis.[113]

Organisms existing in biofilms are much more resistant to antimicrobial agents because the drugs have difficulty penetrating the biofilm layer. The biofilm-associated organisms also grow much more slowly than organisms in suspension. As a result, antimicrobial agents such as penicillins and cephalosporins, which act on rapidly dividing organisms, are not very effective in treating device-related infections. Rifampin and ciprofloxacin, on the other hand, may be more effective because they are active against organisms in the stationary phase of growth.[114,115] Recent research efforts have focused on ways to exploit this natural phenomenon of biofilm formation. The field of probiotics utilizes nonpathogenic bacteria to compete with pathogenic organisms. In the case of prosthetic devices, coating of polymers with *Lactobacillus acidophilus* decreases the adherence of *S. epidermidis* and *E. coli* to surfaces of prosthetic material.[116] The mechanism of action appears to be competition and interference with adhesion.

Treatment of late prosthetic joint infections requires a combination of antibiotics with the removal of the orthopedic device. Failure to remove the infected prosthesis is associated with an unacceptably high rate of relapse, probably related to biofilm formation on the orthopedic implant. Removal of the joint prosthesis, débridement of infected bone, and placement of a new prosthesis during the same operation is associated with a high rate of recurrence of infection.[117,118] The treatment of choice is a two-stage process involving 1) removal of the infected prosthesis and débridement of infected bone; 2) stabilization of the joint using an antibiotic-impregnated methylmethacrylate spacer; 3) 6 weeks of IV antibiotics; followed by 4) reimplantation of a second orthopedic implant.[119] Using this approach the success rate is approximately 80 to 90 percent. Rarely, antibiotic treatment is continued indefinitely in the patient in whom the risk of removing the infected prosthesis is too great, the prosthesis is not loose, and the organism responsible for the infection can be reasonably suppressed by the use of an oral antibiotic agent.

In summary, the pathogenesis of bacterial infection in native and prosthetic joints is complex. There are anatomic, virulence, and host factors. An understanding of these interactions may lead to novel therapeutic and preventive strategies such as vaccines against capsule antigens or surface adhesins in patients undergoing elective joint replacements.

Prevention of Prosthetic-Joint Infection

There is consensus that preoperative evaluation of the patient for occult infection, such as periodontal disease or bacteriuria, is warranted, and corrective steps to eradicate any infection are essential before joint replacement. There is also consensus that perioperative antibiotic prophylaxis significantly reduces the rate of early postoperative infection, and this practice is routine. However, the role of antibiotic prophylaxis to prevent late prosthetic-joint infection prior to diagnostic or therapeutic procedures that lead to transient bacteremia, especially dental treatment, is highly controversial.

In 1997, the American Dental Association and the American Academy of Orthopedic Surgeons jointly published an advisory on antibiotic prophylaxis for dental patients with total joint replacements.[120] It stated that antibiotic prophylaxis is not routinely indicated for most dental patients with total joint replacements. However, all patients with a total joint replacement within 2 years of the implant procedure, and some immunocompromised patients with total joint replacements who may be at higher risk for hematogenous infections, should be considered to receive antibiotic prophylaxis before undergoing dental procedures with a higher bacteremic risk. Other orthopedic and oral and maxillofacial surgeons have argued that there is "no scientific evidence to support the view that patients with arthroplasties, even in the high-risk groups, require antibiotic prophylaxis during dental treatment."[121]

Professional societies take opposing positions citing evidence from clinical experience, descriptive studies, and reports of expert committees.[122-124] Surveys of physicians and dentists have shown that most are in favor of the use of antibiotic prophylaxis prior to bacteremia-producing procedures to prevent prosthetic joint infection.[125-127] Proponents feel the prevention of prosthetic joint infection is analogous to the prevention of bacterial endocarditis.[128] Other reasons are fear of litigation and previous experience of dealing with the catastrophe of a late prosthetic-joint infection. Opponents to prophylactic antibiotic use cite the lack of data to support a clear-cut relationship between transient bacteremia and infection of a prosthetic joint. Others object because of the concern for antibiotic resistance in bacteria from the excessive use of antibiotics and the cost and consequences of unnecessary drug use. There is no data from randomized controlled trials, cohort or case-control studies, or multiple time series with or without the intervention. In the absence of good evidence-based data, opting for antibiotic for the purpose of prophylaxis is not an unreasonable choice of the well informed.[129]

The incidence of late infection of a prosthetic joint as a result of procedure-related bacteremia is extremely low, between 10 to 100 cases per 100,000 patients with total joint replacement per year. The cost of providing antibiotic prophylaxis to all patients with prosthetic joints before all procedures that are associated with transient bacteremia is substantial. The efficacy of such antibiotic prophylaxis is unknown. Cost-effective analyses have shown mixed results.[130-133] These discrepancies are due to the lack of reliable data and the different assumptions used in the calculations. In the patient with the greatest risk of infection, an invasive procedure that leads to bacteremia can sometimes result in an infected total joint replacement. Counseling these patients on the risks and benefits of antibiotic prophylaxis will lead to an informed decision that the patient and the doctor can agree on.[45]

Arthritis Secondary to Bacterial Components

Reactive arthritis must be distinguished from postinfectious arthritis, which is a sterile synovitis that fol-

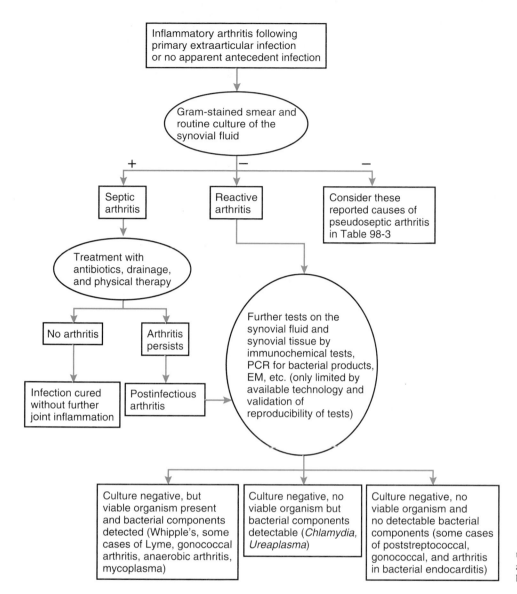

FIGURE 98–3 · Algorithm for the evaluation and classification of arthritis associated with bacteria or bacterial components.

lows treated and cured septic arthritis. The rate of the latter complication is not known, but it is probably rare. Clinically these two conditions differ substantially but they may share similarities in that bacterial components may be involved in the pathogenesis of the synovitis. In the case of reactive arthritis, components of *Chlamydia* and *Ureaplasma* have been detected in the synovial fluid of patients with Reiter's syndrome.[134,135] In staphylococcal septic arthritis, bacterial DNA may persist for several days after the Gram-stained smear and culture have converted to negative with treatment.[136,137] PCR techniques have also been employed to detect microbial DNA in synovial tissue and fluid from patients with RA,[138-140] a painful prosthetic joint,[141] and other infectious and postinfectious arthritis.[142] The sterile arthritis associated with gonococcal disease and the culture-negative

inflammatory arthritis associated with bacterial endocarditis may be other conditions in which bacterial components are involved in the pathogenesis. Additional examples may include poststreptococcal arthritis and reactive arthritis associated with bacterial meningitis,[143] intestinal bypass surgery, hidradenitis suppurativa, acne, cystic fibrosis, and after many bacterial, viral, and parasitic infections.[144] Speculations on the immune pathogenesis of some of these entities have existed since their clinical characterization. Figure 98–3 offers an algorithm to evaluate and classify arthritis associated with bacteria or their components. Although PCR is a very sensitive and powerful tool in molecular biology, its usefulness and cost effectiveness in the diagnosis and management of septic arthritis await further studies on the significance, reproducibility, and validation of test results.

REFERENCES

1. Kaandorp CJE, Dinant HJ, van de Laar MAFJ, et al: Incidence and sources of native and prosthetic joint infection: A community based prospective survey. Ann Rheum Dis 56:470, 1997.
2. Goldenberg DL: Bacterial arthritis. Curr Opin Rheumatol 6:394, 1994.
3. Kaandorp CJ, Van Schaardenburg D, Krijnen P, et al: Risk factors for septic arthritis in patients with joint disease: A prospective study. Arthritis Rheum 38:1819, 1995.
4. Gillespie WJ: Epidemiology in bone and joint infection. Infect Dis Clin North Am 4:361, 1990.
5. Roberts WN Jr, Hauptman HW: Joint aspiration or injection: Complications. In Rose BD (ed): UpToDate, Wellesley, Mass., UpToDate, 2002.
6. Ho G Jr.: Bacterial arthritis. Curr Opin Rheumatol 13:310, 2001.
7. Esterhai JL Jr, Gelb I: Adult septic arthritis. Orthop Clin North Am 22:503, 1991.
8. Armstrong RW, Bolding F, Joseph R: Septic arthritis following arthroscopy: Clinical syndromes and analysis of risk factors. Arthroscopy 8:213, 1992.
9. Babcock HM, Matava MJ, Fraser V: Postarthroscopy surgical site infections: Review of the literature. Clin Infect Dis 34:65, 2002.
10. Centers for Disease Control: Septic arthritis following anterior cruciate ligament reconstruction using tendon allografts-Florida and Louisiana, 2000. MMWR Morb Mortal Wkly Rep 50:1081, 2001.
11. Ram S, Mackinnon FG, Gulati S, et al: The contrasting mechanisms of serum resistance of Neisseria gonorrhoeae and group B Neisseria meningitidis. Mol Immunol 36:915, 1999.
12. Goldenberg DL, Reed JI, Rice PA: Arthritis in rabbits induced by killed Neisseria gonorrhoeae and gonococcal lipopolysaccharide. J Rheumatol 11:3, 1984.
13. Herrmann, M, Vaudaux PE, Pittet D, et al: Fibronectin, fibrinogen, and laminin act as mediators of adherence of clinical staphylococcal isolates to foreign material. J Infect Dis 158:693, 1988.
14. Patti JM, Allen BL, McGavin MJ, et al: MSCRAMM-mediated adherence of microorganisms to host tissues. Annu Rev Microbiol 48:585, 1994.
15. Patti JM, Bremell T, Krajewska-Pietrasik D, et al: The Staphylococcus aureus collagen adhesin is a virulence determinant in experimental septic arthritis. Infect Immun 62:152, 1994.
16. Greene C, McDevitt D, Francois P, et al: Adhesion properties of mutants of Staphylococcus aureus defective in fibronectin-binding proteins and studies on the expression of fnb genes. Mol Microbiol 17:1143, 1995.
17. Novick RP, Muir TW: Virulence gene regulation by peptides in staphylococci and other Gram-positive bacteria. Curr Opin Microbiol 2:40, 1999.
18. Winzer K, Williams P: Quorum sensing and the regulation of virulence gene expression in pathogenic bacteria. Int J Med Microbiol 291:131, 2001.
19. Hudson MC, Ramp WK, Nicholson NC, et al: Internalization of Staphylococcus aureus by cultured osteoblasts. Microb Pathog 19:409, 1995.
20. Gemmell CG, Goutcher SC, Reid R, et al: Role of certain virulence factors in a murine model of Staphylococcus aureus arthritis. J Med Microbiol 46:208, 1997.
21. Albus A, Arbeit RD, Lee JC: Virulence of Staphylococcus aureus mutants altered in type 5 capsule production. Infect Immun 59:1008, 1991.
22. Buxton TB, Rissing JP, Horner JA, et al: Binding of a Staphylococcus aureus bone pathogen to type I collagen. Microb Pathog 8:441, 1990.
23. Vandenesch F, Projan SJ, Kreiswirth B, et al: Agr-related sequences in Staphylococcus lugdunensis. FEMS Microbiol Lett 111:115, 1993.
24. Nilsson IM, Lee JC, Bremell T, et al: The role of staphylococcal polysaccharide microcapsule expression in septicemia and septic arthritis. Infect Immun 65:4216, 1997.
25. Shinefield H, Black S, Fattom A, et al: Use of a Staphylococcus aureus conjugate vaccine in patients receiving hemodialysis. N Engl J Med 346:491, 2002.
26. Bremell T, Tarkowski A: Preferential induction of septic arthritis and mortality by superantigen-producing staphylococci. Infect Immun 63:4185, 1995.
27. Renno T, Hahne M, MacDonald HR: Proliferation is a prerequisite for bacterial superantigen-induced T cell apoptosis in vivo. J Exp Med 181:2283, 1995.
28. Nilsson IM, Verdrengh M, Ulrich RG, et al: Protection against Staphylococcus aureus sepsis by vaccination with recombinant staphylococcal enterotoxin A devoid of superantigenicity. J Infect Dis 180:1370, 1999.
29. Kimura M, Matsukawa A, Ohkawara S, et al: Blocking of TNF-alpha and IL-1 inhibits leukocyte infiltration at early, but not at late stage of S. aureus-induced arthritis and the concomitant cartilage destruction in rabbits. Clin Immunol Immunopathol 82:18, 1997.
30. Zhao YX, Nilsson IM, Tarkowski A: The dual role of interferon-gamma in experimental Staphylococcus aureus septicemia versus arthritis. Immunology 93:80, 1998.
31. Epstein JH, Zimmermann B III, Ho G Jr: Polyarticular septic arthritis. J Rheumatol 13:1105, 1986.
32. Smith JW: Infectious arthritis. Mandel GL, Douglas RG Jr., Bennett JE (eds): Principles and Practice of Infectious Diseases, 3rd ed. New York, Churchill Livingston, 1990, pp 911-918.
33. O'Brien JP, Goldenberg DL, Rice PA: Disseminated gonococcal infection: A prospective analysis of 49 patients and a review of pathophysiology and immune mechanisms. Medicine 62:395, 1983.
34. Goldenberg DL: Septic arthritis and other infections of rheumatologic significance. Rheum Dis Clin North Am 17:149, 1991.
35. Bennet OM, Mannyak SS: Acute septic arthritis of the hip joint in infancy and childhood. Clin Orthop 281:123, 1992.
36. Gupta MN, Sturrock RD, Field M: A prospective 2-year study of 75 patients with adult-onset septic arthritis. Rheumatology Oxford 40:24, 2001.
37. Petersen BH, Lee TJ, Snyderman R, et al: Neisseria meningitidis and Neisseria gonorrhoeae bacteremia associated with C6, C7, or C8 deficiency. Ann Intern Med 90:917, 1979.
38. Franz A, Webster AD, Furr PM, et al: Mycoplasmal arthritis in patients with primary immunoglobulin deficiency: Clinical features and outcome in 18 patients. Br J Rheumatol 36:661, 1997.
39. Nolla JM, Gomez-Vaquero C, Fiter J, et al: Pyarthrosis in patients with rheumatoid arthritis: A detailed analysis of 10 cases and literature review. Semin Arthritis Rheum 30:121, 2000.
40. Gardner GC, Weisman MH: Pyarthrosis in patients with rheumatoid arthritis: A report of 13 cases and a review of the literature from the past 40 years. Am J Med 88:503, 1990.
41. Goldenberg DL: Infectious arthritis complicating rheumatoid arthritis and other chronic rheumatic disorders. Arthritis Rheum 32:496, 1989.
42. Mateo Soria L, Miquel Nolla Sole J, Rozadilla Sacanell A, et al: Infectious arthritis in patients with rheumatoid arthritis. Ann Rheum Dis 51:402, 1992.
43. Ostensson A, Geborek P: Septic arthritis as a non-surgical complication in rheumatoid arthritis: Relation to disease severity and therapy. Br J Rheumatol 30:35, 1991.
44. Shmerling RH, Delbanco TL, Tosteson ANA, et al: Synovial fluid tests. What should be ordered? JAMA 264:1009, 1990.
45. Ho G Jr.: Septic arthritis. In Klippel JH (ed): Primer on the Rheumatic Diseases, 12th ed. Atlanta, Arthritis Foundation, 2001, pp 259-264.
46. Perez-Ruiz F, Testillano M, Gastaca MA, et al: Pseudoseptic pseudogout associated with hypomagnesemia in liver transplant patients. Transplantation 71:696, 2001.
47. Pioro MH, Mandell BF: Septic arthritis. Rheum Dis Clin North Am 23:239, 1997.
48. Goldenberg DL: Septic arthritis. Lancet 351:197, 1998.
49. Liebling MR, Arkfeld DG, Michelini GA, et al: Identification of Neisseria gonorrhoeae in synovial fluid using the polymerase chain reaction. Arthritis Rheum 37:702, 1994.
50. Muralidhar B, Rumore PM, Steinman CR: Use of the polymerase chain reaction to study arthritis due to Neisseria gonorrhoeae. Arthritis Rheum 37:710, 1994.
51. von Essen R: Culture of joint specimens in bacterial arthritis: Impact of blood culture bottle utilization. Scand J Rheumatol 26:293, 1997.

52. Yagupsky P, Press J: Use of the isolator 1.5 microbial tube for culture of synovial fluid from patients with septic arthritis. J Clin Microbiol 35:2410, 1997.

53. Hughes JG, Vetter EA, Patel R, et al: Culture with BACTEC Peds Plus/F bottle compared with conventional methods for detection of bacteria in synovial fluid. J Clin Microbiol 39:4468, 2001.

54. Atkins BL, Bowler IC: The diagnosis of large joint sepsis. J Hosp Infect 40:263, 1998.

55. Adams WG, Deaver KA, Cochi SL, et al: Decline of childhood *Haemophilus influenzae* type b Hib. disease in the Hib vaccine era. JAMA 269:221, 1993.

56. Broadhurst LE, Erickson RL, Kelley PW: Decreases in invasive *Haemophilus influenzae* disease in US Army children, 1984-1991. JAMA 269:227, 1993.

57. Brewer GF, Davis JR, Grossman M: Gonococcal arthritis in an adolescent girl. Am J Dis Child 122:253, 1971.

58. Goldenberg DL, Cohen AS: Acute infectious arthritis. Am J Med 60:369, 1976.

59. Shattner A, Vosti KL: Bacterial arthritis due to beta-hemolytic streptococci of serogroups A, B, C, F, and G: Analysis of 23 cases and review of the literature. Medicine 77:122,1998.

60. Duggan JM, Georgiadis G, VanGorp C, et al: Group B streptococcal prosthetic joint infections. J South Orthop Assoc 10:209, 2001.

61. Straus C, Caplanne D, Bergemer AM, et al: Destructive polyarthritis due to a group B streptococcus. Rev Rhum Engl Educ 64:339,1997.

62. Pischel KD, Weisman MH, Cone RO: Unique features of group B streptococcal arthritis in adults. Arch Intern Med 145:97, 1985.

63. Goldenberg DL, Brandt K, Cathcart E, et al: Acute arthritis caused by gram-negative bacilli: A clinical characterization. Medicine 53:197, 1974.

64. Dubost J, Fis I, Denis P, et al: Polyarticular septic arthritis. Medicine 72:296, 1993.

65. Ho G Jr: Bacterial arthritis. *In* McCarty DJ, Koopman WJ (eds): Arthritis and Allied Conditions, 12th ed. Philadelphia, Lea and Febiger, 1993, pp 2003-2023.

66. Gutierrez KM: Infectious and inflammatory arthritis. *In* Long SL, Pickering LK, Prober CG (eds): Principles and Practice of Pediatric Infectious Diseases. New York, Churchill Livingstone, 1997, pp 537-545.

67. Gilad J, Borer A, Riesenberg K, et al: Polymicrobial polyarticular septic arthritis: a rare clinical entity. Scand J Infect Dis 33:381, 2001.

68. San Miguel VV, Lavery JP, York JC, et al: *Achromobacter xylosidans* septic arthritis in a patient with systemic lupus erythematosus. Arthritis Rheum 34:1484, 1991.

69. Melendez PR, Johnson RH: Bacteremia and septic arthritis caused by *Moraxella catarrhalis*. Rev Infect Dis 13:428, 1991.

70. Mader R, Blake R, Gladman D: Isolated septic meningococcal arthritis. Clin Exp Rheumatol 9:411, 1991.

71. Booth LV, Richards RH, Chandran DR: Septic arthritis caused by *Corynebacterium xerosis* following vascular surgery. Rev Infect Dis 13:548, 1991.

72. Quinn AG, Comaish JS, Pedler SJ: Septic arthritis and endocarditis due to group G-2 coryneform organism. Lancet 338:62, 1991.

73. Richette R, Pizzuti P, Quillard A, et al: A definite case of spondylodiscitis caused by *Streptococcus equisimilis*. Clin Exp Rheumatol 19:587, 2001.

74. Johnson RW, Arnett FC: A fatal case of *Vibrio vulnificus* presenting as septic arthritis. Arch Intern Med 161:2616, 2001.

75. Mandell GA: Imaging in the diagnosis of musculoskeletal infections in children. Curr Probl Pediatr 26:218, 1996.

76. Sanchez RB, Quinn SF: MRI of inflammatory synovial processes. Magn Reson Imaging 7:529, 1989.

77. Widman DS, Craig JG, Van Holsbeeck MT: Sonographic detection, evaluation and aspiration of infected acromioclavicular joints. Skeletal Radiol 30:388, 2001.

78. Espinoza LR: Infectious arthritis. *In* Goldman L, Bennett JC (eds): Cecil Textbook of Medicine, 21st ed. Philadelphia, WB Saunders, 2000, pp 1507-1509.

79. Gilbert DN, Moellering RC, Sande MA (eds): The Sanford Guide Hyde Park. Vermont, Antimicrobial Therapy, Inc., 2002.

80. Goldenberg DL, Sexton DJ: Bacterial (nongonococcal) arthritis. In Rose BD (ed): UpToDate, Wellsley, Mass., UpToDate, 2002.

81. Nicolau DP, Freeman CD, Belliveau PP, et al: Experience with a once-daily aminoglycoside program administered to 2184 adult patients. Antimicrob Agents Chemother 39:650, 1995.

82. Smith JW, Hasan MS: Infectious arthritis. *In* Mandell GL, Bennett JE, Dolin R (eds): Principles and Practice of Infectious Diseases, 5th ed. Philadelphia, Churchill Livingstone, 2000, pp 1175-1182.

83. Ho G Jr: How best to drain an infected joint. Will we ever know for certain? J Rheumatol 20:2001, 1993.

84. Dubost JJ, Soubrier M, De Champs C, et al: No change in the distribution of organisms responsible for septic arthritis over a 20 year period. Ann Rheum Dis 61:267, 2002.

85. Ho G Jr, Su EY: Therapy for septic arthritis. JAMA 247:797, 1982.

86. Yu LP, Bradley JD, Hugenberg ST, et al: Predictors of mortality in non-post-operative patients with septic arthritis. Scand J Rheumatol 21:142, 1992.

87. Kaandorp CJE, Krijnen P, Moens HJB, et al: The outcome of bacterial arthritis: a prospective community-based study. Arthritis Rheum 40:884, 1997.

88. Gelberman RH, Menon J, Austerlitz MS, et al: Pyogenic arthritis of the shoulder in adults. J Bone Joint Surg Am 62:550, 1980.

89. Leslie BM, Harris JM III, Driscoll D: Septic arthritis of the shoulder in adults. J Bone Joint Surg Am 71:1516, 1989.

90. Lossos IS, Yossepowitch O, Kandel L, et al: Septic arthritis of the glenohumeral joint A report of 11 cases and review of the literature. Medicine 77:177, 1998.

91. Ho G Jr: Bacterial arthritis. Curr Opin Rheumatol 3:603, 1991.

92. Abbott GT, Carty H: Pyogenic sacroiliitis, the missed diagnosis? Br J Radiol 782:120, 1993.

93. Bohay DR, Gray JM: Sacroiliac joint pyarthrosis. Orthop Rev 22:817, 1993.

94. Parker VS, Malhotra CM, Ho G Jr, et al: Radiologic appearance of the sternomanubrial joint in arthritis and related conditions. Radiology 153:343, 1984.

95. Leighty SM, Spach DH, Myall RW, et al: Septic arthritis of the temporomandibular joint: Review of the literature and report of two cases in children. Int J Oral Maxillofac Surg 22:292, 1993.

96. Bounds G: Septic arthritis of the temporomandibular joint: a problematic diagnosis. Br J Oral Maxillofac Surg 25:61, 1987.

97. Spanierman C: Animal Bites. eMedicine Journal. Volume 3, Number 4, April 25, 2002.

98. Garcia VR: Animal bites and Pasturella infections. Pediatr Rev 18:127, 1997.

99. Goldstein EJC: Bite wounds and infection. Clin Infect Dis 14:633, 1992.

100. Byington CL, Basow RD: *Streptobacillus moniliformis* rat bite fever. *In* Feigin RD, Cherry JD (eds): Textbook of Pediatric Infectious Diseases 4 ed. Vol 2. Philadelphia, WB Saunders, 1998, pp 1509-1512.

101. Young EJ: Brucella species Brucellosis. *In* Long SL, Pickering LK, Prober CG (eds): Principles and Practice of Pediatric Infectious Diseases. New York, Churchill Livingstone 1997, pp 972-976.

102. Mousa AR, Muhtaseb SA, Almudallal DS, et al: Osteoarticular complications of brucellosis: A study of 169 case. Rev Infect Dis 9:531, 1987.

103. Lubani M, Sharda D, Helin I: Brucella arthritis in children. Infection 14:233, 1986.

104. Gotuzzo E, Alarcon GS, Bocanegra TS, et al: Articular involvement in human brucellosis: A retrospective analysis of 304 cases. Semin Arthritis Rheum 12:245, 1982.

105. Gotuzzo E, Carrillo C, Guerra J, et al: An evaluation of diagnostic methods for brucellosis: The value of bone marrow cultures. J Infect Dis 153:122, 1986.

106. Darouiche RO: Device-associated infections: A macroproblem that starts with microadherence. Clin Infect Dis 33:1567, 2001.

107. Berbari EF, Hanssen AD, Duffy MC, et al: Risk factors for prosthetic joint infection: case-control study. Clin Infect Dis 27:1247, 1998.

108. Zimmerli W, Waldvogel FA, Vaudaux P, et al: Pathogenesis of foreign body infection: Description and characteristics of an animal model. J Infect Dis 146:487, 1982.

109. Roisman FR, Walz DT, Finkelstein AE: Superoxide radical production by human leukocytes exposed to immune complexes:

Inhibitory action of gold compounds. Inflammation 7:355, 1983.

110. Wang JY, Wicklund BH, Gustilo RB, et al: Prosthetic metals impair murine immune response and cytokine release in vivo and in vitro. J Orthop Res 15:688, 1997.

111. Donlan RM: Biofilms: microbial life on surfaces. Emerg Infect Dis 8:881, 2002.

112. Veenstra GJ, Cremers FF, van Dijk H, et al: Ultrastructural organization and regulation of a biomaterial adhesin of *Staphylococcus epidermidis.* J Bacteriol 178:537, 1996.

113. Shiro H, Muller E, Gutierrez N, et al: Transposon mutants of *Staphylococcus epidermidis* deficient in elaboration of capsular polysaccharide/adhesin and slime are avirulent in a rabbit model of endocarditis. J Infect Dis 169:1042, 1994.

114. Widmer AF, Frei R, Rajacic Z, et al: Correlation between in vivo and in vitro efficacy of antimicrobial agents against foreign body infections. J Infect Dis 162:96, 1990.

115. Widmer AF, Wiestner A, Frei R, et al: Killing of nongrowing and adherent *Escherichia coli* determines drug efficacy in device-related infections. Antimicrob Agents Chemother 35:741, 1991.

116. Hawthorn LA, Reid G: Exclusion of uropathogen adherence to polymer surfaces by *Lactobacillus acidophilus.* J Biomed Mater Res 24:39, 1990.

117. Brandt CM, Sistrunk WW, Duffy MC, et al: *Staphylococcus aureus* prosthetic joint infection treated with debridement and prosthesis retention. Clin Infect Dis 24:914, 1997.

118. Raut, VV, Siney, PD, Wroblewski, BM: One-stage revision of total hip arthroplasty for deep infection: Long term followup. Clin Orthop 321:202, 1995.

119. Brandt CM, Duffy MCT, Berbari, EF, et al: *Staphylococcus aureus* prosthetic joint infection treated with prosthesis removed and delayed reimplantation arthroplasty. Mayo Clin Proc 74:553, 1999.

120. American Dental Association: American Academy of Orthopedic Surgeons Advisory statement: Antibiotic prophylaxis for dental patients with total joint replacements. JADA 28:1004, 1997.

121. Sandhu SS, Lowry JC, Morton ME, et al: Antibiotic prophylaxis, dental treatment and arthroplasty: Time to explode a myth. J Bone Joint Surg Br 79-B:521, 1997.

122. American Society for Gastrointestinal Endoscopy: Antibiotic prophylaxis for gastrointestinal endoscopy. Gastrointest Endosc 42:630, 1995.

123. American Society of Colon and Rectal Surgeons: Practice parameters for antibiotic prophylaxis to prevent infective endocarditis or infected prosthesis during colon and rectal endoscopy. Dis Colon Rectum 35:277, 1992.

124. Working Party of the British Society for Antimicrobial Chemotherapy: Case against antibiotic prophylaxis for dental treatment of patients with joint prostheses. Lancet 339:301, 1992.

125. Howell RM, Green JG: Prophylactic antibiotic coverage in dentistry: A survey of need for prosthetic joints. Gen Dent 33:320, 1985.

126. Meyer GW, Artis AL: Antibiotic prophylaxis for orthopedic prostheses and GI procedures: Report of a survey. Am J Gastroenterol 92:989, 1997.

127. Shrout MK, Scarbrough F, Powell BL: Dental care and the prosthetic joint patient: A survey of orthopedic surgeons and general dentists. JADA 125:429, 1994.

128. Dajani AS, Taubert KA, Wilson W, et al: Prevention of bacterial endocarditis: Recommendations by the American Heart Association. JAMA 277:1794, 1997.

129. Mason JC: Hammersmith Staff Rounds: An infected prosthetic hip. Is there a role for prophylactic antibiotics? BMJ 305:300, 1992.

130. Jacobson JJ, Schweitzer SO, Kowalski CJ: Chemoprophylaxis of prosthetic joint patients during dental treatment: A decision-utility analysis. Oral Surg Oral Med Oral Pathol 72:167, 1991.

131. Jaspers MT, Little JW: Prophylactic antibiotic coverage in patients with total arthroplasty: Current practice. JADA 111:943, 1985.

132. Krijnen P, Kaandorp CJE, Steyerberg EW, et al: Antibiotic prophylaxis for haematogenous bacterial arthritis in patients with joint disease: A cost effective analysis. Ann Rheum Dis 60:359, 2001.

133. Tsevat J, Durand-Zaleski I, Pauker SG: Cost-effectiveness of antibiotic prophylaxis for dental procedures in patients with artificial joints. Am J Public Health 79:739, 1989.

134. Li F, Bulbul R, Schumacher HR Jr., et al: Molecular detection of bacterial DNA in venereal-associated arthritis. Arthritis Rheum 39:950, 1996.

135. Vittecoq O, Schaeverbeke T, Favre S, et al: Molecular diagnosis of Ureaplasma urealyticum in an immunocompetent patient with destructive reactive polyarthritis. Arthritis Rheum 40:2084, 1997.

136. Canvin JM, Goutcher SC, Hagig M, et al: Persistence of Staphylococcus aureus as detected by polymerase chain reaction in the synovial fluid of a patient with septic arthritis. Br J Rheumatol 36:203, 1997.

137. van der Heijden IM, Wilbrink B, Vije AE, et al: Detection of bacterial DNA in serial synovial samples obtained during antibiotic treatment from patients with septic arthritis. Arthritis Rheum 42:2198, 1999.

138. van der Heijden IM, Wilbrink B, Tchetverikov I, et al: Presence of bacterial DNA and bacterial peptidoglycans in joints of patients with rheumatoid arthritis and other arthritides. Arthritis Rheum 43:593, 2000.

139. Gerard HC, Wang Z, Wang GF, et al: Chromosomal DNA from a variety of bacterial species is present in synovial tissue from patients with various forms of arthritis. Arthritis Rheum 44:1689, 2001.

140. Stahl HD, Hubner B, Seidl B, et al: Detection of multiple viral DNA species in synovial tissue and fluid of patients with early arthritis. Ann Rheum Dis 59:342, 2000.

141. Mariani BD, Martin DS, Levine MJ, et al: The Coventry Award: Polymerase chain reaction detection of bacterial infection in total knee arthroplasty. Clin Orthop 331:11, 1996.

142. Louie JS, Liebling MR: The polymerase chain reaction in infectious and post-infectious arthritis: A review. Rheum Dis Clin North Am 24:227, 1998.

143. Whittle HC, Abdullahi MT, Fakunle FA, et al: Allergic complications of meningococcal disease. I. Clinical aspects. Br Med J 2:733, 1973.

144. Khan MA: Update on Spondyloarthropathies. Ann Intern Med 136:896, 2002.

99 Lyme Disease

LEONARD H. SIGAL

Lyme arthritis was initially described as a distinct entity in 1975, after the identification of an epidemic of what appeared to be "juvenile rheumatoid arthritis" (pauciarthritis and monarthritis) in adults and children near Old Lyme, Connecticut. Subsequent association with a distinct rash, erythema (chronicum) migrans (EM), and other multisystem features of the syndrome led to the description of Lyme disease (LD). A distinct organism, *Borrelia burgdorferi*, was identified in deer ticks (*Ixodes scapularis*) and from clinical specimens and acknowledged as the causative agent; very similar but distinct organisms are the cause of a similar syndrome in Europe. The term *Lyme borreliosis* is more commonly used in Europe and is interchanged with LD.

LD is a complex, multisystem disease (Table 99–1) resulting from infection with the spirochete *B. burgdorferi sensu lato*; within this are included *B. burgdorferi sensu stricto* (the only species isolated in the United States and also found in Eurasia) and *B. garinii* and *B. afzelii* (each found in Eurasia). There may be other genotypes capable of causing LD. Differences in the spectrum of LD seen in Europe compared to the United States may be due to differences in the organism and the ambient immunogenetics of the populations affected. How *B. burgdorferi* causes damage or dysfunction is unclear but probably involves inflammatory response to the spirochete at the site of infection and immunologically mediated damage; direct toxicity of the organism for host cells may also play a role.[1] LD has become a social phenomenon in certain areas,[2,3] with public concern exceeding the true severity and magnitude of the epidemic. Overdiagnosis and overtreatment rival the true disease in their potential for causing debility and distress.

Ecology and Epidemiology of Lyme Disease

LD is a reportable infectious disease in all 50 of the United States and has been reported from at least 46 states. However, LD is not endemic throughout the United States; most sporadic cases in nonendemic regions are "imported" (i.e., acquired on a trip to endemic areas). More than 85 percent of cases in the United States are reported from southern New England, the mid-Atlantic states (into Maryland and Virginia), the upper Midwest (Wisconsin and Minnesota), and northern California. Within these regions, there are focal endemic areas, such as Suffolk and Westchester counties in New York; coastal southern New England; Cape Cod, Nantucket, and Martha's Vineyard, Massachusetts; and

TABLE 99–1 · CLINICAL MANIFESTATIONS OF LYME DISEASE

Early Localized Disease

Occurs 1 day to a month (mean, 7 to 10 days) after the tick bite
Erythema migrans (EM) in up to 90% of patients; multiple in approximately 10% of patients with EM
Fatigue, malaise, lethargy
Headache
Myalgia
Arthralgias
Regional, generalized lymphadenopathy

Early Disseminated Disease*

Occurs days to 10 months after the tick bite
Carditis (8 to 10% of *untreated* patients)
    Conduction defects
    Mild cardiomyopathy
Neurologic (10 to 12% of *untreated* patients)
    Meningitis
    Cranial neuropathy (most often facial, which can be bilateral)
    Peripheral neuropathy or radiculopathy
    Encephalitis
    Myelitis
Musculoskeletal (approximately 50% of *untreated* patients)
    Migratory polyarthralgias, polyarthritis, or both
Cutaneous: lymphadenosis benigna cutis (lymphocytoma)
Lymphadenopathy: regional or generalized
Ophthalmologic: conjunctivitis, iritis, choroiditis
Hepatic: liver function test abnormalities, hepatitis
Renal: microhematuria, proteinuria

Late Disease*

Occurs months to years after the tick bite
Musculoskeletal
    About 50% of *untreated* patients develop migratory polyarthritis
    About 10% of *untreated* patients develop chronic monoarthritis, usually of the knee
    Neurologic disease
    Chronic, often subtle, encephalopathy
    Chronic, often subtle, peripheral neuropathy
    Ataxia, dementia, sleep disorder
Cutaneous
    Acrodermatitis chronica atrophicans
    Morphea (?), localized scleroderma-like lesions

*May occur in the absence of prior features of Lyme disease.

Hunterdon, Ocean, Monmouth, and Morris counties in New Jersey. Extension of endemicity into the mid-Hudson River valley in New York and south along the Atlantic coast may be explained by increases in deer populations and spread of infected ticks by migrating birds (along the Atlantic and Mid-American flyways) and deer (via riparian migration).

Evidence suggests that the disease may be entering urban centers, perhaps maintained by an enzootic cycle of *B. burgdorferi* in rats.[4] Changes in local ecology in the last century (e.g., regrowth of forest on previously farmed land) have increased deer populations, now protected from predators, human and otherwise.[5] Commercial and residential development of such lands, with an emphasis on maintenance of forest land surrounding new human incursion, creates a high risk of infection for recent human arrivals into areas previously inhabited only by animals.

The number of cases in the United States meeting Centers for Disease Control and Prevention (CDC) epidemiologic criteria has grown steadily, increasing nearly 36-fold from 497 in 1982 to over 17,707 in 2001, more than 92 percent of which occurred within the established endemic areas; 18,101 cases were reported in 2002 as of December 28, and it is likely that 2003 will see more than 20,000 reported cases. Thus, CDC figures for the new millennium suggest a slow but steady increase in the total number of cases of LD in the United States. The number of reported cases is a significant underestimate of the total number of cases in society; the strict CDC surveillance criteria are useful for determining changes in numbers and location of cases but are not meant to be all inclusive nor designed for diagnostic purposes. There also have been reports of an EM-like illness in North Carolina and Missouri,[6] now called STARI (Southern tick-associated rash illness) and polymerase chain reaction (PCR) evidence of another *Borrelia* species (tentatively named *Borrelia lonestarii*[7]) in Lone Star ticks, although no organism has been cultured. There may be other infectious agents, perhaps borrelial, that mimic the LD epidemic. As well, it is important to recall that the ticks that spread LD also carry other organisms (e.g., *Anaplasma phagocytophila* [previously known as the human granulocytic ehrlichia], *Babesia microti*, and *Bartonella hensellae*). These coinfections may be the cause of remarkable constitutional symptoms in early LD and must be considered, especially because antibiotic, especially for *B. microti*, may differ from that which is appropriate for LD.

Ticks and Lyme Disease

LD is spread by the bite of infected Ixodid ticks (the *Ixodes ricinus* complex includes *Ixodes scapularis* [deer tick] in the Northeastern, Southeastern, and Midwestern United States [previously called *I. dammini* in the Northeast]; *I. pacificus* in California; *I. ricinus* in Europe; and *I. persulcatus* in Asia). Claims that other ticks, such as *Dermacentor variabilis* (the dog tick) and *Amblyomma americanum* (the Lone Star tick), spread LD are unproved, but even if they are competent vectors of *B. burgdorferi*, these ticks account for few or no cases. There is no evidence that mosquitoes or other hematophagous insects spread *B. burgdorferi*.

The *I. scapularis* egg mass is laid in the leaf clutter at the bottom of the forest. Larvae emerge in the summer and fall. Larvae and nymphs require a blood meal (usually obtained from *Peromyscus leucopus*, the white-footed field mouse, in the Northeast and Midwest) to proceed with their 2-year life cycle (egg–larva–nymph–adult). Larvae do not seem to survive if they *burgdorferi;* they acquire the organism with their blood meal. After its meal the tick falls off and molts, emerging as the nymph. It then actively seeks its blood meal in late spring, summer, and early fall, again usually from a white-footed field mouse. With its blood meal, an infected nymph can pass the organism to an uninfected mouse; these mice maintain a persistent, asymptomatic spirochetemia for life. A single infected mouse can then play host to and infect dozens of ticks of the next feeding generation. This may help explain the spread of LD: A single tick in a new site, perhaps having hitched a ride on a bird, can infect multiple larvae in the next generation. The Ixodid nymph seeks a blood meal, usually obtained from a mouse, in the mid spring to early fall (the very time of year people are most active outdoors and wearing the least clothing); "LD season" is defined by the time of year the "questing nymph" is searching for its blood meal; nymphs are responsible for 90 percent or more of all cases of LD.

After its postprandial metamorphosis from nymph, the adult emerges in the fall and winter. Females feed on white-tailed deer (*Odocoileus virginianus*), the blood meal providing nutrients to make eggs. Deer do not maintain a spirochetemia; they are not a "competent reservoir" of *B. burgdorferi* (a function served by the mouse). Only about 10 percent of all LD cases are spread by adult deer ticks, probably because they are active when people are not outdoors and if so are more fully clothed. The larger adult tick is more likely to be seen, felt, and removed before it can bite. Nonetheless, LD can be spread in early winter, if there has not been a killing frost, so precautions should still be taken even after Thanksgiving.

Ticks are found on low-lying grass and shrubs and are attracted to warm, carbon dioxide–exhaling animals. If these stimuli are detected, the tick attaches. It takes up to 24 hours for the tick to find its dining site, preferring one that is warm and moist, such as behind the knee, the groin, the midriff, or axilla and begin feeding. Blood reaches the tick's midgut (where *B. burgdorferi* has lain dormant) about 24 hours after the start of the meal. Spirochetes proliferate, change the pattern of coat proteins produced, escape the gut, and ultimately reach the tick's salivary glands. During its meal the tick rids itself of excess water in the blood meal by pumping fluid from the salivary glands back into the feeding cavity; this is how the tick spreads *B. burgdorferi* from its salivary glands into the unsuspecting host. The longer the duration of tick attachment and the more the tick has enlarged during feeding, the greater is the likelihood of transmission of *B. burgdorferi*.[8] It should be clear from this that the long time between first contact with the tick and spread of the organism offers ample opportunity of removing the tick and avoiding LD.

Clinical Features of Lyme Disease

LD is divided into three stages, defined broadly by the duration of infection. Some patients may not have had EM or other features of early LD and can present with later features. Most manifestations of *B. burgdorferi* infection can be defined as early, localized LD; early, disseminated LD; or late LD (see Table 99–1). Other problems have been ascribed to LD and may represent atypical cases or coincidental clinical findings in a seropositive individual.

Another area of major concern is the ramifications of LD in pregnancy. Early case reports and small series suggested an adverse effect. Studies of tissue from abortuses found no inflammation associated with the organisms, in marked contrast to the case in another spirochetal disease, congenital syphilis. No "congenital LD syndrome" has been identified. Studies suggest the outcome of pregnancy complicated by LD is usually good if the woman is treated appropriately for her features of LD.

EARLY LOCALIZED LYME DISEASE

EM, the pathognomonic skin lesion of LD, follows the tick bite by a mean of 1 week (Fig. 99–1), with the bite recalled by only about 30 percent of patients. In earlier series, EM was present or recalled by only 50 to 70 percent of patients, but recent evidence suggests that upward of 90 percent of patients have or had EM. EM is an expanding red papule or macule, usually in the inguina, axilla, midriff, or behind the knee. There may be central clearing; only about 30 percent of cases have the pattern called a bull's eye. EM is usually asymptomatic, although it may be pruritic or burn.[9] Even without antibiotic therapy, EM usually fades spontaneously within 4 weeks. An erythema at the site of a tick bite lasting only a few hours to 2 days is probably a reaction to the tick bite. In contrast, spider bites cause a nearly immediate painful, erythematous lesion, often with necrosis. Spirochetemia occurs soon after tick bite and can result in multiple secondary EM lesions. In early studies, up to 50 percent of patients with EM had multiple lesions; more recent experience suggests this is far less common. Multiple EM implies dissemination of infection, but is not necessarily an indication that the patient will do poorly or require more aggressive therapy.

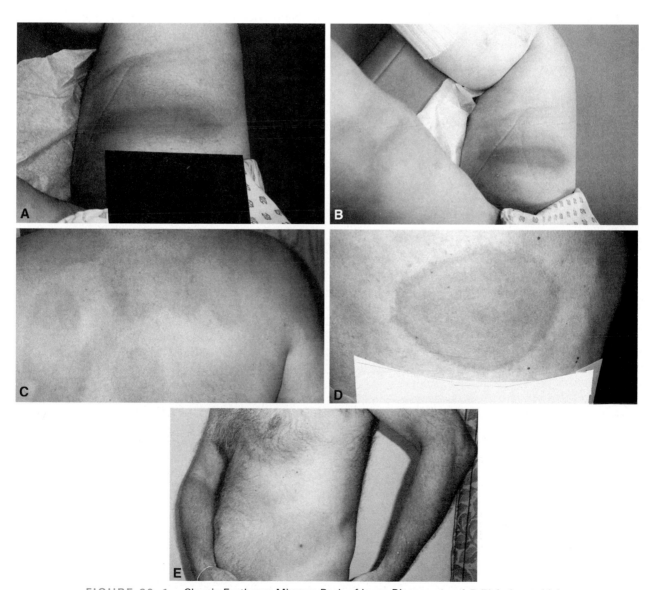

FIGURE 99–1 · Classic Erythema Migrans Rash of Lyme Disease. *A* and *B*, Right inner thigh. *C*, Multiple lesions on back. *D*, Right lateral posterior thorax ("bull's eye"). *E*, Anterior side.

Features of early LD are listed in Table 99–1. Coryza and gastrointestinal complaints are notable by their absence. The symptoms of early LD may resemble a viral syndrome, but even in endemic areas, most such syndromes are viral and not borrelial. Other than EM, there are no findings specific for early LD; "symptoms compatible with LD" is a nonspecific and, therefore, meaningless phrase. The presence of high fevers, extreme constitutional complaints, liver function test abnormalities, cytopenias, or some combination of these should suggest possible coexposure to *Babesia microti* or to *Anaplasma phagocytophila*, both of which can be cotransmitted with *B. burgdorferi* by the Ixodid tick vector.

In the evaluation of a patient with apparent later features of LD it is extraordinarily important to reexamine the initial diagnosis of LD. Often, patients fallaciously acquire a diagnosis of LD, and all that follows is ascribed to this mistaken diagnosis. Commonly the initial diagnosis was a diagnosis of exclusion or was made based on low-level serologic reactivity, or even on misinterpretation of a demonstrably negative serologic result. There should also be doubt of the initial diagnosis of LD if the purported later features of LD follow a lack of response to initial, seemingly, adequate therapy; lack of response to adequate therapy is very commonly due to initial misdiagnosis.

EARLY DISSEMINATED LYME DISEASE

Spirochetemia causes seeding of many organs early in the evolution of LD. The two most common features of early disseminated LD are cardiac and neurologic, both of which occur weeks to as many as 9 months after the EM (if it occurs) and often while the rash persists. However, early disseminated disease may occur in patients without knowledge of a preceding EM rash. Unless the early disseminated LD occurs very early in the course of the infection, such patients should be seropositive.

Cardiac Features

The classic cardiac manifestation of LD is atrioventricular heart block at various levels. Less commonly, patients may experience mild pericarditis and mild left ventricular dysfunction (the latter usually subclinical, apparent only on echocardiogram or chest radiograph). Syncope, dizziness, shortness of breath, substernal chest pain, or palpitations are rare and imply the patient has a higher degrees of block. Rarely, such patients require a temporary pacemaker. Heart block often resolves even before institution of antibiotic therapy, although some patients have slow resolution of second-degree block or gradual decrease in the PR interval. There are very rare cases of persistent of high-degree heart block requiring a permanent pacemaker. The appearance of what appears to be "Lyme carditis" many years after treated and cured LD suggests either another etiology of the carditis or a second episode of acute *B. burgdorferi* infection.

Neurologic Features

The neurologic features of early disseminated LD include cranial neuritis (usually facial palsy, which may be bilateral and rarely is accompanied by "polyneuropathy cranialis"), lymphocytic meningitis, and radiculoneuritis, often multifocal with motor and sensory findings. Lymphocytic pleocytosis and elevated protein levels with oligoclonal bands may be seen in meningitis, but spinal fluid may be unremarkable in isolated neuropathy or radiculoneuritis. The combination of lymphocytic meningitis, cranial neuropathy, and peripheral radiculoneuropathy due to *B. burgdorferi* is known as Bannwarth syndrome. Spinal fluid (and concomitant serum) should be tested for the presence of anti–*B. burgdorferi* antibodies. In patients with "isolated" facial or other cranial neuropathies, spinal fluid analysis should be performed if there is even a hint of other neurologic damage; an abnormal spinal fluid mandates intravenous (IV) rather than oral therapy. Neurologic features also may begin to resolve before the institution of antibiotic therapy.

LATE LYME DISEASE

Neurologic Features

Late neurologic features may appear years after tick bite or EM, but late LD may be the initial presentation of *B. burgdorferi* infection, without antecedent EM or any other feature of LD. Neurologic damage may include subacute encephalopathy, axonal polyneuropathy, and leukoencephalitis[10]; another term for this constellation of neurologic findings is *tertiary neuroborreliosis*, an appellation drawing on the analogy of LD with syphilis. Mild progressive cognitive dysfunction may be the sole feature of the latter. Given the frequency of such complaints in society (e.g., due to sleep disturbance, chronic stress, or fibromyalgia), it is important not to rush to the diagnosis of central nervous system (CNS) LD in patients who complain of isolated or predominant fatigue as a feature of "chronic" lyme disease patients with CNS LD are usually strongly seropositive, and spinal fluid should be examined for specific antibodies to prove that the clinical problems result from *B. burgdorferi*; isolated seropositivity cannot be taken as proof of causality. The spinal fluid of patients with tertiary neuroborreliosis typically contains an elevated protein and specific antibodies to *B. burgdorferi*; a lymphocytic pleocytosis, as would be expected in meningitis, would be most unusual. Some CNS features of LD may result from the elaboration of toxic chemicals produced by monocytes or macrophages in the periphery that enter the neuraxis; thus, a patient with LD can have CNS dysfunction without having CNS infection.[11]

Lyme Arthritis and Other Musculoskeletal Features of Lyme Disease

Musculoskeletal features of LD can be seen at any point in the infection and include arthralgia; intermittent episodes of migratory arthritis, usually monarthritis or asymmetric oligoarthritis; and chronic arthritis, usually of the knees.[12,13] Arthralgia, and even rarely arthritis, can start in the first days of infection. Later in infection a chronic arthritis may occur, often following arthralgia or migratory arthritis; chronic arthritis typically occurs months to years after the start of infection. It is important to recall that Lyme arthritis may be the first and only feature of *B. burgdorferi* infection, without preceding rash, neurologic, or cardiac disease.

Patients often complain more of stiffness than pain. Large effusions are common and reaccumulate rapidly after arthrocentesis, resembling reactive arthritis. The fluid is inflammatory, with 10,000 to 25,000 white blood cells (WBCs)/mm^3, and contains mostly neutrophils. All such fluids should be tested, along with concomitant blood samples, for anti–*B. burgdorferi* antibodies; arthritis of long-duration seropositivity is to be expected, and its absence should introduce some doubt as to the correct diagnosis. Small joint inflammation is quite unusual and suggests other causes of arthritis. I have seen a few cases of symmetric, small joint arthritis compatible with rheumatoid arthritis (RA) (rheumatoid factor [RF] positive) after apparently successful antibiotic treatment of early LD. In no case was a causal relationship established; subsequent treatment was for RA, and, therefore, not with further antibiotics.

Chronic LD arthritis may be intermittent, each episode lasting days to several months. Even untreated, the process typically remits after up to 8 years, with a progressive decrease in the number and the duration of flares. Antibiotic-refractory arthritis is more likely in individuals carrying the human leukocyte antigen (HLA)-DRB1*0401 allele or having immunoglobulin G (IgG) anti-Outer surface protein A, OspA, antibodies.[14-16] Studies have shown that an OspA epitope cross-reacts with an epitope within human lymphocyte-function associated antigen-1 (LFA-1), an integrin also known as CD18/CD11a.[17] This example of molecular mimicry has been cited as an explanation for "antibiotic-resistant Lyme arthritis," but its true role in the pathogenesis of Lyme arthritis is not established; it may be an in vitro phenomenon of no in vivo consequence. Certainly, there is never a clinical reason to test HLA-DR haplotypes, as they are obviously irrevocable and represent correlation not causality in any event untreatable. Furthermore, the commercially available assays are serologic—the linkage noted previously is based on nucleotide sequences of individual HLA-DR markers, detected only by PCR technology, which is not generally available. I have elsewhere reviewed factors that may be involved in the immunopathogenesis of LD and arthritis.[1]

B. burgdorferi has been proposed as a cause of reactive arthritis and seronegative spondyloarthropathy, based on a European case report and a series in which immunologic evidence suggested an association. No such cases have been reported in the United States. It may be that this feature of LD is unique to European LD. European Lyme arthritis appears to resemble that reported in the United States and may be more common than was appreciated previously. An epidemiologic study from Wurzburg, Germany, suggests a yearly incidence rate of 1 case per 1000 total population and a higher prevalence of Lyme arthritis than of neuroborreliosis in that highly endemic district.[18,19]

Patients with prior LD may develop sleep disorder, even in early LD; the precise frequency with which this occurs and how commonly it reverts with antibiotics is currently a matter of study. Fibromyalgia is not caused by ongoing infection and does not respond to antibiotics, even if the patient has not previously been antibiotically treated.

Fibromyalgia has been misdiagnosed as chronic LD arthritis (although there is no joint inflammation) and as tertiary neuroborreliosis (although spinal fluid is normal and neurocognitive testing patterns do not suggest LD).[20,21] Responses to standard regimens for fibromyalgia are similar to those seen for idiopathic fibromyalgia and such patients do not experience a robust response to antibiotics, even of long duration. Pediatric and adolescent post-LD fibromyalgia patients usually respond better than do adults. Much of the post-LD syndrome[22-24] may be caused by the sleep disorder and associated fibromyalgia or "chronic fatigue syndrome" that may follow LD; these do not represent active infection. Anxiety about having "chronic LD" or "antibiotic-resistant LD," suggesting that the patient has an incurable and, therefore, lifelong illness, may be a cause of major debility. In some patients obstructive sleep apnea may be at the root of fibromyalgia; there is no reason to believe that LD in any way predisposes to this syndrome, although some patients may have remarkable weight gain following LD, due to inactivity, depression, or both.

Pediatric LD arthritis is typically less severe and more responsive to antibiotics than adult arthritis.[19,25,26] Pediatric LD resembles that in adults, with 98 percent of children having arthralgias early in the course of LD. In one study, the arthritis started a median of 3.4 months into the LD. Joints were swollen and warm but often only mildly painful. In 78 percent, diffuse or localized lymphadenopathy accompanied episodes of arthritis, and in 40 percent, there was recrudescence of symptoms reminiscent of the initial illness. In a later series, only 26 percent of patients had prior early LD. A mean of five episodes of arthritis occurred in the first year (range of 1 to 15), each resolving within 1 to 3 weeks. There was an increase in the duration of bouts during the second and third years, but, with time, the number of recurrent episodes and bouts per child diminished. A direct correlation was observed between the age at the onset of LD and the duration of arthritis. All patients were IgG seropositive during the first year, and many were persistently IgM positive. The study by Gerber and associates[26] found 51 percent of patients had only one episode of arthritis; only 2 percent went on to chronic synovitis; and the prognosis for children treated with appropriate antibiotics was excellent.

In another cohort of pediatric LD arthritis, keratitis developed in a few patients. Subtle encephalopathy (i.e., memory changes, headache, and fatigue) occurred in two patients 1 and 12 years after the onset of LD and 7 and 9 years after the resolution of arthritis. In both, there was intrathecal production of specific anti–*B. burgdorferi* antibodies, and successful treatment was achieved with IV ceftriaxone. Another two patients had a later onset of neurologic problems, one with demyelinating syndrome and the other with a complex seizure disorder, but neither had concentration of specific antibodies in spinal fluid, and neither responded to IV antibiotics; the authors excluded them from the late neuroborreliosis group analysis.

▌Diagnosis

The diagnosis of LD should *never* be based solely on serologic evidence of exposure to *B. burgdorferi*. The diagnosis of LD should be entertained when a patient has clinical (historic and physical) features suggesting the diagnosis. In such a setting, serologic evidence can be used to enhance the a priori likelihood. There is no such thing as a "Lyme disease test," a "Lyme test," or "Lyme serologies." These serologic tests measure anti–*B. burgdorferi* antibodies, nothing more, nothing less. Although containing more syllables, the term, *anti*–B. burgdorferi *antibody assay* contains less bias and fewer inappropriate expectations.

SEROLOGIC TESTING FOR THE CONFIRMATION OF LYME DISEASE

The diagnosis of LD should be based on specific historic and objective physical features explicitly suggesting the diagnosis. Laboratory testing can confirm but should never be the sole criterion for the diagnosis of LD.[27] Enzyme-linked immunosorbent assay (ELISA) is the most widely available serologic test. Recent exposure can usually be confirmed by finding IgM antibodies in the serum; IgG antibodies develop later. Test results may be negative in early LD. Initially in early infection IgM may occasionally not be detectable for 4 or more weeks, and IgG levels may not be measurable for up to 8 weeks. Early, even inadequate, antibiotic therapy may block antibody responses; such patients may remain seronegative despite having active infection. IgM seroreactivity can persist for more than 1 year.[28,29]

It is important to remember that seroreactivity of any isotype is merely a marker of prior exposure; even persisting IgM is not a marker of active infection. Testing is of very limited use in the aftermath of treatment. If a patient responds well to therapy, follow-up testing should not be done; in such a cured patient, persisting seropositivity is not a marker of ongoing disease. In the rare patient with clinical findings thought to be new features of LD or unabated persistence of old findings, a follow-up test showing increase in ELISA signal, expansion of the immunologic repertoire (i.e., new borrelial protein bands bound on immunoblot), or both may be evidence of ongoing infection, demanding further evaluation.

Cross-reactive antibodies causing a false-positive ELISA result can occur in nonspirochetal bacterial endocarditis,[30] other spirochetal infections (e.g., borrelial gingivitis, syphilis), *Anaplasma phagocytophila* infection, parvovirus B19 and Epstein-Barr virus infections, RA, and systemic lupus erythematosus (SLE)[31] and in some normal individuals. Of note, *B. burgdorferi* infection can cause cross-reactivity that suggests Epstein-Barr virus infection.

All positive or equivocal ELISA results must be corroborated by immunoblot (also known as Western blot or protein blot); an unverified positive ELISA is a false-positive ELISA result that does not confirm exposure. In nonendemic areas, 5 percent or more of normal sera have false-positive ELISA results. ELISA measures antibodies to *B. burgdorferi* that may be of low avidity (e.g., cross-reactive with other organisms), whereas Western blot is more stringent (see Fig. 99–2). Certain *B. burgdorferi* proteins, such as flagellin (41-kD protein) and heat-shock proteins (58-, 60-, 66-, and 74-kD), strongly immunologically resemble those of other pathogenic microorganisms and of normal flora. Cross-reacting anti-

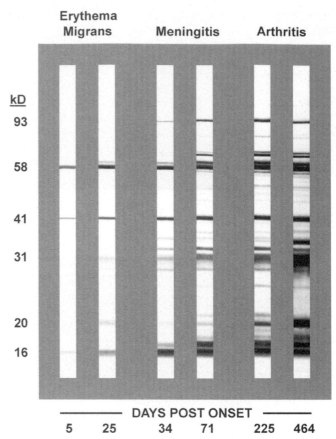

FIGURE 99–2 · Western blot immunoglobulin G(IgG) responses to *B. burgdorferi* in six serial serum specimens from one untreated patient with Lyme disease. The patient presented initially with erythema migrans (EM) (5 days), subsequently developed meningitis (day 34), and later developed synovitis (day 225). The patient had a second episode of Lyme arthritis on day 464. Days post onset are the time points of the collection of each sample following the appearance of erythema migrans. (Courtesy of I MUGEN, Inc.)

bodies may produce a positive ELISA result that is not indicative of *B. burgdorferi* infection. There are criteria for interpretation of Western blots (Table 99–2), but neither ELISA nor immunoblot has been standardized, so comparisons among laboratories remain problematic.[32] Advances in seroconfirmatory testing for LD include the use of recombinant proteins,[33] individual epitopes from borrelial proteins,[34] and perhaps immune complexes[34-36] as the source of antibodies to be tested.

Finding antibodies within spinal or synovial fluid that are not represented in the serum (by immunoblot) or higher levels of specific antibodies in the fluid (by ELISA) is evidence of local production of antibody, tantamount to proof of local infection; similarly, in CNS LD oligoclonal bands imply a local humoral immune response, although in this test no specificity can be demonstrated. Lymphocytic pleocytosis is expected in LD meningitis, but there may be only an elevated protein without pleocytosis in peripheral neuropathy or tertiary neuroborreliosis.

MOLECULAR BIOLOGIC TESTING FOR THE CONFIRMATION OF LYME DISEASE

PCR has allowed the detection of *B. burgdorferi* DNA in clinical specimens, including skin, blood, spinal and

TABLE 99–2 • CRITERIA FOR POSITIVE WESTERN BLOT (IMMUNOBLOT) ANALYSIS IN THE SEROLOGIC CONFIRMATION OF INFECTION WITH BORRELIA BURGDORFERI

Duration of Disease	Isotype Tested	Bands To Be Considered
First few weeks of infection	IgM	Two of the eight following: 18, 21, 28, 37, 41, 45, 58, 93 *or* Two of the three following: ospC (23), 39, 41*
After first weeks of infection	IgG	Five of the 10 following: 18, 21, 28, 30, 39, 41, 45, 58, 66, 93

*Alternate criteria for IgM reactivity, proposed by a Centers for Disease Control and Prevention conference, Dearborn, MI, August 1994. IgM criteria should not be used in the confirmation of purported infection of more than a few weeks' duration.

Data from Dressler F, Whalen JA, Reinhardt BN, Steere AC: Western blotting in the serodiagnosis of LD. J Infect Dis 167:392, 1993.

Abbreviations: IgG, immunoglobulin G.

synovial fluid, urine, and synovial tissue.[37,38] Synovial tissue is more likely to be positive than fluid[39] (Table 99–3). PCR is more sensitive than culture, more specific than ELISA, and may detect spirochetemia before antibodies are detected. PCR positivity in inflammatory fluid suggests that the neurologic or articular findings result from local *B. burgdorferi* infection. The examiner can reasonably expect PCR to become negative after treatment; a persisting signal in subsequent fluid specimens suggests persistence of infection and that further antibiotic treatment may be needed.[40]

PCR is not recommended for routine clinical use because it is not yet standardized. False-positive results can occur due to contamination of samples at the time they are obtained or processed by the laboratory. *B. burgdorferi* does not remain in the fluid phase for long, so a negative PCR result from synovial or spinal fluid or serum and plasma does not rule out the diagnosis of LD.

TABLE 9–3 • *BORRELIA BURGDORFERI* IDENTIFIED IN ORGANS INVOLVED WITH LYME DISEASE

Early Localized Disease

Skin—by culture, polymerase chain reaction (PCR), immunochemistry.

Early Disseminated Disease

Heart—by culture, immunochemistry
Cerebrospinal fluid—by culture, PCR, immunochemistry
Peripheral nerve—not identified
Eye—by culture, immunochemistry

Late Disease

Joint fluid—by culture, PCR, immunochemistry
Joint tissue—by culture, PCR, immunochemistry
Brain—by culture, immunochemistry
Peripheral nerve—not identified
Skin—by culture, PCR, immunochemistry

OTHER TESTS OFTEN USED IN LYME DISEASE

Neuropsychologic testing, electrophysiologic testing (cardiac and neurologic), and brain magnetic resonance imaging (MRI) can be useful in documenting objective abnormalities, but there is no pattern of changes in any of these modalities specific for LD. Evaluation of neurocognitive complaints of patients with LD arthritis may be invaluable in documenting unsuspected or overlooked CNS infection.[10] Although there are no patterns on such tests that allow a specific diagnosis of CNS LD to be made, there are typical patterns of abnormalities that can suggest that diagnosis. In the evaluation of patients with cognitive dysfunction such testing can help differentiate LD from depression, other psychologic disorders, hypochondriasis, anxiety, hypervigilance, and malingering. An added value of neurocognitive testing is that it can be used as a benchmark to document improvement following therapy and as a means to plan rehabilitation strategies. Spinal fluid analysis is mandated if neuropsychologic or electrophysiologic results suggest CNS infection (see Table 99–2).

Urinary antigen testing is of no proven value in the diagnosis or management of LD[41]; its use should be discouraged until and unless studies demonstrate this technology has any validity.

RADIOGRAPHIC FEATURES OF LYME ARTHRITIS

Lawson and Steere[42] studied radiographic evaluation of 25 patients with chronic arthritis of the knees for a median duration of 9 months. Effusions were present in 15, three had soft tissue swelling, six had edema of the infrapatellar fat pad, and five had enthesopathy. Loss of cartilage was found in six knees and in the hips and one shoulder of one patient, calcification of cartilage (in two cases), or of menisci (in one case). Among 14 patients, six had bone changes compatible with inflammatory joint disease, four had osteoarthritis (OA), and another four had inflammation and OA. Erosions were seen in five knees and in both hips and one shoulder of another patient (who also had subarticular bone cysts near the joints); seven had osteophytosis (four with subchondral sclerosis); and eight had osteoporosis, usually juxta-articular.

Treatment and Prevention

The goal of treatment is to cure the current features of LD and prevent progression to later features of the disease. Currently recommended regimens, tailored to the different disease features, are successful in the vast majority of cases (Table 99–4). About 10 percent of patients experience a short-lived and self-limited worsening of their complaints within the first days of *initial* treatment of early LD—this is called a Jarisch-Herxheimer reaction.[10] It is important to warn patients of the possibility of developing such a reaction. Reports of recurrent "Herxheimer reactions" with institution of subsequent therapies or many days after the start of therapy should be greeted with skepticism. Diagnosis based on such "reactions" as the sole evidence of LD are overwhelmingly apocryphal.

◼ TABLE 99–4 · RECOMMENDATIONS FOR THERAPY IN LYME DISEASE (LD)

Oral Therapy for Early Localized Lyme Disease

Adults

Doxycycline*	100 mg PO bid	2 to 4 weeks§
Tetracycline*, †	250 to 500 mg PO qid	2 to 4 weeks§
Amoxicillin†, ‡	250 to 500 mg PO qid	2 to 4 weeks§

Children

Amoxicillin	40 mg/kg/day, divided dose	2 to 4 weeks§
Erythromycin	30 mg/kg/day, divided dose	2 to 4 weeks§
Penicillin G	25 to 50 mg/kg/day, divided dose	2 to 4 weeks§

Intravenous (IV) Therapy for Early Disseminated and Late Lyme Disease

Adults

Third-generation cephalosporins		
Ceftriaxone	2 g qd or 1 g bid	2 to 4 weeks
Cefotaxime	3 g bid	2 to 4 weeks
Penicillin		
Penicillin G	20 million units in 6 divided doses	2 to 4 weeks
Chloramphenicol	50 mg/kg/day in 4 divided doses	2 to 4 weeks

Children

Third-generation cephalosporins		
Ceftriaxone	75 to 100 mg/kg/day	2 to 4 weeks
Cefotaxime	90 to 180 mg/kg/day, in 2 or 3 divided doses	2 to 4 weeks
Penicillin		
Penicillin G	300,000 units/kg/day in 6 divided doses	2 to 4 weeks

*No studies comparing doxycycline with tetracycline have been done.
†Dosage determined by size of patient.
‡No studies comparing amoxicillin with amoxicillin plus probenecid have been done; cefuroxime axetil and azithromycin have also been studied in LD, but neither has been found to be superior to either doxycycline or amoxicillin, although cefuroxime axetil is the equivalent of doxycycline in one large study.
§There is no proof that this is the optimal duration of therapy or that more than 10 to 14 days of treatment is necessary.
‖There is no proof that isolated facial nerve palsy or carditis must be treated with IV therapy. Oral doxycycline for early Lyme neuroborreliosis has been shown to be effective in a European study. Especially in children, oral treatment for Lyme arthritis may suffice. Many treat late central nervous system (CNS) disease and refractory arthritis for 4 weeks, using 2-week regimens for carditis or meningitis, but there are no published controlled trials that address optimal duration of IV or oral therapy.

Adapted from Sigal LH: Current drug therapy recommendations for the treatment of LD. Drugs 43:683, 1992.

Oral therapy is effective for EM, isolated facial palsy (no other neurologic signs or symptoms and a normal spinal fluid), mild carditis, and as initial therapy for Lyme arthritis. The use of IV antibiotics should be reserved for CNS disease, severe carditis, or arthritis not responding to prior oral therapy.[43-45] In patients with nonspecific complaints in whom the diagnosis of LD is in doubt, improvement after antibiotics should not be taken as evidence that the original complaints were related to LD; antibiotics do much more than merely kill microbes, and many have direct effects on mammalian cells, especially cells of the immune system.[46] Some patients with synovitis benefit from intra-articular corticosteroid injections, hydroxychloroquine, or synovectomy.[13] There is no proof that intra-articular steroids lead to chronic arthritis or a poor prognosis. Therapy for LD complicating pregnancy should be as is appropriate for the features of LD, although some clinicians treat all such women parenterally.

Many patients have lingering mild, self-limited, and progressively diminishing complaints such as headache, fatigue, myalgia, and arthralgia. As long as these continue to improve, albeit slowly, and there are no objective findings of inflammation, there is no cause for concern and no reason to institute further antibiotic therapy. These are common (nearly 50% in some reports) and the astute clinician will warn patients about this in advance.

The therapeutic regimens listed in Table 99–4 are of proven efficacy. Although all have been employed for the treatment of hypothesized long-duration or "chronic" LD, there is no evidence that any of the following is of any use: longer-duration IV therapy,[47] oral therapy in the aftermath or IV antibiotic therapy, combination oral therapies, weekly intramuscular or IV "pulse therapy," addition of metronidazole, hydroxychloroquine, or any other agent as a "potentiator" of oral therapies, or hyperbaric oxygen therapy. In the distant past, some LD practitioners utilized malariotherapy (giving the patient an infusion of malarial blood and then treating the resulting parasitemia only after high fevers had been induced); enthusiasm for this approach waned after some of these practitioners admitted it was useless.

All studies suggest the risk of contracting LD from a known tick bite is small (about 1 percent if the tick is not engorged), and prophylactic therapy, therefore, is not recommended.[48,49] Factors suggesting that a tick bite may have transferred *B. burgdorferi* and, therefore, favoring the use of prophylaxis are duration of attachment more than 48 hours and full engorgement of the attached tick. A recent study documents the efficacy of single-dose prophylaxis after tick bite,[50] but the necessity of this approach is still being debated.[51] Major concerns raised are that overreliance on prophylaxis will decrease personal precaution strategies and that many of these people will be repeatedly prophylaxed over the summer, raising questions about toxicity and side effects. Post-LD fibromyalgia does not respond to antibiotics and should be treated as is warranted for primary fibromyalgia.[20]

Prevention is the best treatment. Clinicians in and near endemic areas need to learn about their local ecologies to educate and prepare their patients to avoid LD. People should learn how to identify at-risk areas and then dress and act accordingly by wearing light-colored clothing and high socks and placing the trouser cuffs inside socks whenever possible. A thorough tick check should be performed after time spent in regions where there is potential exposure. If a tick is found, prompt removal represents the most efficient means of preventing LD. Most cases of LD are acquired around the patients' homes. Thus, modification of the "peridomestic" environment can be crucial. Ticks can only survive in areas of higher humidity, such as the leaf clutter on the forest floor. By cleaning out the leaf clutter and low-lying shrubs that commonly constitute the boundary between the forest and their lawn people can eliminate the preferred dwelling site for field mice that are often laden with ticks. Placing a yard width of wood chips at the boundary provides a dry barrier to tick and mouse intrusion; acaricides can be used on the wood chips but need not be applied to sun-drenched lawns, which are dry and, therefore, inhospitable to ticks. Old stone walls are often inhabited by mice, and with the mice come ticks, so such older stone structures should be considered at-risk areas. After time spent in "at risk" areas a shower using a washcloth can dislodge ticks from the body before the tick can attach. Ticks in one's clothing can be killed by placing the clothes in a dryer and running it for 10 to 15 minutes.

As noted previously, LD season starts in mid spring and ends in the mid fall. However, until a killing frost, ticks may still be looking for a blood meal in the winter. These will be adults, which are larger and more easily seen and removed before they can do any harm, but it is important to note that LD can be spread past Thanksgiving should a potential host venture outside and not take appropriate precautions.

Permethrin repellents can be applied to outer clothing and *N,N*-diethyl-*m*-toluamide (DEET) to exposed skin, but the most important precaution is to search for and remove ticks after potential exposure. Acaricides can be used to treat tick-infested domestic animals and can be applied to soil, although if other houses in the community do not use these agents, the efficacy is remarkably reduced.[52] As noted previously, this kind of chemical warfare is not necessary if the environment has been altered appropriately.

The recombinant OspA vaccine was well tolerated and effective,[53,54] but its production ceased prior to the beginning of the 2002 LD season. Its role in the overall public health strategy was never established; were new LD vaccines to be developed, they should certainly not replace personal strategies. Ticks spread other infections, such as those caused by *Babesia microti* and *Anaplasma phagocytophila*,[55,56] and abandoning personal precautions may increase the risk of acquiring one of these other tick-borne infections.

Chronic Lyme Disease

Despite the fact that there is no established definition of, or criteria for the diagnosis of "chronic LD"[57] and that many students of the disease dispute its very existence,[58] there has been great concern about "chronic LD" as a cause of lack of response of LD to antibiotics.[59-61] It is imperative that the consultant seeing a patient with "chronic LD" meticulously examines the initial diagnosis of LD; often the diagnosis was made by faulty interpretation of serologies (often isolated testing without an appropriate clinical context), as a diagnosis of exclusion, or because "my symptoms were classic for LD." The unbiased observer will note that there may be many symptoms associated with LD, but no single complaint nor constellation of features is in any way diagnostic of LD. Once the diagnosis of LD is made, it can take on a life of its own.[62] Commonly, these patients are referred to specialists for evaluation of neurologic and musculoskeletal complaints; if the referring doctor's diagnosis of "chronic LD" precedes the patient, it is common for the "chronic LD" label to be attached to the complaints being evaluated, despite there being no explicit evidence of causality. We must start with the premise that these patients are not well; their complaints are made no less real by the lack of objective findings. As doctor after doctor fails to make a diagnosis leading to successful therapy, as test after test fails to elucidate their plight, they begin to lose faith and hope; this sense of confusion with a lack of any perceived path to personal healing is called "aporia." From confusion comes frustration, anxiety, desperation, and depression. When a clinician is found who makes a diagnosis that is promised to explain all the patient's suffering, that patient may cling to and be fiercely defensive of both diagnosis and chosen clinician. Thus, patients with chronic LD may not be amenable to having the diagnosis changed, antibiotics stopped, or testing terminated.[27,63] Chronic LD is now one of the many explanations for "medically unexplained symptoms."

The literature is now full of reports of patients with chronic LD who had other, potentially remediable problems; in our clinic we have seen antiphospholipid antibody syndrome, multiple sclerosis, partial complex seizure disorder, Parkinson's disease, brain tumors, lupus, ankylosing spondylitis, patellofemoral joint dysfunction, OA, RA, hypermobility, chronic hepatitis C virus infection, and subacute bacterial endocarditis misdiagnosed as chronic LD. Additionally, patients have experienced side effects from long-term antibiotic therapy, including allergic reactions, pseudomembranous colitis, biliary sludging or stones, bone marrow damage (rarely requiring marrow transplant), indwelling catheter–associated thrombosis, line sepsis, and death.

TABLE 99–5 • WARNINGS ON OVERUSE AND MISUSE OF TESTING IN EVALUATING LYME DISEASE

Antibodies may be detectable long after Lyme disease (LD) has been cured; follow-up testing may be misleading. Currently in development, immune complex–based assays may be able to differentiate between persisting seropositivity of no significance and a result indicative of ongoing infection.

Seropositivity is virtually universal in late Lyme disease; "seronegative LD" may occur but is rare and should be subjected to scrutiny.

Seropositivity does not prove causality; a patient may have had LD (or may have a false-positive ELISA) and develop a non-LD problem. Especially in endemic areas, remember the post hoc ergo propter hoc logical fallacy.

Testing inflammatory fluids can provide evidence of local infection.

The Borreliacidal Antibody Assay (the Gundersen Assay) has not been corroborated by another laboratory. It may prove useful, but its role is not well defined.

The Lyme urinary antigen test (LUAT) is of no proven value in the evaluation or management of patients.

Testing antigen-specific T cell proliferative responses has not translated well from the research laboratory to the clinic. False positives and false negatives results and a lack of standardization persists.

There is no role for autoantibody testing in the evaluation or management of patients with LD.

Although there may be long-term consequences,[61] most patients with true LD respond well to standard antibiotic regimens. Post-LD syndromes do occur (e.g., fibromyalgia, depression, cognitive dysfunction). However, overdiagnosis and overtreatment of LD represents a major problem.[27,64,65] In circumstances in which a poorly substantiated diagnosis of chronic LD has been made to explain persisting antibiotic-refractory vague or nonspecific complaints with no objective evidence of *B. burgdorferi* infection (Table 99–5) the clinician must seek alternative explanations and try to guide the patient out of confusion.

Summary

LD is treatable and curable and can be diagnosed with attention to the precise details of the syndrome. Laboratory testing, although not perfect, is certainly valuable when used to help confirm a diagnosis of LD based on explicit and suggestive historic and physical findings. The diagnosis of LD should never be based on isolated test results or made in a patient with "symptoms compatible with LD" without objective findings (i.e., a diagnosis of exclusion). The cause of chronic post-LD complaints is often unclear, but they usually do not indicate ongoing infection. There is no role for long-term or combination antibiotic regimens or novel medications. There is no definable chronic LD syndrome, and this diagnosis should be viewed with skepticism; alternative explanations should be actively pursued, and if resolution is not obtained, referral to an academic center where many such patients are seen should be entertained.

REFERENCES

1. Sigal LH: The immunology and potential mechanisms of immunopathogenesis of Lyme disease. Annu Rev Immunol 15:63, 1997.
2. Barbour AG, Fish D: The biological and social phenomena of Lyme disease. Science 260:1610, 1993.
3. Aronowitz RA: Lyme disease: The social construction of a new disease and its social consequences. Millbank Q 69:79, 1991.
4. Matuschka F-R, Endepols S, Richter D, et al: Risk of urban Lyme disease enhanced by the presence of rats. J Infect Dis 174:1108, 1996.
5. Cronin W: Changes in the Land. New York, Farrar, Straus & Giroux, 1983.
6. Kirkland KB, Klimko TB, Meriwether RA, et al: Erythema migrans–like rash illness at a camp in North Carolina: A new tick-borne disease. Arch Intern Med 157:2635, 1997.
7. Barbour AG, Maupin GO, Teltow GJ, et al: Identification of an uncultivatable *Borrelia* species in the hard tick *Amblyomma americanum*: Possible agent of a Lyme disease-like illness. J Infect Dis 403:173, 1996.
8. Falco RC, Fish D, Piesman J: Duration of tick bites in a Lyme disease–endemic area. Am J Epidemiol 143:187, 1996.
9. Nadelman RB, Wormser GP: Erythema migrans and early Lyme disease. Am J Med 98:15s, 1995.
10. Logigian EL, Kaplan RF, Steere AC: Chronic neurologic manifestations of Lyme disease. N Engl J Med 323:1438, 1990.
11. Halperin J, Heyes MP: Neuroactive kynurenines in Lyme borreliosis. Neurology 42:43, 1992.
12. Sigal LH: Lyme arthritis. Rheum Dis Clin North Am 24:323, 1998.
13. Steere, AC, Schoen RT, Taylor E: The clinical evolution of Lyme arthritis. Ann Intern Med 107:725, 1987.
14. Kalish R, Leong JM, Steere AC: Association of treatment-resistant chronic Lyme arthritis with HLA-DR4 and antibody reactivity to ospA and ospB of *Borrelia burgdorferi*. Infect Immun 61:2774, 1993.
15. Kamradt T, Krause A, Burmester G-R: A role for T cells in the pathogenesis of treatment-resistant Lyme arthritis. Mol Med 1:486, 1995.
16. Lengl-Janssen B, Strauss AF, Steere AC, Kamradt T: The T helper cell response in Lyme arthritis: Differential recognition of *Borrelia burgdorferi* outer surface protein A in patients with treatment-resistant or treatment-responsive Lyme arthritis. J Exp Med 180:2069, 1994.
17. Gross DM, Forsthuber T, Tary-Lehmann M, et al: Identification of LFA-1 as a candidate autoantigen in treatment-resistant Lyme arthritis. Science 281:703, 1998.
18. Bohme M, Standaert SM, Karch H, et al: Lyme Borreliosis: Second most common bacterial disease in Germany. Arthritis Rheum 40:S124, 1997.
19. Huppertz HI, Karch H, Suschke HJ, et al: Lyme arthritis in European children and adolescents. Arthritis Rheum 38:361, 1995.
20. Szer IS, Taylor E, Steere AC: The long-term course of Lyme arthritis in children. N Engl J Med 325:159, 1991.
21. Hsu V, Patella SJ, Sigal LH: "Chronic Lyme disease" as the incorrect diagnosis in patients with fibromyalgia. Arthritis Rheum 36:1493, 1993.
22. Sigal LH, Patella SJ: Lyme arthritis as the incorrect diagnosis in fibromyalgia in children and adolescents. Pediatrics 90:523, 1992.
23. Asch E, Bujak DI, Weiss M, et al: Lyme disease: An infectious and postinfectious syndrome. J Rheumatol 21:454, 1994.
24. Bujak D, Weinstein A, Dornbush RL: Clinical and neurocognitive features of the post Lyme disease syndrome. J Rheumatol 23:1392, 1996.
25. Gaudino EA, Coyle PK, Krupp LB: Post-Lyme syndrome and chronic fatigue syndrome: Neuropsychiatric similarities and differences. Arch Neurol 54:1372, 1997.
26. Gerber MA, Zemel LS, Shapiro ED: Lyme arthritis in children: Clinical epidemiology and long-term outcome. Pediatrics 102:905, 1998.
27. Sigal LH: Special article: Pitfalls in the diagnosis and management of Lyme disease. Arthritis Rheum 41:195, 1998.
28. Hilton E, Tramontano A, DeVoti J, Sood SK: Temporal study of immunoglobulin M seroreactivity to *Borrelia burgdorferi* in patients treated for Lyme Borreliosis. J Clin Microbiol 35:774, 1997.

29. Aguero-Rosenfeld M, Nowakowski J, Bittker S, et al: Evolution of the serologic response to *Borrelia burgdorferi* in treated patients with culture-confirmed erythema migrans. J Clin Microbiol 34:1, 1996.

30. Kaell A, Redecha PR, Elkon KB, et al: Occurrence of antibodies to *Borrelia burgdorferi* in patients with nonspirochetal subacute bacterial endocarditis. Ann Intern Med 119:1079, 1993.

31. Weiss NL, Phillips MR, Sadock VA, Sigal LH, Merryman PF, Abramson SB. False positive seroreactivity to *B. burgdorferi* in systemic lupus erythematosus rheumatic: The value of immunoblotting. Lupus 1995; 4:131-137.

32. Centers for Disease Control: Recommendations for test performance and interpretation from the Second National Conference on Serologic Diagnosis of Lyme Disease. MMWR 44:590-591, 1995.

33. Magnarelli L, Fikrig E, Padula SJ, et al: Use of recombinant antigens of *Borrelia burgdorferi* in serologic tests for diagnosis of Lyme Borreliosis. J Clin Microbiol 34:237, 1996.

34. Brunner M, Stein S, Mitchell PD, Sigal LH: IgM capture assay for the serologic confirmation of early Lyme disease: Analyzing immune complexes with biotinylated *Borrelia burgdorferi* sonicate enhanced with flagellin peptide epitope. J Clin Microbiol 36:1074, 1998.

35. Brunner M, Sigal LH: Immune complexes from Lyme disease sera contain *Borrelia burgdorferi* antigen and antigen-specific antibodies: Potential use for improved testing. J Infect Dis 182:534-539, 2000.

36. Brunner M, Sigal LH: Use of serum immune complexes in a new test that accurately confirms early Lyme disease and active infection with *Borrelia burgdorferi*. J Clin Microbiol 39:3213-3321, 2001.

37. Persing D, Rutledge BJ, Rys PN, et al: Target imbalance: Disparity of *Borrelia burgdorferi* genetic material in synovial fluid from Lyme arthritis patients. J Infect Dis 169:668, 1994.

38. Bradley J, Johnson RC, Goodman JL: The persistence of spirochetal nucleic acids in active Lyme disease. Ann Intern Med 120:487, 1994.

39. Jaulhac B, Chary-Valckenaere I, Sibilia J, et al: Detection of *Borrelia burgdorferi* by DNA amplification in synovial tissue samples from patients with Lyme arthritis. Arthritis Rheum 39:736, 1996.

40. Malawista S, Barthold SW, Persing DH: Fate of *Borrelia burgdorferi* DNA in tissues of infected mice after antibiotic treatment. J Infect Dis 179:1312, 1994.

41. Klempner MS, Schmid CH, Hu L, et al. Intralaboratory reliability of serologic and urine testing for Lyme disease. Am J Med 110:217-219, 2001.

42. Lawson JP, Steere AC: Lyme arthritis: Radiographic features. Radiology 154:37, 1985.

43. Rahn D, Malawista S: Treatment of Lyme disease. *In* Mandell GL, Bone RC, Cline MJ, et al (eds): 1994 Year Book of Medicine. St. Louis, Mosby, 1994, pp xxi-xxxvi.

44. Luft BJ, Dattwyler RJ, Johnson RC, et al: Azithromycin compared with amoxicillin in the treatment of erythema migrans: A double-blind, randomized, controlled trial. Ann Intern Med 124:785, 1996.

45. Dattwyler RJ, Luft BJ, Kunkel MJ, et al: Ceftriaxone compared with doxycycline for the treatment of acute disseminated Lyme disease. N Engl J Med 337:289, 1997.

46. Sigal LH: Use of antibiotics in rheumatologic syndromes. Rheum Dis Clin North Am 25:861, 1999.

47. Klempner MS, Hu LT, Evans J, et al: Two controlled trial of antibiotic treatment in patients with persistent symptoms and a history of Lyme disease. N Engl J Med 345:85-92, 2001.

48. Magid D, Schwartz B, Craft J, Schwartz J: Prevention of Lyme disease after tick bite: A cost-effectiveness analysis. N Engl J Med 327:534, 1992.

49. Warshafsky S, Nowakowsky J, Nadelman RB, et al: Efficacy of antibiotic prophylaxis for prevention of Lyme disease. J Gen Intern Med 11:329, 1996.

50. Nadelman RB, Nowakowski J, Fish D, et al: Prophylaxis with single-dose doxycycline for the prevention of Lyme disease after *Ixodes scapularis* tick bite. N Engl J Med 345:79-84, 2001.

51. Shapiro ED: Doxycycline for tick bites: Not for everyone. N Engl J Med 345:133-134, 2001.

52. Fish D: Environmental risk and prevention of Lyme disease. Am J Med 98(Suppl 4A):2S, 1995.

53. Sigal LH, Zahradnik JM, Lavin P, et al: A vaccine consisting of recombinant *Borrelia burgdorferi* outer-surface protein A to prevent Lyme disease. N Engl J Med 339:216, 1998.

54. Steere AC, Sikand VK, Meurics F, et al: Vaccination against Lyme disease with recombinant *Borrelia burgdorferi* outer-surface lipoprotein A with adjuvant. N Engl J Med 339:209, 1998.

55. Magnarelli LA, Ijdo JW, Anderson JF, et al: Human exposure to a granulocytic *Ehrlichia* and other tick-borne agents in Connecticut. J Clin Microbiol 36:2823, 1998.

56. Mitchell P, Reed KD, Hofkes JM: Immunoserologic evidence of co-infection with *Borrelia burgdorferi*, *Babesia microti*, and human granulocytic *Ehrlichia* species in residents of Wisconsin and Minnesota. J Clin Microbiol 34:724, 1996.

57. Wormser GP, Nadelman RB, Dattwyler RJ, et al: Practice guidelines for the treatment of Lyme disease. Clin Infect Dis 31:S1-S14, 2000.

58. Sigal LH: The existence of "chronic Lyme disease". Curr Treat Opt Infect Dis 3:263-265, 2001.

59. Sigal LH: Persisting complaints attributed to Lyme disease: Possible mechanisms and implications for management. Am J Med 96:365, 1994.

60. Sigal LH: The Lyme disease controversy: The social and financial costs of the mismanagement of Lyme disease. Arch Intern Med 156:1493, 1996.

61. Shadick N, Phillips C, Logigian E, et al: The long-term clinical outcomes of Lyme disease: A population-based retrospective cohort study. Ann Intern Med 121:560, 1994.

62. Sigal LH: Misconceptions about Lyme disease: Focusing on ill-chosen terminology to focus on confusion. Ann Intern Med 136:413-419, 2002.

63. Sigal LH, Hassett AL: Contributions of societal and geographical environments to "Chronic Lyme disease": The psychopathogenesis and aporology of a new "medically unexplained symptoms" syndrome—Environmental Health Perspectives: Environmental Factors in Medically Unexplained Physical Symptoms and Related Syndromes. 110(Suppl 4):607-611, 2002.

64. Steere A, Taylor E, McHugh G, Logigian E: The overdiagnosis of Lyme disease. Environmental Health Perspectives JAMA 269:1812, 1993.

65. Lightfoot RW Jr, Luft BJ, Rahn DW, et al: Treatment of "possible Lyme disease": A practical policy position of the American College of Rheumatology and the Infectious Disease Society of America based on cost-benefit analysis. Ann Intern Med 119:503, 1993.

Mycobacterial and Fungal Infections

J. TIMOTHY HARRINGTON

The epidemiology of tuberculosis and other mycobacterial and fungal infections continues to evolve rapidly in both developed and developing countries. In the United States and other developed countries, the resurgence of tuberculosis during the 1980s and early 1990s has since abated, leading to the lowest rate in U.S. history by 2000 (5.8 cases per 100,000 population)[1] (Fig. 100–1). This improvement, as a result of more effectively implemented public health strategies and improved treatment of infected individuals, does not diminish the need for continuing vigilance, especially with regard to tuberculosis reactivation in both United States–born and foreign-born persons with latent disease.[2-4] This risk is reflected in the high incidence of tuberculosis, often with atypical disease presentations, in aging adults (22 cases per 100,000) and in rheumatoid arthritis (RA) patients treated with tumor necrosis factor (TNF)-neutralizing agents.[5-7]

In contrast, tuberculosis continues to ravage the populations of developing countries, in whom it causes 8 million new cases and 1.9 million deaths each year.[8] About one third of the world's population is infected with tuberculosis, providing a reservoir that will continue to complicate its global control.[9] In many areas, multidrug-resistant disease, coincident human immunodeficiency virus (HIV) infection, and poor nutrition and living conditions magnify the challenge of disease control.[10-12] In addition, a report suggests that some outbreaks may be caused by unusually virulent strains of *Mycobacterium tuberculosis*.[13] Worldwide public health initiatives, more reliable diagnostic tests, new treatment regimens, and more effective vaccines are being developed to address these daunting realities.[14-17]

Skeletal tuberculosis makes up about 1 to 2 percent of all cases and about 10 percent of extrapulmonary cases in the United States. In about 50 percent of these cases, no pulmonary involvement can be detected.[18] By 1991, 21 percent of extrapulmonary tuberculosis cases in the United States were acquired immune deficiency syndrome (AIDS) associated. In developing countries, the HIV pandemic has led to marked increases in osteoarticular tuberculosis coinfection.[19] These cases are distinguished by disseminated multifocal disease suggestive of hematogenous spread, rapid progression, and more common coexistence with pulmonary infection.[20,21]

developed countries where their low incidence leads to a low index of suspicion.[22,23] They typically manifest with chronic indolent localized involvement of the bones, spine, peripheral joints, or soft tissues that produces a focus of nonspecific pain and, less often, swelling. In infections initiated by direct tissue inoculation, the traumatic event is often trivial or remote in time from the onset of clinical disease. Diagnosis may be delayed for months to years, in part because of minimal early symptoms and also through attribution of the problem to a noninfectious disorder until disease progression and disability prompt more aggressive diagnostic investigation.

Constitutional symptoms are typically subtle or absent, and laboratory indicators of inflammation are often normal. Synovial effusion is often minimal, and the fluid, even if it is obtainable, shows nonspecific inflammation. Radiographic abnormalities may be delayed in appearance, although newer imaging techniques have aided in the earlier detection of abnormalities and the distinction of tuberculosis from other infections and neoplasm.[24,25] Characteristic pulmonary or extrapulmonary findings are not always present; for example, more than 50 percent of osteoarticular tuberculosis manifests without evidence of past or present pulmonary disease. Tuberculin and other skin tests may provide useful clues to etiology, but results are not invariably positive, especially in debilitated or immunosuppressed patients. Correct diagnosis is highly dependent, in most cases, on demonstration of the infectious agent by microscopic examination and culture of affected tissue. The role of nucleic acid amplification (NAA) tests in diagnosing these infections is still being defined, and they must be interpreted with caution in extrapulmonary tissue specimens and when the clinical suspicion of infection is low.[26-28]

In HIV-infected patients, these infections are often diagnosed before AIDS and may lead to its recognition.[29] Atypical pulmonary tuberculosis and extrapulmonary (often multifocal) infection are common; extrapulmonary infection occurs in 60 to 70 percent of such cases, compared to 16 percent of all tuberculosis patients.

This review focuses on the musculoskeletal presentations of tuberculosis and other mycobacterial and fungal infections and the principles of their diagnosis and treatment. More general information about these infectious diseases is available elsewhere.[30]

▌ Diagnostic Perspectives

Musculoskeletal infections caused by mycobacteria and fungi are often a diagnostic challenge, particularly in

▌ Osteoarticular Tuberculosis

The clinical patterns of skeletal tuberculosis include spondylitis, osteomyelitis, peripheral joint infection, and

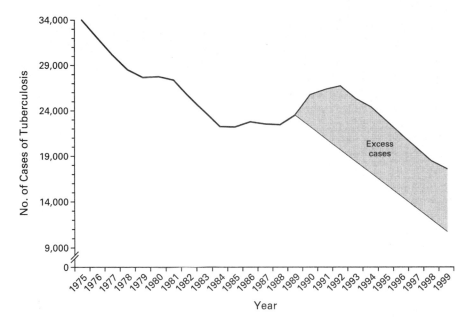

FIGURE 100–1 · Reported Cases of Tuberculosis in the United States from 1975 to 1999. The shaded area represents the 67,000 cases that would not have occurred if earlier plans for the elimination of the disease had been successfully implemented. (From N Engl 3 Med 2001, 345(3). 190)

soft tissue abscess. In a series of 230 consecutive cases of tuberculosis from the preantibiotic era, 5.2 percent had skeletal involvement; the spine was affected in 60 percent of cases.[31] The incidence of extrapulmonary and osteoarticular disease has risen during the last decade at a rate exceeding that of lung involvement.

In nonendemic areas, skeletal tuberculosis usually occurs in elderly, debilitated patients, most often in the form of solitary osteolytic lesions in the axial skeleton. The development of skeletal disease is often remote from the initial infection, which strongly implies reactivation of previous subclinical disease. Patients may have a negative tuberculin test result and long-term corticosteroid use or coexisting debilitating diseases, such as RA, alcoholism, or chronic renal failure, that compromise resistance.[32,33] The occurrence of spinal disease in children has largely been eliminated by effective medical therapy of pulmonary infection.

In contrast, in endemic areas with high infectivity rates, those infected are more commonly children and young to middle-aged adults. These individuals have a higher incidence of multifocal skeletal involvement in the ribs, pelvis, vertebral appendages, cervical spine, feet, and long bone diaphyses, and they show positive tuberculin reactivity.[34] Bony seeding occurs through hematogenous spread, sometimes secondarily from another extrapulmonary site. When pulmonary findings are present, a miliary pattern is typical. Spread to bone may also occur from infected nodes, either by direct extension or through draining lymph channels.[35]

A recently published symposium draws on the experience of experts from high-incidence countries to provide insights into the diagnosis and management of osteoarticular tuberculosis.[36]

SPONDYLITIS

The spine is the dominant site of involvement in skeletal tuberculosis, accounting for 50 to 60 percent of cases.[35]

From 48 to 67 percent of lesions occur in the lower thoracic and thoracolumbar spine in HIV-negative patients, whereas the lumbar spine is most commonly involved in HIV-positive patients.[20] The cervical spine is less often involved. Unilateral sacroiliac involvement is not uncommon. Infection usually begins in the anterior subchondral bone of a single vertebra adjacent to the intervertebral disk (Fig. 100–2). Progression to bone changes takes 2 to 5 months and begins with extension, first from cancellous to cortical bone and then across the disk space to adjacent vertebrae (Fig. 100–3). Bone destruction may lead to vertebral collapse. Isolated neural arch involvement and intraspinal abscess may also occur.

Paravertebral abscess begins with the extension of infection under the anterior longitudinal ligament. In the thoracic spine, this may extend into the pleural space and lung parenchyma. In the cervical region, it may present in the posterior cervical triangle or retropharyngeal space. In the lumbar spine, a cold abscess characteristically produces lateral displacement of the psoas muscle and may dissect along its length to present as a mass in the inguinal triangle, gluteal muscle, or upper thigh. In isolated cases, a cold abscess occurs with inapparent bone involvement. A particular variant of this presentation is subligamentous tuberculosis, in which infection spreads up and down the spine beneath the longitudinal ligament, producing scalloping of multiple anterior vertebral bodies without disk involvement. This pattern is more common in the cervical spine.[37]

The clinical presentation of spinal tuberculosis usually consists of localized pain, often accompanied by low-grade fever, weight loss, chills, and nonspecific constitutional symptoms. Patients may also present initially with abscess formation or kyphosis, or there may be symptoms of spinal cord or nerve root involvement. Paraparesis and paraplegia are reported in 1 to 27 percent of various series. In comparison to pyogenic and brucellar vertebral osteomyelitis, spinal tuberculosis

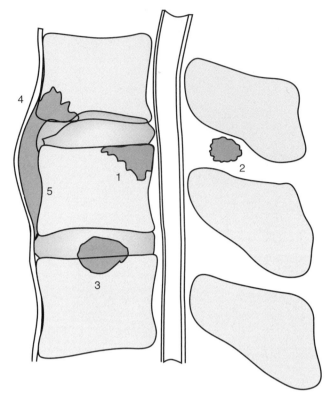

more often presents with a prolonged clinical course, thoracic segment involvement, absence of fever, spinal deformity, neurologic deficit, and paravertebral or epidural masses.[38] On occasion, tuberculous spondylitis may present with chronic inflammatory-type back pain more typical of the spondyloarthropathies.[39]

Conventional radiography, including tomography, is generally a useful approach for defining bone destruction, the extent of disease, and adjacent soft tissue lesions.[40] Magnetic resonance imaging (MRI) is more effective in identifying early disease, may help to distinguish tuberculosis from other infections and neoplasm, and can aid in evaluating the extent of disease.[25,41] Scintiscans with technetium and gallium may also be helpful in localizing bone and soft tissue lesions, but early false-negative findings are not uncommon.[42] Computed tomography (CT) can be helpful in guiding diagnostic needle biopsy. Fine-needle biopsy is an acceptable alternative to core-needle biopsy and open biopsy in the diagnosis of osteoarticular tuberculosis in both the axial and peripheral skeleton, and it has the advantage of obviating general anesthesia.[43,44] Both CT and MRI may also be helpful in monitoring therapy.[45]

Mycobacterial colony counts in bone biopsy specimens are relatively low. Only 40 percent of smears and cultures from psoas abscesses are positive. Of patients meeting strict clinical and radiographic criteria in one series, between 73 and 82 percent had compatible histologic features on biopsy; of these, 80 to 95 percent had positive culture results.[35] The differential diagnosis, which is extensive, includes pyogenic and fungal osteomyelitis, primary and metastatic tumors, sarcoidosis, multiple myeloma, and eosinophilic granuloma.

A consensus approach to therapy is the institution of three-drug treatment, even with neurologic involvement.[46] The main determinent of successful outcome is the duration of infection before treatment is initiated. Important considerations include ensuring patient compliance, coexistence of HIV infection, and emergence of secondary resistance. The traditionally recommended duration of chemotherapy has been 18 months, but the low colony counts in spinal lesions and reports of success with 6-month protocols suggest that briefer treatment may be equally effective.[47] Bed rest provides no advantage over ambulatory chemotherapy.[48] Radical resection and anterior spinal fusion should be strongly considered if neurologic complications do not improve within 4 to 6 weeks of therapy, are severe below the level of infection, or worsen on treatment.[49,50] Otherwise, initial débridement should not be undertaken except for diagnosis if needle biopsy and aspiration are nondiagnostic. Progress of spinal deformity is influenced by the severity of the angle before treatment, the level of the lesion, and the age of the patient.[51] Children with "at risk" radiologic signs are subject to worsening deformity during the growth spurt after infection is controlled. Surgery to prevent deformity must be done early in high-risk patients to achieve satisfactory results. Procedures may be individualized using MRI to evaluate the presence of anterior and posterior vertebral involvement.[52]

Cervical spine involvement is relatively rare, amounting to only 0.4 to 1.2 percent of cases of extrapulmonary tuberculosis in the United States.[53] The most common presenting symptoms are neck pain and stiffness, although hoarseness, dysphagia, torticollis, fever, anorexia, and neurologic disorders may also occur. Spinal involvement can progress to myelopathy because of delays in diagnosis. Radiographs may show characteristic osteolysis of the anterior vertebral body with sparing of the posterior portion, gibbus deformity, disk involvement, and a partially calcified paraspinous mass. CT or MRI is useful for assessing compromise of the spinal canal. Retropharyngeal infection may extend into the craniocervical junction, and if not promptly recognized, it may cause atlantoaxial dislocation and neurologic complications.[54,55]

The sacroiliac joint is involved in up to 10 percent of cases of skeletal tuberculosis, often without other evidence of disease.[56] Infection, and tuberculosis in particular, should be suspected in all cases of unilateral sacroiliitis. Emigration from an endemic area and a past history of tuberculosis increase the likelihood of this cause. Buttock pain on the involved side is the presenting symptom and is often accompanied by proximal leg or radicular pain. Examination reveals sacroiliac tenderness to palpation and stress maneuvers. Sacroiliac films show joint widening and erosion in all cases. An elevated erythrocyte sedimentation rate (ESR) and anemia are common, and a positive tuberculin reaction is typical.

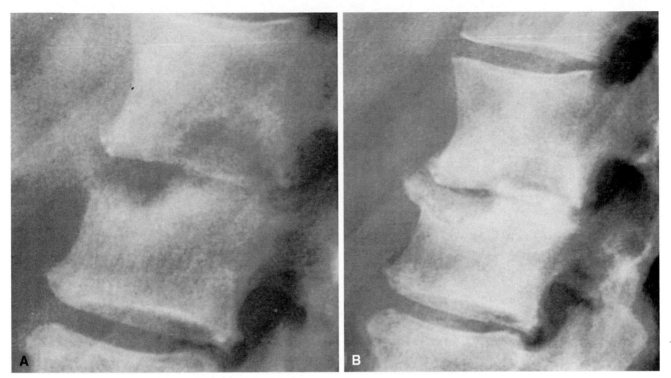

FIGURE 100–3 · Tuberculous Spondylitis: Diskovertebral Lesion. *A,* The initial radiograph reveals subchondral destruction of two vertebral bodies with mild surrounding eburnation and loss of intervertebral disk height. The appearance is identical to that in pyogenic spondylitis *B,* Several months later, osseous response is evident. Note the increased sclerosis. Osteophytosis and improved definition of the osseous margins can be seen. (From Resnick D: Diagnosis of Bone and Joint Disorders, 3rd ed. Philadelphia, WB Saunders, 1995, p 2465.)

Biopsy of the sacroiliac joint shows granulomatous histologic features or nonspecific inflammation and a positive culture in most cases. Treatment for 12 to 18 months is associated with gradual reduction in symptoms and improved function. Needle biopsy showing granulomatous histopathologic features is an appropriate indication for instituting treatment before culture results are available.

Atypical spinal lesions, which occur in about 10 percent of cases, may lead to delayed diagnosis and treatment. Atypical radiographic presentations in single vertebrae include concentric collapse, sclerotic foci, and selective involvement of the vertebral arches and costotransverse joints. Multiple vertebrae may be involved either in continuity or as skipped lesions. Atypical clinical presentations may suggest a herniated intervertebral disk, failed back syndrome, spinal tumor, meningeal granuloma, or cold abscess without vertebral distruction.[37,57]

TUBERCULOUS OSTEOMYELITIS

Bone lesions begin with hematogenous implantation of organisms in the medullary area. Metaphyseal involvement is most common, and lesions may spread through the growth plate to involve the adjacent joint, usually late in the disease course. Lesions are typically destructive.

Tuberculous osteomyelitis occurs in both children and adults.[48,58] Although any bone may be involved, the femur and tibia are most commonly affected. Dactylitis

may also occur in children. In one large series from an endemic area,[59] such cases represented 19 percent of bone and joint tuberculosis and 15 percent of cases of osteomyelitis of hematogenous origin. Bone pain was the most common presentation; a draining sinus, abscess formation, and local swelling and tenderness were also common. The average delay before diagnosis was 28 months.

Multifocal osteoarticular tuberculosis is a less common variant of the disease,[60] but tuberculosis should be considered in all patients from endemic areas who present with multiple destructive skeletal lesions.

For a definitive diagnosis of osteoarticular tuberculosis, a biopsy specimen of an affected site needs to be isolated.[32] Soft tissue lesions characteristically demonstrate rim enhancement on CT examination. CT may also facilitate percutaneous needle biopsy or abscess drainage.[61] Histologic examination generally reveals granulomatous inflammation. In one series, biopsy showed a positive culture in 40 cases, granulomatous histologic features in 56 cases, and both in 25 cases.[59]

Radiographic findings include cavity formation with a thin adjacent layer of sclerosis in about 50 percent of cases, sometimes containing a sequestrum. The true extent of bone involvement may be difficult to detect because of clinically silent lesions. Bone imaging with technetium-99, although more sensitive than conventional radiographs, provides false-negative information in some cases of early, indolent, or highly destructive disease. Tuberculin test reactions are positive in 92 percent of cases.

Treatment with chemotherapy is generally effective. In a minority of cases, surgical débridement is required for healing. Initiation of therapy on the basis of histologic findings is appropriate pending culture results. Sinus cultures are commonly positive for pyogenic bacteria both before and after antituberculous therapy. Healing is associated with sclerosis at the margin of lesions. Misdiagnosis of the condition as pyogenic osteomyelitis may lead to unnecessary surgery or to delayed antituberculous treatment, with resulting extension of infection into the joint and chronic disability.

SEPTIC ARTHRITIS

Tuberculous joint involvement is second in frequency to vertebral infection.[37] The typical pattern is a monarticular arthritis involving the large and medium joints, most commonly the hip and knee.[62,63] Other joints commonly involved include the sacroiliac, shoulder, elbow, ankle, carpal, and tarsal joints. Infection begins in the synovium, with progression of destructive changes being slower than in pyogenic septic arthritis.

Tuberculous arthritis is an often-missed diagnosis. A consecutive series spanning the years 1970 to 1984 emphasizes typical features.[64] Of 23 cases of musculoskeletal tuberculosis, 9 involved the spine; 1 the hip; and the remaining 13 the peripheral joints. Most patients were men older than 50 years. The history of tuberculosis or exposure was generally forgotten. In all cases, presenting symptoms were joint pain and swelling. Four patients had evidence of active pulmonary tuberculosis, and in two patients with sterile pyuria, *M. tuberculosis* grew from the urine. Only 5 of 10 patients tested had a positive tuberculin reaction. Radiographs showed changes of erosive arthritis in 7 and no changes in four of 11 joints studied. The median delay in diagnosis was 8 months.

Arriving at a correct diagnosis requires vigorous pursuit and usually includes synovial biopsy and culture. Initial studies are often misleading and may contribute to delayed diagnosis or misdiagnosis. Synovial fluid findings are variable and do not distinguish this arthropathy from other inflammatory or septic arthritides.[65] Cell counts more often suggest inflammatory rather than septic arthritis and contain a preponderance of neutrophils. Synovial fluid glucose tends to be low and more than 10 mg/dl below fasting serum levels, but nonfasting determinations are often misleading. The diagnosis may be facilitated if the organism is observed on an acid-fast smear of synovial fluid, but only 19 percent of cases are positive. In contrast, 79 percent of synovial fluid cultures are positive. One report has suggested that a synovial fluid lymphocyte proliferation assay using tuberculin protein may have diagnostic value.[66] Radiographic changes are similar to those seen in other septic arthritides, beginning with juxta-articular bone demineralization and progressing to marginal bone erosion and articular cartilage destruction (Fig. 100–4).

With the open-biopsy technique, granulomatous histologic features and positive cultures are present in 94

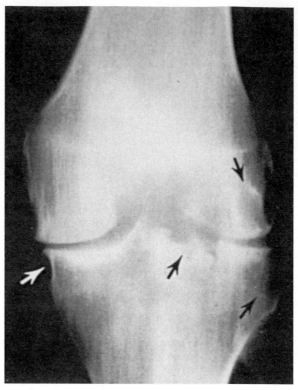

FIGURE 100–4 · Tuberculous Arthritis: Knee. On a conventional computed tomogram, (CT) typical marginal and central osseous erosions (*arrows*) accompany tuberculous arthritis. Osteoporosis is not prominent. (From Resnick D: Diagnosis of Bone and Joint Disorders, 3rd ed. Philadelphia, WB Saunders, 1995, p 2480.)

percent of cases. No data are available for direct amplification tests in mycobacterial arthritis, but their use should be considered in suspected cases to provide earlier diagnosis. The histologic examination alone may be confusing because granulomatous synovitis may also be found in atypical mycobacterial infection, sarcoidosis, erythema nodosum, brucellosis, Crohn's disease, and foreign body reaction. A synovial acid-fast smear is of limited value; only 10 percent of reported cases are positive. Tuberculous arthritis is also reported in children, at times early in the disease course; synovial biopsy and culture are recommended in patients with monarthritis and a positive tuberculin reaction.[67]

Tuberculosis must be considered among the possible causes of septic arthritis occurring in patients with pre-existing RA,[68] although it is not widely seen in developed countries.[68,69] Conversely, rheumatoid factor (RF) may be present in tuberculosis, leading to diagnostic confusion in the presence of monarthritis.[69]

SOFT TISSUE ABSCESS

Tuberculosis only rarely involves skeletal muscle but must be considered in the differential diagnosis of enlarging muscle lesions.[70-74] Isolated cases involving tendons,[75] the trochanteric bursa,[76] and fascia lata[77] illustrate the variety of possibilities. Biopsy and culture are required for diagnosis. Imaging studies do not distinguish tuberculosis from neoplasm.

DRUG TREATMENT

The drugs available for treatment of tuberculosis are classified as standard, or first-line, and reserve, or second-line, drugs[78] (Table 100–1). They may also be bactericidal or bacteriostatic. Generally, the standard drugs are more effective and less toxic, and the reserve drugs are used only when the standard drugs can not be included.

The rationale for using multiple drugs in tuberculosis therapy is that different agents kill multiplying organisms by different mechanisms.[79-81] In addition, pyrazinamide potentiates the activity of isoniazid and rifampin. Streptomycin and ethambutol accelerate killing when they are added to isoniazid and rifampin. Isoniazid and rifampin eliminate the slowly multiplying "persisters" that most often cause late relapses. Pyrazinamide is effective against intracellular organisms in macrophages, another source of relapse.

The increasing incidence of drug-resistant tuberculosis complicates the selection of appropriate drug treatment.[82-84] The likelihood of isoniazid resistance increases in patients who have a relapse after initial treatment that has not included both isoniazid and rifampin. The prevalence of isoniazid resistance is high in many developing countries and generally among Asians and Hispanics. In patients more likely to have drug-resistant strains, therapy should be initiated with at least two drugs that have not been previously used and, preferably, with three or four drugs for at least 24 months. Directly observed therapy is also widely advocated to reduce the spread of infection and frequency of drug-resistant tuberculosis.[85]

The optimal duration of therapy for extrapulmonary tuberculosis, including osteoarticular disease, is an unsettled matter.[79] Reluctance to use the short-duration protocols proven effective for pulmonary disease is based on the unfavorable prognosis associated with extrapulmonary infection before highly effective antimicrobial agents became available.

Recently recommended regimens for osteoarticular tuberculosis caused by susceptible organisms include 6 to 9 months of multidrug treatment; longer durations are used for cases of relapse and infection with resistant organisms. Reports suggest that failure and relapse rates are comparable to those for pulmonary infection, but the success of briefer treatment may depend, in part, on surgical drainage of abscess areas.

Dutt and Stead[79] used daily treatment for 1 month with isoniazid (300 mg) and rifampin (600 mg) followed by isoniazid (900 mg) and rifampin (600 mg) twice weekly for 8 months. They obtained a cure rate of 95 percent in 348 cases of extrapulmonary tuberculosis, including 65 of 66 cases of bone and joint disease, the one failure being a late relapse in vertebral osteomyelitis. With suspected isoniazid resistance, the addition of pyrazinamide (25 to 30 mg/kg/day) and either streptomycin (10 to 15 mg/kg/day) or ethambutol (25 mg/kg/day) for 2 months, followed by 7 months of isoniazid and rifampin, is recommended. Alternatively, in suspected or proven isoniazid-resistant cases, an intensive schedule may be used for 2 months with streptomycin (0.5 to 1.0 g, 5 days/week) or ethambutol (25 mg/kg), plus pyrazinamide (25 to 30 mg/kg), isoniazid (300 mg), and rifampin (600 mg) daily, followed by another 4 months of isoniazid and rifampin (either 300 and 600 mg daily or 900 and 600 mg twice weekly).

In comprehensive reviews of tuberculosis treatment,[80,86] two first-line regimens recommended by the American Thoracic Society and the Centers for Disease Control and Prevention (CDC) are outlined: 1) isoniazid and rifampin for 6 months, supplemented by an initial 2 months of pyrazinamide; or 2) isoniazid and rifampin for 9 months, with ethambutol in the initial 2 months. The second protocol is recommended for individuals with epidemiologic characteristics suggesting a higher likelihood of drug resistance.

Other Tuberculosis-Related Musculoskeletal Syndromes

PONCET'S DISEASE

In individuals with active tuberculosis or family exposure, isolated, apparently rare examples of nonsuppurative reactive arthritis are described that are clinically distinct from septic arthritis and resolve with antituberculous chemotherapy (Poncet's disease).[87] A similarity to other reactive arthritides is implied by the detection of human leukocyte antigen (HLA)-B27 in some cases.

BACILLE CALMETTE-GUÉRIN–ASSOCIATED RHEUMATIC SYNDROMES

Granulomatous bone and joint lesions may also develop after immunization or therapy for bladder cancer with bacille Calmette-Guérin.[87,88] In several reports, 0.5 to 5 percent of patients treated with bacille Calmette-Guérin had polyarthralgia arthritis, typically a self-limited, seronegative, reactive arthritis responsive to nonsteroidal agents. Several patients had presented with other features of Reiter's syndrome as well, including conjunctivitis, fever, urethritis, pericarditis, and epididymitis.

Osteoarticular Infections Caused by Other Mycobacteria

The existence of a wide variety of other mycobacterial species has been known since shortly after the discovery of M. tuberculosis by Koch in the 1880s.[89] These organ-

TABLE 100–1 · CHEMOTHERAPEUTIC AGENTS FOR TUBERCULOSIS

	Bactercidal	Bacteriostatic
Standard	Isoniazid Rafampicin Streptomycin Pyrazinamide	Ethambutol Thiacetazone
Reserve	Capreomycin Kanamycin	Ethionamide Cycloserine Para-amino salicylic acid

isms are ubiquitous in nature and may contaminate clinical specimens or colonize body surfaces without being the cause of clinical disease. Awareness of their importance in human infection was established in the 1950s[90] and has since expanded, in part as a result of improved microbiologic techniques but also because of these species' role in clinical infection in immunocompromised hosts, with about 50 species now recognized as possible causes of disease.[91-93]

The classification of mycobacterial organisms was based until recently on several aspects of their behavior in culture (Runyon Grouping).[94] With expanding use of more rapid molecular identification methods, nontuberculous mycobacteria are now divided more simply into rapidly, intermediately, and slowly growing groups.[93,95] Months may still be necessary for specific identification of some species due to their slow growth rate.[96,97]

Clinical disease produced by nontuberculous mycobacteria most commonly involves the lungs, and results after aspiration of aerosolized organisms from an environmental reservoir. These may disseminate through the blood stream to other sites.[91] Alternatively, some infections are initiated by direct inoculation into tissues. Human-to-human transmission has not been well documented, and only some of the species isolated from the environment have been shown to play a significant role in human disease.[93]

Three distinct patterns of musculoskeletal involvement are reported: tenosynovitis, synovitis, and osteomyelitis.[98,99] Tenosynovitis typically presents as chronic unilateral hand and wrist swelling.[100] Synovitis typically presents as chronic indolent asymmetric swelling in a knee, hand, or wrist. Spondylitis is uncommon, in contrast to M. tuberculosis infection.[101,102] A number of species have been associated with these syndromes (Table 100–2), and the number isolated from immunosuppressed patients is growing.[29] Predisposing factors, in addition to immunosuppression and direct inoculation, include environmental exposure[108] and preexisting joint disease.[118]

Correct diagnosis usually necessitates tissue biopsy and culture. Synovial fluid, when it is obtainable, is typically inflammatory, and a culture can be helpful only if

mycobacterial and fungal techniques are requested. Identification of acid-fast bacteria on smear and granulomatous inflammation from a tissue biopsy specimen often provides direction for appropriate microbiologic investigations, but histologic features do not consistently demonstrate granuloma formation. With compatible clinical presentation and histologic findings, mycobacterial culture, including special techniques for *Mycobacterium marinum*, should be requested. Direct amplification testing may be useful for more rapid identification of mycobacterial species in tissue specimens, but data from musculoskeletal cases are limited.[26,114] Granulomatous synovitis, in fact, may be caused by all of the infectious agents discussed in this chapter as well as by brucellosis, sarcoidosis, inflammatory bowel disease (IBD), and nonmetallic foreign bodies. Mycobacteria other than M. tuberculosis are responsible for a significant proportion of these cases.[101]

Mycobacterium avium has become the most common mycobacterial infectious agent in AIDS patients, in whom it has a greater tendency to cause disseminated disease.[29] The incidence of M. avium disease is estimated to be 17 to 28 percent, according to studies of living AIDS patients, and about 50 percent from autopsy cultures. Clinical manifestations of M. avium infection in AIDS patients may be difficult to distinguish from the underlying HIV infection itself, as well as from other opportunistic infections or side effects of treatment. The organism is commonly cultured from multiple sites, including blood, and histologic examination of tissue shows copious organisms with macrophages and histiocytes.

The clinician must judge whether a nontuberculous mycobacterial isolate is a contaminant, represents insignificant colonization, or is the cause of disease, unlike the case for tuberculosis, in which isolation of the organism is always clinically significant. Certain guidelines have proved useful in this respect[93,133-135]:

1. The illness should be consistent with one or more syndromes associated with mycobacterial infection.
2. Other causes of disease, such as tuberculosis and fungi, should be excluded.
3. A mycobacterial species should be isolated that is associated with human disease, the most significant being those that are not common environmental contaminants (M. kansasii, M. marinum, M. simiae, M. szulgai, and M. ulcerans).
4. The site of isolation of the organism should favor true infection over contamination or colonization.
5. Heavier growth suggests significant infection.
6. With significant disease, multiple isolations of the responsible organism are the rule.

Because laboratory identification of the organism and sensitivities may take weeks to months, initial therapy often includes multiple drugs to cover both tuberculosis and other mycobacteria. Surgical débridement of infected tissue plays an important role in treatment, especially for resistant organisms. In the treatment of localized disease, surgical débridement alone may be sufficient. More commonly, the most efficacious drugs remain controversial, prolonged treatment is

TABLE 100–2 • NONTUBERCULOUS MYCOBACTERIA ASSOCIATED WITH OSTEOARTICULAR INFECTION

Growth Rate	Species	Clinical References
Rapidly growing (within 7 days)	M. fortuitum	100,103,104
	M. chelonae	100, 105
	M. absessus	100, 102
Intermediately growing (7 to 10 days)	M. marinum	100, 106-110
Slow growing (more than 7 days)	M. asiaticum	111
	M. avium	100,102,112-114
	M. haemophilum	115
	M. kansasii	100,116-121
	M. malmoense	100, 122-124
	M. szulgai	100,125,126
	M. terrae	100, 127
	M. xenopi	100,128-132

often necessary, and relapses are not uncommon. Detailed current recommendations for treatment of individual organisms are available.[93,100,136-138] Interferon-γ (IFN-γ) may also have a role in the treatment of refractory disseminated nontuberculous mycobacterial infection,[139] and antiretroviral therapy–induced increases in CD4+ lymphocytes may reduce susceptibility to mycobacterial infections.[140]

Leprosy is caused by *Mycobacterium leprae*. It is associated with symmetric inflammatory peripheral arthritis, with onset months to years after the onset of infection.[141] Sacroiliitis is also common.[142] Because of the high frequency of RF in leprosy patients without arthritis, the distinction of this arthropathy from rheumatoid disease is based on the lack of nodules, the male preponderance, the high frequency of this syndrome in leprosy, and complete resolution with antileprosy therapy. This arthritis is distinguishable from acute arthritis occurring with erythema nodosum leprosum reactions. Bone island is also reported to be associated with leprosy.[143]

◼ Fungal Infections of the Bones and Joints

Osteomyelitis and arthritis caused by fungal infections are generally diagnosed by histologic examination or culture of involved tissues. The epidemiology and clinical features of individual deep mycoses may suggest the diagnosis in some cases, but their indolent symptoms may be misleading. Paradoxically, infection may be acute and overwhelming in immunocompromised patients for whom disseminated fungal infections are a major risk. Fungal diseases that commonly cause osteomyelitis include coccidioidomycosis, blastomycosis, cryptococcosis, candidiasis, and sporotrichosis. Fungal arthritis is less common and is most often associated with sporotrichosis, coccidioidomycosis, blastomycosis, candidiasis, and, occasionally, other species. Spinal actinomycosis may occur rarely through spread from adjacent internal-organ infection.[144]

COCCIDIOIDOMYCOSIS

Coccidioides immitis, a soil fungus, generally causes a primary respiratory illness that is often inapparent, is generally self-limited, and only infrequently becomes chronic. Coccidioidomycosis is endemic to the southwestern United States and areas of Central and South America, but cases are increasingly diagnosed in nonendemic areas because of travel, infection from fomites, and reactivation of remote infection.[145] Direct human-to-human transmission is rare.

Extrapulmonary infection is almost always caused by hematogenous spread from an initial pulmonary focus. The bones and joints are frequent sites of dissemination, particularly in immunocompromised hosts.

Septic arthritis of the knee is common, generally arising from direct infection of the synovium. Other joint infections are caused by spread from a contiguous osteomyelitis involving the vertebrae, wrists, hands, ankles, feet, pelvis, and long bones. The onset is characterized by gradually increasing pain and joint stiffness, with lesser swelling but early radiographic changes. In one series, arthritis was the only manifestation of disseminated coccidioidomycosis in 51 of 57 patients and was an aspect of more generalized disease in the remaining six patients.[146]

Diagnostic confusion is also common in osteoarticular coccidioidomycosis because of the delay of dissemination for months to years after primary infection and because of atypical clinical presentations. The criteria for diagnosis include compatible clinical features, serologic studies, histologic examination, and culture. Most patients have a coccidioidin-positive skin test reaction. Complement fixation serologic values are in a range indicative of disseminated disease in a majority of patients and show a significant decrease with effective treatment. The definitive diagnosis is most commonly made by demonstration of granulomatous synovitis and typical spherules in a biopsy specimen, confirmed in some cases by positive culture and direct amplification testing. Synovial fluid, when it is obtainable, is culture positive in less than 5 percent of cases.

With early diagnosis of effusive synovitis, antifungal treatment alone is appropriate. Indications for combined medical and surgical treatment include 1) more chronic joint inflammation with pannus formation and progressive disease during medical treatment, 2) involvement of contiguous bone, 3) rising complement fixation titers, and 4) extra-articular dissemination. Combined antifungal and surgical treatment is superior to either medical or surgical treatment alone.[146,147] A high priority for combined treatment is identified by a complement fixation titer at or above 1:128. Treatment of skeletal infections with itraconazole is more effective than fluconazole and has been successful in some patients who had relapse after previous treatment with amphotericin or ketoconazole.[148,149]

Coccidioidal synovitis may also be of a noninfectious inflammatory variety that may complicate either primary pulmonary or disseminated disease and is typically a polyarthritis. It is accompanied by fever, erythema nodosum or multiforme, eosinophilia, and hilar adenopathy, and it abates in 2 to 4 weeks.[150-152]

BLASTOMYCOSIS

Blastomycosis, caused by *Blastomyces dermatitidis*, is endemic in the north central and southern United States. Infection most commonly produces sporadic or clustered cases of pulmonary disease and is induced by exposure to soil or dust containing decomposed wood and, presumably, contaminated with the organism.[153] Affected individuals do not appear to have any distinguishing or predisposing characteristics except for exposure to the organism during work or recreation. Clinical presentation includes high fever and other constitutional symptoms, pulmonary and skin involvement, and a significant mortality rate. Hematogenous dissemination is common; skin disease and osteoarticular disease occur most frequently. Bone involvement occurs in 25 to 60 percent of disseminated cases, and arthritis is estimated to occur in 3 to 5 percent.[154] The skeletal areas most commonly affected are the long bones, vertebrae, and ribs.[155-157]

Arthritis is usually monarticular in the knee, ankle, or elbow, but may rarely be polyarticular.[154,158] Joint infection is an isolated skeletal disorder in only a few cases; joint radiographs more commonly show punched-out bone lesions. Synovial fluid is commonly purulent, and organisms are evident on microscopic examination as well as by culture. The synovial histologic examination shows epithelioid granulomas with budding yeast forms. The diagnosis is also commonly made from involved nonarticular sites. The therapeutic response to amphotericin B or itraconazole is generally favorable.[159,160]

CRYPTOCOCCOSIS

Cryptococcus neoformans, the fungus causing cryptococcosis, is geographically ubiquitous and is found in pigeon feces; it is also associated with certain types of eucalyptus trees in tropical climates. It is a common pathogen only in association with defects in cell-mediated host defense, including HIV infection,[161] transplantation,[162] lymphoreticular malignant neoplasms, and corticosteroid therapy. Currently, AIDS is the predisposing factor in 80 to 90 percent of cryptococcal infections.

Cryptococcosis varies in acuity, usually affecting the lungs in its primary form, but it sometimes disseminates hematogenously to a wide variety of sites, including the central nervous system (CNS) and skin. Although bone infection is common, causing osteolytic lesions in 5 to 10 percent of cases, articular involvement is only rarely reported.[163] Bone lesions may be confused with metastatic neoplasm (Fig. 100–5).

Cryptococcal arthritis is an indolent monarticular arthritis in about 60 percent of reported cases and a polyarthritis in the remainder.[164,165] The knee is most commonly involved. A single case of tenosynovitis with carpal tunnel syndrome has been recognized. The majority of the few cases reported from the pre-AIDS era also demonstrated radiographic evidence of periarticular osteomyelitis. These patients were young adults, did not have debilitating disease or show other evidence of dissemination, and had pulmonary involvement in only 50 percent of cases. Synovial tissue showed acute and chronic synovitis, multinucleate giant cells, prominent granuloma formation, and large numbers of budding cryptococci with special stains. Most recently reported cases are associated with immunosuppression and disseminated infection. The choice of treatment for cryptococcal disease depends on both the anatomic sites of involvement and the host's immune status, with amphoteracin and fluconazole being considered most effective.[165,166]

CANDIDIASIS

Candida species are widely distributed yeasts. *Candida albicans* is a normal commensal of humans, and other species can probably live in nonanimal environments such as soil. Since the advent of antibiotic therapy in the 1940s, and related to the common use of immunosuppression and parenteral lines, candidiasis has been responsible for an increasing incidence of mucocutaneous and deep-organ infections.[167]

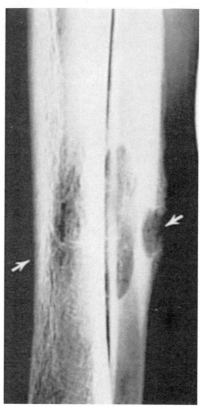

FIGURE 100–5 · Cryptococcosis (Torulosis). Discrete osteolytic foci with surrounding sclerosis and, in some places, periosteal reaction are seen (*arrows*). This involvement of bone protuberances, such as the calcaneus, is not unexpected in this disease. The resulting appearance simulates that of other fungal diseases, especially coccidioidomycosis, as well as neoplastic disorders. (From Resnick D: Diagnosis of Bone and Joint Disorders, 3rd ed. Philadelphia, WB Saunders, 1995, p 2507.)

Osteomyelitis, although rarely reported, is a potentially serious complication of hematogenous dissemination in both adults and children.[168,169] It may also occur from direct tissue inoculation during surgery or by injection of contaminated heroin,[170] and bone infection may emerge after successful amphotericin B treatment of other sites. Infection is commonly located in two adjacent vertebrae[171] or in a single long bone. Surgical inoculation has occurred in the sternum, spine, and mandible. A few patients have had multiple sites of involvement.

The clinical presentation is localized pain. Other symptoms and laboratory abnormalities vary. Bone changes of osteomyelitis are commonly demonstrated by radiographs of the symptomatic site. Diagnosis is established by culture of involved bone obtained by either open or needle biopsy and has identified a variety of *Candida* species. Use of direct amplification testing has been reported.[26] Treatment with ketoconazole, itraconazole, or amphotericin B is effective.[172] Consideration of surgical débridement must be individualized. With vertebral involvement but no neurologic complications, medication alone has been effective.

Candidiasis is an uncommon cause of monarticular arthritis.[173-177] Reported cases commonly involve a knee, occur in the context of multifocal extra-articular *Candida* infection, and are accompanied by constitutional symptoms. Both children and adults have been affected. Predisposing conditions include gastrointestinal and pulmonary disorders, narcotic addiction, intravenous (IV) catheters, leukopenia, immunosuppressive treatment, broad-spectrum antibiotics, and corticosteroids. Some involved joints have previously been affected by arthritis, and infection has followed arthrocentesis in isolated cases. In most cases, radiographs reveal coincident osteomyelitis. *Candida* species have been cultured from synovial fluid in all cases but are not commonly identified on smear. Histologic studies of synovium show nonspecific chronic inflammation rather than granulomas. Muscle infection by *Candida* has also been reported in neutropenic patients, either in the form of diffuse myositis or as localized abscess.[178-180]

SPOROTRICHOSIS

Sporotrichosis is caused by *Sporothrix schenckii*, a saprophyte found widely in soil and plants. Infection in humans occurs through inoculation of the skin or, rarely, by inhalation into the respiratory tract, a source of infection of agricultural workers in tropical and subtropical areas. It most commonly involves the skin and lymphatics but may disseminate to the lungs, CNS, eye, bone, and joints. In immunocompetent hosts, a single site is typically involved; in immunocompromised hosts, multifocal disease may occur.

In contrast to the relatively common occurrence of skin infection, articular sporotrichosis is a rare disorder.[181,182] In 84 percent of patients in one series, there was no accompanying skin involvement, suggesting entry through the lungs. Sporotrichosis most often occurs in individuals with a chronic illness that alters host defense, such as alcoholism or a myeloproliferative disorder. Sporotrichosis arthritis is most often indolent and infects a single joint or multiple joints in equal proportions. The knee, hand, wrists, elbow, and shoulder are most frequently involved; hand and wrist involvement distinguishes this from other fungal arthritides. Articular infection shows a propensity to spread to adjacent soft tissues, forming draining sinuses. Constitutional symptoms are unusual.

Radiographic changes vary from juxta-articular osteopenia to the commonly observed punched-out bone lesions. When it is obtainable, synovial fluid is inflammatory. Synovitis is characterized on gross evaluation by destructive pannus and on microscopic examination by granulomatous histologic features or, less frequently, by nonspecific inflammation. Organisms are difficult to identify in tissue, and diagnosis is often made by positive culture of joint fluid or involved tissue. In a small number of cases, sporotrichosis may disseminate to cause a potentially fatal infection characterized by low-grade fever, weight loss, anemia, osteolytic bone lesions, arthritis, skin lesions, and involvement of the eyes and CNS.[183-186] These cases occur in immunosuppressed patients with either hematologic malignant neoplasia or HIV infection.

In 44 cases reported in 1979,[181] treatment was optimal with combined joint débridement and high-dose IV amphotericin B (11 of 11 cured) and slightly less effective with amphotericin alone (14 of 19 cured). Oral potassium iodide (5 of 15 cured) and other forms of treatment were not adequate. More recently, itraconazole has been proven effective for initial therapy of most patients, with amphotericin B being reserved for those with extensive involvement and for itraconazole failures. In contrast, fluconazole has demonstrated only modest success in osteoarticular sporotrichosis.[187,188]

ASPERGILLOSIS

Aspergillus species are ubiquitous, but infection occurs only rarely in normal individuals. In contrast, invasive infection is an important life-threatening complication in immunocompromised hosts.[189,190] It may spread directly from the lung to adjacent vertebrae, disk spaces, and ribs (more often in children) or through the blood stream.[191,192] Rare cases of monarthritis with adjacent osteomyelitis are also reported.[193] The organism may be observed in infected tissue. Treatment with combined surgical débridement and antifungal therapy remains an ongoing challenge.[190,192]

HISTOPLASMOSIS

Histoplasma capsulatum is a soil fungus that causes endemic disease in the midwestern and southeastern United States.[164,194] Bone and joint involvement in histoplasmosis is rare but has been reported in the knee, wrist, and ankle. Disseminated histoplasmosis is predisposed by immunosuppression, including use of TNF-α antagonists, and may be confused clinically with sarcoidosis, tuberculosis, and reactive inflammatory conditions.[195,196] Diagnosis depends on appropriate use of fungal staining and culture methods, antigen detection, and serologic antibody testing.[197] A case report emphasizes the rare occurrence of fungal prosthetic-joint arthritis.[198] The more common osteoarticular involvement with histoplasmosis is a hypersensitivity syndrome accompanying acute pulmonary infection; it is characterized by self-limited polyarthritis, erythema nodosum, and erythema multiforme. Amphotericin is the preferred treatment for severe infection and itraconazole for less severe cases.[199,200]

SCEDOSPORIOSIS

Scedosporium inflatum, a newly described fungal pathogen, has been associated with focally invasive infection after cutaneous inoculation.[201] Both septic arthritis and osteomyelitis have been reported, and infections were difficult to eradicate with antifungal agents.

TREATMENT OF FUNGAL INFECTION

Antifungal chemotherapy has improved during the last 35 years, first with the introduction of amphotericin B and more recently with the development of oral antifungal agents including flucytosine, ketoconazole, fluconazole, and itraconazole. For detailed treatment guidelines, several excellent reviews are available.[202-210] A new class of antifungal drugs, the echinocandins

TABLE 100–3 • DRUG TREATMENT OF OSTEOARTICULAR MYCOTIC INFECTIONS

Infection	Drug Recommended*	Infection-Specific References
Coccidioidomycosis	Itraconazole	146–149
Blastomycosis	Itraconizole	159,160
Cryptococcosis	Fluconazole	165,166
Candidiasis†	Itraconazole, Fluconazole	172–177
Sporotrichosis	Itraconazole	181,187,188
Aspergillosis	Itraconazole	190,192
Histoplasmosis	Itraconazole	199,200
Scedosporiosis	Undetermined	201

*Amphoteracin B is indicated for severe infections.
†Species *Candida krusei* and *C. glabrata* are resistant.

(caspofungin, micafungin, and anidulafungin), are being studied as less toxic alternatives to amphoteracin B for treating invasive candidiasis and aspergillosis.[211] In choosing an appropriate drug (Table 100–3) and course of treatment, the clinician must consider the infecting agent, clinical manifestations of the disease, immune status of the host, antimicrobial resistance, drug side effect profile, and direct and indirect costs of treatment. Treatment has become more complex because of immune system compromise in infected patients being treated for transplant rejection, autoimmune disorders, malignant disease, and AIDS. In AIDS-related cases, after the initial control of infection, lifelong oral suppressive therapy is mandated by the high frequency of recurrence, although successful antiretroviral therapy may modify this risk.[140]

Itraconazole has become the first consideration for treatment of the endemic mycoses—blastomycosis, histoplasmosis, and sporotrichosis. The initial dose is 200 mg/day, which should be increased to twice daily if a clinical response is not obtained in 2 to 3 weeks. At least 6 months of treatment is required, and some patients may need up to a year of therapy. For cryptococcosis, fluconazole is the recommended azole.[165,166] Amphotericin B is the preferred drug for meningeal and life-threatening infections. Specific treatment protocols and detailed side effect profiles are presented in reviews 202-210 and infection-specific references (Table 100-3).

REFERENCES

1. Small PM, Fujiwara PI: Management of tuberculosis in the United States. N Engl J Med 345:189-200, 2001.
2. Cohn DL: Treatment of latent tuberculosis infection: Renewed opportunity for tuberculosis control. Clin Infect Dis 31:120, 2000.
3. Geng E, Kreiswirth B, Driver C, et al: Changes in the transmission of tuberculosis in New York City from 1990 to 1999. N Engl J Med 346:1453-1458, 2002.
4. Jasmer RM, Nahid P, Hopewell PC: Latent tuberculosis infection. N Engl J Med 347:1860, 2002.
5. Centers for Disease Control: Tuberculosis, final data: United States, 1986. MMWR Morb Mortal Wkly Rep 36:817, 1988.

6. Rajagopalan S: Tuberculosis and aging: A global health problem. Clin Infect Dis 33:1034, 2001.
7. Keane J, Gershon S, Wise RP, et al: Tuberculosis associated with infliximab, a tumor necrosis α-neutralizing agent. N Engl J Med 345:1098, 2001.
8. Wallis RS, Johnson JL: Adult tuberculosis in the 21st century: Pathogenesis, clinical features, and management. Curr Opin Pulm Med 7:124, 2001.
9. Bloom BR: Tuberculosis-the global view. N Engl J Med 346:1434, 2002.
10. Horsburgh RC: The global problem with drug-resistant tuberculosis: The genie is out of the bottle. JAMA 283:2575, 2000.
11. Espinal MA, Laszlo A, Simonsen L, et al: Global trends in resistance to antituberculous drugs. N Engl J Med 344:1294, 2001.
12. Schluger NW, Burzynski J: Tuberculosis and HIV infection: Epidemiology, immunology, and treatment. HIV Clin Trials 2:356, 2001.
13. Khatri GR, Frieden TR: Controlling tuberculosis in India. N Engl J Med 347:1420, 2002.
14. Valway SE, Sanchez MPC, Shinnick TF, et al: An outbreak involving extensive transmission of a virulent strain of *Mycobacterium tuberculosis*. N Engl J Med 338:633, 1998.
15. Mazurek GH, LoBue PA, Daley CL, et al: Comparison of a whole-blood interferon γ assay with tuberculin skin testing for detecting latent Mycobacterium tuberculosis infection. JAMA 286:1740, 2001.
16. Lietman T, Blower SM: Potential impact of tuberculosis vaccines as epidemic control agents. Clin Infect Dis 30(Suppl 3):S316, 2000.
17. Espinal MA, Kim SJ, Suarez PG, et al: Standard short-course chemotherapy for drug-resistant tuberculosis: Treatment outcomes in 6 countries. JAMA 283:2537, 2000.
18. Reider HL, Snider DE Jr, Cauthen GM: Extrapulmonary tuberculosis in the United States. Am Rev Respir Dis 141:347, 1990.
19. Shafer RW, Kim DS, Weiss JP, et al: Extrapulmonary tuberculosis in patients with human immunodeficiency virus infection. Medicine (Baltimore) 70:384, 1991.
20. Jellis JE: Human immunodeficiency virus and osteoarticular tuberculosis. Clin Orthop 398:27, 2002.
21. Havlir DV, Barnes PF: Tuberculosis in patients with human immunodeficiency virus infection. N Engl J Med 340:367, 1999.
22. Walker CF: Failure of early recognition of skeletal tuberculosis. BMJ 1:682, 1968.
23. Tuli SM: General principles of osteoarticular tuberculosis. Clin Orthop 398:11, 2002.
24. Moore SL, Rafii M: Imaging of musculoskeletal and spinal infections: Imaging of musculoskeletal and spinal tuberculosis. Radiol Clin North Am 39:329, 2001.
25. Griffith JF, Kumta SM, Leung PC, et al: Imaging of musculoskeletal tuberculosis: A new look at an old disease. Clin Orthop 398:32, 2002.
26. Harrington JT: The evolving role of direct amplification tests in diagnosing osteoarticular infections caused by mycobacteria and fungi. Curr Opin Rheumatol 11:289, 1999.
27. Catanzaro A, Perry S, Clarridge JE, et al: The role of clinical suspicion in evaluating a new diagnostic test for active tuberculosis: Results of a multicenter prospective trial. JAMA 283:639, 2000.
28. Woods GL: Molecular techniques in mycobacterial detection. Arch Pathol Lab Med 125:122, 2001.
29. American Thoracic Society and the Centers for Disease Control: Mycobacterioses and the acquired immunodeficiency syndrome. Am Rev Respir Dis 136:492, 1987.
30. Mandell GL, Bennett JE, Dolin R (eds): Mandell, Douglas, and Bennett's Principles and Practice of Infectious Diseases. Philadelphia, Churchill Livingston, 2000.
31. La Fond EM: An analysis of adult skeletal tuberculosis. J Bone Joint Surg Am 40:346, 1958.
32. Alvarez S, McCabe WR: Extrapulmonary tuberculosis revisited: A review of experience at Boston City and other hospitals. Medicine (Baltimore) 63:25, 1984.
33. el-Shahawy MA, Gadallah MF, Campese VM: Tuberculosis of the spine (Pott's disease) in patients with end-stage renal disease. Am J Nephrol 14:55, 1994.
34. Jacobs P: Osteo-articular tuberculosis in coloured immigrants: A radiologic study. Clin Radiol 15:59, 1964.

35. Gorse GJ, Pais MJ, Kusske JA, Cesario TC: Tuberculous spondylitis. Medicine (Baltimore) 62:178, 1983.
36. Babhulkar S (ed): Symposium: Osteoarticular tuberculosis. Clin Orthop 398:1-120, 2002.
37. Chapman M, Murray RD, Stoker DJ: Tuberculosis of bones and joints. Semin Roentgenol 14:266, 1985.
38. Colmenero JD, Jimenez-Mejias ME, Sanchez-Lora FJ, et al: Pyogenic, tuberculous, and brucellar vertebral osteomyelitis: A descriptive and comparative study of 219 cases. Ann Rheum Dis 56:709, 1997.
39. Cantini F, Salvarani C, Olivieri I, et al: Tuberculous spondylitis as a cause of inflammatory spinal pain: A report of 4 cases. Clin Exp Rheum 16:305, 1998.
40. Resnick D: Osteomyelitis, septic arthritis, and soft tissue infection. In Resnick D (ed): Diagnosis of Bone and Joint Disorders, 4th ed. Philadelphia, WB Saunders, 2002, pp 2510-2624.
41. Gupta RK, Gupta S, Kumar S, et al: MRI in intraspinal tuberculosis. Neuroradiology 36:39, 1994.
42. Lifeso RM, Weaver P, Harder EH: Tuberculous spondylitis in adults. J Bone Joint Surg Am 67:1405, 1985.
43. Mondal A: Cytological diagnosis of vertebral tuberculosis with fine-needle aspiration biopsy. J Bone Joint Surg Am 76:181, 1994.
44. Masood S: Diagnosis of tuberculosis of bone and soft tissue by fine-needle aspiration biopsy. Diagn Cytopathol 8:451, 1992.
45. Omari B, Robertson JM, Nelson RJ, Chiu LC: Pott's disease: A resurgent challenge to the thoracic surgeon. Chest 95:145, 1989.
46. Shembekar A, Babhulkar S: Chemotherapy of osteoarticular tuberculosis. Clin Orthop 398:20, 2002.
47. Van Loenhout-Rooyackers JH, Verbeek ALM, Jutte PC: Chemotherapeutic treatment for spinal tuberculosis. Int J Tuberc Lung Dis 6:259, 2002.
48. Shih HN, Hsu RW, Lin TY: Tuberculosis of the long bone in children. Clin Orthop 335:246, 1997.
49. Vidyasagar C, Murthy HK: Management of tuberculosis of the spine with neurological complications. Ann R Coll Surg 76:80, 1994.
50. Jain AK: Treatment of tuberculosis of the spine with neurologic complications. Clin Orthop 398:75, 2002.
51. Rajasekaran S: The problem of deformity in spinal tuberculosis. Clin Orthop 398:85, 2002.
52. Metha JS, Bhojraj SY: Tuberculosis of the thoracic spine: A classification based on the selection of surgical strategies. J Bone Joint Surg Br 83-B:859, 2001.
53. Slater RR Jr, Beale RW, Bullitt E: Pott's disease of the cervical spine. South Med J 84:521, 1991.
54. Krishnan A, Patkar D, Patankar T, et al: Craniovertebral junction tuberculosis: A review of 29 cases. J Comput Assist Tomogr 25:171, 2001.
55. Bhojraj SY, Shetty N, Shah PJ: Tuberculosis of the craniocervical junction. J Bone Joint Surg Br 83-B:222, 2001.
56. Pouchot J, Vinceneus P, Barge J, et al: Tuberculosis of the sacroiliac joint: Clinical features, outcome, and evaluation of closed needle biopsy in 11 consecutive cases. Am J Med 84:622, 1988.
57. Pande KC, Babhulkar SS: Atypical spinal tuberculosis. Clin Orthop 398:64, 2002.
58. Babhulkar SS, Pande SK: Unusual manifestations of osteoarticular tuberculosis. Clin Orthop 398:114, 2002.
59. Martini M, Adjrad A, Boudjemaa A: Tuberculous osteomyelitis: A review of 125 cases. Int Orthop 10:201, 1986.
60. Muradali D, Gold WL, Vellend H, Becker E: Multifocal osteoarticular tuberculosis: Report of four cases and review of management. Clin Infect Dis 17:204, 1993.
61. Coppola J, Muller NL, Connell DG: Computed tomography of musculoskeletal tuberculosis. J Can Assoc Radiol 38:199, 1987.
62. Babhulkar S, Pande S: Tuberculosis of the hip. Clin Orthop 398:93, 2002.
63. Hoffman EB, Allin J, Campbell JAB, Leisegang FM: Tuberculosis of the knee. Clin Orthop 398:100, 2002.
64. Evanchick CC, Davis DE, Harrington TM: Tuberculosis of peripheral joints: An often missed diagnosis. J Rheumatol 13:187, 1986.
65. Wallace R, Cohen AS: Tuberculous arthritis: A report of two cases with a review of biopsy and synovial fluid findings. Am J Med 61:277, 1976.
66. Choy EH, Chieco-Bianchi F, Panayi GS, Kingsley GH: Synovial fluid lymphocyte proliferation to tuberculin protein product derivative: A novel way of diagnosing tuberculous arthritis. Clin Exp Rheumatol 12:187, 1994.
67. Jacobs JC, Li SC, Ruzal-Shapiro C, et al: Tuberculous arthritis in children: Diagnosis by needle biopsy of the synovium. Clin Pediatr 33:344, 1994.
68. Sorio LM, Sole JMN, Sacanell AR, et al: Infectious arthritis in patients with rheumatoid arthritis. Ann Rheum Dis 51:402, 1992.
69. Davidson PT, Horowitz I: Skeletal tuberculosis; a review with patient presentations and discussion. Am J Med 48:77, 1970.
70. Ashworth MJ, Meadows TH: Isolated tuberculosis of a skeletal muscle. J Hand Surg Br 17:235, 1992.
71. Hasan N, Baithun S, Swash M, Wagg A: Tuberculosis of striated muscle. Muscle Nerve 16:984, 1993.
72. Indudhara R, Singh SK, Minz M, et al: Tuberculous pyomyositis in a renal transplant recipient. Tuber Lung Dis 73:239, 1992.
73. George JC, Buckwalter KA, Braunstein EM: Tuberculosis presenting as a soft tissue forearm mass in a patient with a negative tuberculin skin test. Skeletal Radiol 23:79, 1994.
74. Abdelwahab IF, Kenan S, Hermann G, et al: Tuberculous gluteal abscess without bone involvement. Skeletal Radiol 27:36, 1998.
75. Albornoz MA, Mezgarzedeh M, Neumann CH, et al: Granulomatous tenosynovitis: A rare musculoskeletal manifestation of tuberculosis. Clin Rheumatol 17:166, 1998.
76. King AD, Griffith J, Rushton A, et al: Tuberculosis of the greater trochanter and the trochanteric bursa. J Rheumatol 25:391, 1998.
77. Chen W-S: Tuberculosis of the fascia lata. Clin Rheumatol 17:77, 1998.
78. Sembekar A, Babhulkar S: Chemotherapy for osteoarticular tuberculosis. Clin Orthop 398:20, 2002.
79. Dutt AK, Stead WW: Treatment of extrapulmonary tuberculosis. Semin Respir Infect 4:225, 1989.
80. American Thoracic Society: Treatment of tuberculosis and tuberculosis infection in adults and children. Am J Respir Crit Care Med 149:1359, 1994.
81. Alangaden GJ, Lerner SA: The clinical use of fluoroquinolones for the treatment of mycobacterial diseases. Clin Infect Dis 25:1213, 1997.
82. Hannachi MR, Martini M, Boulahal F, et al: A comparison of three daily short-course regimens in osteoarticular tuberculosis in Algiers. Bull Int Union Tuberc 57:46, 1982.
83. Parsons LM, Driscoll JR, Taber HW, et al: Antimicrobial resistance: Drug resistance in tuberculosis. Infect Dis Clin North Am 11:906, 1997.
84. Bradford WZ, Daley CL: Emerging infectious diseases: Multiple drug-resistant tuberculosis. Infect Dis Clin North Am 12:157, 1998.
85. Chaulk CP, Kazandjian VA: Directly observed therapy for treatment completion of pulmonary tuberculosis: Consensus Statement of the Public Health Tuberculosis Guidelines Panel. JAMA 279:943, 1998.
86. Perez-Stable EJ, Hopewell PC: Current tuberculosis treatment regimens: Choosing the right one for your patient. Clin Chest Med 10:323, 1989.
87. Keat A: TB or not TB? That is the question. Br J Rheumatol 32:769, 1993.
88. Xerri B, Chretien Y, Le Parc JM: Reactive polyarthritis induced by intravesical BCG therapy for carcinoma of the bladder [Letter]. Eur J Med 8:503, 1993.
89. Koch M, Rabinowitsch I: Die Tuberculose der Vogel und ihre Beziehungen zur Sangertiertuberculose. Virchows Arch Pathol Anat 190:246, 1907.
90. Timpe A, Runyon EH: Relationship of "atypical" acid-fast bacilli to human disease: Preliminary report. J Lab Clin Med 44:202, 1954.
91. Wolinsky E: Nontuberculous mycobacteria and associated diseases. Am Rev Respir Dis 119:107, 1979.
92. Wolinsky E: Mycobacterial diseases other than tuberculosis. Clin Infect Dis 15:1, 1992.
93. Brown BA, Wallace RJ: Infections due to nontuberculous mycobacteria. In Mandell GL, Bennett JE, Dolin R (eds): Mandell, Douglas, and Bennett's Principles and Practice of Infectious Diseases. Philadelphia, Churchill Livingston, 2000, pp 2630-2636.
94. Runyon EH: Anonymous mycobacteria in pulmonary disease. Med Clin North Am 43:273, 1959.
95. Richter E, Niemann S, Rusch-Gerdes S, Hoffner S: Identification of Mycobacterium kansasii by using a DNA probe (AccuProbe) and molecular techniques. J Clin Microbiol 37:964, 1999.

96. Woods GL, Washington JA II: Mycobacteria other than *Mycobacterium tuberculosis:* Review of microbiologic and clinical aspects. Rev Infect Dis 9:275, 1987.

97. Vestal AL: Procedures for the Isolation and Identification of Mycobacteria. CDC Publication No. 76-8230. Washington DC, Department of Health, Education and Welfare, 1975.

98. Kelly PJ, Karlson AG, Weed LA, et al: Infection of synovial tissues by mycobacteria other than *Mycobacterium tuberculosis.* J Bone Joint Surg Am 49:1521, 1967.

99. Marchevsky AM, Damsker B, Green S, Tepper S: The clinico-pathological spectrum of non-tuberculous mycobacterial osteoarticular infections. J Bone Joint Surg Am 67:925, 1985.

100. Zenone T, Boibieux A, Tigaud S, et al: Non-tuberculous mycobacterial tenosynovitis: A review. Scand J Infect Dis 31:221, 1999.

101. Sutker WL, Lankford LL, Tompsett R: Granulomatous synovitis: The role of atypical mycobacteria. Rev Infect Dis 1:729, 1979.

102. Chan ED, Kong P-M, Fennelly K, et al: Vertebral osteomyelitis due to infection with nontuberculous mycobacterium species after blunt trauma to the back: 3 examples of the principle of locus minoris resistentiae. Clin Infect Dis 32:1506, 2001.

103. Butt AA, Janney A: Arthritis due to *Mycobacterium fortuitum.* Scand J Infect Dis 30:525, 1998.

104. Lazzarini L, Amina S, Wang J, Calhoun JH: *Mycobacterium tuberculosis* and *Mycobacterium fortuitum* osteomyelitis of the foot and septic arthritis of the ankle in an immunocompetent patient. Eur J Clin Microbiol Infect Dis 21:468, 2002.

105. Suttner NJ, Adhami Z, Aspoas AR: *Mycobacterium chelonae* lumbar spinal infection. Br J Neurosurg 15:265, 2001.

106. Bailey JP, Stevens S, Bell WM, et al: *Mycobacterium marinum* infection. JAMA 247:1314, 1982.

107. Jones MW, Wahid IA, Matthews JP: Septic arthritis of the hand due to *Mycobacterium marinum.* J Hand Surg Br 13:333, 1988.

108. Clark RB, Spector H, Friedman DM: Osteomyelitis and synovitis produced by *Mycobacterium marinum* in a fisherman. J Clin Microbiol 28:2570, 1990.

109. Barton A, Bernstein RM, Struthers JK, et al: *Mycobacterium marinum* infection causing septic arthritis and osteomyelitis. Br J Rheumatol 36:1207, 1997.

110. Aubry A, Chosidow O, Caumes E, et al: Sixty-three cases of *Mycobacterium marinum* infection. Arch Intern Med 162:1746, 2002.

111. Foulkes GD, Floyd JCP, Stephens JL, et al: Flexor tensosynovitis due to *Mycobacterium asiaticum.* J Hand Surg Am 23:753, 1998.

112. Hoffman GS, Myers RL, Stark FR, Thoen CO: Septic arthritis associated with *Mycobacterium avium:* A case report and literature review. J Rheumatol 5:2, 1978.

113. Blumenthal DR, Zucker JR, Hawkins CC: *Mycobacterium avium* complex induced septic arthritis and osteomyelitis in a patient with acquired immunodeficiency syndrome [Letter]. Arthritis Rheum 33:757, 1990.

114. Weigl JAI, Haas WH: Postoperative *Mycobacterium avium* osteomyelitis confirmed by polymerase chain reaction. Eur J Pediatr 159:64, 2000.

115. Shah MK, Sebti A, Kiehn TE, et al: *Mycobacterium haemophilim* in immunocompromised patients. Clin Infect Dis 33:330, 2001.

116. Dorff GJ, Frerichs L, Zabransky RJ, et al: Musculoskeletal infections due to *Mycobacterium kansasii.* Clin Orthop 136:244, 1978.

117. Sherer R, Sable R, Sonnenberg M, et al: Disseminated infection with *Mycobacterium kansasii* in the acquired immunodeficiency syndrome. Ann Intern Med 105:710, 1986.

118. Glickstein SL, Nashel DJ: *Mycobacterium kansasii* septic arthritis complicating rheumatic disease: Case report and review of the literature. Semin Arthritis Rheum 16:231, 1987.

119. Carpenter JL, Parks JM: *Mycobacterium kansasii* infections in patients positive for human immunodeficiency virus. Rev Infect Dis 13:789, 1991.

120. Bernard L, Vincent V, Lortholary O, et al: *Mycobacterium kansasii* septic arthritis: French retrospective study of 5 years and review. Clin Infect Dis 29:1455, 1999.

121. Nakamura T, Yamamura Y, Tsuruta T, et al. *Mycobacterium kansasii* arthritis of the foot in a patient with systemic lupus erythematosus. Intern Med 40:1045, 2001.

122. Prince H, Ispahani P, Baker M: A *Mycobacterium malmoense* infection of the hand presenting as carpal tunnel syndrome. J Hand Surg (Br) 13:328, 1988.

123. Gabl M, Pechlaner S, Kreczy A, Went P. Flexor tenosynovitis in the hand caused by *Mycobacterium malmoense:* A case report. J Hand Surg (Am) 22:338, 1997.

124. Syedd AA, O'Flanagan J: *Mycobacterium malmoense* infection: An unusual cause of wrist swelling. J Hand Surg (Br) 23:811, 1998.

125. Maloney JM, Gregg CR, Stephens DS, et al: Infections caused by *Mycobacterium szulgai* in humans. Rev Infect Dis 9:1120, 1987.

126. Hurr H, Sorg T: *Mycobacterium szulgai* osteomyelitis. J Infect 37:191, 1998.

127. Smith DS, Lindholm-Levy P, Huitt GA, et al: *Mycobacterium terrae:* Case reports, literature review, and in vitro antibiotic susceptibility testing. Clin Infect Dis 30:444, 2000.

128. Rutten MJCM, van den Berg JC, van den Hoogen FHJ, et al: Nontuberculous mycobacterial bursitis and arthritis of the shoulder. Skeletal Radiol 27:33, 1998.

129. Prigogine T, Stoffels G, Fauville-Dufaux M, et al: Primary psoas muscle abscess due to *Mycobacterium xenopi.* Clin Infect Dis 26:221, 1998.

130. Yuen K, Fam AG, Simor A: *Mycobacterium xenopi* arthritis. J Rheum 25:1016, 1998.

131. Danesh-Clough T, Theis J-C, van der Linden A: *Mycobacterium xenopi* infection of the spine: A case report and literature review. Spine 25:626, 2000.

132. Astagneau P, Desplaces N, Vincent V, et al: *Mycobacterium xenopi* spinal infections after discovertebral surgery: Investigation and screening of a large outbreak. Lancet 358:747, 2001.

133. Wolinsky E: When is an infection disease? Rev Infect Dis 3:1025, 1981.

134. Wallace RJ Jr, O'Brien R, Glassroth J, et al: Diagnosis and treatment of disease caused by nontuberculous mycobacteria. Am Rev Respir Dis 142:940, 1990.

135. Ahn CH, McLarty JW, Ahn SS, et al: Diagnostic criteria for pulmonary disease caused by *Mycobacterium kansasii* and *Mycobacterium intracellulare.* Am Rev Respir Dis 125:388, 1992.

136. Havlir DV, Ellner JJ: *Mycobacterium avium* complex. *In* Mandel GL, Bennett JE, Dolin R (eds): Mandell, Douglas, and Bennett's Principles and Practice of Infectious Diseases. Philadelphia, Churchill Livingston, 2000, pp 2616-2630.

137. Tartaglione T: Treatment of nontuberculous mycobacterial infections: Role of clarithromycin and azithromycin. Clin Ther 19:626, 1998.

138. Gillespie SH, Morrissey I, Everett D: A comparison of the bactericidal activity of quinolone antibiotics in a *Mycobacterium fortuitum* model. J Med Microbiol 50: 565, 2001.

139. Holland SM, Eisenstein EM, Kuhns DB, et al: Treatment of disseminated nontuberculous mycobacterial infection with interferon gamma: A preliminary report. N Engl J Med 330:1348, 1994.

140. Currier JS, Williams PL, Koletar SL, et al: Discontinuation of *Mycobacteriam avium* complex prophylaxis in patients with anti-retroviral therapy-induced increases in CD4+ cell count: A randomized, double-blind, placebo-controlled trial. Ann Intern Med 133:493, 2000.

141. Atkin SL, El-Ghobarey A, Kamel M, et al: Clinical and laboratory studies of arthritis in leprosy. BMJ 298:1423, 1989.

142. Cossermelli-Messina W, Neto CF, Cossermelli W: Articular inflammatory manifestations in patients with different forms of leprosy. J Rheumatol 25:111, 1998.

143. Carpintero P, Garcia-Frasquet A, Tarradas E, et al: Bone island and leprosy. Skeletal Radiol 27:330, 1998.

144. Voisin L, Vittecoq O, Mejjad O, et al: Spinal abscess and spondylitis due to actinomycosis. Spine 23:487, 1998.

145. Galgiani JN: Coccidioidomycosis. West J Med 159:153, 1993.

146. Bayer AS, Guze LB: Coccidioidal synovitis: Clinical, diagnostic, therapeutic, and prognostic considerations. Semin Arthritis Rheum 8:200, 1979.

147. Bried JM, Galgiani JN: *Coccidioides immitis* infections in bones and joints. Clin Orthop 211:235, 1986.

148. Galgaini JN, Catanzaro A, Cloud GA, et al, for the National Institute of Allergy and Infectious Diseases-Mycoses Study Group: Comparison of oral fluconazole and itraconaxole for progressive, nonmeningeal coccidioidomycosis: A randomized, double-blind trial. Ann Intern Med 133:676, 2000.

149. Graybill JR, Stevens DA, Galgiani JN, et al: Itraconazole treatment of coccidioidomycosis. Am J Med 89:282, 1990.

150. Fiese MJ: Coccidioidomycosis. Springfield, Ill, Charles C Thomas, 1958.

151. Smith CE: Coccidioidomycosis. Pediatr Clin North Am 39:109, 1955.

152. Rosenberg EF, Dockerty EF, Meyerding HW: Coccidioidal arthritis. Arch Intern Med 69:238, 1942.

153. Chapman SW: *Blastomyces dermatitidis. In* Mandell GL, Bennett JE, Dolin R (eds): Mandell, Douglas, and Bennett's Principles and Practice of Infectious Diseases. Philadelphia, Churchill Livingston, 2000, pp 2733-2746.

154. Bayer AS, Scott VJ, Guze LB: Fungal arthritis. IV. Blastomycosis arthritis. Semin Arthritis Rheum 9:145, 1979.

155. MacDonald PB, Black GB, MacKenzie R: Orthopaedic manifestations of blastomycosis. J Bone Joint Surg Am 72:860, 1990.

156. Pritchard DJ: Granulomatous infections of the bones and joints. Orthop Clin North Am 6:1029, 1975.

157. Saccente M, Abernathy RS, Pappas PG, et al: Vertebral blastomycosis with paravertebral abscess: Report of eight cases and review of the literature. Clin Infect Dis 26:413, 1998.

158. Abril A, Campbell MD, Cotten VR, et al: Polyarticular blastomycotic arthritis. J Rheumatol 25:1019, 1998.

159. Bradsher RW: Therapy of blastomycosis. Semin Respir Infect 12:263, 1997.

160. Chapman SW, Bradsher RW Jr, Campbell DG, et al: Practice guidelines for the management of patients with blastomycosis. Clin Infect Dis 30:697, 2000.

161. Levitz SM: The ecology of *Cryptococcus neoformans* and the epidemiology of cryptococcosis. J Infect Dis 13:1153, 1991.

162. Aulakh HS, Straus SE, Kwon-Chung KJ: Genetic relatedness of *Filobasidiella neoformans* (*Cryptococcus neoformans*) and *Filobasidiella bacillispora* (*Cryptococcus bacillispora*) as determined by deoxyribonucleic acid-base composition and sequence homology studies. J Syst Bacteriol 31:97, 1981.

163. Behrman RE, Masci JR, Nicholas P: Cryptococcal skeletal infections: Case report and review. Rev Infect Dis 12:181, 1990.

164. Bayer AS, Choi C, Tillman DB, Guze LB: Fungal arthritis: V. Cryptococcal and histoplasmal arthritis. Semin Arthritis Rheum 9:218, 1980.

165. Bruno KM, Farhoomand L, Libman BS, et al: Cryptococcal arthritis, tendonitis, tenosynovitis, and carpal tunnel syndrome: Report of a case and review of the literature. Arthritis Care Res 47:104, 2002.

166. Saag MS, Graybill RJ, Larsen RA: Practice guidelines for the management of cryptococal disease. Infectious Diseases Society of America. Clin Infect Dis 30:710, 2000.

167. Edwards JE Jr: *Candida* species. *In* Mandell GL, Bennett JE, Dolin R (eds): Mandell, Douglas, and Bennett's Principles and Practice of Infectious Diseases. Philadelphia, Churchill Livingston, 2000, pp 2656-2674.

168. Gathe JC, Harris RL, Garland B, et al: *Candida* osteomyelitis: A review of five cases and review of the literature. Am J Med 82:927, 1987.

169. McCullers JA, Flynn PM: *Candida tropicalis* osteomyelitis: Case report and review. Clin Infect Dis 26:1000, 1998.

170. Lafont A, Olive A, Gelman M, et al: *Candida albicans* spondylodiscitis and vertebral osteomyelitis in patients with intravenous heroin drug addiction: Report of 3 new cases. J Rheumatol 21:953, 1994.

171. Almekinders LC, Greene WB: Vertebral candida infections: A case report and review of the literature. Clin Orthop 267:174, 1991.

172. Martin MV: The use of fluconazole and itraconazole in the treatment of *Candida albicans* infections: A review. J Antimicrob Chemother 44:429, 1999.

173. Bayer AS, Guze LB: Fungal arthritis: I. *Candida* arthritis: Diagnostic and prognostic implications and therapeutic considerations. Semin Arthritis Rheum 8:142, 1978.

174. Barson WJ, Marcon MJ: Successful therapy of *Candida albicans* arthritis with a sequential intravenous amphotericin B and oral fluconazole regimen. Pediatr Infect Dis J 15:1119, 1996.

175. Weers-Pothoff G, Havermans JF, Kamphuis J, et al: *Candida tropicalis* arthritis in a patient with acute myeloid leukemia successfully treated with fluconazole: Case report and review of the literature. Infection 25:109, 1997.

176. Evdoridou J, Roilides E, Bibashi G, et al: Multifocal osteoarthritis due to *Candida albicans* in a neonate: Serum level monitoring

177. Fraucher J-F, Thiebaut M-M, Reynes J, et al: Unusual outcome of disseminated candidiasis treated with fluconazole: A matter of pharmacodynamics. Clin Infect Dis 26:197, 1998.

178. Arena FP, Perlin M, Brahman H: Fever, rash, and myalgias of disseminated candidiasis during antifungal therapy. Arch Intern Med 14:1233, 1981.

179. Fornadley JA, Parker GS, Rickman LS, et al: *Candida* myositis manifesting as a discrete neck mass. Otolaryngol Head Neck Surg 102:74, 1990.

180. Behar SM, Chertow GM: Olecranon bursitis caused by infection with *Candida lusitaniae.* J Rheumatol 25:598, 1998.

181. Bayer AS, Scott VJ, Guze LB: Fungal arthritis. III. Sporotrichal arthritis. Semin Arthritis Rheum 9:66, 1979.

182. Crout JE, Brewer NS, Tompkins RB: Sporotrichosis arthritis: Clinical features in seven patients. Ann Intern Med 86:294, 1977.

183. Wilson DE, Mann JJ, Bennett JE, Utz JP: Clinical features of extracutaneous sporotrichosis. Medicine (Baltimore) 46:265, 1967.

184. Lynch PJ, Voorhees JJ, Harrell ER: Systemic sporotrichosis. Ann Intern Med 73:23, 1970.

185. Oscherwitz SL, Rinaldi MG: Disseminated sporotrichosis in a patient infected with human immunodeficiency virus. Clin Infect Dis 15:568, 1992.

186. Al-Tawfiq JA, Wools KK: Disseminated sporotrichosis and *Sporothrix schenckii* fungemia as the initial presentation of immunodeficiency infection. Clin Infect Dis 26:1403, 1998.

187. Sharkey-Mathis PK, Kauffman CA, Graybill JR, et al: Treatment of sporotrichosis with itraconazole: NIAID Mycoses Study Group. Am J Med 95:279, 1993.

188. Kauffman CA, Hajjeh R, Chapman SW for the Mycoses Study Group: Practice guidelines for management of patients with sporotirchosis. Clin Infect Dis 30:684, 2000.

189. Cuellar ML, Silveira LH, Espinoza LR: Fungal arthritis. Ann Rheum Dis 51:690, 1992.

190. Kontoyiannia DP, Bodey GP: Invasive aspergillosis in 2002: An update. Eur J Microbiol Infect Dis 21:161, 2002.

191. Pasic S, Abinun M, Pistignjat B, et al: *Aspergillus* osteomyelitis in chronic granulomatous disease: Treatment with recombinant gamma-interferon and itraconazole. Pediatr Infect Dis J 15:833, 1996.

192. Vinas FC, King PK, Diaz FG: Spinal *aspergillus* osteomyelitis. Clin Infect Dis 28:1223, 1999.

193. Steinfeld S, Durez P, Hauzeur J-P, et al: Articular aspergillosis: Two case reports and review of the literature. Br J Rheumatol 36:1331, 1997.

194. Wheat J: Histoplasmosis: Recognition and treatment. Clin Infect Dis 19(Suppl 1):S19, 1994.

195. Weinberg JM, Ali R, Badve S, Pelker RR: Musculoskeletal histoplasmosis: A case report and review of the literature. J Bone Joint Surg Am 83: 1718, 2001.

196. Lee J-H, Slifman NR, Gershon SK, et al: Life-threatening histoplasmosis complicating immunotherapy with tumor necrosis factor α antagonists infliximab and etanercept. Arthritis Rheum 46:2565, 2002.

197. Wheat LJ: Laboratory diagnosis of histoplasmosis: Update 2000. Semin Respir Infect 16:131, 2001.

198. Fowler VG, Nacinovich FM, Alspaugh JA, et al: Prosthetic joint infection due to *Histoplasma capsulatum*: Case report and review. Clin Infect Dis 26:1017, 1998.

199. Wheat J, Sarosi, McKinsey D, et al: Practice guidelines for management of patients with histoplasmosis. Clin Infect Dis 30:688, 2000.

200. Mocherla S, Wheat JL: Treatment of histoplasmosis. Semin Respir Infect 16:141, 2001.

201. Wilson CM, O'Rourke EJ, McGinnis MR, Salkin IF: *Scedosporium inflatum*: Clinical spectrum of a newly recognized pathogen. J Infect Dis 161:102, 1990.

202. Terrell CL, Hughes CE: Antifungal agents used for deep-seated mycotic infections. Mayo Clin Proc 67:69, 1992.

203. Sarosi GA, Davies SF: Therapy for fungal infections. Mayo Clin Proc 69:1111, 1994.

204. Meier JL: Mycobacterial and fungal infections of the bones and joints. Curr Opin Rheumatol 6:408, 1994.

205. Martino P, Girmenia C: Are we making progress in antifungal therapy? Curr Opin Oncol 9:314, 1997.
206. Perez-Gomez A, Prieto A, Torresano M, et al: Role of the new azoles in the treatment of fungal osteoarticular infections. Semin Arthritis Rheum 27:226, 1998.
207. Rapp RP, Gubbins PO, Evans ME: Amphotericin B lipid complex. Ann Pharmacother 31:1174, 1997.
208. Alexander BD, Perfect JR: Antifungal resistance trends toward the year 2000. Drugs 54:657, 1997.
209. Espinel-Ingroff A: Clinical relevance of antifungal resistance. Infect Dis Clin North Am 11:929, 1997.
210. Summers KK, Hardin TC, Gore SJ, et al: Therapeutic drug monitoring of systemic antifungal therapy. J Antimicrob Chemother 40:753, 1997.
211. Mara-Duarte J, Bettis R, Rotstein C, et al, for the Caspofungin Invasive Candidaisis Study Group: Comparison of caspofungin and amphoteracin B for invasive candidiasis. N Engl J Med 347:2020, 2002.

Rheumatic Manifestations of Human Immunodeficiency Virus Infection

JOHN D. REVEILLE

Nearly 23 years have passed since the first descriptions of patients with human immunodeficiency virus (HIV) infection. By the end of 2002, the World Health Organization (WHO) estimated 42 million people to be living with HIV infection, with 3.1 million deaths due to acquired immune deficiency syndrome (AIDS) and 5 million newly infected people in 2002 alone (http://www.who.int/hiv/pub/epidemiology/epi2002/en/). More than 95 percent of new cases were in developing countries, with most rapid rates of new infection in Africa and Central and Southern Asia (where 84% of new cases occurred).

Although the principal caregivers for HIV-infected individuals have been primary care practitioners and infectious disease specialists, complications of HIV infection (and its treatment) have required the input and care of nearly every subspecialty of internal medicine, including the rheumatologist. Indeed, one of the biggest paradoxes of HIV infection is the finding of certain rheumatic diseases—such as the diffuse infiltrative lymphocytosis syndrome (DILS), reactive arthritis (Reiter's syndrome), or inflammatory myopathy—occurring in the face of immunodeficiency, which possibly gives a clue to their very pathogenesis. Alternately, other rheumatic diseases, such as rheumatoid arthritis (RA) and systemic lupus erythematosus (SLE), have been reported as improving in the face of the cell determinant (CD)4+ lymphocyte depletion associated with this disease. On the whole, however, rheumatic symptoms appear to occur more commonly in HIV-positive individuals.[1,2] Table 101–1 lists the spectrum of rheumatic diseases associated with HIV infection. In this chapter, the spectrum of rheumatic diseases occurring in patients with HIV infection is explored, including classic diseases, such as reactive arthritis and polymyositis, and some novel diseases peculiar to HIV-infected individuals, such as DILS and HIV-associated arthritis.

Human Immunodeficiency Virus–Associated Joint Disease

HUMAN IMMUNODEFICIENCY VIRUS–ASSOCIATED ARTHRALGIA

HIV outpatient clinics report the frequency of otherwise unexplained arthralgia to be as high as 45 percent, although this figure varies widely among different groups[1-6] (Table 101–2), probably reflecting differences in the mode of ascertaining symptoms. Whether the arthralgia can be attributed to circulating viral and host immune

TABLE 101–1 · RHEUMATIC DISEASES ASSOCIATED WITH OR OCCURRING IN PATIENTS WITH HUMAN IMMUNODEFICIENCY VIRUS (HIV) INFECTION

Unique to HIV Infection	Found in HIV-Infected Patients	Ameliorated by HIV Infection
Diffuse infiltrative leukocytosis syndrome (DILS)	HIV-associated Reiter's syndrome	Rheumatoid arthritis (RA)
HIV-associated arthritis	Polymyositis	Systemic lupus erythematosus (SLE)
Zidovudine (ZDV)-associated myopathy	Psoriatic arthritis	
Painful articular syndrome	Polyarteritis nodosa (PAN)	
	Giant cell arteritis (GCA)	
	Hypersensitivity angiitis	
	Wegener's granulomatosis (WG)	
	Schönlein-Henoch purpura	
	Behçet's syndrome	
	Infectious arthritis (bacterial, fungal)	

complexes due to HIV infection per se or to other infections (e.g., hepatitis C) has not been determined. Most patients presenting with arthralgia alone do not progress to inflammatory joint disease. The most appropriate treatment, along with non-narcotic analgesics such as acetaminophen or tramadol, is reassurance.

Painful Articular Syndrome

A self-limited syndrome usually lasting less than 24 hours, accompanied by few objective clinical findings, and characterized by extremely painful bone and joint pain has been described in patients from the United States with HIV infection.[3-6] This same disorder has been described in Africans with HIV infection, with frequencies as high as 10 percent.[7-9] The etiology of this disorder is unknown, and there is no evidence of synovitis in these patients. The treatment is symptomatic.

HUMAN IMMUNODEFICIENCY VIRUS–ASSOCIATED ARTHRITIS

Epidemiology

The first reports of a seronegative arthritis associated with HIV infection appeared in 1988,[10-12] with frequencies as

TABLE 101–2 • DISTRIBUTION OF VARIOUS RHEUMATIC DISEASES FROM VARIOUS SITES

Feature	Cincinnati, Ohio, USA[77]	Houston, Texas, USA*[10]	Madrid, Spain[4]
Number of patients	1100	4467	556
HIV-associated arthralgia	NA	0.7%	1.6%
Myalgia	0.7%	0.6%	4.5%
PsA/Reiter's syndrome	0.5%	0.6%	0.5%
HIV-associated arthritis	0%	0.47%	0.4%
DILS/Sjögren's syndrome	NR	3-4%[†57]	NR

*Prevalences represent patients referred to a HIV subspecialty clinic within the acquired immune deficiency syndrome (AIDS) clinic divided by the clinic census between 1994 and 2001.
†Prevalence determined from systematic survey of 522 patients attending the county AIDS clinic.

Abbreviations: DILS, diffuse infiltrative lymphocytosis syndrome; HIV, human immunodeficiency virus; NA, not applicable; NR, not reported; PsA, psoriatic arthritis.

high as 12 percent (see Table 101–2). HIV-associated arthritis appears to be more common in sub-Saharan Africa, where HIV infection is pandemic. In series of patients seen in rheumatology clinics in the Democratic Republic of Congo,[7] Zimbabwe,[8] and Rwanda,[9] HIV-associated arthritis occurred at least as frequently, and sometimes more commonly, than HIV-associated spondyloarthropathy.

Clinical Features

The arthritis associated with HIV infection was initially described as an oligoarthritis, predominantly lower extremity in distribution, which tended to be self limited, lasting less than 6 weeks[10-12] (Table 101–3). This is consistent with a recent report that has suggested that HIV-associated arthritis shares many of the clinical characteristics of other viral arthritidies.[12] However, some patients have been reported as having a longer course with joint destruction.[10] The synovial fluid leukocyte count is lower than that seen in HIV-associated reactive arthritis. The etiology is unclear. There is no association with human leukocyte antigen (HLA)-B27 or any other

known genetic factor. Synovial fluid cultures are typically sterile, although one report described the presence of tuboreticular inclusions, suggesting a viral etiology, possibly HIV itself.[12] Further evidence for a direct role of HIV was the isolation of HIV virus from one synovial fluid sample and electron microscopy showing particles resembling retrovirus.[11] Radiographs of the affected joints are usually normal, except in uncommon cases with prolonged symptoms, in which joint-space narrowing can occur.[10]

Treatment

The treatment of HIV-associated arthritis included nonsteroidal anti-inflammatory drugs (NSAIDs) and, in more severe cases, low-dose glucocorticoids. Hydroxychloroquine has also been reported as being effective in this setting,[13] as has sulfasalazine.

HUMAN IMMUNODEFICIENCY VIRUS–ASSOCIATED REACTIVE ARTHRITIS

Epidemiology

The first paper on the coexistence of HIV infection and reactive arthritis[14] occurred the same year (1987) that zidovudine was shown as being effective in treating HIV infection. Data from this reporting center, in New York City,[15] suggested that reactive arthritis occurred more commonly in the setting of HIV infection. Another conclusion from this was that the perturbation in the CD4 lymphocyte counts and CD4 to CD8 ratios may be involved in the pathogenesis of reactive arthritis, at least in HIV-positive individuals. Subsequently, however, two population-based surveys, in San Francisco and Baltimore, failed to find an association of reactive arthritis with HIV infection per se, but instead suggested that the increased frequency of reactive arthritis was due to the sexually active nature of the population at highest risk for HIV infection.[15,16]

These data are contradicted by studies from Africa. HLA-B27 is virtually absent in most of the sub-Saharan Africa populations, and prior to the outbreak of the HIV epidemic, reports of patients with seronegative spondyloarthropathy were rare.[10,17] However, with the arrival of HIV infection in sub-Saharan Africa in recent

TABLE 101–3 • CONTRASTING FEATURES OF HUMAN IMMUNODEFICIENCY VIRUS (HIV)-ASSOCIATED ARTHRITIS AND REITER'S SYNDROME

Feature	HIV-Associated Arthritis	HIV-Associated Reiter's Syndrome
Joint involvement	Asymmetric oligopolyarthritis	Asymmetric oligopolyarthritis
Mucocutaneous involvement	Absent	Present
Enthesopathy	Absent	Frequent
Synovial fluid white blood cell count	500-2000/μl	2000-10,000/μl
Synovial fluid cultures	Negative	Negative
Microorganisms in synovial membranes	?HIV-1 virus	*Chlamydia**
HLA-B27 association	Absent	70 to 90%[†]

*Demonstrated in non–HIV-associated Reiter's syndrome. Reports of such infections in those with HIV-associated Reiter's syndrome are lacking.
† In whites.

years has been associated with a dramatic upsurge in the prevalence of spondyloarthropathies other than ankylosing spondylitis (AS), primarily reactive arthritis and undifferentiated spondyloarthropathy, and less often psoriatic arthritis,[10,17] suggesting a pathogenic role of HIV infection in spondyloarthropathy. Similarly, in Thailand, reactive arthritis and other spondyloarthropathies are well-described complications of HIV infection.[5]

Clinical Presentation

The most typical presentation is that of a seronegative peripheral arthritis predominantly involving the lower extremities, usually accompanied by enthesitis (sausaging of toes or fingers, Achilles tendinitis, and plantar fasciitis). Mucocutaneous features are common, especially keratoderma blennorrhagicum (Fig. 101–1) and circinate balanitis. The latter is frequently not observed by the patient and must be sought by the examining physician. Psoriaform skin rashes are likewise common and can be extensive. The clinical overlap makes it difficult at times to distinguish HIV-associated reactive arthritis from psoriatic arthritis, leading to the speculation that these entities represent a "disease continuum."[18] Urethritis occurs in similar frequency as in HIV-negative reactive arthritis. Axial involvement and uveitis appear to be uncommon, but they do occur.

HLA-B27 is found in 80 to 90 percent of those with HIV-associated reactive arthritis, at least in whites.[18] However, studies of Africans with HIV-associated reactive arthritis have found the majority to be negative for HLA-B27.[9,10,17] Of particular interest are studies from large series of HIV-infected individuals that have suggested that the presence of HLA-B27 antigen may slow the progression to AIDS.[19] A study of asymptomatic

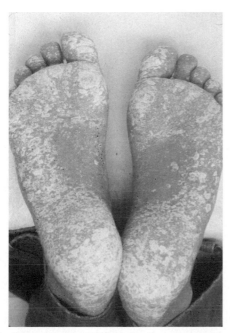

FIGURE 101–1 · Keratoderma blennorrhagicum in a patient with Reiter's syndrome as well as human immunodeficiency virus (HIV) infection.

HIV-infected, HLA-B27–positive individuals found their cytotoxic T lymphocyte response to be dominated by recognition of a *gag*-encoded p24 protein epitope that was not seen in HLA-B27–negative, HIV-positive individuals.[20] Other HLA class I antigens that have been associated with a better outcome in HIV infection have also been implicated in psoriasis and psoriatic arthritis and include HLA-B13 and HLA-B17 (B57).[19]

Treatment

The treatment is much the same as for HIV-negative patients with reactive arthritis. NSAIDs are the mainstay of treatment. Indomethacin, in particular, is recommended, not only for its efficacy but also for its inhibition of HIV replication (observed in vitro) that appears to be unique to this NSAID.[21] Phenylbutazone, rarely used now because of its high side-effect profile, may be useful in refractory cases. Patients frequently have an inadequate response to NSAIDs alone, and these drugs are frequently used in combination with other antiarthritic agents. Sulfasalazine has been shown to be effective in some studies at doses of 1.5 to 2 g/day,[22,23] and in fact, one study suggested that it ameliorated HIV infection.[23] Methotrexate (MTX) was initially felt to be contraindicated because of its immunosuppressive effect. Its use in early reports was associated with the development of *Pneumocystis carinii* pneumonia and other opportunistic infections.[15] However, with careful monitoring of HIV viral loads and CD4 counts, as well as the patient's clinical status, more recent studies have suggest a place for MTX in the treatment of reactive arthritis and psoriatic arthritis occurring in the setting of HIV infection.[24] Hydroxychloroquine has also been reported to be as efficacious not only in treating HIV-associated reactive arthritis[14] but also in reducing HIV replication in vitro and in reducing HIV viral loads in vivo.[25] Both the arthritis and the cutaneous lesions of HIV-associated reactive arthritis and psoriatic arthritis have been found to respond to etretinate (0.5 to 1 mg/kg/day).[26]

In one case of refractory reactive arthritis associated with HIV infection in which infliximab was given, the patient tolerated the drug well and improved clinically.[27] However, given the known tendency for infection, especially mycobacterial infections in HIV-negative individuals receiving infliximab, this drug should be used with extreme caution and only in patients with otherwise refractory disease in patients with HIV-associated reactive arthritis and spondyloarthopathy. Clearly more studies are necessary before tumor necrosis factor (TNF) blockers can be routinely recommended in patients with HIV-associated reactive arthritis.

PSORIASIS AND PSORIATIC ARTHRITIS

Psoriasis, psoriatic arthritis, and reactive arthritis occur most often in those with advanced HIV disease.[18,28,29] In fact, one study found that the appearance of psoriasis in an HIV-positive patient heralded subsequent opportunistic infection, such as *P. carinii* pneumonia.[30] The psoriatic rash can be extensive (Fig. 101–2), especially in

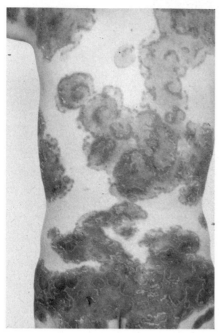

FIGURE 101-2 · Disseminated psoriasis vulgaris in a patient with human immunodeficiency virus (HIV)-associated psoriasis.

patients not taking antiretroviral treatment. Despite early suggestive data, it is not entirely clear that psoriasis per se occurs more commonly in Caucasians with HIV infection.

Psoriasis and psoriatic arthritis were extremely uncommon in Africa prior to the arrival of HIV.[10,17,30] However, a recent report from Zambia found 27 of 28 African patients with psoriatic arthritis to be HIV positive (out of 702 new patients attending an outpatient rheumatology clinic in a 40-month period).[30] The arthritis was predominantly polyarticular, lower limb, and progressive. In contrast to the early reports in Caucasians, amelioration was noted with onset of AIDS. Psoriasis was commonly an extensive guttate-plaque admixture and, unlike the articular disease, was non-remittive with onset of AIDS.[30]

Antiretroviral treatment has been shown to be effective in treating both HIV-associated psoriasis and its associated arthritis.[31] Phototherapy may improve the skin rash, but it may also enhance viral replication and worsen HIV disease.[31] Other agents reported as efficacious include cyclosporine[32] (although renal function must be carefully monitored) and etretinate.[27] MTX can also be used, albeit with caution. One report of the use of etanercept in patients with refractory psoriatic arthritis suggested the drug to be efficacious for both skin and joint disease, with no deterioration in the immunologic and viral parameters, although frequent polymicrobial infections while taking the drug resulted in its discontinuation.[33]

UNDIFFERENTIATED SPONDYLOARTHROPATHY

Also frequently encountered are stigmata of reactive arthritis or psoriatic arthritis in patients who do not otherwise develop full-blown disease, such as enthesopathy (plantar fasciitis, Achilles tendinitis). The treatment is symptomatic (NSAIDs, intralesional corticosteroid injections, when indicated), although sulfasalazine should be considered in patients with more extensive disease.

AVASCULAR NECROSIS OF BONE

Recent reports have suggested that patients with HIV infections are at increased risk for developing avascular necrosis. This has been attributed to metabolic complications of protease-inhibitor treatment such as hyperlipidemia or to other causes such as high-dose glucocorticoid usage or antiphospholipid antibodies.[11,35]

■ Human Immunodeficiency Virus–Associated Muscle Disease

Muscle involvement in HIV infection runs the gamut of disorders, ranging from uncomplicated myalgias and fibromyalgia or asymptomatic creatine kinase elevation to severe, disabling HIV-associated polymyositis or pyomyositis.[36-54] HIV seroconversion can also coincide with myoglobinuria and acute myalgia, suggesting that myotropism for HIV may be symptomatic early in the infection. One series of skeletal muscle biopsies obtained from 92 adults with HIV infection at autopsy found atrophy to be the most common finding (in 51 of 92), followed by the finding of inflammatory skeletal muscle infiltrates (in 8 of 92), necrosis (in 8 of 92), and infection in (3 of 92).[38] Creatine kinase elevation is commonly encountered in the outpatients with HIV infection,[36,37] either due to HIV per se, behaviors associated with higher risk for HIV infection (such as cocaine use), or due to HIV treatment itself (see following). In most patients these elevations are transient and of little consequence, but they require careful follow-up.

MYALGIA AND FIBROMYALGIA

Series of HIV-positive outpatients have revealed myalgias to occur in up to a third of HIV-infected patients.[2-7] Fibromyalgia is associated with myalgia and arthralgia, but not with age, duration of HIV infection, or zidovudine (ZDV) therapy.[39] In another series of 140 patients attending an outpatient, inner-city HIV facility in Boston, Massachusetts,[40] 15 were found to have fibromyalgia, which was associated with longer disease duration and a history of depression. Treatment is similar to that for fibromyalgia in the non-HIV setting (see Chapter 31).

NONINFLAMMATORY NECROTIZING MYOPATHY AND HUMAN IMMUNODEFICIENCY VIRUS–RELATED WASTING SYNDROME

A noninflammatory necrotizing myopathy of unclear pathogenesis has been described in patients with HIV infection.[39,40] It has been described in as many as 42 percent of those diagnosed with myopathy.[41] In some, it has been attributed to the poorly characterized HIV-related wasting syndrome,[41] but a necrotizing myopathy has been recognized in those without significant wasting. Despite the lack of inflammation seen, an immune-mediated pathogenesis is favored by most investigators,[42] although this has been recently contested in those with HIV-related wasting syndrome, in whom metabolic or nutritional factors have been implicated.[41] Corticosteroids have been reported to restore muscle strength and mass.[41]

HUMAN IMMUNODEFICIENCY VIRUS–ASSOCIATED POLYMYOSITIS

Considered the most common of the myopathies occurring in the setting of HIV-1 infection,[44] HIV-associated polymyositis most typically manifests early in the course of HIV infection. The most common manifestation is that of a subacute, progressive proximal muscle weakness occurring in the setting of an elevated creatine kinase.[37,45] As in HIV-negative polymyositis, myalgia is not a prominent presenting feature. Electromyographic studies reveal myopathic motor unit potentials with early recruitment and full interference patterns, as well as fibrillation potentials, positive sharp waves, and complex repetitive discharges indicative of an irritative process.[45] Light microscopy of muscle biopsies demonstrates interstitial inflammatory infiltrates of variable intensity accompanied by degenerating and regenerating myofibrils, similar to those seen in polymyositis without HIV-1 (Fig. 101–3). Concomitant vasculitis rarely occurs. In specimens from both HIV-positive and HIV-negative patients with myositis, the predominant cell populations were CD8+ T cells and macrophages invading or surrounding healthy muscle fibers that express major histocompatibility complex (MHC) class I antigens on their cell surfaces.[42] The endomysial infiltrates in specimens from HIV-positive patients differed from patients with polymyositis without HIV infection only by a significant reduction of CD4+ cells.[44]

The cause of HIV-associated polymyositis is unclear. Whether the HIV virus per se directly contributes to inflammatory myopathy is controversial. One study sought HIV proviral DNA and amplified sequences in the muscle biopsies of patients with HIV-associated polymyositis and found integrated HIV sequences only in the surrounding lymphoid cells but not within the muscle fibers, suggesting that HIV-associated polymyositis was not due to persistent infection of the muscle fiber by the HIV virus.[46] In another study, however, amplified HIV-1 nucleic acids were found primarily in macrophages but also in myocyte nuclei, bringing the authors to the opposite conclusion.[47] Nutritional factors have also been implicated in HIV-associated myopathy.[42]

The treatment of HIV-associated polymyositis is similar to that for other inflammatory myopathies. Both the creative kinase (CK) elevation and the muscle weakness respond to moderate-dose glucocorticoids. Refractory cases may require immunosuppressive agents such as MTX or azathioprine. There is little evidence to suggest a role for intravenous immunoglobulin (IVIg).[37] These agents should be used with caution with careful monitoring of the patient's clinical status, CD4+ counts, and HIV mRNA levels. In a recent longitudinal study of 13 patients with biopsy-proven myositis, eight were treated with prednisone (60 mg/day) with five attaining complete resolution of myositis. The remaining three patients received immunosuppressive therapy (azathioprine or MTX and IVIg) and had normalization of strength and CK. Four patients had spontaneous resolution of their myositis without treatment. No evidence of adverse outcome on the HIV infection by treatment of polymyositis was seen in this cohort,[37] suggesting that with careful management, the overall prognosis of HIV-associated polymyositis is favorable.

Whether asymptomatic patients with CK elevation will eventually develop HIV-associated polymyositis is unclear. We have followed two such individuals for more than 5 years, and they have not shown any clinical deterioration. This suggests that asymptomatic patients with isolated, unexplained, persistent CK elevation can be followed carefully for any sign of clinical deterioration before electrodiagnostic and biopsy studies are undertaken.

NEMALINE ROD MYOPATHY

This rare disorder has been described as occurring in a number of settings, including congenitally, as an acquired disorder in adults, and as a complication of certain rheumatic diseases, such as SLE or polymyositis. It has also rarely been described in HIV-infected individuals.[48] Nemaline rod myopathy is a nonspecific myofibrillar alteration resulting from Z band disruption. Studies of HIV-associated nemaline rod myopathy have shown marked intrasarcoplasmic changes, including small vacuoles and granular degeneration.[49]

MYOPATHY ASSOCIATED WITH TREATMENT

Within a year of the introduction of ZDV for the treatment of HIV, reports of a diffuse myopathy attributed to its use began to appear.[42,50,51] The syndrome is characterized by the insidious onset of myalgias, muscle tenderness, and proximal muscle weakness after a mean duration of therapy of 11 months. ZDV myopathy

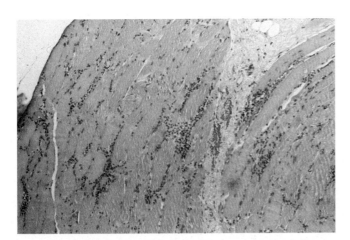

FIGURE 101–3 · Muscle biopsy from a patient with human immunodeficiency virus (HIV)-associated polymyositis.

tends to be dose-related, being associated with long-term ZDV usage, and is associated with mitochondrial dysfunction.[51] Both clinically, and by EMG or muscle biopsy, it can be difficult to distinguish ZDV myopathy from HIV-associated polymyositis, although the inflammatory infiltrates tend to be much less severe (and often absent) in patients taking ZDV. The mitochondrial abnormalities originally attributed to ZDV were ultimately described in all patients with HIV-associated myopathy,[42] although they tend to be more severe in those taking ZDV. In one study, tuboreticular inclusions were identified in capillary endothelial cells in patients with HIV-associated myopathy regardless of ZDV usage, suggesting that ZDV caused myopathy only when an underlying HIV-associated myopathy was present. The symptoms tend to improve as the drug is discontinued,[42,50,51] with CK levels returning to normal within 4 weeks of discontinuing the drug and muscle strength returning within 8 weeks. Myalgias associated with ZDV use respond to NSAIDs.[2] Repeat muscle biopsies on those who improved clinically after discontinuation of ZDV showed remarkable histologic improvement. Thus, in any HIV-infected patient presenting with an elevated CK, especially when symptoms of myalgia or muscle weakness are present, the ZDV should be discontinued for 4 weeks and the patient reevaluated before EMG or muscle biopsies are undertaken.

PYOMYOSITIS

Rarely seen in developed countries, infectious myositis (pyomyositis) nonetheless remains an important complication of HIV infection in areas most endemic for HIV, such as Africa and India. A case-control study from Uganda found a highly significant association of pyomyositis with HIV infection.[52] *Staphylococcus aureus* remains the most common pathogen,[53] although other organisms have been identified, including *Salmonella enteritidis*, *Microsporum*, and *Toxoplasma*.[54] Concomitant HTLV-I viral infection has also been reported in HIV-positive patients with myositis[55] (usually associated with a myelopathy).

▌ Diffuse Infiltrative Lymphocytosis Syndrome

Although a number of groups described a syndrome resembling Sjögren's syndrome occurring in HIV-positive patients in the mid-1980s, diffuse infiltrative lymphocytosis syndrome (DILS) as we now recognize it was categorized as a discrete syndrome by Itescu and coworkers[56] more than 13 years ago. DILS is characterized by salivary gland enlargement and peripheral CD8 lymphocytosis often accompanied by sicca symptoms and extraglandular features found in HIV-positive individuals.

EPIDEMIOLOGY

Two studies were undertaken to define the prevalence of DILS. In one, the prevalence of DILS, parotid enlargement, and sicca symptoms were determined in 522 HIV-positive outpatients in an urban Texas HIV clinic.[57] There, DILS was defined by the presence of parotid enlargement accompanied by a positive minor salivary gland biopsy or positive ^{67}Ga scintigraphy. The prevalence of DILS was 3 to 4 percent in HIV-positive outpatients. In another study, 77 HIV-positive outpatients were examined for xerophthalmia and xerostomia,[58] and positive responders underwent minor salivary gland biopsy and technetium scintigraphy. In this study from Greece, the prevalence of DILS was 7.8 percent. African Americans are more frequently affected than other ethnic groups.[57,58] A recent report has suggested a significantly higher prevalence of DILS in HIV-positive West African individuals, although this may be explained by differences in patient selection; 30 HIV-positive individuals underwent a minor salivary gland biopsy, and 48 percent had more than 1 lymphocytic focus in a minor salivary gland (primarily CD8+).[59]

PATHOGENESIS

The primary immunogenetic association has been with HLA-DRB1 alleles expressing the *ILEDE* amino acid sequence in the third diversity region, most usually *HLA-DRB1*1102*, *DRB1*1301*, and *DRB1*1302*.[56] The delayed progression to AIDS in patients with DILS has been attributed to delay in the evolution of the HIV-1 virus from the less aggressive M-tropic strain to the more rapidly replicating T-tropic strain caused by a more effective CD8 lymphocyte response.[60] This has been attributed, at least in part, to the finding of sequence homology of a six-residue epitope shared by HLA-DRB1 alleles associated with DILS with a V3 loop on M-tropic HIV strains. Studies of immunophenotypes of circulating and tissue-infiltrating lymphocytes and salivary gland T cell receptor (TCR) sequence analysis suggested that DILS represents an MHC-restricted, antigen-driven, oligoclonal selection of CD8+, CD29– lymphocytes that express selective homing receptors and infiltrate the salivary glands, lungs, and other organs, where they are postulated to suppress HIV-1 replication.[61]

PATHOLOGY

Minor salivary gland biopsies show a focal sialadenitis, similar to that observed in Sjögren's syndrome, although there tends to be less destruction of the salivary glands (Fig. 101–4). CD8+ lymphocytes constitute most of the inflammatory infiltrate,[59,62-64] in contrast to that seen in primary (non–HIV-associated) Sjögren's syndrome. Lymphoepithelial cysts are frequently seen in the parotid glands of patients with DILS, leading to inspissated salivary secretions that may be painful. Histologically, the cysts demonstrate follicular hyperplasia, cystic dilatation of the ducts lined by pseudostratified squamous epithelium, and lymphocytic infiltrate.[66]

CLINICAL PRESENTATION

The characteristic, if not defining, presentation of DILS is that of painless parotid enlargement, often massive

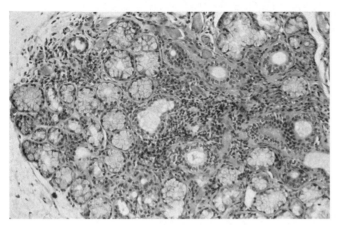

FIGURE 101-4 · Minor Salivary Gland Biopsy from a Patient with Diffuse Infiltrative Lymphocytosis Syndrome (DILS). Note the relative preservation of the glandular architecture, even with significant interstitial inflammation.

(Fig. 101-5). The mean period of time between the discovery of HIV seropositivity to the onset of symptoms in one study was 3.4 years.[62] The physical disfigurement associated with this is often distressing to the patient. Submandibular and lacrimal gland enlargement often occur concomitantly. This enlargement is accompanied by sicca symptoms in more than 60 percent of patients. Those with DILS have lower mean stimulated parotid salivary flow rates than HIV-positive patients without parotid enlargement, and this reduction in flow rates remains stable over time despite ZVD therapy.[64] Longitudinal studies have shown that the parotid enlargement also persists over time in most patients.

Although parotid and submandibular enlargement is nearly universal in this disorder, accompanied by sicca symptoms in more than 60 percent of cases, certain extraglandular features are also prominent[56,62-64] (Table 101-4). Early reports noted a frequency of lymphocytic interstitial pneumonitis (LIP) as high as 25 to 50 percent in patients with DILS.[63-65] Since the introduction of protease inhibitors, this complication occurs much less commonly. Neurologic disease also figures prominently in the presentation of DILS. Probably the most common neurologic complication is cranial nerve VII palsy, usually due to mechanical compression of the nerve by inflamed parotid tissue, although peripheral neuropathy has also been described. Other extraglandular complications of DILS include renal tubular acidosis, polymyositis, lymphocytic hepatitis, and lymphoma, the latter associated with an especially poor prognosis.[64] Two groups have suggested that patients with DILS have a better prognosis than other HIV patients, as they progress to opportunistic infection and death at half the rate as others.[58,63] The influence of protease inhibitors and other newer HIV therapies on this protection from progression, however, remains to be determined, although of particular note is the report of parotid lipomatosis in patients taking protease inhibitors that can resemble DILS.[65]

DILS and Sjögren's syndrome share both similarities and striking differences (Table 101-5). Parotid enlargement occurs in less than one third of those with Sjögren's syndrome, whereas it occurs in nearly all those with DILS.[63,65] Extraglandular manifestations, such as LIP and facial nerve VII palsies, occur uncommonly in patients with Sjögren's syndrome. Autoantibodies characteristically found in those with Sjögren's syndrome, such as antinuclear antibodies (ANA), rheumatoid factor (RF), and anti-Ro (SS-A) and anti-La (SS-B) are not characteristically found in those with DILS.

The sicca complex has also been reported in as many as 8 percent of patients with chronic hepatitis C infection, which frequently coexists with HIV infection. Patients

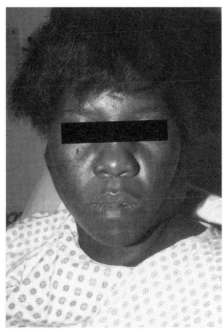

FIGURE 101-5 · Massive Bilateral Asymmetric Salivary Gland Enlargement in a Patient with Diffuse Infiltrative Lymphocytosis Syndrome (DILS). This was the presenting feature of her human immunodeficiency virus (HIV) infection. Computed tomography (CT) scanning revealed this to be a solid mass. At follow-up 2-years after this photograph was taken, the gland had not changed in size.

TABLE 101-4 · EXTRAGLANDULAR FEATURES OF DIFFUSE INFILTRATIVE LYMPHOCYTOSIS SYNDROME (DILS)

Pulmonary
    Lymphocytic interstitial pneumonitis (LIP)
Neurologic
    Cranial nerve VII palsy
    Aseptic lymphocytic meningitis
    Peripheral neuropathy
Gastrointestinal
    Lymphocytic hepatitis
Renal
    Renal tubular acidosis
    Interstitial nephritis
Musculoskeletal
    Peripheral arthritis
    Polymyositis
Hematologic
    Lymphoma

TABLE 101–5 • SIMILARITIES AND DIFFERENCES BETWEEN DIFFUSE INFILTRATIVE LYMPHOCYTOSIS SYNDROME (DILS) AND SJÖGREN'S SYNDROME

Feature	DILS	Sjögren's Syndrome
Parotid swelling	Ubiquitous	Uncommon
Sicca symptoms	Common	Very common
Extraglandular symptoms	Common	Uncommon
Autoantibodies (antinuclear antibodies, anti-Ro/La)	Rare	Common
Human leukocyte antigen (HLA) class II association	DRB1*1102, 1301, 1302	DRB1*0301, DQA1*0501, DQB1*0201

with hepatitis C–associated sicca complex also have less prominence of parotid glandular enlargement and more severe sicca symptoms.[66] Patients with DILS should be screened for a concomitant diagnosis of hepatitis C.

DIAGNOSTIC MEASURES

Diagnostic criteria have been proposed for DILS as follows: The subject 1) must be HIV-seropositive by enzyme-linked immunosorbent assay (ELISA) and Western blot analysis, 2) must have bilateral salivary gland enlargement or xerostomia persisting for more than 6 months, and 3) must have histologic confirmation or salivary or lacrimal gland lymphocytic infiltration in the absence of granulomatous or neoplastic enlargement.[64] Minor salivary gland biopsies are usually positive[62,64] (see Fig. 101–4). Gallium Ga67 scintigraphy[67] (Fig. 101–6) of the salivary glands has been used when lip biopsy was not feasible (hemophiliacs) or biopsy results were equivocal. Technetium pertechnetate scanning, on the other hand, offers little diagnostic help. Recently, we have been utilizing scintigraphy as a primary diagnostic aid in patients on protease inhibitors, because we found that minor salivary gland biopsies were rarely positive in patients taking protease inhibitors. Computed tomography (CT) scan-

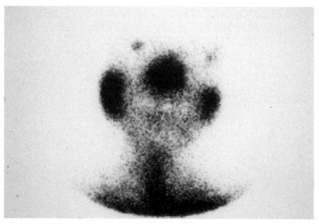

FIGURE 101–6 • The "Snowman" Sign. [67]Ga scintigraphy of the parotid glands of a patient with diffuse infiltrative lymphocytosis syndrome (DILS) occurring in the setting of hemophilia.

ning has also been utilized to determine the extent of glandular swelling, as well as in the evaluation of parotid cysts and possible salivary glandular malignancy.[68]

TREATMENT (TABLE 101–6)

A number of patients with DILS are not bothered by the glandular swelling, and the sicca symptoms are frequently mild or even absent. For these individuals, observation alone can suffice. The first reports of DILS predated the use of ZDV therapy in HIV patients. However, antiretroviral treatment soon was described as effective in treating the glandular swelling and sicca symptoms associated with DILS,[64] as well as complications such as neuropathy. We have found also that moderate doses of corticosteroids (30 to 40 mg of prednisone per day) are effective in treating both the glandular swelling and sicca symptoms of DILS without adversely affecting either the frequency of opportunistic infections, raising the viral loads, or depressing the CD4 counts, although the effect is transient. LIP may require higher doses of corticosteroids (up to 60 mg/day of prednisone), sometimes for extended periods. In another study, low-dose radiotherapy was successful in reducing parotid enlargement in all 12 patients treated,[69] but the improvement only lasted for a mean of 9.5 months. Retreatment gave much less favorable results; cranial nerve VII palsy tends to respond poorly to treatment of any sort.

Combination antiretroviral therapy also has been reported as effective in resolving parotid epithelial cysts,[70] although when refractory, they can be managed by aspiration and instillation of 1 ml of a deposteroid into the cyst (Fig. 101–7). The clinician should be careful to avoid the facial nerve as it exits the cranium just below the earlobe. Frequent recurrence may necessitate surgical excision.

Vasculitis Associated with Human Immunodeficiency Virus Infection

A wide spectrum of inflammatory vascular diseases has been described in patients with HIV infection.[1,71] One series found 34 (23 percent) of 148 "symptomatic" HIV-positive patients to have vasculitis.[71] Of these, 11 met American College of Rheumatologists (ACR) criteria for a distinct category of vasculitis, including hypersensitivity vasculitis in six, polyarteritis nodosa (PAN) in four, and

TABLE 101–6 • TREATMENT OF THE DIFFUSE INFILTRATIVE LYMPHOCYTOSIS SYNDROME (DILS)

Reassurance and education
Regular dental care
No specific treatment for asymptomatic individuals
Effective antiretroviral treatment
Pilocarpine (5 to 10 mg) or cevimeline (30 mg PO tid) for sicca symptoms
Systemic glucocorticoids
Drainage and instillation of corticosteroids into parotid lymphoepithelial cysts
Radiation of parotid cysts

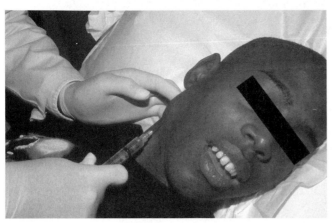

FIGURE 101-7 · Aspiration of a parotid epithelial cyst in a patient with diffuse infiltrative lymphocytosis syndrome (DILS).

Schönlein-Henoch purpura in one. A number of other series have also described PAN in patients with HIV infection.[72,73] Behçet's syndrome occurring in the setting of HIV infection has also been described.[74] A rapidly progressive, focal, necrotizing vasculitis of the aorta and large arteries with aneurysm formation and rupture has been described among Africans with HIV infection.[75] Kawasaki's disease has been reported in both children and adults who are HIV positive.[76] Giant cell arteritis (GCA) has likewise been described in patients with HIV infection.[77] Patients with isolated central nervous system (CNS) angiitis usually present with organic brain syndromes and neurologic deficit.[78] Although imaging studies (e.g., magnetic resonance imaging [MRI], angiography) may be of assistance, brain biopsy may be necessary to establish the diagnosis. Although this syndrome is rarely encountered clinically, perivascular mononuclear cell infiltrates have been described in brain tissue specimens collected at autopsy from five of six children with AIDS.[79]

Corticosteroids remain the mainstay of treatment of HIV-associated vasculitis, although cytotoxic agents have been employed in refractory cases.[71] Painful neuropathy due to vasculitis responds well to high-dose glucocorticoids,[80] although the common peripheral neuropathy associated with HIV infection does not. Our own experience with glucocorticoid therapy for vasculitis in three patients, two with Wegener's granulomatosis (WG) and a third with isolated CNS angiitis (confirmed by brain biopsy) is that all patients responded well to high-dose glucocorticoids and were doing well at 5-years follow-up (though one patient with WG did require a brief course of oral cyclophosphamide after 4 years).

Primary Pulmonary Hypertension

A number of reports have shown an association of primary pulmonary hypertension with HIV infection.[81] The predominant histopathologic finding has been a plexogenic pulmonary arteriopathy,[82] although thromboembolic changes have also been reported. One group[82] found an association with *HLA-DRB1*1301* and *DRB1*1302*, as well

with the linked allele *DRB3*0301*. In a recent review of 131 reviewed cases of pulmonary hypertension associated with HIV infection, the interval between the diagnosis of HIV disease and the diagnosis of pulmonary hypertension was 33 months. Presenting symptoms were progressive shortness of breath, pedal edema, nonproductive cough, fatigue, syncope or near syncope, and chest pain. Pulmonary-function tests demonstrated mild restrictive patterns with variably reduced diffusing capacities. The responses to vasodilator agents and antiretroviral therapy were variable. The median length of time from diagnosis to death was 6 months.[83] Subsequent reports have demonstrated a favorable response to sildenafil.[84]

Human Immunodeficiency Virus–Associated Musculoskeletal Infections

BACTERIAL ARTHRITIS

There are no data to suggest that bacterial infections of bones or joints due to the usual infectious agents, such as *S. aureus*, occur more frequently in patients with HIV infection.[85] One study of 4023 HIV-infected patients admitted to a large Italian university hospital between 1985 and 1996 found that *S. aureus* was the most common infectious agent encountered, but that parenteral drug use, and not HIV infection per se, accounted for these. In studies from Africa, septic arthritis occurred much less frequently than HIV-associated aseptic arthritis.[8-10]

Atypical Mycobacterial Infections

Musculoskeletal infections due to atypical mycobacterial species are distinctly unusual in nonimmunosuppressed individuals. Atypical mycobacterial species most commonly implicated in causing septic arthritis or osteomyelitis include *Mycobacterium avium intracellulare* complex (MAI), *M. kansasii*, *M. haemophilum*, *M. terrae*, and *M. fortuitum*. *M. haemophilum* has been most frequently implicated in skeletal infection, accounting for more than half of cases, and *M. kansasii* is second, accounting for an additional 25 percent. These are systemic infections and often involve several joints or skeletal sites. Cutaneous lesions, such as nodules, ulcers, and draining sinus tracts, occur in approximately 50 percent of patients infected with atypical mycobacterial species.[86]

These infections tend to occur late in the course of HIV, usually when the CD4+ T lymphocyte count is less than 100/μl.[86] On the other hand, *M. tuberculosis* arthritis appears to be no more frequent in HIV-positive than in HIV-negative individuals.[85] Along with standard antituberculosis therapy, clarithromycin has been reported as effective in most atypical mycobacterial bone and joint infections.

FUNGAL INFECTIONS

In addition to bacterial infections, patients with advanced HIV infection (CD4+ T lymphocyte count below 100/μl) are at high risk for fungal musculoskeletal infections, particularly those due to *Candida albicans*[6,87] and *Sporotrichosis schenkii*.[88] The latter can manifest with oligoarticular or even polyarticular involvement, with tendon sheath effusions (Fig. 101–8), and can be particularly difficult to eradicate, requiring chronic suppressive antifungal therapy.

Response of Other Rheumatic Diseases to Human Immunodeficiency Virus Infection

Early reports suggested that RA went into remission in the face of HIV infection.[89] More recent studies, however, have suggested that active RA may coexist with HIV infection.[90] In one histopathologic study, progressive joint destruction caused by proliferating synovium that lacked T cells occurred in an HIV-infected patient despite clinical symptomatic improvement.[91] Likewise, early reports suggested that HIV infection might reduce lupus activity, particularly at times of low CD4+ T cell counts.[92] One interesting result of the better control of HIV infection with highly active antiretroviral treatment (HAART) and immune reconstitution may be the recurrence of activity of RA and SLE. Recent reports of RA and SLE developing de novo in patients after HIV infection had come under control with HAART treatment further underscores this concern.[93,94]

Rheumatologic Complications of Human Immunodeficiency Virus Treatment

Although the benefits of HAART treatment for patients with HIV infections in terms of better disease control

and increased survival can hardly be argued, the side effects (most notably lipodystrophy) can be distressing to the patient. The myopathy associated with nucleoside transcriptase inhibitors such as ZDV has already been discussed, as has osteonecrosis and parotid lipomatosis associated with the use of protease inhibitors. Rhabdomyolysis (at times causing acute renal failure) has been reported with the use of protease inhibitors, particularly when used in combination with statin drugs (themselves used for treatment of dyslipidemia, complicating protease inhibitor treatment), hence this combination should be used with extreme care. In addition to this, cases of adhesive capsulitis, Dupuytren's contractures, tenosynovitis, and temporomandibular joint dysfunction have been reported as a consequence of indinivir treament.[95] A recent survey of 878 HIV-positive individuals suggested that patients taking protease inhibitors have an increased frequency of arthralgia.[95]

Laboratory Abnormalities Associated with Human Immunodeficiency Virus Infection

The most common laboratory abnormality is polyclonal hyperglobulinemia, found in up to 45 percent of HIV-positive individuals.[96] This reflects, at least in part, the increased level of circulating immune complexes that are commonly found in HIV-positive individuals, which are rarely of clinical consequence; hypocomplementemia is rare.[96] Autoantibodies are more frequently described in HIV-positive individuals.[2] RF and ANAs, usually in low titer, have been described in up to 17 percent of those with HIV infection in some series,[2,96] but not in others.[96] Of particular note is the finding of immunoglobulin G (IgG) anticardiolipin antibodies in up to 95 percent of patients with AIDS, particularly in those with advanced

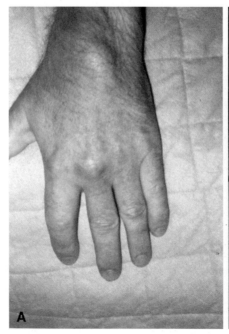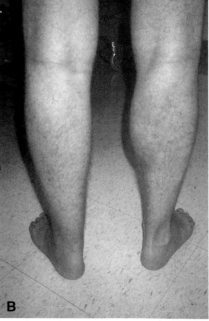

FIGURE 101–8 · *A*, Third metacarpophalangeal synovitis and common extensor digitorum longus tendon sheath effusion at the dorsal surface of the wrist. *B*, Dissecting a Backer's cyst in the same patient with disseminated *Sporotrichosis schenkii* infection (organism cultured from synovial fluid obtained from both sites).

disease,[2,3,97] and in 20 to 30 percent overall in HIV-positive individuals. These changes are rarely of clinical significance. The presence of circulating cryoglobulins are rarely of clinical consequence and usually represent the concomitant presence of hepatitis C infection.[98] Antineutrophil cytoplasmic antibodies (ANCAs), both cANCA and pANCA, have been described in the serum of HIV-positive individuals,[99] in frequencies up to 43 percent by ELISA and 18 percent by indirect immunofluorescence. Reactivity against myeloperoxidase and neutrophil elastase has been described,[99] although without any stigmata of vasculitis. Autoantibodies directed against circulating lymphocytes have likewise been described in up to 75 percent of HIV-positive individuals. These antibodies may contribute to the functional impairment of CD4+ T lymphocytes and ultimately to the CD8+ T lymphocyte depletion observed late in the disease.[100]

▌Conclusions

The impact of the global HIV pandemic continues to grow, hence the need for the rheumatologist to keep aware of the wide spectrum of rheumatic diseases that has been described in HIV-positive individuals. Most of these are typical of what is encountered in non–HIV-positive populations (soft tissue rheumatism, reactive arthritis, polymyositis). Others represent entities that may be particular to the setting of HIV (DILS, HIV-associated arthritis). Effective antiretroviral treatment improves the clinical signs and symptoms of many HIV-associated rheumatic diseases (reactive arthritis, DILS). On the other hand, some drugs used in the treatment of the rheumatic diseases (indomethacin, hydroxychloroquine, and sulfasalazine) also appear to have antiretroviral properties. The introduction of HAART therapy has not only prolonged the lives of patients with HIV infection but has introduced a new spectrum of diseases that must be considered by the practicing clinician (arthralgia, rhabdomyolysis, osteonecrosis), and effective immune reconstitution may reactivate certain rheumatic diseases that HIV infection itself may have caused to remit (RA, SLE). The spectrum of rheumatic disease associated with HIV infection and its treatment is an evolving story, which will continue for the indefinite future.

REFERENCES

1. Medina-Rodriguez F, Guzman C, Jara LJ, et al: Rheumatic manifestations in human immunodeficiency virus positive and negative individuals: A study of 2 populations with similar risk factors. J Rheumatol 20:1880, 1993.
2. Berman A, Espinoza LR, Diaz JD, et al: Rheumatic manifestations of human immunodeficiency virus infection. Am J Med 85:59, 1988.
3. Buskila D, Gladmann DD, Langevitz P, et al: Rheumatologic manifestations of infection with the human immunodeficiency virus (HIV). Clin Exp Rheumatol 8:567, 1990.
4. Munoz Fernandez S, Cardenal A, Balsa A, et al: Rheumatic manifestations in 556 patients with human immunodeficiency virus infection. Semin Arthritis Rheum 21:30, 1991.
5. Louthrenoo W: Musculoskeletal manifestations of HIV infection in Thailand: An analysis of 100 cases. J Clin Rheumatol 3: 258, 1997.
6. Reveille JD: The changing spectrum of rheumatic disease in human immunodeficiency virus infection. Semin Arthritis Rheum 30:147, 2000.
7. Bileckot R, Mouaya A, Makuwa M: Prevalence and clinical presentations of arthritis in HIV-positive patients seen at a rheumatology department in Congo-Brazzaville. Rev Rhum Engl 64:60, 1997.
8. Stein CM, Davis P: Arthritis associated with HIV infection in Zimbabwe. J Rheumatol 23:506, 1996.
9. Blanche P, Taelman H, Saraux A, et al: Acute arthritis and human immunodeficiency virus infection in Rwanda. J Rheumatol 20:2123, 1993.
10. Mody GM, Parke F, Reveille JD: Articular manifestations of human immunodeficiency virus infection. Baillieres Clin Rheum, in press, 2003.
11. Rynes RI, Goldenberg DL, DiGiacomo R, et al: Acquired immunodeficiency syndrome-associated arthritis. Am J Med 84:810, 1988.
12. Berman A, Cahn P, Perez H, et al: Human immunodeficiency virus infection associated arthritis: clinical characteristics. J Rheumatol 26:1158, 1999.
13. Ornstein MH, Sperber K: The anti-inflammatory and antiviral effects of hydroxychloroquine in two patients with acquired immunodeficiency syndrome and active inflammatory arthritis. Arthritis Rheum 39:157, 1996.
14. Winchester R, Bernstein DH, Fischer HD, et al: The co-occurrence of Reiter's syndrome and acquired immunodeficiency. Ann Intern Med 106:19, 1987.
15. Clark MR, Solinger AM, Hochberg MC: Human immunodeficiency virus infection is not associated with Reiter's syndrome: Data from three large cohort studies: Rheum Dis Clin North Am 18:267, 1992.
16. Hochberg MC, Fox R, Nelson KE, Saah A: HIV infection is not associated with Reiter's syndrome: Data from the Johns Hopkins Multicenter AIDS cohort study. AIDS 4:1149, 1990.
17. Mijiyawa M, Oniankitan O, Khan MA: Spondyloarthropathies in sub-Saharan Africa. Curr Opin Rheumatol 12:281, 2000.
18. Reveille JD, Conant MA, Duvic M: HIV-associated psoriasis, psoriatic arthritis and Reiter's syndrome: A disease continuum? Arthritis Rheum 33:1574, 1990.
19. Kaslow RA, Carrington M, Apply R, et al: Influence of combinations of human major histocompatibility complex genes on the course of HIV-1 infection. Nature Med 2:395, 1996.
20. Goulder PJR, Phillips RE, Colbert RA, et al: Late escape from an immunodominant cytotoxic T-lymphocyte response associated with progression to AIDS. Nature Med 3:212, 1997.
21. Bourinbaiar AS, Lee-Huang S: The non-steroidal anti-inflammatory drug, indomethacin, as an inhibitor of HIV replication. FEBS Lett 360:85, 1995.
22. Youssef PP, Bertouch W, Jones PD: Successful treatment of human immunodeficiency virus-associated Reiter's syndrome with sulfasalazine. Arthritis Rheum 35:723, 1992.
23. Disla E, Rhim HR, Reddy A, Taranta A: Improvement in CD4 lymphocyte count in HIV-Reiter's syndrome after treatment with sulfasalazine. J Rheumatol 21:662, 1993.
24. Masson C, Chennebault JM, Leclech C: Is HIV infection a contraindication to the use of methotrexate in psoriatic arthritis? J Rheumatol 22:2191, 1995.
25. Sperber K, Kalb TH, Stecher VJ, et al: Inhibition of human immunodeficiency virus type I replication by hydroxychloroquine in T cells and monocytes. AIDS Res Human Retrovir 9:91, 1993.
26. Louthrenoo W: Successful treatment of severe Reiter's syndrome associated with human immunodeficiency virus infection with etretinate: Report of 2 cases. J Rheumatol 20:1243, 1993.
27. Gaylis N: Infliximab in the treatment of an HIV positive patient with Reiter's syndrome. J Rheumatol 30:407, 2003.
28. Duvic M, Johnson TM, Rapini RP: Acquired immunodeficiency syndrome-associated psoriasis and Reiter's syndrome. Arch Dermatol 123:1622, 1987.
29. Espinoza LR, Berman AVFB: Psoriatic arthritis and acquired immunodeficiency syndrome. Arthritis Rheum 31:1034, 1988.
30. Njobvu P, McGill P: Psoriatic arthritis and human immunodeficiency virus infection in Zambia. J Rheumatol 27:1699, 2000.
31. Duvic M, Crane MM, Conant M, et al: Zidovudine improves psoriasis in human immunodeficiency-positive males. Arch Dermatol 130:447, 1994.

32. Tourne L, Durez P, Van Vooren JP, et al: Alleviation of HIV-associated psoriasis and psoriatic arthritis with cyclosporine. J Am Acad Dermatol 37:501, 1997.

33. Aboulafia DM, Bundow D, Wilske K, Ochs UI: Etanercept for the treatment of human immunodeficiency virus-associated psoriatic arthritis. Mayo Clin Proc 75:1093, 2000.

34. McGonagle D, Reade S, Marzo-Ortega H, et al: Human immunodeficiency virus associated spondyloarthropathy: pathogenic insights based on imaging findings and response to highly active antiretroviral treatment. Ann Rheum Dis 60:696, 2001.

35. Glesby MJ, Hoover DR, Vaamonde CM: Osteonecrosis in patients infected with human immunodeficiency virus: a case-control study. J Infec Dis 184:519, 2001.

36. Manfredi R, Motta R, Patrono D, et al: A prospective case-control survey of laboratory markers of skeletal muscle damage during HIV disease and antiretroviral therapy. AIDS 27(16):1969, 2002.

37. Johnson RW, Williams FM, Kazi S, et al: Human immunodeficiency virus-associated polymyositis: A longitudinal study of outcome. Arthritis Rheum 49:172, 2003.

38. Wrzolek MA, Sher JH, Kozlowski PB, Rao C: Skeletal muscle pathology in AIDS: An autopsy study. Muscle Nerve 13:508, 1990.

39. Buskila D, Gladman D, Langevitz P, et al: Fibromyalgia in human immunodeficiency virus infection. J Rheumatol 17:1202, 1990.

40. Simms RW, Zerbini CAF, Ferrante N, et al: Boston City Hospital Clinical AIDS Team: Fibromyalgia syndrome in patients infected with human immunodeficiency virus. Am J Med 92:368, 1992.

41. Simpson DM, Bender AM, Farraye J, et al: Human immunodeficiency virus wasting syndrome may represent a treatable myopathy. Neurology 40:535, 1990.

42. Gonzales MF, Olney RK, So YT, et al: Subacute structural myopathy associated with human immunodeficiency virus. Arch Neurol 45:585, 1988.

43. Miro O, Pedrol E, Cebrian M, et al: Skeletal muscle studies in patients with HIV-related wasting syndrome. J Neurol Sci 150:153, 1997.

44. Illa I, Nath A, Dalakas M: Immunocytochemical and virological characteristics of HIV-associated inflammatory myopathies: Similarities with seronegative polymyositis. Ann Neurol 29:474, 1991.

45. Simpson DM, Bender AN: Human immunodeficiency virus-associated myopathy: Analysis of 11 patients. Ann Neurol 24:79, 1988.

46. Leon-Monzon M, Lamperth L, Dalakas M: Search for HIV proviral DNA and amplified sequences in the muscle biopsies of patients with HIV polymyositis. Muscle Nerve 16:408, 1992.

47. Seidman R, Peress NS, Nuovo GJ: In situ detection of polymerase chain reaction-amplified HIV-1 nucleic acids in skeletal muscle in patients with myopathy. Mod Pathol 7:369, 1994.

48. Dalakas MC, Pezeshkpour GH, Flaherty M: Progressive nemaline (rod) myopathy associated with HIV infection. N Engl J Med 317:1602, 1987.

49. Feinberg DM, Spiro AJ, Weidenheim KM: Distinct light microscopic changes in human immunodeficiency virus-associated nemaline myopathy. Neurology 50:529, 1998.

50. Besson LJ, Greene JB, Louie E, et al: Severe polymyositis-like syndrome associated with zidovudine therapy of AIDS and ARC. N Engl J Med 318:708, 1988.

51. Mhiri MD, Baudrimont M, Bonne G, et al: Zidovudine myopathy: A distinctive disorder associated with mitochondrial dysfunction. Ann Neurol 29:606, 1991.

52. Ansaloni L, Acaye GL, Re M: High HIV seroprevalence among patients with pyomyositis in northern Uganda. Trop Med Int Health 1:210, 1996.

53. Jellis J: Orthopaedic surgery and HIV disease in Africa. Int Orthop 20:253, 1996.

54. Gherardi R, Baudrimont M, Lionnet F, et al: Skeletal muscle toxoplasmosis in patients with acquired immunodeficiency syndrome: A clinical and pathological study. Ann Neurol 32:535, 1992.

55. Wiley CA, Nerenberg M, Cros D, Soto-Aguilar MC: HTLV-I polymyositis in a patient also infected with the human immunodeficiency virus. N Engl J Med 320:992, 1989.

56. Itescu S, Brancato LJ, Buxbaum J, et al: A diffuse infiltrative CD8 lymphocytosis syndrome in human immunodeficiency virus (HIV) infection: A host immune response associated with HLA-DR5. Ann Intern Med 112:3, 1991.

57. Williams FM, Cohen PR, Jumshyd J, Reveille JD: Prevalence of the diffuse infiltrative lymphocytosis syndrome among human immun-odeficiency virus type 1-positive outpatients. Arthritis Rheum 41:863, 1998.

58. Kordossis T, Paikos S, Aroni K, et al: Prevalence of Sjögren's-like syndrome in a cohort of HIV-1-positive patients: descriptive pathology and immunopathology. Br J Rheumatol 37:691, 1998.

59. McArthur CP, Subtil-DeOliveira A, Palmer D, et al: Characteristics of salivary diffuse infiltrative lymphocytosis syndrome in West Africa. Arch Pathol Lab Med 124:1773, 2000.

60. Itescu S, Simonelli PF, Winchester RJ, Ginsberg HS: Human immunodeficiency virus type 1 strains in the lungs of infected individuals evolve independently from those in peripheral blood and are highly conserved in the C-terminal region of the envelope V3 loop. Proc Natl Acad Sci U S A 91:11378, 1994.

61. Itescu S, Dalton J, Zhang HZ, Winchester R: Tissue infiltration in a CD8 lymphocytosis syndrome associated with human immunodeficiency virus-1 infection has the phenotypic appearance of an antigenically driven response. J Clin Invest 91:2216, 1993.

62. Kazi S, Cohen PR, Williams F, et al: The diffuse infiltrative lymphocytosis syndrome: Clinical and immunogenetic features in 35 patients. AIDS 10:385, 1996.

63. Schiodt M, Dodd CL, Greenspan D, et al: Natural history of HIV-associated salivary gland disease. Oral Surg Oral Med Oral Pathol 74:326, 1992.

64. Itescu S, Winchester R: Diffuse infiltrative lymphocytosis syndrome: A disorder occurring in human immunodeficiency virus-1 infection that may present as a sicca syndrome. Rheum Dis Clin North Am 18:683, 1992.

65. Olive A, Salavert A, Manriquez M, et al: Parotid lipomatosis in HIV positive patients: a new clinical disorder associated with protease inhibitors. Ann Rheum Dis 57:749, 1998.

66. Barrett S, Goh J, Coughlan B, et al: The natural course of hepatitis C virus infection after 22 years in a unique homogenous cohort: spontaneous viral clearance and chronic HCV infection. Gut 49:423, 2001.

67. Rosenberg ZS, Joffe SA, Itescu S: Spectrum of salivary gland disease in HIV-infected patients: Characterization with Ga-67 citrate imaging. Radiology 184:761, 1992.

68. Holliday RA, Cohen WA, Schinella RA, et al: Benign lymphoepithelial parotid cysts and hyperplastic cervical adenopathy in AIDS-risk patients: A new CT appearance. Radiology 168:439, 1988.

69. Beitler JJ, Vikram B, Silver CE, et al: Low-dose radiotherapy for multicystic benign lymphoepithelial lesions of the parotid gland in HIV-positive patients: Long-term results. Head Neck 17:31, 1995.

70. Craven DE, Duncan RA, Stram JR, et al: Response of lymphoepithelial parotid cysts to antiretroviral treatment in HIV-infected adults. Ann Intern Med 128:455, 1998.

71. Gherardi R, Belec L, Mhiri C, et al: The spectrum of vasculitis in human immunodeficiency virus-infected patients: A clinico-pathologic evaluation. Arthritis Rheum 36:1164, 1993.

72. Libman BS, Quismorio FP Jr., Stimmler MM: Polyarteritis nodosa-like vasculitis in human immunodeficiency virus infection. J Rheumatol 22:351, 1995.

73. Font C, Miro O, Pedrol E, et al: Polyarteritis nodosa in human immunodeficiency virus infection: Report of four cases and review of the literature. Br J Rheumatol 35:796, 1996.

74. Buskila D, Gladmann DD, Gilmore J, Salit IE: Behçet's disease in a patient with immunodeficiency virus infection. Ann Rheum Dis 50:115, 1991.

75. Chetty R, Batitang S, Nair R: Large artery vasculopathy in HIV-positive patients: another vasculitic enigma. Hum Pathol 31:374, 2000.

76. Bayrou O, Phlippoteau C, Artigou C, et al: Adult Kawasaki syndrome associated with HIV infection and anticardiolipin antibodies. J Am Acad Dermatol 29:663, 1993.

77. Solinger AM, Hess EV: Rheumatic diseases and AIDS: Is the association real? J Rheumatol 20:678, 1993.

78. Brannagan T: Retroviral-associated vasculitis of the nervous system. Neuro Clin 15:927, 1997.

79. Katsetos CD, Fincke JE, Legido A, et al: Angiocentric CD3(+) T-cell infiltrates in human immunodeficiency virus type 1–associated central nervous system disease in children. Clin Diagn Lab Immunol 6:105, 1999.

80. Bradley WG, Verma A: Painful vasculitic neuropathy in HIV-1 infection: Relief of pain with prednisone therapy. Neurology 47:1446, 1996.

81. Coplan NL, Shimony RY, Ioachim H, et al: Primary pulmonary hypertension associated with human immunodeficiency viral infection. Am J Med 89:96, 1990.
82. Morse JH, Barst RJ, Itescu S, et al: Primary pulmonary hypertension in HIV infection: An outcome determined by particular HLA class II alleles. Am J Resp Crit Care Med 153:1299, 1996.
83. Mehta NJ, Khan IA, Mehta RN, Sepkowitz DA: HIV-Related pulmonary hypertension: analytic review of 131 cases. Chest 118:1133, 2000.
84. Schumacher YO, Zdebik A, Huonker M, Kreisel W: Sildenafil in HIV-related pulmonary hypertension. AIDS 15:1747, 2001.
85. Vassilopoulos D, Chalasani P, Jurado RL, et al: Musculoskeletal infections in patients with human immunodeficiency virus infection. Medicine (Baltimore) 76:284, 1997.
86. Hirsch R, Miller SM, Kazi S, et al: Human immunodeficiency virus–associated atypical mycobacterial skeletal infarctions. Semin Arthritis Rheum 25:347, 1996.
87. Edelstein H, McCabe R: Candida albicans septic arthritis and osteomyelitis of the sternoclavicular joint in a patient with human immunodeficiency virus infection. J Rheumatol 18:110, 1991.
88. Heller HM, Fuhrer J: Disseminated sporotrichosis in patients with AIDS: Case report and review of the literature. AIDS 5:1243, 1991.
89. Bijlsma JS, Derksen RW, Huber-Bruning O, Borleffs JC: Does AIDS "cure" rheumatoid arthritis. Ann Rheum Dis 47:350, 1988.
90. Orustein MH, Kerr LD, Spiera H: A re-examination of the relationship between active rheumatoid arthritis and the acquired immunodeficiency syndrome. Arthritis Rheum 38:1701, 1995.
91. Muller-Ladner U, Kriegsmann J, Gay RE, et al: Progressive joint destruction in a human immunodeficiency virus–infected patient with rheumatoid arthritis. Arthritis Rheum 38:1328, 1995.
92. Fernandez-Miranda C, Rubio R, Pulido F: Development of acquired immune deficiency syndrome in a patient with systemic lupus erythematosus. J Rheumatol 22:347, 1995.
93. Wegrzyn J, Livrozet JM, Touraine JL, Miossec P: Rheumatoid arthritis after 9 years of human immunodeficiency virus infection: possible contribution of tritherapy. J Rheumatol 29:2232, 2002.
94. Diri E, Lipsky PE, Berggren RE: Emergence of systemic lupus erythematosus after initiation of highly active antiretroviral therapy for human immunodeficiency virus infection. J Rheumatol 27:2711, 2000.
95. Florence E, Schrooten W, Verdonck K, et al: Rheumatological complications associated with the use of indinavir and other protease inhibitors. Ann Rheum Dis 61:82, 2002.
96. Kaye BR: Rheumatologic manifestations of infection with human immunodeficiency virus (HIV). Ann Intern Med 111:158,1989.
97. Canoso RT, Zon LI, Groopman JE: Anticardiolipin antibodies associated with HTLV-III infection. Br J Haematol 65:495, 1987.
98. Fabris P, Tositti G, Giordani MT, et al: Prevalence and clinical significance of circulating cryoglobulins in HIV-positive patients with and without co-infection with hepatitis C virus. J Med Virol 69:339, 2003.
99. Klaassen RJ, Goldschmeding R, Dolman KM, et al: Anti-neutrophil cytoplasmic autoantibodies in patients with symptomatic HIV infection. Clin Exp Immunol 87:24, 1992.
100. Wang ZQ, Horowitz HW, Orlikowsky T, et al: Lymphocyte-reactive autoantibodies in human immunodeficiency virus type 1–infected persons facilitate the deletion of CD8 T cells by macrophages. J Infect Dis 178:404, 1998.

102

Viral Arthritis

STANLEY J. NAIDES

Arthralgia and arthritis are prominent features of certain viral infections. Viruses have been candidate etiologic agents for various rheumatic diseases. Understanding how viruses cause arthritis and the nature of virus-host cell interactions may suggest how viruses may precipitate, establish, or maintain chronic inflammatory arthritis such as rheumatoid arthritis (RA).

Viral effects in a given host may depend on host factors including age, gender, genetic background, infection history, and immune response. The ability of a given virus to infect a host may also depend on viral mode of host entry, tissue tropism, replication strategy, cytopathologic affects, ability to establish persistent infection, viral expression of host-like antigens, and ability to alter host antigens. Infected cells may die by classic cell necrosis, programmed cell death (i.e., apoptosis), or initiation of an immune response to virally encoded antigens on the cell surface. The antibody response may generate immune complexes that deposit locally at the site of viral infection or systemically with deposition of circulating immune complex in synovium. Alternatively, cells may survive with their behavior altered by expression of viral genes. Transactivation of cellular genes by viral gene products may induce the cell cycle or cytokines that elicit or perpetuate an immune response targeting host cells. Molecular mimicry of host autoantigens by viral proteins may break immune tolerance or elicit "danger signals" that trigger an immune response.[1,2]

◼ Parvovirus B19

Human parvovirus B19 is a member of the family *Parvoviridae*, subfamily *Parvoviridae*, genus erythrovirus, consisting of the small, single-stranded DNA viruses that autonomously replicate in erythroid precursors. B19 has no envelope and is approximately 23 nm in diameter. Productive infection occurs in erythroid precursors, hence the name *erythrovirus*. Infection of nonerythroid tissues does occur but is restricted, meaning that assembly of virions may occur but is inefficient, or that some but not all viral genes are expressed without virion assembly. Parvoviruses are species specific and not known to readily cross species barriers. The common canine parvovirus does not infect humans.

EPIDEMIOLOGY

B19 infection is common and occurs worldwide. B19 is typically transmitted by respiratory secretions but may also be transmitted via pooled blood products. Outbreaks commonly occur in late winter and spring, when close quartering is most common, although epidemics may also occur in summer and fall. Most B19 infections, especially in children, remain asymptomatic or are diagnosed as nonspecific viral illness. Outbreaks tend to occur in 3- to 5-year cycles, representing the time required for a new cohort of susceptible children to enter school. Up to 60 percent of adults have serologic evidence of past B19 infection.[3] Susceptible adults in occupations with multiple exposures to children, such as school teachers and pediatric nurses, are at greatest risk (up to 50 percent) of acquiring infection during outbreaks.[4,5] Sporadic cases do occur during nonepidemic periods. The diagnosis should be entertained even in the absence of surveillance data to suggest an outbreak.

PATHOGENESIS

The onset of joint symptoms and rash is associated temporally with appearance of serum anti-B19 immunoglobulin M (IgM) antibody.[6] Although there is little evidence of circulating virus in patients who have chronic joint symptoms, B19 DNA may be found in the bone marrow and synovium of patients with chronic B19 arthropathy. Persistence in chronic B19 arthropathy may be facilitated by failure to develop IgG antibodies to the N-terminal region of the minor capsid protein, VP1, known to encode neutralizing epitopes.[7] Presence of antibody to the B19 nonstructural protein (NS1) in some cases of chronic B19 arthropathy probably reflects immune response to NS1 on the surface of B19 virions or NS1 spilled during cell death.[8] NS1 protein itself, however, may play a pathogenic role in perpetuating chronic B19 arthropathy through its interaction with cellular genes. NS1 protein upregulates in vitro transcription from the interleukin-6 (IL-6) promoter and from the human immunodeficiency virus (HIV) LTR in the presence of tat and an intact *tar* element.[6] A high prevalence of B19 DNA and proteins in synovium from RA patients was reported in association with enhanced synovial production of IL-6 and tumor necrosis factor-α (TNF-α). These findings remain controversial. B19 may induce apoptosis through NS1, which is known to be toxic to cells.[10] Production of NS1 in nonpermissive synoviocytes could theoretically induce autoimmunity by disrupting normal patterns of cell interactions and intercellular regulation.[11]

DIAGNOSIS

Clinical Features

B19 causes transient aplastic crisis in the setting of chronic hemolytic anemia.[6] In otherwise healthy children, B19 causes erythema infectiosum, or fifth disease, characterized by bright red "slapped cheeks" and a macular or maculopapular eruption on the torso and extremities. Up to 70 percent of infected children may be asymptomatic, but others may have mild flu-like symptoms, including fever, headache, sore throat, cough, anorexia, vomiting, diarrhea, and arthralgia. In adults, the rash tends to be subtler. The slapped-cheek rash is usually absent. Uncommon dermatologic manifestations include vesicular or hemorrhagic vesiculopustular eruptions, purpura with or without thrombocytopenia, Henoch-Schönlein purpura, and a "socks and gloves" acral erythema. B19 infection may be associated with paresthesias in the fingers and, rarely, with numbness of the toes. Progressive arm weakness has been associated with mild nerve conduction slowing and decreased motor and sensory potential amplitudes. B19 may cross the placenta to infect the fetus, which may develop hydrops fetalis on the basis of B19-induced anemia or viral cardiomyopathy. B19 has been reported to less commonly cause pancytopenia, isolated anemia, thrombocytopenia, leukopenia, myocarditis, neuropathy, or hepatitis.[12] Reports have suggested that B19 may be associated with vasculitis, including giant cell arteritis (GCA).[13]

Patients with congenital or acquired immunodeficiencies, including prior chemotherapy or acquired immune deficiency syndrome (AIDS) due to HIV infection, may develop persistent B19 infection with chronic or recurrent anemia, thrombocytopenia, or leukopenia. B19 infection is the leading cause of pure red cell aplasia in patients with AIDS.[14]

In a study of an outbreak of erythema infectiosum in Port Angeles, Washington, in which subjects were identified on the basis of rash, arthralgia, and joint swelling, symptoms occurred with increasing incidence with age[15] (Table 102–1). In adults, a severe, flu-like illness consisting of fever, chills, malaise, and myalgias may precede or accompany sudden-onset, moderately severe, symmetric polyarthritis in a rheumatoid-like distribution. The arthritis is characterized by prominent involvement of the finger proximal interphalangeal, metacarpophalangeal, wrist, knee, and ankle joints. Within 24 to 48 hours of onset, all affected joints become involved. Axial skeleton involvement is uncommon. Joint symptoms are usually self-limited.

After the initial infection, objective joint swelling, heat, and erythema, when present, tend to resolve over several weeks. A minority have prolonged symptoms that fall into one of two patterns. Approximately two thirds have continuous morning stiffness and arthralgias with intermittent flares. The other third are symptom free between flares. Chronic B19 arthropathy may last months to years. Pain remains a prominent feature during flares and patients commonly continue to report morning stiffness. Approximately 12 percent of patients presenting with "early synovitis" have B19 infection, most of whom are women.[6]

Laboratory Tests

The incubation period from B19 infection to symptoms is 7 to 18 days. Viremia lasts 5 to 6 days and is associated with absence of reticulocytosis and, in the otherwise normal individual, minimal decreases in the concentrations of hemoglobin, neutrophils, and lymphocytes. Flu-like symptoms may occur during viremia. An IgM antibody response follows the initial viremia in 4 to 6 days and is associated with clearing of viremia and cessation of nasal shedding of virus.

The antibody response is associated with the second phase of clinical illness characterized by rash and joint symptoms. Onset of the anti-B19 IgG antibody response occurs almost concurrently with the IgM response. The two clinical phases of illness often overlap. Low to moderate titers of rheumatoid factor (RF) and anti-DNA, antilymphocyte, antinuclear, and antiphospholipid antibodies may be present initially.

During viremia, immune electron microscopy may detect virions in serum. However, this is not a method readily available to clinicians. B19 DNA may be detected during viremia. However, because adult patients usually present after onset of joint symptoms, the most useful diagnostic test is anti-B19 IgM serology. Radioimmunoassays and enzyme-linked immunosorbent assays (ELISAs) have been used to detect B19 antigen and specific antibody to B19 capsid.[6] The anti-B19 IgM antibody response is usually positive for 2 months after the acute illness and may wane shortly thereafter. In some patients, anti-B19 IgM may be detected for 6 months or longer. A positive anti-B19 IgG antibody test in the absence of anti-B19 IgM is usually not diagnostically helpful because of the high seroprevalence of anti-B19 IgG in the adult population. Reports of B19 DNA in normal synovium suggests that testing for B19 DNA in these tissues is of little clinical utility in the absence of anti-B19 IgM.[16]

Differential Diagnosis

Many patients with B19 arthropathy meet the American Rheumatism Association criteria for a diagnosis of

---

TABLE 102–1 · PREVALENCE OF JOINT SYMPTOMS IN FIFTH DISEASE RASH BY AGE IN AN OUTBREAK IN PORT ANGELES, 1961–1962

Symptoms	Prevalence (%) by Age (years)		
	0–9	10–19	>20
Pain	5.1	11.5	77.2
Swelling	2.8	5.3	59.6

Data from Ager EA, Chin TDY, Poland JD: Epidemic erythema infectiosum. N Engl J Med 275:1326, 1966.

RA: morning stiffness lasting more than 1 hour; symmetric involvement; involvement of at least three joints; and involvement of the finger proximal interphalangeal, metacarpophalangeal, and wrist joints. RF in low to moderate titer may be present. Absence of rheumatoid nodules and joint destruction differentiates B19 arthropathy from classic, erosive RA.

Occasionally, B19 may present with features of systemic lupus erythematosus (SLE). Whether this represents a clinical mimic or B19 plays a role in initiating or precipitating SLE in these patients remains to be determined.[6]

Rubella in the adult may present with rash and symmetric polyarthralgia or polyarthritis that is clinically indistinguishable from B19 infection. A history of prenatal rubella testing, prior rubella vaccination, or rubella exposure may aid in choosing appropriate diagnostic serologies.

MANAGEMENT AND PROGNOSIS

There is no specific treatment or vaccine for B19 infection. Treatment remains symptomatic, with nonsteroidal anti-inflammatory drugs (NSAIDs). Intravenous immunoglobulin (IVIg) has been successful in the treatment of bone marrow suppression and B19 persistence in immunocompromised patients,[14] but initial studies suggest that this is not applicable to chronic arthropathy patients. Long-term prognosis is good. Although subjective arthralgias and morning stiffness may be prolonged, joint destruction is not a feature of chronic B19 arthropathy.

▌ Togaviruses

The family *Togaviridae* includes the rubivirus and alphavirus genuses.

RUBELLA VIRUS

Rubella virus is the sole member of the genus rubivirus, family *Togaviridae*, and consists of enveloped, single-stranded RNA viruses. The rubella virion is spherical and measures 50 to 70 nm in diameter, with a 30 nm, dense core. Envelope glycoproteins form 5- to 6-nm spike-like projections that contain hemagglutination activity.[17]

Epidemiology

Transmission is by nasopharyngeal secretions, with peak incidence in late winter and spring. Vaccination has reduced the incidence of rubella outbreaks and shifted the demographic profile from children to college students and adults. The incubation period from infection to rash is 14 to 21 days. Viremia precedes rash by 6 to 7 days, peaks just before onset of rash, and clears within 48 hours after the onset of rash. Nasopharyngeal shedding of virus is detectable from 7 days before rash until 14 days after the rash's appearance, but it is maximal from just before the rash until 5 to 6 days later.[17]

Pathogenesis

Rubella virus can persistently infect synoviocytes and chondrocytes in vitro. An inadequate humoral immune response to specific rubella envelope glycoprotein epitopes may allow rubella virus to persistently infect synovium and lymphocytes in chronic rubella arthritis patients. The onset of rash and arthritis is concurrent with antibody production, suggesting a role for antibody or immune complexes.[17] Concentrations of rubella antibody are higher in synovial fluid than in serum. Synovial lymphocytes from infected individuals spontaneously secrete rubella antibody in vitro, suggesting that there is also an immune response to rubella infection in the joint.[18]

Diagnosis

Clinical Features

Asymptomatic infection occurs in children and adults. Low-grade fever, malaise, coryza, and prominent lymphadenopathy involving posterior cervical, postauricular, and occipital nodes may precede a rash by 5 days. A morbilliform facial rash may initially appear on the face and then spread to the torso, upper extremities, and lower extremities over 2 to 3 days. The facial rash may coalesce and clear as the extremities become involved. In some cases, the rash is only a transient blush.

Joint symptoms commonly occur in women beginning 1 week before or 1 week after onset of the rash. Symmetric or migratory arthralgias are more common than synovitis. Morning stiffness is prominent. Joint symptoms usually resolve over a few days to 2 weeks. Proximal interphalangeal, metacarpophalangeal, wrist, elbow, ankle, and knee joints are most frequently affected. Periarthritis, tenosynovitis, and carpal tunnel syndrome may be seen. In some patients, symptoms may persist for months to years.[19-21]

Live, attenuated rubella vaccines have caused a high frequency of postvaccination myalgia, arthralgia, arthritis, and paraesthesias—symptoms similar to those in natural infection—beginning 2 weeks after inoculation and lasting less than a week. However, in some patients, symptoms may persist for more than a year. RA27/3, the vaccine strain in current use, may cause postvaccination joint symptoms in 15 percent or more of recipients.[19-21]

Two rheumatologic syndromes may complicate natural infection or vaccination in children. In the catcher's crouch syndrome, a lumbar radiculoneuropathy causes popliteal fossa pain on arising in the morning. Exacerbation of the pain by knee extension encourages assumption of a catcher's crouch position (Fig. 102–1). The pain gradually subsides through the day but recurs the next morning. In the arm syndrome, brachial neuropathy causes arm and hand pain and dysesthesias that are worse at night. Both syndromes may occur beginning 1 to 2 months after infection or after vaccination, with the initial episode lasting up to 2 months. Episodes recur for up to 1 year but eventually resolve without long-term sequelae.[21,22]

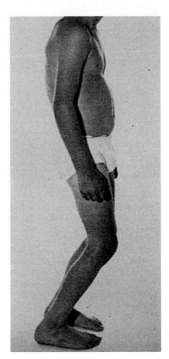

FIGURE 102–1 · Typical Stance of a Child with Post–Rubella Vaccination "Catcher's Crouch" Syndrome. (From Schaffner W, Fleet WF, Kilroy AW, et al: Polyneuropathy following rubella immunization: A follow-up study and review of the problem. Am J Dis Child 127:684, 1974.)

Laboratory Tests

Although rubella may be cultured from tissues and body fluids, including throat swabs, detecting anti-rubella IgM antibody usually makes the diagnosis of acute rubella infection. Diagnosis by anti-IgG antibody seroconversion requires paired acute and convalescent sera. IgM and IgG are usually present at onset of joint symptoms. IgM antibody levels peak 8 to 21 days after symptom onset, but wane by 5 weeks. Anti-rubella IgG rises rapidly over a period of 1 to 3 weeks and is long lived. A single positive IgG serum sample or a set of untitered IgG positive–screens only documents immunity.[17]

Differential Diagnosis

Rubella arthritis needs to be differentiated from other viral arthritides and from inflammatory arthritides, including RA. It may be confused with parvovirus B19 infection.

Management and Prognosis

NSAIDs are useful for control of symptoms. Some investigators have suggested use of low to moderate doses of steroids to control symptoms and viremia.[20] Long-term prognosis is good.

ALPHAVIRUSES

The members of the genus alphavirus, family *Togaviridae*, are enveloped, single-stranded RNA viruses transmitted by mosquitoes.[23] Several cause acute febrile arthropathy, and their names reflect local appreciation of their clinical impact. For example, chikungunya means "that which twists or bends up" (Tanzania). The related O'nyong-nyong virus means "joint breaker" in the Acholi (Uganda) dialect. Igbo ora is "the disease that breaks your wings."

Epidemiology

Chikungunya, O'nyong-nyong, and Igbo Ora viruses form a serologically related group. Chikungunya virus was isolated during an epidemic of febrile arthritis in Tanzania between 1952 and 1953. Similar epidemics probably occurred in Africa, Asia, India, Indonesia, and possibly the southern United States as early as 1779.[23] Mosquitoes responsible for transmission to humans define its geographic distribution (Table 102–2).

Chikungunya fever occurs endemically and in epidemics.[24] A large-scale outbreak of the serologically related O'nyong-nyong virus occurred in the Acholi province of northwestern Uganda in February 1959, and spread through Uganda and the surrounding region within 2 years, affecting more than 2 million and spreading at a rate of 2 to 3 kilometers daily.[25] After the initial O'nyong-nyong epidemic, clinical disease was not detected again until it reemerged in the Acholi region in 1996.[26] Despite the absence of outbreaks in the intervening years, serologic surveys demonstrated that O'nyong-nyong virus is endemic.[27,28]

Weber's line is a hypothetic demarcation separating the Australian and Asiatic geographic zones. Antibodies to Chikungunya virus are found west of Weber's line, and Ross River virus antibodies are found only east of it. Ross River virus causes epidemics of fever and rash in Australia, New Zealand, and the western Pacific islands.[29] In the Fiji Islands from 1979 to 1980, Ross River virus affected more than 40,000 with febrile polyarthritis.[30] In Australia, endemic cases and epidemics occur in tropical and temperate regions annually.[31] Most cases occur in Queensland and New South Wales territories, where high rainfall leading to increases in mosquito populations usually precedes epidemic periods. Infection rates in Australia range from 0.2 to 3.5 percent per year. Male and female infection rates are similar, but there is a female predominance in presenting cases. Most adults infected are symptomatic; the case rate for children is lower. Barmah Forest virus, another alphavirus in Australia, may manifest in a fashion similar to Ross River virus.[32]

Sindbis virus infection occurs predominately in individuals involved in outdoor activities or occupations in forested areas in Sweden, Finland, and the neighboring Karelian isthmus of Russia, where it is known as Okelbo disease, Pogosta disease, or Karelian fever, respectively.[33] Birds are the intermediate host.[34,35] It has also been reported in Central Africa, Zimbabwe, South Africa, and Australia in sporadic cases or in small outbreaks.[23]

TABLE 102–2 • MOSQUITO VECTORS AND RESERVOIRS OF ALPHAVIRUSES

Virus	Mosquito	Reservoir	Disease Occurrence
Chikungunya virus	*Aedes* species *Mansonia africana*	Baboons, monkeys, *Scotophilis* bat species	Africa, Asia
O'nyong-nyong virus	*Anopheles funestus* *Anopheles gambiae*	Unknown	Africa
Igbo ora virus	*Anopheles funestus* *Anopheles gambiae*	Unknown	Ivory Coast
Ross River virus	*Aedes vigilax* *Aedes camptorbynchus* *Culex annulirostris* *Mansonia uniformus* *Aedes polynesiensis* *Aedes aegypti*	Rodents, marsupials, domestic animals	Australia, New Zealand, Papua New Guinea, Pacific islands
Barmah forest virus	*Aedes* species *Anopheles* species *Culex* species	Unknown	Australia
Sindbis virus	*Aedes* species *Culex* species *Culista* species	Unknown	Sweden, Finland, Karelian isthmus of Russia
Mayaro virus	*Haemogogus janthinomys*	Marmosets	Bolivia, Brazil, Peru

Mayaro virus, first recognized in Trinidad in 1954, is endemic in the tropical rain forests of Bolivia, Brazil, and Peru. Cases have been imported into the United States.[36] The reemergence of *Aedes aegypti* and *Aedes albopictus* mosquitoes in the western hemisphere raises the specter of a widened alphavirus geographic range.[37]

Diagnosis

Clinical Features

Chikungunya fever presents with explosive onset of high fever and severe arthralgia after a 1- to 12-day incubation period. Fever lasts 1 to 7 days. Typically, a macular or maculopapular, sometimes pruritic, rash on the torso, extremities, and occasionally the face, palms, and soles occurs on day 2 to 5 of illness as the patient defervesces. Rash may last 1 to 5 days and may recur with fever. Isolated petechiae and mucosal bleeding may occur. In some patients, involved skin desquamates.[38] Chemosis is prominent. Headache, photophobia, retroorbital pain, pharyngitis, anorexia, nausea, vomiting, and abdominal pain may be present. Diffuse myalgia, and back and shoulder pain are common. Migratory polyarthralgia, stiffness, and swelling predominantly affects the small joints of the hands, wrists, feet, and ankles. Large joints are less severely affected. Previously injured joints may be disproportionately affected. Large effusions are uncommon. Symptoms in children tend to be milder. Low-titerRF may be found in those with long-standing symptoms. O'nyong-nyong fever is clinically similar to chikungunya fever.[39,40] In 1984, Igbo Ora caused an epidemic of fever, myalgias, arthralgias, and rash in four villages of Ivory Coast. Sequencing the isolates from the 1996 outbreak of O'nyong-nyong fever suggested that Igbo Ora virus is a variant of O'nyong-nyong virus.[26]

Ross River virus polyarthralgia is severe, incapacitating, and often migratory and asymmetric.[41] Symptoms follow a 7- to 11-day incubation period. Finger interphalangeal and metacarpophalangeal joints, wrists, knees, ankles, shoulders, elbows, and toes are often involved. Polyarticular swelling and tenosynovitis are common. Arthralgias are worse in the morning and after inactivity. Rash is macular, papular, or maculopapular and may be pruritic. Vesicles, papules, or petechiae are typically seen on the trunk and extremities. The palms, soles, and face may be involved. Rash typically appears 1 to 2 days before joint symptoms but may range from 11 days before to 15 days after onset of arthralgias, and it resolves by fading to a brownish discoloration or by desquamation. One half of patients have no fever, and those who do may have only modest fevers lasting 1 to 3 days. Nausea, headache, and myalgia are common. Respiratory symptoms, mild photophobia, and lymphadenopathy may occur. Up to a third have paraesthesias and palm or sole pain. Carpal tunnel syndrome may be seen. In Barmah Forest virus infection, found in Australia and having epidemiologic features similar to Ross River virus infection, arthritis is less common and less prominent than in Ross River virus infection, but the rash is more common and florid.[32,34,43]

Rash and arthralgia are the presenting symptoms in Sindbis virus infection, although one may precede the other by a few days. Constitutional symptoms are usually mild and include low-grade fever, headache, fatigue, malaise, nausea, vomiting, pharyngitis, and paresthesias. A macular rash typically begins on the torso and then spreads to the arms and legs, palms, soles, and occasionally the head. Macules evolve to form papules that tend to vesiculate. Vesiculation is prominent on pressure points, including the palms and soles. As the rash fades, a brownish discoloration is left. Vesicles on the palms and soles may become hemorrhagic. The rash may recur during convalescence.[44]

A Mayaro virus outbreak in Belterra, Brazil, in 1988 was characterized by sudden onset of fever, headache, dizziness, chills, and arthralgias in the wrists, fingers, ankles, and toes. The clinical attack rate was 80 percent.

Joint swelling, unilateral inguinal lymphadenopathy, and leukopenia may be present. A maculopapular rash on the trunk and extremities lasts about 3 days.[45] Mayaro virus is endemic in the tropical rain forest area where Brazil, Bolivia, and Peru intersect. Visitors to that area have presented in the United States after acquiring infection shortly before returning home.[46]

Laboratory Tests

The diagnosis of alphavirus infection requires laboratory confirmation. Any febrile patient residing in or returning from an endemic area should have a laboratory investigation. Chikungunya virus may be isolated from serum during days 2 through 4 of illness.[47] Neutralizing antibody, hemagglutination inhibition activity, and complement fixation tests may be used to detect antibodies. Chikungunya virus specific IgM antibodies may be found for 6 months or longer.[48] O'nyong-nyong virus may be isolated by intracerebral injection into suckling mice, in which it produces alopecia, rash, and runting. Hemagglutination inhibition or complement fixation tests identify O'nyong-nyong virus.[49] Because Chikungunya and O'nyong-nyong viruses are serologically closely related, mouse antisera raised to Chikungunya virus or O'nyong-nyong virus react equally well with O'nyong-nyong virus, but O'nyong-nyong antisera does not react well with Chikungunya virus. Molecular detection methods have improved specific diagnosis.[50-53]

In Chikungunya fever, synovial fluid shows decreased viscosity, poor mucin clot, and 2000 to 5000 white blood cells (WBCs)/mm³. Ross River virus has been isolated only from antibody-negative sera. In the Australian epidemics before 1979, patients were antibody positive at the time of presentation. In contrast, patients in the Pacific Island epidemics of 1979 to 1980 remained viremic and seronegative for up to 1 week after onset of the symptoms. Synovial fluid cell counts range from 1500 to 13,800 cells per mm³, predominately monocytes and vacuolated macrophages.[54] Barmah Forest virus infection is confirmed by rising titers of specific IgG.[42] Diagnosis of Sindbis virus infection is confirmed by specific serology.

Pathogenesis

Little is known about the pathogenesis of Chikungunya fever or arthritis. Involved skin shows erythrocyte extravasation from superficial capillaries and perivascular cuffing. The virus adsorbs to human platelets, causing aggregation and suggesting a mechanism for bleeding. Synovitis probably results from direct viral infection of synovium. In one patient with chronic arthropathy, the synovium appeared atrophic on arthroscopy and was histologically normal.[55] The mechanisms of O'nyong-nyong virus pathogenesis are unknown. Ross River virus antigen may be detected early in monocytes and macrophages by immunofluorescence, but intact virus is not identifiable by electron microscopy or cell culture.[56] Erythematous and purpuric rashes show mild dermal perivascular mononuclear cell infiltrates, mostly T lymphocytes. Purpuric areas also show erythrocyte extravasation. Viral antigen may be detected in epithelial cells in erythematous and purpuric skin lesions and in perivascular zones in erythematous lesions.[57] Sindbis virus has been isolated from a skin vesicle in the absence of viremia. Skin lesions show perivascular edema, hemorrhage, lymphocytic infiltrates, and areas of necrosis. Anti-Sindbis virus IgM may persist for years, raising the possibility that Sindbis virus arthritis is associated with viral persistence.[58]

Management and Prognosis

Management is supportive. NSAIDs are useful, but aspirin should be avoided in view of the tendency for alphavirus rashes to develop a hemorrhagic component. Chloroquine has been used in Chikungunya fever when NSAIDs failed.[59] During the acute attack, range-of-motion exercises may decrease stiffness. In general, alphavirus infection management is symptomatic.

Patients recover without sequelae. After acute Chikungunya fever, symptoms may persist for months before resolution. Approximately 10 percent of patients have joint symptoms at 1 year after infection.[55] A few patients may develop chronic arthralgia. Case reports suggest that a few patients with chronic arthropathy develop destructive joint lesions, but a second process cannot be ruled out. For persons with Ross River virus arthritis, mild exercise tends to improve joint symptoms. One half of all patients are able to resume their daily activities within 4 weeks, although residual polyarthralgia may be present. Joint symptoms may recur.[60] Arthralgia, myalgia, and lethargy may continue for at least 6 months in up to one half of patients.[42] Relapsing episodes gradually resolve, but joint symptoms have been reported in a few patients for up to 3 years.[41,61] Nonerosive chronic arthropathy is common after Sindbis virus infection, with up to one third of patients having arthropathy 2 years or longer after onset. A smaller number had symptoms as long as 5 to 6 years.[58] Mayaro virus–infected patients have persistent arthralgias for months.

Hepatitis B Virus

Hepatitis B virus (HBV), a member of the family *Hepadnaviridae*, genus orthohepadnavirus, is an enveloped, double-stranded, icosahedral DNA virus measuring 42 nm in diameter.[62-64]

EPIDEMIOLOGY

HBV occurs worldwide and is transmitted by parenteral and sexual routes. Prevalence is highest in Asia, the Middle East, and sub-Saharan Africa. In China, prevalence is as high as 10 percent, compared to 0.01 percent in the United States. In endemic regions, infection occurs at an early age, frequently perinatally. Early HBV infection is usually asymptomatic. Rates of HBV carriage and specific antibody positivity decline with age. In the West, most infections are acquired during adulthood through sexual or needle exposures, leading to acute hepatitis. Of those with hepatitis, 5 to 10 percent develop persistent infection. In endemic regions, HBV is a common cause of chronic liver disease and a leading cause of hepatocellular carcinoma.[63]

CLINICAL FEATURES

The time from infection to clinical hepatitis is usually 45 to 120 days. A preicteric prodromal period lasts several days to a month and may be associated with fever, myalgia, malaise, anorexia, nausea, and vomiting. Joint involvement is usually sudden in onset and often severe, with symmetric and simultaneous involvement of several joints at onset. Alternatively, arthritis may be migratory or additive.[65] The joints of the hand and knee are most often affected, but wrists, ankles, elbows, shoulders, and other large joints may be involved as well. Fusiform swelling occurs in the small joints of the hand. Morning stiffness is common. Arthritis and urticaria may precede jaundice by days to weeks and may persist several weeks after jaundice, but they usually subside soon after onset of clinical jaundice. Arthritis is usually limited to the preicteric prodrome. Those who develop chronic active hepatitis or chronic HBV viremia may have recurrent polyarthralgia or polyarthritis.[66] Polyarteritis nodosa (PAN) may be associated with chronic hepatitis B viremia[67] (see Chapter 84).

DIAGNOSIS

Urticaria in the presence of polyarthritis should suggest the possibility of HBV infection. Acute hepatitis may be asymptomatic, but elevated bilirubin and transaminases are usually present when the arthritis appears. At the onset of arthritis, peak levels of serum hepatitis B surface antigen (HBsAg) are detectable. Virions, viral DNA, polymerase, and hepatitis B antigen may be detectable in serum. Anti–hepatitis B core antigen IgM antibodies indicate acute HBV infection rather than past or chronic infection.[68]

PATHOGENESIS

Significant viremia occurs early in infection. Soluble immune complexes with circulating HBsAg form as anti-HBsAg antibodies are produced. An immune complex–mediated arthritis usually results, with immune-complex deposition in synovium. Immune complexes containing HBsAg, antibody and complement components may be detected.

▮ Hepatitis C Virus

Hepatitis C virus (HCV), a member of the family *Flaviviridae*, is an enveloped, single-stranded, spherical RNA virus measuring 38 to 50 nm in diameter.[69]

EPIDEMIOLOGY

HCV infection occurs worldwide. Like HBV infection, seroprevalence is higher in Africa and Asia, where it may cause one fourth of acute and chronic hepatitis cases. In Japan, up to 50 percent of hepatitides may be caused by HCV.[70] In the United States, an estimated 2.7 million individuals are infected.[71,72]

HCV is transmitted by the parenteral route. Sexual transmission may occur but is uncommon.[73] More than one half of all cases of non-A, non-B hepatitis are attributable to HCV infection.[74] Multiple HCV genotypes and quasispecies are organized into six major groups, or clades. They differ in their pathogenicity, severity of disease, and response to interferon (IFN).[74-77]

CLINICAL FEATURES

Acute HCV infection is usually benign. Up to 80 percent of post-transfusion infections are anicteric and asymptomatic. Liver enzyme elevations are usually minimal when present. Normal transaminase levels do not exclude HCV infection. Community-acquired cases may present more symptomatically and with significant transaminase elevations. However, fulminant HCV hepatitis is rare. Acute HCV infection may be accompanied by acute-onset polyarthritis in a rheumatoid distribution, including the small joints of the hand, wrists, shoulders, knees, and hips.[78]

HCV is often associated with mixed (type II and III) cryoglobulinemia. Essential mixed cryoglobulinemia, a triad of arthritis, palpable purpura, and cryoglobulinemia, is associated with HCV infection in most cases. HCV infection is also seen in nonessential secondary cryoglobulinemia, although less commonly.[79] Cryoglobulinemia may be associated with necrotizing vasculitis. The presence of anti-HCV antibodies in essential mixed cryoglobulinemia is associated with more severe cutaneous involvement, such as Raynaud's phenomenon, purpura, livedo, distal ulcers, and gangrene.[80] HCV RNA may be found in 75 percent of cryoprecipitates from patients with essential mixed cryoglobulinemia and anti-HCV antibodies.[81]

DIAGNOSIS

Serologic tests use an array of antigens in an enzyme immunoassay. A recombinant antigen strip immunoblot assay (RIBA) is confirmatory.[70,79] Polymerase chain reaction (PCR)-based diagnostics allow confirmation of HCV viremia, viral load, and genotype.[75,76] A minority of patients may have HCV RNA detectable by PCR amplification methods in the absence of a positive serologic findings.[76,82-86] A liver biopsy for staging of liver disease is indicated in patients who have serum anti-HCV antibody or RNA, even in the setting of normal liver enzymes because the liver enzymes do not reflect liver histology.

PATHOGENESIS

HCV infection persists despite antibody response to viral epitopes. A high rate of mutation in the envelope protein is responsible for emergence of neutralization-escape mutants and quasispecies.[87] HCV may contain an IgG fragment crystallizable (Fc) binding region on its surface; humoral immune response to HCV would, by epitope spreading, also target bound Ig Fc structures. Chronic HCV infection leads to cirrhosis, end-stage liver failure, and hepatocellular carcinoma after a period of

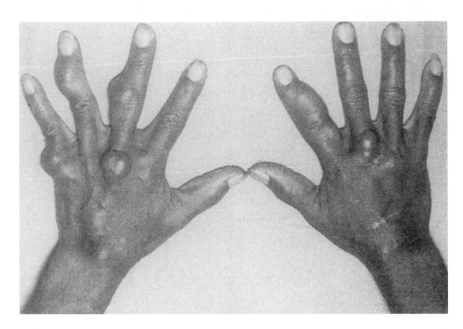

FIGURE 102–2 · Nodular Synovitis Associated with HTLV-I Infection. (From Yancey WB Jr., Dolson LH, Oblon D, et al: HTLV-I-associated adult T-cell leukemia/lymphoma presenting with nodular synovial masses. Am J Med 89:676, 1990. Copyright 1990, with permission from Excerpta Medica, Inc.)

up to 20 years, but the frequency of these sequelae is controversial and the mechanisms by which they occur are unknown.[88]

MANAGEMENT

IFN-α2b at a dose of 3 million units three times weekly for 6 months suppresses viral titers and ameliorates HCV liver disease in about one half of patients and may benefit HCV-associated cryoglobulinemia.[89] Relapse after completion of the initial course of therapy is common. Use of pegylated IFNs to increase drug half-life and decrease clearance and the addition of ribavirin has improved outcomes.[90] There is controversy about whether IFN therapy precipitates autoimmune diseases such as autoimmune thyroiditis.[91,92] Those with cryoglobulinemia failing IFN therapy require immunosuppressive therapy when vasculitis is present.

▮ Human T Lymphocyte Leukemia Virus Type 1

Human T lymphocyte leukemia virus type 1 (HTLV-1), a retrovirus, is endemic in southern Japan, where it has been associated with oligoarthritis and a nodular rash (Fig. 102–2). Anti-HTLV serology is positive. Type C viral particles are found in skin nodules. Synovial tissue is infiltrated by leukemic T lymphocytes with lobulated nuclei.[93]

▮ Other Viruses

There are a host of commonly encountered viral syndromes, in addition to those described previously, in which joint involvement occasionally occurs. Children with varicella rarely develop brief monoarticular or pauciarticular arthritis. Mumps in adults is occasionally associated with small- or large-joint synovitis preceding or after parotitis by up to 4 weeks. Mumps arthritis may last several weeks. Infection with adenovirus and coxsackieviruses A9, B2, B3, B4, and B6 have been associated with recurrent episodes of polyarthritis, pleuritis, myalgia, rash, pharyngitis, myocarditis, and leukocytosis. Epstein-Barr virus (EBV)-induced mononucleosis is frequently accompanied by polyarthralgia, but monoarticular knee arthritis sometimes occurs. A few cases of polyarthritis, fever, and myalgias due to echovirus 9 infection have been reported. Arthritis associated with herpes simplex virus or cytomegalovirus infections are rare, but a severe cytomegalovirus polyarthritis has been described in several immunocompromised bone marrow transplant recipients. *Herpes hominis* occasionally causes arthritis of the knee in wrestlers, a condition referred to as herpes gladiatorum. Knee arthritis after vaccinia inoculation has been reported in two cases.

REFERENCES

1. Pennisi E: Teetering on the brink of danger. Science 271:1665, 1996.
2. Albert LJ, Inman RD: Molecular mimicry and autoimmunity. N Engl J Med 341:2068-2074, 1999.
3. Gillespie SM, Cartter ML, Asch S, et al: Occupational risk of human parvovirus B19 infection for school and day-care personnel during an outbreak of erythema infectiosum. JAMA 263:2061, 1990.
4. Bell LM, Naides SJ, Stoffman P, et al: Human parvovirus B19 infection among hospital staff members after contact with infected patients. N Engl J Med 321:485, 1989.
5. Anderson MJ, Higgins PG, Davis LR, et al: Experimental parvoviral infection in humans. J Infect Dis 152:257, 1985.
6. Naides SJ: Rheumatic manifestations of parvovirus B19 infection. Rheum Dis Clin North Am 24:375, 1998.
7. Von Poblotzki A, Hemauer A, Gigler A, et al: Antibodies to the nonstructural protein of parvovirus B19 in persistently infected patients: Implications for pathogenesis. J Infect Dis 172:1356, 1995.
8. Peterlana D, Puccetti A, Beri R, et al: The presence of parvovirus B19 VP and NS1 genes in the synovium is not correlated with rheumatoid arthritis. J Rheumatol 30:1907-1910, 2003.

9. Takahashi Y, Murai C, Shibata S, et al: Human parvovirus B19 as a causative agent for rheumatoid arthritis. Proc Natl Acad Sci USA 95:8227, 1998.

10. Moffatt S, Yaegashi N, Tada K, et al: Human parvovirus B19 nonstructural (NS1) protein induces apoptosis in erythroid lineage cells. J Virol 72:3018, 1998.

11. Ray NB, Nieva DRC, Seftor EA, et al: Human parvovirus B19 induces an invasive phenotype in normal human synovial fibroblasts. Arthritis Rheum 44:1582-1586, 2001.

12. Karetnyi YV, Beck PR, Markin RS, et al: Human parvovirus B19 infection in acute fulminant liver failure. Arch Virol 144:1713-1724, 1999.

13. Gabriel SE, Espy M, Erdman DD, et al: The role of parvovirus B19 in the pathogenesis of giant cell arteritis: A preliminary evaluation. Arthritis Rheum 42:1255, 1999.

14. Frickhofen N, Abkowitz JL, Safford M, et al: Persistent B19 parvovirus infection in patients infected with human immunodeficiency virus type 1 (HIV-1): A treatable cause of anemia in AIDS. Ann Intern Med 113:926, 1990.

15. Ager EA, Chin TDY, Poland JD: Epidemic erythema infectiosum. N Engl J Med 275:1326, 1966.

16. Söderlund M, von Essen R, Haapasaari J, et al: Persistence of parvovirus B19 DNA in synovial membranes of young patients with and without chronic arthropathy. Lancet 349:1063, 1997.

17. Chantler J, Wolinsky JS, Tingle A: Rubella. In Knipe DM, Howley PM, et al (eds): Fields Virology, 4th ed. New York, Lippincott Williams & Wilkins, 2001, pp 963-990.

18. Mims CA, Stokes A, Grahame R: Synthesis of antibodies, including antiviral antibodies, in the knee joints of patients with arthritis. Ann Rheum Dis 44:734, 1985.

19. Smith CA, Petty RE, Tingle AJ: Rubella virus and arthritis. Rheum Dis Clin North Am 13:265-274, 1987.

20. Mitchell LA, Tingle AJ, Shukin R, et al: Chronic rubella vaccine-associated arthropathy. Arch Intern Med 153:2268, 1993.

21. Howson CP, Katz M, Johnston RB Jr, et al: Chronic arthritis after rubella vaccination. Clin Infect Dis 15:307, 1992.

22. Schaffner W, Fleet WF, Kilroy AW, et al: Polyneuropathy following rubella immunization: A follow-up study and review of the problem. Am J Dis Child 127:684, 1974.

23. Griffin DE: Alphaviruses. In Knipe DM, Howley PM, et al (eds): Fields Virology, 4th ed. New York, Lippincott Williams & Wilkins, 2001, pp 917-962.

24. Halstead SB, Nimmannitya S, Margiotta MR: Dengue and chikungunya virus infection in man in Thailand, 1962–1964. II. Observations on disease in outpatients. Am J Trop Med Hyg 18:972, 1969.

25. Williams MC, Woodall JP, Gillett JD: O'nyong-nyong fever: An epidemic in East Africa. VII. Virus isolations from man and serological studies up to July 1961. Trans R Soc Trop Med Hyg 59:186, 1965.

26. Lanciotti RS, Ludwig ML, Rwaguma EB, et al: Emergence of epidemic O'nyong-nyong fever in Uganda, after a 35 year absence. Virology 252:258, 1998.

27. Blumer C, Roche P, Spencer J, et al: Australia's notifiabl diseases status, 2001: Annual report of the National Notifiable Diseases Surveillance System. Commun Dis Intell 27:1-78, 2003.

28. Marshall TF, Keenlyside RA, Johnson BK, et al: The epidemiology of O'nyong-nyong in the Kano Plain, Kenya. Ann Trop Med Parasitol 76:153, 1982.

29. Harley D, Sleigh A, Ritchie S: Ross River virus transmission, infection, and disease: a cross-disciplinary review. Clin Microbiol Rev 14:909-932, 2001.

30. Bennett NM, Cunningham AL, Fraser JR, et al: Epidemic polyarthritis acquired in Fiji. Med J Aust 1:316, 1980.

31. Mudge PR, Aaskov JG: Epidemic polyarthritis in Australia, 1980-1981. Med J Aust 2:269, 1983.

32. Lindsay MDA, Johansen CA, Broom AK, et al: Emergence of Barmah Forest virus in western Australia. Emerg Infect Dis 1:1, 1995.

33. Brummer-Korvenkontio M, Vapalahti O, Kuusisto P, et al: Epidemiology of Sindbis virus infections in Finland 1981-96: possible factors explaining a peculiar disease pattern. Epidemiol Infect 129:335-345, 2002.

34. Kelly-Hope LA, Kay BH, Purdie DM, Williams GM: The risk of Ross River and Barmah Forest virus disease in Queensland: implications for New Zealand. Aust N Z J Public Health 26:69-77, 2002.

35. Kelly-Hope LA, Purdie DM, Kay BH: Risk of mosquito-borne epidemic polyarthritis disease among international visitors to Queensland, Australia. J Travel Med 9:211-213, 2002.

36. Tesh RB, Watts DM, Russell KL, et al: Mayaro virus disease: An emerging mosquito-borne zoonosis in tropical South America. Clin Infect Dis 28:67, 1999.

37. Moore CG: Aedes albopictus in the United States: current status and prospects for further spread. J Am Mosq Control Assoc 15:221-227, 1999.

38. Halstead SB, Udomsakdi S, Singharaj P, et al: Dengue and chikungunya virus infection in man in Thailand, 1962–1964. III. Clinical, epidemiologic, and virologic observations on disease in non-indigenous white persons. Am J Trop Med Hyg 18:984, 1969.

39. Sanders EJ, Rwaguma EB, Kawamata J, et al: O'nyong-nyong fever in south-central Uganda, 1996-1997: description of the epidemic and results of a household-based seroprevalence survey. J Infect Dis 180:1436-1443, 1999.

40. Kiwanuka N, Sanders EJ, Rwaguma EB, et al: O'nyong-nyong fever in south-central Uganda, 1996-1997: clinical features and validation of a clinical case definition for surveillance purposes. Clin Infect Dis 29:1243-1250, 1999.

41. Fraser JRE: Epidemic polyarthritis and Ross River virus disease. Clin Rheum Dis 12:369, 1986.

42. Flexman JP, Smith DW, Mackenzie JS, et al: A comparison of the diseases caused by Ross River virus and Barmah Forest virus. Med J Aust 169:159, 1998.

43. Passmore J, O'Grady KA, Moran R, et al: An outbreak of Barmah Forest virus disease in Victoria. Commun Dis Intell 26:600-604, 2002.

44. Julkunen I, Brummer Korvenkontio M, Hautanen A, et al: Elevated serum immune complex levels in Pogosta disease, an acute alphavirus infection with rash and arthritis. J Clin Lab Immunol 21:77, 1986.

45. Pinheiro FP, Freitas RB, Travassos da Rosa JF, et al: An outbreak of Mayaro virus disease in Belterra, Brazil. I. Clinical and virological findings. Am J Trop Med Hyg 30:674, 1981.

46. Tesh RB, Watts DM, Russell KL, et al: Mayaro virus disease: an emerging mosquito-borne zoonosis in tropical South America. Clin Infect Dis 28:67-73, 1999.

47. Nimmannitya S, Halstead SB, Cohen SN, et al: Dengue and chikungunya virus infection in man in Thailand, 1962-1964. I. Observations on hospitalized patients with hemorrhagic fever. Am J Trop Med Hyg 18:954, 1969.

48. Nakitare GW, Bundo K, Igarashi A: Enzyme-linked immunosorbent assay (ELISA) for antibody titers against chikungunya virus of human serum from Kenya. Trop Med 25:119, 1983.

49. Williams MC, Woodall JP, Porterfield JS: O'nyong-nyong fever: An epidemic virus disease in east Africa. V. Human antibody studies by plaque inhibition and other serological tests. Trans R Soc Trop Med Hyg 56:166, 1962.

50. Hasebe F, Parquet MC, Pandey BD, et al: Combined detection and genotyping of Chikungunya virus by a specific reverse transcription-polymerase chain reaction. J Med Virol 67:370-374, 2002.

51. Pfeffer M, Linssen B, Parke MD, Kinney RM: Specific detection of chikungunya virus using a RT-PCR/nested PCR combination. J Vet Med B Infect Dis Vet Public Health 49:49-54, 2002.

52. Corwin A, Simanjuntak CH, Ansari A: Emerging disease surveillance in Southeast Asia. Ann Acad Med Singapore 26:628-631, 1997.

53. Junt T, Heraud JM, Lelarge J, et al: Determination of natural versus laboratory human infection with Mayaro virus by molecular analysis. Epidemiol Infect 123:511-513, 1999.

54. Aaskov JG, Mataika JU, Lawrence GW, et al: An epidemic of Ross River virus infection in Fiji, 1979. Am J Trop Med Hyg 30:1053, 1981.

55. Brighton SW, Prozesky OW, De la Harpe AL: Chikungunya virus infection: A retrospective study of 107 cases. South Afr Med J 63:313, 1983.

56. Fraser JR, Cunningham AL, Clarris BJ, et al: Cytology of synovial effusions in epidemic polyarthritis. Aust N Z J Med 11:168, 1981.

57. Fraser JR, Ratnamohan VM, Dowling JP, et al: The exanthem of Ross River virus infection: histology, location of virus antigen and nature of inflammatory infiltrate. J Clin Pathol 36:1256, 1983.

58. Niklasson B, Espmark A, Lundstrom J: Occurrence of arthralgia and specific IgM antibodies three to four years after Ockelbo disease. J Infect Dis 157:832, 1988.

59. Brighton SW: Chloroquine phosphate treatment of chronic chikungunya arthritis: An open pilot study. South Afr Med J 66:217, 1984.

60. Mylonas AD, Brown AM, Carthew TL, et al: Natural history of Ross River virus-induced epidemic polyarthritis. Med J Aust 177:356-360, 2002.

61. Laine M, Luukkainen R, Jalava J, et al: Prolonged arthritis associated with Sindbis-related (Pogosta) virus infection. Rheumatology (Oxford) 41:829-830, 2002.

62. Robinson WS: Hepatitis B viruses: General features (human). *In* Webster RG, Granoff A (eds): Encyclopedia of Virology. San Diego, Academic Press, 1994, pp 554-559.

63. Hollinger FB, Liang TJ: Hepatitis B virus. *In* Knipe DM, Howley PM, Griffin DE, Lamb RA, et al (eds): Fields Virology. Philadelphia, Lippincott Williams & Wilkins, 2001, pp 2971-3036.

64. Bendinelli M, Pistello M, Maggi F, Vatteroni ML: Blood-borne hepatitis viruses: Hepatitis B, C, D, and G viruses and TT virus. *In* Specter S, Hodinka RL, Young SA (eds): Clinical Virology Manual. Washington, DC, ASM Press, 2000, pp 306-337.

65. Alarcon GS, Townes AS: Arthritis in viral hepatitis: Report of two cases and review of the literature. Johns Hopkins Med J 132:1, 1973.

66. Csepregi A, Rojkovich B, Nemesanszky E, et al: Chronic seropositive polyarthritis associated with hepatitis B virus-induced chronic liver disease: a sequel of virus persistence. Arthritis Rheum 43:232-233, 2000.

67. Guillevin L, Lhote F, Cohen P, et al: Polyarteritis nodosa related to hepatitis B virus: A prospective study with long-term observation of 41 patients. Medicine (Baltimore) 74:238, 1995.

68. Hoofnagle JH: Serologic markers of hepatitis B virus infection. Ann Rev Med 32:1, 1981.

69. Lindebach BD, Rice CM: *Flaviviridae*: the viruses and their replication. *In* Knipe DM, Howley PM, Griffin DE, Lamb RA, et al (eds): Fields Virology. Philadelphia, Lippincott Williams & Wilkins, 2001, pp 991-1041.

70. Kuboki M, Shinzawa H, Shao L, et al: A cohort study of hepatitis C virus (HCV) infection in an HCV epidemic area of Japan: age and sex-related seroprevalence of anti-HCV antibody, frequency of viremia, biochemical abnormality and histological changes. Liver 19:88-96, 1999.

71. Alter MJ, Mast EE: The epidemiology of viral hepatitis in the United States. Gastroenterol Clin North Am 23:437-455, 1994.

72. Williams I: Epidemiology of hepatitis C in the United States. Am J Med 107:2S-9S, 1999.

73. Neumayr G, Propst A, Schwaighofer H, et al: Lack of evidence for the heterosexual transmission of hepatitis C. QJM 92:505-508, 1999.

74. Bhandari BN, Wright TL: Hepatitis C: An overview. Ann Rev Med 46:309, 1995.

75. Pawlotsky JM: Hepatitis C virus genetic variability: pathogenic and clinical implications. Clin Liver Dis 7:45-66, 2003.

76. Pawlotsky JM: Use and interpretation of hepatitis C virus diagnostic assays. Clin Liver Dis 7:127-137, 2003.

77. Davis GL: Hepatitis C virus genotypes and quasispecies. Am J Med 107:21S-26S, 1999.

78. Siegel LB, Cohn L, Nashel D: Rheumatic manifestations of hepatitis C infection. Semin Arthritis Rheum 23:149, 1993.

79. Arranz FR, Díaz RD, Díez LI, et al: Cryoglobulinemic vasculitis associated with hepatitis C virus infection: A report of eight cases. Acta Derm Venereol (Stockh) 75:234, 1995.

80. Sansonno D, Cornacchiulo V, Iacobelli AR, et al: Localization of hepatitis C virus antigens in liver and skin tissues of chronic hepatitis C virus-infected patients with mixed cryoglobulinemia. Hepatology 21:305, 1995.

81. Munoz-Fernandez S, Barbado FJ, Martin Mola E, et al: Evidence of hepatitis C virus antibodies in the cryoprecipitate of patients with mixed cryoglobulinemia. J Rheumatol 21:229, 1994.

82. Stapleton JT, Klinzman D, Schmidt WN, et al: Prospective comparison of whole-blood-and plasma-based hepatitis C virus RNA detection systems: improved detection using whole blood as the source of viral RNA. J Clin Microbiol 37:484-489, 1999.

83. George SL, Gebhardt J, Klinzman D, et al: Hepatitis C virus viremia in HIV-infected individuals with negative HCV antibody tests. J Acquir Immune Defic Syndr 31:154-162, 2002.

84. Schmidt WN, Klinzman D, LaBrecque DR, et al: Direct detection of hepatitis C virus (HCV) RNA from whole blood, and comparison with HCV RNA in plasma and peripheral blood mononuclear cells. J Med Virol 47:153, 1995.

85. Schmidt WN, Wu P, Cederna J, et al: Surreptitious hepatitis C virus (HCV) infection detected in the majority of patients with cryptogenic chronic hepatitis and negative HCV antibody tests. Infect Dis 176:27-33, 1997.

86. Schmidt W, Stapleton JT: Whole-blood hepatitis C virus RNA extraction methods. J Clin Microbiol 39:3812-3813, 2001.

87. Shimizu YK, Hijikata M, Iwamoto A, et al: Neutralizing antibodies against hepatitis C virus and the emergence of neutralization escape mutant viruses. J Virology 68:1494, 1994.

88. Seeff LB: Natural history of hepatitis C. *In* Liang TJ, Hoofnagle JH (eds): Hepatitis C. San Diego, Academic Press, 2000, pp 85-105.

89. Gish RG: Standards of treatment in chronic hepatitis C. Semin Liver Dis 19(Suppl 1):35, 1999.

90. Baker DE: Pegylated interferon plus ribavirin for the treatment of chronic hepatitis C. Rev Gastroenterol Disord 3: 93-109, 2003.

91. Morisco F, Mazziotti G, Rotondi M, et al: Interferon-related thyroid autoimmunity and long-term clinical outcome of chronic hepatitis C. Dig Liver Dis 33:247-253, 2001.

92. Rocco A, Gargano S, Provenzano A, et al: Incidence of autoimmune thyroiditis in interferon-alpha treated and untreated patients with chronic hepatitis C virus infection. Neuroendocrinol Lett 22:39-44, 2001.

93. Yancey WB Jr., Dolson LH, Oblon D, et al: HTLV-I-associated adult T-cell leukemia/lymphoma presenting with nodular synovial masses. Am J Med 89:676, 1990.

103

Acute Rheumatic Fever and Poststreptococcal Arthritis

ALLAN GIBOFSKY · JOHN ZABRISKIE

Acute rheumatic fever (ARF) is a delayed, non-suppurative sequela of a pharyngeal infection with the group A streptococcus. Following the initial streptococcal pharyngitis, there is a latent period of 2 to 3 weeks. The onset of disease is usually characterized by an acute febrile illness, which may manifest itself in one of three classic ways: 1) The patient may present with migratory arthritis predominantly involving the large joints of the body. 2) There may be concomitant clinical and laboratory signs of carditis and valvulitis. 3) There may be involvement of the central nervous system (CNS), manifesting itself as Sydenham's chorea. The clinical episodes are self limiting, but damage to the valves may be chronic and progressive, resulting in cardiac decompensation and death.

Although there has been a dramatic decline in both the severity and mortality of the disease since the turn of the century, there have been recent reports of its resurgence in this country[1] and in many military installations in the world, reminding us that the disease remains a public health problem even in developed countries. In addition, the disease continues essentially unabated in many of the developing countries: Estimates suggest there will be 10 to 20 million new cases per year in those countries where two thirds of the world population lives.

Epidemiology

The incidence of ARF actually began to decline long before the introduction of antibiotics into clinical practice, decreasing from 250 to 100 patients per 100,000 population from 1862 to 1962 in Denmark.[2] The introduction of antibiotics in 1950 rapidly accelerated this decline, until by 1980, the incidence ranged from 0.23 to 1.88 patients per 100,000, primarily in children and teenagers. A notable exception to this has been in the native Hawaiian and Maori populations (both of Polynesian ancestry), in whom the incidence continues to be 13.4 per 100,000 hospitalized children each year.[3]

Only a few M serotypes (types 5, 14, 18, 24) have been identified with outbreaks of ARF, suggesting that certain strains of group A streptococci may be more "rheumatogenic" than others.[4] In Trinidad, however, types 41 and 11 have been the most common strains isolated from the oropharynx of patients with ARF. In our own series, gathered over a 20-year period (Table 103–1) a large number of different M serotypes were isolated, including six strains that could not be typed. Kaplan and colleagues[5] isolated several M types from patients seen during an outbreak of ARF in Utah, and

these strains were both mucoid and nonmucoid in character. Thus, whether or not certain strains are more "rheumatogenic" than others remains unresolved. What is true, however, is that a streptococcal strain capable of causing a well-documented pharyngitis is generally capable of causing ARF, although some notable exceptions have been recorded.[6]

Pathogenesis

Although there is little evidence for the direct involvement of group A streptococci in the affected tissues of ARF patients, there is a large body of epidemiologic and immunologic evidence indirectly implicating the group A streptococcus in the initiation of the disease process: 1) It is well known that outbreaks of ARF closely follow epidemics of either streptococcal sore throats or scarlet fever.[6] 2) Adequate treatment of a documented streptococcal pharyngitis markedly reduces the incidence of subsequent ARF.[7] 3) Appropriate antimicrobial prophylaxis prevents the recurrences of disease in known patients with acute ARF.[8] 4) If the sera of the majority of ARF patients is tested for three antistreptococcal antibodies (streptolysin "O", hyaluronidase, and streptokinase), the vast majority of ARF patients (whether or not they recall an antecedent streptococcal sore throat) will have elevated antibody titers to these antigens.[9]

A note of caution is necessary concerning documentation (either clinical or microbiologic) of an antecedent

TABLE 103–1 · POSITIVE THROAT CULTURES FOR GROUP A BETA–HEMOLYTIC STREPTOCOCCI AMONG ROCKEFELLER UNIVERSITY HOSPITAL RHEUMATIC FEVER PATIENTS*

M TYPE	RHD	No RHD	TOTAL
Nontypable	1	5	6
1	1	1	2
2	0	1	1
5	1	1	2
6	1	1	2
12	0	2	2
18	2	2	4
19	2	1	3
28	1	0	1
TOTAL	9	11	23

*N = 87

Abbreviations: No RHD, patients without rheumatic heart disease; RHD, patients with rheumatic heart disease.

streptococcal infection. The frequency of isolation of group A streptococci from the oropharynx is extremely low even in populations with limited access to antibiotics. Further, there appears to be an age-related discrepancy in the clinical documentation of an antecedent sore throat. In older children and young adults, the recollection of a streptococcal sore throat approaches 70 percent; in younger children, this rate approaches only 20 percent.[1] Thus, it is important to have a high index of suspicion of ARF in children or young adults presenting with signs of arthritis, carditis, or both even in the absence of a clinically documented sore throat.

Another intriguing, and as yet unexplained, observation has been the invariable association of ARF only with streptococcal pharyngitis. Although there have many outbreaks of impetigo, ARF almost never occurs following infection with these strains. Furthermore, in Trinidad, where both impetigo and ARF are concomitant infections, the strains colonizing the skin are different from those associated with ARF and did not influence the incidence of ARF.[10]

The explanations for these observations remain obscure. It is clear that group A streptococci fall into two main classes based on differences in the C repeat regions of the M protein.[11] One class is clearly associated with streptococcal pharyngeal infection, the other (with some exceptions) is commonly associated with impetigo. Thus, the particular strain of streptococcus may be crucial in initiating the disease process. The pharyngeal site of infection, with its large repository of lymphoid tissue, may also be important in the initiation of the abnormal humoral response by the host to those antigens cross-reactive with target organs. Finally, whereas impetigo

strains do colonize the pharynx, they do not appear to elicit as strong an immunologic response to the M protein moiety as do the pharyngeal strains.[12,13] This may prove to be an important factor, especially in light of the known cross-reactions between various streptococcal structures and mammalian proteins.

▉ Group A Streptococcus

Figure 103–1 is a schematic cross-section of the group A streptococcus. The capsule is composed of equimolar concentrations of N-acetyl glucosamine and glucuronic acid and is structurally identical to hyaluronic acid of mammalian tissues.[14]

Although numerous attempts to produce antibodies to this capsule have been unsuccessful,[15,16] Fillet and coworkers[17] were able to demonstrate high antibody titers to hyaluronic acid using techniques designed to detect nonprecipitating antibodies in the sera of immunized animals. Similar antibodies have been noted in humans.[18] The data establishing the importance of this capsule in human infections has been almost nonexistent, although Stollerman[19] has commented on the presence of a large mucoid capsule as being one of the more important characteristics of certain "rheumatogenic" strains.

With respect to the M protein moiety, investigations by Lancefield and others spanning almost 70 years[20] have established that the M protein molecule (at least 80 distinct serologic types) is perhaps the most important virulence factor in group A streptococcal infections of humans. The protein is a helical coiled-coil structure and bears a striking structural homology to

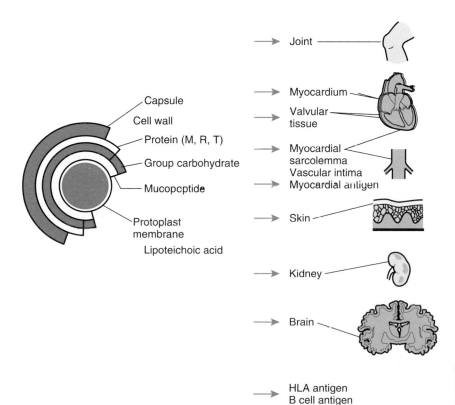

FIGURE 103–1 · Structures of the Group A Streptococcus. Note the wide variety of cross-reactions between its antigens and mammalian tissues.

the cardiac cytoskeletal proteins—tropomyosin and myosin—as well as to many other coil-coiled structures such as keratin, DNA, lamin, and vimentin.

Once the amino acid sequence of a number of M proteins was delineated, it was possible to specifically localize those cross-reactive areas of the molecules. The studies of Dale and Beachey[21] showed that the segment of the M protein involved in the opsonic reaction also cross-reacted with human sarcolemma antigens. Sargent and coworkers[22] more precisely localized this cross-reaction to the M protein amino acid residues 164 through 197.

The evidence implicating these cross-reactions in the pathogenesis of ARF remains scant. Antibodies to myosin have been detected in the sera of ARF patients, but they are also present in a high percentage of the sera obtained from individuals who had a streptococcal infection, but did not subsequently develop ARF.[23] The significance of this observation is unclear, because myosin is an internal protein of cardiac muscle cells and, therefore, not easily exposed to M protein cross-reacting antibodies.

The group-specific carbohydrate of the streptococcus is a polysaccharide chain consisting of repeating units of rhamnose capped by N-acetyl glucosamine molecules. The N-acetyl glucosamine is immunodominant and gives rise to the serologic group-specificity of group A streptococci.[24] The cross reaction between group A carbohydrate and valvular glycoproteins was first described by Goldstein and colleagues,[25] and the reactivity was related to the N-acetyl glucosamine moiety present in both structures. Goldstein and Caravano[26] noted that rheumatoid factor (RF) sera reacted to the heart valve glycoprotein. Fillet (unpublished data) has observed strong reactivity of RF sera with purified proteoglycan material. Thus, these cross-reactions could involve the sugar moiety present in both the proteoglycan portion of the glycoprotein and the carbohydrate.

It has generally been assumed that group A anticarbohydrate antibodies do not play a role in phagocytosis of group A streptococci. However, Salvadori and coworkers[27] demonstrated that human sera containing high titers of anti–group A carbohydrate antibody promoted opsonization and phagocytosis of a number of different M protein–specific strains, and the opsonophagocytic antibodies were directed to the N-acetyl glucosamine moiety of the group A carbohydrate.

The mucopeptide portion of the cell wall is the "backbone" of the organism and, thus, is quite rigid in structure. It is composed of repeating units of muramic acid and N-acetyl glucosamine, cross-linked by peptide bridges.[28] It is particularly difficult to degrade and induces a wide variety of lesions when injected into various species, including arthritis in rats[29] and myocardial granulomas in mice resembling (but not identical to) rheumatic fever Aschoff lesions.[30]

The relationship of cell wall mucopeptides to the pathogenesis of ARF remains obscure. Elevated levels of antimucopeptide antibody have been detected in the sera of patients with ARF, but also in the sera of patients with rheumatoid arthritis (RA) and juvenile rheumatoid arthritis (JRA),[31] but its pathogenetic relationship to clinical disease has been difficult to establish. There is no evidence that cell wall antigens are present either in the Aschoff lesion or in the myocardial tissue obtained from patients with ARF.

Perhaps the most significant cross-reactions lie in the streptococcal membrane structure. We have shown that immunization with membrane material[32] elicited antibodies that bound to heart sections in a pattern similar to that observed with acute RF.

Kingston and Glynn[33] were the first to show that animals immunized with streptococcal antigens developed antibodies in their sera that stained astrocytes. Husby and colleagues[34] demonstrated that sera from ARF patients with chorea exhibited antibodies that were specific for caudate cells. Absorption of the sera with streptococcal membrane antigens eliminated the reactivity with caudate cells.

Numerous other cross-reactions between streptococcal membranes and other organs have also been reported (e.g., renal basement membranes, basement membrane proteoglycans, and skin, particularly keratin). In the context of this chapter, space does not permit an exhaustive discussion of these cross-reactions, and the reader is referred to our previous review[35] for a more detailed discussion. Whether or not these cross-reactions (especially those seen with basement membranes and skin) play a role in the disease awaits further study.

Genetics

The concept that ARF might be the result of a host genetic predisposition has intrigued investigators for more than a century.[36] It has been variously suggested that the disease gene is transmitted in an autosomal dominant fashion,[37] or autosomal recessive fashion with limited penetrance,[38] or that it is possibly related to the genes conferring blood group secretor status.[39]

Renewed interest in the genetics of ARF occurred with the recognition that gene products of the human major histocompatibility complex (MHC) were associated with certain clinical disease states. Using an alloserum from a multiparous donor, an increased frequency of a B cell alloantigen was reported in several genetically distinct and ethnically diverse populations of ARF individuals and was not MHC related.[40]

Most recently, a monoclonal antibody (D8/17) was prepared by immunizing mice with B cells from an ARF patient.[41] A B cell antigen identified by this antibody was found to be expressed on increased numbers of B cells in 100 percent of rheumatics of diverse ethnic origins and only in 10 percent of normal individuals. The antigen defined by this monoclonal antibody showed no association with or linkage to any of the known MHC haplotypes, nor did it appear to be related to B cell–activation antigens.

Studies with D8/17 have been expanded to a larger number of patients with RF (see Table 103–1) of diverse ethnic origins with essentially the same results. As will be discussed later, the presence or absence of elevated levels of D8/17-positive B cells in cases of questionable RF has been helpful in establishing or ruling out the diagnosis.

These studies are in contrast to other reports in which an increased frequency of human leukocyte antigen

(HLA)-DR4 and -DR2 has been seen in Caucasian and black patients with rheumatic heart disease.[42] Other studies have implicated DR1 and DRW6 as susceptibility factors in South African black patients with rheumatic heart disease.[43] Most recently, Guilherme and associates[44] have reported an increased frequency of HLA-DR7 and DW53 in RF patients in Brazil. These seemingly conflicting results concerning HLA antigens and RF susceptibility prompts speculation that these reported associations might be of class II genes close to (or in linkage disequilibrium with) but not identical to the putative RF susceptibility gene. Alternatively, and more likely, susceptibility to ARF is polygenic, and the D8/17 antigen might be associated with only one of the genes (i.e., those of the MHC complex encoding for DR antigens) conferring susceptibility. Although the explanation remains to be determined, the presence of the D8/17 antigen does appear to identify a population at special risk of contracting ARF (Table 103–2).

Etiologic Considerations

Although a large body of evidence, both immunologic and epidemiologic, has implicated the group A streptococcus in the induction of the disease process, the precise pathologic mechanisms involved in the process still remain obscure. At least three main theories have been proposed.

The first theory is concerned with the question of whether persistence of the organism is important. Despite several controversial reports, no investigators have been able to consistently and reproducibly demonstrate live organisms in RF cardiac tissues or valves.[45]

The second theory revolves around the question of whether deposition of toxic products is required. Although an attractive hypothesis, little or no experi-

mental evidence has been obtained to support this concept. For example, Halbert and coworkers[46] have suggested that streptolysin "O" (an extracellular product of group A streptococci) is cardiotoxic and might be carried to the site by circulating complexes containing streptolysin "O" and antibody. However, in spite of an intensive search for these products, no such complexes in situ have been identified.[47,48]

Renewed interest in these extracellular toxins has recently emerged with the observation by Schlievert and colleagues[49] that certain streptococcal pyrogenic toxins (A and C) may act as superantigens. These antigens may stimulate large numbers of T cells through their unique bridging interaction with T cell receptors (TCRs) of specific Vß types and class II MHC molecules. This interaction is clearly distinct from conventional antigen presentation in the context of the MHC complex. Once activated, these cells elaborate tumor necrosis factor (TNF), interferon-γ (IFN-γ), and a number of interleukin (IL) moieties, thereby contributing to the initiation of pathologic damage. Furthermore it has been suggested[50] that in certain disease states, such as RA, autoreactive cells of specific Vß lineage may "home" to the target organ. Although an attractive hypothesis, no data concerning the role of these superantigens in ARF has as yet been forthcoming.

Perhaps the best evidence to date favors the theory of an abnormal host immune response (both humoral and cellular) in an individual genetically susceptible to those streptococcal antigens that are cross-reactive with mammalian tissues. The evidence supporting this theory may be divided into three broad categories:

1. Employing a wide variety of methods, numerous investigators have documented the presence of heart-reactive antibodies in ARF sera. The prevalence of these antibodies has varied from a low of 33 percent to a high of 85 percent in various series. Although these antibodies are seen in other individuals (notably those with uncomplicated streptococcal infections that do not go on to rheumatic fever and patients with poststreptococcal glomerulonephritis), the titers are always lower than that seen in RF and decrease with time during the convalescent period (Table 103–3). An important point, both in terms of diagnosis and prognosis, has been the observation of Zabriskie and coworkers[51] that these heart-reactive antibody titers decline over time. By the end of 3 years, these titers are essentially undetectable in those patients who had only a single attack (Fig. 103–2). This pattern is consistent with the well-known clinical observations that recurrences of rheumatic fever most often occur within the first 2 to 3 years after the initial attack and become rarer 5 years after an initial episode.

   As illustrated in Figure 103–3 this pattern of titers also has prognostic value. During the 2- to 5-year period after the initial attack, patient MP's titers dropped to undetectable levels. However, with a known break in prophylaxis starting in year 6, at least two streptococcal infections occurred, as evidenced by rise in antisteptolysm O (ASO) titers during that period. Of note was the concomitant rise in heart

TABLE 103–2 · THE FREQUENCY OF THE D8/17 MARKER IN PATIENTS WITH RHEUMATIC FEVER, OTHER DISEASES, AND CONTROLS IN VARIOUS GEOGRAPHIC POPULATIONS

Rheumatic Fever Patients	Number	Percent Positive
New York (USA)	43/45	93
New Mexico (USA)	30/31	97
Utah* (USA)	18/18	100
Russia (Georgian)	27/30	90
Russia (Moscow)	50/52	96
Mexico	35/39	89
Chile	45/50	90
Controls		
Russia	4/78	5
New York	6/68	8
Chile	8/50	16
Mexico	6/72	8
Other Diseases		
Rheumatoid arthritis	2/42	4
Ischemic heart disease	0/10	0
Multiple sclerosis	1/25	4
Lupus erythematosus	1/12	9

*Acute patients

TABLE 103–3 • HEART-REACTIVE ANTIBODY TITERS IN THE SERA OF PATIENTS WITH ACUTE RHEUMATIC FEVER (ARF) AS COMPARED TO UNCOMPLICATED STREPTOCOCCAL INFECTIONS AND OTHER ARTHRITIC CONDITIONS

Clinical Disorder	Number of Patients	Serum Dilutions	Average ASO Titer
		1:5, 1:10, 1:20	
Acute rheumatic fever (Gr. I)	34	4+, 2+, +*	700
Uncomplicated streptococcal infections (Gr. II)	40	1+, 0, 0	561
APSGN	20	+/–, 0, 0	520
Rheumatoid arthritis	10	0, 0, 0†	ND
Lupus erythematosus	10	0, 0, 0	ND

*Serum samples obtained at onset of rheumatic fever and at a comparable time in the group with uncomplicated scarlet fever.
†Sera obtained during active disease.
Abbreviations: APSGN, acute poststreptococcal glomerulonephritis; ND, not determined.

reactive antibody titers. The final infection was followed by a clinical recurrence of classic rheumatic carditis, complete with isolation of the organism, elevated heart-reactive antibodies, and acute-phase reactants 11 years after the initial attack.

2. Sera from patients with ARF also contain increased levels of antibodies to both myosin and tropomyosin, as compared to sera from patients with pharyngeal streptococcal infections who do not go on to develop ARF. These myosin-affinity purified antibodies also cross-react with M protein moieties, suggesting this molecule could be the antigenic stimulus for the production of myosin antibodies in these sera.[23,52]

3. Finally, as indicated previously, autoimmune antibodies are a prominent finding in another major clinical manifestation of ARF, chorea, and these antibodies are directed against the cells of the caudate nucleus. The titer of this antibody corresponds with clinical disease activity.[34]

Although it is not necessarily autoimmune in nature, the presence of elevated levels of immune complexes in ARF has been well documented both in the sera and in the joints of ARF patients.[53] Elevated levels of immune complexes, which may be as high as those seen in classic poststreptococcal glomerulonephritis, may be responsible for the immune-complex vasculitis seen in ARF tissues and may provide the initial impetus for vascular damage followed by the secondary penetration of autoreactive antibodies. Support for the concept is the close clinical similarity of rheumatic fever arthritis to experimentally induced serum sickness in animals or the arthritis seen secondary to drug hypersensitivity. Deposition of host immunoglobulin (Ig) and complement is also seen in the cardiac tissues of ARF patients, suggesting autoimmune deposition of Igs in or near the Aschoff lesions.

At a cellular level, there is now ample evidence for the presence of both lymphocytes and macrophages at the site of pathologic damage in the heart in patients with ARF.[54] The cells are predominantly cell determinant (CD)4+ helper lymphocytes during acute stages of the disease (in a ratio of 4:1). The ratio of CD4+ to CD8+ lymphocytes (2:1) more closely approximates the normal ratio in chronic valvular specimens. A majority of these cells express DR antigens. A potentially important finding has been the observation that macrophage-like fibroblasts present in the diseased valves express DR antigens[55] and might be the antigen-presenting cells for the CD4+ positive lymphocytes.

Increased cellular reactivity to streptococcal antigens has also been noted in the peripheral blood mononuclear cell preparations of ARF patients when compared to these cells isolated from nephritis patients.[56] This abnormal reactivity peaks at 6 months after the attack

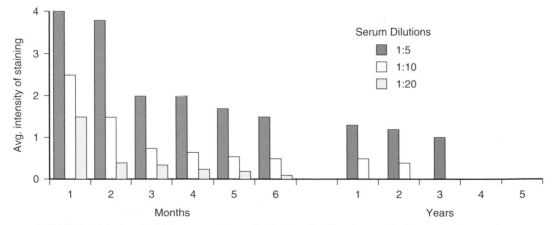

DECLINE OF THE TITER OF HEART REACTIVE ANTIBODY IN THE SERUM OF PATIENTS WITH ACUTE RHEUMATIC FEVER OVER 5-YEAR PERIOD

Serum Dilutions
■ 1:5
□ 1:10
□ 1:20

Avg. intensity of staining

Months   Years

FIGURE 103–2 • Serial heart reactive antibody titers in 40 patients with documented acute rheumatic fever (ARF). Note the slow decline of these titers over the first 2 years after the initial episode and the absence of these antibodies 5 years after the initial attack.

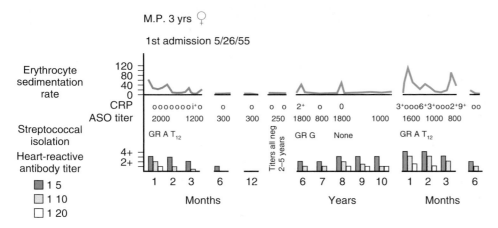

FIGURE 103-3 · Heart-reactive antibody titers and laboratory data obtained from a patient with rheumatic fever who had two well-documented acute attacks 11 years apart. Note absence of the heart-reactive antibody during years 2 to 5 and its reappearance during years 6 to 10 after evidence of two intercurrent streptococcal infections secondary to breaks in penicillin prophylaxis (see ASO titers). High titers of heart-reactive antibody appeared with the second attack. CRP, C-reactive protein.

but may persist for as long as 2 years after the initial episode. Once again, the reactivity was specific only for those strains associated with ARF, suggesting an abnormal humoral and cellular response to streptococcal antigens unique to rheumatic fever–associated streptococci.

Support for the potential pathologic importance of these T cells is further strengthened by the observation that lymphocytes obtained from experimental animals sensitized to cell membranes, but not cell walls, are specifically cytotoxic for syngeneic embryonic cardiac myofibers in vitro.[57] In humans, normal mononuclear cells primed in vitro by M protein molecules from a rheumatic fever–associated strain are also cytotoxic for myofibers, but specificity solely for cardiac cells was lacking in the human studies.[58] Similar studies have not yet been performed using lymphocytes from active ARF patients.

Clinical Features of Acute Rheumatic Fever

The clinical presentation of ARF is quite variable, and the lack of a single pathognomonic feature has resulted in the development of the revised Jones Criteria,[59] as illustrated in Table 103–5, which are used to establish a diagnosis. It should be noted that these criteria were established only as guidelines for the diagnosis and were never intended to be "etched in stone." Thus, depending on the age, geographic location, ethnic population, or some combination of these, emphasis on one criterion for the diagnosis of ARF may be more important than others. Manifestations of rheumatic fever that are not clearly expressed pose a dilemma because of the importance of identifying a first rheumatic attack clearly to establish the need for prophylaxis of recurrences (see following). Some of the isolated manifestations, particularly polyarthritis, may be difficult or impossible to distinguish from other diseases, especially at their onset. The diagnosis can be made, however, when "pure" chorea is the sole manifestation because of the rarity with which this syndrome is due to any other cause (see Tables 103–4 and 103–5).

ARTHRITIS

In the classic untreated case, the arthritis of ARF affects several joints in quick succession, each for a short time. The legs are usually affected first and later the arms. The terms *migrating* and *migratory* are often used to describe the polyarthritis of ARF, but these designations are not meant to signify that the inflammation necessarily disappears in one joint when it appears in another. Rather, the various localizations usually overlap in time, and the onset, as opposed to the full course of the arthritis, migrates from joint to joint.

Joint involvement is more common, and also more severe, in teenagers and young adults than in children. Arthritis is usually the earliest symptomatic manifestation of the disease, although asymptomatic carditis may precede it. Rheumatic polyarthritis may be excruciatingly painful, but it is almost always transient. The pain is usually more prominent than the objective signs of inflammation.

When the disease is allowed to express itself fully, unmodified by anti-inflammatory treatment, more than half of patients studied show a true polyarthritis, with inflammation in anywhere from 6 to 16 joints. Classically, each joint is maximally inflamed for only a few days, or a week at the most; the inflammation decreases, perhaps lingering for another week or so, and then disappears completely. Radiographs at this point may show a slight effusion but most likely will be unremarkable.

In routine practice, however, many patients with arthritis or arthralgias are treated empirically with salicylates or other nonsteroidal anti-inflammatory drugs (NSAIDs). Accordingly, arthritis subsides quickly in the joint(s) already affected and does not migrate to new joints. Thus, therapy may deprive the diagnostician of a useful sign. In a large series of patients with ARF and associated arthritis, most of whom had been treated, involvement of only a single large joint was common (25%). One or both knees were affected in 76 percent and one or both ankles in 50 percent. Elbows, wrists, hips, or small joints of the feet were involved in 12 to 15 percent of patients, and shoulder or small joints of the head were affected in 7 to 8 percent. Joints rarely affected were the lumbosacral (2%), cervical (1%), ster-

TABLE 103–4 • COMPOSITION OF MONONUCLEAR CELLULAR INFILTRATES IN ACUTE AND CHRONIC ACTIVE RHEUMATIC VALVULITIS

Patients	Type of Valve	Type of Valvulitis*	Composition of Infiltrate (%)						
			HLA-DR+	CD1+†	CD20+‡	CD3+§	CD4+¶	CD8+¶	CD4/CD8 Ratio
Acute valvulitis									
1	Mitral	Acute	58.9	42.6	5.1	49.5	75.6	23.0	3.1
2	Mitral	Acute	49.8	43.1	6.9	43.1	58.7	34.3	1.9
	Aortic	Acute	52.7	51.0	3.9	38.1	65.9	26.5	2.3
3	Mitral	Acute	63.9	42.0	5.5	52.4	75.4	18.9	4.0
4	Aortic	Acute	68.1	56.0	7.4	33.7	71.6	22.0	1.9
Chronic valvulitis									
4	Mitral	Chronic active	49.4	47.4	7.4	44.3	53.7	38.8	1.4
5	Mitral	Chronic active	48.8	39.1	1.4	53.9	45.2	51.5	0.9
	Aortic	Chronic active	67.8	35.0	4.0	36.8	47.5	49.1	1.0
6	Mitral	Chronic active	41.8	23.4	8.0	65.9	57.3	33.3	1.7
	Aortic	Chronic active	69.6	48.7	6.2	30.1	58.2	32.6	1.8
7	Mitral	Chronic active	55.4	24.2	8.1	59.8	64.9	24.7	2.6
8	Mitral	Chronic active	80.4	34.1	13.4	44.4	44.8	50.9	0.9
9	Mitral	Chronic active	46.1	29.6	0.8	65.6	61.6	33.3	1.8

*Determined in the frozen valve samples studied
† (63D3) Monocytes/macrophages
‡ (Leu 16) B cells
§ Pan T cells
¶ Helper T cells
¶ Suppressor cells

noclavicular (0.5%), and temporomandibular (0.5%). Involvement of the small joints of the hands or feet alone occurred in only 1 percent of these patients.[60]

Analysis of the synovial fluid in well-documented cases of ARF with arthritis generally reveals a sterile, inflammatory fluid. There may be a decrease of the complement components C1q, C3, and C4, indicating their consumption by immune complexes in the joint fluid.[61]

Poststreptococcal Reactive Arthritis

A number of investigators[62-64] have suggested that poststreptococcal migratory arthritis (both in adults and children) in the absence of carditis might be a distinct entity from acute rheumatic fever for the following reasons:

1. The latent period between the antecedent streptococcal infection and the onset of poststreptococcal reactive arthritis (PSRA) is shorter (1 to 2 weeks) than the 3 to 4 weeks usually seen in classic ARF.
2. The response of PSRA to aspirin and other NSAIDs is poor in comparison to the dramatic response seen in classic ARF.
3. Evidence of carditis is not usually seen in these patients; further, the severity of the arthritis is quite marked.
4. Extra-articular manifestations (such as tenosynovitis and renal abnormalities) are often seen in these patients.

Although these features may be seen (admittedly rarely), migratory arthritis without evidence of other

TABLE 103–5 • REVISED JONES CRITERIA FOR DIAGNOSIS OF ACUTE RHEUMATIC FEVER (ARF)

Major Manifestations	Minor Manifestations	Laboratory Findings
Carditis	Fever	Elevated acute-phase reactants:
Polyarthritis	Arthralgia	a) C-reactive protein (CRP)
Chorea	Previous rheumatic fever or rheumatic heart disease (RHD)	b) Erythrocyte sedimentation rate (ESR)
Erythema marginatum		Prolonged P-R interval rate
Subcutaneous nodules		Supporting evidence of preceding streptococcal infection: a) Increased ASO or other streptococcal antibodies b) Positive throat culture for Group A-hemolytic streptococci c) Recent scarlet fever

From: Jones Criteria update 1992. JAMA 268:2069-2070, 1992.

major Jones Criteria, if supported by two minor manifestations (see Table 103–5) must still be considered ARF, especially in children. Variations in the response to aspirin in these children often are not documented with serum salicylate levels, and an unusual clinical course is not sufficient to exclude the diagnosis of ARF. Thus, appropriate prophylactic measures should be taken.[65] Support for this concept may be found in the work of Crea and Mortimer.[66] In their series of patients with ARF, 50 percent of the children who presented solely with signs of migratory arthritis went on to develop significant valvular damage.

Rheumatic fever in adults also occurs. Although migratory arthritis is a common presenting symptom, a recent outbreak in San Diego Naval Training Camp[67] revealed a 30-percent incidence of valvular damage in these patients.

The importance of clearly defining this reactive arthritis as a rheumatic fever variant has obvious implications for secondary prophylactic treatment. As suggested by some investigators, PSRA is a benign condition without need for prophylaxsis. Yet as these patients by and large do fulfill the Jones Criteria (one major, two minor) they should be considered as having RF and, in our opinion, be treated as such.

CARDITIS

Cardiac valvular and muscle damage can manifest in a variety of signs or symptoms. These manifestations include organic heart murmurs, cardiomegaly, congestive heart failure, or pericarditis. Mild to moderate chest discomfort, pleuritic chest pain, or a pericardial friction rub are indications of pericarditis. On clinical examination, the patient can have new or changing organic murmurs, most commonly mitral regurgitant murmurs and occasionally aortic regurgitant murmurs and systolic ejection murmurs, caused by acute valvular inflammation and deformity. Rarely a Carey-Coombs mid-diastolic murmur caused by rapid flow over the mitral valve is heard. If the valvular damage is severe and there is concurrent cardiac dysfunction, congestive heart failure can occur. Congestive heart failure is the most life-threatening clinical syndrome of ARF and must be treated aggressively and early with a combination of NSAIDs, diuretics and, occasionally, steroids to acutely decrease cardiac inflammation. Electrocardiogram (ECG) abnormalities may include all degrees of heart block, including atrioventricular (AV) dissociation, but first-degree heart block is not associated with a poor prognosis. Second- or third-degree heart block can occasionally be symptomatic. If heart block is associated with congestive heart failure, temporary pacemaker placement may be required. The most common manifestation of carditis is cardiomegaly, as seen on radiograph.

Among patients at the Rockefeller University Hospital (RUH) who were diagnosed with acute ARF between 1950 and 1970 with an average of 20 years of follow-up, 90 percent had evidence of carditis at diagnosis (Table 103–6). In Bland and Jones'[68] classic review of 1000 patients with ARF, only 65 percent were diagnosed with carditis. However, when Doppler sonography was employed in the clinical evaluation of patients during the recent Utah outbreak, 91 percent of patients had

TABLE 103–6 • PHYSICAL SIGNS AND SYMPTOMS OF ACUTE RHEUMATIC FEVER: ROCKEFELLER UNIVERSITY HOSPITAL 1950-1970

	RHD (N = 40)	No RHD (N = 47)	TOTAL (N = 87)	Bland and Jones
Carditis	100%	83.0%	90.1%	65.3%
Arthritis	67.5%	68.1%	67.8%	41.0%
Epistaxis	0	10.6%	5.7%	27.4%
Chorea	5.0%	2.1%	3.4%	51.8%
Pericarditis	2.5%	4.3%	3.4%	13.0%
Nodules	7.5%	0	3.4%	8.8%
Erythema marginatum	0	4.3%	2.3%	7.1%

Abbreviations: No RHD, patients without rheumatic heart disease; RHD, patients with rheumatic heart disease.

carditis,[1] indicating that with more sensitive measurements of cardiac dysfunction, almost all ARF patients have signs of acute carditis.

Rheumatic Heart Disease

Rheumatic heart disease (RHD) is the most severe sequela of ARF. Usually occurring 10 to 20 years after the original attack, it is the most prevalent cause of acquired valvular disease in the world. The mitral valve is mainly involved, and aortic valve involvement occurs less often. Mitral stenosis is a classic RHD finding and can manifest as a combination of mitral insufficiency and stenosis, secondary to severe calcification of the mitral valve. When symptoms of left-atrial enlargement are present, mitral valve replacement may become necessary.

In various studies, the incidence of RHD in patients with a history of ARF has varied. In Bland and Jones' classic follow-up study of patients with ARF,[68] after 20 years, one third of patients had no murmur, another one third had died, and the remaining one third were alive with RHD. A majority of the patients who died had RHD. Although the classic dogma is that patients with RHD have invariably had more than one attack of ARF, recent analysis of our patients at the RUH disproves this notion. The population studied was 87 patients who had only one documented attack of ARF, without any evidence (clinical or laboratory) of a recurrence during a 20-year follow-up under close supervision. More than 80 percent had carditis at admission, and approximately 50 percent now have organic murmurs (see Table 103–6). Thus, valvular damage manifesting as organic murmurs later in life is still likely to occur in 50 percent of patients, particularly if they presented with evidence of carditis at initial diagnosis. All the patients in our population who ended up with RHD had carditis at diagnosis.

CHOREA

Sydenham's chorea, chorea minor, or "St. Vitus dance" is a neurologic disorder consisting of abrupt, purposeless, nonrhythmic, involuntary movements; muscular weakness; and emotional disturbances. Involuntary movements disappear during sleep, but they may occur at rest and may interfere with voluntary activity. Initially, it may be possible to suppress these movements, which may affect all voluntary muscles, with the hands and face usually the most obvious. Grimaces and inappropriate smiles are common. Handwriting usually becomes clumsy and provides a convenient way of following the patient's course. Speech is often slurred. The movements are commonly more marked on one side of the body and are occasionally completely unilateral (hemichorea).

The muscular weakness is best revealed by asking the patients to squeeze the examiner's hands: The pressure of the patient's grip increases and decreases continuously and capriciously, a phenomenon known as relapsing grip, or milking sign.

The emotional changes manifest themselves in outbursts of inappropriate behavior, including crying and restlessness. In rare cases, the psychologic manifestions may be severe and may result in transient psychosis.

The neurologic examination fails to reveal sensory losses or pyramidal tract involvement. Diffuse hypotonia may be present. Chorea may follow streptococcal infections after a latent period, which is longer, on the average, than the latent period of other rheumatic manifestations. Some patients with chorea have no other symptoms, but other patients develop chorea weeks or months after arthritis. In both cases, examination of the heart may reveal murmurs.

A new and potentially very interesting chapter is unfolding concerning this manifestation of rheumatic fever. It has been known for years that often the early symptoms of chorea may present as emotional or behavioral changes in the patient,[69] and only later do the choreiform moter symptoms appear. It was also noted that a number of chorea patients, years after the choreiform symptoms had subsided, would present with behavioral disorders such as tics or obsessive compulsive disorder (OCD).

These earlier observations, sampled with the known presence of antibrain antibodies in the sera of Sydenham's chorea patients, raised the question of whether a prior streptococcal infection (or infection with other microbes) might induce antibodies cross-reactive with brain antigen involved in neural pathways associated with behavior. Two papers[70,71] have indicated that there is a strong association of the D8/17 B cell marker (described previously) with children who have OCD (see Table 103–4). Whereas Swedo and colleagues[70] selected patients on the basis of a strong history of prior streptococcal infections, Murphy and colleagues[71] noted a strong association of the marker with OCD patients without a history of streptococcal infections. These preliminary studies suggest that streptococci, and probably other microbes, may induce antibodies that functionally disrupt the basal ganglia pathways, lending not only to classic chorea but to other more behavioral disorders in these children, without evidence of classic chorea.

SUBCUTANEOUS NODULES

The subcutaneous nodules of ARF are firm and painless. The overlying skin is not inflamed and can usually be moved over the nodules. The diameter of these round lesions varies from a few millimeters to 1 or even 2 cm. They are located over bony surfaces or prominences or near tendons. Their number varies from a single nodule to a few dozen and averages three or four; when numerous, they are usually symmetric. Nodules are rarely present for more than a month. They are smaller and more short lived than the nodules of RA. Although in both diseases the elbows are most frequently involved, the rheumatic nodules are more common on the olecranon, whereas nodules of RA are usually found 3- or 4-cm distal to it. Rheumatic subcutaneous nodules generally appear only after the first few weeks of illness and usually only in patients with carditis.

ERYTHEMA MARGINATUM

Erythema marginatum is an evanescent, nonpruritic skin rash, pink or faintly red, affecting usually the trunk, sometimes the proximal parts or the limbs, but not the face. This lesion extends centrifugally while the skin in the center returns gradually to normal—hence, the name erythema marginatum. The outer edge of the lesion is sharp, whereas the inner edge is diffuse. Because the margin of the lesion is usually continuous, making a ring, it is also known as erythema annulare.

The individual lesions may appear and disappear in a matter of hours, usually to return. A hot bath or shower may make them more evident or may even reveal them for the first time.

Erythema marginatum usually occurs in the early phase of the disease. It often persists or recurs, even when all other manifestations of disease have disappeared. Occasionally, the lesions appear for the first time or, more likely, are noticed for the first time, late in the course of the illness or even during convalescence. This disorder usually occurs only in patients with carditis.

MINOR MANIFESTATIONS

Fever

Temperature is increased in almost all ARF attacks and ranges from 38.4 to 40°C. Usually fever decreases in approximately a week without antipyretic treatment and may become low grade for another week or two. Fever rarely lasts for more than 3 to 4 weeks.

Abdominal Pain

The abdominal pain of ARF resembles that of other conditions associated with acute microvascular mesenteric inflammation and is nonspecific. It usually occurs at or near the onset of the rheumatic fever attack, so other manifestations may not yet be present to clarify the diagnosis. In many cases, it may mimic acute appendicitis.

Epistaxis

In the past, epistaxis occurred most prominently and severely in patients with severe and protracted rheumatic carditis. Early clinical studies reported a frequency as high as 48 percent, but it probably occurs even less frequently now (see Table 103–6). Although epistaxis has been correlated in the past with the severity of rheumatic inflammation, it is difficult to assess retrospectively the possible thrombasthenic effect of large doses of salicylates, which are administered for prolonged periods in protracted attacks.

Rheumatic Pneumonia

Pneumonia may appear during the course of severe rheumatic carditis. This inflammatory process is difficult or impossible to distinguish from pulmonary edema or the alveolitis associated with respiratory distress syndromes due to a variety of pathophysiologic states.

∎ Laboratory Findings

The diagnosis of ARF cannot readily be established by laboratory tests. Nevertheless, such tests may be helpful in two ways: 1) in demonstrating that an antecedent streptococcal infection has occurred and 2) in documenting the presence or persistence of an inflammatory process. Serial chest radiographs may be helpful in following the course of carditis, and the ECG may reflect the inflammatory process on the conduction system.

Throat cultures are usually negative by the time ARF appears, but an attempt should be made to isolate the organism. It is our practice to take three throat cultures during the first 24 hours, prior to administration of antibiotics. Streptococcal antibodies are more useful because 1) they reach a peak titer at about the time of onset of ARF; 2) they indicate true infection rather than transient carriage; and 3) by performing several tests for different antibodies, any significant recent streptococcal infection can be detected. To demonstrate a rising titer, it is useful to take a serum specimen when the patient is first seen and another 2 weeks later for comparison.

The specific antibody tests used to diagnose streptococcal infections most frequently are those directed against extracellular products including antistreptolysin O (ASO), anti-DNAse B, antihyaluronidase (antidiphosphopyridine nucleotide [anti-DPNase]), and antistreptokinase. ASO has been the most widely used test and is generally available in hospitals in the United States.

ASO titers vary with age, season, and geography. They reach peak levels in the young, school-age population. Therefore, titers of 200 to 300 Todd units per milliliter are common in healthy children of elementary-school age. After a streptococcal pharyngitis, the antibody response peaks at about 4 to 5 weeks, which is usually during the second or third week of ARF (depending on how early it is detected). Thereafter, antibody titers fall off rapidly in the next several months and, after 6 months, they decline more slowly. Because only 80 percent of documented ARF patients exhibit a rise in the ASO titer, it is recommended that other antistreptococcal antibody tests be performed in the absence of a positive ASO titer. These include anti-DNAse B, antihyaluronidase, or antistreptozyme (which is a combination of various streptococcal antigens).

Streptococcal antibodies, when increased, support—but do not prove—the diagnosis of ARF, and they are not a measure of rheumatic activity. Even in the absence of intercurrent streptococcal infection, titers decline during the rheumatic attack despite the persistence or severity of rheumatic activity.

ACUTE-PHASE REACTANTS

Acute-phase reactants are elevated during ARF, just as they are during other inflammatory conditions. Both the C-reactive protein (CRP) and erythrocyte sedimentation rate (ESR) are almost invariably elevated during the active rheumatic process, if they are not suppressed by antirheumatic drugs. These may be normal, however, during episodes of pure chorea or persistent erythema marginatum. Particularly when treatment has been discontinued or is being tapered off, the CRP and ESR are useful in monitoring "rebounds" of rheumatic inflammation, which indicate that the rheumatic process is still active. If either the CRP or ESR remain normal a few weeks after discontinuing antirheumatic therapy, the attack may be considered ended unless chorea appears. Usually, there will be no exacerbation of the systemic inflammation, and chorea will be present as an isolated manifestation.

ANEMIA

A mild, normochromic, normocytic anemia of chronic infection or inflammation may be seen during ARF. Suppressing the inflammation usually improves the anemia; thus, hematinic therapy is usually not indicated.

OTHER SUPPORTING TESTS

As noted in Figure 103–3 and Table 103–2, two other tests have, in our experience, been helpful in confirming the diagnosis of acute ARF, especially when the diagnosis is in doubt.

First, clinicians can detect elevated titers of heart-reactive antibodies directed against sarcolemmal antigens in the vast majority of ARF patients. Elevated levels of these antibodies are not seen in either uncomplicated streptococcal infections or acute poststreptococcal glomerulonephritis (APSGN). Using enzyme-linked immunosorbent assay (ELISA), antibodies directed against cytoskeletal constituents such as myosin and tropomyosin are also found to be elevated in ARF patients and might be helpful in determining whether or not cross-reactive antibodies unique to ARF exist.[51]

Secondly, the use of the D8/17 monoclonal antibody mentioned previously has also proved helpful in the differential diagnosis of ARF from other disorders. In our hands, all rheumatic fever patients express abnormal levels of D8/17-positive B cells, especially during the acute attack. In those cases where the diagnosis of ARF has been doubtful, presence of elevated levels of D8/17 positive B cells has proven to be very helpful in establishing the correct diagnosis.[41]

Clinical Course and Treatment of Acute Rheumatic Fever

The mainstay of treatment for ARF has always been NSAIDs, most commonly aspirin. Dramatic improvement in symptoms is usually seen after the initiation of therapy. Usually 80 to 100 mg/kg/day in children and 4 to 8 g/day in adults is required for an effect to be seen. Aspirin levels can be measured, and 20 to 30 mg/dl is the therapeutic range. Duration of NSAID therapy can vary but needs to be maintained until all symptoms are absent and laboratory values are normal. If severe carditis is also present (as indicated by significant cardiomegaly, congestive heart failure, or third-degree heart block), steroid therapy can be instituted. The usual dosage is 2 mg/kg/day of oral prednisone during the first 1 to 2 weeks. Depending on clinical and laboratory improvement, the dosage is then tapered over the next 2 weeks, and during the last week, aspirin may be added in the dosage recommended previously, sufficient to achieve the 20 to 30 mg/dl level.

Whether or not signs of pharyngitis are present at the time of diagnosis, antibiotic therapy with penicillin should be started and maintained for at least 10 days, given in doses recommended for the eradication of a streptococcal pharyngitis. Additionally, all family contacts should be cultured and treated for streptococcal infection, if positive. If compliance is an issue, depot penicillins (i.e., 600,000 units of benzathine penicillin G in children, 1.2 million units in adults) should be given. Recurrences of ARF are most common within 2 years of the original attack but can occur at any time. The risk of recurrence decreases with age. Recurrence rates have been decreasing, from 20 percent to 2 to 4 percent in recent outbreaks. This might be due to better surveillance and treatment.

PROPHYLAXIS

Antibiotic prophylaxis with penicillin should be started immediately following the resolution of the acute episode. The optimal regimen consists of oral penicillin (VK 250,000 twice a day) or parenteral penicillin G (1.2 million units intramuscularly every 4 weeks). One study suggests, however, that injections every 3 weeks are more effective than every-4-week injections at preventing ARF recurrences.[72] If the patient is allergic to penicillin, erythromycin (250 mg/day) can be substituted.

The end point of prophylaxis is unclear; most believe it should continue at least until the patient is a young adult, which is usually 10 years from an acute attack with no recurrence. In our opinion, individuals with documented evidence of rheumatic heart disease should be on continuous prophylaxis indefinitely, because our experience has indicated that ARF recurrences can occur even in the fifth or sixth decade. A potential problem for ARF recurrences are young children in the household who could transmit new group A streptococcal infections to the rheumatic-susceptible individuals.

The alternative to long-term prophylaxis in an individual with ARF will be the introduction of streptococcal vaccines designed not only to prevent recurrent infections in susceptible individuals with previous ARF, but also to prevent streptococcal disease in general.

STREPTOCOCCAL VACCINES

The difficulties in developing a streptococcal vaccine have mainly been related to the numerous reports that streptococcal antigens are known to cross-react with mammalian tissues.[65] In spite of these caveats, recent work indicates progress in this area. Perhaps the most advanced has been the work of Dale and colleagues, who have synthesized short peptides (20 to 30 amino acids) of a number of different M proteins, linked them together, and have shown that they can develop type-specific antibodies that are also opsonic.[73] Little toxicity or cross-reactivity to human tissues has been noted with the antigen or the antibodies. Phase I trials are now in progress.

The second approach revolves around C-repeat region of the M protein moiety, which is common to all group A streptococci. Bessen and Fischetti[74] have used a commensural organism commonly found in the oral mucosa of humans, and by genetic engineering, they have inserted into it the C-repeat of the M protein, which is preferentially displayed on the surface of the organism. This induces IgA antibodies, thereby preventing oral colonization of mice by live group A streptococci. Others[75] have confirmed these results using a different M-type organism. Good and colleagues[76] have used similar methods, except they have added additional amino acids, making their antibodies opsonic. Bessen and Fischetti are now in phase I trials of the safety of *S. gordoni* without the M-protein insert.

Based on the observation by Lancefield[77] that human sera rarely if ever contained more than one type-specific M protein antibody, Salvadori and coworkers[27] have examined other possible streptococcal antigens that might explain the broad-based immunity to streptococcal infections that occurs with increasing age. Their studies indicated that the streptococcal group A carbohydrate (GRA-CHO) might be a good immunogen for the following reasons: Antibodies to GRA-CHO are present in human sera, increase with age, and are opsonic for several distinct M+-type strains. Furthermore, both active and passive immunization with GRA-CHO in mice has demonstrated protection against a live lethal challenge in mice. No cross-reactive antibodies have been detected. Phase I trials will probably commence in the year 2002.

Two other candidates are also under consideration. Cleary and associates have described a surface antigen present on group A streptococci called C5a peptidase. This enzyme specifically cleaves the human serum chemotoxin C5a at the polymorphonuclear binding site. These observations led to experiments in which intranasal inoculation with C5a peptidase resulted in the appearance of antibodies that clearly reduced the potential of several different M+ strains to colonize mice.[78] Finally Musser and colleagues[79] have shown that the presence of SPEB markedly increases the virulence of a given group A streptococcal strain. Inactivation of the SPEB gene markedly decreases the lethality (IP challenge) of at least two strains: type 49 and S43 type 6. The mechanism whereby SPEB-negative strains decrease the lethality of the strain appears to reside in the fact that polymorphonuclear neutrophils were able to clear the mutant strain from the circulation and tissues much more rapidly than the wild-type strain.[80]

■ Conclusion

Despite its disappearance in many areas of the world, ARF continues to be a serious problem in the geographic areas where two thirds of the population live. Even in developed countries with full access to medical care and better nutrition and housing, a recent resurgence of the disease emphasizes the need for continued vigilance of physicians and other health officials in both diagnosing and treating ARF. Whether this resurgence represents a change in the virulence of the organism or failure to recognize the importance and adequate treatment of an antecedent streptococcal infection remains an area of intense debate and will, therefore, require careful and controlled epidemiologic surveillance. The importance of early diagnosis and therapy cannot be overemphasized. Although the joint manifestations are transient and self limiting, the cardiac sequela are chronic and life threatening.

Nevertheless, ARF remains one of the few autoimmune disorders known to occur as a result of infection with a specific organism. The confirmed observation of an increased frequency of a B cell alloantigen in several populations of rheumatics suggests that it might be possible to identify susceptible individuals to ARF at birth. If so, from a public health standpoint: 1) These individuals would be prime candidates for immunization with any streptococcal vaccine that might be developed in the future; (2) careful monitoring of streptococcal disease in the susceptible population could lead to early and effective antibiotic strategies, resulting in disease prevention; and (3) in individuals previously infected who later present with subtle or nonspecific manifestations of the disease, the presence or absence of the marker could be of value in arriving at a diagnosis.

The continued study of ARF as a paradigm for microbal-host interactions also has important implications for the study of autoimmune diseases in general and rheumatic diseases in particular. Further insights into this intriguing host-parasite relationship may shed additional light on those diseases in which the infection is presumed but has not as yet been identified.

REFERENCES

1. Veasy LG, et al: Resurgence of acute rheumatic fever in the intermountain area of the United States. New Engl J Med 316:421-427, 1987.
2. Gordis L: The virtual diappearance of rheumatic fever in the United States: lessons in the rise and fall of disease. Circulation 72:1155-1162, 1985.
3. Pope RM: Rheumatic fever in the 1980s. Bull Rheum Dis 38:1-8, 1989.
4. Markowitz M: Rheumatic fever: recent outbreaks of an old disease. Conn Med 51:229-233, 1987.
5. Kaplan EL, Johnson DR, Cleary PP: Group A streptococcal serotypes isolated from patients and sibling contacts during the resurgence of rheumatic fever in the United States in the mid 1980s. J Infect Dis 159:101-103, 1989.
6. Whitnack E, Bisno AL: Rheumatic fever and other immunologically mediated cardiac diseases. In Parker C (ed): Clinical Immunology. Vol. II. WB Sanders, 1980, pp 894-929.
7. Denny FW Jr., Wannamaker LW, Brink WR, et al: Prevention of rheumatic fever: treatment of the preceding streptococcal infection. JAMA 143:151-153, 1950.
8. Markowitz M, Gordis L: Rheumatic Fever, 2nd ed. Philadelphia, WB Saunders, 1972.
9. Stollerman GH, Lewis AJ, Schultz I, Taranta A: Relationship of the immune response to group A streptococci to the cause of acute, chronic and recurrent rheumatic fever. Am J Med 20:163-169, 1956.
10. Potter EV, Svartman M, Mohammed I, et al: Tropical acute rheumatic fever and associated streptococcal infections compared with concurrent acute glomerulonephritis. J Pediatr 92:325-333, 1978.
11. Bessen D, Jones KF, Fischetti VA: Evidence for the distinct classes of streptococcal M protein and their relationship to rheumatic fever. J Exper Med 169:269-283, 1989.
12. Kaplan EL, Anthony BF, Chapman SS, et al: The influence of the site of infection on the immune response to group A streptococci. J Clin Invest 49:1405-1414. 1970.
13. Bisno AL, Nelson KE: Type-specific opsonic antibodies in streptococcal pyoderma. Infect Immun 10:1356-1361, 1975.
14. Kendall F, Heidelberger M, Dawson M: A serologically inactive polysaccharide elaborated by mucoid strains of group A hemolytic streptococcus. J Biol Chem 118:61-82, 1937.
15. Seastone CV: The virulence of group C hemolytic streptococci of animal origin. J Exper Med 70:361 378, 1939.
16. Quinn RW, Singh KP: Antigenicity of hyaluronic acid. Biochem J 95:290-301, 1957.
17. Fillit HM, McCarty M, Blake M: Induction of antibodies to hyaluronic acid by immunization of rabbits with encapsulated streptococci. J Exper Med 164:762-776, 1986.
18. Faarber P, Capel PJ, Rigke PM, et al: Cross reactivity of anti DNA antibodies with proteoglycans. Clin Exper Immunol 55:402-412, 1984.
19. Stollerman GH: Rheumatic Fever and Streptococcal Infection. Grune and Stratton, 1975, p 70.
20. Fischetti VA: Streptococcal M protein: molecular design and biological behavior. Clini Microbiol Rev 2:285-314, 1989.
21. Dale JB, Beachey EH: Multiple cross reactive epitopes of streptococcal M proteins. J Exper Med 161:113-122, 1985.
22. Sargent SJ, Beachey EH, Corbett CE, Dale JB: Sequence of protective epitopes of streptococcal M proteins shared with cardiac sarcolemmal membranes. J Immunol 139:1285-1290, 1987.
23. Cunningham MW, McCormack JM, Talaber LR, et al: Human monoclonal antibodies reactive with antigens of the group A streptococcus and human heart. J Immunol 141:2760-2766, 1988.
24. McCarty M: The streptococcal cell wall. The Harvey Lectures Series 65:73-96, 1970.
25. Goldstein I, Rebeyrotte P, Parlebas J, et al: Isolation from heart valves of glycopeptides which share immunological properties with streptococcus heamolyticus group A polysaccharides. Nature 219:866-868, 1968.
26. Goldstein I, Caravano R: Determination of anti group A streptococcal polysaccharide antibodies in human sera by an hemagglutination technique. Proc Soc Exper Biol Med 124(4):1209-1212, 1967.
27. Salvadori LG, Blake MS, McCarty M, et al: Group A streptococcus-liposome ELISA antibody titers to group A polysaccharide and opsonophagocytic capabilities of the antibodies. J Infect Dis 171:593-600, 1995.
28. Chetty C, Schwab JH: Chemistry of endotoxins. In Rietschel ET (ed): Handbook of Endotoxin. Vol 1. Elsenier Science BV, 1984, pp 376-410.
29. Cromartie WJ, Craddock JB, Schwab JH, et al: Arthritis in rats after systemic injection of streptococcal cells or cell walls. J Exper Med 146:1585-1602,1977.

30. Cromartie WJ, Craddock JB: Rheumatic-like cardiac lesions in mice. Science 154:285-287, 1966.
31. Heymer B, Schleifer KH, Read SE, et al: Detection of antibodies to bacterial cell wall peptidoglycan in human sera. J Immunol 117:23-26, 1976.
32. Zabriskie JB: Rheumatic fever: the interplay between host genetics and microbe. Circulation 71:1077-1086, 1985.
33. Kingston D, Glynn LE: A cross-reaction between Streptococcus pyogenes and human fibroblasts, endothelial cells and astrocytes. Immunology 21:1003-1016, 1971.
34. Husby G, van de Rijn I, Zabriskie JB, et al: Antibodies reacting with cytoplasm of subthalmic and caudate nuclei neurons in chorea and acute rheumatic fever. J Exper Med 144:1094-1110, 1976.
35. Froude J, Gibofsky A, Buskirk DR, et al: Cross reactivity between streptococcus and human tissue: a model of molecular mimicry and autoimmuntiy. Curr Top Microbiol Immunol 145:5-26, 1989.
36. Cheadle WB: Harvean lectures on the various manifestations of the rheumatic state as exemplified in childhood and early life. Lancet i:821-832, 1889.
37. Wilson MG, Schweitzr MD, Lubschez R: The familial epidermiology of rheumatic fever. J Ped 22:468-482, 1943.
38. Taranta A, Torosdag S, Metrakos JD, et al: Rheumatic fever in monozygotic and dizygotic twins. Circulation 20:778-792, 1959.
39. Glynn LE, Halborrow EJ: Relationship between blood groups, secretion status and susceptibility to rheumatic fever. Arthritis Rheum 4:203, 1961.
40. Patarroyo ME, Winchester RJ, Vejerano A, et al: Association of a B cell alloantigen with susceptibility to rheumatic fever. Nature 278:173-174, 1979.
41. Khanna AK, Buskirk DR, Williams RC Jr., et al: Presence of a non-HLA B cell antigen in rheumatic fever patients and their families as defined by a monoclonal antibody. J Clin Invest 83:1710-1716, 1989.
42. Ayoub EA, Barrett DJ, Maclaren NK, Krischer JP: Association of class II human histocompatibility leucocyte antigens with rheumatic fever. J Clin Invest 77:2019-2026, 1986.
43. Maharaj B, Hammond MG, Appadoo B, et al: HLA-A, B, DR and DQ antigens in black patients with severe chronic rheumatic heart disease. Circulation 765:259-261, 1987.
44. Guilherme L, Weidenbach W, Kiss MH, et al: Association of human leukocyte class II antigens with rheumatic fever or rheumatic heart disease in a Brazilian population. Circulation 83:1995-1998, 1991.
45. Watson RF, Hirst GK, Lancefield RC: Bacteriological studies of cardiac tissues obtained at autopsy from eleven patients dying with rheumatic fever. Arthritis Rheum 4:74-85, 1961.
46. Halbert SP, Bircher R, Dahle E: The analysis of streptococcal infections. V. Cardiotoxicity of streptolysin O for rabbits in vivo. J Exper Med 113:759-784, 1961.
47. Wagner BM: Studies in rheumatic fever. III. Histochemical reactivity of the Aschoff body. Ann N Y Acad Sci 86:992-1008, 1960.
48. Zabriskie JB: Unpublished data, 1959.
49. Schlievert PM, Johnson LP, Tomai MA, Handley JP: Characterization and genetics of group A streptococcal pyrogenic exotoxins. In Ferretti J, Curtisis R (eds): Streptococcal Genetics. Washington, DC, ASM, 1987, pp 136-142.
50. Paliard X, et al: Evidence for the effects of superantigen in rheumatoid arthritis. Science 253(5015):325-329, 1991.
51. Zabriskie JB, Hsu KC, Seegal BC: Heart-reactive antibody associated with rheumatic fever: characterization and diagnostic significance. Clin Exp Immunol 7:147-159, 1970.
52. Khanna AK, Nomura Y, Fischetti VA, Zabriskie JB: Antibodies in the sera of acute rheumatic fever patients bind to human cardiac tropomyosin. J Autoimmun 10:99-106, 1997.
53. van de Rijn I, et al: Serial studies on circulating immune complexes in post-streptococcal sequelae. Clin Exper Immunol 34:318-325, 1978.
54. Kemeny E, Grieve T, Marcus R, et al: Identification of mononuclear cells and T cell subsets in rheumatic valvulitis. Clin Immunol Immunopathol 5:225-237, 1989.
55. Amoils B, et al: Aberrant expression of HLA-DR antigen on valvular fibroblasts from patients with acute rheumatic carditis. Clin Exper Immunol 66:84-94, 1986.
56. Read SE, et al: Serial studies on the cellular immune response to streptococcal antigens in acute and convalescent rheumatic fever patients in Trinidad. J Clin Immunol 6:433-441, 1986.
57. Yang LC, Soprey PR, Wittner MK, Fox EN: Streptococcal induced cell mediated immune destruction of cardiac myofibers in vitro. J Exper Med 146:344-360, 1977.
58. Dale JB, Beachey EH: Human cytotoxic T lymphocytes evoked by group A streptococcal M proteins. J Exper Med 166:1825-1835, 1987.
59. Jones Criteria 1992 update. Guidelines for diagnosis of rheumatic fever. JAMA 268:2069-2070, 1992.
60. Feinstein AR, Spagnulo M: The clinical patterns of rheumatic fever: a reappraisal. Medicine 41:279-305, 1962.
61. Svartman M, Potter EV, Poon-King T: Immunoglobulin components in synovial fluids of patients with acute rheumatic fever. J Clin Invest 56:111-117, 1975.
62. Goldsmith DP, Long SS: Poststreptococcal disease of childhood: a changing syndrome [abstract]. Arthritis Rheum 25:S18, 1982.
63. Arnold MH, Tyndall A: Post-streptococcal reactive arthritis. Ann Rheum Dis 48, 681-688, 1989.
64. Fink CW: The role of streptococcus in post streptococcal reactive arthritis and childhood polyarteritis nodosa. J Rheumatol 18: 14-20, 1991.
65. Gibofsky A, Zabriskie JB: Rheumatic fever: new insights into an old disease. Bulletin on the Rheumatic Disease. Arthritis Found 42(7):5-7, 1994.
66. Crea MA, Mortimer EA: The nature of scarlatinal arthritis. Pediatrics 23:879-884, 1959.
67. Wallace MR, Garst PD, Papadimos TJ, Oldfield EC: The return of acute rheumatic fever in young adults. JAMA 262(18):2557-2561, 1989.
68. Bland EF, Jones TD: Rheumatic fever and rheumatic heart disease: a twenty year report on 1,000 patients followed since childhood. Circulation 4:836-843,1951.
69. Osler W: On Chorea and Choreiform Movements, HK Lewis and Co., 1894.
70. Swedo SE, Leonard HL, Mittleman BB, et al: Children with PANDAS (Pediatric autoimmune neuropsychiatric disorders associated with strep) infections are identified by a marker associated with rheumatic fever. Am J Psychiatry 154:110-112, 1997.
71. Murphy and colleagues, 1997
72. Lue HC, Mil-Wham W, Hsieh KH, et al: Rheumatic fever recurrences: controlled study of 3 week versus 4 week benzathnic penicillin prevention programs. J Ped 108:299-304, 1986.
73. Dale JB, Simmons M, et al: Recombinant, octavalent group A streptococcal M protein vaccine. Vaccine 14(10): 944-948, 1996.
74. Bessen D, Fischetti VA: Influence of intranasal immunization with synthetic peptides corresponding to conserved epitopes of M protein on mucosal colonization by group A streptococci. Infect Immun 56:2666-2672, 1988.
75. Bronze MS, Courtney HS, Dale JB: Epitopes of Group A Streptococcal M protein that evoke cross protection local immune responses. J Immunol 148:888-893, 1992.
76. Good MF, Brandt ER, Currie B, Hayman M: Strategies for developing a Group A streptococcoal vaccine based on the M protein. Presented at the XIV Lancefield International Symposium on Streptococci and Streptococcal Diseases. Auckland, New Zealand. Chapter 053, 1999.
77. Lancefield RC: Persistence of type specific antibodies in man following infection with group A streptococci. J Exper Med 110:271-292, 1959.
78. Ji Y, Carlson B, et al: Intranasal immunization with C5a peptidase prevents nasopharyngeal colonization of mice by the group A Streptococcus. Infect Immun 65(6):2080-2087, 1997.
79. Lukonski 1997.
80. Lukonski 1998.

XVII

Arthritis Accompanying Systemic Diseases

104

Amyloidosis

DAVID C. SELDIN · MARTHA SKINNER

Amyloidosis is a term for diseases that have in common the extracellular deposition of insoluble fibrillar proteins in tissues and organs. These diseases are a subset of a growing group of disorders recognized to be caused by misfolding of proteins; these include Alzheimer's and other neurodegenerative diseases, prion diseases, serpinopathies, and some of the cystic fibroses, among others. A unifying feature of the amyloidoses is that the deposits share a common β-pleated sheet structural conformation that confers unique staining properties. The name "amyloid" is attributed to the pathologist Virchow, who in 1854 thought such deposits in autopsy livers were cellulose because of their peculiar staining reaction with iodine and sulfuric acid.[1] Although the name did not accurately identify the amyloid deposits as proteinaceous, it has persisted and is not entirely inaccurate, because other constituents, including carbohydrates, are found in association with amyloid fibrils.

Classification and Epidemiology

Amyloid diseases are defined by the biochemical nature of the protein in the deposited fibril. The proteins are diverse and unrelated in primary amino acid sequence, causing amyloid diseases to be classified according to whether they are systemic or localized, acquired or inherited, and by their recognized clinical patterns (Table 104–1). Each amyloid disease has a shorthand nomenclature, expressed as A for amyloidosis and an abbreviation for the biochemical nature of the fibrils: For example, AL is amyloid of light-chain origin.[2] Discussion in this chapter is limited to the systemic amyloidoses, as these are the diseases that can involve the joints and are potentially confused with autoimmune rheumatologic disorders. The acquired systemic amyloidoses are AL (immunoglobulin [Ig] light chain, or primary), AA (reactive, secondary), and Aβ2M (β2-microglobulin, dialysis-associated) types. The AL type is most common, although epidemiologic data are limited. One study based on National Center for Health Statistics data estimated the incidence as 4.5 cases per 100,000 population.[3] AL amyloidosis usually begins after age 40 years and is associated with rapid progression, multisystem involvement, and a short survival. AA amyloidosis is rare, occurring in less than 1 percent of persons with chronic inflammatory diseases in the United States and Europe, but is more common in Turkey and the Middle East where it occurs in association with familial Mediterranean fever.[4-6] It may begin within a year after onset of the underlying inflammatory disease or many years later. It is the only type of amyloidosis that occurs in children. Aβ₂M amyloidosis is a frequent chronic rheumatologic complication of long-term dialysis,[7] although a recent reduction in incidence has been attributed to changes in the purity of water used for the dialysate.[8]

The inherited amyloidoses are rare, with an estimated incidence of less than 1 per 100,000.[9] They are autosomal dominant diseases in which a variant plasma protein forms amyloid deposits beginning in midlife. The most common form is caused by variant transthyretin (TTR), of which there are more than 80 associated with amyloidosis.[10] One variant, Val-122-Ile, has a carrier frequency that may be as high as 4 percent of the U.S. black population and is associated with late-onset cardiac amyloidosis.[11] Even wild-type TTR can form fibrils, leading to so-called "senile cardiac" amyloidosis in older patients.[12] Other familial amyloidoses, caused by variant apolipoprotein A-I, A-II, gelsolin, fibrinogen Aα, or lysozyme, have been reported in only a few families worldwide.

Pathology and Pathogenesis of Amyloid Fibril Formation

PATHOLOGIC FEATURES

Amyloid deposits are widespread in AL amyloidosis and can be present in the extracellular spaces and the blood vessels of all organs. Deposits are limited in AA amyloidosis, occurring in the kidneys, liver, and spleen, although widespread deposits can be found late in the course of the

TABLE 104–1 · CLASSIFICATION OF AMYLOIDOSIS

Term	Fibril Composition	Systemic (S) or Localized (L)	Clinical Syndrome
AL	Immunoglobulin light chains (kappa or lambda)	S, L	Primary; myeloma associated; localized in skin, lymph nodes, bladder, tracheobronchial tree
AA	Amyloid A protein	S	Secondary; reactive; familial Mediterranean fever
Aβ₂M	β₂-Microglobulin	S	Long-term hemodialysis or chronic ambulatory peritoneal dialysis
ATTR	Transthyretin (80+ familial variants); wild-type transthyretin (TTR) in senile cardiac amyloidosis	S	Familial amyloidotic polyneuropathy and cardiomyopathy; sporadic senile cardiomyopathy
AApoA	Apolipoprotein AI (variant Arg 26, Arg 50, Arg 60) or Apolipoprotein AII	S	Familial polyneuropathy with nephropathy
AGel	Gelsolin (variant Asn 187, Tyr 187)	S	Familial polyneuropathy with lattice corneal dystrophy, cranial neuropathy, nephropathy
AFib	Fibrinogen Aα (variant Leu 554, Val 526)	S	Familial amyloidosis with nephropathy
ALys	Lysozyme (variant Thr 56, His 67)	S	Familial amyloidosis with nephropathy
Aβ	Amyloid β protein	L	Alzheimer's disease; Down syndrome; cerebral amyloid angiopathy (Dutch)
ACys	Cystatin C (variant form with deletion of N-terminal 10 amino acids and Glu 68)	S	Cerebral amyloid angiopathy (Icelandic)
AIAPP	Islet amyloid polypeptide	L	Diabetes mellitus, type II; insulinoma
ACal	Calcitonin	L	Medullary carcinoma of the thyroid
AANF	Atrial naturetic factor	L	Atrial amyloid; localized

disease. In Aβ2M amyloidosis, deposits tend to occur in synovial membrane, cartilage, and bone, but visceral organs are sometimes affected. In ATTR amyloidosis, the nervous system, heart, and thyroid are frequently affected organs, with only small deposits found elsewhere.

All amyloid deposits stain with Congo red dye and exhibit a unique green birefringence by polarized light microscop,[13] although the deposits also can be recognized on routine hematoxylin and eosin (H&E)-stained sections. Typing of the amyloid deposits can usually be done with conventional immunohistochemical staining. For cases difficult to interpret, additional typing with immunoelectron polarized light microscopy has been used.[14] By electron microscopy, all amyloid fibrils are 8- to 10-nm wide and of varying lengths, with a 2.5- to 3.5-nm filamentous subunit arranged along the long axis of the fibril in a slow twist.[15]

PATHOGENESIS OF AMYLOID FIBRIL FORMATION

The exact mechanism of fibril formation is unknown and may be different among the various types of amyloid.[16,17] However, studies suggest there may be a common underlying mechanism in which a partially unfolded protein intermediate forms multimers and then higher-order polymers. Some of the factors that contribute to fibrillogenesis may include variant or unstable protein structure, extensive β-conformation of the precursor protein, proteolytic processing of the precursor protein, association with components of the serum or extracellular matrix (e.g., amyloid P-component, amyloid enhancing factor, apolipoprotein E, or glycosaminoglycans), and physical properties including pH of the tissue site.

AL amyloidosis is a plasma cell dyscrasia with an excess of clonal plasma cells in the bone marrow and can occur in isolation or along with multiple myeloma. Similar cytogenetic changes have been identified in both plasma cell diseases, suggesting they may have a common molec-ular pathogenesis.[18] The amyloid fibril deposits are composed of intact 23-kD monoclonal Ig light chains or smaller fragments, 11 to 18 kD in size, representing the variable or the variable and a portion of the constant region of the light chain.[19,20] Although all kappa (κ) and lambda (λ) light-chain subtypes have been identified in amyloid fibrils, λ subtypes predominate, and the λ VI subtype appears to have unique structural properties that predispose it to fibril formation,[21] often in the kidney.[22] AL amyloidosis is usually a rapidly progressive disease with amyloid deposits in multiple tissue sites.

The AA type of amyloidosis is a complication of severe, long-standing inflammation, as occurs in rheumatic diseases or infection. The AA amyloid fibrils are usually composed of an 8-kD, 76-amino acid amino-terminal portion of the 12-kD precursor, serum amyloid A (SAA).[23] SAA is a polymorphic protein encoded by a family of SAA genes, which are acute-phase apoproteins synthesized in the liver and transported by high-density lipoprotein, HDL3, in the plasma.[24] Several years of an underlying inflammatory disease causing an elevated SAA usually precedes fibril formation, although infections can produce AA deposition more quickly. AA fibril formation can be accelerated by an amyloid enhancing factor present in high concentration in the spleen (which may be early SAA aggregates or deposits), by basement membrane heparan sulfate proteoglycan, or by seeding with AA or heterologous fibrils.[25,26]

Factors related to β₂M-fibril formation are under investigation. The high prevalence of Aβ₂M disease in patients undergoing long-term dialysis argues against an amyloidogenic variant β₂-microglobulin molecule. Permeability of dialysis membranes may be a factor, as the molecular weight of β₂-microglobulin is 11.8 kD, above the porosity of standard membranes. It has been hypothesized that dialysis membranes may be bioincompatible and induce proinflammatory mediators that stimulate β₂-microglobulin and contribute to fibril formation.[27]

In ATTR (also called familial amyloidotic polyneuropathy), and all other forms of familial amyloidosis, the variant structure of the precursor protein is the most important factor in fibrillogenesis. Fibrillogenesis is hypothesized to occur when the variant structure interferes at certain critical regions with the conformation of the folded β-structured molecule.[28-30] The role of aging is intriguing, because patients with the variant proteins do not have clinically apparent disease until mid- or later life, despite the lifelong presence of the abnormal protein. Further evidence of an age-related "trigger" is that senile cardiac amyloidosis, caused by the deposition of fibrils derived from normal TTR, is exclusively a disease of elderly people.[12]

Diagnosis

A tissue biopsy demonstrating amyloid fibrils is necessary for the diagnosis of amyloidosis (Fig. 104–1). The least invasive biopsy is the abdominal fat aspirate, which is positive in 80 to 90 percent of patients with either AL or ATTR amyloidosis and in 60 to 70 percent of patients with AA amyloidosis.[31,32] It is easy to perform after local injection of anesthetic and has a low rate of infectious or hemorrhagic complications (Fig. 104–12). If the aspirate is negative but clinical suspicion for disease persists, a more invasive tissue biopsy should be done. Although a biopsy of a clinically involved organ is rec-

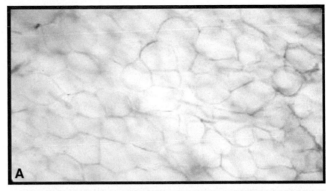
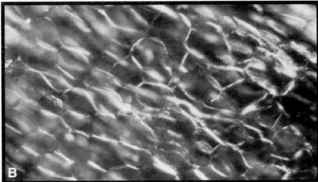

FIGURE 104–2 · Subcutaneous Fat Aspirate Stained with Congo Red. *A,* Sample viewed by light microscopy. *B,* Sample viewed under polarized light (×200). The staining and birefringence is evident in the walls and connective tissue surrounding the adipose cells. (See color plate 44.)

CLINICAL SUSPICION OF AMYLOID DISEASE

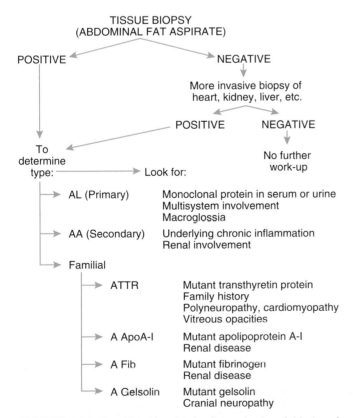

FIGURE 104–1 · Algorithm for the diagnosis of amyloidosis and determination of type.

ommended, almost any tissue biopsy is likely to be positive if the patient has systemic amyloidosis: In a series of 100 patients with AL amyloidosis, 85 percent of 249 tissues biopsied were positive, including all samples from the kidney, heart, and liver.[33] Once the diagnosis of amyloidosis is made, a careful evaluation of the entire clinical picture, including manner of presentation, organ system involvement, underlying diseases, and family history, should provide a clue to the type of amyloid. However, routine laboratory testing is available only for the AL type.

Identification of a plasma cell dycrasia distinguishes AL from other types of amyloidosis (Fig. 104–3). More than 90 percent of patients have a serum or urine monoclonal Ig protein or a free light chain on testing by immunofixation electrophoresis or by a recently available nephelometric assay for free light chains.[34] In addition, there is often an increased percentage of plasma cells in the bone marrow, which are monoclonal on immunohistochemical staining[35] (Fig. 104–4). A monoclonal serum protein by itself is not diagnostic of amyloidosis, because monoclonal gammopathy of uncertain significance (MGUS) is common in older patients. However, when MGUS is present in a patient with biopsy-proven amyloidosis, the AL type is strongly suspected. Immunohistochemical staining may not be that useful, as AL deposits can bind many antisera nonspecifically. Immunoelectron microscopy can be more reliable,[14] but is not widely available. Mass spectrometry–based microsequencing of small amounts of protein extracted from

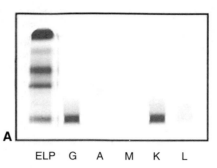

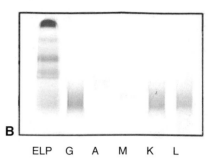

FIGURE 104-3 · A, Pretreatment serum immunofixation electrophoresis shows an immunoglobulin G kappa (IgGκ) monoclonal protein. B, Post-treatment serum immunofixation electrophoresis shows absence of the monoclonal protein.

A   ELP G   A   M   K   L

B   ELP G   A   M   K   L

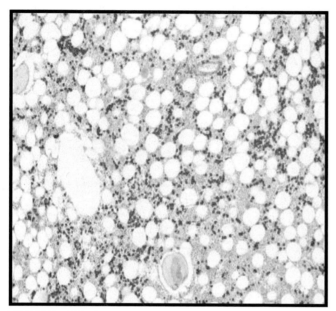

FIGURE 104-4 · Bone marrow biopsy specimen stained with antibody to λ light chain shows preferential staining of plasma cells as well as staining of amyloid deposit around a blood vessel (×400). (See color plate 45.)

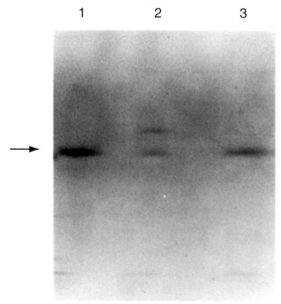

FIGURE 104-5 · Isoelectric focusing of serum samples shows bands of both variant and wild-type transthyretin (TTR) protein (*arrow*) from a patient with ATTR (*lane 2*) and a single band of wild-type TTR in normal subjects (*lanes 1 and 3*). (See color plate 46.)

fibril deposits may ultimately be the most reliable way to identify the components of the fibrils.[36]

AA amyloidosis is suspected in patients with renal amyloidosis and a chronic inflammatory condition or infection. AL and ATTR amyloidosis must be ruled out and confirmation of AA amyloidosis made by immunohistochemical staining for AA protein.

Familial ATTR amyloidosis must be excluded in every patient who does not have a plasma cell dyscrasia or the AA type of amyloidosis. Although the disease has a dominant inheritance, family history may not be apparent when the disease occurs later in life; also, some cases occur through new mutation. Variant TTR proteins can usually be detected by isoelectric focusing (IEF)[37] (Fig. 104-5). An abnormal IEF should prompt genetic testing to determine the precise TTR mutation. Genetic testing should also be employed when screening tests fail to identify the fibril protein. Using polymerase chain reaction, PCR-based sequencing, abnormal fibrinogens and apolipoproteins can be detected.[9]

Clinical Features and Treatment of the Systemic Amyloidoses

AL AMYLOIDOSIS

AL amyloidosis usually occurs in persons of middle age or older, but it can also occur in the third or fourth decade of life. It has a wide spectrum of organ system involvement, and presenting features reflect the organs most prominently affected.[38] Initial symptoms of fatigue and weight loss are frequent, but the diagnosis is rarely made until symptoms referable to a specific organ appear. The kidneys are commonly affected; renal amyloidosis is manifested by proteinuria, sometimes massive, with edema and hypoalbuminemia. Mild renal dysfunction is frequent, but rapidly progressing renal failure is rare. Cardiac involvement, often with congestive heart failure, is a common presentation.[39] The electrocardiogram may show low voltage with a pattern of myocardial infarction. The echocardiogram frequently shows concentrically thickened ventricles and a normal or mildly reduced ejection fraction. Nervous system features include peripheral sensory neuropathy, carpal tunnel syndrome, and autonomic dysfunction with gastrointestinal motility disturbances (early satiety, diarrhea, constipation) and orthostatic hypotension. Macroglossia, a classic feature pathognomonic of AL amyloidosis, is found in 10 percent

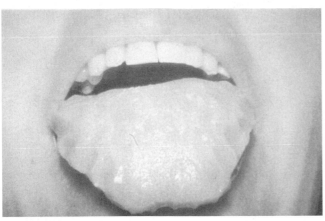

FIGURE 104-6 · Pathognomonic macroglossia in a patient with AL amyloidosis. (See color plate 47.) (See color plate 47.)

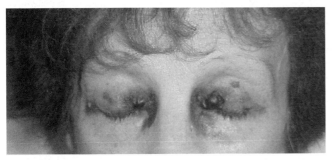

FIGURE 104-7 · Periorbital ecchymoses in a patient with AL amyloidosis. (See color plate 48.) (See color plate 48.)

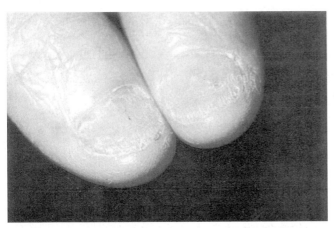

FIGURE 104-8 · Fingernail dystrophy in a patient with AL amyloidosis. (See color plate 49.)

of patients (Fig. 104–6). Hepatomegaly may be massive with mild cholestatic abnormalities of liver function, although liver failure is uncommon, even when hepatomegaly is massive. The spleen is frequently involved, and there may be functional hyposplenism even in the absence of significant splenomegaly. Cutaneous ecchymoses are common, particularly around the eyes, giving the "raccoon-eyes" sign, and appear spontaneously or when provoked by minor trauma (Fig. 104–7). Other findings include nail dystrophy (Fig. 104–8), alopecia, and amyloid arthropathy with thickening of synovial membranes. Timely diagnosis of AL amyloidosis is criti-

cal, and patients with any of these clinical syndromes should have immunofixation electrophoresis performed; the sensitivity of serum or urine protein electrophoresis without immunofixation is inadequate for diagnosis.

Extensive multisystem involvement typifies AL amyloidosis, and median survival with no treatment is usually only about 1 year from diagnosis. Current therapies target the clonal bone marrow plasma cells using chemotherapy approaches employed for multiple myeloma (Table 104–2). Cyclic oral melphalan and prednisone can decrease the plasma-cell burden but produce complete hematologic remission in only a few percent of patients and modestly increase median survival.[33,40]

High-dose intravenous (IV) melphalan followed by autologous stem cell transplantation appears to be far more effective than oral melphalan and prednisone. Of more than 300 patients treated on such protocols at Boston Medical Center, approximately 40 percent of evaluable patients achieve a hematologic complete response, and most of these enjoy significant improvement or stabilization of organ function.[41] Median survival in the treated patients exceeds 4.5 years. Smaller series from other centers have found similar results.[42-45] Unfortunately, only about half of AL amyloidosis patients are eligible for such aggressive treatment, and even at specialized treatment centers, peritransplant mortality is high in these patients because of underlying impaired organ function (14% in the Boston Medical Center series). Some of the factors that contribute to mortality are amyloid cardiomyopathy, nutritional status as measured by weight loss, performance status, and—in some studies—number of involved organs. The bleeding diathesis due to absorption of clotting factor X to amyloid fibrils also confers high mortality during myelosuppressive therapy. However, age alone or renal insufficiency should not exclude patients from such treatment.

For patients with impaired cardiac function or arrhythmias due to amyloid involvement of the myocardium, median survival is only about 6 months without treatment, and stem cell mobilization and high-dose chemotherapy are extremely morbid. In a few such patients, cardiac transplantation has been performed followed by treatment with IV melphalan and stem cell rescue to prevent fibrillogenesis in the transplanted heart or other organs.

Alternative chemotherapy approaches are being investigated. Innovative approaches target the amyloid fibrils themselves or accessory binding proteins. The anthracycline derivative 4'-iodo-4'-deoxydoxorubicin (IDOX) was serendipitously noted to cause resorption of amyloid deposits in model systems, but preliminary trials with single agent IDOX have not produced clinically significant responses.[46,47] R-1-[6-[R-2-carboxy-pyrrolidin-1-yl]-6-oxo-hexanoyl]pyrrolidine-2-carboxylic acid (CPHPC) binds serum amyloid P protein and accelerates clearance from the circulation and from amyloid fibrils;[48] its potential efficacy in promoting fibril resorption and reducing amyloid disease is under study.

Supportive treatment is recommended for patients with all types of amyloidosis (Table 104–3). At times, supportive treatments are lifesaving (e.g., heart or kidney transplantation, renal dialysis, cardiac pacemaker, and nutritional support). It is important to note that

TABLE 104–2 • MAJOR TREATMENT OPTIONS FOR AMYLOIDOSIS

AL (Primary) Amyloidosis

Intravenous (IV) melphalan with autologous stem cell rescue
Granulocyte colony-stimulating factor (G-CSF) mobilized
   peripheral blood stem cell collection
IV melphalan: 140 to 200 mg/m2 during 2 days
Autologous stem cell reinfusion (day 0)
Cyclic oral melphalan and prednisone
Melphalan* 0.15 to 0.25 mg/kg/day for 4 days
Prednisone 0.8 to 1.5 mg/kg/day for 4 days
Repeat administration every 6 weeks as tolerated, up to
   600 mg of melphalan
Other antiplasma cell chemotherapy or immunomodulators
   such as thalidomide
Antifibril drugs (e.g. IDOX, CPHPC) in development

AA (Secondary) Amyloidosis

Aggressive treatment of underlying inflammatory disease
Medical or surgical treatment of underlying infection
Colchicine (1.2 to 1.8 mg/day) for AA amyloidosis secondary to
   familial Mediterranean fever
Antifibril drugs (e.g. Fibrillex) in development

ATTR (Familial) Amyloidosis

Orthotopic liver transplantation
Antifibril drugs (e.g. CPHPC) in development

*White blood cell and platelet counts must be determined every 3 weeks and the dosage of melphalan adjusted so that leukopenia occurs at midcycle and platelets are maintained at more than 100,000/mm³.

digitalis, calcium-channel blockers, and beta blockers are relatively contraindicated as toxicity has been observed at therapeutic levels.

AA AMYLOIDOSIS

AA amyloidosis can occur at any age. The primary clinical manifestation is proteinuria, renal insufficiency, or both.[4] A study from Finland found AA amyloidosis to be the most common cause of nephrotic syndrome in patients with rheumatoid arthritis (RA).[49] Hepatomegaly, splenomegaly, and autonomic neuropathy frequently occur as the disease progresses; cardiomyopathy occurs rarely. With chronic inflammatory diseases, amyloid progression is slow and survival is often more than 10 years, particularly with treatment for end-stage renal disease. In contrast, untreated infections such as osteomyelitis, tuberculosis, or leprosy can produce a more rapidly progressive amyloid syndrome, which will remit with effective medical or surgical treatment of the infection.

The major therapy in AA amyloidosis is treatment of the underlying inflammatory or infectious disease. Treatment that suppresses or eliminates the inflammation or infection also decreases the SAA protein. For familial Mediterranean fever, colchicine in a dose of 1.2 to 1.8 mg/day is the appropriate treatment. Colchicine has not been helpful for AA amyloidosis of other causes or for other amyloidoses. A multicenter trial using a new antiamyloid drug, Fibrillex™, is underway for the treatment of AA amyloidosis. Fibrillex has been

designed to interfere with the interaction of AA amyloid protein with glycosaminoglycans in tissues and, thus, prevent fibril formation and deposition.

Aβ₂M AMYLOIDOSIS

Several distinct rheumatologic conditions are observed in Aβ₂M amyloidosis, including carpal tunnel syndrome, persistent joint effusions, spondyloarthropathy, and cystic bone lesions. Carpal tunnel syndrome is usually the first symptom of disease. Persistent joint effusions accompanied by mild discomfort occur in up to 50 percent of patients on dialysis for more than 12 years. Involvement is bilateral, and large joints (shoulders, knees, wrists, and hips) are more frequently affected. The synovial fluid is noninflammatory, and β₂-microglobulin amyloid deposits can be found if the sediment is examined with Congo red staining. Spondyloarthropathy with destructive changes of the intervertebral disks and paravertebral erosions have occurred in association with β₂-microglobulin amyloid deposits. Cystic bone lesions sometimes leading to pathologic fractures have been described in the femoral head, acetabulum, humerus, tibial plateau, vertebral bodies, and carpal bones. Although less common, visceral β₂-microglobulin amyloid deposits do occasionally occur in the gastrointestinal tract, heart, tendons, and subcutaneous tissues of the buttocks.

The treatment for Aβ₂M amyloidosis is difficult because the 11-kD β₂-microglobulin molecule is too large to pass through a dialysis membrane. However, consistent with a postulated role of copper in initiating Aβ₂M fibrillogenesis,[50] copper-free dialysis membranes appear to reduce the incidence of disease. Furthermore, patients on chronic ambulatory peritoneal dialysis usually have lower plasma levels of β₂-microglobulin than those on hemodialysis and may not develop amyloid deposits as quickly. Symptoms of arthropathy are common and prevalence may approach 100 percent of individuals on dialysis for more than 15 years. Patients who have received kidney transplants after developing Aβ₂M report an improvement in symptoms.

ATTR FAMILIAL AMYLOIDOSIS

The clinical features of ATTR amyloidosis overlap AL amyloidosis such that the diseases cannot be reliably distinguished on clinical grounds alone. A family history makes ATTR more likely, but many patients appear to present sporadically with new mutations. Within each family, disease begins at nearly the same age and symptoms usually include neuropathy, cardiomyopathy, or both. Peripheral neuropathy begins as a lower-extremity sensory and motor neuropathy and progresses to the upper extremities. Autonomic neuropathy includes gastrointestinal symptoms of diarrhea with weight loss and orthostatic hypotension. Patients with TTR Val-30-Met, the most common mutation, have normal echocardiograms but may have conduction system defects and require a pacemaker. Patients with TTR Thr-60-Ala and several other mutations have myocardial thickening similar to that caused by AL amyloidosis, although heart failure is less common and the prognosis is better. Vitreous opacities caused by amyloid deposits are pathognomonic of ATTR amyloidosis.

TABLE 104–3 · SUPPORTIVE TREATMENT FOR ALL TYPES OF AMYLOIDOSIS

Organ System	Symptom	Treatment Options
Cardiac	Congestive failure	Salt restriction of 1 to 2 g/day
		Diuretics: furosemide, spironolactone, metolazone
	Arrhythmia	Pacemaker
		Automatic implantable cardiac defibrillator
		Antiarrhythmics
Renal	Nephrotic syndrome	Salt restriction of 1 to 2 g/day
		Elastic stockings, leg elevation
		Maintain dietary protein
		Angiotensin converting enzyme inhibitor, if blood pressure tolerates
	Renal failure	Dialysis (chronic ambulatory peritoneal dialysis or hemodialysis)
Autonomic nervous	Orthostatic hypotension	Midodrine (ProAmatine)
		Increase dietary salt or add fludrocortisone, depending on edema
		Elastic stockings
	Gastric atony or ileus	Small, frequent feedings (6/day) low in fat
		Oral nutritional supplements
		Jejunostomy tube feeding
		Parenteral nutrition
Gastrointestinal	Diarrhea	Low-fat diet (40 g or less/day)
		Psyllium hydrophilic muciloid (Metamucil)
		Loperamide hydrochloride (Imodium)
		Tincture of opium
		Parenteral nutrition
	Macroglossia	Soft solid diet
		Partial glossectomy (rarely effective)
Peripheral nervous	Sensory neuropathy	Avoid trauma
		Gabapentin (Neurontin): 100 to 300 mg 3 times daily
		Amitriptyline: 25 to 50 mg at bedtime
		Carbamazepine (Tegretol)
	Motor neuropathy	Shoe braces for foot drop
		Physical therapy
Hematologic	Intracutaneous bleeding	Avoid trauma, antiplatelet agents
	Factor X deficiency	Factor replacement (recombinant factor VIIa, prothrombin complex concentrates)
		Consider splenectomy if splenomegaly present

The TTR variant, Val 122 Ile, is a common allele in the black population and appears to be associated with cardiomyopathy. In a large referral population, 25 percent of black patients with amyloidosis had this TTR variant.[51] It is likely that this disease is underdiagnosed due to a lack of physician awareness and the difficulty of distinguishing amyloid and hypertensive cardiomyopathy without an endomyocardial biopsy.[11]

Without intervention, survival after ATTR disease onset is 5 to 15 years. Orthotopic liver transplantation, which removes the major source of variant TTR production and replaces it with normal TTR, is the major treatment for ATTR amyloidosis.[52] Liver transplantation arrests disease progression, and some improvement in autonomic and peripheral neuropathy can occur.[53] Cardiomyopathy has not improved, and in some patients appears to have worsened, after liver transplantation.[54] Long-term outcome and the timing of transplantation are being evaluated.[55] Waiting periods for organ donation are frequently long, and optimal benefit requires transplantation before severe disability occurs.

Summary

Treatment of the amyloidoses begins with recognition of the clinical amyloid syndromes and obtaining appropriate biopsies and screening tests to rule in or out AL amyloidosis. For difficult cases and for identification of variant serum proteins, amyloid referral centers can provide specialized diagnostic techniques. Effective therapy is now available for AL and ATTR amyloidosis. An understanding of the biophysical properties of amyloid proteins and of the mechanisms of protein misfolding in a wide variety of diseases will enable the further development of more specific and less toxic antifibril drugs.

REFERENCES

1. Virchow VR: Ueber einem Gehirn and Rueckenmark des Menchen auf gefundene Substanz mit chemischen reaction der Cellulose. Virchows Arch Pathol Anat 6;135-138, 1854.
2. Westermark P, Benson MD, Buxbaum JN, et al: Amyloid fibril protein nomenclature 2002. Amyloid 9:197-200, 2002.
3. Simms RW, Prout MN, Cohen AS: The epidemiology of AL and AA amyloidosis. Bailliere Clin Rheumatol 8:627-634, 1994.
4. Gertz MA, Kyle RA: Secondary systemic amyloidosis: response and survival in 64 patients. Medicine 70:246-256, 1991.
5. David J, Vouyiouka O, Ansell BM, et al: Amyloidosis in juvenile chronic arthritis: a morbidity and mortality study. Clin Exper Rheumatol 11:85-90, 1993.
6. Livneh A, Langevitz P, Shinar Y, et al: MEFV mutation analysis in patients suffering from amyloidosis of familial Mediterranean fever. Amyloid 6:1-6, 1999.
7. Danesh F, Ho LT: Dialysis-related amyloidosis: history and clinical manifestations. Semin Dialysis 14:80-85, 2001.
8. Schwalbe S, Holzhauer M, Schaeffer J, et al: Beta 2-microgulin associated amyloidosis: a vanishing complication of long-term hemodialysis? Kidney Int 52:1077-1083, 1997.

9. Benson MD: Amyloidosis. *In* Scriver CR, Beaudet AL, Sly WS, Valle D (eds): The Metabolic and Molecular Bases of Inherited Disease. New York, McGraw-Hill, 1999, pp 4159-4191.

10. Connors LH, Richardson AM, Theberge R, Costello CE: Tabulation of transthyretin (TTR) variants as of 1/1/2000. Amyloid: Int J Exp Clin Invest 7:54-69, 2000.

11. Jacobson DR, Pastore RD, Yaghoubian R, et al: Variant-sequence transthyretin (isoleucine 122) in late-onset cardiac amyloidosis in black Americans [see comments]. New Engl J Med 336:466-473, 1997.

12. Kyle RA, Spittell PC, Gertz MA, et al: The premortem recognition of systemic senile amyloidosis with cardiac involvement. Am J Med 101:395-400, 1996.

13. Bennhold H: Eine spezifische Amyloidfarbung mit Kongorot. Munch Med Wochenschr 69:1537-1538, 1922.

14. Arbustini E, Morbini P, Verga L, et al: Light and electrom microscopy immunohistochemical characterization of amyloid deposits. Amyloid: Int J Exp Clin Invest 4:157-170, 1997.

15. Shirahama T, Cohen AS: High-resolution electron microscopic analysis of the amyloid fibril. J Cell Biol 33:679-708, 1967.

16. Westermark P: The pathogenesis of amyloidosis: understanding general principles [comment]. Am J Pathol 152:1125-1127, 1998.

17. Bellotti V, Mangione P, Merlini G: Review: Immunoglogulin light chain amyloidosis–the archetype of structural and pathologic variability. J Struct Biol 130:280-289, 2000.

18. Hayman SR, Bailey RJ, Jalal SM, et al: Translocations involving the immunoglobulin heavy-chain locus are possibly early genetic events in patients with primary systemic amyloidosis. Blood 98:2266-2268, 2001.

19. Glenner GG: Amyloid deposits and amyloidosis: the beta-fibril-loses (second of two parts). New Engl J Med 302:1333-1343, 1980.

20. Wally J, Kica G, Zhang Y, et al: Identification of a novel substitution in the constant region of a gene coding for an amyloidogenic kappa1 light chain. Biochim Biophys Acta 1454:49-56, 1999.

21. Solomon A, Frangione B, Franklin EC: Bence Jones proteins and light chains of immunoglobulins. Preferential association of the V lambda VI subgroup of human light chains with amyloidosis AL (lambda). J Clin Invest 70:453-460, 1982.

22. Comenzo RL, Zhang Y, Martinez C, et al: The tropism of organ involvement in primary systemic amyloidosis. Blood 98:714-720, 2001.

23. Husby G, Marhung G, Dowton B, et al: Serum amyloid A (SAA): biochemistry, genetics, and the pathogenesis of AA amyloidosis. Amyloid: Int J Exp Clin Invest 1:119-137, 1994.

24. Kluve-Beckerman B, Dwulet FE, Benson MD: Human serum amyloid A. J Clin Invest 82:1670-1675, 1988.

25. Kisilevsky R, Gruys E, Shirahama T: Does amyloid enhancing factor (AEF) exist? Is AEF a single biological entity? Amyloid: Int J Exp Clin Invest 2:128-133, 1995.

26. Johan K, Westermark G, Engstrom U, et al: Acceleration of amyloid protein A amyloidosis by amyloid-like synthetic fibrils. Proc Nat Acad Sci U S A 95:2558-2563, 1998.

27. Zingraff J, Drueke T: Beta2-microglobulin amyloidosis: past and future. Artificial Organs 22:581-584, 1998.

28. Serpell LC, Goldstein G, Dacklin I, et al: The "edge strand" hypothesis: prediction and test of a mutational "hot-spot" on the transthyretin molecule associated with FAP amyloidogenesis. Amyloid: Int J Exp Clin Invest 3:75-85, 1996.

29. Kelly JW: Amyloid fibril formation and protein misassembly: a structural quest for insights into amyloid and prion diseases. Structure 5:595-600, 1997.

30. Quintas A, Saraiva MJ, Brito RM: The tetrameric protein transthyretin dissociated to a non-native monomer in solution. A novel model for amyloidogenesis. J Biol Chem 274:32943-32949, 1999.

31. Libbey CA, Skinner M, Cohen AS: Use of abdominal fat tissue aspirate in the diagnosis of systemic amyloidosis. Arch Intern Med 143:1549-1552, 1983.

32. Duston MA, Skinner M, Shirahama T, Cohen AS: Diagnosis of amyloidosis by abdominal fat aspiration. Analysis of four years' experience. Am J Med 82:412-414, 1987.

33. Skinner M, Anderson J, Simms R, et al: Treatment of 100 patients with primary amyloidosis: a randomized trial of melphalan, prednisone, and colchicine versus colchicine only. Am J Med 100: 290-298, 1996.

34. Abraham RS, Clark RJ, Bryant SC, et al: Correlation of serum immunoglobulin free light chain quantification with urinary Bence Jones protein in light chain myeloma. Clin Chem 48: 655-657, 2002.

35. Kyle RA, Gertz MA: Primary systemic amyloidosis: clinical and laboratory features in 474 cases. Semin Hematol 32:45-59, 1995.

36. Lim A, Wally J, Walsh MT, et al: Identification and localization of a cysteinyl posttranslational modification in an amyloidogenic kappa 1 light chain protein by electrospray ionization and matrix-assisted laser desoption/ionization mass spectrometry. Anal Biochem 295:45-56, 2001.

37. Connors LH, Ericsson T, Skare J, et al: A simple screening test for variant transthyretins associated with familial transthyretin amyloidosis using isoelectric focusing. Biochim Biophys Acta 1407:185-192, 1998.

38. Falk RH, Comenzo RL, Skinner M: The systemic amyloidoses [see comments]. New Engl J Med 337:898-909, 1997.

39. Dubrey SW, Cha K, Anderson J, et al: The clinical features of immunoglobulin light-chain (AL) amyloidosis with heart involvement. QJM 91:141-57, 1998.

40. Kyle RA, Gertz MA, Greipp PR, et al: A trial of three regimens for primary amyloidosis: colchicine alone, melphalan and prednisone, and melphalan, prednisone, and colchicine [see comments]. New Engl J Med 336:1202-1207, 1997.

41. Sanchorawala V, Wright D, Seldin D, et al: Use of high dose melphalan with autologous stem cell transplantation for the treatment of AL amyloidosis. Bone Marrow Trans 28:637-642, 2001.

42. Moreau P, Leblond V, Bourquelot P, et al: Prognostic factors for survival and response after high-dose therapy and autologous stem cell transplantation in systemic AL amyloidosis: a report on 21 patients. Br J Haematol 101:766-769, 1998.

43. Gillmore JD, Apperley JF, Craddock C, et al: High-dose melphalan and stem cell rescue for AL amyloidosis. *In* Kyle RA, Gertz MA (eds): Amyloid and Amyloidosis 1998. New York, Parthenon Publishing Group, 1999, pp 102-104.

44. Gertz MA, Lacy MQ, Dispenzieri A: Myeloablative chemotherapy with stem cell rescue for the treatment of primary systemic amyloidosis: a status report. Bone Marrow Trans 25:465-470, 2000.

45. vanGameren II, Hazenberg BPC, Jager PL, et al: AL amyloidosis treated with induction chemotherapy with VAD followed by high dose melphalan and autologous stem cell transplantation. Amyloid: J. Protein Folding Disorders 9:165-174, 2002.

46. Gianni L, Bellotti V, Gianni AM, Merlini G: New drug therapy of amyloidoses: resorption of AL-type deposits with 4'-iodo-4'-deoxy-doxorubicin. Blood 86:855-861, 1995.

47. Gertz MA, Lacy MQ, Dispenzieri A, et al: A multicenter phase II trial of 4'-iodo-4'-deoxydoxorubicin (IDOX) in primary amyloidosis (AL). Amyloid: J Protein Folding Disorders 9:24-30, 2002.

48. Pepys MB, Herbert J, Hutchinson WL, et al: Targeted pharmacological depletion of serum amyloid P component (SAP) for treatment of human amyloidosis. Nature 417:254-259, 2002.

49. Helin HJ, Korpela MM, Mustonen JT, Pasternack AI: Renal biopsy findings and clinicopathologic correlations in rheumatoid arthritis. Arthritis Rheum 38:242-247, 1995.

50. Morgan CJ, Gelfand M, Atreya C, Miranker AD: Kidney dialysis-associated amyloidosis: a molecular role for copper in fiber formation. J Mol Biol 309:339-345, 2001.

51. Berg A, Falk RH, Connors LH, et al: Transthyretin ILE-122 in a series of black patients with amyloidosis. *In* Kyle RA, Gertz MA (eds): Amyloid and Amyloidosis 1998. New York, Parthenon Publishing Group, 1999, 556-558.

52. Holmgren G, Steen L, Ekstedt J, et al: Biochemical effect of liver transplantation in two Swedish patients with familial amyloidotic polyneuropathy (FAP-met30). Clin Genet 40:242-246, 1991.

53. Bergethon P, Sabin T, Lewis D, et al: Improvement in the polyneuropathy associated with familial amyloid polyneuropathy after liver transplantation. Neurology 47:944-951, 1996.

54. Dubrey SW, Davidoff R, Skinner M, et al: Progression of ventricular wall thickening after liver transplantation for familial amyloidosis. Transplantation 64:74-80, 1997.

55. de Carvalho M, Conceicao I, Bentes C, Sales Luis ML: Long-term quantitative evaluation of liver transplantation in familial amyloid polyneuropathy (Portuguese V30M). Amyloid: J Protein Folding Disorders 9:126-133, 2002.

105

Sarcoidosis

YASMINE WASFI · RICHARD MEEHAN · LEE S. NEWMAN

Sarcoidosis is a multisystem, inflammatory disorder characterized by noncaseating granulomas that can infiltrate any organ. Most often occurring in early adulthood, sarcoidosis often presents with hilar lymphadenopathy, pulmonary infiltration, and ocular and skin lesions. With protean clinical manifestations, this disorder can mimic many inflammatory and infectious disorders.[1] Particular targets include the lungs, lymphatics, eyes, skin, liver, bone, and neurologic system. This chapter will emphasize, in particular, the rheumatologic and immunologic aspects of this condition.

The diagnosis of sarcoidosis is based largely on 1) demonstration of noncaseating granulomatous disease (Fig. 105–1), often in more than one affected organ; and 2) exclusion of other conditions that can produce similar pathology, including a panoply of infections, autoimmune disorders, and inhalation diseases, as discussed in the differential diagnosis section.

Epidemiology

Sarcoidosis occurs worldwide and affects people of all racial and ethnic backgrounds.[1] Estimated prevalence rates vary from 1 to 40 per 100,000 population. Similarly, there is a range of age-adjusted annual incidence rates, from 10.9 per 100,000 for whites to 35.5 per 100,000 for African Americans in the United States. Such rates likely underestimate the frequency of this disorder, because many cases may go undiagnosed or misdiagnosed. Familial and twin studies demonstrate much higher prevalence of disease in first-generation relatives of those with sarcoidosis.[2] Highest risks for familial sarcoidosis are in African Americans, women, and patients with active disease, although familial risk has also been demonstrated in whites.

Etiology and Pathogenesis

The cause of sarcoidosis remains unknown. Spatial and temporal clustering of cases, reports of community outbreaks, as well as reports of work-related risk for health care workers, suggest either shared environmental exposure or possibly person-to-person transmission. Careful environmental investigation of new cases sometimes uncovers clusters of disease and may suggest sources of antigen exposures or exposures to known causes of granulomatous disease. However, no single infective agent or antigen has been consistently linked to sarcoidosis. The possibility that an infection, especially due to mycobacteria, causes sarcoidosis has been considered in multiple studies. The published data using available tissue-staining, culture, and molecular-genetic methods are contradictory and by no means compelling.

The prevailing hypothesis is that this disease results from a cell-mediated hypersensitivity response to one or more agents (bacteria, fungi, virus, chemical) in persons with either inherited or acquired predisposition. Current lines of evidence suggest that sarcoidal granulomas form as a result of 1) antigen exposure, 2) an antigen-specific cell-mediated immune response, and 3) inflammatory or innate immune responses that amplify and perpetuate the antigen-specific immunologic reaction.

The disease is mediated primarily through cell determinant (CD)4+ T helper cells and cells derived from the mononuclear phagocytes.[3] These cells accumulate within affected tissue, where they become increasingly organized and form noncaseating granulomas. Recent reviews describe in detail the current state of knowledge on the immune and inflammatory events.[4-6]

The earliest manifestation of sarcoidosis is a mononuclear infiltration of the target organ, which precedes granuloma formation. This infiltrative process is thought to be mediated primarily by CD4+ T lymphocytes and mononuclear phagocytes, although other inflammatory cells (e.g., mast cells, fibroblasts), as well as epithelial and endothelial cells, may contribute to the nonspecific inflammatory response leading to increased tissue permeability and cell migration. The recruitment of mononuclear cells in sarcoidosis is enhanced by the production of chemokines, including "regulated on activation normal T expressed secreted" (RANTES), macrophage chemoattractant protein-1 (MCP-1), macrophage inflammatory protein-1α (MIP-1α, and interleukin-8 (IL-8). Additionally, adhesion molecules, such as intercellular adhesion molecule-1 (ICAM-1), vascular cell adhesion molecule-1 (VCAM-1), and the selectins, are chemoattractant and promote cell binding.

As a consequence of chemoattractant signals, at early stages of sarcoidosis an elevated lymphocyte count and a marked increase in the CD4-to-CD8 T lymphocyte ratio is observed in affected organs, such as the lungs. Effector cells such as dendritic cells and macrophages may function by presenting antigen to T cells and by producing proinflammatory cytokines, such as IL-12 and IL-15. IL-12 induces the differentiation of naïve CD4+ T lymphocytes into T helper type 1 (Th1) cells and promotes the release of interferon-gamma (IFN-γ).

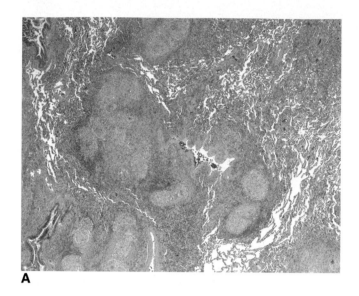

A

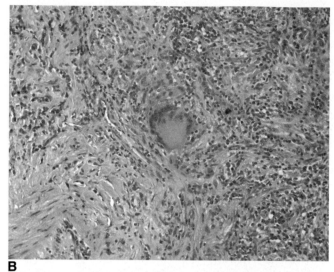

B

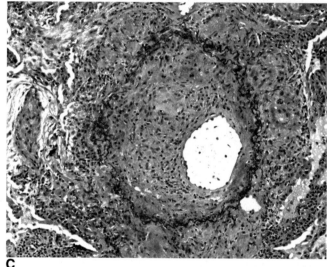

C

FIGURE 105–1 • *A,* The typical pathologic appearance of sarcoidosis consists of non-necrotizing granulomas, which are mononuclear cell infiltrates with varying degrees of adjacent collagen deposition. Shown here is lung tissue (×100, H&E), the most commonly affected organ, infiltrated by multiple noncaseating granulomas adjacent to vessels and bronchioles. *B,* This ×400 photomicrograph demonstrates the classic, but not pathognomonic, features of the noncaseating granuloma, including multinucleated giant cell (at center), abundant lymphocytes, macrophages, epithelioid cells, mast cells, plasma cells, and fibroblasts. *C,* Although uncommon, sarcoidosis can cause a non-necrotizing granulomatous vasculitis in virtually any organ. Shown is a ×200 view of a pulmonary artery using an elastic tissue Verhoeff Van Gieson, (VVG), stain. The elastic lamina (dark stain) is intact. Within the intima is a large area of non-necrotizing granulomatous inflammation producing a narrowing of the vessel lumen. Efforts must be made to exclude other causes of vasculitis, as discussed in the text. Prognosis is generally poor for this form of sarcoidosis. (See color plate 50.)

Th1 cells in sarcoidosis are antigen-activated CD4+ T lymphocytes and produce IFN-γ and IL-2, resulting in a delayed-type hypersensitivity immune response. IL-15 acts synergistically with IL-2 and tumor necrosis factor-alpha (TNF-α) to stimulate T lymphocyte proliferation.

Sarcoidosis antigen–specific T lymphocytes generated during the initial host response play a central role in mediating the subsequent inflammatory events within the lung. Once naïve T lymphocytes are activated, they undergo clonal expansion and differentiation into effector and memory T lymphocytes. In sarcoidosis, most of the T lymphocytes appear to have been previously stimulated, likely in regional lymph nodes, and to have migrated back to the affected organ. Studies of the T lymphocyte antigen–specific receptor (TCR) repertoire in sarcoidosis demonstrate that the disorder is initiated by an antigen-specific immune response, based on observed oligoclonal expansion of T lymphocyte subsets bearing particular, restricted alpha/beta TCR. Lymphocytes bearing gamma/delta TCR are unlikely to play a role in the pathogenesis of this disorder. Of note, a body of work from Sweden demonstrated Vα2.3 CD4+ T lymphocytes within the lungs that correlated with human leukocyte antigen, (HLA), haplotype DR3 in patients with Lofgren's syndrome and with acute, remitting sarcoidosis.[7,8] These data suggest that the combination of a specific T cell antigen receptor and particular HLA antigen-presentation molecule interact with the putative sarcoidosis antigen to trigger this acute form of disease.

CD4+ T lymphocytes from sarcoidosis patients spontaneously proliferate and release IL-2 and IFN-γ in vitro. The IL-2 stimulates further T lymphocyte proliferation, release of more IL-2 and IFN-γ and is chemotactic, as more T lymphocytes are recruited to the affected site. IFN-γ amplifies the immune response through its effects on multiple target cells.

The release of inflammatory cytokines serves to recruit additional peripheral blood monocytes to the affected organ, where they differentiate into exudate macrophages that show enhanced antigen-presenting capacity and release TNF-α and IL-1β, both of which promote granuloma formation. In light of potential immunotherapeutic advances, it is noteworthy that TNF-α upregulates endothelial cell adhesion molecules involved in leukocyte binding, stimulates T lymphocyte release of IFN-γ, and enhances T lymphocyte proliferation. IL-1β may be needed in granuloma formation because it stimulates exudate macrophage production of IL-8 and granulocyte macrophage-colony stimulating factor (GM-CSF). GM-CSF, in turn, promotes monocyte differentiation and resultant macrophage proliferation. The net result is an amplification loop involving antigen recognition, proinflammatory cytokine release, cell activation, cell recruitment, and granuloma formation.

The progression from granulomatous inflammation to increasing amounts of fibrosis may be a prognostically bad sign in sarcoidosis. Factors leading from granuloma to fibrosis are poorly understood, but probably involve changes in local cytokine and growth factor expression, including transforming growth factor-beta (TGF-β) basic fibroblast growth factor (bFGF), insulin-like growth factor-I (IGF-I), and IL-4.

Clinical Features

Sarcoidosis typically affects multiple organs simultaneously. The majority of patients present with systemic symptoms, such as fatigue, fever, anorexia, and weight loss, plus symptoms referable to the most actively inflamed target organs. Usually the disease appears in patients between the ages of 20 and 50; however, both childhood and geriatric cases occur with some regularity. Presentation can be acute or chronic—a determination that can influence decision making regarding treatment.

Acute sarcoidosis has an abrupt onset and transient course and is often associated with erythema nodosum, or other skin lesions such as vesicles or maculopapular rash. Acute iritis, conjunctivitis, and even conjunctival nodules are common. Bell's palsy may occur prior to, or concomitant with, the acute symptoms. In a study of 55 patients with acute sarcoidosis arthritis, Visser and colleagues found that four clinical features—symmetric ankle arthritis, symptoms for less than 2 months, age less than 40, and erythema nodosum—provided a high degree of diagnostic certainty in an outpatient rheumatology practice in the Netherlands.[8] In acute disease, bone cysts are rare; however, hypercalcemia and hypercalciuria may be found in approximately 20 percent of patients. Chest radiographs typically are normal or show significant hilar and mediastinal lymphadenopathy without pulmonary infiltrates. Arrhythmias may occur due to acute granulomatous cardiac involvement. The acute form has a higher probability of spontaneous resolution. Although relapse may occur, it is thought to be less common than in those patients with more chronic presentation. Prognosis is generally good.

Although a true "dividing line" between chronic and acute forms of disease does not exist, certain features of sarcoidosis enhance the likelihood that the disease will persist. Chronic disease is usually insidious in onset and occurs in older patients. Skin lesions are more typically plaques, keloids, nodules within surgical incision lines and scars, or lupus pernio, which is a persistent, disfiguring, violaceous rash over the nose, cheeks, and ears. Chronic eye involvement includes chronic uveitis, cataracts, glaucoma, or keratoconjunctivitis sicca, which can be confused with Sjögren's syndrome. Compared to the acute presentation, bone involvement is much more common in chronic cases, as are pulmonary infiltrates, nephrocalcinosis, and cardiac involvement with cor pulmonale. Persistence of disease and recurrence after treatment are common in the chronic form.

The remainder of this section will focus on more specifically on the rheumatologic manifestations of sarcoidosis.

BONE

Sarcoidal changes in bone are most commonly found in the hands or feet. Bone lesions are reported in approximately 3 to 13 percent of cases. This is likely an underestimation because osseous lesions are typically asymptomatic and imaging procedures not performed routinely.[9] There is a higher prevalence of radiographically evident osseous disease in the progressive, chronic form of sarcoidosis; in patients with pulmonary involvement; among African-American patients; and in those who have granulomatous skin lesions, especially lupus pernio.

Bone involvement is usually bilateral and asymptomatic, but it may present as localized pain, swelling, and stiffness. Lesions are most commonly lytic, sometimes with associated expansion of the shaft, pathologic fractures, and cavitation. Lesions also may be sclerotic, starting with progressive cortical tunneling and remodeling, and are sometimes associated with rapid destruction, periosteal reaction, and secondary involvement of joint surfaces.[10,11] Involvement of the metacarpals, metatarsals, and phalanges of hands and feet are typical, although any bone can be affected, as suggested by recent case reports and case series describing vertebral, iliac, scapular, and even skull sarcoidosis.[9,12-18]

The classic, lacy-reticular (lytic) radiographic appearance of sarcoidosis usually produces little disturbance of adjacent soft tissues, although sometimes subchondral lesions extend into the joint space.[9] Figure 105–2 illustrates the range of radiographic findings in osseous sarcoidosis, from early disease to the more typical abnormalities found in untreated, advanced disease. Bony cysts have also been observed, sometimes large enough to result in pathologic fractures.[19] Periostitis is rare. Recent reports suggest that bone scans using either 99mTc–methylene diphosphonate or 67Ga citrate may detect bone changes not seen on plain radiographic films. However, abnormalities on these scans are not specific for sarcoidosis and may represent other pathology even in a patient with biopsy-proven sarcoidosis elsewhere.[20,21] Magnetic resonance imaging (MRI) may be more sensitive than plain radiographs for detection of osseous sarcoidosis. On MRI, the lesions may appear hypointense on T1-weighted images and hyperintense on T2–weighted images.[22] Scintigraphy may be superior in detecting multiple bone involvement or osteonecrosis associated with glucocorticoid therapy. MRI probably offers the greater precision needed if biopsies are to be performed or if osteonecrosis is suspected.[23,24] When diagnostic biopsies are performed, they can demonstrate noncaseating granulomas in both the bone marrow and bone cortex.[11]

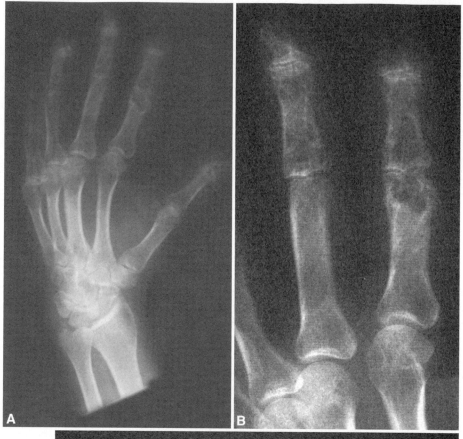

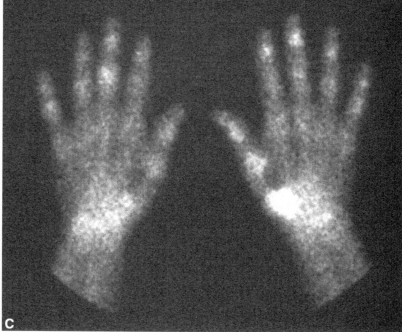

FIGURE 105-2 • *A*, This plain film demonstrates multiple areas of radiolucency, including cystic changes in the small finger metacarpal and proximal phalanx, and index finger proximal and middle phalanx. A destructive process also can be noted in the ulnar styloid, whereas the joint space is well maintained. *B*, A closer view of *A* reveals large cystic lesions involving the subchondral bone adjacent to the proximal interphalangeal joint of the index finger. Similar lesions involve the middle phalanx of the long finger with a reticular pattern of radiolucency. Unrelated osteoarthritis changes can be noted at the proximal and distal interphalangeal joints. *C*, This bone scan demonstrates increased uptake of 99mTc–methylene diphosphonate in the left long finger proximal to the interphalangeal joint region. This corresponds to a subtle lesion visible on the plain film in *D*.

Sarcoid dactylitis is characterized by diffuse soft tissue swelling of the affected digit, and when the terminal phalanx is involved, the proximal nail becomes distorted, thickened, and dystrophic. Dactylitis is often associated with painful stiffness of the adjacent joints and tenderness. The overlying skin may be erythematous. There is marked angular deformity or ankylosis due to bone loss or joint damage in severe cases. Bony involvement may also be associated with a tenosynovitis, as has been reported in several cases involving the wrists.[25-27]

Osteopenia and osteoporosis occur in up to two thirds of patients with sarcoidosis, in part as a consequence of dysregulated calcium metabolism.[28,29] Case series data

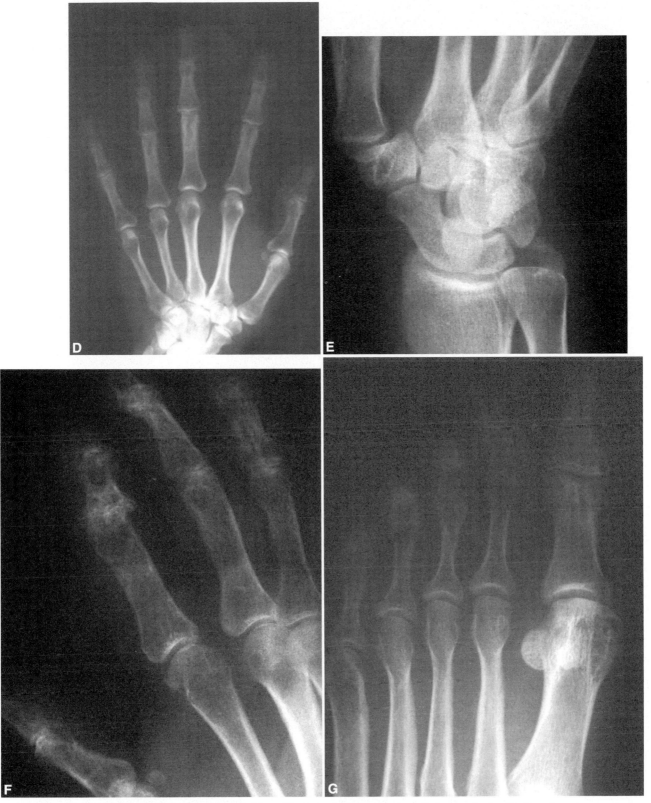

FIGURE 105–2, cont'd · *D,* The subtle lesion is an increase in radiolucency in the distal portion of the long finger proximal phalanx, as well as associated fusiform soft tissue swelling. *E,* This plain film demonstrates an unusual destructive lesion at the ulnar styloid and a sharply demarcated cyst in the trapezium in a patient with sarcoidosis arthritis. *F,* This radiograph highlights advanced destructive sarcoidosis arthritis involving all of the proximal and distal interphalangeal joints. A cystic lesion is present in the head of the long finger metacarpal bone, and a destructive lesion can be noted in the head of the index finger metacarpal bone with preservation of the joint space. *G,* In this study, a cystic region of radiolucency with a reticular pattern on the head of the metatarsal bone of the great toe is associated with destruction of the cortical margin. It is important to note the absence of periarticular osteopenia or uniform joint-space loss, which would be observed in rheumatoid arthritis.

support the existence of bone loss in untreated sarcoidosis, with some authors suggesting that this occurs independent of dysregulated calcium and vitamin D metabolism and is instead related to osteoclast activation by granulomas.[11] Because of the common use of corticosteroids in the disease, patients are also at risk of developing glucocorticoid-related bone loss. This is particularly true of postmenopausal women, whose loss of bone-mineral density is significantly greater than other sarcoidosis patients on prednisone therapy.[30] Although there is no standardized approach to the management of this problem in sarcoidosis, a few small studies have attempted to address this question. One trial randomized 30 sarcoidosis patients who were being started on prednisone therapy to receive either alendronate or placebo. After 1 year of follow-up, the alendronate group demonstrated a slight increase in bone mineral density, whereas the placebo group demonstrated a statistically significant decrease (4.5 percent) in bone mineral density.[31] In a nonrandomized study, a group of glucocorticoid-treated sarcoidosis patients were followed, a subset of whom were treated with salmon calcitonin for 15 months. This additional treatment resulted in significant benefit in terms of maintenance of bone-mineral density. The efficacy of salmon calcitonin is supported by at least one other nonrandomized trial.[32,33] In practice, most sarcoidosis clinics apply the same primary and secondary treatment strategies advocated for management of other patients with glucocorticoid-induced osteoporosis. However, it is particularly important to monitor serum and urinary calcium levels more frequently when introducing therapy with cholecalciferol or bisphosphonates. Calcitriol should be avoided because of the risk of inducing hypercalcemia in sarcoidosis patients receiving corticosteroids, especially in a condition in which pretreatment serum calcitriol levels are usually elevated.

JOINT

Sarcoidal joint involvement produces symmetric arthralgia or arthritis, often with accompanying erythema nodosum. Sarcoidosis most commonly affects the larger joints (ankles, knees, wrists, elbows), although any joint may be involved. Joint pain and stiffness can be the presenting symptoms of the disease. In the acute form of disease presentation, the arthropathy is symmetric, peripheral, and most often associated with erythema nodosum. The majority of these patients report bilateral ankle arthralgias.[8] Within a few weeks to a few months, the arthralgias tend to subside without recurrence or joint deformity. If the joint disease persists, it can result in joint destruction. In such cases, the arthritis is usually accompanied by chronic skin lesions. Arthralgias without erythema nodosum are more common in white males with hilar adenopathy, whereas arthralgias associated with erythema nodosum are more frequent in women. Chronic polyarthritis without involvement of the adjacent bone has been reported mostly in African-American patients. Several cases of spondyloarthropathy associated with sarcoidosis have also been described.[34,35]

Acute sarcoid arthritis is diagnosed mainly on clinical grounds. When obtained, synovial-fluid analysis typically demonstrates a sterile lymphocytosis and elevated protein.[11] Synovial biopsies of involved joints tend to be indeterminate, demonstrating a mild inflammatory synovitis, but often without granulomas.[36-38] Chronic destructive joint disease occurs in a minority of patients. It is often associated with other manifestations of more severe disease, such as lupus pernio and chronic uveitis.[11] Synovial biopsies in this form of arthritis show inflammatory infiltrates of lymphocytes and plasma cells, proliferation of fibroblasts, and noncaseating granulomas.[11]

Lofgren's syndrome is acute erythema nodosum with bilateral hilar lymphadenopathy that may be accompanied by fever, arthralgias or arthritis, anterior uveitis, and lung involvement. In a retrospective review of 187 cases,[39] Mana and colleagues[39] reported a significant seasonal clustering in spring and winter for erythema nodosum and Lofgren's syndrome. Asymptomatic myopathy was common. This disease was self-limited in most cases. In a review of sequential clinical cases of erythema nodosum, Garcia-Porrua and coworkers found that approximately one third were due to sarcoidosis. They emphasize that other causes must be excluded, including nonstreptococcal upper respiratory tract infection and pharmaceutical use, in particular oral contraceptives.[40]

MUSCLE

Muscle involvement is usually subclinical. Symptomatic muscle involvement occurs in less than 0.5 percent of cases.[11] When it does occur, it is often in concert with osseous disease. In systemic sarcoidosis without clinical manifestations of muscle disease, 50 to 80 percent of cases are found to have granulomas on muscle biopsy. Gastrocnemius muscle biopsy has been evaluated as a diagnostic tool in patients presenting with hilar adenopathy but no muscle symptoms. In one series of 22 patients this procedure was 100-percent sensitive and specific for making the diagnosis of sarcoidosis.[41] Other studies have not found muscle biopsy to be as useful in asymptomatic patients, and it is not routinely used to make a diagnosis in this patient population.[11] When clinically evident, sarcoidosis muscle involvement takes one of three major forms. The most common form is a chronic, progressive myopathy of gradual onset. It is associated with proximal muscle wasting in the extremities, trunk, and neck. It must be distinguished from glucocorticoid-induced myopathy. Of note, cardiac involvement is often found concurrently with this form of sarcoid muscle disease.[11] Electromyography (EMG) is often normal, but it can sometimes help distinguish between myopathic and neuropathic disorders.

The nodular form of muscular sarcoidosis is the next most common form and may present as small nodules or as a frank soft tissue mass, often mistaken for a soft tissue neoplasm.[42] Some characteristic findings of this presentation on MRI include the "dark star" sign on axial images, which consists of a star-shaped central structure of decreased signal intensity, and the "three stripes" sign seen on coronal and sagittal images, which consists of an inner stripe of decreased signal intensity and outer stripes of increased signal intensity. 67Gallium scanning may sometimes help distinguish between a sarcoidosis nodule (significantly greater uptake) and a soft tissue mass.[11]

The rarest form of muscle involvement is granulomatous myositis, which typically presents with acute to subacute onset of proximal muscle weakness, muscle pain or tenderness, and weight loss. The majority of these patients are female, African American, have elevated creatine Phosphokinase, (CPK), and erythrocyte sedimentation rate (ESR), and demonstrate a myopathic pattern on EMG.[11] Still rarer clinical presentations have included respiratory muscle weakness and painful ophthalmoplegia due to enlargement of the extraocular muscles.[43-45]

The diagnosis of myositis or myopathy may be suggested by MRI and gallium or technecium scanning; however, the increased uptake during scintigraphy is nonspecific.[46] As noted previously, MRI findings may be more characteristic in the nodular form of the disease. The gold standard for diagnosis in all forms of muscle involvement is muscle biopsy. Biopsies may demonstrate typical noncaseating granulomas, muscle fiber degeneration and regeneration, perivascular inflammation, and occasional vasculitis. Neurogenic atrophy and granulomatous infiltration of nerves is also common in sarcoidal myositis.[47] Fine-needle aspiration biopsies can also be strongly suggestive of the diagnosis, demonstrating multinucleated giant cells, epithelioid histiocytes, or both.[42,48]

VASCULITIS

Systemic vasculitis is a rare but serious form of sarcoidal involvement. Either large or small vessels may be affected in virtually any organ. Biopsies may demonstrate vasculitis associated with noncaseating granulomas[49] (as shown in Fig. 105–1C), or frank necrotizing sarcoidal granulomas. Although the relationship between sarcoidosis and vasculitis is unclear in some cases, associations have been reported between sarcoidosis and such diverse vasculitic processes as Takayasu's arteritis,[50,51] hypersensitivity vasculitis, polyarteritis nodosa, microscopic polyangiitis,[52] and Churg-Strauss syndrome.[53] Significant morbidity and relapse despite corticosteroid therapy are common. Discovery of vasculitis in one organ generally implies involvement elsewhere.

▌ Differential Diagnosis

As discussed earlier, the diagnosis of sarcoidosis is made by exclusion of other conditions. Table 105–1 summarizes the major categories of both infectious and noninfectious disorders that must be considered prior to accepting the idiopathic diagnosis. The most important infectious agents to exclude are mycobacteria, other bacteria, fungi, spirochetes, and protozoa. Diseases caused by occupational and environmental inhaled agents must also be considered, including hypersensitivity pneumonitis due to inhaled organic and inorganic antigens, metal-induced disorders such as chronic beryllium disease[54] and silicosis.[55] Neoplasms can be associated with granulomatous inflammation. Local sarcoidal reactions can occur, especially in skin, but they are not associated with systemic symptoms and lack multiorgan distribution.

Sarcoidosis must be distinguished from inflammatory conditions of unknown etiology, especially the autoimmune disorders, as discussed below. Sarcoidosis has been associated with elevation of various autoantibodies in serum, including nonspecific elevations of rheumatoid factor and ANA. In a recent retrospective study of 34 patients with sarcoidosis, antinuclear antibody, (ANA), positivity was observed in one third of patients, two of whom had antibodies to double-stranded DNA. None of these antibody-positive patients developed systemic lupus erythematosus (SLE) during the 10 to 15 year follow-up.[56] Several researchers have suggested an association between autoimmune endocrinopathies and sarcoidosis. One series demonstrated

---

TABLE 105–1 · DIFFERENTIAL DIAGNOSIS OF GRANULOMATOUS DISEASE

Cause	Disease Examples
Infectious agents	
Mycobacteria	Tuberculosis, atypical mycobacterial infections
Fungi	Histoplasmosis, coccidioidomycosis
Bacteria	Brucellosis
Spirochetes	Syphilis
Metazoa	Schistosomiasis
Parasites	Leishmaniasis, toxoplasmosis
Neoplasms	Carcinoma, sarcomas, malignant nasal granuloma
Hypersensitivity pneumonitis	Farmers' lung, bird fanciers' lung, suberosis, bagassosis
Metals	Chronic beryllium disease, zirconium granulomas, aluminum granulomas
Silicates	Silicosis with granulomatous inflammation
Vasculitic granulomatoses and autoimmune disorders	Wegener's granulomatosis, Churg-Strauss, lymphomatoid granulomatosis, polyarteritis nodosa, bronchocentric granulomatosis, systemic lupus erythematosus, primary biliary cirrhosis, juvenile rheumatoid arthritis
Other conditions	Chronic granulomatous disease (children), Whipple's disease, lymphocytic infiltration after cancer chemotherapy, Blau's syndrome, local sarcoidal reactions

significantly higher levels of antibodies against thyroid peroxidase and purified thyroglobulin, as well as Hashimoto's thyroiditis, in sarcoidosis patients as compared to diseased and nondiseased controls.[57] Similarly, in another series of 78 sarcoidosis patients, nearly 20 percent were found to have evidence of autoimmune endocrine disease, such as polyglandular autoimmune syndromes, Graves' disease, and autoimmune thyroiditis.[58] Finally, a Japanese group found an association between antiphospholipid antibodies and sarcoidosis with 21 of 55 sarcoidosis patients in their series having either immunoglobulin G (IgG) or IgM antiphospholipid antibodies. The antibody-positive subset was found to have significantly more extrathoracic organ involvement and longer persistence of abnormal chest radiographs.[59]

The putative link between sarcoidosis and autoimmunity is supported by cases of concurrent diagnoses, as well as by some of the obvious similarities between sarcoidosis and the autoimmune diseases. Although sarcoidosis is rare in children, when it does occur in preschool children, it may mimic the manifestations of juvenile rheumatoid arthritis with skin, eye, and joint involvement without lung disease. Distinction between the two entities usually requires biopsy of skin, synovium, lymph node, or liver.[60-63] In contrast, the clinical presentations of rheumatoid arthritis and sarcoidosis in adults are quite distinct. Interestingly, the coexistence of the two diseases with biopsy verification of both has been demonstrated in numerous case reports, suggesting a possible etiologic similarity.[64-67] Sjögren's syndrome has also frequently been reported as occurring concurrently with or being difficult to distinguish from sarcoidosis, particularly when there is lung involvement. Both diseases can present with keratoconjunctivitis sicca, parotid swelling, lung involvement, and cutaneous anergy. Some authors suggest that labial minor salivary gland biopsy or lung biopsy can distinguish between the two diseases, but even biopsy findings are sometimes inconclusive.[68-74]

■ Evaluation and Management

Table 105–2 summarizes the recommended baseline and follow-up tests used in the evaluation and management of sarcoidosis.[1] These recommendations are based on the expected major organs targeted by sarcoidosis. Other tests may be appropriate for evaluation and management, depending on which other organs are found to be affected.

As a general principle, because there is no single nor specific diagnostic test for sarcoidosis, the diagnosis depends on establishing the compatible clinicopathologic picture and excluding other granulomatous diseases. Ideally, the evaluation should provide histologic confirmation of disease and negative cultures and special stains for organisms.

Clinical impact of sarcoidosis depends on the extent of granulomatous inflammation and the particular organs affected. In determining the extent and severity of disease, clinicians should use available noninvasive

TABLE 105–2 • RECOMMENDED BASELINE AND FOLLOW-UP CLINICAL EVALUATION FOR SARCOIDOSIS

Baseline
Occupational/environmental history
Medication history
Examination emphasizing lungs, lymphatics, skin, eye, liver, heart, joints
Biopsy of an affected organ, with special stains, cultures
Chest radiography
Pulmonary function tests, including gas exchange
Electrocardiogram
Slit-lamp examination
Liver function tests, renal function tests
Serum calcium
24-Hour urinary calcium excretion
Other tests, depending on clinical/organ system presentation

Follow-up
Monitoring for resolution or progression:
   Track organs previously involved using least invasive methods
   Monitor for new involvement of common disease target organs

tools as much as possible to assess which organs are clinically involved and to assess the extent and severity of organ injury. Asymptomatic organ involvement may be missed, but it is usually of mild or no clinical significance with two significant exceptions: A slit-lamp examination is recommended for all patients with suspected sarcoidosis, to look for clinically undetected uveitis. Subclinical hypercalciuria, even in the absence of hypercalcemia, is associated with nephrolithiasis, and, thus, a baseline 24-hour urine calcium measurement is advisable. Periodic electrocardiograms should also be obtained to screen for rare, but potentially life threatening, cardiac arrhythmias and conduction abnormalities.

Baseline complete blood count (CBC) is recommended to evaluate for anemia, leukopenia, and thrombocytopenia. Serum calcium and liver enzymes may reflect organ involvement meriting treatment. Serum angiotensin converting enzyme activity is frequently elevated in sarcoidosis. It is not specific, but can be of use in monitoring the progression of disease and the response to therapy. Tests of cutaneous anergy may help suggest a diagnosis of sarcoidosis and help rule out tuberculosis, but the anergy panel is neither sensitive nor specific.

In cases that present with arthritic or bone symptoms, by obtaining a chest radiograph or, in some cases, a high-resolution computed tomography (CT) scan of the thorax, the rheumatologist can detect evidence of hilar or mediastinal lymphadenopathy. In the proper clinical setting, this can help make the diagnosis of sarcoidosis and also point to a logical site for biopsy, because the majority of patients with hilar adenopathy are found to have pulmonary granulomas when transbronchial lung biopsies are performed by bronchoscopy.

Kveim-Siltzbach skin testing—using a preparation of sarcoidosis spleen that is intradermally injected—has been used in the past to help establish a diagnosis of sarcoidosis in patients with unexplained erythema nodosum, uveitis, liver granulomas, or hypercalciuria. However, this is not approved for general use in the United States and is not recommended.

67Gallium citrate scanning adds no specificity to the diagnosis of sarcoidosis, except in the case of patients with lacrimal and salivary gland involvement, in which the so-called "panda" sign is observed due to increased uptake in those sites.[75]

Monitoring for disease progress, regression, or response to therapy should be customized, relying on the least invasive markers of disease activity and vital organ involvement. The clinician must remain vigilant, given the tendency of this disorder to relapse and erupt in new or previously subclinical organs.

▌ Treatment

It is not known why some sarcoidosis patients recover and others progress. Even after an apparent recovery, a proportion of patients may relapse months or years later. Factors associated with worse prognosis include older age at time of diagnosis, African-American race, duration of illness longer than 6 months, pulmonary infiltrates, splenomegaly, lupus pernio, and number of organs involved. A more favorable prognosis has been found in patients with acute disease who expressed HLA-DR3 and -DQ2, whether or not erythema nodosum was present.[7,8,76] It is important to recognize that the disease can spontaneously resolve without treatment. Thus, most treatment protocols incorporate a period of observation without treatment whenever possible.

A detailed summary of current pharmacotherapy in sarcoidosis has been the subject of several recent reviews.[4,77,78] This section addresses general treatment of sarcoidosis with emphasis on rheumatologic manifestations where data are available. Oral corticosteroids remain the first-line therapy in most cases; however, there is no consensus as to when corticosteroids should be initiated.[77] The use of oral corticosteroids in sarcoidosis is aimed at the relief of symptoms with intended improvement in quality of life and modulation of disease activity to prevent serious morbidity and mortality related to vital organ damage. It is debatable whether all of these goals can be achieved, especially in light of the side effects of corticosteroids.

In a systematic review, Paramothayan and Jones assessed the beneficial and adverse effects of corticosteroids in sarcoidosis by reviewing all of the randomized trials that included a control group. In synthesizing the data from eight studies that met their requirements for inclusion, the authors concluded that oral corticosteroids improved chest radiographs after 6 to 24 months of treatment and produced a small improvement in lung function and gas exchange. They found no data to suggest that corticosteroid therapy alters long-term disease progression.[77]

Studies examining outcome at more than 2 years suggest no significant benefit from corticosteroid therapy in asymptomatic sarcoidosis patients with more advanced forms of pulmonary involvement.[79-83] In a British Thoracic Society study,[84] patients not meeting the indications for immediate therapy were observed for 6 months. At that point, using a strategy of alternate assignment, they were designated to receive either long-term corticosteroid therapy or to receive corticosteroids only as indicated symptomatically. Analysis of data at 2 years suggested that the long-term therapy group experienced only mild improvements in pulmonary function.

There is no consensus regarding the optimal initial dosage of corticosteroids. The American Thoracic Society consensus statement on sarcoidosis (Anonymous. Statement on sarcoidosis. Joint Statement of the American Thoracic Society (ATS), the European Respiratory Society (ERS) and the World Association of Sarcoidosis and Other Granulomatous Disorders (WASOG) adopted by the ATS Board of Directors and by the ERS Executive Committee, February 1999. *American Journal of Respiratory & Critical Care Medicine. 160(2):736-55, 1999 Aug.*) reports a usual starting dose of 20 to 40 mg of prednisone, or its equivalent, daily or on alternate days. The British Thoracic Society study (reference 84 in existing text) similarly used 30 mg of prednisolone (potency equivalent to prednisone) daily as a starting dose both in their long term and selective therapy groups. We typically start therapy at a dosage of 30 to 40 mg of prednisone daily or on alternate days, although we use higher doses to a maximum of 60 mg daily for severe disease, such as symptomatic cardiac involvement. Patients return to the clinic after 8-12 weeks, at which time clinical, radiologic, physiologic and laboratory assessments are repeated and patients are evaluated for side effects. Those who objectively improve on corticosteroids initiate a taper of corticosteroids to as low a dose as is tolerated without return of symptoms or organ dysfunction – usually 5 to 10 mg daily or on alternate days. The ATS statement recommends that for those who respond to steroids, treatment should be continued for at least 1 year.

Patients with evidence of further disease progression, or who become stable on high-dose corticosteroids but who have yet to improve, are maintained at the same dosage, unless they have developed significant side effects. If intolerable side effects occur, or if the disease worsens, patients are considered candidates for the addition of a second-line immunosuppressive agent. If patients suffer relapse on maintenance therapy, we reinitiate higher-dose prednisone and consider second-line, steroid-sparing options.

Patients who have evidence of a clinical response to corticosteroids are reevaluated using objective measures prior to attempts to completely withdraw immunosuppressive medication. In some patients, the disease remains quiescent off of all corticosteroids. Unfortunately, in others, the disease relapses, requiring that therapy be restarted for purposes of symptomatic relief and clinical control of failing organs.

The use of other immunosuppressive agents in sarcoidosis should be reserved for those patients who experience symptomatic disease progression despite the use of systemic corticosteroids or who require systemic therapy but cannot tolerate steroid side effects. In general, there has been less clinical experience and fewer published studies testing other immunosuppressive agents' efficacy as either single agents or as steroid-sparing agents.

Methotrexate (MTX) has emerged as the preferred second-line drug, especially used as a steroid-sparing agent. There are few published randomized clinical trials of the use of MTX in sarcoidosis.[85] The largest published experience comes from Lower and Baughman, who reported improvement in 33 of 50 patients treated with MTX for a minimum of 2 years.[86] Those with cutaneous and musculoskeletal involvement showed the greatest response. Of 30 patients who were also receiving corticosteroids, 25 were able to decrease corticosteroid dosage. Thirteen discontinued corticosteroids entirely. A follow-up report of 209 patients showed that 52 percent of those on MTX entered remission and 16 percent remained stable, with or without low-dose prednisone.[87] Other reports confirm the beneficial effects of MTX in cutaneous and musculoskeletal sarcoidosis.[88,89] In a study by Kaye and colleagues, low-dose MTX (average 10 mg/week, range 7.5 to 15 mg), when used for an average of 30 months, controlled clinical symptoms in patients with musculoskeletal involvement and helped reduce corticosteroid dose.[89] In most studies, treatment doses of MTX range from 5 to 15 mg per week, usually taken as a single or divided oral dose on one day per week. MTX may take up to 6 months to become fully effective in sarcoidosis. During this period patients are usually maintained on corticosteroids.

Case reports on the benefits of cyclosporin A in sarcoidosis have not been supported by later larger cohort studies.[90-92] The first study to examine cyclosporin in a more rigorous fashion found that cyclosporin, administered at doses that achieved a blood level between 150 and 250 ng/ml, failed to produce clinical improvement in 20 patients who had pulmonary involvement, despite 6 months of therapy.[91] Cyclosporin was undetectable in bronchoalveolar lavage fluid, suggesting poor penetration of cyclosporin into the lung as a reason for its failure. A more recent study, using a standardized treatment protocol, found the combination of prednisone and cyclosporin to be no better and possibly worse than prednisone alone in treating pulmonary sarcoidosis.[92]

Despite anecdotal reports and frequent use of azathioprine, there are few published studies examining the drug's efficacy in sarcoidosis. One group reported objective improvement in 7 of 10 patients with pulmonary sarcoidosis after receiving 150 mg/day of azathioprine for 6 months.[93] Some data suggest that it may be efficacious for extrapulmonary disease,[94] although side effects often limit the acceptance of this option.

Two more recent case series evaluated combined therapy with azathioprine and corticosteroids in patients with chronic pulmonary sarcoidosis. A retrospective review of 10 patients demonstrated sustained improvement in lung function in only 2 patients, but a prospective evaluation of 11 patients demonstrated symptomatic relief and improvement in lung physiology and radiographic abnormalities in 9 after an average of 20 months of therapy. Thus, azathioprine may be an effective second-line agent in a subset of sarcoidosis patients. (Lewis, S. J., G. M. Ainslie, and E. D. Bateman. 1999. Efficacy of azathioprine as second-line treatment in pulmonary sarcoidosis. *Sarcoidosis Vasc Diffuse Lung Dis* 16(1):87-92; Muller-Quernheim, J., K. Kienast, M. Held, S. Pfeifer, and U. Costabel. 1999. Treatment of chronic sarcoidosis with an azathioprine/prednisolone regimen. *Eur Respir J* 14(5):1117-1122.)

Chloroquine has proven effective in treating cutaneous manifestations of sarcoidosis,[95] hypercalcemia and hypercalciuria associated with sarcoidosis, and steroid-refractory neurosarcoidosis.[96,97] Generally, chloroquine therapy is initiated at a dosage of 500 mg/day and may be titrated up to a maximum of 1000 mg/day and decreased to a low of 250 mg/day. Hydroxychloroquine is used at a dosage of 200 to 400 mg/day. The British Tuberculosis Association performed the first controlled sarcoidosis trial on the use of antimalarials.[98] They observed some benefit early in attenuating symptoms of pulmonary sarcoidosis but showed little effect on disease outcome when comparing treatment and control groups at 6 months.

A more recent trial examined the efficacy of chloroquine therapy in chronic pulmonary sarcoidosis. During an initial run-in phase, all subjects received chloroquine therapy for 6 months and demonstrated a significant improvement in several lung physiologic parameters. During the subsequent randomization phase, subjects were assigned to receive maintenance therapy with low dose (250 mg/day) chloroquine or to be observed. With a mean of 19.7 months of follow up, the maintenance group demonstrated significantly slower decline in lung function and a trend toward fewer relapses. (Baltzan, M., S. Mehta, T. H. Kirkham, and M. G. Cosio. 1999. Randomized trial of prolonged chloroquine therapy in advanced pulmonary sarcoidosis. *Am J Respir Crit Care Med* 160(1):192-197.) Thus, while chloroquine or hydroxychloroquine are more commonly employed for extrathoracic disease, there may be a role for these agents in pulmonary disease as well.

Cyclophosphamide is employed in selected cases of corticosteroid-refractory sarcoidosis.[99,100] It appears beneficial for both cardiac and neurosarcoidosis, in the latter case, even following both corticosteroid and MTX failure. If used, oral cyclophosphamide is given at a dose of 1 to 2 mg/kg/day to a maximum dose of 150 mg/day. Therapy is maintained for several months before tapering. In one open-label study, the investigators used intravenous pulse cyclophosphamide therapy for the treatment of neurosarcoidosis at a dosage of 0.75 to 1.5 g monthly.[100]

Based on our present understanding of cytokine expression in sarcoidosis, it is logical to expect that anti–TNF-α therapies, such as etanercept, infliximab, adalimumab, thalidomide, and pentoxifylline should prove effective. There are individual published cases and small case-series data supporting the use of thalidomide in treatment of patients with cutaneous sarcoidosis and lupus pernio.[101-105] Pentoxifylline, at high doses, improved lung function in a group of patients with mild pulmonary sarcoidosis.[106] Clinical trials are underway examining the safety and efficacy of inflixin in pulmonary and extrathoracic sarcoidosis. A recent prospective, open-label study examined the treatment of sarcoidosis with etanercept, a protein that binds tumor necrosis factor and makes it biologically inactive.

Seventeen patients with progressive pulmonary sarcoidosis and on no other immunosuppressive agents were enrolled and followed for 3 to 12 months. The study was terminated prior to the full planned enrollment due to excessive treatment failures, defined as a deterioration in two or three of the following: lung function (≥ 10% decline in FEV1, FVC, TLC, or DLCO), dyspnea score and chest radiograph appearance. The authors conclude that etanercept should not be further studied as a therapeutic option for patients with stage II or III pulmonary sarcoidosis. Several shortcomings of this study are worth noting. First, at baseline, all of the mean lung function values were within the normal range. Therefore, this may have been a negative study because the subjects were too healthy to experience a significant benefit from etanercept. Second, patients were not permitted to be on any other immunosuppressive therapy. Since studies in other inflammatory disorders have demonstrated efficacy of TNF blockers in conjunction with other agents, this stipulation may have doomed the study to fail from the outset. Finally, the authors conclude that the drug deserves no further investigation despite the successful responses of nearly one-third of the patients studied. (Utz, J. P., A. H. Limper, S. Kalra, U. Specks, J. P. Scott, Z. Vuk-Pavlovic, and D. R. Schroeder. 2003. Etanercept for the treatment of stage II and III progressive pulmonary sarcoidosis. *Chest* 124(1):177-185.) It is therefore still certainly possible that for a subset of sarcoidosis patients with more significant pulmonary dysfunction and possibly on concomitant immunosuppressive therapy, this therapy will be effective. Thus far, case reports have been published supporting the use of infliximab in treatment of lupus pernio, neurosarcoidosis, and progressive cutaneous sarcoidosis.[107-109] In one case, investigators reported clinical response in a sarcoidosis patient who presented with severe protein-losing enteropathy, hypoalbuminemia, and proximal myopathy.[110]

Combined regimens are coming into increasing favor as treatments for sarcoidosis, although there have been few trials. Most combination treatment regimens for sarcoidosis are corticosteroids plus a second-line agent. The corticosteroid is then slowly tapered over a 3- to 6-month period as allowed by the patient's clinical status, leaving the second drug as the main therapeutic agent. In one study, the combination of cyclosporin plus oral fluocortolone and oral MTX was studied in an open-label, uncontrolled trial in steroid refractory patients.[111] All 11 patients entered remission. These preliminary results need to be confirmed with a larger, prospective, controlled trial.

◼ Summary and Conclusion

Sarcoidosis should be considered in any patient presenting with systemic and multiorgan symptoms, or whenever granulomatous inflammation is discovered on histology. Therapeutic advances based on an understanding of immune mechanisms will likely improve our approaches to medical management of this enigmatic condition.

REFERENCES

1. Newman LS, Rose CS, Maier LA: Medical progress: Sarcoidosis. N Engl J Med 336:1224-1234, 1997.
2. Baughman RP, Teirstein AS, Judson MA, et al: Clinical characteristics of patients in a case control study of sarcoidosis. Am J Respir Crit Care Med 164:1885-1889, 2001.
3. Hunninghake GW, Gadek JE, Kawanami O, et al: Inflammatory and immune processes in the human lung in health and disease: Evaluation by bronchoalveolar lavage. Am J Pathol 97:199-206, 1979.
4. Vourlekis JS, Sawyer RT, Newman LS: Sarcoidosis: developments in etiology, immunology, and therapeutics. Adv Intern Med 45:209-257, 2000.
5. Agostini C, Adami F, Semenzato G: New pathogenetic insights into the sarcoid granuloma. Curr Opin Rheumatol 12:71-76, 2000.
6. Moller DR, Chen ES: What causes sarcoidosis? Curr Opin Pulm Med 8:429-434, 2002.
7. Grunewald J, Janson CH, Eklund A, et al: Restricted Va2.3 gene usage by CD4+ T lymphocytes in bronchoalveolar lavage fluid from sarcoidosis patients correlates with HLA-DR3. Eur J Immunol 22:129-135, 1992.
8. Visser H, Vos K, Zanelli E, et al: Sarcoid arthritis: clinical characteristics, diagnostic aspects, and risk factors. Ann Rheum Dis 61:499-504, 2002.
9. Wilcox A, Bharadwaj P, Sharma OP: Bone sarcoidosis. Curr Opin Rheumatol 12:321-330, 2000.
10. Atanes A, Gomez N, de Toro FJ, et al: [The bone manifestations in 94 cases of sarcoidosis]. An Med Interna 8:481-486, 1991.
11. Zisman DA, Shorr, AF, Lynch JP: Sarcoidosis involving the musculoskeletal system. Semin Resp Crit Care Med 23:555-570, 2002.
12. Rua-Figueroa I, Gantes MA, Erausquin C, et al: Vertebral sarcoidosis: clinical and imaging findings. Semin Arthritis Rheum 31:346-352, 2002.
13. Cohen NP, Gosset J, Staron RB, Levine WN: Vertebral sarcoidosis of the spine in a football player. Am J Orthop 30:875-877, 2001.
14. Andres E, Loth F, Orion B, et al: Iliac bone defects revealing systemic sarcoidosis. Joint Bone Spine 68:74-75, 2001.
15. Sundaram M, Place H, Shaffer WO, Martin DS: Progressive destructive vertebral sarcoid leading to surgical fusion. Skeletal Radiol 28:717-722, 1999.
16. Franco M, Passeron C, Tieulie N, et al: Long-term radiographic follow-up in a patient with osteosclerotic sarcoidosis of the spine and pelvis. Rev Rhum Engl Ed 65:586-590, 1998.
17. Finelli DA, Christopherson LA, Rhodes RH, et al: Leptomeningeal and calvarial sarcoidosis: CT and MR appearance. J Comput Assist Tomogr 19:639-642, 1995.
18. Marymont JV, Murphy DA: Sarcoidosis of the axial skeleton. Clin Nucl Med 19:1060-1062, 1994.
19. Zisman LS, Abraham WT, Meixell GE, et al: Angiotensin II formation in the intact human heart: Predominance of the angiotensin-converting enzyme pathway. J Clin Invest 95:1490-1498, 1995.
20. Matsuoka S, Uchiyama K, Shima H, et al: Positivity of extrapulmonary Ga-67 uptake in sarcoidosis: thyroid uptake due to chronic thyroiditis and bone uptake due to fibrous dysplasia. Ann Nucl Med 15:537-539, 2001.
21. Milman N, Lund JO, Graudal N, et al: Diagnostic value of routine radioisotope bone scanning in a series of 63 patients with pulmonary sarcoidosis. Sarcoidosis Vasc Diffuse Lung Dis 17:67-70, 2000.
22. Fisher AJ, Gilula LA, Kyriakos M, Holzaepfel CD: MR imaging changes of lumbar vertebral sarcoidosis. AJR Am J Roentgenol 173:354-356, 1999.
23. Shorr A: Osseous sarcoidosis: clinical, radiographic and therapeutic observations. J Clin Rheumatol 4:186-192, 1998.
24. Shorr AF, Murphy FT, Gilliland WR, Hnatiuk W: Osseous disease in patients with pulmonary sarcoidosis and musculoskeletal symptoms. Respir Med 94:228-232, 2000.
25. Gonzalez del Pino J, Diez Ulloa A, Lovic A, Relea MF: Sarcoidosis of the hand and wrist: a report of two cases. J Hand Surg [Am] 22:942-945, 1997.

26. Katzman BM, Caligiuri DA, Klein DM, et al: Sarcoid flexor tenosynovitis of the wrist: a case report. J Hand Surg [Am] 22:336-337, 1997.

27. Larsen TK: Tenosynovitis as initial diagnosis of sarcoidosis. Case report. Scand J Plast Reconstr Surg Hand Surg 30:157-159, 1996.

28. Rizzato G, Fraioli P, Sabbioni E, et al: Multi-element follow up in biological specimens of hard metal pneumoconiosis. Sarcoidosis 9:104-117, 1992.

29. Conron M, Young C, Beynon HL: Calcium metabolism in sarcoidosis and its clinical implications. Rheumatology (Oxford) 39:707-713, 2000.

30. Montemurro L, Fraioli P, Riboldi A, et al: Bone loss in prednisone treated sarcoidosis: a two-year follow-up. Ann Ital Med Int 5:164-168, 1990.

31. Gonnelli S, Rottoli P, Cepollaro C, et al: Prevention of corticosteroid-induced osteoporosis with alendronate in sarcoid patients. Calcif Tissue Int 61:382-385, 1997.

32. Rizzato G, Tosi G, Schiraldi G, et al: Bone protection with salmon calcitonin (sCT) in the long-term steroid therapy of chronic sarcoidosis. Sarcoidosis 5:99-103, 1988.

33. Montemurro L, Schiraldi G, Fraioli P, et al: Prevention of corticosteroid-induced osteoporosis with salmon calcitonin in sarcoid patients. Calcif Tissue Int 49:71-76, 1991.

34. Kremer P, Gallinet E, Benmansour A, et al: Sarcoidosis and spondylarthropathy: Three case-reports. Rev Rhum Engl Ed 63:405-411, 1996.

35. Kotter I, Durk H, Saal JG: Sacroiliitis in sarcoidosis: case reports and review of the literature. Clin Rheumatol 14:695-700, 1995.

36. Kremer JM: Histologic findings in siblings with acute sarcoid arthritis: association with the B8,DR3 phenotype. J Rheumatol 13:593-597, 1986.

37. Palmer DG, Schumacher HR: Synovitis with non-specific histological changes in synovium in chronic sarcoidosis. Ann Rheum Dis 43:778-782, 1984.

38. Scott DG, Porto LO, Lovell CR, Thomas GO: Chronic sarcoid synovitis in the Caucasian: an arthroscopic and histological study. Ann Rheum Dis 40:121-123, 1981.

39. Mana J, Gomez-Vaquero C, Montero A, et al: Lofgren's syndrome revisited: a study of 186 patients. Am J Med 107:240-245, 1999.

40. Garcia-Porrua C, Gonzalez-Gay MA, Vazquez-Caruncho M, et al: Erythema nodosum: etiologic and predictive factors in a defined population. Arthritis Rheum 43:584-592, 2000.

41. Andonopoulos AP, Papadimitriou C, Melachrinou M, et al: Asymptomatic gastrocnemius muscle biopsy: an extremely sensitive and specific test in the pathologic confirmation of sarcoidosis presenting with hilar adenopathy. Clin Exp Rheumatol 19:569-572, 2001.

42. Yamamoto T, Nagira K, Akisue T, et al: Aspiration biopsy of nodular sarcoidosis of the muscle. Diagn Cytopathol 26:109-112, 2002.

43. Ost D, Yeldandi A, Cugell D: Acute sarcoid myositis with respiratory muscle involvement: Case report and review of the literature. Chest 107:879-882, 1995.

44. Dewberry RG, Schneider BF, Cale WF, Phillips LH II: Sarcoid myopathy presenting with diaphragm weakness. Muscle Nerve 16:832-835, 1993.

45. Cornblath WT, Elner V, Rolfe M: Extraocular muscle involvement in sarcoidosis. Ophthalmology 100:501-505, 1993.

46. Otake S, Ishigaki T: Muscular sarcoidosis. Semin Musculoskelet Radiol 5:167-170, 2001.

47. Prayson RA: Granulomatous myositis: Clinicopathologic study of 12 cases. Am J Clin Pathol 112:63-68, 1999.

48. Guo M, Lemos L, Baliga M: Nodular sarcoid myositis of skeletal muscle diagnosed by fine needle aspiration biopsy: A case report. Acta Cytol 43:1171-1176, 1999.

49. Diri E, Espinoza CG, Espinoza LR: Spinal cord granulomatous vasculitis: an unusual clinical presentation of sarcoidosis. J Rheumatol 26:1408-1410, 1999.

50. Weiler V, Redtenbacher S, Bancher C, et al: Concurrence of sarcoidosis and aortitis: case report and review of the literature. Ann Rheum Dis 59:850-853, 2000.

51. Schapiro JM, Shpitzer S, Pinkhas J, et al: Sarcoidosis as the initial manifestation of Takayasu's arteritis. J Med 25:121-128, 1994.

52. Fernandes SR, Singsen BH, Hoffman GS: Sarcoidosis and systemic vasculitis. Semin Arthritis Rheum 30:33-46, 2000.

53. Ohori N, Arita K, Ohta M: [A case of Churg-Strauss syndrome overlapping with sarcoidosis]. Rinsho Shinkeigaku 38:631-636, 1998.

54. Newman LS: Metals that cause sarcoidosis. Semin Respir Infect 13:212-220, 1998.

55. Safirstein BH, Klukowicz A, Miller R, Teirstein A: Granulomatous pneumonitis following exposure to the World Trade Center collapse. Chest 123:301-304, 2003.

56. Weinberg I, Vasiliev L, Gotsman I: Anti-dsDNA antibodies in sarcoidosis. Semin Arthritis Rheum 29:328-331, 2000.

57. Nakamura H, Genma R, Mikami T, et al: High incidence of positive autoantibodies against thyroid peroxidase and thyroglobulin in patients with sarcoidosis. Clin Endocrinol (Oxf) 46:467-472, 1997.

58. Papadopoulos KI, Hornblad Y, Liljebladh H, Hallengren B: High frequency of endocrine autoimmunity in patients with sarcoidosis. Eur J Endocrinol 134:331-336, 1996.

59. Ina Y, Takada K, Yamamoto M, et al: Antiphospholipid antibodies: A prognostic factor in sarcoidosis? Chest 105:1179-1183, 1994.

60. Sarigol SS, Hay MH, Wyllie R: Sarcoidosis in preschool children with hepatic involvement mimicking juvenile rheumatoid arthritis. J Pediatr Gastroenterol Nutr 28:510-512, 1999.

61. Sahn EE, Hampton MT, Garen PD, et al: Preschool sarcoidosis masquerading as juvenile rheumatoid arthritis: two case reports and a review of the literature. Pediatr Dermatol 7:208-213, 1990.

62. Ukae S, Tsutsumi H, Adachi N, et al: Preschool sarcoidosis manifesting as juvenile rheumatoid arthritis: a case report and a review of the literature of Japanese cases. Acta Paediatr Jpn 36:515-518, 1994.

63. Sakurai Y, Nakajima M, Kamisue S, et al: Preschool sarcoidosis mimicking juvenile rheumatoid arthritis: the significance of gallium scintigraphy and skin biopsy in the differential diagnosis. Acta Paediatr Jpn 39:74-78, 1997.

64. Fallahi S, Collins RD, Miller RK, Halla JT: Coexistence of rheumatoid arthritis and sarcoidosis: difficulties encountered in the differential diagnosis of common manifestations. J Rheumatol 11:526-529, 1984.

65. Kucera RF: A possible association of rheumatoid arthritis and sarcoidosis. Chest 95:604-606, 1989.

66. Menard O, Petit N, Gillet P, et al: Association of histologically proven rheumatoid arthritis with pulmonary sarcoidosis. Eur Respir J 8:472-473, 1995.

67. Yutani Y, Minato Y, Hirata K, et al: A rare case of sarcoidosis with rheumatoid arthritis. Osaka City Med J 41:85-89, 1995.

68. Justiniani FR: Sarcoidosis complicating primary Sjögren's syndrome. Mt Sinai J Med 56:59-61, 1989.

69. Radenne F, Tillie-Leblond I, Maurage CA, et al: [Sjögren's syndrome and necrotizing sarcoid-like granulomatosis]. Rev Mal Respir 16:554-557, 1999.

70. Giotaki H, Constantopoulos SH, Papadimitriou CS, Moutsopoulos HM: Labial minor salivary gland biopsy: a highly discriminatory diagnostic method between sarcoidosis and Sjögren's syndrome. Respiration 50:102-107, 1986.

71. Miyata M, Takase Y, Kobayashi H, et al: Primary Sjögren's syndrome complicated by sarcoidosis. Intern Med 37:174-178, 1998.

72. Lois M, Roman J, Holland W, Agudelo C: Coexisting Sjögren's syndrome and sarcoidosis in the lung. Semin Arthritis Rheum 28:31-40, 1998.

73. Drosos AA, Voulgari PV, Psychos PN, et al: Sicca syndrome in patients with sarcoidosis. Rheumatol Int 18:177-180, 1999.

74. Gal I, Kovacs J, Zeher M: Case series: coexistence of Sjögren's syndrome and sarcoidosis. J Rheumatol 27:2507-2510, 2000.

75. Oates E, Metherall J: Images in clinical medicine: Sarcoidosis. N Engl J Med 329:1394, 1993.

76. Grunewald J, Olerup O, Persson U, et al: T-cell receptor variable region gene usage by CD4+ and CD8+ T cells in bronchoalveolar lavage fluid and peripheral blood of sarcoidosis patients. Proc Natl Acad Sci U S A 91:4965-4969, 1994.

77. Paramothayan S, Jones PW: Corticosteroid therapy in pulmonary sarcoidosis: a systematic review. JAMA 287:1301-1307, 2002.

78. Moller DR: Treatment of sarcoidosis-from a basic science point of view. J Intern Med 253:31-40, 2003.

79. Young R: Pulmonary sarcoidosis: a prospective evaluation of glucocorticoid therapy: Ann Int Med 7:207-212, 1970.

80. Harkleroad LE, Young RL, Savage PJ, et al: Pulmonary sarcoidosis. Long-term follow-up of the effects of steroid therapy. Chest 82:84-87, 1982.

81. Israel HL, Fouts DW, Beggs RA: A controlled trial of prednisone treatment of sarcoidosis. Am Rev Respir Dis 107:609-614, 1973.

82. Eule H, Weinecke A, Roth I, Wuthe H: The possible influence of corticosteroid therapy on the natural course of pulmonary sarcoidosis. Late results of a continuing clinical study. Ann N Y Acad Sci 465:695-701, 1986.

83. Zaki MH, Lyons HA, Leilop L, Huang CT: Corticosteroid therapy in sarcoidosis: A five-year, controlled follow-up study. N Y State J Med 87:496-499, 1987.

84. Gibson GJ, Prescott RJ, Muers MF, et al: British Thoracic Society Sarcoidosis study: effects of long term corticosteroid treatment. Thorax 51:238-247, 1996.

85. Baughman RP, Winget DB, Lower EE: Methotrexate is steroid sparing in acute sarcoidosis: results of a double blind, randomized trial. Sarcoidosis Vasc Diffuse Lung Dis 17:60-66, 2000.

86. Lower EE, Baughman RP: Prolonged use of methotrexate for sarcoidosis. Arch Intern Med 155:846-851, 1995.

87. Baughman R, Lower E: Alternative to corticosteroids in the treatment of sarcoidosis. Sarcoidosis 14:121-130, 1997.

88. Webster GF, Razsi LK, Sanchez M, Shupack JL: Weekly low-dose methotrexate therapy for cutaneous sarcoidosis. J Am Acad Dermatol 24:451-454, 1991.

89. Kaye O, Palazzo E, Grossin M, et al: Low-dose methotrexate: An effective corticosteroid-sparing agent in the musculoskeletal manifestations of sarcoidosis. Br J Rheumatol 34:642-644, 1995.

90. Rebuck AS, Stiller CR, Braude AC, et al: Cyclosporin for pulmonary sarcoidosis. Lancet 1:1174, 1984.

91. Martinet Y, Pinkston P, Saltini C, et al: Evaluation of the in vitro and in vivo effects of cyclosporine on the lung T-lymphocyte alveolitis of active pulmonary sarcoidosis. Am Rev Respir Dis 138:1242-1248, 1988.

92. Wyser CP, van Schalkwyk EM, Alheit B, et al: Treatment of progressive pulmonary sarcoidosis with cyclosporin A: A randomized controlled trial. Am J Respir Crit Care Med 156:1371-1376, 1997.

93. Pacheco Y, Marechal C, Marechal F, et al: Azathioprine treatment of chronic pulmonary sarcoidosis. Sarcoidosis 2:107-113, 1985.

94. Hof D, Hof P, Godfrey W: Long-term use of azathioprine as a steroid-sparing agent for chronic sarcoidosis. Am J Respir Crit Care Med 153:A870, 1996.

95. Zic JA, Horowitz DH, Arzubiaga C, King LE Jr: Treatment of cutaneous sarcoidosis with chloroquine: Review of the literature. Arch Dermatol 127:1034-1040, 1991.

96. O'Leary TJ, Jones G, Yip A, et al: The effects of chloroquine on serum 1,25-dihydroxyvitamin D and calcium metabolism in sarcoidosis. N Engl J Med 315:727-730, 1986.

97. Sharma OP: Effectiveness of chloroquine and hydroxychloroquine in treating selected patients with sarcoidosis with neurological involvement. Arch Neurol 55:1248-1254, 1998.

98. British. Chloroquine in the treatment of sarcoidosis: A report from the Research Committee of the British Tuberculosis Association. Tubercle 48:257-272, 1967.

99. Demeter SL: Myocardial sarcoidosis unresponsive to steroids: Treatment with cyclophosphamide. Chest 94:202-203, 1988.

100. Lower EE, Broderick JP, Brott TG, Baughman RP: Diagnosis and management of neurological sarcoidosis. Arch Intern Med 157:1864-1868, 1997.

101. Carlesimo M, Giustini S, Rossi A, et al: Treatment of cutaneous and pulmonary sarcoidosis with thalidomide. J Am Acad Dermatol 32:866-869, 1995.

102. Rousseau L, Beylot-Barry M, Doutre MS, Beylot C: Cutaneous sarcoidosis successfully treated with low doses of thalidomide. Arch Dermatol 134:1045-1046, 1998.

103. Lee JB, Koblenzer PS: Disfiguring cutaneous manifestation of sarcoidosis treated with thalidomide: a case report. J Am Acad Dermatol 39:835-838, 1998.

104. Oliver SJ, Kikuchi T, Krueger JG, Kaplan G: Thalidomide induces granuloma differentiation in sarcoid skin lesions associated with disease improvement. Clin Immunol 102:225-236, 2002.

105. Baughman RP, Judson MA, Teirstein AS, Moller DR, Lower EE: Thalidomide for chronic sarcoidosis. chest 122:227-232, 2002.

106. Zabel P, Entzian P, Dalhoff K, Schlaak M: Pentoxifylline in treatment of sarcoidosis. Am J Respir Crit Care Med 155:1665-1669, 1997.

107. Baughman RP, Lower EE: Infliximab for refractory sarcoidosis. Sarcoidosis Vasc Diffuse Lung Dis 18:70-74, 2001.

108. Pettersen JA, Zochodne DW, Bell RB, et al: Refractory neurosarcoidosis responding to infliximab. Neurology 59:1660-1661, 2002.

109. Mallbris L, Ljungberg A, Hedblad MA, et al: Progressive cutaneous sarcoidosis responding to anti-tumor necrosis factor-alpha therapy. J Am Acad Dermatol 48:290-293, 2003.

110. Yee AM, Pochapin MB: Treatment of complicated sarcoidosis with infliximab anti-tumor necrosis factor-alpha therapy. Ann Intern Med 135:27-31, 2001.

111. Pia G, Pascalis L, Aresu G, et al: Evaluation of the efficacy and toxicity of the cyclosporine A-flucortolone-methotrexate combination in the treatment of sarcoidosis. Sarcoidosis Vasc Diffuse Lung Dis 13:146-152, 1996.

106

Iron Storage Disease

R. ELAINE LAMBERT

Iron storage diseases may be divided into genetic hemochromatosis (previously primary or idiopathic) and secondary iron-overload states. Genetic hemochromatosis is an autosomal recessive disease characterized by inappropriately high intestinal iron absorption that results in the pathologic deposition of iron in parenchymal cells of many organs. Secondary iron overload refers to a variety of conditions associated with increased iron availability from parenteral or oral routes, ineffective erythropoiesis, or inherited defects[1] (Table 106-1). *Hemosiderosis* is a term used by pathologists to describe excessive iron stain in tissues without regard to the underlying cause or the specific target cell involved.[2]

Etiology

In genetic hemochromatosis, the excess iron is deposited in parenchymal cells with relatively little uptake by the reticuloendothelial system (RES). In secondary iron overload, especially when administered parenterally, large amounts of iron are found within the cells of the RES, with variable deposition in other organ tissues.[2] The dyserythropoietic anemias, such as thalassemia major and sideroblastic anemias, may demonstrate at an early age a pattern of organ involvement that is indistinguishable from genetic hemochromatosis.[1]

Patients with alcoholic cirrhosis and secondary iron overload may be difficult to distinguish from patients with genetic hemochromatosis. Both may have hepatomegaly, hypogonadism, carbohydrate intolerance, hyperpigmentation, and increased intestinal iron absorption in association with elevated plasma ferritin concentrations and transferrin saturations. In comparison with genetic hemochromatosis, the histologic examination in alcoholic cirrhosis demonstrates less overall hemosiderin and a predominance of the iron stain within the Kupffer cells rather than in the parenchymal cells.[3] The excess hepatic iron found in alcoholic cirrhosis rarely exceeds 3 g as compared with the total pool of 15 to 35 g of iron in hemochromatosis.[4]

The development of marked siderosis from excessive absorption of medicinal or dietary iron is distinctly rare. However, certain groups of black Africans absorb excessive exogenous iron as a result of the leaching of this metal from steel drums used in brewing alcoholic drinks. The iron-containing beverage produced has a low pH, resulting in more iron bioavailability than usual.[3] The pathologic pattern of hepatic iron overload in these Africans is distinct from both alcoholic liver disease and genetic hemochromatosis.[5,6] A recent pedigree study suggests that in African dietary iron overload an inborn error of metabolism that is distinct from the hemochromatosis gene (HFE) may lead to iron loading in homozygotes and make possible a genotype-by-environment interaction in which heterozygotes who ingest increased amounts of dietary iron in traditional beer also develop iron overload.[5,7]

About 75 percent of patients with porphyria cutanea tarda (PCT) have excessive stainable iron in the liver.[8] A study in patients with PCT demonstrated that mutations in the HFE gene were present in 73 percent, and the prevalence of hepatitis C viral infection was also increased at 56 percent.[9] Even in minor tissue levels, iron may act as a cofactor in potentiating cell injury in other liver diseases. Patients with chronic hepatitis C who are heterozygous for HFE develop more liver fibrosis despite relatively minor increases in iron stores.[10] Other rare, congenital iron-storage disorders include ceruloplasmin deficiency, transferrin deficiency or atransferrinemia, and neonatal iron overload in which liver damage begins in utero. Hemodialysis patients may be predisposed to severe hemosiderosis from repeated transfusions, chronic iron administration, and hematologic abnormalities, as well as the concomitant presence of heterozygosity for genetic hemochromatosis.[11]

Normal Iron Metabolism

To understand the altered iron metabolism in hemochromatosis, it is necessary to review normal iron metabolism. The average total body iron content is 3 to 4 g in the adult; approximately 60 percent is present as hemoglobin, 10 percent is present as myoglobin, 5 percent is present in other proteins and enzymes, and the remaining 25 percent is distributed in the storage proteins ferritin and hemosiderin. Ferritin is the primary and most readily available iron storage protein. The serum ferritin concentration directly reflects reticuloendothelial ferritin. As the intracellular level increases, ferritin is taken up by secondary lysosomes and is then denatured and hydrolyzed into relatively inert hemosiderin deposits.

Only about 7 mg of iron is distributed within the extracellular fluid, with 50 percent (3.5 mg) being bound to the primary transport protein in plasma, transferrin.[2] Normally, 20 to 50 percent of transferrin is saturated with iron. Absolute levels of transferrin increase during iron deficiency and decrease during iron overload.

The typical Western diet contains 10 to 20 mg of iron a day. Usually 1 to 2 mg of iron are absorbed daily by

TABLE 106–1 · CAUSES OF IRON STORAGE DISEASE

Disorder	Mechanism(s) of the Iron Overload
Hereditary hemochromatosis	Recessive inheritance of increased intestinal iron absorption (HFE* gene defect)
Iron-loading anemias	Ineffective erythropoiesis, with or without red blood cell (RBC) transfusions
Thalassemia syndromes	
Sideroblastic anemias	
Congenital dyserythropoietic anemias	
Excessive iron intake	
RBC transfusions	Infusion of hemoglobin iron
Elemental iron	Prolonged ingestion of medicinal iron
Iron dextran	Prolonged parenteral iron therapy
African iron overload	Ingestion of excessive dietary iron plus a genetic factor (?)
Defects of iron transport and metabolism	
Hereditary atransferrinemia	Shunting of iron to nonerythroid tissues, increased absorption
Hereditary ceruloplasmin deficiency	Impaired oxidation of iron, increased intestinal absorption
Porphyria cutanea tarda	Associated inheritance of hereditary hemochromatosis allele
Hereditary hemolytic anemias (some)	Associated inheritance of hereditary hemochromatosis allele
Liver disease	Increased intestinal absorption of dietary iron (?)
Alcoholic liver disease	
Nonalcoholic steatohepatitis	
Viral hepatitis C	
Portacaval shunt	
Neonatal hemochromatosis	Unknown

*HFE is the designation for the gene defective in hereditary hemochromatosis.

Adapted from Bottomly SS: Secondary iron overload disorders. Semin Hematol 35:77, 1998.

the duodenal mucosa, which balances the loss of iron from exfoliated gastrointestinal mucosal cells.[2] Iron homeostasis is maintained by control of intestinal iron absorption; there is no effective physiologic mechanism to alter excretion once absorption is deranged.

Pathogenesis

Genetic hemochromatosis is characterized by continued inappropriate gastrointestinal iron absorption in the face of expanded iron stores. Excess absorption usually ranges from 1 to 3 mg of iron per day, which results in a total accumulated pool of 15 to 35 g of iron over a 35- to 60-year period.[4] In genetic hemochromatosis, levels of duodenal epithelial cell ferritin are inappropriately low,[12] and regulation of the transferrin receptor is aberrant.[13] This failure in duodenal cell iron regulation may result in inappropriate iron absorption.

The precise mechanisms by which chronic iron overload leads to tissue injury are not known. Several mechanisms have been proposed, including:

Increased lysosomal fragility
Iron-induced lipid peroxidation of mitochondrial and microsomal membranes14
A direct effect of iron on collagen biosynthesis, which leads to fibrosis15
Iron-stimulated depletion of vitamin E and C stores16

In 1996, Feder and coworkers presented HFE as a strong candidate gene for hemochromatosis.[17] The gene, which is located more than 3 Mb from human leukocyte antigen (HLA)-A on the short arm of chromosome 6, encodes a 343–amino acid protein expressed on the cell surface. Mutation of residue 282 prevents cell surface expression. HFE forms a stable cell surface complex with the transferrin receptor, decreasing the affinity of the receptor for transferrin.[18] Three mutations have been described: C282Y, H63D, and S65C.[19] In 178 typical hemochromatosis subjects, 83.2 percent were homozygous for C282Y, 4.5 percent for compound heterozygotes C282Y/H63D, 0.6 percent were homozygous for H63D, 6.7 percent heterozygotes for either C282Y or H63D, and 6.7 percent had neither mutation.[17] A recent study in Norway demonstrated that C282Y/S65C compound heterozygotes had a higher incidence of phenotypic hemochromatosis than the wild-type group. Many additional studies have confirmed these findings in hemochromatosis populations in the United States, United Kingdom, Canada, Australia, France, and Italy, with the percentage of cases homozygous for C282Y ranging from 60 to 100 percent.[21]

With the availability of testing for HFE, more accurate prevalence figures for hemochromatosis can be established. A recent large cross-sectional study reported a carrier rate among European-Americans of 6 percent for C282Y and 15 percent for H63D. These gene mutations were less common among persons of Asian, Hispanic, or African descent.[19] Hemochromatosis remains one of the most common genetic diseases in populations derived from a European heritage. The expression of homozygous hemochromatosis is variable and may be influenced by sex, age, alcohol intake, dietary habits, and other factors, including modifier genes.[23] Thus, clinical disease frequency rates would be lower than the 1 to 5 per 1000 population indicated by genetics and biochemical markers.

Compound heterozygotes (C282Y/H63D and C282Y/S65C) typically exhibit increased transferrin saturation but do not often develop clinically significant iron overload. C282Y heterozygotes without abnormal iron tests do not require special follow-up. Asymptomatic compound heterozygotes and homozygotes can be monitored with the aim of prophylactically treating them prior to the development of overt disease.

In joints, as well as in the other various target organs of hemochromatosis, tissue damage reflects both the amount and duration of iron deposition. The arthropathy of hemochromatosis is characterized by hemosiderin deposition found in synovium and chondrocytes.[25] The presence of iron in these synthetic cells may lead to altered production of critical enzymes or substrates. Additionally, synovial fibroblasts incubated with iron have been reported to produce increased amounts of collagenase and prostaglandin E_2.[26] Ferritin may also function as a source of iron for the promotion of superoxide-dependent lipid peroxidation, which can contribute to damage to chondrocytes.[27]

Chondrocalcinosis due to calcium pyrophosphate dihydrate (CPPD) or apatite deposition is a frequent finding in the arthropathy of hemochromatosis.[25,28] Ferrous iron inhibits pyrophosphatase in vitro.[28] Inhibition of this enzyme in chondrocytes could lead to CPPD crystal formation. However, these data do not account for the progressive CPPD deposition, which has occurred despite effective iron depletion by phlebotomy in some cases of hemochromatosis. Articular damage may result from iron-mediated alteration of glycosaminoglycanscomplexes[29] or by increased lipid peroxidation, resulting in membrane and lysosomal damage to chondrocytes[14] (Fig. 106–1).

Clinical Features

EXTRA-ARTICULAR FEATURES

Typically, the clinical manifestations of genetic hemochromatosis appear in persons between the ages of 40 and 60 years; this timing corresponds to the 20- to 30-fold expansion of total body iron in these patients. Symptomatic disease develops at a male-to-female ratio of approximately 5 to 10:1. The pattern of organ development in hemochromatosis does not follow a predictable sequence, and the classic triad of cirrhosis, diabetes mellitus, and pigmentation (i.e., bronze diabetes) rarely occur together and are late complications.[10]

The common target organs in iron storage disease are the liver, pancreas, heart, skin, joints, and pituitary gland. Table 106–2 lists the frequency of clinical symptoms and signs at the time of diagnosis in 251 patients with genetic hemochromatosis.[30] The liver is typically involved because it is a major site of iron storage. In addition to the hemosiderin-granule deposition, hepatocyte degeneration and varying degrees of fibrosis are characteristically observed. In advanced disease, macronodular cirrhosis may be present. Excess alcohol consumption greatly increases the prevalence of cirrhosis in hemochromatosis, likely due to the synergistic profibrogenic effect of iron and alcohol on the liver.[31] The incidence of hepatocellular carcinoma in genetic hemochromatosis is increased 200-fold.[32] Typically, hepatocellular carcinoma occurs only in cirrhotic livers, although its incidence is not altered despite successful phlebotomy therapy.[30,33]

Hyperpigmentation of the skin is related to increased deposition of melanin and dermal iron. Coloration can vary from slate gray to brown and is most prominent in exposed areas, external genitals, nipple areola, and flexion folds.[4] Diabetes usually results from insulin

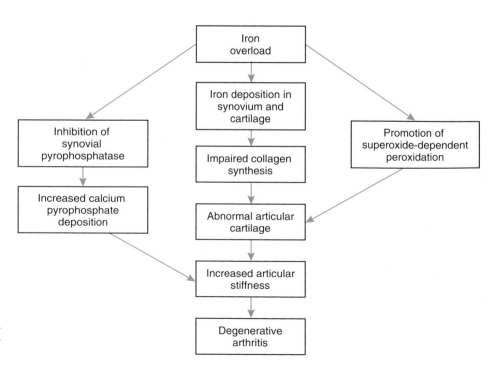

FIGURE 106–1 • Proposed mechanisms for the development of arthropathy in iron-overload states.

TABLE 106–2 · FREQUENCY OF CLINICAL FEATURES AT THE TIME OF DIAGNOSIS IN PATIENTS WITH GENETIC HEMOCHROMATOSIS

Symptoms and Findings	Percentage of Patients*
Weakness, lethargy	82 (205)
Abdominal pain	56 (140)
Arthralgia	44 (111)
Loss of libido or sexual potency	36 (81/224)
Amenorrhea, secondary	15 (4/27)
Dyspnea on exertion	12 (31)
Neurologic symptoms†	4 (11)
Hepatomegaly	81 (203)
Pigmentation	72 (181)
Loss of body hair	16 (39)
Splenomegaly	10 (26)
Peripheral edema	9 (23)
Jaundice	8 (19)
Gynecomastia	7 (15/224)
Ascites	5 (13)
Electrocardiographic changes	35 (88)
Esophageal varices	12 (29)

*Percentage of all patients (n = 251).
†These symptoms consist of disorientation (n = 3), depression (n = 2), marked lethargy (n = 2), and Parkinson-like hearing loss (n = 1).

Adapted with permission from Niederau C, Fischer R, Purschel A, et al: Long-term survival in patients with hereditary hemochromatosis. Gastroenterology 110:1107, 1996.

depletion, although resistance to insulin can also occur. In the pancreas, iron is selectively deposited in islet beta cells, which impairs insulin, but not glucagon, secretion.[34,35] Cardiac involvement in hemochromatosis typically presents as a dilated cardiomyopathy with associated dysrhythmia and heart failure.

Impotence and loss of libido are often prominent symptoms in patients with hemochromatosis. Iron deposition in gonadotropic cells of the pituitary gland leads to deficient gonadotropin secretion with resultant testicular atrophy and low testosterone levels in affected men.[36] Secondary amenorrhea has been described in women with hemochromatosis.[30,37]

Osteoporosis has been described in patients with hemochromatosis, especially if hypogonadism is present. Both trabecular and cortical bone can be lost. Hypogonadal men who do not undergo phlebotomy tend to experience the lowest bone density, but untreated eugonadal men also have insufficient osteoblastic activity.[38,39] In hypogonadal patients, increased bone resorption is combined with low bone formation to result in low bone density. Indeed, bone mineral density can be improved in some hypogonadal men with hemochromatosis by treatment with both phlebotomy and testosterone.[38]

ARTICULAR FEATURES

The arthropathy of genetic hemochromatosis has been recognized as an increasingly important feature of the disease and as having the greatest impact on quality of life.[40] However, arthropathy is uncommon in other forms of iron storage disease.[6] In hemochromatosis, arthritis is present in 50 percent, or more, of cases,[41,42] and it may be the initial symptom in as many as one third of cases.[42,43] Moreover, the extent of articular disease does not correlate with the severity of other organ involvement.[43] The spectrum of joint disease ranges from arthralgia to symmetric polyarticular arthritis, although unilateral disease, especially in weight-bearing joints, has also been described. Joint symptoms predominate in the hands and wrists, but knees, hips, ankles, feet, and shoulders are also common areas of involvement.[43,44] Progressive degenerative arthropathy with joint-space narrowing, subchondral sclerosis, and cyst formation at these joints is typical. The increased incidence of hip arthropathy in 25 percent of a surveyed 112 cases of hemochromatosis emphasized that joint destruction was severe enough that 37 percent of patients with hip involvement required surgery.[45] Analysis of femoral heads in patients requiring hip arthroplasty has revealed a distinctive wedge-shaped radioluscent zone in the subchondral bone, correlating to a separation of articular cartilage from bone.[45]

Chondrocalcinosis has been found in 20 to 50 percent of patients diagnosed with hemochromatosis.[41,42] Chondrocalcinosis in hemochromatosis occurs primarily in the hands and wrists. Deposition in the triangular fibrocartilage above the ulnar styloid and in the metacarpophalangeal (MCP) joints in most characteristic.[46] Widespread chondrocalcinosis may also be present in elbows, shoulders, hips, knees, ankles, feet, the symphysis pubis, intervertebral disks, and periarticular soft tissues. Typically, chondrocalcinosis in hemochromatosis is associated with CPPD or hydroxyapatite (HA) crystals. However, crystals and articular damage have been demonstrated in some joints without obvious chondrocalcinosis by radiography.[25] The degenerative arthropathy of hemochromatosis is similar to that of pyrophosphate arthropathy and osteoarthritis (OA). However, the proclivity to affect MCP joints and wrists is not typical of OA[47] (Table 106–3). Idiopathic CPPD arthropathy and the arthropathy in hemochromatosis both commonly affect the index and middle MCP

TABLE 106–3 · CLINICAL AND RADIOGRAPHIC DIFFERENCES BETWEEN OSTEOARTHRITIS AND ARTHROPATHY ASSOCIATED WITH HEMOCHROMATOSIS

Feature	Osteoarthritis	Hemochromatosis
Age of onset	> 50 years	< 50 years
Association with chondrocalcinosis	Low	Moderate (20 to 50%)
Metacarpophalangeal (MCP) involvement	Rare	Typically present
MCP hook-type osteophytes	Rare	Typically present
Radiocarpal narrowing	Rare	Common

joints (so-called victory or peace sign, designating involvement of those MCP joints) leading to symmetric joint-space narrowing, subchondral cysts, sclerosis, and squaring of the metacarpal heads. Hemochromatosis may be distinguished from idiopathic CPPD deposition disease in other ways as well. Hemochromatosis has 1) increased severity of MCP joint involvement, 2) likely involvement of the MCP joints of the ring and little fingers, 3) increased prevalence of hook- or beak-like osteophytes on the radial aspect of metacarpal heads, 4) minimal radiocarpal joint-space narrowing, 5) presentation at an earlier age, and 6) association with juxta-articular osteopenia[46,47] (Fig. 106–2).

The arthropathy of hemochromatosis often results in pain and stiffness prior to objective enlargement of the joint. Final stages include limitation of movement, increased pain with use, progressive deformity, and bone spur formation. Synovial thickening, warmth, and erythema are characteristically absent. The joint effusions are noninflammatory unless acute inflammation due to CPPD or HA crystals occurs.[43] The involvement of MCP joints and the occasional finding of subcutaneous nodules may lead to the erroneous diagnosis of rheumatoid arthritis (RA). However, the radiographic appearance described previously is atypical for RA, and

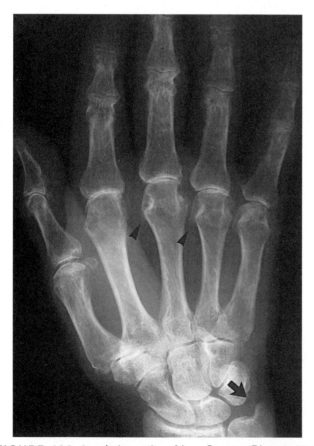

FIGURE 106–2 · Arthropathy of Iron Storage Disease. This radiograph demonstrates advanced arthritis present in a 66-year-old man with genetic hemochromatosis. Note the joint-space narrowing and subchondral sclerosis of the metacarpophalangeal (MCP) joints and hooklike osteophytes of the metacarpal heads (*arrow heads*), most pronounced in the index and middle fingers. Subtle chondrocalcinosis is present in the triangular fibrocartilage above the ulnar styloid (*arrow*).

the histopathologic examination of the nodules demonstrates iron deposition within noncaseating granulomas.[42,48] Degenerative MCP arthritis has been described in patients with type II diabetes mellitus in the absence of chondrocalcinosis with the same radiographic appearance as seen in hemochromatosis.[49]

The patient who presents with unexplained chondrocalcinosis, premature OA (before 50 years of age), OA in atypical joints (e.g., shoulder or ankle), or degenerative changes in MCP joints warrants an evaluation for hemochromatosis as well as for other diseases associated with CPPD deposition disease, such as hypothyroidism, hyperparathyroidism, acromegaly, Wilson's disease, ochronosis, gout, and diabetes mellitus (see Table 106–3).

■ Laboratory Features

When the diagnosis of hemochromatosis is suspected, transferrin saturation and serum ferritin levels are useful for screening. Normally, the percentage of saturation of transferrin—calculated by dividing serum iron concentration by total iron-binding capacity multiplied by 100—is 20 to 50 percent. In homozygotes with overt hemochromatosis, transferrin saturation is typically 80 to 100 percent.[2] Serum iron levels should be measured while the patient is in a fasting state because they may be elevated after a meal. In general, serum ferritin concentration is an accurate peripheral measure of iron stores, although acute liver injury, systemic inflammation, and neoplasia may also increase ferritin levels. Normal levels of ferritin are 20 to 300 ng/ml in men and 15 to 250 ng/ml in women, whereas levels greater than 500 ng/ml are typically found in individuals with symptomatic hemochromatosis.[2] The combination of an increased serum ferritin level and transferrin saturation of greater than 50 percent is approximately 95-percent sensitive and 85-percent specific for the diagnosis of genetic hemochromatosis.[50]

Other laboratory results may be abnormal in patients with hemochromatosis, depending on the severity of disease. Hyperglycemia, hepatic transaminase elevation, hypoalbuminemia, elevated alkaline phosphatase levels, and hyperbilirubinemia are examples.

The definitive diagnosis of hemochromatosis is made by the direct measurement of iron in a liver biopsy specimen. Quantitative biochemical iron concentration using atomic absorption should also be employed.[2] As emphasized earlier, the distribution of stainable iron in genetic hemochromatosis is located primarily in the hepatocytes, whereas in alcoholic cirrhosis, iron is most prominent in the Kupffer cells.[3] The hepatic iron index—calculated by dividing hepatic iron by age—has predictive value in distinguishing homozygotes for the hemochromatosis gene from heterozygotes. It also allows the differentiation of patients with other liver diseases associated with increased hepatic iron (e.g., alcoholic siderosis) from patients with hemochromatosis.[51,52] The measurement of stainable hepatic iron using microcomputerized image analysis has demonstrated a linear relationship to biochemical iron measurements. This rapid method can be accurately applied to liver biopsies that were obtained previously and embedded in paraffin.[53]

Noninvasive hepatic imaging procedures have been proposed as alternative means of estimating the degree of iron overload in iron storage diseases. With magnetic resonance imaging (MRI), a decrease in hepatic signal intensity occurs in the presence of iron overload as shown by alterations in magnetic T_2 relaxation rates[54] (Fig. 106–3). Among MRI techniques to determine iron overload, gradient echo T_2-weighted sequences have shown high sensitivity (91%) and specificity (88%) when compared with liver iron concentrations.[55] MRI may also identify extrahepatic iron deposition in the spleen, pancreas, lymph nodes, pituitary gland, and heart.[54,56]

The synovial fluid is typically noninflammatory except in patients in whom acute inflammation develops in association with CPPD or HA deposition disease. The synovium obtained at arthroplasty may demonstrate mild to moderate cellular proliferation, minimal to no inflammation, and occasional intracellular hemosiderin deposits.[43]

Screening

The high prevalence, extent of the morbidity and mortality rates, and benefit of early diagnosis and treatment make hemochromatosis a prime target for disease screening techniques.[57] Screening of patients for hemochromatosis is aimed at making the diagnosis in the precirrhotic and presymptomatic stage. Phlebotomy initiated early in the course of disease can prevent progression and decrease the mortality rate. Most patients with

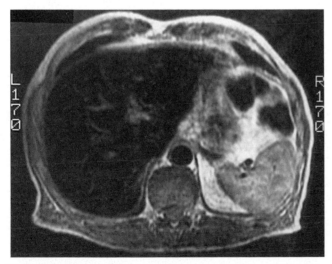

FIGURE 106–3 · Magnetic Resonance Imaging (MRI) in Iron Storage Disease. This MRI is a coronal section of the abdomen of a 58-year-old man with genetic hemochromatosis who presented with calcium pyrophosphate dihydrate (CPPD) arthropathy of his wrists and ankles, a transferrin saturation of 95 percent, and a serum ferritin level of 1494 ng/ml. This figure demonstrates the very low signal intensity of the liver consistent with the paramagnetic effects of excess iron deposition, which was quantitatively measured on a liver biopsy specimen as an iron concentration of 21,903 μg/g dry weight. The patient required 70 phlebotomized units to normalize his serum ferritin level. The MRI was obtained at 1.5 tesla with an echo time of 20 msec and a repetition time of 800 msec. (Courtesy of Dr. Lester Miller, Santa Cruz, California.)

hemochromatosis do not become symptomatic until after 40 years of age; thus, the optimal group to screen using biochemical studies would be young, asymptomatic, white adults.[57] Recent screening studies have proved cost effective, especially in rheumatology clinic populations and in patients with extreme fatigue, arthralgia, and loss of libido.[58,60] Use of transferrin saturation thresholds of 50 percent for women and 60 percent for men provides fewer false-negative results; repeating the value after an overnight fast reduces the number of false-positive results.[57] Unsaturated iron binding capacity (UIBC) has equal reliability in predicting hemochromatosis at a threshold of 143mcg/dl and can be used as an inexpensive alternative to transferrin saturation.[59]

Even though the HFE gene mutations have been identified in a high percentage of hemochromatosis cases (60 to 100 percent), they should not be used to screen populations because of the uncertainties about genotype-phenotype correlations and possible discrimination due to genetic typing. Also, cost-benefit analysis does not favor genetic testing over lower-priced iron studies.[19]

Patients with any disease manifestation suggestive of hemochromatosis should be screened for transferrin saturation and serum ferritin levels. Because clinical manifestations take decades to develop and are often subtle, a high index of suspicion for this disorder must be maintained. In most cases, hemochromatosis is detected during the management of incidental illness or is discovered during periodic health examinations.

Once a case of hemochromatosis is identified, genetic typing for HFE mutations can be employed. If two HFE mutations are identified in the proband (i.e., C282Y/C282Y, C282Y/H63D), siblings at risk to develop hemochromatosis can be identified by testing for these mutations. Homozygotes for H63D do not typically develop iron overload.

Children of a proband and children of heterozygotes will not be affected by the disease unless the spouse is also a heterozygote for hemochromatosis. Heterozygotes occasionally exhibit abnormal serum iron indices but are not at risk for development of the disease and, therefore, can be reassured. Figure 106–4 offers a clinical algorithm to use in diagnosis of hemochromatosis.

Screening is recommended for all first-degree relatives of individuals with hemochromatosis using transferrin saturation, serum ferritin determinations, and HFE typing starting at the age of 20 years.[2,61] If a homozygote C282Y or heterozygote C282Y/H63D for the disease is identified, yearly biochemical iron testing should be followed. A recent study found that the combination of a ferritin level of greater than or equal to 1000 ng/ml, platelets less than or equal to 200,000/uL, and AST above the upper limit of normal led to the correct diagnosis of cirrhosis in 81 percent of C282Y homozygous hemochromatosis patients, reducing the need for liver biopsy.[62]

Treatment and Prognosis

The primary treatment of genetic hemochromatosis is to remove excess iron by phlebotomy. Removal of 500 ml of blood, equivalent to 250 mg of iron, on a

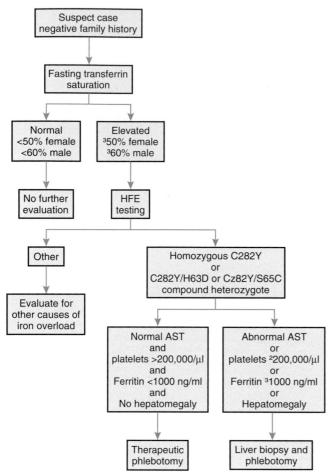

FIGURE 106-4 · Clinical Algorithm for Diagnosis of Hemochromatosis.

weekly basis will eliminate 10 to 13 g of iron in a year. Depletion of iron stores in advanced cases may require phlebotomy for 2 or 3 years, followed by maintenance phlebotomy four to six times annually to counteract continued excessive iron absorption.[4] The serum ferritin level declines progressively during phlebotomy, whereas serum iron levels and transferrin saturation remain high until iron depletion has occurred.[63] Hemoglobin and hematocrit levels fall when iron deficiency develops and can be used as a monitor of adequacy of therapy during phlebotomy. Once the hemoglobin falls to 11 g/dl or the hematocrit falls to 34 percent, maintenance phlebotomy can be instituted to keep transferrin saturation at about 50 percent, approximately 4 to 8 times a year for life.[2,64]

Phlebotomy has also been used effectively in various forms of secondary iron overload but is not feasible as treatment in diseases associated with anemia. Deferoxamine, an iron-chelating agent, may be administered by subcutaneous or intravenous (IV) infusion to remove excess iron in these patients. In cardiomyopathy secondary to iron overload, chelation therapy with deferoxamine combined with phlebotomy may be warranted to maximize iron removal. Red cell apheresis removes excess iron twice as fast as manual whole blood phlebotomy and could be considered as an alternative procedure if phlebotomy is contraindicated.[65]

The effectiveness of phlebotomy therapy varies with the severity and degree of organ dysfunction in individuals with hemochromatosis. Hepatic function may improve with phlebotomy, but regression of the fibrosis or cirrhosis is unusual.[33,66] Liver neoplasms, including both hepatocellular carcinoma and intrahepatic bile duct carcinoma, are life-threatening complications that occur in approximately 30 percent of patients with cirrhosis.[30] Unfortunately, the successful depletion of hepatic iron may not decrease the incidence of subsequent liver cancer.[30] Similarly, only one third of patients experience improvement in their diabetes mellitus to the degree that they no longer require insulin therapy.[66] With hypogonadism, iron depletion alone can occasionally restore libido, potency, or reversal of amenorrhea, but most individuals will require supplemental hormone therapy to replace depleted testosterone or estrogen.[37] Testosterone injections plus phlebotomy may also be effective therapy for improving bone mineral density (BMD) in adult males with associated osteoporosis.[39]

In general, phlebotomy does not alleviate symptoms of arthralgia and loss of joint mobility in patients with established arthropathy associated with hemochromatosis. In fact, arthritis may progress despite phlebotomy.[41,43] Nonsteroidal anti-inflammatory drugs (NSAIDs) may be of some symptomatic benefit in managing chronic arthritis. In patients with recurrent, acute episodes of CPPD crystal deposition, joint aspiration, intra-articular corticosteroids, and prophylaxis with colchicine may be beneficial. If progressive joint destruction occurs, arthroplasty may be appropriate in selected cases.

The prognosis of patients with genetic hemochromatosis depends on the amount and the duration of iron excess. The presence of cirrhosis and diabetes at the time of diagnosis is a poor prognostic indicator.[30] In a 1996 study, the cumulative survival of 251 patients treated with phlebotomy was 93 percent at 5 years, 77 percent at 10 years, 62 percent at 15 years, 55 percent at 20 years, 46 percent at 25 years, and 20 percent at 30 years (mean survival of 21 years).[30] Compared with the norm, hemochromatosis demonstrates a 119 times more frequent liver cancer rate, a 14 times more frequent rate for cardiomyopathy, a 10 times more frequent rate for cirrhosis, and a 14 times more frequent rate for diabetes.[30] In contrast, patients who are identified in the precirrhotic stage and are treated by adequate phlebotomy have a normal life expectancy.[30,67]

ACKNOWLEDGEMENT

I wish to acknowledge Dr. James L. McGuire (1948–1997), my mentor and friend, for his contribution to this chapter and to my life.

REFERENCES

1. Bottomly SS: Secondary iron overload disorders. Semin Hematol 35:77, 1998.
2. Tavill AS, Bacon BR: Hemochromatosis: Iron metabolism and the iron overload syndromes. *In* Zakim D, Boyer TD (eds): Hepatology:

A Textbook of Liver Disease, 2nd ed. Philadelphia, WB Saunders, 1990.

3. Bothwell TH, Charlton RW: Hemochromatosis. *In* Schiff L, Schiff ER (eds): Diseases of the Liver, 6th ed. Philadelphia, JB Lippincott, 1987.

4. Smith LH Jr.: Overview of hemochromatosis. West J Med 153:96, 1990.

5. Gordeuk VR: Hereditary and nutritional iron overload. Baillieres Clin Hematol 5:169, 1992.

6. Gordeuk VR, McLaren GD, Samowitz W: Etiologies, consequences and treatment of iron overload. Crit Rev Clin Lab Sci 31:89, 1994.

7. Gordeuk V, Mukiibi J, Hasstedt SF, et al: Iron overload in Africa—interaction between a gene and dietary iron content. N Engl J Med 326:95, 1992.

8. Grossman ME, Bickers DR, Poh-Fitzpatrick MB, et al: Porphyria cutanea tarda: Clinical and laboratory findings in 40 patients. Am J Med 67:277, 1979.

9. Bonkovsky HL, Poh-Fitzpatrick M, Pimstone N, et al: Porphyria cutanea tarda, hepatitis C, and HFE gene mutations in North America. Hepatology 27:1661, 1998.

10. Smith BC, Grove J, Guzail MA, et al: Heterozygosity for hereditary hemochromatosis is associated with more fibrosis in chronic hepatitis C. Hepatology 27:1695, 1998.

11. Hakim RM, Stivelman JC, Schulman G, et al: Iron overload and mobilization in long-term hemodialysis patients. Am J Kidney Dis 10:293, 1987.

12. Francanzani AL, Fargion S, Romeno R, et al: Immuno-histochemical evidence for a lack of ferritin in duodenal absorptive epithelioid cells in idiopathic hemochromatosis. Gastroenterology 96:1071, 1989.

13. Lombard M, Bomford AB, Polson RJ, et al: Differential expression of transferrin receptor in duodenal mucosa in iron overload: Evidence for a site-specific defect in genetic hemochromatosis. Gastroenterology 98:976, 1990.

14. Bacon BR, Britton RS: The pathology of hepatic iron overload: A free-radical mediated process? Hepatology 11.127, 1990.

15. Weintraub LR, Goral A, Grasso J: Pathogenesis of hepatic fibrosis in experimental iron overload. Br J Hepatol 59:321, 1985.

16. von Herbay A, DeGroot H, Hegi U, et al: Low vitamin E content of patients with alcoholic liver disease, haemochromatosis and Wilson's disease. J Hepatol 20:41, 1993.

17. Feder JN, Gnirke A, Thomas W, et al: A novel MHC class I–like gene is mutated in patients with hereditary hemochromatosis. Nat Genet 13:399, 1996.

18. Feder JN, Penny DM, Irrinki A, et al: The hemachromatosis gene product complexes with the transferrin receptor and lowers its affinity for ligand binding. Proc Natl Acad Sci USA 95:1472, 1998.

19. Beutler E, Felitti V, Gelbart T, et al: The effect of HFE genotypes on measurements of iron overlaod in patients attending a health appraisal conference. Ann Intern Med 133:329, 2000.

20. Asberg A, Thorstensen K, Hveem K, Bjerve KS: Hereditary hemochromatosis: the clinical significance of the S65C mutation. Genet Test 6:59, 2002.

21. Burke W, Thomson E, Khoury MJ, et al: Hereditary hemochromatosis: Gene discovery and its implications for population-based screening. JAMA 280:172, 1998.

22. Porto G, Vicente C, Fraga J, et al: Importance of establishing appropriate local reference values for the screening of hemochromatosis: A study of three different control populations and 136 hemochromatosis family members. J Lab Clin Med 119:295, 1992.

23. Britton RS, Fleming RE, Parkkila S, et al: Pathogenesis of hereditary hemochromatosis: genetics and beyond. Semin Gastrointest Dis 13:68, 2002.

24. Moirand R, Guyader D, Mendler MH, et al: HFE based re-evaluation of heterozygous hemochromatosis. Am J Med Genet 111:356, 2002.

25. Schumacher HR: Articular cartilage in the degenerative arthropathy of hemochromatosis. Arthritis Rheum 25:1460, 1982.

26. Okazaki I, Brinckerhoff CE, Sinclair JF, et al: Iron increases collagenase production by rabbit synovial fibroblasts. J Lab Clin Med 97:396, 1981.

27. Thomas CE, Morehouse LA, Aust SD: Ferritin and superoxide-dependent lipid peroxidation. J Biol Chem 260:3275, 1985.

28. McCarty DJ, Pepe PF: Erythrocyte neutral inorganic pyrophosphatase in pseudogout. J Lab Clin Med 79:277, 1972.

29. De Seye S, Solnica J, Mitrovic D, et al: Joint and bone disorders and hypoparathyroidism in hemochromatosis. Semin Arthritis Rheum 2:71, 1972.

30. Niederau G, Fischer R, Purschel A, et al: Long-term survival in patients with hereditary hemochromatosis. Gastroenterology 110:1107, 1996.

31. Fletcher LM, Dixon JL, Purdie DM, et al: Excess alcohol greatly increases the prevalence of cirrhosis in hereditary hemochromatosis. Gastroenterology 122:281, 2002

32. Bradbear RA, Bain C, Siskind V, et al: Cohort study of internal malignancy in genetic hemochromatosis and other chronic non-alcoholic liver diseases. J Natl Cancer Inst 75:81, 1985.

33. Tiniakos G, Williams R: Cirrhotic process, liver cell carcinoma and extrahepatic malignant tumors in idiopathic haemochromatosis: Study of 71 patients treated with venesection therapy. Appl Pathol 6:128, 1988.

34. Rahier J, Loozen S, Goebbels RM, et al: The haemochromatotic human pancreas: A quantitative immunohistochemical and ultrastructural study. Diabetologia 30:5, 1987.

35. Muller WA, Berger M, Cüppers HJ, et al: Plasma glucagon in diabetes of haemochromatosis: Too low or too high? Gut 20:200, 1979.

36. Stremmel W, Niederau C, Berger M, et al: Abnormalities in estrogen, androgen, and insulin metabolism in idiopathic hemochromatosis. Ann N Y Acad Sci 526:209, 1988.

37. Meyer WR, Hutchinson-Williams KA, Jones EE, DeCherney AH: Secondary hypogonadism in hemochromatosis. Fertil Steril 54:740, 1990.

38. Diamond T, Stiel D, Posen S: Effects of testosterone and venesection on spinal and peripheral bone mineral in six hypogonadal men with hemochromatosis. J Bone Miner Res 6:39, 1991.

39. Sinigaglia L, Fargion S, Francanzani AL, et al: Bone and joint involvement in genetic hemochromatosis: Role of cirrhosis and iron overload. J Rheumatol 24.1809, 1997.

40. Adams PC, Speechley M: The effect of arthritis on the quality of life in hereditary hemochromatosis. J Rheumatol 23:707, 1996.

41. Hamilton EBD, Bomford AB, Laws JW, Williams R: The natural history of arthritis in idiopathic haemochromatosis. Q J Med 50:321, 1981.

42. Huaux JP, Geubel A, Koch MC, et al: The arthritis of hemochromatosis: A review of 25 cases with special reference to chondrocalcinosis, and a comparison with patients with primary hyperparathyroidism and controls. Clin Rheumatol 5:317, 1986.

43. Schumacher HR: Haemochromatosis. Bailleres Best Pract Res Clin Rheumatol 14:277, 2000.

44. Bailey EJ, Gardner AB: Hemochromatosis of the foot and ankle: Report of three cases and review of the literature. Clin Orthop Res 349:108, 1998.

45. Axford JS, Bomford A, Revell P, et al: Hip arthropathy in genetic hemochromatosis: Radiographic and histologic features. Arthritis Rheum 34:357, 1991.

46. Adamson TC III, Resnik CS, Guerra J Jr., et al: Hand and wrist arthropathies of hemochromatosis and calcium pyrophosphate deposition disease: Distinct radiographic features Radiology 147:377, 1983.

47. Atkins CJ, McIvor J, Smith PM, et al: Chondrocalcinosis and arthropathy: Studies in haemochromatosis and in idiopathic chondrocalcinosis. Q J Med 39:71, 1970.

48. Bensen WG, Laskin CA, Little HA, Fam AG: Hemochromatotic arthropathy mimicking rheumatoid arthritis: A case with subcutaneous nodules, tenosynovitis and bursitis. Arthritis Rheum 21:844, 1978.

49. McCarthy GM, Rosenthal AK, Carrera GF: Hemochromatosis-like arthropathy in diabetes mellitus without hemochromatosis. J Rheumatol 23:1453, 1996.

50. Bassett ML, Halliday JW, Ferris RA, et al: Diagnosis of hemochromatosis in young subjects: Predictive accuracy of biochemical screening tests. Gastroenterology 87:628, 1984.

51. Adams PC: Hepatic iron in hemochromatosis. Dig Dis Sci 35:690, 1990.

52. Summers KM, Halliday JW, Powell LW: Identification of homozygous hemochromatosis subjects by measurement of hepatic iron index. Hepatology 12:20, 1990.

53. Olynyk J, Hall P, Sallie R, et al: Computerized measurement of iron in liver biopsies: A comparison with biochemical iron measurement. Hepatology 12:26, 1990.

54. Johnston DL, Rice L, Vick W III, et al: Assessment of tissue iron overload by nuclear magnetic resonance imaging. Am J Med 87:40, 1989.

55. Ernst O, Sergent G, Bonvarlet P, et al: Hepatic iron overload: Diagnosis and quantification with MR imaging. AJR 168:1205, 1997.

56. Housman JF, Chezmar JL, Nelson RC: Magnetic resonance imaging in hemochromatosis: Extrahepatic iron deposition. Gastrointest Radiol 14:59, 1989.

57. Adams PC, Gregor JC, Kertesz AE, Valberg LS: Screening blood donors for hereditary hemochromatosis: Decision analysis model based on a 30-year database. Gastroenterology 109:177, 1995.

58. Olynyk J, Hall P, Ahern M, et al: Screening for genetic haemochromatosis in a rheumatology clinic. Aust N Z J Med 24:22, 1994.

59. Murtagh LJ, Whiley M, Wilson S, et al: Unsaturated iron binding capacity and transferrin saturation are equally reliable in detection of HFE hemochromatosis. Am J Gastroenterol 97:2093, 2002.

60. McDonnell SM, Preston SL, Jewell SA, et al: A survey of 2,851 patients with hemochromatosis: symptoms and response to therapy. Am J Med 106:619, 1999.

61. Adams PC, Kertesz AE, Valberg LS: Screening for hemochromatosis in children of homozygotes: prevalence and cost-effectiveness. Hepatology 22:1720, 1995.

62. Beaton M, Guyader D, Deugnier Y, et al: Noninvasive prediction of cirrhosis in C282Y-linked hemochromatosis. Hepatology 36:673, 2002.

63. Edwards CO, Cartwright GE, Skolnick MH, et al: Homozygosity for hemochromatosis: Clinical manifestations. Ann Intern Med 93:519, 1980.

64. Fox IH: Iron storage disease. *In* Kelley WN, Harris ED Jr., Ruddy S, Sledge CB (eds): Textbook of Rheumatology, 3rd ed. Philadelphia, WB Saunders, 1989.

65. Muncunill J, Vaquer P, Galmes A, et al: In hereditary hemochromatosis, red cell aphresis removes excess iron turice as fast as manual whole blood phlebotomy. J Clin Apheresis 17:88, 2002.

66. Bomford A, Williams R: Long-term results of venesection therapy in idiopathic haemochromatosis. Q J Med 45:611, 1976.

67. Wojcik JP, Speechley MR, Kertesz AE, et al: Natural history of C282Y homozygotes for hemochromatosis. Can J Gastroenterol 16:297, 2002.

107

Hemophilic Arthropathy

KATHERINE S. UPCHURCH · DOREEN B. BRETTLER

Although spontaneous joint hemorrhage has been described in a variety of inherited disorders of coagulation[1-3] and in the setting of anticoagulation therapy,[4] it occurs most frequently in hemophilia. Bleeding into the joints is, in fact, the complication of hemophilia that most often requires therapeutic intervention and, when it is recurrent, can lead to chronic, deforming arthritis that is independent of bleeding episodes.

Hemophilia refers to a group of inherited diseases in which there is a functional deficiency of a specific clotting factor. The most common are hemophilia A (classic hemophilia) and hemophilia B (Christmas disease), the deficient factors being factor VIII and factor IX, respectively. The incidence and severity of hemorrhagic complications of hemophilia are directly related to the severity of the underlying coagulation defect.

Although the intrinsic pathway of coagulation is severely impaired in hemophilia, the extrinsic tissue-dependent pathway remains intact[5] and is probably the major hemostatic regulatory system. It is of interest that normal synovial tissue and cultures of synovial fibroblasts have been found to be deficient in tissue factor,[6,7] which suggests that in synovium-lined joints, hemophiliacs have functional inactivity of both intrinsic and extrinsic coagulation pathways. This may explain the marked propensity toward hemorrhage in joints compared to other tissue sites in these patients.

Clinical Features

The spectrum of articular disease in hemophiliacs has been the subject of numerous comprehensive reviews[8-15] and includes acute hemarthrosis, subacute or chronic arthritis, and end-stage hemophilic arthropathy. The usual distribution of joint involvement is shown in Figure 107-1. Involvement of the small joints of the hands and feet may also occur, although infrequently.

ACUTE HEMARTHROSIS

Nearly all patients with severe hemophilia A or B (less than 1 percent activity of the deficient factor) and up to half[15] of patients with moderate disease activity experience hemarthrosis. Acute hemarthroses generally first occur when a child begins to walk and continues, usually cyclically, into adulthood, when the frequency diminishes. Patients frequently have premonitory symptoms, such as stiffness or warmth in the affected joint,

followed by intense pain, which may be due in part to rapid joint-capsule distension.

Pain is accompanied by objective clinical findings of warmth, a tense effusion, tenderness, limitation of motion, and a joint that is often held in a flexed position. Joint pain responds rapidly to replacement of the deficient clotting factor. If hemostasis is achieved early after onset of hemarthrosis, full joint function may be regained within 12 to 24 hours. If the hemorrhage is more advanced, however, blood is resorbed slowly during 5 to 7 days, and full joint function is regained within 10 to 14 days.

SUBACUTE OR CHRONIC ARTHRITIS

Recurrent hemarthroses, particularly in patients with severe factor deficiency, may lead to a self-perpetuating condition in which joint abnormalities persist in intervals between bleeding episodes. The involved joint is chronically swollen, although painless and only slightly warm. Chronic synovitis, including prominent synovial proliferation with or without effusion, may be present. There may be mild limitation of motion, often with a flexion deformity. Factor replacement does not modify these findings.

END-STAGE HEMOPHILIC ARTHROPATHY

Long-standing end-stage hemophilic arthropathy has features in common with both degenerative joint disease and advanced rheumatoid arthritis (RA). The joint appears enlarged and "knobby," owing to osteophytic bone overgrowth. Synovial thickening and effusion, however, are not prominent. Range of motion is severely restricted, and fibrous ankylosis is common. Subluxation, joint laxity, and malalignment are frequently present. Hemarthroses decrease in frequency, however.

SEPTIC ARTHRITIS

Until the early 1980s, septic arthritis rarely occurred in hemophiliac patients. With the widespread occurrence of human immunodeficiency virus (HIV) infection as a result of contaminated factor concentrates, the incidence of this complication has risen significantly.[16,17] Septic arthritis is seen more often in adult than in pediatric hemophiliacs and is most commonly monarticular, usually involving the knee. In contrast to spontaneous hemarthrosis, septic arthritis is significantly associated with a temperature higher than 38°C within 12 hours of

Percentage joints with:

Any hemarthrosis	Many hemarthroses	Chronic pain	Synovitis	Limitation of motion	Any radiologic abnormality
34.5	13.3	13.9	—	16.9	21.6
54.0	38.5	13.8	9.8	27.0	52.6
28.6	8.0	5.4	—	19.8	18.8
63.1	50.9	26.8	11.6	27.0	50.2
60.8	42.8	15.2	2.2	34.2	52.4

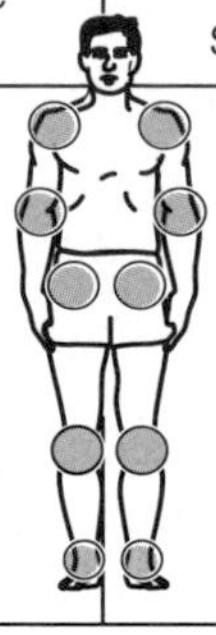

FIGURE 107–1 · Distribution of Acute Hemarthrosis Based on a Study of 139 Patients with Hemophilia. Clinical and radiologic features of chronic arthritis in hemophilia. (Adapted from Steven MM, Yogarojah S, Madhok R, et al: Haemophilic arthritis. Q J Med 58:181, 1986.)

presentation and articular pain that does not improve with replacement therapy.[16] Peripheral leukocyte count may not be elevated, particularly in HIV-positive patients.[17] A predisposing factor other than hemophilic arthropathy is often identifiable, including previous arthrocentesis or arthroplasty, intravenous (IV) drug use, and infected indwelling venous-access catheters. Even in HIV-infected patients, *Staphylococcus aureus* is the most frequently identified organism, followed by *Streptococcus pneumoniae*.[18]

MUSCLE AND SOFT TISSUE HEMORRHAGE

Bleeding into muscles and soft tissue is common in hemophiliacs and may be more insidious than hemarthrosis because of the lack of premonitory symptoms. Bleeding into the iliopsoas and gastrocnemius muscles and the forearm results in well-described syndromes with which the rheumatologist should be familiar. Iliopsoas hemorrhage produces acute groin pain with marked pain on hip extension and a hip flexion contracture. Rotation is preserved, in contrast to intra-articular hemorrhage. If untreated, the expanding soft tissue mass may compress the femoral nerve, causing signs and symptoms of femoral neuropathy.[14,19] Bleeding into the gastrocnemius muscle can cause an equinus deformity from heel cord contracture.[14] Finally, hemorrhage into closed compartments can cause acute muscle necrosis and nerve compression.[20] Of particular importance is bleeding into the volar compartment of the forearm, which can cause flexion deformities of the wrist and fingers. If a compartment syndrome is suspected, compartment pressures should be measured to confirm the diagnosis.

A large intramuscular hemorrhage uncommonly results in the formation of a simple muscle cyst, which clinically appears to be an encapsulated soft tissue area of swelling overlying muscle. Cyst formation in this setting is confined by the muscular fascial plane and most likely results from inadequate resorption of blood and clot. Subperiosteal or intraosseous hemorrhage, in contrast, may lead to a rare skeletal complication of hemophilia, a pseudotumor. Hemophilic pseudotumors are of two types: the adult type, which occurs proximally,

usually in the pelvis or femur; and the childhood type, which occurs distal to the elbows or knees and carries a better prognosis.[21,22]

Conservative early management of both muscle cysts and childhood-type pseudotumors is indicated, including immobilization and factor replacement. In adult-type pseudotumors, which are usually refractory to conservative therapy, and in progressive childhood pseudotumors, surgical removal is indicated[22] to prevent serious complications, such as spontaneous rupture, fistula formation, neurologic or vascular entrapment, and fracture of adjacent bone. Aspiration of a pseudotumor or cyst is contraindicated.

▌ Diagnostic Imaging

RADIOGRAPHS

The earliest radiographic changes in hemophilic arthropathy are confined to the soft tissue and reflect acute hemarthrosis. The joint capsule is distended with displacement of fat pads, and there is an increased hazy density caused by intra-articular blood. Hemarthrosis before epiphyseal plate closure may result in epiphyseal overgrowth and irregularity. On occasion, premature epiphyseal closure is seen.

With the progression of chronic proliferative synovitis, irreversible radiologic changes appear. These reflect both the inflammatory and the degenerative nature of chronic hemophilic arthropathy (Table 107–1 and Fig. 107–2A). Certain changes unique to hemophilic arthropathy occur as well (see Table 107–1 and Fig. 107–2B).

OTHER IMAGING METHODS

Magnetic resonance imaging (MRI) is now routinely used to accurately stage hemophilic arthritis, both to determine optimal treatment and to follow response to therapy.[23] A scoring system based on MRI has recently been proposed.[24] Additionally, MRI and ultrasonography are useful in both the detection and the quantitation of soft tissue bleeding, cysts, and pseudotumors.[25,26]

TABLE 107–1 • RADIOLOGIC MANIFESTATIONS OF CHRONIC HEMOPHILIC ARTHROPATHY

Characteristic	Also Seen in
Periarticular soft tissue swelling	RA
Periarticular demineralization	RA
Marginal erosions	RA
Subchondral irregularity and cyst formation	RA, OA
Decreased joint space	OA
Osteophyte formation	CPPD*
Chondrocalcinosis	
Specific	
Femoral intercondylar notch widening	
Squaring of distal patellar margin (lateral view)	
Proximal radial enlargement (see Fig. 107–2B)	
Talar flattening ±ankle ankylosis†	

*From Jensen PS, Putnam CE: Chondrocalcinosis and hemophilia. Clin Radiol 28:401, 1977.

†From Schreiber RR: Musculoskeletal system: radiologic findings. *In* Brinkhous KM, Hemker HC (eds): Handbook of Hemophilia. I. New York, American Elsevier, 1975, pp. xxx.

Abbreviations: CPPD, calcium pyrophosphate deposition disease; OA, osteoarthritis; RA, rheumatoid arthritis.

Pathologic Features and Pathogenesis

Pathologic studies of human hemophilic arthropathy have been limited to synovial specimens obtained at surgery[27,28] or at postmortem examination and, thus, reflect changes of advanced disease only. Studies of experimentally produced hemarthrosis in animals,[29,30] post-traumatic hemarthrosis in nonhemophilic humans,[31] and hemophilia A in dogs[32] have provided an understanding of the earliest changes induced by acute hemarthrosis and, in the last case, their evolution to chronic arthritis.

A single synovial hemorrhage induces serial changes in the synovial membrane, including early focal villous synovial proliferation and subsynovial diapedesis of erythrocytes, followed by the appearance of perivascular inflammatory cells, patchy subsynovial fibrosis, and intracellular iron accumulation in both synovial cells and subsynovial macrophages. With repeated hemarthroses, the synovium becomes grossly hypertrophied and hyperpigmented, with eventual organization into a pannus that invades and erodes marginal cartilage. On histologic examination, villous hypertrophy and subsynovial fibrosis progress, but inflammatory cells are scarce[28] (Fig. 107–3). Up to 75 percent of synoviocytes contain siderosomes (electron-dense, iron-filled deposits within lysosomes), in contrast to 10 percent in normal synovium and 25 percent in rheumatoid synovium.[33]

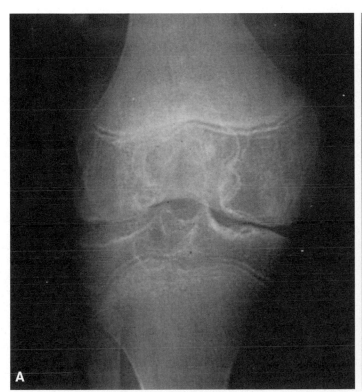
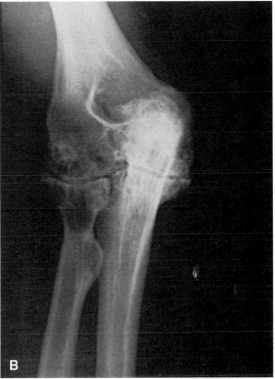

FIGURE 107–2 • Roentgenographic Changes of Hemophilic Arthropathy. *A*, Early arthritis of the knee, showing soft tissue swelling, widening of the femoral condyles and tibial plateau, irregularity of the distal femoral epiphysis, and a few subchondral bone cysts. *B*, More advanced arthritis involving the elbow, demonstrating almost complete loss of joint space and extensive subchondral cyst formation. The widening of the proximal radius is characteristic of hemophilic arthropathy.

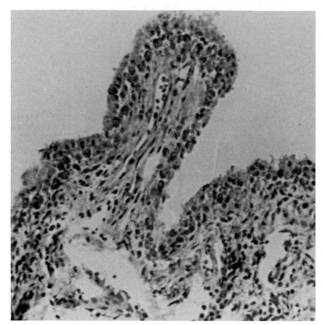

FIGURE 107–3 • Proliferative Synovitis of Hemophilia. Villous hypertrophy of synovium with pigment deposition in superficial cells. The reaction is mainly synovial cell hyperplasia. Infiltrating inflammatory cells are scarce (H&E, ×2500).

The articular cartilage is grossly and microscopically abnormal in the setting of recurrent hemarthrosis.[29] There are areas of cartilaginous fissuring and rarefaction exposing sclerotic bone. The remaining cartilage is thin and unevenly distributed, often freely protruding into the joint cavity. Bone erosions appear at weight-bearing surfaces. There is loss of matrix glycosaminoglycan, which is also seen in degenerative arthritis.[28,34]

Current studies suggest that recurrent hemarthrosis induces joint destruction in hemophilic arthropathy through direct and indirect effects of iron on the synovium[35,36] and cartilage,[34,37] by the degradative effect of the proliferative synovium,[38] and through an alteration in cartilage biochemical composition similar to that seen in degenerative arthritis.

Diagnosis

In most cases of congenital coagulopathy, the diagnosis will have been made before presentation to a rheumatologist. In the case of hemophilia, if there is an affected family member, prenatal diagnosis is possible. Because the spontaneous mutation rate in hemophilia is significant, the diagnosis may not be suspected until infancy, when recurrent, large ecchymoses or sustained oral hemorrhages commonly develop in most affected patients. In the case of hemophilia A or B, hemarthrosis is usually a later manifestation but may be the initial symptom of other, less severe coagulopathies, even in adult life. When a coagulopathy is suspected, baseline screening tests, including prothrombin time, activated partial thromboplastin time, and platelet count, should be performed. In patients with hemophilia, the prothrombin time and platelet count are normal and the activated partial thromboplastin time is prolonged, denoting a defect in the intrinsic clotting cascade. Referral to a hematologist, who will obtain the appropriate factor assays, is the next step.

Individuals with factor VIII or IX levels of 1 percent or less of the normal level have joint and muscle hemorrhages requiring therapy four or five times per month on the average. Such patients are classified as having severe hemophilia.

Individuals with factor VIII or IX levels greater than 5 percent of normal are considered to have mild hemophilia and usually hemorrhage only with trauma or at surgery. Occasional "spontaneous" hemarthrosis may occur in such patients, especially in joints damaged by previously undertreated hemorrhage.

Patients whose factor VIII or IX levels fall between these two ranges are considered to have moderately severe hemophilia, and their clinical picture falls somewhere between the extremes. If such patients have had multiple untreated or suboptimally treated hemarthroses with subsequent joint damage, the anatomic instability of these joints will cause frequent and severe bleeding, and the condition will, thus, appear clinically more severe than the factor VIII or IX assay might suggest.

Treatment of Hemophilia

Until recent years, in most hemophilia centers factor replacement therapy has been given on demand; that is, factor concentrate has been infused at the earliest sign of a hemorrhage. With the introduction of highly purified, safe concentrates, prophylactic treatment is now much more common in countries where this product is available, especially in pediatric patients.[23,39] Instead of being infused when a hemorrhage has occurred, factor concentrate is given regularly three times per week to prevent bleeds. Prophylaxis is started before any joint damage has occurred, usually at approximately 2 years of age, with the goal of minimizing bleeding episodes to no more than 4 to 6 per year. Indwelling catheters, such as Port-A-Cath and Hickman lines, are required for factor administration, because frequent venipunctures are painful and cumbersome. Recent data suggest that the institution of prophylactic factor infusion will significantly decrease the long-term joint sequelae of hemophilia and, thus, decrease lifetime disability.[40-42]

With adequate factor replacement, all types of surgery, including joint replacements, can be done. However, surgical intervention in a person with hemophilia should be done only at specialized centers with blood bank and coagulation laboratory support, as well as with the participation of a hematologist who specializes in clotting disorders. A surgeon who feels comfortable operating on patients with clotting disorders is also essential. Constant-infusion techniques for administering factor concentrate during and after surgery have made adequate factor levels easier to maintain and have decreased overall perioperative use of factor concentrates.[43] Many types of commercial factor VIII concentrate are available, manufactured either from plasma pools or recombinant technology.

FACTOR VIII REPLACEMENT

All factor concentrates are virally inactivated by various methods, including exposure to solvent detergent, heat, and pasteurization. Several recombinant factor VIII concentrates, manufactured by inserting the human factor VIII gene into a mammalian cell line, are also currently available.[44,45] Because human plasma is not used in their production, transfusion-transmitted diseases, such as hepatitis and HIV-1, are no longer a risk. Recombinant concentrates at doses similar to those of plasma-derived concentrates have been efficacious in the treatment of hemorrhages. Half-life and recovery times for the infused factor VIII are similar to those for plasma-derived concentrates. Current prices range from $0.35 to $0.90 per unit for factor VIII plasma-derived concentrates and from $1.00 to $1.20 per unit for recombinant factor VIII. In most hemophilia centers in the United States, recombinant factor concentrates are the only concentrates used, although high-purity plasma-derived concentrates are still available. Because these concentrates have made early and intensive home therapy possible, overall costs of health care have greatly declined for patients treated with these materials.

Arginine vasopressin (desmopressin), a vasopressin analogue, can be used in the treatment of mild hemophilia A to raise the endogenous factor VIII level. Desmopressin raises the baseline factor VIII level about threefold, so a baseline level of at least 10 percent is required for efficacy.[46] Because this is not a blood product, it poses no danger of transmitting blood-borne viruses. Although cryoprecipitate contains factor VIII, its use has been discouraged because it is not virally inactivated. Thus, it is less safe than concentrates.

FACTOR IX REPLACEMENT

Factor IX is not found in either cryoprecipitate or factor VIII concentrate; thus, these two materials are totally ineffective for the treatment of hemophilia B. Fresh-frozen plasma does contain factor IX and has been used in the past. However, most fresh-frozen plasma products are not virally inactivated and, therefore, are less safe than factor IX concentrates.

The principles of treatment are similar to those for factor VIII replacement. However, because the half-life of factor IX is longer, it can be given less frequently. Demand therapy is still commonly used; as for factor VIII deficiency, however, prophylaxis is beginning to be used in pediatric patients. Several factor IX concentrates are available, all virally inactivated. In the past, all such concentrates also contained factors II, VII, and X (prothrombin complex concentrates). Currently, only pure factor IX concentrates are used to treat factor IX deficiency. As with factor VIII concentrates, a recombinant factor IX concentrate is available and is widely used. However, recovery is less than that of its plasma-derived counterpart, and higher doses (approximately 1.5 times calculated levels) must be infused to reach appropriate levels.

COMPLICATIONS OF FACTOR-REPLACEMENT THERAPY

Inhibitor Antibodies

Inhibitor antibodies may develop after exposure to factor concentrate. They occur most often in persons with severe hemophilia after 9 to 30 exposures of replacement therapy, usually before the age of 5 years. There may be a familial predisposition to the development of this complication. Because bleeding cannot be reliably controlled in patients with inhibitor antibodies, elective surgery in these patients should be done only after careful deliberation.

Inhibitor antibodies in factor VIII–deficient hemophiliacs are immunoglobulin G (IgG) antibodies (usually IG4) and may have an unpredictable natural history. At times, low titer and clinically weak antibodies are easily neutralized by factor VIII and do not undergo anamnestic rises in titer after multiple factor VIII challenges. Such antibodies may rarely become high in titer. In other patients, antibody titers rise after each exposure to factor VIII. Still other patients appear to spontaneously lose antibody despite multiple subsequent factor VIII challenges. The type of antibody response to factor VIII infusion and the patient's clinical response dictate therapy.

Therapy for patients with inhibitor antibodies ranges from total avoidance of all exposure to factor VIII in some centers to aggressive megadose factor VIII replacement in others. Prothrombin complex concentrates, possibly because of their variable contamination with activated factor X and procoagulant phospholipids, are often efficacious. Activated prothrombin complex concentrates have been useful in certain patients with inhibitor antibodies who have not responded to treatment. Porcine factor VIII, which does not cross-react with the human antibody, is another valuable therapy. The use of immunosuppressives or glucocorticoids has been abandoned in most centers owing to lack of efficacy in this condition and serious side effects. Regimens of regular factor VIII infusions for induction of tolerance have been successful in eliminating the antibody.[47] It has been suggested by some groups that an immune tolerance regimen be started as early as possible after an inhibitor develops.

Inhibitor antibodies against factor IX are exceedingly rare. There is no generally accepted efficacious therapy. Treatment usually includes large and frequent doses of factor IX concentrate. Induction of immune tolerance with elimination of the antibody has also been used but with less success than with antibodies to factor VIII. Using large doses of purified factor IX concentrate in some patients with inhibitor antibodies to factor IX has resulted in anaphylactic reactions and nephrotic syndrome secondary to immune complex formation and deposition in the kidney.[48,49]

Human Immunodeficiency Virus

HIV was introduced into the American blood supply in the 1970s.[50] By the late 1970s, factor concentrate was widely contaminated. By 1982, approximately 50 percent of patients with hemophilia were infected with HIV.[51] Currently, approximately 20 percent of American hemophiliacs are infected with HIV. As with other infected individuals, cell determinant (CD)4 lymphocyte counts and HIV titers are used to guide treatment regimens. Since 1985, in the manufacture of plasma-derived concentrates a triple barrier to viral contamination of plasma-derived concentrates has been employed: 1) self exclusion for donors, 2) donor screening with serologic tests for HIV, and 3) viral inactivation during concentrate production. Recombinant concentrates are also now widely available. Thus, acquisition of HIV-1 through factor concentrate in persons with hemophilia has been virtually nonexistent since 1985.

Viral Hepatitis

A second infectious side effect of either cryoprecipitate or factor concentrate is hepatitis, which may be a result of parenterally transmitted hepatitis B virus, hepatitis C virus, hepatitis A virus, hepatitis G virus, cytomegalovirus, or other as yet unidentified pathogens. In most series, the majority of persons with hemophilia treated before the 1980s have plasma levels of hepatitis B virus surface antibody, and a minority (2 to 5 percent) carry hepatitis B virus surface antigen. Approximately 80 percent of hemophiliacs transfused before 1990 have antibody to hepatitis C virus,[52] which, unlike hepatitis B virus antibody, is a marker for ongoing infection. Virucidal concentrate treatment methods have reduced, but not eliminated, parenteral transmission of hepatitis B and C viruses. Transmission of hepatitis A and G viruses has also been reported with the use of plasma-derived concentrates. Vaccination against hepatitis B and hepatitis A is now recommended for infants with hemophilia. Transmission of hepatitis has decreased dramatically because almost all pediatric patients are treated with recombinant products.

THERAPY FOR MUSCULOSKELETAL COMPLICATIONS OF HEMOPHILIA

Acute Hemarthrosis

The most important measure in therapy for acute hemarthrosis is prompt correction of the clotting abnormality by administration of the deficient factor. Arthrocentesis, if it is accomplished within 24 hours of the onset of symptoms (but after factor replacement), may be symptomatically beneficial in advanced acute hemarthrosis; however, for diagnostic and potentially therapeutic purposes, it should be considered mandatory at any time if suspicion of infection is high.[16,17] Analgesia and brief joint immobilization for no more than 2 days often aid in pain control. Subsequently, passive range-of-motion isometric exercise should be initiated to reduce the likelihood of joint contracture.

Chronic Hemophilic Arthropathy

Conservative

A variety of conservative measures can bring remarkable benefit in the setting of chronic hemophilic arthropathy.[53-56] These include the following:

Prophylactic factor infusions
Intensive physical therapy for muscle building and increased joint stability
Periods of avoidance of weight-bearing to allow regression of synovitis
Correction of flexion contractures by wedging casts, night splints, or the judicious use of traction
Training in sports to allow future maintenance of muscle mass

In modern treatment programs, aspiration of joints with chronic synovial effusions is rarely necessary or of lasting benefit. Failure of these conservative modalities to relieve symptoms or produce regression of synovitis should prompt consideration of other options, including local corticosteroid injections (which have recently been described as useful),[57] the use of nonsteroidal anti-inflammatory drugs (NSAIDs), synovectomy, and joint replacement in the end stage.

Despite the obvious theoretical contraindications to the use of NSAIDs in hemophilia (namely, the antiplatelet effects), several NSAIDs may be used safely for short periods as adjuncts to the conservative regimen. Ibuprofen, salsalate, and choline magnesium salicylate have been shown in small numbers of patients to be safe and efficacious in reducing joint pain and analgesic dependence,[58,59] although long-term regression of synovitis and modification of the course of chronic hemophilic arthropathy have not been demonstrated with any NSAID. The new class of NSAIDs, cyclooxygenase-2 (COX-2) inhibitors, do not have significant antiplatelet effects[57] and theoretically should be safer than conventional NSAIDs in patients with hemophilia. They have not been specifically tested in this setting, however, and they, as well as other NSAIDs should be used with caution.

Synovectomy

Synovectomy in the setting of hemophilic arthritis has been shown to reduce the incidence of recurrent hemarthrosis and the severity of synovitis. This procedure can be accomplished surgically, arthroscopically, or through intra-articular injections of radioactive colloids. Patients should be considered for synovectomy if, despite aggressive conservative measures as outlined previously, persistent hemarthroses continue with ongoing chronic synovitis. In our center, specific indications for synovectomy include persistence of at least two hemarthroses per month in the same joint accompanied by symptoms and signs of chronic synovitis despite at least 4 months of conservative therapy, including intensive factor replacement. The major drawback to surgical synovectomy remains the observation, confirmed in most series,[60,61] that joint motion is reduced postoperatively compared to preoperative baseline joint motion, despite intensive rehabilitation.

To overcome this finding, as well as the high cost of hospitalization and factor replacement therapy attendant with surgical synovectomy, arthroscopic synovectomy has been employed in chronic hemophilic arthritis in recent years. Most follow-up series report that this technique is as successful as surgical synovectomy and results in less loss of motion,[62-64] particularly when continuous passive motion is used in the postoperative period.[65] The total cost of the procedure is less than that of surgical synovectomy, as is the rehabilitation period. Postoperative bleeding after arthroscopic synovectomy has been associated with poor results.[66,67]

An alternative to surgical or arthroscopic synovectomy is ablation of the synovium using either radioisotopic or chemical agents, as recently reviewed.[23,68,69] Such a nonoperative approach has been successful in patients with hemophilia and is especially useful in those with circulating factor inhibitors, in whom surgery is generally contraindicated. Commonly used radioisotopes include colloidal P32 chromic phosphate,[70] yttrium 90, dysprosium 165 (by C. B. Sledge in conjunction with the authors (unpublished)), and radioactive gold. Theoretical long-term carcinogenic and teratogenic effects remain the major concerns associated with this technique in most patients who may have long life expectancies and are still of reproductive age. Chemical synovectomies using osmic acid, rifampicin, and hyaluronic acid have been attempted in some European centers with modest success, especially in children.[68-72] The short-term results of radioactive and chemical synovectomies are similar, although long-term outcomes may be superior in radioisotopic synovectomy.[23] Radioactive and chemical synovectomies remain experimental in the United States. Both offer the advantages of being minimally invasive, requiring little factor replacement, and resulting in little morbidity, and both are much less expensive than operative procedures.

Total Joint Replacement

Total joint replacement has been safely and successfully employed in end-stage hemophilic arthropathy,[73-76] the primary indication being pain in the involved joint that is refractory to all conservative measures. Of concern, however, is that most hemophilic patients in need of total joint replacement are young and may, if they are not infected with HIV, have a long life expectancy; this virtually ensures the need for one or more revisions during the patient's lifetime. In addition, patients are at risk for complications of surgery because of their underlying coagulopathy, and loosening is observed more commonly than in nonhemophilic patients in long-term follow-up. Finally, hemophilic patients with HIV infections have an above-average incidence of postoperative infections and poor results. These findings suggest that total joint replacement should be reserved for the most severe cases of hemophilic arthropathy. A comprehensive recent review details the many orthopedic procedures that are now available for alleviating the pain and deformity resulting from hemophilic arthropathy.[77]

∎ Conclusion

The best therapy for hemophilic arthropathy remains its prevention, and prevention is now clearly achievable. With improvement in the safety and availability of factor concentrates, prophylactic infusion is now feasible. Through a combination of prevention of hemarthrosis or correction of the hemostatic defect at the earliest symptom of joint hemorrhage, education of the patient, application of comprehensive care, and emphasis on the importance of physical activity to maintain muscle mass, the incidence of new or progressive arthropathy can be significantly reduced.

REFERENCES

1. Roberts HR, Jones MR: Hemophilia and related conditions: Congenital deficiencies of prothrombin (factor II), factor V, and factors VII to XII. *In* Williams WJ, Beutler E, Erslev AJ, Lichtman MA (eds): Hematology. New York, McGraw-Hill, 1990.
2. Larrieu JM, Caen JP, Meyer DO, et al: Congenital bleeding disorders with long bleeding time and normal platelet count. II. Von Willebrand's disease (report of thirty-seven patients). Am J Med 45:354, 1968.
3. Ahlberg A, Silwer J: Arthropathy in von Willebrand's disease. Acta Orthop Scand 41:539, 1970.
4. Wild JH, Zvaifler NJ: Hemarthrosis associated with sodium warfarin therapy. Arthritis Rheum 19:98, 1976.
5. Astrup T, Brakman P: Tissue Repair and Vascular Disease in Hemophilia. I. New York, American Elsevier, 1975.
6. Astrup T, Sjolin KE: Thromboplastic and fibrinolytic activity of the synovial membrane and fibrous capsular tissue. Proc Soc Exp Biol Med 97:852, 1958.
7. Green D, Ryan C, Malandruccuolo N, et al: Characterization of the coagulant activity of cultured human fibroblasts. Blood 37:47, 1971.
8. Ramgren O: Hemophilia in Sweden. III. Symptomatology, with special reference to differences between hemophilia A and B. Acta Med Scand 171:237, 1962.
9. Duthie RB, Matthews JM, Rizza CE, Steel WM: The Management of Musculoskeletal Problems in the Haemophilias. Oxford, UK, Blackwell Scientific, 1972.
10. Hilgartner MW: Hemophilic arthropathy. Adv Pediatr 21:1939, 1975.
11. Gilbert MS: Musculoskeletal manifestations of hemophilia. Mt Sinai J Med 44:339, 1977.
12. Steven MM, Madhok SY, Forbes CD, Sturrack RD: Hemophilic arthritis. Am J Med 58:181, 1986.
13. Rodriguez-Merchan EC: Pathogenesis, early diagnosis, and prophylaxis for chronic hemophilic synovitis. Clin Ortho Rel Res 343:6, 1997.
14. Gilbert MS: Musculoskeletal manifestations of hemophilia. Mt Sinai J Med 44:339, 1977.
15. Steven MM, Madhok SY, Forbes CD, Sturrack RD: Hemophilic arthritis. Am J Med 58:181, 1986.
16. Ellison RT, Reller LB: Differentiating pyogenic arthritis from spontaneous hemarthrosis in patients with hemophilia. West J Med 144:42, 1986.
17. Gilbert MS, Aledort LM, Seremetis S et al: Long term evaluation of septic arthritis in hemophilic patients. Clin Orthop 388:54, 1996.
18. Rodriguez-Merchan EC, Magallon M, Manso F et al: Septic arthritis in HIV positive haemophiliacs. Int Orthop 16:302, 1992.
19. Helm M, Horoszowski H, Seligsohn U, et al: Iliopsoas hematoma: Its detection, and treatment with special reference to hemophilia. Arch Orthop Trauma Surg 99:195, 1982.
20. Madigan RP, Hanna WT, Wallace SL: Acute compartment syndrome in hemophilia. J Bone Joint Surg Am 63:1327, 1981.
21. Ahlberg A: On the natural history of hemophilia pseudotumor. J Bone Joint Surg Am 57:1133, 1975.
22. Gilbert MS, Kreel I, Hermann G: The hemophilic pseudotumor. *In* Hilgartner MW, Pochedly C (eds): Hemophilia in the Child and Adult. New York, Raven Press, 1989.
23. Hilgartner MW: Current treatment of hemophilic arthropathy. Curr Opin Ped 14:46, 2002.
24. Soler R, Lopez-Fernandez F, Rodriguez E, et al: Hemophilic arthropathy: A scoring system for magnetic resonance imaging. Eur Radiol 12:836, 2002.

25. Wilson DA, Prince JR: MR imaging of hemophilic pseudotumors. Am J Roentgenol 150:349, 1988.
26. Wilson DJ, McLardy-Smith PD, Woodham CH, et al: Diagnostic ultrasound in haemophilia. J Bone Joint Surg Br 69:103, 1987.
27. Ghadially FN, Ailsby RL, Yong NK: Ultrastructure of the hemophilic synovial membrane and electron-probe x-ray analysis of hemosiderin. J Pathol 120:201, 1976.
28. Roosendaal G, Mauser-Bunschoten EP, De Kleijn P, et al: Synovium in hemophilic arthropathy. Haemophilia 4:502, 1998.
29. Roy S, Ghadially FN: Pathology of experimental hemarthrosis. Ann Rheum Dis 25:402, 1966.
30. Hoaglund FT: Experimental hemarthrosis. J Bone Joint Surg Am 49:285, 1967.
31. Roy S, Ghadially FN: Ultrastructure of synovial membrane in human hemarthrosis. J Bone Joint Surg Am 49:1636, 1967.
32. Swanton MC, Wysocki GP: Pathology of joints in canine hemophilia A. In Brinkhous KM, Hemker HC (eds): Handbook of Hemophilia. Part I. New York, American Elsevier, 1975.
33. Morris CJ, Blake DR, Wainwright AC, Steven MM: Relationship between iron deposits and tissue damage in the synovium: An ultrastructural study. Ann Rheum Dis 45:21, 1986.
34. Hough AJ, Banfield WG, Sokoloff L: Cartilage in hemophilic arthropathy. Arch Pathol Lab Med 100:91, 1976.
35. Okazaki I, Brinckerhoff CE, Sinclair JF, et al: Iron increases collagenase production by rabbit synovial fibroblasts. J Lab Clin Med 97:396, 1981.
36. Wen FQ, Jabbar AA, Chen YX, et al: c-myc protooncogene expression in hemophilic synovitis: in vitro studies of the effects of iron and ceramide. Blood 100:912, 2002.
37. Choi YC, Hough AJ, Morris GM, et al: Experimental siderosis of articular chondrocytes cultured in vitro. Arthritis Rheum 24:809, 1981.
38. Mainardi CL, Levine PH, Werb Z, et al: Proliferative synovitis in hemophilia: Biochemical and morphologic observations. Arthritis Rheum 21:137, 1978.
39. Berntorp E: Methods of haemophilia care delivery: Regular prophylaxis versus episodic treatment. Haemophilia 1(Suppl 1):3, 1995.
40. Nilsson IM, Berntorp E, Lofquist T, Pettersson H: Twenty five years' experience of prophylactic treatment in severe haemophilia A and B. J Intern Med 232:25, 1992.
41. Astermark J, Petrini P, Tengborn L, et al: Primary prophylaxis in severe haemophilia should be started at an early age but can be individualized. Br J Haemataol 105:1109, 1999.
42. Fischer K, van der Born J, Mauser-Bunschoten EP, et al: The effects of postponing prophylactic treatment on long-term outcome in patients with severe hemophilia. Blood 99:2337, 2002.
43. Varon D, Martinowitz U: Continuous infusion in hemophilia. Haemophilia 4:431, 1998.
44. White GC, MacMillan CW, Kingdon HS, Shoemaker CB: Use of recombinant hemophilic factor in the treatment of two patients with classic hemophilia. N Engl J Med 320:166, 1989.
45. Schwartz RS, Agilgaard CF, Aledort LM, et al: Human recombinant DNA derived antihemophilic factor (factor VIII) in the treatment of hemophilia A. N Engl J Med 323:1800, 1990.
46. Mannucci PM: DDAVP in haemophilia. Lancet 2:1171, 1977.
47. van Leeuwen EF, Mauser-Bunschoten EP, van Dijken PM, et al: Disappearance of factor VIII:C antibodies in patients with haemophilia A upon frequent administration of factor VIII in intermediate or low dose. Br J Haematol 64:291, 1986.
48. Warrier I: Factor IX antibody and immune tolerance. Vox Sanguinis 77:70, 1999.
49. Ewenstein B, Takemoto C, Warrier I, et al: Nephrotic syndrome as a complication of immune tolerance in hemophilia B [Letter]. Blood 89:1115, 1997.
50. Levine PH: The acquired immune deficiency syndrome in persons with hemophilia. Ann Intern Med 13:723, 1985.
51. Eyster MG, Goedert JJ, Sarngadharan MG, et al: Development and early natural history of HTLV-III antibodies in persons with hemophilia. JAMA 253:2219, 1985.
52. Brettler DB, Forsberg JL, Dienstag JL, et al: The prevalence of antibody to HCV in a cohort of hemophilic patients. Blood 76:254, 1990.
53. Miser AW, Miser JS, Newton WA: Intensive factor replacement for management of chronic synovitis in hemophilic children. Am J Pediatr Hematol Oncol 8:66, 1986.
54. Buzzard BM: Physiotherapy for prevention and treatment of chronic hemophilic synovitis. Clin Orthop 343:42, 1997.
55. Schumacher P: Discussion paper: Orthotic management in hemophilia. Ann N Y Acad Sci 240:344, 1975.
56. Atkins RM, Henderson NJ, Duthie RB: Joint contractures in the hemophilias. Clin Orthop 219:97, 1987.
57. Fernandez-Palazzi F, Caviglia HA, Salazar JR, et al: Intraarticular dexamethasone in advanced chronic synovitis in hemophilia. Clin Orthop 343:25, 1997.
58. Thomas P, Hepburn B, Kim HC, Saich P: Non-steroidal anti-inflammatory drugs in the treatment of haemophilic arthropathy. Am J Hematol 12:131, 1982.
59. Inwood MJ, Killackey B, Startup SJ: The use and safety of ibuprofen in the haemophiliac. Blood 61:709, 1983.
60. Steven MM, Small M, Pinkerton L, et al: Non-steroidal anti-inflammatory drugs in haemophilic arthritis. Haemostasis 15:204, 1985.
61. Cryer B, Dubois A: The advent of highly selective inhibitors of cyclooxygenase: a review. Prostaglandins Other Lipid Mediat 56:341, 1998.
62. Montane I, McCollough NC, Lian EC-Y: Synovectomy of the knee for hemophilic arthropathy. J Bone Joint Surg Am 68:210, 1986.
63. Post M, Watts G, Telfer M: Synovectomy in hemophilic arthropathy: A retrospective review of 17 cases. Clin Orthop 202:139, 1986.
64. Weidel JD: Arthroscopic synovectomy for chronic hemophilic synovitis of the knee. Arthroscopy 1:205, 1985.
65. Weidel JD: Arthroscopic synovectomy of the knee in hemophilia. 10- to 15-year follow-up. Clin Orthop 328:46, 1996.
66. Klein KS, Aland CM, Kin HC, et al: Long-term follow-up of arthroscopic synovectomy for chronic hemophilic synovitis. Arthroscopy 3:231, 1987.
67. Limbird TJ, Dennis SC: Synovectomy and continuous passive motion (CPM) in hemophiliac patients. Arthroscopy 3:74, 1987.
68. Heim M: The treatment of intra-articular synovitis by the use of chemical and radioactive substances. Haemophilia 8:369, 2002.
69. Molho, P, Vernier P, Stielties N, et al: A retrospectives study on chemical and radioactive synovectomy in severe haemophilia patients with recurrent hemarthrosis. Haemophilia 5:115, 1999.
70. Siegel HJ, Luck JV Jr, Siegel, et al: Phosphate-32 colloid radiosynovectomy in hemophilia: outcome in 125 patients. Clin Orthop 392:409, 2001.
71. Ayral X: Chemical synovitis with osmic acid in haemophilia. Haemophilia 7:20, 2001.
72. Caviglia HA, Fernadez-Palazzi G, Galatro G, et al: Chemical synovitis with rifampicin in haemophilia. Haemophilia 7:26, 2001.
73. Birch NC, Ribbans WJ, Goldman E, et al: Knee replacement in haemophilia. J Bone Joint Surg 76B:165, 1994.
74. Kelley SS, Lachiewicz PF, Gilbert MS, et al: Hip arthroplasty in hemophilic arthropathy. J Bone Joint Surg Am 77:828, 1995.
75. Thomason HC, Wilson FC, Lachiewicz PF, et al: Knee arthroplasty in hemophilic arthropathy. Clin Orthop 360:169, 1999.
76. Norian, JM, Ries, MD, Karp S, et al: Total knee arthroplasty in hemophilic arthopathy. J Bone Joint Surg 84A:1141, 2002.
77. Rodriquez-Merchan EC: Orthopedic surgery of haemophilia in the 21st century: An overview. Haemophilia 8:360, 2002.

108

Hemoglobinopathies and Arthritis

H. RALPH SCHUMACHER, JR.

Musculoskeletal manifestations are common in the hemoglobinopathies. Problems can be seen not only in homozygous sickle cell (hemoglobin SS) disease but also in sickle C hemoglobin and sickle-thalassemia diseases. Patients with sickle cell disease and high circulating levels of hemoglobin F tend to have milder disease.[1] Rheumatic manifestations appear to be rare in sickle trait (hemoglobin AS) but have been reported in β-thalassemia.

Hemoglobin S, which is most common in African Americans, results from a unique DNA base-pair substitution (β^s) in the sixth codon of the *β-globin* gene leading to the substitution of a single amino acid in the β-chain of hemoglobin.[2] Glutamic acid, which is normally present, is replaced by valine. This change produces systemic disease, manifested by sickling of the erythrocytes in small vessels, which is the presumed basis for the painful crises with important interactions between erythrocytes and vascular endothelium.[3] Complex interactions of sickled cells with endothelium can induce red cell binding to the endothelial cell–receptor complex of glycoproteins, Ib, Ix, and V, endothelial CD36; and vascular cell adhesion molecule-1 (VCAM-1)[4] providing potential targets for therapy. Occlusive microvascular disease is also the basis for many of the musculoskeletal syndromes described in the following paragraphs (Table 108-1).

Other manifestations are hemolytic anemia, hyposthenuria, leg ulcers, hyporegenerative crises, increased infections—especially with salmonellae—and the bone and joint problems to be discussed. The diagnosis is suspected when sickled cells are identified in vitro through the use of reducing agents such as metabisulfite. Diagnosis of the homozygous disease is by starch or cellulose acetate hemoglobin electrophoresis showing 76 to 100 percent hemoglobin S or with allele-specific oligonucleotide probes.[5]

Hemoglobin C disease is less common and is caused by the substitution of lysine for glutamic acid in the β-chains. The pure disease produces some hemolysis and many target cells, but this abnormal hemoglobin is most important when combined with hemoglobin S.

β-Thalassemia refers to another inherited disorder that is especially common in persons of Mediterranean background. A variety of mutations result in reduced or absent β-chains, producing an unstable hemoglobin with formation of Heinz bodies. There are high levels of hemoglobin F. Patients with β-thalassemia have hemolytic anemia (which is severe and transfusion dependent in homozygotes), splenomegaly, and hyperplastic bone marrows, producing changes on skeletal radiographs. Patients with a combination of β-thalassemia and hemoglobin S often have increased hemoglobin A2. This hemoglobinopathy clinically combines features of thalassemia and homozygous sickle cell disease.

Sickle Cell Disease

BONE TRABECULAR CHANGES ASSOCIATED WITH EXPANSION OF THE BONE MARROW

Sickle cell disease and other hemoglobinopathies associated with hemolysis cause characteristic expansion of the bone marrow, producing wider intertrabecular spaces with coarser trabeculations; these are most evident in the axial skeleton in which red (hematopoietic) marrow is most plentiful (Fig. 108–1). In patients with SC hemoglobin, hemolysis tends to be less, and there are fewer bone trabecular changes.[6] Scattered increased densities can interrupt trabecular patterns and are probably attributable to areas of marrow infarction.[7] In vertebral bodies, coarsened trabeculae are most often vertical, and the bodies of the vertebrae can have a characteristic deep, central, cuplike indentation (Fig. 108–2). Vertebral compression can occur, with resulting accentuated dorsal kyphosis and lumbar lordosis. Osteophytes occasionally develop, and vertebrae may even fuse.

HAND-FOOT SYNDROME

The hand-foot syndrome may develop in children 6 months to 2 years of age. It involves dramatic, diffuse, symmetric, very tender, warm swelling of the hands, feet, or both[8] (Fig. 108–3). Hematologic signs and fever may be absent, or fever may be present with peripheral blood leukocytosis up to 55,000 cells/mm^3. Swelling lasts 1 to 3 weeks. Infarction of marrow, cortical bone, periosteum, and periarticular tissues is probably the underlying mechanism. Radiographs may be normal, especially during the first week, but later show marrow densities, lytic areas, or periosteal elevation. Most of the periosteal changes are no longer identifiable in 1 to 4 months.

TABLE 108–1 · MUSCULOSKELETAL MANIFESTATIONS OF SICKLE CELL DISEASE

Bone trabecular changes	Joint effusions
Hand-foot syndrome	Erosions and chronic inflammation
Hyperuricemia and gout	Bone infarctions
Osteomyelitis	Avascular necrosis
Septic arthritis	Others, including muscle necrosis

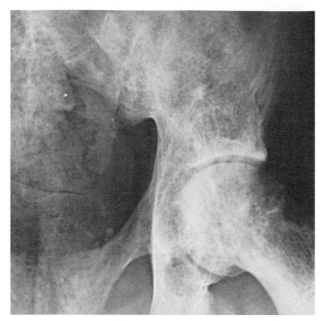

FIGURE 108–1 • Radiograph showing coarsened trabeculae from marrow expansion in severe sickle cell anemia. Some focal densities may be a result of bone infarctions.

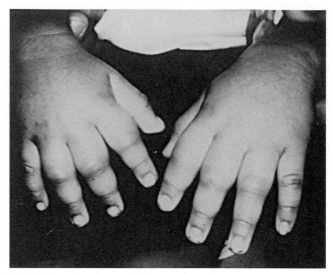

FIGURE 108–3 • Diffusely swollen hands as seen in the hand-foot syndrome of young children with sickle cell disease.

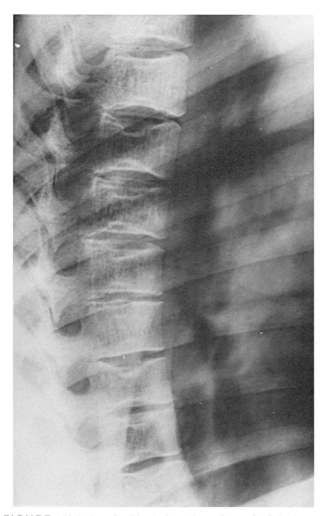

FIGURE 108–2 • Cuplike indentation of vertebral bodies in radiograph of patient with sickle cell disease.

Hematopoiesis in the small finger and toe bones of children is presumably a factor in the restriction of this syndrome to childhood.

The frequency of hand-foot syndrome varies from 17 percent in a study of African Americans to 80 percent in a group of African children. Five examples have been described in Saudi Arabians with SS hemoglobin, a reminder that the various manifestations of sickle cell disease can affect other racial groups.[9] Hand-foot syndrome has also been reported in children with SC hemoglobin disease and S thalassemia. Analgesics, anti-inflammatory agents, and hydration have been used for therapy. Osteomyelitis can also occur in children and must always be kept in mind.

HYPERURICEMIA AND GOUT

Approximately 40 percent of adults with sickle cell disease are hyperuricemic (most often 6.5 to 11 mg/dl), whereas only occasionally do affected children younger than 13 years of age have elevated serum uric acid levels. Overproduction of uric acid associated with increased red blood cell (RBC) turnover seems initially to be associated with hyperuricosuria.[10] In young people, urate clearance maintains a normal serum uric acid; in older patients, however, uric acid excretion often diminishes and results in hyperuricemia. Diagnosis is by synovial fluid analysis. Clinical gout with typical crystals of monosodium urate was found in eight patients in one review.[11] Attacks may be polyarticular and associated with fever, so they could be confused with sickle cell crises unless crystals are carefully sought. Treatment is the same as for idiopathic gout.

OSTEOMYELITIS

Patients with sickle cell disease are especially susceptible to bacterial infection. The frequency of osteomyelitis, which is caused by a variety of organisms (but predominantly salmonellae), is more than 100 times that seen in normal populations.[12,13] More than 80 percent of hematogenous osteomyelitis in persons without hemoglobinopathies is attributable to staphylococci, but more than 50 percent of osteomyelitis in sickle cell patients is caused by salmonellae. Most other organisms have also been gram-negative.[14]

Multiple sites of osteomyelitis may be seen in infected patients. Onset may not be dramatic, and bone infection apparently has been overlooked for years. Osteomyelitis may be difficult to distinguish from the results of bone infarction with radiography or magnetic resonance imaging (MRI).[15] Progression or other signs of infection are often needed for diagnosis; scans with indium-labeled leukocytes may suggest the diagnosis.[16]

Acute osteomyelitis is more common in children. The medullary cavities of diaphyses or epiphyses of long bones are often involved. Both crisis and infection may present with bone pain, fever, and leukocytosis. Persistent fever must increase the concern about osteomyelitis. Infection rarely extends from bones into joints, although this seemed more common in a Nigerian series.[14] Exploration or demonstration of the organism from a draining site is needed for diagnosis. Treatment generally includes splinting severely involved bones to prevent pathologic fracture. *Salmonella* bone infection seems to respond well to several antibiotics, including quinolones, without much development of chronic osteomyelitis. Surgical drainage is not necessary in most cases.

SEPTIC ARTHRITIS

Septic arthritis occurs but, fortunately, is not especially common[17] and is much less frequent than osteomyelitis. Multiple joints are involved in some cases. A variety of organisms are seen, including staphylococci, *Escherichia coli*, *Enterobacter*, and especially *Salmonella*. High leukocyte counts and sedimentation rates helped identify infection in one series.[18] Five of six cases in one group of children had *Streptococcus* pneumonia.[19] Antibiotic therapy and drainage are usually successful. Impaired synovial capillary flow caused by sickling was suggested as a factor in poor responses to therapy in two patients, and exchange transfusion has been suggested as an adjunct to treatment.[20]

JOINT EFFUSIONS

Far more common than gout or septic arthritis are other joint effusions that appear to be attributable to sickle cell disease. Effusions are often, but not invariably, associated with fever, leukocytosis, and other manifestations of crises.[17,21] There generally is warmth and tenderness, which may also involve the periarticular areas. Knees are by far the most commonly involved joints, but effusions have also often been found in elbows, ankles, and other joints. Usually, only one or two joints are involved. Effusions generally subside in 2 to 14 days.

Radiographs in most of these patients at the time of effusion have shown only the results of previous cortical or medullary infarcts. Radioisotope scans have shown areas of decreased marrow uptake adjacent to many effused joints and at other areas of bone infarctions, suggesting small marrow infarctions.[22] MRI may show increased signal on T2-weighted images.[24]

If the erythrocyte sedimentation rate (ESR) is being used in evaluation of the effusion, one should be aware that the ESR is usually abnormally low between crises. It may rise with crises or inflammation.

Synovial effusions have often been "noninflammatory," that is, clear, with most synovial fluid leukocyte counts less than 1000 cells/mm^3 and with a low percentage of polymorphonuclear leukocytes. Similar noninflammatory effusions have been seen in sickle-thalassemia.[17,25] Other effusions in sickle cell disease are cloudy and contain higher leukocyte counts in the inflammatory range.[21,26] Effusions with leukocyte counts of up to 126,000 with 90 to 97 percent polymorphonuclear cells have been described.[27] Crystals or organisms were not found, but some of the patients were given antibiotics. Diggs[7] reported "purulent exudates" in knee joints, which produced negative results for bacteria on direct examination and culture. Synovial fluid complement levels have not been depressed,[21] and synovial fluid glucose levels have been normal.[17] Needle-like clumps of sickled hemoglobin can be phagocytized.[26] Heme from lysed erythrocytes can be inflammatory.[28] Sickled erythrocytes can be seen in effusions, but this shows only that the patient has sickle hemoglobin because sickled cells can also be seen in persons with sickle cell trait and arthritis of other causes.

Needle synovial biopsies[17] at the time of acute joint effusions have shown only focal lining cell proliferation and a few chronic inflammatory cells. Small vessels have been congested or have had definite microvascular thrombosis. Electron microscopy of synovium has confirmed the presence of occluded vessels, with some vessel lumens containing erythrocytes with the characteristic 18-nm diameter rods or "tactoids" of typical sickled hemoglobin. Infarction of bone adjacent to joints with effusions or pain may also contribute to joint manifestations.

No specific treatment is required for the joint effusions. Local steroids have not been useful. Treatment of associated painful crises generally involves the use of analgesics, including narcotics if needed, plus hydration. Limited-exchange transfusion can eliminate many abnormal cells and help to terminate prolonged crises. Alkali can be given to prevent acidosis, which can aggravate sickling. Transfusion programs to maintain a level of hemoglobin S below 30 percent and hydroxyurea therapy, which increases hemoglobin F, may decrease the frequency of crises.[29] Hydroxyurea given daily by mouth is approved for use in those over age 13 and is well tolerated, but it can cause occasional marrow suppression or changes in liver function tests.[30] Counseling can be important for patients and families as crises and effusions often affect school attendance and performance.

EROSIONS AND CHRONIC INFLAMMATION

Occasional chronic synovitis with cartilage destruction or erosion has been mentioned in patients with sickle cell disease and no other evident cause for arthritis.[31,32] Erosions have been described at wrists, metacarpal heads, and calcanei. Lymphocytic and plasma cell infiltration of synovium can occur. Although chronic inflammation is nonspecific, immunologic mechanisms might possibly be involved. Immune complexes have been implicated as factors in the nephropathy of sickle cell disease and in the leg ulcers.[33] Johnston and associates[34] reported an abnormality of the alternate pathway of complement activation in sickle cell disease. Defects in cell-mediated immunity have also been reported.[35] Cases with rheumatoid arthritis (RA) or juvenile RA (JRA) and sickle cell disease have been reported.[36] Patients with such chronic synovitis may need anti-inflammatory agents including disease-modifying antirheumatic drugs (DMARDs).

BONE INFARCTIONS AND AVASCULAR NECROSIS

Bone infarctions occur most commonly in persons with SS hemoglobin, but they may also be seen in SC hemoglobin disease and S thalassemia. Localized deformities and failure of bone growth can result from infarction of the epiphyseal plate of growing children. This is common in both SS hemoglobin and SC hemoglobin disease.[6] The chronic anemia itself can cause some general retardation of growth. Infarctions in cortical bone are thought to be the cause of periosteal elevation, irregular cortical thickening, and sclerosis. Infarctions in the erythropoetic bone marrow produce fibrosis, lysis, sclerosis, new bone formation, and calcified dense marks on radiographs. Radiographs taken at the time of acute bone pain do not show changes from that infarction. Small infarcts may never produce radiographic changes.

Radioisotope studies using technetium colloid have shown areas of decreased marrow uptake at sites of bone pain, whereas radiographs of the same sites were normal. MRI might be the most sensitive technique for detection of acute or chronic infarcts.[37] The basis for bone infarcts is presumed to be sickling and thrombosis in small vessels. The bone pains in sickle cell crises are thought to be largely a result of such infarctions. Infarcts that involve only the medulla often produce pain without local tenderness.

When bone infarction occurs from occlusion of end arteries so that necrotic bone is at the articular margin, collapse of the periarticular bone and cartilage occurs. Based on pathologic studies after hip disintegration, Sherman[38] suggested that both small hemorrhages and local damage to small blood vessels were significant factors. One study revealed positive cultures in five of nine patients undergoing operation for osteonecrosis, suggesting that some such necrosis is actually septic.[39]

Aseptic necrosis of the head of the femur is a common finding and is the most disabling musculoskeletal complication of sickle cell disease. Incidence ranges have been from 2 to 4.5 cases per 100 patient-years.[40] Similar aseptic necrosis occurs at the humeral head, tibial condyles, and at other sites, including ribs and spine.[41] Cases have occurred in children as young as 5 years. Radiographs are similar to those of aseptic necrosis from other causes. Initially, there is local sclerosis near the joint margin. Patchy lucencies then develop and may include a lucency between the sclerotic bone and the intact bone. Flattening, separation of the necrotic fragment, and secondary osteoarthritis (OA) may later be seen.

Radioisotope studies or MRI can suggest infarction before the development of detectable aseptic necrosis.[22] Technetium pyrophosphate bone scans show increased uptake at sites of infarction. Marrow scans with colloids may show decreased uptake. Aseptic necrosis of the femoral head is relatively rare in children and can be followed by remodeling, probably because the artery in the ligamentum teres femoris is patent, giving the femoral head a dual blood supply.

Early treatment can be attempted with prevention of weight-bearing or with cement injection into the femoral head[42] to try to allow healing without the resultant distortion of bone. Young people seem better able to replace necrotic bone. Replacement of the femoral head with a prosthesis or total hip replacement is the treatment of choice once articular breakdown has become well established,[43] although results have been variable and failure rates appear to be increased.[42] Osteotomies have also been used to try to alter the line of weight-bearing. Surgical core decompression was helpful in a patient with aseptic necrosis of both calcanei[44] and is being studied for the femoral head.[45] Bracing has been needed for collapsed vertebrae.[41]

Aseptic necrosis of the humeral head produces much less difficulty and often needs no treatment. Shoulder prostheses have been inserted in two patients with good early results. Preoperative transfusions have been used to diminish the chances of sickling. Tourniquets can be avoided to reduce anoxia and stasis. Good hydration and special efforts during anesthesia to avoid hypoxia and acidosis are merited.

Aseptic necrosis can occur in SC hemoglobin disease and is believed by some to be even more common than in SS hemoglobin disease. This is possibly because many patients with SS hemoglobin die at a younger age of other complications. Diggs[7] explained the prominence of infarcts in SC hemoglobin disease on the basis of greater viscosity of the blood. Aseptic necrosis has also been reported in S thalassemia, with SF hemoglobin.

OTHER MUSCULOSKELETAL ASPECTS

Bony ankylosis of hips[7] and spine[46] has been reported, but it is not certain whether it was caused by sickle cell disease alone or whether infection also played a role. There can be incompletely explained protrusio acetabuli.[47] Irregular sclerosis of sacroiliac joints superficially mimicking the changes of ankylosing spondylitis (AS) has been reported[17] and is probably a result of bone infarctions at the joint.

Acute, painful, localized muscle swelling with necrosis can be seen with crises.[48] Local intramuscular injections may be a factor in some muscle injury. Myonecrosis has been demonstrated and has even required fasciotomy for pain relief. Fibrosis may result.[49] MRI can be used to detect such soft tissue lesions.[50]

Leukemia has occasionally occurred in patients with sickle cell disease. One such patient had elbow pain due to leukemic infiltration.[51]

▮ Thalassemia

In β-thalassemia (major, intermedia, and occasionally minor), there is increased erythrocyte destruction, causing osteopenia, expansion of the marrow with wide medullary spaces, coarse trabeculations, thin cortices, and fractures. However, aseptic necrosis is not characteristic. In a series of 50 thalassemic patients,[52] 25 patients (aged 5 to 33 years) had ankle pain that was exacerbated by weight-bearing and relieved by rest. There was diffuse ankle and foot tenderness and occasional ankle effusions. Radiographs of the ankles of one patient showed subchondral sclerosis suggestive of microfractures. Pathologic studies on two autopsy specimens and on a specimen obtained from a femoral osteotomy showed expansion of hematopoietic marrow into the small bones, osteopenia, increased osteoid, and a striking number of microfractures, findings generally confirmed at other sites.[53] All the patients studied by Gratwick and colleagues[52] had received multiple transfusions, and iron deposition was prominent in the marrow, in osteoid, at cement lines, and in synovial lining cells. Iron was not mentioned in osteocytes or chondrocytes, but slight articular cartilage erosion was reported. Similar osseous iron deposition was reported[54] along with signs of impaired mineralization.

Leg length discrepancies, limb deformities, and metaphyseal abnormalities have been described in younger patients despite or perhaps even due to early use of desferrioxamine.[55] Growth hormone therapy might have exaggerated deformities in those cases. An increased incidence of scoliosis has been reported.[56] In one study, 17 of 19 young Turkish patients with thalassemia major or intermedia (aged 2 to 17 years) had joint manifestations.[57] Shoulders were prominently involved. Periarticular bone cysts were also prominent. No therapy has yet been found effective, but rest gives temporary relief. Transfusion therapy may decrease excessive erythropoiesis and bone loss in patients with severe expansion of the marrow.

Patients with thalassemia and repeated transfusions have experienced chronic iron overload[58] and arthropathy with iron deposition in the synovium, as occurs in idiopathic hemochromatosis. Patients with iron overload should have chelation therapy with deferoxamine. Transfusion-dependent patients have also developed hepatitis C infection with cryoglobulinemia.[59] Hyperuricemia with gout[60] and septic arthritis[61] can occur in thalassemia.

Reports of otherwise unexplained monarticular or oligoarticular disease in thalassemia minor have appeared. Joint effusions have been noninflammatory or mildly inflammatory. Large and small joints have been involved. In one recent study, symptoms such as arthralgias were noted in 52 percent of patients with thalassemia minor but also in 54 percent of healthy controls.[62] Mechanisms of any arthropathy in these patients are still unclear. Other potentially confusing causes of leg pains in thalassemic patients include claudication-like pain when severely anemic and a postural, pulsating pain believed to be in some cases related to high intraosseous pressure.[63]

Patients with homozygous β-thalassemia now can have successful stem cell or allogeneic bone marrow transplantations.[64] Some of the risks of these procedures and the attendant immunosuppression may affect muscles and joints.

REFERENCES

1. Miller BA, Oliver N, Salameh M, et al: Molecular analysis of the high-hemoglobin F phenotype in Saudi Arabian sickle-cell anemia. N Engl J Med 316:255, 1987.
2. Bunn HF: Pathogenesis and treatment of sickle cell disease. N Engl J Med 337:762, 1997.
3. Belcher JD, Marker PH, Webber JP, et al: Activated monocytes in sickle cell disease: potential role in the activation of vascular endothelium and vasco-occlusion. Blood 96:2451, 2000.
4. Hebbel RP: Blockade of adhesion of sickle cells to endothelium by monoclonal antibodies. N Engl J Med 342:1911, 2000.
5. Saiki RK, Chang C-A, Levenson CH, et al: Diagnosis of sickle cell anemia and beta thalassemia with enzymatically amplified DNA and non-radioactive allele-specific oligonucleotide probes. N Engl J Med 319:537, 1988.
6. Barton CJ, Cockshott WP: Bone changes in hemoglobin SC disease. AJR 88:523, 1962.
7. Diggs LW: Bone and joint lesions in sickle cell disease. Clin Orthop 52:119, 1967.
8. Watson RJ, Burko H, Megas H, Robinson M: Hand-foot syndrome in sickle cell disease in young children. Pediatrics 31:975, 1963.
9. Perrine RP, Pembry ME, John P, et al: Natural history of sickle cell anemia in Saudi Arabs: A study of 270 subjects. Ann Intern Med 88:1, 1978.
10. Reynolds MD: Gout and hyperuricemia associated with sickle-cell anemia. Semin Arthritis Rheum 12:404, 1983.
11. Leff RD, Aldo-Benson MA, Fife RS: Tophaceous gout in a patient with sickle cell-thalassemia: Case report and review of the literature. Arthritis Rheum 26:928, 1983.
12. Barrett-Connor E: Bacterial infection and sickle cell anemia: An analysis of 250 infections in 166 patients and a review of the literature. Medicine 50:97, 1971.
13. Chambers JB, Forsythe DA, Bertrand SL, et al: Retrospective review of osteoarticular infections in a pediatric sickle cell age group. J Pediatr Orthop 20:682, 2000.
14. Ebong WW: Acute osteomyelitis in Nigerians with sickle cell disease. Ann Rheum Dis 45:911, 1986.
15. Umans H, Haramati N, Flusser G: The diagnostic role of gadolinium enhanced MRI in distiguishing between acute medullary bone infarct and osteomyelitis. Magn Reson Imaging 18:255, 2000.
16. Fernandez-Ullos M, Vasavada PJ, Black RR: Detection of acute osteomyelitis with indium-111-labelled white blood cells in a patient with sickle cell disease. Clin Nucl Med 14:97, 1989.
17. Schumacher HR, Andrews R, McLaughlin G: Arthropathy in sickle cell disease. Ann Intern Med 78:203, 1973.
18. Dalton GP, Drummond S, Davidson RS, et al: Bone infarction versus infection in sickle cell disease in children. J Pediatr Orthop 16:540, 1996.
19. Syrogiannopoulos GA, McCracken GH, Nelson JD: Osteoarticular infections in children with sickle cell disease. Pediatrics 78:1090, 1986.
20. Palmer DW, Ellman MH: Septic arthritis and Reiter's syndrome in sickle cell disorders: Case reports and implications for management. South Med J 69:902, 1976.
21. deCeulaer K, Forbes M, Roper D, Serjeant GR: Non-gouty arthritis in sickle cell disease: Report of 37 consecutive cases. Ann Rheum Dis 43:599, 1984.
22. Alavi A, Schumacher HR, Dorwart BB, Kuhl DE: Bone marrow scan evaluation of arthropathy in sickle cell disorders. Arch Intern Med 136:436, 1976.
23. Skaggs DL, Kim SK, Greene NW, et al: Differentiation between bone infarction and acute osteomyelitis in children with sickle-cell disease with use of sequential radionuclide bone-marrow and bone scans. J Bone Joint Surg Am 83-A:1810, 2001.

24. Mankad VN, Williams JP, Harpen MD, et al: Magnetic resonance imaging of bone marrow in sichle cell disease: clinical, hematologic, and pathologic correlations. Blood 75:274, 1990.

25. Crout JE, McKenna CH, Petit RM: Symptomatic joint effusion in sickle cell–beta-thalassemia disease: Report of a case. JAMA 235:1878, 1976.

26. Mann D, Schumacher HR: Pseudoseptic inflammatory knee effusions caused by phagocytosis of sickled erythrocytes after fracture into the knee joint. Arthritis Rheum 38:284, 1995.

27. Orozco-Alcala J, Baum J: Arthritis during sickle cell crisis. N Engl J Med 288:420, 1973.

28. Wagener FA, Abraham NG van Kooyk Y, et al: Heme-induced cell adhesion in the pathogenesis of sickle-cell disease and inflammation. Trends Pharmacol Sci 22:52, 2001.

29. Goldberg MA, Bugnara C, Dover GJ, et al: Treatment of sickle cell anemia with hydroxyurea and erythropoietin. N Engl J Med 323:366, 1990.

30. Ferster A, Tahrir P, Vermylen C, et al: Five years of experience with hydroxyurea in children and young adults with sickle cell disease. Blood 97:3628, 2001.

31. Schumacher HR, Dorwart BB, Bond J, et al: Chronic synovitis with early cartilage destruction in sickle cell disease. Ann Rheum Dis 36:413, 1977.

32. Rothschild BM, Sebes JI: Calcaneal abnormalities and erosive bone disease associated with sickle cell anemia. Am J Med 71:427, 1981.

33. Morgan AG, Venner AM: Immunity and leg ulcers in homozygous sickle cell disease. J Clin Lab Immunol 6:51, 1981.

34. Johnston RB, Newman SL, Struth AG: An abnormality of the alternate pathway of complement activation in sickle cell disease. N Engl J Med 288:803, 1973.

35. Glassman AB, Deas DV, Berlinsky FS, et al: Lymphocyte blast transformation and peripheral lymphocyte percentages in patients with sickle cell disease. Ann Clin Lab Sci 10:9, 1980.

36. Nistala K, Murray KJ: Co-existent sickle cell disease and juvenile rheumatoid arthritis: Two cases with delayed diagnosis and severe destructive arthropathy. J Rheumatol 28:2125, 2001.

37. Rao VM, Fishman M, Mitchell DG, et al: Painful sickle cell crisis: Bone marrow patterns observed with MR imaging. Radiology 161:211, 1986.

38. Sherman M: Pathogenesis of disintegration of the hip in sickle cell anemia. South Med J 52:632, 1959.

39. Shah A, Mukherjee A, Moreau PG: Nine knee arthroplasties for sickle cell disease. Acta Orthop Scand 64:150, 1993.

40. Milner PF, Kraus AP, Sebes JI, et al: Sickle cell disease as a cause of osteonecrosis of the femoral head. N Engl J Med 325:1476, 1991.

41. Roger E, Letts M: Sickle cell disease of the spine in children. Can J Surg 42:289, 1999.

42. Hernigou P, Bachir D, Galacteros F: Avascular necrosis of the femoral head in sickle cell disease. J Bone Joint Surg 75B:875, 1993.

43. Moran MC, Huo MH, Garvin KI, et al: Total hip arthroplasty in sickle cell hemoglobinopathy. Clin Orthop Rel Res 294:140, 1993.

44. Allen BJ, Andrews BS: Bilateral aseptic necrosis of calcanei in an adult male with sickle cell disease treated by a surgical coring procedure. J Rheumatol 10:294, 1983.

45. Castro FP Jr., Barrack RL: Core decompression and conservative treatment for avascular necrosis of the femoral head: a meta-analysis. Am J Orthop 29:187, 2000.

46. Kanyerezi BR, Ndugwa C, Owor R, et al: The spinal column in sickle cell disease. J Rheumatol 1(Suppl):21, 1974.

47. Martinez S, Apple JS, Baber C, et al: Protrusio acetabuli in sickle-cell anemia. Radiology 151:43, 1984.

48. Schumacher HR, Murray WM, Dalinka MK: Acute muscle injury complicating sickle cell crisis. Semin Arthritis Rheum 19:243, 1990.

49. Valeriano-Marcet J, Kerr LD: Myonecrosis and myofibrosis as complications of sickle cell anemia. Ann Intern Med 115:99, 1991.

50. Feldman F, Zwass A, Staron RB, Haramiti H: MRI of soft tissue abnormalities: A primary cause of sickle cell crisis. Skeletal Radiol 22:501, 1993.

51. Ludmerer KM, Kissane JM: Left elbow pain and death in a young woman with sickle-cell anemia. Am J Med 73:268, 1982.

52. Gratwick GM, Bullough PG, Bohne WHO, et al: Thalassemic arthropathy. Ann Intern Med 88:494, 1978.

53. Rioja L, Girot R, Garabedian M, Cournot-Witmer G: Bone disease in children with homozygous beta-thalassemia. Bone Miner 8:69, 1990.

54. deVernejoul MC, Girot R, Gueris J, et al: Calcium phosphate metabolism and bone disease in patients with homozygous thalassemia. J Clin Endocrinol Metab 54:276, 1982.

55. Williams BA, Morris LL, Toogood IR, et al: Limb deformity and metaphyseal abnormalities in thalassemia major. Am J Pediatr Hematol Oncol 14:197, 1992.

56. Korovessis P, Papanastasiou D, Tiniakou M, et al: Incidence of scoliosis in beta thalassemia and follow-up evaluation. Spine 21:1798, 1996.

57. Arman MI: Gelenk beteiligung bei Hamoglobinopathien. Akt Rheumatol 15:17, 1990.

58. Wayne AS, Zelicof SB, Sledge CB: Total hip arthroplasty in beta thalassemia: Case report and review of the literature. Clin Orthop 294:149, 1993.

59. Dessi C, Clemente MG, Diana G, et al: Cyoglobulinemia in transfusion dependent thalassemia major. Clin Exp Rheum 13:149, 1995.

60. Kumar V, Gruber B: To phaceons gout in a patient with thalassemia. J Clin Rheumatol. 9:380-384, 2003.

61. Schlumpf U, Gerber N, Bunzli H, et al: Arthritiden bei Thalassemia minor. Schweiz Med Wochenschr 107:1156, 1977.

62. Arman MI, Butun B, Doseyen A, et al: Frequency and features of rheumatic findings in thalassemia minor: A blind controlled study. Br J Rheum 31:197, 1992.

63. Finterbush A, Ferber I, Mogle P: Lower limb pain in thalassemia. J Rheumatol 12:529, 1985.

64. Boulard F, Gardina P, Gillo A, et al: Bone marrow transplantation for homozygous beta thalassemia: The Memorial Sloan Kettering experience. Ann N Y Acad Sci 850:498, 1998.

109 Arthritis Accompanying Endocrine and Metabolic Disorders

JOHN S. SERGENT

A rheumatologist or primary care physician must always be cognizant of the many ways that systemic diseases affect muscles and joints. These may be manifest in a number of ways:

1. A primary endocrine or metabolic disorder may present with important musculoskeletal problems (e.g., proximal muscle weakness in Cushing's syndrome, carpal tunnel syndrome in diabetes mellitus, and acromegaly).
2. A patient with long-standing endocrine or metabolic disease may develop musculoskeletal complications (e.g., diabetic stiff-hand syndrome).
3. A patient with a well-established rheumatic disease may develop an endocrine disorder (e.g., hypothyroidism in scleroderma).
4. An endocrine or metabolic disorder may develop as a result of therapy for a rheumatic disease (e.g., iatrogenic Cushing's syndrome).

Many of these disorders can be subtle when occurring in previously normal individuals. When they occur in association with preexisting rheumatic disease, or when their manifestations are atypical, considerable skill is often necessary to establish the diagnosis.

Diabetes Mellitus

Diabetes mellitus is associated with a wide variety of complications involving joints. In many of these complications there is a direct cause; in others, there is a reported epidemiologic association, although the actual cause-and-effect relationship is unproved (Table 109–1).

The hand is an important target for diabetic complications. The diabetic stiff-hand syndrome, also known as diabetic cheirarthropathy and the limited joint-mobility syndrome, is a common complication of both type I and type II diabetes mellitus[1] (Fig. 109–1). The condition is believed to be caused by excessive glycosylation of collagen in the skin, blood vessels, and periarticular structures[2] and to decreased collagen degeneration and removal,[3] resulting in thick, inelastic tissues. In its advanced stages the fingers remain permanently contracted at the metacarpophalangeal (MCP) and proximal interphalangeal (PIP) joints, and the thick, shiny skin may resemble that of scleroderma.[4] This complication, usually only bothersome but not disabling, increases in association with the duration of the disease.[5] As might be expected, it is predictive of renal, retinal, and other diabetic complications[6,7] and occurs in up to 30 percent of patients with long-standing diabetes.[8]

TABLE 109–1 · JOINT COMPLICATIONS OF DIABETES MELLITUS

Manifestation	Typical Joint Involved
Diabetic stiff-hand syndrome	Metacarpophalangeal, proximal interphalangeal joints
Dupuytren's contractures	Fourth (and other) flexion tendons
Trigger fingers	Flexor tendons
Adhesive capsulitis	Shoulders
Reflex sympathetic dystrophy	Shoulders, hands
Carpal tunnel syndrome	First four fingers
Charcot's arthropathy	Foot, ankle
Diffuse idiopathic skeletal hyperostosis	Spine
Osteomyelitis	Foot
Diabetic angotrophy	Shoulder, back, thighs

Therapy with aldose reductase inhibitors has been reported to be beneficial for the stiff-hand syndrome[9] and has improved nerve conduction in diabetic neuropathy,[10] but further use has been limited by side effects.

Dupuytren's contractures may be seen in patients with diabetic stiff-hand syndrome, or they may occur independently. It is thought that the pathogenesis is similar to stiff-hand syndrome, with glycosylation and increased collagen deposition both playing a role. Unlike most cases of stiff-hand syndrome, Dupuytren's contractures may be seen relatively early in the course of the disease. The prevalence of Dupuytren's contractures in adult diabetics is about 30 percent.[8]

Trigger fingers, a catching and snapping of the fingers, occasionally painful, is also frequent in diabetic patients and is due to flexor tenosynovitis and believed to have the same pathogenesis as stiff-hand syndrome.[11]

Adhesive capsulitis of the shoulders, with or without calcific tendinitis, is well established as a complication of diabetes.[12,13] It can be associated with reflex-sympathetic dystrophy.[14] Although sometimes associated with recurrent painful tendinitis and bursitis, the loss of motion can be painless and insidious.

Carpal tunnel syndrome occurs in about 25 percent of individuals with diabetes mellitus[8] and can be quite subtle, especially in patients with preexisting peripheral neuropathy. Because nocturnal paresthesias are common in both, the clinician must be alert to the possibility of carpal tunnel syndrome to intervene early in disease to prevent thenar muscle atrophy.

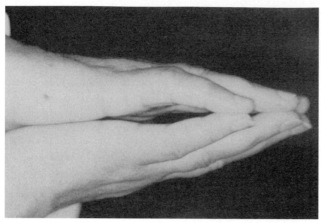

FIGURE 109-1 · The "Prayer Sign" in the Diabetic Stiff-Hand Syndrome. As a result of progressive thickening of tendons, joint capsules, and subcutaneous tissues, progressive stiffness and flexion contractures develop in these patients.

Charcot's arthropathy in diabetes usually involves the ankle or midfoot and invariably occurs in persons with sensory neuropathy.[15] The onset can be sudden,[16] occasionally in association with minor trauma. The abrupt onset, with swelling and radiographs showing the bone fragments and disorganization, can lead the unwary clinician on an unnecessary search for infection. As with Charcot joints of other causes, treatment is generally unsatisfactory, with little more to offer than splinting and bracing.

Diffuse idiopathic skeletal hyperostosis (DISH) is strongly association with diabetes. This complication is most prominently seen in obese patients with type II diabetes. It has also been seen in nondiabetic individuals with abnormal insulin responses to hyperglycemia.[17] It is manifest by proliferative new bone formation at joint margins, particularly in the axial skeleton. Clinically, patients may suffer from diminished mobility similar to that seen in anklyosing spondylitis (AS). There is no evidence to date that diabetic control improves the condition or delays DISH, although no careful studies have yet been performed to evaluate the relationship. The pathophysiologic mechanism of the condition has also not yet been elucidated, although it may be related more to hyperlipidemia and other metabolic factors than to diabetes itself.[18,19]

Osteomyelitis in the foot is a major problem in long-standing diabetics. Because of the peripheral sensory neuropathy, foot injuries and pressure ulcers tend to be underappreciated, and patients may not realize anything is seriously wrong until advanced osteomyelitis has developed. In addition, subcutaneous foreign bodies, such as needles and splinters, can be present for weeks or months before the diabetic patient is aware of them. There is good evidence that infections and other complications of these problems can be markedly diminished by meticulous foot care.[20,21]

Diabetic amyotrophy is a rare condition associated with the abrupt onset of pain and rapid atrophy in large muscle groups, usually the thighs, the perispinous muscles, and the shoulder girdle.[22,23] Fasciculations are often prominent, and electromyography reveals a neuropathic picture. Severe pain is the most frequent complaint, although profound weakness of the affected muscles is also a problem. This problem slowly resolves in the majority of cases.

▌ Parathyroid Disorders

Hyperparathyroidism has major effects on the skeleton, the most important of which is osteopenia (see Chapter 90). The most important joint manifestation of primary hyperparathyroidism is chondrocalcinosis with associated calcium pyrophosphate dihydrate (CPPD) deposition disease[24] (see Chapter 88). Although the most common arthritic manifestation is acute pseudogout, the entire spectrum of arthropathies associated with CPPD may be seen in this disorder, including a crippling and slowly progressive polyarthritis.[25]

Most patients with long-standing hyperparathyroidism have proximal muscle weakness, a condition rapidly reversed by removal of the parathyroid adenoma.[26,27] In these patients, the muscle enzymes are normal, and electromyography and muscle biopsy show a picture most consistent with denervation.

Patients with secondary hyperparathyroidism associated with advanced renal disease have a number of abnormalities in the bones and joints. The changes of renal osteodystrophy due to secondary hyperparathyroidism include an erosive arthritis in the hands,[28] resorption of the distal clavicle,[29] and erosions in the axial skeleton.[30] In children, the widespread bone deformities of osteitis fibrosa cystica can be crippling.[31] Other musculoskeletal manifestations of advanced renal failure include aluminum-induced osteomalacia[32] and β_2-microglobulin amyloidosis (see Chapter 90).

Hypoparathyroidism, usually due to surgical removal of the parathyroid glands, most commonly causes proximal muscle weakness related to the degree of hypocalcemia. This condition responds dramatically to treatment with vitamin D and calcium. Idiopathic hypoparathyroidism is a rare disorder, usually seen as part of the DiGeorge syndrome with thymic hypoplasia.

Pseudohypoparathyroidism, known as Albright's hereditary osteodystrophy, is due to end-organ resistance to the effect of parathyroid hormone. These patients have persistent hypocalcemia and hyperphosphatemia, but parathyroid hormone levels are consistently elevated.

Type Ia pseudohypoparathyroidism, which is autosomal dominant, is associated with short stature, calcification of the perispinal ligaments, and, usually, mental retardation. Most patients have an impressive shortening of the fourth metacarpal and metatarsal bones that can be demonstrated by having the patient clench the fist. Instead of the usual knuckle appearance over the fourth metacarpal head, these individuals have a dimple. Patients with type Ib pseudohypoparathyroidism also have resistance to parathyroid hormone but have normal phenotype.

Patients with pseudohypoparathyroidism have a defect in the genes encoding the alpha subunit of the cell membrane–associated guanine nucleotide stimulating unit (GS2) of adenyl cyclase.[33] Type Ia pseudohypoparathyroidism is almost always inherited maternally,[34] and type Ib is inherited paternally.[35]

The musculoskeletal manifestations of osteomalacia and rickets are covered in Chapter 90.

Thyroid Disorders

Hyperthyroidism (Graves' disease) may affect the musculoskeletal system in several ways. The most common complication is osteopenia and frank osteoporosis, which can be a major problem either with idiopathic Graves' disease or in patients with iatrogenic hyperthyroidism.[36] Failure to recognize the declining need for thyroid replacement with age is an important cause of iatrogenic hyperthyroidism in older women. For that reason, patients with hypothyroidism who are on both thyroid hormone and estrogen therapy should have TSH levels monitored and the dose readjusted to keep the TSH level within the normal range.[37,38] Bone density has been shown to increase after correction of the hyperthyroid state.[39]

Pretibial myxedema is a syndrome of painless nodules that occur over the pretibial areas. Virtually all affected patients have concomitant Graves' ophthalmopathy.[40] The lesions can be variable in size, ranging from nodules of 1-cm diameter to very large lesions covering most of the pretibial surface. They are variably colored, ranging from pink to a light-purple hue, and can mimic erythema nodosum. However, unlike erythema nodosum, these lesions are painless. They are caused by the accumulation of hyaluronic acid in the skin,[41] and in some cases have a shiny appearance resembling scleroderma or morphea.

Hyperthyroidism can also be associated with a number of changes in the nails,[42] including onycholysis, or elevation of the nail from the nail bed, and clubbing. Clubbing is usually part of the condition known as thyroid acropachy, a rare manifestation of hyperthyroidism also associated with periostitis around the metacarpal joints and distal soft tissue swelling of the digits. The condition is not clearly related to the levels of thyroid hormone, as it may be seen after the patient has reverted to the euthyroid state.

Proximal muscle weakness is a common complication of hyperthyroidism and is present in the vast majority of patients. Most of these patients will have lost weight and have other evidence of loss of muscle mass. The proximal muscle weakness corrects rapidly with correction of the hyperthyroid state.[43] Perhaps related to the proximal myopathy, adhesive capsulitis of the shoulder seems to be increased in patients with hyperthyroidism. In these patients, the condition can be quite insidious and, therefore, difficult to treat, often presenting with frozen-shoulder syndrome as the initial manifestation.

There are strong relationships between both Graves' and Hashimoto's diseases and other rheumatic diseases. From 75 to 90 percent of patients with Graves' disease,[44] and a smaller percentage of patients with Hashimoto's thyroiditis, have antinuclear antibodies (ANAs), and many have anti-DNA antibodies as well, despite the fact that overt systemic lupus erythematosus (SLE) is relatively uncommon. There is a true increased incidence of hypothyroidism in patients with scleroderma, and there is some evidence that other rheumatic diseases are also associated with an increased incidence as well, including SLE, rheumatoid arthritis (RA), mixed connective tissue disease, Sjögren's syndrome, and polymyositis.

Graves' disease is associated with human leukocyte antigen (HLA)-B8, HLA-A1, HLA-Cw7, and HLA-DR3, and combinations of these antigens correlate with persistent disease.[45] Hashimoto's disease is associated with HLA-B8, HLA-DR3 HLA-Aw30, and HLA-DR5. Not surprisingly, these diseases occur in increased frequency in individuals with other autoimmune diseases that are associated with these HLA antigens.[46]

Hypothyroidism in its idiopathic form is almost always caused by Hashimoto's thyroiditis and can be associated with a very unusual arthropathy. Patients present with swelling and stiffness in large joints, usually the knees. However, the hands may also be involved, and this is often very impressive in joints previously involved with osteoarthritis (OA). Examination of the swollen joint reveals a thick, gelatinous sensation that causes a very slow fluid wave (bulge sign). Synovial thickening on palpation can be very impressive. Aspiration of the fluid from patients with the arthropathy of myxedema reveals noninflammatory fluid that is extremely viscous with very high hyaluronic acid levels. CPPD crystals may be present, but inflammation is not.[47] This arthropathy resolves very quickly with correction of the hypothyroid state.

The myopathy of hypothyroidism can be quite confusing. Many patients have proximal muscle weakness; however, some complain only of generalized lassitude and fatigue. In one study, 25 percent of hypothyroid patients had muscle symptoms, although creatine kinase levels were usually normal.[48] Occasionally, levels can be quite elevated and rhabdomyolysis has been reported.[49] Muscle biopsies are usually normal, although moderate inflammatory changes are sometimes present.[50] This condition can resemble either polymyalgia rheumatica or polymyositis, depending on the predominance of stiffness versus weakness.

Carpal tunnel syndrome is increased in patients with hypothyroidism, and in one study hypothyroidism was present in 7 percent of patients with carpal tunnel syndrome.[51] It is frequent enough that most patients with idiopathic carpal tunnel syndrome should be screened for early myxedema.

Because of all these considerations, the clinician facing patients with musculoskeletal complications must always keep thyroid disorders in mind. Many of these conditions can be quite subtle, and the musculoskeletal manifestations, ranging from myopathy to pretibial myxedema to frank arthropathies, can be the presenting manifestation of thyroid disorders.

Adrenal Disorders

Iatrogenic Cushing's syndrome due to exogenous glucocorticoid therapy of an underlying inflammatory disease is the most common condition involving adrenal hormones seen in patients with rheumatic diseases (see Chapter 57). However, a few complication of iatrogenic Cushing's syndrome deserve special comment.

Osteonecrosis is a common late complication of glucocorticoid therapy[52] and may first become evident months or years after glucocorticoid therapy has been discontinued. However, it can also be seen following short courses of therapy, or from intermittent high-dose intravenous (IV) therapy.[53] Because many of the patients receiving glucocorticoid therapy have diseases associated with joint pain, the clinician must be alert to this condition. When it affects the hip, which is the most common joint involved, the pain is usually dull, located in the groin, increased by weight-bearing, and progressive. An increased incidence of osteonecrosis has been seen in patients on replacement glucocorticoid therapy, pointing out the need to treat with the lowest acceptable dose of the drug.[54]

Steroid myopathy can be particularly perplexing in patients being treated for primary or secondary inflammatory myopathies. Steroid myopathy is characteristically more severe in the pelvic girdle and can be so severe that patients are bedridden. It may come on gradually or abruptly, heralded by weakness and muscle aching. Biopsies show type II fiber atrophy, and muscle enzymes are normal. There is evidence that longer acting and fluorinated compounds are more likely to cause myopathy.[55] Once myopathy has developed, it usually requires nearly total discontinuation of the glucocorticoids before any improvement is seen, and even then it may be weeks or months before strength begins to return.

Osteopenia (see Chapters 57 and 90) is related both to the dose and the duration of glucocorticoid therapy. No "safe" dose has yet been established. Because osteoporosis can develop rapidly after beginning glucocorticoid therapy, prophylaxis is recommended in most patients. Regimens shown to be effective at preventing or treating glucocorticoid-induced osteoporosis include calcium and vitamin D_3,[56] calcitonin,[57] and bisphosphonates.[58,59]

Idiopathic Cushing's syndrome may be confused with primary musculoskeletal disease. Over 50 percent of patients will have muscle weakness and a similar percentage will have back pain, often due to osteoporotic fractures. In patients with Cushing's syndrome due to ectopic ACTH production, glucocorticoid levels may be extremely high, resulting in profound myopathy and other features such as steroid psychosis. Because weight loss, rather than typical centripetal obesity, is often present in these patients, the appearance may not be typical of idiopathic Cushing's syndrome of pituitary origin.

Other effects of glucocorticoids on the musculoskeletal system are less well understood. Some patients complain of intense joint pain, usually most severe in the knees, when high doses of glucocorticoids are first administered. This pain typically resolves even if the dose is left unchanged.

The so-called steroid withdrawal syndrome consists of widespread arthralgias, myalgias, malaise, and sometimes low-grade fever.[60] It may be seen when glucocorticoids have been used for nonrheumatic conditions, such as asthma or inflammatory bowel disease, and does not necessarily require suppression of the pituitary-adrenal axis.

Finally, the abrupt reduction of the dose of a glucocorticoid can cause a severe rebound flare in the underlying disease. This may be seen even though the dose of the glucocorticoid remains in the pharmacologic range.

Idiopathic Addison's disease presents with weakness, weight loss, abdominal pain, hyperpigmentation, nausea, and hypotension. Iatrogenic Addison's disease, on the other hand, can be much more subtle. Because mineralocorticoids are still being produced, salt wasting, hyperkalemia, and postural hypotension are usually less impressive, and hyperpigmentation is not seen because the pituitary is suppressed. Moreover, as in idiopathic Addison's disease, the features may not be impressive unless the individual undergoes a second exogenous stress, such as surgery or an infection. In that setting, addisonian crisis has been seen, even in individuals still receiving physiologic or "replacement" doses of glucocorticoids. Thus, it should be assumed that people taking glucocorticoids at more than the equivalent of 5 mg/day of prednisone have a pituitary-adrenal axis unable to respond to severe stress, and appropriate increases in the glucocorticoid dose should be considered. In addition, the development of idiopathic Addison's disease in individuals receiving low-dose glucocorticoids can result in similar diagnostic difficulty.[61]

■ Acromegaly

Growth hormone levels tend to decline with age, and there is evidence that treatment of the elderly with growth hormone will increase muscle mass[62] and, in some cases, increase bone density as well. However, at this point in time the most important musculoskeletal manifestations related to growth hormones are those seen in acromegaly.

Growth hormone is secreted primarily in nocturnal pulses, and it stimulates hepatocytes to produce somatomedin C, or insulin-like growth factor (IGF). Somatomedin C has variable effects on adult tissues, but osteocytes, chondrocytes, and fibroblasts are all responsive in the adult. Acromegaly, caused by an adenoma in the anterior pituitary gland, is a very insidious disease, and often, years have passed before the diagnosis is made. During those years, a variety of musculoskeletal consequences have usually developed.

Carpal tunnel syndrome occurs in about half of the patients with acromegaly and is one of the few musculoskeletal manifestations that may develop relatively early in the disease course.[63] It is due to enlargement of the nerve and to expansion of the transverse carpal ligament and other soft tissues. Raynaud's phenomenon due to compression of the distal arteries by soft tissues occurs in about one third of patients with acromegaly.

If the diagnosis is not made early, and it rarely is, premature OA almost inevitably develops. The knee is the joint most frequently involved, followed by the hip and the spine. The hypertrophied cartilage tends to fissure and ulcerate, and the ligaments of the knee become elongated and lax. This combination of instability and abnormal cartilage can lead to severe disability.[64] Other areas affected include the temporomandibular joints and the small joints of the hands and feet. The reason that glove size increases in acromegalics is not because bones grow; it is because cartilage in each joint increases in thickness and the soft tissues proliferate.

The early radiographic picture of acromegalic joints shows joint-space widening due to cartilage hypertrophy. In the spine, disk spaces may also be widened. Later, as the inevitable degeneration occurs, the changes are indistinguishable from those of idiopathic OA.

Back pain is a particularly troubling feature of acromegaly. Most patients complain of dull, diffuse pain in the lumbar spine. The pain does not radiate into the legs and is often present both at rest and with activity. These changes are caused by several factors, including disk-space enlargement, osteophyte production, and ligamentous calcifications. Some patients improve when growth hormone levels are lowered following surgery, radiation, or treatment with a somatostatin analogue.[65]

The majority of acromegalic patients develop proximal muscle weakness, which is occasionally an early symptom. Muscle enzymes are normal, and biopsies show no inflammation but do reveal abnormal variations in fiber size.

▌ Pregnancy

The pregnant state produces a complex series of musculoskeletal changes in normal individuals. Probably the most common is the near-universal problem of low back pain, especially during the third trimester. This pain is felt to be primarily mechanical in nature and is due to the increased lumbar lordosis. In addition, the increased mobility of the sacroiliac and other joints of the pelvic girdle, under the influence of the hormone relaxin, may be a factor in many women.

Carpal tunnel syndrome is also common in the last trimester, due primarily to increased fluid retention. It is usually mild and responsive to wrist splints. It resolves quickly after delivery.

Pregnancy has impressive effects in patients with inflammatory rheumatic diseases. Virtually all the rheumatic diseases, especially RA and SLE, have been reported to develop in the early postpartum period.

There is evidence that rheumatoid factor (RF) positivity during pregnancy predicts subsequent RA.[66] This finding could be interpreted in several ways, but a likely interpretation is that the pregnant state itself has delayed the clinical onset of the disease until the postpartum period. In other words, the true incidence of RA may be unaffected by pregnancy, but the time of its onset is. This observation would be compatible with the well-known improvement in the course of RA in about three fourths of patients when they become pregnant. This improvement usually begins in the first trimester, but virtually all patients relapse in the first 3 or 4 months postpartum. There have been a number of attempts to explain this amelioration of the disease during the pregnant state. HLA incompatibilities in DRB1, DQA1, and DQB1 have all been associated with a greater likelihood of disease improvement during pregnancy.[67] In addition, cytokines are affected by the pregnant state. Interleukin-2 (IL-2) production is decreased, and production of soluble tumor necrosis factor (TNF) receptors is increased.[68]

In other rheumatic diseases, the situation during pregnancy is more complex. In SLE, fetal wastage is increased, and there is some evidence that the disease is more apt to flare during the postpartum period. The relationship between SLE and pregnancy is discussed in detail in Chapter 76.

The use of hormone therapy to treat rheumatic diseases has had a rather stormy history. Based in part on murine studies showing that SLE can be made worse by estrogen and improved by androgen,[69] SLE has been the subject of extensive study. Persons with SLE metabolize the active metabolite of estrogen (i.e., estrone) preferentially to the feminizing metabolites 16-hydroxyestrone and estriol.[70] In addition, there is some evidence that testosterone levels are lower and that inactive forms predominate.[71] This has led to some interest in using dehydroepiandrosterone (DHEA), which has also been reported to be low in patients with SLE, in treatment of fatigue and other manifestations of the disease.[72]

The role of birth control pills has also been investigated. Studies have suggested that oral contraceptive use diminishes the lifetime risk of RA.[73] In contradistinction, SLE may flare more often in women taking birth control pills containing estrogen.[74] However, if progesterone-only birth control pills are used, SLE activity may actually be decreased. At this point it is safe to say that the decision to use oral contraceptives in patients with SLE requires careful considerations of the risks, which are probably small, versus the benefits. If an oral contraceptive is chosen, the lowest effective dose of estrogen or a progesterone-only preparation should be used.[75] There is no evidence, incidentally, to suggest that postmenopausal hormone replacement therapy with estrogen adversely affects the course of SLE.

REFERENCES

1. Kapoor A, Sibbitt WL Jr: Contractures in diabetes mellitus: The syndrome of limited joint mobility. Sem Arthritis Rheum 18:168, 1989.
2. Sheetz MJ, King GL: Molecular understanding of hyperglycemia adverse effects for diabetic complications. JAMA 288:2579, 2002.
3. Seibold JR, Uitto J, Dorwart BB, et al: Collagen synthesis and collagenase activity in dermal fibroblasts from patients with diabetes and digital sclerosis. J Lab Clin Med 105:664, 1985.
4. Iwasaki T, Kohama T, Houjou S, et al: Diabetic scleroderma and scleroderma-like changes in a patient with maturity onset type diabetes of young people. Dermatology 188:228, 1994.
5. Gamstedt A, Holm-Glad J, Ohlson CG, et al: Hand abnormalities are strongly associated with the duration of diabetes mellitus. J Intern Med 234:189, 1993.
6. Lawson PM, Maneschi F, Kohner EM: The relationship of hand abnormalities to diabetes and diabetic retinopathy. Diabetes Care 6:140, 1983.

7. Rosenbloom AL, Silverstein JH, Lezotte DC, et al: Limited joint mobility in diabetes mellitus indicating increased risk for microvascular disease. N Engl J Med 305:191, 1981.

8. Chammas M, Bousquet P, Renard E, et al: Dupuytren's disease, carpal tunnel syndrome, trigger finger, and diabetes mellitus. J Hand Surg Am 20:109, 1995.

9. Eaton P, Sibbitt WL Jr., Harsh A: The effect of an aldose reductase inhibiting agent on limited joint mobility in diabetic patients. JAMA 253:1437, 1985.

10. Goto Y, Hotta N, Shigeta Y, et al: Effects of an aldose reductase inhibitor, Epalrestat, on diabetic neuropathy. Biomed Pharmacother 49:296, 1995.

11. Benedetti A, Noacco C, Simonatti M, et al: Diabetic trigger finger. N Engl J Med 306:1552, 1982.

12. Arkkila PE, Kantola IM, Viikari JS, et al: Shoulder capsulitis in type I and II diabetic patients: Association with diabetic complications and related diseases. Ann Rheum Dis 55:907, 1996.

13. Boyle-Walker KL, Gabard DL, Bietsch E, et al: A profile of patients with adhesive capsulitis. J Hand Ther 10:222, 1997.

14. Lequesne M, Dang N, Benasson M, et al: Increased association of diabetes mellitus with capsulitis of the shoulder and shoulder-hand syndrome. Scand J Rheumatol 6:53, 1997.

15. Serra F, Mancini L, Ghirlanda G, et al: Charcot's foot. RAYS 22:524, 1997.

16. Armstrong DG, Lavery LA: Acute Charcot's arthropathy of the foot and ankle. Phys Ther 78:74, 1998.

17. Julkunen H, Heinonen OP, Pyorala K: Hyperostosis of the spine in an adult population: Its relationship to hyperglycemia and obesity. Ann Rheum Dis 30:605, 1971.

18. Daragon A, Mejjad O, Czernichow P, et al: Vertebral hyperostosis and diabetes mellitus: A case-control study. Ann Rheum Dis 54:375, 1995.

19. Vezyroglou G, Mitropoulos A, Antoniadis C: A metabolic syndrome in diffuse idiopathic skeletal hyperostosis: A controlled study. J Rheumatol 23:672, 1996.

20. Suico JG, Marriott DJ, Vinicor F, et al: Behaviors predicting foot lesions in patients with non–insulin-dependent diabetes mellitus. J Gen Int Med 13:482, 1998.

21. Rith-Najarian S, Branchaud C, Beulieu O, et al: Reducing lower-extremity amputations due to diabetes: Application of the staged diabetes management approach in a primary care setting. J Family Pract 47:127, 1998.

22. Thomas PK: Classification, differential diagnosis, and staging of diabetic peripheral neuropathy. Diabetes 46(Suppl 2):S54, 1997.

23. Naftulin S, Fast A, Thomas M: Diabetic lumbar radiculopathy: Sciatica without disc herniation. Spine 18:2419, 1993.

24. Rynes RI, Merzig EG: Calcium pyrophosphate crystal deposition disease and hyperparathyroidism: A controlled, prospective study. J Rheumatol 5(4):460, 1978.

25. Resnick DL: Erosive arthritis of the hand and wrist in hyperparathyroidism. Radiology 110(2):263, 1974.

26. Frame B, Heinze EG, Block M, et al: Myopathy in primary hyperparathyroidism: Observations in 3 patients. Ann Intern Med 68:1022, 1968.

27. Nudelman I, Deutsch AA, Reiss R: Surgical treatment of primary hyperparathyroidism in the elderly patient. Isr J Med Sci 19(2):150, 1983.

28. Rubin LA, Fam AG, Rubenstein J, et al: Erosive azotemic osteoarthropathy. Arthritis Rheum 27:1086, 1984.

29. Pecovnik-Balon B, Kramberger S: Tumoral calcinosis in patients on hemodialysis: Care report and review of the literature. Am J Nephrol 17(1):93, 1997.

30. Kuntz D, Navean B, Bardin T, et al: Destructive spondyloarthropathy in hemodialyzed patients. Arthritis Rheum 27:369, 1984.

31. Dabbagh S: Renal osteodystrophy. Curr Opin Pediatrics 10(2):190, 1998.

32. Pei Y, Hercz G, Greenwood C, et al: Risk factors for renal osteodystrophy: A multivariant analysis. J Bone Miner Res 10(1):149, 1995.

33. Ringel MD, Schwindinger WF, Levine MA: Clinical implications of genetic defects in G proteins: The molecular basis of McCune-Albright syndrome and Albright hereditary osteodystrophy. Medicine 75(4):171, 1996.

34. Hayward BE, Kamiya M, Strain L, et al: The human GNAS1 gene is imprinted and encodes distinct paternally and biallelically expressed G proteins. Proc Natl Acad Sci U S A 95(17):10038, 1998.

35. Juppner H, Schipani E, Bastepe M, et al: The gene responsible for pseudohypoparathyroidism type Ib is paternally imprinted and maps in four unrelated kindreds of chromosome 20Q13.3. Proc Natl Acad Sci U S A 95(20):11798, 1998.

36. Jodar E, Munoz-Torres M, Escobar-Jimenez F, et al: Bone loss in hyperthyroid patients and in former hyperthyroid patients controlled on medical therapy: Influence of etiology and menopause. Clin Endocrinol 47(3):279, 1997.

37. Chiovato L, Mariotti S, Pinchera A: Thyroid diseases in the elderly. Baillieres Clin Endocrinol Metab 11(2):251, 1997.

38. Shetty KR, Duthie EH Jr.: Thyroid disease and associated illness in the elderly. Clin Geriatric Med 11(2):311, 1995.

39. Rosen CJ, Alder RA: Longitudinal changes in lumbar bone density among thyrotoxic patients after attainment of euthyroidism. J Clin Endocrinol Metab 75:1531, 1992.

40. Fatourechi V, Pajouhi M, Fransway AF: Dermopathy of Graves disease (pretibial myxedema): Review of 150 cases. Medicine 73(1):1, 1994.

41. Kriss JP: Pathogenesis and treatment of pretibial myxedema. Endocrinol Metab Clin North Am 16(2):409, 1987.

42. Nixon DW, Samols E: Acral changes associated with thyroid diseases. JAMA 212(7):1175, 1970.

43. Ramsey ID: Muscle dysfunction in hyperthyroidism. Lancet 2:931, 1966.

44. Katakura M, Yamada T, Aizawa T, et al: Presence of antideoxyribonucleic acid antibody in patients with hyperthyroidism of Graves' disease. J Clin Endocrinol Metab 64:405, 1987.

45. Baldini M, Pappalettera M, Lecchi L, et al: Human lymphocyte antigens in Graves' disease: Correlation with persistent course of disease. Am J Med Sci 309:43, 1995.

46. Torfs CP, King M, Huey B, et al: Genetic interrelationship between insulin-dependent diabetes mellitus, the autoimmune thyroid diseases, and rheumatoid arthritis. Am J Hum Gen 38:170, 1986.

47. Dorwart BB, Schumacher HR: Joint effusions, chondrocalcinosis and rheumatic manifestations of hypothyroidism. Am J Med 59:780, 1975.

48. Hartl E, Finsterer J, Grossegger C, et al: Relationship between thyroid function and skeletal muscle involvement in subclinical and overt hypothyroidism. Endocrinologist 11:217, 2001.

49. Bhansazi A, Chandran V, Ranesh J, et al: Acute myoedema: an unusual presenting manifestation of hypothyroid myopathy. Postgrad Med J 76:99, 2000.

50. Mastaglia FL, Ojeda VJ, Sarnat HB, et al: Myopathies associated with hypothyroidism: A review based upon 13 cases. Aust N Z J Med 18(6):799, 1988.

51. Katz JN, Larson MG, Sabra A: The carpal tunnel syndrome: Diagnostic utility of the history and physical examination findings. Ann Intern Med 112:321, 1990.

52. Weiner ES, Abeles M: Aseptic necrosis and glucocorticosteroids in systemic lupus erythematosus: A reevaluation. J Rheumatol 16(5):604, 1989.

53. Wollheim FA: Acute and long-term complications of corticosteroid pulse therapy. Scand J Rheumatol Suppl 54:27, 1984.

54. Vreden SG, Hermus AR, van Liessum PA, et al: Aseptic bone necrosis in patients on glucocorticoid replacement therapy. Neth J Med 39(3-4):153, 1991.

55. Lane RJ, Mastaglia FL: Drug-induced myopathies in man. Lancet 2:562, 1978.

56. Buckley LM, Leib ES, Cartularo KS, et al: Calcium and vitamin D_3 supplementation prevents bone loss in the spine secondary to low dose corticosteroids in patients with rheumatoid arthritis. Ann Intern Med 125:961, 1996.

57. Adachi JD, Bensen WG, Bell MJ, et al: Salmon calcitonin nasal spray in the prevention of corticosteroid-induced osteoporosis. Br J Rheumatol 36:255, 1997.

58. Saag KG, Emkey R, Schnitzer TJ, et al: Alendronate for the prevention and treatment of glucocorticoid-induced osteoporosis. N Engl J Med 339:292, 1998.

59. Adachi JD, Bensen WG, Brown J, et al: Intermittent etidronate therapy to prevent corticosteroid-induced osteoporosis. N Engl J Med 337:382, 1997.

60. Dixon RB, Nicholas PC: On the various forms of corticosteroid withdrawal syndrome. Am J Med 68:224, 1980.

61. Cronin CC, Callaghan N, Kearney PJ, et al: Addison disease in patients treated with glucocorticoid therapy. Arch Intern Med 157:456, 1997.

62. Schwartz RS: Trophic factor supplementation: Effect on the age-associated changes in body composition. J Gerontol Series A 50(Spec. No.):151, 1995.

63. Baum H, Ludecke DK, Herrmann HD: Carpal tunnel syndrome and acromegaly. Acta Neurochirurg 83:54, 1986.

64. Bluestone R, Bywaters EG, Hartog M, et al: Acromegalic arthropathy. Ann Rheum Dis 30:243, 1971.

65. Layton MW, Fudman EJ, Barkan A, et al: Acromegalic arthropathy: Characteristics and response to therapy. Arthritis Rheum 31:1, 1990.

66. Iijima T, Tada H, Hidaka Y, et al: Prediction of postpartum onset of rheumatoid arthritis. Ann Rheum Dis 57:460, 1998.

67. Van der Horst-Bruinsma IE, de Vries RR, de Buck PD, et al: Influence of HLA-class II incompatibility between mother and fetus on the development and course of rheumatoid arthritis of the mother. Ann Rheum Dis 57(5):286, 1998.

68. Russell AS, Johnston C, Chew C, et al: Evidence for reduced Th1 function in normal pregnancy: A hypothesis for the remission of rheumatoid arthritis. J Rheumatol 24(6):1045, 1997.

69. Van Vollenhoven RF, McGuire JL: Estrogen, progesterone, and testosterone: Can they be used to treat autoimmune diseases? Cleve Clin J Med 61:276, 1994.

70. Lahita RG: The role of sex hormones in systemic lupus erythematosus. Curr Opin Rheumatol 11:352, 1999.

71. Lahita RG, Bradlow HL, Ginzler E, et al: Low plasma androgens in women with systemic lupus erythematosus. Arthritis Rheum 30:241, 1987.

72. Van Vollenhoven RF, Morabito LM, Engleman EG, et al: Treatment of systemic lupus erythematosus with dehydroepiandrosterone: 50 patients tested up to 12 months. J Rheumatol 25:285, 1998.

73. Hazes JM, Dijkmans BA, Vandenbroucke JP, et al: Reduction of the risk of rheumatoid arthritis among women who take oral contraceptives. Arthritis Rheum 33:173, 1990.

74. Julkunen HA: Oral contraceptives in systemic lupus erythematosus: Side effects and influence on the activity of SLE. Scand J Rheumatol 20:427, 1991.

75. Buyon JP: Oral contraceptives in women with systemic lupus erythematosus. Ann Med Interne 147:259, 1996.

Hypertrophic Osteoarthropathy

ROY D. ALTMAN · JERRY TENENBAUM

Hypertrophic osteoarthropathy (HOA) is a syndrome of chronic periostitis of bones, clubbing, and synovitis.[1] Clubbing was described in the writings of Hippocrates[2] and HOA was described more than a century ago in Central America.[3] The association of clubbing and arthritis with chronic lung and heart disease was noted by von Bamburger and Marie[4,5] and a familial form of HOA has been described.[6] The triad of periostitis, clubbing, and arthritis has been associated with numerous intrathoracic and extrathoracic diseases.

Classification

HOA is classified as either primary (hereditary or occasionally idiopathic, in adults) or secondary (often associated with neoplastic or infectious diseases)[7-31] (Table 110-1). Isolated clubbing may be familial or associated with chronic diseases such as bronchitis, pneumoconiosis, or bacterial endocarditis.[9] Thyroid acropachy is a

rare and unique form of HOA associated with long-standing hyperthyroidism.[28]

Clinical Syndromes

PACHYDERMOPERIOSTOSIS

Primary HOA, or pachydermoperiostosis, occurs most often within families. Symptoms commonly begin in boys about 1 year old or around the time of puberty and often decline within 10 to 20 years. Transmission is probably through an autosomal dominant gene with variable expression.

Primary HOA is characterized by the insidious development of clubbing with "spade-like" enlargement of hands and feet. Complaints include cosmetic unsightliness and decreasing dexterity or awkwardness in using the fingers.[32] There may be vague bone pain, and joint pain with swelling may be exacerbated by alcohol.

There may be prominent clubbing with cylindrical thickening of forearms and legs—these often correspond with radiographic periosteal thickening.[6,7] Recurrent, mildly symptomatic joint effusions may be accompanied by acro-osteolysis, particularly with resorption of distal phalanges of hands and feet. Facial features may be thickened and furrowed with deep nasolabial folds and a corrugated scalp, known as "leonine" facies (Fig. 110-1). The skin of the face, scalp, hands, and feet may show excessive sweating and a "greasy" feel. Other features may include gynecomastia, female hair distribution, striae, acne vulgaris, and cranial suture defects.[33]

TABLE 110-1 · CLASSIFICATION OF HYPERTROPHIC OSTEOARTHROPATHY

Primary
Pachydermoperiostosis[7]
Idiopathic[7] hypertrophic osteothropathy
Clubbing (familial,[8] idiopathic[9])

Secondary
Pulmonary Diseases
Neoplasms (bronchogenic carcinoma[10])
Infections (chronic bronchitis,[9] bronchiectasis[11])
Other (cystic fibrosis,[12] pulmonary fibrosis,[13] pneumoconiosis,[9] sarcoidosis[14])
Cardiovascular Diseases
Bacterial endocarditis[15]
Cyanotic congenital heart disease[16]
Patent ductus arteroisus[17]
Other (aortic aneurysm,[18] aortic prosthesis[19])
Gastrointestinal Diseases
Neoplasms (carcinoma of esophagus,[20] liver,[21] colon[9])
Infections[11] (amebic dystentery[9])
Hepatobiliary Diseases[11] (biliary cirrhosis,[9] cirrhosis[12])
Other (inflammatory bowel disease,[22] Whipple's disease[23])
Neoplasms (often with intrathoracic metastases such as lymphomas[24,25])
Miscellaneous (connective tissue diseases,[26] POEMS syndrome[27])
Thyroid acropachy[28]
Acquired immune deficiency syndrome (AIDS)[29-31]

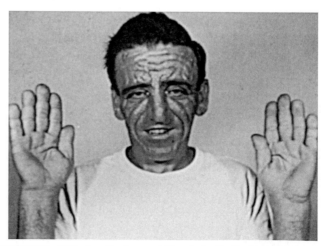

FIGURE 110–1 · Facies and Hands in Pachydermoperiostosis. Note coarse facial features and diffusely enlarged hands.

CLUBBING

The term *clubbing* is descriptive of the appearance of the fingers or toes (Figs. 110-2 and 110-3). There is initially a softening of the nail bed, giving a "rocking" sensation when the nail bed is palpated. This is accompanied by periungual erythema and telangiectasias. Subsequently, there is a loss of the normal 7- to 11-degree angle between the nail and the soft tissue of

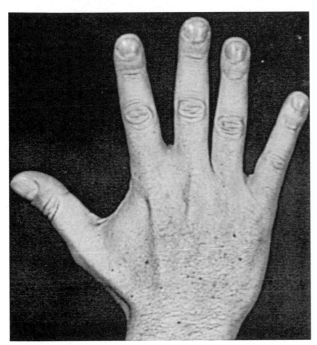

FIGURE 110–2 · Dorsal view of the hand shows clubbing, with widening of the fingertips replacing the normally tapered appearance of the digits.

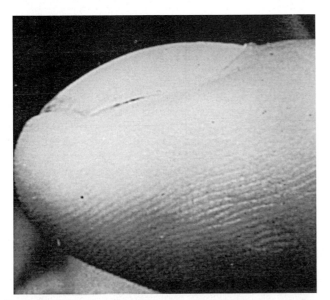

FIGURE 110–3 · A lateral view of the index finger demonstrates clubbing with loss of the normal 15-degree angle between the nail and the cuticle due to accentuated convexity of the nail. There is also enlargement of the distal finger pad and shininess of the nail and adjacent skin.

the nail bed (cuticle).[34] As the nail grows, it develops a convexity. The fingertip then develops a clubbed appearance with local warmth and sweating. Finally, the nail and adjacent skin develop a shiny or glossy appearance with longitudinal striations of the nail. Eponychia, paronychia, friability, and "hangnails" with accelerated nail or cuticle growth may occur. The adjacent distal interphalangeal joints may become hyperextensible.

Measurement of the interphalangeal and distal phalangeal distance have recently been suggested to define a digital clubbing index.[35] Reversal of the ratio of these distances predicts a risk of lung cancer relative risk, (RR) (RR 3.9) or inflammatory bowel disease (IBD) (RR 2.8 to 3.7).[34] Digital photography with computerized analysis may reduce some of the differences in diagnosis caused by different examiners.[34,36]

Clubbing most often emerges insidiously over a prolonged period and is asymptomatic other than for its unsightliness. Most cases of isolated clubbing are idiopathic and may be hereditary (no genetic pattern has been established) with delayed expression. More rapid onset is associated with chronic infections (e. g., bacterial endocarditis).[15] Unilateral clubbing is reported with aneurysmal dilation of large thoracic arteries, apical lung and axillary neoplasms, aortic insufficiency, hemiplegia, and other conditions.[9]

Clubbing is less common in connective tissue disease-related interstitial pneumonitis than in idiopathic interstitial pneumonia.[37] The presence of clubbing is one of several predictors of a poor prognosis in idiopathic pulmonary fibrosis or the hepatopulmonary syndrome, suggesting the need for lung transplantation.[38,39] Clubbing is more common in non–small cell carcinoma of the lung than in small cell carcinoma of the lung.[40] Growth hormone-releasing hormone has been present in non–small cell cancer of the lung, suggesting a pathogenic role.[41]

SECONDARY HYPERTROPHIC OSTEOARTHROPATHY

Secondary HOA occurs most often in adults, with age and gender distributions corresponding to those of the underlying disease. Disease progression may be rapid, and the underlying disease is usually already apparent. Unusually, clinical features of HOA may precede symptoms of the associated disease by more than a year.[10]

Periostitis causes acute, severe burning pain of the involved distal extremities. In the legs, it is often accentuated by dependency and relieved with elevation. The feet and legs may feel hot and may swell. The patient often complains of finger dysesthesia, heat, sweating, clumsiness, and stiffness. Arthralgia or severe symmetric pain of large and small joints as well as a low-grade fever and muscular weakness may occur.

Physical examination may reveal mild pitting edema with warmth and tenderness to pressure over the feet, legs, and forearms. The skin may glisten and be erythematous. Clubbing is often apparent and the periungual tissues are commonly injected, edematous, and warm. The tips of the digits may show dusky discoloration, whereas the nails may rock, loosen, or break. Severely clubbed fingers may resemble drumsticks. Joints may be mildly symptomatic, cool, and show small effusions, or they may be more painful, tender, and warm with larger effusions and limited range of motion. Symmetric involvement of large and small joints resembles rheumatoid arthritis (RA).[42] In far-advanced cases, ankylosis may occur. Subcutaneous tissues around active joints may be thickened and indurated, with hypopigmented skin suggestive of scleroderma. Hand function may be reduced and gait may be awkward. Whereas insidious emergence of clubbing with mild bone and joint pain suggests infectious disease, rapid progression of clubbing with severe bone and joint symptoms suggests an underlying malignant disease. Signs and symptoms of HOA may precede any symptoms of neoplasia, so a complete assessment must include a chest radiograph.

In childhood, secondary HOA is often related to pulmonary infections,[43] congenital heart disease,[19] or osteosarcoma metastatic to lung. HOA related to cyanotic congenital heart disease has been reported in as many as 31 percent of cases, and the severity is directly related to the degree of bypass of the lungs.[44] The degree of digital clubbing is directly related to the severity of pulmonary disease in cystic fibrosis.[45]

In the adult, neoplastic or infectious intrathoracic conditions are most common. HOA was described in 9.2 percent of 1879 patients, with pulmonary neoplasms with bronchogenic carcinoma being most common.[10] HOA is reported uncommonly in association with hepatobiliary and gastrointestinal diseases. Symptoms may flare with alcohol use.

Clubbing alone or HOA restricted to the lower extremities occurs in patients with patent ductus arteriosus who have developed right-to-left shunting of blood flow secondary to pulmonary hypertension,[17] infected aortic grafts,[46] or intra-abdominal fistula formation.[47] HOA may begin during pregnancy and may remit postpartum; it occurs most often in patients with other illnesses.[48] Clubbing has been associated with fibrosing alveolitis in RA patients, in patients with diffuse interstitial pulmonary fibrosis, and in the immunocompromised host with pneumonitis (e.g., acquired immune deficiency syndrome [AIDS]).[29,30]

THYROID ACROPACHY

Thyroid acropachy is an uncommon condition characterized by clubbing and asymptomatic periosteal proliferation of the bones of the hands and feet. It is associated with prior or active hyperthyroidism, exophthalmos, and pretibial myxedema.[28]

▌ Laboratory Findings

Laboratory findings in primary and secondary HOA are similar. The erythrocyte sedimentation rate (ESR) may be elevated. Blood and urine tests, including serum complement levels, are normal. Other serologic tests (e.g., rheumatoid factor [RF], antinuclear antibody [ANA]) are negative. When there is considerable new bone formation, serum alkaline phosphatase may be elevated. Synovial fluid is characteristically noninflammatory, with low white count characterized by mononuclear cells and with low protein and normal complement component levels.

▌ Imaging

The radiographic findings of HOA may occur in the absence of any clinical findings in both primary and secondary forms. Periosteal thickening occurs along the shafts of long and short bones, appearing first in the musculotendinous insertion site and in the distal diaphyseal regions of the long bones. It appears less often in the phalanges (Fig. 110-4). Periosteal changes appear as a continuous, thin, sclerotic line of new bone at the distal end of the diaphysis of the long bones. The periosteum is separated from the bony cortex by a narrow, radiolucent line. Periosteal new bone thickens and with time fuses with the cortex. Involvement progresses proximally and symmetrically with prominence of subperiosteal new bone. Still later, the cancellous protion of the involved bone may become osteopenic with cortical thinning. Changes are most often seen in the tibia, radius, ulna, fibula, and femur and occasionally in the clavicles.[9]

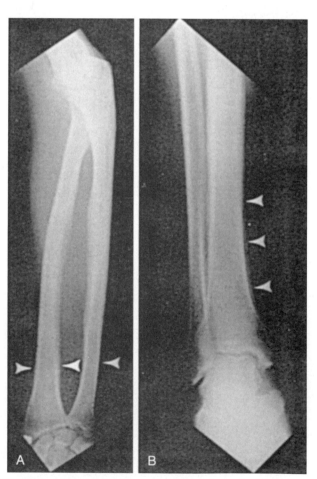

FIGURE 110-4 • Radiographs of long bone in hypertrophic osteoarthropathy demonstrate periosteal new bone formation (*arrow heads*). *A,* Distal radius and ulna. *B,* Distal tibia.

Tufting of the terminal processes of the phalanges may occur followed by osteophytosis in the more advanced stages of clubbing. Acro-osteolysis may occur in younger patients.[49] Uncommonly, radiographs are normal in the presence of florid clinical disease. Angiography demonstrates hypervascularization of the fingerpads associated with arteriovenous anastomoses and rapid filling of veins.[50] Magnetic resonance imaging (MRI) findings have been described for HOA.[51]

Radionuclide polyphosphate bone scan[52] (Fig. 110-5) often demonstrates a pericortical linear concentration of nuclide along the involved bone shafts with periarticular uptake, emphasizing the presence of periostitis and synovitis. The clubbed phalanges may accumulate radionuclide, giving the digital tips a "string of lights" appearance. The bone scan may be positive prior to onset of symptoms.

MRI of a patient with pachydermoperiostosis revealed fluffy periosteal new bone formation that encroached upon the medullary cavity with expansion of the diaphysis. The skull showed thickening of the diploe with diminished signal to the intradiploic fat and thickening of the scalp with furrowing.[53]

Pathology

The periosteal lesion is characterized by subperiosteal cancellous new bone formation at the level of the distal diaphysis of tubular bones. Subperiosteal edema results in periosteal elevation. This is followed by deposition of new osteoid beneath the periosteum. The osteoid mineralizes, resulting in a new layer of bone distally in the long bones. The process, with time, advances proximally. Associated osteoclastic activity results in weakening of the subperiosteal bone, and pathologic fractures uncommonly occur.

Synovial involvement is often contiguous to the subperiosteal changes. Synovium may be normal or may show pannus formation with cartilage erosion and damage. Thickening of subsynovial blood vessels may be accompanied by mild synovial cellular hyperplasia. Edematous synovium becomes mildly infiltrated with lymphocytes, plasma cells, and occasional polymorphonuclear leukocytes.[54,55] Immunohistologic stains are negative,[46] whereas electron microscopic studies reveal occasional electron-dense subendothelial deposits in vessel walls,[46,47] occasionally containing hyaline-like material.[55] There is concentric increase in basement membrane-like lamellae with intervening cytoplasmic processes.

The clubbing distal portion of the digit results from an increase in the connective tissue of the nail bed, as well as from a proliferation of the distal digital soft tissues. The collagen bundles of the dermis are swollen, with enlargement of the rete pegs and narrowing of the epidermal papillae. Lymphocytic infiltrates and fibroblast proliferation with dilation and thickening of blood vessel walls occurs.

Differential Diagnosis

Whenever HOA is diagnosed, it is critical to search for an associated disease. A chest radiograph should be accompanied by an assessment of the cardiopulmonary and gastrointestinal systems.

The triad of clubbing, periostitis, and joint symptoms may occur together or in different combinations over a time interval. Isolated clubbing may present as a distinct entity or as a prodrome of HOA. Nail spooning associated with iron-deficiency anemia should be distinguished from clubbing. Other conditions that involve the digits also must be distinguished from clubbing (e.g., acromegaly, scleroderma with calcinosis, and sarcoidosis).

Periostitis may occur with a bone tumor, osteomyelitis, subperiosteal hemorrhage, juvenile chronic polyarthri-

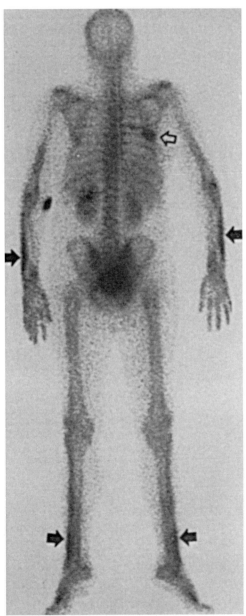

FIGURE 110-5 · Total-body radionuclide bone scan in hypertrophic osteoarthropathy demonstrates localization of the nuclide to the periosteal area of the tibiae and ulnae (*closed arrows*). The primary lesion, a bronchogenic carcinoma, also accumulated the nuclide (*open arrow*).

tis, Reiter's syndrome, psoriatic arthritis, syphilis, lymphangitis, and scurvy. Long-bone pain may occur with peripheral neuritis, Paget's disease of bone, or radioculopathy. Pretibial edema may occur with thrombophlebitis, venous stasis, or pretibial myxedema. Simultaneous appearance of synovial metastases with the development of HOA has been reported.[18]

RA and other polyarthritides must be distinguished from HOA when the primary presentation is a symmetric polyarthritis.

Pachydermoperiostosis can usually be differentiated from secondary HOA on the basis of family history and age of onset. The periostitis in pachydermoperiostosis is less symptomatic and is radiographically thicker, smoother, and more dense than in secondary HOA.

Thyroid acropachy is associated with long-standing hyperthyroidism and exophthalmos. Periostitis is limited to the phalanges despite the associated pretibial myxoedema.

Etiology and Pathogenesis

The etiology of HOA is unknown. The role that intrathoracic malignant or infectious diseases play in HOA remains speculative. The success of vagotomy in reversing or improving HOA suggests a role for reflex vagal stimulation.[56] Growth factors[41,57,58] and hormonal[59] and immune mechanisms have been proposed.[55] Platelet-endothelial interaction with production of von Willebrand factor (vWf) antigen has been implicated in the pathogenesis of HOA.[60,61] It has been suggested that HOA may be caused by vascular thrombi caused by platelets[62] or antiphospholipid antibodies.[63] A pathogenic role has been suggested for Prostaglahdin E-1, (PGE-1), as it induced HOA during infusions, with remission upon withdrawal, in a prospective heart-transplant patient in congestive heart failure.[57]

Lung cancers may be related to an elevation of circulating levels of vascular endothelial growth factor (VEGF), suggesting a pathogenic role in HOA for that cytokine.[58]

Management

The most effective treatment for the pain and discomfort of secondary HOA is cure of the underlying condition. Tumor ablation or chemosuppressive therapy of an associated malignancy often results in prompt reversal of sympotms.[10] Radiotherapy to a primary tumor[64] or to a metastatic lesion[65] may result in relief of joint symptoms. With recurrence of metastases or tumor progression, joint pain may or may not recur. Vagotomy[56] or percutaneous vagus nerve block[66] is sometimes helpful in reducing symptoms. Treatment of infections with antimicrobial therapy or with drainage has resulted in disease remission. Symptoms may resolve with successful treatment of bacterial endocarditis. Pamidronate has been used successfully to reduce pain of HOA[67] and pachydermoperiostosis,[32] whereas treatment of resistant pain with subcutaneous octreotide[68] has helped

some patients. Nonsteroidal anti-inflammatory drugs (NSAIDs),[69] glucocorticoids,[42] and colchicine[70] have reduced joint pain and swelling in some patients. Hepatic-induced HOA may respond to liver transplantation.[71]

Familial HOA and clubbing are often asymptomatic and uncommonly require treatment.

Course and Prognosis

The course of primary HOA is self limited in the adolescent. Recurrent synovial effusions may occur. The course of secondary HOA varies, reflecting the nature and activity of the associated primary disease. Symptoms may wax and wane concomitant with the progress of the primary condition. After lung tumor resection or lung abscess drainage, symptoms and signs of arthropathy may subside rapidly, whereas radiographic changes may remit over weeks and months. Without treatment of the primary condition, symptoms of HOA may result in a chronic, painful demise.

REFERENCES

1. Martinez-Lavin M, Martucci-Cerinic M, Jajic I, Pineda C: Hypertrophic osteoarthropathy: Consensus on its definition, classification, assessment and diagnostic criteria. J Rheumatol 20:1386, 1993.
2. Hippocrates: The Book of Prognostics. In Adams F (trans): The Genuine Works of Hippocrates. Vol 1. London, Sydenham Society, 1849.
3. Martinez-Lavin M, Mansilla J, Pineda C, et al: Evidence of hypertrophic osteoarthropathy in human skeletal remains from pre-Hispanic Mesoamerica. Ann Intern Med 120:238-241, 1994.
4. von Bamburger E: Uber Knochenveranderungen bei chronischen Lungenund Herzkrankenheiten. Ztschr Klin Med 18:193, 1890-1891.
5. Marie P: De l'osteo-arthropathie hypertrophiante pneumique. Rev Med (Paris) 10:1, 1890.
6. Touraine A, Solente G, Golé L: Un syndrome osteodermopathique: La pachydermie plicaturee avec pachyperiostose des extremites. Presse Med 43:1820, 1935.
7. Vogl A, Goldfischer S: Pachydermoperiostosis: Primary or idiopathic hypertrophic osteoarthropathy. Am J Med 33:166, 1962.
8. Seaton DR: Familial clubbing of fingers and toes. Br Med J 1:614, 1938.
9. Mendlowitz M: Clubbing and hypertrophic osteoarthropathy. Medicine 21:269, 1942.
10. Vogl A, Blumenfeld S, Gutner LB: Diagnostic significance of pulmonary hypertrophic osteoarthropathy. Am J Med 18:51, 1955.
11. Wierman WH, Clagett OT, McDonald JR: Articular manifestations in pulmonary diseases: Analysis of their occurrence in 1,024 cases in which pulmonary resection was performed. JAMA 155:1459, 1954.
12. Matthay MA, Matthay RA, Mills DM, et al: Hypertrophic osteoarthropathy in adults with cystic fibrosis. Thorax 31:572, 1976.
13. Galko B, Grossman RF, Day A, et al: Hypertrophic pulmonary osteoarthropathy in four patients with interstitial pulmonary disease. Chest 88:94, 1985.
14. Alloway JA, Nashel DJ, Rohatgi PK: Sarcoidosis and hypertrophic osteoarthropathy. J Rheumatol 19:180-181, 1992.
15. Cotton TF: Clubbed fingers as a sign of subacute infective endocarditis. Heart 9:347, 1921-1922.
16. McLaughlin GE, McCarty DJ, Downing DF: Hypertrophic osteoarthropathy associated with cyanotic congenital heart disease. Ann Intern Med 67:579, 1967.
17. Williams B, Ling J, Leight L, McGaff CJ: Ductus arteriosus and osteoarthropathy. Arch Intern Med 111:346, 1963.
18. Shapiro S: Hypertrophic osteoarthropathy. Arch Intern Med 98:700, 1956.

19. Pascuzzi CA, Parkin TW, Bruwer AJ, Edwards JE: Hypertrophic osteoarthropathy associated with primary rhabdomyosarcoma of the heart. Mayo Clin Proc 32:30, 1957.

20. Peirce TH, Weir DG: Hypertrophic osteoarthropathy associated with a non-metastasizing carcinoma of the oesophagus. J Ir Med Assoc 66:160, 1973.

21. Morgan AG, Walker WC, Mason MD, et al: A new syndrome associated with hepatocellular carcinoma. Gastroenterology 63:340, 1972.

22. Kitis G, Thompson H, Allan RN: Finger clubbing in inflammatory bowel disease: Its prevalence and pathogenesis. Br Med J 2:825, 1979.

23. Marie I, Levesque H, Levade MH, et al: Hypertrophic osteoarthropathy can indicate recurrence of Whipple's disease Arthritis Rheum 42:2002-2006, 1999.

24. Lofters WS, Walker TM: Hodgkin's disease and hypertrophic pulmonary osteoarthropathy. West Indian Med J 28:227, 1978.

25. McNeil MM, Sage RE, Dale BM: Hypertrophic osteoarthropathy complicating primary bone lymphoma: Association with invasive *Phycomyosis* and *Aspergillus* infections. Aust N Z J Med 11:71, 1981.

26. Mackie RM: Lupus erythematosus in association with finger-clubbing. Br J Dermatol 89:533, 1973.

27. Martinez-Lavin M, Vargas AS, Cabre J, et al: Features of hypertrophic osteoarthropathy in patients with POEMS Syndrome: a metaanalysis. J Rheumatol 24(11):2267-2268, 1997.

28. Fatourechi V, Ahmed DD, Schwartz KM: Thyroid acropachy: report of 40 patients treated at a single institution in a 26-year period. J Clin Endocrinol Metab 87:5435, 2002.

29. Biviji AA, Paiement GD, Steinbach LS: Musculoskeletal manifestations of human immunodeficiency virus infection. Am Acad Orthop Surg 10:312, 2002.

30. Simmank K, Meyers T, Galpin J, et al: Clinical features and T-cell subsets in HIV-infected children with and without lymphocytic interstitial pneumonitis. Ann Trop Paediatr 21:195-201, 2001.

31. Carreiro-Rodriguez M, Hernandez-Blanca D, Fernandez LM, et al: Hypertrophic pulmonary osteoarthropathy in acquired immunodeficiency syndrome: Case report and review. Invest Clin 4:267-276, 1999.

32. Guyot-Drouot MH, Solau-Gervais E, Cortet B, et al: Rheumatologic manifestations of pachydermoperiostosis and preliminary experience with bisphosphonates J Rheumatol 27:2418-2423, 2000.

33. Reginato A Jr., Schinpachasse Y, Guerrero R: Familial idiopathic hypertrophic osteoarthropathy and cranial suture defects in children. Skeletal Radiol 8:105, 1982.

34. Myers KA, Farquhar DR: Does the patient have clubbing? JAMA 286:341, 2001.

35. Baughman RP, Gunther KL, Bucksbaum JA, Lower EE: Measurement of the interphalangeal and distal phalangeal distance have been used to define a digital clubbing index. Clin Exp Rheum 16(1):21-26, 1998.

36. Husarik D, Vavricka SR, Mark M, et al: Assessment of digital clubbing in medical inpatients by digital photography and computer analysis. Swiss Med Wkly 132:132, 2002.

37. Ishioka S, Nakamura K, Maeda A, et al: Clinical evaluation of idiopathic interstitial pneumonia and interstitial pneumonia associated with collagen vascular disease using logistic regression analysis. Intern Med 39:213, 2000.

38. King TE Jr., Tooze JA, Schwarz MI, et al: Predicting survival in idiopathic pulmonary fibrosis: scoring system and survival model. Am J Respir Crit Care Med 164:1171, 2001.

39. Martinez GP, Barbera JA, Visa J, et al: Hepatopulmonary syndrome in candidates for liver transplantation. J Hepatol 34:651, 2001.

40. Sridhar KS, Lobo CF, Altman RD: Digital clubbing and lung cancer. Chest 114:1535, 1998.

41. Mito K, Maruyama R, Uenishi Y, et al: Hypertrophic pulmonary osteoarthropathy associated with non-small cell lung cancer demonstrated growth hormone-releasing hormone by immunohitochemical analysis. Intern Med 40:532, 2001.

42. Sega AM, MacKenzie AH: Hypertrophic osteoarthropathy: A ten year retrospective analysis. Semin Arthritis Rheum 12:220, 1982.

43. Cavanaugh JJA, Holman GH: Hypertrophic osteoarthropathy in childhood. J Pediatr 66:27, 1965.

44. Martinez-Lavin M, Bobadilla M, Casanova J, et al: Hypertrophic osteoarthropathy in cyanotic congenital heart disease. Arthritis Rheum 25:1186, 1982.

45. Nakamura CT, Ng GY, Paton JY, et al: Correlation between digital clubbing and pulmonary function in cystic fibrosis. Pediatr Pulmonol 33:332, 2002.

46. Sorin SB, Askari A, Rhodes RS: Hypertrophic osteoarthropathy of the lower extremities as a manifestation of arterial graft sepsis. Arthritis Rheum 23:768, 1980.

47. Stein HB, Little HA: Localized hypertrophic osteoarthropathy in the presence of an abdominal aortic prosthesis. Can Med Assoc J 118:947, 1978.

48. Borden EC, Holling HE: Hypertrophic osteoarthropathy and pregnancy. Ann Intern Med 71:577, 1969.

49. Pineda C, Fonseca C, Martinez-Lavin M: The spectrum of soft tissue and skeletal abnormalities of hypertrophic osteoarthropathy. J Rheumatol 17:626, 1990.

50. Jajic I, Pecina M, Kostulovic B, et al: Primary hypertrophic osteoarthropathy (PHO) and changes in the joints. Scand J Rheumatol 9:89, 1980.

51. Capelastegui A, Astigarraga E, Garcia-Iturraspe C: MR findings in pulmonary hypertrophic osteoarthropathy. Clin Radiol 55:72-75, 2000.

52. Rosenthall L, Kirsh J: Observations on radionuclide imaging in hypertrophic pulmonary osteoarthropathy. Radiology 120:359, 1976.

53. Demirpolat G, Sener RN, Stun EE: MR imaging of pachydermoperiostosis. Neuroradiol 26:61, 1999.

54. Vidal AF, Altman RD, Pardo D, Schultz D: Structural and immunologic changes of synovium of hypertrophic osteoarthropathy. Arthritis Rheum 20:139, 1977.

55. Schumacher HR: Articular manifestations of hypertrophic pulmonary osteoarthropathy in bronchogenic carcinoma. Arthritis Rheum 19:629, 1976.

56. Yacoub MH: Cervical vagotomy for pulmonary osteoarthropathy. Br J Dis Chest 59:28, 1965.

57. Crevenna R, Quittan M, Hulsmann M, et al: Hypertrophic osteoarthropathy caused by PGE1 in a patient with congestive heart failure during cardiac rehabilitation. Wien Klin Wochenschr 114:115, 2002.

58. Silvereira LH, Martinez-Lavin M, Pineda C, et al: Vascular endothelial growth factor and hypertrophic osteoarthropathy. Clin Exp Rheumatol 18:57, 2000.

59. Ginsburg J, Brown JB: Increased oestrogen excretion in hypertrophic pulmonary osteoarthropathy. Lancet 2:1274, 1961.

60. Silver F, DeAngelis R, Argentati F, et al: Hypertrophic osteoarthropathy: endothelium and platelet function. Clin Rheumatol 15:435-439, 1996.

61. Silveira LH, Martinez-Lavin M, Pineda C, et al: Vascular endothelial growth factor and hypertrophic osteoarthropathy Clin Exp Rheumatol 18:57-62, 2000.

62. Dickenson CJ: The aetiology of clubbing and hypertrophic osteoarthropathy. Eur J Clin Invest 23:330-338, 1993.

63. Harris AW, Harding TAC, Gaitonde MD, Maxwell JD: Is clubbing a feature of the anti-phospholipid antibody syndrome? Postgrad Med J 69:748-750, 1993.

64. Steinfeld AD, Munzenrider JE: The response of hypertrophic pulmonary osteoarthropathy to radiotherapy. Radiology 113:709, 1974.

65. Rao GM, Gurupoakash GH, Poulose KP, Blaskar G: Improvement in hypertrophic pulmonary osteoarthropathy after radiotherapy to metastasis. Am J Radiol 133:944, 1979.

66. Dam WH, Hagelsten JO: Blocking of the vagus nerve relieving osteoarthropathy in lung disease. Dan Med Bull 11:131, 1964.

67. Garske LA, Bell SC: Pamidronate results in symptom control of hypertrophic pulmonary osteoarthropathy in cystic fibrosis. Chest 121:1363, 2002.

68. Johnson SA, Spiller PA, Faull CM: Treatment of resistant pain in hypertrophic pulmonary osteoarthropathy with subcutaneous ocreotide. Thorax 52(3):297-298, 1997.

69. Leung FW, Williams AJ, Fan P: Indomethacin therapy for hypertrophic pulmonary osteoarthropathy in patients with bronchogenic carcinoma. West J Med 142:345, 1985.

70. Matucci-Cerinic M, Fattorini L, Gerini G, et al: Colchicine treatment in a case of pachydermoperiostosis with acroosteolysis. Rheumatol Int 8:185, 1988.

71. Taillandier J, Alemanni M, Samuel D, Bismuth H: Hepatic hypertrophic osteoarthropathy: the value of liver transplantation. Clin Exp Rheumatol 16:80-81, 1998.

Musculoskeletal Syndromes in Malignancy

ELIZA F. CHAKRAVARTY · MARK C. GENOVESE

There are a variety of ways in which musculoskeletal syndromes appear to be associated with malignancy. However, cause and effect are difficult to define clearly in many situations. Certain rheumatic diseases have been associated with an increased risk of the subsequent development of malignancy; one such example is the development of lymphoma in an individual with primary Sjögren's syndrome. The converse situation also exists, in that certain rheumatic diseases are seen more frequently in the presence of an underlying malignancy such as dermatomyositis (DM). Little is understood regarding the pathogenesis of connective tissue disease in association with neoplastic disease. Of course, other factors can contribute to the association of musculoskeletal syndromes and malignancy. Many of the medications used to treat the rheumatic diseases modulate the immune system and may directly or indirectly be associated with an increased risk for the subsequent development of malignancy. In unusual circumstances, musculoskeletal involvement occurs as a paraneoplastic process defined as a hormonal, neurologic, hematologic, or biochemical disturbance associated with malignancy but not directly related to invasion by the neoplasm or its metastases.[1]

■ Paraneoplastic Syndromes

Musculoskeletal syndromes can develop as a manifestation of a paraneoplastic process and can occasionally be the first presentation of an underlying malignancy. Hematologic malignancies, lymphoproliferative disorders, and solid tumors are associated with a wide variety of paraneoplastic rheumatic syndromes. Older age of onset, atypical features of rheumatic disease, and absence of response to glucocorticoids or other conventional therapy may be suggestive of a paraneoplastic process. The knowledge of the associations with rheumatic syndromes and underlying malignancy is critical when caring for these patients. Hypertrophic osteoarthropathy, amyloidosis, and secondary gout are reviewed in Chapters 87, 104, 110, respectively. In Table 111–1, the more common paraneoplastic associations are listed.

CARCINOMATOUS POLYARTHRITIS

Carcinomatous polyarthritis is a term used to describe the development of arthritis in association with malignancy, but it is distinct from arthritis associated with metastasis or direct tumor invasion. Common features of carcinomatous polyarthritis are listed in Table 111–2. It generally develops in patients who are older in age, has an explosive onset, and often develops in close temporal correlation with the discovery of the malignancy. Although it can have various presentations and may mimic the appearance of rheumatoid arthritis (RA),[2] it is more often a seronegative asymmetric disease with predominant involvement of the lower extremities and some sparing of the small joints of the hands. There is no evidence of direct tumor extension or metastasis and no specific identifying histologic or radiographic appearance. Carcinomatous polyarthritis can occur in association with many types of malignancy but has been reported in the greatest frequency in association with breast, colon, lung, and ovarian cancers, as well as with lymphoproliferative disorders.[3] The underlying pathogenesis of this process has not been elucidated; however, the arthritic symptoms may be improved with successful treatment of the malignancy.[4]

VASCULITIS

Vasculitis in association with malignancy is uncommon and has a reported prevalence of only up to 8 percent of patients with malignancy.[5] The association appears significantly higher with lymphoproliferative and myeloproliferative disorders than with solid tumors, and it commonly predates the identification of malignancy. The vasculitic process is most often small vessel and cutaneous and only rarely demonstrates significant organ involvement. Treatment often requires the use of glucocorticoids and therapy directed against the underlying malignancy, although it appears this is often ineffective. Table 111–1 shows malignancies associated with vasculitis. In the setting of malignancy, it is believed that the persistent antigen stimulation from the tumor results in T cell activation or immune-complex formation and deposition.

The development of small vessel vasculitis has been reported to both antedate and postdate the development of both lymphoproliferative and myeloproliferative diseases. One group looked at 222 patients with vasculitis retrospectively and identified 11 who had developed an associated malignancy. Of these 11 patients, seven had hematologic neoplasia, and four suffered from solid malignant tumors. Nine of the patients manifested cutaneous vasculitis, and the remaining two had vasculitic involvement in the bowel. In four of the patients, the development of vasculitis antedated the diagnosis of malignancy.[6] Similar findings were seen by investigators who found an underlying malignancy in eight of 192 patients with cutaneous vasculitis.

TABLE 111–1 · PARANEOPLASTIC SYNDROMES

Connective Tissue Disease	Malignancy	Clinical Setting	Clinical Alert
Carcinomatous polyarthritis	Multiple types of solid tumors, including breast; lymphoproliferative disorders	See Table 111-2	See Table 111-2
Vasculitis	Lymphopoetic and hematopoetic malignancies	Cuteneous vasculitis most common; systemic vasculitis rare	Vasculitis not related to infections, medications, or autoimmune disease
Mixed cryoglobulinemia	Non-Hodgkin's lymphoma	Immune complex–mediated disease with cutaneous vasculitis, neuropathy, fatigue, and visceral organ involvement	Usually appears 5 to 10 years after diagnosis of cryoglobulinemia
Panniculitis	Hematologic malignancies; pancreatic, breast, and prostate cancers	Induration of skin and deeper tissues; eosinophilia often present	Usually refractory to prednisone
Fasciitis	Ovarian, breast, gastric, and pancreatic cancers	Palmar fasciitis with inflammatory polyarthritis; similar in presentation to RSD	Bilateral presentation; severe fibrosis and contractures; aggressive course
Reflex sympathetic dystrophy syndrome, (RSD)	Multiple cancer types; Pancoast tumors	Tumors may invade stellate ganglion or brachial plexus on affected side	Absence of typical antecedent factors; failure to respond to conventional therapies
Erythromelalgia	Myeloproliferative disorders	Often seen in setting of thrombocytosis	
Atypical PMR	Renal, lung, and colon cancer; multiple myeloma		Age younger than 50 years; asymmetric involvement; poor response to prednisone
Digital necrosis	Gastrointestinal and pulmonary tumors	Severe Raynaud's phenomenon with onset after age 50	Asymmetric features; digital necrosis
Remitting seron egative symmetric synouitis with pitting edema, (RS3PE)	Several tumor types	Abrupt onset of arthritis and edema surrounding wrists and small joints of hands	Presence of fever, weight loss; poor response to prednisone
Multicentric reticulohistiocytosis	Lung, stomach, breast, cervix, colon, and ovarian carcinomas		
Lupus-like syndromes	Variety of solid tumors and lymphoproliferative disorders		Rare associations with malignancy limited to case reports
Antiphospholipid antibodies	Multiple cancer types	Association between antibodies, cancer, and risk of thrombosis unclear	Higher presence of antibodies found in patients with malignancy
Osteogenic osteomalacia	Solid tumors and tumors of mesenchymal origin	Bone pain and muscle weakness	Diligent search is indicated in all patients with late-onset apparent idiopathic osteomalacia
Sarcoidosis	Cervical, bladder, gastric, lung, breast, and renal cancers and cutaneous and pulmonary squamous cell carcinomas	Highest incidence of "malignancy" during first 4 years after detection of granulomas	Malignant tumors can cause sarcoid-like tissue reactions leading to mistaken diagnosis of sarcoidosis before recognition of malignancy
Lymphomatoid granulomatosis	Lymphoma	Unusual granulomatous form of vasculitis with angiodestructive infiltration of various tissues	

TABLE 111–2 · FEATURES OF CARCINOMATOUS POLYARTHRITIS

Close temporal relationship between onset of arthritis and discovery of malignancy
Late age of onset of arthritis
Asymmetric joint involvement
Explosive onset
Predominant lower extremity involvement with sparing of wrists and small joints of hands
Absence of rheumatoid nodules
Absence of rheumatoid factor (RF)
No family history of rheumatoid disease
Nonspecific histopathologic appearance of synovial lining
No periosteal reaction

The majority of malignancies were hematologic (six of eight) and predated (five of eight) the diagnosis of cancer.[7]

Systemic vasculitis is much less commonly associated with underlying malignancy. Case reports and small series have found antineutrophil cytoplasmic antibody (ANCA)-negative and ANCA-positive vasculitis associated with hematologic malignancies.[8–10] Wegener's granulomatosis (WG) has likewise been associated with the development of several types of malignancies, including lymphoproliferative disorders, bladder cancer, and renal cell carcinoma.[11,12] In some cases, the malignancy was diagnosed within months of diagnosis of cancer,[11] and in other reports, cancer developed many years after diagnosis and treatment of vasculitis,[12] making it unclear whether the malignancies were a result of the vasculitis or the treatment.

Vasculitis associated with underlying malignancy is often poorly responsive to conventional therapy directed against the vasculitis. In one series of 13 patients with both cutaneous vasculitis and lympho- or myeloproliferative disorders, symptoms of vasculitis were poorly responsive to therapy with nonsteroidal anti-inflammatory drugs (NSAIDs), glucocorticoids, antihistamines, and antiserotonin agents. Although the investigators reported a lessening of the severity of the vasculitis following chemotherapy directed against the malignancy, they generally found chemotherapy to be ineffective. Of the 13 patients identified, 10 died as a direct result of the malignancy.[13]

CRYOGLOBULINEMA

Cryoglobulins are immunoglobulins that precipitate at reduced temperature. Cryoglobulinemia can be characterized by hyperviscosity symptoms or by vasculitis. Patients often suffer from fatigue, arthralgia or arthritis, cutaneous vasculitis or purpura, neuropathy, digital ischemia, and visceral organ involvement (renal or pulmonary). There are three types of cryoglobulins:

Type I: Monoclonal immunoglobulin (Ig), either IgG or IgM; this type is associated with lymphoproliferative disorders.
Type II: Monoclonal IgM directed against polyclonal IgG; type II cryoglobulins were initially thought to be idiopathic and, thus, were known as mixed essential cryoglobulinemia. With the identification of hepatitis C virus, it has been discovered that the majority of these patients have hepatitis C infection that is directly involved in the pathogenesis of the cryoglobulins. Specific epitopes of hepatitis C antigens are recognized by IgG components of immune complexes and viral particles are found in cryoprecipitate.[14] Approximately 5 to 8 percent of patients with mixed cryoglobulinemia may go on to develop non-Hodgkin's lymphoma, usually after 5 to 10 years of cryoglobulinemia.[15,16] At this time, prediction of the subset of patients with mixed cryoglobulinemia who will develop lymphoma cannot be determined.
Type III: Mixed polyclonal IgG and IgM; type III cryoglobulins are commonly seen with a variety of illnesses, including connective tissue diseases (systemic lupus erythematosus [SLE] and RA) and infections.

PANNICULITIS

The fasciitis-panniculitis syndrome, which includes eosinophilic fasciitis, is characterized by swelling and induration of the skin that extends into deeper subcutaneous tissues and is associated with fibrosis and chronic inflammation. Patients may develop arthritis and subcutaneous nodules similar to those seen in erythema nodosum. The arthropathy appears secondary to periarticular fat necrosis, can be monoarticular or polyarticu-

lar,[17] and may mimic RA or juvenile RA (JRA).[18] Blood and tissue eosinophilia is commonly, but not always, present.[19] This syndrome can be idiopathic and have a benign course, or it can be secondary to a variety of infectious, vascular, or traumatic etiologies.[19] In a small number of patients, the fasciitis-panniculitis syndrome is associated with an underlying malignancy. Hematologic malignancies are most often associated with this syndrome and are usually diagnosed concurrently or within the first year.[20,21] Pancreatic cancer, as well as pancreatitis, can also be associated with this syndrome.[17,18] Patients with cancer-associated fasciitis-panniculitis syndrome are predominantly female and are generally refractory to prednisone.[20] Occasionally, fasciitis will regress with treatment of the underlying malignancy.[22]

PALMAR FASCIITIS

Palmar fasciitis and arthritis is a syndrome characterized by progressive bilateral contractures of the digits, fibrosis of palmar fascia, and inflammatory polyarthritis.[22,23] The metacarpophalangeal and proximal interphalangeal joints are most commonly affected, but other affected joints include the elbows, wrists, knees, ankles, and feet. Palmar fasciitis is almost uniformly associated with the presence of an underlying malignancy, most often ovarian, breast, gastric, and pancreatic tumors.[23-25] Although initially thought to be an atypical variant of reflex-sympathetic dystrophy, the severity of manifestations, bilateral presentation, and strong association with occult malignancy suggest that, in these cases, palmar fasciitis is a distinct entity that behaves as a paraneoplastic syndrome. Glucocorticoids, chemotherapy, or both do not appear to result in improvement.[26]

REFLEX-SYMPATHETIC DYSTROPHY SYNDROME

Reflex-sympathetic dystrophy and a variant, shoulder-hand syndrome, are characterized by regional pain, swelling, vasomotor instability, and focal osteoporosis in a given limb; this condition is thought to be caused by sympathetic dysfunction. The absence of associated antecedent factors such as stroke, myocardial infarction, or trauma, as well as failure to respond to conventional therapy, warrant a search for an underlying malignancy. A variety of malignancies have been associated with the development of reflex-sympathetic dystrophy or its variants.[27] Pancoast tumor of the lung apices or other malignancies that infiltrate the stellate ganglion or brachial plexus have been described with the development of reflex-sympathetic dystrophy.[28-30] Therapy directed against the underlying malignancy may lead to some amelioration of symptoms associated with reflex-sympathetic dystrophy.

ERYTHROMELALGIA

Erythromelalgia is an enigmatic condition characterized by attacks of severe burning, erythema, and warmth of the extremities with symptoms predominantly involving the feet.[31] Symptoms are often exacerbated when the extremities are placed in a dependent position, during ambulation, or during exposure to increased temperatures. Relief can be obtained in part through elevation or cooling of the extremity. This disorder can occur idiopathically (60%) or as a secondary form of the disease (40%).[31,32] Myeloproliferative disorders, including polycythemia vera and essential thrombocytosis, are a common secondary cause and have been found to precede the diagnosis of erythromelalgia by several years.[33] The underlying pathophysiology of this disease is unknown; however, it is often associated with thrombocythemia. In the largest published retrospective cohort, 168 patients at the Mayo Clinic were identified with this diagnosis between 1970 and 1994.[34] The authors found that after a mean follow-up of 8.7 years, 31.9 percent of patients reported worsening of disease, 26.6 percent reported no change, 30.9 percent reported improvement, and 10.6 percent reported complete resolution of symptoms. Kaplan-Meier survival curves revealed a significant decrease in survival when compared to controls. A history of myeloproliferative disease was found in 15 of 168 patients. The exact cause of the symptoms remains unclear, but microvascular arteriovenous shunting has been hypothesized.[35] The most effective therapy appears to be the use of daily aspirin, leading to a significant relief of symptoms, which is believed to be related to inhibition of cyclooxygenase-1 (COX-1). A host of other therapies have been tried with varying success.[35] Given the association with myeloproliferative diseases, routine monitoring with complete blood counts (CBCs) is prudent.

POLYMYALGIA RHEUMATICA

Polymyalgia rheumatica is a disorder affecting older adults that manifests with discomfort and stiffness in the shoulder and hip girdle, fatigue, anemia of chronic disease, and elevated erythrocyte sedimentation rate (ESR). Classically, this condition responds to moderate doses of prednisone within 48 hours. A variety of other conditions can have presentations that mimic polymyalgia rheumatica, including other rheumatic disorders, systemic infections, and malignancy.[36] The association between polymyalgia rheumatica and malignancy has been controversial. However, atypical features of polymyalgia rheumatica may be suggestive of the presence of occult malignancy. These include age less than 50 years, limited or asymmetric involvement of typical sites, ESR less than 40 or greater than 100, severe anemia, proteinuria, and poor or delayed response to 10 mg daily prednisone. Kidney, lung, or colon cancer and multiple myeloma are most often found in patients presenting with atypical polymyalgia rheumatica.[37-40] In contrast, several prospective studies have shown that patients who present with classic polymyalgia rheumatica do not appear to have an increased risk of developing malignancy over age-matched controls.[41,42]

DIGITAL NECROSIS

The development of digital necrosis or profound Raynaud's phenomenon may suggest the presence of infection, inflammatory disease, or an underlying malignancy. In patients over the age of 50 years, the development of Raynaud's phenomenon, particularly in an asymmetric fashion or in association with digital necrosis, should raise the possibility that this is a paraneoplastic process. These features often antedate the diagnosis of the malignancy by an average of 7 to 9 months.[43,44] A variety of solid tumors and lymphoproliferative disorders have been associated with this syndrome.[43-48] Mechanisms proposed include cryoglobulinemia, immune complex–induced vasospasm, hypercoagulability, marantic endocarditis with emboli, and necrotizing vasculitis.[46]

Interestingly, therapy with interferon-alpha (IFN-α) has also been reported in association with the development of Raynaud's phenomenon and digital necrosis.[49-50]

REMITTING SERONEGATIVE SYMMETRIC SYNOVITIS WITH PITTING EDEMA

Remitting seronegative symmetric synovitis with pitting edema (RS3PE) is an uncommon disorder primarily affecting the metacarpophalangeal joints and the wrists. Although the underlying etiology and pathogenesis of this illness remain unclear, lymphoma, myelodysplastic syndrome, and several solid tumors, mostly adenocarcinoma, have all been reported in association with it.[51-54] Characteristics suggestive of possible underlying malignancy include the presence of systemic features (such as fever or weight loss) and a poor response to glucocorticoids.[53,54]

MULTICENTRIC RETICULOHISTIOCYTOSIS

Multicentric reticulohistiocytosis is a rare condition characterized by the presence of cutaneous papules; it is often associated with a destructive arthritis. The papules are flesh colored to brown-yellow and are classically present in the periungal region and on the dorsal hands and face. Arthritis mutilans may develop in up to 50 percent of cases. The characteristic histologic appearance of tissue infiltration with histiocytes and multinucleated giant cells can be found in affected skin, joints, and occasionally internal organs.[55] Multicentric reticulohistiocytosis has been reported in association with hyperlipidemia, malignancies, and autoimmune diseases. Malignancy has been associated in 25 to 31 percent of cases.[56] The most frequently seen malignancies include carcinoma of the lung, stomach, breast, cervix, colon, and ovary.[55]

LUPUS-LIKE SYNDROMES

Lupus-like syndromes are rarely associated with underlying malignancy. Isolated case reports have described lupus-like syndromes with ovarian carcinoma[57,58] and hairycell leukemia[59]; subacute cutaneous lupus was reported in a patient with breast carcinoma.[60] Studies on the presence of antinuclear antibodies (ANAs) in patients with cancer have had mixed results. Two studies were unable to find a significantly increased rate of ANAs in patients with solid tumors or lymphomas when compared to healthy controls.[61-62] In contrast, one smaller study found an increased prevalence of ANAs in patients with non-Hodgkin's lymphoma compared to controls (21% vs. 0).[63] There do not appear to be any predictive features suggestive of occult malignancy in patients presenting with lupus-like syndromes or positive ANAs.

ANTIPHOSPHOLIPID ANTIBODIES

Antiphospholipid antibodies and their association with thromboses have been described as a primary syndrome as well as a secondary phenomenon in autoimmune diseases, primarily SLE. More recently, antiphospholipid antibodies have been associated with a variety of malignancies. However, correlations between antiphospholipid antibodies in cancer patients and thromboembolic events have been less clear.

Several studies have shown the presence of antiphospholipid antibodies in patients with both solid tumors and lymphoproliferative disorders at a higher frequency than the 1 to 5 percent seen in the general population.[64,65] An early study of 216 consecutive patients with cancer found 22 percent positive for anticardiolipin antibodies compared to 3.4 percent in controls. This study found a two-fold increase in the development of thromboembolism in patients with positive antibodies compared to those with negative serologies; it also indicated that the majority of thromboembolic events occurred in patients with higher antibody titers.[67] Other studies have confirmed the association between malignancy and antiphospholipid antibodies (12.5 to 68%) but have been unable to show a correlation with thromboembolic events.[63,64,68-70] Furthermore, a correlation between antibody titer and disease activity has been shown in some case reports[70] and studies.[67,69-70]

Studies of the prevalence of antiphospholipid antibodies in unselected patient populations have again shown an association with underlying malignancy. A prospective study in France found that 7 percent of 1014 consecutive patients admitted to a medicine ward had antiphospholipid antibodies.[71] In antibody-positive patients, cancer was the most frequently associated disease. A more recent study in patients presenting with their first ischemic stroke found a significantly higher rate of development of cancer within 12 months in patients who had positive anticardiolipin antibodies (19% vs. 5%).[72]

OSTEOMALACIA

Osteomalacia is the softening of bones often associated with the failure of adequate calcification secondary to renal dysfunction or a lack of vitamin D. Osteomalacia has been associated with solid tissue and mesenchymal tumors, both benign and malignant. Octreotide scintigraphy may be a useful tool for identifying occult tumors.[73,74] With removal of the tumor, there appears to be resolution of the osteomalacia.[75,76]

SARCOIDOSIS

Noncaseating granulomas can occur in numerous settings and are not necessarily pathognomonic for sarcoidosis. Granulomas resembling those of sarcoidosis may be found in lymph nodes that drain sites with malignancy. These tumor-related tissue reactions resulting in granuloma formation have been described with many types of malignant lesions, including solid tumors and lymphomas.[77,78] The clinical and radiographic presentation of sarcoidosis and cancer can be virtually indistinguishable, making it important to pursue aggressive evaluation in the patient with sarcoidosis.[79]

The risk of malignancy developing in patients with established diagnoses of sarcoidosis remains controversial. Some studies have shown an increased risk of developing lung cancer and lymphoma, whereas others have shown no increased risk of cancer over the general population.[79]

LYMPHOMATOID GRANULOMATOSIS

Lymphomatoid granulomatosis is a rare disorder with angiodestructive and lymphoproliferative features that involves the lung and, less often, the skin and central nervous system (CNS). Although lymphocytic infiltration of vessels is a hallmark of the disease, lymphomatoid granulomatosis now appears to fall within the spectrum of lymphoproliferative disorders. Despite the predominance of T cells within inflammatory infiltrates, recent studies have suggested that an Epstein-Barr virus (EBV)-associated B cell proliferation may underlie the pathogenesis of the disease.[80,81] Prognosis is generally poor with a median survival from diagnosis of 14 months.[82] Lymphomas evolve in as many as 25 percent of cases.[83]

Inflammatory Myopathies

The inflammatory myopathies in adult populations encompass a group of illnesses characterized by an idiopathic immune-mediated attack of skeletal muscle that results in muscle weakness. There have been many associations between the inflammatory myopathies and the presence of malignancy, but the character of the association remains controversial.[84] DM has classically been associated with occult malignancies, whereas the associations between polymyositis (PM) and inclusion body myositis are less clear. Of issue as well is whether the inflammatory myopathy predates the malignancy and can be considered a primary rheumatic disease with known risks of developing malignancy or whether it simply represents a manifestation of a paraneoplastic process.

On average, the prevalence of malignancy in association with the inflammatory myopathies has been approximately 25 percent. However, frequency of malignancy has ranged from 6 to 60 percent, in patients with DM, to 0 to 28 percent, in patients with PM.[84] Other estimates have placed the incidence of cancer in patients with inflammatory myopathies at five to seven times that of the general population.[84]

DM has been associated with a wide range of malignancies. Most common are ovarian, lung, and gastric tumors in European populations, and nasopharyngeal malignancies in Asian populations. Recent studies have confirmed a strong association between DM and malignancy. Hill and colleagues studied a pooled cohort of patients from Sweden, Denmark, and Finland and found 198 cases of cancer in 618 patients with DM.[85] The standardized incidence ratio (SIR) for malignancy with DM was 3.0. Similar results were found in a Scottish cohort of 286 patients with DM.[86] Seventy-seven patients were found to have underlying malignancies, with a SIR of 3.3 to 7.7. Buchbinder and coworkers used strict histopathologic criteria to classify myositis in patients from Victoria, Australia.[87] This group found 36 cases of cancer in 85 patients diagnosed with DM and a SIR of 4.3 to 6.2.

In contrast to the previous work, studies of Asian populations have shown a higher association of nasopharyngeal carcinomas with DM. In a Taiwanese study, 18 percent of 91 patients with DM were found to have an underlying malignancy, the most common of which was nasopharyngeal cancer, followed by lung cancer.[88] In a smaller study, 66.6 percent of 15 DM patients in Singapore had malignancies, the majority of which were nasopharyngeal carcinoma.[89]

In PM, the relative risk for developing internal malignancies appears to be lower than that for DM, but it is consistently increased over that expected in the general population. Recent studies have found a 14- to 30-percent prevalence of cancer among patients with PM with SIRs increased to 1.2 to 2.1.[85-88] Small numbers of many types of cancers were found in these studies.

These recent studies confirm results found in previous large studies of Swedish and Finnish populations, as well as a 1994 meta-analysis of all published case-control and cohort studies of malignancy and myositis that identified an odds ratio for the association of cancer with DM of 4.4 and of cancer with PM of 2.1.[90]

In amyopathic DM, a variant of DM in which typical cutaneous manifestations are present with subclinical or no identifiable muscle disease, the association with underlying malignancy remains controversial, and published reports are limited to small groups of patients.[89,91-93]

Far less is known about the association of inclusion body myositis and underlying malignancy. In Buchbinder's study from Northern Europe, 52 patients were identified with inclusion body myositis. Of those, 12 were found to have internal malignancies, with a standardized incidence ration of 2.4. The numbers of each type of cancer seen were too small to find specific associations.[88]

Not all studies concur regarding the association between the inflammatory myopathies and malignancy.[94,95] In a study done at the Mayo Clinic, patients with myositis did not appear to be at a statistically significant risk for the development of malignancy. As well, no clinical differences were seen between patients who developed a malignancy and those who did not.[95]

Despite the negative results of some studies, it appears that the majority of work supports the notion of an increased risk of malignancy in association with DM and PM. For patients in whom an inflammatory myopathy has been diagnosed, a workup for the presence of malignancy should be undertaken. The extent of this workup has been debated, however, as extensive undirected searches often result in a very low yield. It is probably rare for an undirected workup to yield evidence of malignancy in the PM and DM population[96]; thus, any workup should be tailored to the individual patient's age, symptoms, and signs. Recent studies have suggested that imaging of the chest, abdomen, and pelvis may increase the potential for discovery of underlying malignancy.[97,98] Malignancies associated with inflammatory myopathies have been known to develop many years after the diagnosis of muscle disease, so continued vigilance and repeated screening for malignancy is warranted.

There are certain cohorts in whom the risk of malignancy may be higher, including patients who have active DM but exhibit a normal creatine kinase level. They may have a higher risk of malignancy and a worse outcome.[99] Patients with myositis-associated autoantibodies may be at less risk for the development of malignancy.[100] More-recent work has suggested that the presence of leukocytoclastic vasculitis further increases the risk of underlying malignancy.[101]

Although the pathogenesis is unknown, the types of malignancy associated with the inflammatory myopathies have been varied, including adenocarcinomas of the breast, ovaries, and stomach. Most cases of DM and malignancy appear to occur within 1 year of each other, with myositis diagnosed first in the majority of cases.[84] When identified, removal of the malignancy may, in fact, result in improvement of the myopathic process, which further supports the paraneoplastic nature of myositis in some cases.[102]

▌ Risks of Developing Lymphoproliferative Disorders in Rheumatic Diseases

Since the 1980's, there have been increasing reports of the association between rheumatic diseases and the development of malignancies, particularly lymphoproliferative disorders. Table 111–3 shows preexisting connective tissue diseases that have been associated with malignancy. Much of what is known about associations between rheumatic disease and malignancy is drawn from retrospective and prospective cohort studies, registry-linkage studies, small series, and case reports. In addition, certain confounding factors need to be considered when assessing the risk of the development of malignancy. These factors must include the potential oncogenic properties of many of the immunosuppressive and cytotoxic medications prescribed to treat autoimmune diseases. The development of lymphoproliferative disorders has been seen in patients with rheumatic diseases as well as in post–solid organ transplantation recipients treated with immunosuppressive agents. Certainly EBV has been implicated in the development of lymphoid neoplasia in the immunosuppressed population. In the following sections, many of the rheumatic diseases and the therapies used to treat them are covered.

SJÖGREN'S SYNDROME

Sjögren's syndrome is characterized by a benign lymphocytic infiltrate of salivary and lacrimal glands that

TABLE 111–3 • PREEXISTING CONNECTIVE TISSUE DISEASES ASSOCIATED WITH MALIGNANCY

Connective Tissue Disease	Malignancy	Associated Factors	Clinical Alert
Sjögren's syndrome	Lymphoproliferative disorders	Glandular features: lymphadenopathy, parotid or salivary enlargement Extraglandular features: purpura, vasculitis, splenomegaly, lymphopenia, low C4 cryoglobulins	Clues to progression from pseudolymphoma to lymphoma include worsening of clinical features, disappearance of rheumatoid factor (RF), and decline of immunoglobulin M (IgM)
Rheumatoid arthritis (RA)	Lymphoproliferative disorders	Presence of paraproteinemia, greater disease severity, longer disease duration, immunosuppression, Felty's syndrome	Rapidly progressive, refractory flare in long-standing rheumatoid disease may suggest an underlying malignancy
Systemic lupus erythematosus (SLE)	Lymphoproliferative disorders		Non-Hodgkin's lymphoma should be considered in SLE patients who develop adenopathy or masses; lymphoma of the spleen is another cause of splenic enlargement in SLE
Discoid lupus erythematosus	Squamous cell epithelioma	Found in oldest plaques, 20 years or more after onset of discoid lesion, primarily in men aged 30 to 60 years	A poorly healing skin lesion within discoid plaques should be evaluated
Systemic sclerosis (scleroderma)	Alveolar cell carcinoma	Pulmonary fibrosis, interstitial lung disease	Annual chest radiograph after fibrosis is detected
	Nonmelanoma skin cancer	Areas of scleroderma and fibrosis in the skin	Change in skin features or poorly healing lesions should be evaluated
	Adenocarcinoma of the esophagus	Barrett's metaplasia	Esophagoscopy and biopsy, if indicated, of distal esophageal constricting lesions
Paget's disease of bone	Osteogenic sarcoma	Development of severe pain; increasing incidence with age	Swelling and bone destruction in preexisting Paget's disease may be sarcoma; diagnosis may require biopsy
Dermatomyositis	Ovarian, lung, and gastric cancer in Western populations; nasopharyngeal carcinoma in Asian populations	Older in age, normal creatinine kinase levels, presence of cutaneous vasculitis; less likely in setting of myositis-specific antibodies	Malignancy evaluation needs to be tailored to the individual patient's age, symptoms, and signs

leads to the development of sicca syndrome (keratoconjunctivitis and xerostomia). The development of lymphoproliferative disorders in the setting of Sjögren's syndrome is perhaps the prototypic example of chronic autoimmune disease and an increased risk of malignancy. In 1964, investigators first reported the development of four cases of lymphoproliferative disorders in a cohort of 58 patients with Sjögren's syndrome.[103] In 1978, seven of 136 patients with sicca syndrome were identified as having developed non-Hodgkin's lymphoma. Compared to the expected incidence of cancer among women of the same age range, there was a 44-fold increased risk of developing non-Hodgkin's lymphoma.[104] These findings have been reproduced numerous times in other cohorts. Lymphoproliferative disorders complicate approximately 4 to 10 percent of cases of primary Sjögren's syndrome.[105-109] The relative risk (RR) for development of lymphoproliferative disorder in patients with primary Sjögren's syndrome ranges from 13 to 44.[104,110,111] The majority of lymphoproliferative disorders were non-Hodgkin's lymphoma, specifically low-grade B cell lymphoma and lymphoma of mucosa-associated lymphoid tissue (MALT). Waldenström's macroglobulinemia, chronic lymphocytic leukemia, and multiple myeloma were more rarely reported.[104,108,109,111] In these studies, several features appear to be associated with or predictive of development of lymphoproliferative disorders. Generally, the development of lymphoma is a late manifestation of Sjögren's syndrome, often seen after 6.5 years of disease.[106,107,112] Other features associated with development of lymphoma include palpable purpura,[103,108,109] cutaneous ulcerations,[105] cryoglobulinemia,[109] low C_4,[108,109] monoclonal gammopathies,[113] cytopenias,[103] splenomegaly,[103] and adenopathy.[105] Progression to high-grade lymphoma portends a poor prognosis.[107-109,112] In contrast, the incidence of other malignancies was not increased in patients with Sjögren's syndrome compared to the general population.[111] It is believed that chronic B cell stimulation may lead to the malignant transformation of clonal lines characteristic of Sjögren's syndrome. The presence of a viral trigger accounting for malignant transformation is one possible theory. EBV among others has been implicated, but studies have failed to find EBV or other viral particles in lymphoma specimens associated with Sjögren's syndrome.[114] There also have been reports of chromosomal translocations being present with increased frequency in patients with Sjögren's syndrome who have developed lymphoma. One group of investigators identified the presence of translocations of proto-oncogene bcl-2[115,116] in five of seven patients with Sjögren's syndrome and lymphoma by the use of polymerase chain reaction (PCR). Conversely, no evidence of bcl-2 translocations was present in 50 salivary-gland biopsies of patients with Sjögren's syndrome without evidence of lymphoma.[117] Interestingly, analysis of biopsies taken before the development of lymphoma from the seven patients previously mentioned showed no evidence of bcl-2 translocation. Translocation appeared to correlate with the development of lymphoma in at least a subset of patients with Sjögren's syndrome, and the use of PCR technology may allow for early detection of malignant transformation.[117,118]

RHEUMATOID ARTHRITIS

The data from several studies are persuasive that the presence of RA appears to convey an increased risk for the development of lymphoproliferative disorders and may convey a decreased risk for the development of colorectal tumors. When a group of Swedish investigators looked at the cancer risk in 11,683 RA inpatients, they found an increased risk for the development of lymphomas and a decreased risk for the occurrence of cancers of the colon and stomach.[119] This finding agrees with findings from a similar Danish study.[120] The Swedish group also identified high inflammatory activity (defined by ESR, swollen and tender joint counts, and the physician's global assessment of disease activity) as a significant risk factor, with an odds ratio of 25.8 compared to low disease activity. No association between any specific drug and the development of lymphoma was identified; however, the cohort examined was treated between 1965 and 1983, and very few of these patients were apparently treated with immunosuppressive drugs, making the lack of association less certain.[121]

Similarly, Canadian investigators identified an increased risk for the development of lymphoma and myeloma when compared to that for a control group. The risk appeared to be four-fold greater in the RA group when disease-modifying antirheumatic drug (DMARD) use was not controlled for and 3.4-fold greater when the study was controlled for individual DMARD use.[122] Another group found a similar moderate increase in malignancy with DMARD use.[123] In general, lymphomas in patients with RA do not appear to be different with respect to grade, histology, or immunophenotype than those seen in the general population.[124]

However, not all studies concur, as a different group of Canadian investigators failed to find evidence of an increased risk of malignancy associated with RA when they compared the incidence of cancer in patients with RA with the expected cancer incidence rates of age- and sex-matched controls. Although 168 cases of cancer were expected, only 136 were identified in this study. The incidence of colorectal malignancy was significantly reduced in the RA study population, and the incidence of Hodgkin's disease and non-Hodgkin's lymphoma was not found to be significantly different from that of the general population. However, a signif-

icant excess in the incidence of leukemia was found. The decreased risk of colorectal cancer was thought to be related to the long-term use of NSAIDs, and the increased risk of leukemia was postulated to be related to persistent immune stimulation associated with RA itself. Overall, the risk of malignancy was reduced in this RA cohort despite the treatment with potentially oncogenic agents.[125]

Patients with Felty's syndrome (a variant of RA) were found in a Veterans Affairs study of 906 men to have a two-fold increase in total cancer incidence but a 12-fold increase in risk of non-Hodgkin's lymphoma.[104,126]

The majority of studies have suggested that increased disease activity of RA carries a higher risk for the development of lymphoma. Patients with active RA often exhibit elevated immunoglobulin levels. In most cases, this is polyclonal in origin and may reflect the presence of rheumatoid factor (RF). However, the possibility exists that the paraprotein may be of monoclonal B cell origin and may reflect the early development of a lymphoproliferative disorder. The incidence of monoclonal gammopathy in patients with RA has been estimated at 1 to 2 percent.[127] The development of IgA paraproteins has been reported to carry a higher risk than that of IgG for the subsequent development of a lymphoproliferative disorder.[128,129] Other factors, such as the presence of secondary Sjögren's syndrome or the presence of urinary free light chains, appear to be of less prognostic significance for the development of a lymphoproliferative disorder.[128]

Methotrexate (MTX) has become the most commonly utilized disease-modifying agent for the treatment of RA. The recognition that erosion and joint destruction begin very early has increased utilization of disease-modifying agents earlier in the course of disease. A number of long-term clinical studies have shown no excessive risk of lymphoproliferative diseases specifically related to treatment with MTX in patients with RA. However, more than 50 cases of non-Hodgkin's lymphoma in RA patients treated with MTX have been cited in the literature.[130] The majority of these patients have been reported to have B cell lymphoma, and extranodal involvement is common. Only 17 of these cases were assayed for the presence of EBV, of which 7 (or 41 percent) were positive.[130] This rate is less than that seen in post-transplantation patients or in patients with acquired immunodeficiency syndrome (AIDS) who develop lymphoma, but it is still significantly higher than that for lymphoma in the general population.[131] A more recent study, although unable to show an increase risk of non-Hodgkin's lymphoma, has demonstrated an increased risk for the development of Hodgkin's disease (SIR 7.4) in a cohort of French RA patients treated with MTX; EBV was detected in five of seven of these tumors.[131] It has been postulated that, although MTX may carry a small risk of EBV-associated lymphoma in patients with RA, its ability to reduce disease activity of RA (which is an established risk factor for development of lymphoproliferative disorders) may in time lead to an overall reduction in the rate of malignancies seen in the RA population.[132]

Of the 50 original cases of B cell lymphoma cited in the literature, eight patients have been reported to experience spontaneous remission after stopping MTX; of these, four patients were positive for EBV.[130] However, of the patients who developed Hodgkin's disease in the French study, none treated with withdrawal of MTX alone achieved remission.[131] This suggests that, in at least in a very small number of patients with non-Hodgkin's lymphoma, the lymphoma might spontaneously go into remission and that a brief period of observation without immunosuppressive therapy might be considered, particularly in those patients found to be EBV positive.[130,132]

The mechanisms by which lymphoma may develop in RA patients and be potentiated by MTX include persistent immunologic stimulation, which might lead to clonal selection and malignant transformation of CD5+ B cells; proliferation of latent infection with EBV; direct oncogenic action; decreased apoptosis of infected B cells; or decreased natural killer (NK) cell activity.[130]

SYSTEMIC LUPUS ERYTHEMATOSUS

The risks of developing malignancy in association with SLE are difficult to estimate. Small series and cohort studies have noted that patients with SLE might be at increased risk for malignancy, including non-Hodgkin's lymphomas, sarcomas, and breast carcinoma.[133-137] However, other small series have not found differences[138] or have found infrequent associations[139] in numbers or types of malignancy between patients with lupus and the general population.[138] Conflicting results are also seen in case control studies of larger groups of patients, with some cohorts demonstrating an increased overall risk of malignancy,[140-142] whereas others have failed to do so.[143-146] However, some studies that did not find an increased risk of overall malignancies in patients with lupus have shown an increased risk of lymphoproliferative disorders.[144-146] Some confounding factors complicating interpretation of these studies include possible incomplete ascertainment of malignancies, inclusion of nonrepresentative cohorts of patients with SLE, and selection of inappropriate control populations.[147]

To more adequately determine whether individuals suffering from SLE are in fact at an increased risk, systematic reviews and meta-analyses of pooled data are necessary. The SIR of individual studies has ranged from 1.1 to 2.6.[148] A recent meta-analysis of six of the clinical cohort studies found a slightly increased risk of overall malignancies in cohorts of patients with SLE, with a SIR of 1.58.[149] This analysis was able to demonstrate an increased risk of lymphomas in these cohorts, with a SIR of 3.57 for non-Hodgkin's lymphoma and 2.35 for Hodgkin's disease. Individual hospital discharge database studies have shown a consistently higher risk of non-Hodgkin's lymphoma (SIR 3.72 to 6.7), but these studies examined only hospitalized patients with SLE.[148] Pooled analysis showed a slightly elevated risk for the development of breast cancer, with a SIR of 1.53, but they did not find an increased risk of lung or colorectal cancers in these patients.[149] Again, the same confounding factors influencing the individual studies are a factor in interpreting these pooled data. Large, multicenter cohort studies are needed to further define the relationship between SLE and malignancy.[147]

Although the exact etiology of the association is not known, several theories have arisen to explain the possible connection between SLE and malignancy, especially B cell lymphoma. Some authors have postulated that certain immunologic defects may predispose patients to both SLE and B cell lymphoma, including apoptosis dysfunction, chronic antigenic stimulation, and overexpression of bcl-2 oncogene.[148,150] Viruses, EBV in particular, have also been postulated as part of the development of both SLE and lymphoma.[148,150] However, studies have not conclusively validated any of these theories to date.

Overall, it appears that the presence of SLE carries a small increased risk for the development of lymphoproliferative disorders, particularly non-Hodgkin's lymphoma. The underlying etiology of this association is not known. The association does not appear to be related to the use of immunosuppressive or cytotoxic agents.[133,144,146,148] Questions also have been raised regarding a possible increased risk of breast and lung malignancies.

SYSTEMIC SCLEROSIS

Individuals suffering from systemic sclerosis are at an increased risk for developing malignancy. The malignancies that have been implicated are often in organs affected by inflammation and fibrosis, including the lung, breast, esophagus, and skin. The SIR of malignancy in the scleroderma population appears to be 1.5 to 5.1 when compared to that of the general population.[151-154] There is an increase in the observed number of cases of lung cancers that appears to occur in the setting of pulmonary fibrosis but not in association with tobacco use.[155] There also appears to be a temporal correlation between the onset of systemic sclerosis and the development of breast cancer, although not necessarily an increased incidence of breast cancer.[151] Older age at the time of diagnosis with systemic sclerosis appears to be a significant risk factor for the development of cancer.[152]

Although the SIR for malignancy is 1.5 to 2.4, the incidence ratio for lung cancer can be as high as 7.8 and for non-Hodgkin's lymphoma as high as 9.6. Cases of non-Hodgkin's lymphoma appear to be more likely to occur within the first year of the diagnosis of systemic sclerosis.[153] Elevations in incidence were also found for other specific cancers, including nonmelanoma skin cancers (4.2), primary liver cancers (3.3), and hematopoietic cancers (2.3)—all having a higher incidence than that in the general population. The greatest risk appears to correspond to areas commonly affected by fibrosis, particularly the lung and skin. Interestingly, localized scleroderma does not appear to convey an increased risk.[156]

▌ Primary Tumors and Metastatic Disease

PRIMARY MUSCULOSKELETAL TUMORS

This section is not designed to provide in-depth knowledge of the primary tumors of the musculoskeletal system. Rather, it provides a reference to the most common primary malignant musculoskeletal tumors and symptoms that may arise in association with them. Additional insight into the primary tumors of bone, including both benign and malignant tumors, can be found in Chapter 113.

A primary malignant bone cancer is any neoplasm that develops from the tissues or cells found within bone and has the ability to metastasize. Many types of cells are present within the bone. Neoplasms may develop or arise from osteoblasts, chondrocytes, adipose and fibrous tissue, vascular cells, hematopoietic cells, and neural tissue.[157] A neoplasm developing from any of these tissues is referred to as a sarcoma, which signifies that it is derived from mesenchymal tissue. The bone sarcomas are then named for the predominant differentiated tissue type such as osteosarcomas, chondrosarcomas, liposarcomas, and angiosarcomas.[157] The most common manifestation of these tumors is the development of pain in the area of the lesion, which may be accompanied by a sympathetic effusion or stiffness in the surrounding joint. This discomfort does not appear to be activity related and is often worse at night. These tumors can, however, manifest as painless masses or as pathologic fractures. Systemic features such as fatigue, malaise, weight loss, fevers, and night sweats are rare with all of these tumors, with the exception of Ewing's sarcoma.[157]

Primary malignant bone tumors are relatively uncommon, particularly in comparison to other types of cancer. They have their highest incidence in childhood and adolescence and constitute 9.2 percent of childhood malignancies that occur before the age of 15 years. The incidence has been reported in this age-group as 3 per 100,000 people.[158] These tumors commonly arise out of areas of rapid growth, with the most common site of primary bone sarcomas being the metaphysis near the growth plate.[158]

The most common types of primary malignant bone tumors are listed in Table 111–4. Osteosarcoma is the most common of the tumors and generally occurs in the second decade of life. It can also occur secondary to radiation therapy delivered as treatment for other malignancies. Paget's disease of bone can rarely (less than 1% of cases) proceed to malignant transformation. Severe pain in the setting of Paget's disease may signal transformation to osteogenic sarcoma. Tumors most frequently affect the femur, humerus, skull, and pelvis and can result in pathologic fractures. Survival is usually less than 1 year. Differentiating malignancy from Paget's disease may require a biopsy.[159]

Chondrosarcoma has been reported as the second most common of the malignant bone tumors. This tumor may occur as a primary tumor or as a malignant transformation in the setting of benign lesions such as the enchondroma or osteochondroma. Fibrosarcoma is significantly less common than the previously mentioned tumors, as it accounts for less than 4 percent of primary malignant bone tumors.[160]

As a group, the round cell tumors include primary lymphomas of bone, Ewing's sarcoma, and metastatic neuroblastoma. Ewing's sarcoma is a relatively common primary bone tumor of childhood. Giant cell tumors as a group account for 4.5 percent of bone tumors. They usually arise from the metaphysis or epiphysis of long bones, generally around the knee. Most are benign, but a small number are malignant lesions, usually arising out of a previously irradiated benign giant cell tumor.[157]

In addition to the primary malignancies of bone, there are a plethora of malignant tumors that can arise from mesenchymal connective tissue; these are also known as sarcomas.[160] They can result in joint complaints but more often result in soft tissue complaints. They are very rare, and consequently, little time is devoted to this group. Of note, rhabdomyosarcoma is a malignant tumor arising from muscle tissue. It is the fourth most common solid tumor in children and is responsible for more than half of all soft tissue sarcomas in children. It rarely occurs in adults. It can appear at any site, and the symptoms are most often referable to the site involved. Most commonly, rhabdomyosarcoma affects the orbits, genitourinary tract, limbs, head and neck, and parameningeal areas. It commonly metastasizes to the lymph nodes, lungs, and bone.[158]

METASTATIC DISEASE

When bone lesions are identified, primary tumors need to be considered, although the majority of malignant lesions in bone are metastatic. Metastasis rarely affects muscles, joints, or adjacent connective tissue. More commonly it affects bone. The most common sites of metastasis are the spine and pelvis. It is uncommon to find metastatic lesions distal to the elbow, and, although rare, metastasis to the foot is more common than to the hand.[161] When distal or acral metastasis is identified, it is often associated with lung cancer.[162] Primary tumors generally associated with metastases to bone include those in the prostate, thyroid, lung, breast, and kidney.[158] Although the majority of skeletal metastases do not produce pain, one of the most common causes of cancer pain is the infiltration of bone. The pain can be intense and stabbing or dull. It is often constant rather than intermittent, worse at night, and often worse with weight-bearing and movement.[163] Rheumatic or arthritic complaints can often occur before lesions are easily identified on radiographs. Arthritis associated with metastatic carcinoma is most commonly monarticular and most commonly affects the knee. Metastases to the hip, ankle, wrist, hand, and foot have been reported but occur less frequently. Breast and lung carcinomas are present in the majority of patients.[164] Metastases to the extremities can simulate gout, osteomyelitis, tenosynovitis, or acro-osteolysis. The development of joint involve-

TABLE 111–4 · PRIMARY BONE TUMORS

Nonosseous Tumors	Osseous Tumors
Multiple myeloma	Osteosarcoma
Round cell tumors	Chondrosarcoma
	Giant cell tumors
	Fibrosarcoma

TABLE 111–5 • FREQUENT FEATURES OF ARTHRITIS RESULTING FROM METASTATIC CARCINOMA

Presence of constitutional symptoms
Prior history of malignancy
Protracted clinical course
Negative culture results, negative crystal analysis
Medical therapeutic failure
Rapid reaccumulation of hemorrhagic noninflammatory effusion
Radiologic evidence of destructive process

ment can be related to direct synovial implantation, or involvement of the juxta-articular or subchondral bone.[165] Table 111–5 elaborates the clinical features suggestive of underlying metastases.

Radiographic features of bone tumors can be of significance when interpreting the duration of disease and the type of malignancy. Lesions may in fact be lytic or blastic, and patterns of destruction often reflect the aggressiveness of tumors. Well-circumscribed lesions may be more indicative of slower growth, whereas a "moth-eaten" pattern with evidence of cortical destruction typically signifies a more rapid rate of growth. What has been described as a permeative pattern is suggestive of an extremely rapid rate of destruction and is often associated with an extraosseous soft tissue mass.[157] Computed tomography (CT), magnetic resonance imaging (MRI), and radionucleotide imaging can also provide significant information for diagnosis, staging, prognosis, and therapy.

POSTCHEMOTHERAPY RHEUMATISM

Several rheumatic or musculoskeletal manifestations can develop in patients following the administration of chemotherapy for the treatment of malignancy. Postchemotherapy rheumatism has been best described in patients treated for breast cancer but has also been described in other malignancies including ovarian cancer and non-Hodgkin's lymphoma.[166,167] The phenomena has been described as a noninflammatory, self-limited, migratory arthropathy. Typically, symptoms develop several weeks to several months following the completion of chemotherapy and often include myalgia, stiffness, arthralgia, and arthritis involving the small joints of the hands, ankles, and knees.[167] It can be mistaken for RA based on its symptoms; however, most patients have little or no evidence of synovial thickening and have no radiographic or serologic evidence to suggest RA. The pathogenesis of this process is unknown; however, it is self-limited, usually lasting less than 1 year, and is best treated in a conservative fashion. Evaluation should be performed to exclude recurrent carcinoma or another inflammatory condition. The medications most frequently associated with this phenomena include cyclophosphamide, 5-flourouracil, MTX, and tamoxifen.[168,169]

Other immunomodulatory agents also have been linked to the development of musculoskeletal findings. Tamoxifen use has been associated with the develop-ment of an acute inflammatory arthritis similar to RA.[169] Use of interleukin-2 (IL-2) can result in spondyloarthritis or inflammatory arthritis. IFN-α administration can result in seropositive nodular RA, as well as myalgia and arthralgia.[172] The use of IFN-α and IFN-γ for the treatment of neoplastic disorders can additionally result in rheumatic manifestations including myalgia, arthralgia, autoantibody formation, and features suggestive of SLE and autoimmune thyroid disease.[171,172]

Lymphoproliferative and Myeloproliferative Diseases

LEUKEMIA

Leukemia can result in the development of musculoskeletal complaints. Bone pain is the most common musculoskeletal manifestation, and it has been reported to occur in 50 percent of adults suffering from leukemia.[173] Bone pain is more common in children, whereas axial pain is more common in adults. Generally, the bone pain is more common in the lower than the upper extremities.[174] Overt synovitis can develop in association with both acute and chronic leukemia and can result in the development of monoarticular or polyarticular arthritis.[51] The pathogenesis appears to be leukemic infiltration of the synovium and subperiosteal tissue. Bleeding or hemorrhage in the joint may also be associated with the process. The majority of cases of arthritis associated with leukemia are seen in children—14 to 50 percent compared to 4 to 16.5 percent in adults.[175,176]

In a series of adult patients with acute leukemia studied over a 10-year period, 5.8 percent (8 of 139) of the patients presented with rheumatic manifestations. On average, symptoms of arthritis preceded the diagnosis of leukemia by a period of 3.25 months.[177] The most common patterns of presentation were of asymmetric large joint involvement in association with low back pain, followed by symmetric polyarthritis mimicking early RA. Rheumatic manifestations included morning stiffness, low back pain, nonarticular bone pain, pain out of proportion to objective findings, low-grade fever, and elevation of the ESR. The response to NSAIDs, glucocorticoids, and conventional antirheumatic therapy was reportedly poor, but tumor-directed chemotherapy resulted in substantial improvement of the rheumatic manifestations. Patients with these manifestations also were more likely to exhibit early osteopenia or lytic bone lesions. Ultimately, it appears that prognosis and mortality rates were no different between those patients presenting with or without rheumatic manifestations.[177] In contrast, a large retrospective study of children with leukemia found 21.4 percent (36 of 168) with acute lymphoblastic leukemia, and 10.5 percent (6 of 57) with acute nonlymphoblastic leukemia developed symptoms associated with their bones and joints. Thirteen of these patients with acute lymphoblastic leukemia had evidence of bony lesions on radiographs.[178] Many of these children had been incorrectly treated for JRA or osteomyelitis before the diagnosis of leukemia. On a whole, the group with bone lesions appeared to do very well, and their condition might fall into a subgroup of childhood leukemia that has a better prognosis.[51,178]

MULTIPLE MYELOMA

Multiple myeloma is a neoplastic proliferation of plasma cells, a nonosseous malignant tumor arising in the marrow. Unlike the other primary tumors of bone, which have their highest incidence in children and adolescents, myeloma is a tumor of adults, occurring most commonly in the fifth and sixth decades of life. The most common musculoskeletal feature of this disease is the development of bone pain. Other hallmark features are diffuse pain and stiffness. Patients characteristically develop osteopenia, and osteolytic lesions are seen on radiographs. The lytic lesions, which can occur in any area of the skeleton, are produced by focal accumulations of plasma cells. However, osteosclerotic lesions have also been reported.[179] True arthritis is rare, but cases of arthritis secondary to articular and periarticular invasion with malignant cells have been reported in multiple myeloma and in Waldenström's macroglobulinemia.[180] A secondary feature of the disease, which can often lead to additional musculoskeletal complaints, is the development of hyperuricemia and secondary gout. Sjögren's syndrome has recently been described in association with multiple myeloma.[181,182]

LYMPHOMA

Musculoskeletal symptoms have been reported in up to 25 percent of cases of non-Hodgkin's lymphoma.[183] The most common musculoskeletal problem associated with lymphoma is the development of bone pain associated with metastases or lymphoma in the bone. By report, more than 50 percent of patients have evidence of bone lesions at autopsy; however, very few patients actually present with arthritis or bone pain.[51,184] Nonetheless, non-Hodgkin's lymphoma has been reported to manifest as a seronegative arthritis with or without other features such as lymphadenopathy and hepatomegaly typically seen with this disease. Both monoarticular and polyarticular involvement can occur. Cases have been reported of polyarthritis simulating RA in the setting of non-Hodgkin's lymphoma.[185] Although it is unusual to see direct involvement of the synovium, this also has been reported. There have been cases with radiographic evidence of bone destruction associated with non-Hodgkin's lymphomatous arthropathy.[186] Suspicion of lymphoma should be heightened in patients in whom severe constitutional symptoms appear out of proportion to the degree of arthritis, especially in those who are RF negative.[183]

ANGIOIMMUNOBLASTIC LYMPHADENOPATHY

Angioimmunoblastic lymphadenopathy is a rare, lymphoproliferative disorder marked by the clinical features of lymphadenopathy, hepatosplenomegaly, rash, and hypergammaglobulinemia. Patients can develop a nonerosive, symmetric, seronegative polyarthritis concurrent with other features or as an initial complaint of the disease.[187,188] Similar features have been reported

TABLE 111–6 · MUSCULOSKELETAL MANIFESTATIONS OF HEMATOLOGIC MALIGNANCY

Malignancy	Pathogenesis
Leukemia	Infiltration of synovium
Lymphoma	Metastases or invasion of bone, rarely joint
Antioblastic lymphadenopathy	Vasculitis, cryoglobulinemia
Multiple myeloma	Metastasis or invasion of bone, hyperuricemia

with intravascular lymphoma, with a report of a patient presenting with a symmetric polyarthritis accompanied by fever.[189] Table 111–6 lists musculoskeletal complaints found with hematologic malignancy.

GRAFT-VERSUS-HOST DISEASE

Graft-versus-host disease is a complication of bone marrow transplantation and a major cause of morbidity and mortality in the transplant population. A number of musculoskeletal complaints arise in the setting of acute graft-versus-host disease (lasting 0 to 3 months) and in chronic graft-versus-host disease (lasting more than 3 months following transplantation). The most frequent manifestation is the involvement of the skin, which in many cases can progress to resemble the sclerodermatous changes of systemic sclerosis. Skin changes consistent with eosinophilic fasciitis have also been reported.[174] Graft-versus-host disease can lead to symptoms of keratoconjunctivitis sicca and xerostomia resembling Sjögren's syndrome. Other features including arthralgias, arthritis, myositis, Raynaud's phenomena, and serositis have also been reported.[174,190]

Association of Immunomodulatory Agents with Malignancy

Many of the medications used to treat the rheumatic diseases are modulators of the immune system. As such, they may be associated directly or indirectly with an increased risk of the subsequent development of malignancy associated with the underlying disorder. An individual agent may confer this risk through direct mutagenesis of DNA, through generalized immunosuppression with the risk of developing an EBV-associated lymphoproliferative disorder, or through injury to an unintended organ system, such as the bladder with the use of cyclophosphamide. Longer duration of use of these agents has been associated with increasing risk of developing subsequent malignancies.[191] However, it is often difficult to adequately differentiate the individual risk of an agent, particularly in the background of an autoimmune disease that itself can convey an increased risk for the development of malignancy. Table 111–7 provides an overview of the potential oncologic risks of various immunomodulatory therapies.

TABLE 111–7 • IMMUNOMODULATORY AGENTS AND RISK OF MALIGNANCY

DMARD	Risk of Malignancy
Cyclophosphamide	Non-Hodgkin's lymphoma, leukemia, bladder cancer, skin cancer
Azathioprine	Non-Hodgkin's lymphoma
Cyclosporine	Immunosuppression-associated lymphoma
Methotrexate (MTX)	Immunosuppression-associated lymphoma
Gold salts	None known
Hydroxychloroquine	None known
Penicillamine	None known
Sulfasalazine	None known
Leflunomide	None known
Biologic response modifiers	Unknown, possible lymphoma

Abbreviation: DMARD, disease-modifying antirheumatic drug.

CYCLOPHOSPHAMIDE

Cyclophosphamide is an alkylating agent that kills both resting and cycling cells and, thus, has cytotoxic, mutagenic, and carcinogenic potential. It is used predominantly for the treatment of vasculitis, glomerulonephritis, and other life- or organ-threatening manifestations of rheumatic disease. The use of cyclophosphamide in RA appears to result in an increased risk of the development of bladder cancer, skin cancer, and hematologic malignancies including non-Hodgkin's lymphoma and leukemia.[192,193] Risk factors for the development of neoplasia include higher total dosage, longer duration of therapy, and tobacco use.[194] The overall relative risk of developing malignancy appears to be 1.5 to 4.1 for those treated, compared to controls, and the increased risk of bladder cancer continues more than 17 years after cyclophosphamide therapy.[193,194] The increased risk for the development of bladder cancer is believed to be a direct result of high concentrations of active metabolites in the bladder, such as acrolein. The overall risks of bladder cancer may be less with pulsed, intravenous (IV) treatment than with daily oral cyclophosphamide. In general, the use of cyclophosphamide is restricted to life- or organ-threatening disease in which the risks associated with treatment often outweigh the serious effects of untreated rheumatic disease.

METHOTREXATE

MTX is one of the most commonly used agents in the treatment of rheumatic diseases and generally has a favorable side-effect profile. Like many other immunomodulatory agents, questions have been raised regarding the oncogenic potential of MTX when used to treat autoimmune or inflammatory disorders. There has been no strong evidence to suggest that MTX conveys an increased risk for the development of solid tumors. However, there have been reports of a relationship between MTX use and the development of lymphomas. Epidemiologic data have failed to support the postulated increased risk for the development of lymphoproliferative disorders in patients with RA treated with MTX. Cohorts of patients with RA treated with MTX have been compared to RA patients who never received MTX to ascertain the association between increased risk of malignancy and exposure to MTX. Of the several cohort studies performed, none have been able to confirm an increased risk of lymphoproliferative disorders with the use of MTX.[132,195] In fact, data published in abstract form in 1998 suggest that MTX may actually improve long-term RA outcome. The effect of DMARDs on mortality was studied in 1842 patients during a 25-year period. The investigators suggested that there was a reduction in mortality in individuals who had been treated with MTX.[196] Although this work may not directly address questions regarding the use of MTX in RA and the risk of developing malignancy, it helps to answer the overall question of whether this agent's benefits outweigh its risks.

Some interesting studies have been published regarding the possible association of MTX use in the treatment of RA and the development of lymphoproliferative disorders associated with EBV, as was previously mentioned in the section on RA-associated malignancies. EBV has been reported in non-Hodgkin's lymphoma, Hodgkin's disease, and T cell lymphomas in RA patients treated with MTX.[131,132,197,198]

One set of investigators reviewed all reported cases of lymphoproliferative disorders in RA patients treated with MTX.[199] They subsequently identified most of the cases as non-Hodgkin's B cell lymphomas, either large-cell or diffuse-mixed type. In many of the cases there was extranodal involvement. In patients tested, 46 percent showed evidence of EBV infection, and in 14 patients treated solely by withdrawal of MTX, eight achieved full remission.[199] The rate of EBV association is less than that seen in post-transplantation patients or in patients with AIDS who develop lymphoma, but it is nevertheless higher than that for lymphoma in the general population.[199]

Further investigation into the association of immunomodulatory agents for the treatment of rheumatic diseases and the development of lymphoproliferative disorders has shown an association with EBV. After analyzing 10 EBV-associated lymphoid neoplasms in patients with RA or DM with the PCR, investigators found that these lymphoproliferative disorders can harbor EBV strain type A or B, with type A being the most prevalent. This is similar to what has been reported in post–solid organ transplantation immunosuppression-associated lymphoproliferative disorders. As well, EBV-latent membrane protein-1 deletions appear to occur in as many as one third of the cases but are not required for the neoplasm to develop.[200]

It is possible that, although not increasing the overall risk for the development of lymphoproliferative disorders, treatment with MTX may carry a small risk for the development of EBV-associated lymphoid malignancies akin to those seen in other immunosuppressed individuals. A subset of these patients may respond with regression of the tumor following discontinuation of MTX.

AZATHIOPRINE

Azathioprine is a purine analogue that leads to both inhibition of purine synthesis and direct cytotoxic effects. The use of azathioprine is associated with an increased risk of both lymphoma and nonlymphoproliferative cancers.[193,201-203] Compared to the risk to the general population, azathioprine treatment can result in a 10-fold increased risk for the development of lymphoproliferative disorders.[203] This amounts to one case of lymphoma per 1000 patient-years of azathioprine treatment.[202] Again, a correlation between the cumulative dose of azathioprine used and the incidence of cancer has been seen.[192,203] Leukemia has also been reported in association with azathioprine use.[204,205]

CYCLOSPORINE

Cyclosporine is currently utilized for the treatment of RA and SLE, particularly for lupus nephritis. Based on experience with solid organ transplantation in which post-transplantation lymphoproliferative disorders are well recognized as complications arising in allograft recipients treated with immunosuppressive drugs, there has been a concern for an increased risk for the development of malignancy, especially lymphoproliferative disorders with cyclosporine treatment of rheumatic diseases. Although cyclosporine has been used formally in the treatment of RA since the 1980s, there have not been sufficient numbers of patients followed longitudinally for sufficient time to determine whether the drug may convey an increased risk for the development of malignancy. Cyclosporine has been associated with the development of EBV-associated lymphomas in some patients with RA[206]; however, a retrospective study looked at more than 1000 RA patients treated with cyclosporine in clinical trials and concluded that the use of cyclosporine did not increase the potential risk for the development of malignancy or the type of malignancy beyond that seen with the use of other DMARDs.[207] In addition, a second retrospective and case-control study found that cyclosporine treatment in RA patients does not increase the risk of malignancies in general or the risk of malignant lymphoproliferative disorders.[208] This may be, at least in part, due to the lower doses generally used for the treatment of rheumatic diseases compared to allograph recipients.[196]

LEFLUNOMIDE

Leflunomide is a selective inhibitor of de novo pyrimidine synthesis and leads to cell cycle arrest in rapidly replicating cell lines, such as activated T cells in RA. At the time of this writing it does not appear that leflunomide conveys an increased risk for the development of malignancy. As is so important with the introduction of any new medication, long-term safety studies and postmarketing surveillance will be necessary to ascertain whether there is increased risk at 10 and 20 years.

Biologic Response Modifiers

These agents are covered in detail in Chapter 61 on anticytokine therapy and Chapter 62 on emerging therapies, but as a group they include biologic agents such as tumor necrosis factor (TNF) inhibitors, and IL-1 antagonists. One case series reported on the development of 26 cases of lymphoproliferative disorders following treatment with TNF inhibition. While no clear causal relationship could be established, in two instances, lymphoma regression was observed following discontinuation of anti-TNF treatment.[209] Although the potential exists to decrease tumor surveillance, it does not appear at this point that these agents have resulted in a substantially increased risk for the development of malignancy. Of the products currently available on the market (etanercept, infliximab, adalimumab, anakinra), none have been shown to result in a significantly greater risk for the induction of malignancy. Based on clinical trial data and postmarketing surveillance, the incidence of both lymphoproliferative and solid-tumor malignancies appear comparable to what would be expected based on age- and sex-matched controls from the National Cancer Institute's surveillance, epidemology, and end results, (SEER), data base. However, it is important to recognize that these drugs have been commercially available for less than 10 years and continued vigilance is warranted.

RADIATION

Radiation therapy is no longer used for the treatment of inflammatory arthritis. Its use in ankylosing spondylitis (AS) in the early part of the twentieth century resulted in significant increases in the presence of malignancy, including leukemia, lymphoma, myeloma, and esophageal, colon, pancreas, lung, bones, soft tissue, prostate, bladder, and kidney cancers. It also resulted in an increased relative risk of mortality of 1.3 when compared to expected deaths. There were clear dose-response relationships between the amount of radiation and the development of individual cancers.[210,211]

Conclusion

A plethora of factors contribute to the development of musculoskeletal syndromes in the setting of autoimmune disease and malignancy. Clearly, there are a great many autoimmune disorders, and, for the majority, the underlying etiology and pathogenesis have not been elucidated. It is this incredible diversity that often makes understanding the relationship between associated symptoms very difficult. To make any generalizations regarding association between an autoimmune disorder and the subsequent development of malignancy, very large numbers of patients must be studied longitudinally for exceptionally long periods of time. Of course, other confounders complicate the picture. Many of the agents used in the treatment of connective tissue and autoimmune disorders modulate the immune system. These agents may have direct carcinogenic potential, whereas others may affect the immune system in a way that may decrease tumor surveillance and subsequently lead to the development of a neoplasm. Intricately entwined are the unique differences of individual immune systems not only in healthy individuals, but also in those whose immune systems are already altered based on an underlying autoimmune disorder. Although not common, it is plausible that virtually any of the autoimmune-based diseases and the agents used to treat them might, in certain circumstances, be associated with malignancy. Most important, when musculoskeletal symptoms arise, malignancy or paraneoplastic syndromes should be considered in the differential diagnosis, especially when patients present with atypical features of autoimmune disease or are refractory to conventional treatment. In addition, the potential for any agent to induce a neoplastic process must be weighed against its proposed benefits before initiating it as therapy.

REFERENCES

1. Stedman's Medical Dictionary, 26th ed. Baltimore, Williams & Wilkins, 1995.
2. Caldwell DS: Carcinoma polyarthritis: Manifestations and differential diagnosis. Med Grand Rounds 1:378,1982.
3. Chan MK, Hendrickson CS, Taylor KE: Polyarthritis associated with breast carcinoma. West J Med 137:132, 1982.
4. Stummvoll GH, Aringer M, Machold KP, et al: Cancer polyarthritis resembling rheumatoid arthritis as a first sign of hidden neoplasms. Scand J Rheumatol 30:40, 2001.
5. Gonzalez-Gay MA, Garcia-Porrua C, Salvarani C, Hunder GG: Cutaneous vasculitis and cancer: a clinical approach. Clin Exp Rheumatol 18:305, 2000.
6. Sanchez-Guerrero J, Gutierrez-Urena S, Vidaller A, et al: Vasculitis as a paraneoplastic syndrome: Report of 11 cases and review of the literature. J Rheumatol 17:1458, 1990.
7. Garcia-Porrua C, Gonzalez-Gay MA: Cutaneous vasculitis as a paraneoplastic syndrome in adults. Arthritis Rheum 41:1133, 1998.
8. Hamidou MA, Derenne S, Audrain MAP, et al: Prevalence of rheumatic manifestations and antineutrophil cytoplasmic antibodies in haematological malignancies: a prospective study. Rheumatology 39:417, 2000.
9. Hamidou MA, Boumalassa A, Larroche C, et al: Systemic medium-sized vessel vasculitis associated with chronic myelomonocytic leukemia. Sem Arthritis Rheum 31:119, 2001.
10. Hamidou MA, El Kouri D, Audrain M, Grolleau JY: Systemic antineutrophil cytoplasmic antibody vasculitis associated with lymphoid neoplasia. Ann Rheum Dis 60:295, 2001.
11. Tatsis E, Reinhold-Keller E, Steindorf K, et al: Wegener's granulomatosis associated with renal cell carcinoma. Arthritis Rheum 42:751, 1999.
12. Knight AM, Ekbom A, Askling J: Cancer risk in a population based cohort of patients with Wegener's granulomatosis [Abstract 1677]. Arthritis Rheum 44:S332, 2001.
13. Greer JM, Longley S, Edwards NL, et al: Vasculitis associated with malignancy: Experience with 13 patients and literature review. Medicine (Baltimore) 67:220, 1988.
14. Dammacco F, Sansonno D, Piccoli C, et al: The cryoglobulins: an overview. Eur J Clin Invest 31:628, 2001.
15. La Civita L, Zignego AL, Monti M, et al: Mixed cryoglobulinemia as a possible preneoplastic disorder. Arthritis Rheum 38:1859, 1995.
16. Ramos-Casals M, Garcia-Carrasco M, Trejo O, et al: Lymphoproliferative diseases in patients with cryoglobulinemia: clinical description of 27 cases. Arthritis Rheum 44:S58, 2001.
17. Virshup AM, Sliwinski AJ: Polyarthritis and subcutaneous nodules associated with carcinoma of the pancreas. Arthritis Rheum 16:388, 1973.
18. Marhaug G, Hvidsten D: Arthritis complicating acute pancreatitis: a rare but important condition to be distinguished from juvenile rheumatoid arthritis. Scand J Rheumatol 12:397, 1988.
19. Naschitz JE, Boss JH, Misselevich I, et al: The fasciitis-panniculitis syndromes: clinical and pathologic features. Medicine (Baltimore) 75:6, 1996.
20. Naschitz JE, Yeshurun D, Zucherman E, et al: Cancer-associated fasciitis panniculitis. Cancer 73:231, 1994.
21. Masuoka H, Kikuchi K, Takahashi S, et al: Eosinophilic fasciitis associated with low-grade T-cell lymphoma. Br J Dermatol 139:928, 1998.
22. Pfinsgraff J, Buckingham RB, Killian PJ, et al: Palmar fasciitis and arthritis with malignant neoplasms: A paraneoplastic syndrome. Semin Arthritis Rheum 16:118, 1986.
23. Enomoto M, Takemura H, Suzuki M, et al: Palmar fasciitis and polyarthritis associated with gastric carcinoma: complete resolution after total gastrectomy. Intern Med 39:754, 2000.
24. Saxman SB, Seitz D: Breast cancer associated with palmar fasciitis and arthritis. J Clin Oncol 15:3515, 1997.
25. Medsger TA, Dixon JA, Garwood VF: Palmar fasciitis and polyarthritis associated with ovarian carcinoma. Ann Intern Med 96:424, 1982.
26. Michaels RM, Sorber JA: Reflex sympathetic dystrophy as a probable paraneoplastic syndrome: Case report and literature review. Arthritis Rheum 27:1183, 1984.
27. Olson WL: Reflex sympathetic dystrophy associated with tumour infiltration of the stellate ganglion. J Royal Soc Med 86:482, 1993.
28. Derbekyan V, Novales-Diaz J, Lisbona R: Pancoast tumor as a cause of reflex sympathetic dystrophy. J Nucl Med 34:1992, 1993.
29. Ku A, Lachmann E, Tunkel R, Nagler W: Upper limb reflex sympathetic dystrophy associated with occult malignancy. Arch Phys Med Rehabil 77:726, 1996.
30. Kalgaard OM, Seem E, Kvernebo K: Erythromelalgia: a clinical study of 87 cases. J Intern Med 242:191, 1997.
31. Kraus A, Alarcon-Segovia D: Erythermalgia, erythromelalgia, or both? Conditions neglected by rheumatologists. J Rheumatol 20:1, 1993.
32. Babb RR, Alarcon-Segovia D, Fairbairn JF II: Erythermalgia. Circulation 19:136, 1964.
33. Davis MD, O'Fallon WM, Rogers RS III, Rooke TW: Natural history of erythromelalgia: presentation and outcome in 168 patients. Arch Dermatol136:330, 2000.
34. Mork C, Asker CL, Salerud EG, Kvernebo K: Microvascular arteriovenous shunting is a probable pathogenic mechanism in erythromelalgia. J Invest Dermatol 43:841, 2000.
35. Cohen JS: Erythromelalgia: new theories and new therapies. J Am Acad Dermatol 43(5 Pt 1):841, 2000.
36. Gonzalez-Gay MA, Garcia-Porrua C, Salvarani C, et al: Polymyalgia manifestations in different conditions mimicking polymyalgia rheumatica. Clin Exp Rheum 18:755, 2000.
37. Kohli M, Bennett RM: An association of polymyalgia rheumatica with myelodysplastic syndromes. J Rheumatol 21:1357, 1994.
38. Naschitz JE, Slobodin G, Yeshurun D, et al: Atypical polymyalgia rheumatica as a presentation of metastatic cancer. Arch Intern Med 157:2381, 1997.
39. Gonzalez-Gay MA, Garcia-Porrua C, Calvarani C, et al: The spectrum of conditions mimicking polymyalgia rheumatica in northwestern Spain. J Rheumatol 27:2179, 2000.
40. Haga HJ, Eide GE, Brun J, et al: Cancer in association with polymyalgia rheumatica and temporal arteritis. J Rheumatol 20:1335, 1993.
41. Myklebust G, Gran JT: A prospective study of 287 patients with polymyalgia rheumatica and temporal arteritis: clinical and laboratory manifestations at onset of disease and at time of diagnosis. Br J Rheum 35:1161, 1996.
42. Legrain S, Raguin G, Piette JC: Digital necrosis revealing ovarian cancer. Dermatology 199:183, 1999.
43. DeCross AJ, Sahasrabudhe DM: Paraneoplastic Raynaud's phenomenon. Am J Med 92:571, 1992.
44. Chow SF, McKenna CH: Ovarian cancer and gangrene of the digits: case report and review of the literature. Mayo Clin Proc 71:253, 1996.
45. Petri M, Fye KH: Digital necrosis: a paraneoplastic syndrome. J Rheumatol 12:800, 1985.

46. Ohtsuka T, Yamakage A, Yamazaki S: Digital ulcers and necroses: novel manifestations of angiocentric lymphoma. Br J Dermatol 142:1013, 2000.
47. D'Hondt L, Guillaume T, Humblet Y, Symann M: Digital necrosis associated with chronic myeloid leukemia: a rare paraneoplastic phenomenon . . . and not a toxicity of recombinant interferon. Acta Clin Belg 52:49, 1997.
48. Courtney PA, Sandhu S, Gardiner PV, Bell AL: Resolution of digital necrosis following treatment of multiple myeloma. Rheumatology (Oxford)39:1163, 2000.
49. Bachmeyer C, Farge D, Gluckman E, et al: Raynaud's phenomenon and digital necrosis induced by interferon-alpha. Br J Dermatol 135:481, 1996.
50. Reid TJ III, Lombardo Fa, Redmond J III, et al: Digital vasculitis associated with interferon therapy. Am J Med 92:702, 1992.
51. Ehrenfeld M, Gur H, Shoenfeld Y: Rheumatologic features of hematologic disorders. Curr Opin Rheumatol 11:62, 1999.
52. Cantini F, Salvarani C, Olivieri I: Paraneoplastic remitting seronegative symmetrical synovitis with pitting edema. Clin Exp Rheumatol 17:741, 1999.
53. Olivieri I, Salvarani C, Cantini F: RS3PE syndrome: an overview. Clin Exp Rheumatol 18(4 Suppl 20):S53, 2000.
54. Paira S, Graf C, Roverano S, Rossini J: Remitting seronegative symmetrical synovitis with pitting oedema: a study of 12 cases. Clin Rheumatol 21:146, 2002.
55. Campbell DA, Edwards NL: Multicentric reticulohistiocytosis: Systemic macrophage disorder. Baillieres Clin Rheumatol 5:301, 1991.
56. Snow JL, Muller SA: Malignancy-associated multicentric reticulo-histiocytosis: a clinical, histological, and immunophenotypic study. Br J Derm 133:71, 1995.
57. Freundlich B, Makover D, Maul GG: A novel antinuclear antibody associated with a lupus-like paraneoplastic syndrome. Ann Int Med 109:295, 1988.
58. Chtourou M, Aubin F, Savariault I, et al: Digital necrosis and lupus-like syndrome preceding ovarian carcinoma. Dermatology 196:348, 1998.
59. Strickland RW, Limmani A, Wall JG, Krishnan J: Hairy cell leukemia presenting as a lupus-like syndrome. Arthritis Rheum 31:566, 1988.
60. Schewach-Millet M, Shpiro D, Ziv R, Trau H: Subacute cutaneous lupus erythematosus associated with breast carcinoma. J Am Acad Dermatol 19:406, 1988.
61. Swissa M, Amital-Teplizki H, Haim N, et al: Autoantibodies in neoplasia: an unresolved enigma. Cancer 65:2554, 1990.
62. Armas JB, Dantas J, Mendonca G, et al: Anticardiolipin and anti-nuclear antibodies in cancer patients: a case control study. Clin Exp Rheumatol 18:227, 2000.
63. Timuragaoglu A, Duman A, Ongut G, et al: The significance of autoantibodies in non-Hodgkin's lymphoma. Leuk Lymphoma 40:119, 2000.
64. Petri M: Epidemiology of the antiphospholipid antibody syndrome. J Autoimmun 15:145, 2000.
65. Asherson RA: Antiphospholipid antibodies, malignancy and paraproteinemias. J Autoimmun 15:117, 2000.
66. Zuckerman E, Toubi E, Dov Golan T, et al: Increased thromboembolic incidence in anti-cardiolipin-positive patients with malignancy. Br J Cancer 72:447, 1995.
67. Ozguroglu M, Arun B, Erzin Y, et al: Serum cardiolipin antibodies in cancer patients with thromboembolic events. Clin Appl Thromb Hemost 5:181, 1999.
68. Stasi R, Stipa E, Masi M, et al: Antiphospholipid antibodies: prevalence, clinical significance and correlation to cytokine levels in acute myeloid leukemia and non-Hodgkin's lymphoma. Thromb Haemostas 70:568, 1993.
69. Lossos IS, Bogomolski-Yahalom V, Matzner Y: Anticardiolipin antibodies in acute myeloid leukemia: prevalence and clinical significance. Am J Hematol 57:139, 1998.
70. Malnick SDH, Geltner D, Sthoeger Z: Anticardiolipin antibody associated with renal carcinoma. J Rheumatol 22:2007, 1995.
71. Schved JF, Dupuy-Fons C, Biron C, et al: A prospective epidemiological study on the occurrence of antiphospholipid antibody: The Montpellier Antiphospholipid (MAP) study. Haemostasis 24:175, 1994.
72. Tanne D, D'Olhaberriague L, Trivedi AM, et al: Anticardiolipin antibodies and mortality in patients with ischemic stroke: a perspective follow-up study. Neuroepidemiology 21:93, 2002.
73. Seufert J, Ebert K, Muller J, et al: Octreotide therapy for tumor induced osteomalacia. New Engl J Med 345:1883, 2001.
74. Paglia F, Dionisi S, Minisola S: Octreotide therapy for tumor induced osteomalacia. New Engl J Med 346:1478, 2002.
75. Ioakimidis DE, Dendrinos GK, Frangia KB, et al: Tumor-induced osteomalacia. J Rheumatol 21:1162, 1994.
76. Cai Q, Hodgson SF, Kao PC, et al: Brief report: Inhibition of renal phosphate transport by a tumor product in a patient with oncogenic osteomalacia. N Engl J Med 330:1645, 1994.
77. Moder KG, Litin SC, Gaffey TA: Renal cell carcinoma associated with sarcoid-like tissue reaction. Mayo Clin Proc 65:1498, 1990.
78. Rawlings DJ, Bernstein B, Rowland JM, et al: Prolonged course of illness in a child with malignant lymphoma mimicking sarcoidosis. J Rheumatol 20:1583, 1993.
79. Bouros D, Hatzakis K, Labrakis H, Zeibecoglu K: Association of malignancy with diseases causing interstitial pulmonary changes. Chest 121:1278, 2002.
80. Nicholson AG, Wotherspoon AC, Diss TC, et al: Lymphomatoid granulomatosis: evidence that some cases represent EBV-associated B-cell lymphoma. Histopathology 29:317, 1996.
81. Jaffe ES, Wilson WH: Lymphomatoid granulomatosis: pathogenesis, pathology and clinical implications. Cancer Surveys 30:233, 1997.
82. Katzenstein AA, Carrington CB, Liebow AA: Lymphomatoid granulomatosis: a clinicopathologic study of 152 cases. Cancer 43:360, 1979.
83. Carson S: The association of malignancy with rheumatic and connective tissue diseases. Semin Oncol 24:360, 1997.
84. Barnes B: Dermatomyositis and malignancy: A review of the literature. Ann Intern Med 84:68, 1976.
85. Hill CL, Zhang Y, Sigurgeirsson B, et al: Frequency of specific cancer types in Dermatomyositis and polymyositis: a population based study. Lancet 357:96, 2001.
86. Stockton D, Doherty VR, Brewster DH: Risk of cancer in patients with dermatomyositis or polymyositis, and follow-up implications: a Scottish population-based cohort study. Br J Cancer 85:41, 2001.
87. Buchbinder F, Forbes A, Hall S, et al: Incidence of malignant disease in biopsy-proven inflammatory myopathy. Ann Intern Med 134:1087, 2001.
88. Chen YJ, Wu CY, Shen JL: Predicting factors of malignancy in dermatomyositis and polymyositis: a case-control study. Br J Derm 144:825, 2001.
89. Ang P, Sugeng MW, Chua SH: Classical and amyopathic dermatomyositis seen at the National Skin Centre of Singapore: a 3-year retrospective review of their clinical characteristics and association with malignancy. Ann Acad Med Singapore 29:219, 2000.
90. Zantos D, Zhang Y, Felson D: The overall and temporal association of cancer with polymyositis and dermatomyositis. J Rheumatol 21:1855, 1994.
91. Jorizzo JL: Dermatomyositis: practical aspects. Arch Dermatol 138:114, 2002.
92. Caproni M, Cardinali C, Parodi A, et al: Amyopathic dermatomyositis: a review by the Italian Group of Immunodermatology. Arch Dermatol138:23, 2002.
93. el-Azhari RA, Pakzad SY: Amyopathic dermatomyositis: retrospective review of 37 cases. J Am Acad Dermatol 46:560, 2002.
94. Medsger TA Jr., Dawson WN Jr, Masi AT: The epidemiology of polymyositis. Am J Med 48:715, 1970.
95. Lakhanpal S, Bunch TW, Ilstrup DM, Melton LJ III: Polymyositis-dermatomyositis and malignant lesions: Does an association exist? Mayo Clin Proc 61:645, 1986.
96. Callen JP: Relationship of cancer to inflammatory muscle diseases: Dermatomyositis, polymyositis and inclusion body myositis. Rheum Dis Clin North Am 20:943, 1994.
97. Callen JP: When and how should the patient with dermatomyositis or amyopathic dermatomyositis be assessed for possible cancer? Arch Dermatol 138:969, 2002.
98. Sparsa A, Liozon E, Herrmann F, et al: Routine versus extensive malignancy search for adult dermatomyositis and polymyositis: a study of 40 patients. Arch Dermatol 138:885, 2002.

99. Fudman EJ, Schnitzer TJ: Dermatomyositis without creatine kinase elevation: A poor prognostic sign. Am J Med 80:329, 1986.

100. Love LA, Leff RL, Fraser DD, et al: A new approach to the classification of idiopathic inflammatory myopathy: Myositis-specific autoantibodies define useful homogeneous patient groups. Medicine (Baltimore) 70:360, 1991.

101. Hunger RE, Durr C, Brand CU: Cutaneous leukocytoclastic vasculitis in dermatomyositis suggests malignancy. Dermatology 202:123, 2001.

102. Hidano A, Kaneko K, Arai Y, et al: Survey of the prognosis for dermatomyositis with special reference to its association with malignancy and pulmonary fibrosis. J Dermatol 13:233, 1986.

103. Talal N, Bunim J: The development of malignant lymphoma in the course of Sjögren's syndrome. Am J Med 36:529, 1964.

104. Kassan SS, Thomas TL, Moutsopoulos HM, et al: Increased risk of lymphoma in sicca syndrome. Ann Intern Med 89:888, 1978.

105. Sutcliffe N, Inanc M, Speight P, Isenberg D: Predictors of lymphoma development in primary Sjögren's syndrome. Semin Arthritis Rheum 28:80, 1998.

106. Zufferey P, Meyer OC, Grossin M, Kahn MF: Primary Sjögren's syndrome (SS) and malignant lymphoma: A retrospective cohort study of 55 patients with SS. Scand J Rheumatol 24:342, 1995.

107. Voulgarelis M, Dafni RG, Isenberg DA, Moutsopoulos HM: Malignant lymphoma in primary Sjögren's syndrome: a multicenter, retrospective, clinical study by the European concerted action on Sjögren's syndrome. Arthritis Rheum 42:1765, 1999.

108. Skopouli FN, Dafni U, Ioannidis JPA, Moutsopoulos HM: Clinical evolution, and morbidity and mortality of primary Sjögren's syndrome. Semin Arthritis Rheum 29:296, 2000.

109. Ioannidis JPA, Vassiliou VA, Moutsopoulos HM: Long-term risk of mortality and lymphoproliferative disease and predictive classification of primary Sjögren's syndrome. Arthritis Rheum 46:741, 2002.

110. Valesini G, Priori R, Bavoillot D, et al: Differential risk of non-Hodgkin's lymphoma in Italian patients with primary Sjögren's syndrome. J Rheumatol 24:2376, 1997.

111. Pertovaara M, Pukkala E, Laippala P, et al: A longitudinal cohort study of Finnish patients with primary Sjögren's syndrome: clinical, immunological, and epidemiological aspects. Ann Rheum Dis 60:467, 2001.

112. Biasi D, Caramaschi P, Ambrosetti A, et al: Mucosa-associated lymphoid tissue lymphoma of the salivary glands occurring in patients affected by Sjögren's syndrome: report of 6 cases. Acta Haematol 105:83, 2001.

113. Moutsopoulos HM, Costello R, Drosos AA, et al: Demonstration and identification of monoclonal proteins in the urine of patients with Sjögren's syndrome. Ann Rheum Dis 44:109, 1985.

114. Mariette X: Lymphomas in patients with Sjögren's syndrome: review of the literature and physiopathologic hypothesis. Leukemia Lymphoma 33:93, 1999.

115. Banks PM, Witrak GA, Conn DL: Lymphoid neoplasia developing after connective tissue disease. Mayo Clin Proc 54:104, 1979.

116. Jacobsen S, Petersen J, Ullman S, et al: A multicentre study of 513 Danish patients with systemic lupus erythematosus. II. Disease mortality and clinical factors of prognostic value. Clin Rheumatol 17:478, 1998.

117. Pisa EK, Pisa P, Kang HI, Fox RI: High frequency of t(14;18) translocation in salivary gland lymphomas from Sjögren's syndrome patients. J Exp Med 174:1245, 1991.

118. De Vita S, Ferraccioli G, De Re V, et al: The polymerase chain reaction detects B cell clonalities in patients with Sjögren's syndrome and suspected malignant lymphoma. J Rheumatol 21:1497, 1994.

119. Gridley G, McLaughlin JK, Ekbom A, et al: Incidence of cancer among patients with rheumatoid arthritis. J Natl Cancer Inst 85:307, 1993.

120. Mellemkjaer L, Linet MS, Gridley G, et al: Rheumatoid arthritis and cancer risk. Eur J Cancer 32A:1753, 1996.

121. Baecklund E, Ekbom A, Sparen P, et al: Disease activity and risk of lymphoma in patients with rheumatoid arthritis: Nested case-control study. BMJ 317(7152):180, 1998.

122. Tennis P, Andrews E, Bombardier C, et al: Record linkage to conduct an epidemiologic study on the association of rheumatoid arthritis and lymphoma in the province of Saskatchewan, Canada. J Clin Epidemiol 46:685, 1993.

123. Matteson EL, Hickey AR, Maguire L, et al: Occurrence of neoplasia in patients with rheumatoid arthritis enrolled in a DMARD Registry: Rheumatoid Arthritis Azathioprine Registry Steering Committee. J Rheumatol 18:809, 1991.

124. Kamel OW, Holly EA, van de Rijn M, et al: A population based, case control study of non-Hodgkin's lymphoma in patients with rheumatoid arthritis. J Rheumatol 26:1676, 1999.

125. Cibere J, Sibley J, Haga M: Rheumatoid arthritis and the risk of malignancy. Arthritis Rheum 40:1580, 1997.

126. Gridley G, Klippel JH, Hoover RN, Fraumeni JF Jr.: Incidence of cancer among men with the Felty syndrome. Ann Intern Med 120:35, 1994.

127. Kelly C, Sykes H: Rheumatoid arthritis, malignancy, and paraproteins. Ann Rheum Dis 49:657, 1990.

128. Kelly CA: Paraproteins in rheumatoid arthritis and related disorders. Int J Clin Lab Res 21:288, 1992.

129. Kelly CA, Baird G, Foster H, et al: Prognostic significance of paraproteinaemia in rheumatoid arthritis. Ann Rheum Dis 50:290, 1991.

130. Georgescu L, Quinn GC, Schwartzman S, Paget SA: Lymphoma in patients with rheumatoid arthritis: Association with the disease state or methotrexate treatment. Semin Arthritis Rheum 26:794, 1997.

131. Mariette X, Cazals-Hatem D, Warszawki J, et al: Lymphomas in rheumatoid arthritis patients treated with methotrexate: a 3-year prospective study in France. Blood 99:3909, 2002.

132. Starkebaum G: Rheumatoid arthritis, methotrexate, and lymphoma: risk substitution, or cat and mouse with Epstein-Barr virus? J Rheumatol 28:2573, 2001.

133. Pettersson T, Pukkala E, Teppo L, Friman C: Increased risk of cancer in patients with systemic lupus erythematosus. Ann Rheum Dis 51:437, 1992.

134. Canoso JJ, Cohen AS: Malignancy in a series of 70 patients with systemic lupus erythematosus. Arthritis Rheum 17:383, 1974.

135. Lewis RB, Castor CW, Knisley RE, Bole GG: Frequency of neoplasia in systemic lupus erythematosus and rheumatoid arthritis. Arthritis Rheum 19:1256, 1976.

136. Green JA, Dawson AA, Walker W: Systemic lupus erythematosus and lymphoma. Lancet 2(8093):753, 1978.

137. Menon S, Snaith ML, Isenberg DA: The association of malignancy with SLE: An analysis of 150 patients under long-term review. Lupus 2:177, 1993.

138. Lopez Dupla M, Khamashta M, Pintado Garcia V, et al: Malignancy in systemic lupus erythematosus: A report of five cases in a series of 96 patients. Lupus 2:377, 1993.

139. Sulkes A, Naparstek Y: The infrequent association of systemic lupus erythematosus and solid tumors. Cancer 68:1389, 1991.

140. Ramsey-Goldman R, Mattai SA, Schilling E, et al: Increased risk of malignancy in patients with systemic lupus erythematosus. J Invest Med 46:217, 1998.

141. Mellemkjaer L, Andersen V, Linet MS, et al: Non-Hodgkin's lymphoma and other cancers among a cohort of patients with systemic lupus erythematosus. Arthritis Rheum 40:761, 1997.

142. Bjornadal L, Lofstrom B, Yin L, et al: Increased cancer incidence in a Swedish cohort of patients with systemic lupus erythematosus. Scand J Rheumatol 31:66, 2002.

143. Sweeney DM, Manzi S, Janosky J, et al: Risk of malignancy in women with systemic lupus erythematosus. J Rheumatol 22:1478, 1995.

144. Abu-Shakra M, Gladman DD, Urowitz MB: Malignancy in systemic lupus erythematosus. Arthritis Rheum 39:1050, 1996.

145. Nived O, Bengtsson A, Jonsen A, et al: Malignancies during follow-up in an epidemiologically defined systemic lupus erythematosus inception cohort in southern Sweden. Lupus 10:500, 2001.

146. Sultan SM, Ioannou Y, Isenberg A: Is there an association of malignancy with systemic lupus erythematosus? An analysis of 276 patients under long-term review. Rheumatology 39:1147, 2000.

147. Ramsey-Goldman R, Clarke AE: Double trouble: are lupus and malignancy associated? Lupus 10:388, 2001.

148. Bernatsky S, Clarke A, Ramsey-Goldman R: Malignancy and systemic lupus erythematosus. Curr Rheum Reports 4:351, 2002.

149. Bernatsky S, Boivin J, Clarke A, Rajan R: Cancer risk in SLE: a meta-analysis. Arthritis Rheum 44:S244 2001.
150. Xu Y, Wiernik PH: Systemic lupus erythematosus and B-cell hematologic neoplasm. Lupus 10:841, 2001.
151. Roumm AD, Medsger TA Jr.: Cancer and systemic sclerosis: An epidemiologic study. Arthritis Rheum 28:1336, 1985.
152. Abu-Shakra M, Guillemin F, Lee P: Cancer in systemic sclerosis. Arthritis Rheum 36:460, 1993.
153. Rosenthal AK, McLaughlin JK, Linet MS, Persson I: Scleroderma and malignancy: An epidemiological study. Ann Rheum Dis 52:531, 1993.
154. Higuchi M, Horiuchi T, Ishibashi N, et al: Anticentromere antibody as a risk factor for cancer in patients with systemic sclerosis. Clin Rheumatol 19:123, 2000.
155. Hesselstrand R, Scheja A, Akesson A: Mortality and causes of death in a Swedish series of systemic sclerosis patients. Ann Rheum Dis 57:682, 1998.
156. Rosenthal AK, McLaughlin JK, Gridley G, Nyren O: Incidence of cancer among patients with systemic sclerosis. Cancer 76:910, 1995.
157. Rosier RN, Konski A, Boros L: Bone tumors. In Rubin P (ed): Clinical Oncology: A Multidisciplinary Approach for Physicians and Students, 7th ed. Philadelphia, WB Saunders, 1993, pp 509-530.
158. Arndt CA, Crist WM: Common musculoskeletal tumors of childhood and adolescence. N Engl J Med 341:342, 1999.
159. Hadjipavlou A, Lander P, Srolovitz H, Enker IP: Malignant transformation in Paget's disease of bone. Cancer 70:2802, 1992.
160. Rosier RN, Constine LS III: Soft tissue sarcoma. In Rubin P (ed): Clinical Oncology: A Multidisciplinary Approach for Physicians and Students, 7th ed. Philadelphia, WB Saunders, 1993, pp 487-507.
161. Spjut, HJ, Dorfman, HD, Fechner RE, Ackerman LV: Tumors of Bone and Cartilage. Washington, DC, Armed Forces Institute of Pathology, 1983.
162. Mirra JM: Bone Tumors: Diagnosis and Treatment. Philadelphia, JB Lippincott, 1989.
163. Patt RB: Basic and advanced methods of pain control. In Rubin P (ed): Clinical Oncology: A Multidisciplinary Approach for Physicians and Students, 7th ed. Philadelphia, WB Saunders, 1993, pp 709-733.
164. Murray GC, Persellin RH: Metastatic carcinoma presenting as monarticular arthritis: A case report and review of the literature. Arthritis Rheum 23:95, 1980.
165. Dunne C, Illidge T: Arthritis and carcinoma. Ann Rheum Dis 52:86, 1993.
166. Raderer M, Scheithauer W: Postchemotherapy rheumatism following adjuvant therapy for ovarian cancer. Scand J Rheumatol 23:291-292, 1994.
167. Loprinzi CL, Duffy J, Ingle JN: Postchemotherapy rheumatism. J Clin Oncol 11:768-770, 1993.
168. Creamer P, Lim K, George E, Dieppe P: Acute inflammatory polyarthritis in association with tamoxifen. Br J Rheumatol 33:583-585, 1994.
169. Warner E, Keshavjee al-N, Shupak R, Bellini A: Rheumatic symptoms following adjuvant therapy for breast cancer. Am J Clin Oncol 20:322, 1997.
170. Passos de Souza E, Evangelista Segundo PT, Jose FF, et al: Rheumatoid arthritis induced by alpha-interferon therapy. Clin Rheumatol 20:297, 2001.
171. Wandl UB, Nagel-Hiemke M, May D, et al: Lupus like autoimmune disease induced by interferon therapy for myeloproliferative disorders. Clin Immunol Immunopathol 65:70, 1992.
172. Ronnblom LE, Alm-GV, Oberg KE: Autoimmunity after alpha-interferon therapy for malignant carcinoid. Ann Intern Med 115:178, 1991.
173. Thomas LB, Forkner CE, Frei E III, et al: The skeletal lesions of acute leukemia. Cancer 14:608, 1961.
174. Rennie JAN, Auchterlonie IA: Leukaemias and GVH disease. Baillieres Clin Rheumatol 5:231, 1991.
175. Silverstein MN, Kelly P: Leukemia with osteoarticular symptoms and signs. Ann Intern Med 59:637, 1963.
176. Spilberg I, Meyer GJ: The arthritis of leukemia. Arthritis Rheum 15:630, 1972.
177. Gur H, Koren V, Ehrenfeld M, Sidi Y. Rheumatic manifestations preceding adult acute leukemia: Characteristics and implication on course and prognosis. Acta Haematol 101:1, 1999.
178. Kai T, Ishii E, Matsuzaki A, et al: Clinical and prognostic implications of bone lesions in childhood leukemia at diagnosis. Leuk Lymphoma 23:119, 1996.
179. Lacy MZ, Gertz MA, Hanson CA, et al: Multiple myeloma associated with diffuse osteosclerotic bone lesions: A clinical entity distinct from osteosclerotic myeloma (POEMS syndrome). Am J Hematol 56:288, 1997.
180. Roux S, Fermand JP, Brechignac S, et al: Tumoral joint involvement in multiple myeloma and Waldenström's macroglobulinemia: report of 4 cases. J Rheumatol 23:2175, 1996.
181. Terpos E, Angelopoulou MK, Variami E, et al: Sjögren's syndrome associated with multiple myeloma. Ann Hematol 79:449, 2000.
182. Fadilah SA, Cheong SK: Multiple myeloma presenting as Sjögren's syndrome. Am J Hematol 61:217, 1999.
183. Hermaszewski RA, Ratnavel RC, Denman DJ, et al: Immunodeficiency and lymphoproliferative disorders. Baillieres Clin Rheumatol 5:277, 1991.
184. Falcini F, Bardare M, Cimaz R, et al: Arthritis as a presenting feature of non-Hodgkin's lymphoma. Arch Dis Child 78:367, 1998.
185. Nishiya K, Tanaka Y: Co-existence of non-Hodgkin's lymphoma in the leukemic phase and polyarthritis simulating rheumatoid arthritis. Intern Med 36:227, 1997.
186. Dorfman HD, Siegel HL, Perry MC, Oxenhandler R: Non-Hodgkin's lymphoma of the synovium simulating rheumatoid arthritis. Arthritis Rheum 30:155, 1987.
187. Davies PG, Fordham JN: Arthritis and angioimmunoblastic lymphadenopathy. Ann Rheum Dis 42:516, 1983.
188. Layton MA, Musgrove C, Dawes PT: Polyarthritis, rash and lymphadenopathy: Case reports of two patients with angioimmunoblastic lymphadenopathy presenting to a rheumatology clinic. Clin Rheumatol 17:148, 1998.
189. von Kempis J, Kohler G, Herbst FW, Peter HH: Intravascular lymphoma presenting as symmetric polyarthritis. Arthritis Rheum 41:1126, 1998.
190. Tichelli A, Duell T, Weill M, et al: Late-onset keratoconjunctivitis sicca syndrome after bone marrow transplantation: incidence and risk factors—European Group or Blood and Marrow Transplantation (EBMT) Working Party on Late Effects. Bone Marrow Transplant 17:1105, 1996.
191. Asten P, Barrett J, Symmons D: Risk of developing certain malignancies is related to duration of immunosuppressive drug exposure in patients with rheumatic diseases. J Rheumatol 26:1705, 1999.
192. Baltus JA, Boersma JW, Hartman AP, Vandenbroucke JP: The occurrence of malignancies in patients with rheumatoid arthritis treated with cyclophosphamide: A controlled retrospective follow-up. Ann Rheum Dis 42:368, 1983.
193. Kinlen LJ: Incidence of cancer in rheumatoid arthritis and other disorders after immunosuppressive treatment. Am J Med 21(78):44, 1985.
194. Radis CD, Kahl LE, Baker GL, et al: Effects of cyclophosphamide on the development of malignancy and on long-term survival of patients with rheumatoid arthritis: A 20-year follow-up study. Arthritis Rheum 38:1120, 1995.
195. Beauparlant P, Papp K, Haraoui B: The incidence of cancer associated with the treatment of rheumatoid arthritis. Semin Arthritis Rheum 29:148, 1999.
196. Wolfe F, Hawley DJ, Pincus T: Methotrexate alters the course of rheumatoid arthritis (RA). Increased survival of methotrexate-treated RA patients: A 25-year study of 1,842 patients. Arthritis Rheum 41(Suppl S188):9, 1998.
197. Liote F, Pertuiset E, Cochand-Priollet B, et al: Methotrexate-related B lymphoproliferative disease in a patient with rheumatoid arthritis: Role of Epstein-Barr virus infection. J Rheumatol 22:1174, 1995.
198. Bachman TR, Sawitzke AD, Perkins SL, et al: Methotrexate-associated lymphoma in patients with rheumatoid arthritis: Report of two cases. Arthritis Rheum 39:325, 1996.
199. Sibilia J, Liote F, Mariette X: Lymphoproliferative disorders in rheumatoid arthritis patients on low-dose methotrexate. Rev Rhum Engl Ed 65:267, 1998.

200. Natkunam Y, Elenitoba-Johnson KS, Kingma DW, Kamel OW: Epstein-Barr virus strain type and latent membrane protein 1 gene deletions in lymphomas in patients with rheumatic diseases. Arthritis Rheum 40:1152, 1997.

201. van Wanghe P, Dequeker J: Compliance and long-term effect of azathioprine in 65 rheumatoid arthritis cases. Ann Rheum Dis 41(Suppl 1):40, 1982.

202. Silman AJ, Petrie J, Hazleman B, Evans SJ: Lymphoproliferative cancer and other malignancy in patients with rheumatoid arthritis treated with azathioprine: a 20-year follow-up study. Ann Rheum Dis 47:988, 1988.

203. Pitt PI, Sultan AH, Malone M, et al: Association between azathioprine therapy and lymphoma in rheumatoid disease. J R Soc Med 80:428, 1987.

204. Vasquez S, Kavanaugh AF, Schneider NR, et al: Acute nonlymphocytic leukemia after treatment of systemic lupus erythematosus with immunosuppressive agents. J Rheumatol 19:1625, 1992.

205. Seidenfeld AM, Smythe HA, Ogryzlo MA, et al: Acute leukemia in rheumatoid arthritis treated with cytotoxic agents. J Rheumatol 11:586, 1984.

206. Zijlmans JM, van Rijthoven AW, Kluin PM, et al: Epstein-Barr virus–associated lymphoma in a patient with rheumatoid arthritis treated with cyclosporine. N Engl J Med 326:1363, 1992.

207. Arellano F, Krupp P: Malignancies in rheumatoid arthritis patients treated with cyclosporin A. Br J Rheumatol 32(Suppl 1):72, 1993.

208. van den Borne BE, Landewe RB, Houkes I, et al: No increased risk of malignancies and mortality in cyclosporin A–treated patients with rheumatoid arthritis. Arthritis Rheum 41:1930,1998.

209. Brown SL, Greene MH, Gershon SK, et al: Tumor necrosis factor antagonist therapy and lymphoma development. Arthritis Rheum 46(12):3151, 2002.

210. Darby SC, Doll R, Gill SK, et al: Long-term mortality after a single course with x-rays in patients treated for ankylosing spondylitis. Br J Cancer 55:179, 1987.

211. Weiss HA, Darby SC, Doll R: Cancer mortality following x-ray treatment for ankylosing spondylitis. Int J Cancer 59:327, 1994.

Familial Autoinflammatory Syndromes

ANNA SIMON · JOS W.M. VAN DER MEER · JOOST P.H. DRENTH

Definition

The familial autoinflammatory syndromes, often referred to as hereditary periodic fever syndromes, form a group of rare disorders with a common phenotype of lifelong, recurrent inflammatory episodes, with fever and usually accompanied by other inflammatory symptoms such as abdominal pain, diarrhea, rash or arthralgia, and separated by symptom-free intervals.[1] Between the fever episodes, patients feel healthy and function normally. Routine laboratory investigations during a fever attack invariably reveal a severe acute-phase response with a high erythrocyte sedimentation rate (ESR), leukocytosis, and high concentrations of acute-phase proteins such as C-reactive protein (CRP), serum amyloid A (SAA), and several proinflammatory cytokines. The episodes of fever come on without an obvious trigger, although some patients note a relationship to physical stimuli (exposure to cold), emotional stress, or with the menstrual cycle. They resolve spontaneously in days or weeks. Patients with periodic fever often go undiagnosed for years, generating a high level of discouragement and frustration for patients and physicians when no diagnosis is made.[2,3] The term *autoinflammatory*, coined by McDermott and colleages in 1999 for these disorders,[4] adequately describes the phenotype of recurrent, acute inflammatory responses. It is preferable to "autoimmune" in these cases, because autoimmune phenomena are not found.

Four distinct subtypes of hereditary periodic fever are recognized. Despite the common phenotype described previously, these genetically distinct subtypes can often be differentiated clinically by a number of specific characteristics, in particular by the mode of inheritance, age of onset, average duration of the fever episodes and the fever-free interval, geographic region of origin of the patient's family, and occurrence of long-term complications such as amyloidosis or deafness (Table 112–1, Fig. 112–1).

Since the end of the 1990s, when three of these subtypes were genetically characterized (the fourth followed in 2001), a positive diagnosis became possible instead of a diagnosis per exclusionem. However, a significant number of patients with periodic fever phenotypes exist who do not fit into this genetically based classification, probably representing additional (genetic) defects that can lead to periodic fevers. Another disappointment is the lack of efficacious therapy for these disorders. There is hope that further characterization of the distinct pathogenetic mechanisms in the near future will provide clues for treatment of these debilitating disorders.

In this chapter, we will describe the six major subtypes of familial autoinflammatory syndromes:

- Familial Mediterranean fever (FMF)
- Hyper–immunoglobulin D (IgD) and periodic fever syndrome (HIDS)
- Tumor necrosis factor (TNF)-receptor–associated periodic syndrome (TRAPS)
- Familial cold autoinflammatory syndrome (FCAS)
- Muckle-Wells syndrome (MWS)
- Chronic infantile neurologic cutaneous and articular syndrome (CINCA), which is known as the neonatal-onset multisystemic inflammatory disease (NOMID) in English literature

Recently, it has been proposed to include a number of other syndromes in the group of autoinflammatory disorders. These include Crohn's disease, Blau syndrome, and the inherited syndromes known as pyogenic sterile arthritis, pyoderma gangrenosum, and acne (PAPA syndrome).[5]

Differential Diagnosis

When a patient has had recurrent fever episodes for more than 2 years, it is increasingly unlikely that these are caused by an infection or a malignant disorder. The differential diagnosis at that time may include numerous inflammatory disorders such as juvenile rheumatoid arthritis (JRA), adult-onset Still's disease, inflammatory bowel disease (IBD), Blau syndrome, Schnitzler syndrome, and Behçet's disease, in addition to the hereditary periodic fever syndromes (Table 112–2). Because the hereditary syndromes are rare (except for FMF in people with a distinct ethnic background), the more common diagnoses should be excluded first.

The mainstay of the diagnosis of hereditary periodic fever is clinical assessment, with a detailed medical and family history, and preferably at least one observation of the patient during a fever episode, because physical examination of the patient in a period of remission is seldom abnormal. This clinical assessment will often yield enough information to build a differential diagnosis of the specific familial autoinflammatory syndromes (see Table 112–1). To make a specific diagnosis within the group of familial autoinflammatory syndromes is important.

TABLE 112-1 • DIFFERENTIAL DIAGNOSIS OF FAMILIAL AUTOINFLAMMATORY SYNDROMES

	Familial Mediterranean Fever (FMF)	Mevalonate Kinase Deficiencies			Tumor Necrosis Factor (TNF)-Receptor-Associated Periodic Syndrome (TRAPS)	Cryopyrin Diseases		
		Classic Hyper-Immunoglobulin D syndrome (HIDS)	Mevalonic Aciduria	Variant HIDS		Familial Cold Autoinflammatory Syndrome (FCAS)	Muckle-Wells Syndrome (MWS)	Chronic Infantile Neurologic Cutaneous and Articular Syndrome (CINCA)
Mode of inheritance	Autosomal recessive	Autosomal recessive	Autosomal recessive	?	Autosomal dominant	Autosomal dominant	Autosomal dominant	Autosomal dominant
Age at onset (yrs)	<20	<1	<1	<10	<20	<1	<20	<1
Duration of attack (days)*	<2	4-6	4-5	6-8	>14	<2	1-2	?
Cutaneous involvement	Erysipelas-like erythema	Maculopapular rash	Morbilliform rash	Maculopapular rash	Migratory rash, overlying area of myalgia	Cold-induced urticaria-like lesions	Urticaria-like rash	Urticaria-like lesions
Musculoskeletal involvement	Monoarthritis common	Arthralgia, occasional oligoarthritis	Arthralgia common	Arthralgia	Severe myalgia common; occasional frank monoarthritis	Arthralgia common; occasional mild myalgia	Lancing limb pain, arthralgia common; arthritis can occur	Epiphyseal bone formation
Abdominal involvement	Sterile peritonitis common	Splenomegaly, severe pain common	Splenomegaly, pain may occur	may occur	Severe pain very common	None	May occur	Hepatosplenomegaly
Eye involvement	Uncommon	Uncommon	Uncommon	Uncommon	Conjunctivitis and periorbital edema very common	Conjunctivitis	Conjunctivitis, sometimes optic nerve elevation	Papilledema with possible loss of vision, uveitis
Distinguishing clinical symptoms	Erysipelas-like erythema	Prominent cervical lymphadenopathy	Dysmorphic features, neurological symptoms	Lymphadenopathy may occur	Migratory nature of myalgia and rash, periorbital edema	Cold-induced urticaria-like lesions	Sensorineural hearing loss	Chronic aseptic meningitis, sensorineural hearing loss, arthropathy
Gene involved	MEFV	MVK	MVK	?	TNFRSF1A	CIAS1	CIAS1	CIAS1
Protein involved	Pyrin (marenostrin)	Mevalonate kinase	Mevalonate kinase	?	Type 1 TNF-receptor	Cryopyrin	Cryopyrin	Cryopyrin

*Duration may be variable; this is a typical duration.

Adapted from Hull KM, Shoham N, Chae JJ, et al: The expanding spectrum of systemic autoinflammatory disorders and their rheumatic manifestations. Curr Opin Rheumatol 15:61-69, 2003.

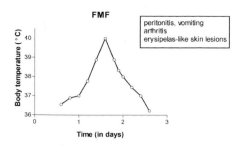

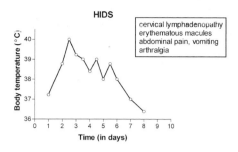

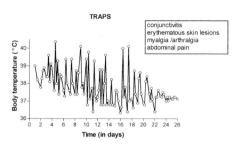

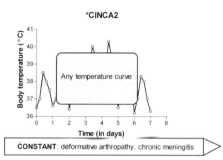

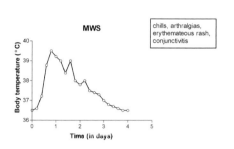

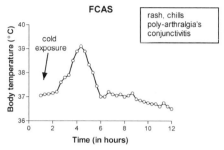

FIGURE 112–1 · Characteristic patterns of body temperature during inflammatory attacks in the familial autoinflammatory syndromes. However, there is considerable interindividual variability for each syndrome, and even for the individual patient, the fever pattern may vary greatly from episode to episode. Please note the different time scales on the x-axes.

■ Familial Mediterranean Fever

EPIDEMIOLOGY

FMF (Mendelian Inheritance in Men, (MIM) 249100) is the most prevalent disorder among the hereditary autoinflammatory syndromes, with more than 10,000 patients affected worldwide. It occurs primarily in people originating from the Mediter-ranean basin, including Armenians, Sephardic Jews, Arabs, and Turks. FMF is an autosomal recessively inherited disorder. Most families reported with an apparent autosomal dominant inheritance pattern of FMF[6] represent examples of pseudodominant inheritance due to consanguinity combined with the high carrier frequency of FMF mutations in certain populations[6-8]; however, at least three families studied do seem to show a true dominant inheritance, even after extensive genetic analysis.[8]

ETIOLOGY

In 1997, two groups independently traced the genetic background of FMF to a hitherto unknown gene on the short arm of chromosome 16, dubbed the MEditerranean FeVer (*MEFV*) gene. At least 67 disease-linked mutations in the *MEFV* gene have been described so far, most of which are clustered in the tenth exon of this gene. The majority are missense mutations that produce a single amino acid change in the protein (Fig. 112–2). There are

TABLE 112–2 · DIFFERENTIAL DIAGNOSIS OF PERIODIC FEVER

1. Hereditary (see Table 112–1)
2. Nonhereditary
   a. Infectious
      i. Hidden infectious focus (e.g., aorta-enteral fistula, Caroli syndrome)
      ii. Recurrent reinfection (e.g., chronic meningococcemia, host defense defect)
      iii. Specific infection (e.g., Whipple's disease, malaria)
   b. Noninfectious inflammatory disorder
      i. Adult-onset Still's disease
      ii. Juvenile chronic rheumatoid arthritis (RA)
      iii. Periodic fever, aphtous stomatitis, pharyngitis, and adenitis (PFAPA)
      iv. Schnitzler syndrome
      v. Behçet's syndrome
      vi. Crohn's disease
      vii. Sarcoidosis
      viii. Extrinsic alveolitis
      ix. Humidifier lung, polymere fume fever
   c. Neoplastic
      i. Lymphoma (e.g., Hodgkin's disease, angioimmunoblastic lymphoma [AILD])
      ii. Solid tumor (e.g., pheochromocytoma, myxoma, colon carcinoma)
   d. Vascular
      i. Recurrent pulmonary embolism
   e. Hypothalamic
   f. Psychogenic periodic fever[87]
   g. Factitious or fraudulent

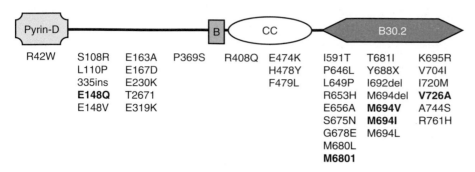

R42W	S108R	E163A	P369S	R408Q	E474K	I591T	T681I	K695R	
	L110P	E167D			H478Y	P646L	Y688X	V704I	
	335ins	E230K			F479L	L649P	I692del	I720M	
	E148Q	T2671				R653H	M694del	**V726A**	
	E148V	E319K				E656A	**M694V**	A744S	
						S675N	**M694I**	R761H	
						G678E	M694L		
						M680L			
						M6801			

FIGURE 112–2 • Schematic representation of pyrin (marenostrin) protein, with four conserved domains, including a pyrin domain, a coiled-coil domain, and a B30.2 domain. Indicated are the mutations as found in familial Mediter-ranean fever (FMF), with the five most common missense mutations in bold type.

six common mutations, accounting for almost 99 percent of all FMF chromosomes; these are M694V (occurring in 20 to 65% of cases, depending on the population examined[9]), V726A (in 7 to 35%), M680I, M694I, V694I, and E148Q. For the first three mutations mentioned here, a founder effect has been established,[10] pointing to common ancestors at least 2500 years ago. The high frequency of the mutated *MEFV* gene in more than one Middle Eastern population has led to the hypothesis that heterozygous carriers have an as-yet-unknown advantage, possibly a heightened (inflammatory) resistance to an as-yet-unidentified endemic pathogen of the Mediterranean basin.[10] The *MEFV* gene encodes for a protein of 781 amino acids, known as pyrin or marenostrin, which is expressed as a cytoplasmic protein in mature neutrophils and monocytes[11] in association with microtubules.[12] The expression of pyrin is induced by inflammatory mediators such as interferon-γ (IFN-γ) and TNF.[13] The pyrin domain is shared by a number of proteins involved in apoptosis and inflammation and is a member of the six-helix bundle death-domain superfamily that includes death domains, death-effector domains, and caspase-recruitment domains. Pyrin binds specifically to other proteins that contain a pyrin domain. There is increasing evidence for a function of pyrin as mediator of apoptosis.[14] Another hypothesis on pathogenesis of FMF implicates a specific inhibitor of chemotaxis, a serine protease that inactivates the complement factor C5a and interleukin-8 (IL-8), that can be found in peritoneal and synovial fluids.[14-16] It is thought that this inhibitor acts to prevent inappropriate inflammation.[15] Activity of this C5a-inhibitor was found greatly reduced in serosal fluid from FMF patients.[14,16] The hypothetic relationship between pyrin and C5a-inhibitor has not been established so far.

CLINICAL FEATURES

In approximately 90 percent of FMF patients, symptoms start before the age of 20 years.[17] The inflammatory attacks of FMF usually last only 1 to 3 days, and their frequency can be very variable. Two to 4 weeks is the most common interval (see Fig. 112–1). Fever is the principal symptom in FMF and is usually accompanied by symptoms of serositis (either peritonitis, pleuritis, or synovitis). Abdominal pain of 1 or 2 days' duration occurs in 95 percent of patients,[18] varying in severity from severe peritonitis resembling an acute abdomen to only mild abdominal pain without overt peritonitis.[19] Arthritis (rarely destructive) is often confined to one large joint, such as the knee, ankle, or wrist, and may also be the only symptom. Chest pain due to pleuritis is usually unilateral and associated with a friction rub or transient pleural effusion. Skin involvement occurs in

approximately 30 percent of patients, most often as erysipelas-like skin lesions on the shins or feet[20] (Fig. 112–3). Other, more uncommon, symptoms are pericarditis, occurring in less than 1 percent[21]; acute scrotal swelling and tenderness[22]; aseptic meningitis; and severe protracted myalgia, especially of the legs.

Recurrent attacks of peritonitis may lead to intra-abdominal or pelvic adhesions, resulting in complications such as small bowel obstruction or reduced fertility in female patients. Another serious long-term complication of FMF is Amyloid A (AA) amyloidosis, primarily in the kidneys but also in the gastrointestinal tract, liver, and spleen, and eventually in the heart, testes, and thyroid. The prevalence of amyloidosis is variable, especially according to the population, but is high in untreated patients. It is common among Sephardic Jews but rare in Ashkenazi Jews.[23]

EVALUATION AND MANAGEMENT

No specific biologic marker for FMF is available. During an inflammatory attack there will be a polymorphonu-

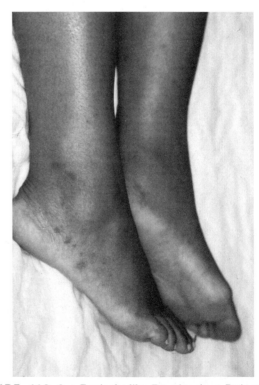

FIGURE 112–3 • Erysipelas-like Eruption in a Patient with a Familial Mediterranean Fever (FMF) Attack. (Picture courtesy of Professor A. Livneh, Heller Institute of Medical Research, Tel Hashomer, Israel.)

clear leukocytosis. Acute-phase reactants such as SAA, CRP, and plasma fibrinogen are elevated. Proteinuria in patients with FMF is highly suggestive of amyloidosis.[19]

FMF is a clinical diagnosis; there is a set of validated diagnostic criteria[24] (Table 112–3) with a reported sensitivity and specificity of 96 to 99 percent. However, this was validated in a population with a very high prevalence of FMF and low prevalence of the other autoinflammatory disorders, and it is not known whether these criteria also apply to other populations.[1]

Because the location of FMF mutations is known, it is possible to establish a molecular diagnosis of FMF.[1] Genetic laboratories usually screen for the five most common mutations, and those that are more rare will be missed. Furthermore, *MEFV* mutations occur on both alleles in only 70 percent of typical cases,[25] whereas in the remaining 30 percent, only one or no mutation can be detected, even after sequencing. There is also evidence of reduced penetrance. Despite these limitations, molecular testing can be used as a confirmatory test in cases in which there is a high index of suspicion. Whether or not the results are positive, treatment with colchicine is warranted in symptomatic cases fulfilling the diagnostic criteria.[26-29]

Fertility problems are encountered in FMF. For a variety of reasons, including peritoneal adhesions and ovulatory dysfunction, subfertility in women is not rare.[30] In men, subfertility due to azoospermia (sometimes secondary to testicular amyloidosis) or impairment of sperm penetration has been found.[31]

TREATMENT

Colchicine is the first-line of treatment for patients with FMF. Its efficacy was established in two controlled clinical trials in 1974.[28,29] Colchicine will prevent inflammatory attacks in 60 percent of patients, and it significantly reduces the number of attacks in an additional 20 to 30 percent.[17] The average dose in adults is 1 mg daily, but this may be increased to up to 3 mg in cases in which no response is seen at the lower dose. This regimen is usually well tolerated, and gastrointestinal side effects, including diarrhea or abdominal pain, will generally resolve with dose reduction. More serious side effects, such as myopathy, neuropathy and leukopenia, are rare and occur primarily in patients with renal or liver impairment. During a fever attack, oral or intramuscular nonsteroidal anti-inflammatory drugs (NSAIDs) can be used for pain relief. Glucocorticoids have limited efficacy.

Compliance with colchicine use is very important, because colchicine has been shown to prevent the occurrence of amyloidosis. Since the introduction of colchicine therapy, the incidence of amyloidosis in FMF has dropped dramatically, whereas in areas with a high prevalence of FMF where colchicine is not routinely available, such as Armenia, amyloidosis is still common.

Colchicine's principal effect at the cellular level is to depolymerize microtubules by interacting with tubulin, thereby inhibiting motility and exostosis of intracellular granules. Furthermore, it has a powerful antimitotic effect, causing metaphase arrest. Therefore, it has been speculated, in cases of infertility in patients treated with colchicine, that this medication causes azoospermia. However, colchicine does not have a significant adverse effect on sperm production or function.[32] Unfounded fear of teratogenic effects of colchicine often wrongly leads to cessation of this drug in young women who wish to get pregnant, with a subsequent increased frequency and severity of attacks, which enhances problems with fertility and pregnancy. Colchicine has proven safe, even in early pregnancy, and treatment should not be interrupted for this reason[30,33]; it can also be used while breast feeding.[31]

TABLE 112–3 · DIAGNOSTIC CRITERIA FOR DIAGNOSIS OF FAMILIAL MEDITERRANEAN FEVER*

Major Criteria
Typical attacks† with peritonitis (generalized)
Typical attacks with pleuritis (unilateral) or pericarditis
Typical attacks with monarthritis (hip, knee, ankle)
Typical attacks with fever alone
Incomplete abdominal attack

Minor Criteria
Incomplete attacks‡ involving chest pain
Incomplete attacks involving monarthritis
Exertional leg pain
Favorable response to colchicine

*Requirements for diagnosis of FMF are one or more major criteria or two or more minor criteria.
†Typical attacks are defined as recurrent (three or more of the same type), febrile (38° C or higher) and short (lasting between 12 hours and 3 days).
‡Incomplete attacks are defined as painful and recurrent attacks not fulfilling the criteria for a typical attack.
From Livneh A, Langevitz P, Zemer D, et al: Criteria for the diagnosis of familial Mediterranean fever. Arthritis Rheum 40:1879-1885, 1997.

Hyper–Immunoglobulin D Syndrome

EPIDEMIOLOGY

HIDS (MIM 260920) is also an autosomal recessively inherited disorder, but it is far less prevalent than FMF. The International Hyper-IgD Syndrome Registry, based in Nijmegen, the Netherlands, in which clinical information is actively collected from physicians worldwide, currently holds data on some 190 patients. More than 80 percent of these stem from Western Europe, and 55 percent originate from the Netherlands and France. Almost all of the HIDS patients are of Caucasian origin. These observations can, at least in part, be explained by a founder effect.[34] In the Netherlands, the carrier frequency of a hyper-IgD mutation is estimated to be 1:530[34a]. There are equal numbers of men and women affected. Based on the genotype and phenotype, we now distinguish classic HIDS and variant HIDS.[35]

ETIOLOGY

HIDS in its classic form is caused by mutations in the gene encoding for the enzyme mevalonate kinase, located on the long arm of chromosome 12.[35-37] Mevalonate kinase is part of the isoprenoid pathway; it is involved in the next step after 3'5'-hydroxy methyl glutaryl coenzyme A (HMG CoA) reductase by phosphorylating mevalonic acid. The isoprenoid pathway has a number of very diverse end products that include cholesterol, dolichol, and ubiquinone, and it also leads to isoprenylation of proteins, a post-translational modification directing these proteins, such as Rho and Ras, to the cell membrane.[38]

Patients with classic HIDS are most often compound heterozygotes for two different missense mutations in the mevalonate kinase gene (Fig. 112–4). Two mutations (leading to a valine-to-isoleucine change, V377I, and to a isoleucine-tyrosine change, I268T) account for more than 85 percent of the patients described to date.[38,39] The mutations lead to a constantly diminished activity of mevalonate kinase to about 5 to 15 percent of normal levels, and these drop even further during a fever attack.[40]

Because of this reduced enzyme activity, the substrate mevalonic acid accumulates in serum and urine. Higher levels are found during the episodes of fever. There does not appear to be a dramatic shortage of any specific end product; concentrations of cholesterol, ubiquinone, and dolichol in patients are normal to low-normal. How this metabolic defect in the isoprenoid pathway leads to the inflammatory phenotype of HIDS is still unknown. The cause of the characteristic high serum concentrations of IgD in this syndrome, which have led to its name, are also still unexplained.

Another syndrome was already linked to mutations in the mevalonate kinase gene before the discovery of HIDS.[41] Mevalonic-aciduria patients carry specific mutations that cause a more severe reduction of mevalonate kinase enzyme activity, often reducing it to undetectable levels. These patients constantly produce large amounts of mevalonic acid and often have more than 1000 times as much mevalonic acid in their urine than do HIDS patients.[42] They also have a more severe phenotype, which will be described later. Evidence is emerging that mevalonic aciduria and HIDS are two extremes of a continuous spectrum of disease related to mevalonate kinase deficiency[42a].

Not all patients with HIDS appear to have an increased urinary excretion of mevalonic acid and a gene defect of mevalonate kinase. We have designated these patients as variant HIDS[35] (see Table 112–1).

CLINICAL FEATURES

Ninety percent of patients with classic HIDS will experience their first fever episode in the first year of life,[43] and these episodes will become most frequent in childhood and adolescence. The high fevers may lead to seizures, especially in young children. Vaccination, minor trauma, surgery, and physical or emotional stress are factors that provoke a fever episode, although often a triggering factor is not obvious. The fevers often begin with cold chills and a sharp rise in body temperature[1]. They are almost always accompanied by (cervical) lymphadenopathy and abdominal pain with vomiting and diarrhea. Other frequent symptoms are headache, myalgia, and arthralgia. Apart from the lymphadenopathy, physical signs frequently consist of splenomegaly and a skin rash with erythematous macules and papules (Fig. 112–5) or petechia[44] (Fig. 112–6). Sometimes there are also signs of frank arthritis (principally large joints) and hepatomegaly. About 40 percent of patients report painful aphthous ulcers in the mouth, vagina, or scrotum (Fig. 112–7). The fever will disappear spontaneously after 3 to 5 days, although it may take longer before the symptoms in joints or skin disappear completely. These inflammatory attacks occur, on average, once every 4 to 6 weeks, although this may be variable from patient to patient or in an individual patient. The phenotype of variant HIDS differs slightly from and is milder than that of classic HIDS.[35]

Patients with mevalonic aciduria, the metabolic disorder that is also caused by mevalonate kinase gene mutations, experience similar inflammatory episodes as HIDS patients, but these are often of lesser importance in comparison to the severity of the rest of the phenotype, which consists of psychomotor retardation, ataxia, failure to thrive, cataracts, and dysmorphic facies. These unfortunate patients usually die in early childhood.[42]

The long-term outcome in both classic and variant HIDS is relatively benign. No cases of amyloidosis have been reported in the literature, nor has this occurred in the 190 patients in the International Nijmegen HIDS registry since its initiation in 1992.[1] There is no excess mortality in this patient group. In many patients, the fever episodes occur less frequently and become less severe later in life. Joint destruction is extremely rare. Abdominal adhesions are frequently seen, resulting from repeated abdominal inflammation or (unnecessary) diagnostic laparotomy because of suspected acute abdomen.

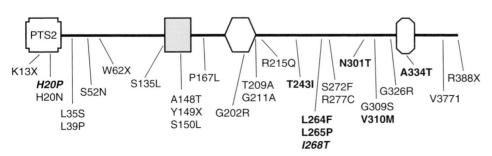

FIGURE 112–4 · Mevalonate kinase, with four conserved domains represented by colored boxes. Indicated are the missense mutations, nonsense mutations, and two deletions, which have been identified in mevalonate kinase deficiency. In bold are mutations found in mevalonic aciduria patients; in bold and italic are mutations found in both classic HIDS and mevalonic aciduria.

EVALUATION AND MANAGEMENT

HIDS is diagnosed based on a combination of characteristic clinical findings and continuously elevated IgD concentrations (more than 100 IU/ml) (Table 112–4). However, IgD values may be normal in very young patients (especially those less than 3 years old),[45] and persistently low levels have been reported in a small number of patients with typical clinical findings and the genotype for HIDS.[37] More than 80 percent of HIDS patients combine a high concentration of IgD with high IgA levels.[45,46] During fever attacks, a brisk acute-phase response is observed, including leukocytosis, high levels of SAA and CRP, and activation of the cytokine network.[47] The diagnosis of classic HIDS can be confirmed by DNA analysis of the mevalonate kinase gene. The best approach is to start with screening for the two most prevalent mutations, V377I and I268T. If this screening is negative but the clinical suspicion remains very high, sequencing of the entire gene can be considered. An alternative is the measurement of urinary mevalonic acid concentrations during an attack, which are slightly elevated. However, gas chromatography–mass spectroscopy is necessary to detect this slight increase.[48] The measurement of mevalonate kinase enzyme activity is complicated and time-consuming and should be reserved for research purposes.

TREATMENT

There is no good therapy for HIDS. Some individual patients have been reported to have benefited from treatment with corticosteroid, colchicine, intravenous

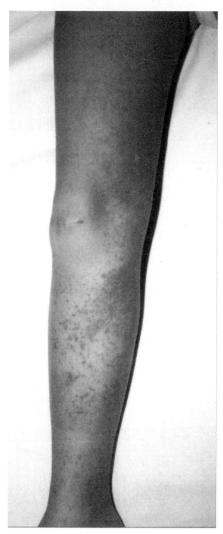

FIGURE 112–6 · Petechiae on the leg of a hyper–immunoglobulin D syndrome (HIDS) patient during a febrile attack.

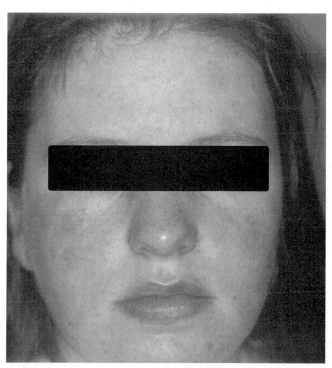

FIGURE 112–5 · Facial erythematous macules and papules in a hyper–immunoglobulin D syndrome (HIDS) patient during an attack.

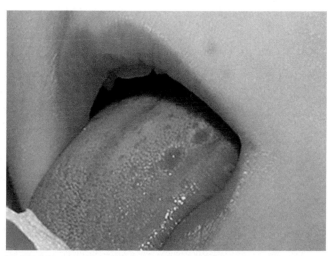

FIGURE 112–7 · Aphthous Ulceration Detected on the Tongue of a Patient with Hyper–Immunoglobulin D Syndrome (HIDS). (Picture courtesy of Dr. K. Antila, North Carelian Central Hospital, Joensuu, Finland.)

TABLE 112–4 • DIAGNOSTIC INDICATORS OF HYPER–IMMUNOGLOBULIN D SYNDROME (HIDS)

At Time of Attacks

Elevated erythrocyte sedimentation rate (ESR) and leukocytosis
Abrupt onset of fever (38.5° C or higher)
Recurrent attacks
Lymphadenopathy (cervical)
Abdominal distress (e.g., vomiting, diarrhea, pain)
Skin manifestations (e.g., erythematous macules and papules)
Arthralgias and arthritis
Splenomegaly

Constantly Present

Elevated immunoglobulin D (IgD) (100 units/ml or more)
  measured on two occasions at least 1 month apart*
Elevated IgA (2.6 g/L or more)

Classic HIDS Only

Mutations in mevalonate kinase gene
Decreased mevalonate kinase enzyme activity

*Extremely high serum concentrations of IgD are characteristic but not obligatory.

immunoglobulin (IVIg), or cyclosporine, but these results can not be repeated in the majority of patients.[43] Thalidomide did not have an effect on disease activity in a recent placebo-controlled trial.[49] Results of a double-blind, placebo-controlled trial we performed with the HMG-CoA reductase inhibitor simvastatin on a small group of HIDS patients indicate a beneficial effect of this drug, reducing the number of days illness in five out of six patients[49a].

Tumor Necrosis Factor Receptor–Associated Periodic Syndrome

EPIDEMIOLOGY

TRAPS (MIM 142680) has an autosomal dominant inheritance pattern. It was originally described in a large family from Irish and Scottish descent as "familial Hibernian fever."[50] It is primarily found in patients originating from northwestern Europe but has also been described in families from Australia, Mexico, Puerto Rico, Portugal, and the Czech Republic.[51] It is clear that any ethnic group may be affected. Other previous nomenclature for this syndrome includes "autosomal dominant familial periodic fever"[52] and "familial perireticular amyloidosis."[53]

ETIOLOGY

Mutations are found in the gene for the type I TNF-receptor (TNFRSF1A), which is located on the short arm of chromosome 12.[4] These are mainly single-nucleotide missense substitutions, located in exons 2, 3, and 4, which encode for the extracellular domain of TNFRSF1A. Many of these mutations disrupt one of the highly conserved cysteine residues involved in extracellular disulfide bonds of the 55-kD TNF receptor protein (Fig. 112–8). These mutations are supposed to be gain-of-function mutations, leading to increased TNF-α signaling through the TNF-receptor. TNF-α is a pleiotropic molecule, which induces cytokine secretion, activation of leukocytes, fever, and cachexia.[54] Activation of the receptor by TNF-α causes cleavage and shedding of its extracellular part into the circulation, where it acts as an inhibitor of TNF-α. It has been suggested that the muta-

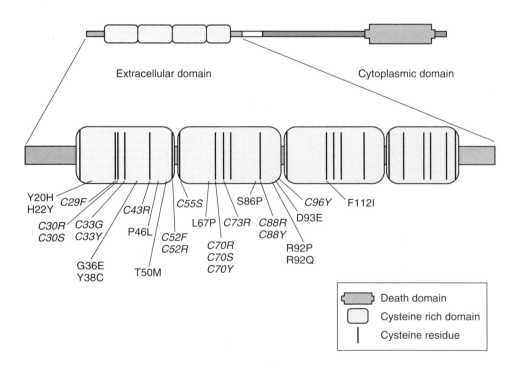

FIGURE 112–8 · Schematic representation of the tumor necrosis factor (TNF)-receptor type 1 protein (*TNFRSF1A*), depicting all mutations found in TNF-receptor–associated periodic syndrome (TRAPS) up to this time (except for one intron mutation affecting a splice site). Mutations disrupting cysteine residues are in blue italics.

tions in the TNFRSF1A found in TRAPS interfere with receptor shedding, leading to continuous TNF-α signaling and, hence, uncontrolled inflammation. An in vitro shedding defect has been demonstrated in the case of a number of TRAPS mutations, but not in all of them.[4,55] Also, serum concentrations of the shedded soluble TNFRSF1A in TRAPS patients during periods without symptoms are often found to be significantly reduced compared to normal subjects,[51,55,56] but not in all cases. Thus, the hypothesis of reduced shedding, although attractive by its simplicity, is not supported as the sole cause of the fever attacks in TRAPS, and additional mechanisms seem to be at work.

There are some general genotype-phenotype correlations, especially when mutations are grouped in cysteine and noncysteine mutations. Noncysteine mutations have, overall, a lower penetrance than cysteine mutations, and amyloidosis is seen far more often in association with cysteine mutations.[55] Two missense mutations in TNFRSF1A, P46L and R92Q, have a particularly low penetrance and are found in approximately 1 percent of control chromosomes.[55] Interestingly, R92Q has been observed in higher prevalence in, for example, a group of patients with arthritis. It is thought that the clinical manifestations of patients with an R92Q mutation depend on other so-far-unidentified modifying genes, environmental factors, or both.[55,55]

CLINICAL FEATURES

The clinical features can vary much more between individual TRAPS patients than is generally seen in FMF or HIDS.[51] The age of onset can be variable, even within the same family, with a documented range of 2 weeks to 53 years of age.[51,57] There is also a large variation in duration and frequency of the fever episodes in TRAPS. On average, attacks last 3 to 4 weeks and recur 2 to 6 times each year, but episodes may also be limited to a few days (see Fig. 112–1). Although the index patient, through whom the diagnosis is made, often displays well-defined inflammatory attacks, affected family members may suffer from less-typical symptoms, such as episodic mild arthritis.

During inflammatory attacks, a high, spiking fever can be accompanied by skin lesions, myalgia and arthralgia, abdominal distress, and ocular symptoms. The most common cutaneous manifestation is a centrifugal, migratory, erythematous patch, which may overlie a local area of myalgia[58] (Fig. 112–9), but urticarial plaques may also be seen. Myalgia is often located primarily in the muscles of the thighs, but it may also migrate during the fever episode, affecting all of the limbs, as well as the torso, face, and neck.[51] Arthralgia primarily affects large joints, including hips, knees, and ankles. Frank synovitis is more rare, and when it does occur it is nonerosive, asymmetric, and monoarticular.[51] Abdominal pain occurs in 92 percent of TRAPS patients during inflammatory attacks; other gastrointestinal symptoms often seen include vomiting and constipation. Ocular involvement is characteristic in TRAPS, and it may involve conjunctivitis, periorbital edema, or periorbital pain in one or both eyes. Severe

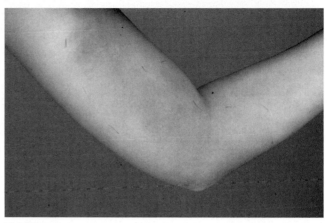

FIGURE 112–9 · Migrating erythematous rash during a tumor necrosis factor–receptor–associated periodic syndrome (TRAPS) attack. (Picture courtesy of Dr. T. Fiselier, University Medical Center St. Radboud, Nijmegen, The Netherlands.)

uveitis and iritis has been described, and any TRAPS patient with ocular pain should be examined for these complications.[51,58] Other less frequently observed symptoms during fever attacks in TRAPS are chest pain, breathlessness, pericarditis, and testicular and scrotal pain, which may be caused by inflammation of the tunica vaginalis.[51,57] It has been suggested from observation in one of the first families with TRAPS that this disorder is associated with an increased incidence of indirect inguinal hernias,[56] but this has not been demonstrated in other patients. Lymphadenopathy is rare in TRAPS.

Reactive AA amyloidosis is the principal systemic complication of TRAPS. It occurs in about 15 to 25 percent of patients[55,59] and generally leads to renal impairment. Amyloidosis in a patient with TRAPS places other affected family members at high risk for this complication. It is principally associated with TNFRSF1A mutations affecting cysteine residues.[55]

EVALUATION AND MANAGEMENT

As in the other familial autoinflammatory syndromes, laboratory investigations during inflammatory attacks show a clear acute-phase response, and again, even in between fever attacks, such an inflammatory response may be measured. Autoantibodies are generally not detected in TRAPS. The IgD level may be elevated, but the value is almost always less than 100 IU/ml.[56,57] Most patients exhibit a significantly lower concentration of soluble TNFRSF1A, most prominently in symptom-free intervals, compared to appropriate controls,[56] although this does not appear to be a universal rule.[51] Also, because soluble TNFRSF1A is cleared by the kidneys, TRAPS patients with renal insufficiency (e.g., due to renal amyloidosis) may have normal or elevated plasma concentrations of this protein.[60]

A set of clinical diagnostic criteria was proposed by Hull and colleagues[51] as indicators of TRAPS (Table 112–5). These are not validated by epidemiologic measures but may be used as a first step in evaluation of

TABLE 112–5 • DIAGNOSTIC INDICATORS OF TUMOR NECROSIS FACTOR (TNF) RECEPTOR–ASSOCIATED PERIODIC SYNDROME (TRAPS)

1. Recurrent episodes of inflammatory symptoms spanning a period of more than 6 months' duration (several symptoms generally will occur simultaneously)
   a. Fever
   b. Abdominal pain
   c. Myalgia (migratory)
   d. Rash (erythematous macular rash occurs with myalgia)
   e. Conjunctivitis or periorbital edema
   f. Chest pain
   g. Arthralgia or monoarticular synovitis
2. Episodes last more than 5 days on average (although variable)
3. Responsive to glucocorticosteroids but not colchicine
4. Affects family members in autosomal dominant pattern (although may not always be present)
5. Any ethnicity may be affected

From Hull KM, Drewe E, Aksentijevich I, et al: The TNF receptor-associated periodic syndrome (TRAPS): emerging concepts of an autoinflammatory disorder. Medicine (Baltimore) 81:349-368, 2002.

patients. TRAPS is ultimately a genetic diagnosis, defined by a missense mutation in the gene for TNFRSF1A. However, it must be borne in mind that clinical penetrance of TRAPS mutations is not 100 percent, even for cysteine mutations, and asymptomatic carriers are not uncommon.

Because proteinuria is the initial manifestation of renal amyloidosis, it is advisable to screen urine samples from TRAPS patients regularly by dipstick examination, especially affected family members of a TRAPS patient with amyloidosis.

TREATMENT

Both NSAIDs and glucocorticoids in relatively high doses (more than 20 mg oral prednisone per day) are able to alleviate the symptoms of fever and inflammation in most TRAPS patients, although they do not alter the frequency of attacks. They can be used beneficially at times of attack, and glucocorticoids usually can be tapered in the course of 1 or 2 weeks, as tolerated. There is no response to colchicine or immunosuppressive drugs such as azathioprine, cyclosporine, thalidomide, or cyclophosphamide.[51]

With regard to the pathogenesis of TRAPS, intravenous (IV) infusion of a synthetic TNFRSF1A fusion protein was tried in one patient by Drewe and coworkers,[51] but this seemed to provoke a severe attack. Use of etanercept, a fusion product of TNFRSF1B (the receptor that is *not* defective) has been more successful.[51,55,61] A pilot study with twice-weekly administration of etanercept (25 mg for adults or 0.4 mg/kg for children) in nine TRAPS patients with various mutations revealed an overall 66-percent reponse rate as determined by decreased number of attacks over a 6-month period.[51] A similar regimen of etanercept reversed the nephrotic syndrome in a patient

with amyloidosis.[62] We have shown that use of etanercept (25 mg at the time of an attack) may abort the symptoms and induce a long-lasting remission.[60] Drewe and colleagues have described one patient whose symptoms were resistant to administration of etanercept, who responded favorably to use of oral sirolimus (4 to 6 mg daily).[60a] Infliximab, a monoclonal antibody against TNF, has been shown to be less effective than etanercept in TRAPS.[60a]

Muckle-Wells Syndrome, Familial Cold Autoinflammatory Syndrome, and Chronic Infantile Neurologic Cutaneous and Articular Syndrome

These three syndromes have all been traced to mutations in one common gene, but their phenotypes differ, at least to some degree. After the recognition of the genetic defect it became clear that there is considerable overlap between these three disorders. Most notably, families have been described with features of both MWS and FCAS.[63] It has been suggested that FCAS, MWS, and CINCA (or NOMID) appear to represent a spectrum of disease, with FCAS the mildest and CINCA the most severe form. Given their common genotype, they will be discussed under one heading here.

EPIDEMIOLOGY

All three are rare, autosomal dominantly inherited syndromes. Since its original description in 1940, FCAS has been described in some 20 published reports. Most articles describe large families from Europe and Northern America with extensive pedigrees, but sporadic cases have been described. There appears to be a founder effect in American families of Northern European extraction.[64] MWS was described for the first time in 1962, and has since been described in large families, although it does occur in isolated cases and small nuclear families. Most affected families come from France and the United Kingdom.[65] CINCA is rare and, to date, some 70 cases, and only a few families, have been described. Most patients stem from France and Argentina, but cases are also seen in other European countries and the United States.[66,67]

ETIOLOGY

The first indications that MWS and FCAS are allelic stem from early linkage studies demonstrating that both FCAS and MWS were linked to the same region on the long arm of chromosome 1 (1q44).[65,68] In 2001, the gene for FCAS and MWS was identified. In a large-scale, positional cloning effort using three families with FCAS and one family with MWS, missense mutations in a new gene were found. This gene, CIAS1 (synonyms are *NALP3* and *PYPAF*), encodes for a protein denoted as cryopyrin, which consists of three recognized protein domains, including an N-terminal pyrin domain, a central nucleotide binding site (NBS) domain, and a leucine-rich repeat domain.[69] The protein is predominantly expressed in granulocytes and monocytes. It has been shown that overexpressed cryopoyrin interacts with apoptosis-associated specklike protein, activates nuclear factor kappa B (NFκB) and caspase 1, suggesting a proinflammatory effect. Later studies demonstrated that CIAS1 mutations were also associated with CINCA.[67,70] All mutations ascertained so far can be found in exon 3 of the CIAS1 gene, which encodes the NBS domain of crypopyrin, lending support to the suggestion that this domain is crucial in cryopyrin function. So far, 21 missense mutations have been identified in these three disorders.[71] Some mutations occur in MWS as well as in FCAS (R260W) or in both MWS and CINCA (D303N) [67] (Fig. 112–10).

CLINICAL FEATURES

Familial Cold Autoinflammatory Syndrome

FCAS (MIM 120100) is characterized by episodes of rash, fever, and arthralgia after generalized exposure to cold (see Fig. 112–1). The disease occurs in large families as an autosomal dominant inherited disorder with an almost complete penetrance.[64] The rash usually starts on the exposed extremities and, in most episodes, extends to the remainder of the body. It consists of erythematous macules and plaques (Figs. 112–11 and 112–12), urticarial lesions, and sometimes petechiae[72] and can cause a burning or itchy sensation. In some cases, localized edematous swelling of extremities is reported. The arthralgias, present in 93 percent of cases, most often affect the hands, knees, and ankles but can also involve feet, wrists, and elbows.[73] Frank arthritis is not seen. The majority of patients (84%) also report conjunctivitis during a fever episode. Other symptoms can include myalgia, profuse sweating, drowsiness, headache, extreme thirst, and nausea.

A typical feature of FCAS is the requirement of cold exposure to trigger the symptoms. The delay between cold and onset of symptoms, as reported in a study by Hoffman and coworkers,[73] varied from 10 minutes to 8 hours. The subsequent fever attack can be variable in length, depending on the degree of cold exposure; generally it will last a few hours to a maximum of 3 days. These episodes start at an early age, with 95 percent of patients having had their first fever episode in the first year of life—60% even within the first days of life. The symptoms tend to become less severe with advancing age.[72] Type AA amyloidosis complicated by renal insufficiency has been described in three FCAS families.[73]

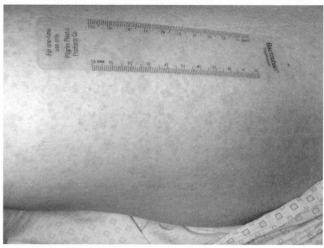

FIGURE 112–11 · Fine, confluent, erythematous macules on the upper leg of a patient with familial cold autoinflammatory syndrome (FCAS). (Picture courtesy of Dr. Johnstone, Medical College of Georgia, Augusta, Georgia, USA.)

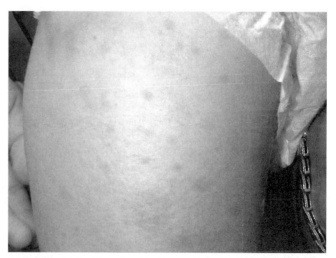

FIGURE 112–12 · Detail of upper leg with fine, confluent, erythematous macules in familial cold autoinflammatory syndrome (FCAS). (Picture courtesy of Dr. Johnstone, Medical College of Georgia, Augusta, Georgia, USA.)

Muckle-Wells Syndrome

MWS (MIM 191900) is a rare autosomal dominant inflammatory disorder with incomplete penetrance. Patients suffer from recurrent episodes of fever, abdominal pain, myalgia, urticarial rash (Figs. 112–13 and 112–14), and

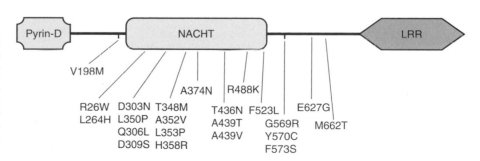

FIGURE 112–10 · Cryopyrin protein, containing an N-terminal pyrin domain, a nucleotide binding site (NACHT), and a leucine-rich repeat (LRR) domain. Indicated are the missense mutations identified in patients with familial cold autoinflammatory syndrome (FCAS), Muckle-Wells syndrome (MWS), or chronic infantile neurologic cutaneous and articular syndrome (CINCA), and mutations found in common in two or all of these clinical syndromes.

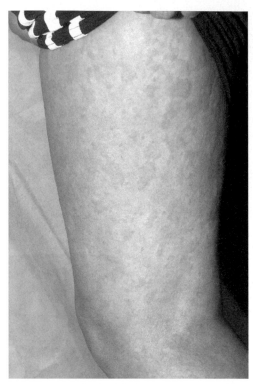

FIGURE 112-13 · Urticarial skin rash in a Muckle-Wells syndrome (MWS) patient. (Picture courtesy of Dr. D.L. Kastner, National Institute of Health, Bethesda, Maryland, USA.)

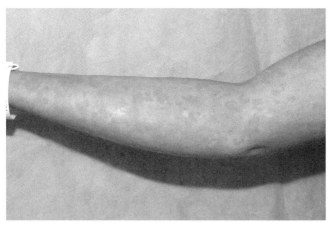

FIGURE 112-14 · Urticarial skin rash on the arm of a Muckle-Wells syndrome (MWS) patient. (Picture courtesy of Dr. D.L. Kastner, National Institute of Health, Bethesda, Maryland, USA.)

conjunctivitis, frequently accompanied by arthralgias, arthritis with limb pain, or both. Attacks start in adolescence and can be provoked by hunger, tiredness, and sometimes by exposure to cold.[74] The inflammatory episodes generally last 24 to 48 hours (see Fig. 112–1) and start with ill-defined malaise and transient chills and rigor, followed by aching or lancinating pains in the distal limbs and larger joints. Arthralgia is a common feature of the attacks, but synovitis of the large joints is less common.[75] The rash consists of usually aching and sometimes pruritic erythematous papules 1 to 7 cm in diameter. In a few cases

genital and buccal aphthous ulcers have been seen.[76] Ocular symptoms can include uveitis and conjunctivitis. Symptoms typically start in adolescence, although their debut at earlier age has been reported. Late-onset development of perceptive deafness is common in MWS. Bone involvement, such as clubbing of nails and pes cavus, can be seen as well. Most often, patients have a positive family history for the disease, which is indicative of autosomal dominant inheritance, but isolated cases have been reported. The most feared complication of the inflammatory attacks is type AA amyloidosis, which affects the kidneys first, leading to proteinuria and subsequent rapid progression to renal failure.

Chronic Infantile Neurologic Cutaneous and Articular Syndrome

CINCA (MIM 607115) is a rare congenital disorder defined by the presence of the triad of: 1) neonatal-onset skin lesions, 2) chronic aseptic meningitis, and 3) recurrent fever along with joint symptoms.[77] CINCA appears to be an autosomal dominant inherited disorder.[67] The key clinical feature of CINCA is a skin rash accompanied by peculiar joint manifestations and central nervous system (CNS) involvement. The symptoms in CINCA begin right after birth or in the first months of life with a generalized skin rash. The disease follows an unpredictable course with persistent nonpruritic and migratory rash with fever, hepatosplenomegaly, and lymphadenopathies. CNS involvement is not obvious from the outset, although occasional patients will present with seizures, spasticity, or transient episodes of hemiplegia. In the majority of patients there are signs of chronic persistent aseptic meningitis.[78] Cerebral-fluid analysis may show mild pleiocytosis, and there may be an increased intracranial pressure. Brain imaging shows mild ventricular dilatation, prominent sulci, and central atrophy and, in long-standing cases, calcifications of faulx and dura. In older children, headache is often a prominent feature as a sign of chronic meningitis. There is mental retardation in almost all cases. Progressive sensoneural impairment leading to high-frequency hearing loss can be seen in a minority. Ocular manifestations are prominent, with optic disk changes such as optic disk edema, pseudopapilledema, and optic atrophy, and anterior segment manifestations such as chronic anterior uveitis.[66] These symptoms may lead to visual impairment. Hoarseness, especially in older children, is typical. Joint and bone symptoms are a prominent feature of CINCA, and these present as bone inflammation, which gives rise to major arthropathies due to epiphyseal and metaphyseal disorganization. Growth-cartilage alterations, such as enlarged epiphyses and patellar overgrowth, can be an impressive feature of the disease (Figs. 112–15 and 112–16). Erosive changes occur, especially in the phalanges of hands and feet. There are typical dysmorphic features, such as frontal bossing and a saddle nose. These common physical features are the reason CINCA patients give the impression that (totally) unrelated patients are siblings. The prognosis of these patients is grave, as 20 percent die in childhood because of infections, vasculitis, and amyloidosis.[77]

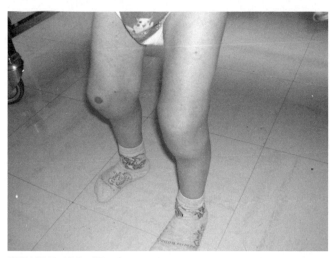

FIGURE 112–15 · Severe deformative arthropathy of the knees in a patient with chronic infantile neurologic cutaneous and articular syndrome (CINCA). (Picture courtesy of Dr. A.M. Prieur, Hôpital Necker-Enfants Malades, Paris, France.)

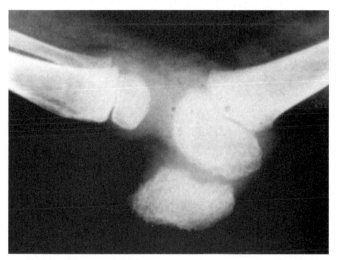

FIGURE 112–16 · Radiograph of the knee in a patient with chronic infantile neurologic cutaneous and articular syndrome (CINCA) showing greatly enlarged epiphyses and patella with punctate increased density. (Picture courtesy of Dr. A.M. Prieur, Hôpital Necker-Enfants Malades, Paris, France.)

EVALUATION AND MANAGEMENT

Again, most important for diagnosis are patient and family history (see Table 112–1). Hoffman and coworkers suggested a set of diagnostic criteria for FCAS[73] after studying six large families with this syndrome (Table 112–6), but these have not been validated in an independent cohort. Laboratory examination during a fever episode in FCAS, but also MWS and CINCA, will show an acute-phase response with polymorphonuclear leukocytosis and raised ESR, but this will not differentiate among the periodic fever disorders. Symptoms such as an urticarial rash after cold exposure highly favor a diagnosis of FCAS. The ice cube test (i.e., holding an ice cube to a patch of skin to provoke urticaria), which is diagnostic in acquired cold urticaria, is negative in FCAS. Typical facial

TABLE 112–6 · DIAGNOSTIC CRITERIA FOR FAMILIAL COLD AUTOINFLAMMATORY SYNDROME (FCAS)

1. Recurrent intermittent episodes of fever and rash that primarily follow generalized cold exposures
2. Autosomal dominant pattern of disease inheritance
3. Age of onset younger than 6 months
4. Duration of most attacks less than 24 hours
5. Presence of conjunctivitis associated with attacks
6. Absence of deafness, periorbital edema, lymphadenopathy, and serositis

From Hoffman HM, Wanderer AA, Broide DH: Familial cold autoinflammatory syndrome: phenotype and genotype of an autosomal dominant periodic fever. J Allergy Clin Immunol 108:615-620, 2001.

features, such as frontal bossing, and a long pediatric history, including chronic aseptic meningitis, will point to CINCA. There appears to be genetic heterogeneity in CINCA because not all patients have CIAS1 mutations.

TREATMENT

Treatment with Anakinra has emerged as beneficial for patients suffering from MWS and CINCA. No specific treatment can be offered for patients suffering from FCAS. In FCAS, some patients benefit from high-dose corticosteroids, and NSAIDs may be effective in selective cases.[73] Most effective is the avoidance of precipitating factors such as exposure to cold. In MWS, colchicine was effective in controlling arthritic events in one patient[79] but failed in other patients.[74,80] Oral corticosteroids may provide relief of skin and joint symptoms, but the role for azathioprine and cyclosporine is less clear.[74,81] CINCA is a chronic remitting disease, and whereas corticosteroids may have a beneficial effect on fever, pain, and general well-being, they will not induce a remission. NSAIDs, disease-modifying antirheumatic drugs (DMARDs), and cytotoxic drugs do not help.

Other Familial Autoinflammatory Syndromes

Two recent suggested additions to the group of familial autoinflammatory syndromes are Blau syndrome and PAPA syndrome.

BLAU SYNDROME

Blau syndrome (MIM 186580) is an autosomal dominant disorder characterized by recurrent granulomatous inflammation with a varying age of onset.[82] Typical granulomatous inflammations are acute anterior uveitis, arthritis, and skin rash; other symptoms include camptodactyly, cranial neuropathies, fever, and arteritis.[83] Blau syndrome is caused by mutations in the nucleotide-binding oligomerization domain z/caspase recruitment domain 15, (NOD2/CARD15) gene.[83,84] The NOD2/CARD15 protein is thought to have a function in regulation of apoptosis. Polymorphisms in the same NOD2/CARD15 gene on chromosome 16 are associated with a susceptibility to Crohn's disease[85]; the risk of developing Crohn's disease is increased up to 40-fold in persons homozygous for these polymorphisms. There are certainly some shared features between the two diseases: Both are characterized by granulomatous inflammation, and whereas bowel inflammation is not seen in Blau syndrome, Crohn's disease can present with uveitis, arthritis, and skin rash.

PYOGENIC STERILE ARTHRITIS, PYODERMA GANGRENOSUM, AND ACNE SYNDROME

PAPA syndrome (MIM 604416) is an autosomal dominant disorder first described by Lindor and colleagues.[86] The episodic inflammation in this syndrome leads to eventual destruction of joints, muscle, and skin. Wise and coworkers identified mutations in the CD2-binding protein 1 (CD2BP1) gene linked with PAPA syndrome.[5] CD2BP1 has a role in actin reorganization during cytoskeletal-mediated events and as such is hypothesized to have a functional relationship with pyrin.

■ Summary and Conclusion

The familial autoinflammatory syndromes are characterized by recurrent episodes of fever and inflammation. This group of disorders should be considered in a patient with a history of years of such inflammatory attacks with symptom-free intervals in between (except for CINCA, in which some symptoms and morphologic features will persist).

The discovery of the causative genes has had an enormous impact in the field of periodic fevers. This has been made possible only because of the accurate phenotypic characterization of patients with periodic fever. Careful analysis and proper clustering of these patients is indispensable to allow the elucidation of the genetic background, as well as the evaluation of possible treatment options. Central periodic fever registries have afforded the opportunity to appreciate previously unrecognized symptoms, to give insight into the long-term prognosis, and to allow better evaluation of drug regimens. Despite these efforts at classification, however, many periodic fever patients do not fall in one of the previously mentioned disease categories. It is to be expected that in the future other periodic fever syndromes and corresponding genes will be discovered.

REFERENCES

1. Drenth JPH, van der Meer JWM: Hereditary periodic fever. N Engl J Med 345:1748-1757, 2001.
2. Knockaert DC, Vanneste LJ, Bobbaers HJ: Recurrent or episodic fever of unknown origin: review of 45 cases and survey of the literature. Medicine (Baltimore) 72:184-196, 1993.
3. de Kleijn EM, Vandenbroucke JP, van der Meer JWM: Fever of unknown origin (FUO). I A. prospective multicenter study of 167 patients with FUO, using fixed epidemiologic entry criteria. The Netherlands FUO Study Group. Medicine (Baltimore) 76:392-400, 1997.
4. McDermott MF, Aksentijevich I, Galon J, et al: Germline mutations in the extracellular domains of the 55 kDa TNF receptor, TNFR1, define a family of dominantly inherited autoinflammatory syndromes. Cell 97:133-144, 1999.
5. Wise CA, Gillum JD, Seidman CE, et al: Mutations in CD2BP1 disrupt binding to PTP PEST and are responsible for PAPA syndrome, an autoinflammatory disorder. Hum Mol Genet 11:961-969, 2002.
6. Yuval Y, Hemo-Zisser M, Zemer D, et al: Dominant inheritance in two families with familial Mediterranean fever (FMF). Am J Med Genet 57:455-457, 1995.
7. Aksentijevich I, Torosyan Y, Samuels J, et al: Mutation and haplotype studies of familial Mediterranean fever reveal new ancestral relationships and evidence for a high carrier frequency with reduced penetrance in the Ashkenazi Jewish population. Am J Hum Genet 64:949-962, 1999.
8. Booth DR, Gillmore JD, Lachmann HJ, et al: The genetic basis of autosomal dominant familial Mediterranean fever. QJM 93:217-221, 2000.
9. Touitou I: The spectrum of familial Mediterranean fever (FMF) mutations. Eur J Hum Genet 9:473-483, 2001.
10. The International FMF Consortium: ancient missense mutations in a new member of the RoRet gene family are likely to cause familial Mediterranean fever. Cell 90:797-807, 1997.
11. Tidow N, Chen X, Muller C, et al: Hematopoietic-specific expression of MEFV, the gene mutated in familial Mediterranean fever, and subcellular localization of its corresponding protein, pyrin. Blood 95:1451-1455, 2000.
12. Mansfield E, Chae JJ, Komarow HD, et al: The familial Mediterranean fever protein, pyrin, associates with microtubules and colocalizes with actin filaments. Blood 98:851-859, 2001.
13. Centola M, Wood G, Frucht DM, et al: The gene for familial Mediterranean fever, MEFV, is expressed in early leukocyte development and is regulated in response to inflammatory mediators. Blood 95:3223-3231, 2000.
14. Richards N, Schaner P, Diaz A, et al: Interaction between pyrin and the apoptotic speck protein (ASC) modulates ASC-induced apoptosis. J Biol Chem 276:39320-39329, 2001.
15. Matzner Y, Abedat S, Shapiro E, et al: Expression of the familial Mediterranean fever gene and activity of the C5a inhibitor in human primary fibroblast cultures. Blood 96:727-731, 2000.
16. Matzner Y, Brzezinski A: C5a-inhibitor deficiency in peritoneal fluids from patients with familial Mediterranean fever. N Engl J Med 311:287-290, 1984.
17. Ben Chetrit E, Levy M: Familial Mediterranean fever. Lancet 351:659-664, 1998.
18. Sohar E, Gafni J, Pras M, Heller H: Familial Mediterranean fever: a survey of 470 cases and review of the literature. Am J Med 43:227-253, 1967.
19. Livneh A, Langevitz P: Diagnostic and treatment concerns in familial Mediterranean fever. Baillieres Best Pract Res Clin Rheumatol 14:477-498, 2000.
20. Majeed HA, Quabazard Z, Hijazi Z, et al: The cutaneous manifestations in children with familial Mediterranean fever (recurrent hereditary polyserositis): a six-year study. Q J Med 75:607-616, 1990.
21. Kees S, Langevitz P, Zemer D, et al: Attacks of pericarditis as a manifestation of familial Mediterranean fever (FMF). QJM 90:643-647, 1997.
22. Eshel G, Vinograd I, Barr J, Zemer D: Acute scrotal pain complicating familial Mediterranean fever in children. Br J Surg 81:894-896, 1994.
23. Grateau G: The relation between familial Mediterranean fever and amyloidosis. Curr Opin Rheumatol 12:61-64, 2000.
24. Livneh A, Langevitz P, Zemer D, et al: Criteria for the diagnosis of familial Mediterranean fever. Arthritis Rheum 40:1879-1885, 1997.
25. Chen X, Fischel-Ghodsian N, Cercek A, et al: Assessment of pyrin gene mutations in Turks with familial Mediterranean fever (FMF). Hum Mutat 11:456-460, 1998.
26. Livneh A, Langevitz P, Shinar Y, et al: MEFV mutation analysis in patients suffering from amyloidosis of familial Mediterranean fever. Amyloid 6:1-6, 1999.
27. Shohat M, Magal N, Shohat T, et al: Phenotype-genotype correlation in familial Mediterranean fever: evidence for an association between Met694Val and amyloidosis. Eur J Hum Genet 7:287-292, 1999.

28. Zemer D, Revach M, Pras M, et al: A controlled trial of colchicine in preventing attacks of familial mediterranean fever. N Engl J Med 291:932-934, 1974.

29. Dinarello CA, Wolff SM, Goldfinger SE, et al: Colchicine therapy for familial mediterranean fever: a double-blind trial. N Engl J Med 291:934-937, 1974.

30. Ehrenfeld M, Brzezinski A, Levy M, Eliakim M: Fertility and obstetric history in patients with familial Mediterranean fever on long-term colchicine therapy. Br J Obstet Gynaecol 94:1186-1191, 1987.

31. Ben Chetrit E, Levy M: Colchicine: 1998 update. Semin Arthritis Rheum 28:48-59, 1998.

32. Haimov-Kochman R, Ben Chetrit E: The effect of colchicine treatment on sperm production and function: a review. Hum Reprod 13:360-362, 1998.

33. Rabinovitch O, Zemer D, Kukia E, et al: Colchicine treatment in conception and pregnancy: two hundred thirty-one pregnancies in patients with familial Mediterranean fever. Am J Reprod Immunol 28:245-246, 1992.

34. Simon A, Mariman EC, van der Meer JWM, Drenth JPH: A founder effect in the hyperimmunoglobulinemia D and periodic fever syndrome. Am J Med 114:148-152, 2003.

34a. Houten SM, Van Woerden CS, Wijburg FA, et al: Carrier frequency of the V3771 (1129G>A) MVK mutation, associated with Hyper-IgD and periodic fever syndrome, in the Netherlands. Eur J Hum Genet 11(2): 196-200, 2003.

35. Simon A, Cuisset L, Vincent MF, et al: Molecular analysis of the mevalonate kinase gene in a cohort of patients with the hyper IgD and periodic fever syndrome: its application as a diagnostic tool. Ann Intern Med 135:338-343, 2001.

36. Drenth JPH, Cuisset L, Grateau G, et al: Mutations in the gene encoding mevalonate kinase cause hyper-IgD and periodic fever syndrome. International Hyper-IgD Study Group. Nat Genet 22:178-181, 1999.

37. Houten SM, Kuis W, Duran M, et al: Mutations in MVK, encoding mevalonate kinase, cause hyperimmunoglobulinaemia D and periodic fever syndrome. Nat Genet 22:175-177, 1999.

38. Houten SM, Wanders RJ, Waterham HR: Biochemical and genetic aspects of mevalonate kinase and its deficiency. Biochim Biophys Acta 1529:19-32, 2000.

39. Cuisset L, Drenth JPH, Simon A, et al: Molecular analysis of MVK mutations and enzymatic activity in hyper-IgD and periodic fever syndrome. Eur J Hum Genet 9:260-266, 2001.

40. Houten SM, Schneiders MS, Wanders RJA, Waterham HR: Regulation of isoprenoid/cholesterol biosynthesis in cells from mevalonate kinase-deficient patients. J Biol Chem 278:5736-5743, 2003.

41. Schafer BL, Bishop RW, Kratunis VJ, et al: Molecular cloning of human mevalonate kinase and identification of a missense mutation in the genetic disease mevalonic aciduria. J Biol Chem 267:13229-13238, 1992.

42. Hoffmann GF, Charpentier C, Mayatepek E, et al: Clinical and biochemical phenotype in 11 patients with mevalonic aciduria. Pediatrics 91:915-921, 1993.

42a. Simon A, Kremer HP, Wevers RA, et al. Mevalonate kinase deficiency: Evidence for a phenotypic continuum. Neurology 62(6):994-997, 2004.

43. Drenth JPH, Haagsma CJ, van der Meer JWM: Hyperimmunoglobulinemia D and periodic fever syndrome: the clinical spectrum in a series of 50 patients. International Hyper-IgD Study Group. Medicine (Baltimore) 73:133-144, 1994.

44. Drenth JP, Boom BW, Toonstra J, van der Meer JW: Cutaneous manifestations and histologic findings in the hyperimmunoglobulinemia D syndrome. International Hyper IgD Study Group. Arch Dermatol 130:59-65, 1994.

45. Haraldsson A, Weemaes CM, de Boer AW, et al: Immunological studies in the hyper-immunoglobulin D syndrome. J Clin Immunol 12:424-428, 1992.

46. Klasen IS, Goertz JH, van de Wiel GA, et al: Hyper-immunoglobulin A in the hyperimmunoglobulinemia D syndrome. Clin Diagn Lab Immunol 8:58-61, 2001.

47. Drenth JPH, van Deuren M, van der Ven-Jongekrijg J, et al: Cytokine activation during attacks of the hyperimmunoglobulinemia D and periodic fever syndrome. Blood 85:3586-3593, 1995.

48. Kelley RI, Herman GE: Inborn errors of sterol biosynthesis. Ann Rev Genomics Hum Genet 2:299-341, 2001.

49. Drenth JPH, Vonk AG, Simon A, et al: Limited efficacy of thalidomide in the treatment of febrile attacks of the hyper-IgD and periodic fever syndrome: a randomized, double-blind, placebo-controlled trial. J Pharmacol Exp Ther 298:1221-1226, 2001.

49a. Simon A, Drewe E, van der Meer JW, et al. Simvastatin treatment for inflammatory attacks of the hyperimmunoglobulinemia D and periodic fever syndrome. Clin Pharmacol Ther 75(5):476-483, 2004.

50. Williamson LM, Hull D, Mehta R, et al: Familial Hibernian fever. Q J Med 51:469-480, 1982.

51. Hull KM, Drewe E, Aksentijevich I, et al: The TNF receptor-associated periodic syndrome (TRAPS): emerging concepts of an autoinflammatory disorder. Medicine (Baltimore) 81:349-368, 2002.

52. Mulley J, Saar K, Hewitt G, et al: Gene localization for an autosomal dominant familial periodic fever to 12p13. Am J Hum Genet 62:884-889, 1998.

53. Bergman F, Warmenius S: Familial perireticular amyloidosis in a Swedish family. Am J Med 45:601-606, 1968.

54. Beutler B, Cerami A: Cachectin: more than a tumor necrosis factor. N Engl J Med 316:379-385, 1987.

55. Aksentijevich I, Galon J, Soares M, et al: The tumor-necrosis-factor receptor-associated periodic syndrome: new mutations in TNFRSF1A, ancestral origins, genotype-phenotype studies, and evidence for further genetic heterogeneity of periodic fevers. Am J Hum Genet 69:301-314, 2001.

56. McDermott EM, Smillie DM, Powell RJ: Clinical spectrum of familial Hibernian fever: a 14-year follow-up study of the index case and extended family. Mayo Clin Proc 72:806-817, 1997.

57. Dode C, Andre M, Bienvenu T, et al: The enlarging clinical, genetic, and population spectrum of tumor necrosis factor receptor-associated periodic syndrome. Arthritis Rheum 46:2181-2188, 2002.

58. Toro JR, Aksentijevich I, Hull K, et al: Tumor necrosis factor receptor-associated periodic syndrome: a novel syndrome with cutaneous manifestations. Arch Dermatol 136:1487-1494, 2000.

59. McDermott MF: Autosomal dominant recurrent fevers: clinical and genetic aspects. Rev Rhum Engl Ed 66:484-491, 1999.

60. Simon A, Dode C, van der Meer JWM, Drenth JPH: Familial periodic fever and amyloidosis due to a new mutation in the TNFRSF1A gene. Am J Med 110:313-316, 2001.

60a. Drewe E, Powell RJ. Novel treatment for tumour necrosis factor receptor associated periodic syndrome (TRAPS): case history of experience with infliximab and sirolimus post etanercept. Clin Exp Rheumatol 20(suppl. 26)(4):S71, 2002.

61. Simon A, van Deuren M, Tighe PJ, et al: Genetic analysis as a valuable key to diagnosis and treatment of periodic fever. Arch Intern Med 161:2491-2493, 2001.

62. Drewe E, McDermott EM, Powell RJ: Treatment of the nephrotic syndrome with etanercept in patients with the tumor necrosis factor receptor-associated periodic syndrome. N Engl J Med 343:1044-1045, 2000.

63. Aganna E, Martinon F, Hawkins PN, et al: Association of mutations in the NALP3/CIAS1/PYPAF1 gene with a broad phenotype including recurrent fever, cold sensitivity, sensorineural deafness, and AA amyloidosis. Arthritis Rheum 46:2445-2452, 2002.

64. Hoffman HM, Gregory SG, Mueller JL, et al: Fine structure mapping of CIAS1: identification of an ancestral haplotype and a common FCAS mutation, L353P. Hum Genet 112:209-216, 2003.

65. Cuisset L, Drenth JPH, Berthelot JM, et al: Genetic linkage of the Muckle-Wells syndrome to chromosome 1q44. Am J Hum Genet 65:1054-1059, 1999.

66. Dollfus H, Hafner R, Hofmann HM, et al: Chronic infantile neurological cutaneous and articular/neonatal onset multisystem inflammatory disease syndrome: ocular manifestations in a recently recognized chronic inflammatory disease of childhood. Arch Ophthalmol 118:1386-1392, 2000.

67. Aksentijevich I, Nowak M, Mallah M, et al: De novo CIAS1 mutations, cytokine activation, and evidence for genetic heterogeneity in patients with neonatal-onset multisystem inflammatory disease (NOMID): a new member of the expanding family of pyrin-associated autoinflammatory diseases. Arthritis Rheum 46:3340-3348, 2002.

68. Hoffman HM, Wright FA, Broide DH, et al: Identification of a locus on chromosome 1q44 for familial cold urticaria. Am J Hum Genet 66:1693-1698, 2000.

69. Hoffman HM, Mueller JL, Broide DH, et al: Mutation of a new gene encoding a putative pyrin-like protein causes familial cold autoinflammatory syndrome and Muckle-Wells syndrome. Nat Genet 29:301-305, 2001.

70. Feldmann J, Prieur AM, Quartier P, et al: Chronic infantile neurological cutaneous and articular syndrome is caused by mutations in CIAS1, a gene highly expressed in polymorphonuclear cells and chondrocytes. Am J Hum Genet 71:198-203, 2002.

71. Hull KM, Shoham N, Chae JJ, et al: The expanding spectrum of systemic autoinflammatory disorders and their rheumatic manifestations. Curr Opin Rheumatol 15:61-69, 2003.

72. Doeglas HM, Bleumink E: Familial cold urticaria: clinical findings. Arch Dermatol 110:382-388, 1974.

73. Hoffman HM, Wanderer AA, Broide DH: Familial cold autoinflammatory syndrome: phenotype and genotype of an autosomal dominant periodic fever. J Allergy Clin Immunol 108:615-620, 2001.

74. Watts RA, Nicholls A, Scott DG: The arthropathy of the Muckle-Wells syndrome. Br J Rheumatol 33:1184-1187, 1994.

75. Schwarz RE, Dralle H, Linke RP, et al: Amyloid goiter and arthritides after kidney transplantation in a patient with systemic amyloidosis and Muckle-Wells syndrome. Am J Clin Pathol 92:821-825, 1989.

76. Berthelot JM, Maugars Y, Robillard N, et al: Autosomal dominant Muckle-Wells syndrome associated with cystinuria, ichthyosis, and aphthosis in a four-generation family. Am J Med Genet 53:72-74, 1994.

77. Prieur AM: A recently recognised chronic inflammatory disease of early onset characterised by the triad of rash, central nervous system involvement and arthropathy. Clin Exp Rheumatol 19:103-106, 2001.

78. Prieur AM, Griscelli C, Lampert F, et al: A chronic, infantile, neurological, cutaneous and articular (CINCA) syndrome: a specific entity analysed in 30 patients. Scand J Rheumatol Suppl 66:57-68, 1987.

79. Schwarz RE, Neumann KH, Dralle H: Colchicine in the treatment of systemic amyloidosis of Muckle-Wells-type. J Rheumatol 15:1736, 1988.

80. Bustorff MM, Oliveria JP, Moura C, et al: Muckle-Wells syndrome nephropathy: lack of response to colchicine therapy. Nephrol Dial Transplant 10:709-710, 1995.

81. Fuger K, Fleischmann E, Weber M, Mann J: Complications in the course of the Muckle-Wells syndrome. Dtsch Med Wochenschr 117:256-260, 1992.

82. Blau EB: Familial granulomatous arthritis, iritis, and rash. J Pediatr 107:689-693, 1985.

83. Wang X, Kuivaniemi H, Bonavita G, et al: CARD15 mutations in familial granulomatosis syndromes: a study of the original Blau syndrome kindred and other families with large-vessel arteritis and cranial neuropathy. Arthritis Rheum 46:3041-3045, 2002.

84. Miceli-Richard C, Lesage S, Rybojad M, et al: CARD15 mutations in Blau syndrome. Nat Genet 29:19-20, 2001.

85. Hugot JP, Chamaillard M, Zouali H, et al: Association of NOD2 leucine-rich repeat variants with susceptibility to Crohn's disease. Nature 411:599-603, 2001.

86. Lindor NM, Arsenault TM, Solomon H, et al: A new autosomal dominant disorder of pyogenic sterile arthritis, pyoderma gangrenosum, and acne: PAPA syndrome. Mayo Clin Proc 72:611-615, 1997.

87. Timmerman RJ, Thompson J, Noordzij HM, van der Meer JW: Psychogenic periodic fever. Neth J Med 41:158-160, 1992.

XVIII

The Common Ground of Rheumatology and Orthopaedic Surgery

113 Tumors and Tumor-like Lesions of the Joints and Related Structures

ANDREW E. ROSENBERG

The joint is a common site for the development of tumor-like lesions, such as synovial cysts and loose bodies, and is infrequently involved by benign or malignant neoplasms. Neoplasms of the joint can be divided into those that arise de novo and those that secondarily invade it from neighboring bone or soft tissues or from distant sites via the vascular system. Theoretically, any type of mesenchymal neoplasm can originate in a joint; however, the majority recapitulate the phenotype of periarticular tissues, including synovium, fat, blood vessels, fibrous tissue, and cartilage. Primary joint neoplasms almost always arise within the synovium and not the other articular structures, and the benign tumors greatly outnumber the malignancies. This chapter discusses the clinicopathologic features of tumor-like conditions and neoplasms of joints and related structures and incorporates the recent advances in cell biology that have increased our understanding of synovial neoplasia.

Non-Neoplastic Lesions

SYNOVIAL AND GANGLION CYSTS

Cysts are defined as closed compartments or sacs lined by epithelium and frequently filled with fluid. Thus, neither the synovial cyst nor the ganglion cyst is considered a true cyst, as each lacks an epithelial lining.

Synovial cysts are relatively common and develop from continuation or herniation of the synovial lining of a joint through the joint capsule into the neighboring periarticular tissues. They arise in association with a variety of joint disorders including trauma, osteoarthritis (OA), crystal arthopathies, infection, and rheumatoid arthritis (RA) or one of its variants.[1] Synovial cysts may develop from any joint, but most originate from the posterior aspect of the knee, where they are known as a popliteal or Baker's cysts, followed in frequency by shoulder and hip locations.[2] Synovial cyst of the posterior knee joint has been identified in 2.4 percent of asymptomatic children.[2]

Synovial cysts usually become distended with synovial fluid, and it is by this mechanism that they gradually enlarge.[1-4] Consequently, they may present as periarticular masses, cause progressive joint pain and swelling, limit joint mobility, and compress adjacent neurovascular structures. An example of the latter occurs in the spine, where synovial cysts arise from facet joints and impinge upon spinal nerves, producing radicular pain.[5] Other complications of synovial cysts, which can sometimes produce dramatic clinical findings, are acute rupture and secondary infection.

A variety of radiographic techniques has been used to image synovial cysts. Those that provide the most diagnostic information include arthrography, ultrasonography, computed tomography (CT), and magnetic resonance imaging (MRI).[1-4] All of these modalities diagnose synovial cysts as simple or septated thin-walled structures that arise from joints and are filled with fluid whose density is similar to that of water (Fig. 113–1).

Grossly, synovial cysts usually range in size from 1 to 10 cm in diameter. Their inner surface is smooth, glistening, and translucent; however, prior hemorrhage or secondary infection may distort it by virtue of an attached blood clot, granulation tissue, and inflammatory debris. The cyst wall is composed of an inner surface of flattened, or cuboidal, synoviocytes that are arranged one or several layers thick and are surrounded by an outer sheath of fibrous tissue (Fig. 113–2). Sometimes the synovial lining cells may be hyperplastic and form papillary fronds, and occasionally there are scattered subsynovial collections of hemosiderin-laden macrophages, which are indicative of previous microscopic hemorrhage.

The treatment of synovial cysts is variable and depends on their location and associated symptomatology. They may be successfully treated with conservative therapy; however, in certain situations surgical excision is required.[1-5]

Ganglion cysts have been recognized for centuries; Hippocrates described them as being composed of "mucoid flesh."[6] They are more common than synovial cysts and arise from tendon sheaths, ligaments, menisci, joint capsules, and bursae.[6] Occasionally, they develop de

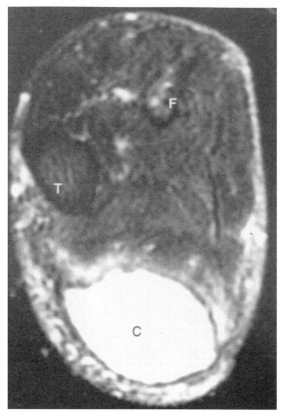

FIGURE 113-1 · Magnetic resonance image (MRI) showing high T2 signal intensity of large, oval-shaped, synovial cyst that extends from the knee joint into the posterior calf. F, fibula; C, synovial cyst; T, tibia.

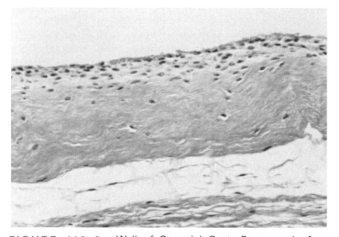

FIGURE 113-2 · Wall of Synovial Cyst, Composed of an Inner Lining of Synoviocytes Overlaying a Layer of Dense, Fibrous Tissue.

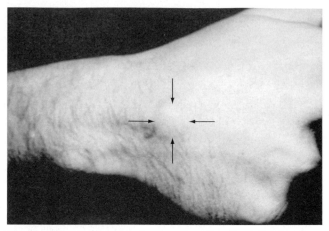

FIGURE 113-3 · Round, Firm Ganglion Cyst Bulging from the Dorsal Aspect of the Hand.

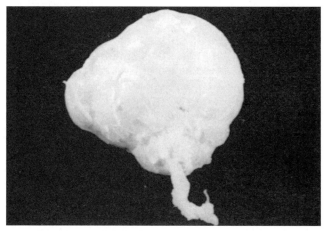

FIGURE 113-4 · Intact Ganglion Cyst with Threadlike Pedicle that Attaches to a Periarticular Structure.

novo in the subchondral areas of bone, and rarely, they develop within skeletal muscle without communication with a joint. Ganglion cysts are distinguished from synovial cysts by virtue of the fact that they lack a surface lining and do not directly communicate with a joint cavity or synovial lining.[1] A variety of hypotheses has been developed to explain their pathogenesis; however, none of the hypotheses has been proven.[6] The most accepted theory is that ganglion cysts develop from mucoid cystic degeneration of periarticular structures.

Most ganglion cysts arise along the dorsal and volar aspects of the wrists, fingers, and dorsum of the feet.[6,7] They may be associated with repetitive-use activities, inflammatory arthritides, and trauma.[1] They are usually asymptomatic and most present as a slowly growing, firm mass (Fig. 113–3). Ganglion cysts may be painful if traumatized and can compress adjacent neurovascular structures, producing a variety of symptoms. Their radiographic characteristics are similar to those of synovial cysts, and they manifest as relatively small cystic structures filled with fluid.[1,7]

Macroscopically, most ganglion cysts are round; however, they may form elongated, cylindrical structures if they track along a tendon sheath. Ganglion cysts are uni- or multiloculated, have thin walls, and are filled with translucent mucoid fluid (Figs. 113–4 and 113–5). The cyst surface lacks a cellular lining and is composed of either fibrous tissue or loose connective tissue, the latter of which may contain muciphages (Fig. 113–6). Dense fibrous tissue accounts for the bulk of the cyst wall, and it, in turn, is usually surrounded by areolar tissue.

Once ganglion cysts form, they may remain stable for years or spontaneously resolve; those that disappear may reform at a later time. Because they are relatively innocuous, it is not surprising that their treatment is frequently conservative.[1] Occasionally, they may require aspiration

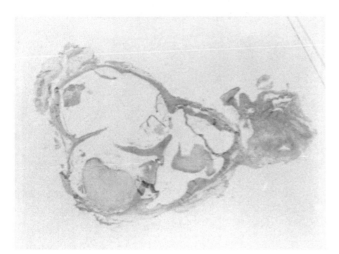

FIGURE 113-5 · Multiloculated Ganglion Cyst Containing Remnants of Proteinaceous Cyst Fluid.

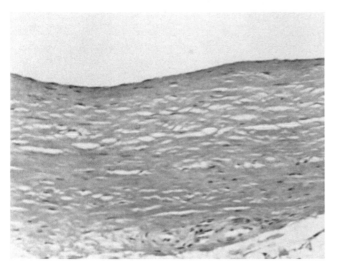

FIGURE 113-6 · Ganglion cyst wall composed of scattered, flattened fibroblasts on the luminal surface and a well-formed layer of dense, fibrous tissue.

or surgical excision, especially those that are intraosseous in location and symptomatic.

LOOSE BODIES

Loose bodies, or joint mice, are generic terms for free-floating structures within a joint cavity. They may be exogenous, such as fragments of a bullet, or endogenous, such as pieces of articular cartilage, menisci, ligaments, or bone.[8,9] When not otherwise specified, "loose bodies" refers to pieces of articular cartilage, subchondral bone, or both that have become detached and lie free within the joint or that have become secondarily embedded in the synovium. Loose bodies are the most common tumor-like lesion of the joint.

Osteoarticular loose bodies result from fractures or destruction of the joint in the setting of OA or other arthritides. The sloughed articular cartilage remains viable because it receives its nourishment from the synovial fluid; but the bone dies because it is supplied only by blood vessels. As the loose body tumbles in the joint, its edges become round and smooth, and eventu-

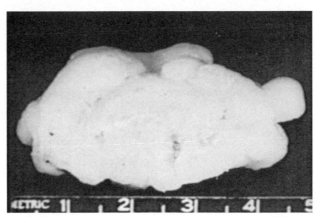

FIGURE 113-7 · Large, nodular loose body formed from a semilunar-shaped piece of articular cartilage surrounded by newly formed cartilage.

ally it becomes embedded within the synovium (Fig. 113–7). At this stage it may be resorbed or may stimulate a proliferative response in which the loose body serves as scaffolding for the deposition of newly formed fibro and hyaline cartilage, which may undergo enchondral ossification. The newly formed cartilage and bone surrounds the loose body like cambium layers of a tree (Fig. 113–8). As the loose body enlarges, the deeper portions of cartilage can no longer be supported by diffusion of synovial fluid, so it dies and becomes calcified. This combination of events produces the dense speckled and ring-like calcifications seen on radiographs (Fig. 113–9). In addition, it is in this fashion that the loose body becomes larger than the initial osteochondral defect from which it originated. Loose bodies can be painful and limit the range of joint motion. Radiographically and histologically, the differential diagnosis includes synovial chondromatosis. Treatment is simple excision, which can be performed arthroscopically.[9]

INTRA-ARTICULAR OSSICLES

Small bony nodules normally occur in the knees of some rodents[10] and other mammals and may rarely occur in humans.[11,12] In rodents, they are constantly found in the anterior portions of the joint and frequently in the posterior portions as well. In humans they develop within the substance of the meniscus adjacent to its tibial attachments.

The exact etiology of such structures is unknown, although most probably they are either true sesamoid bones, as seen in rodents, or represent ossification secondary to local injury. This latter possibility is supported by the fact that previous knee trauma has been present in a number of reported cases. The symptoms are usually pain after some sort of exertion, such as walking or prolonged standing, with relief when the knee is at rest. Radiographs of the involved knee may reveal what appears to be a loose body.[12] MRI shows the ossicle to be a corticated, marrow-containing structure that has increased signal intensity on T1-weighted images and decreased signal intensity on T2-weighted images.[11,12] The differential diagnosis usually includes a loose body and a torn meniscus. At surgery, the joint

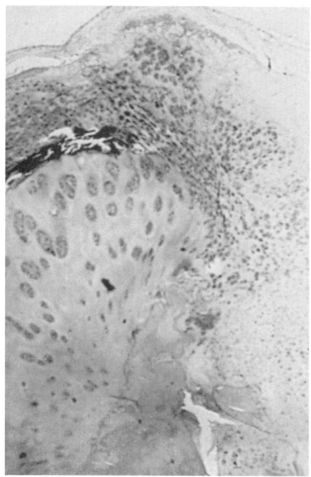

FIGURE 113-8 · Osteoarticular Loose Body Embedded Within Synovium. Note that the piece of articular cartilage and attached subchondral bone are surrounded by newly formed layers of metaplastic cartilage and bone derived from synovial tissue.

surface will be intact and neither a loose body nor a torn meniscus will be found unless there have been other joint problems. The ossicle, however, will be found within either the lateral or medial meniscus and appear as a small (about 1.0 cm in diameter) palpable bony nodule (Fig. 113-10). If the ossicle is symptomatic, it should be excised; however, if it is an incidental finding it can be managed conservatively.[11]

▌ Neoplasms

FATTY LESIONS OF THE SYNOVIUM

Although the subsynovial connective tissue of diarthrodial joints is rich in fat, a true lipoma of the synovium is rare. Lipomas have been described in the knee and ankle joints[13,14] and the synovial sheaths of tendons of the hands, ankles, and feet in which they affect the extensor more frequently than the flexor synovial sheaths. Synovial lipoma can be sessile or pedunculated and, similar to a lipoma arising in the subcutis, it is composed of lobules of mature adipocytes delineated by a thin fibrous capsule. Pedunculated lipomas may produce pain if they twist on their stalks and become ischemic.

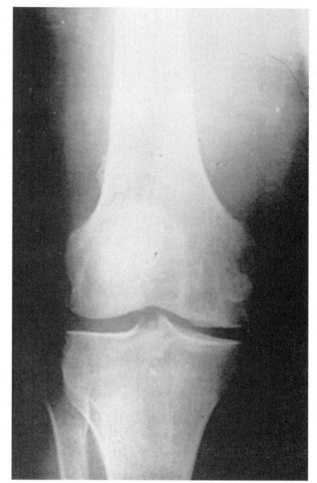

FIGURE 113-9 · Knee Joint with Several Mineralized Loose Bodies.

A more common but still unusual fatty lesion of the joint is lipoma arborescens, also known as villous lipomatous proliferation of the synovium.[15,16] This disorder is characterized by a diffuse increase in the quantity of subsynovial fat, which bulges the overlying synovial lining and produces a villous architecture. It is not certain

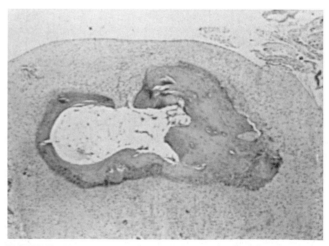

FIGURE 113-10 · An intra-Articular Ossicle Embedded in the Fibrocartilage of the Meniscus. The bone is lamellar, and the marrow is fatty. The interface between the fibrocartilage and bone resembles a tendinous insertion, including Sharpey's fibers.

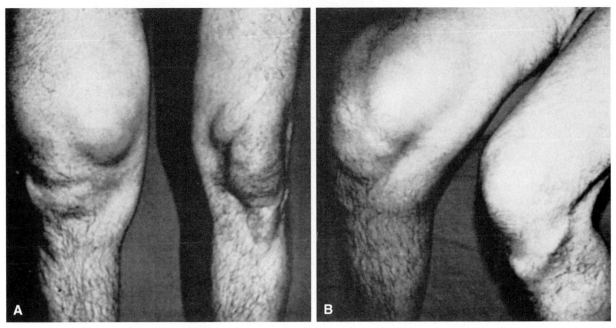

FIGURE 113–11 · *A*, Lipoma arborescens presenting as a suprapatellar mass. *B*, It is easily seen on flexion of the knee.(Courtesy of Drs. C. Rowe and B. Zarins.)

whether the proliferating fat is neoplastic (lipomatosis) or a manifestation of a hyperplastic or reactive process. Lipoma arborescens usually involves the suprapatellar portion of the knee joint (Fig. 113–11); however, it has also been observed in the hip, ankle, and wrist. Although the process is usually localized to one joint, several cases of bilateral knee involvement have been reported.[16] Affected patients tend to be middle-aged males who usually present with a history of variable pain, swelling, and limitation of motion.[16,17] The duration of symptoms is usually long, and they may be present for up to 30 years; however, acute onset has been documented. Plain films typically show joint fullness and changes of OA of the involved joint. This combination of findings produces speculation regarding the relationship between these two disease processes. Arthrography reveals multiple lobulated filling defects, CT scans show a low-density villonodular mass, and by MRI they have the density of fat.[18] Laboratory studies are unremarkable, and the joint effusions consist of clear, yellow fluid that is free of crystals.[16] At surgery, the effected synovium has a prominent villous or villonodular architecture and is tan-yellow (Fig. 113–12). Histologically, the lesion is composed of sheets of mature adipocytes admixed with nutrient blood vessels, all of which are partially compartmentalized by fibrous septa and covered on the intra-articular surface by several layers of synovial cells. Synovectomy may relieve the symptoms and prevent effusions; however, the associated OA may be progressive.[16] The clinicopathologic differential diagnosis includes pigmented villonodular synovitis (PVNS), synovial chondromatosis, and synovial hemangioma. These lesions can be easily distinguished from lipoma arborescens by their distinct histologic features. Another disorder that should be included in the differential is Hoffa's disease, a condition of irritation, inflammation, and hyperplasia of the

synovial lining in regions where fat is normally present, such as adjacent to the patella or patellar ligament.[19]

VASCULAR LESIONS OF THE SYNOVIUM

Benign vascular tumors of the synovium are very uncommon, and only about 160 cases have been described in the literature. They are subclassified according to their growth pattern into localized and diffuse variants. Both tend to predominate in adolescence and young adulthood; however, symptoms frequently can be traced back to childhood.[20] Synovial hemangiomas produce a variety of symptoms, including unilateral, intermittent joint pain and enlargement, which may result in limitation of motion, locking or buckling, and hemarthrosis, especially after minimal trauma.[21] Classically, the affected joint diminishes in size if sufficiently elevated to allow

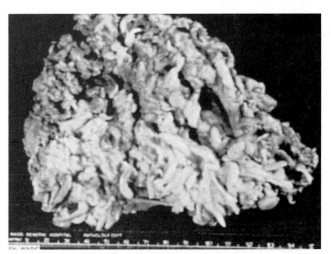

FIGURE 113–12 · Lipoma Arborescens Represented As A Diffuse, Fatty Polypoid Mass Covered By A Thin, Glistening Synovium.

the blood to drain out of the lesion. The joint most commonly involved is the knee; however, hemangiomas have been described in the elbow, ankle, tarsometatarsal and temporomandibular joints, and the tendon sheaths of the wrist and ankle.[21,22] Unusual complications of synovial hemangiomas include a secondary destructive arthritis and Kasabach-Merritt syndrome.

On physical examination, the joint is swollen and doughy, and nearby cutaneous hemangiomas may be evident. Joint aspiration frequently yields bloody fluid. Preoperative diagnosis of the localized hemangioma is very difficult. Its differential diagnosis includes localized nodular synovitis and, in the knee, a diskoid meniscus, meniscal tears, cysts, and ossicles.[22] The diffuse hemangioma is more easily identified, but it can mimic PVNS and hemophilic arthropathy.

Radiographic evaluation may show nothing more than a vague soft tissue shadow indicative of a swollen synovium, and distended joint capsule or regional osteoporosis in patients who have had long-term symptoms and recurrent hemarthrosis. Rarely, calcified phleboliths are apparent; however, they are more often associated with a soft tissue arteriovenous malformation with secondary joint involvement than an isolated intra-articular hemangioma (Fig. 113–13). Arthrography may demonstrate an intra-articular filling defect, and arteriography may be negative in small, localized capillary hemangiomas, but contrast may collect in the more diffuse lesions that contain cavernous or large ectatic vascular spaces (Fig. 113–14). CT may reveal a lobulated soft tissue mass with

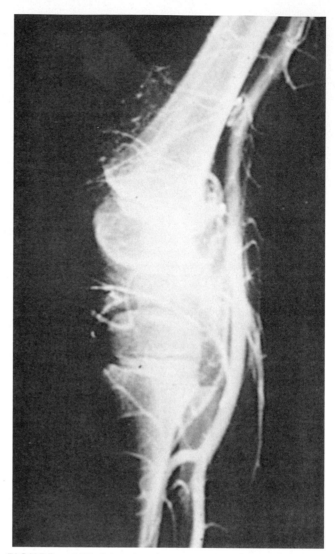

FIGURE   113–14 · Arteriogram of an Arteriovenous Malformation in the Soft Tissues of the Thigh and Leg with Involvement of the Knee Joint. The extensive vascular blush in the knee indicates aberrant synovial and capsular vasculature.

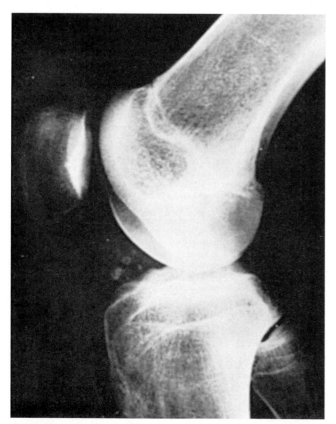

FIGURE   113–13 · A Localized Synovial Hemangioma with Phleboliths Prominently Seen in the Joint. The patient is 16 years old with many years' history of painful swelling when standing and relief of this pain when the knee is flexed.

mild enhancement after contrast injection.[22,23] MRI may show the tumor to have a low signal on T1-weighted images and high signal intensity on T2-weighted images.[23]

Macroscopically, the localized hemangioma tends to be small, but larger lesions up to 8.0 cm in diameter have been documented. It may be sessile or stalked, is well circumscribed, and ranges in color from red to blue (Fig. 113–15). Microscopically, the hemangioma is usually of the cavernous or venous type with large, dilated, blood-filled vessels lined by cytologically benign endothelial cells. In the diffuse form, the entire synovium may be edematous and beefy red, or stained brown by hemosiderin, and usually contains prominent tortuous congested vessels that may penetrate the joint capsule and extend into the neighboring soft tissues. Histologically, the vessels recapitulate arteries, veins, and capillaries; have abnormal interconnections; and are arranged in a disorganized tangle.[22]

Therapy for a localized hemangioma is marginal surgical excision, which usually is curative. Diffuse lesions are frequently difficult to eradicate because of their

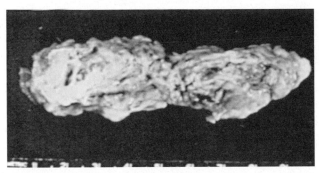

FIGURE 113–15 · A diffuse form of hemangioma of the synovium with an edematous, beefy synovium and large, dilated vascular channels. In life these channels were filled with blood, and the synovium was markedly thickened.

extensive nature. Therefore, incomplete excision or debulking may be the only surgical option. Radiation therapy is not indicated.

FIBROMA OF THE TENDON SHEATH

Fibroma of the tendon sheath is an uncommon benign lesion that clinically mimics giant cell tumor of the tendon sheath but is morphologically distinct. Fibroma of the tendon sheath was first identified as a clinicopathologic entity in 1936, and since that time more than 220 cases have been reported.[24,25] Although it is uncertain whether this lesion is some sort of reactive process, hyperplasia, or a benign neoplasm, recent cytogenetic abnormalities identified in this tumor support the concept that the lesion is neoplastic.

Fibroma of the tendon sheath usually arises from the tendons and sheaths of the flexor surfaces of the distal extremities, and approximately 70 percent involve the fingers or hand. Of the fingers, the thumb is most frequently involved, followed by the index and middle fingers.[24] Less commonly, large diarthrodial joints, such as the knee and rarely the elbow and ankle, are sites of origin.[24,25] The patients range in age from infants to the elderly, but the median age of onset is in the early fourth decade of life.[24,25] Most series report a male predominance with the largest study of 138 cases having a male-to-female ratio of 3:1.[24] Patients present with a slow-growing, painless mass that has usually been noted for several months to a year.[25] In 6 to 10 percent of cases there is a history of antecedent trauma.

Plain radiographs show soft tissue fullness, and rarely is there evidence of bony erosion.[24] An MRI or CT demonstrates a solid, well-circumscribed mass of soft tissue density. At surgery, the tumors are usually found to be attached directly to the tendon or tendon sheath. They are oblong, well circumscribed or encapsulated, and average 1.5 to 1.8 cm in their greatest dimension.[24,25] Grossly, they are nodular and have a tan-white cut surface with a rubbery consistency.

Microscopically fibroma of the tendon sheath is multilobular with synovial-like clefts interposed between adjacent lobules (Fig. 113–16). The lobules are composed of spindle and stellate fibroblasts enmeshed in a collagenous and sometimes myxoid stroma. Immunohistochemically, the tumor cells have the staining profile of

FIGURE 113–16 · A Fibroma of Tendon Sheath Composed of a Hypocellular Collagenous Mass, which is Well Demarcated from the Underlying Tendon.

myofibroblasts, and ultrastructurally, the cells have features of fibroblasts and myofibroblasts.[26]

The natural history of fibroma of the tendon sheath is a slow growth, which eventually ceases. Treatment of choice is surgical excision, which is associated with a 24 percent recurrence rate.[24]

SYNOVIAL CHONDROMATOSIS

Synovial chondromatosis is an uncommon condition characterized by the formation of multiple nodules of hyaline cartilage within the subsynovial connective tissue. If the cartilage nodules undergo enchondral ossification, the term *synovial osteochondromatosis* is used. It is unclear whether the proliferating cartilage is metaplastic or neoplastic; however, recent cytogenetic abnormalities involving chromosome 6 in these lesions support a neoplastic process.[27] Regardless, synovial chondromatosis is benign and never metastasizes. Removal of the involved synovium results in a good prognosis, although there may be local recurrences.

Location

Synovial chondromatosis typically arises in large diarthrodial joints. The knee is affected in more than 50 percent of the cases, usually as a monoarticular condition.[28] Other common sites include the hip, elbow, shoulder, and ankle. Infrequently, synovial chondromatosis arises in the small joints of the hands and feet[29] and the temporomandibular joint.[30] When the cartilage nodules develop in the synovial lining of bursae, tendons, and ligaments, this is known as extra-articular synovial chondromatosis.[31,32] The extra-articular variant most commonly affects the fingers, followed by the toes, hand, wrist, foot, and ankle.[31] More than one synovial sheath may be involved.

Age and Sex Distribution

This condition is most common in middle-aged males, and the average age is the fifth decade of life.[28] Interestingly, middle-aged females, more than males, are likely to develop the disease in the temporomandibular joint. In hand and foot involvement, there seems to be an equal distribution of the sexes, and the patients are usually in their sixth decade of life.

Symptoms and Signs

Patients commonly complain of joint pain, swelling, stiffness, crepitence, and limitation of motion with a locking or grating feeling upon movement.[28] The symptoms are usually long-standing, recurrent, and progressive.

Radiographic Findings

The plain radiographic findings largely depend on whether the cartilage nodules are calcified or ossified and if they erode the adjacent bony structures. Visible calcifications are absent in 5 to 33 percent of cases; however, in the majority, there are multiple oval intra-articular radiodensities that range in size from a few millimeters to several centimeters[33] (Figs. 113–17 and 113–18). The pattern of mineralization varies and may appear as irregular flecks that represent calcified cartilage or demonstrate a trabecular architecture, which is a manifestation of enchondral ossification. Lesions that are not mineralized are best visualized on an arthrogram, as they produce multiple filing defects.[33] In approximately 11 percent of cases, the nodules erode the neighboring skeleton, especially along the anterior

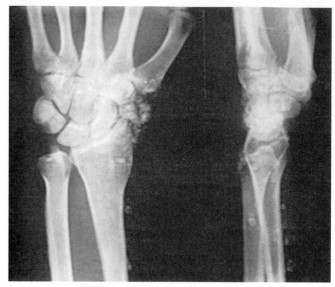

FIGURE 113–17 · Radiographs of the Wrist with Multiple Prominent Calcified Bodies of Varying Sizes in the Soft Tissues of the Wrist and Extending along the Forearm. These bodies have smooth surfaces and a lucent centers, some of which have a trabeculated pattern rather than an amorphous, densely calcified texture. The diagnosis is synovial osteochondromatosis.

aspect of the distal femur. CT examination may show mass-like areas in the synovium that have a density similar to skeletal muscle. CT can also detect small calcifications and erosions before they are apparent on plain films.[33] MRI shows that the nodules of cartilage have low signal intensity on T1-weighted sequences and high intensity on T2-weighted sequences, which reflects the high water content of hyaline cartilage.[33] Areas of calcification or mineralized bone have a low signal intensity on both T1- and T2-weighted sequences. Both CT and MRI scans are helpful in identifying the intra-articular source of the lesion and its anatomic extent. In long-standing disease, the involved joints may also be osteoporotic and show changes of secondary OA (see Fig. 113–18).

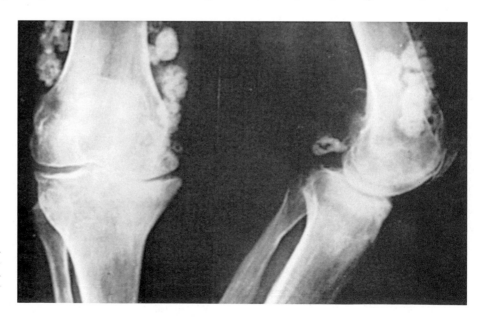

FIGURE 113–18 · Synovial osteochondromatosis of the knee with narrowing of the joint space and multiple large, calcified bodies filling the joint space and suprapatellar pouch.

The cartilage in extra-articular synovial chondromatosis has similar radiographic changes. The nodules of cartilage are more frequently mineralized and may appear as a linear arrangement of small calcific densities that are aligned along the sheath and can span a number of joints.

The radiographic differential diagnosis of synovial chondromatosis includes osteochondritis dissecans, OA with loose bodies, tuberculosis, hemopathic arthropathies, pseudogout with extensive synovial calcification, and synovial tumors. In many instances, the clinical story and radiographic picture should lead to the correct diagnosis. However, there are a significant number of cases in which the radiographs and clinical picture are vague, so only a biopsy will remove all doubts about the diagnosis.

Pathology

Characteristic of synovial chondromatosis is a thickened synovium containing numerous opalescent, firm nodules of cartilage that bulge from the surface in a cobblestone pattern (Fig. 113–19). The nodules are usually less than 5 cm in size and frequently lose their attachment to the synovium and form loose bodies, sometimes hundreds of them. The calcified cartilage is white, and areas of ossification manifest as gritty, tan trabeculae, which may house fatty marrow (Fig. 113–20). The synovium adjacent to the cartilage may demonstrate reactive changes such as edema, hyperemia, and villous transformation.

The cartilage develops in the connective tissue of the subsynovial compartment (Fig. 113–21). The mesenchymal cells give rise to uniformly small, round chondrocytes, which produce the hyaline matrix and eventually form individual nodules that blend peripherally with the surrounding tissues (Fig. 113–22). In some cases, however, the cartilage may be hypercellular, and the chondrocytes may be binucleate, large, and hyperchromatic, similar to those in chondrosarcoma

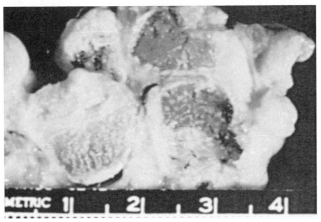

FIGURE 113–20 · Synovial Osteochondromatosis. The smooth-surfaced nodules are seen merging with the synovium, rather than appearing as implanted pieces of cartilage that may easily separate from the synovium, and they have irregular, roughened surfaces. Prominent bone trabeculae and a fatty marrow are easily seen within each nodule.

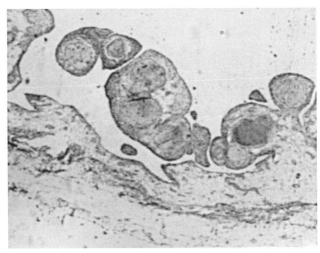

FIGURE 113–21 · Synovial Chondromatosis with Metaplastic Hyaline Cartilage Nodules in the Synovium. The adjacent noncartilaginous synovium is normal.

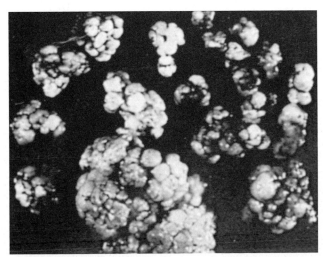

FIGURE 113–19 · Synovial chondromatosis with innumerable cartilage nodules forming a cobblestone-like appearance of the synovial lining. (Courtesy of Dr. C. Campbell.)

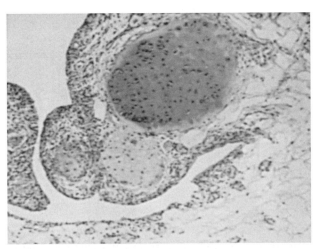

FIGURE 113–22 · A higher-power microscopic view of chondromatosis illustrating the continuity between synovial tissue and metaplastic hyaline-cartilage nodules.

(Fig. 113–23). Despite these ominous histologic findings, experience has shown that lesions with atypical chondrocytes usually behave in a benign fashion. Infrequently, the disease manifests as a single extremely large nodule of cartilage, which may undergo partial enchondral ossification. This giant intra-articular osteochondroma can severely limit joint motion and may be clinically confused with other types of neoplasms.[34]

Ultrastructurally, the chondrocytes in synovial chondromatosis have abundant rough endoplasmic reticulum, prominent Golgi structures, and peripheral aggregates of glycogen. These features are very similar to those present in the chondrocytes of normal articular cartilage and other benign cartilaginous tumors and have supported the interpretation that synovial chondromatosis, even with atypical cartilage, is benign.

Over time, the nodules of cartilage attached to the synovium are invaded by blood vessels. This results in enchondral ossification with woven and lamellar bone formation and even the development of a medullary cavity with fatty marrow (Fig. 113–24). If these nodules lose their synovial attachments and become free-floating, they may continue to increase in size because the cartilage derives its nourishment from synovial fluid, although the osseous portion and marrow will die.

Flow cytometry has been performed in a small number of cases of synovial chondromatosis, and all have shown a diploid pattern.[35]

Clinical Course and Prognosis

The treatment of choice for synovial chondromatosis is excision of the involved synovium and removal of all loose bodies. The prognosis is very good, although there may be recurrences if removal is incomplete. Most recurrences develop in the setting of diffuse involvement of the synovium.

Synovial chondromatosis rarely undergoes malignant transformation into chondrosarcoma, although in one series this phenomenon occurred in 5 percent of cases. It should be noted, however, that a significant percentage of the small number of reported cases of synovial chondrosarcomas have shown evidence of underlying synovial chondromatosis.[36,37]

CHONDROMA OF THE TENDON SHEATH AND PERIARTICULAR STRUCTURES

The solitary soft tissue chondroma is considered to be a benign neoplasm. It commonly arises in tendon sheaths and infrequently involves joint capsules or other periarticular structures.

Tendon sheath chondromas usually arise in the flexor tendon sheaths of the distal extremities and are about three times more common in the hands than in the feet.[38,39] They affect the sexes equally and are detected in early to mid adulthood as they present as a painless, slowly growing, firm mass.[40] Radiographically, they appear as extraosseous, well-delineated soft tissue masses that contain calcifications that are either punctate or ring-like in 33 to 70 percent of cases.[41] Grossly, the tumors are ovoid, firm, blue-white, well-circumscribed masses of hyaline cartilage that are usually 1 to 2 cm in dimension and, unlike synovial chondromatosis, are solitary. Histologically, the hyaline cartilage is well formed with occasional small foci of myxoid change. The cartilage can be cellular, and the chondrocytes may demonstrate cytologic atypia that causes confusion with chondrosarcoma.[42] Treatment of choice is simple excision. Although these tumors may recur in a minority of cases, they are benign and do not metastasize.[38-40]

The intracapsular or periarticular regions are uncommon sites for soft tissue chondromas. When they occur, they usually originate in the anterior infrapatella region of the knee[43] (Fig. 113–25). In this location the chondroma can achieve a large size (8 cm in diameter) and mechanically interfere with knee motion. Their morphology and biologic behavior are similar to soft tissue chondromas that arise elsewhere. Interestingly, intracapsular chondromas have been reported in knees of three members of a family with familial dysplasia epiphysealis hemimelica.[44] There have been two other cases described in which cartilaginous hamartomas of the volar plates of the proximal and distal interphalangeal joints of the hands and feet

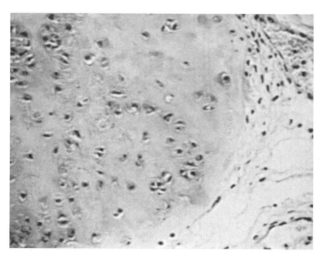

FIGURE 113–23 · Synovial Chondromatosis with Cellular Atypicality and Binucleate Cells.

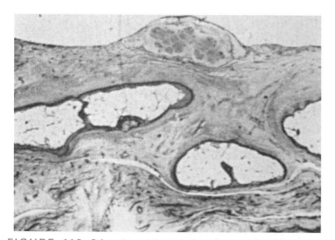

FIGURE 113–24 · Synovial osteochondromatosis with a metaplastic hyaline-cartilage nodule near the synovial surface and bony nodules deeper in the synovium. Note the fatty marrow inside the osseous nodules.

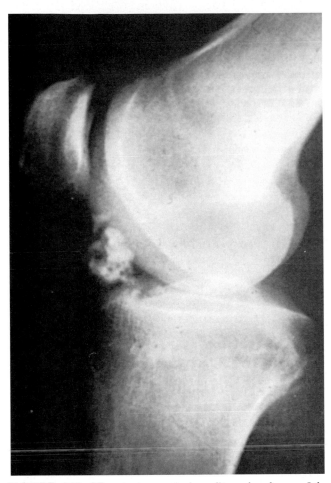

FIGURE 113-25 · An intra-articular solitary chondroma of the knee in the infrapatellar region; it is a well-delineated mass with amorphous dense calcification, suggesting mineralized cartilage. (Courtesy of Dr. C. Campbell.)

were associated with peculiar hypertrophic skin lesions of the hand and hemihypertrophy of the limb. It is possible that these peculiar cartilaginous lesions represent an abnormality in which primitive cartilage tissue persists in joint sites, much akin to the involvement of bones in multiple enchondromatosis (Ollier's disease).

VILLONODULAR SYNOVITIS

Villonodular synovitis is comprised of a group of benign tumors that affect the synovial lining of joints, tendon sheaths, and bursae. Included in this group are PVNS, localized or nodular synovitis, localized or nodular tenosynovitis, and the rare localized nodular bursitis. The diffuse variants may be locally aggressive and invade into bone, joint capsules, tendons, and adjacent soft tissues. However, despite their destructive potential, they do not metastasize.

The common histologic denominator of these lesions is the exuberant proliferation of synovial lining cells that may spread along the synovial surface and invade downward into the subsynovial connective tissue. The growing cells expand the subsynovial compartment, producing finger-like extensions, villi, and redundant folds. These projections often fuse into nodules and form convoluted lobulated masses admixed with a tangle of hair-like villi. The process may be a local phenomenon involving only part of the synovial lining, or it may be extensive with the whole synovial surface affected.

Until recently, the etiology of villonodular synovitis was a mystery. Experimental animal models produced lesions that morphologically resembled the human condition, but biologically they were self limited and resolved when the inducing factor, usually a blood-serum component or iron, was stopped.[45,46] Therefore, the role of trauma and repeated episodes of hemorrhage is probably not important. Also, neither hemophilic patients nor patients with other bleeding disorders are prone to develop villonodular synovitis despite frequent bouts of intra-articular hemorrhage and resultant secondary OA and joint destruction.

Cytogenetic studies have recently shown a variety of aberrant chromosomal findings. Trisomy 7 was found in three cases of PVNS, and six consistent chromosome rearrangements were found in one case of localized nodular tenosynovitis.[47,48] In another series of 44 cases of PVNS and giant cell tumors of tendon sheath in 35 patients, the most common chromosomal abnormality was rearrangement of the short arm of chromosone one (1p11 through 13).[49] These results help validate that each member of this family of lesions develops from a clonal proliferation of cells and, hence, should be considered a benign neoplasm.[47-49]

Pigmented Villonodular Synovitis

This condition is also known as synovial xanthoma, synovial fibroendothelioma, synovial endothelioma, benign fibrous histiocytoma, and xanthomatous giant cell tumor.

The prototype of the villonodular synovitis group is PVNS, which diffusely involves the synovial lining of a joint or tendon sheath. The term *localized nodular synovitis* (see following) is used if the disease presents as a solitary nodule confined to a clearly delineated focus in the synovium.

Age and Sex

Although PVNS may occur in all age groups, spanning children to the elderly, most affect young adults in the third to fourth decades of life.[50] The sexes tend to be equally affected, although some series have reported a predominance of either males or females.[50-52]

Sites

Unilateral involvement of the knee is most commonly seen and occurs in about 80 percent of cases.[50,52] The next most common sites are the hip, ankle, calcaneocuboid joints, elbow, and the tendon sheaths of fingers and sometimes toes. Occasionally involvement is seen in the palm, sole of the foot, and unusual locations such as the temporomandibular joint and posterior elements of the spine. Bursal involvement is rare, but when it occurs it usually develops in the popliteal and iliopectineal bursae and the bursa anserina. Occasionally, the disease affects large tendon sheaths proximal to the ankle and wrist and produces a periarticular soft tissue mass.[53,54] It is thought that these lesions dissect through either a joint capsule or tendon sheath and extend along fascial planes to produce a soft tissue mass.

In the vast majority of the cases, PVNS is monoarticular. Bilaterality or involvement of multiple, separate sites has been infrequently reported.[52] Interestingly, some patients with polyarticular disease have also had significant congenital anomalies.

Invasion of bone on either side of a joint can be seen with intra-articular, bursal, or tendon sheath involvement.[55] This most frequently occurs when the tumor involves "tight" joints such as the hip, elbow, wrist, and feet.[56] Rarely, only one bone may be invaded by an intra-articular lesion, and this may mimic a primary bone tumor.[57]

Symptoms

PVNS usually presents as a monoarticular arthritis. The main complaints include pain and mild, intermittent or repeated bouts of swelling. The symptoms develop insidiously and slowly progress over a long period of time, ranging from months to years.[52] The involved area may be stiff, swollen, and warm, and a palpable mass can sometimes be appreciated. Point tenderness can be detected in approximately 50 percent of patients.[52] Anatomic instability of the involved joint is uncommon.

Joint aspiration frequently yields blood-tinged, brown fluid that lacks diagnostic abnormalities.[58] Synovial fluid analysis may show a low glucose content, minimally elevated protein level, and a fair mucin clot.[52] The inflammatory cell count is usually low but may be elevated.[52] Similar findings can also be seen in trauma, Charcot joint, bleeding disorders, sickle cell disease, and Ehlers-Danlos syndrome.[52]

Radiologic Features

In at least two thirds of cases, a soft tissue density, which is due to the tumor, effusion, or both can be visualized on a plain film.[59] Joint narrowing or calcification is uncommon. Arthrography may demonstrate numerous nodular filling defects that extend into an expanded joint space. Arteriograms are unusually striking, owing to the prominent vascularity of the tumor. There tends to be an inverse correlation between the degree of vascularity and the amount of fibrosis or scarring of the lesion.

CT and MRI scans are useful in delineating the extent of disease and can detect both intralesional lipid and hemosiderin deposits that are important diagnostic features.[59-63] Extension into the bone manifests radiographically as multiple subchondral, well-marginated, cyst-like lucencies or juxtacortical, oval pressure erosions[55,60] (Figs. 113–26 and 113–27). In the knee, the femoral area underlying the intercondylar region is the most frequently invaded by tumor, as the tumor grows along ligamentous insertions. Periarticular osteopenia, joint destruction, and periosteal reactions are unusual. The joint space is preserved until late in the course of the disease.[60]

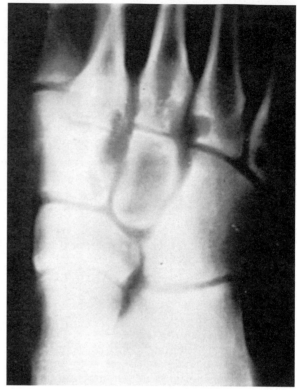

FIGURE 113-26 · Pigmented villonodular synovitis (PVNS) involving the small joints of the foot with multiple bone erosion. There is no clacification present in the lesion.

The differential diagnosis of a given case includes 1) tuberculosis, which generally has more osteopenia and joint destruction; 2) hemophilia, which is also associated with more extensive joint destruction; 3) synovial chondromatosis, which frequently has calcified radiopaque bodies; and 4) RA, which demonstrates more severe osteopenia and joint narrowing.

Arthroscopic Findings

Although arthroscopy is not a required procedure in evaluating patients with PVNS, the lesion has been identified unexpectedly using this method. In these instances, the synovium is red-brown and distorted by numerous hypertrophic villi and nodular projections.

Pathology

Grossly, the synovium in PVNS is red-brown to mottled orange-yellow and looks like a plush angora rug (Fig. 113–28). Matted masses of villous projections and synovial folds are prominent and are admixed with sessile or pedunculated, rubbery to soft nodules (0.5- to 2-cm diameter) enmeshed within the synovial tissue. The synovial membrane is thick and succulent and is often coated with a fibrinous exudate. Red-brown or golden-brown tissue may extend deep into subsynovial structures or invade the joint capsule. If a tendon sheath is involved, a sausage-shaped mass may be evident, as the sheath is distended by the proliferating tumor. If the joint capsule is invaded, adjacent soft tissue structures, including nerves and vessels, may be covered by wispy, red-brown tissue. If soft tissue invasion is extensive, the lesion may present as a soft to rubbery, red-brown mass with foci of hemorrhagic cysts. Similar tissue may be present near the chondro-osseous junc-tion or wrapped around vascular and ligamentous attachments to bone surfaces, which represent entrance points into the bone interior. Although other conditions such as hemochromatosis and hemosidero-sis may similarly stain the synovium brown, the nodular component is usually absent, and, in addition, micro-scopic features are definitive for separating these enti-ties (see following).

Microscopic examination reveals marked synovial cell hyperplasia with surface proliferation and, more impor-tant, subsynovial invasion by masses of polygonal or round cells with pink cytoplasm and round nuclei (Fig. 113–29). Included among the invading synovial cells are multinucleated giant cells (of the osteoclast, Touton, or foreign body type), hemosiderin-laden macrophages, and fibroblasts (Fig. 113–30). Hemosiderin can also be seen between cells, in synovial lining cells, and in polyg-onal cells. Foci of hemorrhage are common and are sur-rounded peripherally by the giant cells and macrophages. Scattered collections of foamy macrophages (xanthoma

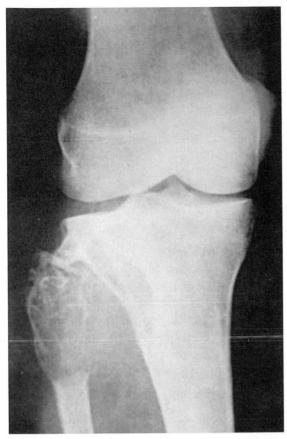

FIGURE 113–27 · Pigmented villonodular synovitis (PVNS) involving the tibiofibular joint with an adjacent extensive soft tissue mass and eccentric erosion of the both bones, simulating a primary bone tumor. The knee joint is normal.

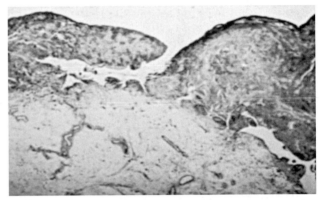

FIGURE 113–29 · A low-power microscopic view of a synovium that is thickened and thrown into papillary folds by invading synovial lining cells, a characteristic feature of pigmented villonodular synovi-tis (PUNS).

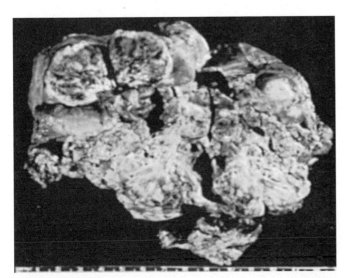

FIGURE 113–28 · This gross specimen shows a large, bulky, soft tissue mass that is mottled from red to yellow, soft, and focally hem-orrhagic. The lesion totally obscures the fibular head and pushes into the soft tissue as a lobulated mass.

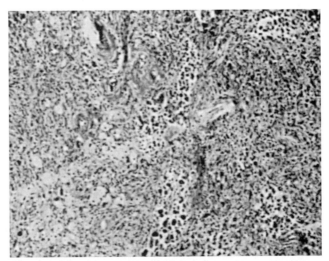

FIGURE 113–30 · Pigmented villonodular synovitis (PVNS) with polygonal and round synovial-type cells, hemosiderin-laden macrophages, prominent vascularity, and scattered foam cells (macrophages).

cells) filled with lipid are also common. These cell populations fill the distended synovial villi and cause them to fuse with adjacent ones, forming nodules. Slits or clefts between villi are present owing to the persistence of some areas that have not fused and are still lined by the residual synovial cells. In some nodules, there may be massive collagen deposition with interlacing bands of fibroblasts and hyalinized foci with little cellular activity except for a few scattered giant cells and macrophages. Often a scant, diffuse chronic inflammatory component is seen, particularly near hemorrhagic foci. Occasional mitoses may be present in the proliferating cells, but cytologic criteria for malignancy are absent.

If there is bone erosion, the tumor enters the bone along vascular foramina or ligamentous and synovial attachments. A biopsy taken from an intraosseous focus may cause much confusion, because giant cell tumor of bone may be offered as a diagnostic possibility. This diagnosis should be ruled out by clinical suspicion coupled with the absence of the histologic features typical of giant cell tumor such as random distribution of osteoclastic-type giant cells, the characteristic stromal cells, and the similarity of the nuclei of the giant cells and stromal cells.

PVNS can be distinguished from hemosiderotic synovitis of a variety of causes by the presence of the proliferating polyhedral cells that invade into the subsynovial connective tissue. These cells are absent in hemosiderotic synovitis, and in hemosiderotic synovitis, the hemosiderin is usually limited to synovial lining cells and some superficially located macrophages.

Immunohistochemical studies of these tumors have not yielded consistent results and have been interpreted to support both a synovial cell or fibrohistiocytic phenotype.[26,64] Flow cytometric analyses have shown that some of these tumors, especially those that have large extra-articular soft tissue components, may be aneuploid and have high proliferative indices.[54] Although these flow cytometric findings may help predict which cases of PVNS will behave more locally aggressively, examples of PVNS with these attributes have not been shown to metastasize.[54]

Treatment and Outcome

The treatment of PVNS has not been standardized and has included radiation therapy, total synovectomy, arthrodesis, bone-grafting, and primary arthroplasty.[52] Although no single therapy has been consistently successful, currently, wide synovectomy is the recommended treatment.[65] However, it is difficult to perform an actual complete synovectomy; therefore, residual involved synovium frequently remains, causing a local recurrence rate of 16 to 48 percent.[65] Tumors in the knee have a higher rate of recurrence compared to tumors in other joints.[66] Rarely, recurrent disease or tumors with large extra-articular components may require more radical surgery, such as ray resection or even amputation.[54] Recent studies have shown that moderate doses of radiation may control and even cure patients with such extensive disease, thereby, possibly obviating the need for radical surgery or amputation.

Malignant Pigmented Villonodular Synovitis

Malignant PVNS is a very rare lesion with only a handful of cases reported.[67,68] The knee is the joint most commonly affected, and in a significant number of cases, there was coexisting benign-appearing PVNS. In malignant PVNS, the neoplastic cells are cytologically malignant. These tumors have the capacity to behave aggressively, as almost 50 percent of patients have died from metastatic disease.[67]

Localized Nodular Synovitis

The term localized nodular synovitis refers to the focal expression of pigmented villonodular synovitis in which only a discrete area of the synovium is involved. This condition is also known as benign giant cell synovioma or benign synovioma. Histologically, it is identical to the nodules of PVNS. The main difference is that the prominent synovial villi present in PVNS are absent or sparse. The localized variant usually consists of a single sessile or pedunculated, sometimes lobulated, nodule or mass that ranges from 1 to 8 cm in diameter (Fig. 113–31). Most commonly it is unilateral, arises in the knee (Fig. 113–32), and is equally distributed between the sexes.[69]

Symptoms are similar to those of PVNS except in the localized variant, there is a lower incidence of pain and stiffness[51] and a higher frequency of joint locking as the mass interferes with motion. A minority of patients may present with acute, severe joint pain caused by torsion and infarction of the tumor (Fig. 113–33). Effusions are common, but the synovial fluid tends to be less bloody than in PVNS and may even be clear.

Imaging studies show a heterogeneous nodular mass that contains lipid and hemosiderin deposits (Fig. 113–34). In the knee joint, the tumor frequently arises between the meniscus and joint capsule, as well as the intercondylar fossa adjacent to the patella.[26] There is usually no bone invasion. Marginal excision is usually curative[50] and small lesions can be extirpated arthroscopically.

Localized Nodular Tenosynovitis

Localized nodular tenosynovitis arises from the tendon sheath and usually involves the hand or wrist and less frequently the foot or ankle.[51] In fact, localized nodular tenosynovitis is the most common soft tissue tumor of the hand. This condition may also be known as giant cell tumor of the tendon sheath or fibroxanthoma of the tendon sheath. It usually arises from the flexor tendon sheaths of the fingers. The index finger is most commonly affected, followed by the middle finger, ring finger, little finger, and thumb.[50]

Finger tumors predominate in females by a ratio of at least 2:1[51,70] and tumors of the toes have an equal sex distribution.[51] On average, patients are in their third to fifth decades of life and present with a painless, palpable, firm mobile mass.

Clinically, the mass is usually solitary and located on the flexor surface, but it may bulge into the extensor or lateral aspects of the digits (Fig. 113–35). The tumors are slow

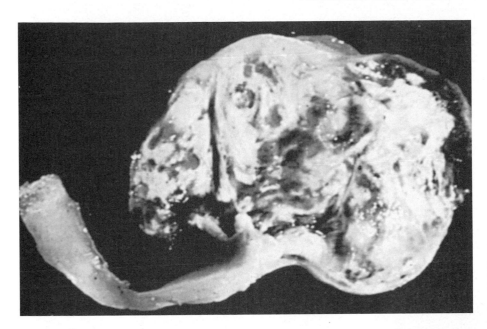

FIGURE 113–31 · Localized nodular synovitis on cross section with mottled, hemorrhagic, yellow soft tissue, similar to a nodule of pigmented villonodular synovitis (PVNS), with a long stalk. This is typical for this lesion. (Courtesy of Dr. C. Campbell.)

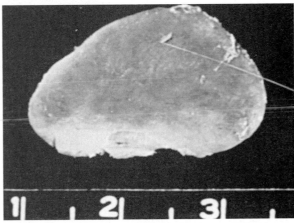

FIGURE 113–33 · An infarcted, localized nodular synovitis that has twisted on its stalk. Histologically, it is composed of dense collagen and necrotic hemorrhagic tissue. Grossly, the lesion is bright red.

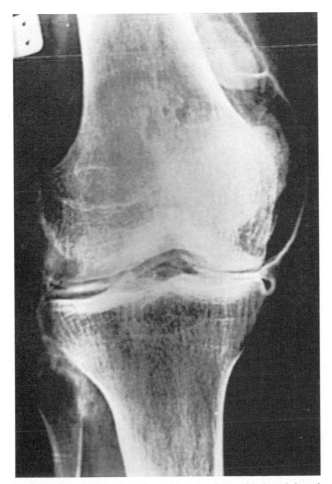

FIGURE 113–32 · Localized Nodular Synovitis Involving the Suprapatellar Portion of the Knee. The lesion is a large, elliptical, intra-articular soft tissue density.

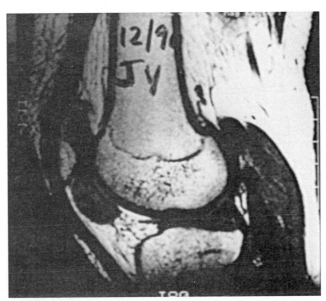

FIGURE 113–34 · Magnetic Resonance Image (mri) Of Knee Showing Localized Nodular Synovitis.

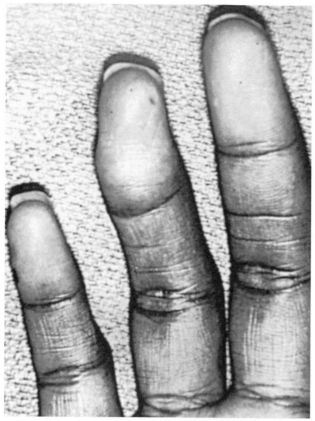

FIGURE 113-35 · Localized nodular tenosynovitis of the distal flexor surface of the fourth finger. Note the distended, flattened overlaying skin. The mass straddles the distal interphalangeal joint. (Courtesy of Dr. C. Campbell.)

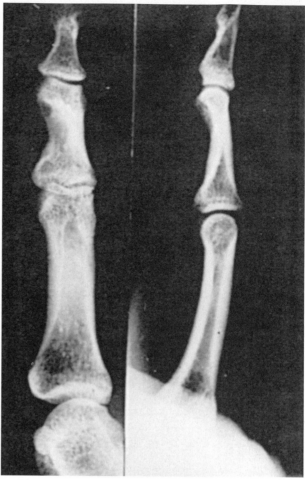

FIGURE 113-36 · A localized nodular tenosynovitis of the index finger with pressure erosion of the flexor aspect of the middle phalanx. There is a scalloped, well-marginated bone lesion, including a more distal subcortical cyst.

growing and the interval between detection and surgical treatment has ranged from several weeks to greater than a decade with an average of slightly more than 2 years.[51,70]

Radiographically tumors appear as well-circumscribed soft tissue masses, and in about 25 percent of cases there is adjacent extrinsic excavation of the cortical bone that has a sclerotic margin[51,70] (Fig. 113–36). MRI reveals the lesions to have a hypointense signal on T1-weighted images and either a hypo- or hyperintense signal on T2-weighted images; these findings are helpful in distinguishing giant-cell tumor of the tendon sheath from other soft tissue tumors.[71]

The gross pathology is that of a multinodular, round, rubbery mass, generally not larger than 5 cm in diameter, which is firmly attached to but easily peeled off of the involved tendon. At surgery, the lesion may "pop out" of the incision as a well-circumscribed mass. Careful attention should be paid to the external surface of the mass because the tumor may not be truly encapsulated and may infiltrate the adjacent structures. The cut surface ranges from hues of yellow to orange-brown, depending on the amount of lipid and blood pigments present. Often there are bands, or septae, of white, fibrous tissue that divide the lesion. Cystic spaces are unusual. Microscopically, the cell types present are identical to those in PVNS and may be mitotically active[72] (Fig. 113–37). Ultrastructurally, the proliferating cells have features similar to both type A and type B synovial lining cells.[70-73] Their antigenic and enzymatic profiles have suggested a

synovial or monocyte and macrophage lineage, the latter being similar to osteoclasts.[70,74] Flow cytometry has been performed on a small number of cases, and all have been diploid.[54] Cytogenetics show that many of these tumors

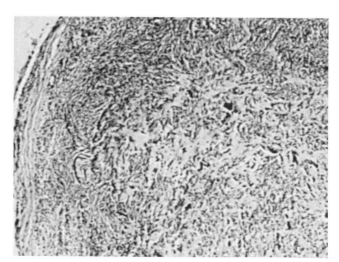

FIGURE 113-37 · A low-power microscopic view of localized nodular tenosynovitis to emphasize the relatively clear delineation of the mass from adjacent soft tissue and the broad bands of collagen traversing the lesion. Note the scattered osteoclast-type giant cells.

have a structural rearrangement in the region of chromosome 1p11 through 13.[75]

These tumors are benign and do not metastasize. Rarely have malignant giant cell tumors of the tendon sheath been reported.[76] The treatment of choice is conservative surgical excision, which is usually curative. There may be local recurrence if the tumor is incompletely excised.[51,70]

■ Malignant Tumors of the Joint

Malignant tumors of joints are uncommon and are classified into primary and secondary types. Primary malignancies are virtually always sarcomas. The sarcomas usually arise within the synovium of large diarthrodial joints, and the vast majority are either chondrosarcomas or synovial sarcomas. Rarely, other sarcomas arise within joints, and we have experience with intra-articular malignant fibrous histiocytoma and angiosarcoma (Fig. 113–38). Secondary malignant tumors of joints, by definition, originate beyond the confines of the joint, and most are sarcomas that extend from neighboring bones or surrounding soft tissues. Although synovial tissue is very vascular, metastases or involvement of the synovium by carcinoma, lymphoma, or leukemia is relatively uncommon.

PRIMARY SARCOMAS OF JOINTS

Chondrosarcoma

Chondrosarcoma arising in the synovium is unusual, and fewer than 50 cases have been reported in the English-language literature.[36,37,78,79] In approximately 50 percent of these cases, the chondrosarcoma arose in

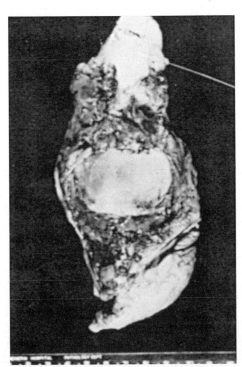

FIGURE 113–38 · Angiosarcoma arising in the knee of a 76-year-old man as friable red-tan tissue replacing the synovium, crawling over the patella, and filling up all synovial recesses. The patient died 8 months later with microscopic lung metastases.

association with preexisting synovial chondromatosis.[36,37,79] The patients are usually in their fifth to seventh decade of life and have an equal sex distribution.[79] Typically, they present with a progressively enlarging mass in the joint that may cause mechanical dysfunction, pain, and stiffness. In patients who have preexisting synovial chondromatosis, the duration of symptoms is usually long-standing and in some instances may be present for as many as 25 years.[79] Most chondrosarcomas arise in the knee joint, followed by the hip and elbow joints.

Radiographic studies usually demonstrate a periarticular soft tissue mass that may have dense irregular or ring-like calcifications. Occasionally, invasion into the medullary cavity of adjacent bone is present. The radiographic differential diagnosis varies according to the presence of calcification and includes synovial chondromatosis, synovial sarcoma, PVNS, and chronic synovitis.[79]

Grossly, the involved joint is filled with synovium massively thickened by innumerable nodules of opalescent blue-white cartilage. The nodules of cartilage vary in size and may be free-floating in the joint cavity. In several cases, the tumor has extended into the adjacent soft tissue and bone.

Microscopically the tumor is usually composed of malignant hyaline and myxoid cartilage. Rarely, the matrix is entirely myxoid and has the features of extraskeletal myxoid chondrosarcoma.[80] The neoplastic cartilage is cellular and contains cytologically atypical chondrocytes. The periphery of the lobules of cartilage is typically the most cellular, and it is in this region that some of the tumor cells are spindled. Other findings include myxoid change of the matrix, necrosis, and permeation of invaded bone.[79] Coexisting synovial chondromatosis can be identified by the presence of well-formed nodules of hyaline cartilage that re less cellular, contain cytologically banal–appearing chondrocytes, and a matrix that is frequently mineralized.

Treatment is usually surgical extirpation with consideration given for chemotherapy in high-grade lesions or those that have metastasized. Inadequate surgical removal virtually ensures local recurrence that may necessitate future radical excision. Metastases have occurred in approximately one third of the reported patients with the lung being the most common site for systemic spread.[79]

Synovial Sarcoma

Synovial sarcoma is a relatively common sarcoma and accounts for approximately 6 to 10 percent of soft tissue sarcomas. It usually develops in the deep soft tissues and rarely arises in joints, but it may secondarily invade articular synovium from neighboring soft tissues (Fig. 113–40). Earlier descriptions of this tumor attest to its wide spectrum of morphology because such names as adenosarcoma and synovial fibrosarcoma were used until the term *synovial sarcoma*, first introduced in 1936, became commonplace. The morphology of synovial sarcoma mimics a joint in its early stage of development in that it contains cleft-like spaces and glands delineated by large polygonal (epithelioid) cells surrounded by fascicles of spindle cells. The clefts and glands simulate a microscopic "joint space" that is bounded by synovial lining cells

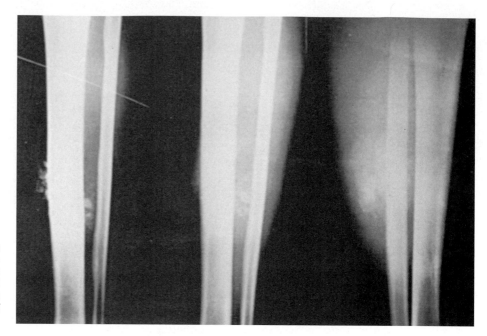

FIGURE 113-39 · Synovial sarcoma in the soft tissues of the calf is shown in these multiple views as a large, soft tissue density with amorphous speckled and nodular calcifications. There is slight pressure erosion of the medial aspect of the fibula.

and supported by subsynovial mesenchymal cells. Because either the epithelioid or spindle cells may predominate, synovial sarcoma has been subtyped into biphasic and monophasic spindle cell and epithelioid types.

Age

Synovial sarcoma commonly affects adolescents and young adults. In a series of 121 cases, the age range was 9 to 74 years with a median age of 34 years; however, synovial sarcoma occurs in children with significant frequency.[81,82]

Sites

Although the term *synovial sarcoma* implies that the tumor originates from the synovium, less than 10 percent of cases actually are intra-articular or in continuity with a synovial lining.[83,84] The fact that many synovial sarcomas arise near joints was also misconstrued as supporting its synovial origin.[85] Approximately 60 to 70 percent of synovial sarcomas arise in the extremities, especially the lower limb, in the vicinity of large joints, particularly the popliteal area of the knee and foot.[86] Regions of the thigh, hand, leg, and digits may be affected, and in the distal extremities, the tumors often are adjacent to joint capsules, tendon sheaths or both. In the upper limb, distal involvement is more common than arm or elbow sites. Tumors have also been reported in the neck, torso, craniofacial region, retroperitoneum, orbit, tongue, mediastinum, soft palate, kidney, lung, pleura, and prostate. These latter sites suggest an undifferentiated mesenchymal cell of origin for synovial sarcoma because they are not near joints or synovium.

Clinical Data

There are no clinical features related to synovial sarcoma that distinguish it from other sarcomas. The most common complaint is the development of a slowly enlarging, deep-seated, palpable mass that is painful in about 50 percent of cases.[82,86] Symptoms may be present for unusually long periods of time before medical evaluation is sought; this time period has ranged from months to 25 years, with an average of about 6 months to 2.5 years.[82,86] Delay in diagnosis is more frequent with tumors located in the deep soft tissues compared to those based in the more superficial and clinically noticeable regions. In some cases involving the knee region, vague mild pain over several months may occur before a mass is appreciated, and it if the tumor reaches a large size, limitation of motion may finally occur. Head and neck lesions produce symptoms related to their specific sites, such as hoarseness and breathing or swallowing difficulties. Rarely, a patient may present with symptoms secondary to pulmonary metastases, such as hemoptysis.[86]

Radiographic Findings

Classically, the plain film findings of synovial sarcoma are a well-circumscribed, deep-seated soft tissue mass. Synovial sarcoma is one of the few primary soft tissue tumors that frequently calcifies. Approximately 30 to 50 percent of cases will have radiographically detectable calcifications that can have a fine, stippled, or dense appearance[87] (Fig. 113–39). The calcification may be focal or present throughout most of the tumor.[88] Adjacent periosteal reaction is elicited in approximately 20 percent of cases, but the tumors infrequently erode into bone.

CT scanning is important in delineating the anatomic extent of the tumor and is more sensitive than plain radiographs in demonstrating calcification or periosteal reaction. MRI usually shows a large inhomogeneous mass with areas of hemorrhage[89] (see Fig. 113–40). Angiography is not very helpful because synovial sarcomas may be hyper- or hypovascular; however, it does show the relation of the tumor to important vessels. The radi-

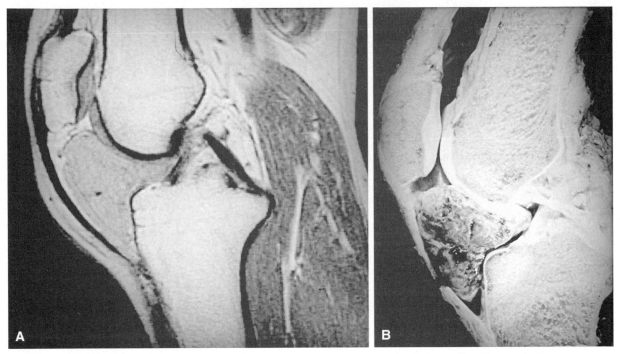

FIGURE 113–40 · *A*, Magnetic resonance imaging (MRI) scan of a rare example of intra-articular synovial sarcoma. The infrapatellar tumor is well circumscribed and has a focal inhomogeneous appearance. *B*, The gross specimen shows that the tan, hemorrhagic tumor bulges into the joint but is covered by synovium.

ographic differential diagnosis includes hemangioma, lipoma, synovial chondromatosis, soft tissue chondrosarcoma or osteosarcoma, myositis ossificans, aneurysms, and other sarcomas.

Pathology

The gross pathology of synovial sarcoma is invariably a well-demarcated, pink-tan, rather fleshy mass that easily detaches or "shells out" from its tumor bed. The cut surface is usually uniform, gray-yellow, and rubbery (see Fig. 113–40). If calcification is present, the tumor may be gritty. In larger tumors, areas of hemorrhage, necrosis, or both with cystification and gelatinous breakdown of tissue may also be seen. Occasionally, the tumors interdigitate between tendons, muscle, and fascial planes or wrap around neurovascular bundles. Extension into a joint is very uncommon.

Synovial sarcoma is subtyped into three patterns on the basis of predominant microscopic findings. The categories are as follows:

- Monophasic spindle cell
- Monophasic epithelioid
- Biphasic synovial sarcoma

Obviously, there is some subjectivity in the use of such a classification system, because many of these tumors have a variable histologic picture. A useful differential observation is that marked cellular pleomorphism and atypia are usually not present in synovial sarcoma, and when they are present, they tend to point to some other type of neoplasm such as a high-grade malignant fibrous histiocytoma or fibrosarcoma. Microscopically, the hall-mark of the more common biphasic synovial sarcoma is the two different populations of neoplastic cells, consisting of epithelioid and spindle cells (Fig. 113–41). The epithelioid cells may be cuboidal or columnar and, like true epithelium, have well-defined cytoplasmic borders. These cells may form gland-like spaces, line papillae, form cleft-like spaces, or grow in cohesive groups. The epithelioid cells are usually surrounded by the other cell type, namely small, plump spindle cells. The spindle cells grow in densely cellular fascicles that may be arranged in a "herringbone" pattern. In most biphasic synovial sar-

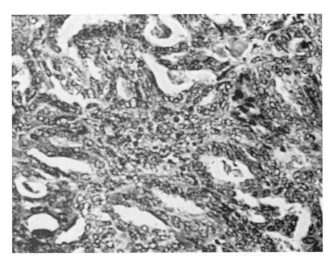

FIGURE 113–41 · Synovial sarcoma with a biphasic pattern of spindle cells and epithelioid cells arranged around gland-like spaces. Mitoses are evident, and the lumina of the pseudoglands contain hyaluronic acid.

comas, the spindle cell component predominates; and it is in the spindle-cell regions that calcification of hyalinized stroma most frequently occurs. Some tumors may have bone formation, which may be present in the spindle or epithelioid areas. In the monophasic variants, either the spindle or epithelioid cells predominate (Figs. 113–42 and 113–43). Pure epithelioid synovial sarcomas are extraordinarily rare.

Electron microscopy and tissue-culture observations indicate some unifying and common features of both cell types composing synovial sarcoma. These include a distinct basal lamina between epithelioid and spindle cells and specialized cell junctions, such as desmosomes and maculae adherents, which are present mostly between the epithelioid cells but also between some spindle cells. The epithelioid cells may also have microvilli, intercellular spaces, free ribosomes, arrays of endoplasmic reticulum, prominent Golgi apparatuses, and small vesicles (Figs. 113–44 and 113–45).

The spindle cells possess microfibrils and secrete amorphous extracellular fibrils. There are usually few recognizable collagen fibrils. Because most of these features are nonspecific and may be found in many cells of the body, they do not necessarily support the

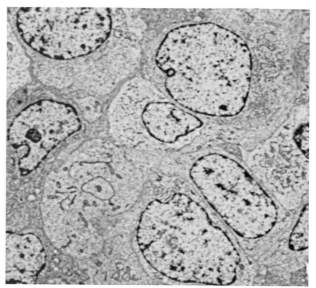

FIGURE 113–44 · Lower-Power Electron Microscopic Print of a Synovial Sarcoma. The neoplastic cells are polygonal, slightly elongated, and have abutting cell borders. There is a high nuclear-cytoplasmic ratio, and prominent nucleoli are sometimes visible.

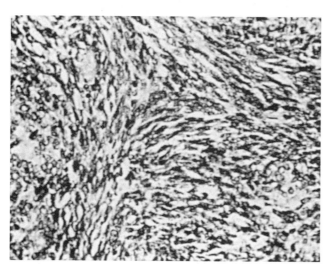

FIGURE 113–42 · Synovial sarcoma of the monophasic spindle cell type, with interdigitating fascicles of spindle cells. The cells have plump nuclei, little cytoplasm, and very little collagen production.

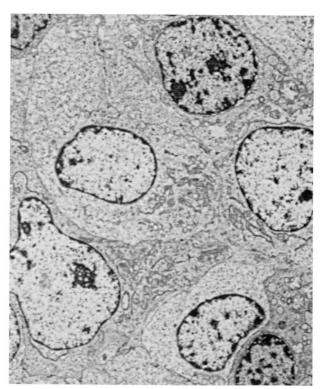

FIGURE 113–45 · Higher-power electron microscopic print of synovial sarcoma. The abutting cell borders have frequent junctions. The cytoplasm contains a background of free ribosomes and scattered microfilaments. Moderate numbers of mitochondria and cisternae of rough endoplasmic reticulum are localized in one end of the cell, and cisternae are slightly dilated and contain a material of medium electron density.

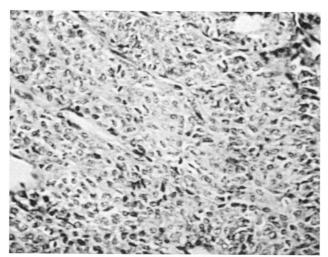

FIGURE 113–43 · Synovial sarcoma composed of monophasic epithelioid cells with sheets of polygonal or oval cells with indistinct cytoplasmic borders. There is slight nuclear pleomorphism.

view that synovial sarcoma represents a neoplasm of a primitive ancestor cell committed to modulate into synovial tissue. In tissue culture, both cell types make mucopolysaccharides, a feature that synovium shares with other mesenchymal tissues.

Immunohistochemistry has shown that both the epithelioid and spindle-cell components may stain with antibodies to keratin, epithelial membrane antigen, and carcinoembryonic antigen, which are usually associated with epithelial neoplasms.[90-92] This pattern of reactivity has helped make it possible to separate synovial sarcoma from other morphologically similar tumors, such as fibrosarcoma and malignant peripheral nerve sheath tumor. As well, it has provided evidence that synovial sarcoma does not arise from or recapitulate the synovium because normal synovial cells do not stain with these antibodies.[93]

Cytogenetic studies of synovial sarcomas have detected a consistent translocation in almost all cases, regardless of whether the tumor is biphasic or monophasic.[94] This finding provides insight into the genesis of synovial sarcoma and can be used as a diagnostic feature. There is no consensus regarding its utility in providing prognostic information.

Prognosis and Therapy

The prognosis of synovial sarcoma is not very good. In one recent study of 121 patients, the 5-, 10-, and 15-year survival rates were 60, 50, and 45 percent, respectively.[82] There is some evidence to suggest that more modern modes of therapy, which combine surgery and chemotherapy, improve outcome.[95]

A number of factors influence prognosis. Tumors that are small (less than 5 cm in diameter), arise in persons less than 25 years of age, and have clearly differentiated areas have a high rate of cure.[82] In contrast, large tumors (5-cm diameter or greater) that arise in persons 25 years or older and contain poorly differentiated areas have a dismal outcome.[82] The impact of histologic subtype has been controversial. Some studies have indicated that the monophasic spindle-cell variant behaves the most aggressively, and those patients whose tumors have a predominate glandular component, are heavily calcified,[88] and have a diploid pattern by flow cytometry do the best.

The natural history of synovial sarcoma is local recurrence, which may be repetitive. Most recurrences manifest within 2 years after initial treatment; however, intervals longer than 10 years are not exceptional. Ultimately, metastases develop in most patients and involve regional lymph nodes in 10 to 23 percent of patients,[96] with other common sites being the lungs and skeleton. About 10 percent of patients die within 1 year after diagnosis of metastatic disease, and 90 percent of these will have massive pulmonary metastases.

Treatment must contend with issues involved with both local and systemic therapy. Successful local control can usually be achieved by limb-salvage surgery combined with radiation. Because the regional lymph nodes are commonly involved, their status should be carefully evaluated, and they should be treated if enlarged. Systemic treatment consists of various chemo-

therapy regimens, some of which have been shown to be beneficial.[95]

SECONDARY MALIGNANT TUMORS OF THE JOINT

Sarcomas

Primary bone sarcomas, such as chondrosarcoma and osteosarcoma, infrequently invade through the joint capsule or articular surface and involve the synovium. When this occurs it may be difficult to distinguish based on histologic features alone primary from secondary sarcomas.

Primary soft tissue sarcomas rarely destroy joint capsules and invade the synovium. However, certain soft tissue sarcomas have a propensity to grow along tendon sheaths for significant distances from the main mass. Because of this pattern of spread and certain microscopic features, these sarcomas—namely, clear cell sarcoma, epithelioid sarcoma, extraskeletal myxoid chondrosarcoma, and synovial sarcoma—were believed to have a common histogenesis and were lumped together to form the entity "tendosynovial sarcoma." However, subsequent clinical, immunohistochemical, and ultrastructural studies have shown these tumors to be distinct clinicopathologic entities. For instance, clear cell sarcoma is now known to be a malignant melanoma that arises in the soft tissues,[97] and the phenotype of extraskeletal myxoid chondrosarcoma is now being questioned. Epithelioid sarcoma appears to be unique, and its normal tissue counterpart has not been identified. Therefore, the term *tendosynovial sarcoma* is no longer appropriate.

Metastatic Carcinoma

The synovium, unlike other richly vascular tissues, is rarely the site of metastatic carcinoma. This may reflect the fact that only clinical cases in which joint symptoms prevail are reported, because at autopsy joints are not routinely examined. Most of the carcinomas that have metastasized to the synovium originate in the lung, followed by the gastrointestinal tract and breast.[98] The affected patients are usually elderly, and the joint most frequently involved is the knee. In many of the reported cases, the underlying bone has also contained metastatic deposits.

Malignant Lymphoproliferative Disease

The various types of malignant lymphoproliferative diseases, including leukemia, lymphoma, and myeloma, can involve the synovium and produce osteoarticular symptoms.[99-101] This complication occurs most frequently in leukemia and is seen in both the acute and chronic forms.[101] Joint symptoms have been observed in 12 to 65 percent of childhood leukemia and in 4 to 13 percent of adult patients with leukemia.[101] The arthritis can develop at any time during the disease course and can even be the presenting complaint. Large joints are affected more commonly than small joints, and the arthritis is often pauciarticular, asymmetric, migratory, and severe. The symptoms may result from leukemic infiltration of the synovium or irritation of the neighboring periosteum. When arthritis is the major presenting symptom, it may cause confusion with septic arthritis, rheumatic fever, subacute bacterial endocarditis, or RA.

REFERENCES

1. Treadwell EL: Synovial cysts and ganglia: the value of magnetic resonance imaging. Semin Arthritis Rheum 24:61-70, 1994.
2. Seil R, Rupp S, Jochum M, et al: Prevalence of popliteal cysts in children: A sonographic study and review of the literature. Arch Orthop Trauma Surg 119:73-75, 1999.
3. Hall FM: Baker cysts. Radiology 203:577-578, 1997.
4. Torreggiani WC, Al-Ismail K, Munk PL, et al: The imaging spectrum of Baker's (popliteal) cysts. Clin Radiol 57:681-691, 2002.
5. Radatz M, Jakubowski J, Cooper J, Powell T: Synovial cysts of the lumbar spine: a review. Br J Neurosurg 11:520-524, 1997.
6. McEvedy BV: Simple ganglia. Br J Surg 49:40, 1962.
7. Thornburg LE: Ganglions of the hand and wrist. J Am Acad Orthop Surg 7:231-238, 1999.
8. Milgram JW: The classification of loose bodies in human joints. Clin Orthop 124:282-291, 1977.
9. Kumar VP, Satku K: Arthroscopic retrieval of loose bodies. Arthroscopy 10:696-697, 1994.
10. Cooper G, Schiller AL: Anatomy of the Guinea Pig. Cambridge, Mass, Harvard University Press, 1975.
11. Martinoli C, Bianchi S, Spadola L, Garcia J: Multimodality imaging assessment of meniscal ossicle. Skeletal Radiol 29:481-484, 2000.
12. Schnarkowski P, Tirman PF, Fuchigami KD, et al: Meniscal ossicle: Radiographic and MR imaging findings. Radiology 196:47-50, 1995.
13. Pudlowski RM, Gilula LA, Kyriakos M: Intraarticular lipoma with osseous metaplasia: radiographic-pathologic correlation. AJR Am J Roentgenol 132:471-473, 1979.
14. Coventry MB, Harrison EG Jr, Martin JF: Benign synovial tumors of the knee: a diagnostic problem. J Bone Joint Surg Am 48:1350-1358, 1966.
15. Allen PW: Lipoma arborescens. In Allen PW (ed): Tumors and Prolif-erations of Adipose Tissue. Chicago, Year Book Medical Publishers, 1981, p 129.
16. Kloen P, Keel SB, Chandler HP, et al: Lipoma arborescens of the knee. J Bone Joint Surg Br 80:298-301, 1998.
17. Martinez D, Millner PA, Coral A, et al: Case report 745: synovial lipoma arborescens. Skeletal Radiol 21:393-395, 1992.
18. Martin S, Hernandez L, Romero J, et al: Diagnostic imaging of lipoma arborescens. Skeletal Radiol 27:325-329, 1998.
19. Hoffa A: The influence of the adipose tissue with regard to the pathology of the knee joint. JAMA 43:795, 1904.
20. Devaney K, Vinh TN, Sweet DE: Synovial hemangioma: a report of 20 cases with differential diagnostic considerations. Hum Pathol 24:737-745, 1993.
21. Lichtenstein L: Tumors of synovial joints, bursae, and tendon sheaths. Cancer 8:816-830, 1955.
22. Greenspan A, Azouz EM, Matthews J II, Decarie JC: Synovial hemangioma: Imaging features in eight histologically proven cases, review of the literature, and differential diagnosis. Skeletal Radiol 24:583-590, 1995.
23. Cotten A, Flipo RM, Herbaux B, et al: Synovial haemangioma of the knee: A frequently misdiagnosed lesion. Skeletal Radiol 24:257-261, 1995.
24. Chung EB, Enzinger FM: Fibroma of tendon sheath. Cancer 44:1945-1954, 1979.
25. Pulitzer DR, Martin PC, Reed RJ: Fibroma of tendon sheath: A clinicopathologic study of 32 cases. Am J Surg Pathol 13:472-479, 1989.
26. Maluf HM, DeYoung BR, Swanson PE, Wick MR: Fibroma and giant cell tumor of tendon sheath: A comparative histological and immunohistological study. Mod Pathol 8:155-159, 1995.
27. Buddingh EP, Krallman P, Neff JR, et al: Chromosone 6 abnormalities are recurrent in synovial chondromatosis. Cancer Genet Cytogenet 140:18-22, 2003.
28. Davis RI, Hamilton A, Biggart JD: Primary synovial chondromatosis: A clinicopathologic review and assessment of malignant potential. Hum Pathol 29:683-688, 1998.
29. Hettiaratchy SP, Nanchahal J: Synovial chondromatosis of the metacarpophalangeal joint. J Hand Surg [Br] 27:104-106, 2002.
30. von Lindern JJ, Theuerkauf, I, Niederhagen B, et al: Synovial chondromatosis of the temperomandibular joint: Clinical, diagnostic, and histomorphologic findings. Oral Surg Oral Med Radiol Endod 94:31-38, 2002.
31. Sim FH, Dahlin DC, Ivins JC: Extra-articular synovial chondromatosis. J Bone Joint Surg Am 59:492-495, 1977.
32. Jones WA, Ghorbal MS: Benign tendon sheath chondroma. J Hand Surg [Br] 11:276-278, 1986.
33. Crotty JM, Monu JU, Pope TL Jr: Synovial osteochondromatosis. Radiol Clin North Am 34:327-342, xi, 1996.
34. Edeiken J, Edeiken B, Ayala G, et al: Giant solitary synovial chondromatosis. Skeletal Radiol 23:23-9, 1994.
35. Coughlan B, Feliz A, Ishida T, et al: p53 expression and DNA ploidy of cartilage lesions. Hum Pathol 26:620-624, 1995.
36. Taconis WK, van der Heul RO, Taminiau AM: Synovial chondrosarcoma: report of a case and review of the literature. Skeletal Radiol 26:682-685, 1997.
37. Ontell F, Greenspan A: Chondrosarcoma complicating synovial chondromatosis: Findings with magnetic resonance imaging. Can Assoc Radiol J 45:318-323, 1994.
38. Dahlin DC, Salvador AH: Cartilaginous tumors of the soft tissues of the hands and feet. Mayo Clin Proc 49:721-726, 1974.
39. Chung EB, Enzinger FM: Chondroma of soft parts. Cancer 41:1414-1424, 1978.
40. Fletcher CDM, Krausz T: Cartilaginous tumors of soft tissue. Appl Pathol 6:208, 1986.
41. Zlatkin MB, Lander PH, Begin LR, Hadjipavlou A: Soft-tissue chondromas. AJR Am J Roentgenol 144:1263-1267, 1985.
42. Lichtenstein L, Goldman RL: Cartilage tumors in soft tissues, particularly in the hand and foot. Cancer 17:1203, 1964.
43. Steiner GC, Meushar N, Norman A, Present D: Intracapsular and paraarticular chondromas. Clin Orthop 303:231-236, 1994.
44. Hensinger RN, Cowell HR, Ramsey PL, Leopold RG: Familial dysplasia epiphysealis hemimelica, associated with chondromas and osteochondromas: Report of a kindred with variable presentations. J Bone Joint Surg Am 56:1513-1516, 1974.
45. Young JM, Hudacek AG: Experimental production of pigmented villonodular synovitis in dogs. Am J Pathol 30:799, 1954.
46. Singh R, Grewal DS, Chakravarti RN: Experimental production of pigmented villonodular synovitis in the knee and ankle joints of rhesus monkeys. J Pathol 98:137-142, 1969.
47. Fletcher JA, Henkle C, Atkins L, et al: Trisomy 5 and trisomy 7 are nonrandom aberrations in pigmented villonodular synovitis: Confirmation of trisomy 7 in uncultured cells. Genes Chromosomes Cancer 4:264-266, 1992.
48. Rowlands CG, Roland B, Hwang WS, Sevick RJ: Diffuse-variant tenosynovial giant cell tumor: a rare and aggressive lesion. Hum Pathol 25:423-425, 1994.
49. Sciot R, Rosai J, Dal Cin P, et al: Analysis of 35 cases of localized and diffuse tenosynovial giant cell tumor: A report from the Chromosomes and Morphology (CHAMP) study group. Mod Pathol 12:576-579, 1999.
50. Rydholm U: Pigmented villonodular synovitis. Acta Orthop Scand 69:203-210, 1998.
51. Rao AS, Vigorita VJ: Pigmented villonodular synovitis (giant-cell tumor of the tendon sheath and synovial membrane): A review of eighty-one cases. J Bone Joint Surg Am 66:76-94, 1984.
52. Flandry F, Hughston JC: Pigmented villonodular synovitis. J Bone Joint Surg Am 69:942-949, 1987.
53. Arthaud JB: Pigmented nodular synovitis: report of 11 lesions in non-articular locations. Am J Clin Pathol 58:511-517, 1972.
54. Abdul-Karim FW, el-Naggar AK, Joyce MJ, et al: Diffuse and localized tenosynovial giant cell tumor and pigmented villonodular synovitis: A clinicopathologic and flow cytometric DNA analysis. Hum Pathol 23:729-735, 1992.
55. Kindblom LG, Gunterberg B: Pigmented villonodular synovitis involving bone: Case report. J Bone Joint Surg Am 60:830-832, 1978.
56. Cotten A, Flipo RM, Chastanet P, et al: Pigmented villonodular synovitis of the hip: review of radiographic features in 58 patients. Skeletal Radiol 24:1-6, 1995.

57. Jergesen HE, Mankin HJ, Schiller AL: Diffuse pigmented villon-odular synovitis of the knee mimicking primary bone neoplasms: A report of two cases. J Bone Joint Surg Am 60:825-829, 1978.

58. Myers BW, Masi AT: Pigmented villonodular synovitis and tenosynovitis: a clinical epidemiologic study of 166 cases and literature review. Medicine (Baltimore) 59:223-238, 1980.

59. Lin J, Jacobson JA, Jamadar DA, Ellis JH: Pigmented villonodular synovitis and related lesions: the spectrum of imaging findings. AJR Am J Roentgenol 172:191-197, 1999.

60. Goldman AB, DiCarlo EF: Pigmented villonodular synovitis: diagnosis and differential diagnosis. Radiol Clin North Am 26:1327-1347, 1988.

61. Burk DL Jr., Mitchell DG, Rifkin MD, Vinitski S: Recent advances in magnetic resonance imaging of the knee. Radiol Clin North Am 28:379-393, 1990.

62. Hughes TH, Sartoris DJ, Schweitzer ME, Resnick DL: Pigmented villonodular synovitis: MRI characteristics. Skeletal Radiol 24:7-12, 1995.

63. Flandry F, Hughston JC, McCann SB, Kurtz DM: Diagnostic features of diffuse pigmented villonodular synovitis of the knee. Clin Orthop 298:212-220, 1994.

64. O'Connell JX, Fanburg JC, Rosenberg AE: Giant cell tumor of tendon sheath and pigmented villonodular synovitis: immunophenotype suggests a synovial cell origin. Hum Pathol 26:771-775, 1995.

65. Flandry FC, Hughston JC, Jacobson KE, et al: Surgical treatment of diffuse pigmented villonodular synovitis of the knee. Clin Orthop 300:183-192, 1994.

66. Adem C, Sebo TJ, Riehle DL, et al: Recurrent and non-recurrent pigmented villonodular synovitis 1. Ann Pathol 22:448-452, 2002.

67. Bertoni F, Unni KK, Beabout JW, Sim FH: Malignant giant cell tumor of the tendon sheaths and joints (malignant pigmented villonodular synovitis). Am J Surg Pathol 21:153-163, 1997.

68. Layfield LJ, Meloni-Ehrig A, Liu K, et al: Malignant giant cell tumor of synovium (malignant pigmented villonodular synovitis). Arch Pathol Lab Med 124:1636-1641, 2000.

69. Fraire AE, Fechner RE: Intra-articular localized nodular synovitis of the knee. Arch Pathol 93:473-476, 1972.

70. Ushijima M, Hashimoto H, Tsuneyoshi M, Enjoji M: Giant cell tumor of the tendon sheath (nodular tenosynovitis): A study of 207 cases to compare the large joint group with the common digit group. Cancer 57:875-884, 1986.

71. Jelinek JS, Kransdorf MJ, Shmookler BM, et al: Giant cell tumor of the tendon sheath: MR findings in nine cases. AJR Am J Roentgenol 162:919-922, 1994.

72. Monaghan H, Salter DM, Al-Nafussi A: Giant cell tumour of tendon sheath (localised nodular tenosynovitis): clinicopathological features of 71 cases. J Clin Pathol 54:404-407, 2001.

73. Alguacil-Garcia A, Unni KK, Goellner JR: Giant cell tumor of tendon sheath and pigmented villonodular synovitis: an ultrastructural study. Am J Clin Pathol 69:6-17, 1978.

74. Wood GS, Beckstead JH, Medeiros LJ, et al: The cells of giant cell tumor of tendon sheath resemble osteoclasts. Am J Surg Pathol 12:444-452, 1988.

75. Nilsson M, Hoglund M, Panagopoulos I, et al: Molecular cytogenetic mapping of recurrent chromosomal breakpoints in tenosynovial giant cell tumors. Virchows Arch 441:475-480, 2002.

76. Castens HP, Howell RS: Maglignant giant cell tumor of tendon sheath. Virchows Arch A Pathol Anat Histol 382:237-243, 1979.

77. Bertoni F, Unnik K, Beabout JW, sim FH: Malignant giant cell tumor of the tendon sheaths and joints (malignant pigmented villondular synovitis). Am J surrg Pathol 21:153-163, 1997.

78. Perry BE, McQueen DA, Lin JJ: Synovial chondromatosis with malignant degeneration to chondrosarcoma: Report of a case. J Bone Joint Surg Am 70:1259-1261, 1988.

79. Bertoni F, Unni KK, Beabout JW, Sim FH: Chondrosarcomas of the synovium. Cancer 67:155-162, 1991.

80. Kindblom LG, Angervall L: Myxoid chondrosarcoma of the synovial tissue: A clinicopathologic, histochemical, and ultrastructural analysis. Cancer 52:1886-1895, 1983.

81. Okcu MF, Munsell M, Treuner J, et al: Synovial sarcoma of childhood and adolescence: A multicenter, multivariate analysis of outcome. J Clin Oncol 21:1602-1611, 2003.

82. Bergh P, Meis-Kindblom JM, Gherlinzoni F, et al: Synovial sarcoma: identification of low and high risk groups. Cancer 85:2596-2607, 1999.

83. Dardick I, O'Brien PK, Jeans MT, Massiah KA: Synovial sarcoma arising in an anatomical bursa. Virchows Arch A Pathol Anat Histol 397:93-101, 1982.

84. McKinney CD, Mills SE, Fechner RE: Intraarticular synovial sarcoma. Am J Surg Pathol 16:1017-1020, 1992.

85. DeSanto DA, Tennant R, Rosahn P: Synovial sarcomas in joints, bursae, and tendon sheaths. Surg Gynecol Obstet 72:951, 1961.

86. Cadman NL, Soule EH, Kelly PJ: Synovial sarcoma: An analysis of 134 tumors. Cancer 18:613-627, 1965.

87. Milchgrub S, Ghandur-Mnaymneh L, Dorfman HD, Albores-Saavedra J: Synovial sarcoma with extensive osteoid and bone formation. Am J Surg Pathol 17:357-363, 1993.

88. Varela-Duran J, Enzinger FM: Calcifying synovial sarcoma. Cancer 50:345-352, 1982.

89. Blacksin MF, Siegel JR, Benevenia J, Aisner SC: Synovial sarcoma: frequency of nonaggressive MR characteristics. J Comput Assist Tomogr 21:785-789, 1997.

90. Corson JM, Weiss LM, Banks-Schlegel SP, Pinkus GS: Keratin proteins and carcinoembryonic antigen in synovial sarcomas: An immunohistochemical study of 24 cases. Hum Pathol 15:615-621, 1984.

91. Fisher C: Synovial sarcoma. Diag Pathol 1:13-18, 1994.

92. Lopes JM, Bjerkehagen B, Holm R, et al: Immunohistochemical profile of synovial sarcoma with emphasis on the epithelial-type differentiation: A study of 49 primary tumours, recurrences and metastases. Pathol Res Pract 190:168-177, 1994.

93. Miettinen M, Virtanen I: Synovial sarcoma: A misnomer. Am J Pathol 117:18-25, 1984.

94. Kawai A, Woodruff J, Healey JH, et al: SYT-SSX gene fusion as a determinant of morphology and prognosis in synovial sarcoma. N Engl J Med 338:153-160, 1998.

95. Van Glabbeke M, van Oosterom AT, Oosterhuis JW, et al: Prognostic factors for the outcome of chemotherapy in advanced soft tissue sarcoma: An analysis of 2,185 patients treated with anthracycline-containing first-line regimens—a European Organization for Research and Treatment of Cancer Soft Tissue and Bone Sarcoma Group Study. J Clin Oncol 17:150-157, 1999.

96. Hajdu SI, Shiu MH, Fortner JG: Tendosynovial sarcoma: a clinicopathological study of 136 cases. Cancer 39:1201-1217, 1977.

97. Chung EB, Enzinger FM: Malignant melanoma of soft parts: A reassessment of clear cell sarcoma. Am J Surg Pathol 7:405-413, 1983.

98. Younes M, Hayem G, Brissaud P, et al: Monoarthritis secondary to joint metastases: Two case reports and literature review. Joint Bone Spine 69:495-498, 2002.

99. Ehrenfeld M, Gur H, Shoenfeld Y: Rheumatologic features of hematologic disorders. Curr Opin Rheumatol 11:62-67, 1999.

100. Gur H, Koren V, Ehrenfeld M, et al: Rheumatic manifestations preceding adult acute leukemia: Characteristics and implication in course and prognosis. Acta Haematol 101:1-6, 1999.

101. Evans TI, Nercessian BM, Sanders KM: Leukemic arthritis. Semin Arthritis Rheum 24:48-56, 1994.

MARCO RIZZO · JAMES R. URBANIAK

Osteonecrosis is defined as the death of bone marrow and bone elements due to either repeated interruptions or a single large disruption of its blood supply. The process may occur in any bone, and it commonly occur in the small bones of the hands (e.g., lunate, scaphoid), femoral head, femoral condyles, and humeral head. Multiple etiologies have been described and are summarized in Table 114–1. When the process affects subchondral bone, the supporting trabeculae may fracture, leading to collapse of the articular cartilage, incongruity of the joint, and subsequent osteoarthritis (OA). This process of subarticular collapse has been described in many joints, but it is most common in the femoral head (hip joint), distal femur (knees), and humeral head (shoulder). Once subchondral fracture and collapse occurs, the damage is irreversible, as spontaneous bony union of the necrotic subarticular bone is nearly impossible, and the incongruent articular surfaces progress to arthritis. Osteonecrosis is recognized as a prevalent cause of arthritis of the hip, accounting for more than 10 percent of total hip arthroplasties performed in the United States annually.[1] Because osteonecrosis frequently affects patients in the third, fourth, and fifth decades of life, the potential for long-term physical disability and pain is high.

Osteonecrosis of the Femoral Head

ETIOLOGY AND PATHOGENESIS

The etiology of osteonecrosis is associated with interruption of the bone's blood supply. This may be due to a single traumatic disruption, such as hip fracture or dislocation, or repeated (microvascular) interruptions, which can occur through a variety of systemic, local, and hematologic factors. The fracture that occurs following bone death is secondary to either fatigue failure of the nonviable bone or fracture through weakened, revascularized bone (Fig. 114–1).

The microanatomy of the circulation for subchondral bone is composed of a system of end arteries with absent collaterals. In the femoral head, these end arteries are supplied by several groups of vessels: 1) an extracapsular arterial ring at the base of the femoral neck, 2) the artery of the ligamentum teres, 3) ascending cervical branches that arise from the extracapsular ring at the base of the femoral neck, and 4) intramedullary arteries of the femoral neck[2,3] (Fig. 114–2). The extracapsular ring is formed posteriorly by a branch of the medial femoral circumflex artery and anteriorly by branches of the lateral femoral circumflex artery. The inferior gluteal artery may have minor contributions to the ring as well. The ascending cervical branches arise from the ring along the intertrochanteric line and posterior femoral neck, and they run toward and penetrate the articular cartilage rim of the epiphysis. During their course, the ascending cervical branches, or retinacular arteries, are intracapsular and give off metaphyseal branches that penetrate the femoral neck. At the margin of the cartilage, the ascending branches form a subsynovial intra-articular ring, which may be complete or incomplete, depending on anatomic variation. From this ring, epiphyseal arterial branches arise and penetrate the head of the femur and supply the epiphysis. The epiphyseal arteries are terminal arterioles with little collateral circulation between one another. The artery of the ligamentum teres is a branch of the obturator artery or medial femoral circumflex artery. It gives rise to the medial epiphyseal arteries, which enter the femoral head at the fovea. The latcral epiphyseal arteries provide the bulk of the blood supply to the femoral head in most individuals, with only about one third having substantial perfusion of the head through medial epiphyseal vessels arising from the ligamentum teres. Collateral blood supply within the head is usually limited, so occlusion or destruction of the lateral retinacular or lateral epiphyseal arteries routinely results in the devascularization of and necrosis of a significant portion of the epiphysis.

TABLE 114–1 · ETIOLOGY OF OSTEONECROSIS

Atraumatic Causes
Corticosteroids
Immunosuppression
Systemic lupus erythematosus (SLE)
Rheumatoid arthritis (RA)
Ethanol abuse
Hemoglobinopathy
Coagulopathy
Myeloproliferative disorders
Radiation
Dysbarism
Pregnancy
Gout
Chronic pancreatitis
Gaucher's disease
Asthma

Traumatic Causes
Femoral-neck fracture
Hip dislocation

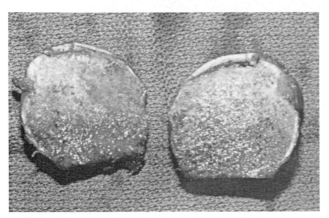

FIGURE 114–1 · Gross specimen of a divided femoral head showning an osteonecrotic lesion and a subchondral fracture.

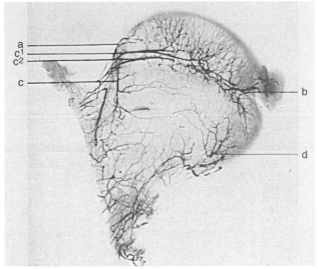

FIGURE 114–2 · Injection study demostrating lateral epiphyseal vessels(a) and medial epiphyseal vessels(b), C, lateral retinacular vessels; d, medial retinacular vessels. (From Trueta J, Harrison MHM: The normal vascular anatomy of the femoral head in adult man. J Bone Joint Surg 35B:445, 1953.)

POST-TRAUMATIC OSTEONECROSIS

Fractures of the femoral neck are the most common cause of post-traumatic osteonecrosis of the femoral head.[4,5] Hip dislocations and femoral neck fractures result in mechanical disruption of the blood supply, leading to osteonecrosis of some or all of the femoral head.[3] Displaced femoral neck fractures result in total or subtotal devascularization of the femoral head in 60 to 80 percent of cases.[2,5,6] The incidence of post-traumatic avascular necrosis of the femoral head has been reported to range from 15 to 86 percent.[7-13] The blood supply to the superolateral aspect of the femoral head is almost uniformly interrupted in this group, either by tearing of the lateral retinacular vessels or by a more proximal subcapital fracture that results in the destruction of the lateral epiphyseal vessels in their

intraosseous location. Because the majority of vessels that supply the femoral head are both intracapsular and extraosseous, blood flow may become impaired by hematoma and subsequent tamponade.[14]

Fortunately, late segmental collapse of the femoral head is not uniformly disabling. In elderly patients, some data suggest that they may maintain acceptable levels of function years after collapse.[15,16] However, in younger patients who have greater functional demands, the effects of femoral head collapse are more clinically relevant and often lead to significant disability. Late segmental collapse occurs through the necrotic segment of the femoral head, usually in the superior and superolateral aspects of the head where the hip is subject to the greatest mechanic and weight-bearing loads.[17] This collapse is thought to occur secondary to fatigue failure of the dead bone, which is incapable of remodeling, or through weakened, remodeling bone.

Despite the fact that most femoral heads undergo substantial, if not total, necrosis following displaced femoral neck fracture, late segmental collapse is not a certainty.[7,8,18,19] The absence of late segmental collapse in most femoral heads, even after significant necrosis, is a consequence of the head's potential to rapidly revascularize through the medial epiphyseal artery of the ligamentum teres and the remaining medial retinacular blood supply. The rapidity of revascularization and the likelihood of avoiding late segmental collapse may, therefore, be primarily a function of the initial relative contribution of the medial epiphyseal artery to the perfusion of the head and the adequacy of the development of collaterals to revascularize the superolateral segment.[4,20]

ATRAUMATIC OSTEONECROSIS

A wide variety of conditions and exposures have been associated with the development of atraumatic osteonecrosis[21] (see Table 114–1). In contrast to traumatic osteonecrosis, the relationship between cause and effect within this group is less clearly understood. Only a minority of patients with a given risk factor goes on to develop symptomatic osteonecrosis. The failure to produce an experimental model of atraumatic osteonecrosis by exposing animals to reputed risk factors underscores our incomplete understanding of the basic biology of this process. Depending on the risk factor, injury may occur through intravascular coagulation,[22] a thromboembolic event, vessel wall injury, or vessel compression.[1] The size and location of a lesion in a given patient most likely reflect this unique pattern of blood supply to the femoral head and the watershed areas most vulnerable to vascular insult. The most commonly affected area is the superolateral femoral head.

In most large series of patients with atraumatic osteonecrosis of the hip, alcohol abuse and corticosteroid use account for 60 to 90 percent of the cases.[23-25] The prevalence of this disease in alcoholic populations is between 2 and 5 percent.[26,27] The threshold for developing osteonecrosis of the hip has been estimated to require consumption of 150 liters of 100-percent alcohol at a rate of 400 ml or more per week.[23] Similarly, the risk from corticosteroids appears to depend both on the dose and the duration of exposure.[28] A cumulative dose of 2000 mg of prednisone administered over an uninterrupted time course appears to be an important threshold for developing osteonecrosis.[23] For each 20-mg increase in the daily dose of prednisone, the risk of osteonecrosis increases 5 percent. It is difficult, however, to define an absolutely safe dose of corticosteroids. Anecdotal reports have been made of osteonecrosis of the femoral head developing after small corticosteroid exposures. The prevalence of osteonecrosis in renal-transplant patients on chronic steroid therapy has been reported to be 20 to 50 percent.[28,29] Similarly high rates of osteonecrosis of the femoral head have been reported in association with systemic lupus erythematosus (SLE) and rheumatoid arthritis (RA) patients treated with corticosteroids. In contrast, the incidence of osteonecrosis of the hip is significantly lower in patients treated with steroids after cardiac transplantation (3%).[30] The variable occurrence of osteonecrosis, even in populations with high steroid exposure, suggests that other patient-specific risk factors affect the likelihood of developing osteonecrosis.[31] Dysbaria, compression sickness associated with either deep water descent or high attitudes, has been associated with increased risk of osteonecrosis, with rates of radiographically apparent disease reported to be as high as 50 percent.[32] The mechanism appears to be related to the formation of gas bubbles within tissues of the body and their subsequent intravascular and extravascular effects.[33] Sickle cell anemia and other hemoglobinopathies are also associated with osteonecrosis. Radiographic signs of osteonecrosis have been reported in 4 to 12 percent of patients with the SS genotype and 20 to 60 percent of individuals with the SC genotype.[34] The hemoglobinopathies have two principal effects on bone: osteoporosis due to erythroid hypoplasia and bone infarction secondary to sluggish capillary flow.

The lack of a simple dose-response relationship between duration and magnitude of ethanol and corticosteroid exposure and the development of osteonecrosis suggests that other patient-specific risk factors play a role. Identification of conditions, such as coagulation abnormalities predisposing to osteonecrosis, may help understand as well as promote the development of nonsurgical treatment options for patients at risk. Statistically higher incidences of vascular abnormalities in hips of patients with osteonecrosis compared to control groups have been reported.[35] Patients with collagen vascular disease and antiphospholipid antibodies have been shown to be at greater risk for osteonecrosis.[36-40] The rates of symptomatic osteonecrosis in patients with SLE is approximately 13 percent.[37] In analyzing predictive factors in lupus for the development of osteonecrosis, it appears that steroid therapy, the presence of arthritis, and the use of cytotoxic medications are independent risk factors for the development of necrosis.[41] Hypofibrinolysis is also associated with osteonecrosis.[42-45] Populations of patients with osteonecrosis have a far greater incidence of abnormalities in coagulation than the general population.[45] Clinical studies attempting to prevent and treat this problem with pharmacologic correction of the thrombotic abnormalities are well under way.[46]

HISTOPATHOLOGY OF OSTEONECROSIS

A layer of articular cartilage, which receives its nourishment from the synovial fluid of the hip joint, covers the femoral head. Directly beneath the cartilage is a layer of supportive compact bone referred to as the subchondral plate. The remainder of the core of the femoral head is made up of an interlacing framework of trabecular bone. The normal hip joint is subjected to forces two to four times the person's body weight. Loads are transmitted from the cartilage to the subchondral bone, and then to the major trabecular tracts of cancellous bone. The orientation and thickness of the seams of trabecular bone are determined by the magnitude and direction of the load transmitted across the cartilage surface and subchondral plate. The main weight-bearing portion of the femoral head is located beneath the dome of the acetabulum. The stress-to-strength ratio of a normal femoral head is about 0.02 in the subchondral bone and 0.35 in the primary weight-bearing trabeculae.[17] The bone has sufficient strength to resist the forces encountered in normal activities of daily living, work, and recreation.

In atraumatic osteonecrosis, a metabolic or vascular event occurs and leads to necrosis of the marrow elements, trabecular bone, and subchondral bone. Microscopically, the zone of necrosis is initially invaded by an inflammatory cell infiltrate and lipophages.[47] At the margin of the infarct, the necrotic marrow is infiltrated and then replaced by a fibrovascular repair tissue. In the trabecular portion of bone, pluripotential mesenchymal cells within this tissue differentiate into osteoblasts, which begin to lay down new bone over the necrotic trabeculae.[48] In the subchondral bone, the repair process proceeds in such a way that necrotic bone initially is resorbed prior to laying down of new bone in a cycle of osteoclastic resorption and osteoblastic deposition. Grossly, the femoral head remains round. The articular cartilage is not affected because it receives nourishment from the synovial fluid. On cut sections of the femoral head, there is a wedge-shaped zone of infarct that begins in the trabecular bone and then widens as it extends to the subchondral plate. Typically, the infarct occurs in the anterolateral aspect of the femoral head. Radiographs appear normal or nondiagnostic. Magnetic resonance imaging (MRI) scan and scintigraphy are abnormal. These histopathologic and imaging findings correspond to stage I in the modified Steinberg classification system (see later discussion).

For unknown reasons, the reparative response stalls at its leading edge and changes both in quality and quantity.[49] As the time from initial injury and the distance from the margin of the necrotic zone increase, the cellular makeup of the repair tissue within the necrotic trabecular bone changes. The necrotic marrow tends to be replaced by avascular fibrous tissue, which contains areas of dystrophic calcification.[47] Differentiation of mesenchymal cells into osteoblasts ceases. Along the trailing edge of the reparative zone, there is some evidence of creeping substitution with osteoclastic resorption. At the lateral margins of the necrotic zone, resorption proceeds faster than new bone deposition. Grossly, the femoral head remains round and the cartilage continues to be unaffected. On cut sections of the femoral head, there is a rim of bony thickening or sclerosis at the margin of the infarct zone. Radiographs show an area of mixed lucent and sclerotic changes. MRI scan and scintigraphy results are abnormal. These histopathologic and imaging findings correspond to stage II in the classification system.

Most osteonecrotic lesions within the weight-bearing portion of the femoral head go on to develop a subchondral fracture. Despite the maintenance of normal geometry of the femoral head, the repair process itself compromises the local structure of the bone and alters its material properties and loading characteristics.[50] Femoral heads with osteonecrosis retrieved during surgery for total hip arthroplasty demonstrated a 50-percent reduction in strength and 75-percent reduction in modulus of elasticity.[51] Based on theoretical models, the stress-to-strength ratio of the necrotic trabecular bone now approaches 0.75 with normal gait, a level at high risk for fracture.[17] The necrotic bone lacks the intrinsic ability to repair itself and eventually fatigues at physiologic levels of loading. Cumulative microfractures eventually lead to a macrofracture, which propagates and becomes visible grossly as well as radiographically. The fracture tends to start laterally and propagates centrally along the interface between the subchondral plate and underlying necrotic bone,[50] where there is a stress riser or significant mismatch in the modulus of elasticity between the two layers. Microscopically, there is no repair response at the fracture site. Grossly, the femoral head remains spherical, but there is often a wrinkle or dimple in the cartilage overlying the fracture site. Upon probing, this area of cartilage is ballotable, but does not collapse. Radiographs show the classic "crescent sign." These changes correspond to stage III in the classification system.

Because the subchondral fracture does not heal, repetitive loading of the femoral head eventually causes fragmentation of the underlying necrotic subchondral bone, leading first to flattening of the femoral head and later to collapse or subsidence of the overlying cartilage segment (stage IV). Once the head becomes aspherical, there is progressive erosion and loss of cartilage above and adjacent to the site of collapse. This begins a cycle of further subchondral collapse, cartilage loss, and progressive deformity. As congruency is lost between the joint surfaces, degenerative changes become apparent on the acetabular side (stage V), eventually leading to an end-stage joint (stage VI).

In post-traumatic osteonecrosis, the overall mechanisms leading to collapse of the femoral head are similar, but not identical, to atraumatic osteonecrosis.[2,48-50] Following fracture of the femoral neck or dislocation of the hip, the disruption of the blood supply causes necrosis of the marrow and trabecular elements throughout the femoral head. The repair front begins within the femoral neck and proceeds proximally. It does not have the tendency to stall, as occurs in atraumatic osteonecrosis. If a given hip receives a significant portion of its blood supply through the ligamentum teres, a second repair front extends from the medial portion of the femoral head. As revascularization proceeds and the repair front advances, the material properties of the bone are altered, and the head is unable to resist normal load demands. Fractures and segmental collapse tend to occur along stress risers, which exist at the subchondral-trabecular bone interface and along a plane proximal and parallel to the original fracture site. Unlike atraumatic osteonecrosis, there is a rudimentary attempt to heal the fracture site with formation of new woven bone. However, few of these fractures go on to heal, probably because of repetitive microfracture at the site. Loss of sphericity can lead either to segmental collapse or massive collapse, depending on the pattern of revascularization and propagation of the secondary fracture.

DIAGNOSIS

Patients usually present with complaints of deep hip pain that localizes to the groin. They may also describe pain that radiates down the thigh to the knee. Symptoms are exacerbated with physical activity and weight-bearing and are relieved by rest. On physical examination, range of motion of the affected hip often is limited and painful, especially with flexion and internal rotation. Their gait pattern may be antalgic or may demonstrate a gluteus medius lurch. A careful history should be obtained to identify etiologic risk factors, the most common being steroid use and alcohol abuse, along with other conditions associated with osteonecrosis.

Imaging studies should begin with anteroposterior (AP) and frog-leg lateral radiographs of the affected hip (Fig. 114–3). Both radiographs demonstrate the location and extent of the necrotic lesion. Subchondral fracture of the femoral head typically is seen more clearly on the frog-leg lateral radiograph because the overlapping margins of the acetabulum are eliminated. If the radiographs show definitive evidence of osteonecrosis, no further imaging studies are necessary. However, radiographs of the contralateral hip should be obtained to rule out asymptomatic disease.

For the symptomatic patient with nondiagnostic radiographs, the study of choice is the MRI scan. MRI is the most sensitive and specific modality for imaging precollapse stages of osteonecrosis, and it will reveal stage I lesions not seen on radiographs.[51] Studies comparing MRI findings to biopsy specimens have shown excellent correlation, eliminating the need for invasive diagnostic techniques.[18] In addition, quantitative estimates of the size of the necrotic lesion are easily obtained and reproducible. The study should include T1- and T2-weighted images in both the coronal and sagittal planes. For stage I disease, the images will show a pattern of focal bone marrow edema appearing low signal on T1-weighted images and high signal on T2-weighted images.[52] This correlates with the histologic pattern of marrow and bone necrosis and early invasion by fibrovascular repair tissue. For stage II disease, the subchondral necrotic lesion with show a variable pattern, but the border of the lesion will show changes path gnomonic for osteonecrosis. On T1-weighted images, the lesion will be surrounded by a low-signal band, which histologically represents new bone formation at the reactive interface. On T2-weighted images, a

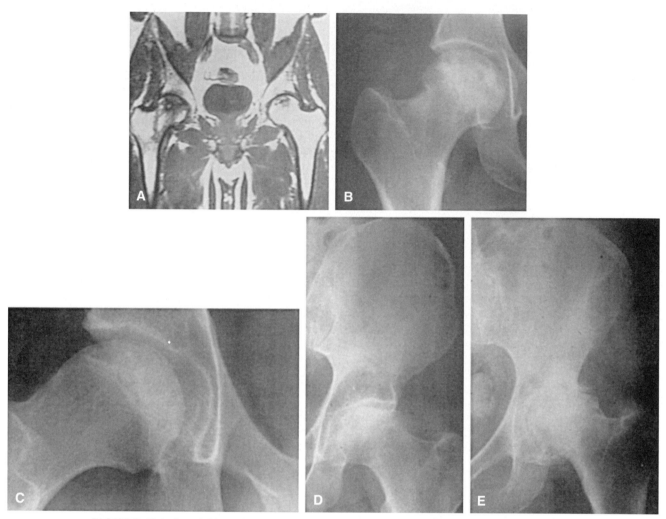

FIGURE 114–3 · *A,* Magnetic resonance image showing bilateral osteonecrosis of the hip, stage IC osteonecrosis of the right hip and stage IA osteonecrosis of the left hip. *B,* Anteroposterior (AP) radiograph of the hip demonstrating stage IIIC osteonecrosis, *C,* Frog-lateral radiograph of the hip demostrating stage IIIC osteonecrosis with subchondral fracture or the "crescent sign." *D,* AP radiograph of the hip demostrating collapse of the femoral head, stage IVC. *E,* AP radiograph of the hip demonstrating stage V osteonecrosis with arthrosis of the joint.

high-signal line central to the low-signal line can be visualized, producing the "double line sign."[51] Histologically, the outer dark line represents the sclerotic new bone formation at the reactive interface, and the lighter inner line represents the hypervascularity of the leading edge of the repair front. For stage III lesions, MRI scan is not as sensitive as computed tomography (CT) scan or plain radiographs for identifying a subchondral fracture. Penetration of joint fluid into the subchondral fracture gap may produce a high-intensity line: the MRI crescent sign.[51] For stage IV lesions and beyond, MRI scan will demonstrate secondary changes consistent with degenerative changes as well as the original underlying necrotic lesion. Postoperative MRI scans have not been helpful in demonstrating revascularization, as there are persistent abnormalities in the marrow signal despite apparent clinical success.[53]

Bone scintigraphy is not as sensitive or specific as MRI in assessing early-stage osteonecrotic lesions. Bone scan is useful as a screening study to diagnose multifocal disease

or when MRI is not available. Standard technique should include three-phase scintigraphy using ⁹⁹ᵐTechnetium-99, (Tc). Increased uptake indicates high bone metabolism or increased bone formation and resorption. Decreased uptake indicates decreased bone metabolism, decreased blood flow, or both. For stage I lesions, there is typically decreased uptake or radiotracer, with a photopenic "cold spot" in the femoral head. This finding is nonspecific and can be seen in other marrow disorders. For stage II lesions and some stage I lesions, there is increased radiotracer uptake involving the femoral head. This is the most commonly observed finding in patients with osteonecrosis, but still is nonspecific. A study in which an area of decreased tracer uptake is surrounded by an area of increased tracer uptake, the "cold in hot spot," is pathognomonic for osteonecrosis but is only found in 25 to 50 percent of patients.[54] Bone scans are not necessary or useful in diagnosing stage III lesions or higher.

CT is more useful for detecting occult subchondral fracture and distinguishing between stage II and stage

III lesions. Between 15 and 30 percent of stage II lesions were upgraded to stage III on the basis of comparison of radiographs and CT scans.[55] A standard study should utilize high-resolution, contiguous axial imaging. CT scan should not be used as a screening study, because it fails to detect most stage I lesions. For stages II and III, a scan will demonstrate a distinct sclerotic rim surrounding a mottled area of both sclerosis and osteolysis. The disadvantage of CT is that it may fail to detect small lesions in the superior head because of volume averaging artifacts. CT scan is not necessary for diagnosing or distinguishing between stage IV lesions and higher.

Classification

Currently, there is no universally accepted classification system for osteonecrosis of the hip, a fact that has hampered research efforts and comparisons of treatment modalities. The earliest classification systems used a combination of radiographs, invasive tests, biopsy, and clinical symptoms to segment patients into different stages.[56,57] The main prognostic variable was whether the femoral head lesion was precollapse, postcollapse, or postcollapse with degenerative changes. Newer classification schemes have evolved to reflect improvements in noninvasive imaging studies and to recognize the importance of lesion size and location.[58,59] Patients are now staged using imaging criteria alone, with no additional invasive tests or biopsy. Furthermore, patients are segmented within stages on the basis of quantitative measurements of lesion size,[58] amount of collapse,[58] and location of lesion.[59] Large lesions (greater than 30- to 40-percent involvement of the femoral head) and lesions located under the weight-bearing portion of the acetabulum (lateral and central) have a greater propensity to progress to collapse than smaller lesions and lesions located under the non–weight-bearing portion of the acetabulum (medial).

We currently favor a modified Steinberg classification system to stage patients with osteonecrosis of the hip (Table 114–2). This system differs from its predecessor, which was originated by Marcus and Enneking, by stratifying patients within a given stage on the basis of quantitative measurements of the percentage of involvement of the head and amount of subchondral collapse.[57] We use both MRI and radiographs to determine those measurements. We have modified the original Steinberg classification system in two ways: Stage IV lesions are stratified on the basis of both the amount of collapse and the percentage of involvement of the femoral head. We also have omitted stage 0, which represents high-risk patients who are asymptomatic and have normal imaging studies, but have previously diagnosed disease of the contralateral hip. Neither the original Steinberg system nor our modified version incorporates lesion location because the overwhelming majority of our patients present with necrotic lesions involving the central and lateral portion of the femoral head.

The other commonly used staging system is the one originated by Ficat and Arlet.[56] This system uses four stages to stratify patients. Stage I patients have negative

TABLE 114–2 · THE MODIFIED STEINBERG CLASSIFICATION SYSTEM FOR STAGING OSTEONECROSIS

I. **Normal radiograph; abnormal bone scan, magnetic resonance imaging (MRI), or both; percentage of head involvement as follows**
  A. Mild (1 to 25%)
  B. Moderate (26 to 50%)
  C. Severe (greater than 50%)
II. **Lucent and sclerotic changes in femoral head; percentage of head involvement as follows**
  A. Mild (1 to 25%)
  B. Moderate (26 to 50%)
  C. Severe (greater than 50%)
III. **Subchondral fracture (crescent sign) without flattening; percentage of head involvement as follows**
  A. Mild (1 to 25%)
  B. Moderate (26 to 50%)
  C. Severe (greater than 50%)
IV. **Subchondral fracture with flattening depression of femoral head; percentage of head involvement as follows**
  A. Mild (1 to 25%)
  B. Moderate (26 to 50%)
  C. Severe (greater than 50%)
V. **Joint narrowing, acetabular changes, or both**
VI. **Advanced degenerative changes**

radiographs, but abnormal MRI, bone scan, or functional tests. Stage II patients have abnormal radiographs that show sclerotic changes and abnormal MRI and bone scan. Stage III patients have radiographs that show femoral head flattening or subchondral collapse. Stage IV patients have radiographs that show joint-space narrowing and degenerative changes. The Association of Research Circulation Osseous (ARCO) has proposed a modification of this system, which adds a stage 0 for high-risk patients with negative imaging studies and quantitative stratification of patients in stages I to III on the basis of lesion location, lesion size, and amount of collapse.[60]

Our staging system, as well as others, will need to be validated on the basis of prospective studies. Efforts should be made to simplify the staging system as much as possible to facilitate communication between clinicians and improve accuracy. Existing classification schemes have been criticized because of poor inter- and intraobserver reliability. The most difficult lesions to differentiate have been stage III and stage IV lesions. Arthroscopy has been suggested as a more reliable method for differentiating these stages than MRI and radiography.[61] In addition, many subchondral fractures are occult by radiograph, but are demonstrated on CT scan, suggesting the misclassification of a portion of stage III lesions as stage II.

NATURAL HISTORY

Because atraumatic osteonecrosis of the hip typically is asymptomatic in the earliest stages of the disease process, it has been difficult to establish the definitive natural history. Much of the information on natural history is derived from screening studies of asymptomatic high-risk patients or from symptomatic patients presenting with stage II or III disease. Eighty percent of patients who present with symptomatic osteonecrosis of the hip progress to end-stage osteonecrosis over the course of 3 to 5 years in the absence of surgical intervention.[62] Predictors of collapse include an advanced stage of disease on presentation, a necrotic lesion occupying greater than 50 percent of the femoral head, and a necrotic lesion located in the anterolateral aspect of the femoral head. Predictors for a more benign course include a necrotic lesion involving less than 15 percent of the femoral head and a necrotic lesion located in the medial aspect of the femoral head.

The prevalence of osteonecrosis of the hip is unclear because there may be a cohort of patients with asymptomatic disease that spontaneously heals or never progresses to become symptomatic. The incidence of osteonecrosis has been estimated to be 10,000 to 15,000 new cases per year, based on the reported pathology of patients undergoing total hip arthroplasty.[1] Screening MRI studies of asymptomatic patients receiving corticosteroid therapy following renal transplant have identified a 6- to 14-percent prevalence of osteonecrosis of the hip, with only 0 to 4 percent of patients going on to develop symptomatic disease.[63] In one study, 30 percent of asymptomatic stage I lesions spontaneously healed.[63]

The overall rate of bilateral osteonecrosis of the hip has been reported to be as high as 72 percent.[64] At the time of presentation, 42 percent of patients with symptomatic disease in one hip will have asymptomatic disease present in the contralateral hip. In patients with eventual bilateral disease, the duration of the asymptomatic period for the second hip averages 4.6 to 5.5 years. For patients with asymptomatic unilateral osteonecrosis and no evidence of disease in the contralateral hip by MRI at the time of presentation, 2 to 7.8 percent will go on to develop symptomatic disease in the second hip over the next 5 years.[64]

TREATMENT

The ideal treatment for osteonecrosis of the hip would provide complete pain relief and a stable joint for the duration of the patient's life span. Total hip arthroplasty can successfully achieve these goals in older patients with excellent long-term clinical results. The results in younger patients with osteonecrosis, however, have been disappointing, with a high rate of aseptic implant loosening and revision surgery. No current treatment method has shown the ability to cure osteonecrosis, completely relieve pain, or last the 40 to 60 years necessary for a young patient afflicted with osteonecrosis. Therefore, we view the various treatment approaches for osteonecrosis of the hip as bridging strategies to maintain the native hip as long as possible, with conversion to a total hip arthroplasty if necessary.

There are three fundamental approaches to treating atraumatic osteonecrosis of the femoral head: nonoperative management, femoral head–preserving procedures, and femoral head–resurfacing or –sacrificing procedures. Femoral head–preserving procedures attempt to modify the biologic or biomechanic environment to facilitate healing of the osteonecrotic lesion. The main

modalities are core decompression, electrical stimulation, intertrochanteric osteotomy, nonvascularized bone grafts, and vascularized bone grafts. Femoral head resurfacing and sacrificing procedures substitute a load-bearing mechanic implant for the compromised cartilage surface. The main modalities are surface-replacement arthroplasty, hemiarthroplasty, and total hip arthroplasty. Should a femoral head develop osteonecrosis following fracture reduction and internal fixation, many of the general principles of treatment for atraumatic osteonecrosis can be extended for the treatment of traumatic osteonecrosis. For a general description of the acute treatment of femoral neck fractures or hip dislocations, the reader is referred to textbooks of orthopedic fracture care.[65]

Methods of nonoperative treatment have varied, including weight-bearing as tolerated, partial weight-bearing with crutches, and no weight-bearing. A meta-analysis of published reports (21 studies) from 1960 to 1993 reported a successful clinical result in only 22.7 percent of hips (182 of 819) followed for an average of 34 months.[62] Hip survival rates stratified by Ficat stage were 35 percent for stage I, 31 percent for stage II, and 13 percent for stage III. There was no difference in outcome for different degrees of weight-bearing. In more recent reports, stratification of patients on the basis of lesion size and location suggests that small lesions located in the medial portion of the femoral head have a much lower tendency to progress to collapse, with survival rates approaching 80 to 100 percent.[59] In general, conservative treatment does not appear to alter the natural history of progressive collapse and arthrosis. Long-term prospective studies are needed to validate whether the subset of patients with small lesions located in the non–weight-bearing portion of the femoral head can be managed with observation and symptomatic treatment.

Core decompression is a surgical procedure in which a core of bone is removed from the femoral neck and head. The femur is opened along the lateral cortex below the greater trochanter, and the biopsy tract or core tract is directed along the femoral neck into the osteonecrotic lesion. The tract stops short of the subchondral bone. The rationale for performing core decompression is to provide pain relief by decreasing intraosseous hypertension and to improve revascularization of the necrotic lesion by stimulating angiogenesis and providing a channel for vascular ingrowth. Proponents of this procedure have recommended it for stage I and stage II lesions.[21] The majority of patients have immediate relief of their pain following this procedure. The degree of revascularization in femoral heads retrieved at the time of total hip arthroplasty, however, has been variable. Performance of core decompression does not technically complicate a total hip arthroplasty procedure should it become necessary.

The clinical efficacy of core decompression remains controversial. There has been significant variability reported in different surgical series. Comparison of outcomes is difficult because of the use of different staging systems, different surgical techniques, and varying study sizes. Biomechanic studies suggest that variations in surgical technique can markedly affect outcomes, with an improperly placed core tract hastening collapse of the necrotic segment.[17] A meta-analysis of 24 reports published between 1960 and 1993 showed a successful clinical result in 63.5 percent of hips (741 of 1166) followed for an average of 30 months.[62] The average hip survival stratified for Ficat stages was 84 percent for stage I, 65 percent for stage II, and 47 percent for stage III. For studies with longer follow-up, survival of stage III hips decreased to 20 to 30 percent at 5 years and beyond.[66,67] Two randomized, prospective studies comparing core decompression to nonoperative treatment have shown markedly different outcomes, with one study showing no benefit to the surgical procedure whereas the other study did demonstrate a benefit.[68,69]

Electrical stimulation has been used both as a primary treatment modality and as adjunctive therapy in combination with core decompression and bone grafting. The rationale for the use of electrical stimulation is that it enhances osteogenesis and neovascularization and leads to a net increase of bone substance by altering the balance between bone resorption by osteoclasts and bone production by osteoblasts. Proponents of this therapy have recommended it for patients with precollapse lesions or subchondral fracture. Three different methods for administering electric stimulation have been described: direct current, capacitance-coupled current, and pulsed electromagnetic fields (PEMF). For direct current stimulation, a cathode is placed within the femoral head after core decompression, with the anode placed in the adjacent soft tissues. When used in conjunction with core decompression and bone grafting, direct-current electric stimulation led to improved clinical function and decreased radiographic progression but no increase in hip survival when compared to core decompression and bone grafting alone.[70] For capacitance coupled current, an electric field is generated through electrodes placed on the skin over the femoral head. When used in conjunction with core decompression and bone grafting, capacitance-coupled current showed no difference in clinical function, radiographic progression, and hip survival when compared to core decompression and bone grafting alone.[71] For PEMF, a time-varied electric field is generated from a coil, and an external generator is placed on the skin over the femoral head. A retrospective study comparing PEMF to core decompression at 6 years of follow-up found improved hip survival (81% vs. 52% for Ficat stage II and 45% vs. 0% for Ficat stage III), decreased radiographic progression, and increased clinical success.[72] The patients making up each group were not studied concurrently or prospectively and came from different institutions. The results of PEMF are promising, and its use as a primary of adjunctive modality awaits further testing in the United States pending Food and Drug Administration (FDA) approval of the device.

Structural bone grafting is a surgical technique whereby a corticocancellous bone graft is inserted through a core decompression tract into the necrotic lesion of the femoral head. The technique was originally described for treatment of nonunion of femoral neck fractures but was extended for treatment of atraumatic osteonecrosis of the femoral head. Both autologous and allogeneic grafts harvested from the tibia or fibula have been used. Placement of the graft is critical, and it should come within millimeters of the overlying subchondral bone.[73] The rationale for the procedure is that the bone graft will provide structural support to the overlying subchondral bone, thereby preventing collapse. In addition, pain relief as well as vascular ingrowth is enhanced from the core decompression. Femoral heads retrieved from patients undergoing total hip arthroplasty have shown that the structural graft will unite with the surrounding bone, but there is often incomplete revascularization of the entire necrotic lesion. Proponents of this technique recommend it for treatments of stage I and stage II lesions.

Marcus and coworkers have described the results of structural bone grafting in 11 asymptomatic patients with stage I and stage II lesions and in 37 patients with symptomatic stage III and stage IV lesions with a follow-up of 2 to 4 years.[57] Seven of 11 patients with stages I and II lesions had satisfactory results (pain relief, lack of radiographic progression or collapse), and all the patients with stages III and IV lesions had poor results (progressive collapse and degenerative disease). Failure in the stages I and II groups was related to poor graft placement or ongoing exposure to etiologic risk factors (alcohol abuse, steroid use). In a follow-up study from the same institution, Buckley and associates reported on 20 hips in 19 patients with asymptomatic stages I and II lesions treated with structural bone grafting.[73] Patients were considered candidates for the procedure if they no longer had ongoing exposure to etiologic risk factors for osteonecrosis. At an average 8-year follow-up, 18 hips in 17 patients had a satisfactory clinical result with no hip pain or progression of the lesion. Two hips in two patients went on to collapse, with poor graft placement considered the cause of failure. No difference in graft survival was found between allogeneic and autogenous grafts or between lesions with greater than or less than 50 percent involvement of the femoral head. Nelson and Clark reported on structural grafting of 52 symptomatic hips in 40 patients with a 2-year follow-up.[74] They described radiographic progression of at least one stage in the vast majority of the patients in their series, with 76 percent progressing from stage II (13 of 17), 64 percent progressing from stage III (7 of 11), and 86 percent progressing from stage IV (19 of 22).

Vascularized structural bone grafting is a surgical procedure in which a corticocancellous bone graft with its vascular pedicle is inserted into the femoral neck and head through a core decompression tract. The vascular pedicle of the graft is then anastomosed to a nearby vessel. The most common sources for the graft are the fibula or iliac crest. The most commonly used vessels to create the anastomosis are branches of the lateral femoral circumflex artery, profunda femorus artery, or inferior gluteal artery. The rationale for the procedure is that revascularization of the necrotic lesion and union between the graft and surrounding bone will be enhanced by the addition of blood supply to the structural graft (Fig. 114–4). The drawbacks of the procedure are the requirement of microvascular

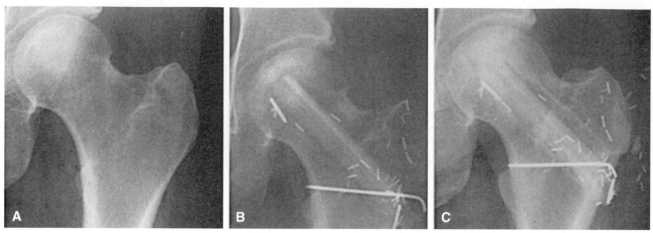

FIGURE 114–4 • *A*, Preoperative anteroposterior(AP) radiograph of a hip with stage II disease, *B*, AP radiograph immediately after placement of a vascularized autogenous fibular graft. *C*, AP radiograph of left hip 7 years postoperatively.

surgical skills to perform the anastomosis and the development of donor site morbidity following harvesting of the graft. Conversion to total hip arthroplasty requires excavation of the intramedullary portion of the fibular graft prior to the use of conventional instrumentation.

Urbaniak and colleagues reported the results of vascularized fibula grafting for 103 hips in 89 patients with Marcus stages II to V hip disease.[75] The 5-year hip survival rate was 89 percent (17 of 19) for stage II disease, 77 percent (18 of 22) for stage III disease, 57 percent (23 of 40) for stage IV disease, and 68 percent (15 of 22) for stage V disease. In a subsequent report from the same institution that incorporated the original series, Scully and associates published the results of vascularized fibula grafting for 614 hips in 480 patients with symptomatic Ficat stages II and III disease.[66] The 5-year survival rate for Ficat stage II and Ficat stage III disease was 89 percent (99 of 111) and 81 percent (405 of 500), respectively. Similar rates of hip survival have been reported by others for stages II and III hip disease.[76,77] Vail and Urbaniak reported donor site morbidity in 24.3 percent of patients at 5 years who had undergone vascularized fibula grafting, with pain at sites other than the ankle, ankle pain, and sensory deficits being the most common complaints.[78] The patency of the vascular anastomosis in the immediate postoperative period has been high (87 to 90%) as assessed by digital subtraction angiography[75] and the use of a reporter skin paddle supplied by the same vessels as the bone graft.

Femoral osteotomy is a surgical procedure whereby a cut is made in the proximal femur to allow the osteonecrotic lesion to be rotated or flexed out of the weight-bearing region of the acetabulum. Because most lesions involve the anterosuperior head, rotational or redirection osteotomies can bring the relatively well-preserved posterior head underneath the weight-bearing dome of the acetabulum. The rationale for the procedure is that it facilitates healing by eliminating direct shear forces on the necrotic lesion, and it restores apposition of congruent joint surfaces.[79] Proponents have recommended

osteotomy for lesions with early subchondral collapse and no acetabular degeneration (stage III and IV). The main drawbacks of the procedure are the need for an extended period of non–weight-bearing or protected weight-bearing for the operative extremity and the technical difficulty of performing the procedure. The most important predictors for success are lesions that involve less than one third of the femoral head, complete or near-complete rotation of the necrotic lesion out of the weight-bearing region of the acetabulum, and discontinuation of steroid use by affected patients.[79-83] Failures have been due to femoral neck fracture, osteotomy nonunion, and progressive collapse of lesions that are not adequately rotated. Conversion to total hip osteotomy is technically more challenging and requires hardware removal, but osteotomy does not appear to compromise the results.[81,84]

Sugioka and coworkers have described a transtrochanteric rotational osteotomy in which rotation occurs about the longitudinal axis of the femoral neck.[85] They have reported a 10-year follow-up for 136 hips in 98 patients with Japanese stage II (Steinberg II, III, and early IV stages), stage III (late Steinberg stage IV), and stage IV (Steinberg stage V) disease. Survival rates of 95 percent for stage II disease (56 of 60), 86.9 percent for stage III disease (37 of 47), and 79.3 percent for stage IV disease (22 of 29) were noted. Femoral head collapse tended to occur within 3 years of the osteotomy, and secondary degenerative changes occurred much later. Complete healing of the necrotic lesion has been demonstrated for lesions completely rotated out of the weight-bearing region of the acetabulum. Other investigators have been unable to match this level of success and have reported high complication rates and conversion to total hip arthroplasty of 40 to 83 percent at 5-year follow-up. Dean and Cabanela have sugggested ethnic origin and differences in hip capsular anatomy and blood supply may explain the apparent success of this procedure in Japan compared to Europe and the United States.[86] Mont and associates reported a 76-percent survival rate (28 of 37 hips in 34 patients) of Ficat stages II and III hip disease with an average follow-up of 11.5 years for patients undergoing varus or flexion intertrochanteric osteotomy.[81] Scher and Jakim reported an 87-percent hip survival rate (39 of 45 hips in 43 patients) at 5 years for Ficat stage III hips undergoing valgus or flexion intertrochanteric osteotomy, sequestrectomy, and cancellous bone grafting.[80] Indications for osteotomy must be critically addressed; a recent study comparing rotational and flexion osteotomy reported, at a mean 7-year follow-up, that 27 of 29 in the rotational osteotomy group and 36 of 63 hips in the flexion osteotomy group required conversion to total hip arthroplasty.[83] They also noted a significant complication rate of more than 55 percent in the rotational osteotomy group compared to 17.5 percent in the patients who underwent flexion osteotomy. Most series that have used redirectional osteotomies have not been as successful as Scher and Mont, who restricted their studies to patients who had discontinued steroid use and had less than one-third involvement of the femoral head.

Resurfacing arthroplasty is a surgical procedure in which a metal or ceramic shell is cemented over the surface of a femoral head that has been prepared with débridement of necrotic material and reaming. Modern components use either a cemented shell alone (precision fit surface hemiarthroplasty, toal hip articular replacement using internal eccentric shells, (THARIES), design)[87] or a spherical articular portion with a small intramedullary stem (surface replacement hemiarthroplasty, TARA design).[88] Proponents of this procedure have recommended it for patients with femoral-head collapse (stage IV). The rationale for the procedure is that it relieves pain and preserves femoral-neck bone stock in anticipation of later conversion to total hip arthroplasty. Early designs were plagued with mismatch between component and acetabular size, aseptic loosening, and acetabulum protrusio. The original designs do not incorporate resurfacing of the acetabulum. In a series of 33 procedures in 25 patients, the total articular replacement arthroplasty, (TARA), design has shown 91-percent survival rate for the prosthesis at 5 years and 62-percent survival rate at long-term follow-up (average 10.5 years).[88] The primary reason for revision to total hip arthroplasty was progressive degeneration of acetabular cartilage. In a series of 27 procedures in 25 patients, long-term follow-up for the THARIES design has shown an 83-percent survival rate at 5 years and 53-percent survival rate at 12 years.[87] The design has fared poorly in patients with sickle cell disease, with a 100 percent early failure rate in one series. Both prosthetic designs have provided excellent pain relief early in the postoperative course, with less relief over time with acetabular changes. Problems with the acetabulum have led to the development of a design that resurfaces the acetabulum as well as the femoral head. We await the preliminary results with this new design. Both types of resurfacing arthroplasty can be converted to a total hip replacement with little modification of standard techniques.

Hemiarthroplasty is a surgical procedure in which the femoral head is replaced by a prosthetic head mounted on an endoprosthesis, which is fixed within the proximal femoral canal. The head of a unipolar prosthesis articulates directly with the acetabulum. A bipolar prosthesis has a bearing interposed between the prosthesis and the surface of the prosthetic head, with movement theoretically occurring at the bearing rather than the prosthetic head–acetabulum interface. Use of both unipolar and bipolar prostheses for the treatment of stage IV and stage V disease has largely been abandoned because of high rates of mechanical failure, acetabulum protrusio, groin pain, and acetabular wear. Failure rates for unipolar prostheses were as high as 50 to 60 percent within 3 years. Although mechanical failure rates for bipolar designs were lower (7 to 17%) at 5- to 10-year follow-up, the rate of groin pain from acetabular wear ranged from 20 to 44 percent.[89]

Total hip arthroplasty is a surgical procedure in which both the femoral head and acetabular surface are replaced with prosthetic components. The femoral endoprosthesis and the acetabular cup are fixed, using cement or by means of bone ingrowth. The interface between the two components is either metal on polyethylene, ceramic on polyethylene, or ceramic on ceramic. The reasons to select total hip arthroplasty to treat osteonecrosis are predictable pain relief and improved function. The drawbacks of the procedure are the high rates of aseptic failure and the likely need for at least one revision during the patient's lifetime. For multiple revisions, there is progressive loss of bone stock and increased difficulty in successfully reconstructing the hip joint. The earliest published reports of total hip arthroplasty in patients with osteonecrosis showed dismal results, with early rates of aseptic loosening of 37 to 50 percent within 10 years. With improvements in prosthetic design and the advent of cementless prostheses, rates of clinical and radiographic aseptic loosening have decreased but do not approach those found in older patients or aged-matched control subjects with OA. Capello and colleagues summarized the results of reports published between 1983 and 1995 on patients with osteonecrosis treated with both cemented and cementless total hip arthroplasty.[90] The average rate of clinical and radiographic aseptic loosening was 14.3 percent for cemented stems at an average of 6.25 years and 13.2 percent for cementless stems at an average of 5.75 years. The main reasons cited for premature failure of total hip arthroplasty in patients with osteonecrosis are younger patient age, increased functional demands, and poor bone quality secondary to renal disease, steroid use, and alcohol abuse.[90] Results for patients with renal failure and sickle cell disease are especially poor, with infection rates of 20 percent and aseptic loosening of 40 percent at follow-up less than 5 years.

AUTHORS' PREFERRED METHOD OF TREATMENT

Valid comparisons among different treatment strategies or a single treatment performed by different surgeons at different institutions are difficult to make. As seen by the preceding descriptions, results are not reported in a systematic way, with different authors using different staging systems and varying definitions of a successful clinical result. Lesion size and location, important predictors of disease progression, have only recently been recognized and have not been used to stratify results. Results for a given treatment method tend to be best at high-volume institutions, suggesting the importance of proficiency in patient selection and technical execution of the procedure. Most important, there are few prospective, randomized, controlled studies to compare different treatment modalities directly with one another.

We believe that the treatment of choice for stage I through stage IVB disease is the vascularized fibula graft. We acknowledge that the choice of treatment for precollapse osteonecrosis is controversial, and some advocate core decompression or nonvascularized structural bone grafts. Core decompression is an acceptable treatment option, but it has not shown the same degree of long-term durability as the vascularized fibula graft, especially for stage III disease. Although nonvascularized structural bone grafts have performed well in a small number of asymptomatic patients with stages I and II disease, their success has been poor for stage III and higher disease. In our opinion, the high rates of long-term hip survival with vascularized bone grafting justify the donor site morbidity associated with fibula harvest. We currently offer this procedure to symptomatic patients younger than 50 years. We extend the indications for surgery to some patients under age 20 years with stage V disease secondary to trauma or Perthes' disease. For patients with stage IVC and higher disease, we have recommended total hip arthroplasty when their symptoms were sufficiently severe to warrant surgery. For those patients with small lesions (stage IIIA and B, stage IVA and B), osteotomy is an appropriate choice when performed at an experienced center. Although promising, femoral resurfacing arthroplasty has not been used in sufficiently large numbers to be recommended on a routine basis. We are currently exploring the use of bone growth factors and bisphosphonates as adjunctive therapy for use with vascularized fibula grafting. For patients with asymptomatic disease, we recommend close follow-up, with radiographs every 3 months, and MRI scan every 6 to 12 months to monitor disease progression.

Bone Marrow Edema Syndrome

Bone marrow edema syndrome (BMES) or transient osteoporosis is a self-limited, transitory clinical entity characterized by hip pain, osteopenia on radiographs, and bone marrow edema on MRI.[91] The disorder typically affects women, almost exclusively during the third trimester of pregnancy, and middle-aged men. Patients present with progressive hip pain, an antalgic gait pattern, and functional disability of the affected extremity that is out of proportion to the amount of stated pain. Range of motion of the affected hip is not limited but often is painful at the extremes of motion. Symptoms and changes on imaging studies last an average of 6 months. Usually one hip is involved at a time, but 40 percent of patients may have recurrence of the process or involvement of the other hip or other joints.[92]

The typical clinical course includes three phases.[92] The initial phase lasts for 4 weeks, with acute onset of pain and increasing functional disability. Radiographs appear normal. A bone scan will show increased radiotracer uptake involving the entire femoral head and neck and extending down to the intertrochanteric line.[92] MRI scan will show signal changes in the same distribution as the bone scan, which will appear low signal on T1-weighted images and high signal on T2-weighted images. In addition, an effusion is often seen within the joint. Changes can be seen on both MRI and bone scan as early as 48 hours after the onset of hip pain. The second phase, or plateau phase, lasts for 1 to 2 months. Symptoms stabilize, and radiographs show diffuse osteopenia involving the femoral head and neck, which occasionally extends to the acetabulum. There is no evidence of subchondral fracture, dense sclerosis, or degenerative changes, which are the hallmarks of osteonecrosis. The third phase, or regression phase, lasts for an additional 4 to 6 months. Radiographs show reconstitution of normal bone density and symptoms abate in their entirety.

The etiology of BMES is unknown. Speculative theories include a nontraumatic form of reflex sympathetic dystrophy, a virally mediated increase in osteoclastic activity, or a transient ischemic event that causes selective marrow necrosis but not bony necrosis.[91] Those that support the last hypothesis believe that BMES represents a reversible precursor of osteonecrosis in which the ischemic episode is of a limited duration. Functional testing of affected patients has shown markedly elevated intraosseous pressure within the femoral head and abnormal contrast clearance.[93] Biopsy samples of the femoral head and neck obtained within 3 weeks of the onset of symptoms demonstrate diffuse interstitial edema between marrow elements, fragmentation of fatty marrow cells, and intense new bone formation.[91] There are continuous seams of osteoid laid down upon normal bony trabeculae, which contain live osteocytes. Bone mass is not lost, but there is a shift toward relative undermineralization with an increased ratio of osteoid to mineralized bone. This is reflected in the osteopenic appearance of the femoral head on radiographs.

Patients with BMES should be treated symptomatically with protective weight-bearing and analgesics.[94] Although core decompression will provide acute pain relief, the risks of the procedure are not warranted for this self-limited condition. There have been rare reports of pregnant women with BMES who have fallen and suffered a femoral neck fracture, requiring reduction and internal fixation. Because the changes seen on radiographs, bone scan, and MRI are not pathognomonic, other conditions such as an infiltrative tumor, bone bruise, and infection should be ruled out.[95]

Osteonecrosis of the Lunate (Kienbock's Disease)

ETIOLOGY

The cause and pathogenesis of Kienbock's disease are not completely understood but most likely are multifactorial. Anatomic, vascular, and traumatic factors have been described. Although still debated, there appears to be an association between negative ulnar variance (short ulna) and osteonecrosis of the lunate.[96,97] The shortened ulna is thought to cause increased forces and load transmission across the radiolunate joint of the wrist.[98,99] Other associated anatomic factors include smaller lunate size and increased radial inclination.[100] Variations in the vascularity of the lunate have been explored as potential predisposing factors for osteonecrosis. Most lunates have both volar and dorsal blood supply.[101] However, intraosseous vascularity demonstrates a 20-percent incidence of a single nutrient artery, poorly organized intraosseous anastomoses, or both, potentially predisposing to osteonecrosis.[102] There is a relationship between repetitive (micro) traumatic fracture and the development of Kienbock's disease, but it is unclear whether this is a cause or effect. However, investigators have noted that greater than 80 percent of lunates had fractures in patients with lunatmalacia.[103,104]

DIAGNOSIS

Osteonecrosis of the lunate most commonly affects males between second and fifth decades of life and involves the dominant hand.[105] There is an association with manual labor. Clinically, the patients will present with pain of insidious onset localized to the radiolunate joint, weakness, and diminished wrist range of motion. The pain is increased with activity and relieved with rest. The differential diagnosis includes ulnocarpal impaction syndrome, post-traumatic transient bone ischemia, intraosseous ganglions, and lunate fractures.

RADIOGRAPHIC FINDINGS AND STAGING

Much like femoral head osteonecrosis, plain films do not demonstrate early lunate disease. However, plain radiographs demonstrate possible other pathologies and anatomic predisposing factors, such as ulnar minus variance, and, thus, are an essential first study in patients with wrist pain. Additional studies include bone scintigraphy and MRI, which are more sensitive in detecting early disease and allow for earlier intervention.[106] CT, tomograms, arthroscopy, or some combination of these have been advocated by some authors in cases of obvious fragmentation and collapse as a more precise method of characterizing the amount of destruction.[103,107,108]

A staging system to be utilized in classifying Kienbock's disease was originated by Stahl and is based on AP radiographic findings.[109] This was later modified by Lichtman to include four stages and is now the most common system for grading progression of the disease[110,111] (Table 114–3). Despite flaws in quantifying collapse with plain films, the staging system is helpful in guiding treatment. The treatment for precollapse disease (stages I and II) differs than that for collapsed-lunate (stages IIIa, IIIb, and IV) osteonecrosis.

NATURAL HISTORY

The natural history of Kienbock's disease is poorly understood because there are so few studies analyzing benign neglect. Although most experts agree that left untreated, lunate collapse and subsequent arthritis is inevitable, a clinical correlation is not absolute. One study found that 80 percent of patients followed for an

TABLE 114–3 • STAHL-LICHTMAN CLASSIFICATION OF KIENBOCK'S DISEASE

Stage I:	Normal radiographs, positive bone scan and magnetic resonance imaging (MRI)
Stage II:	Plain films demonstrate increased lunate density; lunate integrity maintained
Stage III:	Lunate collapse with partial or complete sclerosis; proximal carpal row remains normally aligned; proximal carpal row malaligned and destabilized
Stage IV:	Lunate disintegrated, degenerative changes in the radiocarpal joints, midcarpal joints, or both

average of 20 years had no pain or pain only with hard labor activity.[112] However, all 49 of the wrists examined progressed radiographically with a significant number (two thirds) demonstrating arthritis. Another report showed nonoperative treatment was unsuccessful, with 60 percent of patients having daily pain and seven patients required to change jobs.[113]

TREATMENT

Multiple treatments for Kienbock's have been described, with a failure to reach concensus regarding the best option. As demonstrated in natural history, the radiographic deformities do not always correlate with poor clinical outcome. Unfortunately, adequate comparison studies are difficult as most studies involve a small number of patients with often-inadequate follow-up. The treatment options include immobilization, joint-leveling procedures, radial osteotomy, vascularized and nonvascularized bone grafting, partial carpal arthrodesis, capitate shortening, and salvage procedures (for arthritic wrists).

Immobilization and anti-inflammatory pharmacologic therapy has been recommended in patients with early disease.[109] However, as mentioned previously, not all patients have fared well with conservative therapy, and radiographic progression is likely.[113]

Joint-leveling procedures for patients with negative ulnar variance (short ulna) aim to reduce forces across the radiolunate joint. Both ulnar lengthening and radial shortening have been described and have been shown to decrease load transmission across the radiolunate joint.[114,115] Good results, including improved pain, strength, and range of motion, with both procedures have been reported for all stages except advanced stage IV disease.[104,116-119] Increased nonunion rates have been reported with ulnar lengthening.[104]

In cases of neutral ulnar variance, lateral closing wedge osteotomy of the radius has been advocated.[119-122] This effectively unloads the radiolunate joint and forces across the lunate, increasing contact area of the scaphoid on the radius and transferring forces to the radioscaphoid joint.[119] Recent long-term (average 14 years) follow-up has shown good clinical results despite radiographic progression of the disease in 8 of 13 wrists.[121] Acceptable results, with four of seven patients having good outcomes, have also been reported in treating late stages (IIIb and IV) of Kienbock's disease.[122]

Vascularized bone grafting utilizing pedicled bone grafts locally or free vascularized bone grafts have gained popularity as a means to address the theory that vascular insufficiency is the culprit in the development of osteonecrosis of the lunate. A variety of anatomic sources have been suggested, including the second dorsal metacarpal artery,[123] a pedicled vascularized pisiform,[124] a pronator quadratus bone flap,[125] a variety of vascularized bone grafts from the dorsum of the distal radius,[126,127] nonvascularized bone grafting with core revascularization,[128] and free vascularized grafts (e.g., iliac crest).[129] The pedicled bone grafting is technically easier than free vascularized bone transfer. Good results have been reported, with disappearance or reduction of pain and increased strength, but much like joint-leveling procedures, radiographic progression was noted in up to 20 percent of patients and frank arthritis in 10 percent.[122] A potential problem is collapse and fragmentation of the lunate during the healing phase.[129] This can be prevented with pinning of the scaphocapitate joint or external fixation across the wrist during revascularization. A major concern is clotting of the vascular pedicle following implantation within the lunate before adequate capillary anastomoses can occur.[130] Despite this possibility, medium-term results have been encouraging in early disease, especially when combined with other procedures such as joint leveling, partial carpal arthrodesis, or external fixation.[122,128,129] Nonvascularized bone grafting has been reported in early disease with small localized areas of fragmentation.[131]

Partial wrist fusions such as scaphoid-trapezium-trapezoid (STT) and scaphoid-capitate (SC) arthrodeses function to unload the lunate and shift the forces across the wrist toward the radioscaphoid articulation.[114] STT fusion is the most commonly described. In addition to unloading the lunate, it carries the benefit of preventing a progressive scaphoid rotatory subluxation and collapse.[132,133] SC arthrodesis has been described with success similar to STT fusions, and although less motion was reported with SC fusion, the nonunion rate was approximately half that of STT arthrodesis.[134] However, in cadaveric studies, both fusions produced similar reduction in global wrist motion.[135]

Capitohamate (CH) fusion has been reported but is more controversial as a treatment for Kienbock's.[136] Experimental studies have demonstrated that this fusion does not successfully unload the lunate.[98,115]

Salvage procedures such as proximal row carpectomy, total wrist arthroplasty, or wrist arthrodesis have been advocated for late-stage disease.[137,138] The advantage of proximal row carpectomy and arthroplasty are preservation of motion, whereas arthrodesis provides improved strength.

Osteonecrosis of the Scaphoid

ETIOLOGY AND PATHOGENESIS

Like osteonecrosis of the femoral head, scaphoid avascular necrosis may be traumatic or atraumatic. The most common cause of partial scaphoid osteonecrosis is a fracture. However, this is beyond the scope of this chapter and we will limit our discussion to osteonecrosis without associated fracture of the scaphoid, or Preiser's disease.

Preiser's disease is rare and has no universally accepted definition, no generally accepted etiologic theory, and no established treatment.[139] Theoretical causes include microtrauma, steroid therapy, and terminal vessel thrombosis.[140-142] Associations with SLE and systemic sclerosis have been reported.[143,144] The vascularity of the scaphoid is tenuous and vulnerable to osteonecrosis, especially following injury.[145,146] An etiologic classification for Preiser's disease has been proposed and includes: 1) traumatic, 2) systemic, 3) congenital abnormalities, and 4) idiopathic.[139]

The clinical presentation of Preiser's disease includes radial-sided wrist pain of insidious onset without history of specific trauma. Examination findings include weakness, limitation of motion, swelling, and tenderness localized to the radioscaphoid joint on the dorsoradial aspect of the wrist. Radiograph presentation is similar to the findings of femoral head and lunate osteonecrosis. In early disease, no obvious plain radiograph pathology is noticeable. MRI and bone scan are sensitive in detecting early disease. As the disease progresses, radiographic findings reveal sclerosis, fragmentation, collapse, and subsequent arthritis.[139] Herbert and Lanzetta have presented a classification system based on radiographic findings[147] (Table 114–4).

Much like Kienbock's disease, treatment options for scaphoid osteonecrosis are mainly dependent on the stage of disease. Because there are so few cases reported for Preiser's, no conclusions regarding best treatment options can be made. Stage I, II, and early III disease (precollapse) include immobilization,[139] drilling of the proximal pole,[139] arthroscopic débridement,[148] vascularized bone grafting,[123,149] excision of part or all of the scaphoid with or without silicone replacement,[147] and radial osteotomy.[147] Although not an identical entity, successful treatment of scaphoid nonunion and avascular necrosis has been reported with vascularized bone grafting by multiple investigators.[150-152] For cases that involve fragmentation and collapse, treatments include scaphoid excision and replacement,[147] limited carpal arthrodesis,[153] proximal row carpectomy,[139] or total wrist fusion.[139]

Osteonecrosis in Other Joints

HUMERAL HEAD

Osteonecrosis may involve the bone supporting any diarthrodial joint. After the femoral head, the most fre-

TABLE 114–4 • STAGES OF PREISER'S DISEASE

Stage I:	Normal radiographs; positive bone scan
Stage II:	Increased density of proximal pole; generalized osteoporosis
Stage III:	Fragmentation of the proximal pole with or without pathologic fracture
Stage IV:	Carpal collapse, osteoarthritis (OA)

From Herbert TJ, Lanzetta: Idiopathic avascular necrosis of the scaphoid. J Hand Surg 19B:174-182, 1993.

quently affected sites in adult atraumatic osteonecrosis are the humeral head and the femoral condyles. As in the case of osteonecrosis of the femoral head, osteonecrosis of the humeral head may occur as a complication of proximal humerus fractures or dislocations. The principles of diagnosis and treatment of humeral head osteonecrosis closely parallel those for disease involving the femoral head.[154] Diagnosis is best made with MRI, and core decompression may provide symptomatic relief. The functional consequences of humeral head osteonecrosis are more variable than osteonecrosis of the femoral head, possibly because the humeral head is subjected to lower activity demands than the femoral head. Furthermore, unlike the hip, patients may compensate for pain and dysfunction in the glenohumeral joint by various means. Little experience has been documented with regard to humeral head–salvage procedures, and patients are most often offered replacement arthroplasty when symptoms are sufficiently severe to warrant it.

FEMORAL CONDYLES

Although generally not as debilitating as osteonecrosis of the femoral head, osteonecrosis of the femoral condyles is usually symptomatic and progressive.[155] Diagnosis can be confirmed by a bone scan or MRI. The disease process occurs in two distinct forms. One form occurs in relatively young patients in association with previously described risk factors for atraumatic osteonecrosis of the femoral head. The lesions tend to be large. A second form is idiopathic and occurs in elderly patients. These lesions tend to be small and to involve the medial femoral condyle more frequently than the lateral femoral condyle. Attempts at joint salvage using core decompression, arthroscopic débridement, tibial osteotomy, and osteochondral allograft replacement have been described with variable results. Unicompartmental and total knee arthroplasty are offered as a last resort to younger patients because of the high lifetime risk for aseptic loosening and revision; however, they are reliable surgical options in elderly patients with advanced arthrosis. Three treatments appear to provide the best results: 1) conservative treatment for small lesions with no collapse, 2) core decompression for relief of pain and possible delay in structural collapse in the patients with steroid-induced osteonecrosis, and 3) unicompartmental or total knee arthroplasty in patients whose bones have collapsed.[156]

▌ Summary

Osteonecrosis is defined as ischemic death of bone. When it occurs at or near subchondral bone of a diarthrodial joint, it can lead to subchondral fracture, collapse of the articular cartilage, joint incongruity, and OA. The process may be caused by multiple factors, including trauma; corticosteroid use, ethanol abuse, or both; or it may be idiopathic. Increasing evidence points to microvascular thrombosis playing an essential role in the pathogenesis of osteonecrosis. The natural history of the disease is variable but usually progressive and particularly disabling when

the disease occurs in large, weight-bearing joints. Treatment for osteonecrosis remains an unsolved problem. Attempts to restore the joint are significantly more difficult following subchondral collapse. A variety of surgical techniques has attempted to prevent disease progression. Some have produced promising results, but none is uniformly successful. Further insight into the pathogenesis of the disease may lead to promising preventive therapies or nonsurgical solutions for this most difficult problem.

REFERENCES

1. Mankin JH: Nontraumatic necrosis of bone (osteonecrosis). N Engl J Med 326:1473-1479, 1992.
2. Catto M: A histological study of avascular necrosis of the femoral head after transcervical fracture. J Bone Joint Surg Br 47: 749-776,1965.
3. Crock HV: A revision of the anatomy of the arteries supplying the upper end of the human femur. J Anat 99:77, 1965.
4. Bachiller FG, Caballer AP, Portal LF: Avascular necrosis of the femoral head after femoral neck fracture. Clin Orthop 399: 87-109, 2002.
5. Sevitt S: Avascular necrosis and revascularization of the femoral head after intracapsular fracture. J Bone Joint Surg Br 46: 270-96, 1964.
6. Catto M: The histological appearances of late segmental collapse of the femoral head after transcervical fracture. J Bone Joint Surg Br 47:777-791, 1965.
7. Lu-Yao GL, Keller RB, Littenberg B, Wennberg JE: Outcomes after displaced fractures of the femoral neck: a meta-analysis of one hundred and six published reports. J Bone Joint Surg Am 76:15-25, 1994.
8. Askin SR, Bryan RS: Femoral neck fractures in young adults. Clin Orthop 114:259-264, 1976.
9. Barnes R, Brown JT, Garden RS, Nicoll EA: Subcapital fractures of the femur. J Bone Joint Surg Br 58:2-24, 1976.
10. Garden RS: The structure and function of the proximal end of the femur. J Bone Joint Surg Br 43:576-589, 1961.
11. Dedrick DK, Mackenzie JR, Burney RE: Complications of femoral neck fractures in young adults. J Trauma 26:932-937, 1986.
12. Protzman RB, Burkhalter WE: Femoral neck fractures in young adults. J Bone Joint Surg Am 58:689-695, 1976.
13. Zetterberg CH, Irstam L, Andersson GBJ: Femoral neck fratures in young adults. Acta Orthop Scand 53:427-435, 1982.
14. Soto-Hall R, Johnson LH, Johnson R: Variations in the intra-articular pressure of the hip joint in injury and disease. J Bone Joint Surg Am 46:509, 1964.
15. Calandruccio RA, Anderson WE: Post-fracture avascular necrosis of the femoral head: correlation of experimental and clinical studies. Clin Orthop 152:49-84, 1980.
16. Phemister DB: Fractures of the neck of the femur, dislocation of the hip and obscure vascular disturbances producing aseptic necrosis of the head of the femur. Surg Gynecol Obstet 59:415-440, 1934.
17. Brown TD, Pederson DR, Baker KJ: Mechanical consequences of core drilling and bone-grafting on osteonecrosis of the femoral head. J Bone Joint Surg Am 75:1358-1367, 1993.
18. Arnold WD, Lydon JP, Minkoff J: Treatment of intracapsular fractures of the femoral neck. J Bone Joint Surg Am 56:254-262, 1974.
19. Brown JT, Abrami G: Transcervical femoral neck fractures. J Bone Joint Surg Br 46:648-663, 1964.
20. Sevitt S, Thompson RG: The distribution and anastomoses of arteries supplying the head and neck of the femur. J Bone Joint Surg 47B:560-573, 1965.
21. Mont MA, Hungerford DS: Current concepts review: Non traumatic avascular necrosis of the femoral head. J Bone Joint Surg Am 77:459-474, 1995.
22. Jones JP Jr., Urbaniak JR (eds): Osteonecrosis: Etiology, Diagnosis, and Treatment. Rosemont, Ill., American Academy of Orthopaedic Surgeons, 1997, pp 89-96.
23. Jones JP: Concepts of etiology and early pathogenesis of osteonecrosis. Instr Course Lect 43:499-512, 1994.

Jones Jp: Risk factors potentially activating intravascular congulation and causing nontraumatic osteonecrosis

24. Cruess RL: Steroid induced osteonecrosis: a review. Canadian J Surg 24:567-571, 1981.

25. Hungerford DS, Zizic TM: Alcoholism associated ischemic necrosis of the femoral head. Early diagnosis and treatment. Clin Orthop 130:144-153, 1978.

26. Nashi H, Coda K, Nakazima N: Idiopathic avascular necrosis of the femoral head and chronic alcoholism. In Nishi A (ed): Annual Report of Idiopathic Avascular Necrosis of the Femoral Head Research Committee. Fukuoka, Japan, Ministry of Health and Welfare, 1980, p 65.

27. Orlic D, Jovanovic D, Auticevic D, Zecevic J: Frequency of idiopathic aseptic necrosis in medically treated alcoholics. Int Orthop 14:383-386, 1990.

28. Felson DT, Anderson JS: A cross-study evaluation of association between steroid dose and bolus steroids and avascular necrosis of bone. Lancet 1:902-906, 1987.

29. Brazil M, Lindeser RS, Dickhaus JJ, Garvin PJ: Aseptic hip necrosis after renal transplantation. Arch Surg 121:803-806, 1986.

30. Bradbury G, Benjamin J, Thompson J, et al: Avascular necrosis of bone after cardiac transplantation. J Bone Joint Surg Am 76:1385-1388, 1994.

31. Ono K, Tohjima T, Komazawa T: Risk factors of avascular necrosis of the femoral head in patients with SLE under high dose corticosteroid therapy. Clin Orthop 277:89-97, 1992.

32. Ota Y, Matsunga H: Bone lesions in divers. J Bone Joint Surg Br 56:3-16, 1974.

33. Kawashima M, Torisu T, Hayashi K, Kitano M: Pathologic review of osteonecrosis in divers. Clin Orthop 130:107-117, 1978.

34. Chung SMK, Ralston EL: Necrosis of the femoral head associated with sickle-cell anemia and its genetic variants. J Bone Joint Surg Am 51:33-58, 1969.

35. Wheeless CR, Lins RE, Knelson MH, Urbanisk JR: Digital subtraction angiography in patients with osteonecrosis of the femoral head. In Jones JP, Urbaniak JR (eds): Ostconccrosis: Etiology, Diagnosis and Treatment. Rosemont, Ill., American Academy of Orthopaedic Surgeons, 1997, pp 241-245.

36. Yoshida T, Kanayama Y, Okamura M, et al: Long-term observation of avascular necrosis of the femoral head in systemic lupus erythematosus: an MRI study. Clin Exp Rheumatol 20:525-530, 2002.

37. Gladman DD, Chaudhry-Ahluwalia V, Ibanez D, et al: Outcomes of symptomatic osteonecrosis in 95 patients with systemic lupus erythematosus. J Rheumatol 28:2226-2229, 2001.

38. Asherson RA, Liote F, Page B, et al: Avascular necrosis of bone and antiphospholipid antibodies in systemic lupus erythematosus. J Rheumatol 20:284-288, 1993.

39. Nagasawa K, Tsukamoto H, Tada Y, et al: Imaging study on the mode of development an dchanges in avascular necrosis of the femoral head in systemic lupus erythematosus: Long-term observations. Br J Rheumatol 33:343-347, 1994.

40. Vela P, Battle E, Salas E, Marco P: Primary antiphospholipid syndrome and osteonecrosis (letter). Clin Exp Rheumatol 9:545-546, 1991.

41. Gladman DD, Urowitz MB, Chaudhry-Ahluwalia V, et al: Predictive factors for symptomatic osteonecrosis in patients with systemic lupus erythematosus. J Rheumatol 28:2365-2366, 2001.

42. Glueck CJ, Freiberg RA, Fontaine RN, et al: Hypofibrinolysis, thrombophilia, osteonecrosis. Clin Orthop 386:19-33, 2001.

43. Glueck CJ, Glueck HI, Mieczkowski L, et al: Familial high plasminogen activatorinhibitor with hypofibrinolysis: a new pathophysiologic cause of ostenecrosis? Thromb Haemost 69:460-465, 1993.

44. Glueck CJ, Fontaine RN, Gruppo R, et al: The plasminogen activator inhibitor-1 gene, hypofibrinolysis, and osteonecrosis. Clin Orthop 366:133-146, 1999.

45. Glueck CJ, Freiberg RA, Glueck HI, et al: Hypofibrinolysis: a common, major cause of osteonecrosis. Am J Hematol 45:156-166, 1994.

46. Glueck CJ, Freiberg RA, Fontaine RN, et al: Anticoagulant therapy for osteonecrosis associated with heritable hypofibrinolysis and thrombophilia. Expert Opin Investig Drugs 10:1309-1316, 2001.

47. Enneking WF: Classification of nontraumatic osteonecrosis of the femoral head. In Jones JP Jr., Urbaniak JR (eds): Osteonecrosis: Etiology, Diagnosis, and Treatment. Rosemont, Ill., American Academy of Orthopaedic Surgeons, 1997, pp 269-284.

48. Glimcher MJ, Kenzora JE: The biology of osteonecrosis of the human femoral head and its implications. I. Tissue biology. Clin Orthop 138:284-309, 1979.

49. Glimcher MJ, Kenzora JE: The biology of osteonecrosis of the human femoral head and its clinical implications. II. The pathologic changes in the femoral head as an organ and in the hip joint. Clin Orthop 139:283-312, 1979.

50. Glimcher MJ, Kenzora JE: The biology of osteonecrosis of the human femoral head and its clinical implications. III. Discussion of the etiology and genesis of the pathological sequelae: Comments on treatment. Clin Orthop 140:273-312, 1979.

51. Mitchell DG, Steinberg ME, Dalinka MK, et al: Magnetic resonance imaging of the ischemic hip: alterations within the osteonecrotic, viable, and reactive zones. Clin Orthop 244:60-77, 1989.

52. Mitchell DG, Rao VM, Dalinka MK, et al: Femoral head avascular necrosis: correlation of MR imaging, radiographic staging, radionuclide imaging, and clinical findings. Radiology 162:709-715, 1987.

53. Chan TW, Dalinka MK, Steinberg ME, Kressel HY: MRI appearance of femoral head osteonecrosis following core decompression and bone grafting. Skeletal Radiol 20:103-107, 1991.

54. Kramer J, Hofmann S, Imhof H: The non-traumatic femur head necrosis in the adult. II. Radiologic diagnosis and staging. Radiology 34:11-20, 1994.

55. Magid D, Fishman EK, Scott WW Jr., et al: Femoral head avascular necrosis: CT assessment with multiplanar reconstruction. Radiology 157:751-756, 1985.

56. Ficat RP: Idiopathic bone necrosis of the femoral head: Early diagnosis and treatment. J Bone Joint Surg Br 67:3-9, 1985.

57. Marcus ND, Enneking WF, Massam RA: The silent hip in idiopathic aseptic necrosis: Treatment by bone-grafting. J Bone Joint Surg Am 55:1351-1366, 1973.

58. Steinberg ME, Hayken GD, Steinberg DR: A quantitative system for staging avascular necrosis. J Bone Joint Surg Br 77:34-41, 1995.

59. Sugano N, Takaoka K, Ohzono K, et al: Prognostication of nontraumatic avascular necrosis of the femoral head: Significance of location and size of the necrotic lesion. Clin Orthop 303:155-164, 1994.

60. Gardeniers JWM: ARCO international classification of osteonecrosis. ARCO Newsletter 5:79, 1993.

61. Sekiya JK, Ruch DS, Hunter DM, et al: The role of arthroscopy in the diagnosis and staging of osteonecrosis. In Jones JP Jr., Urbaniak JR (eds): Osteonecrosis: Etiology, Diagnosis, and Treatment. Rosemont, Ill., American Academy of Orthopaedic Surgeons, 1997, pp 253-260.

62. Mont MA, Carbone JJ, Fairbank AC: Core decompression versus nonoperative management for osteonecrosis of the hip. Clin Orthop 324:169-178, 1996.

63. Kopecky KK, Braunstein EM, Brandt KD, et al: Apparent avascular necrosis of the hip: appearance and spontaneous resolution of MR findings in renal allograft recipients. Radiology 79:523-527, 1991.

64. Davidson JJ, Coogan PG, Gunneson EE, Urbaniak JR: The asymptomatic contralateral hip in osteonecrosis of the femoral head. In Jones JP Jr., Urbaniak JR (eds): Osteonecrosis: Etiology, Diagnosis, and Treatment. Rosemont, Ill, American Academy of Orthopaedic Surgeons, 1997, pp 231-246.

65. Baumgaertner MR, Higgins TF: Femoral neck fractures. In Bucholz RW, Heckman JD (eds): Rockwood and Green's Fractures in Adults. Philadelphia, Lippincott-Raven, 2001, pp 1579-1634.

66. Scully SP, Aaron RK, Urbaniak JR: Survival analysis of hips treated with core decompression or vascularized fibular grafting because of avascular necrosis. J Bone Joint Surg 80A:1270-1275, 1998.

67. Fairbank AC, Bhatia D, Jinnah RH, et al: Long-term results of core decompression for ischaemic necrosis of the femoral head. J Bone Joint Surg Br 77:42-49, 1995.

68. Stulberg BN, Dais AW, Bauer TW, et al: Osteonecrosis of the femoral head: A prospective randomized treatment protocol. Clin Orthop 268:140-151, 1991.

69. Koo KH, Kim R, Ko GH, et al: Preventing collapse in early osteonecrosis of the femoral head: a randomized clinical trial of core decompression. J Bone Joint Surg Br 77:870-874, 1995.

70. Steinberg ME, Brighton CT, Corces A, et al: Osteonecrosis of the femoral head: results of core decompression and grafting with and without electrical stimulation. Clin Orthop 249:199-208, 1989.

71. Steinberg ME, Brighton CT, Bands RE, Hartman KM: Capacitive coupling as an adjunctive treatment for avascular necrosis. Clin Orthop 261:11-19, 1990.

72. Aaron RK, Cimobor DM: Electrical stimulation of bone induction and grafting. *In* Habal MB, Reddi AH (eds): Bone Grafts and Bone Substitutes. Philadelphia, WB Saunders, 1992, pp 192-205.

73. Buckley PD, Gearen PF, Petty RW: Structural bone-grafting for early atraumatic avascular necrosis of the femoral head. J Bone Joint Surg Am 73:1357-1364, 1991.

74. Nelson LM, Clark CR: Efficacy of Phemister bone grafting in non-traumatic aseptic necrosis of the femoral head. J Arthroplasty 8:253-258, 1993.

75. Urbaniak JR, Coogan PG, Gunneson EB, Nunley JA: Treatment of osteonecrosis of the femoral head with free vascularized fibular grafting: a long-term follow-up study of one hundred and three hips. J Bone Joint Surg Am 77:681-694, 1995.

76. Sotereanos DG, Plakseychuk AY, Rubash HE: Free vascularized fibula grafting for the treatment of osteonecrosis of the femoral head. Clin Orthop 344:243-256, 1997.

77. Brunelli G, Brunelli G: Free microvascular fibular transfer for idiopathic femoral head necrosis: Long-term follow-up. J Reconstruct Microsurg 7:285-295, 1991.

78. Vail TP, Urbaniak JR: Donor-site morbidity with use of vascularized autogenous fibular grafts. J Bone Joint Surg Am 78:204-211, 1996.

79. Hosokawa A, Mohtai M, Hotokebuchi T, et al: Transtrochanteric rotational osteotomy for idiopathic and steroid-induced osteonecrosis of the femoral head. *In* Jones JP Jr., Urbaniak JR (eds): Osteonecrosis: Etiology, Diagnosis, and Treatment. Rosemont, Ill., American Academy of Orthopaedic Surgeons, 1997, pp 309-314.

80. Scher MA, Jakim I: Intertrochanteric osteotomy and the autogenous bone-grafting for avascular necrosis of the femoral head. J Bone Joint Surg Am 75:1119-1133, 1993.

81. Mont MA, Fairbank AC, Drackow DA, Hungerford DS: Corrective osteotomy for osteonecrosis of the femoral head. J Bone Joint Surg Am 78:1032-1038, 1996.

82. Koo KH, Song HR, Yang JW, et al: Trochanteric rotational osteotomy for osteonecrosis of the femoral head. J Bone Joint Surg Br 83:83-89, 2001.

83. Schneider W, Aigner N, Pinggera O, Knahr K: Intertrochanteric osteotomy for avascular necrosis of the head of the femur. Survival probability of two different methods. J Bone Joint Surg Br 84:817-824, 2002.

84. Gallinaro P, Masse A: Flexion osteotomy in the treatment of avascular necrosis of the hip. Clin Orthop 386:79-84, 2001.

85. Sugioka Y, Hotokebuchi T, Tsutsui H: Transtrochanteric anterior rotational osteotomy for idiopathic and steroid-induced necrosis of the femoral head: Indications and long-term results Clin Orthop 277:111-120, 1992.

86. Dean MT, Cabanela ME: Transtrochanteric anterior rotational osteotomy for avascular necrosis of the femoral head: Long-term results. J Bone Joint Surg Br 75:597-601, 1993.

87. Amstutz HC, Noordin S, Campbell PA, Schmarlzried TP: Precision fit surface hemiarthroplasty for femoral head osteonecrosis. *In* Jones JP Jr., Urbaniak JR (eds): Osteonecrosis: Etiology, Diagnosis, and Treatment. Rosemont, Ill., American Academy of Orthopaedic Surgeons, 1997, pp 373-383.

88. Hungerford MW, Mont MA, Scott R, et al: Surface replacement hemiarthroplasty for the treatment of osteonecrosis of the femoral head. J Bone Joint Surg Am 80:1656-1664, 1998.

89. Cabanela ME: Bipolar versus total hip arthroplasty for avascular necrosis of the femoral head: a comparison. Clin Orthop 261:59-62, 1990.

90. Capello WN, Colyer RA, Gemlick BF, Feinberg JR: The use of cementless stems in the treatment of osteonecrosis. *In* Jones JP Jr., Urbaniak JR (eds): Osteonecrosis: Etiology, Diagnosis, and Treatment. Rosemont, Ill., American Academy of Orthopaedic Surgeons, 1997, pp 397-403.

91. Plenk H, Hofmann S, Eschberger J, et al: Histomorphology and bone morphometry of the bone marrow edema syndrome of the hip. Clin Orthop 334:73-84, 1997.

92. Schapira D: Transient osteoporosis of the hip. Semin Arthritis Rheum 22:98-105, 1992.

93. Hofmann S, Engel A, Neuhold A, et al: Bone-marrow oedema syndrome and transient osteoporosis of the hip: An MRI-controlled study of treatment by core decompression. J Bone Joint Surg Br 75:210-216, 1994.

94. Guerra JJ, Steinberg ME: Distinguishing transient osteoporosis from avascular necrosis of the hip. J Bone Joint Surg Am 7A:616-624, 1995.

95. Hayes CW, Conway WF, Daniel WW: mR imaging of bone marrow edema pattern: transient osteoporosis, transient bone marrow edema syndrome, or osteonecrosis. Radiographics, 13:1001-11, 1993.

96. Gelberman RH, Salamon PB, Jurist JM, Posch JL: Ulnar variance in Kienbock's disease. J Bone Joint Surg Am 57:674-676, 1975.

97. Bonzar M, Firrell JC, Hainer M, et al: Kienbock disease and negative ulnar variance. J Bone Joint Surg Am 80:1154-1157, 1998.

98. Horii E, Garcia-Elias M, Bishop AT, et al: Effect on force transmission across the carpus in procedures used to treat Kienbock's disease. J Hand Surg 15A:393-400, 1990.

99. Werner FW, Palmer AK: Biomechanical evaluation of operative procedures to treat Kienbock's disease. Hand Clin 9:431-443, 1993.

100. Tsuge S, Nakamura R: Anatomic risk factors for Kienbock's disease. J Hand Surg Br 18:70-75, 1993.

101. Gelberman RH, Bauman TD, Menon J, Akeson WH: The vascularity of the lunate bone and Kienbock's disease. J Hand Surg 5:272-278, 1980.

102. Williams CS, Gelberman RH: Vascularity of the lunate: anatomy studies and implications for the development of osteonecrosis. Hand Clin 9:391-398, 1993.

103. Beckenbaugh RD, Shives TC, Dobyns JH, Linscheid RL: Kienbock's disease: The natural history of Kienbock's disease and consideration of lunate fractures. Clin Orthop 149:98-106, 1980.

104. Trial IA, Linscheid RL, Quenzer DE, Scherer PA: Ulnar lengthening and radial recession procedures for Kienbock's disease: Long-term clinical and radiographic follow-up. J Hand Surg Br 21:169-176, 1996.

105. Linscheid RL: Kienbock's disease. J Hand Surg 10A:1-3, 1985.

106. Hashizume H, Asahara H, Nishida K, et al: Histopathology of Kienbock's disease: Correlation with magnetic resonance and other imaging techniques. J Hand Surg Br 21:169-176, 1996.

107. Menth-Chiari WA, Poehling GG, Wiesler ER, Ruch DS: Arthroscopic debridément for the treatment of Kienbock's disease. Arthroscopy 15:12-19, 1999.

108. Quenzer DE, Linscheid RL, Vidal MA, et al: Trispiral tomographic staging of Kienbock's disease. J Hand Surg Am 22:396-403, 1997.

109. Stahl F: On lunatomalacia (Kienbock's disease): A clinical and roentgenological study, especially on the pathogenesis and late results of immobilization treatment. Acta Chir Scand 95(Suppl): 126, 1947.

110. Lichtman DM, Alexander AH, Mack GR, Gunther SF: Kienbock's disease: The role of silicone replacement arthroplasty. J Bone Joint Surg Am 59:899-908, 1977.

111. Lichtman DM, Degnan GG: Staging and its use in the determination of treatment modalities for Kienbock's disease. Hand Clin 9:409-416, 1993.

112. Kristensen SS, Thomassen E, Christensen F: Kienbock's disease: late results of non-surgical treatment. J Hand Surg Br 11:422-425, 1986.

113. Mikkelsen SS, Gelineck J: Poor function after nonoperative treatment of Kienbock's disease. Acta Orthop Scand 58:241-243, 1987.

114. Trumble T, Glisson RR, Seaber AV, Urbaniak JR: A biomechanical comparison of the methods for treating Kienbock's disease. J Hand Surg Am 11:88-93, 1986.

115. Masear VR, Zook EG, Pichora DR, et al: Strain-gauge evaluation of lunate unloading procedures. J Hand Surg Am 17:437-443, 1992.

116. Tillberg B: Kienbock's disease treated with osteotomy to lengthen ulna. Acta Orthop Scand 39:359-368, 1968.

117. Nakamura R, Horii E, Imaeda T: Excessive radial shortening in Kienbock's disease. J Hand Surg Br 15:46-49, 1990.

118. Weiss AP, Weiland AJ, Moore JR, Wilgis EFS: Radial shortening for Kienbock's disease. J Bone Joint Surg Am 73:384-391, 1991.

119. Nakamura R, Tsuge S, Watanabe K, Tsunoda K: Radial wedge osteotomy for Kienbock's disease. J Bone Joint Surg Am 73:1391-1396, 1991.

120. Miura H, Uchida Y, Sugioka Y: Radial closing wedge osteotomy for Kienbock's disease. J Hand Surg Am 21:1029-1034, 1996.

121. Wada A, Miura H, Kubota H, et al: radial closing wedge osteotomy for Kienbock's disease:An over 10 year clinical and radiographic follow-up. J Hand Surg Br 27:175-179, 2002.

122. Soejima O, Lida H, Komine S, et al: Lateral closing wedge osteotomy of the distal radius for advanced stages of Kienbock's disease. J Hand Surg Am 27:31-36, 2002.

123. Hori Y, Tamai S, Okuda H, et al: Blood vessel transplantation to bone. J Hand Surg 4:23-33, 1979.

124. Sheetz KK, Bishop AT, Berger RA: The arterial blood supply of the distal radius and ulna and its potential use in vascularized pedicled bone grafts. J Hand Surg 20:902-914, 1995.

125. Braun RM: Viable pedicle bone grafting in the wrist. *In* Urbaniak JR (ed): Microsurgery for Major Limb Reconstruction. St Louis, Mosby, 1987, pp 220-229.

126. Zaidenberg C: A new vascularized bone graft for scaphoid nonunion. J Hand Surg Am 16:474-478, 1991.

127. Shin AY, Bishop AT: Treatment of Kienbock's disease with dorsal distal radius pedicled vascularized bone grafts. Atlas Hand Clin ***:91-118, 1999.

128. Bochud RC, Buchler U: Kienbock's disease, early stage 3–height reconstruction and core revascularization of the lunate. J Hand Surg Br 19:466-478, 1994.

129. Gabl M, Lutz M, Reinhart C, et al: Stage 3 Kienbock's disease: reconstruction of the fractured lunate using a free vascularized iliac bone graft and external fixation. J Hand Surg 27:369-73, 2002.

130. Aspenburg P, Wang JS, Jonsson K, Hager CG: Experimental osteonecrosis of the lunate: revascularization may cause collapse. J Hand Surg Br 19:565-569, 1994.

131. Zelouf DS, Ruby LK: External fixation and cancellous bone grafting for Kienbock's disease: a preliminary report. J Hand Surg Am 21:746-753, 1996.

132. Watson HK, Ryu J, Dibella A: An approach to Kienbock's disease: Triscaphe arthrodesis. J Hand Surg Am 10:179-187, 1985.

133. Watson HK, Monacelli DM, Milford RS, Ashmaed D: Treatment of Kienbock's disease with scaphotrapeziotrapezoid arthrodesis. J Hand Surg Am 21:9-15, 1996.

134. Sennwald GR, Ufenast H: Scaphocapitate srthrodesis for the treatment of Kienbock's disease. J Hand Surg Am 20:506-510, 1995.

135. Garcia-Elias M, Cooney WP, An KN, et al: Wrist kinematics after limited intercarpal arthrodesis. J Hand Surg Am 14:791-799, 1989.

136. Inoue G: Capitate-hamate fusion for Kienbock's disease: good results in 8 cases followed for 3 years. Acta Orthop Scand 63:560-562, 1992.

137. Begley BW, Engber WD: Proximal row carpectomy in advanced Kienbock's disease. J Hand Surg Am 19:1016-1018, 1994.

138. Imbriglia JE, Broudy AS, Hagberg WC, McKernan D: Proximal row carpectomy: Clinical evaluation. J Hand Surg Am 15:426-430, 1990.

139. Vidal MA, Linscheid RL, Amadio PC, Dobyns JH: Preiser's disease. Ann Hand Surg 10:227-236, 1991.

140. Milgram JW, Riley LH: Steroid induced avascular necrosis of bones in 18 sites. Bull Hosp Joint Dis 37:11-23, 1976.

141. Allen PR: Idiopathic avascular necrosis of the scaphoid. J Bone Joint Surg Br 65:333-335, 1983.

142. Ferlic DC, Morin P: Idiopathic avascular necrosis of the scaphoid: Preiser's disease? J Hand Surg Am 14:13-16, 1989.

143. Urman JD, Abeles M, Hoghton AN, Rothfield NF: Aspetic necrosis presenting as wrist pain in SLE. Arthritis Rheum 20:825-828, 1977.

144. Kawai H, Tsuyuguchi Y, Yonenobu K, et al: Avascular necrosis of the carpal scaphoid associated with progressive systemic sclerosis. Hand 15:270-273, 1983.

145. Gelberman RH, Menon J: The vascularity of the scaphoid bone. J Hand Surg 5:508-513, 1980.

146. Freedman DM, Botte MJ, Gelberman RH: Vascularity of the carpus. Clin Orthop 383:47-59, 2001.

147. Herbert TJ, Lanzetta M: Idiopathic avascular necrosis of the scaphoid. J Hand Surg Br 19:174-182, 1994.

148. Menth-Chiari WA, Poehling GG: Preiser's disease: arthroscopic treatment of avascular necrosis of the scaphoid. Arthroscopy 16:208-213, 2000.

149. Riley LH, Moore JR, Weiland AJ: Presier's disease: a report of ten cases. Presented at the 45th Annual Meeting of the Society for Surgery of the Hand. Toronto, Ontario. September 24-27, 1990.

150. Straw R, Davis T, Dias J: Scaphoid nonunion: treatment with a pedicled vascularized bone graft based on the 1,2 intercompartmental supraretinacular branch of the radial artery. J Hand Surg Br 27:413-416, 2002.

151. Steinmann SP, Bishop AT, Berger RA: Use of the 1,2 intercompartmental supraretinacular artery as a vascularized pedicle bone graft for difficult scaphoid nonunion. J Hand Surg Am 27:391-401, 2002.

152. Waters PM, Stewart SL: Surgical treatment of nonunion and avascular necrosis of the proximal part of the scaphoid in adolescents. J Bone Joint Surg Am 84:915-920, 2002.

153. Gerwin M, Weiland AJ: Avascular necrosis of the carpals. *In* Peimer CA (ed): Surgery of the Hand and Upper Extremity. New York, McGraw Hill, 1996, pp 759-769.

154. Mont MA, Maar DC, Urquhart MW, et al: Avascular necrosis of the humeral head treated by core decompression: A retrospective review. J Bone Joint Surg Br 75:785-788, 1993.

155. Lotke PA, Ecker JL: Osteonecrosis of the knee. J Bone Joint Surg Br 73:470-473, 1988.

156. Lotke PA, Battish R, Nelson CL: Treatment of osteonecrosis of the knee. Instr Course Lect 50:483-488, 2001.

115

Introduction to Surgical Management of Patients with Arthritis

CLEMENT B. SLEDGE

The various forms of arthritis eventually produce similar consequences in involved joints—pain, loss of function, and cartilage destruction—all of which are progressive. Reconstructive surgery may be indicated to relieve any or all of these disabilities. In selected situations, surgery may be indicated to prevent these consequences. Although the ultimate damage to the joint may be similar, there are significant differences between osteoarthritis (OA) and rheumatoid arthritis (RA); indeed, there are unique surgical aspects to many of the rheumatoid variants. In some instances, these unique features place the patient at risk from surgery and in others they jeopardize the eventual result.

Inflammatory arthritis presents itself in the various joints in unique ways, and an understanding of the various manifestations is important in the outcome of surgery. Additionally, either surgeon or rheumatologist should understand the spectrum of surgical treatments available to the patient so he or she can provide the patient and family with advice. In Europe and in some other parts of the world, there exists the field of "rheumasurgery." Those who practice this specialty cross the usual divisions of surgical specialization, hand surgery, spine surgery, and joint replacement, among others, and treat the spectrum of arthritis as it presents itself in different patients. The value of this approach is that one person is in a position to help the patient decide which procedures to have and in what sequence. The argument on the other side centers on the increased expertise a specialist in hand surgery or spine surgery may bring to the surgical decision and procedure. Given the degree of subspecialization in North America and many parts of the Western world, perhaps the best situation is to have an experienced surgeon or surgeons working closely with a rheumatologist. For optimal care, the rheumatologist should understand the basic aspects of surgical treatment of the various joints.

The characteristic features of RA in various joints are discussed in the preoperative evaluation section, with emphasis on the following two philosophic points:

1. The surgeon who operates on arthritic patients, especially rheumatoid patients, should be familiar with the special technical aspects necessitated by the unusual requirements of the patient with multiple joint involvement.
2. The surgeon should be part of a team that is composed of rheumatologists, nurses, therapists, social workers, and—most important—the patient. At first glance it may seem foolish to list the patient as part of the team. To do so recognizes that the surgical

patient with RA is frequently weak and discouraged and must look forward to a series of operations before reasonable functional independence is achieved. Often the patient has excessive expectations regarding the outcome of surgery.[1] By participating in the planning and staging of the surgical events, the patient can better understand the duration of treatment, the necessity of prolonged physical therapy, and the ultimate realistic goals of the procedure or procedures.

Because pain relief is the most consistent achievement of reconstructive surgery, pain is the primary indication for operative intervention. Restoration of motion and function are less predictable and require careful assessment of each patient's disability before improvement can be potentially offered.[2] Some surgical procedures in RA are as much prophylactic as therapeutic (e.g., synovectomy, fusion of the first and second cervical vertebrae, fusion of the base of the thumb). The patient should understand the preventive aspects so there will not be disappointment when the therapeutic result does not seem to justify the pain and inconvenience of surgery. Often these "prophylactic" procedures, such as synovectomy of the elbow,[3] knee,[4] or hand tendons,[5] can have long-term symptomatic benefit but may not prevent deterioration of cartilage.[6]

In addition to pain relief and improved function, societal and socioeconomic goals must be considered. The patient with RA tends to have a longer duration of stay for each surgical procedure and often requires multiple major procedures. The economic costs are considerable, even when everything proceeds without complication. If a deep infection occurs after a hip replacement, the costs may rise exponentially. Even without complications, it may seem difficult to justify the costs of these major procedures; most patients coming to multiple joint replacement surgeries either have left the workforce because of disability or have postponed surgery until they are ready for retirement. Many are women who have not worked outside the home. These factors make calculation of a cost-benefit ratio difficult.

Without putting a dollar value on the "quality of life," can such extensive procedures be justified? One study of 16 patients undergoing bilateral hip and knee replacement showed that none of those patients returned to work after this expensive series of operations, which involved an average of 3 months of hospitalization.[7] Precise data are not available, but preliminary quality-of-life studies strongly suggest that society does benefit in terms of decreased need for home help, home modifications, hospitalization, or confinement to an institution because of loss of independent functional capacity.[8,9] Additionally, release of the spouse from his or her helping role allows return to the workforce or independent activity. For many individual patients, however, the goal must be relief of pain, restoration of functional independence, and a qualitative improvement in existence without the hope of pure economic justification.[10-12] Part of the difficulty in assessing the potential benefit of a surgical procedure, to the patient or to society, is the lack of uniform methods of assessment before and after surgery. Few studies have reported critical assessment of the outcome in patients with RA who have joint replacement; definitive studies await adoption and general application of uniform criteria of assessment.[13]

Certainly, the major single advance in the care of patients with arthritis was the development of the total hip replacement by Charnley in 1979.[14] The concepts initially involved in replacement of the arthritic hip have been expanded to cover most of the other joints. For patients with OA, there are numerous alternatives to joint replacement, many of which are preferable, especially in younger patients. In patients with RA, procedures such as arthrodesis, synovectomy, repair of ruptured tendons, and other "nonprosthetic" procedures still play an important role. For predictable relief of pain and restoration of function, however, joint replacement surgery has revolutionized the outlook for patients with multiple joint involvement.[2,11,15] The following sections emphasize joint replacement surgery in patients with RA and its variants; when appropriate, however, alternative procedures are mentioned, as are certain features pertinent to the patient with OA.

▮ Preoperative Evaluation

GENERAL CONSIDERATIONS

The first consideration is whether a painful joint in a patient with RA necessitates surgery or not. If synovitis is the cause of the patient's pain and disability, continued medical management with drugs and physical methods is appropriate. If it can be determined that structural damage to the joint is the problem, medication will probably not be sufficient. A trial of anti-inflammatory medication and physical therapy is appropriate, particularly for the weight-bearing joints, where the use of crutches may allow the acute disabling symptoms to subside to an acceptable level, even in the presence of structural damage. If these measures fail, and structural damage can be demonstrated on physical examination or by radiographic examination, arthrodesis or arthroplasty can be considered. It is better to perform surgery on each joint as it becomes structurally destroyed than to wait until the patient has multiple destroyed joints, which would require prolonged hospitalization, multiple anesthetics, and a series of debilitating surgical procedures.

General operative risk should be assessed, especially from the point of view of the systemic manifestations of the rheumatic diseases.[10] The patient should be in optimal medical condition and, when taking glucocorticoids, should be receiving the lowest possible maintenance dose. Obvious sources of infection should be identified and eradicated to prevent postoperative hematogenous seeding of the operative site. Carious teeth should be treated before surgery on the joints, and urinary tract infections should be identified and treated. Many female patients have asymptomatic bacteriuria, and a urine culture before surgery is helpful in identifying and treating such patients. In male patients, prostatic hypertrophy, if severe, should be treated before surgery to avoid postoperative catheterization with its attendant risk of infection and bacterial seeding. It is useful to determine whether the patient can void in the supine position. Frequently, preoperative practice at supine voiding facilitates recovery in the postoperative period. Airway problems are frequent, and preoperative assessment by the anesthesiologist is useful[16,17] (Table 115–1).

Most difficult to evaluate is the patient's motivation and ability to participate meaningfully in the postoperative program. Evaluation by physical and occupational

TABLE 115–1 • EXTUBATION CONSIDERATIONS IN CERTAIN TYPES OF INFLAMMATORY ARTHRITIS

Anatomic/Technical Problem	Rheumatoid Arthritis	Juvenile Rheumatoid Arthritis	Ankylosing Spondylitis	Scleroderma	Systemic Lupus Erythematosus
Narrow nares		✓			
Limited jaw opening	✓	✓	✓	✓	
		Temporomandibular joint		Tense skin	
Overbite		✓			
Flexed or fused neck	✓	✓	✓	✓	
				Tense skin	
Rotational deformity of neck	✓	✓			
		Prepubertal onset			
Laryngeal pathology	✓	✓		✓	✓
Difficult intubation	✓	✓	✓		
Tendency for acute airway obstruction during extubation	✓	✓	✓	✓	✓

From Sharrock NE: Anesthetic considerations. In Kelley WN, Ruddy S, Harris ED Jr, Sledge CB (eds): Textbook of Rheumatology, 5th ed. Philadelphia, WB Saunders, 1997, p 1641.

therapists should be carried out, both to assess the patient's ability to participate in the program and to determine what specific requirements might apply in the postoperative period. Instruction in crutch ambulation before surgery shortens the postoperative hospital period. If multiple procedures are envisioned, it is often useful to perform a simple procedure first so the ability of the patient to follow the postoperative program can be assessed. If surgery is required for both the hip and the knee, the hip can be used for this assessment. The relief of pain and improvement in function following hip arthroplasty are essentially independent of the patient's cooperation. The postoperative period is characterized by minimal pain. If the patient cannot cooperate with a therapy program after hip replacement, it is unlikely that he or she will be able to participate in the extensive postoperative program required after knee arthoplasty.

The patient with RA or its variants poses special problems that may affect the results and risks of surgery. Multiple joints are usually involved, and these patients undergo surgery, on average, 10 years earlier than patients with OA undergoing similar procedures; they, therefore, have the potential to live longer with a prosthetic joint and have more time for complications such as delayed infection, late loosening, and wear of the component parts to appear.

Much has been written of the increased susceptibility to infection in patients with RA, and our experience documents that the patient undergoing joint replacement in RA does have a significantly increased risk of late hematogenous seeding of the prosthetic joint.[18] Drug actions and interactions should also be considered because of the possibility of an adverse effect on the postoperative recovery. Some patients coming to surgery are still on maintenance therapy with glucocorticoids, and this regimen may increase the risk of infection. Aspirin and nonsteroidal anti-inflammatory drugs (NSAIDs) used by almost all patients may produce difficulties with intraoperative and postoperative bleeding and should probably be discontinued before surgery, especially if anticoagulation prophylaxis with heparin or warfarin is planned.[19] Some patients are receiving chronic immunosuppressive treatment, and the effect of these drugs on postoperative infection must be considered.[20] Methotrexate (MTX) is thought by some to increase susceptibility to postoperative infections, and they recommend it be discontinued 2 weeks before surgery and not reinstituted until wound healing is ensured[21,22] (see also Chapter 59). Recent studies of risk factors, however, have failed to find any association between MTX and postoperative infections.[20,23] Although there is controversy regarding the relationship between penicillamine treatment and wound healing,[24,25] most experienced surgeons feel that wound healing is definitely delayed in patients receiving penicillamine. This may delay the postoperative rehabilitation program. A recent study of complications following surgery on patients with RA found that "penicillamine, indomethacin, cyclosporin, hydroxychloroquine, chloroquine, and prednisolone all did significantly increase the risk of infection or surgical complication after elective orthopedic surgery."[23]

Clinical experience suggests that the rheumatoid process is perpetuated in a given joint by retention of articular cartilage. Whether this is because of sequestered antigen-antibody complexes, the continued release of cartilage breakdown products, or other factors is unknown. It has been a frequent observation, however, that patients undergoing total knee replacement, if the patellar cartilage is retained, may have involvement of that joint in subsequent systemic flares, whereas patients in whom all cartilage has been removed rarely experience involvement of the operated knee in such flares.

The quality of bone in patients with RA is frequently poor. This may be because of direct involvement of the subchondral trabecular bone by rheumatoid granulation tissue, or it may be related to the catabolic effects of chronic steroid use, the bone resorption related to excessive production of prostaglandins by rheumatoid synovium, or release of tumor necrosis factor (TNF) and other cytokines in these patients[26] (see also Chapter 25). Regardless of the cause, the quality of bone is of great concern with regard to the long-term fixation of prosthetic components. Many prosthetic devices transfer the enormous joint reactive forces directly to the bone-cement interface, which may be unable to withstand these forces over time. For this reason, it is desirable to use prosthetic devices that are minimally constrained and to transfer forces away from the bone-cement interface to the more compliant and forgiving soft tissues.

Most patients with chronic inflammatory arthritis are anemic, sometimes to the extent that they cannot predeposit autologous blood for intraoperative and postoperative use. Because it is advantageous to have autologous blood available, the clinician should consider the use of erythropoietin to increase hemoglobin levels before surgery.[27,28]

SPECIAL CIRCUMSTANCES

The patient with juvenile rheumatoid arthritis (JRA) (see Chapter 96) presents certain unique features that bear directly on the results to be expected from surgical intervention. As in patients with ankylosing spondylitis (AS), there appears to be a much greater involvement of the soft tissues surrounding the joint, with the result that the ultimate range of motion achieved after joint arthroplasty is less than would be predicted from the range achieved at surgery.[29] In the days and weeks following arthroplasty, there may be a progressive loss of motion in these patients, and the effect of this loss on ultimate functional capacity must be anticipated. The young age at which patients with JRA undergo arthroplasty exposes their prosthetic joints to both greater functional demands and a longer period of exposure to late complications, such as infection and loosening. In addition, these patients often have severe micrognathia, which may make intubation difficult or produce postoperative respiratory problems.[30,31]

Patients with AS (see Chapter 70) also have unique risk factors.[32] Because they have diminished chest excursion, they are at greater risk for postoperative pulmonary problems and may require chest physical therapy to minimize these problems. Because of rigidity of the cervical spine, intubation is extremely difficult, sometimes requiring preoperative tracheostomy before an anesthetic agent can be delivered. Ossification in the spinal ligaments can produce great difficulty in carrying out spinal anesthesia. In addition, atlantoaxial dislocation has been reported as a presenting finding in this disease[33]; it is, therefore, essential that the anesthesiologist carefully assess the patient when choosing the appropriate type and route of anesthetic and in anticipating difficulties.[34]

After total hip replacement, the patient with AS may not achieve the same range of motion that patients with RA or OA achieve.[35] This is due not only to the increased involvement of the periarticular soft tissues seen in this disease but also to an increased frequency of heterotopic ossification in the muscles and capsule surrounding the hip joint. Although the range of motion achieved may be only 65 degrees of hip flexion, this often makes a significant improvement in the patient's function and independence. If warned of this preoperatively, the patient can make a more informed decision regarding the desirability of surgery and is less likely to experience disappointment with the outcome.

Patients with gout, either as the primary diagnosis or as a secondary diagnosis, often experience painful postoperative flares that require skillful management, because these attacks of gouty arthritis are more difficult to treat than the usual spontaneous gouty attack (see Chapter 87).

In patients with psoriatic arthritis, the skin may be affected in the area of the proposed surgical incision (see Chapter 72). Several papers have reported the frequent contamination of psoriatic skin with microorganisms and have suggested an increased risk of infection after incision through such skin.[36] It is desirable to clear up the skin in the operative site by appropriate local therapy before surgery. The arthropathies related to inflammatory bowel disease (IBD) pose a special threat of postoperative infection because of both late hematogenous seeding from a focus of infection in the bowel and the occasional source of contamination from a colostomy in proximity to the incision for hip replacement.

Patients with systemic lupus erythematosus (SLE) (see Section X) may develop osteonecrosis (see Chapter 114) of hips or knees; this presents a very difficult problem for both the patient and the physician. The patients are often young and receiving large doses of glucocorticoids, and they may have a near normal life expectancy when osteonecrosis develops. Implanting a prosthetic joint in a young patient invites long-term failures related to wear and loosening; doing so in a patient receiving long-term glucocorticoid treatment adds the further risk of infection. The presence of renal involvement in these patients may affect their life expectancy. In the young patient with a limited life expectancy, prosthetic replacement may well be justified to relieve pain and improve the quality of life for the remaining years; in the patient with a normal life expectancy, however, there will almost certainly be problems in the third and fourth decades after joint replacement. These patients often present with avascular necrosis of a femoral condyle with pain, deformity, and functional loss. It may be better to accept the lesser result produced by a tibial osteotomy than to carry out joint

replacement surgery with the high probability of eventual complication.

In patients with Reiter's syndrome (see Chapter 71), as well as in those with AS (see Chapter 70), the rate of occurrence of cardiac involvement is significant. Careful preoperative cardiac assessment should be carried out in such patients.

In addition to the systemic problems presented by patients with RA, the involvement of multiple joints presents special problems. Because the patient will require crutches after lower-extremity surgery, it is essential preoperatively to evaluate the patient's ability to use crutches. If there is extensive involvement of the shoulder, elbow, or wrist, axillary crutches may not be appropriate. Forearm crutches are sometimes a suitable alternative, particularly if involvement of the wrist or elbow makes the use of axillary crutches painful (see Chapter 55).

Occasionally, it will be necessary to complete arthrodesis or arthroplasty of the wrist before surgery on the lower extremities so the patient will be able to use forearm crutches in the postoperative period. Patients who do not have 110 degrees of knee flexion find it difficult to rise from a seated position without assistance from the upper extremities.[37] If the upper extremities are unable to cope with these forces, special attention must be directed to obtaining maximal hip and knee flexion after surgery to minimize the need for upper-extremity assistance. The major joints of the upper extremity—the elbow and shoulder—require arthroplasty less often than the weight-bearing joints of the lower extremity. Indeed, relieving the patient of the need to use crutches by performing arthroplasties of the hips and knees often diminishes shoulder pain to a tolerable level. In some patients, shoulder pain and lack of motion produce difficulty in placing the hand in a functional position, and surgical treatment may be indicated. In the elbow, synovectomy (with or without radial head excision) may be adequate. If pain relief is not adequate after synovectomy, or if motion is inadequate, elbow replacement may be appropriate[38,39] The shoulder achieves great compensatory motion by virtue of the mobile scapula. Unremitting pain, however, may suggest shoulder arthroplasty.[40]

Patients with RA usually have early involvement of the hips.[41] In children, hip involvement is often painless but produces functional disability because of loss of motion. In such situations, soft tissue releases may be worthwhile to restore an adequate range of motion of the hip and avoid or delay the consequences of hip flexion deformity.[42] In the adult, although only one hip may be symptomatic on initial presentation, involvement of both is usually inevitable. Involvement of the contralateral hip will handicap the patient's postoperative recovery and may diminish the ultimate range of motion achieved in the operated hip. If it is obvious that both hips will require arthroplasty, it is preferable to carry out both procedures during the same hospitalization to facilitate functional recovery. Except under unusual circumstances, such as extremely difficult and hazardous intubation, it is not routine in most institutions to perform bilateral total hip replacements during the same period of anesthesia, although several studies report no decrease in quality of outcome or increase in complications with simultaneous procedures. Simultaneous bilateral knee replacements are common.[43]

Patients undergoing hip or knee arthroplasty are sometimes disappointed to find that painful foot deformities prevent comfortable ambulation after extensive surgical procedures. In addition, the plantar surface of the feet and dorsum of the toes are subject to skin breakdown because of rheumatoid deformities. These may become sources of bacterial contamination after arthroplasty to more proximal joints. These areas of skin breakdown should be healed before surgery on proximal joints to prevent proximal spread of infection. This can often be achieved by satisfactory shoe modifications and protective footwear, but surgical correction may be necessary.[44-46] Such surgery should be carried out before hip and knee arthroplasty so that problems of skin breakdown and infection, frequent after foot surgery, will not compromise the results of arthroplasties of the proximal joint. The temporomandibular joint is frequently involved in patients with J sRA as well as adult RA. In the juvenile, involvement of the temporomandibular joint combined with micrognathia may produce difficulties with intubation and respiration after extubation.[31] Careful preoperative analysis by the anesthesiologist can prevent some of these difficulties, and fiberoptic intubation will minimize trauma and postoperative laryngeal edema (Table 115–2). The cervical spine is significantly involved in 30 to 40 percent of patients with RA.[47,48] Usually, this involvement is asymptomatic and unknown by the patient, but it should be sought in the preoperative evaluation to avoid the potentially disastrous consequences of excessive manipulation of the neck during intubation. Whether or not every patient with RA about to undergo anesthesia should have preoperative radiographs is debated, but the frequency of unsuspected instability suggests that the clinician should maintain a low threshold for such studies.[49] The patient with marked C1-C2 instability may sustain damage to the medullary respiratory center and long spinal tracts when the neck is manipulated during intubation. When spinal anesthesia is being administered, the patient is often asked to

"curl up" to facilitate insertion of the spinal needle. Flexion of the cervical spine in the presence of C1-C2 instability should be avoided during this maneuver. Recently, fiber optic intubation has been shown to be useful in preventing postoperative airway obstruction in patients undergoing cervical spine fusion for RA.[17]

In addition to these general considerations, specific interactions between adjacent joints may jeopardize the technical aspects of surgery. For example, involvement of the ipsilateral hip and knee usually leads to the performance of hip arthroplasty first. The position of the flexed knee is used as a guide for insertion of the femoral component in the hip arthroplasty. In the presence of severe knee instability, valgus deformity, or both, proper placement of the hip component will be compromised.[50] If the component is placed in retroversion, postoperative dislocation of the hip becomes more common. Similarly, if the hip has been arthrodesed, the position of knee components must be suitably altered depending on the degree of abduction or adduction of the hip.

Postoperative Management

The role of physical therapy in the postoperative management of patients undergoing joint replacement surgery has not been clearly defined (see Chapter 55). Controlled prospective studies are notably lacking. In their place is the nearly universal acceptance of the importance of postoperative physical therapy, which in my case is an acceptance based on personal experience. The requirements for such therapy appear to vary from joint to joint. For example, Charnley did not advocate postoperative physical therapy for patients undergoing hip replacements.[14] His early and late follow-up studies suggest that physical therapy may play a minimal role in the rehabilitation of these patients. At the other extreme is the clear advantage of careful and prolonged therapy after surgery of the hand. Regardless of the lack of scientific evidence, essentially all surgeons with experience in the field of joint replacement surgery are convinced that the active participation of both the patient and the physical therapist in a postoperative exercise program will improve muscle strength, increase motion,

TABLE 115–2 · AIRWAY PROBLEMS RELEVANT TO ANESTHESIA

Anatomic/Technical Problem	Rheumatoid Arthritis	Juvenile Rheumatoid Arthritis	Ankylosing Spondylitis	Scleroderma	Systemic Lupus Erythematosus
Narrow nares		✓		✓	
Limited jaw opening	✓	✓	✓	✓	
		Temporomandibular joint		Tense skin	
Overbite		✓			
Flexed or fused neck	✓	✓	✓	Tense skin	
Rotational deformity of neck	✓				
Laryngeal pathology	✓	✓		✓	✓
Difficult intubation	✓	✓	✓	✓	
Tendency for acute airway obstruction following extubation	✓	✓	✓	✓	✓

and educate the patient in the proper protection of operated and unoperated joints.

Radiographic evaluation, critical in the preoperative assessment of the need for surgery and proper technical approach, is the mainstay of postoperative evaluation (see Chapter 51). Parameters to be assessed are the alignment of the prosthetic components, adequacy of cement fixation, restoration of joint alignment, and detection of postoperative loosening, as indicated by the development of a radiolucent zone between the implant and the bone. Studies of prosthetic placement in the hip have indicated the undesirability of a varus configuration to the femoral component, as well as increased frequency of loosening in patients with incomplete filling of the proximal femur with methacrylate, voids in the methacrylate, and increased rates of dislocation with retroverted femoral components or excessively abducted acetabular components. In the knee, late loosening has been correlated with faulty alignment of the prosthetic components, and the early development of a radiolucent line, particularly at the bone-cement interface on the tibial side, has given early warning that certain prosthetic designs are inappropriate.

Because loosening is a time-related complication, and infection may make its appearance late, prolonged follow-up of patients undergoing joint arthroplasty is necessary. If early signs of loosening develop, a decrease in joint loading by appropriate use of crutches and avoidance of strenuous activities may prevent or slow the progress of such loosening. Because of evidence that patients with artificial joints continue to be at some increased risk for hematogenous infection, careful attention must be devoted to the prevention of infection anywhere in the body and its prompt recognition and treatment if it does occur. I recommend that patients utilize prophylactic antibiotics before dental or urologic procedures and that they be aware of the potential danger of untreated infections and seek early medical attention. However, there are those who disagree.[51,52]

▮ Conclusion

Despite the dramatic advances in joint replacement surgery since the 1980's, all such procedures must still be considered evolving. Changes in design, surgical technique, and materials continue, with improvements coming rapidly for some joints and more slowly for other joints, such as the ankle and wrist. For this reason, such surgery should be delayed as long as possible in patients who continue to function at a satisfactory level with tolerable discomfort. There is mounting evidence that if surgery is delayed to the point that severe functional deterioration occurs, the ultimate outcome for patients is compromised and they will never reach the level of function they would have had surgery been carried out earlier.[53,54]

The old, reliable procedures such as fusion and osteotomy should be used when appropriate, especially in younger patients. One clear lesson gained from experience with joint replacements is that the more anatomic the replacement, the greater its long-term success is likely to be. It is also clear that there is a close and obvious relationship between the technical expertise with which an arthroplasty is performed and its immediate and ultimate functional result.

New materials for prosthetic replacement and for the fixation of prosthetic devices to bone will certainly be developed. Whether it is better to fix implants with bone cement or rely on biologic fixation has yet to be determined by long-term studies, although in the intermediate term, cement appears to be most effective.[55] Clearer understanding of normal joint anatomy and function will result in improved anatomic designs with greater life expectancy. Functional analysis of large numbers of patients who have undergone arthroplasty will determine the appropriate indications for surgery and choice of prosthetic designs, but medical judgment in selecting patients for surgery, along with precise surgical technique in carrying out the operation, will remain the dominant aspects in the surgical management of arthritis. Increased awareness of the negative effect of prolonged delay in obtaining surgical treatment places new responsibility on the health care team to carefully monitor patient function and complete surgical treatment in a timely manner.

REFERENCES

1. Burton K, Wright V, Richards J: Patients' expectations in relation to outcome of total hip replacement surgery. Ann Rheum Dis 38:471, 1979.
2. Kirwan J, Currey H, Freeman M, et al: Overall longterm impact of total hip and knee joint replacement surgery on patients with osteoarthritis and rheumatoid arthritis. Br J Rheumatol 33:357, 1994.
3. Tulp N, Winia W: Synovectomy of the elbow in rheumatoid arthritis: Longterm results. J Bone Joint Surg Br 71:664, 1989.
4. Jensen C, Poulsen S, Ostergren M, Hansen K: Early and late synovectomy of the knee in rheumatoid arthritis. Scand J Rheumatol 20:127, 1991.
5. Wheen D, Tonkin M, Green J, et al: Longterm results following digital flexor tenosynovectomy in rheumatoid arthritis. J Hand Surg Am 20:790, 1995.
6. Doets H, Bierman B, von Soesbergen R: Synovectomy of the rheumatoid knee does not prevent deterioration: 7 year followup of 83 cases. Acta Orthop Scand 60:523, 1989.
7. Liang M, Cullen K, Larson M, et al: Cost effectiveness of total joint arthroplasty in osteoarthritis. Arthritis Rheum 29:937. 1975
8. Walker D, Usher K, O'Morchoe M, et al: Outcome from multiple joint replacement surgery to the lower limbs. Br J Rheumatol 28:139, 1989.
9. Wolfe F, Zwillich S: The long-term outcomes of rheumatoid arthritis: a 23-year prospective, longitudinal study of total joint replacement and its predictors in 1,600 patients with rheumatoid arthritis. Arthritis Rheum 41:1072, 1998.
10. Corbett M, Dalton S, Young A, et al: Factors predicting death, survival and functional outcome in a prospective. Br J Rheumatol 32:717, 1993.
11. Shields RK, Enloe LJ, Leo KC: Health related quality of life in patients with total hip or knee replacement. Arch Phys Med Rehabil 80:572-579, 1999.
12. March L, Cross M, Tribe K, et al: Cost of joint replacement surgery for osteoarthritis: the patients' perspective. J Rheumatol 29:1006-1014, 2002.
13. Katz J, Phillips C, Poss R, et al: The validity and reliability of a total hip arthroplasty outcome evaluation questionnaire. J Bone Joint Surg Am 77:1528, 1995.
14. Charnley J: Low Friction Arthroplasty of the Hip: Theory and Practice. Berlin, Springer-Verlag, 1979.

15. Kageyama Y, Miyamoto S, Ozeki T, et al: Outcomes for patients undergoing one or more total hip and knee arthroplasties. Clin Rheumatol 17:130, 1998.
16. Skues M, Welchew E: Anaesthesia and rheumatoid arthritis. Anaesthesia 48:989, 1993.
17. Wattenmaker I, Concepcion M, Hibberd P, Lipson S: Upper airway obstruction and perioperative management of the airway in patients managed with posterior operations on the cervical spine for rheumatoid arthritis. J Bone Joint Surg Am 76:360, 1994.
18. Wilson M, Kelley K, Thornhill T: Infection as a complication of total knee replacement arthroplasty: Risk factors and treatment in sixty seven cases. J Bone Joint Surg Am 72:878, 1990.
19. Weinblatt M: Antirheumatic drug therapy and the surgical patient. In Sledge C, Ruddy S, Harris EJ, Kelley W (eds): Arthritis Surgery. Philadelphia, WB Saunders, 1994, p 669.
20. Escalante A, Beardmore TD: Risk factors for early wound complications after orthopedic surgery for rheumatoid arthritis. J Rheumatol 22:1844-1851, 1995.
21. Perhala R, Wilke W, Clough J, et al: Local infectious complications following large joint replacement in rheumatoid arthritis patients treated with methotrexate versus those not treated with methotrexate. Arthritis Rheum 34:146, 1991.
22. Sany J, Anaya J, Canovas F, et al: Influence of methotrexate on the frequency of postoperative infectious complications in patients with rheumatoid arthritis. J Rheumatol 20:1129, 1993.
23. Grennan DM, Gray J, Loudon J, Fear S: Methotrexate and early postoperative complications in patients with rheumatoid arthritis undergoing elective orthopaedic surgery. Ann Rheum Dis 60: 214-217, 2001.
24. Schorn D, Mowat A: Penicillamine in rheumatoid arthritis: Wound healing, skin thickness and osteoporosis. Rheumatol Rehabil 16:223, 1977.
25. Garner R, Mowat A, Hazelman B: Wound healing after operations on patients with rheumatoid arthritis. J Bone Joint Surg Br 55:134, 1973.
26. Bertolini D, Nedwin G, Bringham T, et al: Stimulation of bone resorption and inhibition of bone formation in vitro by human tumour necrosis factor. Nature 319:516, 1986.
27. Mercuriali F, Gualtieri G, Sinigaglia L, et al: Use of recombinant human erythropoietin to assist autologous blood donation by anemic rheumatoid arthritis patients undergoing major orthopedic surgery. Transfusion 34:501, 1994.
28. Saikawa I, Hotokebuchi T, Arita C, et al: Autologous blood transfusion with recombinant erythropoietin treatment: 22 arthroplasties for rheumatoid arthritis. Acta Orthop Scand 65:15, 1994.
29. Maric Z, Haynes D: Total hip arthroplasty in juvenile rheumatoid arthritis. Clin Orthop 290:197, 1993.
30. Sugahara T, Mori Y, Kawamoto T, et al: Obstructive sleep apnea associated with temporomandibular joint destruction by rheumatoid arthritis: Report of case. J Oral Maxillofac Surg 52:876, 1994.
31. Pedersen T, Gronhoj J, Melsen B, et al: Condylar condition and mandibular growth during early functional treatment of children with juvenile chronic arthritis. Eur J Orthod 17:385, 1995.
32. Lakatos J, Csakanyi L: Comparison of complications of total hip arthroplasty in rheumatoid arthritis, ankylosing spondylitis and osteoarthritis. Orthopedics 14:55, 1991.
33. Kremer P, Despaux J, Benmansour A, et al: Spontaneous fracture of the odontoid process in a patient with ankylosing spondylitis:

34. Winkler M, Marker E, Hetz H: The peri-operative management of major orthopaedic procedures. Anaesthesia 2:37, 1998.
35. Walker L, Sledge C: Total hip arthroplasty in ankylosing spondylitis. Clin Orthop 262:198, 1991.
36. Lambert J, Wright V: Surgery in patients with psoriasis and arthritis. Rheumatol Rehab 18:35, 1979.
37. Jergesen H, Poss R, Sledge C: Bilateral total hip and knee replacement in adults with rheumatoid arthritis: An evaluation of function. Clin Orthop 137:120, 1978.
38. Morrey B, Adams R: Semiconstrained arthroplasty for the treatment of rheumatoid arthritis of the elbow. J Bone Joint Surg Am 74:479, 1992.
39. Ewald F, Simmons E, Sullivan J, et al: Capitellocondylar total elbow replacement in rheumatoid arthritis: Longterm results. J Bone Joint Surg Am 75:498, 1993.
40. Friedman R, Thornhill T, Thomas W, et al: Nonconstrained total shoulder replacement in patients who have rheumatoid arthritis and class IV function. J Bone Joint Surg Am 71:494, 1989.
41. Eberhardt K, Fex E, Johnsson K, et al: Hip involvement in early rheumatoid arthritis. Ann Rheum Dis 54:45, 1995.
42. Witt J, McCullough C: Anterior soft tissue release of the hip in juvenile chronic arthritis. J Bone Joint Surg Br 76:267, 1994.
43. Stanley D, Stockley I, Getty C: Simultaneous or staged bilateral total knee replacements in rheumatoid arthritis: A prospective study. J Bone Joint Surg Br 72:772, 1990.
44. Mann R, Schakel MN: Surgical correction of rheumatoid forefoot deformities. Foot Ankle Int 16:1, 1995.
45. Donatto K: Ankle arthrodesis in patients with rheumatoid arthritis. Clin Orthop 349:81-92, 1998.
46. Haber D, Goodman S: Arthritis and arthrodesis of the hindfoot. J Arthroplasty 13:259, 1998.
47. Boden S, Dodge L, Bohlman H, et al: Rheumatoid arthritis of the cervical spine: A longterm analysis with predictors of paralysis and recovery. J Bone Joint Surg Am 75:1282, 1993.
48. Clark C: Rheumatoid involvement of the cervical spine: An overview. Spine 19:2257, 1994.
49. Campbell R, Wou P, Watt I: A continuing role for preoperative cervical spine radiography. Clin Radiol 50:157, 1995.
50. Harris W, Sledge C: Total hip and total knee replacement. N Engl J Med 323:725, 1990.
51. Tsevat J, Durand Z, Pauker S: Cost effectiveness of antibiotic prophylaxis for dental procedures in patients with artificial joints. Am J Public Health 79:739, 1989.
52. Wahl M: Myths of dental-induced prosthetic joint infections. Clin Infect Dis 20:1420, 1995.
53. Fortin PR, Clarke AE, Joseph L, et al: Outcomes of total hip and knee replacement: preoperative functional status predicts outcomes at six months after surgery. Arthritis Rheum 42:1722-1728, 1999.
54. Hajat S, Fitzpatrick R, Morris R, et al: Does waiting for total hip replacement matter? Prospective cohort study. J Health Serv Res Policy 7:19-25, 2002.
55. Mehlhoff M, Sledge C: Comparison of cemented and cementless hip and knee replacements. Arthritis Rheum 33:293, 1990.

Nonunion responsible for compression of the upper cervical cord. Rev Rhum Engl 62:455, 1995.

116

Principles of Reconstructive Surgery for Arthritis

CLEMENT B. SLEDGE

THE HAND AND WRIST

The hand has significant functional and psychologic importance; it is our extension to the environment, the means of livelihood for most, and a means of survival and hygiene for all. As important as those functions are, the hand is also a major part of our self image. It is not unusual to see a patient with rheumatoid arthritis (RA) sitting in a doctor's waiting room performing fine hand-work, such as knitting, while she waits to see the doctor about her "hand problem." Function has been maintained, but the appearance of the hand and its importance in self-image have led the patient to seek improvement. Because the hand and wrist are commonly affected in many rheumatologic conditions, all caregivers should have some understanding of the various types of involvement and their natural history.

As in other aspects of arthritis care, a multidisciplinary team approach involving the rheumatologist, hand surgeon, hand therapist, and others is crucial for adequately attending to the many needs of these patients. Many pathologic processes can be significantly improved or even prevented when dealt with early, whereas prolonged attempts at avoiding surgery may lead to further disease progression, greater joint and tendon destruction, and deterioration of function. The inherent anatomic complexities of the hand and wrist can make not only treatment but also initial evaluation of a patient's problem challenging. However, with a clear understanding of anatomy and a systematic approach to evaluating the patient, a rational plan of treatment can be generated.

■ Patient Evaluation

As with any anatomic system, a thorough history and physical examination are paramount. The most important questions regarding hand function are targeted toward both symptoms and function.

Physical examination of a severely deformed hand and wrist can at times be overwhelming, and, thus, it is important to develop a systematic framework for looking at specific joints, tendons, and their functions. First, the wrist should be evaluated for localized areas of tenderness, as well as for swelling indicative of synovitis. Range of motion compared over time is important when looking for disease progression. Next, the thumb should be eval-

uated; the carpometacarpal (CMC) joint, metacarpophalangeal (MCP) joint, and interphalangeal (IP) joint should be evaluated separately for deformity and for active and passive range of motion. The MCP joints, proximal interphalangeal (PIP), and distal interphalangeal (DIP) joints of the index through the small finger then should be evaluated for swelling, deformity, and range of motion. Function of the various wrist and digit flexors and extensors should be evaluated for function. Finally, sensation and strength should be assessed and recorded.[1]

The conditions discussed in the following sections commonly have hand or wrist involvement, or both. Because of the progressive nature of many of these diseases, it is helpful to consider treatment options in different categories: nonsurgical treatment, prophylactic surgery, and reconstructive or salvage surgery.

■ Rheumatoid Arthritis

Swelling on the dorsum of the hand, secondary to synovitis of the extensor tendons, is often the presenting complaint in patients with RA. Eventually, most patients with RA will experience problems in the hand and wrist that may benefit from medical and surgical interventions.

NONSURGICAL TREATMENT

Rest, exercise, splinting, and injections play a critical role not only initially but also during all stages of the disease.

Rest and Exercise

The patient with RA should understand the principles of rest and exercise and their practical application. In no other area is patient education more important. Patients use their hands hundreds of times a day for eating, turning doorknobs, opening jars, and so on. They must learn to regulate their activities to minimize symptoms and progression of deformity. There are many useful adaptive devices available, such as modified doorknobs and jar openers, and an occupational therapist or hand therapist can be very helpful in guiding the patient to these environmental modifications.

Diseased joints require exercise to prevent stiffness and maintain motion; active motion is needed to maintain tendon gliding and muscle strength. Conversely, inflamed, painful, swollen joints require rest to lessen acute synovitis. Therefore, when a joint is warm, painful, and inflamed, exercise must be reduced and rest increased. As the inflammatory process subsides, exercise can be resumed. Short, frequent periods of exercise are more beneficial than long, vigorous ones, which can aggravate the synovial inflammation. A hand therapist is invaluable in working with patients and teaching them how much exercise and activity they can carry out. Patients must learn to monitor their own activity. If, after a particular activity, hands become swollen, painful, or stiff, the activity has been too strenuous and it should be modified.

Splinting

Splints alleviate pain, may decrease the progression of deformity during the active stages of the disease, and aid in postoperative management. Resting splints are especially effective for wrist pain and allow patients to use their hand while wearing the splint. Full hand-wrist-thumb splints also alleviate pain but restrict function and are often used mainly at night. Various types of dynamic splints are used to stretch out fixed deformities. Dynamic splinting is used mainly after reconstructive surgery, especially after MCP joint arthroplasty.[2]

Corticosteroid Injections

The judicious use of local injections of corticosteroids often lessens active synovitis and tenosynovitis. Corticosteroids can be used for symptomatic carpal tunnel syndrome, flexor and dorsal tenosynovitis, and any painful joint that does not respond to medical treatment. Because of the concern that frequent, repeated administration to the same area may cause tendon ruptures and corticosteroid-induced arthropathies, the clinician should probably not inject one joint or one tendon sheath more than two or three times a year.[1] If the local disease persists or increases after this time, surgical intervention is indicated.

PREVENTIVE OR PROPHYLACTIC SURGERY

Tenosynovitis

Tenosynovitis is a frequent manifestation of rheumatoid hand disease and results from a proliferation of the tenosynovium that surrounds the extensor or flexor tendons of the wrist and hand.

Dorsal tenosynovitis may be the presenting sign in RA, and RA is the primary diagnosis to rule out when dorsal tenosynovitis is present. It produces a soft, initially nonpainful mass, which may be located along any or all of the extensor compartments; accompanying pain should alert the clinician to underlying radiocarpal or radioulnar involvement.

It is important to identify dorsal tenosynovitis early, as it may lead to extensor tendon ruptures, either from attrition or from infiltrative disease. The surgical repair of such ruptures is less than perfect and involves a significant postoperative rehabilitation. Although the clinician cannot predict which patients will experience ruptured tendons, there are certain helpful guidelines for predicting which patients are at risk: dorsal dislocation of the distal ulna, radiographic evidence of wrist involvement with irregular bony surfaces under the tendons, distal radioulnar involvement with erosion of the radius, a previous tendon rupture, and patients in whom the tenosynovitis has persisted for 6 months or longer.[3,4]

Tenosynovectomy is recommended for patients with persistent tenosynovitis who have not responded to a 4- to 6-month period of conservative therapy. Earlier tenosynovectomy is indicated for patients who are at risk for tendon ruptures.[2]

Of all surgical procedures on the rheumatoid hand and wrist, tenosynovectomy is one of the most rewarding. The surgical technique is safe and effective, and the morbidity is low. The procedure can be done on an outpatient basis with regional anesthesia. Postoperative immobilization is short and patients generally have little problem regaining their range of motion. Recurrence after dorsal tenosynovectomy is low (5 to 6%),[4] and future extensor tendon rupture is effectively prevented.

Extensor Tendon Rupture

If dorsal tenosynovitis is ignored or inadequately controlled medically, extensor tendons may rupture. The most frequent tendons to rupture are the extensors to the small and ring fingers (Fig. 116–1) and the extensor pollicis longus.[4] In severe destructive disease, multiple digital extensor tendons may rupture. Even the wrist extensor tendons can rupture, with resultant severe flexion deformity of the wrist. Diagnosis and early surgical treatment are important to repair the tendons or perform tendon transfers, and a tenosynovectomy may prevent further tendon rupture.

Single extensor tendon ruptures may be difficult to diagnose given the cross-connections between the tendons of the extensor digitorum communis. As the disease progresses and more tendons rupture, however, diagnosis becomes easier. Generally, the patient experiences a loss of active MCP extension and loses the tenodesis effect when flexing and extending the wrist. It is important, however, to know that other conditions may mimic extensor tendon rupture: 1) ulnarly subluxated tendons with extensor hood attenuations secondary to MCP synovitis; 2) posterior interosseous nerve palsy, usually secondary to elbow synovitis; and 3) MCP joint destruction and contracture, not allowing relocation of the joints and extension of the fingers.

Because the results of tendon transfer are inversely proportional to the number of tendon ruptures, prompt diagnosis and early treatment are important. In addition, the morbidity and the results are directly proportional to the number of tendons ruptured plus the status of the adjacent joints. Because much of the hand must be immobilized for 4 weeks after surgery to allow for tendon healing, joint stiffness may develop, and, therefore, rehabilitation requires more time. Because of this, both patient and physician should be alerted to the complications of

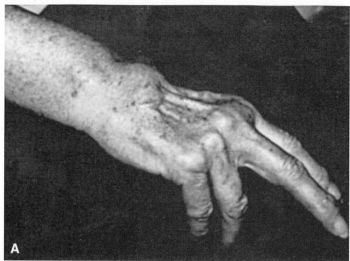

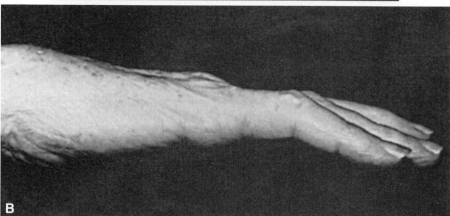

FIGURE 116-1 • Patient with Dorsal Tenosynovitis and Double Tendon Rupture.

dorsal tenosynovitis so that early tenosynovectomy can be carried out before tendon rupture occurs.

Flexor Tenosynovitis

Flexor tenosynovitis is a result of a proliferation of the tenosynovium that lines the flexor tendons. The signs and symptoms of flexor tenosynovitis differ with the anatomic location: wrist, palmar, or digital flexor tenosynovitis. As with dorsal tenosynovitis, early diagnosis and prompt treatment of flexor tenosynovitis prevent the complications of tendon rupture or permanent damage from prolonged median nerve compression.

Wrist Flexor Tenosynovitis

Wrist flexor tenosynovitis may present with signs and symptoms of carpal tunnel syndrome, because the swelling within the carpal tunnel causes compression of the median nerve. Some patients may have limited active digital flexion owing to impairment of flexor tendon excursion. On physical examination, unless there is limited active range of motion, the signs will be minimal. Because the wrist flexor tendons are covered by thick fascia, flexor tenosynovitis does not produce noticeable swelling, in contrast to dorsal tenosynovitis. If the volar surface of the wrist is observed carefully, loss of skin wrinkles and lack of venous markings can sometimes be observed. Additionally, evidence of thenar muscle atrophy can sometimes be noted, especially with long-standing median nerve compression.

The treatment for early wrist flexor tenosynovitis is steroid injection, wrist splinting, and medical management. For persistent wrist flexor tenosynovitis or prolonged median nerve symptoms, carpal tunnel release and tenosynovectomy should be carried out early to prevent permanent median nerve damage, restore active digit flexion, and prevent tendon rupture; this can be done either by open surgery or arthroscopically.[5]

Palmar Stenosing Tenosynovitis

Palmar stenosing tenosynovitis (trigger finger) occurs when proliferating tenosynovium within the proximal portion of the palm results in snapping and locking as the tendon slides within the tendon sheath. Patients can usually flex the digit fully, but as the digit extends, the nodule catches on the proximal edge of the tendon sheath and the digit snaps into extension. Sometimes the digit becomes acutely locked in flexion and cannot be extended actively. A painful snap occurs as the digit is passively extended. On examination, the flexor tendon nodule can often be palpated and the clinician can feel crepitation as the patient actively flexes and extends the digit.

The initial treatment is steroid injection into the flexor sheath. If the patient does not improve after two injections, flexor tenosynovectomy with or without release of the tendon sheath should be performed.

Digital Flexor Tenosynovitis

In contrast to stenosing tenosynovitis, digital flexor tenosynovitis is due to proliferation of tenosynovium within the digit. The most common finding in this condition is loss of active digital flexion with preserved passive digital flexion. This is a result of impairment of tendon excursion within the narrow tendon sheath. Additionally, crepitation and locking can be seen as the tendon nodule slides within the sheath, and a fullness can sometimes be felt and observed on the volar surface of the digit.[6]

A less common but important manifestation of digital flexor tenosynovitis is stiffness of the PIP joints. This occurs because the patient is unable to flex the digits actively, and this, plus the associated PIP joint synovitis and pain, leads to joint stiffness. The initial treatment is flexor sheath injection and, if there is no response, digital flexor tenosynovectomy.[6] If the patient has associated PIP stiffness, joint manipulation or release followed by vigorous postoperative hand therapy can restore considerable range of motion.

Flexor Tendon Rupture

Flexor tendon rupture can occur within the carpal tunnel, palm, or digit. Fortunately it is not common, as the results of treatment for multiple palmar and digital flexor tendon ruptures are not as good as those for their extensor counterparts.

At the wrist, attritional ruptures of the flexor pollicis longus or the flexors of the index finger are caused by a bony spur of the scaphoid that protrudes volarly. Additionally, flexor tendon rupture within the carpal tunnel can occur from infiltrative flexor tenosynovitis.

Within the palm and digit, flexor tendon ruptures are less common because there are no bony spurs that lead to attritional ruptures, and the symptoms of locking and snapping cause the patient to seek earlier medical attention, which usually results in earlier diagnosis and treatment.

Flexor tendon rupture in the wrist is treated with tenosynovectomy, removal of the scaphoid spur, and either tendon repair (if recognized early) or grafting or tendon transfer. If the thumb IP joint is destroyed, arthrodesis is usually recommended. If a single rupture is diagnosed within the digit or palm, prompt flexor tenosynovectomy is advisable to prevent a rupture of the remaining intact tendons. If a flexor digitorum profundus rupture occurs, either tenodesis to an adjacent tendon or arthrodesis of the DIP joint is indicated. For flexor digitorum superficialis rupture, only tenosynovectomy is indicated to protect the intact flexor digitorum profundus.

Synovectomy

In contrast to tenosynovectomy, which is an established surgical procedure, the case for synovectomy in the small joints of the wrist and hand is less well defined. There are limited data to show that synovectomy will appreciably alter the natural course of the disease, but it may have some definite, although narrow, indications in the hand.

The primary indications for synovectomy of the wrist or digital joint are found in the small group of patients with smoldering, slowly progressive disease who are responding to systemic medication but who continue to show synovitis in one or more joints. Typically, these patients will have responded to three steroid injections over a 6- to 12-month period but continue to have recurrent synovitis, sometimes with pain. Radiographs show minimal involvement with little evidence of progression. Synovectomy can alleviate pain and, ideally, delay or prevent further joint destruction.

Synovectomy can be performed in almost any joint of the hand or wrist. It is occasionally carried out in the wrist to relieve pain, and it may be useful in the PIP joints to prevent progressive boutonnière deformities. Arthroscopic synovectomy of the wrist has shown encouraging results with regard to pain and grip strength, and it avoids most postoperative stiffness.[5] Synovectomy is less frequently indicated in the MCP joints because progression of the usual deformity is frequently not altered by this procedure.

RECONSTRUCTIVE AND SALVAGE SURGERY

In spite of early recognition, splinting, and prophylactic surgery, the natural progression of RA often leads to destructive changes in the joints of the hand and wrist. The late effects include loss of articular cartilage, stretching of the supporting joint structures, and bone loss. The clinical aspects of these changes include pain, instability, and deformity with subsequent loss of function. After these changes have occurred, it is no longer possible to restore the joint to its former state. The surgeon must then resort to either reconstructive or salvage surgery to relieve pain and to provide stability and motion. The surgeon has one of two choices in the management of destroyed joints: arthrodesis or arthroplasty. Each of these procedures has benefits and drawbacks and, therefore, represents a compromise with full function. Choosing between these two operations takes judgment and experience.

Wrist

The wrist is the foundation on which hand function is built. A painful, unstable wrist reduces hand function even without digital involvement and may itself be a primary factor in producing digital deformities. Deformities of the wrist result from several factors. Early synovial involvement between the carpal bones may lead to stretching of the intercarpal and radiocarpal ligaments allowing the carpus to shift ulnarward and volarly in relation to the radius. The carpus can then dislocate volarly or ulnarward, or both, and displace proximally. There may also be dorsal tenosynovitis and extensor tendon ruptures. Chronic synovitis of the distal radioulnar joint stretches the supporting ligaments, allowing dorsal displacement of the ulna. With radial rotation of the carpus, the metacarpals become angulated radially in relationship to the radius, and this, in turn, is followed by ulnar deviation of the digits at the MCP joints. Patients who have this "zigzag" deformity are poor candidates for MCP arthroplasties to correct the ulnar deviation until the wrist alignment has been restored. The rough bony edge of the ulna that protrudes dorsally can wear away the adjacent extensor tendons to the fingers.

Surgical options to realign the wrist and alleviate pain include total or partial fusion and arthroplasty. The choice between these procedures depends on many factors, including the condition of the wrist extensors, the amount of bone resorbed in the carpus, and the status of the hand, the opposite wrist, and even the lower extremities.

Wrist arthrodesis accomplishes several things. It eliminates pain, provides stability for hand function, and corrects alignment.[7] Although the patient gives up flexion and extension motions, forearm supination and pronation are preserved. The position of fusion is important. Although arthrodesis in 15 to 20 degrees of dorsiflexion is preferable in traumatic arthritis, the same is not usually true in patients with RA; neutral or slight flexion may be preferable.[8] With the use of intramedullary fixation technique, there is a high likelihood of successful union, and the period of immobilization is quite limited. The great advantages of a solid wrist fusion are stability and dependability. Disease is arrested at this site and is no longer a source of pain. Progression or recurrence of deformity is halted. If the patient has lower-extremity problems that require a cane or crutch support, the fused wrist provides the necessary support. The benefits of a single fused wrist far outweigh the disadvantages of loss of flexion and extension, and especially in young vigorous patients, this is a reliable solution to the problem of a destroyed wrist joint.

Although wrist fusion has been an accepted treatment for the severely involved wrist, there are many patients in whom the major changes are limited to the radiocarpal joints, whereas the midcarpal area is preserved. In these patients, limited fusion restores the anatomy to a more normal situation and can preserve significant motion.[9] A theoretical benefit of these limited arthrodeses is that by restoring the wrist to a more normal anatomic position, the midcarpal joints are protected. Another option is excision of the proximal row of carpal bones; motion is preserved and pain is relieved. It has been suggested, however, that these limited procedures may not prevent disease progression.[10,11]

Wrist Arthroplasty

Wrist involvement is usually bilateral, and the loss of motion produced by arthrodesis in both wrists can create a functional loss for the patient. In patients whose major difficulty with the wrist is pain, yet significant motion is still present, arthroplasty may be appropriate.[12]

After the success of metal-to-plastic prostheses in other joints, similar devices have been developed for the wrist. These can be inserted with or without methyl methacrylate fixation. Their early use was marked by difficulty in balancing the wrist. Although this problem has been largely overcome, painful loosening has become more

apparent with time. Although long-term studies are not yet available, in properly selected patients, wrist arthroplasty has a definite role.[13] Arthrodesis, however, is still the mainstay of treatment.

Distal Radioulnar Joint

One of the consequences of wrist involvement is progressive prominence of the distal ulna, which disrupts wrist function and jeopardizes the overlying extensor tendons. The standard treatment has been distal ulna resection (Darrach procedure).[14] Although alternative procedures have been proposed to avoid some late problems, such as carpal shift and snapping of the resected ulna against the radius, the standard procedure remains distal ulna resection. If adequate soft tissues are preserved, the remaining ulna, although mobile, does not cause symptoms, and the risk of extensor tendon rupture is minimized.

Thumb

The thumb is frequently involved with RA and can, as a result of muscular imbalance or joint destruction, assume bizarre deformities.[15] The most common deformity seen is the boutonnière deformity (MCP flexion and IP hyperextension). This originates at the MCP joint, which assumes a flexed position secondary to stretching out or loss of the extensor force. As sequela of this, the IP joint assumes a hyperextended position, and the patient tends to adduct the first metacarpal to substitute for the lack of extension. This thumb deformity is made worse with each pinch of the thumb against the other digits. The reverse deformity (swan neck), with MCP hyperextension and IP flexion, is usually secondary to changes at the CMC joint from synovitis. The CMC joint subluxates, and the first metacarpal adducts. The patient then hyperextends the MCP joint to substitute for the lost abduction. With the tendon imbalance produced, the IP joint often assumes a flexed position. Other deformities can occur as a result of collateral ligament or tendon ruptures occurring in combination with joint changes.

As is true with other deformities of the rheumatoid hand, early reconstruction is generally more satisfying than late salvage procedures. The distal joint of the thumb (IP joint) is usually treated by fusion. It is usually fused in the straight or slightly flexed position to restore a stable pinch (Fig. 116–2). At the MCP-joint level, the clinician can choose between fusion or arthroplasty. With isolated MCP joint disease, a fusion in 15 degrees of flexion gives excellent results with little functional loss. With associated IP joint disease, however, an arthroplasty is preferred at the MCP level to avoid fusion of two adjacent joints. The silicone implant gives excellent results with good pain relief, about 25 degrees of motion, and good stability, but long-term follow-up studies demonstrate a high percentage of problems, which have lead some surgeons to abandon the procedure.[16] At the CMC-joint level, it is important to maintain motion. A fusion here could become quite disabling if subsequent instability developed and the patient required fusions distally.

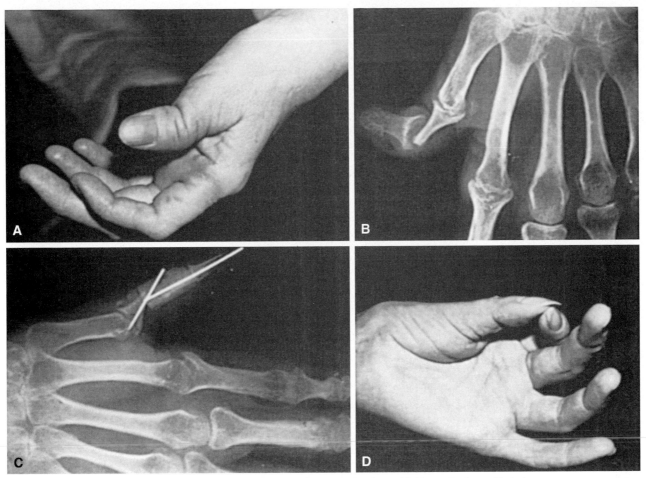

FIGURE 116-2 · Unstable Distal Joint Treated by Fusion with Bone Graft. *A*, Clinical appearance of the thumb with collapse of interphalangeal (IP) joint. *B*, Radiograph shows significant absorption of the distal end of the proximal phalanx. *C*, Postoperative radiograph shows use of bone graft to restore length and facilitate joint fusion. *D*, Note stable "pulp pinch" between lengthened thumb and index finger. Distal joint fused in slight flexion.

Generally, a resection arthroplasty has been preferred over trapezium implant in patients with RA.

Metacarpophalangeal Joints

The MCP joints of the hand allow 80 to 90 degrees of flexion, as well as rotary and lateral motions. They play an important role in positioning the fingers; if they are fixed in poor position, hand function is greatly reduced. Unfortunately, MCP joint involvement is common in RA. The capsular laxity, which gives the joints varied mobility, makes subluxation and dislocation common late sequelae of synovitis. The extensor tendons pass precariously across the joints and, with stretching of the supporting attachments, often deviate ulnarward and then slip between the metacarpal heads. Once this has occurred, all extensor force is lost and progressive flexion of the MCP joints occurs. As the patient tries to extend the joints, they deviate ulnarward instead. Similarly, with flexor tenosynovitis the sheath stretches, allowing a change in alignment of the flexor tendons, which now become a deforming force. There is often a stretching of the radial collateral ligaments and subsequent shortening of the ulnar collateral ligaments and intrinsic muscles. The end result may appear as dislocated MCP joints with the fingers fixed in flexion or severely deviated ulnarward. The result is a significant loss of hand function, such as the ability to grasp large objects. With ulnar deviation, the fingers are beyond the reach of the thumb, and the ability to complete precision activities requiring thumb-digit opposition is lost.

MCP Arthroplasty

Arthroplasty is the treatment of choice to restore function at the MCP level. In the late 1960s and early 1970s, prostheses made of silicone rubber were developed.[2] The prosthesis acts as a flexible implant or spacer between the resected bone ends. Other designs involving metal and plastic, either with or without cement fixation, have not yet proven as reliable as silicone implants. Because the silicone implant has provided the most predictable results, it remains the most widely employed choice for arthroplasty.

Numerous factors affect the ultimate result, including the condition of the surrounding soft tissues, the strength and mobility of the controlling muscles, the status of the adjacent joints, the use of postoperative splinting and exercise, and, certainly, the motivation of the patient. With proper surgical technique, it is possible to realign the digit, relieve pain, and maintain between 30 and 60 degrees of motion, with an average of 45 degrees[17,18] (Fig. 116–3).

Implant fracture can occur, but its frequency is less than 5 percent with the high-performance silicone rubber used today. Within several months following implant insertion, encapsulation has already taken place; if implant fracture does occur, it is often asymptomatic, noted only on radiograph, and may not significantly affect the result.

Infections around the implant occur in less than 1 percent of the joints inserted. Usually an isolated joint is involved and removal of the implant combined with appropriate antibiotic coverage is sufficient to control the infection. Removal of the implant converts the arthroplasty to a resection type, and although some loss of motion is anticipated, function may remain good.

Performing surgery earlier is considerably easier than postponing surgical intervention to the point where the patient has severe deformity, significant bony erosions, severe ulnar drift, and flexion contractures. The Silastic prosthesis (Dow-Corning) is excellent for pain relief and improvement of both appearance and positioning of the fingers, but it does not restore full motion or significantly improve grip or pinch strength. Despite this, patient satisfaction is high.[17]

Proximal Interphalangeal Joints

The PIP joints are hinge joints with motion from full extension to 110 degrees of flexion. This mobility, although only slightly greater than that at the distal joint, is far more important in bringing the fingertip to the palm. Therefore, loss of motion at the PIP level is more of a hardship for the patient, and efforts to preserve it are more frequently indicated (Fig. 116–4). In addition to motion, lateral stability is important, especially in

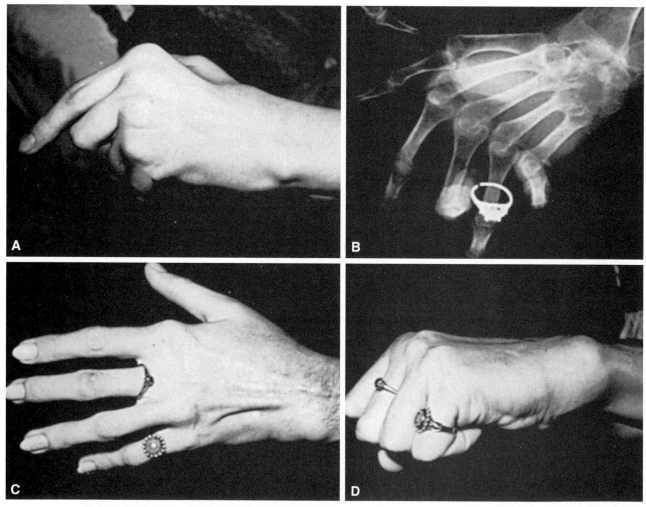

FIGURE 116–3 · Metacarpophalangeal (MCP) Arthroplasty to Improve Joint Function and the Appearance of Rheumatoid Hand Deformity. *A*, Preoperative digital extension. Note MCP joint subluxations with associated boutonnière deformity of middle finger. *B*, Preoperative radiograph shows advanced wrist involvement in addition to MCP and proximal interphalangeal (PIP) joint deformities. *C*, Note improved function and appearance of hand and wrist following second-stage wrist fusion and MCP arthroplasties. *D*, Excellent postoperative digital flexion.

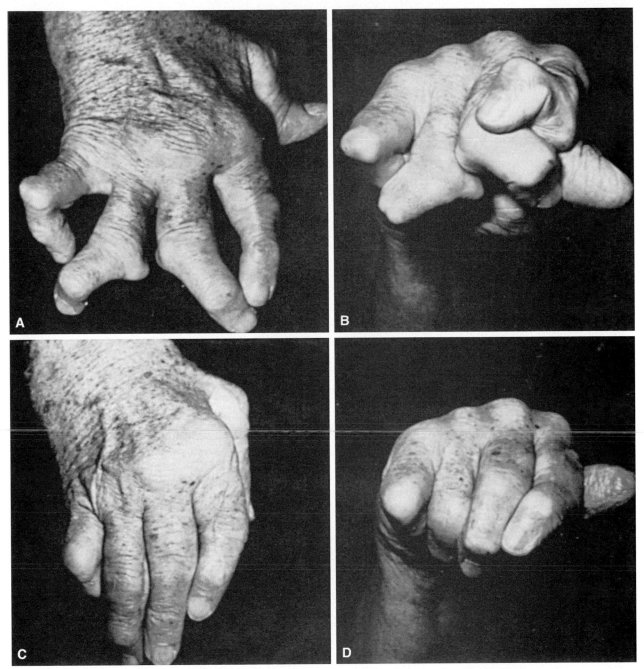

FIGURE 116–4 · Proximal Interphalangeal (PIP) Joint Arthroplasties for Severe Deformities. *A,* Preoperative view of hand with fingers in extension. Note severe lateral deformities of PIP joints. *B,* Patient's fingers overlap on attempted flexion. Grasping ability is poor. *C,* Postoperative extension following PIP arthroplasties. *D,* Postoperative flexion.

activities involving pinch. Unlike the situation of the distal joints, in which fusion is the procedure of choice in salvage conditions, the surgeon has a choice between a fusion or flexible implant arthroplasty at the PIP level. Factors to consider in making this decision include the type or severity of deformity, the digit involved, the condition of adjacent joints, and the status of the extensor and flexor apparatus. Because a stable index finger is needed for pinch, PIP stability is more important than motion and, thus, arthrodesis is often indicated for this joint.

The ability to flex the PIP joints becomes increasingly important from the index finger to the small digit. In the ring and small fingers, acute flexion of the PIP joint is needed to grasp small objects firmly. For this reason, arthroplasty is likely to be chosen over fusion in these digits. If fusion is selected, the position chosen is in more flexion than that chosen for the index finger.

Digital Deformities

Digital deformities are classified as boutonnière or swan neck deformities.[19] Boutonnière deformities are flexion of the PIP joint and hyperextension of the DIP joint (Fig. 116–5). The cause of boutonnière deformities is synovi-

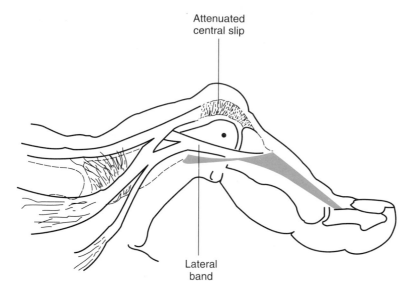

FIGURE 116-5 · Diagram of the Boutonnière Deformity. Stretching of the dorsal capsule and central slip allows the lateral bands to slip toward the palmar surface, producing flexion at the proximal interphalangeal (PIP) joint and hyperextension at the distal interphalangeal (DIP) joint. (From Rizio L, Belsky MR: Finger deformities in rheumatoid arthritis. Hand Clin 12:531, 1996.)

tis with subsequent attenuation of the dorsal capsule of the PIP joint and the overlying central tendon, which allows the lateral bands to slide palmarly with subsequent extension of the DIP joint. Initially, the boutonnière deformity is passively correctable, although full extension can rarely be achieved with the amount of synovitis present. With time, because of changes within the joint and shortening of the capsular structures on the palmar aspect, the deformities become fixed.

Surgical correction of the boutonnière deformity should be carried out only after the MCP joints have been attended to. The procedures can be done in conjunction with one another (e.g., MCP joint arthroplas-

ties with PIP joint fusions). The passively correctable or minimally deformed fingers can be corrected with a soft tissue procedure, consisting of a synovectomy and mobilization of the lateral bands; a terminal tenotomy may be required if there is a fixed deformity at the DIP joint. If the joint is destroyed, a PIP arthroplasty along with soft tissue reconstruction is indicated.

With fixed boutonnière deformities of more than 50 degrees, the patient and surgeon should seriously consider arthrodeses in the appropriate position, depending on the digit (Fig. 116–6).

Swan neck deformities are the result of hyperextension of the PIP joint and subsequent flexion of the DIP

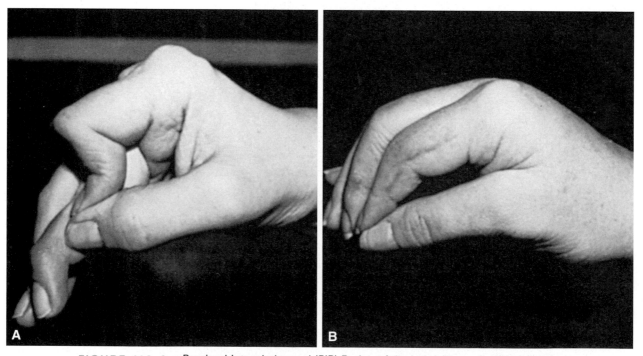

FIGURE 116-6 · Proximal Interphalangeal (PIP) Fusion of the Index Finger for Fixed-flexion Deformity. A, Note poor pinch posture because of severe flexion contracture of the index PIP joint. B, Improved function obtained by fusion of the PIP joint in 25-degree flexion.

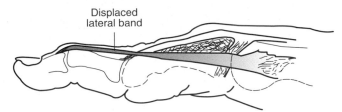

FIGURE 116-7 · Diagram of the Swan Neck Deformity. Lateral bands have displaced dorsal to the axis of the proximal interphalangeal (PIP) joint, where they extend the joint and allow the distal interphalangeal (DIP) joint to flex. (From Rizio L, Belsky MR: Finger deformities in rheumatoid arthritis. Hand Clin 12:531, 1996.)

joint (Fig. 116–7). Again, the cause is synovitis, although this time the structures that are attenuated are more palmar than dorsal. The primary disease is in the PIP joint, with DIP joint changes occurring as a result of the changes proximally. As with boutonnière deformities, all MCP deformities must be corrected before the swan neck deformity is approached surgically. Fixed deformities at the MCP joints are often the cause of swan neck deformities, and if the MCP flexion deformities are not corrected, swan neck deformities will recur in the PIP joint.

The results of either manipulation and fixation or arthroplasty are modest. At best, a range of 30 to 50 degrees of motion can be expected, ideally from a fixed-flexion deformity position of approximately 10 degrees.

In general, the results of arthroplasty at the PIP joint level are better with swan neck deformity than with boutonnière deformity. Although long-term follow-up has not shown a significant increase in range of motion from the preoperative level, pain relief has been good.[20]

Distal Interphalangeal Joints

The DIP joints of the digits normally allow 70 to 80 degrees of flexion. With intact collateral ligaments, the joints are quite stable against lateral stresses. As a result of RA, the cartilaginous joint surfaces can be destroyed, producing pain and limitation of motion. As a result of these changes, an unsightly deformity develops that not only is painful but also results in decreased function.

Unfortunately, it is not possible to restore the damaged DIP joint to its former state, and the goal becomes relief of pain, correction of deformity, and restoration of useful function. Of the two salvage procedures at the DIP, fusion and arthroplasty, fusion is the treatment preferred by most surgeons. Wilgis, however, reports good pain relief and function at 10 years in patients with silastic arthroplasty of the DIP joints.[21]

The best position for arthrodesis of the DIP joint is 0 to 10 degrees of flexion. In this position, the digit has a relatively normal appearance when the fingers are extended, and when the patient makes a fist, the lack of distal joint motion is of little functional significance. Picking up or holding objects between the thumb and the involved digit is not compromised, with the distal joint being almost straight. This position enhances "pulp-to-pulp" pinch, which is more useful than "tip" pinch, which requires distal joint mobility.

Arthritis Mutilans

Some patients have such marked involvement that severe deformity and instability coexist with severe bone loss. Generally, arthrodesis with bone grafting is the only salvage procedure available for these patients.

▌ Juvenile Rheumatoid Arthritis

Nearly all patients with juvenile rheumatoid arthritis (JRA) have some involvement of the hands and wrists.[22] Although many of the deformities are similar to those in RA in adults, there are important differences regarding both treatment and progression. Additionally, although the surgical indications are generally similar to those in adult RA (namely, pain, deformity, and the progressive nature of the disease), timing may be different in children.

SIGNS AND SYMPTOMS

Examination may show a loss of wrist extension with ulnar deviation of the carpus and metacarpals. Loss of flexion and radial deviation of the MCP joints is in contrast to the deformity seen in adults. The fingers become stiff. General radiographic findings in the hand are those of diminished joint space, accelerated epiphyseal maturation, and diminished size of the small tubular bones of the hand. In the carpus, there is premature ossification, and the bones appear crenated. Bony diameter may increase or decrease depending on the degree of periostitis present. Severe periostitis has been associated with more severe eventual deformity. Local synovitis can result in epiphyseal overgrowth, undergrowth, or premature physeal closure around affected joints. Later radiographic findings are those of osteoporosis and bony erosion.

PRINCIPLES OF MANAGEMENT

The goal of treatment is to prevent deformity or to promote return of function in the safest, simplest manner. Maintaining as normal a lifestyle as possible and achieving independence should be foremost. In addition to rest, splinting, and medical management, steroid injections may be useful for persistent involvement of joints and tendon sheaths.

The priorities and goals for surgery in JRA are similar to those in adults, keeping in mind that skeletal immaturity must be considered when planning to either perform, or unduly delay, a surgical procedure.

SYNOVECTOMY

The role of synovectomy is not completely agreed on, but some authors believe that early synovectomy has prophylactic value. The timing is also a dilemma, because it is preferable to perform synovectomy before there is severe destruction and fixed deformity, yet there may be a possibility of spontaneous remission. In general, surgery is considered after 6 months of persistent synovitis despite adequate medical management. Furthermore, synovectomy may be indicated sooner if there is persistent synovitis adjacent to an open physis, because this may cause premature physeal closure. Results show good relief of pain, but range of motion has not significantly improved.

TENOSYNOVECTOMY

In contrast to adult RA, in which extensor rather than flexor tenosynovitis is more common, patients with JRA more often have flexor rather than extensor tenosynovitis. In children, as in adults, the indication for flexor tenosynovectomy is triggering or decreased active flexion. Triggering can be more severe than standard stenosing tenosynovitis, because the digits can become locked in either flexion or extension and persistence may result in contracture. Often the pathologic changes are distal to the A1 pulley or throughout the digit and, thus, generally all tenosynovium must be removed. Patients regain motion well 6 to 8 weeks postoperatively, and the recurrence rate is low.

Extensor tenosynovitis is less common in children than in adults. Tendon ruptures and entrapment neuropathies have generally not been a problem in children. Should any of these problems occur, however, indications for tenosynovectomy are the same as those in adults.

SPECIFIC DEFORMITIES

Wrist

Differential epiphyseal growth may lead to distal radioulnar joint incongruity secondary to the shortened ulna, which contrasts with the prominent ulna in adults. Also, given open physes, hemiresection or lengthening are preferred to distal ulnar resection when surgery is indicated.[23]

The radiocarpal joint is more susceptible to ulnar and volar subluxation, whereas the midcarpal and CMC joints are less susceptible to instability and collapse. They are, therefore, actually more at risk for spontaneous ankylosis. Consequently, juvenile patients more commonly require corrective osteotomy to put the wrist in a more functional position after a spontaneous fusion has occurred, rather than formal surgical fusion as in the case of an adult. At present arthroplasty of the child's wrist is not indicated.[22]

Thumb

The deformities at the CMC, MCP, and IP joints are similar to those in the adult. In addition, persistent synovitis and periostitis are associated with bony overgrowth or, the opposite, undergrowth if synovitis causes premature physeal closure. Also, severe erosive changes may lead to a "flail thumb."

Metacarpophalangeal Joints

Synovectomy alone is performed more commonly in children than in adults to control pain, slow progression of deformity, and prevent physeal closure. Silastic arthroplasty has a role in treating MCP joints with severe erosive changes.[22]

Interphalangeal Joints

Boutonnière deformities are relatively common, whereas swan neck deformities are rare, and early PIP synovectomy or flexor tenosynovectomy is preferred to prevent fixed deformities. Proximal IP joint arthroplasty is not indicated in JRA.

Systemic Lupus Erythematosus

CLINICAL FEATURES

Systemic lupus erythematosus (SLE) often has musculoskeletal involvement. (see Chapter 75) The joints most often involved are the knees, but the smaller joints of the hands and the wrists are also frequently affected. The most typical pattern of involvement is one of migratory arthralgias.

Hand involvement in lupus is generally more benign than that seen in RA. Bleifield and Inglis[24] reported some hand involvement in 86 percent of 50 randomly examined patients with lupus. Most patients reported evanescent arthralgias, although some described definitive evidence of swelling and synovitis. The most common cause of symptoms in the hand is Raynaud's phenomenon, occurring in 50 percent of patients. Deformities can affect any joint in the hand and can mimic any of the rheumatoid deformities.

In contrast to patients with RA or OA, patients with lupus do not have articular cartilage involvement, and unless there is a secondary degenerative type of arthritis from the ligamentous laxity, the articular cartilage is completely normal. Because of the ligamentous laxity, however, some of the most severe unstable digital deformities can be seen in these patients. Because of this, early reconstructive surgery prior to severe dislocations and severe fixed deformities is indicated.[25]

SPECIFIC DEFORMITIES

Wrist

Wrist involvement is a frequent radiographic manifestation of the lupus hand but usually is asymptomatic. The most common findings are those of ligamentous laxity. This results in dorsal subluxation of the distal ulna, which can result in pain and limited rotation. Ulnar translocation of the carpus is common, and intercarpal dissociation manifested by an increased scapholunate gap and rotation of the scaphoid is also seen. These generally are asymptomatic, and even in the more significant collapse patterns pain is unusual.

Digital Deformities

The most common digital deformities seen in SLE are secondary to ulnar subluxation of the extensor tendons at the MCP joint and their subsequent overpull at the PIP joints. This picture of MCP flexion deformity with mild ulnar deviation combined with PIP hyperextension and DIP flexion (or swan neck deformity) is known as Jaccoud's syndrome. Initially, these deformities are passively correctable, but eventually they become fixed.

At the PIP joints, swan neck deformities are most common but boutonnière and lateral deformities also occur. Initially, these deformities are supple, but with time they become fixed, and secondary degenerative changes develop.

The type of surgery performed for lupus deformities depends on whether destructive changes have occurred. With Jaccoud's syndrome, attention must be directed to both the MCP and PIP joints. This surgery, although extensive, has relatively good results if it is done when all the joints are fully passively correctable. Once fixed deformities occur, arthroplasty generally yields the best results.[25]

Thumb

The lupus thumb deformity most commonly results from involvement of all three joints. Initially, the clinician sees an extension lag at the MCP joint, with hyperextension at the IP joint. Even at this early stage, a laxity at the CMC joint can be noted. As the laxity increases to dorsal radial subluxation and ultimately dislocation, the thumb deformity abruptly changes to one with adduction of the first metacarpal and hyperextension of the MCP joint and flexion at the IP joint (Fig. 116–8).

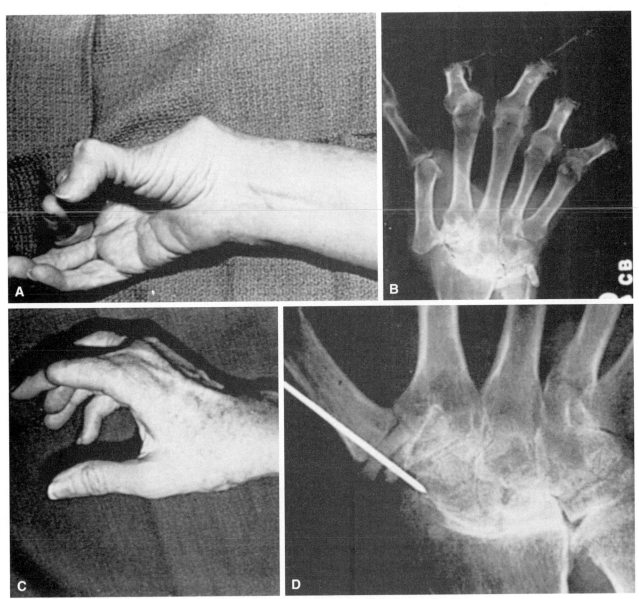

FIGURE 116–8 · Advanced Systemic Lupus Erythematosus (SLE) Thumb Deformity. *A*, Dislocated carpometacarpal (CMC) joint with adduction deformity of metacarpal and hyperextension deformity of the metacarpophalangeal (MCP) joint. *B*, Radiograph of patient in A. Also note collapsed deformity of wrist, dislocation of MCP joints, and lateral dislocation of index proximal interphalangeal (PIP) joint. *C*, Postoperative status after hemiarthroplasty of the CMC joint and soft tissue reconstruction of MCP joint. *D*, Radiograph demonstrating hemiarthroplasty utilizing silicone prosthesis, with Kirschner wire used for temporary prosthetic fixation.

As in other areas, surgery is most effective when performed early. CMC ligamentous stabilization, using a portion of the flexor carpi radialis, has been successful in maintaining stabilization of the joint. Reinforcement of the MCP joint with a rerouted extensor pollicis longus for supple flexion deformity is helpful. For dislocated CMC joints or CMC joints with articular changes, arthrodesis or arthroplasty is carried out. As discussed previously, appropriate distal surgery, such as MCP ligamentous stabilization or fusion, must be included. Interphalangeal fusion is frequently needed for marked instability of the IP joint.

▌ Psoriasis

CLINICAL FEATURES

Approximately 5 percent of patients with psoriasis have arthritis, predominantly involving the small bones of the hands and feet. Generally, arthropathy develops in patients with severe skin involvement, although 20 percent of psoriatic patients present with arthritis prior to development of skin changes. Unlike RA, psoriasis rarely presents with an exuberant proliferative synovitis or tenosynovitis. Characteristically, there is more diffuse involvement of all soft tissues, which predisposes to scarring.

SPECIFIC DEFORMITIES

Digital Deformities

Digital stiffness from involvement of the skin is common. Patients classically present with a "sausage digit" (finger, toe, or both). Articular cartilage and metaphyseal bony changes most often involve the DIP and PIP joints. At the DIP level, the severity of arthritis frequently parallels the degree of nail deformities, such as pitting, ridging, thickening, or detachment. Radiographically, erosive articular destruction in the IP joints (PIP more than DIP) predominates. Pencil-in-cup deformities are characteristic (Fig. 116–9). Progressive distal phalangeal osteolysis with tuft resorption is highly suggestive of psoriatic arthropathy. Severe resorption may result in an "opera-glass hand" with skin collapse over resorbed phalanges.

With psoriatic arthritis, spontaneous fusion of the DIP and intercarpal joints often occurs in a functional position and, thus, surgical intervention is not needed. The PIP joint is involved most severely, and often flexion contractures greater than 90 degrees develop. The radiographs frequently show a narrowed but not completely destroyed joint space; however, the articular cartilage usually is involved more significantly than expected, and joint release usually fails. In addition, there may be an adhesive tenosynovitis that prevents good flexor tendon function, predisposing to recurrent contracture or stiffness. Unless there are significant flexion deformities or pain, surgery usually is not advisable. If either is present, arthrodesis in a functional position is advocated.

Arthroplasty at the MCP and PIP levels is reserved for patients with severe involvement. MCP arthroplasties are performed for the same indications as in RA, that is, pain, deformity, stiffness, and lack of function (Fig. 116–10). However, the rate of infection is slightly higher

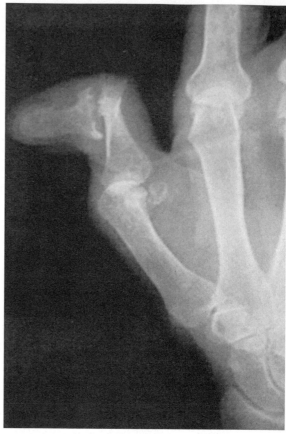

FIGURE 116–9 • Psoriatic pencil-in-cup deformity of the thumb interphalangeal (IP) joint that has progressed to instability and subluxation.

than in patients with RA and lupus, and the eventual range of motion is smaller.[26]

Wrist

Involvement of the wrist includes carpal erosions, joint-space narrowing, and spontaneous intercarpal fusions but generally affects only patients with severe IP involvement. Although surgery is required less frequently at the wrist, the indications and procedures are the same as in RA. Arthrodesis is the procedure of choice.

Thumb

Arthritic thumb involvement of the IP, MCP, and CMC joints can occur, with the CMC joint affected most severely (see Fig. 116–9). CMC destruction with stiffness and decreased opposition may occur. Swan neck deformities are rarer than in RA. At the CMC level, resection arthroplasty should be performed.

At the thumb MCP level, either silastic arthroplasty or arthrodesis can be performed. Arthroplasty, which can be done at the same time as CMC arthroplasty, may be the preferred treatment (see Fig. 116–8c and 116–8d) except when a swan neck deformity is present. When swan neck deformities are present, there is a tendency toward recurrent hyperextension at the MCP level and a resultant "collapse" deformity at the CMC and IP levels. In this situation, MCP arthrodesis has yielded the best results.

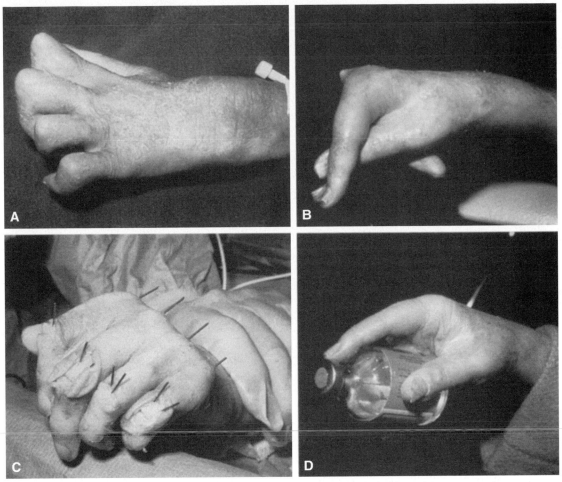

FIGURE 116–10 · Severe Hand Deformities in Psoriatic Arthritis. *A*, Fixed metacarpho-phalangeal (MCP) joint hyperextension with severe flexion deformities of the fingers. *B*, Fixed MCP joint flexion with stiff straight fingers and adducted thumb. *C*, Postoperative appearance of the hand. *D*, Illustration of function after surgery. (From Nalebuff EA: Surgery of psoriatic arthritis of the hand. Hand Clin 12:608, 1996.)

Arthroplasties at the IP level yield very little motion, with a tendency toward hyperextension; joint releases also result in very little motion. For arthrodesis, the interosseous screw has been of great value. To date, the fusion rate has been near 100 percent, with limited postoperative immobilization needed.

As in all arthritides, the results in patient satisfaction are best with thumb and wrist surgery as compared to finger surgery.

Scleroderma

Scleroderma may present as progressive systemic sclerosis or the CREST (*c*alcinosis, *R*aynaud's syndrome, *e*sophageal dysfunction, *s*clerodactyly, *t*elangiectasis) syndrome. Initial hand involvement is usually with Raynaud's syndrome, skin sclerosis, and decreased digital motion. More than 75 percent of patients have calcinosis, usually in areas of chronic stress, such as in the radial aspect of the index fingers, over bony prominences, and in the dominant hand. Sclerosis of the soft tissues is associated with distal tuft resorption in a conical shape and PIP joint contractures. Aggressive synovitis is uncommon. Thumb CMC involvement includes trapezial resorption with metacarpal dorsoradial subluxation and intra-articular calcification. Tenosynovitis is rare and is seen predominantly in patients with progressive systemic sclerosis.

Severe acrosclerosis may result in PIP flexion contractures and thumb metacarpal adduction contractures from sclerosis of the skin, collateral ligaments, joint capsule, and tendon sheaths. At the PIP level, severe progressive flexion contractures may result in attenuation of the central slip and dorsal skin, which may ulcerate and potentially cause septic arthritis. In these situations, PIP arthrodesis allows dorsal skin healing and improved digital function. However, the position for the arthrodesis is often as much as 60 degrees because the severe soft tissue contracture prevents further correction. Arthroplasty has limited indications, yielding little increased range of motion because of the skin sclerosis (average 30 degrees range of motion), and carries the risk of delayed healing and infection.

Calcinosis is more common in CREST syndrome than in diffuse disease and frequently involves the volar aspect of the thumb, index finger, and long fingers. Colchicine may reduce the incidence of calcification. Surgical debulking is indicated when the lesions interfere with hand function or result in skin breakdown and potential infection.

In patients with scleroderma, Raynaud's syndrome may be severe and result in foci of digital ischemic necrosis. The lesion of arterial spasm and stenosis is more common in the proper digital artery than in the common digital artery. If these ischemic lesions are not infected, they can be treated with dressing changes.[27] It may be 3 to 4 months before they heal. The patient is advised to avoid exposure to cold and to discontinue cigarette smoking and other tobacco use.

When medical treatment fails, digital sympathectomy to treat ischemic pain, with or without fingertip ulceration, has proved quite successful. Healing is generally seen by 6 weeks postoperatively. If patients have not healed in 3 months with the use of medical therapy (including dressing changes, cessation of all vasoconstrictive agents, systemic medications, and bupivacaine wrist blocks), digital sympathectomy may be indicated.[27,28] Palmar synovectomy has also been reported to relieve symptoms.[29] Cervical sympathectomy has been less successful. Microvascular reconstruction has recently been reported to be successful in a few cases.[30] Attempts at skin grafting of the ulcers have been complicated by poor healing and sclerodermatous transformation of the graft.

Ignored or improperly treated, these ulcers may progress to gangrene. Autoamputation of the distal digits is occasionally allowed to progress if there is minimal pain and no infection. During the period of autoamputation, meticulous wound care is advised. These lesions of ischemic necrosis may become secondarily infected with *Staphylococcus* and *Pseudomonas*. When there is associated severe pain, septic arthritis, or extensive gangrene, digital amputation is recommended.

Congenital scleroderma is even rarer. Unlike scleroderma in adults, congenital scleroderma in children is less a vascular problem and more a problem of contractures. The progressive collagenization of the soft tissues in a growing child results in severe deformities. Correction is difficult to achieve and maintain, and useful motion is unlikely. Amputations often are necessary.[31]

Sarcoidosis

Sarcoidosis is a systemic granulomatous disease that involves muscular structures. Although not common, involvement of the hand—especially the proximal and middle phalanges—is possible.[32,33] Bone, tendon sheath, skin, and muscle can all be affected. Typically, the hand involvement is either 1) dactylitis, 2) osteolytic bony lesions, 3) tenosynovitis, or 4) soft tissue granulomas. Although usually occurring in patients with a diagnosed sarcoidosis, the various lesions can be confused with many other processes, including malignancy, tuberculosis, and other granulomatous diseases, infections, and hyperparathyroidism.

Sarcoid dactylitis is a rare manifestation of the disease and is characterized by osseous lesions and soft tissue granulomas.[33] A concerted effort to combine maximal medical therapy with surgical excision is generally needed, as progressive deformity and a predilection to nonunion may occur. Isolated bone lesions may go on to pathologic fracture and nonunion, and they typically respond poorly to bone grafting. Therefore, excision with intramedullary cement and stable fixation is warranted. Tenosynovitis is best treated with tenosynovectomy and systemic medical therapy. Isolated soft tissue lesions may require excision.[32]

Gout

Medical management is certainly the cornerstone of treatment for most afflictions secondary to gout (see Chapter 87); however, sometimes surgical intervention is indicated (e.g., to reduce pain, control infection, decompress a nerve, or permit the wearing of gloves and rings).[34] Additionally, gouty tenosynovitis may best be treated with surgical decompression to improve tendon gliding, increase range of motion, and ameliorate pain.[35]

Calcium Pyrophosphate Dihydrate Deposition Disease

Patients with calcium pyrophosphate dihydrate (CPPD) deposition disease have the same hand manifestations as seen in patients with gout (see Chapter 88). One of the earliest findings is calcification of the triangular fibrocartilaginous complex. This and other radiographic findings may not correlate with symptoms and, therefore, it is important to treat the patient and not the radiographs.

If a patient is symptomatic, as in cases of advanced arthropathy, nerve compression, or recalcitrant pain, surgery may be indicated. Common findings in CPPD deposition disease are MCP disease and wrist scapholunate ligament attenuation, leading to a "scapholunate advanced collapse pattern" of wrist involvement.[36] If the patient is symptomatic, either reconstructive (as with MCP joint arthroplasty) or salvage (arthrodesis in wrist arthropathy) procedures are performed, as previously outlined.

Osteoarthritis

CLINICAL FEATURES

OA of the hand is characterized not by synovial hypertrophy but by a gradual loss of articular cartilage. Relating to the hand and wrist, this condition is most prevalent in postmenopausal women but can appear at a younger age in men, especially those in whom previous joint trauma is thought to be a contributing factor. The onset of this condition is slow, with pain being the chief symptom. Radiographic examination of the involved joints initially shows a loss of joint space followed by the appearance of osteophytes. Sclerosis of adjacent bone is also seen. With loss of collateral ligament support, or as a result of stretching of the extensor mechanism, these joints become deformed with decreased functional capacity.

Although any joints in the hand or wrist may be involved with the various rheumatologic conditions, there are four sites where OA is frequently seen: the DIP and PIP joints of the fingers (and IP joint of the thumb), the CMC joint of the thumb, and the wrist (radiocarpal) joint.

SPECIFIC DEFORMITIES

Distal Interphalangeal Joint

The DIP joint is the most common location of OA, and the typical patient with symptomatic involvement at this level is the postmenopausal woman. The patient seeks medical attention because of pain or unhappiness with the appearance of the distal joints of the fingers. Osteophyte formation at the margins of the joints (Heberden's nodes) is a typical physical finding, as is mild radial or ulnar deviation. There is a loss of joint motion noted on clinical examination, but this is seldom of concern to the patient. In fact, as the joint loses motion, pain decreases. In these patients with distal joint arthritis, small mucous cysts may develop on the dorsal aspect of the distal phalanx, which gradually enlarge and stretch the overlying skin. Although the cysts originate from the joint, they may appear at the base of the fingernail, where pressure against the nail matrix causes irregular nail growth.

The treatment of arthritis of the DIP joint and the IP joint of the thumb includes splinting, analgesics for mild pain, and arthroplasty or arthrodesis with spur removal for unstable and unsightly joints. Bothersome mucous cysts are treated with local excision and removal of any underlying bony spurs that are thought to be contributing factors to their development. Recurrence of mucous cysts is occasionally seen and can be eliminated by joint fusion. Distal IP joint arthrodesis is a good operation for pain or instability, and the lost motion is not a problem functionally.

Recently there has been limited enthusiasm for DIP arthroplasty instead of arthrodesis.[21] Although patients often have an extensor lag of about 10 degrees, pain relief is excellent, the average active range of motion is 30 degrees, and patients feel that they have more dexterity than with arthrodesis.

Proximal Interphalangeal Joint

At the PIP joint level, the gradual loss of joint motion assumes major significance, with the patient finding it difficult to grasp small objects. The joints enlarge with spur formation (Bouchard's nodes) and become unsightly. Pain may also be noted with loss of joint articular cartilage. Lateral deformities of this joint are common, with stretching of the collateral ligaments and bone resorption. This leads to overlapping of the fingers and considerable loss of functional ability. The pain at this level can be controlled by splinting, but restoration of

motion can be achieved only by arthroplasty. The use of flexible implants has been worthwhile in this regard; however, clinicians cannot expect to achieve more than an average of 50 degrees of motion with this procedure initially. Long-term follow-up may show an additional loss of 5 to 10 degrees. When patients are being considered for PIP joint arthroplasties because of OA, attention should be directed toward the distal joints. If there is distal joint involvement, it is advisable to combine fusion of the distal joint with arthroplasty of the PIP joint.

Thumb Carpometacarpal Joint

The third area of common hand involvement in OA is the CMC joint of the thumb. This is the joint that most commonly requires surgery in the OA hand. Patients present with increasing pain at the base of the thumb. The joint space between the first metacarpal and trapezium narrows with loss of articular cartilage. Rotary motions of the joint are particularly painful. With a gradual lateral subluxation of the joint, the typical patient develops a "shoulder," or a prominence, at the base of the thumb. The patient has increasing difficulty applying pressure with the thumb, thus making any activity requiring pinch painful. A simple activity, such as opening a car door, becomes difficult and painful. Secondary deformities include adduction of the metacarpal and MCP hyperextension; these can cause further limitation in function, especially in activities involving grasp.

Resting and splinting are frequently helpful in relieving pain and certainly should be tried before surgery is contemplated. Many of these patients respond to a conservative program with relief of pain that is long-lasting in spite of advanced radiographic findings. In patients who do not respond to conservative treatment, arthroplasty affords an excellent solution. Three surgical approaches have been successful. The most simple procedure is osteotomy of the first metacarpal, which can provide satisfactory pain relief in 80 percent of patients.[37] In another procedure, the trapezium is removed and replaced by autogenous soft tissue, such as joint capsule or tendon (resection arthroplasty). In the third approach, the trapezium is replaced by a prosthesis.

Resection arthroplasty gives predictable relief of pain but some loss of pinch power and some residual proximal migration of the metacarpal. The advantage of this technique is simplicity of surgery and consistency of satisfactory results. Other resection techniques may use a tendon sling to prevent proximal migration or to preserve the proximal half of the trapezium.[38]

Trapezium replacement arthroplasties can also be used to maintain space and thumb alignment. The results of this technique, mainly using the silastic trapezium prosthesis, were initially encouraging. However, this approach is surgically more demanding and longer follow-up has shown increasingly frequent reports of prosthetic erosion or breakage or silastic synovitis and deterioration of results.[39] Thus, in most cases, complete trapezial resection with autogenous tissue interposition, with or without ligamentous reconstruction, is the procedure of choice.

CMC fusion can be successful in restoring stability and relieving pain in these patients but should be used only in patients who have localized CMC joint involvement and in whom MCP flexion is maintained. CMC fusion is currently advised only in traumatic arthritis in the young patient. This procedure requires 10 to 12 weeks of postoperative casting and has become less frequently used since the introduction of successful arthroplasties.

Wrist

Primary OA of the wrist is extremely rare. Degenerative changes occur as a result of a traumatic injury, that is, ligamentous disruption with subsequent carpal collapse, or after a displaced fracture. Splinting, therapy, and nonsteroidal anti-inflammatory drugs (NSAIDs) may provide benefit in certain situations, whereas surgical intervention is indicated in others. It is beyond the scope of this chapter to discuss these rare conditions.

REFERENCES

1. Millender L, Nalebuff E: Evaluation and treatment of early rheumatoid hand involvement. Orthop Clin North Am 6:697, 1975.
2. Swanson A: Flexible Implant Resection Arthroplasty in the Hand and Extremities. St. Louis, Mosby, 1973.
3. Ryu J, Saito S, Honda T, et al: Risk factors and prophylactic tenosynovectomy for extensor tendon ruptures in the rheumatoid hand. J Hand Surg Br 23:658, 1998.
4. Williamson S, Feldon P: Extensor tendon ruptures in rheumatoid arthritis. Hand Clin 11:449, 1995.
5. Adolfsson L, Frisen M: Arthroscopic synovectomy of the rheumatoid wrist: A 3.8 year follow-up. J Hand Surg Br 22:711, 1997.
6. Wheen D, Tonkin M, Green J, et al: Long-term results following digital flexor tenosynovectomy in rheumatoid arthritis. J Hand Surg Am 20:790, 1995.
7. Millender L, Nalebuff E: Arthrodesis of the rheumatoid wrist: An evaluation of sixty patients and a description of a different surgical technique. J Bone Joint Surg Am 55:1026, 1973.
8. O'Driscoll S, Horli E, Ness R, et al: The relationship between wrist position, grasp size and grip strength. J Hand Surg Am 17:169, 1992.
9. Ishikawa H, Hanyu T, Saito H, et al: Limited arthrodesis for the rheumatoid wrist. J Hand Surg Am 17:1103, 1992.
10. DellaSanta D, Chamay A: Radiologic evolution of the rheumatoid wrist after radiolunate arthrodesis. J Hand Surg Br 20:46, 1995.
11. Doets HC, Raven EE: A procedure for stabilising and preserving mobility in the arthritic wrist. J Bone Joint Surg Br 81:1013, 1999.
12. Jolly S, Ferlic D, Clayton M, et al: Swanson silicone arthroplasty of the wrist in rheumatoid arthritis: A long-term follow-up. J Hand Surg Am 17:142, 1992.
13. Carlson J, Simmons B: Total wrist arthroplasty. J Am Acad Orthop Surg 6:308, 1998.
14. Nanchahal J, Sykes P, Williams R: Excision of the distal ulna in rheumatoid arthritis: Is the price too high? J Hand Surg Br 21:189, 1996.
15. Nalebuff E: Diagnosis, classification and management of rheumatoid thumb deformities. Bull Hosp Joint Dis 29:119, 1968.
16. van Cappelle HG, Deutman R, van Horn JR: Use of the Swanson silicone trapezium implant for treatment of primary osteoarthritis: long-term results. J Bone Joint Surg Am 83:999, 2001.
17. Kirschenbaum D, Schneider L, Adams D, et al: Arthroplasty of the metacarpal phalangeal joints with use of silicone rubber implants in patients who have rheumatoid arthritis: Longterm results. J Bone Joint Surg Am 75:3, 1993.
18. Rothwell A, Cragg K, O'Neill L: Hand function following Silastic arthroplasty of the metacarpophalangeal joints in the rheumatoid hand. J Hand Surg Br 22:90, 1997.
19. Rizio L, Belsky M: Finger deformities in rheumatoid arthritis. Hand Clin 12:531, 1996.
20. Lin H, Wyrick J, Stern P: Proximal interphalangeal joint silicone replacement arthroplasty: Clinical results using an anterior approach. J Hand Surg Am 20:123, 1995.
21. Wilgis E: Distal interphalangeal joint silicone interpositional arthroplasty of the hand. Clin Orthop 342:38, 1997.
22. Simmons B, Nutting J, Bernstein R: Juvenile rheumatoid arthritis. Hand Clin 12:573, 1996.
23. Mink van der Molen A, Hall M, Evans D: Ulnar lengthening in juvenile chronic arthritis. J Hand Surg Br 23:438, 1998.
24. Bleifield C, Inglis A: The hand in systemic lupus erythematosus. J Bone Joint Surg Am 56:1207, 1974.
25. Nalebuff E: Surgery of systemic lupus erythematosus arthritis of the hand. Hand Clin 12:591, 1996.
26. Nalebuff E: Surgery of psoriatic arthritis of the hand. Hand Clin 12:603, 1996.
27. Ward W, Van Moore A: Management of finger ulcers in scleroderma. J Hand Surg Am 20:868, 1995.
28. Ruch DS, Holden M, Smith BP, et al: Periarterial sympathectomy in scleroderma patients: intermediate-term follow-up. J Hand Surg Am 27:258, 2002.
29. Tomaino MM, Goitz RJ, Medsger TA: Surgery for ischemic pain and Raynaud's phenomenon in scleroderma: a description of treatment protocol and evaluation of results. Microsurgery 21:75, 2001.
30. Tomaino MM, King J, Medsger T: Rationale for and efficacy of digital arterial reconstruction in scleroderma: report of two cases. J Reconstr Microsurg 18:263, 2002.
31. Floyd W, Simmons B, Griffin P: Focal scleroderma affecting the hand. J Bone Joint Surg Am 67:637, 1985.
32. Adelaar R: Sarcoidosis of the upper extremity: Case presentation and literature review. J Hand Surg Am 8:492, 1983.
33. Rodriguez-Gomez M, Fernandez-Sueiro JL, Willisch A, et al: Multifocal dactylitis as the sole clinical expression of sarcoidosis. J Rheumatol 27:245, 2000.
34. Ertugrul Sener E, Guzel VB, Takka S: Surgical management of tophaceous gout in the hand. Arch Orthop Trauma Surg 120:482, 2000.
35. Moore J, Weiland A: Gouty tenosynovitis in the hand. J Hand Surg Am 10:291, 1985.
36. Chen C, Chandnani V, Kang H, et al: Scapholunate advanced collapse: A common wrist abnormality in calcium pyrophosphate dihydrate crystal deposition disease. Radiology 177:459, 1990.
37. Hobby J, Lyall H, Meggitt B: First metacarpal osteotomy for trapeziometacarpal osteoarthritis. J Bone Joint Surg Br 80:508, 1998.
38. Damen A, van der Lei B, Robinson P: Carpometacarpal arthritis of the thumb. J Hand Surg Am 21:807, 1996.
39. Sollerman C, Herrlin K, Abrahamsson S, et al: Silastic replacement of the trapezium for arthrosis: A twelve year followup study. J Hand Surg Br 13:426, 1988.

THE ELBOW
CLEMENT B. SLEDGE

Function of the Elbow

The function of the elbow joint consists primarily of allowing enough motion to position the hand in space, from the perineum to the mouth. It is obvious that the status of the associated joints—the shoulder, wrist, and hand—is important in analyzing elbow function. Amis and colleagues[1] studied a group of 200 patients being followed in a rheumatology clinic. Among those with elbow symptoms, 83 percent complained of shoulder involvement and 92 percent had problems with the hand and wrist. Thus, the clinician may expect the elbow to be an isolated problem in 10 percent or fewer of patients presenting with rheumatoid arthritis (RA).

Compromised shoulder motion reduces the effectiveness of the elbow and places greater significance on elbow function. Similarly, wrist pathology can markedly alter the ability to pronate and supinate the hand independent of the status of the elbow joint. In some patients, particularly those with RA, the status of these adjacent joints should be specifically examined.

MOTION

Associated motion of the neck, hip, and knee may compensate for lost elbow flexion and extension. Limited forearm pronation can be compensated for to some extent by shoulder abduction, although patients may complain of fatigue with this compensatory position. The one motion loss that is not readily compensated for is supination, because the shoulder is not able to readily adduct to accommodate for this loss. It has been shown that the amount of motion required for routine daily activities is approximately 100 degrees of flexion and extension, from 30 to 130 degrees, and approximately 100 degrees of forearm rotation, equally divided between pronation and supination[2] (Fig. 116–11).

STRENGTH

The strongest position of elbow flexion is at 90 degrees, with the forearm in neutral position or supination; strength of extension is only approximately 70 percent that of flexion owing to the mechanic advantage and size of the muscles in each group. Supination strength is about 10 percent greater than pronation strength. Males tend to be stronger than females, on average, by a factor of 2, and the dominant extremity is about 5- to 7-percent stronger than the nondominant extremity.[3]

STABILITY

Because stability is important for the elbow to serve as an effective link, or fulcrum, marked instability even without associated pain may be incapacitating and may become an indication for surgical intervention.

Arthritic Disorders

RA is the most common affliction of the elbow joint that prompts consultation with a rheumatologist. Post-traumatic arthritis is an uncommon presentation, with patients usually visiting an orthopedic surgeon. Because the elbow is vulnerable to sepsis, hematogenous septic arthritis, especially in patients on steroids with RA, is an occasional but serious problem. Direct spread from an infected olecranon bursa is a concern in those with RA. Hence, a swollen olecranon bursa with pain is assumed to be infected and is aspirated, with a course of antibiotics initiated after the aspiration. In the noninfected patient, the bursa may become quite large but is not painful, an important point of the differential diagnosis. Postoperative infection is also more common in patients with elbow involvement, compared to similar surgeries on the hip, knee, and shoulder.[4]

In addition to these conditions, the elbow may be afflicted with hemophilia and inflammatory processes such as gout and pseudogout, but there are no particular distinguishing features concerning elbow involvement in these disease states.

RHEUMATOID ARTHRITIS

A radiographic classification system, based on that used in the knee, has been proposed by Morrey.[4] The scheme proposes four rather simple and readily defined groups (Fig. 116–12):

Stage 1: No gross articular alteration. Osteoporosis is present. Joint mechanics are normal. Synovitis is the prominent pathologic process.
Stage 2: Joint narrowing is present, but the contour of the joint is not badly disrupted. Osteoporosis is usually present. Bone cysts may have developed, but they are not a prominent feature.
Stage 3: The joint architecture has been altered, and the contour of the joint is lost. The joint is somewhat unstable. The olecranon, as viewed on the lateral projection, is thinned. Cystic formation is common.
Stage 4: Gross joint destruction. The articular surface has been resorbed. Mechanical dysfunction and gross instability are characteristic.

Within 2 years of first symptoms in the elbow, 35 percent of patients will show deterioration in elbow function.[5] Because of compensatory motion in adjacent joints, the most common indication for surgery is pain. Instability justifies surgical intervention in about 10 to

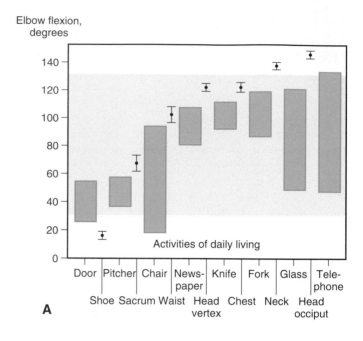

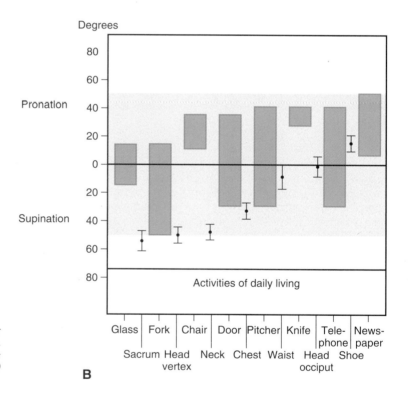

FIGURE 116–11 • *A*, The functional arc of flexion for selected activities of daily living is about 30 to 130 degrees. *B*, The functional arc of pronation and supination for these activities is also 100 degrees: 50 degrees of pronation and 50 degrees of supination.

15 percent of patients. Motion is generally in the functional range. Strength loss is related to pain and instability and, thus, is not generally a primary indication for reconstructive surgery.

POST-TRAUMATIC ARTHRITIS

Unlike the situation of the patient with RA, loss of motion is a typical complaint and prompts a surgical opinion in the patient with post-traumatic arthritis. Pain is not usually a major complaint. The elbow stability of

patients with post-traumatic arthritis is generally good, as is strength. The major complaint of patients with post-traumatic elbow arthritis is limitation of motion incompatible with the activities of daily living, with or without significant pain. In selected cases, elbow replacement can produce good results.[6]

OSTEOARTHRITIS

Osteoarthritis (OA) of the elbow is being recognized with increased frequency in North America and is also

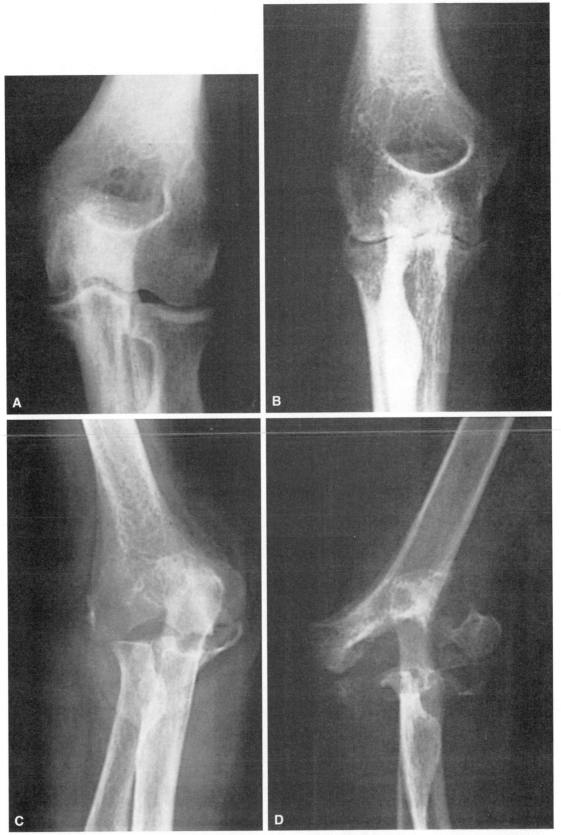

FIGURE 116–12 · Mayo Clinic Classification of Rheumatoid Involvement of the Elbow. *A*, Stage 1: Synovitis; radiograph is normal or shows osteoporosis only. *B*, Stage 2: Synovitis; some mechanical symptoms. Radiograph shows joint narrowing and subchondral changes; the contour is not destroyed. *C*, Stage 3: Less synovitis; mild to moderate instability. Radiograph shows architectural changes. *D*, Stage 4: Grossly unstable; radiograph shows gross destruction. (reproduced with permission of Mayo Foundation.)

well recognized in Asia, particularly Japan.[7] This process appears to be a form of post-traumatic, overuse arthritis. The typical early presentation of the joint with primary degenerative arthritis is loss of extension. Limitation of flexion is noted later, with complaints of pain at the extremes of flexion and extension. The patient tends to seek attention with loss of about 30 degrees of extension and 10 to 20 degrees of flexion. Radiographically, osteophytes are noted anteriorly and posteriorly (Fig. 116–13). Loose bodies occur in about 25 percent of patients. Treatment to date has been symptomatic or limited to arthroscopic procedures. In some instances, removal of osteophytes is indicated to relieve the impingement pain that is noted at the extremes of flexion and extension.[8] An extensive decompression procedure has been successful in about 90 percent of cases.

▌ Indications for Surgical Treatment

As in other joints with arthritis, the primary aim of surgery on the elbow is to restore joint function or relieve pain.

PAIN

Pain is the most common primary indication for elbow surgery, and pain relief is most predictable and complete after prosthetic replacement, especially for RA; however, interposition or distraction arthroplasty should be considered for post-traumatic arthritis.

RESTRICTED MOTION

Distraction and interposition arthroplasty are the two procedures specifically directed at improving motion. If more than 60 degrees of flexion contracture is present, and if this markedly limits the patient's occupational or daily activities, surgical release is considered. Flexion of

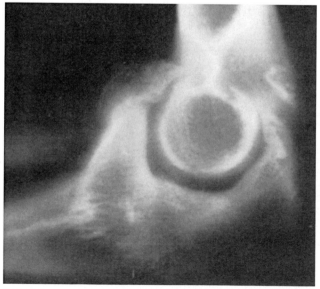

FIGURE 116–13 · Lateral tomogram of an elbow with primary degenerative arthritis shows the characteristic osteophytes from the tip of the olecranon and the coronoid process.

less than 100 degrees does not allow the patient to reach the mouth or head. Thus, surgical intervention is appropriate for such patients as well. In most instances, prosthetic joint replacement is effective at restoring a functional arc of motion, but severe limitation of motion, distinct from pain, is generally found in younger patients in whom prosthetic arthroplasty may not be appropriate.

INSTABILITY

In patients with gross instability from RA, tumor resection, or traumatic bone loss, articulated total joint replacement is effective.[8]

WEAKNESS

Prosthetic joint replacement may help to improve strength by virtue of its elimination of the reflex inhibition associated with pain. Strength is generally remains decreased in the stiff or ankylosed elbow after interposition or distraction arthroplasty.

▌ Surgical Options

SYNOVECTOMY

Synovectomy with radial head excision has been performed for many years. Synovectomy is the accepted procedure for early stages of RA (stages 1 and 2) with chronic refractory synovitis and pain. Concurrent removal of the radial head was recommended by most authorities in the past, but today the radial head is preserved if it is not severely involved and producing pain with pronation or supination. Arthroscopic synovectomy is being performed increasingly, particularly if removal of the radial head is not required.

For RA, the indication for synovectomy is primarily relief of pain. It has been a successful operation with good results lasting about 3 years in most patients. However, the results deteriorate with time.[9] In one series, an initial satisfactory rate of 93 percent at 6 months decreased to about 60 percent at 3 years.[4] The best results are to be anticipated in patients whose elbows have less structural damage. This is not an operation to be offered for limitation of flexion or extension, because that motion is variably affected by the procedure. In approximately half of the patients, flexion arc is not changed by the operation. In approximately 30 percent, there is some improvement, and in 20 percent, motion may be lost after the procedure.[4] The best predictors of success are severe limitation of pronation and supination (less than 80 degrees), flexion and extension of more than 60, and a short duration of symptoms.[9] In patients who otherwise qualify for elbow synovectomy but have severe flexion deformity, anterior release of the elbow capsule can provide increased extension.[10]

In addition to the decrease in satisfactory results over time, the radiographic changes of the disease process may progress after synovectomy, even in the face of decreased symptoms (Fig. 116–14). When elbow replacement is required in this situation, the results are not as

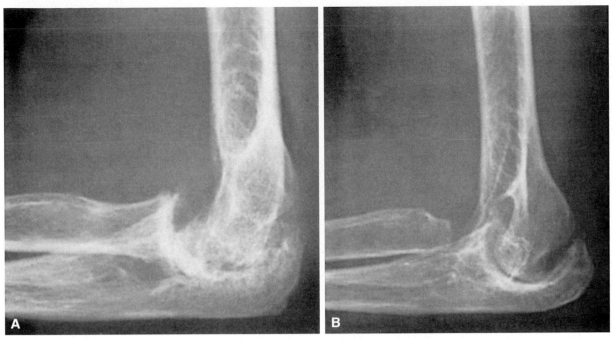

FIGURE 116–14 · *A*, Patient with stage 2 rheumatoid involvement of the elbow and painful synovitis refractory to medical management. *B*, Three years after radial head excision and synovectomy, patient has no pain and 120 degrees of flexion and is pleased with the early result.

good as in patients without preceding synovectomy and radial head excision.[11] Whether this situation will be changed in patients who do not have the radial head excised or who have nonsurgical synovectomy remains to be seen. Nevertheless, caution should be exercised in recommending this procedure in light of the good long-term results of elbow replacement.

More recently, arthroscopic elbow synovectomy has been reported with results that are similar to those achieved by open synovectomy.[12] Given the short-term results described previously, the less intrusive arthroscopic procedure has merit.

INTERPOSITION ARTHROPLASTY

Interposition arthroplasty is rarely carried out today. At present, the indication for this operation is quite limited, but it may be useful in the younger individual in whom reasonably heavy demands are placed on the joint.[13]

Morrey has employed fascial interposition arthroplasty in association with a distraction device in patients undergoing correction of ankylosis following trauma.[14] This procedure, although demanding, does have a limited but definite role in reconstructive surgery of the elbow. Adjunctive use of the distraction device, described in the following section, has broadened the application of this procedure.

DISTRACTION ARTHROPLASTY

Complications of unpredictable pain relief and instability with the interposition resection arthroplasty prompted investigators to consider alternative techniques to obtain

the same functional results. In 1975, Volkov and Oganesian reported their experience with the use of an external fixator.[15] This device employs a pin through the axis of rotation of the elbow joint, and the serial application of traction through additional pins allows the elbow joint to be mobilized, often without additional or significant surgical release. Many pathologies have been treated with this device, including failed excision arthroplasty, post-traumatic contracture, chronic dislocations, and non-united distal humeral fractures.

As a result of Volkov and Oganesian's report, the technique was introduced to North America by Sledge and coworkers.[16] The Volkov-Oganesian distraction apparatus was modified, which led to the development of a similar device at the Mayo Clinic. Their results in 50 patients, with an average follow-up of 40 months, revealed that the mean preoperative arc of motion of 33 degrees was improved to a mean postoperative arc of motion of 98 degrees.[4] Ninety percent of the patients were satisfied with the procedure. Although this may represent a valuable option for the treatment of a young person with a stiff elbow, it is not, at this time, considered a surgical procedure that is universally available to most orthopedic surgeons, owing to its complexity and the infrequency of appropriate indications.

PROSTHETIC JOINT REPLACEMENT

History

Total elbow arthroplasty was developed rather late in the history of modern joint replacement operations—after hip, knee, and shoulder replacement. Several unsatisfactory, highly constrained devices were tried but failed because of loosening of fixation or mechanic problems with the device itself.[17] As built-in mechanic constraint diminished and knowledge of the role of the soft tissues increased, success became more predictable.[18]

Indications

RA is responsible for the vast majority of surgical candidates for elbow replacement. In general, inability to use the extremity for functions of daily living because of pain, motion loss, or instability constitutes the basic indication for elbow joint replacement. In a given patient, several components of disability may be present, although pain is the most common primary indication. Significant cartilage loss or gross deformity should be present before this surgical option is considered. Extensive motion loss is rather uncommon in rheumatoid patients, with the exception of juvenile rheumatoid patients, in whom marked joint motion loss or even ankylosis is typical. In these particular patients, motion limitation may persist even after total elbow arthroplasty.[19,20]

Post-traumatic painful loss of motion in patients younger than 60 years of age should probably be treated with distraction arthroplasty if the patient will return to a high level of demand on the elbow. In the patient older than 60 years and in patients with low demand, elbow arthroplasty may still be appropriate, and the results with recent designs have been gratifying.[21]

Instability, observed with advanced RA and certain post-traumatic conditions, serves as a secondary indication for elbow joint replacement. Such pathology usually dictates the selection of a semiconstrained prosthesis, but good results have been reported with less constrained devices that offer the possibility of surviving in a mechanically testing environment.[6]

Contraindications

Active infection from any source should delay surgery for a minimum of 6 months after treatment and after all evidence of infection has resolved. A previously infected elbow, except in the most unusual circumstances, is a reasonably firm contraindication to elbow joint replacement. Soft tissue contracture or paralysis of the flexor or extensor musculature compromises the anticipated outcome and is a relative contraindication to total elbow arthroplasty. Elbow arthrodesis or painful ankylosis in a satisfactory position is also considered a relative contraindication for elbow replacement at this time because of the unpredictable motion obtained. Most patients who will place significant physical demands on the elbow do not qualify for replacement.[6]

Joint Replacement Options

Currently, both resurfacing and semiconstrained designs are viable options. The resurfacing devices are designed to remove a minimal amount of bone and to replicate the articular anatomy of the distal humerus and proximal ulna and, thus, are considered the "conservative" option.[18] Stability is provided by the integrity of the soft tissue as well as by the inherent design of the prosthesis. Long-term results have demonstrated to durability of the design concept and dependability of pain relief.[22]

Semiconstrained elbow devices provide inherent stability by virtue of the articular design, which is usually a hinge (see Fig. 116–15).[23-25] The semiconstrained devices provide some "play" in the articulation. This relaxation of the articular constraint has dramatically decreased the loosening rate of these devices, which now is only 3 to 5 percent with follow-up exceeding 5 years.[25]

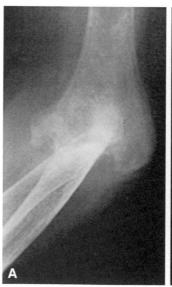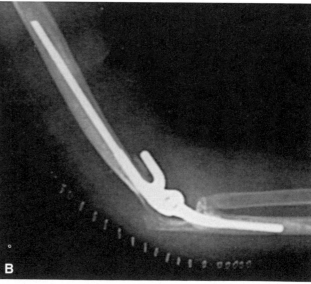

FIGURE 116–15 · *A*, Extensive joint changes and instability from stage 4 rheumatoid arthritis (RA). B, Appearance after treatment with a Mayo-modified Coonrad (III) device.

Postoperative Management

Generally elbow motion is allowed as tolerated, and strengthening exercises are avoided until complete wound healing, usually 3 to 6 weeks. Most patients spontaneously attain an arc of motion of about 50 to 110 degrees after 10 to 14 days with gentle physical therapy or self-treatment by an educated patient. A recent helpful adjunct to attaining this goal has been the use of continuous motion machines. Continuous motion for approximately a week, either in the hospital or at home, generally is effective in allowing the patient to obtain and maintain motion.[4] Motion of 40 to 120 degrees is typical at 3 weeks, and little motion is gained after 3 months. Overaggressive active or passive motion or strength exercises can elicit an inflammatory response, followed by soft tissue scarring, which will not only retard the rehabilitation program and lengthen the period of disability but may compromise the result as well. Generalized swelling is rather common during the early period, but gradually resolves over a 3- to 6-month period, allowing further motion improvement.

Results

Results for the capitellocondylar implant[22] (Fig. 116–16) and for the Mayo-modified Coonrad device[26] indicate that these must be considered the standards for their respective implant categories, with essentially equal results.[27] Ewald and colleagues[22] followed 202 capitellocondylar total elbow replacements an average of 69 months (range, 24 to 178 months). The most improvement occurred in the categories of pain relief, functional status, and range of motion in all planes except extension; these improvements did not deteriorate with time. The average preoperative arc of motion at the elbow ranged from −37 degrees of extension to 118 degrees of flexion. The average postoperative arc of motion at the elbow ranged from −30 degrees of extension to 135 degrees of flexion. Supination improved from 45 degrees preoperatively to 64 degrees postoperatively; pronation improved from 56 degrees preoperatively to 72 degrees postoperatively. Revision of the prosthesis was necessary in three elbows (1.5%) because of loosening without infection and in three additional elbows because of dislocation of the prosthesis. Complications included deep infection in three elbows (1.5%); problems related to the wound in 15 elbows (7%); permanent, partial-sensory ulnar nerve palsy in five elbows (2.5%); permanent, partial-motor ulnar nerve palsy in one elbow (0.5%); and dislocation in seven elbows (3.5%∧).[22] Results with the more constrained Mayo-Coonrad implant have been quite similar. A review of results in 41 patients with minimum 10-year follow-up revealed that 97 percent of patients reported that the elbow was not painful, and all patients considered the outcome satisfactory; range of motion was similar to that reported by Ewald and colleagues. Complications occurred in 14 percent of elbows and required reoperation in all but one of these patients.[28]

Relief of Pain

Typically, more than 90 percent of patients with either the resurfacing or semiconstrained device note virtually complete relief of pain, which is consistent with other total joint replacements. The presence of pain is almost always associated with loosening, subluxation, primary or secondary (reactive) synovitis, or infection.

Motion

For both classifications of devices, a functional arc of flexion is almost universally reported, averaging about 30

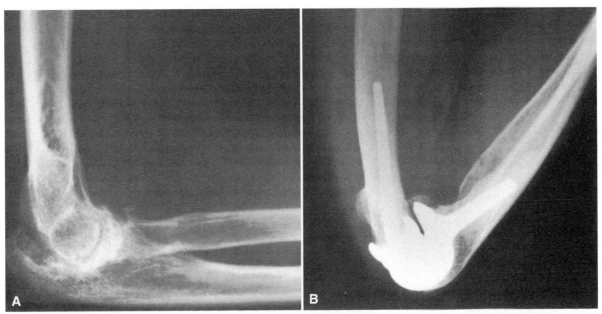

FIGURE 116–16 · *A*, Severe destruction of the elbow with rheumatoid arthritis. *B*, Six years after elbow replacement with the capitellocondylar implant, the elbow is functional without pain. The radiograph shows maintainance of component fixation. (Courtesy of F.C. Ewald)

to 130 degrees. To help ensure stability with the resurfacing devices, extension past 30 degrees is restricted. Without diligence in the postoperative period, this may progress to further extension loss.

Forearm rotation averages greater than 60 degrees of pronation and 60 degrees of supination, again generally independent of the design. Based on the reports to date, postoperative motion correlates most closely with the preoperative state of the soft tissue. The mean extent of motion observed is adequate for most activities of daily living.

Complications

Complications after total elbow arthroplasty (excluding loosening) have been reported in a larger percentage of patients than with other joint replacements. The elbow is a complex joint prone to involvement in RA and post-traumatic arthritis. Both of these operative diagnoses are associated with a higher rate of complications than other joint replacements. The subcutaneous location of the joint makes it more likely to experience delayed wound healing and infection. The intimate relationship of the ulnar nerve at the elbow and the frequent involvement of the nerve with vasculitis in patients with RA all conspire to produce frequent, but usually minor, complications.

Infection

Deep infection is probably more common after elbow replacement compared to other joints and is reported to be as high as 11 percent in some reports.[29] The incidence seems to be reduced by the use of antibiotic-impregnated cement. Morrey found no infection in patients after approximately 50 consecutive procedures when antibiotics were added to the cement, and his overall infection rate is now about 3 percent.[30]

Neurapraxia

The ulnar nerve is particularly vulnerable at the elbow, and the incidence of ulnar-nerve involvement after surgery has averaged about 7 percent.[22] The etiology of this complication involves several factors, including excessive traction, exposure trauma, perineural hematoma, mechanical pressure, possibly thermal damage from the polymethyl methacrylate, and even translocation causing devascularization or constriction. The subclinical neuropathy that occasionally occurs with patients with RA might be aggravated at the time of a surgical procedure. Knowledge of the frequency of this complication has led surgeons to take extreme care of the ulnar nerve during the procedure, and the incidence of this complication has been decreased.[31]

Impaired Wound Healing

Wound healing has been a problem in 3 to 5 percent of patients, yet 75 percent of these required no additional surgical procedure.[29] Careful handling of the tissues, well-designed incisions, proper hemostasis and drainage, and careful postoperative management are helpful adjuncts to prevent this problem.

Loosening

Loosening is uncommon with the resurfacing devices and the semiconstrained hinged devices currently being used. The rigidly linked devices develop loosening in more than 25 percent of patients with long-term follow-up.[17]

Instability

Instability is a unique complication of the resurfacing, or snap-fit, implants. Dislocation or subluxation of resurfacing designs usually occurs soon after surgery. Inadequate soft tissue balance, either from the collateral ligaments or dynamically from the pull of the triceps, is the basic cause of this complication. Currently, the incidence of instability is less than 5 percent with suitable designs in experienced hands.[22,23,25] This again underscores the precise technical requirements of elbow replacement surgery.

REFERENCES

1. Amis A, Hughes S, Miller J, et al: A functional study of the rheumatoid elbow. Rheum Rehab 21:151, 1982.
2. Morrey B, Askew L, An K, et al: A biomechanical study of normal functional elbow motion. J Bone Joint Surg Am 63:872, 1981.
3. Askew L, Morrey B, An K: Isometric strength patterns of the normal elbow. Clin Orthop 222:261, 1987.
4. Morrey B: The elbow. In Kelley WN, Harris ED Jr, Ruddy S, Sledge CB (eds): Textbook of Rheumatology. Philadelphia, WB Saunders, 1997, p 1675.
5. Eberhardt K, Fex E: Functional impairment and disability in early rheumatoid arthritis–development over 5 years. J Rheumatol 22:1037, 1995.
6. Schneeberger A, Adams R, Morrey B: Semiconstrained total elbow replacement for the treatment of post-traumatic osteoarthrosis. J Bone Joint Surg Am 79:1211, 1997.
7. Oka Y, Ohta K, Saitoh I: Débridement arthroplasty for osteoarthritis of the elbow. Clin Orthop 351:127, 1998.
8. Morrey B: Primary degenerative arthritis of the elbow. Treatment by ulnohumeral arthroplasty. J Bone Joint Surg Br 74:409, 1992.
9. Gendi N, Axon J, Carr A, et al: Synovectomy of the elbow and radial head excision in rheumatoid arthritis: Predictive factors and long-term outcome. J Bone Joint Surg Br 79:918, 1997.
10. Lonner J, Stuchin S: Synovectomy, radial head excision, and anterior capsular release in stage III inflammatory arthritis of the elbow. J Hand Surg Am 22:279, 1997.
11. Schemitsch E, Ewald F, Thornhill T: Results of total elbow arthroplasty after excision of the radial head and synovectomy in patients who had rheumatoid arthritis. J Bone Joint Surg Am 78:1541, 1996.
12. Lee B, Morrey B: Arthroscopic synovectomy of the elbow for rheumatoid arthritis: A prospective study. J Bone Joint Surg Br 79:770, 1997.
13. Ljung P, Jonsson K, Larsson K, et al: Interposition arthroplasty of the elbow with rheumatoid arthritis. J Shoulder Elbow Surg 5:81, 1996.
14. Morrey B: Distraction arthroplasty. In Morrey BF (ed): The Elbow and Its Disorders. Philadelphia, WB Saunders, 1993, p 433.
15. Volkov M, Oganesian O: Restoration of function in the knee and the elbow with the hinged distractor apparatus. J Bone Joint Surg Am 75:591, 1975.
16. Deland J, Walker P, Sledge C, et al: Treatment of posttraumatic elbows with a new hinge-distractor. Orthopedics 6:732, 1983.

17. Gschwend N, Simmen B, Matejovsky Z: Late complications in elbow arthroplasty. J Shoulder Elbow Surg 5:86, 1996.
18. Ewald F, Scheinberg R, Poss R, et al: Capitellocondylar total elbow arthroplasty: Two to five year followup in rheumatoid arthritis. J Bone Joint Surg Am 62:1259, 1980.
19. Connor P, Morrey B: Total elbow arthroplasty in patients who have juvenile rheumatoid arthritis. J Bone Joint Surg Am 80:678, 1998.
20. Mansat P, Morrey BF: Semiconstrained total elbow arthroplasty for ankylosed and stiff elbows. J Bone Joint Surg Am 82:1260-1268, 2000.
21. Kozak T, Adams R, Morrey B: Total elbow arthroplasty in primary osteoarthritis of the elbow. J Arthroplasty 13:837, 1998.
22. Ewald F, Simmons E Jr, Sullivan J, et al: Capitellocondylar total elbow replacement in rheumatoid arthritis: Long-term results. J Bone Joint Surg Am 75:498, 1993.
23. Ikavalko M, Lehto MU, Repo A, et al: The Souter-Strathclyde elbow arthroplasty: A clinical and radiological study of 525 consecutive cases. J Bone Joint Surg Br 84:77-82, 2002.
24. Rozing P: Souter-Strathclyde total elbow arthroplasty. J Bone Joint Surg Br 82:1129-1134, 2000.
25. Tanaka N, Kudo H, Iwano K, et al: Kudo total elbow arthroplasty in patients with rheumatoid arthritis: a long-term follow-up study. J Bone Joint Surg Am 83:1506-1513, 2001.
26. Hildebrand KA, Patterson SD, Regan WD, et al: Functional outcome of semiconstrained total elbow arthroplasty. J Bone Joint Surg Am 82:1379-1386, 2000.
27. Wright TW, Wong AM, Jaffe R: Functional outcome comparison of semiconstrained and unconstrained total elbow arthroplasties. J Shoulder Elbow Surg 9:524-531, 2000.
28. Gill D, Morrey B: The Coonrad-Morrey total elbow arthroplasty in patients who have rheumatoid arthritis: A ten to fifteen-year follow-up study. J Bone Joint Surg Am 80:1327, 1998.
29. Ljung P, Bornmyr S, Svensson H: Wound healing after total elbow replacement in rheumatoid arthritis: Wound complications in 50 cases and laser-Doppler imaging of skin microcirculation. A. Acta Orthop Scand 66:59, 1995.
30. Morrey B, Adams RA: Semiconstrained arthroplasty for rheumatoid arthritis. J Bone Joint Surg Am 74:479, 1992.
31. Ljung P, Ahlmann S, Knutson K, et al: Intraoperative monitoring of ulnar nerve function during replacement of the rheumatoid elbow via the lateral approach. Acta Orthop Scand 66:132, 1995.

THE SHOULDER
CLEMENT B. SLEDGE

The shoulder is often ignored by patients and physicians. In patients with rheumatoid arthritis (RA), other problems with greater pain or functional impairment relegate the shoulder to the background. In addition, there is general lack of awareness of the benefits of surgical treatment of the shoulder.

The shoulder is not commonly involved by osteoarthritis (OA) and, when it is, underlying causes should be suspected: old injury, recurrent dislocations, or massive tear of the rotator cuff. Of all the arthritides, six categories account for more than 95 percent of the diseases requiring reconstructive shoulder surgery:

OA
RA or other, much less common inflammatory arthritides
Post-traumatic arthritis (arthritis due to past injuries)
Humeral-head osteonecrosis
Cuff-tear arthritis
Revision surgical procedures for failed prior surgical treatment

In some instances, destruction of the glenohumeral joint articular surfaces is the only pathologic abnormality. In more complex situations there may be rotator cuff contracture or deficiency, manifested by weakness and per-

haps instability. Some cases of traumatic arthritis may have associated neurologic compromise. Finally, there may be problems in adjacent articulations—the acromioclavicular joint, sternoclavicular joint, or scapulothoracic interval. These combinations of problems make diagnosis and treatment in this area often confusing and difficult. Careful clinical and radiographic evaluation is necessary to arrive at a correct anatomic diagnosis and treatment plan. A shoulder function assessment (SFA) scale has been developed that can filled out in 3 minutes and provides a reliable, validated means of assessing shoulder function.[1]

Clinical Evaluation

The patient history, physical examination, and various forms of standard radiography are the keys in diagnosis, possibly supplemented by other testing such as ultrasound and magnetic resonance imaging (MRI).

The pain can be focal, as is usually the case in patients with acromioclavicular joint disease, or it can be more general over the deltoid region. Shoulder pain may be referred down the arm and into the dorsoradial aspect of the proximal forearm. If the hand is also painful, the clinician should look for neural or vascular disease or consider the existence of a second problem in the hand. Pain can also be referred proximally to the trapezius and periscapular area and sometimes to the base of the neck. However, if neck pain is also present, probably a cervical spine problem is present.

Pain in the shoulder, as in other musculoskeletal areas, is often improved by rest and worsened with use; in the shoulder specifically, it is usually intensified by overhead activities. Patients with shoulder pain are characteristically concerned about night pain with interruption of sleep.

Muscle atrophy about the shoulder girdle may be noted if the disease is of long duration, as it often is before coming to the attention of the physician. In OA of the glenohumeral joint, the shoulder may be subluxated slightly posterior and appear flattened on the anterior aspect, with the posterior aspect more full and rounded. In RA, there may be enormous prominence of the shoulder related to synovitis and effusion. The shoulder may be subluxated forward and slightly upward, or there may be bony resorption with a medial displacement of the upper end of the humerus producing an undue prominence of the acromion and distal clavicle.

Patients with early glenohumeral arthritis, rotator cuff disease, or both often experience pain in the mid range of abduction or flexion. If the arm is elevated by the examiner and the patient is asked to lower it slowly, the arm often "drops" when it reaches the painful midrange. Patients with inflammatory changes in the shoulder capsule and rotator cuff usually have pain at the extremes of motion. When there is significant rotator cuff disease, active motion is less than passive motion, particularly in elevation. The wide range of motion provided by the mobile scapula may conceal significant loss of glenohumeral motion.

Radiographic interpretation of shoulder disorders has been difficult for a variety of reasons: the standard shoulder films are anteroposterior (AP) views taken in reference to the thorax, producing an oblique view of the glenohumeral space; radiographs taken with the patient relaxed and standing show an apparent joint space when there may be none; the important soft tissues, such as the rotator cuff, are not seen with standard radiographs.

If the rotator cuff or other soft tissues are thought to need further evaluation, there are several choices: ultrasonography, contrast arthrography or MRI. Ultrasound has been widely used in Europe, but less so in North America. It is both equipment and operator dependent. In experienced hands, however, synovitis of the glenohumeral joint, biceps tendinitis, and changes in the supraspinatus tendon of the rotator cuff can be identified.[2]

Arthrography is the best test for establishing the presence or absence of a full-thickness rotator cuff tear and is also the best study for outlining the characteristics of the synovium. With films taken in various positions, arthrography allows estimation of the size of rotator cuff tears.[3]

MRI has proved useful in the evaluation of rotator cuff pathology. For optimally defining the characteristics of the rotator cuff, MRI, with or without contrast, is the imaging modality of choice.

A comparison of plain radiography, ultrasound, and MRI showed the superiority of the latter two in demonstrating small erosion and soft tissue changes and the superiority of MRI in assessing overall damage to the joint.[4] In addition, MRI can be useful in demonstrating osteonecrosis before there is collapse evident on plain films.

Because of the accuracy of the noninvasive imaging techniques, arthroscopy has not proved very useful in the evaluation of the shoulder with arthritis.

Computed tomography (CT) is useful in defining the bony anatomy before undertaking shoulder replacement.

◼ Characteristics of Shoulder Arthritis

OSTEOARTHRITIS

OA, primary or secondary, has a rather typical presentation in the shoulder. Pain and crepitus are early findings. Plain films reveal a typical appearance with loss of joint space, peripheral osteophytes, and varying mixtures of disuse osteopenia and subchondral sclerosis (Fig. 116–17). The glenoid is often eroded and may provide a clue to the etiology of arthritis secondary to trauma such as recurrent posterior dislocations. The rotator cuff is usually intact, allowing restoration of the anatomic and functional relationships of the shoulder at the time of shoulder replacement (Fig. 116–18).

RHEUMATOID ARTHRITIS

RA is the prototype for the inflammatory arthropathies; in fact, there is seldom a need for reconstructive shoulder surgery in other inflammatory arthropathies in the shoulder, such as ankylosing spondylitis (AS) or psoriatic arthritis. The rotator cuff in patients with RA may be involved, and evidence for this should be sought because of its influence on the outcome of shoulder replacement. By the time such involvement is detected, the articular surfaces are usually destroyed. Rather than simply considering cuff repair, shoulder replacement and simultaneous repair of the cuff can be undertaken.[5]

With progressive disease in the shoulder, changes in the rotator cuff and associated shoulder capsule can lead to joint subluxation. In RA, this is often superior or anterior and superior (Fig. 116–19). Subluxation may be associated with gross, full-thickness rotator cuff tearing or may be related to stretching and thinning of these soft tissues.

If shoulder involvement is detected early in the course of disease, the joint may be painful but show preservation of glenohumeral cartilage. Synovectomy has been considered in this situation. Even with the availability of arthroscopic surgery, this operation is not commonly performed in North America, but good results have been reported in patients with early, minimally erosive disease.[6] Radioisotope synovectomy is even more rarely performed. Patients with preserved glenohumeral cartilage are usually treated medically, and patients with loss of glenohumeral cartilage are treated with total shoulder arthroplasty.

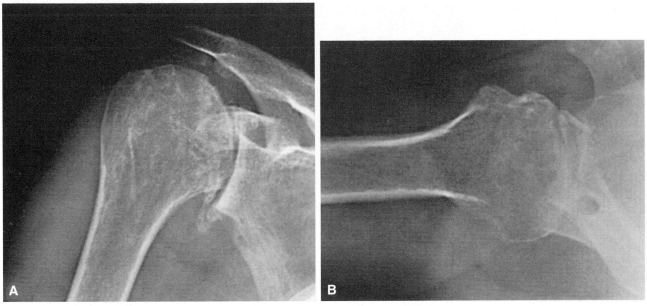

FIGURE 116–17 · Osteoarthritis (OA) of the shoulder with loss of glenohumeral cartilage, some subchondral cyst formation, posterior-central glenoid erosion, and posterior humeral subluxation. The amount of subchondral sclerosis and osteophyte formation is somewhat less than in the typical case of OA.

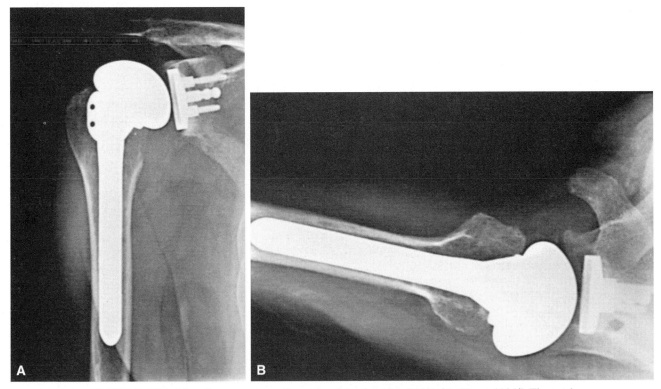

FIGURE 116–18 · Postoperative radiographs of the shoulder depicted in Figure 116-17. The total joint arthroplasty has been positioned so the joint is balanced, eliminating much of the tendency for posterior humeral subluxation.

Approximately one third to one half of patients with RA who require prosthetic shoulder arthroplasty will be found to have major tears of the rotator cuff.[7] Repair is possible in only about half of these instances.[5] If repair is not possible, hemiarthroplasty without glenoid replacement is probably indicated[8] (Fig. 116–20). Because there is a significant functional difference in the outcome of shoulder replacement depending on whether the cuff is intact or not, early intervention, before irreparable cuff tear occurs, is important.[9] However, even ARA class IV

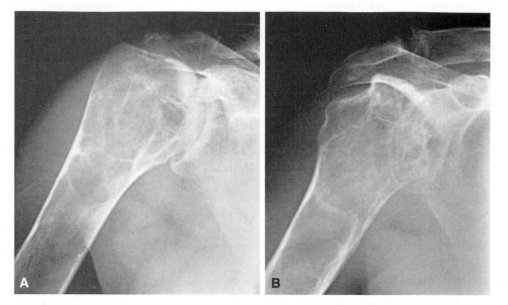

FIGURE 116–19 • *A*, Rheumatoid arthritis (RA) of the shoulder with osteopenia and some cyst formation in the humeral head; there is also loss of glenohumeral cartilage. *B*, On the internal rotation view, marginal joint erosions are readily visible.

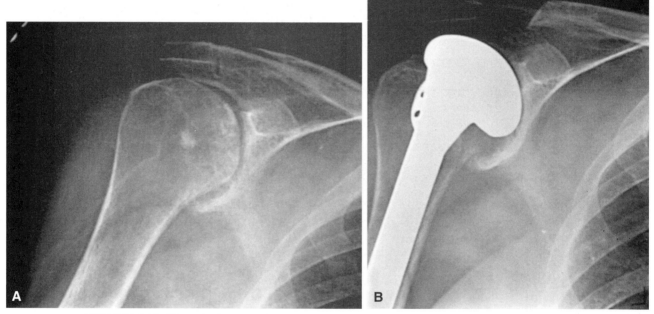

FIGURE 116–20 • *A*, Rheumatoid arthritis (RA) of the shoulder with central resorption of the glenoid. *B*, Humeral-head replacement was performed because there was not enough bone remaining to securely place a glenoid component.

patients with irreparable cuff tears have significant functional and symptomatic improvement following shoulder replacement.[10] The major functional difference is in overhead activities; without a cuff, arm elevation above the horizontal is unlikely.[11]

Special concerns apply to those with juvenile rheumatoid arthritis (JRA). These individuals often have long-standing involvement of the joint and surrounding soft tissue structures and have a notable tendency to be stiff. Reconstructive prosthetic arthroplasty can, of course, resurface the joint and relieve pain. Releases at surgery can achieve more movement, but, owing to tissue stiffness, this range of motion is seldom retained. In these patients,

postoperative motion at follow-up is often approximately half of normal.

POST-TRAUMATIC ARTHRITIS

Arthritis may develop secondary to shoulder instability, either after recurrent subluxations or dislocations or as a result of a chronic dislocation. Arthritis is an uncommon development of recurrent shoulder instability, but it does occur and has been associated with surgical repair of anterior structures, in which healing leads to overtightening and creates posterior humeral subluxation and the resulting features of OA.

In chronic shoulder dislocation that has been present for 6 months or more, the cartilage on the humeral head may be lost and replaced by fibrous tissue. If the impaction fracture of the humeral head that often accompanies traumatic dislocation of the shoulder occupies one third or more of the head substance, the humeral head may need to be replaced by a prosthesis. The same is true for long-standing dislocations in which severe humeral-head osteopenia may result in an inability to withstand the usual joint forces.

In fractures of the proximal humerus, the humeral head may be directly damaged, or it may lose its blood supply with subsequent osteonecrosis. The fracture pattern in some instances may suggest such a high likelihood of osteonecrosis that primary humeral-head replacement is indicated. In some instances, the fracture may unite successfully but with the articular surface malpositioned. Humeral-head replacement or total joint arthroplasty is a reasonable consideration to relieve pain and improve motion.

OSTEONECROSIS

Osteonecrosis of the subchondral bone of the humeral head is often associated with trauma, particularly four-part humeral-head fractures and, occasionally, humeral head fractures with lesser degrees of fragment displacement. A number of conditions have been implicated in the development of nontraumatic osteonecrosis, including corticosteroid use, alcoholism, sickle cell disease, decompression sickness, hyperuricemia, Gaucher's disease, pancreatitis, familial hyperlipidemia, renal or other organ transplantation, lymphoma, systemic lupus erythematosus (SLE), and therapeutic radiation.

For treatment, it is useful to stage osteonecrosis of the humeral head, and the staging system utilized for the femoral head is applicable.[12] In stage I, the plain roentgenogram is normal, but abnormalities appear on the bone scan or MRI. Stage II is characterized by a change in the trabecular bone pattern of the humeral head (Fig. 116–21D). Stage III is associated with a subchondral fracture—a so-called crescent sign with no or minimal collapse of the articular surface. In stage IV, there is segmental collapse of the humeral head. In stage V, there are associated glenoid arthritic changes.

The course of humeral-head osteonecrosis is not completely clear. Cofield studied a group of patients with osteonecrosis and determined that in stage II or early stage III disease, clinical progression may or may not occur; in patients with stage IV or V disease, however, symptomatic progression is likely. He recommends conservative treatment for stage I, stage II, and early stage III disease and recommends considering surgery for severely symptomatic stage III, stage IV, or stage V disease.[12]

Patients with osteonecrosis usually do well following prosthetic arthroplasty because the rotator cuff and

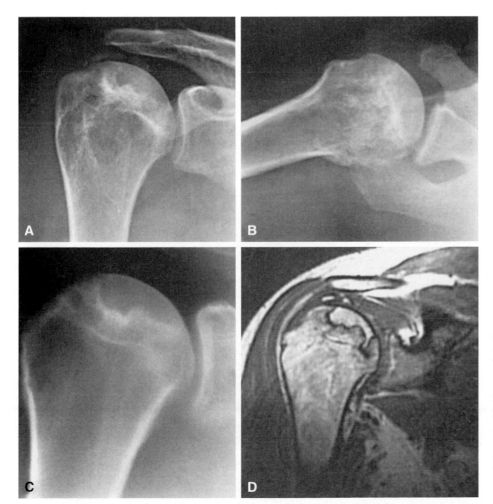

FIGURE 116–21 · A and B, Standard radiographic views of a shoulder with osteonecrosis. C, An anteroposterior tomogram shows the lesion somewhat more clearly but does not demonstrate a fracture at the junction between the osteonecrotic segment and the remaining bone of the humeral head. D, A magnetic resonance image (MRI) shows the osteonecrotic fragment more clearly. It is not clear on any of these films whether there is a fracture separating the necrotic segment from the remainder of the humeral head.

shoulder capsule are normal and the glenoid is usually not eroded. The glenoid cartilage may be injured by the irregular humeral-head surface and require resurfacing; in the absence of damage to the glenoid, hemiarthroplasty is usually chosen.

CUFF-TEAR ARTHROPATHY

A peculiar condition in the shoulder is marked by a loss of glenohumeral cartilage, often loss of bone substance in the humeral head or glenoid, destruction of a large portion of the rotator cuff and shoulder capsule, glenohumeral instability, and sometimes even erosion of the acromion process and distal clavicle (Fig. 116–22). This condition has been given a variety of designations. Robert Adams perhaps first defined this as a disease process.[13] It has been called cuff tear arthropathy by Neer and colleagues, who described a series of patients with this presentation.[14,15] They felt that this condition represented a very advanced stage of chronic rotator-cuff disease, with tearing and chronic instability leading to the secondary features. McCarty and coworkers termed this the *Milwaukee shoulder* and subsequently identified a number of joints with arthropathy associated with basic calcium phosphate crystals.[16] The radiographic and clinical features of Milwaukee shoulder are similar, if not identical, to those of cuff-tear arthropathy. Clinically, women are affected more often than men, and the condition usually occurs in elderly patients. Bilaterality is common. A large effusion may be present, and patients occasionally develop recurrent hemorrhages.

There are no pathognomonic features; it is useful to develop a differential diagnosis in patients presenting with this problem and consider a variant of OA, RA, infection, osteonecrosis, or neuroarthropathy.

Surgical treatment for this condition is extraordinarily difficult. It is possible, of course, to replace the joint surfaces, but it is essentially impossible to perform rotator-cuff repair. There is, therefore, a strong ten-dency for the shoulder to become unstable following surgery. It is generally recommended that surgical treatment be avoided for these patients. If that is not possible, hemiarthroplasty with infraspinatus transfer superiorly is probably the treatment of choice.[15]

▌ Surgical Management

Usually, surgery is performed for the combination of pain and functional limitations. Pain is the major factor leading to the decision of whether or not to perform surgery.

The inflammatory arthropathies often involve multiple joints, many with severe pain and limitation of function. Although opinions vary as to treatment, it is generally agreed that if patients have severe upper- and lower-extremity symptomatology, serious consideration should be given to performing surgery first on the major lower-extremity joints. This allows the patient to ambulate more effectively and to put lesser demands on the upper extremities, leading overall to large functional gains for the patient. Thus, if a patient has both severe hip arthritis and severe shoulder arthritis, the performance of hip surgery before shoulder surgery is generally advised.

With involvement of multiple joints in the upper extremity, the timing of hand surgery can be judged on its own merit. The combination of hand surgery with major shoulder or elbow surgery is probably too much at one setting, unless the hand procedure is quite limited. Thus, if significant gains are expected from hand surgery, it can be performed either before or after the shoulder or elbow surgery; the sequence is not critical.

If the decision must be made between performing shoulder or elbow surgery, most surgeons feel that the more proximal surgery should be performed earlier. There is some referral of shoulder pain to the elbow and a lesser referral of elbow pain to the shoulder. Relieving the shoulder pain and thereby improving motion may, in fact, alleviate the need for elbow surgery. Before elbow

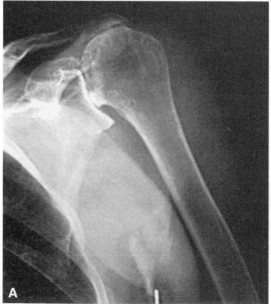
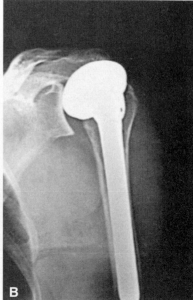

FIGURE 116–22 · *A,* Rotator-cuff tear arthritis with glenohumeral cartilage loss and a large rotator cuff tear. *B,* Treatment with a humeral-head prosthesis gives the patient reduced pain and allows more adequate function of the shoulder, but it does not address the significant muscle weakness produced by loss of the rotator cuff.

arthroplasty, it is helpful to have ample arm rotation available by means of a reconstructed shoulder joint than a somewhat stiff shoulder joint causing more stresses to be placed on the operated elbow.

ARTHRODESIS

In the past, there were many indications for arthrodesis, including arthritis of various types in the shoulder. Currently, however, shoulder arthrodesis is largely limited to individuals who have significant neurologic damage compromising the deltoid and rotator cuff muscles or to those who have infection of the shoulder joint with cartilage loss. Occasionally, arthrodesis is used for patients with a condition such as old trauma who have loss of glenohumeral cartilage, considerable distortion of bone, stiffness and partial destruction of the capsule and rotator cuff about the shoulder, and incomplete nerve lesions. These features together suggest that arthroplasty may not be a good choice, and a fusion is then considered, particularly in younger men who wish to be quite vigorous in their activities.

The outcome of shoulder arthrodesis is well established. Union across the glenohumeral joint is attained in between 90 and 95 percent of cases.[17] Approximately nine tenths of arm rotation occurs via the glenohumeral joint, and this motion will be eliminated with fusion. Approximately two thirds of overhead movement occurs via the glenohumeral joint, and this also will be lost following shoulder arthrodesis. The functional limitations following arthrodesis are significant, but in individuals with substantial paralysis or the residuals of infection, function may, in fact, be improved following operation. If the fusion is positioned appropriately, the patient can have the arm come comfortably to the side, and it can be raised approximately 70 degrees. It is difficult following a fusion for the patient to place the hand behind the trunk, but typically he or she can touch the perineum, the abdomen, and the face. Outward rotation is usually to neutral at best.

PROSTHETIC ARTHROPLASTY

Surgical Options

There are many designs for prosthetic arthroplasty for the shoulder. In North America, the prototype was developed by Neer in the late 1940s and became available for general use in the early 1950s.[18] This was initially intended for use in patients with proximal humeral fractures and gradually was extended to include patients with the various arthritic diseases.

A variety of shoulder arthroplasty designs have been used, incorporating metal, high-density polyethylene, and bone cement. Neer was responsible for the first commonly used design incorporating these rather simple features (Fig. 116–23). This has been followed by many other similar designs, and a number of reports are available in the literature.

The newer implant designs vary more in details than in principle. Some systems have better instrumentation than the early designs and come in a large variety of

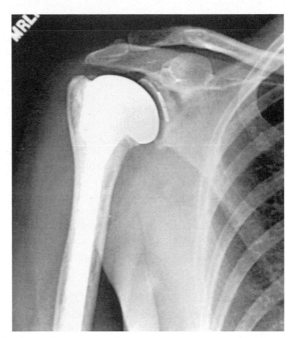

FIGURE 116–23 · Radiograph of a typical Neer-type total shoulder arthroplasty performed in the late 1970s. A small lucent line has developed around the glenoid component, but it has remained stable, and the patient has experienced excellent pain relief for more than 15 years following the surgical procedure.

sizes. In addition, a few designs incorporate tissue ingrowth capabilities, as in the case of implants developed for the hip and knee.

Results

Approximately 90 percent of patients who have undergone total shoulder arthroplasty achieve satisfactory pain relief, not unlike the rate for total hip or total knee arthroplasty.[19] Also similar to the situation in total hip or knee arthroplasty, the average return of motion is two thirds of normal. However, this varies considerably depending on the condition of the soft tissues. In OA, in which soft tissue involvement is limited, patients typically regain three quarters of normal motion or more.[20] In RA, motion following reconstruction varies between one third and two thirds of normal, with only a few patients who have excellent soft tissues attaining more motion than this. In patients with traumatic arthritis and abundant scarring, average motion following arthroplasty approaches one half to two thirds of normal. In patients with osteonecrosis, motion may be normal but averages between two thirds and three quarters of normal. In patients with cuff-tear arthropathy who have extensive rotator-cuff deficiency, average movement following surgery is between one third and one half of normal. Younger patients undergoing shoulder arthroplasty, regardless of diagnosis, seem to have poorer outcomes and require more frequent revisions.[21]

Although advice varies, many surgeons allow patients who have undergone this procedure to perform ordinary daily activities, do lighter forms of yard work, play golf, play recreational tennis, do recreational swimming, and enjoy similar activities. Typically, it is suggested that these patients avoid activities that involve repetitive impact loading, undertake only occasional heavy lifting, and avoid extremely repetitive arm movements.

The need for revision surgery has been infrequent; in general, it approximates 1 percent a year and is additive. Thus, for a group of patients 10 years after shoulder arthroplasty, 90 percent would still be functioning satisfactorily, and 10 percent would have required some form of reoperation. A review of results from the literature for nearly 1500 unconstrained total shoulder arthroplasties revealed that, at an average of 3.9 years of follow-up (range 1.7 to 10 years), 90 percent of patients reported little or no pain and had, on average, 98 degrees of shoulder elevation. Complications occurred in 13.7 percent overall, but most did not lead to revision.[19,22]

▊ Conclusions and Recommendations

Imaging methods are now available to help the physician understand the structural changes that occur in the shoulder as a result of rheumatologic conditions. Conservative management may be rewarding but in advanced disease is often inadequate. A variety of operative treatments are available, but prosthetic arthroplasty is now the treatment of choice. Humeral-head replacement alone is considered for patients with humeral-head disease in the absence of glenoid involvement or with a large amount of glenoid bone destruction that precludes support for a glenoid component. An additional indication for humeral-head replacement is the patient with a massive tear of the rotator cuff.[23] Otherwise, total shoulder arthroplasty, with replacement of both the humeral head and the glenoid surface, is usually considered the optimal treatment for advanced arthritic conditions.

Although many forms of prosthetic arthroplasty are available, most designs are quite similar in concept and vary only in the details. Both cemented and tissue-ingrowth designs are available. Cement fixation for the glenoid is probably more desirable, and tissue-ingrowth fixation for the humerus is perhaps reasonable in this anatomic location, although some express a preference for cement fixation.[24]

The indications for shoulder arthroplasty are found less commonly than for arthroplasty for the hip or the knee; however, the shoulder parallels those other major joints in many respects. The indications for surgery are similar, the modes of conservative management are almost identical, the operative treatment options are similar, and the outcome of prosthetic arthroplasty is comparable. What distinguishes the shoulder so dramatically is the enormous variability in the characteristics of the different forms of shoulder arthritis and the great heterogeneity of adjunctive procedures needed at the time of surgery. Also, more attention must be directed toward integration of the surgical findings, operative repair, and postoperative rehabilitation. The postoperative rehabilitation is not complicated, but it is prolonged and requires considerable patient cooperation. The ability of the patient to protect the shoulder following surgery yet still accomplish the rehabilitation is a delicate balance and perhaps the biggest challenge of treatment in this area.

REFERENCES

1. van Den Ende C, Rozing P, Dijkmans B, et al: Assessment of shoulder function in rheumatoid arthritis. J Rheumatol 23:2043, 1996.
2. Alasaarela E, Alasaarela E: Ultrasound evaluation of painful rheumatoid shoulders. J Rheumatol 21:1642, 1994.
3. Hattrup S, Cofield R, Berquist T, et al: Shoulder arthrography for determination of the size of rotator cuff tear. J Shoulder Elbow Surg 1:98, 1992.
4. Alasaarela E, Suramo I, Tervonen O, et al: Evaluation of humeral head erosions in rheumatoid arthritis: A comparison of ultrasonography, magnetic resonance imaging, computed tomography and plain radiography. Br J Rheumatol 37:1152, 1998.
5. Rozing P, Brand R: Rotator cuff repair during shoulder arthroplasty in rheumatoid arthritis. J Arthroplasty 13:311, 1998.
6. Wakitani S, Imoto K, Saito M, et al: Evaluation of surgeries for rheumatoid shoulder based on the destruction pattern. J Rheumatol 26:41, 1999.
7. Hirooka A, Wakitani S, Yoneda M, et al: Shoulder destruction in rheumatoid arthritis: Classification and prognostic signs in 83 patients followed 5-23 years. Acta Orthop Scand 67:258, 1996.
8. Sanchez-Sotelo J, Cofield RH, Rowland CM: Shoulder hemiarthroplasty for glenohumeral arthritis associated with severe rotator cuff deficiency. J Bone Joint Surg Am 83:1814, 2001.
9. Koorevaar R, Merkies N, de Waal Malefijt M, et al: Shoulder hemiarthroplasty in rheumatoid arthritis: 19 cases reexamined after 1-17 years. Acta Orthop Scand 68:243, 1997.
10. Friedman R, Thornhill T, Thomas W, et al: Non-constrained total shoulder replacement in patients who have rheumatoid arthritis and class-IV function. J Bone Joint Surg Am 71:494, 1989.
11. Nwakama AC, Cofield RH, Kavanagh BF, et al: Semiconstrained total shoulder arthroplasty for glenohumeral arthritis and massive rotator cuff tearing. J Shoulder Elbow Surg 9:302, 2000.
12. Hattrup S, Cofield R: Osteonecrosis of the humeral head: Relationship of disease stage, extent, and cause to natural history. J Shoulder Elbow Surg 8:559, 1999.
13. McCarty D: Robert Adams' rheumatic arthritis of the shoulder: "Milwaukee shoulder" revisited. J Rheumatol 16:668, 1989.
14. Neer C, Craig E, Fukuda H: Cuff-tear arthropathy. J Bone Joint Surg Am 65:1232, 1983.
15. Zeman C, Arcand M, Cantrell J, et al: The rotator cuff-deficient arthritis shoulder: Diagnosis and surgical management. J Am Acad Orth Surg 6:337, 1998.
16. McCarty D, Halverson P, Carrera G, et al: "Milwaukee shoulder"—association of microspheroids containing hydroxyapatite crystals, active collagenase, and neutral protease with rotator cuff defects. I. Clinical aspects. Arthritis Rheum 24:464, 1981.
17. Richards R, Beaton D, Hudson A: Shoulder arthrodesis with plate fixation: Functional outcome analysis. J Shoulder Elbow Surg 2:225, 1993.
18. Neer C: Replacement arthroplasty for glenohumeral osteoarthritis. J Bone Joint Surg Am 56:1, 1974.
19. Torchia M, Cofield R, Settergren C: Total shoulder arthroplasty with the Neer prosthesis: long-term results. J Shoulder Elbow Surg 6:495, 1997.
20. Goldberg BA, Smith K, Jackins S, et al: The magnitude and durability of functional improvement after total shoulder arthroplasty for degenerative joint disease. J Shoulder Elbow Surg 10:464, 2001.
21. Sperling J, Cofield R, Rowland C: Neer hemiarthroplasty and Neer total shoulder arthroplasty in patients fifty years old or less. Long-term results. J Bone Joint Surg Am 80:464, 1998.
22. Lynch N, Cofield R, Silbert P, et al: Neurologic complications after total shoulder arthroplasty. J Shoulder Elbow Surg 5:53, 1996.
23. Boyd AD, Thomas W, Scott R, et al: Total shoulder arthroplasty versus hemiarthroplasty. Indications for glenoid resurfacing. J Arthroplasty 5:1990, 1998.
24. Stewart M, Kelly I: Total shoulder replacement in rheumatoid disease: 7- to 13-year follow-up of 37 joints. J Bone Joint Surg Br 79:1997, 1997.

THE CERVICAL SPINE
CLEMENT B. SLEDGE

Rheumatoid Arthritis

Rheumatoid arthritis eventually affects the cervical spine in most patients with long-standing disease.(see Fig. 116-24)[1] The thoracic and lumbar spine are seldom involved. Radiographic involvement in the cervical area varies from 43 to 86 percent, depending on the duration of the disease, and appears after a mean duration of 16 years.[2] The clinician should be aware of the possibility of spine involvement and should ensure that before manipulation of the neck, such as occurs during general anesthesia, the stability of the spine and safety of the spinal cord are determined.[3] Neurologic compromise occurs in 11 to 58 percent of these patients[4] and is correlated to levels of C-reactive protein (CRP), peripheral joint involvement, and carpal collapse.[5]

PATHOPHYSIOLOGY OF SUBLUXATIONS

Involvement of the cervical spine results in destruction of joints, ligaments, and bone by synovitis, which produces subluxations, nerve compression, and, in certain instances, basilar impression and sudden death.[4] In addition, the vertebral artery may be involved due to subluxation, proliferative synovial tissues, or both. These pathophysiologic changes in the cervical spine may produce either subluxation, usually of C1-C2 (atlantoaxial subluxation [AAS], seen in approximately 50% of patients) (Fig. 116–24), basilar impression (atlantoaxial impaction [AAI], seen in approximately 35% of patients) (Fig. 116–25), or subaxial involvement of facet joints and intervertebral disks (seen in approximately 15% of patients).

The activity of RA in the cervical spine appears to begin early in the disease and progresses in relation to peripheral involvement. The severity of cervical spine damage strongly correlates with that of peripheral erosive disease, and subluxation is more likely in patients with progressive peripheral erosions, a history of medical therapy with glucocorticoids, seropositivity, elevated CRP levels, male gender, the presence of rheumatoid subcutaneous nodules, and the presence of erosive and mutilating articular disease.[5,6]

ANATOMY OF SUBLUXATIONS

Atlantoaxial Subluxation

Atlantoaxial stability is dependent on the transverse, alar, and apical ligaments. Anterior subluxation of more than 10 to 12 mm implies destruction of the entire ligamentous complex and reduces the space available for the spinal cord. Most anterior AASs in RA are of this magnitude. An atlantodental distance of greater than 3.5 mm is considered abnormal in an adult. Using that criterion, 43 to 86 percent of RA patients exhibit subluxations.[7]

Atlantoaxial Impaction

AAI, also known as cranial settling, pseudobasilar invagination, vertical subluxation of the axis, and superior migration of the odontoid (SMO) (Fig. 116–26), is a consequence of bone and cartilage loss from the occipitoatlantal and atlantoaxial joints. AAI is found in 5 to

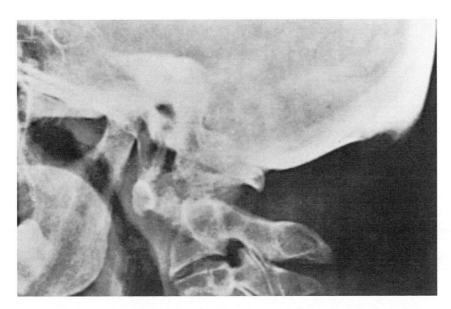

FIGURE 116–24 • Rheumatoid arthritis (RA) with forward displacement of the atlas. The odontoid process is in the center of the C1 ring. (From Fielding JW: Rheumatoid arthritis of the cervical spine. *In*: The American Academy of Orthopaedic Surgeons: Instructional Course Lectures. Vol XXXII. St. Louis, Mosby, 1983, pp 114.)

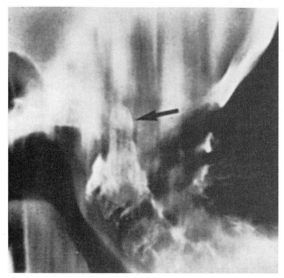

FIGURE 116-25 · Advanced destruction of the atlantoaxial articulation with upward displacement of the odontoid. (From Fielding JW: Rheumatoid arthritis of the cervical spine. *In*: The American Academy of Orthopaedic Surgeons: Instructional Course Lectures. Vol XXXII. St. Louis, Mosby, 1983, pp 114. Courtesy of Harvey L. Barish, MD.)

32 percent of rheumatoid patients and accounts for 22 percent of all upper cervical subluxations.[7] AAI has been measured in a variety of ways; using McGregor's line, the height of the tip of the odontoid above a line from the hard palate to the occiput on a lateral view (Fig. 116–27), is probably the most traditional.[8] Ranawat and colleagues defined a more useful index that relies on the actual settling of C1 on C2.[9] This index avoids the difficulty of defining the hard palate, which is often not included in the radiograph, and the eroded odontoid[10] (Fig. 116–28).

The subaxial cervical spine (Fig. 116–29) is affected through involvement of the facets, interspinous ligaments, and intervertebral disks (spondylodiskitis).[11]

CLINICAL FINDINGS

The clinical manifestations of cervical RA are pain, neurologic disturbance, and, rarely, death.[12,13] Pain is typically in the neck and occipital area and is accompanied by stiffness and crepitus. The Sharp/Purser test, in which the flexed head is forced into extension while the spinous process of C2 is held fixed, has been reported to be positive in 20 to 44 percent of patients with anterior AAS.[6] Neurologic changes, found in 11 to 58 percent of

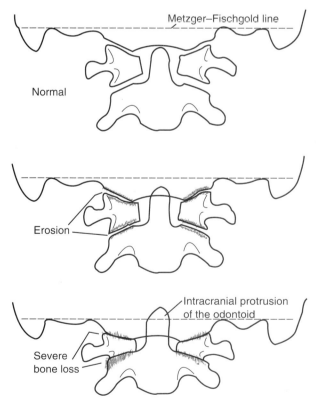

FIGURE 116-26 · Stages in destruction of the atlantoaxial articulation with resultant settling of the skull and upward displacement of the odontoid process into the foramen magnum. Fischgold and Metzger's line (a line drawn between the two digastric grooves on the anteroposterior laminogram of the skull) will pass well above the odontoid tip (10.7 mm). It can be used to determine the degree of upper displacement of the odontoid process. (From Fischgold H, Metzger J: Etude radiotomographique de l'impression basilaire. Rev Rhum Mal Osteoartic 19:261, 1952.)

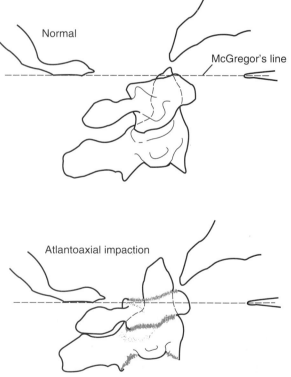

FIGURE 116-27 · Schematic representation of the normal relationship of the odontoid to the base of the skull and upward displacement of the odontoid incident to destruction of the atlantoaxial articulation. McGregor's line can be used for routine screening. Normally, the tip of the odontoid process should be no more than 4.5 mm above McGregor's line, which is drawn from the upper surface of the posterior edge of the hard palate to the most caudal portion of the occipital curve of the skull. (From McGregor M: The significance of certain measurements of the skull in the diagnosis of basilar impression. Br J Radiol 21:171, 1948.)

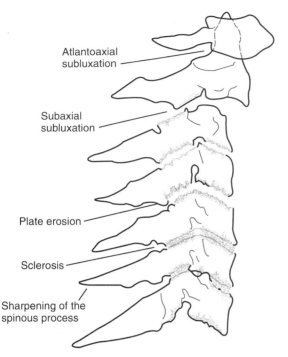

FIGURE 116-28 · Schematic representation of the effects of the rheumatoid process on the cervical spine. (From Fielding JW: Rheumatoid arthritis of the cervical spine. *In*: The American Academy of Orthopaedic Surgeons: Instructional Course Lectures. Vol XXXII. St. Louis, Mosby, 1983, pp 114. Courtesy of William Park.)

patients with radiographic involvement, may be vague and are often misinterpreted as entrapment neuropathy or rheumatoid peripheral neuropathy. Occipital neuralgia is commonly observed, and pyramidal tract involve-

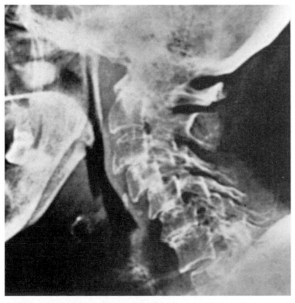

FIGURE 116-29 · Subaxial Rheumatoid Involvement. The disk spaces are markedly narrowed without significant sclerosis. The endplates collapse into one another, and the vertebral spines are thinned and "sharpened." Subluxation from C3 to C6 has occurred in "stepladder" fashion. (From Fielding JW: Rheumatoid arthritis of the cervical spine. *In*: The American Academy of Orthopaedic Surgeons: Instructional Course Lectures. Vol XXXII. St. Louis, Mosby, 1983, pp 114. Used by permission.)

ment is manifest in upper motor neuron signs and pathologic reflexes. Vertebrobasilar insufficiency may cause a loss of equilibrium, tinnitus, vertigo, visual disturbances, and diplopia. Subjective sensation may be altered, yielding paresthesias, numbness, and sensations of hot and cold. Bulbar disturbances can be paroxysmal and fatal. They may occur as abnormalities in swallowing and phonation. Sphincter disturbance usually presents as urinary retention and then incontinence. It may be difficult to interpret symptoms and signs in the face of severe, crippling polyarticular disease; somatosensory-evoked potentials (SSEP) and transcranial Doppler (TCD) may be helpful.[14] Sleep apnea is a rare and potentially lethal syndrome seen with severe AAI.[13]

Natural History

As indicated previously, cervical spine involvement in RA appears to start early in the course of the disease and correlates with the extent and severity of the disease process elsewhere. This circumstance underlines the importance of early, aggressive, continued medical intervention. Pain, neurologic disturbance, and death are the main concerns. Pain is found in 40 to 88 percent of affected patients.[7] The rate of neural compromise because of cervical instability ranges from 11 to 58 percent.[4] Even asymptomatic patients who are to under general anesthesia should be carefully screened to avoid manipulation of an unstable cervical spine, which can have grave neurologic consequences.[3,15]

Worsening of existing radiologic subluxations over time was reported to occur in 80 percent of cases in one report.[7] Neurologic progression is less certain and correlates with severity of the disease process in peripheral joints and the degree of cervical involvement as revealed radiographically.[16] Once cervical myelopathy is established, death is imminent.[1,2] Only surgical stabilization of the spine, usually with decompression, offers prolonged survival and continued function.

In summary, patients with cervical RA are at risk for premature, spontaneous death and are at risk when undergoing general anesthesia. Subluxation can worsen with time, but neurologic progression is less marked. Once cervical myelopathy is established, the natural history without surgical intervention is grave.[17] Careful neurologic examination, usually supplemented by magnetic resonance imaging (MRI) and, occasionally employing SSEP and TCD, is needed to detect threatening neural involvement and institute timely treatment.

Radiographic Imaging

The usefulness of plain radiographs with flexion and extension views cannot be overemphasized because they permit initial assessment of involvement, instability, and the areas likely to need further study. On the basis of plain radiographs, Weissman and coworkers defined risk factors that predisposed to cord compression and neurologic involvement.[6] The concept of impending neurologic deficit has been used to describe a patient with marked instability in whom neurologic deterioration is likely. This group includes patients who, despite the absence of clinical signs of myelopathy, have one of the following:

- Atlantodental distance of more than 8 mm and cord compression on neuroradiologic studies
- Subaxial subluxation of more than 4 mm and cord compression on neuroradiologic studies
- AAI with the dens through the foramen magnum and spinal cord or brain stem compression on neuroradiologic studies

Computed tomography (CT) can show the extent of erosions and spinal cord compression and the axial and sagittal relationships.[10] The degree of medullary compression seen on the CT scan in anterior AAS correlates with the presence of upper motor neuron signs but underestimates the situation because of the failure to visualize soft tissue pannus, which can further decrease available space for the cord; this shortcoming can be overcome by adding intrathecal contrast material to demonstrate the pannus.

MRI is adding further definition to the pathologic anatomy of the cervical spine in RA.[18] It has the advantage of requiring no contrast material and can be reformatted in any plane. The craniomedullary junction and the entire length of the cervical cord can be visualized. T_2-weighted images display a myelographic image demonstrating occlusion of the subarachnoid space, whereas T_1-weighted images show the cord itself. Erosion, pannus, and inflammation of soft tissues can be demonstrated.[18,19] MRI has been used in a functional evaluation of the spinal cord, with the cord in a flexed position to demonstrate compression when it is absent with the neck in neutral or extension.[20] In one study of 34 patients with AAS, 22 had more than 3 mm of pannus behind the dens, and 12 had myelopathic signs. The spinal-cord diameter was decreased from 7.4 to 6.5 mm in flexion.[21]

Demonstration of such radiologic parameters may further allow early clinical definition of the patient at risk for neurologic deterioration. Because of the expense of MRI studies, several authors have suggested the clinical and plain radiographic findings that indicate the need for MRI.[18,22] Reiter and Boden have suggested that all patients with cervical spine abnormalities and neurologic deficits have an MRI scan; patients with contraindications to MRI scanning should have a CT scan with intrathecal contrast.[11]

Nonsurgical Management

Medical management aimed toward reduction of synovitis is the cornerstone of nonsurgical treatment of cervical RA. The remaining treatment is symptomatic. Cervical collars are commonly used and, when coupled with patient education, have been reported to reduce symptoms of AAS.[23,24] Collars are used for psychologic support, pain relief, warmth, and a feeling of stability, with some instances of improvement in subluxation. Rigid orthoses have no special advantage and are not well tolerated. Patient education is critical to successful conservative management.

Surgical Management

The indications for surgery are intractable pain and neurologic abnormality. The presence of a subluxation is not an indication, because subluxations are common and are not necessarily a clinical problem. Progression of instability is a relative indication for surgery; a spinal cord diameter of less than 6 mm at C1-C2, a posterior atlantodental interval of less than 14 mm, and cranial migration of greater the 31.5 mm have been proposed as indications for surgical intervention.[11] Patients with rheumatoid disease tend to be severely affected, with debilitation, crippling, poor skin, and difficult airways for anesthetic intubation. They are further compromised by an unstable neck, susceptibility to infection, and poor wound-healing capability. These circumstances present preoperative, intraoperative, and postoperative challenges reflected by significant morbidity and mortality. Preoperative skeletal traction is necessary to reduce subluxation and myelopathic changes. Constant skeletal traction is recommended by most surgeons.[9]

Stabilization through posterior fusion is the most common surgical procedure. The use of internal fixation may allow the rapid mobilization of the patient and the avoidance of cumbersome halo casts. Surgical series are usually mixes of subluxations at different levels and combinations of subluxations in a given patient. Current guidelines are to select patients who are at risk and operate on them early to prevent progressive neurologic deficits, which may be irreversible. The results of surgical stabilization are good, with pain relief reported in 92 percent and improved neurologic function in 89 percent in one series of 26 patients.[25] Another series reported less satisfactory results: "Overall, 67 percent felt that surgery had been successful. Surgery was more successful in producing symptomatic relief in patients with neck or radicular pain than in those with neurologic deficit, but did prevent progression of neurologic symptoms".[26] In a series of 10 patients over the age of 70, the results of cervical fusion were comparable to a series in younger patients.[27]

The postoperative mortality rate is 0 to 33 percent, but the trend in the more recent reports is toward less than 10 percent mortality, possibly because of earlier intervention and improved anesthetic and perioperative management.[28]

Transoral decompression has been advocated for irreducible AAS and in situations in which pannus behind the dens causes persistent compression.[29-31]

Complications of fusion of any type include, but are not limited to, infections in up to 25 percent of patients, wound dehiscence, and occasional quadriplegia. Late subaxial subluxation below previous fusion has been reported, and previously asymptomatic levels can develop subluxation below rigid spinal segments so that long-term follow-up is necessary.

In the subaxial area, subluxations are usually stabilized by wired posterior fusions.

At all levels, the surgical goal is alignment of the spine, decompression where necessary, and the stabilization of the segments involved.

Ankylosing Spondylitis

Unlike RA, which results in joint destruction, ankylosing spondylitis (AS) results in joint fusion. Spine involvement usually begins in the lumbar area, with later involvement of the thoracic and cervical regions. In the cervical region, this involvement often produces ankylosis from the occiput downward (Fig. 116–30).

CLINICAL SIGNS

In the cervical region, the pain, stiffness, and limitation of motion associated with a flexion deformity usually cause patients to seek medical advice. To compensate for the cervical deformity, they may simultaneously flex the hips and knees to obtain a horizontal "line of sight."

SURGICAL MANAGEMENT

If the patient's head position is satisfactory, and the cervical spine is completely fused, there is little surgery can offer. Surgical intervention may be necessary in unacceptable cervical flexion deformities, in fractures, and in threatening atlantoaxial displacements.

The most common spinal complication of AS is spontaneous fusion of the spine, often with unacceptable fixed flexion (Fig. 116–31). If the deformity is maximal in the cervical or cervicothoracic junction, cervical osteotomy provides satisfactory correction. Simmons recommends that the procedure be performed using local anesthetic, with the patient in the sitting position and a halo ring and halo jacket applied.[32] A laminectomy is performed at the C7 level; the spine is then manually fractured at the C7-D1 level by backward pressure on the head, and correction is obtained.[33] Osteotomy of the spine at this level is recom-

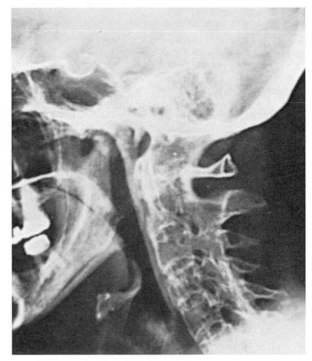

FIGURE 116–30 · Ankylosing Spondylitis (AS) with Solid Fusion from the Occiput Down.

mended because the vertebral canal is wider in this region and also because the vertebral arteries enter the foramen transversarium at C6, above the osteotomy site. Most patients benefit from the procedure with reduced pain, improved ability to look forward, and improved neurologic complaints.[33] (Fig. 116–32). In some instances the maximum deformity is in the lumbar area, and osteotomy

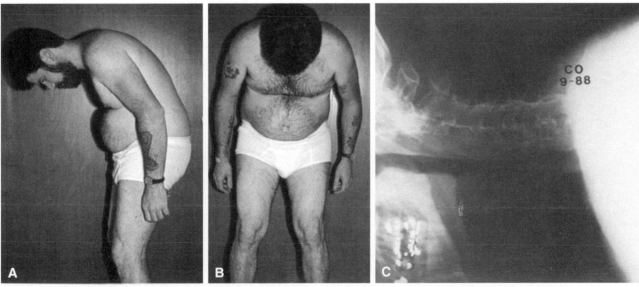

FIGURE 116–31 · Ankylosing Spondylitis (AS) with Severe Deformity. *A,* View of the patient from the side. *B,* View of the patient from the front. Both views show how severe the deformity is; it gives the patient virtually no ability to see much ahead of his feet. *C,* Lateral radiograph of the solidly fused spine showing that most of the deformity is at the cervicothoracic junction. (From Bohlman HH, Dabb B: Anterior and posterior cervical osteotomy. *In* Bradford DS (ed): The Spine. New York, Raven Press, 1997, pp 85.)

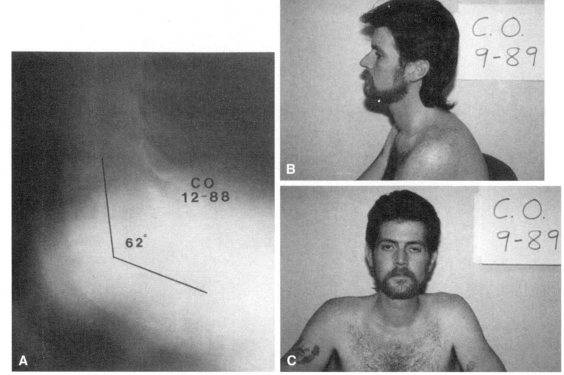

FIGURE 116–32 • Same patient as in Figure 116–31 seen 3 months after a corrective osteotomy at C-7 and T-1. *A*, The amount of correction was 62 degrees, giving the patient the ability to direct his gaze forward (B and C). (From Bohlman HH, Dabb B: Anterior and posterior cervical osteotomy. *In* Bradford DS (ed): The Spine. New York, Raven Press, 1997, pp 86.)

at that level is indicated.[34,35] At either cervical or lumbar area, corrective spine surgery in AS is a formidable procedure; the patient should be informed of the neurologic and other hazards before the operation to aid him or her in making an informed decision about treatment.

FRACTURES

The rigidity of the spondylitic cervical spine, unprotected by ribs or normal musculature, renders it particularly vulnerable to trauma. The force of a blow cannot be absorbed by mobile cervical segments, and the ankylosed spine may behave in a manner similar to a long bone. Because there is also a degree of osteoporosis, the spine may fracture easily with minimal pain, and the patient may not recall the injury. The fractures are usually transverse, occur at the level of a disk space, and are generally at the midportion of the neck.

Not all fractures of the ankylosed cervical spine are benign; some are associated with a poor prognosis. The normal flexibility of the neck is eliminated by the ankylosing process. Therefore, all motion takes place at the fracture site and frequently results in a nonunion with exuberant callus and symptoms of pain and neurologic involvement. Because of the fused segments above and below the fracture it is difficult to control motion and allow the fracture to heal. Surgery to stabilize the spine is often necessary.[36] The radiographic appearance may suggest a tumor unless the true nature of the condition is understood.

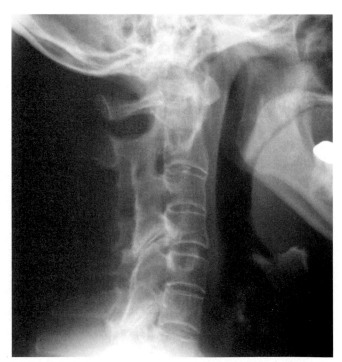

FIGURE 116–33 • Juvenile rheumatoid arthritis (JRA) with early onset that has resulted in complete ankylosis of the cervical spine.

Juvenile Rheumatoid Arthritis

The cervical spine is involved in many children with juvenile rheumatoid arthritis (JRA) who experience disease onset in infancy or adolescence, often without symptoms. Involvement is usually manifest as stiffness with occasional spontaneous fusion of the posterior arches (Fig. 116–33). In patients with later onset, the cervical spine is involved with about the same frequency as in adults with RA. MRI may detect involvement in patients who are asymptomatic. One study demonstrated involvement in 13 of 18 patients of whom only four had changes on plain radiographs: Because "the early diagnostic ability of MRI in JRA allows early therapeutic intervention, every patient with a probable diagnosis of JRA would benefit from MRI."[38]

REFERENCES

1. Clark C: Rheumatoid involvement of the cervical spine: An overview. Spine 19:2257, 1994.
2. Falope ZF, Griffiths ID, Platt PN, Todd NV: Cervical myelopathy and rheumatoid arthritis: a retrospective analysis of management. Clin Rehabil 16:625-629, 2002.
3. Kwek T, Lew T, Thoo F: The role of preoperative cervical spine X-rays in rheumatoid arthritis. Anaesth Intensive Care 26:636, 1998.
4. Rawlins BA, GFaB-AO: Rheumatoid arthritis of the cervical spine. Rheum Dis Clin North Am 24:55, 1998.
5. Fujiwara K, Fujimoto M, Owaki H: Cervical lesions related to the systemic progression in rheumatoid arthritis. Spine 23:2052, 1998.
6. Weissman B, Aliabadi P, Weinfeld M: Prognostic features of atlantoaxial subluxation in rheumatoid arthritis. Radiology 144:745, 1982.
7. Pellicci P, Ranawat C, Tsairis P: A prospective study of the progression of rheumatoid arthritis of the cervical spine. J Bone Joint Surg Am 63:342, 1981.
8. McGregor M: The significance of certain measurements of the skull in the diagnosis of basilar impression. Br J Radiol 21:171, 1948.
9. Ranawat C, O'Leary P, Tsairis P: Cervical fusion in rheumatoid arthritis. J Bone Joint Surg Am 61:1003. 1979
10. Riew KD, Hilibrand AS, Palumbo MA, Sethi N, Bohlman HH. Diagnosing basilar invagination in the rheumatoid patient: The reliability of radiographic criteria. J Bone Joint Surg Am 83-A: 194-200, 2001.
11. Reiter M, Boden S: Inflammatory disorders of the cervical spine. Spine 23:2755, 1998.
12. Mikulowski P, Wolheim F, Rotmil P: Sudden death in rheumatoid arthritis with atlantoaxial dislocation. Acta Med Scand 198:445, 1975.
13. Drossaers-Bakker K, Hamburger H, Bongartz E: Sleep apnea caused by rheumatoid arthritis. Br J Rheumatol 37:889, 1998.
14. Babic-Naglic D, Nesek-Madaric V, Potocki K: Early diagnosis of rheumatoid cervical myelopathy. Scand J Rheumatol 26:247, 1997.
15. Casey AT, Crockard HA, Pringle J, et al: Rheumatoid arthritis of the cervical spine: Current techniques for management. Orthop Clin North Am 33:291-309, 2002.
16. Paimela L, Laasonen L, Kankaanpaa E: Progression of cervical spine changes in patients with early rheumatoid arthritis. J Rheumatol 24:1280, 1997.
17. Hamilton JD, Johnston RA, Madhok R, Capell HA: Factors predictive of subsequent deterioration in rheumatoid cervical myelopathy. Rheumatology (Oxford) 40:811-815, 2001.
18. Einig M, Higer H, Meairs S: Magnetic resonance imaging of the craniocervical junction in rheumatoid arthritis: Value, limitations, indications. Skeletal Radiol 19:341, 1990.
19. Jacobsen EA, Riise T: MRI of cervical spine with flexion and extension used in patients with rheumatoid arthritis. Scand J Rheumatol 29:249-254, 2000.
20. Allmann K, Uhl M, Uhrmeister P: Functional MR imaging of the cervical spine in patients with rheumatoid arthritis. Acta Radiol 39:543, 1998.
21. Dvorak J, Grob D, Baumgartner H: Functional evaluation of the spinal cord by magnetic resonance imaging in patients with rheumatoid arthritis and instability of the upper cervical spine. Spine 10:1057, 1989.
22. Reijnierse M, Bloem J, Dijkmans B: The cervical spine in rheumatoid arthritis: relationship between neurologic signs and morphology of MR imaging and radiographs. Skeletal Radiol 25:113, 1996.
23. Kauppi M, Anttila P: A stiff collar for the treatment of rheumatoid atlantoaxial subluxation. Br J Rheumatol 35:771-774, 1996.
24. Kauppi M, Leppanen L, Heikkila S: Active conservative treatment of atlantoaxial subluxation in rheumatoid arthritis. Br J Rheumatol 37:417-420, 1998.
25. Eyres K, Gray D, Robertson P: Posterior surgical treatment for the rheumatoid cervical spine. Br J Rheumatol 37:756, 1998.
26. McRorie E, McLoughlin P, Russell T: Cervical spine surgery in patients with rheumatoid arthritis: an appraisal. Ann Rheum Dis 55:99, 1996.
27. Mizutani J, Tsubouchi S, Fukuoka M, et al: Surgical treatment of the rheumatoid cervical spine in patients aged 70 years or older. Rheumatology (Oxford) 41:910-916, 2002.
28. van Asselt KM, Lems WF, Bongartz EB, et al: Outcome of cervical spine surgery in patients with rheumatoid arthritis. Ann Rheum Dis 60:448-452, 2001.
29. Brattstrom H, Elner A, Granholm L: Transoral surgery for myelopathy caused by rheumatoid arthritis of the cervical spine. Ann Rheum Dis 32:578, 1973.
30. Crockard H, Calder I, Ransford A: One-stage transoral decompression and posterior fixation in rheumatoid atlanto-axial subluxation. J Bone Joint Surg Am 72:682, 1990.
31. Kerschbaumer F, Kandziora F, Klein C, et al: Transoral decompression, anterior plate fixation, and posterior wire fusion for irreducible atlantoaxial kyphosis in rheumatoid arthritis. Spine 25:2708-2715, 2000.
32. Simmons E: The surgical correction of flexion deformity of the cervical spine in ankylosing spondylitis. Clin Orthop Rel Res 86:132, 1972.
33. McMaster M: Osteotomy of the cervical spine in ankylosing spondylitis. J Bone Joint Surg Br 79:197, 1997.
34. Berven SH, Deviren V, Smith JA, et al: Management of fixed sagittal plane deformity: Results of the transpedicular wedge resection osteotomy. Spine 26:2036-2043, 2001.
35. Kim KT, Suk KS, Cho YJ, et al: Clinical outcome results of pedicle subtraction osteotomy in ankylosing spondylitis with kyphotic deformity. Spine 27:612-618, 2002.
36. Hitchon PW, From AM, Brenton MD, et al: Fractures of the thoracolumbar spine complicating ankylosing spondylitis. J Neurosurg 97:218-222, 2002.
37. Martel W: Pathogenesis of cervical discovertebral destruction in rheumatoid arthritis. Arthritis Rheum 20:1217, 1977.
38. Oren B, Oren H, Osma E: Juvenile rheumatoid arthritis: cervical spine involvement and MRI in early diagnosis. Turk J Pediatr 38:189, 1996.

THE HIP

CLEMENT B. SLEDGE

Since the development of "low-friction arthroplasty" by John Charnley in the 1960s,[1] total hip arthroplasty has become a highly reliable, successful operation with a wide array of indications. The techniques developed for total hip arthroplasty have been expanded to replacement procedures for the other major joints of the extremities. These procedures have been particularly beneficial for patients with rheumatoid arthritis (RA). For them, surgery can mean the difference between being completely disabled, wheelchair-bound, and reliant on others and being independent, ambulatory, and able to carry on with daily activities, hobbies, and work.

Biomechanics of the Hip Joint

A basic knowledge of the mechanics of the hip joint is helpful in understanding the manifestations of hip diseases and their treatment (Fig. 116–34). Biomechanically, the hip can be thought of as a balance scale, with the femoral head acting as the fulcrum.[2] The weight of the person is counterbalanced by the force exerted by the abductor muscles. Because the center of gravity of the body is twice the distance from the femoral head fulcrum, compared to the insertion of the abductor muscles, the force exerted by the muscles must be twice that through the center of gravity. The resultant force acting on the hip joint is a combination of the weight of the body and the pull of the muscles and is three times body weight during single-leg stance. Direct measurement of the forces across the hip joint during level walking have corroborated this mathematic calculation.[3] Consideration

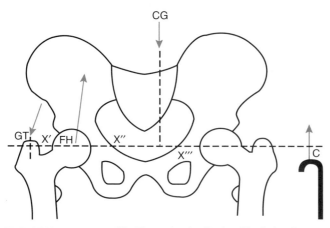

FIGURE 116–34 · Hip Biomechanics During Single-leg Stance. The center of gravity (*point CG*), is approximately twice the horizontal distance (*X*) from the center of the femoral head (*point FH*) than is the abductor muscle insertion (*point GT; distance X*). Therefore, the force exerted by the abductor muscles must be twice that of the center of gravity. The resultant force experienced at the hip joint is approximately three times body weight.

of the biomechanical forces about the hip allows the clinician to understand how force reduction across the hip joint can be accomplished to decrease hip pain. When a hip joint is painful, a person instinctively seeks to diminish the symptoms by leaning toward the painful side. In this way, the center of gravity is brought closer to the femoral head fulcrum and less force is required from the abductor muscles. The net effect is a reduction of the forces across the hip, which reduces pain. It is also clear how important simple weight loss can be, in that a reduction of 10 pounds of body weight will produce a reduction of 30 pounds in the load borne by the hip.[4]

The benefit of a cane also can be understood using this biomechanical model. When a cane is used, part of the body weight is borne by the arm, which reduces the force of the body weight acting on the hip and, therefore, reduces the necessary abductor muscle force. The cane is effective when held in the contralateral hand. Because of the large lever arm, a force of 20 pounds on a cane reduces the force acting on the contralateral hip joint by more than 160 pounds.[4]

Pathologic Conditions of the Hip Joint

Because of the large contact area between the femoral head and acetabulum, forces across the hip joint are widely distributed, and the cartilage can last a lifetime. Given the large forces acting on the joint, however, even a small deformity in the articulating surfaces can predispose to mechanic overload of cartilage and bone with resulting degenerative arthritis.

Chronic irritation arising in the hip can cause a decrease in the range of motion. With time, this can result in secondary contractures of the hip joint capsule and of the muscles around the hip joint. Osteophytes of the femoral head and acetabular margin may produce impingement in certain positions, also limiting hip motion.

OSTEOARTHRITIS

Osteoarthritis (OA) of the hip is likely a culmination of many different events with a similar end result of cartilage destruction. Studies have shown that 76 to 79 percent of patients with hip OA had evidence of previously unrecognized childhood hip disease.[5,6] In other patients, occupational[7,8] or recreational activities[9,10] can be shown to increase the incidence of hip arthritis. Running does not appear to be a risk factor.[11] Regardless of the etiology, progressive OA results in the eventual destruction of the articular cartilage, with osteophytes forming on the femoral head and acetabulum and as cystic changes in the subchondral bone.[12] Patients who undergo replacement of one hip for OA have a

47-percent likelihood of having the other hip replaced within 10 years—a 15-fold increase over the likelihood of hip replacement in the general population.[13]

DEVELOPMENTAL DYSPLASIA OF THE HIP

Hip dysplasia is one of the most common causes of OA in young adults.[14] In this developmental disease, the acetabular fossa remains shallow and provides insufficient coverage for the femoral head. The forces that are normally distributed throughout the acetabular roof are concentrated on the lateral aspect of the acetabulum, resulting in mechanical overload. The proximal femur may also have a deformity consisting of an excessively vertical (valgus) femoral neck with an abnormal rotation that accentuates the abnormal distribution of forces. Eventually, the repetitive overload of the cartilage of the hip may result in arthritis.

AVASCULAR NECROSIS

Avascular necrosis of the femoral head is a significant cause of hip disease in younger patients. Pain may occur from the necrotic process or from collapse of the subchondral bone. This collapse produces a painful synovitis acutely, and the incongruity that is created in the joint usually results in arthritis.

RHEUMATOID ARTHRITIS

Patients with RA have a 25-percent likelihood of undergoing hip replacement within 20 years or more of disease onset.[15] In addition to this high probability of needing a joint replacement, patients with RA and other inflammatory diseases of the hip present a unique situation: Soft tissue deformity is common, and other joints are also affected. Soft tissue contractures of the hip are extremely common, with the usual deformity being flexion and adduction. Involvement of other joints will affect the functional outcome after the hip is treated.

Osteoporosis of the juxta-articular bone is a well-known finding in RA and is related to inflammation with increased local blood flow and, probably, local release of cytokines from the inflamed synovium. The situation is made worse by the immobility caused by the joint stiffness and pain. The chronic use of corticosteroids may worsen this tendency to osteoporosis. As a result of these factors, hips affected by RA are predisposed to protrusio deformity, in which the femoral head deforms the acetabular fossa and progressively enters the confines of the true pelvis (Fig. 116–35).

LABRAL TEARS

In recent years, tears of the acetabular labrum have been increasingly implicated in the etiology of obscure hip pain.[16,17] The patient is usually young and active with no recollection of a specific incident that began the hip pain. Physical examination may reveal a "click" or "clunk" when the hip is flexed, adducted, and internally rotated (producing impingement between the femoral head and the anteriosuperior acetabulum). The diagnosis may be confirmed by arthrography, arthroscopy, or magnetic resonance imaging (MRI), with or without contrast.[2,3]

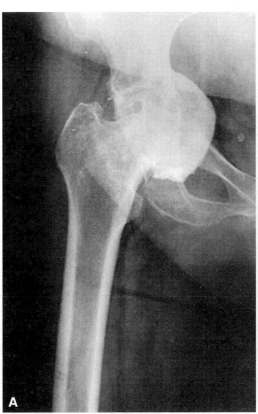
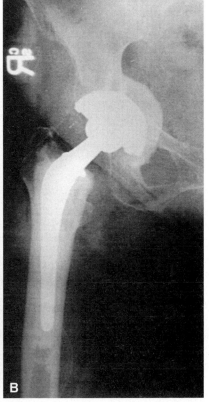

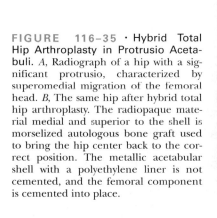

FIGURE 116–35 · Hybrid Total Hip Arthroplasty in Protrusio Acetabuli. *A,* Radiograph of a hip with a significant protrusio, characterized by superomedial migration of the femoral head. *B,* The same hip after hybrid total hip arthroplasty. The radiopaque material medial and superior to the shell is morselized autologous bone graft used to bring the hip center back to the correct position. The metallic acetabular shell with a polyethylene liner is not cemented, and the femoral component is cemented into place.

Treatment can sometimes be accomplished arthroscopically but may require open surgery to correct other pathology such as acetabular dysplasia.[16]

Evaluation of Hip Pain

HISTORY

The patient with hip arthritis may be affected by pain, stiffness, and a limp. Pain about the hip is thought to arise from the richly innervated synovium and capsule of the hip joint. The time course of the pain should be noted; slowly progressive pain is more often seen in OA of the hip. Acute flares of pain may relate to a subchondral fracture, fracture of an osteophyte, acute synovitis, infection, or hemarthrosis.

The location of the pain may offer clues to its etiology. Classically, pain from the hip joint is felt in the groin. Pain may also be present in the buttock and over the hip abductor musculature and lateral thigh. Because the obturator nerve has sensory innervation to both the hip and knee, pain may be referred to the knee joint as well.

A patient complaining of "hip pain" may actually have pain referred from the low back and sacroiliac joints. Many patients with so-called "trochanteric bursitis" actually have referred pain from the lower back. Sacroiliac joint pain is usually localized to the region directly over the sacroiliac joints without radiation. The various forms of low back pain, including facet joint arthritis, disk herniation, and spinal stenosis, all have well-described pain symptoms differentiating them from true hip pain. Hip pathology does not cause pain extending below the knee. A patient with "hip pain" radiating beyond the knee often has pathology in the lower back as the cause of the symptoms. If it is unclear whether the pain is originating in the hip, injection of an analgesic agent into the hip joint under fluorooscopic control may be helpful.[18] Ablation or diminution of the pain after such treatment is strongly suggestive that the hip is actually the source of the pain; a negative result is less helpful.

It is important to assess the impact of hip arthritis on the patient's life. Validated measures such as the SF-36 and WOMAC should be obtained when the patient is first seen so the overall impact of the disease can be measured and followed over time (See chapter 29). The ability of the patient to ambulate and the need to use assistive devices should be noted. The patient should also be questioned regarding specific activities such as the ability to put on shoes and socks, cut toenails, get into a bathtub, sit down on a toilet, drive or ride in a car, use public transportation, ride a bicycle, and climb and descend stairs with or without the use of a banister. If the patient is contemplating surgery, a realistic estimate can be given regarding the restoration of these functional deficits.

The patient's medical history may shed more light onto the cause of the hip pain. A history of diabetes increases the possibility of avascular necrosis of the hip or of diabetic neuropathy causing a Charcot hip. It is also important to note previous treatments. Even a short course of prednisone may precipitate avascular necrosis

of the hip. Radiation osteonecrosis of the hip is a well-documented sequela of pelvic radiotherapy.

PHYSICAL EXAMINATION

The evaluation of the patient's gait is an essential part of the physical examination. The presence and severity of a limp should be noted. The patient should also be examined in a standing position, and any pelvic tilt should be noted. Blocks placed under the patient's short leg may determine the degree of functional leg length inequality. At this time, the back can be examined for scoliosis. The spine should be placed through a full range of motion and pain evaluated carefully.

With the patient supine on the examining table, the range of motion of each lower extremity joint should be noted. Pain in the groin or lower back or buttock with the Patrick test (for which the foot of the involved side is placed on the contralateral distal thigh with the involved hip flexed, maximally abducted, and externally rotated) is indicative of hip joint or sacroiliac joint pathology, which can be further differentiated by the location of the pain produced. The Patrick test is also an excellent screening test for hip arthritis because it measures a combined range of motion of the hip. This motion is limited in patients with hip arthritis and can be quantified by measuring the distance from the involved knee to the examining table. Straight-leg raising tests are useful in differentiating pain originating in the back and hip. Supine leg lengths may be measured at this time from the anterior superior iliac spine to the medial malleolus.

RADIOGRAPHIC EVALUATION

Plain Radiographs

Radiographs of the hip should be obtained in any patient who presents complaining of significant hip pain. The standard views include a standing anteroposterior (AP) view of the pelvis and AP and frog-lateral views of the involved hip. These films should be carefully evaluated for changes in the joint space, juxta-articular changes, extra-articular changes, and any abnormalities of the bones.

Computed Tomography

Computed tomography (CT) is of limited use in the evaluation of a painful hip. It is useful for preoperative planning of total hip surgery when the bony anatomy is abnormal, such as in dysplasia. In addition, CT scan may help to elucidate intra-articular fractures of the femoral head and acetabulum, the degree of deformity in avascular necrosis, and the extent of neoplastic lesions.

Magnetic Resonance Imaging

MRI generally does not add any clinically useful information when plain radiographs reveal evidence of hip arthritis or avascular necrosis with bony collapse. MRI can be useful in evaluating hip pain when radiographs appear normal. Early avascular necrosis can be diagnosed by

MRI before changes are apparent on plain films. Intra-articular soft tissue pathology, such as inflammatory synovitis, pigmented villonodular synovitis, and labral tears, are best demonstrated by MRI, with or with gadolinium enhancement. The technique is also useful in evaluating soft tissue lesions about the hip joint and to evaluate possible neoplastic lesions.

Bone Scans

Technetium bone scanning is useful in investigating occult femoral neck fractures, metastatic and neoplastic diseases of the hip, and avascular necrosis. Bone scanning can also be helpful in the evaluation of suspected osteomyelitis. Unfortunately, a positive bone scan is not specific and must be correlated with the patient's history, physical examination, and other radiologic tests.

Arthrography and Hip-Joint Aspiration

In the adult, hip arthrography has largely been replaced by the noninvasive techniques of CT and MRI studies. It is mainly used to confirm needle placement in the hip joint. Aspiration of the hip joint may be useful in diagnosing septic arthritis and septic loosening of a hip prosthesis. In addition, the administration of local anesthetic following hip aspiration may help to differentiate pain of hip origin from pain of spinal origin.[18]

Nonoperative Management of Hip Pathology

Unless the symptoms are so debilitating that early surgery is indicated, a patient with hip arthritis should initially be treated nonoperatively. Conservative management can consist of pharmacologic treatment combined with methods to reduce forces at the hip joint such as crutches or a cane.

Surgical Treatment of Hip Pathology

ARTHROSCOPY

Arthroscopy of the hip has a limited role in the hip compared to the broad role it plays in the knee and shoulder. A role may exist for synovial biopsies and for the detection of intra-articular pathology that has eluded conventional diagnostic tests. Arthroscopy can be useful in the removal of intra-articular loose bodies from the hip and in the resection of a torn acetabular labrum.[19] In such cases, the ability to remove the offending structure through a small incision makes arthroscopy of the hip attractive.

ARTHRODESIS

Arthrodesis of the hip creates a bony union between the femur and the acetabulum, eliminating all motion. It can provide durable relief of arthritic hip pain in a young patient who is not a candidate for arthroplasty.

Follow-up studies have shown up to 70 percent patient satisfaction at 30 years.[20,21] Prerequisites for consideration of an arthrodesis include a stable spine and ipsilateral knee with no significant arthritis. These joints will be excessively stressed after the hip is fused and a significant number of patients who have undergone arthrodesis of the hip develop arthritis of the spine (55 to 60%), ipsilateral knee (45 to 60%), and contralateral hip (25%).[20] The ideal candidate is an active young adult who performs manual labor. This type of patient places high demands on the hip joint, making total hip arthroplasty a less-attractive option.

OSTEOTOMY

Osteotomy of either the pelvis or proximal femur can be performed to correct a deformity of the hip before significant arthritis develops. The rationale for osteotomies is that by correcting a deformed hip, the clinician may lessen symptoms and alter the abnormal mechanical situation, thereby delaying or even preventing arthritis. Prior to the widespread use of total hip replacement, osteotomy of the proximal femur was used to treat OA and, in some patients, is still an appropriate choice.[22,23] Candidates include young, active patients with evidence of underlying anatomic abnormality such as the sequellae of childhood avascular necrosis (Legg-Perthes disease) or developmental dysplasia. One study of femoral osteotomy at 25 years follow-up revealed that 18 percent of patients required no further surgery, whereas those who had undergone subsequent hip replacement had received almost 10 years of satisfactory service from the osteotomy.[24] Osteotomy of the pelvis has been used to treat early arthritis associated with acetabular dysplasia. Patients with mild to moderate arthritis associated with dysplasia have had significant pain relief and improvement in function from pelvic osteotomy.[25] Those with advanced arthritis usually require hip replacement.

TOTAL HIP ARTHROPLASTY

Indications

The most predictable treatment for end-stage arthritis of the hip joint is total hip arthroplasty. The principal indication for total hip arthroplasty in patients with hip arthritis is severe pain or functional disability despite optimal medical management. Many hip-disease processes can be treated with total hip arthroplasty, but even in a patient with one of these conditions, other sources of the hip pain must always be ruled out. In addition, there should be objective physical and radiographic evidence of hip pathology.

The following conditions, among others, can produce hip dysfunction that can be corrected by total hip arthroplasty:

OA[26]
Inflammatory arthritis[15]
Hip dysplasia[27,28]
Osteonecrosis[29]

Synovial chondromatosis[30]
Paget's disease[31]
Metastatic disease of the hip[32]
Intracapsular hip fracture[33]
Ochronosis[34]
Ankylosing spondylitis (AS)[35]
Infection of a previous hip replacement[36]

Contraindications

Absolute contraindications to primary total hip replacement surgery include the presence of active infection in the hip region or at a distant site, as well as medical conditions that would contraindicate anesthesia or surgery. Relative contraindications to hip replacement include poor local skin condition, impaired vascularity to the extremity, previous sepsis in the involved joint, and arthritis secondary to a neuropathic hip joint. Results are less favorable in patients who are obese, young, and who perform heavy manual labor or participate in demanding sports.

Medical Considerations

Most patients undergoing total joint arthroplasty are either older or have concurrent systemic illnesses; a thorough preoperative assessment is, therefore, imperative. It is important to evaluate the patient for potential sources of occult bacteremia, because prosthetic joints are particularly susceptible to bacterial seeding. Any source of infection must be eradicated before surgery. If the patient requires extensive dental work, it should be done before the implantation of an artificial joint.

Deep-vein thrombosis (DVT) and pulmonary embolism (PE) are relatively common complications after total hip surgery, and the risk factors for thromboembolic disease and anticoagulation should be carefully assessed. History of hematologic disorders, previous intracranial hemorrhage, peptic ulcer disease, or other gastrointestinal bleeding conditions should be noted. To avoid excessive intraoperative blood loss, the patient should discontinue nonsteroidal anti-inflammatory drugs (NSAIDs) 3 days prior to surgery. Because of the risk of transfusion reactions and blood-borne viral illnesses, the patient may be given the option to donate autologous blood before surgery.

In patients who have been receiving corticosteroids, adrenal function may be suppressed. In such cases, perioperative medical management should include appropriate additional doses of corticosteroids to meet the requirements imposed by the metabolic stress of surgery. Patients being treated with methotrexate (MTX) may need to have their dose schedule modified. The decreased renal blood flow that may accompany surgery can diminish renal clearance and increase the chance of MTX toxicity. Additionally, wound complications are felt to be more common in patients on MTX. Because of these risk factors and the ability of most patients to tolerate a short period without MTX, treatment can be delayed for several days before surgery and reinstituted when the patient is homeostatically stable and the incision is healing (see Chapter 59).

Patients with RA have significant involvement of the cervical spine in 30 to 40 percent of cases Flexion and extension radiographs of the cervical spine are usually obtained preoperatively to determine whether instability is present. These patients may also have deformity or loss of flexibility of the cervical spine, as well as arthritis of the temporomandibular joint. These conditions may necessitate the use of special techniques, such as fiberoptic intubation, if general anesthesia is being used. Although we generally use epidural anesthesia during hip replacement surgery, the cervical spine in all rheumatoid patients should be evaluated preoperatively in case general anesthesia becomes necessary intraoperatively.

Rheumatoid patients often have arthritis of multiple upper- and lower-extremity joints. If the upper-extremity function is sufficient to allow the use of a walker or crutches after lower-extremity surgery, it is preferable to operate on the lower extremities first to avoid crutch use with recent upper-extremity arthroplasties. If this is not the case, it may be necessary to first perform upper-extremity arthroplasty to gain enough function in the upper extremities to use the ambulation aids needed for lower-extremity rehabilitation.

In a rheumatoid patient with involvement of multiple joints in the lower extremities, the clinician must evaluate the entire lower extremity. The first priority is with the feet and ankles. The patient must have stable, plantigrade feet to ambulate and must have no areas of skin breakdown, which can become a source of infection. Once the feet and ankles are in satisfactory condition, hip and knee replacement surgery may be considered.

When a patient requires ipsilateral hip and knee replacements, the more painful joint should be operated on first. If the level of pain is equal in both joints, the hip operation is performed first, unless there is such a severe flexion contracture or instability of the knee that rehabilitation would be difficult after total hip arthroplasty. Hip surgery is performed before knee surgery because rehabilitation after hip arthroplasty requires less knee motion than the hip motion required for rehabilitation after knee replacement.

Prosthesis Selection

Much controversy in the literature surrounds the best type of prosthesis to use. An in-depth discussion of this is beyond the scope of this review. The surgeon can use cemented (Fig. 116–36), cementless (Fig. 116–37), or a combination of the two techniques known as a hybrid hip (Fig. 116–38).

Polymethylmethacrylate cement secures the prostheses to the bone by interdigitating into the interstices of the cancellous bone. The advantages of using cement are immediate stable fixation of the prostheses and proven long-term reliability with more than 20 years of experience.[37] Disadvantages of cement include the possibility that particles of the cement may be released from a loose prosthesis and participate in bone resorption, increase wear of the polyethylene, or both.

Cementless prostheses have a porous, coated-metallic surface that provides a three-dimensional sponge into

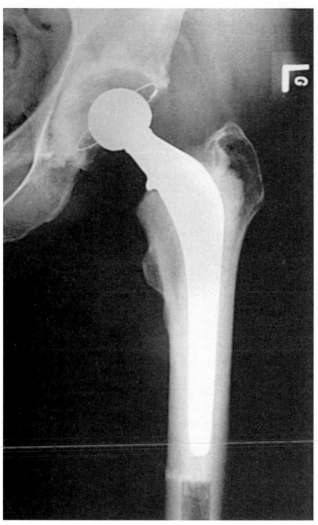

FIGURE 116-36 · Cemented Total Hip Arthroplasty. Both the femoral and acetabular components are cemented into place. The acetabular component is made of polyethylene and is, therefore, not visible radiographically except for the metallic wire located at its rim. The cement mantle is clearly visible around the stem and ends abruptly distally because of a nonopaque cement plug.

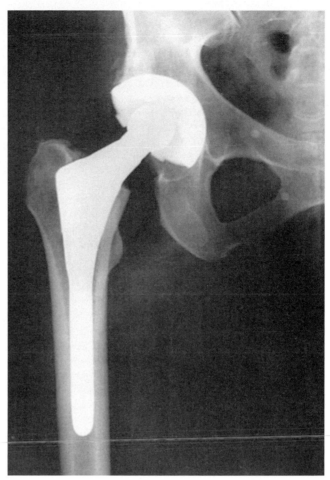

FIGURE 116-37 · Noncemented Total Hip Arthroplasty. Both the cup and stem are inserted without cement. The entire exterior surface of the acetabular shell has a porous, bone-ingrowth coating. This particular stem is proximally porous coated, with the bone ingrowth surface visible radiographically as a less distinct medial and lateral border.

which bone may grow. Another alternative is to coat the prosthesis with hydroxyapatite (HA) allowing bone to adhere directly to the implant.[38] Advantages of cementless systems include direct fixation of bone to the prostheses without an intermediary substance and, possibly, greater preservation of bone stock if revision should become necessary. The disadvantages of cementless femoral components include the observation that their use is associated with a higher incidence of postoperative thigh pain, which, although usually mild, may in rare instances persist for years.[39] Additionally, cementless techniques have been in use for only a little more than a decade, so the long-term results are not yet known. Cementless acetabular cups, on the other hand, have demonstrated better survivorship at 10 years than cemented cups.[40,41] This has led to the common use of the "hybrid hip," which has a cemented femoral component and an uncemented acetabular component.[41]

In adults with RA, current data supports the use of the hybrid hip. This combination provides immediate fixation of the femoral component in a femoral canal that is osteopenic and often patulous and difficult to fit with a cementless sstem. The use of cement results in a low rate of postoperative thigh pain. The uncemented acetabular component provides stable fixation with reduced migration in the osteopenic pelvic bone.[41] For younger patients with good bone stock, many clinicians use a cementless system with a proximally porous-coated femoral component and a porous-coated, metal-backed acetabular component.

Postoperative Regimen

Because infection is a particularly worrisome complication of joint-replacement surgery, prophylactic antibiotics should be administered before surgery.[43] My preference is cefazolin administered shortly before the procedure and continued for 48 hours postoperatively. Vancomycin or clindamycin can be used for patients allergic to cephalosporins. Secondary means utilized to decrease the infection rate include improved operating room air,

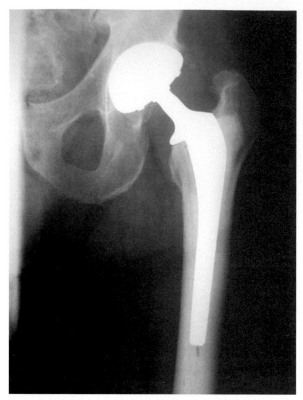

FIGURE 116–38 · Hybrid Hip Replacement. The cup is not cemented but relies on bone ingrowth into its porous surface for fixation. The stem is fixed with cement. (Courtesy of John Sledge MD.)

either by use of ultraviolet lights or laminar flow enclosures, and body exhaust systems ("space suits") for the operating team.

Prophylaxis against venous thromboembolic disease should be undertaken, either by mechanical means (compression leg devices), pharmacologic means (heparin or related substances), or warfarin. My preference is low-dose warfarin therapy begun on the evening of surgery and continued for 4 weeks. The dosage is adjusted to maintain an international normalized ratio (INR) of 2.0. If anticoagulation is contraindicated, the patient should be placed in pneumatic compression stockings and monitored for signs of DVT both clinically and with Doppler ultrasonography. If the patient is at a significant risk for thrombophlebitis and is a poor candidate for anticoagulation, consideration should be given to preoperative placement of an inferior vena cava filter.

Patients are placed in an abduction sling postoperatively to prevent dislocation. Specific dislocation precautions are also explained. Generally, patients are told not to flex the hip beyond 90 degrees or to adduct or internally rotate the hip beyond neutral. They are instructed to sit on a high chair and use an elevated toilet seat to avoid full hip flexion in the early postoperative period. They are also told to sleep in the supine position with a pillow between their legs until 1 month after the operation.

Physical therapy is begun on the first postoperative day. Patients are allowed to bear full weight on the involved leg using two crutches or a walker in the case of a cemented or hybrid total hip replacement, and to bear partial weight in the case of a cementless replacement.

Patients are usually discharged from the hospital in 5 to 7 days. At that time, they are able to get in and out of bed independently, ambulate for short distances with a walker or crutches, and negotiate stairs. Upon discharge, they are encouraged to ambulate as much as possible and are instructed to perform straight-leg raises to strengthen the hip flexors and abductor exercises. Formal physical therapy is generally not necessary after discharge.

Patients are advanced to a single cane or crutch if they have good abductor strength 1 month after surgery. They are allowed to discard the assistive devices when they can walk without a limp. They may sit in chairs of normal height, use a regular toilet, drive a car, and sleep in any position. Supine and side-lying straight-leg raise exercises are taught, and swimming and the use of a stationary bicycle are encouraged.

After total joint arthroplasty, patients should be followed periodically for the rest of their lives. It is important to continue to monitor the condition of the joint because a doctor may find imminent failure of the implant even when the patient is asymptomatic. In such cases, intervention can be performed before bone is resorbed and the problem becomes a greater one.

Once a total joint is implanted, I recommend that patients be given prophylactic antibiotics before the performance of any invasive medical procedure or dental work for the rest of their lives. For dental work, I recommend two doses of amoxicillin (3 g taken 1 hour prior to the procedure and 1.5 g taken 6 hours after the procedure). Whether or not such prophylaxis is necessary is debated.[44,45,46] Given the cost of an infected hip replacement (both in financial terms and in human terms), many feel prophylaxis is appropriate.[45,47]

Results

Both patients with OA and those with RA generally experience immediate and dramatic relief of their hip pain following total hip arthroplasty. Functional improvement is also apparent in most patients. Women, perhaps because they delay surgery until more functionally handicapped, may realize less-complete restoration of function following surgery.[48] Improvement in the quality of life in patients after hip replacement is both predictable and cost effective.[49]

Cemented Primary Total Hip Arthroplasty

The long-term performance of cemented total hip arthroplasty in OA and RA when implanted using early cementing technique has been reported by numerous authors.[50-67] These studies have consistently shown 95- to 96-percent patient satisfaction with the surgery. Pain relief was excellent, with 91 to 99 percent of the patients having mild or no pain after the procedure. In terms of function, 57 to 65 percent could walk well (for more than 30 minutes or five blocks), and 71 to 75 percent either did not use supportive devices or only occasionally used a cane. Survivorship analysis shows an 80- to 84-percent survival rate of total hip arthroplasty at 20 years after surgery. There were radiographic signs of prosthesis loosening in a significant proportion of cases, especially of the acetabular component, but in older patients with limited activity level and relatively low body weight, clinical results often remained excellent despite the radiographic loosening.

Younger patients, those under 40 or 50, have generally had a higher incidence of failure after cemented hip replacement. Joshi and coworkers[51] reported on patients younger than 40 years of age who had hip replacement surgery. After an average of 16 years, 94 percent of the patients had little or no hip pain, and 69 percent had good function. The 20-year implant survivorship was 75 percent. Although the quality of bone in patients with RA is generally inferior to that in patients with OA, the survivorship in rheumatoid patients was 96 percent compared to 51 percent for OA patients in that study. The most probable explanation for this marked difference in survivorship is that the two groups have different levels of activity. Young patients with monarticular OA of the hip tend to be very active after hip replacement surgery. Rheumatoid patients who require hip arthroplasty at a young age often are debilitated from significant polyarticular and systemic disease.

Other studies of rheumatoid patients undergoing hip arthroplasty have not reported the high survivorship rate obtained by Joshi and associates. Rheumatoid patients appear to be particularly susceptible to loosening of the cemented acetabular component. In one study, a 78-percent incidence of progressive acetabular radiolucencies was noted at an average of 7 years after surgery.[52] This was attributed to the poor quality of bone, the bony deficit in protrusio acetabuli, and excessive bleeding from bone in rheumatoid patients, which resulted in suboptimal fixation of the acetabular component.

Because of the incidence of mechanical failure of about 1 percent per year in patients undergoing hip replacement with the original Charnley technique, methods of improving fixation were developed, leading to so-called second- and third-generation cement techniques. These involve better preparation of the bony surfaces and pressurization of cement during insertion.

Cementless Primary Total Hip Arthroplasty

Cementless hip arthroplasty using porous-coated femoral and acetabular components was developed because of disappointing results with cemented arthroplasty using the first-generation technique, particularly in young patients. This system has surfaces designed to allow bony ingrowth into the pores of the surface of the implant. Good bone quality and proper prosthetic fit are prerequisites for success of these implants because growth of bony interdigitation appears to require intimate contact without motion at the interface. Even when bone ingrowth does not occur, the prosthesis may often be effectively stabilized by fibrous ingrowth.

The results at about 10 years of follow-up appear to be roughly comparable to those achieved with modern cement technique. Engh and coworkers[39] have presented the largest follow-up of cementless total hip arthroplasty. They examined the results of porous-coated femoral stem fixation, with patients followed for a minimum of 10 years. The survivorship of the stems was 97 percent and that of the cups was 92 percent. Radiographically, 89 percent of the stems were classified as having stable bone ingrowth fixation, 8 percent had stable fibrous fixation, and 2 percent had unstable fixation. The outcome of cases with stable fibrous fixation was satisfactory but not as good as that with bone ingrowth fixation. Postoperative pain and limp were present in 27 percent of patients without bony fixation of the implant and in 6 percent of patients demonstrating bone ingrowth. A subgroup of patients under 40 years of age did not do quite as well as the older patients, probably reflecting a higher level of activity after surgery. These results are comparable to those obtained with modern cemented femoral fixation.

Postoperative thigh pain has been reported in 15 to 23 percent of patients undergoing total hip arthroplasty using a cementless femoral stem. In most cases, the pain does not limit activity. Engh[39] has reported that with design modifications of the femoral implant, the incidence of thigh pain decreased from 14 percent to 1.2 percent.

A matter of concern for the long-term is the issue of stress shielding; a rigidly fixed implant with bone ingrowth into the proximal portion of the femoral component effectively shields the bone proximal to the site of ingrowth. The greater trochanter, the site of attachment of the abductor muscles, is at risk. In the results available at 10 years, this is a significant radiographic finding but has not yet become a significant clinical problem.[58] However, trochanteric fractures have been reported.[59]

Hybrid Hip Replacement

Based on the long-term studies (10 years for uncemented devices and 20 or more years for cemented devices), many surgeons have come to the conclusion that a combination of the two techniques is preferred: an uncemented acetabular component and a cemented femoral component. The use of cement on the femoral side allows fitting of the component into the often capacious canal seen in patients with RA and improves implant longevity in nonrheumatoid patients. Intermediate-term results suggest that this combination has the lowest rate of complications, including loosening.[60,61]

Patient Age as a Factor

Young patients present a difficult problem in hip-replacement surgery; they have many years ahead in which to develop complications, they may not always follow requested restrictions of activity, and their bones may still be growing and remodeling. Even in patients in their forties and fifties, the mechanical failure rate has been higher than in the usual population for this procedure, who are 65 years and older.[62,63,64] Young patients with RA have lower failure rates than young patients with OA.[65] The failure rate of the cemented acetabular component is significantly higher than failure of the femoral component (50% vs. 8%).

At the other end of the age spectrum, results in patients over the age of 80 are virtually identical to results in the usual patient (aged 60 to 70 years).[66]

Complications

Death

Death following total hip arthroplasty is very unusual; indeed, the life expectancy after hip replacement exceeds that for an age-matched population, as only those deemed fit for surgery are in the operative group. The mortality rate within 42 days of operation in one large study was 0.91 percent, with half of the deaths due to PE.[67] In another series in which prophylaxis for thromboembolism was used, the mortality rate was 0.27 percent.[68]

Infection

With death following hip replacement an extremely rare event (and half of the deaths due to preventable PE), infection becomes the most serious complication of hip replacement. The incidence of infections following total joint arthroplasty is approximately 1 percent over the lifetime of the prosthesis.[69] Infections that occur within 1 year of surgery are most often due to direct contamination at the time of the operation. Late infections, manifesting more than 1 year postoperatively, are usually from hematogenous seeding of the hip joint from distant sources and are most common in patients with RA.[53]

The most important method to decrease the incidence of infection is to administer prophylactic antibiotics.[43] Other means to lower the risk of infection include unidirectional airflow operating rooms, body exhaust systems, ultraviolet light, and the use of double gloves.

Certain conditions are known to increase the risk of infection after total joint arthroplasty: diabetes, psoriasis, RA, steroid use, genitourinary instrumentation, and, perhaps, extensive dental procedures. In one study, patients on chronic renal dialysis were found to have an exceptionally high incidence (19%) of infection.[70] The infection rate in revision total hip surgery (after a previous complication) is at least twice that of primary hip arthroplasty.

The clinical presentation of an infection following total hip arthroplasty can be extremely variable. Infections in the early postoperative period often present with acute symptoms, including pain, fever, wound drainage, swelling, induration, and erythema. Subacute and late infections tend to present more insidiously, with a gradual onset of pain.

The white blood cell (WBC) count is not specific or extremely sensitive for infection. The erythrocyte sedimentation rate (ESR) is more helpful, as it is elevated over 50 mm/hour in most patients with a documented infection, but it too has a low specificity and can be elevated for 1 year after total hip surgery. The C-reactive protein (CRP) level, which is also elevated during infection, is less affected by surgery, normalizing within 3 weeks after total hip arthroplasty, and is, therefore, quite useful.[71] Although none of the tests is specific, persistent elevation of the ESR and CRP—particularly more than 1 year after surgery—is suggestive of infection.

Radiographs appear normal in the early stages of infection and later generally show changes that are difficult to distinguish from aseptic loosening. Periosteal elevation is suggestive of infection (or neoplasm or fracture) but often is not present. A technetium bone scan has good sensitivity for infection, with a negative bone scan meaning that infection is unlikely.[72] Technetium bone scanning is not specific, however, and studies have shown that an indium scan may be a more accurate test for diagnosing septic arthritis compared to the combination of a technetium bone scan and a gallium scan.[73]

Hip aspiration with arthrography to confirm intra-articular needle placement should be performed if infection is suspected. The diagnosis of infection and the identification of the organism can be made if positive cultures are obtained. Although a negative culture of the aspirate does not rule out infection, when combined with clinical impressions and other laboratory data, hip aspiration is extremely useful.

Staphylococcus aureus and *S. epidermidis* are the two most common organisms isolated in most series, each accounting for 26 percent of the cases. Gram-positive cocci are present in approximately 60 percent of the infections, with streptococci being involved in 9 percent of the cases. Gram-negative rods are found in 21 percent, with *Escherichia coli* accounting for 9 percent and *Pseudomonas aeruginosa* for 6 percent. Anaerobes are responsible for 15 percent of the cases.[74,75]

Treatment of an infected hip arthroplasty generally requires both antibiotics and surgical intervention. Use of antibiotics alone to suppress the infection with retention of the implant may be considered in patients too ill to undergo surgery. If the implants are well fixed and the infection is diagnosed early, treatment with antibiotics and surgical irrigation and débridement of the joint with the implants left in place may be attempted, but this is associated with a high failure rate. If the infection cannot be controlled in this manner, the implant must be removed. Two-stage revision surgery is successful in 86 to 95 percent of the cases.[36] This involves thorough débridement with implant removal and temporary implantation of antibiotic-impregnated beads. The patient is treated with parenteral antibiotics for 6 weeks, after which reimplantation of the prosthesis can be performed if there are no signs of infection. With more virulent organisms, such as gram-negative rods, reimplantation should be delayed longer to ensure that the infection has been eradicated. In some cases of severe or recurrent infection, reimplantation of the prosthesis may never be possible.

Thromboembolic Disease

The incidence of DVT in patients undergoing hip or knee arthroplasty without prophylaxis is approximately 40 to 60 percent, with fatal PE occurring in 0.5 to 2 percent of cases.[76,77] Approximately half of the thrombi have been shown to develop intraoperatively.

The incidence of DVT following hip replacement surgery is increased in patients with a previous history of DVT, varicose veins, or malignancy. Patients with OA are at much greater risk than patients with RA. Lengthy hip-replacement surgery is associated with a significantly higher rate of DVT. Both epidural and spinal anesthesia have lower rates of DVT than general anesthesia.[78]

A DVT can lead to postphlebitic syndrome with chronic leg edema, varicosities, and ulcerations. However, the major concern is the risk of embolization and death. Although there is no conclusive data, the literature indicates that the mortality rate in patients who are not treated prophylactically is 0.3 to 0.4 percent, whereas in those who receive adequate prophylaxis, the rate of fatal PE is less than 0.1 percent.[77] Thromboses that occur proximal to the calf are associated with PE. Calf DVTs are thought to be less worrisome, although one study found that 17 percent of distal DVTs propagated proximally within 2 weeks.[79]

Diagnosis of Deep Venous Thrombosis

Because clinical diagnosis of DVT is unreliable, diagnostic tests should be performed if there is any clinical suspicion of DVT and in high-risk patients. Ascending-contrast venogram is the "gold standard," with high sensitivity and specificity for diagnosing DVT in the entire lower extremity. However, it is a painful procedure with a risk of causing allergic reactions and vein thrombosis.

B-mode duplex ultrasonography is widely used to evaluate patients for DVT. The procedure is highly operator dependent, however, and accuracy will vary among institutions. Following hip or knee arthroplasty, ultrasonography has been shown to range from 62 to 88 percent in sensitivity, 97 to 98 percent specificity, and 66 to 98 percent in positive predictive value, with the higher numbers relating to thrombi in the thigh.[80] Importantly, thrombi missed tend to be small, non-occlusive calf thrombi that pose little risk.[81]

Diagnosis of Pulmonary Embolism

PE may present clinically with pleuritic chest pain, dyspnea, tachypnea, hemoptysis, and lethargy. However, the clinical diagnosis of PE is very unreliable, as a significant number of documented cases of PE occur without any clinical symptoms. In one study, dyspnea was found in only 60 percent of patients with proven PE, chest pain in 80 percent, and both symptoms in only 40 percent. Pleuritic chest pain was seen only with massive PE.[82]

The most useful diagnostic test for PE is the ventilation/perfusion ($\dot{V}/\dot{Q}$) scan. Arterial blood gasses are helpful but are not diagnostic.[83] In a prospective study with pulmonary angiography as the "gold-standard", abnormal $\dot{V}/\dot{Q}$ excluded PE with 96-percent confidence, whereas a high-probability scan was predictive in 88 percent of cases. Combining scans and clinical assessment produces 96-percent agreement when both are positive. A high-probability scan with a low clinical suspicion was found in 56 percent of patients with proven PE; a normal or low-probability scan with a low clinical suspicion makes PE unlikely.[84] Patients with a high-probability ($\dot{V}/\dot{Q}$) scan and those with an intermediate-probability scan or a low-probability scan but with a high clinical suspicion for PE should be evaluated with an angiogram[85] (Fig. 116–39).

Prophylaxis and Treatment of Thromboembolic Disease

Despite of the fact that without prophylaxis 50 percent of patients undergoing hip replacement have a postoperative DVT, 20 percent have a PE, and 0.5 to 2 percent die of a PE,[67] controversy exists regarding the need for chemical prophylaxis. The most commonly used agent for DVT prophylaxis is warfarin. A meta-analysis of DVT prophylaxis methods after total hip replacement showed that warfarin significantly reduced the incidence of distal and proximal vein thrombosis. The incidence of PE with warfarin was 32 percent less than with no prophylaxis, but this difference did not reach statistic significance.[86] Indeed, the major reason controversy exists regarding prophylaxis against DVT is that the incidence of fatal PE is so low that to demonstrate a significant reduction at the 5-percent level would require more than 45,000 patients in a prospective trial.[67] In the United States, most surgeons use a combination of mechanic prophylaxis (compression stockings or foot pumps) and chemical prophylaxis (warfarin or low-molecular-weight [LMW] heparin); in the United Kingdom, opinion regarding the need for prophylaxis is split about 50/50.[87]

LMW heparin has been shown in numerous studies to decrease the rate of DVT after total hip arthroplasty.[86] Few studies have compared the efficacy of LMW heparin to warfarin in preventing DVT after total joint arthroplasty. Hull and associates found that LMW heparin resulted in a significantly lower rate of DVT than warfarin (31.4 vs. 37.4%), but it also had a significantly higher bleeding complication rate (2.8% versus 1.2%).[88,89] Further studies comparing warfarin and LMW heparin are needed to better understand their relative efficacy and complication rates.

Pneumatic compression stockings and foot pumps have also been used for DVT prophylaxis. They appear to significantly reduce the incidence of distal DVT but have less of an effect on proximal DVT. These mechanical devices have an advantage over pharmacologic agents in that they do not cause an increase in bleeding complications.

Patients with documented proximal DVT or PE are treated with intravenous (IV) heparin for 5 days (maintaining the activated partial thromboplastin time [APTT] at 1.5 to 2.0 times control) followed by conversion to warfarin and treatment for 3 months. If anticoagulation is contraindicated or if the patient has a recurrent PE despite anticoagulation, a vena cava filter may be inserted.[83]

Heterotopic Ossification

The cause of heterotopic ossification (HO), the deposition of bone in soft tissue, is not clear, but it is generally felt that trauma to muscle and periosteum is involved. Some degree of HO often develops after total

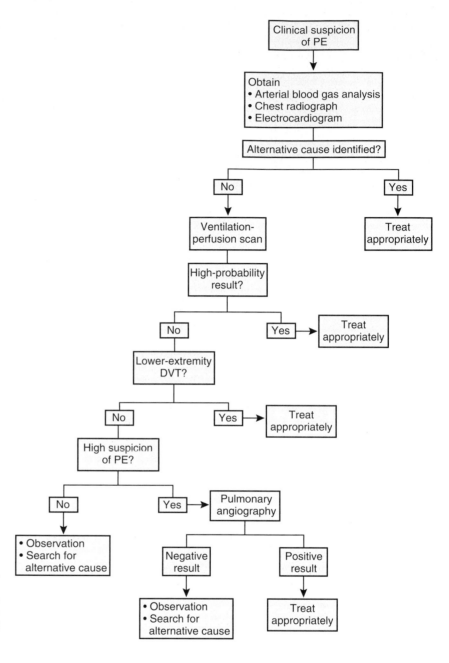

FIGURE 116–39 · Algorithm for Evaluation of Suspected Pulmonary Embolism (PE). (From Della Valle C, Steiger D, DiCesare P: Thrombolism after hip and knee arthroplasty: Diagnosis and treatment. J Am Acad Orthop Surg 6:327, 1998.

hip arthroplasty, but the incidence of significant HO that affects hip joint function is approximately 5 percent. Risk factors for HO include a previous history of HO, hypertrophic OA, AS, and diffuse idiopathic skeletal hyperostosis.[90] The incidence and the severity of HO appear to be greater in men. Patients with RA infrequently develop HO.

Patients with clinically significant HO have a diminished or a progressively decreasing range of motion of the hip. The diagnosis is made by plain radiography. The extent of the ossification generally does not change after 6 to 12 weeks postoperatively, although the bone continues to mature. The functional result after total hip arthroplasty in patients with extensive heterotopic ossification is reduced by virtue of the lost motion.

NSAIDs and radiotherapy are both effective prophylactic measures for preventing HO in patients at risk. Indomethacin has been studied more than any

other pharmacologic agent.[91] The standard regimen of indo-methacin is 25 mg three times daily for 6 weeks, but a recent study found that a 4- to 8-day course may be sufficient.[92] Ibuprofen is also effective.[93] Because indomethacin (and perhaps other NSAIDs) interferes with bone remodeling, there is some concern that its use in cases of noncemented joint arthroplasty might inhibit bone ingrowth. However, this concern has not been substantiated in clinical studies.

Radiation therapy in the perioperative period has been shown to decrease the incidence of HO. A single dose of 600 to 700 centigray given within 3 days postoperatively has been shown to be effective.[94] Because of the potential concern over interference with bony ingrowth in noncemented hip arthroplasty, the periprosthetic region should be shielded when the hip is irradiated. Controlled trials have shown indomethacin and irradiation to be equally effective in preventing HO after hip replacement and in acetabular fractures, and the cost advantage of indomethacin is significant.[60,61]

Heterotopic ossification is treated by surgical excision only if it is symptomatic. Surgery should be delayed for at least 6 months or until Tc-bone scan is negative to avoid recurrence. Postoperatively, early radiotherapy or administration of an anti-inflammatory medication is essential, as there is a high risk of recurrence.

Dislocation

The incidence of hip dislocation after total hip arthroplasty is between 0.5 and 3 percent. After the usual posterior approach, the hip generally dislocates posteriorly (75 to 90%), because of excessive flexion, adduction, and internal rotation of the hip. Anterior hip dislocations occur with extension, adduction, and external rotation. Dislocations are most common during the first few months after surgery and women are 1.5 to 2 times more likely to sustain a hip dislocation than men. Patients who have had previous operations on the hip are twice as likely to have a dislocation. Dislocation is also more likely in patients with neuromuscular disorders or mental confusion.[95,96]

Osteolysis

As discussed previously, death, infection, and PE are rare complications. Dislocations are infrequent and are becoming more so with improved surgical technique. In long-term follow-up, bone resorption around the implants (osteolysis) is the most common and serious complication, occurring in 15 to 20 percent of patients followed for 10 years or more.[97]

The resorption of bone around the implant is attributed to the activation of macrophages by particle ingestion.[98] The particles most commonly responsible are produced by cup wear and are, therefore, most commonly made of polyethylene, but they may also be from ceramic bearing surfaces,[100] metal debris, HA coatings,[101] or bone cement.

Reducing the amount of wear should reduce the incidence of osteolysis. Patients can help reduce wear by keeping their weight down and avoiding excessive physical activity. Implant design may affect access of the inevitable wear debris to the implant-bone interface.[102] Promising techniques are being developed to improve the wear characteristics of polyethylene. Regardless of the etiology, continued surveillance of implant patients is necessary so that osteolysis can be detected before fractures and further bone loss occur; early intervention is cost effective.[103]

Revision Total Hip Arthroplasty

Revision hip replacement is a considerably more involved procedure than the primary operation. The bone stock may be deficient and require supplementation. Fewer landmarks may be present for the placement of the implants, making it more difficult to obtain the proper leg length, implant rotation, and hip-center location. This may result in an unstable hip prone to dislocation.

There may be technical difficulties in removing the old prosthesis and cement and inserting the new prosthesis. It is not surprising that the results of revision hip replacement are inferior to those in primary cases.

Modern cement techniques in revision have a 90-percent clinical or radiographic success rate of the cemented femoral component after 11.7 years.[104]

Porous-coated stems in revision hip surgery have produced results similar to, if not better than, those with modern cemented stems. One study reported a 9-year survivorship of the acetabular and femoral components of 94 percent and 90 percent, respectively.[105]

Impaction Grafting

One of the reasons the results of revision for femoral loosening are no better than they are is that, over time, the femoral canal around a loose component becomes enlarged and thin walled. It is difficult to achieve good fixation with either the usual cement techniques or with an uncemented device. A newer technique for revising patients with loose femoral components is impaction grafting. In this technique, allograft bone is ground into particles that are packed tightly into the enlarged femoral canal. Cement is then inserted under pressure, followed by a polished, tapered femoral component designed to subside slightly into the composite mantle. Early results with this technique are promising, with incorporation of the allograft and reconstitution of the femoral cortex.[106]

REFERENCES

1. Charnley, J: The long term results of low-friction arthroplasty of the hip performed as a primary intervention. J Bone Joint Surg Br 54:61, 1972.
2. Pauwels, F: Biomechanics of the Normal and Diseased Hip: Theoretical Foundation, Technique, and Results: An Atlas. New York, Springer, 1976, p.
3. Davy, D, Kotzar, G, Brown, R, et al: Telemetric force measurements across the hip after total hip arthroplasty. J Bone Joint Surg Am 70:45, 1988.
4. Blount, W: Don't throw away the cane. J Bone Joint Surg Am 38:695, 1956.
5. Murphy, S, Ganz, R and Müller, M: The prognosis in untreated dysplasia of the hip: A study of radiographic factors that predict outcome. J Bone Joint Surg Am 77:985, 1995.
6. Stulberg, S and Harris, W: Acetabular dysplasia and development of osteoarthritis of the hip. In The Hip: Proceedings of the Second Open Scientific Meeting of the Hip Society. St Louis, CV Mosby, 1974, p 82.
7. Reference deleted.
8. Maetzel, A, Makela, M, Hawker, G, et al: Osteoarthritis of the hip and knee and mechanical occupational exposure–a systematic overview of the evidence. J Rheumatol 24:1599, 1997.
9. Cooper, C, Inskip, H, Croft, P, et al.: Individual risk factors for hip osteoarthritis: Obesity, hip injury, and physical activity. Am J Epidemiol 147:516, 1998.
10. Vingard, E, Alfredsson, L and Malchau, H: Osteoarthrosis of the hip in women and its relationship to physical load from sports activities. Am J Sports Med 26:78, 1998.
11. Lane, NE, Oehlert, JW, Bloch, DA, et al.: The relationship of running to osteoarthritis of the knee and hip and bone mineral density of the lumbar spine: A 9 year longitudinal study. J Rheumatol 25:334, 1998.
12. Harrison, M, Schajowicz, F and Trueta, J: Osteoarthritis of the hip: A study of the nature and evolution of the disease. J Bone Joint Surg Br 35:598, 1953.

13. Husted, H, Overgaard, S, Laursen, JO, et al: Need for bilateral arthroplasty for coxarthrosis. 1,477 replacements in 1,199 patients followed for 0–14 years. Acta Orthop Scand 67:421, 1996.

14. Stulberg, S, Cordell, L, Harris, W, et al: Unrecognized childhood hip disease: A major cause of idiopathic osteoarthritis of the hip. In The Hip: Proceedings of the Third Open Scientific Meeting of The Hip Society. St Louis, CV Mosby, 1975, p 212.

15. Wolfe, F and Zwillich, S: The long-term outcomes of rheumatoid arthritis: A 23-year prospective, longitudinal study of total joint replacement and its predictors in 1,600 patients with rheumatoid arthritis. Arthritis Rheum 41:1072, 1998.

16. Fitzgerald, RH, Jr: Acetabular labrum tears. Diagnosis and treatment. Clin Orthop 311:60, 1995.

17. Leunig, M, Werlen, S, Ungersbock, A, et al: Evaluation of the acetabular labrum by MR arthrography [published erratum appears in J Bone Joint Surg Br 79:693, 1997]. J Bone Joint Surg Br 79:230, 1997.

18. Allcock, P: Diagnostic value of intra-articular anaesthetic in primary osteoarthritis of the hip [letter; comment]. J Bone Joint Surg Br 80:934, 1998.

19. Byrd, JW: Labral lesions: An elusive source of hip pain case reports and literature review. Arthroscopy 12:603, 1996.

20. Callaghan, J, Brand, R and Pedersen, D: Hip arthrodesis: A longterm followup. J Bone Joint Surg Am 67:1328, 1985.

21. Tavares, JO and Frankovitch, KF: Hip arthrodesis using the AO modular external fixator. J Pediatr Orthop 18:651, 1998.

22. Iwase, T, Hasegawa, Y, Kawamoto, K, et al: Twenty years' followup of intertrochanteric osteotomy for treatment of the dysplastic hip. Clin Orthop 245, 1996.

23. Poss, R and Younger, A: The Intertrochanteric Osteotomy. In Sledge, CB (Ed.): The Hip. Philadelphia, Lippincott-Raven, 1998, p 183.

24. McGrory, BJ, Estok, DMn and Harris, WH: Follow-up of intertrochanteric osteotomy of the hip during a 25-year period. Orthopedics 21:651, 1998.

25. Trousdale, R, Ekkernkamp, A, Ganz, R, et al: Periacetabular and intertrochanteric osteotomy for the treatment of osteoarthrosis in dysplastic hips. J Bone Joint Surg Am 77:73, 1995.

26. Xenakis, TA, Beris, AE, Malizos, KK, et al: Total hip arthroplasty for avascular necrosis and degenerative osteoarthritis of the hip. Clin Orthop 341:162, 1997.

27. Nagano, H, Inoue, H, Usui, M, et al: Long-term results of Charnley low-friction arthroplasty for coxarthrosis with congenital hip dysplasia. 15 year follow-up study. Bull Hosp Jt Dis 56:197, 1997.

28. Numair, J, Joshi, AB, Murphy, JC, et al: Total hip arthroplasty for congenital dysplasia or dislocation of the hip. Survivorship analysis and long-term results. J Bone Joint Surg Am 79:1352, 1997.

29. D'Antonio, JA, Capello, WN, Manley, MT, et al: Hydroxyapatite coated implants. Total hip arthroplasty in the young patient and patients with avascular necrosis. Clin Orthop 344:124, 1997.

30. Shpitzer, T, Ganel, A and Engelberg, S: Surgery for synovial chondromatosis. 26 cases followed up for 6 years. Acta Orthop Scand 61:567, 1990.

31. Alexakis, PG, Brown, BA and Hohl, WM: Porous hip replacement in Paget's disease. An 8-2/3-year followup. Clin Orthop 350:138, 1998.

32. Algan, SM and Horowitz, SM: Surgical treatment of pathologic hip lesions in patients with metastatic disease. Clin Orthop 332:223, 1996.

33. Lee, BP, Berry, DJ, Harmsen, WS, et al: Total hip arthroplasty for the treatment of an acute fracture of the femoral neck: Long-term results. J Bone Joint Surg Am 80:70, 1998.

34. Dom, K and Pittevils, T: Ochronotic arthropathy: the black hip. Case report and review of the literature. Acta Orthop Belg 63:122, 1997.

35. Brinker, MR, Rosenberg, AG, Kull, L, et al: Primary noncemented total hip arthroplasty in patients with ankylosing spondylitis. Clinical and radiographic results at an average follow-up period of 6 years. J Arthroplasty 11:802, 1996.

36. Salvati, E and Lieberman, J: Secondary Total Hip Arthroplasty: After Infection. In Sledge, CB (Ed.): The Hip. Philadelphia, Lippincott-Raven, 1998, p 283.

37. Wroblewski, BM and Siney, P: Charnley low-friction arthroplasty of the hip. Longterm results. Clin Orthop 292:191, 1993.

38. Geesink, R and Hoefnagels, N: Eight years results of HA-coated primary total hip replacement. Acta Orthop Belg 63 Suppl 1:72, 1997.

39. Engh, CA, Jr., Culpepper, WJn and Engh, CA: Long-term results of use of the anatomic medullary locking prosthesis in total hip arthroplasty. J Bone Joint Surg Am 79:177, 1997.

40. Petersen, MB, Poulsen, IH, Thomsen, J, et al: The hemispherical Harris-Galante acetabular cup, inserted without cement. The results of an eight to eleven-year follow-up of one hundred and sixty-eight hips. J Bone Joint Surg Am 81:219, 1999.

41. Harris, WH: The hybrid total hip replacement. In Sledge, CB (Ed.): The Hip. Philadelphia, Lippincott-Raven, 1998, p 239.

42. Dominkus, M, Wanivenhaus, AH, Morscher, M, et al: Different cup migration in rheumatoid arthritis and arthrosis: a radiographic analysis of 127 uncemented acetabular cups. Acta Orthop Scand 69:455, 1998.

43. Espehaug, B, Engesaeter, LB, Vollset, SE, et al: Antibiotic prophylaxis in total hip arthroplasty. Review of 10,905 primary cemented total hip replacements reported to the Norwegian arthroplasty register, 1987 to 1995. J Bone Joint Surg Br 79:590, 1997.

44. Wahl, M: Myths of dental-induced prosthetic joint infections. Clin Infect Dis 20:1420, 1995.

45. LaPorte, DM, Waldman, BJ, Mont, MA, et al: Infections associated with dental procedures in total hip arthroplasty. J Bone Joint Surg Br 81:56, 1999.

46. Tsevat, J, Durand-Zaleski, I and Pauker, S: Cost/effectiveness of antibiotic prophylaxis for dental procedures in patients with artificial joints. Am J Public Health 79:739, 1989.

47. Drangsholt, MT: Current concepts review. Prophylactic use of antibiotics for procedures after total joint replacement [letter; comment]. J Bone Joint Surg Am 80:1394, 1998.

48. Karlson, EW, Daltroy, LH, Liang, MH, et al: Gender differences in patient preferences may underlie differential utilization of elective surgery. Am J Med 102:524, 1997.

49. Towheed, TE and Hochberg, MC: Health-related quality of life after total hip replacement. Semin Arthritis Rheum 26:483, 1996

50. Shulte, K, Callaghan, J, Kelley, S, et al: The outcome of Charnley total hip arthroplasty with cement after a minimum twentyyear followup. J Bone Joint Surg Am 75:961, 1993.

51. Hartofilakidis, G: Survival of the Charnley low-friction arthroplasty. A 12-24-year follow-up of 276 cases. Acta Orthop Scand Suppl 275:27, 1997.

52. Joshi, A, Porter, M, Trail, I, et al: Long-term results of Charnley low-friction arthroplasty in young patients. J Bone Joint Surg Br 75:616, 1993.

53. Poss, R, Maloney, J, Ewald, F, et al: Six to 11-year results of total hip arthroplasty in rheumatoid arthritis. Clin Orthop 182:109, 1984.

54. Barrack, R, Mulroy, R, Jr and Harris, W: Improved cementing techniques and femoral component loosening in young patients with hip arthroplasty. J Bone Joint Surg Br 74:385, 1992.

55. Ranawat, C, Deshmukh, R, Peters, L, et al: Prediction of the longterm durability of all-polyethylene cemented sockets. Clin Orthop 317:89, 1995.

56. McAuley, JP, Moore, KD, Culpepper, WJn, et al: Total hip arthroplasty with porous-coated prostheses fixed without cement in patients who are sixty-five years of age or older. J Bone Joint Surg Am 80:1648, 1998.

57. Bugbee, WD, Culpepper, WJn, Engh, CA, Jr, et al: Long-term clinical consequences of stress-shielding after total hip arthroplasty without cement. J Bone Joint Surg Am 79:1007, 1997.

58. McAuley, JP, Culpepper, WJ and Engh, CA: Total hip arthroplasty. Concerns with extensively porous coated femoral components. Clin Orthop 355:182, 1998.

59. D'Lima, DD, Oishi, CS, Petersilge, WJ, et al: 100 cemented versus 100 noncemented stems with comparison of 25 matched pairs. Clin Orthop 348:140, 1998.

60. Lewallen, DG and Cabanela, ME: Hybrid primary total hip arthroplasty: a 5- to 9-year followup study. Clin Orthop 335:126, 1996.

61. Smith, SW, Estok, DM and Harris, WH: Total hip arthroplasty with use of second-generation cementing techniques. An eighteen-year-average follow-up study. J Bone Joint Surg Am 80:1632, 1998.

62. Callaghan, JJ, Forest, EE, Olejniczak, JP, et al: Charnley total hip arthroplasty in patients less than fifty years old. A twenty to

twenty-five-year follow-up note. J Bone Joint Surg Am 80:704, 1998.

63. Hartofilakidis, G, Karachalios, T and Zacharakis, N: Charnley low friction arthroplasty in young patients with osteoarthritis. A 12- to 24-year clinical and radiographic followup study of 84 cases. Clin Orthop 341:51, 1997.

64. Sochart, DH and Porter, ML: The long-term results of Charnley low-friction arthroplasty in young patients who have congenital dislocation, degenerative osteoarthrosis, or rheumatoid arthritis. J Bone Joint Surg Am 79:1599, 1997.

65. Sullivan, PM, MacKenzie, JR, Callaghan, JJ, et al: Total hip arthroplasty with cement in patients who are less than fifty years old. A sixteen to twenty-two-year follow-up study. J Bone Joint Surg Am 76:863, 1994.

66. Brander, VA, Malhotra, S, Jet, J, et al: Outcome of hip and knee arthroplasty in persons aged 80 years and older. Clin Orthop 345:67, 1997.

67. Fender, D, Harper, W, Thompson, J, et al: Mortality and fatal pulmonary embolism after primary total hip replacement: results from a regional register. J Bone Joint Surg Br 79:896, 1997.

68. Lieberman, J, Wollaeger, J, Dorey, F, et al: The efficacy of prophylaxis with low dose warfarin for prevention of pulmonary embolism following total hip arthroplasty. J Bone Joint Surg Am 79:319, 1997.

69. Nelson, J: Deep infection following total hip arthroplasty. J Bone Joint Surg Am 59:1042, 1977.

70. Lieberman, J, Fuchs, M, Haas, S, et al: Hip arthroplasty in patients with chronic renal failure. J Arthroplasty 10:191, 1995.

71. Okafor, B and MacLellan, G: Postoperative changes of erythrocyte sedimentation rate, plasma viscosity and C-reactive protein levels after hip surgery. Acta Orthop Belg 64:52, 1998.

72. Mittal, R, Khetarpal, R, Malhotra, R, et al: The role of Tc-99m bone imaging in the management of pain after complicated total hip replacement. Clin Nucl Med 22:593, 1997.

73. Kraemer, W, Saplys, R, Waddell, J, et al: Bone scan, gallium scan, and hip aspiration in the diagnosis of infected total hip arthroplasty. J Arthroplasty 8:611, 1993.

74. Schmalzried, TP, Amstutz, HC, Au, MK, et al: Etiology of deep sepsis in total hip arthroplasty. The significance of hematogenous and recurrent infections. Clin Orthop 280:200, 1992.

75. Nasser, S: Prevention and treatment of sepsis in total hip replacement surgery. Orthop Clin North Am 23:265, 1992.

76. Lieberman, J and Geerts, W: Prevention of venous thromboembolism after total hip and knee arthroplasty. J Bone Joint Surg Am 76:1239, 1994.

77. Sikorski, J, Hampson, W and Staddon, G: The natural history and etiology of deep vein thrombosis following total hip replacement. J Bone Joint Surg Br 63:171, 1981.

78. Davis, F, Laurenson, V, Gillespie, W, et al: Deep vein thrombosis after total hip replacement: A comparison between spinal and general anesthesia. J Bone Joint Surg Br 71:181, 1989.

79. Oishi, C, Grady-Benson, J, Otis, S, et al: The clinical course of distal deep venous thrombosis after total hip and total knee arthroplasty, as determined with duplex ultrasonography. J Bone Joint Surg Am 76:1658, 1994.

80. Grady-Benson, J, Oishi, C, Hanson, P, et al: Postoperative surveillance for deep venous thrombosis with duplex ultrasonography after total knee arthroplasty. J Bone Joint Surg Am 76:1649, 1994.

81. Wells, P, Lensing, A, Davidson, B, et al: Accuracy of ultrasound for the diagnosis of deep venous thrombosis in asymptomatic patients after orthopedic surgery: A meta-analysis. Ann Intern Med 122:47, 1995.

82. Manganelli, D, Palla, A, Donnamaria, V, et al: Clinical features of pulmonary embolism: Doubts and certainties. Chest 107 (suppl 1):25S, 1995.

83. Della Valle, C, Steiger, D and DiCesare, P: Thrombolism after hip and knee arthroplasty: Diagnosis and treatment. J Amer Acad Orthop Surg 6:327, 1998.

84. (no authors listed): Value of ventilation/perfusion scan in acute pulmonary embolism: Results of the prospective investigation of pulmonary embolism diagnosis. The PIOPED investigators. JAMA 263:2753, 1990.

85. Haake, D and Berkman, S: Venous thromboembolic disease after hip surgery: Risk factors, prophylaxis, and diagnosis. Clin Orthop 242:212, 1989.

86. Imperiale, T and Speroff, T: A metaanalysis of methods to prevent venous thromboembolism following total hip replacement. JAMA 271:1780, 1994.

87. Unwin, A, Jones, J and Harries, W: Current UK opinion on thromboprophylaxis in orthopaedic surgery: Its use in routine total hip and knee arthroplasty. Ann R Coll Surg Engl 77:351, 1995.

88. Hull, R, Delmore, T, Genton, E, et al: Warfarin sodium versus low-dose heparin in the long-term treatment of venous thrombosis. N Engl J Med 301:855, 1979.

89. Hull, R, Raskob, G, Pineo, G, et al: A comparison of subcutaneous low molecular-weight heparin with warfarin sodium for prophylaxis against deepvein thrombosis after hip or knee implantation. N Engl J Med 329:1370, 1993.

90. Brooker, A, Bowerman, J, Robinson, R, et al: Ectopic ossification following total hip replacement. J Bone Joint Surg Am 55:1629, 1973.

91. Schmidt, S, Kjaersgaard-Andersen, P, Pedersen, N, et al: The use of indomethacin to prevent the formation of heterotopic bone after total hip replacement: A randomized, doubleblind clinical trial. J Bone Joint Surg Am 70:834, 1988.

92. Dorn, U, Grethen, C, Effenberger, H, et al: Indomethacin for prevention of heterotopic ossification after hip arthroplasty. A randomized comparison between 4 and 8 days of treatment. Acta Orthop Scand 69:107, 1998.

93. Persson, PE, Sodemann, B and Nilsson, OS: Preventive effects of ibuprofen on periarticular heterotopic ossification after total hip arthroplasty. A randomized double-blind prospective study of treatment time. Acta Orthop Scand 69:111, 1998.

94. Healy, W, Lo, T, DeSimone, A, et al: Single-dose irradiation for the prevention of heterotopic ossification after total hip arthroplasty: A comparison of doses of five hundred and fifty and seven hundred centigray. J Bone Joint Surg Am 77:590, 1995.

95. Woo, R and Morey, B: Dislocations after total hip arthroplasty. J Bone Joint Surg Am 64:1295, 1982.

96. Roberts, J, Fu, F, McClain, E, et al: A comparison of the posterolateral and anterolateral approach to total hip arthroplasty. Clin Orthop 187:205, 1984.

97. Schmalzried, TP, Jasty, M and Harris, WH: Periprosthetic bone loss in total hip arthroplasty. Polyethylene wear debris and the concept of the effective joint space. J Bone Joint Surg Am 74:849, 1992.

98. Nakashima, Y, Sun, DH, Traindade, MC, et al: Induction of macrophage C-C chemokine expression by titanium alloy and bone cement particles. J Bone Joint Surg Br 81:155, 1999.

99. Joshi, RP, Eftekhar, NS, McMahon, DJ, et al: Osteolysis after Charnley primary low-friction arthroplasty. A comparison of two matched paired groups. J Bone Joint Surg Br 80:585, 1998.

100. Sedel, L, Nizard, R and Bizot, P: Osteolysis and ceramic bearing surfaces. J Bone Joint Surg Am 82:1519, 2000.

101. Morscher, EW, Hefti, A and Aebi, U: Severe osteolysis after third-body wear due to hydroxyapatite particles from acetabular cup coating J Bone Joint Surg Br 80:267, 1998.

102. Collis, DK and Mohler, CG: Loosening rates and bone lysis with rough finished and polished stems. Clin Orthop 113, 1998.

103. Lavernia, CJ: Cost-effectiveness of early surgical intervention in silent osteolysis. J Arthroplasty 13:277, 1998.

104. Estok, DM and Harris, WH: Long-term results of cemented femoral revision surgery using second-generation techniques. An average 11.7-year follow-up evaluation. Clin Orthop 190, 1994.

105. Lawrence, J, Engh, C, Macalino, G, et al: Outcome of revision hip arthroplasty done without cement. J Bone Joint Surg Am 76:965, 1994.

106. Gie, G, Linder, L, Ling, R, et al: Impacted cancellous allografts and cement for revision total hip arthroplasty. J Bone Joint Surg Br 75:14.

THE KNEE
CLEMENT B. SLEDGE

▮ Nonprosthetic Treatment Options

OSTEOARTHRITIS

The success of total replacement of the knee has overshadowed other procedures that should be considered in patients with arthritis. Artificial devices fail and with each failure there is loss of bone, rendering fixation of the next implant less certain. Additionally, the plastic component is subject to wear, especially with long, heavy use as might be the case in young patients with osteoarthritis (OA). Multiple joint involvement is uncommon, and the patients often are healthy and vigorous, so increased activity following relief of pain may put severe stress on the prosthetic components. These patients are also frequently obese.[1] Unlike the situation in rheumatoid arthritis (RA), however, several alternative procedures can be considered.

Arthrodesis

It is appropriate to consider arthrodesis in a young, active male with post-traumatic arthritis of the knee. This type of patient is likely to subject the implant to severe mechanical stresses leading to wear of the polyethylene surface, loosening of the components, or both. Although a failed arthroplasty can be successfully revised, each revision is accompanied by further loss of supporting bone and increased risks of fracture, infection, and another failure. The ability to stand and walk for long periods without pain can greatly outweigh the awkwardness created by knee stiffness.[2] Nonetheless, even in ideal circumstances, it is almost impossible for the patient to accept the permanent lack of knee motion that results from arthrodesis. Some patients who have a satisfactory and painless arthrodesis request an arthroplasty to return mobility to the knee, but this is seldom advisable.

Débridement

Removal of degenerated menisci and osteophytes, shaving of degenerated articular cartilage, and drilling or microfracture of eburnated bone may be the best approach for young or middle-aged patients with arthritis of the type that may follow athletic injuries. These patients usually retain an interest in sports and wish to participate in some kind of recreational activity. The débridement procedure has been reported as being successful in about two thirds of patients and can be of long-lasting benefit.[3] Débridement is now done arthroscopically, and good results have been reported in retrospective reviews.[4] Prospective studies, however, report that without sign of meniscal tear, arthroscopic débridement is of limited usefulness.[5,6] A recent prospective, controlled study comparing arthroscopic débride-ment to placebo lavage showed no advantage for the more extensive procedure.[7]

Cartilage Repair

Attempts to replace lost articular cartilage, whether from focal OA or traumatic injury, have captured the imagination of clinical investigators since John Hunter, the "father" of modern surgery. Thus far, no method has been found that will predictably replace lost articular cartilage, although there are several promising new techniques. These fall into three categories: attempts to induce repair by local tissue; transplantation of another tissue; and transplantation of cells.

Induction of repair by local tissue has the longest history. Surgical excision of damaged cartilage followed by drilling of the subchondral bone was popularized by Insall, who reported good short-term relief of pain.[3] More recently, the procedure has been carried out arthroscopically, with abrasion of the subchondral bone in place of multiple drill holes.[8] More recently, a technique of arthroscopic "microfracture" has been developed, and there have been reports of good early results.[9] In this technique, as in drilling or abrasion, the goal is to breach the subchondral plate to allow ingrowth of fibroblasts which, under some circumstances, will undergo metaplasia into cartilage.

Transplantation techniques employ periosteum, perichondrium, or articular cartilage. In experimental animals, periosteum was shown to bring about repair of cartilage defects.[10] In humans, however, the reports have been less promising, with early pain relief followed by failure. In one study of 14 patients with osteochondritis dissecans of the femoral condyle treated with periosteal transplantation, nine patients were pain free at 1 year, but all had a poor result at follow-up of 6 to 9 years.[11] Perichondrium has also been used but, in the largest series reported, 21 of 30 patients developed calcification of the new cartilage.[12]

Transplantation of cells, either chondrocytes or precursor cells, has created great excitement since the report of Brittberg and colleagues in 1994.[13] The technique involved taking small biopsies of normal cartilage from the patient and using tissue culture techniques to grow several million chondrocytes. At surgery several weeks after the biopsies, the lesion was débrided and a graft of nearby periosteum was used to create a watertight covering over the defect. One to three million chondrocytes were then injected under the flap into the defect. In the initial report, 14 of 16 patients treated with this technique were reported to have good-to-excellent results at short-term follow-up. The 2- to 9-year follow-up found that 62 percent of patients with lesions on the patella, 89 percent of patients with osteochondritis diseccans, and 92 percent of patients with lesions on the femoral condyle were symptomatically improved.[14] This treatment, although exciting in its possibilities, has certain obvious drawbacks: Some normal cartilage must be sacrificed for the cell culture, and this requires at least an arthroscopic procedure; the creation of a water-tight recipient site is technically difficult, and transplanted cells could easily leak with the first application of weight-bearing force; and, most importantly, true articular cartilage, with its complex architecture of collagen and proteoglycan, has not been demonstrated in late biopsies.[15] Newer techniques with magnetic resonance imaging (MRI) show promise of evaluating the quality of new cartilage formed after chondrocyte transplantation.[16] Efforts are currently underway to improve the procedure by using cells incorporated into either an artificial matrix[17] or a collagen matrix.[18]

Because of the uncertainty of obtaining true articular cartilage after either microfracture, abrasion, or chondrocyte transplantation, transplantation of articular cartilage itself is being tried. The articular cartilage can be either minute pieces of autologous cartilage (so-called mosaicplasty) taken from the same knee[19] or larger osteochondral pieces from cadaver donors.[20] A prospective study comparing chondrocyte transplantation to transplantation of autologous osteochondral grafts suggests that the latter is more effective.[15]

Osteotomy

Primary OA of the knee is usually compartmental and associated with angular deformity (most commonly a varus angulation). Correction of varus malalignment by osteotomy through the upper tibia is a proven and satisfactory operation.[21] The most successful results are obtained in patients who have a relatively small angulation (10 degrees of varus or less) and stable knees. Provided that the correct valgus alignment of 7 to 10 degrees is obtained, the results are satisfactory in about 90 percent of cases.[22] In knees with more severe deformity, which is usually associated with instability, the results are much less satisfactory, because obtaining correct postoperative alignment is more difficult and the ligament instability tends to cause either overcorrection or recurrence of the original varus deformity. The effect of osteotomy is explained by the shifting of weight-bearing stress to the uninvolved lateral compartment and is purely mechanical (Fig. 116–40). When good results are not achieved because of either ligamentous instability or incorrect technique, pain is not relieved.

Tibial osteotomy for the correction of the less-common valgus deformity is less often reported but may produce satisfactory results.[23] Most valgus knees

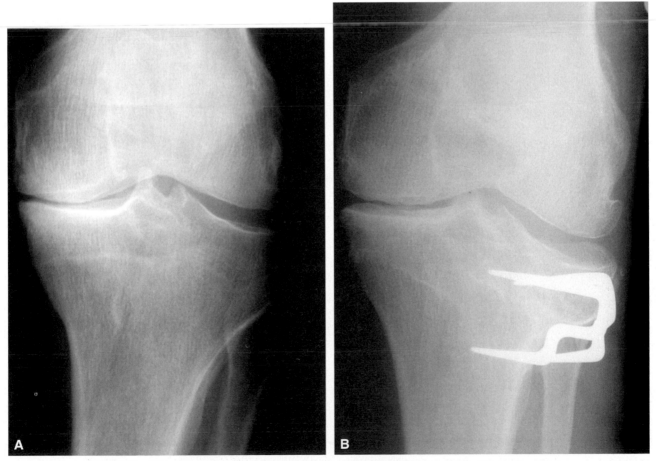

FIGURE 116–40 · Osteoarthritis of the Medial Compartment of the Knee, Treated by Osteotomy of the Proximal Tibia. *A,* Preoperative view. *B,* View following surgery. Note the change of alignment of the limb and opening of the medial joint space.

have a considerable deformity that, if corrected in the tibia, produces a marked joint obliquity that causes medial subluxation of the femur and the development of late varus deformity. For this reason, it is generally preferable to correct valgus knees by distal femoral osteotomy, which preserves the horizontal joint axis.[24] However, femoral osteotomy is associated with a higher morbidity, more frequent nonunion, and sometimes knee stiffness.

RHEUMATOID ARTHRITIS

There are fewer alternatives for patients with RA of the knee. This is unfortunate as knee involvement is common. In a 22-year follow-up of patients with RA, 25 percent underwent a total joint arthroplasty, with replacement of the knee being the most common.[25]

Synovectomy

Synovectomy may temporarily relieve the pain and swelling of RA. It has little effect on the progression of arthritis and is of no value when cartilage erosion has already occurred. The procedure, now usually done by arthroscopy (see Chapter 48) or isotope injection,[26] may defer the need for total replacement in young patients or in those whose symptoms are due primarily to persistent effusion.

▪ Knee Replacement

One or both articular surfaces may be replaced by prosthetic components when severe arthritis or trauma has destroyed the articular cartilage of the knee. Replacement of only one side of the articulation (hemiarthroplasty) is infrequently utilized, although interest has increased in cases of OA in recent years.[27] Modern devices replace both articulating surfaces of the femorotibial and patellofemoral joints. These metal and plastic components attempt to duplicate normal joint surfaces so that motion and stability can be restored.

Total knee arthroplasty with a metal hinge, which sacrifices the knee ligaments and assumes both stability and mobility functions, was popular in the 1960s, but it had a high failure rate. Hinge devices are now only rarely indicated—usually in tumor surgery when the stabilizing soft tissues must be sacrificed. *Interposition arthroplasty*, the term used to describe modern devices that resurface the joint by interposing prosthetic surfaces, requires the preservation of ligamentous support to provide the necessary stability.

A significant advance in knee arthroplasty was made by Gunston.[28] The polycentric arthroplasty was the first attempt to apply to the knee the prosthetic system of high-density polyethylene articulating against metal (either stainless steel or chrome cobalt alloy) bonded to bone by methyl methacrylate cement, which had proved very successful in total hip replacement.

Many implant designs for knee replacement have since appeared. Most are cemented into both the femur and tibia, some are fixed by biologic means (utilizing porous surfaces into which bone may grow), and

some systems combine both techniques into a hybrid system with cement fixation for the tibia and patella and ingrowth for the femur. Although alternative bearing surfaces are being tested, most devices still utilize metal and polyethylene bearing surfaces.

TYPES OF PROSTHESES

Prostheses can be divided into two categories: 1) surface replacements and 2) constrained prostheses.

Surface Replacements

Unicompartmental Replacement

Unicompartmental replacement of the OA knee is widely used in both the United States and Europe.[27,29] The concept has been recommended because only the abnormal joint surfaces are removed, and the total amount of bone excised is minimal. The amount of foreign material used (metal, polyethylene, and cement) is also relatively small. Finally, it has been claimed that less operative time is required, complications are fewer, and the ultimate range of motion is greater than with total replacement of the joint surfaces.[29]

Unicompartmental designs may be used in OA knees in which only one compartment (medial or lateral) is involved (Fig. 116–41). The ligaments, including the cruciates, must all be present and relatively normal; therefore, the prosthesis cannot be used in severely involved arthritic knees with a large deformity, severe instability, or significant flexion contracture. Likewise, the procedure has no place in the treatment of rheu-matoid panarthritis. The indications for unicompartmental replacement in varus OA are essentially the same as those for high tibial osteotomy. For lateral compartment arthritis with valgus deformity, unicompartmental replacement is more attractive, as the only alternatives are total replacement or distal femoral osteotomy.

Bicondylar Replacements

These may be divided into fixed bearing or mobile bearing devices, with either retention of the posterior cruciate ligament or its substitution.

Fixed-Bearing Prostheses

The debate regarding sacrifice or retention of the posterior cruciate has largely been silenced by long-term studies of both types of implants; the results with cruciate preservation or substitution are virtually identical.[30-32]

Mobile-Bearing Prostheses

Mobile-bearing prostheses represent a family of designs that differ from the usual knee prosthesis in that the polyethylene bearing surface is free to move over a metal plate on the upper tibia. The concept is that plastic wear will be reduced by providing more conforming geometry between the femoral and tibial articulations, thereby reducing contact stresses and wear.[33] The lack

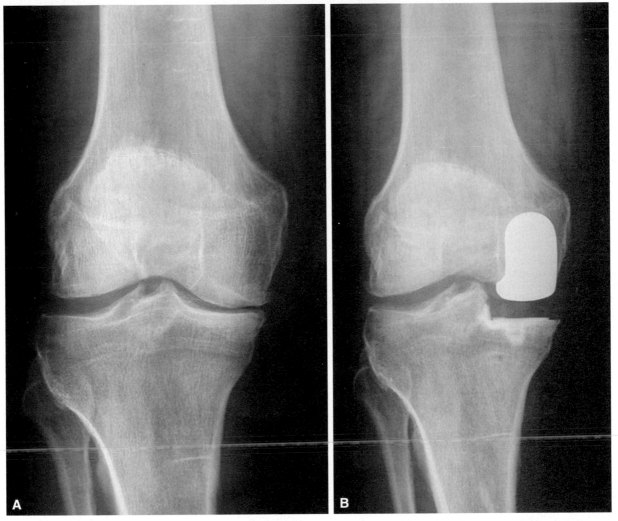

FIGURE 116–41 · This patient had symptoms similar to those of the patient in Figure 116–40 but was elderly, lived alone, and needed maximal range of knee motion for self help. *A,* Preoperative radiograph showing primary involvement of the medial compartment. *B,* Postoperative radiograph following unicompartmental replacement. Knee flexion was 125 degrees, allowing independent foot care and other activities of daily living.

of motion that such constraint would otherwise impose is offset by the ability of the plastic to slide over the almost flat tibial surface; this occurred in half of the cases in one study.[34] Both unicompartmental and total replacement designs are available.[35]

Constrained Prostheses

Constrained prostheses provide all the required knee joint stability; thus, both cruciate and collateral ligaments may be excised or absent. Infection and loosening have been major problems with early fixed-hinge designs. Consequently, their use has now been largely abandoned and newer designs have evolved with metal-on-polyethylene articulations, which allow rotary and gliding movements while providing the necessary stability. Such mechanical constraint is occasionally required for revision surgery and for a few primary cases, especially in tumor surgery in which soft tissue resection may dictate use of such prosthetic constraint.

▌ Indications

Only severe symptoms and disability justify knee joint replacement. Although it is no longer true that a patient should consent to arthrodesis before undergoing an arthroplasty, a frank discussion with the patient concerning the consequences of failure is essential. Medical management should be continued for as long as possible, and alternative treatments, such as tibial osteotomy in OA, should be selected when appropriate.

The indications for total knee replacement in OA are pain and limitation of function to a degree sufficient to interfere with the patient's enjoyment of life (quality of life). A recent study found that preoperative function determines postoperative function; patients in whom self-reported function had decreased below a certain level did not fully return to the functional level expected after surgery.[36] This suggests that an appropriate time for surgery is when the patient's self-reported function, measured sequentially, falls below this threshold. It should also be understood that patients in whom function is close to normal have a high likelihood of decreased function after surgery, especially if pain was not a dominant symptom before surgery.

The patient should understand that failure of the operation, although rare, will be followed by at least one other operation and, in very rare circumstances, may lead to arthrodesis or even amputation.

In the presence of severe and unremitting symptoms, total knee arthroplasty is indicated in the following circumstances:

1. RA with severe cartilage damage, functional limitation, and pain (Fig. 116–42)
2. OA of the knee (The patient's age, occupation, sex, weight, and level of activity all are factors that must be considered [Fig. 116–43]. In general terms, arthroplasty should be avoided in patients younger than 60 years of age, in manual laborers, in athletes, and in those who are grossly overweight; its use in patients under age 60 must be individualized.[37] Arthroplasty should not be selected for patients younger than 60 if a suitable alternative exists. Replacement arthroplasty also is not suitable for persons who wish to engage in sports, except perhaps golf, bicycling, and swimming.

Because of the great long-term success of knee replacement, more young patients are demanding it to relieve their arthritic pain. They should, however, be warned of the limitations imposed by wear, with subsequent bone loss that can develop in a knee that is actively used.)

3. Post-traumatic OA (In rare cases, there may be an indication for knee replacement in the younger patient following intra-articular fractures or other traumatic injuries to the joint, especially if one of the cartilage-restoration operations has failed.)
4. Failure of high tibial osteotomy (When high tibial osteotomy has not relieved symptoms, or when symptoms recur after an interval owing to progressive arthritis, total knee replacement can be performed with good results.)
5. Patellofemoral OA (In most cases, patellofemoral OA is not an indication for total replacement of the joint, and the condition is better managed with other techniques. Evidence of damage to the weight-bearing compartments is usually a prerequisite for joint replacement. However, occasionally an elderly patient presents with severe patellofemoral arthritis without significant femorotibial narrowing, despite a finding of patchy articular degeneration

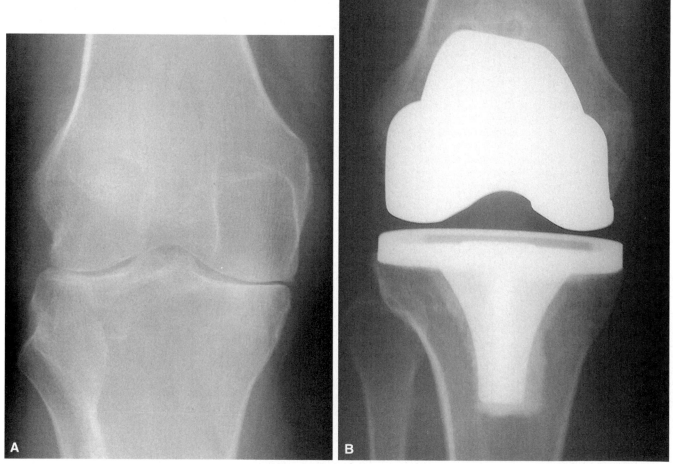

FIGURE 116–42 · Rheumatoid Arthritis (RA) with Severe Involvement of the Knee. *A,* View before surgery. *B,* Anteroposterior (AP) projection following tricompartmental replacement.

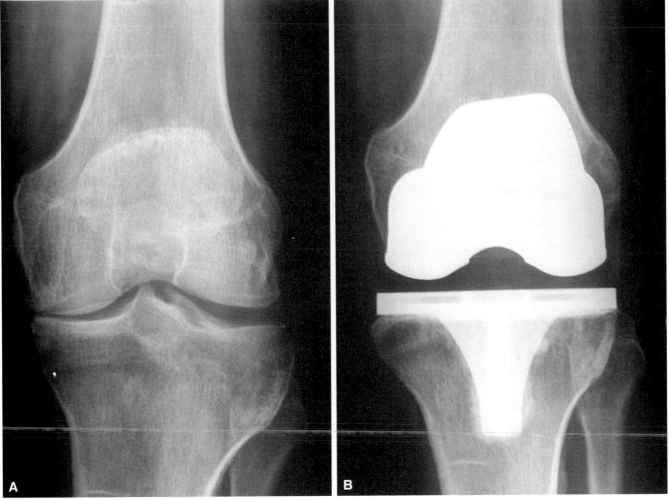

FIGURE 116–43 · Osteoarthritis (OA) with Involvement of all Three Compartments. *A,* View before surgery. *B,* View following tricompartmental replacement.

throughout the joint at arthrotomy. This situation, although rare, is currently best treated with total joint replacement. Attempts to replace just the articular surface of the patella and the opposing femoral groove had been largely unsuccessful.[38])

6. The neuropathic joint (Joint replacement in neuropathic conditions is controversial and represents a technical challenge, as instability and deformity are often extreme, and neuromuscular and proprioceptive loss endanger the prosthetic joint.)

Contraindications

The following are relative contraindications to knee replacement:

1. A sound, painless arthrodesis in good position (The prospects of a successful arthroplasty are not good, and a constrained prosthesis is usually required. Should the arthroplasty fail, another attempt at knee arthrodesis may not succeed.)

2. Genu recurvatum associated with muscular weakness and paralysis (This condition is likely to recur after a surface replacement, and the stresses imposed on a constrained prosthesis will probably loosen it.)

3. Gross quadriceps weakness

4. Active sepsis (When infection is caused by a susceptible organism, thorough débridement and appropriate antibiotic therapy may be followed by a replacement after eradication of infection. Tuberculous joints can be managed in a similar manner. When the infecting organism cannot be treated adequately because of the potential toxicity of the necessary antibiotic therapy or bacterial resistance, arthrodesis is a better choice.)

Surgical Considerations

The success of any total knee replacement depends on patient selection, prosthetic design, prosthetic materials, and surgical technique.

Prosthetic design has evolved to the point where little improvement of the results can be expected from continued design refinement. Current prostheses possess many basic similarities and, if correctly inserted, give satisfactory results. However, although total hip arthroplasty is relatively forgiving of surgical error, whereas total knee replacement is not. Component malposition of 5, 10, or even 20 degrees may not affect the outcome in hip arthroplasty; in knee replacement, a 5-degree error is significant, and a 10-degree error is often catastrophic. Furthermore, even when the components themselves are correctly positioned, the soft tissue tension adjustments must be exactly right for proper arthroplasty function. If these requirements are not met, the arthroplasty will at best be suboptimal and often will be a total failure.

Although some minor degree of postoperative ligament asymmetry or laxity may be tolerated, it is better to obtain nearly perfect stability through surgical technique. Some surgeons have advocated the use of constrained prostheses for unstable knees with greater than 20 degrees of fixed varus or valgus deformity, greater than 30 degrees of fixed flexion deformity, or gross preoperative instability with incompetence of two or more of the major knee ligaments. However, such protheses are very rarely required for a primary knee arthroplasty, although they may be needed in occasional revision cases.

Most surgeons advocate routine patellar resurfacing, although some practice a selective resurfacing in OA and preserve patellae that appear more or less normal with a good surface of articular cartilage.[39] In RA, there is an argument for always resurfacing the patella, so that all articular cartilage (which may be the source of recurrent synovitis) is removed.

Perioperative Care

Intravenous (IV) antibiotics (usually oxacillin or cephalosporin) are administered immediately preoperatively and for 24 hours postoperatively. After successful rehabilitation of the knee, there are times when prophylactic antibiotics are necessary. As prophylaxis for extensive dental procedures, genitourinary tract instrumentation, or other surgery in which there is a possibility of bacteremia, antibiotic coverage is recommended by most surgeons. The appropriate antibiotic, determined by likely contaminants in the area to be manipulated, are given 1 hour before the procedure and again 6 hours after the procedure.[40]

The prevention of thrombophlebitis should be a major goal of every orthopedic surgeon who performs total knee arthroplasty. In one study of patients undergoing total knee arthroplasty, 64 percent had evidence of thrombophlebitis, as indicated by a positive venogram on the fifth postoperative day.[41] This occurred despite prophylactic anticoagulation treatments including aspirin, dextran, and low-dose heparin. It is commonly accepted that some form of antithrombotic prophylactic treatment should be administered after total knee replacement—be it warfarin, intermittent mechanic compression of the calf, aspirin, or low molecular weight (LMW) heparin. The duration of prophylaxis is controversial; when do the risks of anticoagulation outweigh the danger of late thromboembolism?[42]

Prophylaxis and diagnosis of thromboembolism are discussed more fully in Chapter 116.5.

Total knee arthroplasty patients are allowed to walk on the first postoperative day using a walker or crutches, with weight-bearing as tolerated. Early motion in the recovery room, with a continuous passive motion machine, has been employed with encouraging early results, but long-term studies show minimal, if any, improvement in knee motion.[43] Active assisted flexion exercises are performed under the guidance of a physiotherapist. Many hospitals now employ "critical pathways" to guide the postoperative management of these patients. This has resulted in an average length of stay of 4 or 5 days. Under such circumstances, many patients will not be able to ambulate independently at discharge and must either go to a rehabilitation facility or have home physical therapy to achieve optimal outcomes.

Complications of Knee Replacement

GENERAL

Despite the advanced age of most patients and the frequency of associated medical conditions, complications of knee replacement are relatively few and are consistent with those discussed previously with regard to hip surgery (see Chapter 116.5).

SPECIFIC TO THE OPERATION

Hemarthrosis and minor problems of wound healing are the most common early complications and usually resolve without consequence. Peroneal nerve palsies are uncommon and usually follow correction of severe valgus deformity. These also usually resolve. Wound infection occurs in 0.5 to 1 percent of patients.

Patellar complications are probably the most common problem with all types of knee replacements and may lead to revision in up to 3 to 4 percent of patients within the first 15 years.[39,44] Complications consist of loosening of the patellar component, improper tracking, wear, and fracture of the patella. Patellar fractures are a complication of success, as they are seen in the most active patients with the greatest range of motion, who use the knee arthroplasty in a normal manner for stair climbing, arising from a chair, and other stressful activities. The fracture can usually be treated conservatively unless the patellar button is loosened, in which case the button must be removed.

Inadequate Motion

The motion obtained after arthroplasty depends on several factors, including body habitus, patient motivation, adequacy of physical therapy, and prosthetic design. Probably the most important determinant is the preoperative range of motion.[45] Patients with severe restriction of motion preoperatively will regain nearly full extension but flexion will remain close to the preoperative amount.[46]

Manipulation of the knee is sometimes recommended postoperatively if motion of at least 75 degrees is not regained within the first 3 or 4 weeks following surgery. A general or epidural anesthetic with full muscular relaxation is needed, as the purpose of the manipulation is to overcome articular adhesions with minimum force after quadriceps resistance is eliminated.

Continuous passive motion machines are widely used in an attempt to regain motion after knee arthroplasty. Whether or not these machines are useful in the long term is questionable[43]; they do appear, however, to advance the rate at which patients achieve postoperative functional milestones.

Loosening

Component loosening, usually the tibial component, was the most frequent cause of failure of hinged prostheses and early surface replacements. The high incidence of tibial-component loosening represented a design problem. Modifications to the tibial component in more recent designs have resulted in a marked decrease in loosening. Metal backing of the tibial component, which increases the rigidity of the polyethylene, and improved cement techniques have reduced the incidence of component loosening to almost zero in technically correct arthroplasties.[30,31,47]

Osteolysis

With the increased longevity of surface-replacement designs, polyethylene wear has become a problem. Premature wear may result from poor implant design, thin polyethylene tibial inserts, or manufacturing effects on the polyethylene itself. However, even with proven designs, wear remains an issue. Polyethylene debris has been shown to create a synovitis that can attack bone, resulting in the local loss of bone around the implant and jeopardizing fixation.[48]

Infection

Persistent symptoms after total knee replacement in the absence of a clear mechanical explanation should alert the surgeon to the possibility of infection. Although diagnosis of acute, severe infection poses no particular problems, latent infections can manifest themselves, mainly by knee pain, with mild or no general symptoms. The wound can be benign, and the usual laboratory tests and radiologic findings may prove negative.

Joint infection occurs more commonly in immunologically deficient RA patients. Frequently, these patients have had previous operations, and earlier incisions may predispose them to skin necrosis that may lead to a deep prosthetic infection.

The overall infection rate with surface total knee replacements is less than 1 percent. The recommended procedure for establishing the presence of infection is a knee aspiration, with the joint fluid sent for Gram stain and culture for aerobic, anaerobic, and acid-fast bacilli, as well as for fungus. The aspirate should be inoculated as soon as possible into broth and culture media to increase the detection of indolent organisms.

Deep Infection

Deep or periprosthetic infection, the most serious complication of total joint replacement, may occur either early (within 1 month of surgery) or late (after 1 month).

Early Infection

An early infection, provided that its course is not modified by the injudicious use of antibiotics, usually is not difficult to recognize. The clinical course is abnormal, with prolonged pain, swelling, inflammation, and fever. The white blood cell (WBC) count and erythrocyte sedimentation rate (ESR) remain elevated.

In acute cases, the clinician may attempt a thorough débridement of the knee, leaving the components in situ. Tissue should be sent for frozen section, Gram stain, and culture; the wound is closed over suction drains that remain in place for 24 hours.

IV antibiotic therapy is begun immediately, based on the most likely organism, and is subsequently modified according to the sensitivities of the organism. The wound is reaspirated 2 weeks later, and if cultures are negative, antibiotic therapy is continued for another 4 weeks (6 weeks total). If cultures are positive, the prosthetic components and all cement are removed, followed by at least 6 weeks of IV antibiotic therapy. Even in the optimal situation, wound débridement with retention of the components is successful in only 23 percent of cases.[49]

Treatment of deep infection with antibiotics alone is rarely indicated, because this treatment might suppress the symptoms of infection. Such treatment is indicated only in the most extenuating circumstances, such as when other medical problems are too severe for the patient to undergo surgery. Procrastination with prolonged use of oral antibiotics is ill advised because it will compromise future definitive treatment by masking a subclinical infection and by creating resistant bacterial strains.

Late Infection

Late infection is more common, and diagnosis is usually provided by aspiration. The knee frequently becomes painful and swollen. Any pain with use of a prosthesis for which a cause is not readily apparent should be assumed to be related to infection until proven otherwise.

The treatment for proven or suspected late deep infection consists of incision, drainage, thorough débridement of the involved tissues, and removal of the prosthetic components along with the acrylic cement, if present. This course should be followed, even in suspected cases, because only cultures obtained from the bone-cement interface may be positive.

If the infecting organism is resistant to antibiotic therapy, if there is an undue risk of antibiotic toxicity to the patient, or if the patient does not want a prosthesis out of fear of acquiring another infection, an arthrodesis is performed as a second stage. If the patient is medically fragile, the knee joint may be allowed to stiffen as a pseudarthrosis.

When the organism is susceptible, a new total knee replacement is implanted after a 6-week course of appropriate antibiotic therapy. Frozen tissue sections and Gram-stained tissue cultures are obtained at the time of surgery, and reimplantation proceeds only when these intraoperative tests reveal no evidence of active infection. An adequate selection of prosthetic components with modular metallic augments and stems should be available. Rarely, custom-designed prostheses may be necessary to handle bone deficiency. Patellectomy may prove helpful if the skin closure is too tight. Frequently, both alignment and stability can be restored with a posterior cruciate ligament—substituting surface replacement. Sometimes, constrained condylar posterior-stabilized prostheses are recommended; these have intramedullary stems on both components and restrict varus-valgus, anteroposterior (AP), and rotary motions by means of a centrally positioned peg.[50]

One survey of 38 reimplantations subjected to the previously described two-stage protocol with an average follow-up of 49 months (range 2 to 10 years), showed eradication of the original infection in all but one patient. The clinical results were acceptable and resembled those obtained in the most difficult, aseptic, revision total knee arthroplasties.[51] Reimplantation of a new prothesis was not performed in 14 patients for the following reasons: antibiotic-toxicity risk, medical infirmity, inadequate skin viability, extensive extensor-mechanism necrosis, and patient preference.

Revision of Total Knee Arthroplasty

Revision of a knee arthroplasty is relatively uncommon in the first 10 years following initial surgery. Reported failure rates with designs produced in the last 10 to 15 years range from 3 percent at 2 years[52] to 5 percent at 10 years.[53] More than half of the revisions in most series are carried out because of problems with the patella. Other reasons for revision are infection, ligamentous instability, component loosening, progression of arthritis in unreplaced surfaces (patella or the unreplaced compartment in unicompartmental designs), and polyethylene wear. Component loosening was the major cause of failure with early prosthetic designs, but this is not the case with later models, regardless of whether they are fixed with cement or by ingrowth.

The technical principles of revision surgery are similar to those described for infected cases, except that immediate exchange of components is done. Femoral and tibial bone loss is the major technical problem, and bone deficits, caused by osteolysis, may be built up by metal augments, bone grafts, or custom-designed prostheses. A posterior-stabilized condylar prosthesis is the prosthesis recommended for most revision procedures; however, the posterior cruciate ligament may be still preserved in milder cases of failure. The results of revision are not quite as good as those of the primary operation, and the complete pain relief normally found after knee replacement is not obtained as often in revision cases. Restricted motion has not been a problem, and the average range of motion after revision is almost the same as after the primary operation.

Results of Total Knee Arthroplasty

Results with modern knee prostheses, properly implanted, are at least as good as the excellent results obtained with total hip arthroplasty. Pain relief is either complete or nearly so in more than 95 percent of patients.[54] Functional improvement is somewhat less certain and is related to preoperative functional level, mental health, and the health system.[36] It is important to note that patient satisfaction after knee replacement is often higher than "objective" measures of knee function would suggest.[54-56]

For patients older than 60 years, a knee prosthesis will last for the remainder of life in most cases. For younger, more active patients, the longevity of the implant may be less certain, but one series of patients under the age of 55, with an average age of 43 years, had an implant survival rate at 10 years of 99 percent.[57] The high functional level of some of these younger patients may well produce problems in the long term because of wear of the polyethylene bearing surface.

The use of unicompartmental replacement remains controversial, and the published results of these pros theses are conflicting. Some report excellent results,[27,29,35] and others report failure rates of up to 13 percent at 10 years.[58]

Total knee designs that are currently in use, regardless of whether they retain the posterior cruciate ligament or substitute for it, demonstrate good-to-excellent results in 92 to 96 percent of patients at periods ranging from 10 to 14 years after surgery. The average range of motion is 105 to 110 degrees, and function is greatly improved in all except in those who are most severely disabled before surgery and in those who are depressed.[31,32,47,59-63]

Summary

The patient with localized cartilage defects, whether from trauma or OA, may shortly be able to receive engineered tissue containing chondrocytes and growth factors incorporated into a three-dimensional matrix that will induce repair of the defect with durable articular cartilage. Until that happens, and for those with more advanced OA and RA, prosthetic replacement of the knee offers almost certain relief of pain and improvement of function. Further developments in prosthetic design, such as refinement of the articular surfaces, utilization of a sliding bearing, and improvements in polyethylene, should improve on the already impressive results of replacement of the arthritic knee.

Important determinants of the clinical result include surgical technique, preoperative functional and mental status, and patient motivation.

REFERENCES

1. Sandmark H, Hogstedt C, Lewold S: Osteoarthrosis of the knee in men and women in association with overweight, smoking, and hormone therapy. Ann Rheum Dis 58:151, 1999.
2. Benson E, Resine S, Lewis, C: Functional outcome of arthrodesis for failed total knee arthroplasty. Orthopedics 21:875, 1998.

3. Insall J: Intra-articular surgery for degenerative arthritis of the knee: A report of the work of the late K.H. Pridie. J Bone Joint Surg Br 49:211, 1967.
4. Harwin S: Arthroscopic débridement for osteoarthritis of the knee: predictors of patient satisfaction. Arthroscopy 15:142, 1999.
5. Dervin GF, Stiell IG, Rody K, et al: Effect of arthroscopic débridement for osteoarthritis of the knee on health-related quality of life. J Bone Joint Surg Am 85-A:10, 2003.
6. Hunt SA, Jazrawi LM, Sherman OH: Arthroscopic management of osteoarthritis of the knee. J Am Acad Orthop Surg 10:356, 2002.
7. Moseley JB, O'Malley K, Petersen NJ, et al: A controlled trial of arthroscopic surgery for osteoarthritis of the knee. N Engl J Med 347:81, 2002.
8. Johnson L: Arthroscopic abrasion arthroplasty. In Poehling GG (ed): Operative Arthroscopy. New York, Raven Press, 1991, p 341.
9. Steadman J, Rodkey W, Singleton S: Microfracture technique for full-thickness chondral defects: technique and clinical results. Operative Tech Ortho 7:300, 1997.
10. O'Driscoll S, Salter R: The repair of major osteochondral defects in joint surfaces by neochondrogenesis with autogenous osteoperiosteal grafts stimulated by continuous passive motion: An experimental investigation in the rabbit. Clin Orthop 208:131, 1986.
11. Angermann P, Riegels-Nielsen P, Pedersen H: Osteochondritis dissecans of the femoral condyle treated with periosteal transplantation. Poor outcome in 14 patients followed for 6-9 years. Acta Orthop Scand 69:595, 1998.
12. Hominga G, Bulstra D, Bouwmeester P: Perichondral grafting for cartilage lesions of the knee. J Bone Joint Surg Br 72:1003, 1990.
13. Brittberg M, Lindahl A, Nilsson A: Treatment of deep cartilage defects in the knee with autologous chondrocyte transplantation. N Engl J Med 331:889, 1994.
14. Peterson L: Articular cartilage injuries treated with autologous chondrocyte transplantation in the human knee. Acta Orthop Belg 62:196, 1996.
15. Horas U, Pelinkovic D, Herr G, et al: Autologous chondrocyte implantation and osteochondral cylinder transplantation in cartilage repair of the knee joint: a prospective, comparative trial. J Bone Joint Surg Am 85-A:185, 2003.
16. Recht M, White LM, Winalski CS, et al: MR imaging of cartilage repair procedures. Skeletal Radiol 32:185, 2003.
17. Rahfoth B, Weisser J, Sternkopf F: Transplantation of allograft chondrocytes embedded in agarose gel into cartilage defects of rabbits. Osteoarthritis Cartilage 6:50, 1998.
18. Nehrer S, Breinan H, Ramappa A: Chondrocyte-seeded collagen matrices implanted in a chondral defect in a canine model. Biomaterials 19:2313, 1998.
19. Hangody L, Feczko P, Bartha L, et al: Mosaicplasty for the treatment of articular defects of the knee and ankle. Clin Orthop 391 (Suppl) 5328, 2001.
20. Aubin PP, Cheah HK, Davis AM, et al: Long-term followup of fresh femoral osteochondral allografts for posttraumatic knee defects. Clin Orthop 391:S318, 2001.
21. Coventry M: Osteotomy of the upper portion of the tibia for degenerative arthritis of the knee: A preliminary report. J Bone Joint Surg Am 47:984, 1965.
22. Choi HR, Hasegawa Y, Kondo S, et al: High tibial osteotomy for varus gonarthrosis: a 10- to 24-year follow-up study. J Orthop Sci 6:493, 2001.
23. Marti RK, Verhagen RA, Kerkhoffs GM, et al: Proximal tibial varus osteotomy. Indications, technique, and five to twenty-one-year results. J Bone Joint Surg Am 83-A:164, 2001.
24. Aglietti P, Menchetti PP: Distal femoral varus osteotomy in the valgus osteoarthritic knee. Am J Knee Surg 13:89, 2000.
25. Wolfe F, Zwillich S: The long-term outcomes of rheumatoid arthritis: a 23-year prospective, longitudinal study of total joint replacement and its predictors in 1,600 patients with rheumatoid arthritis. Arthritis Rheum 41:1072, 1998.
26. Barnes C, Shortkroff S, Sledge C: Radiation synovectomy using dysprosium 165 ferric hydroxide macroaggregates: A review. Rheum Rev 1:151, 1992.
27. Robertsson O: Unicompartmental arthroplasty: Results in Sweden 1986-1995. Orthopade 29(Suppl 1):S6, 2000.
28. Gunston F: Polycentric knee arthroplasty: Prosthetic simulation of normal knee movement. J Bone Joint Surg Br 53:272, 1971.
29. Newman J, Ackroyd C, Shah N: Unicompartmental or total knee replacement? Five-year results of a prospective, randomised trial of 102 osteoarthritic knees with unicompartmental arthritis. J Bone Joint Surg Br 80:862, 1998.
30. Archibeck MJ, Berger RA, Barden RM, et al: Posterior cruciate ligament-retaining total knee arthroplasty in patients with rheumatoid arthritis. J Bone Joint Surg Am 83:1231, 2001.
31. Berger RA, Rosenberg AG, Barden RM, et al: Long-term followup of the Miller-Galante total knee replacement. Clin Orthop 388:58, 2001.
32. Rodriguez JA, Bhende H, Ranawat CS: Total condylar knee replacement: a 20-year followup study. Clin Orthop 388:10, 2001.
33. O'Connor J, Goodfellow J: Theory and practice of meniscal knee replacement: designing against wear. Proc Inst Mech Eng 210:217, 1996.
34. Stiehl J, Dennis D, Komistek R: In vivo analysis of a mobile bearing total knee prosthesis. Clin Orthop 345:60, 1997.
35. Murray D, Goodfellow J, O'Connor J: The Oxford medial unicompartmental arthroplasty: a ten-year survival study. J Bone Joint Surg Br 80:983, 1998.
36. Fortin P, Clarke A, Joseph L, et al: Outcomes of total hip and knee replacement: preoperative functional status predicts outcomes at six months after surgery. Arthritis Rheum 42:1722, 1999.
37. Lonner JH, Hershman S, Mont M, et al: Total knee arthroplasty in patients 40 years of age and younger with osteoarthritis. Clin Orthop 380:85, 2000.
38. Tauro B, Ackroyd CE, Newman JH, et al: The Lubinus patellofemoral arthroplasty: A five- to ten-year prospective study. J Bone Joint Surg Br 83:696, 2001.
39. Boyd A, Ewald F, Thomas W, et al: Long term complications after total knee arthroplasty with or without resurfacing of the patella. J Bone Joint Surg Am 75:674, 1993.
40. Drangsholt M: Current concepts review: Prophylactic use of antibiotics for procedures after total joint replacement. J Bone Joint Surg Am 80:1394, 1998.
41. Stulberg B, Insall J, Lewis R: Deep vein thrombosis following total knee replacement: an analysis of 638 arthroplasties. J Bone Joint Surg Am 66:194, 1984.
42. Nurmohamed M, Lems W, Dijkmans B: Risk of post-discharge venous thromboembolism in patients with rheumatoid arthritis undergoing knee or hip arthroplasty: Is prolonged thromboprophylaxis warranted or dangerous? Ann Rheum Dis 58:392, 1999.
43. MacDonald SJ, Bourne RB, Rorabeck CH, et al: Prospective randomized clinical trial of continuous passive motion after total knee arthroplasty. Clin Orthop 380:30, 2000.
44. Barrack RL, Bertot AJ, Wolfe MW, et al: Patellar resurfacing in total knee arthroplasty: A prospective, randomized, double-blind study with five to seven years of follow-up. J Bone Joint Surg Am 83:1376, 2001.
45. Schurman D, Matityahu A, Goodman S, et al: Prediction of postoperative knee flexion in Insall-Burstein II total knee arthroplasty. Clin Orthop 175:84, 1998.
46. Montgomery W, Insall J, Haas S, et al: Primary total knee arthroplasty in stiff and ankylosed knees. Am J Knee Surg 11:20, 1998.
47. Buechel FF Sr., Buechel FF Jr, Pappas MJ, et al: Twenty-year evaluation of meniscal bearing and rotating platform knee replacements. Clin Orthop 388:41, 2001.
48. Fink B, Berger I, Siegmuller C, et al: Recurring synovitis as a possible reason for aseptic loosening of knee endoprostheses in patients with rheumatoid arthritis. J Bone Joint Surg Br 83:604, 2001.
49. Schoifet S, Morrey B: Treatment of infection after total knee arthroplasty by debridement with retention of the components. J Bone Joint Surg Am 72:1383, 1990.
50. Barrack RL: Evolution of the rotating hinge for complex total knee arthroplasty. Clin Orthop 392:292, 2001.
51. Windsor R, Insall J, Urs W, et al: Two-stage reimplantation for the salvage of total knee arthroplasty complicated by infection. J Bone Joint Surg Am 72:272, 1990.
52. Heck D, Melfi C, Mamlin L, et al: Revision rates after knee replacement in the United States. Med Care 36:661, 1998.
53. Robertsson O, Knutson K, Lewold S, et al: Knee arthroplasty in rheumatoid arthritis: A report from the Swedish Knee Arthroplasty Register on 4,381 primary operations 1985-1995. Acta Orthop Scand 68:545, 1997.

54. Heck D, Robinson R, Partridge C, et al: Patient outcomes after knee replacement. Clin Orthop 93:110, 1998.

55. Bullens PH, van Loon CJ, de Waal Malefijt MC, et al: Patient satisfaction after total knee arthroplasty: a comparison between subjective and objective outcome assessments. J Arthroplasty 16:740, 2001.

56. Lingard EA, Katz JN, Wright RJ, et al: Validity and responsiveness of the Knee Society Clinical Rating System in comparison with the SF-36 and WOMAC. J Bone Joint Surg Am 83:1856, 2001.

57. Duffy G, Trousdale R, Stuart M: Total knee arthroplasty in patients 55 years old or younger. 10- to 17-year results. Clin Orthop 356: 22-27, 1998.

58. Bert J: 10-year survivorship of metal-backed, unicompartmental arthroplasty. J Arthroplasty 13:901, 1998.

59. Ewald F, Wright R, Poss R: Kinematic total knee arthroplasty: a 10- to 14-year prospective follow-up review. J Arthroplasty 14:473, 1999.

60. Gill GS, Joshi AB: Long-term results of Kinematic Condylar knee replacement: An analysis of 404 knees. J Bone Joint Surg Br 83:355, 2001.

61. Gill GS, Joshi AB: Long-term results of cemented, posterior cruciate ligament-retaining total knee arthroplasty in osteoarthritis. Am J Knee Surg 14:209, 2001.

62. Laskin RS: The Genesis total knee prosthesis: a 10-year followup study. Clin Orthop 388:95, 2001

63. Parker DA, Rorabeck CH, Bourne RB: Long-term followup of cementless versus hybrid fixation for total knee arthroplasty. Clin Orthop 388:68, 2001.

THE ANKLE AND FOOT
CLEMENT B. SLEDGE

The Ankle

TYPES OF PATHOLOGY

Osteoarthritis

Osteoarthritis (OA) is far less common in the ankle than it is in the knee or the hip. When it does occur, however, it is almost always the result of previous trauma or secondary to malalignment caused by other lower extremity injuries, such as tibial and calcaneal fractures.[1]

Common ankle fractures rarely lead to significant secondary OA when they are treated by anatomic reduction. When the articular cartilage of the roof of the ankle joint—the *plafond* (French)—or the dome of the talus is damaged by a fracture through the cartilage or severe contusion, arthritis may well follow.

The flutelike distal expansion of the tibial shaft, ending in the tibial side of the ankle joint, is frequently referred to as the *pilon* (also a French term) because of its resemblance to the pylons used to support large overhead power cables. Unlike common ankle fractures, pilon fractures are very susceptible to post-traumatic arthritis. The typical mechanism of a pilon fracture includes an axial loading component that crushes the ankle cartilage and produces an intra-articular fracture within the major weight-bearing area. The incidence of post-traumatic arthritis increases greatly when cartilage has been crushed, but satisfactory ankle function is still possible with appropriate surgical reconstruction.

Several other injuries are also associated with ankle arthritis, including fractures of the tibia that have healed with angular deformity, particularly those that have united in varus displacement or extension—a deformity also called posterior angulation in the distal tibia. Similarly, calcaneal fractures that have united in marked varus or valgus displacement can also exert eccentric forces on the ankle and eventually cause arthritis.

Ankle arthritis can occur as a consequence of posterior tibial tendon rupture, a condition commonly seen in patients with rheumatoid arthritis (RA) but that can also occur in others, most notably older women. Rupture of the posterior tibial tendon can result in severe hindfoot valgus and, in due course, slowly progressive ankle arthritis. Subtalar coalitions and surgical subtalar fusions can produce severe stresses in the ankle that can cause slowly progressive arthritis. Normal subtalar motion protects the ankle by absorbing the stresses produced in walking on uneven surfaces; loss of this natural shock absorber increases the magnitude of impact on the ankle and the other lower-extremity joints.

A type of limited arthritis can occur in the anterior ankle. It is a sequela of long-time repetitive ankle dorsiflexion and jumping, as can occur in football, basketball, and soccer (Fig. 116–44). In this type of arthritis, repetitive impingement of the anterior tibial malleolus into the neck of the talus stimulates the development of reactive spurs. The problem is made more likely by preexisting deformity. For example, an old calcaneal fracture can precipitate impaction of a dorsiflexed talus into the calcaneus. It is also possible for callus that formed in an undiagnosed, undisplaced fracture to build up and obliterate the talar neck. If the problem is not recognized and treated, the symptoms can become disabling. Satisfactory results are possible with early surgical intervention because only a small area of the articular weight-bearing surface is involved in the early stages.

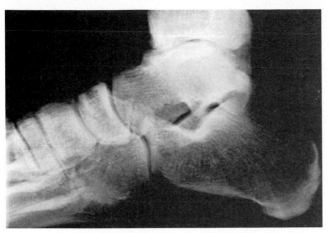

FIGURE 116-44 · Lateral Radiograph Shows Anterior Impingement Arthritis Following an Ankle Fracture with an Intra-articular Extension. Impingement arthritis routinely initiates formation of a lip or spur on the anterior talus, formation of a spur and thickening of the neck of the talus, or both.

Inflammatory Arthritis

Inflammatory arthritides can also occur in the ankle but are less common in this location than in the hip or the knee. When this form of arthritis does occur, the functional disability can be severe.[2]

Inflammatory involvement in the ankle can be attributed to indirect or direct causes. An example of indirect involvement is that due to tenosynovitis, producing rupture of the posterior tibial tendon. This results in valgus malalignment in the foot, which in turn initiates erosion of the fibular and lateral tibial articular surfaces. Direct involvement is characterized by ankle synovitis and subsequent joint destruction; inflammatory changes may involve other joints in the foot as well. Manifestations of inflammatory arthritides are more common in the forefoot, particularly in the metatarsophalangeal joints, than they are in the midfoot or hindfoot. As with ankle involvement, however, the functional implications can be profound, with severe pain and gait limitation.

TREATMENT IMPLICATIONS

Because most cases of OA of the ankle are the result of trauma and subsequent malalignment of the lower extremity and foot, great attention should be paid to prevention of tibial or hindfoot malalignment during primary fracture care. When malalignment occurs following fractures of the tibia or ankle, it can be corrected by an osteotomy. When the deformity is due to rupture of the posterior tibial tendon, correction can be achieved by muscle balancing if the foot is still supple. Subtalar fusion and triple arthrodesis should be reserved for advanced stages of deformity, when these joints become symptomatic.

The late sequelae of unrecognized or poorly treated ankle injuries and tendon ruptures should alert primary care providers and rheumatologists to the importance of early diagnosis and referral. They should be able to diagnose potentially disabling conditions early and should refer patients with impending problems to orthopedic foot and ankle surgeons before serious damage has occurred.

DIAGNOSIS

Diagnosis of arthritis of the ankle should not be difficult if the clinician is alert to the possibility and the patient's shoes and socks are routinely removed for examination. The presenting manifestations—pain and swelling in the ankle with limitation of motion and synovial thickening (usually anterolateral at first)—are readily noted. Plain weight-bearing anteroposterior (AP), mortise, and lateral radiographic views should be obtained to confirm the diagnosis. Tibial malalignment can be seen on AP and lateral tibial radiographs, and foot malalignment can be confirmed on weight-bearing AP, lateral, and axial (heel) radiographs. Because radiologists do not observe the patients standing, alignment parameters in the foot must be understood by the treating physician and appropriate confirmatory radiographs requested.

NONOPERATIVE TREATMENT

In the absence of significant malalignment or deformity, many patients presenting with pain and stiffness in the ankle from arthritis can obtain adequate relief with nonoperative treatment (See chapters 41, 55). Management of symptoms by orthoses may constitute definitive treatment, or the use of an orthosis can be a temporary measure to alleviate symptoms until surgical treatment is undertaken. Modifications made to shoes can compensate for much of the motion normally provided by the ankle during gait. The sole of a well-fitting shoe can be modified with thick cushioning material, and the heel and toe of the shoe can be beveled to create a rocker bottom. Sometimes use of these measures alone is adequate to prevent excessive motion with resultant pain in the arthritic ankle. Additional relief can be provided by immobilization of the ankle with an ankle-foot orthosis, which consists of a posterior plastic device that is placed inside the shoe as a heel cup, with extensions behind the ankle and up the calf. By limiting motion in the ankle and holding the foot in correct alignment, such a device can relieve most if not all symptoms.

SURGICAL TREATMENT

Ankle arthritis can be treated by a variety of surgical procedures including arthrodesis, débridement with realignment by osteotomy, and ankle arthroplasty (total ankle replacement).[2]

Débridement with realignment serves a useful purpose in spite of progressive deterioration in the ankle and the eventual reappearance of symptoms in most cases (Fig. 116-45). This approach can provide temporary relief from pain and postpone the need for an arthrodesis or arthroplasty for 10 years or longer. Fusion of an ankle in optimal alignment provides a satisfactory functional result, but the benefits of arthrodesis are also only temporary. Over time, usually 10 to 20 years, a fused ankle transfers excessive forces to the subtalar and midtarsal joints, leading to changes in

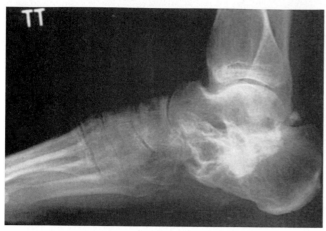

FIGURE 116-45 · Lateral Radiograph Shows Anterior Impingement of the Ankle. Impingement in this case resulted from a previous calcaneal fracture and collapse of the subtalar joint.

those joints. Arthritis eventually develops, and the benefits provided by the fusion are lost. Pain from arthritis in the subtalar and midtarsal joints after ankle fusion can also be alleviated by shoe modifications and activity restrictions, much as in the nonoperative treatment for ankle arthritis.

Ankle arthroplasty is a procedure that is still considered by most authorities to be in evolution. The useful life of current ankle-implant devices appears to be approximately 10 years, and salvage after failure of the prosthesis presents a challenging problem. Failure of an ankle arthroplasty is usually related to subsidence and loosening of the prosthesis. By the time a prosthesis fails and salvage is undertaken, attempts at reconstruction of the foot and ankle are impeded by the presence of a large bone defect that makes arthrodesis difficult.

Ankle Arthrodesis

Numerous techniques for ankle arthrodesis have been devised, suggesting that none is perfect. There is debate regarding the ideal position in which to fuse the ankle. Some authorities favor a neutral position of the foot and ankle in males and slight plantar flexion in females to facilitate wearing shoes with a raised heel. As shoe fashions and activities change, these guidelines need to be reexamined in each case; a position of dorsiflexion or plantar flexion with slight heel valgus is usually appropriate.[3] The foot should be displaced not more than 1 cm posterior to its anatomic position in the sagittal plane to reduce the length of the anterior lever arm and to facilitate smooth gait.

The malleoli are left intact to preserve the normal channels that carry the posterior tibial tendon, the flexor digitorum communis, and the peroneal tendons. These tendons control the subtalar joint as well as position and motion in the midfoot. The malleoli also provide supplementary stabilization for the fused ankle. Minimal bone removal prevents the malleoli from descending and impinging on the shoe. An illustrative case is shown in Figure 116-46.

A cast is applied after surgery and is removed 2 to 3 weeks postoperatively to allow mobilization of the subtalar and the other tarsal joints, as well as for bathing and sleeping, but weight-bearing is limited to 15 pounds until healing is complete. Healing is usually demonstrated at 8 to 12 postoperative weeks, but it can occur in as little as 6 weeks. After solid fusion is obtained, function can be facilitated by the use of a shoe with a "rocker" configuration that has added impact-absorptive capacity in the sole.[4]

Although arthrodesis is a treatment usually used as a last resort, it can restore function in young patients with OA who wish to return to strenuous activities. In patients with RA, the aim is almost always to preserve motion in every joint. In these patients, if arthrodesis of the ankle becomes necessary, most will have adequate function and relief of pain and will be satisfied with the result.[5]

Débridement and Realignment by Osteotomy

Anterior ankle pain accompanied by bone spurs as seen on radiographs is an indication for débridement of the anterior lip of the tibia or of the tibia and the neck of the talus. The procedure, done either as open surgery or arthroscopically, usually improves dorsiflexion and alleviates pain in the anterior ankle.

Ankle malalignment can be corrected by a supramalleolar osteotomy (Fig. 116-47) or, if malalignment is the result of a malunion, by an osteotomy at the malunion site. Varus, valgus, or extension deformities can occur as a consequence of congenital, degenerative, or post-traumatic problems, or from a combination of these conditions. Long-standing hindfoot valgus precipitated by posterior tibial tendon rupture can tilt the talus into the ankle mortise and erode it into the lateral plafond. Delayed treatment of this condition necessitates correction not only of the underlying valgus deformity in the heel but also of the secondary deformity, the tilted talus. The valgus deformity can be realigned by a triple arthrodesis, a subtalar arthrodesis, or a calcaneocuboid arthrodesis with distraction, medial column stabilization, and tendon transfers. The ankle joint is anatomically realigned by a medial closing wedge supramalleolar osteotomy or by a total ankle arthroplasty.

Long-standing tibia vara, which may be a result of tibial fracture or knee arthritis or may represent a genetic anatomic variation, produces a compensatory valgus deformity at the ankle and hindfoot. Correction of the tibial deformity by a total knee arthroplasty may result in a valgus deformity of the ankle. A medial closing wedge supramalleolar osteotomy can be carried out to correct the deformity and minimize the risk of development of secondary arthritis in the foot and ankle.

Ankle Arthroplasty

In spite of extensive research and testing, the same problems that plague other total joint replacements—loosening and subsidence—have occurred with the use of all the ankle implants designed so far.[6-8] Therefore, their use is limited to narrow indications, usually for ankle problems in elderly patients with RA.[7-9]

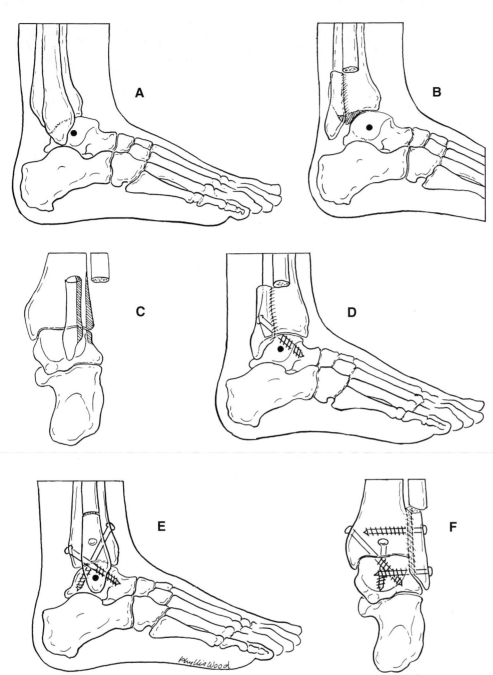

FIGURE 116–46 · *A*, A typical deformity following a pilon fracture. The foot is extruded forward from its normal alignment. *B* and *C*, The fibula is transected and rolled back over the posterior soft tissues to provide an approach to the ankle. The distal segment is left attached to the posterior soft tissues. Damaged cartilage and spurs are débrided, but only a small amount of bone is removed to permit anatomic repositioning. Mobilization of the posterior deltoid ligament may be needed to facilitate moving the talus posteriorly. The alignment is corrected by pushing the foot back into its normal position. *D*, The first screw is placed through the lateral exposure at the back of the tibia and is directed across the joint and into the neck and head of the talus. When it is tightened, it compresses the joint, provides posterior translation, and resists flexion. *E* and *F*, A factor critical to the success of an ankle arthrodesis is precise placement of the compression screws. The screws must be able to resist motion in all planes, namely flexion and extension, inversion and eversion, and translation (shear). The second screw is placed to resist extension forces. It is started laterally or medially from the anterior distal tibia and placed across the joint into the posterior talus. This is a difficult target at which to aim, because the screw must not cross the posterior facet of the subtalar joint. The function of the third screw is to resist eversion. It is inserted percutaneously through the medial malleolus and into the midbody of the talus. The fibula is replaced with the posterior vascular pedicle intact. The apposing surfaces of the tibia and the talus are stripped to cancellous bone before they are joined. Two cortical screws are placed through the fibula to resist inversion. (Copyright Phyllis Wood Associates, Seattle, Washington.)

Arthroplasty allows motion in the ankle joint and protects the other joints in the foot. If the procedure is unsuccessful but marked subsidence has not occurred, replacement with another prosthesis is sometimes possible. Alternatively, the joint may be salvaged by fusion using bone grafts to maintain length.[9,10]

Recommendations

None of the treatments currently recommended for arthritis in the ankle provides a permanent correction. Despite failure after an average of 10 years—from secondary overload and subsequent development of arthritis in the subtalar and midtarsal joints—fusion remains the standard treatment for these conditions, particularly in patients with advanced deformity. There is no reason to assume that ankle arthroplasty will be a permanent solution for this problem, certainly not in young patients with severe ankle disease, although it may be the best alternative for some patients with severe polyarticular RA.

The Foot

THE HINDFOOT AND MIDFOOT

Anatomic Considerations

The hindfoot structures include the talus and the calcaneus along with their ligaments and joints. The midfoot

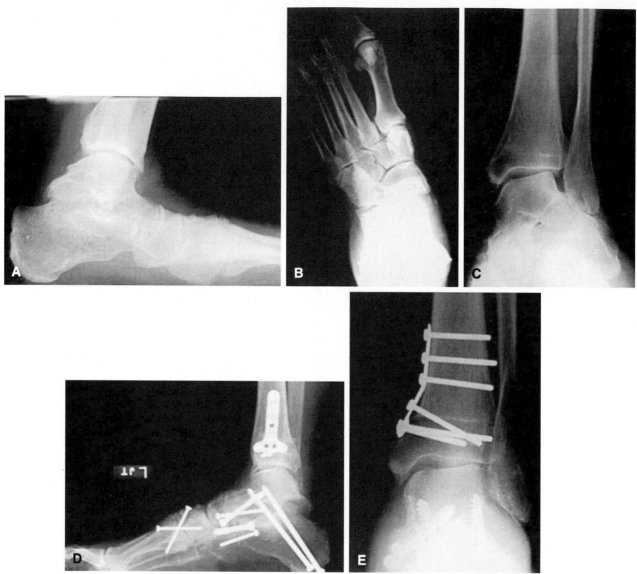

FIGURE 116-47 · Radiographs of a Patient with Long-Standing Posterior Tibial Tendon Rupture. *A*, Lateral weight-bearing view demonstrates anterior ankle arthritis, posterior subtalar arthritis, dorsolateral peritalar subluxation, naviculocuneiform sag and arthritis, and dorsal subluxation of the first metatarsal base on the first cuneiform. *B*, The anteroposterior (AP) radiograph reveals additional findings, including lateral peritalar subluxation and hypertrophy of the second metatarsal. *C*, AP radiograph of the ankle shows the talus tilted laterally in the ankle mortise as a consequence of a long-term valgus deformity in the heel and other foot deformities. Note the loss of cartilage in the lateral ankle joint and the stretched deltoid ligament. *D*, Lateral radiographic view after realignment of the foot by a triple arthrodesis and a first-cuneiform arthrodesis. *E*, AP radiograph of the ankle taken after a closing medial wedge osteotomy was performed at the supramalleolar level to bring the corrected foot under the weight-bearing line of the tibia. Narrowing of the lateral joint cartilage can still be seen.

consists of five bones: the tarsal navicular; the cuboid; and the medial, intermediate, and lateral cuneiform bones, as well as numerous ligaments and joints. The hindfoot and forefoot share a close anatomic relationship, and although traditionally they have been regarded as separate structures, it is somewhat unrealistic to consider them distinct entities.

From a functional standpoint, not all of the joints in the foot are equally important. Of the 28 bones and even more numerous joints in the foot, only a few carry out motion that is indispensable for normal function. The most important attribute in the other bones and joints is stability. The greatest number of functionally important (essential) joints is found in the hindfoot; these joints include the ankle (both the tibiotalar and fibulotalar joints), the subtalar (talocalcaneal) joint, and the talonavicular articulation with the midfoot. The chief functions of the essential joints are to adapt the foot and ankle to uneven surfaces by means of inversion and eversion, to cushion impact by pronation and supination, and to provide stability during late stance. Complete or significant lack of normal motion in these joints can alter gait and place severe stresses on other joints. Significant joint arthritis is uncommon in the hindfoot joints, but it can cause marked disability when it occurs.

Unlike in the hindfoot joints, virtually no motion is required in the midtarsal or tarsometatarsal joints for normal function except for slight translation in the cuboid-fourth metatarsal and cuboid-fifth metatarsal joints and the calcaneocuboid joints. In a normal foot, the nonessential naviculocuneiform, intercuneiform, and cuneiform-metatarsal joints are very stable, and functional impairment is minimal after their fusion. Motion in these joints is a pathologic condition that typically leads to a flatfoot deformity. Just one muscle—the triceps surae, or gastrocsoleus—powers the hindfoot, and only one other—the posterior tibialis—controls the position of the entire five-bone midfoot block.

An understanding of the functions of the various structures in the hindfoot and the midfoot allows the physician or surgeon to infer the extent of damage that has occurred in the ankle and to choose the best methods for managing synovitis, tendinitis, and arthritis. For example, newly developing deformity in the hindfoot is indicative of muscle imbalance caused by contracture or rupture of the posterior tibial tendon or muscle. Contracture of the muscle or tendon produces a cavovarus deformity; rupture causes a planovalgus deformity; and muscle weakness is responsible for progressive flatfoot in valgus.

The function of the posterior tibial muscle is to align the midfoot section in front of the talar head, thereby maintaining a normal arch or medial column. During early stance, the posterior tibial muscle is relaxed and the tibia is internally rotated. The arch is pronated and flat in this attitude, and it can absorb the shocks produced by gait. During midstance, and in successive phases when the foot is planted, the tibia is externally rotated, and it rotates the talus externally through the ankle mortise. With contraction of the posterior tibial muscle, the midfoot moves inferomedially over the head of the talus, lifting the arch and making it rigid. Gastrocsoleus contractions work against the medial column to create a long lever arm and to generate strong push-off.

A deficiency in any element of this system, such as looseness in the ankle mortise, abnormal motion in the subtalar or talonavicular joints, weakness in the posterior tibial muscle, or tightness of the heel cord, can pronate the foot and make it incapable of strong push-off. In functional terms, a foot with any of these abnormalities lacks adequate propulsion for gait, causing the patient to walk with a limp and with the toe pointing out. As deformity progresses, the heel turns toward the valgus and the foot appears to be displaced laterally under the talus.

This type of lateral deviation in the foot frequently occurs in patients with partial or complete rupture of the posterior tibial tendon and can also be caused by inflammatory arthritides. When it is diagnosed promptly, posterior tibial tendinitis is frequently treated by synovectomy or with steroid injections. Synovectomy can reduce pain, but it rarely prevents further deformity and it cannot restore normal anatomy. Steroid injections can increase the potential for rupture. Similarly, augmentation of the posterior tibialis with the flexor digitorum communis may also alleviate symptoms, but it rarely corrects the deformity because the gastrocnemius (or, rarely, the gastrocsoleus) is an extremely strong muscle

that can overpower the weakened posterior tibial tendon. Tightness in the gastrocsoleus muscle tends to produce pronation or an equinus deformity in the foot. This is frequently followed by development of arthritis in the calcaneocuboid joint and, subsequently, forefoot abduction and heel valgus.

An uncommon but not rare condition seen in patients with RA is isolated talonavicular arthritis, often accompanied by spasm in the peroneal muscles. The patient complains of "ankle" pain, but a careful examination of the foot usually reveals the true source of the pain. For this examination, the clinician holds the ankle joint firmly (i.e., with the left hand on the patient's left ankle), and forcibly and rapidly inverts the forefoot. With inflammatory changes in the talonavicular joint, this maneuver produces pain in the joint and reflex spasm in the peroneal muscles. The diagnosis can be confirmed by radiographs. Injection of local anesthetic is not helpful in confirming the diagnosis because of the frequent communication of the ankle joint and talonavicular joints. Fusion of the talonavicular joint is curative in most instances and produces little disability.[11]

Some overweight, middle-aged or elderly persons develop a severely pronated foot that progresses to a rigid flatfoot with arthritis involving several of the midtarsal and tarsometatarsal joints. A similar picture can also be seen after fractures, especially fracture dislocation of the tarsometatarsal joint of Lisfranc. Good long-term results have been reported with fusion of the involved joints.[12]

Surgical Treatment for Posterior Tibial Tendon Insufficiency

Posterior tibial tendon rupture syndrome most commonly occurs in persons with RA, but it is not limited to this patient population. The goal of treatment is to restore alignment, comfort, and function without sacrificing motion in the essential joints.

Various types of arthrodesis—talonavicular, subtalar, double, and triple—have been carried out in an attempt to correct hyperpronation or dorsolateral peritalar subluxation.[13] All of these fusions sacrifice subtalar motion and should be avoided if possible by early recognition of the process and conservative treatment. When arthrodesis is necessary to stabilize a foot that has lost posterior tibial tendon function, isolated subtalar fusion has been reported to give good results.

When arthrodesis is warranted, the hindfoot should be fused with the foot in neutral to slight valgus alignment. This is accomplished by rotating the peritalar joints into their neutral positions and stabilizing them with compression screws. Manipulation of the joints into their anatomic positions becomes more difficult in cases of advanced deformity, but positioning should not be performed by inserting and removing wedges of bone, thereby further altering foot mechanics.

The key to obtaining satisfactory results with reconstructive procedures is early diagnosis and appropriate treatment. The sequence of events leading to pronation and collapse of the arch can be averted altogether when tendinitis, specifically tendinitis caused by tight-

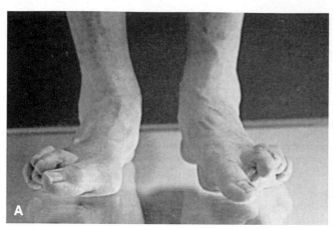
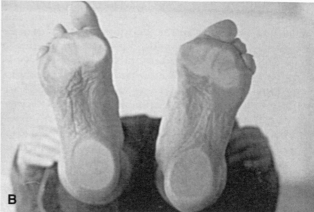

FIGURE 116–48 • *A*, Feet with typical rheumatoid arthritis (RA) deformities. The great toe is in valgus, and the lesser toes are extended and clawed. The deformity is more severe in the second and third toes. *B*, A weight-bearing view from below shows heavily concentrated weight-bearing under the metatarsal heads, which have been displaced downward, stretching the soft tissues in the sole of the foot. Note lack of weight-bearing by all but the great toe on patient's left foot.

ness in the Achilles tendon, is diagnosed early and treated by tendon lengthening and use of orthoses. Likewise, the deformities secondary to rupture of the posterior tibial tendon can be avoided by early recognition and appropriate treatment without sacrifice of foot function. Once a joint has sustained intrinsic damage and the patient experiences pain with daily activity, the only remaining treatment options are likely to sacrifice some aspects of normal foot function.

THE FOREFOOT

Of all the structures in the foot and ankle, the forefoot is the most susceptible to involvement with RA.[14] Indeed, almost every patient with RA will eventually develop involvement of one or more joints of the feet. In the foot, as in the hand, inflammatory synovitis affects the small joints as well as the intrinsic muscles and tendons and frequently causes severe deformity. The most common deformities are hallux valgus, cockup toes, and depressed metatarsal heads.[15] Large rheumatoid nodules are especially troublesome in the feet because they make shoe fitting difficult. Degenerative arthritis occurs most frequently in the great toe metatarsophalangeal (MTP) joint, but it can develop in other forefoot joints after direct trauma.

Synovial destruction of a joint capsule coupled with malalignment of the intrinsic tendons produces a characteristic pattern of deformity. The first cuneiform–first metatarsal joint becomes hypermobile and then elevates and drifts into varus. Elevation of the first metatarsal transfers excessive weight to the other metatarsal joints, accelerating existing synovial damage in the capsules and aggravating the abnormal position of the intrinsic muscles. Development of a hallux valgus deformity soon follows, and the combined deformities disrupt stability in the second toe. The deformity usually progresses laterally, and the second toe begins to show signs of clawing and dislocation from lack of integrity in the intrinsic musculature, capsular destruction, and exces-

sive pull by the extrinsic muscles. The lesser metatarsal heads become increasingly more prominent and overloaded, and they are displaced from their protected positions over the plantar fat pads. They are pushed downward into the sole of the foot, stretching the plantar soft tissues and causing pain in the sole of the foot. Patients frequently describe this pain as being like that from "having rocks in my shoes" (Fig. 116–48). In the past, the standard surgical treatment for this condition has been to remove the metatarsal heads or metatarsal heads and the bases of the proximal phalanges, thereby permanently disrupting normal function in the toes. If recognized early, the deformity can be corrected by soft tissue realignment, similar to that carried out in the hand joints.

Nonoperative Treatment

The use of orthoses does not preclude the need for surgical reconstruction in the future, but wearing shoes of extra depth and custom-molded orthoses can provide satisfactory relief from discomfort and improve function. This type of shoe provides extra room in the toebox to accommodate the bunion, the cocked-up toe, and the clawed toes.[16] A molded orthosis is added to distribute weight evenly under the sole of the foot and to displace weight from underneath the most painful and prominent metatarsal heads. Shoes can be formed to accommodate extra width as well as extra depth. Such shoes are never fashionable, and patients rarely wear them regularly unless they are housebound or have severe pain or dysfunction.

Surgical Treatment

Although commonly performed in the past, synovectomy of the MTP joints is insufficient treatment unless concomitant immunosuppression is successful in quieting the disease process.[17] Early definitive reconstructive procedures can prevent the development of serious deformities, such as complete joint dislocation and soft tissue contracture, if they address the loss of intrinsic musculature and joint instability at the first tarsometatarsal joint level. A series of minor procedures can be carried out to restore alignment and function to the toes and eliminate excessive weight-bearing under the metatarsal heads. Because human toes are not used for grasping, the extrinsic interphalangeal flexors and the extensors can be transferred to replace intrinsic muscle function and restore normal function in the lesser toes (Fig. 116–49). However, all the problems in the hindfoot and midfoot must be corrected to ensure that no underlying primary conditions have been overlooked.

Common associated problems that can overload the forefoot include gastrocnemius tightness, secondary chronic posterior tibial tendinitis, and excessive pronation. Percutaneous lengthening of the heel cord and

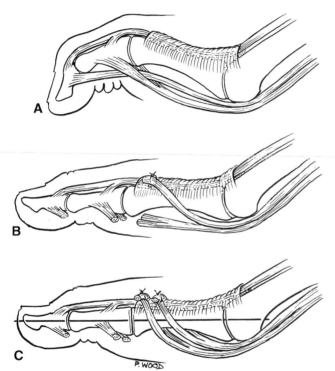

A

B

C

P. WOOD

FIGURE 116–49 · Intrinsicplasty (flexor-to-extensor transfer). *A,* The normal extrinsic flexor tendon arrangement. *B,* The long and short extrinsic flexors are released at the distal and proximal interphalangeal joints, respectively, and the flexor digitorum longus is transferred to the dorsal hood through a medial midline incision. This tendon transfer can be done in toes with excessive flexibility at the interphalangeal joints if there is adequate plantar skin. *C,* A more complex transfer should be done in toes with a fixed flexion deformity and those with contracted plantar skin resulting from a long-standing deformity. Here, 5 to 10 mm of the distal proximal phalanx is resected to straighten and slightly shorten the toe. Both flexors have been released and transferred. After being split, the tendon ends are brought around the proximal phalanx and sutured to the dorsal extensor hood on top of the phalanx. A K wire or small screw is placed through the phalangeal bones to maintain joint alignment for 3 to 5 weeks. This procedure is routinely done concurrently with an extensor transfer and substitution procedure. When combined with or tarsometatarsal stabilization, either with or without lesser metatarsal shortening, much more satisfactory claw toe and metatarsophalangeal (MTP) joint correction is obtained than with internal amputation of the metatarsal heads. (Copyright Phyllis Wood Associates, Seattle, Washington.)

augmentation of the posterior tibial tendon with the flexor digitorum communis may be required as part of the surgical correction. Hypermobility in the first tarsometatarsal joint with a varus deformity in the first metatarsal joint requires correction by joint realignment and a tarsometatarsal arthrodesis (Fig. 116–50). In addition to this, the first MTP joint is aligned and stabilized by an appropriate capsulorrhaphy, and the sesamoid bones are recentered. When required, the flexor hallucis longus can be transferred to the proximal phalanx. Fusion of the first MTP joint in appropriate alignment should be performed when this joint has been destroyed by arthritis. When the great toe interphalangeal joint has been destroyed or displaced by rheumatoid synovitis, it can also be fused without creating any further functional deficit.

A mild clawing deformity in the lesser toes is treated by transfer of the extensor digitorum communis to the peroneus tertius and transfer of the extensor digitorum brevis to the distal extensor digitorum communis tendon. In the absence of contracture, tenodesis of these tendons constitutes adequate treatment. In a final step, the long and short extrinsic flexors are moved over the proximal phalanx and back into the dorsal hood as in the procedure illustrated in Figure 116–49. When the MTP joints are only subluxated or the deformity can be reduced by manual pressure, shortening of the metatarsal shaft will produce relative lengthening of the contracted soft tissues, restore function, and relieve the excessive pressure on the plantar surface of the foot.[18]

Patients with advanced deformities, including dislocation of the lesser toes and contracture of the skin and other soft tissues, require more complex surgery. This approach can take the form of either "classic" resection

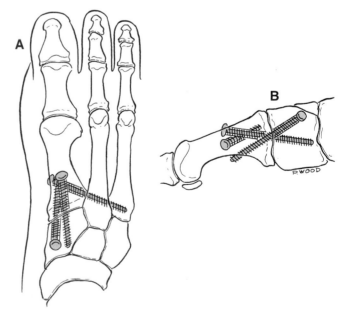

A

B

P. WOOD

FIGURE 116–50 · Recommended Fixation for tarsometatarsal Arthrodesis. *A,* Dorsal view. *B,* Lateral view. As in other arthrodeses, the joint is first prepared by removal of cartilage and deformity and perforation of the subchondral bone. The joint is fixed with the metatarsal in its anatomic position parallel to the second metatarsal. (Copyright Phyllis Wood Associates, Seattle, Washington.)

arthroplasty of the MTP joints[17] or shortening of both the metatarsal shaft and the toes by resection of the interphalangeal joint in addition to the tendon transfers. Recent studies have demonstrated that most patients benefit from MTP joint resection, but the benefits are lost over time. In one study, 60 of 82 cases still exhibited a successful result at an average of 12.8 years after surgery.[19] The most common cause of failure in the long term is recurrence of deformity, usually in the great toe.[20] Results are improved if the first MTP joint is fused rather than resected. The recommended position is in 15 degrees of valgus and 25 to 30 degrees of dorsiflexion.[21] Silicone-rubber implants have been used in the first MTP joint rather than either resection alone or arthrodesis, but the results do not appear to be better than with arthrodesis of the great toe, and there is a danger of particle-induced synovitis from degraded silicone.

Without exception, all foot surgery involving an osteotomy or arthrodesis requires a long healing period with protected weight-bearing. When the use of conventional crutches is precluded by upper-extremity impairment, elbow crutches, a rolling walker, a scooter, or a wheelchair can be used during the healing phase.

Treatment of Hallux Rigidus

Arthritis in the great toe MTP joint, with possible primary or secondary contracture of the plantar fascia, can be a consequence of previous trauma (e.g., "turf toe"), degenerative arthritis, or can be due to a genetic predisposition in joint shape. Excessive length in the proximal phalanx, which is typically a bilateral finding, can aggravate this condition. Discomfort from hallux rigidus can frequently be relieved by wearing shoes with stiff, thick soles and beveled toes, such as wooden clogs.

Surgical treatment includes removal of large dorsal and lateral bony excrescences and a small amount of bone on the dorsal side of the joint. Adhesions in the area of the sesamoid bones and the inferior capsules should be released and an attempt made to release contracted plantar fascia bands. When arthrodesis is indicated, the MTP joint is fused in slight valgus and minimal extension.

After débridement or cheilectomy, the foot is placed in a cast for a brief time (usually about 10 days) to allow the wounds to heal, and the patient then begins a vigorous physical therapy regimen to regain motion. Removal of bony prominences assures significant relief of pain, but the amount of motion that can be recovered varies and cannot be predicted. The benefits of this procedure are temporary but sometimes last several years. An MTP joint fusion should be carried out when the results are no longer satisfactory. Except for women who wear high-heeled shoes, most patients note little additional functional impairment after fusion.

▌ Summary

Modern surgical procedures for arthritic problems of the foot and ankle offer not only relief from pain and decreased deformity but also a more normal gait and the ability to wear normal-looking shoes. Shoes always require some modification after foot surgery, but the corrections are now done in ways that preserve the outward appearance of normal footwear.

The second factor that has shaped the results of foot and ankle surgery is the growing awareness among primary care physicians that many of the problems they see are caused by serious underlying conditions. Many of these physicians now recognize that posterior tibial tendinitis and insufficiency syndrome lead to a unilateral progressive flatfoot deformity and that intrinsic failure in the toes leads to dislocation and metatarsalgia. They recognize that a muscle imbalance, such as occurs with a tight heel cord, can place excessive stress on the posterior tibial tendon and the forefoot and that secondary symptoms can mask the primary causes of dysfunction and deformity. Consequently, they refer patients with developing problems to foot and ankle surgeons soon after making a diagnosis. Satisfactory results can be obtained with the use of fairly simple surgical procedures (such as muscle balancing and osteotomy) in the early stages of deformity, but only complex and functionally limiting operations (such as realignment and arthrodesis) are possible after deterioration of a joint.

The management of patients with rheumatoid involvement of the foot and ankle is complex and requires, in addition to an experienced surgeon, a multidisciplinary team of rheumatologists, anesthesiologists, radiologists, and rehabilitation experts.

REFERENCES

1. Demetriades L, Strauss E, Gallina J: Osteoarthritis of the ankle. Clin Orthop 349:28, 1998.
2. Kirkup J: Rheumatoid arthritis and ankle surgery. Ann Rheum Dis 49:837, 1990.
3. Takakura Y, Tanaka Y, Sugimoto K, et al: Long-term results of arthrodesis for osteoarthritis of the ankle. Clin Orthop 361:178, 1999.
4. Felix N, Kitaoka H: Ankle arthrodesis in patients with rheumatoid arthritis. Clin Orthop 349:58, 1998.
5. Patsalis T, Georgousis H, Gopfert S: Long-term results of forefoot arthroplasty in patients with rheumatoid arthritis. Orthopedics 19:439, 1996.
6. Buechel FF Sr., Buechel FF Jr., Pappas MJ: Eighteen-year evaluation of cementless meniscal bearing total ankle replacements. Instr Course Lect 51:143, 2002.
7. Conti SF, Wong YS: Complications of total ankle replacement. Foot Ankle Clin 7:791, vii, 2002.
8. Easley ME, Vertullo CJ, Urban WC, Nunley JA: Total ankle arthroplasty. J Am Acad Orthop Surg 10:157, 2002.
9. Myerson MS, Mroczek K: Perioperative complications of total ankle arthroplasty. Foot Ankle Int 24:17-21, 2003.
10. Myerson MS, Miller SD: Salvage after complications of total ankle arthroplasty. Foot Ankle Clin 7:191, 2002.
11. Kindsfater K, Wilson M, Thomas W: Management of the rheumatoid hindfoot with special reference to talonavicular arthrodesis. Clin Orthop 340:69, 1997.
12. Mann R, Prieskorn D, Sobel M: Mid-tarsal and tarsometatarsal arthrodesis for primary degenerative osteoarthrosis or osteoarthrosis after trauma. J Bone Joint Surg Am 78:1376, 1996.
13. Cracchiolo A: Rheumatoid arthritis: Hindfoot disease. Clin Orthop 340:58, 1997.
14. Burra G, Katchis S: Rheumatoid arthritis of the forefoot. Rheum Dis Clin North Am 24:173, 1998.

15. Clayton M, Leidholt J, Clark W: Arthroplasty of rheumatoid metatarsophalangeal joints: An outcome study. Clin Orthop 340:48, 1997.

16. Kaye R: The extra-depth toe box: A rational approach. Foot Ankle Int 13:146, 1994.

17. Belt E, Kaarela K, Lehto M: Destruction and arthroplasties of the metatarsophalangeal joints in seropositive rheumatoid arthritis: A 20-year follow-up study. Scand J Rheumatol 27:194, 1998.

18. Hanyu T, Yamazaki H, Murasawa A, et al: Arthroplasty for rheumatoid forefoot deformities by a shortening oblique osteotomy. Clin Orthop 338:131, 1997.

19. Karbowski A, Schwitalle M, Eckhardt A: Arthroplasty of the forefoot in rheumatoid arthritis: Long-term results after Clayton procedure. Acta Orthop Belg 64:401, 1998.

20. Tillmann K: Surgery of the rheumatoid forefoot with special reference to the plantar approach. Clin Orthop 340:39, 1997.

21. Hamalainen M, Raunio P: Long-term followup of rheumatoid forefoot surgery. Clin Orthop 340:34, 1997.

THE SURGICAL MANAGEMENT OF JUVENILE RHEUMATOID ARTHRITIS

CLEMENT B. SLEDGE

The deformities and functional losses produced by juvenile rheumatoid arthritis (JRA) have devastating effects on the physical and emotional development of the child. The physical handicap often evokes cruel comments from peers, condescension from adults, and overprotection by parents. The efforts of physicians, nurses, and therapists should consist of a coordinated attempt to normalize function and thereby facilitate emotional development. In many instances, anti–inflammatory treatment, combined with physical therapy and splinting, is sufficient to maintain function and to prevent deformity.

Occasionally, chronic synovitis interferes with function and threatens to destroy the joint, necessitating synovectomy. Contractures may develop, requiring surgical release. Rarely, joint destruction is so severe that replacement arthroplasty becomes necessary, with the potential for complications with disastrous effects (such as sepsis); the relative lack of long-term results with such procedures is also a concern. Nevertheless, most patients (and their parents) opt for surgery that restores near-normal function during the important formative years, when the pressures of education, spouse-seeking, and career development command maximal attention.

Surgery for rheumatoid arthritis (RA) in children presents some unique problems. In the adult who has RA, pain is usually the primary indication for surgery. The child often denies pain and accepts contracture, so restoration of function is the primary goal. The adult patient has usually been "normal" for much of her or his life, and the surgery attempts to return the person toward this normal state. The young child with severe JRA has never functioned at the level of his or her peers and often suffers from retarded psychologic and social development. Surgery attempts to bring the patient toward a "normal" state that is totally unfamiliar.

Frequently, significant adjustment problems exist in the home and at school. Furthermore, the extreme importance of a continuous vigorous physical therapy program is often not appreciated by the child. Poor patient cooperation can lead to stiffness and contracture requiring surgical therapy; later, that same lack of cooperation can compromise the potential benefits gained from surgery.

Children with JRA have small bones, which may necessitate the use of special prostheses for joint replacement. Their bones are often osteopenic secondary to the disease, as well as to disuse, medication effects, and compromised nutritional status, further complicating surgical reconstruction. The effect of growth and the effect on growth must be carefully considered when surgical procedures are undertaken in the child. Finally, the altered immune status in JRA, whether from the disease process itself or from medication, can adversely affect surgical outcomes.

Surgical procedures in JRA are designed to combat a particular aspect of the disease process, such as joint inflammation, swelling, and stiffness, as well as deformity and joint destruction. Among the procedures to be considered are synovectomy, soft tissue release, epiphysiodesis, osteotomy, and total joint arthroplasty. Arthrodesis is rarely indicated except in advanced disease involving the hand and foot when splinting does not relieve symptoms.

Surgery is quite common in patients with polyarticular JRA. One follow-up study of 44 consecutive patients with JRA found that the most common surgical procedure was total hip replacement, followed by procedures on the foot and ankle and the hand and wrist.[1]

Synovectomy

The indications for synovectomy in the child are similar to those in the adult: persistent synovitis that has not responded to medical management in a joint with adequate articular cartilage. In the adult, 6 months is an acceptable period to wait for a medically induced or spontaneous remission. Because spontaneous remissions are more common in the child, some authorities recommend waiting 18 months, as long as the joint space is well preserved. In addition to systemic medical management, intra-articular corticosteroid injection may help in reducing inflammation, although long-term effects of such treatment are not definitively known. In one study, 300 joints, including 124 knees, were injected in 71 patients with chronic inflammatory arthritis. Of the injected joints, 82 percent went into full remission of pain in the injected joint for more than 6 months.[2]

The task of determining the appropriate treatment for chronic synovitis and the timing of any surgical intervention is difficult because of the frequency of spontaneous remission in JRA. The interpretation of the results of such treatment is also made less straightforward because of the possibility of spontaneous remission. With rapidly occurring loss of motion, altered longitudinal limb growth, and the destruction of joint space in the presence of active disease, however, synovectomy may offer the only chance to prevent permanent contracture, leg length discrepancy, and complete joint destruction.

In reported series, the joints that most frequently required synovectomy were the wrists and metacarpophalangeal (MCP) joints in the upper extremity and the knee in the lower extremity.[3] The tendency today is to avoid synovectomy in the wrists and to manage the patient with vigorous physical therapy and appropriate splinting. Even if the wrist stiffens, it will be functional if it has been held in proper position. Occasionally it may be necessary to lengthen the ulna to maintain a functional position of the wrist.[4] Many physicians have the false impression that upper-extremity surgery is rarely necessary in the patient with JRA. This is because most of these patients do not require surgery until they are adults.

In the child, the knee is the joint most likely to require synovectomy. This likelihood is probably due to its function as a weight-bearing articulation in which inflammation, pain, and contracture cause significant dysfunction. Achieving a successful result after synovectomy requires a motivated and cooperative patient because of the prime importance of postoperative physical therapy. In addition to being less able to cooperate, a younger child who may otherwise benefit from synovectomy may have a more malignant form of disease with systemic illness and multiple joint involvement.

The best results with synovectomy are obtained in older children (more than 7 years of age) with chronic monarticular or oligoarticular disease and a well-preserved joint space. In a large series, knee synovectomy diminished swelling and pain and provided limited improvement in range of motion in children after an average follow-up period of 7.5 years.[5] Improvement tended to deteriorate slowly over time, but the results appear to demonstrate the utility of synovectomy in terms of providing and maintaining an improved functional status.[6] Arthroscopic synovectomy has a success rate similar to that obtained by open means, with less morbidity.[7]

Isolated synovectomy of the hip in JRA has not been frequently reported, and the available results have not been encouraging.[8]

Soft Tissue Release

Prior to consideration of surgical treatment for contracted joints, an aggressive course of medical management, splinting, and traction must be undertaken. Exact determination of the degree of contractures should consist of an examination with the patient under anesthesia, because pain, muscle spasm, and apprehension can give the false appearance of a severely contracted joint. As in the case of synovectomy, patient cooperation is of prime importance, because release of a contracted joint must be followed by a supervised rehabilitation program.[8]

Contractures about the hip and knee often produce the major functional impairment in JRA. Release of contracted iliopsoas and adductor tendons about the hip can reduce pain, increase motion, and improve ambulatory status in appropriately selected patients. At the knee, the release of hamstrings, the long head of the biceps femoris, and the origin of the gastrocnemius, if necessary, has similarly resulted in improved motion and function. More recently, the use of external devices affixed to skeletal pins has been reported to be useful in correcting contractures without the need for an open surgical procedure.[9] To prevent recurrence of the knee-flexion contracture following open or closed treatment, the knee must be splinted in extension when at rest. The role (if any) of soft tissue release, in terms of the ultimate fate of a joint, has not been determined.[10] If advanced joint destruction coexists with contracture, surgical release without arthroplasty is unlikely to give lasting improvement.

Length and Angular Correction

Limb length inequality can develop in JRA secondary to a variety of local and systemic factors. The effects of the disease on growth are often unpredictable, however, and skeletal measurements must be obtained at specific intervals for use in determining the need for and timing of any surgical intervention. The synovitis of JRA appears to stimulate growth in younger children, whereas growth retardation is more common in the older child. Thus, children with onset of asymmetric disease before 5 years of age tend to have a length discrepancy in which the affected limb is the longer limb. Factors such as the chronicity of synovitis, weight-bearing status, surgical procedures, medication effects, nutritional status, and general state of health all can affect growth as well, further contributing to the difficulty in predicting the need for surgical treatment of length discrepancies.

There is wide variation in the amount of length contributed by the various growth plates of the lower extremity: 3 mm from the proximal femoral plate, 12 mm from the distal femoral plate, 9 mm from the proximal tibial plate, and 6 mm from the distal tibial plate. The cumulative growth around the knee is 21 mm (12 from the distal femoral plate and 9 from the proximal tibial plate).[11] Unilateral disease involving the knee is, thus, most likely to produce a significant leg-length discrepancy. With chronic wrist involvement, there may be overgrowth of the radius or undergrowth of the ulna, producing severe wrist deformity that is resistant to splinting. In such cases, ulnar lengthening has been recommended.[4] When found to be of sufficient magnitude to produce either cosmetic or functional disability, the length discrepancies seen in JRA are amenable to correction through physeal growth arrest. Epiphysiodesis for this purpose can be successfully accomplished by open or percutaneous methods.

Angular deformity at the knee generally consists of a genu valgum deformity. This may be treated with asymmetric stapling of the physis to provide temporary growth arrest on the medial side of the joint or, alternatively, with a hemiepiphysiodesis procedure for permanent correction.[12] These procedures require sufficient remaining growth potential to correct the deformity and are limited to correction of varus-valgus deformities.

If there is insufficient growth potential left when an angular deformity is recognized, supracondylar osteotomy of the femur or osteotomy of the proximal tibia may be necessary (Fig. 116–51).

Joint Arthroplasty

Joint-replacement arthroplasty is appropriate for patients with permanent structural damage to the joint and significant pain or deformity. Total joint prostheses are available for use in the hip, knee, shoulder, elbow, and ankle. Prosthetic joint replacement in young patients remains a controversial issue, with questions about prosthetic fixation to bone, wear characteristics, the fatigue properties of materials, and the effects of skeletal growth. The literature contains relatively little long-term experience with total joint arthroplasty in young patients, and even less specifically addressing JRA.[13-17] Most series include young people with many different diseases.

Preoperative pain is not usually the primary indication for total hip arthroplasty or total knee arthroplasty in these young patients. In most cases, functional impairment and deformity are the primary indications. Skeletal immaturity is considered only a relative contraindication to surgery. Clearly, there are advantages to waiting until the epiphyses are closed; the bones are larger, and the patient is older and more able to cooperate fully with the rehabilitation program. Once the patient becomes nonambulatory or fixed contractures occur, however, further delay may worsen the chance of

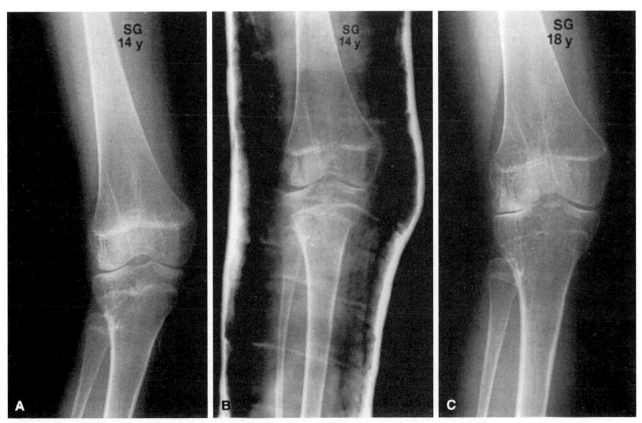

FIGURE 116–51 · *A,* Twenty-three-degree valgus angulation of the right knee in a 14-year-old patient with juvenile rheumatoid arthritis (JRA). *B,* The patient underwent a proximal tibial osteotomy with correction to 10 degrees of valgus. *C,* Four years later, at age 18, correction is maintained, and there is mild lateral compartment degeneration present.

successful restoration of function through replacement of the involved joint.

Other treatments should always be considered prior to joint replacement. Traction, physical therapy, splinting, synovectomy, soft tissue release, and osteotomy may potentially yield only transient improvements, however, in patients with advanced joint destruction.

Often, patients with JRA require replacement of both the hips and knees. In a series of 44 patients followed 10 years into adulthood, all nine patients who required bilateral total knee arthroplasty also underwent bilateral total hip arthroplasty.[1] When both procedures are indicated in the same patient, total hip arthroplasty ought to precede total knee arthroplasty for several reasons. First, hip replacement is usually less painful than knee replacement, thereby promoting the patient's cooperation and bolstering confidence to proceed with further surgery.[18] In addition, patients with multiple joint replacements often report deriving the greatest benefit from total hip arthroplasty. Rehabilitation after a total hip arthroplasty is possible in the presence of a stiff contracted knee joint, but rehabilitation after a total knee arthroplasty is difficult in the presence of a painful and stiff hip joint. Manipulation and casting to gain extension in the contracted knee can be performed while the patient is under general anesthesia for hip replacement. By operating on the hip before the knee, any pain referred from the ipsilateral hip can be resolved. Finally, it is beneficial to correct the soft tissue contractures about the hip and normalize tension in those muscles that cross the hip joint and act on the knee before operating on the knee.

Careful preoperative planning is essential in these patients. In a series of arthroplasties performed at Brigham and Women's Hospital, custom or special miniature prostheses were required in 50 percent of total hip arthroplasties and 40 percent of total knee arthroplasties in patients with JRA.

Hip Replacement

Results of hip replacement in these young patients with JRA are difficult to summarize because of differences in patient populations: age, pauciarticular versus polyarticular involvement, criteria for success, and so on.[19] Overall, the rate of component loosening is higher than that in adults, especially loosening of the cemented acetabulum. Radiographic evidence of loosening of cemented components is found in from 25 percent at 4 years postoperatively (range 8 to 12 years)[16] up to 46 percent in one series.[17] When failure is defined as revision, the results are much better, with implant survival rates of 92 percent at 10 years and 83 percent at 15 years.[15] The length of follow-up with uncemented hip procedures is much shorter, but revision rates at about 4.5 years were one out of 29 hips in one series[13] and 12 percent of 29 hips in another.[14] Functional results are much better than the radiologic results; virtually all series reported greatly improved function and excellent pain relief.

In one large series, the results were evaluated after a minimum follow-up period of 10 years with 66 cemented total hip arthroplasties in 39 patients younger than 30 years of age (average age 19.9 years) who had JRA.[20] After a mean follow-up period of more than 15 years, 12 percent of femoral components and 32 percent of acetabular components had been revised for aseptic loosening. Patients uniformly reported improvement in ambulatory status and reduction in pain, with residual limitations at follow-up secondary to disease in other joints (Fig. 116–52).

The high rate of acetabular revision stems from several causes related to acetabular bone anatomy, in which two types of deficiency are frequently encountered. The first type is acetabular dysplasia resembling that seen in developmental dysplasia of the hip, which is often combined with excessive femoral anteversion. To gain coverage, it is advisable to augment the acetabulum with structural bone grafts, as in other cases of hip dysplasia, rather than through deepening of the socket.[18] The second type of acetabular deficiency is protrusion from upward and inward migration of the femoral head. The amount of protrusion can be alarming, and the process can be rapidly progressive. Bone stock can be restored with various bone-grafting techniques.[27] These problems with the acetabular aspect of the replacement have led to increased interest in cementless fixation of the socket, with good early results.[14]

Knee Replacement

The results of knee arthroplasty in JRA are very similar to those reported for young patients in whom knee replacement was performed for other indications and for adults with RA, with virtual complete relief of pain and increased function. Cemented total knee arthroplasty in JRA has not been associated with the magnitude of difficulties in terms of aseptic loosening found in cemented total hip arthroplasties, and survivorship of the implants is around 95 percent at 5- and 10-year follow-up.[18] As in adult patients with inflammatory arthritis, I recommend patellar resurfacing during total knee arthroplasty in all patients with JRA.

Although cement fixation appears to be tolerated better in the knee than in the hip in JRA, there is still concern about the ultimate potential for loosening, cement failure, and maintenance of bone stock in these young patients. Early results using cementless components in carefully selected patients with JRA have been reported with results comparable to those obtained with use of cemented designs.[21] Until long-term results are available, the use of uncemented implants must be viewed cautiously for the patient with JRA and severe osteopenia.

The range of flexion obtained by knee arthroplasty is largely determined by the preoperative range and is quite accurately predicted by the range achieved by gravity with the patient under general anesthesia at the time of arthroplasty.[22] Preoperative use of traction, physical therapy, and serial casting can reduce flexion deformity and lessen the extent of soft tissue release required at surgery (Fig. 116–53).

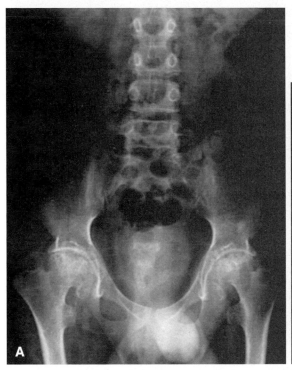
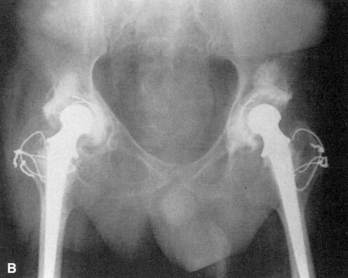

FIGURE 116-52 · *A*, Preoperative radiographs of a patient with juvenile rheumatoid arthritis (JRA). *B*, 15-year postoperative radiograph of same patient after bilateral, cemented total hip arthroplasty. Lucencies can be noted at the cement–bone interface of both acetabuli, whereas the femoral components demonstrate maintenance of excellent fixation.

■ Replacement of Other Joints

Total joint arthroplasty is also used, although less frequently, after arthritic destruction of the shoulder or elbow, or both. In general, such procedures are performed more frequently in adults but occasionally may be required in the child with JRA. In a large series of elbow replacements, only 8 percent were performed in patients with JRA.[23] One study of elbow replacement in JRA reported that 12 (52%) of 23 elbows had an excellent result, 8 (35%) had a good result, and 3 (13%) had a poor result after a minimum follow-up period of 2 years.[24] At later follow-up, the results remained satisfactory.[25]

■ Anesthetic Considerations

Finally, preoperative planning for the surgical treatment of JRA must take into consideration the potential risks of anesthesia unique to these patients. Children with JRA are generally small in stature and possess relatively small airways with an often hypoplastic mandible secondary to the same growth disturbances seen in the extremities.[26] Furthermore, intubation is often made more difficult by stiffness of the cervical spine and the temporomandibular joints. Alternatively, and less frequently, cervical spine laxity with resultant instability may be present. Because of these factors, regional anesthesia in the upper extremity and spinal or epidural anesthesia in the lower extremity have become the anesthetic techniques of choice in patients with in

many instittions. If use of these anesthetic techniques is not possible or if a particular technique is unsuccessful, fiberoptic intubation may be indicated.

Patients with JRA often undergo successive surgical procedures, so they may already have a general understanding of the complex difficulties with anesthesia. If possible, the same anesthesiologist should be involved during each of these procedures to promote optimal patient comprehension and cooperation.

■ Complications

Of special concern in young people who have undergone prosthetic joint replacement are the long-term complications of failure by late metastatic infection, wear, or loosening. Patient, family, physician, and dentist all must be educated about the need for rapid intervention with the use of antibiotics in the treatment of any infectious disease and for the judicious use of prophylactic antibiotics when appropriate (see the earlier section' in this chapter, on hip surgery for discussion).

Articular surface wear has not been a problem in most reported series. The small size of these patients coupled with their relatively low activity level appears to make them less likely to wear down the prosthetic joint surface than the typical adult patient with an arthroplasty.

The most common cause of failure noted in the literature is aseptic loosening. The occurrence of component loosening in adults has been related to a high

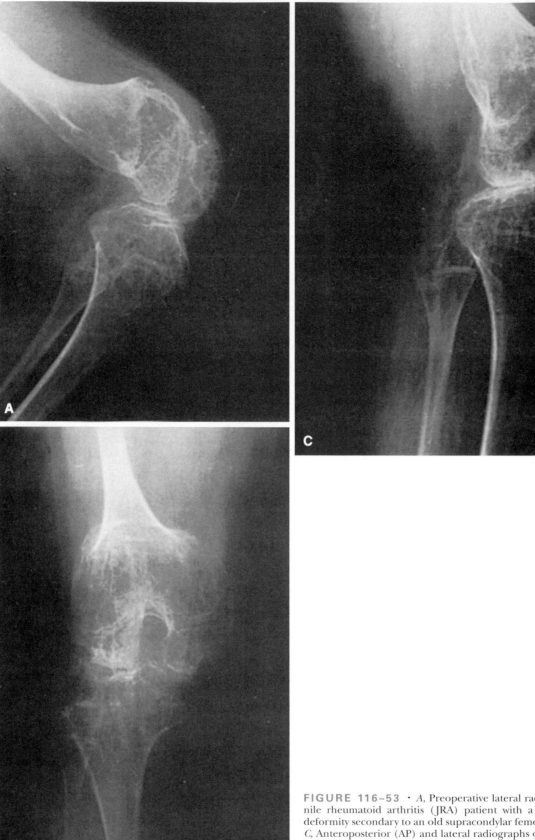

FIGURE 116–53 · *A*, Preoperative lateral radiograph of a juvenile rheumatoid arthritis (JRA) patient with a 90-degree flexion deformity secondary to an old supracondylar femoral fracture. *B* and *C*, Anteroposterior (AP) and lateral radiographs of the same patient following a preoperative program of physical therapy, traction, and serial casts. Long-standing contractures such as this usually do not respond to this program and must be corrected at surgery.

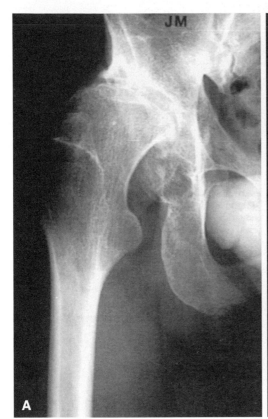
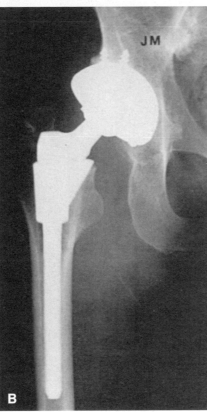

FIGURE 116-54 · *A*, Preoperative radiograph demonstrating hip joint degeneration as well as torsional defomity of the proximal femur: a common finding in juvenile rheumatoid arthritis (JRA). *B*, Reconstruction was performed using a modular, uncemented femoral component, which allowed correction of the torsional deformity. A new, deeper acetabulum was formed using a cementless cup.

activity level, greater than ideal body weight, and monarticular rather than polyarticular disease. Patients with JRA are protected from some of these factors, yet rates of aseptic loosening are about the same as in adults—4 to 8 percent at 10 years. Other aspects of the disease process in JRA probably contribute to the observed rates of aseptic loosening. Among these are potentially poorer bone stock, alterations in immune responsiveness, the anatomic alterations in bone anatomy, and an altered mechanic environment due to local and distant contractures (Fig. 116–54).

REFERENCES

1. Rossouw D, Burnet R, David J, et al: The juvenile arthritic in adult life: A surgical profile. J Orthop Rheum 6:11, 1993.
2. Padeh S, Passwell J: Intra-articular corticosteroid injection in the management of children with chronic arthritis. Arthritis Rheum 41:1210, 1998.
3. Rydholm U, Elborgh R, Ranstam J, et al: Synovectomy of the knee in juvenile chronic arthritis: A retrospective, consecutive follow-up study. J Bone Joint Surg Br 68:223, 1986.
4. Mink van der Molen A, Hall M, Evans D: Ulnar lengthening in juvenile chronic arthritis. J Hand Surg Br 23:438, 1998.
5. Swann M: The surgery of juvenile chronic arthritis. Clin Orthop 259:70, 1990.
6. Paus A, Dale K: Arthroscopic and radiographic examination of patients with juvenile rheumatoid arthritis before and after open synovectomy of the knee joint: A prospective study with a 5-year follow-up. Ann Chir Gynaecol 82:55, 1993.
7. Gattinara M, Lomater C, Paresce E, et al: Arthroscopic synovectomy of the knee joint in the treatment of patients with juvenile chronic arthritis. Acta Univ Carol [Med] (Praha) 40:113, 1994.
8. McCullough C: Surgical management of the hip in juvenile chronic arthritis. Br J Rheumatol 33:178, 1994.
9. Correll J, Truckenbrodt H: Correction of severe joint contractures and leg length discrepancies by external fixation (Ilizarov method): First results in children with rheumatic diseases. Rev Rhum Engl Ed 64:163S, 1997.
10. Moreno Alvarez M, Espada G, Maldonado-Cocco J, et al: Long-term followup of hip and knee soft tissue release in juvenile chronic arthritis. J Rheumatol 19:1608, 1992.
11. Green W, Anderson M: Epiphyseal arrest for the correction of discrepancies in length of the lower extremities. J Bone Joint Surg Am 39:853, 1957.
12. Fraser R, Dickens D, Cole W: Medial physeal stapling for primary and secondary genu valgum in late childhood and adolescence. J Bone Joint Surg Br 77:773, 1995.
13. Haber D, Goodman S: Total hip arthroplasty in juvenile chronic arthritis: A consecutive series. J Arthroplasty 13:259, 1998.
14. Kumar M, Swann M: Uncemented total hip arthroplasty in young patients with juvenile chronic arthritis. Ann R Coll Surg Engl 80:203, 1998.
15. Lehtimaki M, Lehto M, Kautiainen H, et al: Survivorship of the Charnley total hip arthroplasty in juvenile chronic arthritis: A follow-up of 186 cases for 22 years. J Bone Joint Surg Br 79:792, 1997.
16. Williams W, McCullough C: Results of cemented total hip replacement in juvenile chronic arthritis: A radiological review. J Bone Joint Surg Br 75:872, 1993.
17. Maric Z, Haynes R: Total hip arthroplasty in juvenile rheumatoid arthritis. Clin Orthop 290:197, 1993.
18. Scott R, Sledge C: Juvenile rheumatoid arthritis. *In* Steinberg M (ed): The Hip and Its Disorders. Philadelphia, WB Saunders, 1991, p 470.
19. Furnes O, Lie SA, Espehaug B, et al: Hip disease and the prognosis of total hip replacements: A review of 53,698 primary total hip replacements reported to the Norwegian Arthroplasty Register 1987-99. J Bone Joint Surg Br 83:579-586, 2001.
20. Chmell M, Scott R, Thomas W, et al: Total hip arthroplasty with cement for juvenile rheumatoid arthritis: Results at a minimum

of ten years in patients less than thirty years old. J Bone Joint Surg Am 79:44, 1997.

21. Boublik M, Tsahakis P, Scott R: Cementless total knee arthroplasty in juvenile onset rheumatoid arthritis. Clin Orthop 286:88, 1993.

22. Lee D, Kim D, Scott R, et al: Intraoperative flexion against gravity as an indication of ultimate range of motion in individual cases after total knee arthroplasty. J Arthroplasty 13:500, 1998.

23. Ewald F, Simmons E, Sullivan J, et al: Capitellocondylar total elbow replacement in rheumatoid arthritis: Long-term results. J Bone Joint Surg Am 75:498, 1993.

24. Connor P, Morrey B: Total elbow arthroplasty in patients who have juvenile rheumatoid arthritis. J Bone Joint Surg Am 80:678, 1998.

25. Mansat P, Morrey BF: Semiconstrained total elbow arthroplasty for ankylosed and stiff elbows. J Bone Joint Surg Am 82:1260-1268, 2000.

26. Kahnberg KE, Holmstrom H: Augmentation of a retrognathic chin. I. Use of HTR-polymer implants in a long-term prospective clinical and radiographic study. Scand J Plast Reconstr Surg Hand Surg 36:65-70, 2002.

Index

Page numbers followed by "f" denote figures and "t" denote tables